Contents

Essential Clinical Anesthesia

Edited by

Charles A. Vacanti, M.D.
Harvard Medical School and Brigham and Women's Hospital

Pankaj K. Sikka, M.D., Ph.D.
Emerson Hospital

Richard D. Urman, M.D., M.B.A.
Harvard Medical School and Brigham and Women's Hospital

Mark Dershwitz, M.D., Ph.D.
University of Massachusetts Medical School

B. Scott Segal, M.D., M.H.C.M.
Tufts University School of Medicine and Tufts Medical Center

CAMBRIDGE
UNIVERSITY PRESS

CAMBRIDGE UNIVERSITY PRESS
Cambridge, New York, Melbourne, Madrid, Cape Town,
Singapore, São Paulo, Delhi, Tokyo, Mexico City

Cambridge University Press
32 Avenue of the Americas, New York, NY 10013-2473, USA

www.cambridge.org
Information on this title: www.cambridge.org/9780521720205

© Cambridge University Press 2011

First published 2011

Printed in the United States of America

A catalog record for this publication is available from the British Library.

Library of Congress Cataloging in Publication data

Essential clinical anesthesia / edited by Charles Vacanti ... [et al.].
   p. ; cm.
Includes bibliographical references and index.
ISBN 978-0-521-72020-5 (pbk.)
1. Anesthesiology.   2. Anesthesia.   I. Vacanti, Charles.   II. Title.
[DNLM: 1. Anesthesia – methods.   2. Anesthesiology – methods.
3. Anesthetics – administration & dosage.   WO 200]
RD81.E856   2011
617.9′6–dc22   2010028650

ISBN 978-0-521-72020-5 Paperback

Additional resources for this publication at
www.cambridge.org/vacanti

* The appendix entitled "Pre-use checking of anesthesia equipment" and chapters 168–184 can be freely accessed at www.cambridge.org/vacanti.

* The appendix entitled "Pre-use checking of anesthesia equipment" and chapters 168–184 can be freely accessed at www.cambridge.org/vacanti.

Section Editors

Linda S. Aglio, M.D., M.S., *Part 16*

Paul D. Allen, Ph.D., M.D., *Parts 17 and 20*

Angela M. Bader, M.D., *Part 1*

Sascha S. Beutler, M.D., *Part 8*

William R. Camann, M.D., *Part 23*

Mercedes A. Concepcion, M.D., *Part 10*

Mark Dershwitz, M.D., Ph.D., *Parts 6 and 10*

Pradeep Dinakar, M.B., B.S., *Parts 7 and 27*

D. John Doyle, M.D., Ph.D., FRCPC, *Part 21*

Lucinda L. Everett, M.D., *Part 24*

Gyorgy Frendl, M.D., Ph.D., *Part 28*

Simon Gelman, M.D., Ph.D., *Part 14*

Richard M. Kaufman, M.D., *Part 12*

Robert M. Knapp, D.O., J.D., *Part 9*

Bhavani S. Kodali, M.D., M.B., *Parts 4 and 29*

Yasodananda Kumar Areti, M.D., *Part 3*

Stanley Leeson, M.B., B.CH., *Part 14*

Shannon S. McKenna, M.D., *Part 15*

Abdel-Kader Mehio, M.D., *Part 22*

Ross J. Musumeci, M.D., M.B.A., *Part 26*

Beverly K. Philip, M.D., *Part 25*

James H. Philip, M.D., *Part 5*

Selwyn O. Rogers Jr., M.D., M.P.H., *Part 11*

William H. Rosenblatt, M.D., *Part 2*

Edgar L. Ross, M.D., *Part 27*

Warren S. Sandberg, M.D., Ph.D., *Part 18*

B. Scott Segal, M.D., M.H.C.M, *Part 1*

Stanton K. Shernan, M.D., *Part 13*

Gary R. Strichartz, Ph.D., *Part 7*

Balachundhar Subramaniam, M.D., M.P.H., *Part 19*

Kamen V. Vlassakov, M.D., *Part 22*

Contributors

Aakash Agarwala, M.D.
Attending Anesthesiologist
Antelope Valley Medical Center
Palmdale CA

Linda S. Aglio, M.D., M.S.
Associate Professor of Anaesthesia
Harvard Medical School
Brigham and Women's Hospital
Boston MA

Rae M. Allain, M.D.
Assistant Professor of Anaesthesia
Harvard Medical School
Massachusetts General Hospital
Boston MA

Paul D. Allen, Ph.D., M.D.
Professor of Anaesthesia
Harvard Medical School
Brigham and Women's Hospital
Boston MA

Houman Amirfarzan, M.D.
Resident, Anesthesia Department
Tufts Medical Center
Boston MA

Yasodananda Kumar Areti, M.D.
Senior Lecturer
Faculty of Medical Sciences
The University of the West Indies
Queen Elizabeth Hospital
St Michael, BARBADOS

Amit Asopa, M.B., B.S.
Clinical Fellow in Anaesthesia
Harvard Medical School
Beth Israel Deaconess Medical Center
Boston MA

Edwin G. Avery IV, M.D., C.P.I.
Chief, Division of Cardiac Anesthesia
Vice Chairman–Director of Research
Associate Professor of Anesthesiology
Department of Anesthesiology and Perioperative Medicine
University Hospitals Harrington-McLaughlin Heart
    and Vascular Institute
Case Western Reserve University School of Medicine
Cleveland OH

Patricia R. Bachiller, M.D.
Instructor in Anaesthesia
Harvard Medical School
Massachusetts General Hospital
Boston MA

Angela M. Bader, M.D.
Associate Professor of Anaesthesia
Harvard Medical School
Brigham and Women's Hospital
Boston MA

Rana Badr, M.D.
Assistant Professor of Anesthesia
University of Massachusetts Medical School
UMass Memorial Medical Center
Worcester MA

Sibinka Bajic, M.D., Ph.D.
Instructor in Anaesthesia
Harvard Medical School
Brigham and Women's Hospital
Boston MA

David J. Baker, M.Phil., D.M., F.R.C.A.
Emeritus Consultant Anesthesiologist
SAMU de Paris
Hôpital Necker-Enfants Malades
Paris FRANCE

Sheila R. Barnett, M.B., B.S.
Associate Professor of Anaesthesia
Harvard Medical School
Beth Israel Deaconess Medical Center
Boston MA

Rena Beckerly, M.D., M.B.A.
Instructor in Anesthesiology
Northwestern University Feinberg School of Medicine
Northwestern Memorial Hospital
Chicago IL

Lorenzo Berra, M.D.
Clinical Fellow in Anaesthesia
Harvard Medical School
Massachusetts General Hospital
Boston MA

Walter Bethune, M.D.
Cardiothoracic Anesthesiology Fellow
Hospital of the University of Pennsylvania
Philadelphia PA

Sascha S. Beutler, M.D.
Instructor in Anaesthesia
Harvard Medical School
Assistant Program Director
Department of Anesthesiology, Perioperative, and
    Pain Medicine
Brigham and Women's Hospital
Boston MA

Tarun Bhalla, M.D.
Assistant Professor
The Ohio State University College of Medicine
Pediatric Anesthesiologist
Nationwide Children's Hospital
Columbus OH

Edward A. Bittner, M.D., Ph.D.
Instructor in Anaesthesia
Harvard Medical School
Massachusetts General Hospital
Boston MA

Jonathan D. Bloom, M.D.
Associate Director of Medical Affairs
Covidien
Boulder CO

Alina V. Bodas, M.D.
Associate Staff
Pediatric Anesthesiology
Cleveland Clinic Foundation
Cleveland OH

Lina M. Bolanos-Diaz, M.D.
Pediatric Anesthesiologist
Massachusetts Eye and Ear Infirmary
Brigham and Women's Hospital
Boston MA

Ruma R. Bose, M.D., M.B., B.S.
Instructor in Anaesthesia
Harvard Medical School
Beth Israel Deaconess Medical Center
Boston MA

Jan Boublik, M.D., Ph.D.
Instructor in Anesthesiology
New York University School of Medicine
NYU Langone Medical Center
New York NY

John P. Broadnax, M.D.
Clinical Fellow in Anaesthesia
Harvard Medical School
Brigham and Women's Hospital
Boston MA

Jason C. Brookman, M.D.
Fellow in Regional Anesthesia and
    Acute Pain Management
Acute Interventional Perioperative Pain Service
Department of Anesthesiology
University of Pittsburgh Medical Center
Pittsburgh PA

Meredith R. Brooks, M.D., M.P.H.
Pediatric Anesthesiologist
Pediatric Pain Physician
Adult Pain Management Fellow
Stanford University School of Medicine
Stanford CA

Roland Brusseau, M.D.
Instructor in Anaesthesia
Harvard Medical School
Children's Hospital
Boston MA

Ethan O. Bryson, M.D.
Assistant Professor
Department of Anesthesiology
Mount Sinai School of Medicine
New York NY

Linda A. Bulich, M.D.
Assistant Professor of Anaesthesia
Harvard Medical School
Children's Hospital
Boston MA

Kenji Butterfield, M.D.
Staff Anesthesiologist
O'Connor Hospital
San Jose CA

William R. Camann, M.D.
Associate Professor of Anaesthesia
Harvard Medical School
Brigham and Women's Hospital
Boston MA

Denise M. Chan, M.D.
Staff Anesthesiologist
Hasbro Children's Hospital
Providence RI

Theresa S. Chang, M.D.
Staff Anesthesiologist
Specializing in Cardiothoracic Anesthesia
California Pacific Medical Center
San Francisco CA

Jonathan E. Charnin, M.D.
Instructor in Anaesthesia
Harvard Medical School
Massachusetts General Hospital
Boston MA

Mark Chrostowski, M.D.
Department of Anesthesiology
Greenwich Hospital
Greenwich CT

Fred Cobey, M.D.
Attending Cardiac Anesthesiologist
Department of Anesthesiology
Washington Hospital Center
Washington DC

Adam B. Collins, M.D.
Associate Professor
University of California, San Francisco
Department of Anesthesia and Perioperative
   Care
San Francisco General Hospital
San Francisco CA

Mercedes A. Concepcion, M.D.
Associate Professor of Anaesthesia
Harvard Medical School
Brigham and Women's Hospital
Boston MA

Christopher W. Connor, M.D., Ph.D.
Assistant Professor of Anesthesiology and
   Biomedical Engineering
Boston University
Boston Medical Center
Boston MA

Bronwyn Cooper, M.D.
Assistant Professor of Anesthesiology
University of Massachusetts Medical School
UMass Memorial Medical Center
Worcester MA

Jeffrey B. Cooper, Ph.D.
Professor of Anaesthesia
Harvard Medical School
Massachusetts General Hospital
Boston MA

Martha Cordoba-Amorocho, M.D.
Clinical Fellow in Anaesthesia
Harvard Medical School
Brigham and Women's Hospital
Boston MA

Stephen B. Corn, M.D.
Associate Professor of Anaesthesia
Harvard Medical School
Director of Clinical Innovation
Brigham and Women's Hospital
Children's Hospital
Boston MA

Darin J. Correll, M.D.
Assistant Professor of Anaesthesia
Harvard Medical School
Brigham and Women's Hospital
Boston MA

Gregory J. Crosby, M.D.
Associate Professor of Anaesthesia
Harvard Medical School
Brigham and Women's Hospital
Boston MA

Lisa J. Crossley, M.D.
Assistant Professor of Anaesthesia
Harvard Medical School
Brigham and Women's Hospital
Boston MA

Deborah J. Culley, M.D.
Assistant Professor of Anaesthesia
Harvard Medical School
Brigham and Women's Hospital
Boston MA

Tomas Cvrk, M.D., Ph.D.
Staff Anesthesiologist
Lahey Clinic
Burlington MA

Michael N. D'Ambra, M.D.
Associate Professor of Anaesthesia
Harvard Medical School
Brigham and Women's Hospital
Boston MA

Michael Decker, M.D.
Staff Anesthesiologist
Sheridan Healthcare
Aventura Hospital and Medical Center
Miami FL

Daniel F. Dedrick, M.D.
Assistant Professor of Anaesthesia
Harvard Medical School
Brigham and Women's Hospital
Boston MA

Mark Dershwitz, M.D., Ph.D.
Professor and Vice Chair of Anesthesiology
Professor of Biochemistry and Molecular Pharmacology
University of Massachusetts Medical School
Worcester MA

Francis X. Dillon, M.D.
Instructor in Anaesthesia
Harvard Medical School
Massachusetts General Hospital
Massachusetts Eye and Ear Infirmary
Boston MA

Pradeep Dinakar, M.B., B.S.
Instructor in Anaesthesia and Neurology
Harvard Medical School
Brigham and Women's Hospital
Children's Hospital
Boston MA

Alimorad G. Djalali, M.D., Ph.D.
Assistant Professor
Stanford University Medical Center
Department of Anesthesia
Stanford CA

D. John Doyle, M.D., Ph.D., FRCPC
Professor of Anesthesiology
Cleveland Clinic Lerner College of Medicine of Case Western
    Reserve University
Cleveland Clinic Foundation
Cleveland OH

Lambertus Drop, M.D., Ph.D.
Associate Professor of Anaesthesia
Harvard Medical School
Massachusetts General Hospital
Boston MA

Ian F. Dunn, M.D.
Instructor in Surgery
Harvard Medical School
Brigham and Women's Hospital
Department of Neurosurgery
Boston MA

Theodore E. Dushane, M.D., Ph.D.
Cardiac Anesthesiologist
North American Partners in Anesthesia
Melville NY

Sunil Eappen, M.D.
Assistant Professor of Anaesthesia
Harvard Medical School
Chief of Anesthesiology
Medical Director of the Operating Room
Massachusetts Eye and Ear Infirmary
Boston MA

Thomas Edrich, M.D.
Assistant Professor of Anaesthesia
Harvard Medical School
Brigham and Women's Hospital
Boston MA

Jesse M. Ehrenfeld, M.D., M.P.H.
Assistant Professor, Vanderbilt University School of Medicine
Director, Center for Evidence Based Anesthesia
Director, Perioperative Data Systems Research
Department of Anesthesiology
Vanderbilt University
Nashville TN

Jason M. Erlich, M.D.
Clinical Fellow in Anaesthesia
Harvard Medical School
Beth Israel Deaconess Medical Center
Boston MA

Lucinda L. Everett, M.D.
Associate Professor of Anaesthesia
Harvard Medical School
Massachusetts General Hospital
Boston MA

Elliott S. Farber, M.D.
Anesthesiologist
Valley Anesthesiology Consultants
Phoenix AZ

Khaldoun Faris, M.D.
Clinical Associate Professor, Department of Anesthesiology
Associate Director, Surgical Critical Care
University of Massachusetts Medical School

UMass Memorial Medical Center
Worcester MA

Eddy M. Feliz, M.D.
Director of Resident Education
Director of Neurosurgical Anesthesia
Department of Anesthesiology
Boston University Medical Center
Boston MA

Massimo Ferrigno, M.D.
Associate Professor of Anaesthesia
Harvard Medical School
Brigham and Women's Hospital
Boston MA

Richard S. Field, M.D., M.Sc.
North Shore Pain Management
North Shore Anesthesia
Beverly MA

Michael G. Fitzsimons, M.D.
Assistant Professor of Anaesthesia
Harvard Medical School
Massachusetts General Hospital
Boston MA

Hugh L. Flanagan Jr., M.D.
Assistant Professor of Anaesthesia
Harvard Medical School
Brigham and Women's Hospital
Boston MA

Vladimir Formanek, M.D.
Assistant Professor of Anaesthesia
Harvard Medical School
Brigham and Women's Hospital
Boston MA

Amanda A. Fox, M.D., M.P.H.
Assistant Professor of Anaesthesia
Harvard Medical School
Brigham and Women's Hospital
Boston MA

John A. Fox, M.D.
Assistant Professor of Anaesthesia
Harvard Medical School
Brigham and Women's Hospital
Boston MA

Gyorgy Frendl, M.D., Ph.D.
Assistant Professor of Anaesthesia
Harvard Medical School
Brigham and Women's Hospital
Boston MA

Tanja S. Frey, M.D.
Clinical Fellow in Anaesthesia
Harvard Medical School
Brigham and Women's Hospital
Boston MA

Samuel M. Galvagno Jr., D.O.
Assistant Professor
Division of Adult Critical Care Medicine
Department of Anesthesiology and Critical Care
    Medicine
Johns Hopkins Hospital
Baltimore, MD

Edward R. Garcia, M.D.
Cardiothoracic Anesthesiologist
Valley Anesthesiology Consultants
Phoenix AZ

Jonathan D. Gates, M.D.
Assistant Professor of Surgery
Harvard Medical School
Director of Trauma Services
Division of Trauma, Critical Care, and Emergency
    Surgery
Vascular Surgeon
Division of Vascular and Endovascular Surgery
Brigham and Women's Hospital
Boston MA

Cosmin Gauran, M.D.
Instructor in Anaesthesia
Harvard Medical School
Massachusetts General Hospital
Boston MA

Brian J. Gelfand, M.D.
Instructor in Anaesthesia
Harvard Medical School
Brigham and Women's Hospital
Boston MA

Simon Gelman, M.D., Ph.D.
Vandam/Covino Distinguished Professor of Anaesthesia
Harvard Medical School
Brigham and Women's Hospital
Boston MA

Alexander C. Gerhart, M.D.
Anesthesiologist
Newton Wellesley Hospital
Clinical Assistant Professor
Tufts University
Boston MA

Peter Gerner, M.D.
Professor and Chairman
Paracelsus Medical University
Salzburg General Hospital
Salzburg AUSTRIA

Omid Ghalambor, M.D.
Director, Center for Interventional Pain Management
St. Anthony's Memorial Hospital
Effingham IL

Christopher J. Gilligan, M.D.
Instructor in Anaesthesia
Harvard Medical School
Massachusetts General Hospital
Boston MA

Christian D. Gonzalez, M.D., F.I.P.P.
Clinical Director, Wellness Center Multidisciplinary Clinic
Assistant Professor, Department of Anesthesiology
University of Miami
Coral Gables FL

Noah E. Gordon, M.D.
Staff Pediatric Anesthesiologist
California Pacific Medical Center
San Francisco CA

William B. Gormley, M.D.
Instructor in Surgery
Harvard Medical School
Brigham and Women's Hospital
Boston MA

Thomas J. Graetz, M.D.
Fellow in Critical Care
Department of Anesthesiology
Washington University School of Medicine
St. Louis MO

Wendy L. Gross, M.D., M.H.C.M.
Assistant Professor of Anaesthesia
Harvard Medical School
Brigham and Women's Hospital
Boston MA

Amit Gupta, D.O.
Clinical Fellow in Anaesthesia
Harvard Medical School
Brigham and Women's Hospital
Boston MA

James P. Hardy, M.B., B.S.
Clinical Fellow in Anaesthesia
Harvard Medical School

Brigham and Women's Hospital
Boston MA

Seetharaman Hariharan, M.D., F.C.C.M.
Professor, Anesthesia and Intensive Care
Department of Clinical Surgical Sciences
The University of the West Indies, St. Augustine
Trinidad, West Indies

Miriam Harnett, M.D.
Clinical Lecturer
University College Cork
Consultant Anesthetist
Cork University Hospital
Cork IRELAND

Philip M. Hartigan, M.D.
Assistant Professor of Anaesthesia
Harvard Medical School
Brigham and Women's Hospital
Boston MA

Joaquim M. Havens, M.D.
Instructor in Surgery
Harvard Medical School
Brigham and Women's Hospital
Boston MA

Bishr Haydar, M.D.
Instructor in Anaesthesia
Harvard Medical School
Massachusetts General Hospital
Boston MA

Stephen O. Heard, M.D.
Professor of Anesthesiology and Surgery
Chairman, Department of Anesthesiology
University of Massachusetts Medical School
UMass Memorial Medical Center
Worcester MA

James L. Helstrom, M.D., M.B.A.
Staff Anesthesiologist
Fox Chase Cancer Center
Philadelphia PA

David L. Hepner, M.D.
Associate Director, Weiner Center for Perioperative
    Evaluation
Staff Anesthesiologist
Department of Anesthesia, Perioperative, and Pain Medicine
Brigham and Women's Hospital
Associate Professor of Anaesthesia
Harvard Medical School
Boston MA

McCallum R. Hoyt, M.D., M.B.A.
Assistant Professor of Anaesthesia
Harvard Medical School
Brigham and Women's Hospital
Boston MA

Robert N. Jamison, Ph.D.
Associate Professor of Anaesthesia (Psychiatry)
Harvard Medical School
Brigham and Women's Hospital
Boston MA

Karinne Jervis, M.D.
Staff, Cardiothoracic Anesthesiologist
Vice Chair, Department of Anesthesia
Maui Memorial Medical Center
Wailuku HI

Stephanie B. Jones, M.D.
Associate Professor of Anaesthesia
Harvard Medical School
Residency Program Director, Vice Chair for
  Education
Department of Anesthesia, Critical Care and
  Pain Medicine
Beth Israel Deaconess Medical Center
Boston MA

Swaminathan Karthik, M.D.
Instructor in Anaesthesia
Harvard Medical School
Beth Israel Deaconess Medical Center
Boston MA

Richard M. Kaufman, M.D.
Assistant Professor of Pathology
Harvard Medical School
Brigham and Women's Hospital
Boston MA

Shubjeet Kaur, M.D.
Clinical Professor of Anesthesiology
Clinical Vice Chair, Anesthesiology
Medical Director Perioperative Services,
  University Campus
University of Massachusetts Medical
  School
UMass Memorial Medical Center
Worcester, MA

Lee A. Kearse Jr., M.D., Ph.D.
Assistant Professor of Anaesthesia
Harvard Medical School
Brigham and Women's Hospital
Boston MA

John C. Keel, M.D.
Instructor in Orthopedic Surgery
Harvard Medical School
Beth Israel Deaconess Medical Center
Boston MA

Scott D. Kelley, M.D.
Attending Anesthesiologist
Department of Anesthesiology, Perioperative, and Pain
  Medicine
Brigham and Women's Hospital
Vice President, Medical Director
Covidien
Boston MA

Albert H. Kim, M.D., Ph.D.
Clinical Fellow
Department of Neurosurgery
University of Miami Medical Center
Miami FL

Amy L. Kim, M.D.
Clinical Fellow in Anaesthesia
Harvard Medical School
Massachusetts General Hospital
Boston MA

Grace Y. Kim, M.D.
Instructor in Anaesthesia
Harvard Medical School
Brigham and Women's Hospital
Boston MA

Robert J. Klickovich, M.D.
Attending Anaesthesiologist
Harvard Medical School
Brigham and Women's Hospital
Boston MA

Robert M. Knapp, D.O., J.D.
Assistant Professor in Anaesthesia
Harvard Medical School
Brigham and Women's Hospital
Boston MA

Bhavani S. Kodali, M.D., M.B.
Associate Professor of Anaesthesia
Harvard Medical School
Brigham and Women's Hospital
Boston MA

Rahul Koka, M.D.
Instructor in Anaesthesia
Harvard Medical School
Children's Hospital
Boston MA

Alina Lazar, M.D.
Assistant Professor of Anesthesia
Department of Anesthesia and Critical Care
The University of Chicago Hospitals
Chicago IL

Laura H. Leduc, M.D.
Clinical Fellow in Anaesthesia
Harvard Medical School
Children's Hospital
Boston MA

Stanley Leeson, M.B., B.Ch.
Assistant Professor of Anaesthesia
Harvard Medical School
Brigham and Women's Hospital
Boston MA

Lisa R. Leffert, M.D.
Assistant Professor of Anaesthesia
Harvard Medical School
Massachusetts General Hospital
Boston MA

Scott A. LeGrand, M.D.
Pediatric Anesthesiologist
Rockford Memorial Hospital
Rockford IL

Patricio Leyton, M.D.
Instructor in Anaesthesia
Harvard Medical School
Massachusetts General Hospital
Boston MA

J. Lance Lichtor, M.D.
Professor of Anesthesiology and Pediatrics
University of Massachusetts Medical School
Worcester MA

John Lin, M.D.
Clinical Fellow in Anaesthesia
Harvard Medical School
Brigham and Women's Hospital
Boston MA

Alvaro A. Macias, M.D.
Instructor in Anaesthesia
Harvard Medical School
Brigham and Women's Hospital
Massachusetts Eye and Ear Infirmary
Boston MA

Karan Madan, M.B., B.S.
Instructor in Anaesthesia

Harvard Medical School
Brigham and Women's Hospital
Boston MA

Sohail K. Mahboobi, M.D.
Assistant Clinical Professor of
   Anesthesia
Tufts University School of Medicine
Boston MA
Lahey Clinic Medical Center
Burlington MA

Devi Mahendran, M.B., Ch.B.
Clinical Fellow in Anaesthesia
Harvard Medical School
Beth Israel Deaconess Medical Center
Boston MA

Christine Mai, M.D.
Instructor in Anaesthesia
Harvard Medical School
Pediatric Anesthesiologist
Massachusetts General Hospital
Boston MA

Sayeed Malek, M.D.
Instructor in Surgery
Harvard Medical School
Brigham and Women's Hospital
Boston MA

S. Rao Mallampati, M.D.
Assistant Professor of Anaesthesia
Harvard Medical School
Brigham and Women's Hospital
Boston MA

Thomas J. Mancuso, M.D.
Associate Professor of Anaesthesia
Harvard Medical School
Children's Hospital
Boston MA

Ramon Martin, M.D., Ph.D.
Assistant Professor of Anaesthesia
Harvard Medical School
Brigham and Women's Hospital
Boston MA

Matthew C. Martinez, M.D.
Staff Anesthesiologist
Milford Anesthesia Associates, Inc.
Milford Regional Medical Center
Milford MA

J. A. Jeevendra Martyn, M.D., F.R.C.A., F.C.C.M.
Professor of Anaesthesia
Harvard Medical School
Director, Clinical and Biochemical Pharmacology Laboratory
Massachusetts General Hospital
Anesthetist-in-Chief
Shriners Hospital for Children
Boston MA

Kai Matthes, M.D., Ph.D.
Staff Anesthesiologist
Department of Anesthesiology, Perioperative, and
    Pain Medicine
Children's Hospital Boston
Harvard Medical School
Boston MA

Tommaso Mauri, M.D.
Research Fellow in Anesthesiology
University of Milan-Bicocca
San Gerardo Hospital
Monza ITALY

Mary Ellen McCann, M.D.
Assistant Professor of Anaesthesia
Harvard Medical School
Children's Hospital
Boston MA

Shannon S. McKenna, M.D.
Assistant Professor in Anaesthesia
Harvard Medical School
Brigham and Women's Hospital
Boston MA

Dennis J. McNicholl, D.O.
Locum Consultant Anaesthetist
St. Vincent's University Hospital
Dublin IRELAND

Abdel-Kader Mehio, M.D.
Assistant Professor
Department of Anesthesiology
Boston University Medical Center
Boston MA

Thor C. Milland, M.D.
Staff Anesthesiologist
Brooklyn Hospital Center
New York NY

Tonya L. K. Miller, M.D.
Instructor in Anaesthesia
Harvard Medical School
Children's Hospital
Boston MA

John D. Mitchell, M.D.
Assistant Professor of Anaesthesia
Harvard Medical School
Beth Israel Deaconess Medical Center
Boston MA

K. Annette Mizuguchi, M.D., Ph.D., M.M.Sc.
Instructor in Anaesthesia
Harvard Medical School
Brigham and Women's Hospital
Boston MA

Naila Moghul, M.D.
Instructor in Anaesthesia
Harvard Medical School
Brigham and Women's Hospital
Boston MA

David R. Moss, M.D.
Staff Pediatric Anesthesiologist
Tufts Medical Center
Boston MA

Ross J. Musumeci, M.D., M.B.A.
Assistant Professor in Anesthesiology
Boston University Medical School
Boston MA

Naveen Nathan, M.D.
Assistant Professor
Department of Anesthesiology
Assistant Director of Education
Northwestern Memorial Hospital
Chicago IL

Ju-Mei Ng, M.D.
Instructor in Anaesthesia
Harvard Medical School
Brigham and Women's Hospital
Boston MA

Liem C. Nguyen, M.D.
Assistant Clinical Professor
Department of Anesthesiology
Division of Cardiothoracic Anesthesia
University of California, San Diego, Medical
    Center
San Diego CA

Ervant Nishanian, M.D., Ph.D.
Assistant Professor of Cardiothoracic Anesthesia
Columbia University College of Physicians and
    Surgeons

New York–Presbyterian Hospital/Columbia University
   Medical Center
New York NY

Martina Nowak, M.D.
Instructor in Anaesthesia
Harvard Medical School
Brigham and Women's Hospital
Boston MA

Ala Nozari, M.D., Ph.D.
Assistant Professor of Anaesthesia
Harvard Medical School
Massachusetts General Hospital
Boston MA

Michael Nurok, M.B., Ch.B, Ph.D.
Instructor in Anaesthesia
Harvard Medical School
Brigham and Women's Hospital
Boston MA

Arti Ori, M.D.
Clinical Fellow in Anaesthesia
Harvard Medical School
Brigham and Women's Hospital
Boston MA

Rafael A. Ortega, M.D.
Professor of Anesthesia
Boston University School of Medicine
Boston Medical Center
Boston MA

Amy J. Ortman, M.D.
Assistant Professor in Anesthesia
University of Kansas Medical Center
Kansas City KS

David Oxman, M.D.
Instructor in Medicine
Harvard Medical School
Brigham and Women's Hospital
Boston MA

Arvind Palanisamy, M.D.
Instructor in Anaesthesia
Harvard Medical School
Brigham and Women's Hospital
Boston MA

Carlo Pancaro, M.D.
Assistant Professor of Anesthesiology
Tufts University School of Medicine
Tufts Medical Center
Boston MA

Lisbeth Lopez Pappas, M.D.
Pediatric Anesthesiologist
Children's National Medical Center
Washington DC

Benjamin Parish, M.D.
Anesthesiology and Interventional Pain Management
Orthopaedic Center of South Florida
Fort Lauderdale FL

Samuel Park, M.D.
Clinical Fellow in Anaesthesia
Harvard Medical School
Brigham and Women's Hospital
Boston MA

Deborah S. Pederson, M.D.
Instructor in Anaesthesia
Harvard Medical School
Massachusetts General Hospital
Boston MA

Beverly K. Philip, M.D.
Professor of Anaesthesia
Harvard Medical School
Brigham and Women's Hospital
Boston MA

James H. Philip, M.D.
Associate Professor of Anaesthesia
Harvard Medical School
Brigham and Women's Hospital
Boston MA

Silvia Pivi, M.D.
Anesthesiologist
Maurizio Bufalini Hospital
Cesana ITALY

Stephen D. Pratt, M.D.
Assistant Professor of Anaesthesia
Harvard Medical School
Beth Israel Deaconess Medical Center
Boston MA

Douglas E. Raines, M.D.
Associate Professor of Anaesthesia
Harvard Medical School
Massachusetts General Hospital
Boston MA

Stephen L. Ratcliff, M.D.
Associate Professor of Anaesthesia
Harvard Medical School
Beth Israel Deaconess Medical Center
Boston MA

James P. Rathmell, M.D.
Associate Professor of Anaesthesia
Harvard Medical School
Massachusetts General Hospital
Boston MA

J. Taylor Reed, M.D.
Clinical Fellow in Anesthesia
Massachusetts General Hospital
Boston MA

Elizabeth M. Rickerson, M.D.
Clinical Fellow in Anaesthesia
Harvard Medical School
Brigham and Women's Hospital
Boston MA

Selwyn O. Rogers Jr., M.D., M.P.H.
Associate Professor of Surgery
Harvard Medical School
Brigham and Women's Hospital
Boston MA

Thomas M. Romanelli, M.D.
Instructor in Anaesthesia
Harvard Medical School
Massachusetts General Hospital
Boston MA

William H. Rosenblatt, M.D.
Professor of Anesthesiology
Department of Anesthesiology
Yale University School of Medicine
Attending Physician
Yale New Haven Hospital
New Haven CT

Carl E. Rosow, M.D., Ph.D.
Professor of Anaesthesia
Harvard Medical School
Massachusetts General Hospital
Boston MA

Edgar L. Ross, M.D.
Assistant Professor of Anaesthesia
Harvard Medical School
Brigham and Women's Hospital
Boston MA

J. Victor Ryckman, M.D.
Staff Anesthesiologist
Cleveland Clinic Foundation
Cleveland, OH

Mônica M. Sá Rêgo, M.D.
Clinical Director
Instructor in Anaesthesia
Harvard Medical School
Brigham and Women's Hospital
Boston MA

Nicholas Sadovnikoff, M.D.
Assistant Professor of Anaesthesia
Harvard Medical School
Brigham and Women's Hospital
Boston MA

Warren S. Sandberg, M.D., Ph.D.
Professor of Anesthesiology, Surgery, and Biomedical
  Informatics
Chairman, Department of Anesthesiology
Vanderbilt University School of Medicine
Nashville TN

Annette Y. Schure, M.D., D.E.A.A.
Senior Associate in Cardiac Anesthesia
Children's Hospital Boston
Instructor in Anaesthesia
Harvard Medical School
Boston MA

B. Scott Segal, M.D., M.H.C.M.
Professor of Anesthesiology
Tufts University School of Medicine
Chair, Department of Anesthesiology
Tufts Medical Center
Boston MA

Navil F. Sethna, M.B., Ch.B.
Associate Professor of Anaesthesia
Harvard Medical School
Children's Hospital
Boston MA

Swapneel K. Shah, M.D.
Anesthesiologist
Allied Anesthesia Medical Group, Inc.
St. Joseph Hospital
Orange CA

Shaheen F. Shaikh, M.D.
Staff Anesthesiologist
Director of Neuro-Anesthesia
UMass Memorial Hospital
Worcester MA

Fred E. Shapiro, D.O.
Assistant Professor of Anaesthesia

Harvard Medical School
Beth Israel Deaconess Medical Center
Boston MA

Torin D. Shear, M.D.
Attending Anesthesiologist
Department of Anesthesia
Northshore University Healthsystems
Evanston Hospital
Evanston IL

Prem S. Shekar, M.B., B.S.
Assistant Professor of Surgery
Harvard Medical School
Brigham and Women's Hospital
Boston MA

Stanton K. Shernan, M.D.
Associate Professor of Anaesthesia
Harvard Medical School
Brigham and Women's Hospital
Boston MA

Naomi Shimizu, M.D.
Instructor in Surgery
Harvard Medical School
Brigham and Women's Hospital
Boston MA

Douglas C. Shook, M.D.
Instructor in Anaesthesia
Harvard Medical School
Brigham and Women's Hospital
Boston MA

Kamal K. Sikka, Ph.D.
Manager
Electronic Packaging Thermal Mechanical
   Design
IBM Microelectronics
Hopewell Junction NY

Pankaj K. Sikka, M.D., Ph.D.
Staff Anesthesiologist
Emerson Hospital
Concord MA

David A. Silver, M.D.
Instructor in Anaesthesia
Harvard Medical School
Brigham and Women's Hospital
Boston MA

Jeffrey H. Silverstein, M.D., C.I.P.
Professor of Anesthesiology, Surgery, and Geriatrics and
   Palliative Medicine
Vice Chair for Research
Associate Dean for Research
Director, Program for the Protection of Human Subjects
Chair, Embryonic Stem Cell Research Oversight
   Committee
Mount Sinai School of Medicine
New York NY

Emily A. Singer, M.D.
Clinical Fellow in Anaesthesia
Harvard Medical School
Massachusetts General Hospital
Boston MA

Ken Solt, M.D.
Assistant Professor of Anaesthesia
Harvard Medical School
Massachusetts General Hospital
Boston MA

Spiro G. Spanakis, D.O.
Assistant Professor of Anesthesiology and
Pediatrics

University of Massachusetts Medical School
Associate Quality and Safety Officer
Department of Anesthesiology
UMass Memorial Medical Center
Worcester MA

Wolfgang Steudel, M.D.
Assistant Professor of Anaesthesia
Harvard Medical School
Massachusetts General Hospital
Boston MA

Matthias Stopfkuchen-Evans, M.D.
Instructor in Anaesthesia
Harvard Medical School
Brigham and Women's Hospital
Boston MA

Michael P. Storey, CRNA, M.S.
Lawrence General Hospital
Lawrence MA

Gary R. Strichartz, Ph.D.
Professor of Anaesthesia (Pharmacology)
Harvard Medical School
Brigham and Women's Hospital
Boston MA

Balachundhar Subramaniam, M.D., M.P.H.
Assistant Professor of Anaesthesia
Harvard Medical School
Director, Division of Cardiac Anesthesia Research
Beth Israel Deaconess Medical Center
Boston MA

Wariya Sukhupragarn, M.D., F.R.C.A.T.
Assistant Professor in Anesthesiology
Chang Mai University
Maharaj Nakorn Chian Mai Hospital
Chiang Mai, THAILAND
Research Fellow in Airway Management
Yale University School of Medicine
Yale–New Haven Hospital
New Haven CT

John Summers, M.D.
Clinical Fellow in Anaesthesia
Harvard Medical School
Beth Israel Deaconess Medical Center
Boston MA

Shine Sun, M.D.
Cardiothoracic Anesthesiologist
Providence Regional Medical Center
Everett WA

Eswar Sundar, M.B., B.S.
Instructor in Anaesthesia
Harvard Medical School
Beth Israel Deaconess Medical Center
Boston MA

Sugantha Sundar, M.B., B.S.
Assistant Professor of Anaesthesia
Harvard Medical School
Beth Israel Deaconess Medical Center
Boston MA

Neelakantan Sunder, M.B., B.S.
Assistant Professor of Anaesthesia
Harvard Medical School
Massachusetts General Hospital
Boston MA

Faraz Syed, D.O.
Critical Care Fellow
Department of Anesthesiology
University of Chicago Medical School
Chicago IL

Usha B. Tedrow, M.D.
Instructor in Medicine
Harvard Medical School
Brigham and Women's Hospital
Boston MA

Nelson L. Thaemert, M.D.
Instructor in Anaesthesia
Harvard Medical School
Brigham and Women's Hospital
Boston MA

George P. Topulos, M.D.
Associate Professor of Anaesthesia
Harvard Medical School
Brigham and Women's Hospital
Boston MA

Lawrence C. Tsen, M.D.
Associate Professor of Anaesthesia
Harvard Medical School
Brigham and Women's Hospital
Boston MA

Richard D. Urman, M.D., M.B.A.
Assistant Professor of Anaesthesia
Harvard Medical School
Brigham and Women's Hospital
Boston MA

Charles A. Vacanti, M.D.
Vandam/Covino Professor of Anaesthesia
Harvard Medical School
Anesthesiologist-in-Chief
Brigham and Women's Hospital
Boston MA

Francis X. Vacanti, M.D.
Assistant Professor of Anaesthesia
Harvard Medical School
Massachusetts General Hospital
Boston MA

Joshua C. Vacanti, M.D.
Instructor in Anaesthesia
Harvard Medical School
Brigham and Women's Hospital
Boston MA

Assia Valovska, M.D.
Instructor in Anaesthesia
Harvard Medical School
Brigham and Women's Hospital
Boston MA

Ivan T. Valovski, M.D.
Instructor in Anaesthesia
VA Boston Healthcare
Harvard Medical School
Massachusetts General Hospital
Boston MA

Mary Ann Vann, M.D.
Instructor in Anaesthesia
Harvard Medical School
Beth Israel Deaconess Medical Center
Boston MA

Susan Vassallo, M.D.
Assistant Professor of Anaesthesia
Harvard Medical School
Massachusetts General Hospital
Boston, MA

Anasuya Vasudevan, M.D., M.B., B.S.
Anesthesia, Critical Care, and Pain Medicine
Director of Education, Obstetric Anesthesia
Fellowship Director, Obstetric Anesthesia
Department of Anesthesia, Critical Care, and Pain Medicine
Beth Israel Deaconess Medical Center
Boston MA

Kamen V. Vlassakov, M.D.
Assistant Professor of Anaesthesia
Harvard Medical School
Director, Regional and Orthopedic Anesthesia
Brigham and Women's Hospital
Boston MA

Gian Paolo Volpato
Attending Anesthesiologist
Clinica Las Condes
Hospital Mutual de Seguridad
Santiago CHILE

Essi M. Vulli, M.D.
Staff Anesthesiologist
Valley Anesthesiology Consultants
Phoenix AZ

J. Matthias Walz, M.D.
Assistant Professor of Anesthesiology and Surgery
Department of Anesthesiology, Division of Critical
    Care Medicine
University of Massachusetts Medical School
UMass Memorial Medical Center
Worcester MA

Jingping Wang, Ph.D., M.D.
Instructor in Anaesthesia
Harvard Medical School
Massachusetts General Hospital
Boston MA

James F. Watkins, M.D.
Instructor in Surgery
Harvard Medical School
Brigham and Women's Hospital
Boston MA

Maxwell Weinmann, Ph.D., M.B., B.S.
Assistant Professor of Anaesthesia
Harvard Medical School
Brigham and Women's Hospital
Boston MA

Sharon L. Wetherall, M.D.
Anesthesiologist
Physician Anesthesia Services
Lutheran Medical Center
Wheatridge CO

Mallory Williams, M.D., M.P.H.
Associate Professor of Surgery
Chief of the Division of Trauma, Acute Care Surgery, and
    Critical Care
Trauma Medical Director and Director of the
    Surgical ICU
University of Toledo Medical Center
Toledo OH

Sarah H. Wiser, M.D.
Instructor in Anaesthesia
Harvard Medical School
Brigham and Women's Hospital
Boston MA

Zhiling Xiong, Ph.D., M.D.
Instructor in Anaesthesia
Harvard Medical School
Brigham and Women's Hospital
Boston MA

Warren M. Zapol, M.D.
Reginald Jenney Professor of
    Anaesthesia
Harvard Medical School
Massachusetts General Hospital
Boston MA

Jie Zhou, M.D.
Instructor in Anaesthesia
Harvard Medical School
Brigham and Women's Hospital
Boston MA

Preface

Why another basic textbook of anesthesiology? Some of the most classic texts on this topic have been published in many editions and have enjoyed popularity for decades, especially among trainees. Major clinical textbooks have likewise evolved through many editions, providing trainees and practitioners with extensive reference works. Our goal was to develop a text that bridges this gap. *Essential Clinical Anesthesia* is designed to be read cover to cover by trainees, but also to serve as a succinct and compact reference for more experienced practitioners. The format differs from most other texts by featuring a large number of short chapters. The book contains 29 sections and 184 chapters. The majority of these are found in the print version and the remainder, including some of the more advanced topics, can be accessed on the Internet at www.cambridge.org/vacanti. We have endeavored to keep the length of each chapter short enough to be read comfortably in a single sitting yet comprehensive enough to cover the basics as well as the state of the art. References are sufficient to allow the interested reader to delve deeper yet reasonable in number to allow the reader to focus on the most important works on the subject.

We have followed the lead of major textbooks by making this text a multi-authored work. More than 150 authors, all experts in their fields, have written the chapters, and experienced section editors have ensured accuracy and consistency of the format. The astute reader will note that many authors are from Boston teaching hospitals but overall are drawn from institutions nationwide and beyond. We hope this provides a broad perspective on the field of anesthesiology.

The editors wish to express their gratitude to Jerry Buterbaugh, Angela Butler, Jodi Edelstein, Dr. Joseph Garfield, Meghan Hurley, Dr. Robert Pilon, Dr. Matthias Stopfkuchen-Evans, Dr. George Topulos, and Barbara Walthall of Aptara, Inc. for providing valuable editorial assistance, and the editors appreciate the support of Cambridge University Press in the preparation of this textbook. We hope that *Essential Clinical Anesthesia* will prove to be a valuable textbook that will enrich the libraries of our readers and help advance the study of anesthesiology.

Charles A. Vacanti
Pankaj K. Sikka
Richard D. Urman
Mark Dershwitz
B. Scott Segal

Boston, Massachusetts

Foreword

"The practice of medicine is an art based on science."

William Osler

Since William T. G. Morton administered ether to Gilbert Abbott at Massachusetts General Hospital on October 16, 1846, anesthesiology has evolved into one of the most complex disciplines of medicine. The past years have witnessed numerous scientific and technologic advances, resulting in a mountain of information to read and digest. Notable among these are receptor–drug interactions, genes and mutations, and genetic and acquired physiologic variables, to name a few. Variations in these processes among individuals as well as in an individual from time to time serve to explain the wide variations clinicians see in pain perception, stress response, and anesthetic requirements.

While these and other scientific advances provide a strong scientific foundation for clinical practice, art is equally or perhaps more important to produce the best possible clinical outcomes. In this regard, the legacy of William Osler and other giants, who practiced medicine at a time when technologic tools were barely existent, is a constant reminder about the importance of art as well as science in the clinical practice of anesthesiology, a complex branch of medicine.

This book, in an easy-to-access format, is designed to present the essential scientific and non-scientific aspects of the knowledge base. The chapters are written by authors who are well versed in their respective areas of expertise. I am confident that this book will serve readers well in enhancing the art and science of anesthesiology in their clinical practice.

S. Rao Mallampati, M.D.
Boston, Massachusetts

History of anesthesia

Rafael A. Ortega and Christine Mai

It has been said that the disadvantage of not understanding the past is to not understand the present. Knowledge of the history of anesthesia enables us to appreciate the discoveries that shaped this medical field, to recognize the scope of anesthesiology today, and to predict future advancements (Table 1.1).

It is generally agreed that the first successful public demonstration of general inhalation anesthesia with diethyl ether occurred in Boston in the 19th century. Prior to this occasion, all but the simplest procedures in surgery were "to be dreaded only less than death itself." Throughout history, pain prohibited surgical advances and consumed patients. Imagine the sense of awe and pride when William Thomas Green Morton (1819–1868), a dentist from Massachusetts, demonstrated the use of ether to anesthetize a young man for the removal of a tumor. The celebrated demonstration in 1846 at the Massachusetts General Hospital heralded a new era of pain-free operations. As Johann Friedrich Dieffenbach, author of *Ether against Pain*, stated, "Pain, the highest consciousness of our earthly existence, the most distinct sensation of the imperfection of our body, must bow before the power of the human mind, before the power of ether vapor."

Anesthesia prior to ether

The first forays into the field of anesthesiology occurred much earlier than Morton's demonstration. The Greek physician Dioscorides (A.D. 40–90), for instance, reported on the analgesic properties of mandragora, extracted from the bark and leaves of the mandrake plant in the first century. Agents such as ethyl alcohol, cannabis, and opium were inhaled by the ancients for their stupefying effects before surgery. Alchemist and physician Arnold of Villanova (c. 1238–c. 1310) used a mixture of opium, mandragora, and henbane to make his patients insensible to pain.

From the ninth to the 13th century, the "soporific sponge" was used to provide pain relief. These sponges were impregnated with a liquid made from boiling a combination of mandrake leaves, poppies, and herbs. Prior to surgery, the sponge was reconstituted with hot water and placed over the nostrils of the afflicted to deliver the anesthetic. Alcohol fumes also were used in the surgical setting during the Middle Ages, but proved to be of poor value because of their inadequacy both in pain

relief and in minimizing the recollection of unpleasant memories of the surgical procedure.

In the 16th century, Paracelsus (1493–1544) produced laudanum, an opium derivative in the form of a tincture. Laudanum, or "wine of opium," was used as an analgesic but also was inappropriately prescribed for meningitis, cardiac disease, and tuberculosis. Still, alcohol and opium were regarded as of practical value in diminishing the pain of operations by the mid-1800s, despite their relative ineffectiveness.

In 1804, decades before Morton's demonstration, Seishu Hanaoka (1760–1835), a surgeon in Japan, administered general anesthesia. Hanaoka used an herbal concoction containing a combination of potent anticholinergic alkaloids capable of inducing unconsciousness. The patients drank the preparation known as "Tsusensan" before Hanaoka performed surgery. It is also known that Chinese physicians have used acupuncture to ease surgical pain for centuries.

Nitrous oxide

Joseph Priestley (1733–1804), an English clergyman and chemist, first described nitrous oxide's properties as an anesthetic. Like ether, nitrous oxide was known for its ability to produce lightheadedness and inebriation. Sir Humphry Davy (1778–1829) noted the gas's effect on respiration and the central nervous system. In his book *Nitrous Oxide*, Davy commented on its effects of transiently relieving headaches and toothaches and its capability to alleviate physical pain during surgical procedures. The term *laughing gas* was coined by Davy because of its ability to trigger uncontrollable laughter. This gas remains the oldest inhaled anesthetic still used today.

Diethyl ether

The compound diethyl ether has been known for centuries. It may have been first discovered by the Arabian philosopher Jabir ibn Hayyam in the eighth century. Credit also is given to the 13th century European alchemist Raymundus Lullius, who first called it "sweet vitriol." This compound later was renamed *ether*, which in Greek means "the upper, pure bright air." By the 16th century, Paracelsus recognized and recorded the analgesic properties of ether. He noted that it produced drowsiness in chickens, causing them to fall asleep and awaken unharmed.

Table 1.1.   Timeline of the history of anesthesia

First century A.D.	Greek physician Dioscorides reports analgesic properties of mandragora
Ninth–13th century	Soporific sponge method for delivering pain relief
16th century	Paracelsus introduces laudanum, "wine of opium." Spanish conquistadores' account of curare in South America
18th century	
1773	Nitrous oxide first introduced by Joseph Priestley
19th century	
1800	Humphry Davy publishes *Nitrous Oxide*
1804	Seishu Hanaoka of Japan administers general anesthesia
1842	Crawford Long administers diethyl ether inhalational general anesthesia
1844	Horace Wells administers nitrous oxide for dental analgesia
1846	William Morton's public demonstration of diethyl ether at Massachusetts General Hospital
1847	James Young Simpson administers chloroform for general anesthesia in England
1853	John Snow administers chloroform to Queen Victoria for the birth of Prince Leopold
1857	Claude Bernard discovers the effects of curare located at the myoneural junction
1884	Carl Koller introduces the use of cocaine for ophthalmic surgery
1885	William Halsted describes techniques of anesthetizing nerve plexuses using cocaine
1889	August Bier performs the first surgical spinal anesthesia
20th century	
1903	Phenobarbital synthesized by Fischer and von Mering
1905	Procaine introduced as a local anesthetic Long Island Society of Anesthetists founded
1911	Long Island Society of Anesthetists becomes the New York Society of Anesthetists
1927	Ralph Waters establishes first anesthesiology postgraduate training program at the University of Wisconsin–Madison
1932	Thiopental and thiamylal synthesized
1934	Thiopental used by both Waters and Lundy for induction of anesthesia
1935	Emery Rovenstine organizes an anesthesia department at Bellevue Hospital, NY
1936	New York Society of Anesthetists becomes the American Society of Anesthetists
1938	The American Board of Anesthesiology founded
1940	William Lemmon introduces concept of continuous spinal anesthesia
1942	Drug form of curare, intocostrin, introduced
1943	Lidocaine introduced as local anesthetic by Lofgren and Lindquist of Sweden
1944	Edward Tuohy invents the Tuohy needle
1945	American Society of Anesthetists becomes the American Society of Anesthesiologists (ASA)
1949	Daniel Bovet synthesizes succinylcholine
1951	Halothane introduced into clinical practice
1960	Methoxyflurane introduced into clinical practice; its use was limited by nephrotoxicity
1962	Ketamine synthesized
1964	Etomidate synthesized
1965	Isoflurane first introduced; it was marketed in the 1970s
1977	Propofol synthesized
1983	Archie Brain develops the laryngeal mask airway
1985	Anesthesia Patient Safety Foundation established
1986	Standards for basic anesthesia monitoring approved by the ASA House of Delegates
1992	Desflurane introduced into clinical practice
1994	Sevoflurane introduced into clinical practice
1995–present:	The past decade has seen advances in a variety of areas, including refinements in anesthesia delivery apparatus, ultrasound applications for regional anesthesia, transesophageal echocardiography, depth of anesthesia monitors, total intravenous anesthetics, supraglottic airway devices, and other innovations, helping to make the administration of anesthesia safer.

Before ether became known as a general anesthetic, it was marketed as a pain reliever. It also was used as an inexpensive recreational drug during "ether frolics." Many famous British scientists, such as Robert Boyle (1627–1691), Isaac Newton (1643–1728), and Michael Faraday (1791–1867), examined the properties of ether. However, they did not make the connection between its analgesic qualities and the possibility of complete surgical anesthesia. It was not until later that ether was used as a general anesthetic. Crawford Williamson Long (1815–1978), a physician from Georgia, administered ether on March 30, 1842, to James M. Venable for the removal of a neck tumor. Long also conducted comparative trials of procedures, with and without ether, to demonstrate that alleviation of pain was a result of the drug rather than individual pain threshold or hypnotism.

Horace Wells (1815–1848) was first in attempting to publicly demonstrate general anesthesia. Wells, a dentist, knew of the analgesic effects of nitrous oxide and used it for tooth extractions. Understanding its effects, he attempted to demonstrate a painless tooth extraction at Harvard Medical School in 1845. Perhaps because of the low potency of nitrous oxide, during the procedure the subject moved and groaned. Wells was discredited for his display. Deeply disappointed by the

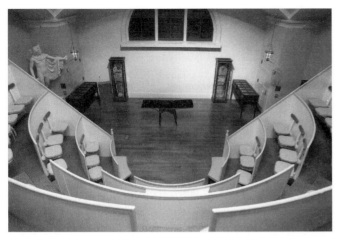

Figure 1.1. The Ether Dome, designed by architect Charles Bulfinch, was originally known as the Surgical Amphitheater of Massachusetts General Hospital.

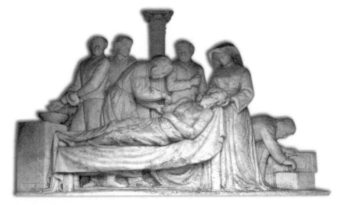

Figure 1.3. Bas-relief on the Ether Monument in Boston representing a surgical procedure in a hospital, with the patient under the influence of ether. To the left, an assistant is washing his hands in a basin, denoting an appreciation for early attempts at antisepsis.

failed demonstration, he committed suicide in 1848. Nevertheless, his idea inspired individuals such as Morton to persist in demonstrating the efficacy of these drugs. On October 16, 1846, Morton administered ether, allowing surgeon John Collins Warren (1778–1856) to painlessly remove a mandible tumor from Edward Gilbert Abbott. This event took place in the surgical amphitheater at Massachusetts General Hospital, which is now known as the Ether Dome, a designated national historical landmark (Fig. 1.1). The account of the ether demonstration appeared the next day in the *Boston Daily Journal*, and within months the discovery of surgical anesthesia was known worldwide.

The ether controversy

Ether anesthesia proved to be controversial from the start. Morton wanted to capitalize on the discovery and initially refused to divulge the identity of the agent in his inhaler (Fig. 1.2). Wells and chemist Charles T. Jackson (1805–1880), Morton's advisor, both claimed the discovery belonged to them. Jackson, a Boston physician and chemistry professor, was well aware of the failed public demonstrations of the past and had advised Morton to use ether rather than nitrous oxide in his historical debut. For this contribution, Jackson adamantly argued it was he who should be credited for the "idea" of administering

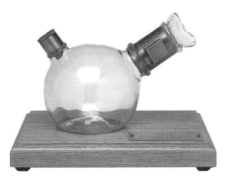

Figure 1.2. A replica of Morton's inhaler as used at the first public demonstration of ether anesthesia on October 16, 1846.

ether-inhaled anesthesia. Wells contended that he had successfully administered general anesthesia with nitrous oxide on several occasions. However, he never convincingly proved it. Long also claimed he had demonstrated the uses of ether in rural areas well before Morton. However, Long did not publish his experiences until 1849, three years after Morton's demonstration. These debates have collectively been referred to as "the ether controversy."

In 1868, to commemorate the first public demonstration of ether in Boston, a monument was erected in the city's Public Garden. The Ether Monument, with its marble and granite images and inscriptions, addresses universal themes such as the suffering caused by war, the desire on behalf of loved ones to relieve pain, and the triumph of medical science (Fig. 1.3 and Fig. 1.4). Perhaps no other monument related to medicine is so rich in history, controversies, and allegories. The Ether Monument, however, makes no mention of any of the claimants to the discovery.

Acceptance of anesthesia in the Western world

In some ways, what matters most is not *who* discovered anesthesia, but rather *where* and *when* it was discovered. Some scholars believe that a spirit of humanitarianism and political freedom were necessary for the development of anesthesia to occur in the 19th century. Initially, there were religious objections to anesthesia. Certain individuals believed it was against the will of God to alleviate pain. The use of anesthesia in labor and delivery was particularly contentious, in part because of the "curse of Eve," which states, "In sorrow thou shalt bring forth children" (Genesis 3:16). Also on biblical grounds, others supported anesthesia, reasoning that God himself performed the first operation under "anesthesia" when he removed Adam's rib: "The Lord God caused a deep sleep to fall upon Adam and he slept…" (Genesis 2:21). Other objections to anesthesia were based on morality rather than the religious implications of pain relief. Some argued that anesthesia's disinhibiting effects threatened

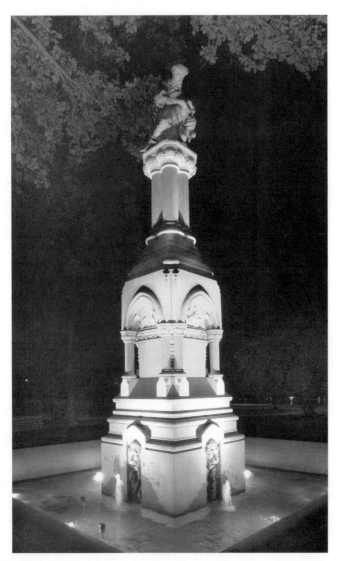

Figure 1.4. The Ether Monument in the Boston Public Garden, with evening illumination and working fountains.

the virtue and decency of women. In 1853, Queen Victoria effectively silenced all opposition when John Snow anesthetized her with chloroform during the birth of Prince Leopold.

Chloroform

Because ether was such a safe anesthetic, its administration was relegated largely to nonphysicians in the United States, whereas in England chloroform quickly became the anesthetic of choice. This preference might have arisen out of a sense of national pride, being that ether anesthesia was introduced in America, which had relatively recently gained its independence. Chloroform, a more dangerous drug than ether, required more skillful and careful titration. The resulting challenges of chloroform administration attracted the attention of brilliant physicians and investigators, including the Scottish obstetrician James Young Simpson (1811–1870) and the English anesthetist John Snow (1813–1858). This may explain why there were few

developments in anesthesia within the United States for many decades after the introduction of ether while in Britain, great progress was made.

Modern inhaled anesthetics

The search for an ideal inhaled anesthetic led to the introduction of many chemicals, including ethyl chloride, ethylene, cyclopropane, and other volatile agents, during the first half of the 20th century. However, their use faded because of varied disadvantages, such as strong pungency, weak potency, and flammability. These agents soon were replaced by fluorinated hydrocarbons. Fluorination made inhaled anesthetics more stable, less combustible, and less toxic. In 1951, halothane was recognized as a superior anesthetic over its predecessors. In the 1960s, methoxyflurane was popular for a decade, until its dose-related nephrotoxicity discouraged its use. Enflurane and its isomer, isoflurane, were introduced in 1963 and 1965, respectively. Enflurane's popularity was limited after it was shown to produce cardiovascular depression and seizures. Isoflurane was more difficult to synthesize and purify than enflurane. However, once the purification process was refined and further trials proved its safety, isoflurane was marketed in the late 1970s and remains a popular anesthetic. For 20 years, no further developments occurred until the release of desflurane in 1992 and sevoflurane in 1994. Today, these three agents, in addition to nitrous oxide, constitute the mainstay of inhalation anesthetics.

Regional anesthesia

Although chloroform and ether provided analgesia for obstetric pain, disadvantages such as inadequate uterine contractions and neonatal respiratory depression were noted. The invention of the hollow needle in 1853 by Alexander Wood allowed for the development of regional anesthesia techniques as an effective alternative to inhaled anesthetics.

In 1884, Carl Koller (1858–1944), an ophthalmologist, introduced the use of cocaine for ophthalmic surgery. Within a year of his reports, injections of cocaine were described to anesthetize nerve trunks and the brachial plexus by William S. Halsted (1852–1922). The idea of spinal anesthesia first was conceived in 1885 by a neurologist, Leonard Corning (1855–1923). Although his writings described the administration of cocaine, the injection was extradural rather than in the subarachnoid space. Corning's technique was improved by the German physician Heinrich Quincke (1842–1922), who described the level below which it was safest to perform a lumbar puncture. In 1899, using Quincke's technique, August Bier (1861–1949) performed the first spinal anesthesia for a surgical procedure. The Swiss obstetrician Oscar Kreis recognized the advantages of regional anesthesia in obstetrics and administered the first spinal anesthesia for control of labor pain at the start of the 20th century.

Early cases of regional anesthesia were noted to have side effects, such as high incidences of postdural puncture headache, vomiting, and the propensity for the those administering it to become addicted to cocaine. The addictive nature of cocaine and its toxicity led to the discovery of safer local anesthetics, such as procaine in 1905 and lidocaine in 1943. In 1940, the introduction of continuous spinal anesthesia was credited to William T. Lemmon, who advocated the administration of repeated small doses of procaine through a malleable needle connected to a rubber tubing and syringe. Four years later, Edward Tuohy (1908–1959) of the Mayo Clinic introduced two important modifications: the invention of the Tuohy needle and the idea of threading a catheter into the epidural space for incremental doses of local anesthetics. A technique for locating the epidural space was made popular by the writings of Achille M. Dogliotti (1897–1966), who identified it using the "loss of resistance."

Over the past 60 years, intrathecal and epidural administration of local anesthetics, opioids, and steroids has become commonplace for analgesia throughout the course of labor and for managing chronic pain. The development of plexus blocks and other regional anesthesia techniques progressed to incorporate the use of nerve stimulators and ultrasound to facilitate locating nerves, thus enhancing the quality of the block.

Neuromuscular blocking agents

Neuromuscular blocking agents were introduced into anesthetic practice nearly a century after the administration of inhalational anesthesia. Curare, the first isolated neuromuscular blocking agent, originally was used in hunting and tribal warfare by natives of South America. Curare alkaloid extracts from lianas (vines) were applied to arrow darts, which natives propelled using blowguns to poison their prey. Accounts of these Amazon jungle poisons by 16th century Spanish conquistadores intrigued the European medical community and triggered early experiments on animals, which determined that the agent paralyzes muscle function. The collaborative work of Benjamin Brodie (1783–1862) and Charles Waterton (1783–1865), demonstrated that animals injected with curare could survive with artificial ventilation. In 1857, Claude Bernard (1813–1878), a French physiologist, determined that the effect of the drug was located in neither the nerve nor the muscle, but at the junction of the two. Initially, there were limited medical applications for curare, such as ameliorating muscle spasms caused by tetanus, reducing trauma during seizure therapy, and treating Parkinson-like muscle rigidity. However, with the advent of tracheal intubation and mechanical ventilation, the use of curare to prevent laryngospasm during laryngoscopy or to relax abdominal muscles during surgery remarkably altered the practice of anesthesia.

On January 23, 1942, the drug form of curare, intocostrin, was introduced into anesthesia practice by anesthesiologist Harold R. Griffith (1894–1985) and his resident, Enid Johnson, at Montreal Homeopathic Hospital. The facilitation of tracheal intubation and abdominal muscle relaxation produced by intocostrin during cyclopropane anesthesia heralded

a new era for neuromuscular blocking agent development. Subsequent muscle relaxants, such as gallamine, decamethonium, and metocurine, were studied. However, their popularity was limited because of undesirable autonomic nervous system effects. In 1949, succinylcholine, a depolarizing neuromuscular agent, was synthesized by Nobel laureate Daniel Bovet (1907–1992). Nondepolarizing neuromuscular drugs, such as the aminosteroids pancuronium, vecuronium and rocuronium and the benzylisoquinoliniums atracurium and cis-atracurium, were introduced in the late 20th century.

Intravenous anesthetics

The first intravenous induction agent was phenobarbital, a barbiturate synthesized by Emil Fischer (1852–1919) and Joseph von Mering in 1903. As a hypnotic, phenobarbital caused prolonged periods of unconsciousness and slow emergence. Hexobarbital, a short-acting oxybarbiturate, was introduced in 1932 but was subsequently replaced by a sulfated barbiturate, thiopental, a potent agent with rapid onset of action and few excitatory side effects. In 1934, both Ralph Waters (1883–1979) at the University of Wisconsin and John Lundy (1894–1973) at the Mayo Clinic successfully administered thiopental as an intravenous anesthetic agent. Furthermore, John Lundy's continued research on intravenous anesthetics popularized its use in clinical practice. His concept of "balanced anesthesia" emphasized combining multiple anesthetic drugs and techniques to provide hypnosis, muscle relaxation, and analgesia. This approach led to the optimization of operating conditions and reduction of side effects, thereby making anesthesia administration safer for patients. The widespread use of thiopental stimulated the development of other classes of intravenous hypnotics, including ketamine (1962), etomidate (1964), and propofol (1977). Benzodiazepines, opioids, antiemetics, and other drugs have enriched the intravenous pharmacologic armamentarium, and their combined use represents an extension of Lundy's approach of balanced anesthesia.

Anesthesiology as a medical specialty

The field of anesthesiology as a recognized medical specialty developed gradually in America during the 20th century. For decades, formal instruction in anesthesia was nonexistent and the field was practiced only by a few self-taught individuals. In the 1910s, Ralph Waters described the environment he encountered in which nurses administered anesthesia because there were few physicians trained as proficient anesthetists. He advocated the development of dedicated anesthesia departments and training programs. Subsequently, several anesthesiologists, including Thomas D. Buchanan and John Lundy, established anesthesia departments at New York Medical College and the Mayo Clinic, respectively. The first anesthesiology postgraduate training program was established by Waters at the University of Wisconsin–Madison in 1927. His department was a milestone in establishing anesthesiology within a university setting. Waters's influence in anesthesiology determined the commitment of this specialty to education and research. Successful application of the Wisconsin model was best reflected by the work of Waters's academic descendants, such as Emery Rovenstine at New York's Bellevue Hospital and Robert Dripps at the University of Pennsylvania.

Modern anesthesiology practice

Although advances were made in the early 1900s, including Sir Robert Macintosh's and Sir Ivan Magill's contributions to airway management, the modern practice of anesthesiology evolved in the latter half of the 20th century with an emphasis on safety. In 1985, the Anesthesia Patient Safety Foundation was established with a mission "to ensure that no patient is harmed by anesthesia." The introduction of additional monitoring tools, such as capnometry and pulse oximetry, remarkably decreased mortality rates during anesthesia. The refinements in current anesthesia delivery systems would have been unimaginable for anesthesiologists of yesteryear.

Today, the practice of anesthesiology in the United States depends on guidelines provided by the American Society of Anesthesiologists (ASA). The stated goals of this professional organization are to establish "an educational, research and scientific association of physicians organized to raise and maintain the standards of anesthesiology and to improve the care of patients."

The history of anesthesiology is vast and complex; this chapter is meant to serve as a brief overview. The best repository for documents and artifacts relating to the history of anesthesia is the Wood Library–Museum at ASA headquarters in Park Ridge, Illinois.

Suggested readings

Bigelow HJ. Insensibility during surgical operations produced by inhalation. *Boston Med Surg J* 1846; 35:309–317.

Ellis T, Narr B, Bacon D. Developing a specialty: J.S. Lundy's three major contributions to anesthesiology. *J Clin Anesth* 2004; 16:226–229.

Frolich MA, Caton D. Pioneers in epidural needle design. *Anesth Analg* 2001; 93:215–220.

Greene NM. Anesthesia and the development of surgery (1846–1896). *Anesth Analg* 1979; 58:5–12.

Griffith HR, Johnson GE. The use of curare in general anesthesia. *Anesthesiology* 1942; 3:418–420.

Keys TE. Paracelsus, 1493–1541. *Anesth Analg* 1972; 51:533.

Knapp H. Cocaine and its use in ophthalmic and general surgery. *Arch Ophthamol Dec* 1834; 1–5.

Lyons AS, Petrucelli RJ. *Medicine: An Illustrated History*. New York: Abradale Press; 1978:530.

McIntyre AR. Historical background, early use and development of muscle relaxants. *Anesthesiology* 1959; 20:409–415.

Ortega RA, Kelly LR, Yee MK, Lewis, KP. Written in Granite: A history of the ether monument and its significance for anesthesiology. *Anesthesiology* 2006; 105: 838–842.

Pierce EC. Anesthesia monitoring guidelines: their origin and development. *ASA Newsletter Sept* 2002; vol. 66(9).

Waters RM. Pioneering in anesthesiology. *Postgrad Med* 1948; 4:265–270.

Waters RM. Why the professional anesthetist? *Journal-Lancet* 1919; 39:32–34.

Waters RM, Hathaway HR, Cassels WH. The relation of anesthesiology to medical education. *JAMA* 1939; 112: 1667–1671.

Preoperative Care and Evaluation

B. Scott Segal and Angela M. Bader, editors

Preoperative anesthetic assessment

Sohail K. Mahboobi and Sheila R. Barnett

The preoperative assessment is a vital part of any procedure requiring anesthesia. The assessment itself may vary considerably, from a simple interview and limited physical examination on the day of surgery to an extensive medical evaluation including invasive cardiac testing and radiologic examinations weeks in advance of the surgery. The choice and type of the preoperative assessment depend on several variables, including the patient's age and medical history as well as the type and degree of risk of procedure planned. Patient and physician preferences should also be considered.

The preoperative assessment

Preoperative assessment provides an evaluation of the patient's anesthetic risk from the proposed procedure and allows recommendations to be made that may minimize risk and ensure a smooth transition from surgical booking to the operating room and beyond. Recommendations may include further testing, consultations, adjustments of medication, or simply reassurance and a consequent reduction of anxiety. Practically, the preoperative assessment may also identify special needs, such as the need for a latex-free environment, special blood products, interpreters, or airway equipment. Failure to plan for these needs may lead to surgical delays. In addition, instructions for fasting and medications, as well as expectations for the day of surgery and postoperative course, should all be provided (Fig. 2.1).

A preoperative assessment should include a medical history focusing on active medical issues, medication usage and past anesthetic and surgical experiences, a limited physical examination, an airway assessment, and additional testing as indicated. The anesthetic risk is derived from the knowledge of the patient and the surgery. The preoperative interview should include a discussion with the patient about the risks and benefits of different anesthetic techniques. Informed consent for anesthesia administration should be obtained. There are several alternative approaches to preoperative assessment (primary physician clearance, telephone interview, preoperative health survey, Internet health quiz), and the choice depends on hospital resources and the type of surgical facility.

The preoperative history

The preoperative history includes a thorough systematic review of the patient's medical problems, including an evaluation of available medical information. Organ systems and selected disorders that have particular impact preoperatively are briefly reviewed, highlighting major issues that should be covered in the course of a preoperative assessment.

Cardiovascular system

Cardiovascular complications may result in significant morbidity and mortality, and a thorough preoperative assessment of cardiovascular status should be part of any routine preoperative evaluation. Questions should be directed at assessing the status of current cardiac problems and eliciting evidence suggesting occult cardiac disease. A complete cardiovascular history also includes assessment of functional capacity (Table 2.1) and ascertains whether symptoms that may indicate significant

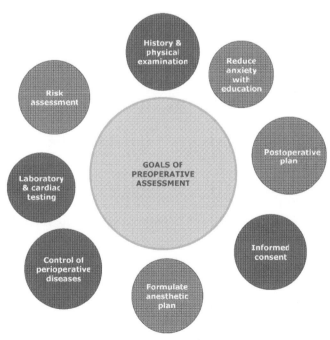

Figure 2.1. Goals of preoperative assessment

Table 2.1. Functional assessment scale

1 MET	Can you take care of yourself? Eat dress, use the toilet? Walk indoors around the house? Walk 1–2 blocks on level ground at 2–3 mph? Do light housework?
4 MET	Climb a flight of stairs? Carry groceries? Walk on level ground at 4 mph? Run a short distance? Do heavy housework? Do moderate sports – golf, dance, doubles tennis?
10 MET	Play competitive sports? Play singles tennis? Ski?

cardiac disease are present. Details about past cardiac events and testing should be requested and reviewed. Past electrocardiograms (ECGs) are critical to obtain in patients found to have an abnormal ECG.

Functional capacity

Functional capacity may be assessed from a careful history in the form of metabolic equivalents. The *metabolic equivalent of task (MET)*, or simply *metabolic equivalent*, is a physiologic concept expressing the energy cost of physical activities as multiples of resting metabolic rate. MET is defined as the ratio of metabolic rate (and therefore the rate of energy consumption) during a specific physical activity to a reference metabolic rate at rest, set by convention to 3.5 ml O_2/kg/min or equivalently, 1 kcal (or 4.184 kJ)/kg/h. By convention, 1 MET is considered the resting metabolic rate obtained during quiet sitting. Patients unable to meet a 4-MET standard are at increased risk for perioperative cardiac risk. Daily activities, such as eating, dressing, walking around the house, and dishwashing, range from 1 to 4 METs. Climbing one flight of stairs, walking on level ground at about 6 km/h, running a short distance, or playing a game of golf range from 4 to 10 METs. Playing tennis, swimming, and playing football exceed 10 METs. This is helpful in assessing cardiac risk and planning preoperative testing (Table 2.1).

The decision to send a patient for further cardiac evaluation is complex and includes consideration of patient comorbidities as well as the level of risk of the planned procedure. The guidelines written by the American College of Cardiology (ACC) and the American Heart Association (AHA) have updated recently and provide excellent algorithms for guidance

in this regard along with various levels of evidence (Table 2.2, Fig. 2.2). Briefly, emergent surgical procedures may not allow further cardiac assessment or treatment. In this case only perioperative medical management and recommendations are required. The patients who are having nonemergency procedures should be evaluated for the presence of active cardiac conditions (Table 2.3). The presence of any of these active cardiac conditions warrants further evaluation prior to procedures of even the lowest risk. If none of these active conditions exists, the patient's functional status should then be assessed.

According to these guidelines, if the patient's functional status is good (>4 MET), even higher-risk procedures (Table 2.4) may be undertaken without further cardiac noninvasive testing. If the functional status is inadequate or cannot be obtained, the presence of five clinical risk factors, as defined by these guidelines, should be ascertained. These clinical risk factors include a history of ischemic cardiac disease, a history of compensated or prior heart failure, diabetes, renal insufficiency, and cerebrovascular disease (Table 2.5). If three or more of these factors are present, and vascular or higher-risk procedures are being contemplated, further cardiac noninvasive testing may be warranted if it is felt this will affect management. Table 2.6 summarizes recommendations for noninvasive stress testing before noncardiac surgery.

Adequate β-blockade should be established perioperatively, if indicated. The recommendations are same for the patients with one or more risk factors going for high-risk vascular or intermediate risk surgery. Patients with no risk factors can proceed with the planned procedure. According to the AHA/ACC guidelines only two groups should be mandated for β-blockade: vascular patients with recent positive provocative cardiac testing (based on Poldermans 1999) and patients already taking β-blockers. Other than that, β blockers are probably recommended for intermediate risk or vascular surgical procedures with the presence of more than one clinical risk factor. Their usefulness is uncertain for patients with no or one risk factor and not already on β blockers. Similarly, patients already receiving calcium channel blockers should continue these medications, including on the day of surgery. Patients taking statins should continue doing so because this has been linked to fewer perioperative cardiac events and improved outcome, presumably by modulating inflammatory pathways. The optimal time for initiation and duration of perioperative statin therapy remains unclear.

There are significant numbers of patients with a history of percutaneous coronary intervention (PCI) in the form

Table 2.2. Levels of evidence

Class I	Class IIa	Class IIb	Class III
Benefit >>> risk Procedure/ treatment should be performed/ administered	Benefit >> risk Additional studies required It is reasonable to perform procedure/ administer treatment	Benefit ≥ risk Additional studies required Procedure/ treatment may be considered	Risk ≥ benefit No additional studies needed Procedure/ treatment should not be performed/ administered because it is not helpful and may be harmful

Table 2.3. Active cardiac conditions as defined by ACC/AHA 2007 guidelines

Unstable coronary syndromes
    Unstable or severe angina
    May include stable angina in unusually sedentary patients
    Recent myocardial infarction (within 30 d)

Decompensated heart failure, worsening or new-onset heart failure

Significant arrhythmias
    Mobitz II atrioventricular block
    Third-degree atrioventricular block
    Symptomatic ventricular arrhythmias
    Supraventricular arrhythmias with uncontrolled ventricular rate
    Symptomatic bradycardia

Severe valvular disease
    Severe aortic stenosis (mean pressure gradient > 40 mm Hg, aortic valve
       area < 1.0 cm^2, or symptomatic)
    Symptomatic mitral stenosis

Table 2.4. Cardiac risk for noncardiac surgery

High risk (>5%)	Intermediate risk (<5%)	Low risk (<1%)
Emergency	Carotid endarterectomy	Endoscopic surgeries
Aortic and major vascular	Head and neck	Superficial procedures
Peripheral vascular	Intraperitoneal and intrathoracic	Cataract surgery
Lengthy procedures with major blood loss or fluid shifts	Orthopedic	Breast procedures
	Prostate	

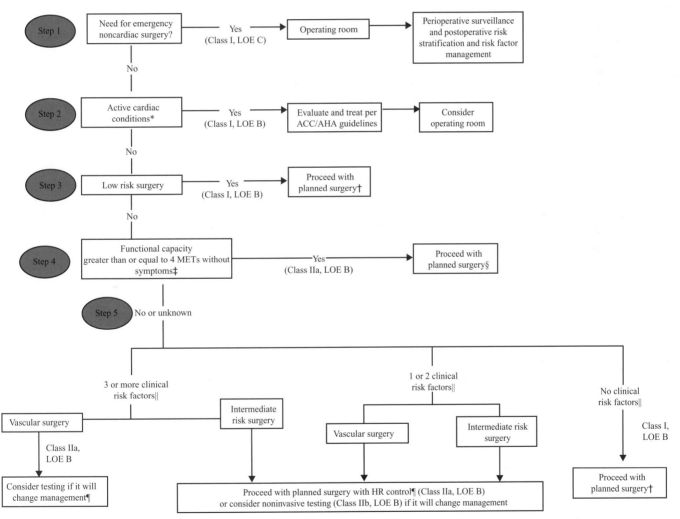

Figure 2.2. Cardiac evaluation and care algorithm for noncardiac surgery based on active clinical conditions, known cardiovascular disease, or cardiac risk factors for patients ≥ 50 years of age. *See Table 2.3 for active clinical conditions. †See class III recommendations in Table 2.6, Noninvasive Stress Testing. ‡See Table 2.1 for estimated MET level equivalent. §Noninvasive testing may be considered before surgery in specific patients with risk factors if it will change management. ||Clinical risk factors include ischemic heart disease, compensated or prior heart failure, diabetes mellitus, renal insufficiency, and cerebrovascular disease. Consider perioperative β-blockade for populations in which this has been shown to reduce cardiac morbidity/mortality. HR, heart rate; LOE, level of evidence. (Modified from Fleisher LA, et al. ACC/AHA 2007 Guidelines on Perioperative Cardiovascular Evaluation and Care for Noncardiac Surgery: Executive Summary: A Report of the American College of Cardiology/American Heart Association Task Force on Practice Guidelines. *Circulation* 2007; 116:1971–1996.)

Table 2.5. Patient clinical risk predictors

Clinical risk factors (formerly known as intermediate risk factors)	Minor risk predictors (have not been proven to increase perioperative risk independently)

History of ischemic heart disease
History of compensated or prior HF
Diabetes mellitus
Renal insufficiency
History of cerebrovascular disease
	Advanced age
	Abnormal ECG
	  • LV hypertrophy
	  • Left bundle-branch block
	  • ST-T abnormalities
	Rhythm other than sinus
	Uncontrolled systemic hypertension

MI, myocardial ischemia; HF, heart failure.

Table 2.6. Recommendations for noninvasive stress testing before noncardiac surgery

Class I	Patients with active cardiac conditions in whom noncardiac surgery is planned should be evaluated and treated per ACC/AHA guidelines before noncardiac surgery
Class IIa	Noninvasive stress testing of patients with 3 or more clinical risk factors and poor functional capacity (less than 4 METs) who require vascular surgery is reasonable if it will change management
Class IIb	Noninvasive stress testing may be considered for patients with at least 1 to 2 clinical risk factors and poor functional capacity (less than 4 METs) who require intermediate-risk or vascular surgery if it will change management.
Class III	• Noninvasive testing is not useful for patients with no clinical factors undergoing intermediate-risk noncardiac surgery • Noninvasive testing is not useful for patients undergoing low-risk noncardiac surgery

of balloon angioplasty, bare metal stents (BMS) or drug-eluting stents (DES). These patients require antiplatelet therapy to avoid thrombosis. According to AHA/ACC recommendations at least four weeks of antiplatelet therapy (clopidogrel) is required for patients with BMS and 12 months of dual antiplatelet therapy (aspirin and clopidogrel) is required for patients with DES. Surgeries during this period of antiplatelet therapy pose a serious challenge. Recommendations are to delay the planned surgical procedures for at least 14 days after balloon angioplasty, 30 to 45 days after BMS placement and 365 days after DES placement. After these periods one can proceed to the operating room with continuation of aspirin (Figure 2.3).

A history of hypertension is common, affecting more than 50% of adult Americans. The preoperative assessment in a patient with hypertension should elicit any history of end-organ disease. Ischemia, myocardial infarction, diastolic dysfunction, renal failure, and cerebrovascular disease all may be consequences of untreated hypertension. Although blood pressure should optimally be controlled at the time of the preoperative visit, the literature suggests there are no absolute contraindications based on systolic or diastolic values that necessitate can-

cellation of an elective procedure. If a patient is seen in the preoperative clinic with poorly controlled hypertension and enough time exists before the procedure, the primary care physician should be contacted to attempt to achieve better medical management.

Pulmonary disease

Chronic pulmonary conditions may increase the risk of postoperative respiratory failure. History taking in patients with chronic obstructive pulmonary disease or asthma should include questions about the type of disease, duration, therapy, and baseline condition. Recent interventions, such as hospitalization, intubation, or changes in medications, such as the addition of steroids or antibiotics, should be documented. Patents may need a steroid pulse prior to surgery, require antibiotics for an acute bacterial process, or they may need arrangements for postoperative chest physiotherapy. Current symptoms may restrict the choice of anesthetic options; for instance, a case

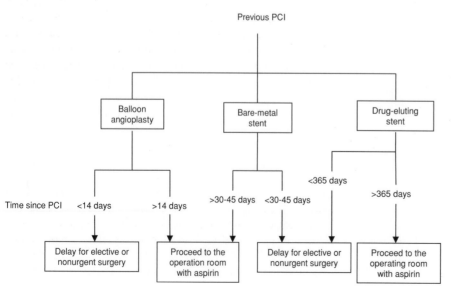

Figure 2.3. Proposed approach to the management of patients with previous percutaneous coronary intervention (PCI) who require non-cardiac surgery. (Modified from Fleisher LA, et al. ACC/AHA 2007 Guidelines on Perioperative Cardiovascular Evaluation and Care for Noncardiac Surgery: Executive Summary: A Report of the American College of Cardiology/American Heart Association Task Force on Practice Guidelines. *Circulation* 2007; 116:1971–1996.)

generally requiring sedation may necessitate the use of general anesthesia in patients with intractable coughing.

Sleep apnea has been associated with poorer postoperative outcomes and increased incidence of apnea and respiratory failure, especially with the administration of opioids. A history of snoring (confirmed by a partner), hypertension, chronic fatigue, and obesity are all associated with significant sleep apnea. It is becoming increasingly common to refer patients with possible sleep apnea for sleep studies and possible intervention preoperatively, to minimize the risk of postoperative apnea. Patients who wear continuous positive airway pressure masks should be instructed to bring the mask with them on the day of surgery.

Airway history frequently is included as part of the pulmonary assessment. If there has been a prolonged intubation or tracheotomy in the past, it is valuable to elicit information regarding etiology and history (for example, whether trauma or pneumonia was a precipitating factor). Residual damage such as symptomatic tracheal stenosis is important to document because the presence of significant stenosis may influence the choice of anesthetic technique. A history of a difficult intubation should be accompanied by an attempt to retrieve medical records and communicate the issues to the anesthetizing team. During the preoperative interview, it may be necessary to spend extra time with patients explaining the goals and procedures surrounding an awake intubation in simple, reassuring language to allow for informed consent and to reduce anxiety.

Gastrointestinal system

Aspiration may result in devastating complications during anesthesia. A positive history of severe, positional reflux may result in a change in the anesthetic plan. For example, endotracheal intubation may be used in cases in which use of a laryngeal mask airway would have been an option. The history of reflux should be carefully documented, and current symptoms and their severity should be quantified. The frequency of the reflux symptoms, the impact of treatment if prescribed, and the onset of symptoms during the night while the patient is lying flat may help distinguish true reflux from the much more common postprandial.

Obesity increases anesthesia risks. In the obese patient, it is valuable to record recent weight changes, body mass index, intubation challenges in the past, and comorbid conditions such as hypertension, diabetes, and sleep apnea. A further important consideration is the practical impact of the patient's weight. These patients may require special equipment in the operating room, including large blood pressure cuffs, wide stretchers, and larger operating room beds.

Neurologic system

Numerous neurologic conditions may affect anesthetic administration. For any patient with a neurologic condition, the diagnosis, medications, and status of current symptomatology should be carefully documented. Many neurologic disorders, especially when severe, have an impact on respiratory status. In patients with epilepsy, preoperative assessment should include a description of the seizure type and frequency. Medications should be continued throughout the perioperative period. Many seizure medications are not available as intravenous formulations, so it is necessary to plan for therapy during prolonged periods when the patient is unable to take oral medicines.

Cerebrovascular disease is common, especially in older patients with peripheral vascular disease and diabetes. If a patient had a prior cerebrovascular accident, it is important to document baseline functional and neurologic impairments. Advanced dementia may prevent the clinician from obtaining a medical history or an informed consent. In such case, an arrangement for a family member or health care proxy will be needed to help obtain the preoperative assessment, and their presence may be needed on the day of surgery. Other less common diseases, such as multiple sclerosis, require a brief description of the symptoms during a relapse and residual damage. Some neurologic diseases, such as myasthenia gravis and myotonic dystrophy, carry significant risks from anesthesia; in these instances, clear documentation and recent neurologic evaluation may be valuable adjuncts to the standard preoperative assessment. Spinal cord injury patients often undergo multiple operations and present many anesthetic challenges. At a minimum, the history should include the level of the lesion, residual damage, and the history of hypertensive crises during procedures.

Endocrine system

Diabetes mellitus is the most common endocrinopathy encountered preoperatively and is associated with many comorbid conditions that increase anesthetic risk. In addition to a description of the type of diabetes and the insulin status, a detailed history should be obtained in all diabetic patients to search for occult cardiac disease, renal impairment, or end organ damage. The hemoglobin A_{1c} level can be used to establish the degree of control. Diabetic comas due to diabetic ketoacidosis are rare but represent an important part of the history of the disease, suggesting poor ("brittle") control and increasing anesthetic challenges. Insulin pumps are becoming more popular for insulin-dependent diabetics. In general, the basal rate of these devices is continued perioperatively, and additional insulin may be added as necessary.

Renal system

Chronic kidney disease affects more than 20 million adults in the United States. Chronic renal failure is a complex systemic disease that may result from many conditions; diabetes mellitus, hypertension, and glomerulonephritis are among the most common causes. For patients on dialysis, the frequency and mode of administration of dialysis should be documented, including a plan for timing of dialysis perioperatively. Volume control is a critical issue in dialysis patients, and the preoperative history should include documentation of volume overload or dialysis-related problems, such as hypotension.

Hepatic system

Both acute and chronic liver disease may increase the risk of surgery. For patients with liver disease, it is important to document the etiology; for example, whether liver disease is infectious, neoplastic, or alcoholic in origin. End-stage liver disease may manifest with ascites, coagulopathies, and encephalopathy, resulting in significant alterations in drug distribution and metabolism.

Reproductive system

Women of childbearing age should be asked if there is any chance of pregnancy, and the date of their last menstrual period should be documented. The literature suggests that routine pregnancy testing is not warranted in patients who are reliable historians.

Rare diseases

Rare illnesses and conditions may require a more detailed history and communication with the patient's primary physician or specialist. Ideally, these evaluations should be coordinated in advance through the surgeon's office and the preoperative testing clinic. This will provide adequate time for additional studies and communication with the assigned anesthesiologist.

Family history

Malignant hyperthermia is a familial disease, and all preoperative assessment discussions should attempt to rule out any disposition for malignant hyperthermia. Other familial diseases relevant to anesthesia include pseudocholinesterase deficiency, which may be suggested by a history of unexplained prolonged weakness or postoperative intubation in otherwise healthy patients. In the event of a positive history of anesthetic issues, efforts should be made to obtain prior anesthetic records in advance of the surgery.

Anesthetic history

The anesthetic history is a key feature of the preoperative assessment. A patient's prior anesthetic experience is extremely important and will greatly influence the patient's attitude (reduce anxiety) toward the upcoming surgery. The history should include a discussion of prior operations, including the type and approximate dates. A history of difficult intubation, prolonged weakness, or intubation should be clearly documented. Prior postoperative nausea or vomiting may predict future difficulties. Other issues that may arise during the discussion include anxiety regarding poor venous access and various

fears surrounding anesthesia, such as a mask "phobia" or claustrophobia.

Allergies and social habits

Documentation of allergies must include the drug and the reaction. A thorough history can sometimes help distinguish a true allergy from a benign reaction or side effect. The preoperative assessment should include details about alcohol intake, smoking, and illegal drug use. A history of drug abuse and alcoholism may result in increased tolerance to anesthetic agents and the potential for unexpected withdrawal following the surgery.

Medications

A detailed list of medications and dosing schedule is part of the preoperative assessment. It is important to document both prescribed and nonprescribed medications, including vitamins and other supplements. The generic names of drugs should be used and the indications recorded. In general, most medications should be continued until the night before surgery. Although there are no clear data on interactions, most institutions recommend discontinuing all alternative and complementary medication supplements prior to the procedure.

Patients on anticoagulants should not have these medications discontinued without a discussion with the cardiologist or primary care physician prescribing them. In addition, the prescribing physician needs to be made aware of the patient's upcoming procedure so that they can ensure that medication is appropriately restarted postoperatively. On the morning of surgery, patients may be advised to hold diuretic medication and nonessential medications and supplements. Angiotensin-converting enzyme inhibitors may result in significant vasodilatation and hypotension after anesthetic induction; holding these medications on the day of surgery has been previously recommended but is now generally done only prior to cardiac surgery. Short-acting insulin is generally held on the morning of surgery, and long-acting insulin is continued at the usual or a reduced (typically half of usual) dose. Chronic pain medication use may result in significant tolerance and create difficulties with pain management in the postoperative period.

Physical examination

A general assessment of the patient is invaluable. Is the patient healthy looking despite a complicated history? Is the patient frail and cachectic? How anxious is the patient? Is the patient able to give his or her own history? These types of observations can help the anesthesia team prepare for their patient encounter.

The physical examination for a preoperative assessment is a targeted examination focusing on the airway and cardiopulmonary system. Blood pressure, pulse, respiratory rate, height, and weight are recorded. Obtaining resting oxygen saturation is recommended, especially in patients with a history of cardiopulmonary illness. Auscultation of the heart and lungs should be done to document the presence or absence of murmurs, abnormalities in cardiac rhythm, and abnormal lung sounds. A brief baseline neurologic examination also is recommended. An examination of the back or the proposed site is recommended if a neuraxial or regional technique is contemplated, as scoliosis and kyphosis may be otherwise unappreciated.

The airway examination should include an assessment of the maximal mouth opening, ability to visualize posterior pharyngeal structures, condition of dentition, degree of neck mobility, and submandibular distance. The presence of prominent incisors, loose or missing teeth, full beard, large tongue, facial and neck obesity, cervical disease, and prior tracheal surgery, neck surgery, or radiation may all contribute to difficult airway management.

Preoperative testing

Many studies have demonstrated that preoperative laboratory testing should be directed by the type of surgery planned and the patient's medical status. Routine screening has not been shown to be advantageous and may lead to excessive cost as well as potential morbidity for further investigation of false-positive results.

A hemoglobin or hematocrit test is indicated if the surgery is associated with significant blood loss potential or if the patient has a complex systemic disease resulting in anemia. Elevated hemoglobin from hemoconcentration may suggest a dehydrated patient. Platelet counts are indicated in patients with a history of low platelets or a disease associated with diminished platelets, such as preeclampsia. Bleeding time is usually not performed as a preoperative screening indicator of platelet function. Coagulation studies are indicated in patients with significant liver disease or known coagulopathic conditions. Generally, patients on anticoagulants such as warfarin should have coagulation studies repeated on the morning of the procedure if warfarin has been discontinued so that normal coagulation parameters can be documented.

Healthy ambulatory patients or those with mild to moderate systemic disease such as hypertension do not need routine electrolyte testing. Patients with chronic renal failure should have electrolytes, blood urea nitrogen, and creatinine tested prior to any significant surgery. Renal dialysis patients should have their potassium tested immediately prior to surgery. An electrocardiogram (ECG) should be obtained in patients with cardiac risk factors and a history of cardiac disease. Many institutions use 50 or 60 years as the age at which screening ECGs are required, but there is no definitive recommendation in this regard. A prior ECG within 3 to 6 months of the surgery in the absence of any ongoing symptoms or changes in cardiac status is generally acceptable. Chest radiographs are not recommended preoperatively unless directed by the history or underlying diagnosis.

Table 2.7. ASA Physical status classification system

ASA Physician Status 1 - A normal healthy patient
ASA Physician Status 2 - A patient with mild systemic disease
ASA Physician Status 3 - A patient with severe systemic disease
ASA Physician Status 4 - A patient with severe systemic disease that is a constant threat to life
ASA Physician Status 5 - A moribund patient who is not expected to survive without the operation
ASA Physician Status 6 - A declared brain-dead patient whose organs are being removed for donor purposes

A "type and screen" should be done prior to surgeries with a potential for significant blood loss. The presence of antibodies may make it difficult and time consuming to find compatible products. Patients may choose to provide autologous blood or donor-specific blood products. These patients should be referred to the blood bank in advance of the scheduled surgery to arrange for donation, as several weeks may be necessary to complete these arrangements. Some patients may refuse blood products for religious or personal reasons. In these instances, the reasons and options must be carefully reviewed and alternatives, such as the use of a cell saver and administration of albumin, explicitly discussed and documented.

American Society of Anesthesiologists classification

After the completion of the preoperative assessment, the anesthesiologist assigns an American Society of Anesthesiologists (ASA) classification (Table 2.7). This reflects the patient's condition and underlying disease complexity. Although the classification is not intended as a measure of risk per se, patients with higher ASA classifications often carry independent diagnoses that lead to increased risk from surgery. An E is added to the physical classification to designate a patient in whom surgery is emergent. The ASA physical classification system is a useful way to communicate about patients and is used by health care providers in other disciplines as well.

Consent and instructions

An important part of the preanesthetic interview is the discussion with the patient about potential risks and benefits of the potential anesthetic options, as well as a preliminary plan for the anesthesia. The final choice of anesthetic can be made only by the anesthesia team caring for the patient during the surgery. Patients may become distressed when promised one type of anesthesia prior to surgery and on the day of surgery find a different anesthesia team with an alternative recommendation.

Patients should be given instructions (Table 2.8) regarding medications as well as expectations regarding the day of procedure and postoperative recovery. At minimum, fasting guidelines should be discussed. In many instances, written instructions should be provided, including a contact phone number if issues arise prior to the day of surgery. Similarly,

Table 2.8. Preoperative instructions

Instructions should be clearly written in simple language
Instructions should be specific, avoiding vague or ambiguous terms such as "maybe"
Directions to exact location in the hospital
Recommendations on clothing and belongings
NPO instructions – written down
Number to call with change in health

patients should receive clear instructions regarding fasting (Table 2.9) and requirements for discharge, such as transportation home.

Inpatient interviews

The inpatient preoperative interview is now uncommon, and patients who undergo them are usually acutely injured or have complicated medical histories. The routine preoperative history should be supplemented with a thorough review of the inpatient chart, as many patients will not be able to adequately explain their hospital course. Recommendations from consultants in specialties should be sought during the admission, if needed. The most recent laboratory information, including radiologic scans and cardiac testing, should be reviewed. NPO (nothing by mouth) recommendations and recommended medications for the day of surgery should be communicated with the nursing and surgical teams.

Outside facilities

The preoperative assessment of institutionalized patients may be especially challenging. It may be difficult or impractical to require these patients to come to a hospital or facility for a preoperative visit. In these instances, a remote preoperative screen may be conducted. If possible, the facility physician should provide a brief history, physical examination, and the results of any laboratory testing done recently. These may be reviewed by the anesthesiology team, who may decide whether more testing is indicated. The preoperative examination may be completed on the day of surgery. Arrangements for consent from a legal guardian or family member should be made in advance to prevent delays on the day of surgery.

Table 2.9. ASA guidelines for NPO status preoperatively

Substance	Minimum fasting period, h
Clear liquids[a]	2
Breast milk	4
Infant formula	6
Nonhuman milk	6
Light meal	6
Fried or fatty foods, meat	8

[a] Include water, fruit juices without pulp, clear tea, carbonated beverages, and black coffee.

Emergency

In extreme cases, it may not be possible to perform more than a very brief preoperative assessment; in these instances, it is important to prioritize the assessment. A few critical facts may be helpful. Is there a family history of anesthetic issues, a history of difficult intubation or tracheotomy, or any allergies? A list of medications may be available, and any laboratory testing should be quickly reviewed.

Cancellations

Sometimes it is necessary to cancel or postpone a procedure based on the results of the preoperative examination, which may cause considerable stress to both the anesthesiologist and the patient. In the event of a cancellation, the anesthesiologist should communicate with the patient and the surgical team and explain why the patient is not ready for surgery and what should be done before the patient is rescheduled. This may mean a cardiology consultation or a recommendation for an adjustment in medications prior to the surgery. Sometimes it is possible for additional tests and consultations to be completed prior to the surgical date, thus avoiding a cancellation. One common cause of day-of-surgery cancellation is a change in the patient's status or a new infection. To prevent these cancellations, patients should be provided with clear guidelines of what to do if they develop an upper respiratory infection or other illness.

Suggested readings

American Society of Anesthesiologists Task Force on Preanesthesia Evaluation. Practice advisory for preanesthesia evaluation: a report by the American Society of Anesthesiologists Task Force on Preanesthesia Evaluation. *Anesthesiology* 2002; 96:485.

American College of Cardiology/American Heart Association Task Force on Practice Guidelines (Writing Committee to Revise the 2002 Guidelines on Perioperative Cardiovascular Evaluation for Noncardiac Surgery); Executive summary of the ACC/AHA task force report: Guidelines for Perioperative Cardiovascular Evaluation for noncardiac surgery. *Anesth Analg* 1996; 82:854–860.

Dasgupta M, Dumbrell AC. Preoperative risk assessment for delirium after noncardiac surgery: a systematic review. *J Am Geriatr Soc* 2006; 54(10):1578–1589.

Dorman T, Breslow MJ, Pronovost PJ, et al. Bundle-branch block as a risk factor in noncardiac surgery. *Arch Intern Med* 2000; 160:1149.

Fischer SP. Development and effectiveness of an anesthesia preoperative evaluation clinic in a teaching hospital. *Anesthesiology* 1996; 85:196–206.

Fleisher LA, et al. ACC/AHA 2007 Guidelines on Perioperative Cardiovascular Evaluation and Care for Noncardiac Surgery: Executive Summary: A Report of the American College of Cardiology/American Heart Association Task Force on Practice Guidelines. *Circulation* 2007; 116(17):1971–1996.

Jacober SJ, Sowers JR. An update on perioperative management of diabetes. *Arch Intern Med* 1999; 159:2405–2411.

Joehl RJ. Preoperative evaluation: pulmonary, cardiac, renal dysfunction and comorbidities. *Surg Clin North Am* 2005; 85(6):1061–1073.

Lawrence VA, Cornell JE, Smetana GW. Strategies to reduce postoperative pulmonary complications after noncardiothoracic surgery: systematic review for the American College of Physicians. *Ann Intern Med* 2006; 144(8):596–608.

Liu LL, Dzankic S, Leung JM. Preoperative electrocardiogram abnormalities do not predict postoperative cardiac complications in geriatric surgical patients. *J Am Geriatr Soc* 2002; 50:1186.

Narr BJ. Outcomes of patients with no laboratory assessment before anesthesia and a surgical procedure. *Mayo Clin Proc* 1997; 72:505–509.

Noordzij PG, Boersma E, et al. Prognostic value of routine preoperative electrocardiography in patients undergoing noncardiac surgery. *Am J Cardiol* 2006; 97(7):1103–1106.

Poldermans D, et al. The effect of bisoprolol on perioperative mortality and myocardial infarction in high risk patients undergoing vascular surgery. *N Engl J Med* 1999; 341:1789–1794.

Schein OD, et al. The value of routine preoperative medical testing before cataract surgery. *N Engl J Med* 2000; 342:168–175.

Smetana GW. Preoperative pulmonary evaluation. *N Engl J Med* 1999; 340:937–944.

Obstructive and restrictive lung disease

Shannon S. McKenna

Introduction

Asthma and chronic obstructive pulmonary disease (COPD) are the two primary obstructive lung diseases that anesthesiologists see on a routine basis. COPD is more common, is more insidious, and poses greater management challenges. Therefore, this chapter focuses on COPD, with only a brief review of asthma.

Restrictive lung disease is fairly uncommon in the operating room setting, but does have specific implications for the anesthesiologist. It is reviewed briefly at the end of the chapter.

Obstructive lung disease
COPD

The significance of COPD

COPD, the most common pulmonary disease encountered in the perioperative setting, afflicts more than 15 million Americans. COPD is now the fourth leading cause of death in the United States. Compared with heart disease, stroke, and cancer, mortality from COPD is increasing rather than decreasing. Tobacco exposure accounts for 85% of all cases.

Definition and classification of COPD

COPD is a chronic disease characterized by airflow limitation that, in contrast to asthma, is not fully reversible. Typically, the airflow limitation progresses over time and is associated with an abnormal inflammatory response in the lung. Classic symptoms include cough, sputum production, dyspnea, and progressive exercise intolerance. Historically, these symptoms were described as either chronic bronchitis or emphysema.

Spirometry is used to confirm the diagnosis and classify the severity of COPD. A postbronchodilator forced expiratory volume in the first second of expiration (FEV_1) < 80% of the predicted value, in the setting of an FEV_1/forced vital capacity (FVC) < 70%, is an accepted criterion for confirming the presence of COPD. The staging systems currently in use classify the severity of disease based on the percent of predicted FEV_1 alone (Table 3.1). A staging system that incorporates clinical status, spirometry, and radiographic features of the disease would be more clinically useful.

Pathogenesis and pathology of COPD

The pathogenesis of COPD is thought to derive from the combined effects of inflammation, increased oxidative stress, and an imbalance in the activity of proteinases and antiproteinases. Smoking, via particulate inhalation, is a primary trigger for lung inflammation. Genetic factors are thought to account for the fact that not all smokers develop COPD.

Pathologic changes of COPD are present throughout the lung and are progressive over time. In the large central airways, mucous glands are enlarged; there is goblet cell hyperplasia, loss of cilia, and decreased ciliary function. The airway walls are affected by inflammatory cell infiltration, accompanied by increased smooth muscle and connective tissue deposition. Small airways are predominantly affected by chronic inflammation leading to collagen deposition and airway remodeling. Emphysema, which is characterized by enlargement of the airspaces distal to the terminal bronchioles, develops in the parenchyma as a result of the destruction of collagen and elastin in alveolar walls. The pulmonary vasculature also is primarily affected. Initial intimal hyperplasia is followed by inflammation of the vessel wall, smooth muscle deposition, and, ultimately, fibrosis.

Pathophysiology of COPD: the intersection of pathology and function

The pathophysiology of COPD is complex and has a wide-ranging impact on functional status and physiologic reserve. Increased mucus production, with abnormal mucus clearance,

Table 3.1. Global Initiative for Chronic Obstructive Lung Disease staging criteria

Stage	Spirometry
Stage 0 (at risk)	FEV_1/FVC $\geq$ 70% $FEV_1 \geq$ 80%
Stage 1 (mild)	FEV_1/FVC < 70% $FEV_1 \geq$ 80%
Stage 2 (moderate)	FEV_1/FVC < 70% FEV_1 50%–80%
Stage 3 (severe)	FEV_1/FVC < 70% FEV_1 30%–50%
Stage 4 (very severe)	FEV_1/FVC < 70% FEV_1 < 30%

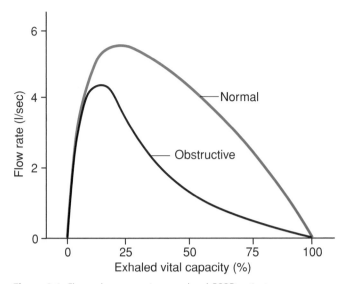

Figure 3.1. Flow-volume curve in normal and COPD patients.

results in the chronic cough and sputum production that are often the first clinical symptoms of COPD.

Expiratory airflow limitation is the pivotal pathophysiologic change. Airflow limitation occurs as a result of the convergence of multiple pathologic processes: airway inflammation and edema, mucus accumulation, airway hyperplasia and fibrosis, bronchospasm, and loss of radial traction as collagen and elastin are destroyed. Expiratory flow is markedly reduced throughout expiration, and expiratory time is increased (Fig. 3.1); hyperinflation occurs. Total lung capacity, functional residual capacity

(FRC), and residual volume are all increased (Fig. 3.2). The result is diaphragmatic flattening, elevation of the ribs, and an overall increase in the cross-sectional area of the thorax. This places the lung at a mechanical disadvantage, causing dyspnea, particularly with exertion – the most significant and limiting symptom of COPD.

Gas exchange is impaired via worsened ventilation–per-fusion (V/Q) matching. There is an increase in both physiologic dead space and shunt. Varying degrees of hypoxemia and hypercarbia occur in different patients, depending on the specific V/Q distribution and an individual patient's metabolic state.

Chronic hypoxia, combined with direct pathologic changes in the pulmonary vasculature, ultimately results in pulmonary hypertension. Late in COPD, as pulmonary hypertension progresses, patients may develop right ventricular dysfunction and frank cor pulmonale.

Treatment of COPD

Treatment of chronic stable COPD

Smoking cessation is the only intervention that slows the progression of COPD. Yearly influenza vaccination has been shown to significantly reduce morbidity and mortality and is recommended for all patients with COPD. Comprehensive, multidisciplinary pulmonary rehabilitation programs may provide sustained improvement in exercise capacity and quality of life for patients with all stages of COPD.

Pharmacologic management is aimed at symptom relief but does not change the progression of disease. It is approached in a stepwise fashion and is tailored to the individual patient's

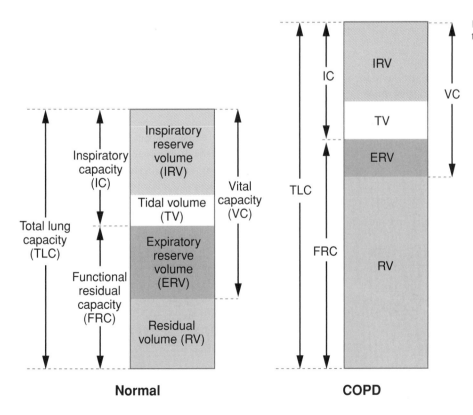

Figure 3.2. Changes in lung volumes and capacities with COPD.

Table 3.2. Commonly used bronchodilator drugs

Drug	Routes	Duration of action, h
β_2 Agonists		
Fenoterol	MDI, Neb	4–6
Albuterol	MDI, Neb, oral	4–6
Levalbuterol	MDI, Neb	4–6
Terbutaline	MDI, Neb, oral	4–6
Formoterol	MDI	12
Salmeterol	MDI	12
Anticholinergics		
Ipratropium bromide	MDI, Neb	6–8
Tiotropium	MDI	24+ hours
Methylxanthines		
Aminophylline	IV, oral	variable
Theophylline	Oral	variable

IV, intravenous; MDI, metered-dose inhaler; Neb, nebulizer.

response (Table 3.2). Short-acting inhaled bronchodilators are used for symptomatic relief in early-stage COPD. For patients with more severe COPD, long-acting inhaled bronchodilators, especially tiotropium, improve lung function, relieve dyspnea, and improve exercise capacity. Inhaled corticosteroids reduce the frequency of exacerbations in patients with severe COPD and may slightly, but not clinically significantly, slow the rate of decline in FEV_1. Use should be limited to patients with frequent acute exacerbations. Recent clinical trials have focused on combination therapy with inhaled long-acting β_2 agonists and inhaled corticosteroids. Combination therapy, in patients with moderate to severe disease, seems to show additive benefits in most trials.

Treatment of acute exacerbations

Acute exacerbations are often triggered by respiratory tract infection. Accompanying symptoms may include worsened dyspnea, wheezing, chest tightness, cough, increased sputum, a change in sputum character, fever, and malaise. Worsened airflow obstruction, with acute hyperinflation, is thought to be the primary cause of the increased dyspnea. Initial management of acute exacerbations includes escalation of bronchodilator therapy and domiciliary oxygen therapy for patients with hypoxia. Antibiotics should be started if there is evidence of bacterial infection. Systemic corticosteroids shorten the recovery time from acute exacerbations and may be indicated in some patients.

Patients with progressive hypoxemia, hypercarbia, respiratory distress, or evidence of new heart failure require hospital admission. Primary management is the same as in the outpatient setting. The development of progressive hypercarbia and respiratory acidosis is associated with the highest risk of mortality. Noninvasive mechanical ventilation may be particularly effective in treating COPD exacerbations, providing a reduction in both mortality and the need for intubation. Patients with severe acidosis, refractory hypoxemia, or respiratory arrest require intubation and conventional mechanical ventilation.

Treatment of end-stage disease

Treatment options for advanced COPD are limited. They include domiciliary oxygen therapy, lung volume reduction surgery (LVRS), and lung transplantation. Oxygen therapy increases exercise capacity and improves survival in patients with chronic respiratory failure. It is recommended for patients with a PaO_2 <55 mm Hg or an arterial oxygen saturation (SaO_2) <89%. If there is evidence of pulmonary hypertension, oxygen therapy may be provided for patients with a PaO_2 <60 mm Hg.

LVRS is an expensive, high-risk palliative treatment. A recent study sponsored by the National Institutes of Health, identified a small subset of patients who may benefit from LVRS. These patients have upper lobe–predominant emphysema with a low exercise capacity. Several risk factors for poor outcome also were identified. Very few patients with end-stage COPD qualify for LVRS. Lung transplantation is the other treatment option for end-stage disease. Currently, the challenge is to correctly identify the patients with a life expectancy short enough that they would benefit from transplantation.

Perioperative care of the patient with COPD
Risk assessment

Patients with COPD have a 2.7- to 4.7-fold increased risk of perioperative pulmonary complications. The degree of risk correlates with the severity of COPD. The most common pulmonary complications are atelectasis, pneumonia, respiratory failure, and acute exacerbation of underlying chronic pulmonary disease. Age greater than 60 years, American Society of Anesthesiologists (ASA) physical status of II or higher, history of congestive heart failure, and current cigarette smoking are additional risk factors. The type of surgery also is important. The highest risk is associated with aortic, thoracic, and upper abdominal procedures. Neurosurgery, head and neck surgery, emergency surgery, and prolonged surgery (>3 hours) also confer increased risk.

Preoperative assessment should focus on the history and physical examination. Patients with severe COPD can be identified easily on this basis alone. Spirometry does not provide effective risk prediction for individual patients; however, it may be used to predict long-term functional status after major lung resection. Current recommendations are to obtain a chest radiograph for patients older than 50 years undergoing high-risk operations, but it is rare for routine preoperative chest radiographs to influence clinical management.

When patients are found to be at increased risk of postoperative pulmonary complications, the potential benefits of the surgery should be weighed against the risk. There is no true pulmonary contraindication to a potential lifesaving surgery. Even within the specific realm of lung resection surgery, there are very few absolute pulmonary contraindications to surgery.

Preoperative optimization

Smoking cessation is a logical preoperative intervention for patients with COPD. Patients undergoing high-risk surgeries who have ceased smoking at least 4 weeks prior to surgery seem to have a lower risk of pulmonary complications. Smoking cessation 24 to 48 hours prior to elective surgery normalizes carboxyhemoglobin levels and corrects the left shift of the oxyhemoglobin dissociation curve, but does not show an improvement in mucociliary function.

Given the significant impact of smoking cessation on the long-term outcome of COPD, all COPD patients should be counseled on smoking cessation, regardless of the type or timing of surgery.

Preoperative optimization of airflow with bronchodilators is thought to decrease perioperative complications. There is no indication, however, for routine preoperative addition of either inhaled or oral corticosteroids. Expert opinion suggests that specific treatment of acute COPD exacerbations preoperatively is beneficial. It may be prudent to delay elective surgery until after full recovery from an acute COPD exacerbation, but there is little evidence available on this issue. The role for routine preoperative pulmonary rehabilitation prior to high-risk surgery is unclear.

Intraoperative management

There is some evidence, of variable quality, available to guide the choice of anesthetic techniques for patients with COPD. One trial of intermediate-acting versus long-acting neuromuscular blockers found a higher rate of residual neuromuscular blockade with the use of long-acting neuromuscular blockers. The rate of postoperative pulmonary complications was three times higher in patients with prolonged blockade. The current recommendation is to use intermediate-acting agents in patients with COPD. There have been several trials comparing neuraxial blockade with general anesthesia and neuraxial analgesia with other postoperative pain relief strategies. Unfortunately, the studies tended to be small and limited by problems with study design or execution; results have been inconsistent. Some of the studies did report lower rates of postoperative pulmonary complications with the use of regional anesthesia and analgesia. Further study is needed; in the interim, it is reasonable to advocate for regional anesthesia and analgesia, when feasible, for patients with significant baseline pulmonary impairment.

Several intraoperative problems may occur during general anesthesia in the setting of underlying COPD. Bronchospasm may cause an abrupt increase in airway resistance and concomitant worsening of airflow obstruction. Acute bronchospasm is best treated with inhaled β_2 agonists or anticholinergics. Increasing the end-tidal concentrations of bronchodilating volatile anesthetics (isoflurane, sevoflurane, halothane, enflurane) also may reverse acute bronchospasm. Rarely, the use of intravenous corticosteroids or low doses of intravenous epinephrine (0.25–0.5 μg/min) via continuous infusion may be necessary to break refractory bronchospasm.

Inspissation of pulmonary secretions may result in acute occlusion of bronchi or even the endotracheal tube itself. Maintaining adequate hydration and humidifying inspiratory gases help prevent desiccation and inspissation of secretions. Use of a large (8.0 mm or larger) endotracheal tube allows for easy endotracheal suctioning and, when necessary, fiberoptic bronchoscopy. On occasion, it may be necessary to instill mucolytics (N-acetylcysteine, dornase alfa) through the bronchoscope into an area of mucus plugging.

V/Q matching, which is impaired at baseline in COPD, is even worse during general anesthesia. This leads to widening of the alveolar–arterial oxygen gradient and also the gradient between end-tidal and arterial carbon dioxide. Consideration should be given to arterial blood gas monitoring for patients with significant COPD undergoing major procedures.

Dynamic hyperinflation is one of the major pitfalls of general anesthesia in patients with significant COPD. It occurs when inspiration is initiated prior to the complete exhalation of the previous tidal volume (Fig. 3.3). End-expiratory volumes and pressures (intrinsic positive end-expiratory pressure [PEEP] or auto-PEEP) rise progressively with each subsequent inhalation until a new steady state is reached. As a result, lung compliance decreases, gas exchange is impaired further because of compression of normal lung, barotrauma and alveolar rupture may occur, and venous return is decreased. The decrease in venous return may be profound enough to cause hypotension, decreased cardiac output, and even pulseless electrical activity. Anesthesiologists should be particularly watchful for dynamic hyperinflation during commencement of assisted ventilation,

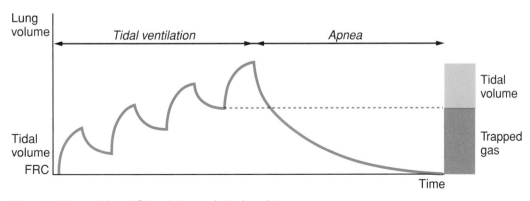

Figure 3.3. Dynamic hyperinflation during mechanical ventilation.

such as at induction. Judicious hydration helps ameliorate the decrease in venous return. Use of a slow respiratory rate, long expiratory time, and the minimum necessary tidal volume to avoid excessive hypercapnia helps prevent the development of dynamic hyperinflation. Extrinsic PEEP can replace 50% to 75% of intrinsic PEEP. Small airways are held open, and more complete exhalation may occur. Unfortunately, there is no easy way to measure intrinsic PEEP in the operating room, so titration of extrinsic PEEP requires clinical judgment and experience. If severe hypotension is thought to be related to dynamic hyperinflation, the most expedient maneuver is to hold ventilation altogether and allow for unobstructed exhalation.

Timely emergence from general anesthesia may be particularly challenging in patients with severe COPD. Patients with COPD are exquisitely sensitive to the respiratory depressant effects of many commonly used medications, including benzodiazepines, narcotics, barbiturates, propofol, and the volatile anesthetics. The long expiratory time-constant, increased dead space, and widened V/Q distribution typical of severe COPD all result in inefficient clearance of volatile agents. Although there are no good randomized trials of specific anesthetic maintenance techniques in the setting of severe COPD, most experts recommend the use of total intravenous anesthesia (TIVA). TIVA allows for timing of emergence independent of underlying lung function. When short-acting agents (e.g., propofol and remifentanil) are used in combination with an approach to postoperative analgesia that does not rely heavily on parenteral opioids, postoperative respiratory depression can be minimized.

Postoperative care

Postoperative care should focus on measures that facilitate the patient's rapid return to baseline levels of pulmonary function. This requires the patient to be extubated, awake, and alert and to have adequate pain control. Lung expansion maneuvers such as deep breathing, chest physiotherapy, and incentive spirometry effectively prevent postoperative pulmonary complications. Early ambulation helps restore baseline lung volumes, facilitate clearance of secretions, and prevent venous thromboembolism. Patients should continue their baseline medical therapy

for COPD. Temporary escalation of bronchodilator therapy and use of intravenous corticosteroids or antibiotics may be necessary for patients who experience an acute COPD exacerbation in the perioperative period.

Asthma

Epidemiology of asthma

Asthma is a chronic inflammatory lung disease characterized by the paroxysmal occurrence of cough, wheezing, and/or dyspnea. The prevalence of asthma has increased over the past three decades and is now about 5% in the United States. The annual mortality rate climbed through the mid-1990s but has declined since then. Currently, roughly 4000 people a year die in the United States from asthma.

Pathology and pathophysiology of asthma

Asthma is a chronic inflammatory disease of the airways that results in airflow obstruction. The pathology includes smooth muscle constriction, airway edema, mucus accumulation, airway inflammation, and abnormal deposition of collagen in basement membranes. The airflow obstruction is reversible, in comparison to COPD. Airway hyperresponsiveness is characteristic of asthma. Triggers may include histamine, cold air, viral infections, and a variety of environmental substances.

Treatment of asthma

Asthma treatment focuses on reducing the frequency and severity of symptoms and associated functional limitations. An additional goal is to reduce the occurrence of long-term morbidity, including loss of lung function and medication side effects. The foundation of management is patient education and identification, avoidance of triggers, and regular monitoring, often done with a handheld peak flow meter.

Pharmacologic management is applied in a stepwise fashion based on the severity of disease. A full description of the classification of severity may be found in the 2007 National Asthma Education and Prevention Program Expert Panel Report. The basics of this approach are summarized in Table 3.3. Acute exacerbations often require systemic glucocorticoid use.

Table 3.3. Stepwise approach to baseline asthma treatment

Asthma severity	Typical features	Recommended treatment
Intermittent (step 1)	Sx 2 d/wk or less; normal FEV_1 at baseline Oral steroids once a year at most	Short-acting inhaled β_2 agonist prn (for step 1 and all other steps)
Mild persistent (step 2)	Sx > 2 d/wk; β agonists use > 2 d/wk; oral steroids twice a year or more	Daily inhaled steroid or alternate controller (leukotriene inhibitor, theophylline, cromoglycates)
Moderate persistent (step 3)	Daily symptoms and β agonist use; some activity limitation; reduced baseline FEV_1	Daily inhaled steroid (or alternate) plus daily long-acting β_2 agonist
Severe persistent (step 4–6)	Sx throughout day; multiple uses of β agonist each day; extreme activity limitation; $FEV_1 < 60\%$	Daily long-acting β_2 agonist plus moderate-dose (step 4) or high-dose (step 5) inhaled steroid; standing oral steroids added (step 6)

prn – as needed; Sx – symptoms.

Perioperative care of the patient with asthma
Preoperative assessment and optimization

There are limited data on the rate of perioperative respiratory complications among asthmatic patients undergoing surgery in the modern era. The data that are available suggest a rate of 1% to 2%. Initial assessment should focus on the patient's asthma history. Elements to assess are frequency and severity of symptoms, baseline activity level, degree of compliance with chronic treatment, and the need over the past year for emergency room treatment, hospital admission, or systemic glucocorticoid use. Patients with moderate persistent or severe persistent asthma should be identified, as presumably they are at higher risk for perioperative complications. Lung auscultation may reveal current airflow obstruction if wheezing or a prolonged expiratory phase is present.

Baseline medications should be continued up until the time of surgery. Patients with poor control of their symptoms should have their treatment optimized by their internist or pulmonologist prior to surgery whenever possible. Patients with moderate to severe asthma might benefit from a short course of oral steroids preoperatively, but the data supporting this approach are limited. Patients at risk for adrenal suppression due to chronic treatment should probably receive stress dose steroids perioperatively, though the magnitude of such risk is unknown.

Intraoperative management

Short-acting bronchodilators may be administered prophylactically immediately before anesthesia. Given that endotracheal intubation may be a major stimulus for bronchospasm, it is prudent to avoid general anesthesia when possible. If endotracheal intubation is needed, it is vital to ensure that sufficient depth of anesthesia to suppress airway reflexes is achieved prior to laryngoscopy. There is some evidence that propofol may be associated with less postintubation wheezing than thiopental. Ketamine is the only induction agent that actually produces smooth muscle relaxation. It may be the induction agent of choice in certain cases. Intravenous lidocaine, 1.5 mg/kg, produces smooth muscle relaxation and may be given prior to induction. Intratracheal lidocaine may be given as well, but if the depth of anesthesia is insufficient, it may trigger bronchospasm.

Keys for intraoperative management are to maintain sufficient depth of anesthesia, avoid histamine-releasing drugs, and monitor for and treat bronchospasm if it occurs. See Table 3.4 for signs of intraoperative bronchospasm. If bronchospasm is confirmed, depth of anesthesia should be reassessed and

a short-acting inhaled β_2 agonist should be administered. Dynamic hyperinflation, as described in the COPD section, may occur and should be managed as previously described. Persistent bronchospasm may necessitate repeat dosing of inhaled bronchodilators, administration of intravenous corticosteroids (though onset of action is delayed), or use of a continuous epinephrine infusion at 0.25 to 0.5 µg/min.

Extubation is another high-risk period. Deep extubation is an option for certain patients. When deep extubation is not an option, pretreatment with an inhaled short-acting β_2 agonist and intravenous lidocaine may help prevent bronchospasm on emergence.

Restrictive lung disease
Definition

Restrictive lung disease impairs lung expansion. It is associated with decreased compliance of the pulmonary system and decreased vital capacity. The causative pathology may be located in the lung parenchyma, pleural space, or chest wall. Additionally, neuromuscular diseases may prevent the respiratory muscles from effectively expanding the thoracic cage and functionally cause restriction. Common etiologies of restrictive disease are summarized in Table 3.5.

Pathology and pathophysiology of restrictive disease

The pathology is variable and specific to the underlying disease process. Primary parenchymal diseases often require biopsy for definitive diagnosis. Pulmonary function testing usually shows

Table 3.4. Signs of bronchospasm during general anesthesia

Wheezing on auscultation
Increased peak airway pressure with unchanged plateau pressure
Decreased expiratory tidal volumes
Upsloping capnography waveform
Failure of expiratory flow to reach zero (flow vs. time waveform)
Hypotension due to impaired venous return (dynamic hyperinflation)

Table 3.5. Causes of restrictive pulmonary physiology

Intrinsic to the lung parenchyma
 Pulmonary edema
 Acute respiratory distress syndrome
 Pneumonia
 Autoimmune and collagen vascular diseases
 Pulmonary fibrosis
 Pneumonitis

Pleural space
 Tumor (mesothelioma)
 Pneumothorax
 Pleural effusion and hemothorax
 Infection and inflammation/fibrosis (empyema)

Chest wall
 Obesity
 Ascites
 Anasarca
 Pregnancy
 Congenital malformations of chest wall/spine
 Circumferential burns

Neuromuscular diseases
 High spinal cord injury
 Muscular dystrophy
 Myasthenia gravis and Eaton-Lambert syndrome
 Guillain-Barré syndrome
 Flail chest

decreased volumes and capacities with a preserved FEV_1/FVC ratio. Clinical symptoms typically include dyspnea and reduced exercise capacity. Other signs and symptoms are specific to the underlying disease process.

Treatment of restrictive diseases

Treatment of restrictive lung disease is specific to the underlying disease. For this reason, it is not unusual to see a patient with restrictive disease present for operative diagnosis. If the disease is localized to the pleural space, operative management may be required.

Perioperative care of the patient with restrictive disease

Appropriate care starts with the recognition that a restrictive process is present. Clues include a restrictive pattern on pulmonary function tests or the presence of a disease or process associated with pulmonary restriction. The next step is to assess severity by evaluating the symptoms and degree of exercise impairment. Oxygen saturation measurement will identify patients with baseline hypoxia. Preoperative exercise testing may be appropriate for a select subset presenting for major pulmonary resection.

Treatable contributors to pulmonary restriction should be addressed preoperatively when possible. These may include pulmonary edema, acute infection, large pleural effusions, or massive ascites. The benefit of specific preoperative treatment of these conditions depends on the operative procedure and the functional reserve of the patient.

Adequate preoxygenation is vital to avoid desaturation during induction, given the decreased FRC. Intraoperative ventilation may require smaller tidal volumes (4–6 ml/kg ideal body weight) at higher rates to avoid excessive inspiratory pressures. Application of PEEP from the beginning of positive pressure ventilation helps maintain FRC and avoid atelectasis. High inspired oxygen concentrations may be needed to avoid hypoxemia. In certain severe cases, use of an intensive care unit ventilator in combination with total intravenous anesthesia may be necessary.

Patients with significant restrictive disease are at increased risk of postoperative respiratory failure. It is important to minimize postoperative respiratory depression, and anesthetic drug choice should be aimed at this goal. Regional anesthesia and analgesia may be quite helpful when the circumstances are amenable. Finally, it is important to remember that many of the parenchymal diseases that cause restrictive pulmonary physiology also are associated with pulmonary hypertension. Care must be taken to avoid worsening pulmonary pressures. In particular, hypoxia, hypercapnia, acidosis, hypothermia, and extreme catecholamine surges should be avoided.

Suggested readings

Ali J, Summer W, Levitzky M. Obstructive lung disease. In: *Pulmonary Pathophysiology.* 2nd ed. New York: Lange Medical Books; 2005:85–104.

American Thoracic Society/European Respiratory Society Task Force. Standards for the Diagnosis and Management of Patients with COPD [Internet]. Version 1.2. New York: American Thoracic Society; 2004:1–222.

Cooper CB, Tashkin DP. Recent developments in inhaled therapy in stable chronic obstructive pulmonary disease. *BMJ* 2005; 330:640–644.

Croxton TL, Weinmann GG, Senior RM, et al. Clinical research in chronic obstructive pulmonary disease: needs and opportunities. *Am J Respir Crit Care Med* 2003; 167:1142–1149.

Fleisher LA. Is there an optimal timing for smoking cessation? In: *Evidenced-Based Practice of Anesthesiology.* Philadelphia: Saunders; 2004:57–61.

Jemal A, Ward E, Hao Y, Thun M. Trends in the leading causes of death in the United States, 1970–2002. *JAMA* 2005; 294:1255–1259.

Lawrence VA, Cornell JE, Smentana GW. Strategies to reduce postoperative pulmonary complications after noncardiothoracic surgery: systematic review for the American College of Physicians. *Ann Intern Med* 2006; 144:596–608.

Litonjua AA, Weiss ST. Epidemiology of asthma. *UpToDate.* Version 16.3. October 2008.

Nathan SD. Lung transplantation: disease-specific considerations for referral. *Chest* 2005; 127:1006–1016.

National Asthma Education and Prevention Program. Expert Panel Report 3: Guidelines for the diagnosis and management of asthma. National Heart Lung and Blood Institute. 2007. Available at: http://www.nih.gov/guidelines/asthma.

National Emphysema Treatment Trial Research Group. A randomized trial comparing lung-volume-reduction surgery with medical therapy for severe emphysema. *N Engl J Med* 2003; 348:2059–2073.

Pauwels RA, Buist AS, Calverley PM, et al. Global strategy for the diagnosis, management, and prevention of chronic obstructive pulmonary disease. NHBLI/WHO Global Initiative for Chronic Obstructive Lung Disease (GOLD) Workshop summary. *Am J Respir Crit Care Med* 2001; 163:1256–1276.

Pierson DJ. Clinical practice guidelines for chronic obstructive pulmonary disease: a review and comparison for current resources. *Resp Care* 2006; 51:277–288.

Qaseem A, Snow V, Fitterman N, et al. Risk assessment for and strategies to reduce perioperative pulmonary complications for patients undergoing noncardiothoracic surgery: a guideline from the American College of Physicians. *Ann Intern Med* 2006; 144:575–580.

Seigne PW, Hartigan PM, Body SC. Anesthetic considerations for patients with severe emphysematous lung disease. *Int Anesthesiol Clin* 2000; 38:1–23.

Smetana GW. A 68-year-old man with COPD contemplating colon cancer surgery. *JAMA* 2007; 297:2121–2130.

West JB. Obstructive diseases. In: *Pulmonary Pathophysiology: The Essentials.* 7th ed. Philadelphia: Lippincott, Williams & Wilkins; 2008:51–79.

Anesthetic goals in patients with myocardial ischemia and heart failure

Sugantha Sundar, Jason M. Erlich, and Eswar Sundar

According to the 2004 statistics compiled by the American Heart Association (AHA), an estimated 79.4 million American adults have cardiovascular disease. The average annual rate of first cardiac event varies by age group, from seven per 1000 in 35- to 44-year-olds to 68 per 1000 in 85- to 94-year-olds. There are approximately 565,000 new and 300,000 recurrent heart attacks per year. Notably, only 18% of new myocardial infarctions (MIs) are preceded by longstanding angina. These statistics demonstrate a necessity to be aware of the scale of the problem in the United States and to understand the underlying mechanisms of coronary artery disease (CAD) leading to myocardial ischemia and its prevention. The pathophysiology of heart failure and its management are discussed in this chapter. The role of ischemic preconditioning in myocardial protection also are briefly discussed.

Pathophysiology of myocardial ischemia

Myocardial metabolism

The myocardium derives energy from lactate, fatty acids, glucose, pyruvate, and acetate and under special circumstances, such as starvation, from fructose, glycogen, and protein. Myocardial oxygen consumption is one of the highest of any organ at 8 to 10 ml oxygen/100 g myocardium/min. The subendocardial requirement is 20% higher than the epicardium, making it particularly susceptible to ischemia.

Myocardial oxygen supply and demand

Myocardial oxygen demand is determined mainly by heart rate, wall tension, and contractility. Oxygen consumption depends on myocardial wall tension, which in turn is directly proportional to the intracavitary pressure and ventricular radius but inversely related to wall thickness. Thus, decreasing ventricular wall distention can decrease oxygen demand. Basal oxygen requirements determine myocardial oxygen demands.

Oxygen supply to the myocardium is determined by the pressure in the aortic root at the end of diastole and the left ventricular end-diastolic pressure. Coronary artery diameter and the arterial oxygen content determine oxygen supply. Immediately after coronary occlusion, two physiologic mechanisms occur in an attempt to correct the stoppage of flow:

- "Reactive hyperemia," in which reperfusion flow increases above preocclusion levels
- "Reactive dilatation," in which large coronaries dilate in an attempt to relieve the occlusion

These physiologic reactions are limited and do not achieve full coronary flow. At >90% occlusion, reactive physiologic dilation is exhausted and normal flow cannot be maintained, necessitating alternative intervention.

Coronary blood flow is maintained mainly based on perfusion pressure and vascular tone of coronary vessels. Postsynaptic β_1, β_2, α_1, and α_2 receptors are present in myocardium. Presynaptic β_2 activation increases norepinephrine release, which is mediated by postsynaptic β_1 receptors. Postsynaptic β_1 receptors predominate, except in the failing and ischemic heart, in which α_1 receptors serve as reserve and high levels of catecholamines down-regulate β_1 expression. Dopaminergic receptors have not been described in the myocardium.

Coronary plaque rupture with thrombosis is an important etiologic mechanism of perioperative MI (PMI). It is very likely that PMI also results from prolonged ischemia (manifest as ST-segment depression on the electrocardiogram [ECG]) in the presence of severe but stable CAD. Data suggest that the risks for perioperative MI include: (1) poor preoperative cardiac status (CAD, history of congestive heart failure), (2) postoperative hypotension, (3) new (long-duration) intraoperative ST-T changes, and (4) increased intraoperative blood loss and transfusion.

There is growing evidence indicating that patients who have recently undergone percutaneous coronary revascularization and stent implantation may be at increased risk for perioperative in-stent thrombosis and MI. The American College of Cardiology/AHA guidelines recommend a delay of at least 2 weeks and ideally 4 to 6 weeks between implantation of a bare metal stent and noncardiac surgery to reduce the risk of PMI. This allows for 4 full weeks of dual-antiplatelet therapy during stent re-endothelialization and 2 weeks for the antiplatelet effect to dissipate after discontinuation of drug therapy. The risk period for in-stent thrombosis is extended further in patients receiving a drug-eluting stent, because the drug that prevents neointimal proliferation delays in-stent endothelialization and anti-platelet therapy is therefore recommended for far longer.

Preoperative testing and risk stratification

Preoperative testing and risk stratification of patients undergoing noncardiac surgery have been topics of debate for many years. The decision to recommend further stratification procedures in each patient must take into account the potential benefit versus the potential risk. The risk of myocardial ischemia is related to three important factors: the extent of the patient's disease, the type of surgery, and the degree of hemodynamic stress associated with the procedure. The duration and intensity of coronary and myocardial stressors may be helpful in estimating the likelihood of perioperative cardiac events, particularly for emergency surgery. See Chapter 2 for in-depth discussion of patient evalution prior to noncardiac surgery, including the latest American College of Cardiology and American Heart Association Guidelines.

Conduct of anesthesia

No one anesthetic is superior to another. There have been no outcome studies to show the superiority of one anesthetic technique over another. It is important to bear in mind that an anesthetic that reduces myocardial oxygen demand and improves coronary blood flow is critical. The choice of anesthetic is determined by the procedure being performed, the clinical condition of the patient, and whether the procedure is an emergency.

The degree of monitoring for ischemia that is warranted is dictated by the clinical situation. Continuous ECG monitoring is the most common method used to detect myocardial ischemia. Monitoring lead V5 can detect up to 82% of ischemic events. Hemodynamic changes, such as hypotension, elevated pulmonary artery pressures, and a decrease in cardiac output are indicators of myocardial ischemia. Regional wall motion abnormalities detected on transesophageal echocardiography may be helpful in determining which coronary artery is involved.

Volatile anesthetics are vasodilators, which could potentially lead to coronary steal in patients with unfavorable anatomy. However, the concern that isoflurane may cause coronary steal has not been validated in human subjects. Reduced serum troponin levels have been documented in cardiac surgical patients receiving volatile anesthetics, possibly reflecting a preconditioning or postconditioning effect. A dose-dependent or class effect of inhalational anesthetics in protecting the myocardium has not been proven in humans.

Neuraxial blockade may be beneficial in certain situations in which sympathectomy is desirable. However, procedures requiring a high dermatomal level of anesthesia may be associated with hemodynamic compromise and may even be detrimental. Use of thoracic epidural anesthesia for postoperative pain control has been associated with fewer pulmonary complications, although the incidence of myocardial infarction or overall mortality is no different.

Monitored anesthesia care was associated with the highest 30-day mortality rate in one large study, possibly because patients who were the sickest were chosen to receive monitored anesthesia care versus general or regional anesthesia. Monitored anesthesia care (MAC) less completely blunts sympathetic nervous system responses to surgical stimulation and hence may be associated with demand ischemia.

Outcome advantages of regional analgesia over patient-controlled analgesia for post-operative pain control have not been documented with sufficient evidence. However, less opioid requirement, better hemodynamic profile, and decreased perioperative hypercoagulable state may be some of the advantages with regional analgesia.

Maintenance of intraoperative normothermia is vital in that patients with core temperatures less than 35°C are at increased risk of developing myocardial ischemia.

Treatment of myocardial ischemia

Treatment of myocardial ischemia is multimodal and depends on the clinical setting.

- In some situations, myocardial ischemia is associated with profound hemodynamic consequences. In this setting, optimizing the blood pressure, reducing the heart rate, and improving preload are crucial.
- Malignant ventricular arrhythmias are not uncommon with severe ischemia. Institution of the Advanced Cardiac Life Support (ACLS) protocols may be necessary when life-threatening arrhythmias occur.
- Nitroglycerin infusion causes coronary vasodilation and improves blood flow to ischemic areas of the myocardium. It also reduces the preload on a failing heart and thus has beneficial effects.
- Calcium channel blockers are given in situations in which coronary vasospasm is suspected.
- Heparin infusion may be indicated to reduce further coronary thrombosis.
- Consideration to stoping surgery and proceeding to the cardiac catheterization laboratory should be given in conjunction with the surgical team. Percutaneous intervention may be necessary with or without the use of thrombolytic therapy. Coronary revascularization may be necessary for a more permanent solution.
- In the interim, placement of an intra-aortic balloon pump (IABP) should be considered to reduce afterload and improve coronary perfusion during diastole.

Ischemic preconditioning and myocardial protection

Ischemic preconditioning (IPC) and myocardial protection have received much attention during the past few years. Ischemic preconditioning is a method by which the target organ is conditioned prior to the ischemic insult to reduce the extent of injury. IPC may be mechanical or pharmacologic. Several studies have shown the beneficial effects of brief limb ischemia in preconditioning the heart, although this is somewhat impractical in an operating room setting. Pharmacologic IPC may be considered in patients at increased risk for myocardial ischemia. Adenosine, endothelial nitrous oxide, free radicals, kinases, opioids, catecholamines, and adenosine triphosphate (ATP)-sensitive potassium channels have been implicated in remote preconditioning. Adenosine is an extracellular molecule that is both a trigger and a mediator of IPC. Several studies implicated volatile anesthetics to be involved in IPC and to exert a myocardial-protectant effect. Volatile anesthetics reduce the amount of myocardial enzyme leak and reduce the size of an infarct following preconditioning. There is an improvement in ventricular function in patients preconditioned with volatile agents. The precise mechanism by which this works is still unclear, but it appears to be multifactorial. This effect depends, at least in part, on anesthetic-induced opening of ATP-sensitive potassium channels. However, the precise dosing and duration of therapy have not been determined.

Pathophysiology and management of heart failure

Each year, 500,000 cases of heart failure are diagnosed in the United States. Extensive myocardial damage from myocardial ischemia may lead to both systolic and diastolic heart failure. The presence of decompensated heart failure is a major predictor of adverse perioperative outcome, whereas compensated heart failure is an intermediate risk factor for adverse perioperative outcome. Symptoms of dyspnea on exertion, orthopnea, edema of the extremities, and end-organ dysfunction are indicators of heart failure.

Systolic heart function may be measured by calculating the ejection fraction on echocardiography or cardiac MRI. In systolic failure, there is impaired left ventricular contractility, and ejection fraction is a measure of the contractile function of the heart. The ability to increase stroke volume via an increase in preload is reduced, and the Starling curve shifts to the right of the normal curve if afterload and inotropy remain unchanged. As Fig. 4.1 demonstrates, any increase in preload in congestive heart failure due to systolic failure results in a smaller increase in stroke volume than in normal ventricles if inotropy and afterload are kept constant. A decrease in afterload or increase in contractility may improve ventricular performance but will not affect filling pressures. A reduction in preload with an increase in inotropic force, a decrease in afterload, or both yields reductions in ventricular filling pressures and improvement in ventricular performance.

Elevated left ventricular end-diastolic pressure is an indicator of poor systolic function of the heart. Use of inotropes to improve systolic function is the first-line treatment for heart failure, although other types of cardiovascular drugs are also useful (Fig. 4.2).

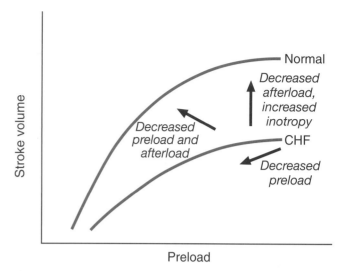

Figure 4.1. Relationship between preload and stroke volume in congestive heart failure. *Source:* Steele L, Webster NR. Altered cardiac function. *J R Coll Surg Edinb* 2001; 46(1):29–34.

Consideration should be given to the placement of an IABP in the absence of adequate response to inotropic medications and adequate treatment of myocardial ischemia.

The IABP is inserted percutaneously through the femoral artery. The balloon tip is situated distal to the origin of the left subclavian artery and should be above the origin of the renal arteries. X-ray and transesophageal echocardiography may be used to aid in optimal positioning of the balloon tip. The IABP inflation and deflation are usually synchronized with the ECG (the QRS complex) or the arterial pressure waveform (Fig. 4.3). It is vital to time the balloon inflation with the dicrotic notch of the arterial waveform. Deflation should be timed when the arterial pressure waveform reaches the lowest level, indicating that the left ventricle is ready for the next contraction. The initial setup of the balloon pump should be at a 1:2 ratio to accurately time the pump, to be followed by a ratio of 1:1 to obtain optimal

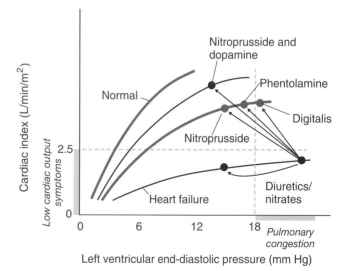

Figure 4.2. Medical management of heart failure.

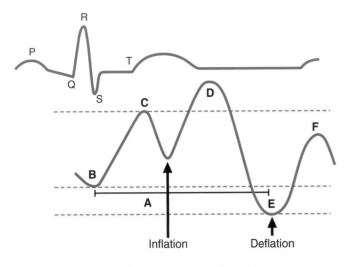

A One complete cardiac cycle
B Unassisted aortic end-diastolic pressure
C Unassisted systolic pressure
D Diastolic augmentation
E Reduced aortic end-diastolic pressure
F Reduced systolic pressure

Figure 4.3. IABP timing: inflation/deflation.

benefits. Some contraindications to placement of an IABP include aortic insufficiency, sepsis, and severe peripheral vascular disease. Cardiovascular effects of the IABP are summarized in Fig. 4.4.

Diastolic heart failure is more challenging to diagnose and manage. It is the inability of the ventricle to adequately relax between contractions, leading to less filling of the ventricle and atrial hypertension. Chronic hypertension is the most common cause of diastolic dysfunction. It leads to left ventricular hypertrophy and increased connective tissue content, both of which decrease cardiac compliance. Diastolic dysfunction is more common in elderly persons, partly because of increased collagen crosslinking, increased smooth muscle content, and loss of elastic fibers. Patients with diastolic dysfunction are highly sensitive to volume changes and preload. Diagnosis can be made using transthoracic and transesophageal echocardiography. Pulsed-wave Doppler examination across the mitral valve during diastole is one modality used to assess diastolic function. In the normal heart, there is an E wave corresponding to early passive filling of the ventricle, followed by an A wave corresponding to atrial contraction leading to ventricular filling. Milder forms of diastolic heart failure are characterized by impaired relaxation, whereas more advanced forms of diastolic heart failure are characterized by a restrictive pattern. More sophisticated imaging modalities such as tissue Doppler and transmitral flow propagation velocities also may be used to fully evaluate diastolic function. Treatment of diastolic heart failure is equally challenging. Maintaining sinus rhythm is vital in this patient population. Slowing the heart rate allows the ventricle time to fill adequately, and β-Blockers are particularly useful. Angiotensin-converting enzyme inhibitors and angiotensin receptor blockers may be beneficial in patients with diastolic dysfunction, especially those with hypertension. Angiotensin-converting enzyme inhibitors and angiotensin receptor blockers directly affect myocardial relaxation and compliance by inhibiting production of, or blocking angiotensin II receptors, thereby reducing interstitial collagen deposition and fibrosis.

Figure 4.4. IABP effects.

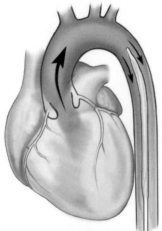

Inflation
•At onset of diastole
•Causes sharp "V" in arterial waveform and increased coronary perfusion

Deflation
•At end of diastole
•Causes reduction in aortic end-diastolic and systolic pressures
•Decreased afterload
•Decreased cardiac work
•Decreased myocardial oxygen consumption
•Increased cardiac output

Conduct of Anesthesia

Anesthetic management of patients who are in heart failure is complex and associated with a high mortality (>10%) and morbidity. These factors should be considered before deciding on a plan:

- Underlying pathophysiology of the heart failure
- Surgery or procedure being planned
- What monitoring is required, and how much time is available to optimize the patient

The majority of heart failure results from loss of inotropy (due to ischemia, valvular regurgitations), increased afterload (due to hypertension, aortic stenosis, coarctation), and fluid overload. Some of these conditions require only gentle afterload reduction. This can be achieved by vasodilators such as nitroglycerine or sodium nitroprusside. In patients with severe heart failure, management with inodilators like milrinone, drugs such as dobutamine, or even placement of an IABP may be required.

Occasionally, heart failure can result from an obstruction to the left ventricular outflow tract for example, systolic anterior motion (SAM) of the mitral leaflet. In these conditions drugs such as phenylephrine and β blockers can help stent open the outflow tract and improve symptoms of heart failure.

Preoperative preparation

Before starting anesthesia on patients with heart failure, drugs must be started to treat the heart failure as discussed above. Oxygenation must be maximized using noninvasive means (CPAP) as far as possible. Intubating a patient in heart failure for a procedure is best done in a highly monitored setting like an operating room or an ICU. An IABP may need to be inserted preoperatively, under local anesthesia in some situations.

Choice of anesthetic depends on the procedure being done. Note that spinals and epidurals often impede the ability of the patient to breathe adequately, although the afterload reduction associated with neuraxial anesthesia can be beneficial. However, general anesthesia may be the only option.

Optimal monitoring in the form of arterial lines, pulmonary artery catheters and transesophageal echocardiograms must be considered, and at least an arterial line may have to be inserted preoperatively.

Intraoperative Management

Induction is often accompanied by a precipitous fall in blood pressure and this can be controlled by titrating induction drugs such as etomidate instead of propofol, and titrating vasoconstrictors and inotropes to maintain blood and pulmonary pressures. Intubation often reverses the hypotension but can cause undesired hypertension that can be extremely detrimental to the forward stroke volume. Hence careful titration and timing of induction and hemodynamic support drugs is vital and so is a slick and quick intubation by an experienced person.

The conduct of anesthesia during heart failure requires constant vigilance with regard to the vital signs, pulmonary pressures, echo findings, blood gases, body temperature, blood loss, coagulation and other parameters. Oxygenation should be maximized, ventilation optimized to blood gases and preferably only blood loss should be replaced with blood, thus avoiding unnecessary fluid administration. Serum calcium levels must be checked if blood products are being administered and corrected appropriately as calcium is an excellent inotrope.

Postanesthetic care

Leaving the patient intubated postoperatively may be prudent to allow heart failure to resolve. However, if the patient is deemed to be suitable for emergence and extubation at the end of the procedure, excellent pain control must be in place. If neuraxial anesthesia has been in place, it may be used to provide not only pain relief but also mild afterload reduction to help with heart failure.

Conclusion

Major noncardiac surgery is associated with significant perioperative mortality and morbidity. Most deaths in this setting are related to cardiac complications such as MI. Survivors of in-hospital perioperative ischemic events such as MI, unstable angina, and postoperative ischemia, warrant more aggressive long-term follow-up and treatment than currently are practiced. MI following coronary artery bypass graft surgery is associated with a significant increase in intensive care unit time, hospital length of stay, and overall costs, which contribute to greater hospital and physician service costs.

Suggested readings

Adesanya AO, de Lemos JA, Greilich NB, Whitten CW. Management of perioperative myocardial infarction in noncardiac surgical patients. *Chest* 2006; 130:584–596.

Barbagallo M, Casati A, Spadini E, et al. Early increases in cardiac troponin levels after major vascular surgery is associated with an increased frequency of delayed cardiac complications. *J Clin Anesth* 2006; 18:280–285.

Ellis JE, Tung A, Lee H, Kasza K. Predictors of perioperative beta-blockade use in vascular surgery: a mail survey of United States anesthesiologists. *J Cardiothorac Vasc Anesth* 2007; 21:330–336.

Mehlhorn U, Kroner A, de Vivie ER. 30 years clinical intra-aortic balloon pumping: facts and figures. *Thorac Cardiovasc Surg* 1999; 47(Suppl 2):298–303.

Ndrepepa G, Braun S, Schomig A, Kastrati A. Accuracy of N-terminal pro-brain natriuretic peptide to predict mortality in various subsets of patients with coronary artery disease. *Am J Cardiol* 2007; 100:575–578.

Schouten O, Poldermans D. Statins in the prevention of perioperative cardiovascular complications. *Curr Opin Anaesthesiol* 2005; 18:51–55.

Wijeysundera DN, Beattie WS. Calcium channel blockers for reducing cardiac morbidity after noncardiac surgery: a meta-analysis. *Anesth Analg* 2003; 97:634–641.

Anesthetic goals in patients with valvular heart disease

Sugantha Sundar, Devi Mahendran, and Eswar Sundar

Valvular heart disease accounts for a significant proportion of patients requiring cardiac surgery. Rheumatic heart disease as a cause of valvular heart disease has become less common with the aggressive use of penicillin to treat streptococcal infections. However, an increasing proportion of adults with congenital heart disease require operations for recurrent valvular lesions or new lesions related to complications from their original surgical procedure.

The anesthetic management of patients with valvular heart disease undergoing noncardiac surgery requires a clear understanding of the pathophysiology and hemodynamic implications of valvular lesions. A patient's physiologic adaptation to his or her valve disease may be acutely disturbed by perioperative events and anesthetic drugs. Hence, the anesthesiologist must be able to manipulate the patient's hemodynamic status to provide the best possible cardiac output to maintain end-organ perfusion.

This chapter summarizes the anesthetic management of valvular heart disease with particular reference to:

- The preoperative evaluation of the patient with valvular heart disease
- The American Heart Association (AHA) recommendations for endocarditis prophylaxis in valvular heart disease
- Management of anticoagulation regimen in the perioperative period
- The etiology, pathophysiology, pressure–volume loops, hemodynamic goals, and anesthetic considerations for each of the major valvular lesions

Evaluating the patient with valvular heart disease

Preoperative evaluation focuses on determining the severity of the valvular lesion and its hemodynamic significance, residual ventricular function, the presence of concomitant coronary artery disease, and the presence of secondary effects on pulmonary, renal, and hepatic function. Table 5.1 demonstrates points to elicit during history taking. The New York Heart Association (NYHA) grades the clinical severity of heart failure and is a prognostic indicator of outcome (Table 5.2). Patients with valvular heart disease may have many physical findings;

Table 5.3 outlines the key physical examination findings in these patients.

Preprocedure investigations

Preprocedure investigations must be tailored to the patient and the procedure in question. It is important to exclude active ischemia, heart failure, arrhythmias, and electrolyte imbalances secondary to medications. A coagulation profile may assume importance if a regional anesthetic is being considered in a patient receiving anticoagulants. Table 5.4 outlines the main investigations that may be considered in patients with valvular heart disease.

Premedication

In general, it is recommended that patients receive their usual medications on the morning of surgery. Premedication with standard doses of commonly used drugs such as midazolam or fentanyl is desirable and well tolerated in patients with normal or near-normal ventricular function. However, patients with poor ventricular function may be highly sensitive to opioids, and premedication should be dose-adjusted in accordance with the severity of ventricular impairment and comorbidities.

Endocarditis prophylaxis

The risk of endocarditis varies according to the valvular abnormality, and antibiotic prophylaxis follows AHA guidelines (Tables 5.5, 5.6, and 5.7).

Prosthetic and mechanical valves

Patients with prosthetic heart valves pose special challenges to the anesthesiologist. The most frequent issue with patients who have a prosthetic valve is the management of systemic anticoagulation in the perioperative period. Prosthetic valves are either bioprosthetic or mechanical. Bioprosthetic valves are usually heterogeneous grafts made from animal tissue and have very low thrombogenic potential. Hence, patients with bioprosthetic valves do not usually need systemic anticoagulation. Aspirin is recommended for all patients with prosthetic heart valves. Aspirin alone is recommended in patients with bioprostheses and no risk factors for thrombosis. However, bioprosthetic

Table 5.1. Points to elicit during history taking

- History of rheumatic fever
- Intravenous drug abuse
- Genetic conditions associated with valvular disease, such as Marfan's syndrome
- Heart surgery in childhood
- Prior valvular surgery, type of prosthetic valve used
- Exercise tolerance
- Fatigability
- Symptoms of dyspnea, orthopnea, dependant edema, chest pain, paroxysmal nocturnal dyspnea, and neurologic symptoms
- A thorough review of medications (e.g., use of digoxin, diuretics, vasodilators, ACE inhibitors, antiarrhythmics, and anticoagulants; if patient is taking digoxin, screen for symptoms of digoxin toxicity)

Table 5.3. Physical findings in valvular heart disease

- Signs of congestive heart failure
  - S_3 gallop
  - Pulmonary rales
  - Elevated jugular venous pressure
  - Hepatojugular reflux
  - Hepatosplenomegaly
  - Pedal edema
- Auscultatory findings specific to individual valvular lesions
- Neurologic deficits secondary to embolic phenomena

valves have a shorter lifespan and are therefore more often placed in elderly patients.

On the other hand, mechanical valves are longer lasting, but patients who have a mechanical valve do need lifelong anticoagulation. All patients with mechanical valves require warfarin therapy. Aspirin is usually combined with warfarin in patients with mechanical heart valves and in high-risk patients with bioprostheses. For high-risk patients who cannot take aspirin, the addition of clopidogrel to warfarin should be considered. Even with the use of warfarin, the risk of thromboembolism is 1% to 2% per year, but the risk is considerably higher without warfarin treatment. Systemic anticoagulation in patients with mechanical valves reduces the risk of thromboembolism by about 75%.

Upon auscultation, patients with mechanical valves may be identified by the high-pitched, crisp opening and closing sounds. Bioprosthetic valves do not have any special auscultatory characteristics. The onset of new murmurs or a change in the quality of murmurs associated with a valve may indicate a problem with the valve or the onset of endocarditis.

Patients presenting for surgery with a prosthetic valve should receive a complete history and physical examination. The anesthesiologist must know what type of valve the patient has and when it was inserted. Preoperatively, transesophageal

echocardiography (TEE) or transthoracic echocardiography can allow excellent visualization of the prosthetic valve and assessment of valvular function. Almost invariably, patients with artificial valves will require perioperative antibiotic prophylaxis for endocarditis.

Patients with mechanical valves taking systemic anticoagulation will require careful management in the perioperative period. The perioperative period is a prothrombotic state, and this danger must be borne in mind when stopping systemic anticoagulation. Intravenous heparin is one method for bridging anticoagulation therapy.

AHA bridging recommendations in patients with mechanical valves who require interruption of warfarin therapy for noncardiac surgery and invasive procedures are as follows:

- In patients at low risk of thrombosis, defined as those with a bileaflet mechanical aortic valve replacement without risk factors, it is recommended that warfarin be stopped 48 to 72 hours before surgery. This will allow the international normalized ratio (INR) to fall to <1.5; warfarin can then be restarted within 24 hours after the procedure. Heparin is usually unnecessary.
- In patients at high risk for thrombosis, defined as those with a mechanical mitral valve or a mechanical aortic valve with any risk factor, therapeutic doses of unfractionated

Table 5.2. The NYHA functional classification of heart disease

Class	Patient symptoms
Class I (mild)	No limitation of physical activity. Ordinary physical activity does not cause undue fatigue, palpitations, or dyspnea.
Class II (mild)	Slight limitation of physical activity. Comfortable at rest, but ordinary physical activity results in fatigue, palpitations, or dyspnea.
Class III (moderate)	Marked limitation of physical activity. Comfortable at rest, but less than ordinary activity causes fatigue, palpitations, or dyspnea.
Class IV (severe)	Unable to carry out any physical activity without discomfort. Symptoms of cardiac insufficiency at rest. If any physical activity is undertaken, discomfort is increased.

Table 5.4. Investigations for patients with valvular heart disease

- ECG for evidence of ischemia, arrhythmias, atrial enlargement, and ventricular hypertrophy
- Serum electrolytes and renal function (mild–moderate hypokalemia is often seen in patients taking diuretics and can exacerbate digoxin toxicity). Hypomagnesemia may cause perioperative arrhythmias. Hyperkalemia may occur in patients taking potassium-sparing diuretics or ACE inhibitors.
- Coagulation studies to check for reversal prior to surgery for patients who have been on anticoagulants
- Arterial blood gases in patients with significant pulmonary symptoms
- A chest radiograph to assess cardiac size and the presence of pulmonary vascular congestion

Special studies can provide important diagnostic and prognostic information about valvular lesions:

- Echocardiography with Doppler technology for evaluating valvular heart diseases
- Cardiac catheterization to identify coexisting coronary artery disease; allows visualization of the cardiac chambers as well as pressure gradients across valves

Table 5.5. AHA recommendations for endocarditis prophylaxis

High- and moderate-risk patients (prophylaxis recommended)	Low-risk patients (prophylaxis not recommended)
• Prosthetic valves or history of infective endocarditis	• Isolated secundum ASD
• Complex cyanotic congenital heart disease	• >6 months after successful surgical or percutaneous repair of an ASD, VSD, or PDA.
• Surgically constructed systemic-pulmonary shunts or conduits	• MVP without MR or thickened leaflets on echocardiography
• Congenital cardiac valve malformations, particularly bicuspid aortic valves, and patients with acquired valvular dysfunction (e.g., rheumatic heart disease)	• Physiologic, functional, or innocent heart murmurs, including aortic valve sclerosis
• A history of surgical valve repair	• Echocardiographic evidence of physiologic MR in the absence of a murmur and with structurally normal valves
• Hypertrophic cardiomyopathy with resting or latent obstruction	• Echocardiographic evidence of physiologic TR and or PR in the absence of a murmur and with structurally normal valves
• MVP and auscultatory evidence of valvular regurgitation and/or thickened leaflets on echocardiography	

ASD, atrial septal defect; PDA, patent ductus arteriosus; VSD, ventricular septal defect.
Source: Wilson W, Taubert KA, Gewitz M, et al; American Heart Association Rheumatic Fever, Endocarditis, and Kawasaki Disease Committee. *Circulation.* 2007; 116(15):1736–1754.

Table 5.6. Indicated and nonindicated procedures for endocarditis prophylaxis

Endocarditis prophylaxis not recommended	Endocarditis prophylaxis recommended
• Respiratory tract	• Respiratory tract
· Endotracheal intubation	· Tonsillectomy/ adenoidectomy
· Flexible bronchoscopy with or without biopsy[a]	· Surgical operations involving respiratory mucosa
· Tympanostomy tube insertion[a]	· Rigid bronchoscopy
• Gastrointestinal tract	• Gastrointestinal tract (prophylaxis for high-risk patients, optimal for moderate risk)
· TEE	
· Endoscopy with or without biopsy[a]	· Sclerotherapy for esophageal varices
• Genitourinary tract	· Esophageal stricture dilation
· Vaginal hysterectomy	· ERCP with biliary obstruction
· Vaginal delivery	· Biliary tract surgery
· Caesarean section	· Surgical operations involving intestinal mucosa
· Urethral catheterization	
· Uterine dilation and curettage	• Genitourinary tract
· Therapeutic abortion	· Prostate surgery
· Sterilization procedures	· Cystoscopy
· Insertion or removal of intrauterine devices	· Urethral dilation
• Other	
· Cardiac catheterization, including balloon angioplasty	
· Implantation of cardiac pacemakers, defibrillators, and coronary stents	
· Incision or biopsy of surgically scrubbed skin	
· Circumcision	

[a] Prophylaxis indicated in high-risk patients.
ERCP, endoscopic retrograde cholangiopancreatography.
Source: Wilson W, Taubert KA, Gewitz M, et al; American Heart Association Rheumatic Fever, Endocarditis, and Kawasaki Disease Committee. *Circulation.* 2007; 116(15):1736–1754.

heparin should be started when the INR falls below 2.0 (typically 48 hours before surgery) and stopped 4 to 6 hours before the procedure. Warfarin is then restarted soon after surgery, as determined by the clinical condition of the patient. Heparin is continued until the INR is back within therapeutic range with warfarin therapy. More recently, low molecular weight heparin (LMWH) has been used, although few studies exist to validate the efficacy and safety of either LMWH or unfractionated heparin in this setting.

• Fresh frozen plasma (FFP) may be given to patients with mechanical valves who require interruption of warfarin therapy for emergency surgery or invasive procedures. FFP is preferable to high-dose vitamin K.

• In patients at high risk for thrombosis, therapeutic doses of unfractionated heparin (15,000 units every 12 hours) or LMWH (100 units/kg every 12 hours) may be considered during the period of subtherapeutic INR.

Risk factors for thrombosis include:

• Atrial fibrillation
• Previous thromboembolism
• Left ventricular (LV) dysfunction
• Hypercoagulable conditions
• Older-generation thrombogenic valves
• More than one mechanical valve

Anesthetic considerations

Choice of anesthetic technique/agents to be employed in patients with valvular heart disease depends on the severity of the valvular lesion, its hemodynamic adaptations, and the proposed procedure. Inhalational agents all produce dose-dependent myocardial depression, which may be accentuated in patients with abnormal hemodynamics secondary to valvular disease. Nitrous oxide is less depressant and maintains peripheral vascular resistance. All inhalational agents cause decreases in blood pressure. Isoflurane, sevoflurane, and desflurane are associated with a decrease in systemic vascular resistance with peripheral vasodilation. Desflurane may cause sympathetic activation that could be detrimental to patients with valvular heart disease. Sevoflurane and isoflurane are both considered safe in patients with cardiac disease. Sevoflurane is reported to have a more stable effect on heart rate and cardiac function than other agents.

Table 5.7. Antibiotic regimens for endocarditis prophylaxis

Dental, oral, respiratory tract, or esophageal procedures

Standard preoperative prophylaxis	Ampicillin	Adults: 2.0 g Children: 50 mg/kg IM/IV
Penicillin allergic	Clindamycin	Adults: 600 mg Children: 20 mg/kg IV
	Cefazolin[b]	Adults: 1 g Children 25 mg/kg IM/IV

Genitourinary/gastrointestinal (excluding esophageal) procedures

High-risk patients	Ampicillin plus gentamicin	Adults: ampicillin, 2.0 g IM/IV, plus gentamicin, 1.5 mg/kg (not to exceed 120 mg); 6 h later, ampicillin 1 g IM/IV
		Children: ampicillin, 50 mg/kg IM/IV (not to exceed 2.0 g), plus gentamicin 1.5 mg/kg; 6 h later, ampicillin 25 mg/kg IM/IV
High-risk patients allergic to penicillins	Vancomycin plus gentamicin	Adults: vancomycin, 1.0 g IV over 1–2 h, plus gentamicin, 1.5 mg/kg (not to exceed 120 mg)
		Children: vancomycin, 20 mg/kg IV over 1–2 h, plus gentamicin, 1.5 mg/kg IM/IV
Moderate-risk patients	Ampicillin	Adults: 2.0 g IM/IV Children: 50 mg/kg IM/IV
Moderate-risk patients allergic to penicillins	Vancomycin	Adults: 1.0 g IV over 1–2 h Children: 20 mg/kg IV over 1–2 h

[a] Total children's dose should not exceed adult dose.
[b] Cephalosporins should not be used in individuals with immediate-type hypersensitivity reaction to penicillin.
IM, intramuscularly; IV, intravenously.
Source: Dajani AS, Taubert KA, Wilson W, et al. Prevention of bacterial endocarditis: recommendations by the American Heart Association. *JAMA.* 1997;277:1794 –1801.

Regional anesthesia may be a consideration for procedures involving extremities, the perineum, and the lower abdomen. Regional anesthetic techniques provide less respiratory and cardiac depression than general anesthesia. However, patients may be very sensitive to the vasodilating effects of spinal and epidural anesthesia. Epidural may be more preferable to spinal anesthesia because of the more gradual onset of sympathetic blockade. A single-shot spinal anesthetic is relatively contraindicated in patients with "fixed" cardiac output states (e.g., critical aortic stenosis [AS]) because these patients are unable to augment their cardiac output in response to the vasodilation and subsequent hypotension that often accompany this technique.

The postoperative management of patients with valvular heart disease should address managing pain control, optimizing fluid therapy, and restarting anticoagulation if necessary. Epidural catheters have been shown to provide excellent postoperative pain relief and should be considered whenever possible in patients with valvular heart disease. Major fluid shifts may occur 48 to 72 hours postoperatively, and patients with severe valvular heart disease require judicious fluid management during this phase, possibly with invasive hemodynamic monitoring. For patients who had been anticoagulated prior to surgery, anticoagulation needs to be restarted, keeping in mind the clinical picture and AHA recommendations.

The anesthetic considerations for valvular heart disease are discussed further in the context of each valvular lesion. Intraoperative monitoring is also tailored to the severity of the valvular disease and the proposed surgery. In addition to the standard American Society of Anesthesiologists monitors, other monitors may be employed intraoperatively include intra-arterial and pulmonary artery catheters, and TEE. Intra-arterial catheters provide beat-to-beat blood pressure measurement as well as the ability to monitor blood gases periodically. TEE can assess the severity of valvular disease accompanying structural or functional abnormalities and also allows evaluation of valve repair as well as function of artificial valves. Pulmonary artery catheters are used to measure cardiac output, mixed venous saturation, and intracardiac pressures (including pulmonary capillary wedge pressure), which are important indices of ventricular function and filling, and are useful for guiding intravenous fluid and inotropic therapy.

Left-sided valvular lesions
Mitral stenosis

Mitral stenosis (MS) occurs most commonly secondary to rheumatic fever and typically is functionally significant within two decades. Most patients are female and have combined stenosis and regurgitation (40%) rather than isolated stenosis (25%).

Pathophysiology

MS results from thickening and immobility of the mitral valve leaflets, which causes an obstruction to blood flow from the left atrium to the left ventricle. As a result, there is an increase in pressure within the left atrium, pulmonary vasculature, and right side of the heart, whereas the left ventricle is underloaded in isolated MS.

There is a significant reduction in preload; hence, a fixed cardiac output state develops. MS markedly affects LV filling, thereby reducing stroke volume and cardiac output. The left atrium undergoes volume overload and stretching, which may result in supraventricular tachycardias, particularly atrial fibrillation, further reducing ventricular filling. Back pressure of blood into the pulmonary circulation causes pulmonary hypertension, leading to right heart failure, hemoptysis, and pulmonary edema. On the systemic side, the reduced cardiac output cannot meet oxygen demands, and organ perfusion is often maintained with a relatively high systemic vascular resistance.

Risk factors for the development of pulmonary edema in MS are:

- Mitral valve area <1.5 cm^2 (the normal mitral valve area is 4–6 cm^2)
- NYHA functional class > II
- Prior adverse cardiac event
- LV ejection fraction (LVEF) < 0.4

Patients with severe MS requiring elective surgery should undergo mitral valvotomy or balloon valvuloplasty prior to their elective procedure, as the presence of pulmonary hypertension is associated with significant morbidity and mortality.

Pressure–volume loop in mitral stenosis

The pressure–volume loop in MS (Fig. 5.1) shows a reduction in end-diastolic, end-systolic, and stroke volume. LV function is normal in most people with MS, but contractility is decreased because of chronic underfilling of the left ventricle.

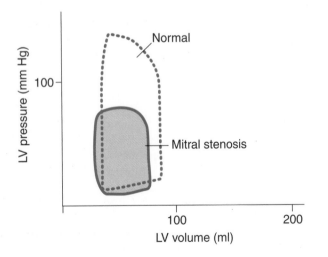

Figure 5.1. Pressure–volume loop in MS.

Table 5.8. Hemodynamic goals for the intraoperative management of valvular heart disease

Lesion	Preload	Systemic vascular resistance	Heart rate	Contractility
Aortic stenosis	↑	↑	↓	→
Hypertrophic cardiomyopathy	↑	↑	↓	↓
Mitral stenosis	↑	→ or ↑	↓	→
Mitral regurgitation	↑	↓	↑	→
Aortic regurgitation	↓	↓	↑	→

Anesthetic considerations in mitral stenosis

The anesthetic considerations in patients with MS are as follows (Table 5.8):

- Maintaining a slightly reduced to normal heart rate facilitates an increase in the time available during diastole, thus improving LV filling.
- Maintaining sinus rhythm facilitates LV filling with the contribution from the atrial kick.
- Maintaining an adequate preload is important to generate an adequate cardiac output. However, fluid therapy should be titrated with care to avoid precipitating pulmonary edema in patients with severe disease.
- Maintaining an adequate afterload is vital to help maintain coronary perfusion.
- Avoiding arterial hypoxemia or hypoventilation that may exacerbate pulmonary hypertension and evoke right ventricular failure is crucial.
- Full hemodynamic monitoring is generally indicated for all major surgical procedures.
- Patients with MS may be very sensitive to the vasodilating effects of spinal and epidural anesthesia.

Mitral regurgitation

Mitral regurgitation (MR) may occur acutely or gradually as a result of several different etiologies. Acute MR may occur in the setting of myocardial ischemia and infarction with papillary muscle dysfunction or chordae tendineae rupture. Chronic MR is usually caused by rheumatic heart disease, ischemia, or mitral valve prolapse (MVP).

Pathophysiology

In MR, a portion of the LV stroke volume is ejected backward into the low-pressure left atrium during systole. As a result, the forward cardiac output into the aorta is less than the left ventricle's total output (forward flow plus regurgitant volume).

The direct consequences of MR include:

- An elevation of left atrial volume and pressure
- A reduction of cardiac output

- Volume-related stress on the left ventricle because the regurgitant volume returns to the left ventricle in diastole along with normal pulmonary venous return

Factors that affect the volume of regurgitant flow include:

- Mitral valve orifice size
- Time available for regurgitant flow with each systolic contraction
- Transvalvular pressure gradient
- Systemic vascular resistance opposing forward LV blood flow
- Left atrial compliance

In acute MR, left atrial compliance undergoes little immediate change and left atrial pressure increases substantially when exposed to the regurgitant volume. This elevated pressure is transmitted backward to the pulmonary circulation and right heart and may precipitate acute pulmonary edema, right-sided heart failure, and pulmonary hypertension.

In chronic MR, the left atrium dilates and its compliance increases to accommodate a larger volume without a substantial increase in pressure. Both the left ventricle and left atrium show volume overload, leading to increased LV end-diastolic volume with a normal end-diastolic pressure. LV end-systolic volume is normal with a high stroke volume. However, forward cardiac output is substantially impaired because the low-pressure left atrium acts as a "sink" for the LVEF. In chronic MR, the LVEF is usually high because of the low resistance against the regurgitation. An LVEF of 50% may indicate significant LV dysfunction.

Pressure–volume loop in mitral regurgitation

The pressure–volume loop in MR shows an increase in end-diastolic volume with high end-diastolic pressure. End-systolic volume is normal or decreased. In chronic MR (Fig. 5.2), the end-diastolic volume is increased with a normal end-diastolic pressure as a result of the chronic dilatation of the left ventricle. The end-systolic volume is normal because of the markedly increased stroke volume.

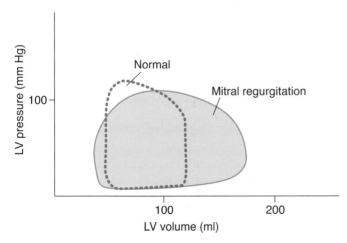

Figure 5.2. Pressure-volume loop in chronic well-compensated mitral regurgitation with normal left ventricular function.

Anesthetic considerations in mitral regurgitation

The main goals are to promote forward cardiac output and minimize regurgitant flow by:

- Medical optimization of MR prior to elective surgery with digoxin, diuretics and vasodilators.
- Maintaining intravascular volume (i.e., an adequate preload) to supply the dilated left ventricle.
- Maintaining normal to high heart rates (80–100 bpm). Higher heart rates promote cardiac emptying and tend to lower LV end-diastolic volume and thus reduce the regurgitant volume during systole. Bradycardia increases the regurgitant volume, decreasing the ejected volume into the aorta.
- Avoiding decreases in contractility. Inotropes with afterload-reducing effects (e.g., milrinone or dobutamine) should be considered.
- Minimizing drug-induced myocardial depression.
- Reducing afterload, because reducing systemic vascular resistance increases forward stroke volume and decreases the regurgitant volume.
- Performing intraoperative monitoring depending on the severity of ventricular dysfunction and the procedure. In patients with severe MR, full hemodynamic monitoring is recommended. Doppler TEE may be used to quantify the severity of the regurgitation and guide therapeutic interventions.
- Noting that patients with mild–moderate MR with well-preserved ventricular function can tolerate most anesthetic techniques without complications. However, patients with higher degrees of MR, especially in the context of atrial fibrillation, may have a high mortality rate.

Mitral valve prolapse

MVP is characterized by an abnormality of the mitral valve support structure that permits prolapse of the valve into the left atrium during contraction of the left ventricle. The estimated prevalence of MVP is 0.6% to 2%. There appears to be an increased incidence of MVP in patients with musculoskeletal abnormalities, including Marfan's syndrome, pectus excavatum, and kyphoscoliosis.

MVP is the most common valvular cause of chronic MR. Approximately 10% of patients with MVP develop progressive MR and will require mitral valve surgery in their lifetime. However, the natural history of MVP is generally benign, and most patients have a normal lifespan, although serious complications may occur; the most common are infective endocarditis, cerebrovascular accidents (due to embolic phenomena), atrial and ventricular arrhythmias, the need for mitral valve surgery, and, rarely, sudden death. Not all patients with MVP need antibiotic prophylaxis, and these patients must have specific auscultatory or echocardiographic features to justify antibiotic prophylaxis (Table 5.5).

Aortic stenosis

LV outflow tract obstruction may be subvalvular, valvular, or supravalvular in nature. The most common etiology of AS is senile calcification and/or fibrosis of a congenital bicuspid valve. In developed countries, rheumatic aortic valvular disease has become very uncommon. However, worldwide, rheumatic fever accounts for a third of all cases of AS.

Pathophysiology

In AS, the narrowed aortic valve creates a resistance to flow and causes a drop in pressure from the left ventricle to the aorta. The pathophysiologic changes in AS are related to the pressure gradient that develops between the left ventricle and aorta. Usually, when the aortic valve opens in systole, there is a minimal gradient between the two chambers. As the stenosis progresses, a resting gradient develops across the aortic valve. As a compensatory mechanism, the left ventricle hypertrophies because of increased wall tension to overcome the stenosis. The increased wall thickness helps normalize wall stress and maintain cardiac output within the normal range. In mild and moderate AS, there is little hemodynamic consequence, and the patient can tolerate this condition for years before the onset of symptoms.

However, with time, LV hypertrophy leads to a decrease in diastolic ventricular compliance (a stiff left ventricle); therefore, end-diastolic pressure must rise to maintain the same end-diastolic volume. The decreased diastolic pressure gradient between the left atrium and left ventricle impairs ventricular filling. The pulmonary capillary bed is usually protected from these diastolic filling abnormalities by a forceful left atrial contraction, which ensures filling of the stiff left ventricle. In AS, the left atrial kick contributes up to 40% (normal, 15%–20%) of ventricular filling. Loss of the atrial kick, as in atrial fibrillation, results in decreased ventricular filling, causing decreased cardiac output or a rise in mean left atrial pressures.

When compensatory LV hypertrophy reaches its limits, muscle degeneration occurs, contractility falls, and the left ventricle dilates to maintain chamber pressure. LV failure ensues, resulting in high pulmonary artery pressures, a low ejection fraction (EF), and reduced cardiac output.

Advanced AS is characterized by a triad of dyspnea on exertion, angina, and orthostatic or exertional syncope. Critical AS is said to exist when the aortic valve orifice is reduced to <0.7 cm^2 (normal, 2.5–3.5 cm^2). With severe AS, patients generate a transvalvular gradient >50 mm Hg at rest with a normal cardiac output and are unable to increase cardiac output appreciably in response to demand. Intraoperatively, the presence of severe AS is associated with an increased risk of acute myocardial infarction, but not death.

Without surgical treatment, most patients with symptomatic AS die within 2 to 5 years. Percutaneous balloon valvuloplasty is generally used for younger patients with congenital AS and for elderly patients who are considered poor surgical candidates for an aortic valve replacement.

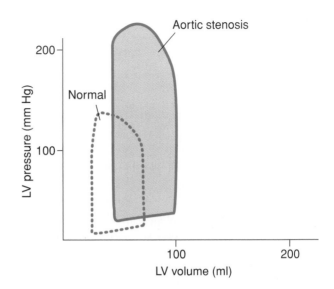

Figure 5.3. Pressure–volume loop in AS.

Pressure–volume loop in aortic stenosis

To generate a normal stroke volume in AS, the intraventricular pressure is high as a result of the pressure gradient across the aortic valve (Fig. 5.3). The end-diastolic pressure is higher than normal in cases of AS because LV hypertrophy leads to reduced LV compliance. High systolic wall tension leads to LV hypertrophy. Initially, LV hypertrophy increases contractility and decreases wall tension during systole. However, in severe AS, the left ventricle stiffens and starts to dilate, resulting in symptoms of LV failure.

Anesthetic considerations in aortic stenosis

Anesthetic considerations in patients with AS are as follows:

- Normal sinus rhythm should be maintained. The ventricle relies on the atrial kick for filling; hence, sinus rhythm is crucial in these patients. Emergent cardioversion is indicated if the patient suffers severe hemodynamic compromise due to arrhythmias.
- Tachycardia or bradycardia should be avoided. Many AS patients behave as though they have a fixed stroke volume, thus cardiac output becomes very rate dependent. High heart rate promotes heart failure by inadequate diastolic filling times and inadequate LV emptying. High heart rate also may aggravate ischemia. Premedication can prevent anxiety-provoked tachycardia. Bradycardia is also poorly tolerated. Heart rates between 60 and 90 bpm are optimal.
- A high normal preload should be maintained because a noncompliant left ventricle requires a high filling pressure to maintain normal end-diastolic volume.
- Sudden decreases in systemic vascular resistance should be avoided. In a normal heart, cardiac output rises when systemic vascular resistance falls; however, in AS, the stenosis limits the rise in cardiac output. Patients with AS are extremely sensitive to vasodilators.

- Myocardial contractility depression should be avoided through prevention of hypercarbia, hypoxia, and acidotic states.
- Concomitant ischemic heart disease worsens an already impaired oxygen delivery system. An adequate aortic diastolic pressure should be maintained using inotropes, vasoconstrictors, and fluid.
- Full hemodynamic monitoring should be considered. TEE can provide useful information for monitoring ischemia, ventricular preload, contractility, valvular function, and the effects of therapeutic interventions.
- Patients with mild to moderate AS may tolerate spinal or epidural anesthesia if it is dosed gradually.
- For general anesthesia, an opioid-based induction technique avoids excessive cardiac depression. Volatile agents should be carefully titrated to avoid excessive vasodilation.

Aortic regurgitation

Aortic regurgitation (AR) may be caused by processes that affect the aortic valve leaflets or the aortic root and valve-supporting structures. Acute AR is most often the result of infective endocarditis, trauma, or an aortic dissection. Chronic AR is usually caused by prior rheumatic valvular heart disease or congenital lesions.

Pathophysiology

Acute AR is characterized by an abrupt regurgitation of blood into a normal left ventricle, leading to a sudden increase in LV volume and a marked elevation of LV end-diastolic pressure. The effective forward stroke volume is reduced because of regurgitant blood flow into the left ventricle during diastole. Systemic arterial blood pressure and systemic vascular resistance are typically low. The decrease in cardiac afterload helps facilitate ventricular ejection. The sudden increase in LV end-diastolic pressure is transmitted to the left atrium and the pulmonary circulation, often producing dyspnea and pulmonary edema. Severe acute AR is an emergency requiring immediate surgery.

In chronic AR, the left ventricle progressively dilates and undergoes eccentric hypertrophy in response to longstanding regurgitation. The dilated left ventricle facilitates the rapid return of blood back to the ventricle during diastole, resulting in a decreased peripheral arterial diastolic pressure. The LV end-diastolic volume and stroke volume gradually increase because the left ventricle receives aortic blood in diastole in addition to blood from left atrium. LV hypertrophy compensates for the increase in LV volume, but over years, decompensation occurs. These changes may ultimately cause arrhythmias, LV impairment, and heart failure.

Most patients with chronic AR remain asymptomatic for 10 to 20 years. For patients with chronic AR, the decision regarding aortic valve replacement surgery is based on the presence of symptoms and should be undertaken before irreversible ventricular dysfunction occurs.

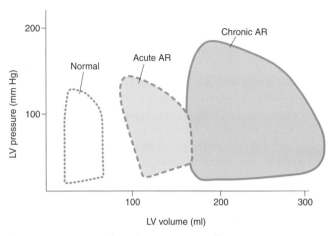

Figure 5.4. Pressure–volume loops in aortic insufficiency.

In chronic AR, aortic valve replacement surgery is indicated for patients with:

- NYHA functional class III to IV symptoms, severe AR, and normal left ventricular systolic function
- NYHA functional class III to IV symptoms with mild to moderate LV dysfunction (EF between 25% and 49%)
- Asymptomatic severe AR with LV dysfunction (EF <50%)
- Severe LV dilation (LV end-systolic volume dimension >55 mm) even in the absence of symptoms

Pressure–volume loop in aortic regurgitation

In acute AR, the end-diastolic volume increases with high end-diastolic pressure (Fig. 5.4). The end-systolic volume is also greater than normal because of regurgitation during isovolumetric relaxation. In chronic AR, the heart may be enormously dilated but the end-diastolic pressure is normal as a result of myocardial remodeling.

Anesthetic considerations in aortic regurgitation

Anesthetic considerations in patients with AR are as follows:

- Preoperative medical therapy should be optimized with digitalis, diuretics, and afterload-reducing agents, particularly angiotensin-converting enzyme (ACE) inhibitors. Decreasing the arterial blood pressure reduces the diastolic gradient for regurgitation.
- Preload should be maintained, but fluids should be titrated carefully to avoid precipitating pulmonary edema.
- Heart rate should be maintained at the upper limit of normal (80–100 bpm). Bradycardia should be avoided because it is associated with increased diastolic filling time, which increases the regurgitant volume. Excessive tachycardia also may contribute to myocardial ischemia.
- A sudden increase in systemic vascular resistance should be avoided because it increases regurgitation.
- Metabolic and drug-induced myocardial depression should be minimized.

- Excessive decreases in diastolic pressure should be avoided so that coronary artery perfusion pressure is maintained.
- Full hemodynamic monitoring may be indicated in patients with acute AR and severe chronic AR.
- Most patients with AR tolerate spinal and epidural anesthesia if intravascular volume is maintained.
- For general anesthesia, the use of isoflurane or desflurane may be beneficial because of its associated vasodilation. In patients with depressed ventricular function, an opioid-based general anesthetic technique should be considered.

Right-sided valvular lesions

Tricuspid stenosis

Tricuspid stenosis is rare and usually coexists with MS, occurring as a sequela of rheumatic heart disease. It is often found in women; it also is seen in association with carcinoid syndrome. The resulting back pressure into the right atrium often results in upper-extremity venous congestion, hepatic enlargement, and ascites. Surgical therapy is usually required (valvuloplasty or valve replacement).

Tricuspid regurgitation

Tricuspid regurgitation (TR) is typically functional rather than structural in that it develops after right ventricular enlargement (e.g., as a result of pressure or volume overload) rather than primary valvular disease. TR also may follow infective endocarditis, rheumatic fever, carcinoid syndrome, or chest trauma or may be a result of Ebstein's anomaly (downward displacement of the tricuspid valve, resulting from abnormal attachment of the valve leaflets). TR is generally well tolerated by most patients in the absence of pulmonary hypertension. Treatment is aimed at the underlying disease process. In moderate to severe TR, tricuspid annuloplasty may be considered.

Pulmonary stenosis

Pulmonary stenosis (PS) is rare and almost always secondary to a congenital deformity of the valve. Severe PS is associated with a peak systolic gradient >80 mm Hg, moderate disease with a gradient of 40 to 80 mm Hg, and mild PS with a transvalvular gradient <40 mm Hg. In moderate to severe PS, transcatheter balloon valvuloplasty should be considered.

Pulmonary regurgitation

Pulmonary regurgitation (PR) refers to diastolic retrograde flow from the pulmonary artery into the right ventricle. Physiologic (trace-to-mild) PR is present in nearly all individuals, particularly in those with advancing age. However, pathologic conditions that produce excessive and clinically significant regurgitation may result in impairment of right ventricular function and eventually clinical manifestations of right-sided volume overload and heart failure.

Incompetence of the pulmonic valve occurs because of one of three pathologic processes: dilatation of the pulmonic valve annulus, acquired alteration of pulmonic valve cusp morphology, or congenital absence or malformation. Congenital PR and congenital absence of the pulmonic valve are rare conditions. Acquired PR may develop in the setting of severe pulmonary hypertension or dilated cardiomyopathy or after surgical or percutaneous relief of PS following repair of tetralogy of Fallot. Treatment options for PR focus on treating the underlying cause. Pulmonic valve replacement is an option if symptoms and signs of right ventricular dysfunction develop, but outcomes and risks are unclear because the need for replacement is so infrequent.

Suggested readings

Chaney MA. Epidural techniques for adult cardiac surgery. In: Chaney MA, ed. *Regional Anesthesia for Cardiothoracic Surgery*. Philadelphia: Lippincott Williams & Wilkins; 2002:59–79.

Christ M, Sharkova Y, Geldner G, Maisch B. Preoperative and perioperative care for patients with suspected or established aortic stenosis facing noncardiac surgery. *Chest* 2005; 128(4):2944–2953.

Cromheecke S, Pepermans V, Hendrickx E, et al. Cardioprotective properties of sevoflurane in patients undergoing aortic valve replacement with cardiopulmonary bypass. *Anesth Analg* 2006; 103(2):289–296.

De Hert SG. Volatile anesthetics and cardiac function. *Semin Cardiothorac Vasc Anesth* 2006; 10(1):33–42.

Fisher JD. New York Heart Association Classification. *Arch Intern Med* 1972; 129(5):836.

Haering JM, Comunale ME, Parker RA, et al. Cardiac risk of noncardiac surgery in patients with asymmetric septal hypertrophy. *Anesthesiology* 1996; 85(2):254–259.

Kearon C, Hirsh J. Management of anticoagulation before and after elective surgery. *N Engl J Med* 1997; 336(21):1506–1511.

Kurup V, Haddadin AS. Valvular heart diseases. *Anesthesiol Clin* 2006; 24(3):487–508, vi.

Lai HC, Lai HC, Lee WL, et al. Mitral regurgitation complicates postoperative outcome of noncardiac surgery. *Am Heart J* 2007; 153(4):712.

Moore RA, Martin DE. Anesthetic management for the treatment of valvular heart disease. In: Hensley FA, Martin DA, Gravlee GP, eds. *A Practical Approach to Cardiac Anesthesia*. 3rd ed. Philadelphia: Lippincott Williams & Wilkins; 2003.

Poliac LC, Barron ME, Maron BJ. Hypertrophic cardiomyopathy. *Anesthesiology* 2006; 104(1):183–192.

Ramakrishna G, Sprung J, Ravi BS, et al. Impact of pulmonary hypertension on the outcomes of noncardiac surgery: predictors of perioperative morbidity and mortality. *J Am Coll Cardiol* 2005; 45(10):1691–1699.

Torsher LC, Shub C, Rettke SR, Brown DL. Risk of patients with severe aortic stenosis undergoing noncardiac surgery. *Am J Cardiol* 1998; 81(4):448–452.

Obesity

Liem C. Nguyen and Stephanie B. Jones

The perioperative management of obese (body mass index [BMI] $\geq$ 30 kg/m^2) and morbidly obese (BMI $\geq$ 35 kg/m^2) patients presenting for surgery carries a significantly higher risk of morbidity and mortality compared with that of nonobese patients. The obese state elicits a complex physiologic response in a variety of organ systems. The comorbidities associated with obesity present a unique challenge to the anesthesiologist, whose expertise in the perioperative management of this group may have a positive impact on surgical outcome. The number of obese patients presenting for surgery has increased markedly over the past decade. It is well known that perioperative risk, including mortality, is directly related to BMI, with the highest risk in patients with a BMI > 40 kg/m^2 (Table 6.1).

Obesity as a physiologic state

Obesity is best described as a physiologic state characterized by an imbalance between energy supply and demand. The thermo-dynamic and physiologic alterations seen in obesity are primar-ily a result of an excess of stored energy in the form of adi-pose cells and the effect of this tissue type on overall cellular metabolism and respiration. On the demand side, the energy requirements can be divided into two categories: energy expen-diture to maintain homeostasis and energy afforded to match physical activity. This is predicated on the fact that each kilo-gram of adipose tissue is supplied by a prerequisite number of blood vessels. The overall result is a cardiovascular system characterized by a volume-avid and high cardiac output state (Fig. 6.1).

Preoperative considerations
Cardiovascular system

The preoperative evaluation of the obese patient begins with a detailed evaluation of the cardiopulmonary system and the airway. The obese patient has an increased prevalence of

Table 6.1. Important indices for diagnosing obesity

BMI	Body weight (kg)/height^2 (m)
Waist circumference	>100 cm (males), > 90 cm (females)
Waist–hip ratio	>1.0
IBW (kg)	Height (cm) – 100

altered cardiorespiratory mechanics predisposing the patient to ventilation–perfusion mismatch and hypoxemia (Table 6.2). It is thus prudent to pay particular attention to the specific signs and symptoms of any compromised cardiopulmonary reserve. The practitioner may be alerted to the presence or absence of symptoms (resting or exertional fatigue, dysp-nea, orthopnea, angina, syncope) and signs of cardiac failure (increased jugular venous distention, adventitious heart or lung sounds, peripheral edema, hepatomegaly). Unfortunately, these symptoms and signs may be obscured by fatty tissue and/or inactivity, necessitating a lower threshold for further cardiac workup.

The electrocardiogram (ECG) may confirm or identify the presence of left or right ventricular hypertrophy, ventricu-lar strain or regional myocardial ischemia, and/or previous myocardial infarction. Chest radiography may reveal signs of pulmonary congestion. The ECG may be invaluable in demon-strating regional wall motion abnormalities, compromised systolic or diastolic function, evidence of ventricular strain or overload, or valvular abnormalities. In fact, the presence of tri-cuspid regurgitation on echocardiography may be the most use-ful confirmation of pulmonary hypertension.

Pulmonary system and airway

The examination of airway anatomy has been studied, and con-sequently a relationship between increased neck circumference and difficult intubation has been proposed. A neck circumfer-ence >60 cm was associated with a 35% chance of "problematic" intubation in one study. An increase in neck circumference or excess pharyngeal soft tissue may indicate a predisposition to upper airway narrowing or collapse and thus difficult mask ven-tilation following induction of anesthesia. Resistance to airflow and patency of the airway in these patients depend on pharyn-geal muscle tone. Airway obstruction may result during admin-istration of sedatives.

With respect to respiratory mechanics, an excess of adipose tissue in the abdomen and thorax generates a significant reduc-tion in diaphragmatic mobility, with a resultant decrease in functional residual capacity (FRC) and total lung capacity. Lung volumes are reduced further in the supine and anesthetized state. This may be ameliorated somewhat by the application of positive end-expiratory pressure (PEEP; described later), but

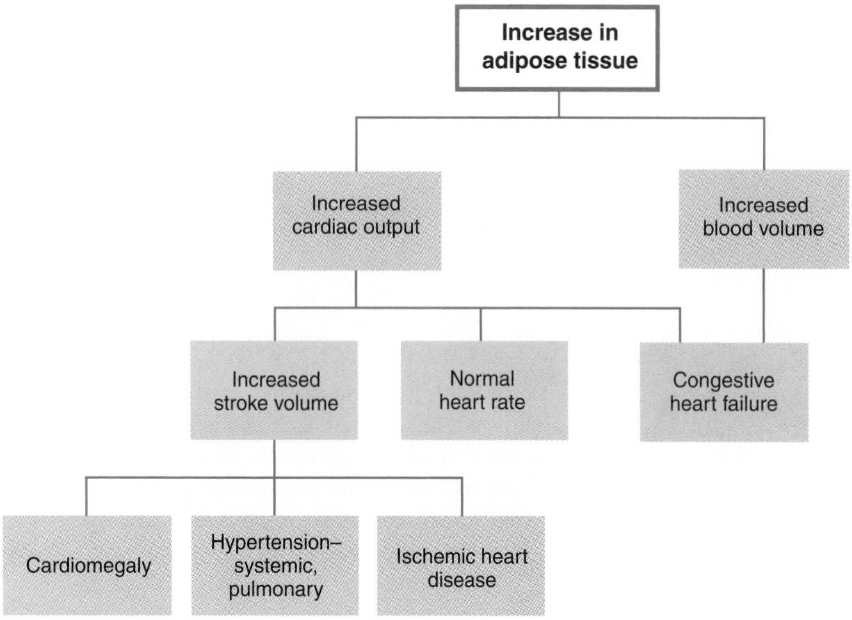

Figure 6.1. Cardiovascular changes in obesity.

possibly to the detriment of cardiac output. The plethora of tissue in the chest cavity also decreases respiratory compliance and increases resistance to airflow, all of which worsen in the anesthetized supine patient. Moreover, obesity increases oxygen consumption and carbon dioxide production because of the abundance of metabolically active adipose cells and the increased energy requirement of the obese state. Mean oxygen consumption is increased by as much as 25% in this population; however, this demand is matched by an overall increase in minute ventilation and cardiac output.

Table 6.2. Obesity and associated comorbidities

Organ system	Comorbidity	Anesthetic implications
Cardiovascular	Hypervolemic state	Increased volume of distribution, hypertension
	High cardiac output state	Cardiomegaly, CHF
	CHF (systolic and diastolic dysfunction)	Increased risk of perioperative CHF
	Ischemic heart disease	Myocardial infarction, heart failure
	DVT	Perioperative thromboembolism, pulmonary embolism, need for DVT prophylaxis
	Hypertension	Myocardial ischemia, LV failure
	Valvular heart disease	Heart failure
	Peripheral vascular disease	Reduced blood flow, limb ischemia, poor wound healing
Pulmonary	OSA	Hypercarbia, respiratory acidosis, polycythemia, difficult ventilation
	Pulmonary hypertension	Right heart failure
	Restrictive lung volumes	Shorter time to hypoxia, difficult oxygenation
	Difficult airway management	Difficult ventilation and intubation, pulmonary aspiration
Endocrine	Diabetes and insulin resistance	Cardiovascular disease, central obesity, perioperative glucose control
	Hypercholesterolemia	Systemic cardiovascular disease
Gastrointestinal	Gastroparesis	Pulmonary aspiration, delayed gastric emptying, PONV?
	GERD	Rapid sequence intubation, risk of pulmonary aspiration
	Fatty liver	Altered liver function
	Hepatobiliary disease	Cholelithiasis, biliary obstruction, hepatic insufficiency
Renal	Increased GFR, RBF	Predisposition to renal insufficiency, greater fluid requirements, altered clearance of drugs; consider discontinuation of ACE inhibitors and/or diuretics
CNS	Hypersensitivity to CNS depressants	Hypersomnolence, central apnea, reduced drug requirement
	Cerebrovascular disease	Decreased cerebral blood flow
Hematologic	Polycythemia	Increased viscosity, poor rheology, platelet aggregation
	Thrombosis	DVT and pulmonary embolus
	Poor wound healing	Wound infections

CHF, congestive heart failure; CNS, central nervous system; GERD, gastroesophageal reflux disease; LV, left ventricular.

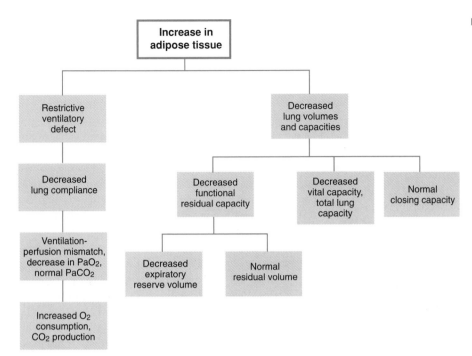

Figure 6.2. Pulmonary changes in obesity.

The incidence of obstructive sleep apnea (OSA), also termed sleep-disordered breathing, in the morbidly obese may be as high as 90% and may be undiagnosed in most cases. The strong association of severe obesity with OSA, altered lung mechanics, and increased oxygen consumption predispose this patient population to rapid development of hypoxemia during periods of apnea (Fig. 6.2). The presence of OSA may signify a higher likelihood of difficult ventilation and/or intubation.

Apnea, which usually lasts 10 seconds or longer, leads to hypoxemia and hypercapnia. The effects of long-term OSA lead to the development of the "obesity-hypoventilation" or "Pickwickian" syndrome, characterized by obesity, hypoxemia, hypercarbia, daytime hypersomnolence, polycythemia, pulmonary hypertension, and right heart failure. Ischemic heart disease and cerebrovascular disease may be associated. There is evidence to indicate that preoperative continuous positive airway pressure (CPAP) treatment may reduce or even reverse some of the cardiovascular changes observed with severe OSA. There also is emerging evidence for the utility of preoperative polysomnography in select patients to identify the presence and severity of OSA.

Renal system

There is an increase in renal blood flow (RBF), glomerular filtration rate (GFR), and tubular reabsorption in the obese state. Glucose intolerance often presents as proteinuria in obese patients. Measured GFR may be increased as much as 40%. This increased RBF and GFR may be related and proportional to the relative increase in blood volume and cardiac output seen in the obese state. As a result, the clearance of renally excreted drugs may be increased. In the perioperative period,

the obese patient may exhibit an increased susceptibility to hypovolemia and prerenal azotemia, especially in the setting of diuretic, angiotensin-converting enzyme (ACE) inhibitor, or nonsteroidal anti-inflammatory drug (NSAID) therapy and/or the presence of cardiac impairment.

Discontinuation of pharmacologic agents that may reduce GFR and RBF may be warranted to minimize the risk of worsening renal insufficiency or precipitating acute renal failure in the perioperative setting. This highlights the importance of volume loading and maintaining euvolemia in these patients throughout the perioperative period to prevent acute tubular necrosis. It also is important to mention that the intraoperative fluid requirements may be significantly greater than calculated for normal-weight patients. The presence of any systolic or diastolic cardiac dysfunction also may require specific adjustment in fluid administration.

Gastrointestinal system

Based on early studies, obesity was considered a risk factor for gastrointestinal reflux and pulmonary aspiration. This concept has been challenged recently, and the increased incidence of a difficult airway and its management may be a significant contributing factor to the risk of aspiration in this population. Nonetheless, the reverse Trendelenburg position may be used during induction and emergence to minimize cephalad displacement of the diaphragm due to intra-abdominal pressure, thereby reducing aspiration risk and improving lung volumes and respiratory mechanics. The pharmacologic use of H_2 antagonists, proton pump inhibitors, and gastric motility agents has been studied in detail. The administration of these agents may reduce the complications of aspiration but most likely does not reduce the risk.

The presence of hepatobiliary disease in the obese state is clearly increased compared with nonobese patients. In fact, fatty infiltration of the liver and cholelithiasis are common findings in this population. Abnormal cholesterol metabolism may predispose obese patients to hepatic dysfunction and postoperative cholelithiasis.

Induction of anesthesia and airway management

Increasing the preparation time for the management of a potentially difficult airway is a crucial but often overlooked safety factor, particularly during the induction of anesthesia in the obese patient. Several specific maneuvers have been shown to provide optimization during the period of nonhypoxic apnea. During the critical preoxygenation phase of induction, it is recommended that the patient be placed in a $30°$ reverse Trendelenburg or sitting position, which has been shown to be more effective than preoxygenation in the supine position.

It is important to note that the use of intubating laryngeal mask airway devices has been shown to be as rapid and effective in securing the airway as conventional direct laryngoscopy in obese patients. Early placement of a laryngeal mask airway prior to muscle paralysis may represent an even quicker and more effective modality for establishing adequate ventilation before intubating the trachea. Such devices improve success rates when attempting ventilation prior to securing the airway and should be immediately available during induction. The immediate availability of additional airway adjuncts, such as an Eschmann stylet, bougie, or a fiberoptic bronchoscope, may further improve success rates in the management of the difficult airway.

Adequate prophylaxis of pulmonary aspiration (aim of gastric volume < 25 ml and pH > 2.5), including metoclopramide and H_2 receptor blockers, may be considered. Rapid sequence induction with cricoid pressure may often be selected in the presence of a normal anticipated airway. Difficult venous access and positioning of extremities with adequate padding also should be considered. In addition, regional anesthesia may be technically difficult in obese patients.

Drug administration

The increased cardiac output and relative hypervolemic state in obesity necessitate changes in drug dosing during the induction and maintenance of anesthesia. The volume of distribution of many of the lipophilic anesthetic agents, such as propofol, thiopental, benzodiazepines, and opioids, is observed to be much greater in obese than nonobese patients because of a greater distribution into the extravascular compartment, mainly adipose tissue. Accordingly, recommended induction or loading doses of lipophilic agents are calculated based on total body weight (TBW) and not ideal body weight (IBW) to achieve an effective plasma concentration.

The pharmacokinetics of remifentanil are similar in obese and lean individuals, and this agent may be an excellent short-acting alternative to other opioids for the obese patient. The unique and predictable metabolism of remifentanil also may be exploited in the setting of renal or hepatic dysfunction because of the renal- and hepatic-independent hydrolysis of this ester compound (metabolized by esterases). In summary, the rational basis for the administration of lipophilic induction agents should be based on TBW because of a proportional increase in the volume of distribution with increased body mass.

In contrast, less lipophilic compounds, such as the nondepolarizing neuromuscular blocking agents, display negligible differences in the volume of distribution in obese versus nonobese patients; therefore, loading doses of cisatracurium and rocuronium by IBW are recommended. This is primarily a function of the relatively homogenous distribution of hydrophilic agents into the plasma compartment, with limited drug distribution into the extravascular fat depot. However, the administration of succinylcholine (hydrophilic) deserves particular attention in that the pseudocholinesterase activity is higher in obese patients, necessitating dosages (1–2 mg/kg) based on TBW and not IBW. Conversely, the loading doses of hydrophilic agents such as muscle relaxants, local anesthetics, and antibiotics should be based on IBW, given their relative confinement to the plasma compartment. With respect to repeated administration of both lipophilic and hydrophilic compounds, an assessment of the patient's IBW and overall renal status should determine dosage requirements. Pharmacokinetic parameters of commonly used anesthetic drugs are outlined in Table 6.3.

Drug elimination is determined primarily by clearance mechanisms, with renal excretion being the most dominant. Repeated administrations or infusion doses of a drug must take into account the increase in GFR in obesity, the presence of renal insufficiency, or the possibility of changing renal function during the perioperative period. Repeated administration or infusion of both lipophilic and hydrophilic compounds therefore should be dictated by the patient's overall renal function (taking into account GFR and renal dysfunction) and IBW (not TBW).

The ideal choice of inhalational anesthetic has been studied prospectively in randomized controlled trials. Desflurane and sevoflurane for maintenance anesthesia have been suggested as the inhaled agents of choice because of their rapid and consistent recovery profile, better hemodynamic control, reduced incidence of postoperative nausea and vomiting (PONV), and overall cost-effectiveness and hospital discharge time compared with isoflurane- or propofol-based techniques. A comparison of the recovery profiles of desflurane versus sevoflurane has shown no clinically significant differences in recovery or emergence times.

Intraoperative considerations

Several methods to improve intraoperative oxygenation in obese patients have been evaluated. Specifically, large tidal volume ventilation has been investigated, and studies indicate that volumes >13 ml/kg do not confer any additional benefit in oxygenation or ventilation. In fact, the risk of volutrauma,

Table 6.3. Pharmacokinetic parameters of the main anesthetic drugs given to obese and nonobese subjects

Drug	Volume of distribution (L)		Volume of distribution (L/kg TBW)		Total body clearance (ml/min)		Terminal elimination half-life		Dose recommendations
	Control	Obese	Control	Obese	Control	Obese	Control	Obese	
Thiopental			1.4	4.7**	197.2	416.3*	6.3 h	27.8 h**	LD reduced
Propofol	13.0	17.9	2.09	1.8	28.3	24.3	4.1	4.05	LD and MD based on TBW
Diazepam	90.1	291.9*	1.533	2.81*	1600	2300	40 h	95 h**	LD adjusted to TBW, MD adjusted to IBW
Lorazepam	77	131*	1.23	1.25	4000	6000**	23.9 h	33.5 h**	LD adjusted to TBW, MD adjusted to IBW
Midazolam	114	311**	1.74	2.66**	530	472	2.27 h	5.94 h**	LD adjusted to TBW, MD adjusted to IBW
Atracurium	8.5	8.6	0.141	0.067	404	444	19.8 min	19.7 min	Dose calculated on TBW
Vecuronium	59.0	44.7	0.99	0.47**	325	260	133 min	119 min	Dose calculated on IBW
Rocuronium			0.14	0.09*	0.45	0.03	70 min	75 min	Reduced infusion rate
Sufentanil	346	547*	4.8	5.8	1780	1990	135 min	208 min*	LD based on TBW, MD reduced
Remifentanil	6.8	7.5	0.1	0.07*	2700	3100			Dosage based on IBW

LD indicates loading dose; MD, maintenance dose.
* $P < 0.05$ vs control group subjects.
** $P < 0.01$ vs control group subjects.
Source: Casati A, Putzu M. Anesthesia in the obese patient: pharmacokinetic considerations. *J Clin Anesth* 2005; 17(2):134–145.

with alveolar injury and pulmonary edema, is a risk of high tidal volume ventilation. Vital capacity or recruitment maneuvers represent an important intraoperative strategy in improving oxygenation. The administration of PEEP also has been examined. Levels up to 15 cm H_2O have been shown to improve FRC and oxygenation; therefore, PEEP may be a more effective strategy than high tidal volume ventilation to improve oxygenation. The beneficial effects of PEEP in increasing intra-alveolar pressure also may reduce lung water content and pulmonary edema. However, the hemodynamic effects of PEEP have to be considered, especially in the setting of surgically induced pneumoperitoneum during laparoscopy and the reverse Trendelenburg position. The avoidance of nitrous oxide (or < 50%) during anesthesia may be beneficial in maintaining oxygenation.

During laparoscopy, the effects of intra-abdominal pressure may deleteriously affect respiratory mechanics and the ventilation–perfusion ratio in the obese state. The abundance of abdominal tissue and cephalad displacement of the diaphragm from pneumoperitoneum, surgical retraction, abdominal packing, or the Trendelenburg position may exert a negative effect on FRC and total lung capacity. Ventilation–perfusion mismatch may worsen in this situation because of compromised diaphragmatic excursion, leading to hypercarbia and hypoxemia. Carbon dioxide absorption from intra-abdominal insufflation may further worsen hypercarbia, acidosis, pulmonary vascular resistance, and right ventricular strain.

Postoperative considerations

The increased prevalence of OSA, increased central sensitivity to respiratory depressants, reduced cardiopulmonary reserve, and risk of thromboembolic complications all may contribute to greater morbidity and mortality in obese patients in the perioperative period. The administration of bilevel positive airway pressure (BiPAP) or CPAP in this patient cohort has proved to be an effective modality to prevent postoperative atelectasis and hypoxia. Early treatment and recognition of postoperative hypoxemia with noninvasive positive pressure ventilation support also may decrease the incidence of respiratory failure, intensive care unit admission, pneumonia, infection, and sepsis.

Obesity is a major risk factor for mortality from acute pulmonary embolism, usually occurring during the postoperative period. The perioperative stress response, as evident by elevated cortisol, antidiuretic hormone, and circulating catecholamines, may further heighten the risk in a group already predisposed to thromboembolism and sudden death, particularly in the setting of immobility. Preoperative administration of heparin subcutaneously and every 12 hours thereafter has been shown to markedly reduce the incidence of deep venous thrombosis (DVT). Low molecular weight heparin at a dosage of 30 mg every 12 hours also has been shown to reduce the incidence of DVT without an increase in bleeding complications.

Postoperative pain management

The physiologic perturbations in obese patients predispose this group to a markedly increased incidence of postoperative cardiopulmonary complications, which has provided the impetus for the generally accepted multimodal and opioid-sparing pain management techniques aimed at minimizing postoperative respiratory depression and improving recovery times.

Consistent with this approach is the administration of NSAIDs, the infiltration of local anesthetics at incision sites, and the use of opioid-free neuraxial epidural analgesia, all of which have been shown to be safe and effective options in reducing opioid requirements and improving pulmonary function postoperatively. More recently, the perioperative administration of pharmacologic adjuncts such as N-methyl-D-aspartate (NMDA) receptor antagonists (ketamine) or α_2-agonists (dexmedetomidine) has shown great promise in decreasing overall opioid consumption in the postoperative period when initiated intraoperatively. Collectively, the aforementioned strategies may be used to deliver more effective perioperative pain management in addition to reducing overall cardiopulmonary morbidity and mortality in this high-risk population.

Suggested readings

ASA practice guidelines for the perioperative management of patients with obstructive sleep apnea. *Anesthesiology* 2006; 104:1081–1093.

Casati A, Putzu M. Anesthesia in the obese patient: pharmacokinetic considerations. *J Clin Anesth* 2005; 17(2):134–145.

Chalhoub V, Yazigi A, Sleilaty G, et al. Effect of vital capacity manoeuvres on arterial oxygenation in morbidly obese patients undergoing open bariatric surgery. *Eur J Anaesthesiol* 2007; 24(3):283–288.

Lemmens HJ, Brodsky JB. The dose of succinylcholine in morbid obesity. *Anesth Analg* 2006; 104:1081–1093.

Ogunnaike BO, Jones SB, Jones DB, et al. Anesthetic considerations for bariatric surgery. *Anesth Analg* 2002; 95(6):1793–1805.

Passannante AN, Rock P. Anesthetic management of patients with obesity and sleep apnea. *Anesthesiol Clin North Am* 2005; 23(3):479–491.

Poirier P, Alpert MA, Fleisher LA, et al. Cardiovascular evaluation and management of severely obese patients undergoing surgery: a science advisory from the American Heart Association. *Circulation* 2009; 120:86–95.

Roizen M, Fleisher L. Anesthetic implications of concurrent diseases. In: *Miller's Anesthesia*. 6th ed. New York: Churchill Livingstone; 2004:1019–27.

Schumann R, Jones SB, Ortiz VE, et al. Best practice recommendations for anesthetic perioperative care and pain management in weight loss surgery. *Obes Res* 2005; 13(2):254–266.

Stoelting RK, Dierdorf SF. Nutritional diseases and inborn errors of metabolism. In: *Anesthesia and Coexisting Disease*. 4th ed. New York: Churchill Livingstone; 2002: 441–470.

Vallejo MC, Sah N, Phelps AL, et al. Desflurane versus sevoflurane for laparoscopic gastroplasty in morbidly obese patients. *J Clin Anesth* 2007; 19(1):3–8.

Chronic renal failure

Edward A. Bittner

It is estimated that 8 million Americans have chronic renal failure (CRF), as defined by an estimated glomerular filtration rate (GFR) <60 ml/min/1.73 m^2 for at least 3 months. Loss of renal function hampers the ability to handle fluids and acid loads, to eliminate potassium and other electrolytes, and to excrete and/or metabolize medications, including anesthetics. Patients with CRF are at high risk for progression of their renal disease in the perioperative period that may be precipitated by otherwise seemingly mild hemodynamic perturbations, nephrotoxins, and hypovolemia. End-stage renal disease (ESRD) is treated by either dialysis or transplantation. A widely used classification divides CRF into stages based on estimated GFR (Fig. 7.1). These stages help facilitate clinical practice guidelines and management approaches.

Etiology

Any disorder that permanently destroys the nephrons may result in chronic renal failure. Common causes of CRF are diabetic nephropathy, hypertensive nephrosclerosis, chronic glomerulonephritis, tubulointerstitial disease, renovascular

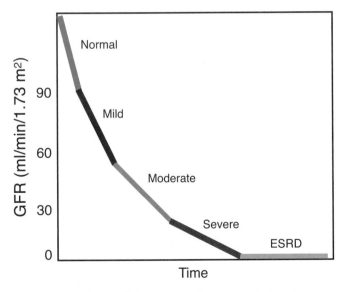

Figure 7.1. Classification of chronic kidney disease: normal >90, mild = 60–89, moderate = 30–59, severe = 15–29, ESRD/dialysis <15. Values are GFR (glomerular filtration rate) in ml/min/1.73 m^2.

disease, and polycystic kidney disease. The cause of the CRF has an impact on management. Patients with primary renal disease (e.g., IgA nephropathy) likely are younger and have good cardiopulmonary reserve. Older patients with CRF due to diabetes mellitus or hypertension also may suffer from diffuse atherosclerosis and heart disease.

Pathophysiology

Azotemia refers to retention of nitrogenous waste products as renal insufficiency develops. *Uremia* refers to more advanced stages of renal insufficiency in which complex, multiorgan system derangements manifest clinically. It results from the inability of the kidney to regulate the volume and composition of extracellular fluid and to excrete waste products. The blood urea nitrogen (BUN) may serve as a marker for uremia but does not cause all the manifestations of the syndrome, and may be elevated independently of renal failure.

Fluid and electrolyte imbalance
Fluid imbalance

Fluid balance in ESRD is difficult to manage because the number of functioning nephrons is too small to either fully concentrate or dilute the urine. A narrow margin for error exists in fluid management, alternating between hypo- and hypervolemia. As little as a positive 500 ml fluid balance may result in hypervolemia. Excessive fluid and sodium intake quickly results in hypervolemia, pulmonary edema, and hypertension.

Metabolic acidosis

Failure to excrete nonvolatile acids (sulfates, phosphates) results in a chronic anion gap metabolic acidosis. In the preoperative period, this metabolic acidosis usually is well compensated (respiratory) but is associated with a markedly diminished buffer base. Minor superimposed acidosis or bicarbonate loss can quickly lead to profound acidemia. Intraoperatively, the metabolic acidosis is unmasked with standard mechanical ventilation. Postoperatively, residual anesthetics and opioids may cause CO_2 retention which will worsen preexisting acidosis. In addition, opioid-induced narcosis may

Table 7.1. Factors contributing to hyperkalemia in CRF

Potassium intake
    Increased dietary intake
    Intravenous supplementation
    Blood transfusion
    GI hemorrhage
Potassium released from intracellular stores
    Increased catabolism from trauma, major surgery, sepsis
    Acute acidosis
    β-Blockers
    Insulin deficiency
    Succinylcholine
    Digitalis toxicity
Impaired potassium excretion
    Acute decrease in GFR
    Constipation
    K^+-sparing diuretics
    Angiotensin-converting enzyme inhibitors
    Heparin

cause CO_2 retention with worsening metabolic acidosis and hyperkalemia.

Electrolyte imbalance

Patients with CRF may present with a wide range of serum K^+ levels. CRF patients can generally maintain potassium excretion at near-normal levels as long as aldosterone secretion and distal tubule flow are maintained. Acute hyperkalemia suppresses cardiac electrical conduction and may result in asystole. Electrocardiographic (ECG) manifestations of hyperkalemia (prolonged PR interval, widened QRS, peaked T waves) are helpful but often not present. Conditions and drugs that can induce acute hyperkalemia in patients with CRF are summarized in Table 7.1. Hypokalemia, although uncommon in patients with CRF, may occur as a result of the effects of malnutrition and aggressive dialysis. Acute hypokalemia lowers the arrhythmia threshold, and these arrhythmias may be refractory to therapy unless hypokalemia is corrected. Caution regarding potassium repletion is essential in patients with CRF, as acute hyperkalemia easily may result.

Hypermagnesemia may result from inadequate dialysis or ingestion of magnesium-containing antacids or cathartics. It is manifested by skeletal weakness and potentiation of nondepolarizing muscle relaxants. Calcium administration may antagonize the effects of hypermagnesemia.

CRF results in impaired phosphate excretion and decreased vitamin D_3 synthesis, resulting in hyperphosphatemia and hypocalcemia. In response, parathyroid hormone is released, resulting in bone resorption and extracellular calcium release (secondary hyperparathyroidism). Elevation of the calcium phosphate product may result in metastatic calcification (calciphylaxis), especially in blood vessels and skin. *Renal osteodystrophy* refers to the changes in mineral metabolism and bone structure that occur in CRF. It manifests as skeletal and joint deformity, osteomalacia, and spontaneous fractures. Treatment of hyperphosphatemia, hypocalcemia, and renal osteodystrophy consists of administration of vitamin D and calcium, phosphate binders, and dietary phosphate restriction. Parathyroidectomy with autograft of parathyroid tissue may be used to treat severe secondary hyperparathyroidism.

Cardiovascular disease

Cardiovascular disease is the leading cause of death in patients with CRF. The increased prevalence of coronary artery disease in patients with CRF derives from both traditional and CRF-related risk factors. CRF-related risk factors include chronic volume overload, anemia, hyperparathyroidism, and chronic inflammation. The combination of hypertension and disordered glucose and fat metabolism in patients results in an accelerated form of atherosclerosis. Conduction blocks also may be encountered in patients with CRF as the result of deposition of calcium in the conduction system.

Abnormal cardiac function, secondary to ischemic myocardial disease and/or left ventricular hypertrophy combined with fluid overload and the increased demands imposed by anemia and hypertension, makes these patients particularly prone to congestive heart failure. In addition, a unique form of pulmonary edema may occur in the absence of fluid overload in patients with ESRD. This "low-pressure" pulmonary edema is the result of increased permeability of alveolar capillary membranes, which usually responds well to dialysis.

Pericarditis is a potentially fatal complication that may develop with uremia. It occurs more often in underdialyzed patients than in patients who undergo regular dialysis. The diagnosis should be considered in any patient with advanced CRF who develops unexplained hypotension. Chest pain or ST elevations characteristic of other causes of pericarditis may not be present, and a friction rub may not be audible if a large effusion is present.

Pulmonary function

Patients with CRF have an increased risk of postoperative pulmonary complications. Low oncotic pressure from hypoalbuminemia in the presence of fluid overload may result in pulmonary edema. Decreased muscle mass and decreased surfactant reduce lung volumes and increase the risk of atelectasis. Impaired immune function results in increased susceptibility to pneumonia. Patients with CRF may depend on increased minute ventilation to compensate for metabolic acidosis, resulting in an increased potential for respiratory failure.

Neurologic alterations

Central nervous system dysfunction from uremic encephalopathy may range from subtle personality changes to drowsiness, asterixis, myoclonus, and seizures. Neurologic signs and symptoms depend on the rapidity of progression of uremia rather than on the absolute level of BUN or serum creatinine. Peripheral neuropathy ("stocking-and-glove" distribution) is common and is an indication for hemodialysis. Autonomic neuropathy likely coexists with peripheral neuropathy and manifests as orthostatic hypotension, impaired circulatory response to anesthesia, potential for silent ischemia, and impaired gastric emptying.

Hematologic alterations

Anemia

CRF frequently is associated with a normochromic, normocytic anemia (hematocrit 25%–28%) due to multiple factors, including decreased erythropoietin production, decreased red cell survival due to dialysis, blood loss via the gastrointestinal (GI) tract, frequent blood sampling, and iron or vitamin deficiencies. Compensatory mechanisms for the chronic anemia include increased cardiac output and a rightward shift of the oxyhemoglobin curve. Treatment of CRF patients with recombinant erythropoietin decreases transfusion requirements, reduces mortality, and improves their quality of life. The anemia of CRF usually is well tolerated for routine/elective surgeries, and the target hemoglobin can be reached through erythropoietin administration and iron supplementation. Transfusion is appropriate for patients with CRF when extensive surgery is planned and there is a potential for excessive blood loss.

Uremic coagulopathy

The pathogenesis of uremic bleeding is multifactorial, but it is caused predominately by alterations in platelet function, including diminished platelet degranulation and reductions in platelet adenosine diphosphate (ADP) and serotonin stores. CRF also results in impaired activation of glycoprotein IIb/IIIa receptors on the platelet membrane, resulting in reduced binding to von Willebrand factor and fibrinogen. Red blood cells improve platelet function through ADP release, inactivation of prostacyclin, and enhancement of platelet–vessel wall interactions. Consequently, anemia is an additional contributor to platelet dysfunction.

The resulting coagulopathy in patients with CRF increases the risk of surgical bleeding and predisposes to GI bleeding, intracerebral hemorrhage, and hemorrhagic pericardial effusion. Diagnosis of uremic coagulopathy may be difficult because the standard coagulation tests – prothrombin time, partial thromboplastin time, and platelet count – usually are normal in patients with CRF. Interventions to reduce bleeding in patients with CRF include a hematocrit goal of 30% for major operations; administration of recombinant erythropoietin, desmopressin acetate (DDAVP), cryoprecipitate, or conjugated estrogens; and intensification of the dialysis regimen using heparin-free or low-dose heparin hemodialysis.

Malnutrition

Malnutrition is prevalent among patients with CRF as a result of multiple factors, including decreased nutritional intake, increased protein catabolism, and dialytic losses. A strong association exists between malnutrition and increased morbidity and mortality in this population. In addition, nutritional status has a well-established impact on wound healing, infection prevention, and recovery following serious illness. A low BUN level does not necessarily indicate that a patient is well dialyzed but may reflect poor protein intake.

Gastrointestinal dysfunction

Urea acts as a mucosal irritant, and uremic enteropathy may result in inflammation of the entire GI tract. Peptic ulcer disease is prevalent in patients with CRF, and occult GI bleeding may occur. Nausea and vomiting are common in patients with severe uremia and predisposes to an increased risk of regurgitation and aspiration with anesthesia.

Infections

Infections are second to cardiovascular disease as the leading cause of death in patients with CRF. The frequency and severity of infections in this population are the result of leukocyte and immune dysfunction caused by uremia, diabetes mellitus, malnutrition, and the inflammatory response to dialysis. In addition, there is an increased exposure to bacterial pathogens through dialysis grafts and catheters, resulting in increased frequency of sepsis, impaired wound healing, dehiscence, fistulas, and pressure ulcers. The diagnosis of infection may be difficult because many patients with ESRD have baseline hypothermia and bacteremia (which may not be associated with fever). The incidence of hepatitis B and C in patients on chronic dialysis is high because of frequent exposure to blood products. All patients on dialysis should be treated as potentially infected, and medical personnel should take precautions against exposure.

Pharmacologic alterations

The pharmacokinetics of many anesthetic and perioperative drugs are altered in CRF. These alterations may be the result of changes in compartment volumes, electrolytes, pH (acidemia resulting in a higher percentage of nonionized drug), decreased serum protein concentration (resulting in increased bioavailability of protein-bound drugs), impaired biotransformation, and rates of excretion. Lipid-soluble drugs are poorly ionized and undergo metabolism by hepatic transformation to water-soluble forms before elimination by the kidney. Ionized drugs tend to be eliminated unchanged by the kidney, and their duration of action may be prolonged with CRF. Respiratory depression is more common with opioids and sedative agents. An altered pharmacodynamic effect also should be anticipated in patients with CRF.

The duration of action of many drugs administered by bolus or short-term infusion is determined by redistribution not elimination. Consequently, the loading dose does not need to be altered significantly in CRF (unless there is altered pharmacodynamic effect). However, with repeated dosing or long-term infusion, the duration of action depends on elimination; therefore, maintenance doses of drugs with significant renal

Table 7.2. Pharmacologic considerations for commonly used perioperative drugs in patients with CRF

Drug Class	Pharmacokinetics	Considerations
Inhalational Anesthetics **Lipid Soluble**	Eliminated primarily by the lungs	Sevoflurane has potentially nephrotoxic metabolite (compound A)
Benzodiazepines	Increased free fraction in CRF	Potentiated clinical effect in CRF Certain metabolites are pharmacologically active and accumulate with repeated dosing
Barbiturates	Free fraction of induction dose is almost doubled in patients with CRF	Exaggerated clinical effect in CRF. Need to reduce induction dose
Propofol	Rapid, extensive hepatic metabolism. Pharmacokinetics unchanged in CRF	Effects are not prolonged in CRF
Etomidate	Increased free fraction in CRF	CRF does not alter clinical effects
Ketamine	Redistribution and hepatic metabolism largely responsible for termination of anesthetic effects. Minimal change in free fraction in CRF.	CFR does not alter clinical effects
Opioids	Primarily metabolized in liver	May have increased and prolonged effect in CRF Active metabolites may prolong action with chronic administration: Morphine– 6-glucuronide (morphine) has potent analgesic and sedative effects. Normeperidine (meperidine) has neurotoxic effects. Hydromorphone –3-glucuronide (hydromorphone) can cause cognitive dysfunction and myoclonus. Fentanyl has no active metabolites
Ionized Drugs Muscle Relaxants	Standard dose of succinylcholine raises serum K+ 0.5–0.8 mEq/L which is unchanged in CRF Many nonpolarizing NMBs result in prolonged effects due to reliance on renal excretion	Succinylcholine is not contraindicated in CRF if the serum K+ is not elevated. Cisatracurium, mivacurium, rocuronium are preferable in CRF.
Cholinesterase inhibitors	Decreased elimination in CRF and half life is prolonged	Half life prolongation is similar or greater than the duration of blockade from long acting NMBs so recurarization is rarely seen
Digoxin	Excreted in urine	Increased risk of toxicity in CRF
Vasoactive Drugs Catecholamines		Catecholamines with a-adrenergic effects constrict renal vasculature and may reduce renal blood flow
Sodium nitroprusside	Metabolized by the kidney and excreted as thiocyanate	Toxicity from thiocyanate accumulation is more likely in CRF
Antibiotics	Penicillins, cephalosporins, aminoglycosides, vancomycin are predominantly dependent on renal elimination	Loading dose is unchanged but maintenance doses are substantially reduced

NMB, neuromuscular blocker.

Table 7.3. Preoperative considerations for patients with CRF

History	Goal is to detect comorbid conditions that might adversely impact morbidity and mortality Etiology of renal disease should be elucidated and renal function should be estimated Based of ACC/AHA guidelines, patients with a Cr > 2 mg/dl have at least an intermediate pretest probability of perioperative cardiovascular risk. This warrants detailed CV surveillance before intermediate or high-risk surgery Elective surgery postponed pending resolution of acute processes
Physical Exam	Thorough physical focused on identifying stigmata of CRF, e.g. HTN, elevated JVP, crackles (volume overload), malnutrition, ecchymoses (platelet dysfunction), pallor (anemia)
Labs	ECG and screening lab tests including CBC, electrolytes and coagulation panel
Preoperative Optimization Preoperative Hemodialysis	Elective surgery should be conducted in the setting of optimized acid/base balance, euvolemia and k+ management with preoperative dialysis within 24 hours of the procedure. HD should be avoided on the day of surgery due to potential problems with rebound anticoagulation, fluid shifts, hypokalemia, hypoxemia and disequilibrium
Transfusion	Transfusion is appropriate for patients with Hb 8–10 g/dL when extensive surgery is planned and there is a potential for excessive blood loss. Blood transfusion may not be indicated for patients with stable chronic anemia and Hb >= 8 g/dL undergoing minor procedures.
Correction of coagulopathy	Maintain higher Hb (with erythropoietin or transfusion), intensify dialysis regimen, administer DDAVP, cryoprecipitate and conjugated estrogens
Control of hypertension	Blood pressure control may be challenging in patients with CRF. Proceeding with elective surgery with moderate chronic hypertension is acceptable but severe or labile BP should be controlled preoperatively
Treatment of hyperkalemia	Increased risk for patients who present for emergency surgery. Treat with $CaCl_2$, $NaCO_3$, insulin/dextrose, kayexalate, dialysis
Prevention of contrast induced nephropathy	For patients not on HD it may be prudent to postpone major elective surgery for a few days after contrast media exposure. Treatment with NAC and sodium HCO_3 infusion before contrast administration may prevent contrast induced nephropathy

ACC, American College of Cardiology; AHA, American Heart Association; CBC, complete blood count; CV, cardiovascular; Hb, hemoglobin; JVP, jugular venous pressure.

Table 7.4. Intraoperative considerations for patients with CRF

Premedication	Minimize premedication because of susceptibility to excess sedation and respiratory depression Histamine H_2 blockers, metoclopramide, citric acid/sodium citrate to reduce gastric acidity and promote emptying
Monitors	ECG, BP cuff, pulse oximeter, capnograph, and thermometer. Invasive monitoring as indicated by comorbid conditions and surgical procedure. No BP cuff on arm with AV fistula or shunt Strict asepsis for all invasive procedures Urinary catheters should not be placed in anuric patients because they may provide a portal for infection
Positioning	Extra care in positioning because these patients are prone to fractures from renal osteodystrophy Patients with sensory neuropathy may not be able to report positional discomfort
Induction	Dose of induction drugs may need to be reduced and rate of administration slowed to avoid hypotension Anticipate hypotension; manage with appropriate preloading of fluid or vasopressors Gastric emptying is delayed in uremic patients; manage as increased risk of aspiration Serum K^+ should be checked before administration of succinylcholine
Maintenance	Ideal technique controls BP with minimal effect on cardiac output Sedative and anesthetic doses should be reduced Avoid renally excreted NMBs
Fluids	Intraoperative fluid and blood administration should not be so restrictive as to permit inadequate organ perfusion, even if postoperative dialysis is required Intraoperative dialysis occasionally is required
Ventilation	Consider controlled ventilation because spontaneous ventilation may result in hypercarbia and exacerbate preexisting acidemia and increase K^+ concentration
Emergence	Anticipate delayed emergence, aspiration, hypertension, respiratory depression, and pulmonary edema Ensure adequate reversal of neuromuscular reflexes
Regional anesthesia	Regional anesthesia may be used in patients with CRF (e.g., brachial plexus block for AV shunt insertion/revision) Preexisting neuropathies should be determined and documented Coagulopathy, which may be present despite normal clotting studies, should be evaluated prior to regional anesthesia Spinal/epidural anesthesia has been used for renal transplantation. It should be used with caution because patients with autonomic neuropathy have increased risk of hypotension with sympathetic block.

AV, atrioventricular; BP, blood pressure; NMB, neuromuscular blocker.

excretion should be reduced. Pharmacologic considerations for commonly used perioperative drugs in patients with CRF are summarized in Table 7.2.

Perioperative management

Preoperative, intraoperative, and postoperative considerations for patients with CRF are outlined in Tables 7.3, 7.4, and 7.5.

Dialysis and transplantation

Hemodialysis uses an artificial semipermeable membrane that separates the patient's blood from the dialysate and allows exchange of solutes by diffusion. Vascular access and anticoagulation often are required. Blood samples taken immediately after hemodialysis may be inaccurate, because the redistribution of fluid and electrolytes takes about 6 hours. Complications of hemodialysis include arteriovenous fistula infection and thrombosis, hypotension, pericarditis, and hypoxemia. Dialysis "disequilibrium syndrome" may occur if fluid and electrolyte shifts are too rapid. Symptoms are weakness, nausea/vomiting, and, more rarely, convulsions and coma.

Peritoneal dialysis uses the patient's peritoneum as the exchange membrane, with the dialysate infused into the peritoneal cavity via an indwelling catheter. Advantages, compared with hemodialysis, include less hypotension or disequilibrium and no need for anticoagulation. However, peritoneal dialysis is less efficient than hemodialysis. Continuous renal

replacement therapies involve either dialysis (diffusion-based solute removal) or filtration (convection-based solute and water removal) operating in a continuous mode. The major advantage is a slower rate of solute/fluid removal that improves hemodynamic stability compared with hemodialysis. Renal transplantation is the treatment of choice for ESRD. A successful renal transplantation improves the quality of life and survival of patients.

Table 7.5. Postoperative considerations for patients with CRF

Monitoring	Monitor for frequent causes of postoperative morbidity (cardiovascular complications, pulmonary edema, hyperkalemia, etc.)
Fluid management	Should consist of isotonic fluids and dextrose until patient can take by mouth Hypertension is a common postoperative problem exacerbated by fluid overload. For those not on dialysis, diuretics and short-acting antihypertensives are effective. Postoperative dialysis may be needed
Laboratory studies	Check hematocrit, electrolytes, BUN, creatinine, ECG (signs of hyperkalemia, ischemia), and chest radiographs (pulmonary edema) Serum creatinine kinase levels are mildly elevated in the absence of myocardial injury in a substantial number of patients with ESRD, but the myocardial (MB) fraction is usually normal. Troponin I is a specific marker of myocardial injury in ESRD, whereas troponin T should not be used.

Suggested readings

ACC/AHA guideline update for perioperative cardiovascular evaluation for noncardiac surgery – executive summary. *J Am Coll Cardiol* 2002; 39:543–553.

Anthony AJ, Cohn SL. Perioperative care of the patient with renal failure. *Med Clin North Am* 2003; 87:193–210.

Dember LM. Critical care issues in the patient with chronic renal failure. *Crit Care Clin* 2002; 18:421–440.

Fort J. Chronic renal failure: a cardiovascular risk factor. *Kidney Int* 2005; 68:S25–S29.

Garwood, S. Renal disease. In: Hines RI, Stoelting, RK, eds. Anesthesia and Coexisting Disease. New York: Churchill Livingstone, 2008: 323–348.

Hines RL, Stoelting RK. Renal diseases. In: *Anesthesia and Coexisting Disease*. Chapter Author: Susan Garwod. New York: Churchill Livingstone; 2002:323–348.

NKF-K/DOQI. Clinical practice guidelines for chronic kidney disease: evaluation, classification, and stratification. *Am J Kidney Dis* 2003; 37(Suppl 1):S1–S266.

O'Hara JF, Cywinski JB, Monk TG. The renal system and anesthesia for urologic surgery. In: Barash PB, Cullen BF, Stoelting RK, eds. *Clinical Anesthesia*. 5th ed. Philadelphia: Lippincott Williams & Wilkins; 2006:1013–1039.

Petroni KC, Cohen NC. Continuous renal replacement therapy: anesthetic implications. *Anesth Analg* 2002; 94:1288–1297.

Sladen RN. Anesthetic considerations for the patient with renal failure. *Anesthesiol Clin North Am* 2000; 18:863–882.

US Renal Data System. USRDS 2006 Annual Data Report: Atlas of End-Stage Renal Disease in the United States, National Institutes of Health, Nation Institute of Diabetes and Digestive and Kidney Diseases, Bethesda, MD, 2006. *Am J Kidney Dis* 2006; 47(Suppl 1): S1.

Yee J, Parasuraman R, Narins RG. Selective review of key perioperative renal-electrolyte disturbances in chronic renal failure patients. *Chest* 1999; 115:149–157.

Liver disease

Jason C. Brookman and Warren S. Sandberg

Anatomy and physiology

The liver is the largest solid organ in the body, weighing about 1500 g. It has two lobes, the larger right and the smaller left. The right lobe has two additional lobes, the caudate and the quadrate lobes. Blood supply to the liver is about 1500 ml/min (25% of cardiac output), about 75% from the portal vein and the rest from the hepatic artery. However, each blood vessel supplies about 50% of the liver's oxygen requirements. Normal portal vein pressure is about 10 mm Hg, and normal hepatic artery pressure is arterial. The liver is supplied by sympathetic nerve fibers (T6–11), which when stimulated result in vasoconstriction of the hepatic artery, thereby decreasing the hepatic blood flow.

Hepatic blood flow is decreased by any cause that lowers systemic blood pressure and cardiac output. These causes include general and regional anesthesia (spinal/epidural), volatile inhalation agents, positive pressure ventilation (and positive end-expiratory pressure [PEEP]), hypoxemia, β-blockers, and α_1-agonists. The liver performs several important functions in the body, including metabolic functions (carbohydrate, fat, protein, and drug metabolism), bile secretion, bilirubin excretion, albumin production, ammonia excretion, and synthesis of all the clotting factors, except factor VIII.

Liver cirrhosis

Care of the patient with liver disease undergoing anesthesia and surgery requires awareness that liver disease is, in reality, a multiorgan disorder that causes a variety of pathophysiologic derangements. Causes of chronic liver disease are multifactorial (Table 8.1) but, regardless of the cause, often may progress to cirrhosis. Cirrhosis is characterized by hepatic cell death, fibrosis, and the formation of regenerative nodules.

Cirrhosis is essentially irreversible and leads to important physiologic disturbances. Portal hypertension is common in patients with significant chronic liver disease and results from increased portal blood flow and/or intrahepatic resistance. It is associated with ascites, portosystemic shunts, hepatic encephalopathy, and splenomegaly. Portosystemic shunts most commonly include esophageal varices or hemorrhoids.

Table 8.1. Major causes of chronic liver disease

Intraparenchymal disease
  Viral infections
    Chronic active hepatitis B
    Chronic active hepatitis C
    Hepatitis D
  Toxins
    Ethanol
  Miscellaneous
    Cystic fibrosis
    Hemochromatosis
    Wilson's disease
    α_1-antitrypsin deficiency
    Metabolic errors of carbohydrate, lipid, and proteins
Cholestatic disease
  Primary biliary cirrhosis
  Primary sclerosing cholangitis

Risk stratification of the cirrhotic patient

A basic assessment of the extent of liver failure is necessary to more fully understand its impact on anesthetic and perioperative management, and on patient outcomes from surgery. Two liver failure classification systems exist for assessing prognosis. The Child-Turcotte-Pugh (CTP) classification is based on five variables and stratifies patients by score to determine their disease prognosis (Table 8.2). The greater the CTP score, the worse the prognosis. The Model for End-Stage Liver Disease (MELD) and its pediatric equivalent (PELD) are used for allocating donor livers for transplantation. The MELD is a statistical model based on serum bilirubin, serum creatinine, and the international normalized ratio (INR) to determine the severity of liver disease and the need for transplantation.

Effects of liver disease
Gastrointestinal

Portal hypertension occurs when pressure in the portal vein is greater than 10 mm Hg. The high portal pressure leads to the development of portovenous collaterals (Fig. 8.1a, b), which commonly are found at the following four sites: gastroesophageal, periumbilical, retroperitoneal, and hemorrhoidal.

Table 8.2. *Child-Turcotte-Pugh classification of liver failure*

	Points (per variable)		
	1	**2**	**3**
Serum bilirubin (mg/dl)	<2	2–3	>3
Serum albumin (g/dl)	>3.5	2.8–3.5	<2.8
Prolongation of PT (sec/control)[a]	<4	4–6	6
Ascites	None	Mild	Moderate
Encephalopathy	None	Minimal	Advanced
Interpretation			
Class	Points	Mortality risk, 3 mo–1 y (%)	
A	5–6	4–10	
B	7–9	14–31	
C	10–15	51–76	

[a] Nutrition (excellent, good, poor) was replaced with prothrombin time by Pugh's modification of the Child-Turcotte classification.
Modified from Rowe P, Mandell MS. Perioperative hepatic dysfunction. In: *Anesthesia Secrets*. Philadelphia: Hanley and Belfus; 2002:289–290, and Garg RK. Anesthetic considerations in patients with hepatic failure. *Int Anesthesia Clin* 2005; 45–63.

Ascites is a hallmark of decompensated liver cirrhosis and is caused by alterations in portal blood flow dynamics, activation of the renin–angiotensin–aldosterone system, and reduction in plasma oncotic pressure. The primary treatment for ascites is sodium and water restriction, administration of diuretics, and abdominal paracentesis, which may lead to intravascular fluid depletion.

Esophageal variceal bleeding is a potentially lethal complication of cirrhosis. Treatment includes β-blockers, vasopressin, somatostatin, variceal banding, sclerotherapy, and transjugular portosystemic shunting. However, portosystemic shunting may cause or worsen existing hepatic encephalopathy. Significant portosystemic shunting also decreases steroid hormone clearance because of impaired extraction via enterohepatic circulation of the unbound steroid molecules. These steroids, specifically androgens, undergo peripheral aromatization to estrogen. Elevated circulating estrogen is responsible for the gonadal and pituitary suppression and feminization commonly seen in advanced liver disease.

Patients with liver disease usually have severe metabolic derangements, including hypoglycemia, hypokalemia, hyponatremia, hypomagnesemia, and hypoalbuminemia.

Hemodynamic

Patients with chronic liver dysfunction and cirrhosis commonly have a hyperdynamic circulation (Table 8.3) with a low peripheral vascular resistance and an increased cardiac index. Hyperdynamic circulation and elevated cardiac output are attributed to increased sympathetic nervous system activity, increased blood volume and preload, and reduced systemic vascular resistance. Often cirrhotic patients develop signs of high-output heart failure (also known as "cirrhotic cardiomyopathy") including impaired cardiac contractility, conduction abnormalities, impaired excitation–contraction coupling, and

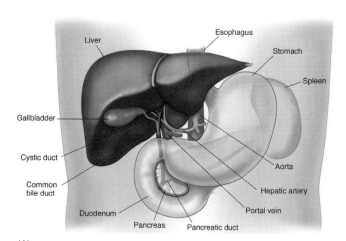

(A)

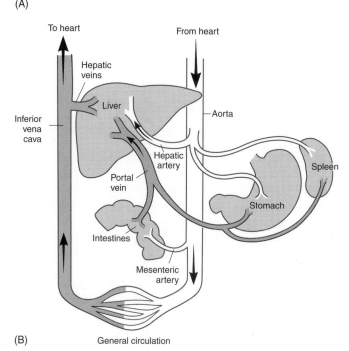

(B)   General circulation

Figure 8.1. (**A**) The liver in relation to the gallbladder and stomach. (**B**) The liver in relation to its circulation.

Table 8.3. Hemodynamic derangements in liver cirrhosis

Decreased systemic vascular resistance
  Peripheral vasodilation
  Arteriovenous shunting
Redirection of blood flow
  Increased pulmonary, splanchnic, muscle, and skin blood flow
  Decreased portal vein flow to liver
  Normal or increased hepatic arterial flow
  Normal to decreased renal blood flow
Increased blood volume
  Decreased serum albumin
  Decreased plasma oncotic pressure
Increased cardiac output
  Apparent cardiomyopathy despite increased output
Decreased arteriovenous O_2 content difference
  Increased venous O_2 content
Decreased responsiveness to catecholamines

decreased β-adrenergic receptor function. Additionally, some patients with a hyperdynamic circulation develop significant left ventricular failure after liver transplantation, possibly as a result of increased peripheral vascular resistance after relief of vasodilation by transplantation. Typical treatment includes inotropes, mechanical ventilation, and supportive care in an intensive care unit.

Hematologic

Hematologic effects include anemia (bone marrow suppression, red cell destruction, blood loss, iron deficiency), thrombocytopenia (splenic sequestration), and coagulopathy. All clotting factors except factor VIII are produced in the liver. Progressive decreasing liver function leads to deficiency of these factors, making patients prone to bleeding. Fresh frozen plasma is used to replace the clotting factors before surgery. A prothrombin time with an INR of <1.4 should be achieved for surgery in these patients. A platelet count of at least 100,000/mm³ is desirable.

Renal

Renal dysfunction is common in patients with liver disease and has at least three major causes: prerenal azotemia, acute tubular necrosis, and hepatorenal syndrome. Prerenal azotemia may result from overuse of diuretics leading to elevated blood urea nitrogen and creatinine, indicative of worsening renal function, and usually responds to reducing the diuretic dose and gentle hydration. Acute tubular necrosis often occurs in the setting of another acute, precipitating factor, such as hypotension, infection, or severe sepsis. Although renal failure commonly develops in the setting of infection in patients with liver disease, renal function tends to recover with the removal of the inciting insult. Hepatorenal syndrome (Table 8.4) is marked by a worsening of renal function as liver disease progresses and does not recover without an improvement in liver function.

Table 8.4. Diagnostic criteria for hepatorenal syndrome[a]

Major criteria
  Low glomerular filtration rate, as indicated by serum creatinine
    >1.5 mg/dl
  Exclusion of shock, ongoing bacterial infection, volume depletion, and
    use of nephrotoxic drugs
  No improvement in renal function after stopping diuretics and volume
    repletion with 1.5 L of normal saline
  No proteinuria or evidence of obstructive uropathy or parenchymal renal
    disease
Minor criteria
  Urine volume <500 ml/d
  Urine sodium <10 mEq/L
  Urine osmolality > plasma osmolality
  Urine RBC <50/high-power field
  Serum sodium <130 mEq/L

[a] Only major criteria are needed to establish the diagnosis; minor criteria provide supporting evidence.
RBC, red blood cells.

Pulmonary

Portopulmonary hypertension

Portopulmonary hypertension affects eligibility for liver transplantation and may complicate hepatic resection if it leads to central venous pressure elevation. Portopulmonary hypertension occurs in 2% to 4% of patients with end-stage liver disease and 5% to 10% of patients evaluated for orthotopic liver transplantation. Clinical predictors of pulmonary hypertension in liver transplantation include systemic hypertension, right ventricular dilatation by echocardiography, estimated pulmonary artery systolic pressure ≥40 mm Hg by transthoracic echocardiography, right ventricular hypertrophy by echocardiography, and/or a right ventricular heave.

Portopulmonary hypertension is characterized by a mean pulmonary artery pressure >25 mm Hg with a normal pulmonary capillary wedge pressure (i.e., <15 mm Hg) and an elevated pulmonary vascular resistance (i.e., >120 dyne·sec/cm⁵) in the setting of portal hypertension. Factors implicated in the etiology of portopulmonary hypertension include (1) increased pulmonary arterial blood flow secondary to an increase in cardiac index, (2) increased circulating blood volume, and (3) vasoconstriction and progressive pulmonary vascular remodeling due to endothelial and smooth muscle cell proliferation. The most common symptom of portopulmonary hypertension is dyspnea on exertion – fatigue, palpitations, chest pain, and syncope are reported less frequently. Diagnosis of portopulmonary hypertension is by noninvasive transthoracic Doppler echocardiography. Figure 8.2 outlines the diagnostic approach to pulmonary hypertension.

Effective management of portopulmonary hypertension is important because it may facilitate hepatic resection. Pulmonary vasodilator treatment also may allow a marginal patient to receive a liver transplant with reduced mortality. Vasodilators, such as epoprostenol, sildenafil, and nitric oxide, can reduce pulmonary vascular resistance.

Hepatopulmonary syndrome

Hepatopulmonary syndrome is defined by the presence of hepatic dysfunction or portal hypertension, an elevated alveolar–arterial oxygen gradient, and intrapulmonary vasodilation. Patients may present with digital clubbing, spider angiomata, arterial hypoxemia, and dyspnea that worsens upon moving from a recumbent to an upright position (orthodeoxia and platypnea). Hepatopulmonary syndrome may contribute to hypoxemia, even when other cardiopulmonary abnormalities are present (Table 8.3).

The diagnosis of hepatopulmonary syndrome in patients with liver disease is confirmed by arterial desaturation, measured by pulse oximetry and arterial blood gas analysis, and pulmonary vasodilation, assessed by contrast echocardiography, lung perfusion scanning, or pulmonary artery catheterization. Other causes of hypoxia also must be excluded. A flow chart outlining the assessment for hepatopulmonary syndrome is shown in Figure 8.3.

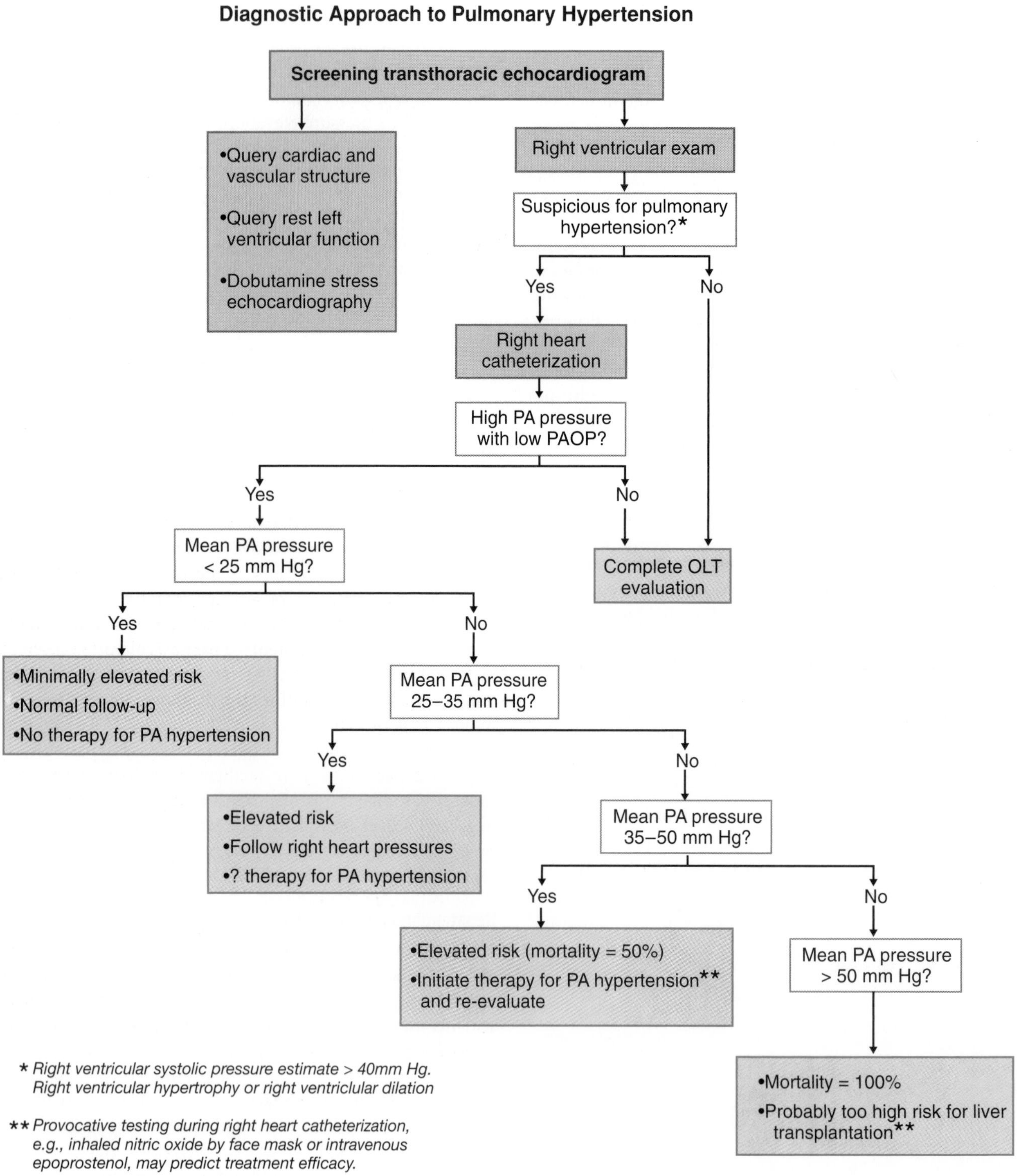

Diagnostic Approach to Pulmonary Hypertension

Figure 8.2. Suggested diagnostic paradigm to exclude or monitor pulmonary hypertension. Although there are many variations, it is important to complete the process with a detailed knowledge of the patient's pulmonary hemodynamics. Normal follow-up: repeat transthoracic echocardiogram or right heart catheterization 1 year after previous test. Elevated risk implies high risk of perioperative mortality. OLT, orthotopic liver transplantation; PA, pulmonary artery.

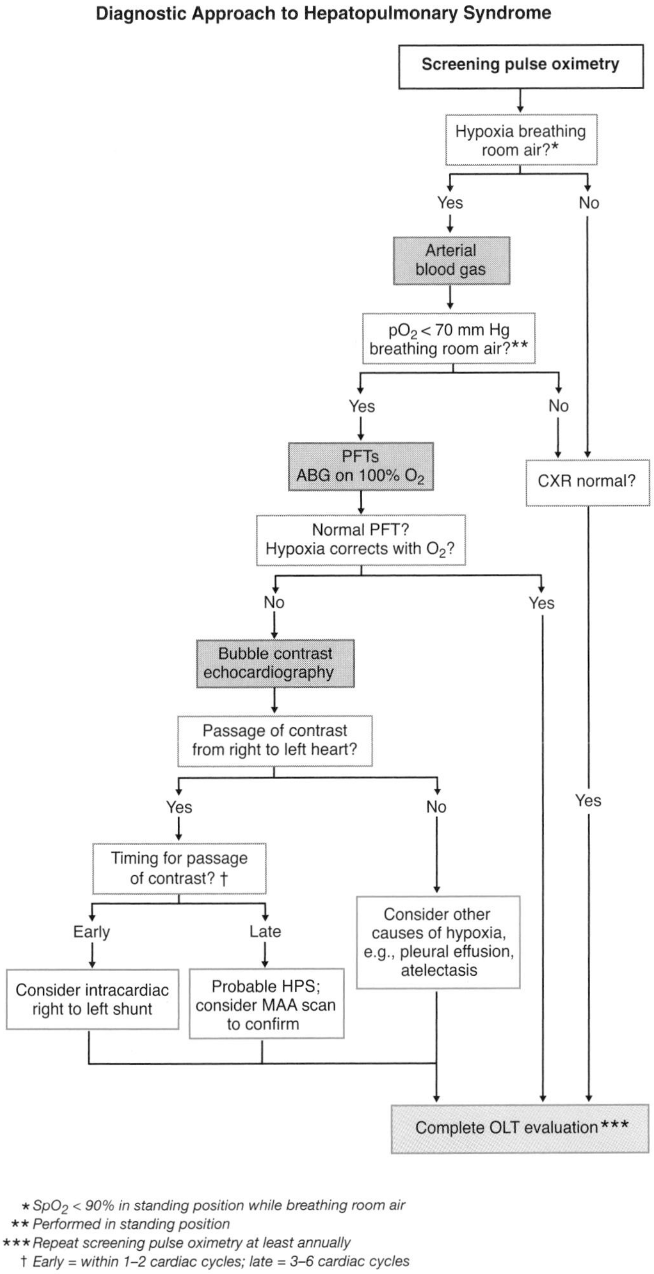

Diagnostic Approach to Hepatopulmonary Syndrome

* $SpO_2 < 90\%$ in standing position while breathing room air
** Performed in standing position
*** Repeat screening pulse oximetry at least annually
† Early = within 1–2 cardiac cycles; late = 3–6 cardiac cycles

Figure 8.3. Diagnostic algorithm for hepatopulmonary syndrome. Some centers extend this algorithm by routinely performing ^{99}Tc macroaggregated albumin scanning, which is very sensitive to intrapulmonary shunts, when other possible right-to-left shunts have been excluded. Screening pulse oximetry should be carried out at every clinic visit and at least annually, as development of hepatopulmonary syndrome shortens life expectancy and is accorded additional MELD points when discovered. PFTs, pulmonary function tests; ABG, arterial blood gas; HPS, hepatopulmonary syndrome; MAA, ^{99}Tc macroaggregated albumin.

There are no effective medical therapies for hepatopulmonary syndrome, although selective inhibition of nitric oxide production has shown theoretic promise. Among matched cirrhotic patients with and without hepatopulmonary syndrome, liver transplantation was the only therapy shown to increase survival compared with medical therapy alone.

Box 8.1. Major causes of hypoxia in patients with liver disease

Ventilation–perfusion mismatching
Premature airway closure
Pulmonary vasodilation
Impaired hypoxic pulmonary vasoconstriction
Diffusion–perfusion deficit
Pulmonary emboli
Compression of lung tissue
Impaired diaphragmatic function due to ascites
Pleural effusion
Pulmonary edema
Pulmonary manifestations of specific liver disease (e.g., α_1-antitrypsin deficiency)
Acute exacerbations of intercurrent chronic lung disease

Neurologic

Hepatic encephalopathy

The cause of hepatic encephalopathy is multifactorial. Elevated ammonia levels are often found in patients with hepatic encephalopathy and may play a role in its development. Activation of γ-aminobutyric acid (GABA) receptors in the brain also may contribute to hepatic encephalopathy, and ammonia has been shown to enhance GABAergic currents, which may explain its role in hepatic encephalopathy. Hepatic encephalopathy resembles many other nonfocal neurologic conditions (Table 8.5), from which it must be differentiated. Many of these occur as comorbid conditions in patients with liver failure. The severity of encephalopathy contributes to the CTP system for stratifying severity of hepatic disease.

Autonomic neuropathy

Autonomic neuropathies are found in up to 50% of patients with chronic liver disease and manifest most commonly as impaired cardiovascular function and gastric motility. In addition, patients with autonomic neuropathies experience a higher incidence of hypotension during general anesthesia. More importantly, autonomic neuropathy predicts increased mortality in cirrhotic patients. The development of autonomic neuropathies does not depend on the etiology of the liver disease,

Table 8.5. Conditions resembling hepatic encephalopathy

Metabolic problems
    Hypoglycemia
    Hyponatremia
    Hypernatremia
Intracranial processes
    Subdural hematoma
    Intracranial hemorrhage
    Intracranial mass lesion
Infectious diseases
    Meningitis

Table 8.6. Major causes of fulminant hepatic failure

Toxins
  Acetaminophen
  Ethanol
  Amanita phalloides
  Halothane
  Phosphorus
Viral infections
  Hepatitis A
  Hepatitis B
  Hepatitis C
  Hepatitis D
Miscellaneous
  Budd-Chiari syndrome
  Acute fatty liver of pregnancy
  Wilson's disease

and they generally resolve with the return of normal liver function after transplantation.

Fulminant hepatic failure

Fulminant hepatic failure is severe hepatic dysfunction that occurs most commonly from drug toxicity, most frequently from acetaminophen (Table 8.6), followed by viral hepatitis, and less often by some unidentifiable agent. Acute hepatic encephalopathy is a prominent clinical feature of fulminant hepatic failure and is associated with progressive brain swelling and an increase in intracranial pressure that may result in brain herniation and death. In patients who are awake and responsive, regular neurologic examinations may be used to exclude dangerous brain swelling.

Treatment of fulminant hepatic failure is supportive, and many patients recover. For those who do not recover, liver transplantation is the treatment of choice. Regardless of the final path to resolution, supportive care aims to reduce the impact of severe encephalopathy and brain swelling. Bacterial infections develop in up to 80% of patients with fulminant hepatic failure and most commonly involve the respiratory and urinary systems. Acute infection may prevent transplantation.

Pharmacologic management in cirrhosis

Cirrhosis and liver failure may affect the distribution, duration of action, elimination, and effect of a variety of drugs by perturbing their normal pharmacokinetics and pharmacodynamics. Cirrhotic patients have a decreased ability to metabolize and clear drugs. Decreases in serum albumin and altered total body water also change the volume of distribution of many drugs. Table 8.7 summarizes these changes. Anesthesiologists need to be cognizant of these changes when administering balanced anesthesia to cirrhotic patients.

Perioperative access and monitoring

Many of the preoperative preparations needed for major surgery in cirrhotic patients are those used for noncirrhotic

Table 8.7. Effect of cirrhosis and liver failure on the administration of drugs used in anesthesia

Drug class	Drug	Effect of liver failure on drug metabolism	Dosing recommendations in cirrhotic patients
Opioids	Morphine Meperidine	Prolonged half-life	Decrease frequency
	Fentanyl	Apparently unchanged	No change for single-dose administration Caution advised for prolonged infusions
	Remifentanil	Unaffected (metabolism by plasma esterases)	No change
Hypnotics	Methohexital	Unchanged clearance ratio	No change for single-dose administration
	Ketamine Etomidate	Prolonged half-life due to increased V_d	
	Propofol	Unchanged clearance (even with extended infusions)	No change
	Benzodiazepines	Decreased clearance ratio	Reduce preanesthetic dose Contraindicated in hepatic encephalopathy
Neuromuscular blockers	Succinylcholine Mivacurium	Significantly prolonged duration of action (because of decreased synthesis of plasma cholinesterases)	Decrease dose in short surgical procedures
	Vecuronium	Decreased clearance Extended duration of action (except in alcoholic cirrhosis)	Decrease dose
	Rocuronium	Increased V_d	Decrease dose
	Pancuronium	Decreased elimination half-life Extended duration of action	Decrease dose
	Atracurium Cisatracurium	Organ independent Hoffmann elimination	No change
Halogenated volatile anesthetics	Halothane	Causes decreased portal blood flow, and decreased hepatic artery blood flow = decreased hepatic perfusion, which may worsen liver damage	Avoid using entirely
	Isoflurane Sevoflurane Desflurane	Decreased portal blood flow; decreased total hepatic blood flow. Compensatory increase in hepatic artery blood flow	No change

V_d, apparent volume of distribution.

patients. Besides the standard ASA (American Society of Anesthesiologists) monitors, and depending on the planned surgical procedure, additional preparation might include use of warming devices, placement of multiple large-bore peripheral intravenous lines, an arterial line for blood pressure monitoring and obtaining serial blood samples during surgery, central or peripheral venous pressure monitoring, pulmonary artery catheter placement for hemodynamic monitoring (especially in patients with portopulmonary hypertension), and/or intraoperative transesophageal echocardiography.

Postoperative care

Ventilatory management is often the main issue one is concerned about in postoperative cirrhotic patients. Intraoperatively in large abdominal operations, pressure control ventilation (PCV) may be needed to prevent dangerously high peak alveolar pressures and PEEP. PCV with permissive hypercapnia of 60 to 70 mm Hg may be used to prevent alveolar barotrauma or volutrauma. In practice, permissive hypercapnia rarely is needed – modern anesthesia machine ventilators are adequate for the ventilatory needs of cirrhotic patients. Nitric oxide may be used to vasodilate the pulmonary vessels in patients with portopulmonary hypertension.

In procedures with a high transfusion requirement, transfusion-related acute lung injury (TRALI) is always a risk. This type of pulmonary edema may manifest between 1 and 3 days postoperatively or, in severe cases, intraoperatively. After lower-risk smaller procedures, these patients generally initially have a higher Fio_2 (fraction of inspired oxygen) requirement stemming from elevated abdominal pressures (i.e., from ascites). Reduced urine output from transient renal insufficiency may occur and is fairly common, occurring in as many as one-third of cirrhotic patients.

Pain management requires special attention in cirrhotic patients with encephalopathy, as opioids may cause undesirable and pronounced sedation. Neuraxial epidural anesthesia may be used as an alternative anesthetic and analgesic method; however, coagulopathy may prevent initial placement, delay catheter removal, and place the patient at increased risk for epidural hematoma and from exposure to foreign blood products if correction of a coagulopathy is necessary to remove a catheter. As such, patient-controlled intravenous analgesia usually is a safer method of postoperative pain control but requires careful attention.

Suggested readings

Fallon MB, Abrams GA. Pulmonary dysfunction in chronic liver disease. *Hepatology* 2000; 32:859–865.

Fernandez-Rodriguez CM, Prieto J, Zozaya JM, et al. Arteriovenous shunting, hemodynamic changes, and renal sodium retention in liver cirrhosis. *Gastroenterology* 1993; 104:1139–1145.

Findlay JY, Harrison BA, Plevak DJ, Krowka MJ. Inhaled nitric oxide reduces pulmonary artery pressures in portopulmonary hypertension. *Liver Transpl Surg* 1999; 5:381–387.

Fleckenstein JF, Frank S, Thuluvath PJ. Presence of autonomic neuropathy is a poor prognostic indicator in patients with advanced liver disease. *Hepatology* 1996; 23:471–475.

Garg RK. Anesthetic considerations in patients with hepatic failure. *Int Anesthesiol Clin* 2005; 43:45–63.

Henriksen JH, Moller S, Ring-Larsen H, Christensen NJ. The sympathetic nervous system in liver disease. *J Hepatol* 1998; 29:328–341.

Hoeper MM, Krowka MJ, Strassburg CP. Portopulmonary hypertension and hepatopulmonary syndrome. *Lancet* 2004; 363:1461–1468.

Martinez G, Barbera JA, Navasa M, et al. Hepatopulmonary syndrome associated with cardiorespiratory disease. *J Hepatol* 1999; 30:882–889.

Moller S, Henriksen JH. Cirrhotic cardiomyopathy: a pathophysiological review of circulatory dysfunction in liver disease. *Heart* 2002; 87:9–15.

Pham PT, Pham PC, Rastogi A, Wilkinson AH. Review article: current management of renal dysfunction in the cirrhotic patient. *Aliment Pharmacol Ther* 2005; 21:949–961.

Robalino BD, Moodie DS. Association between primary pulmonary hypertension and portal hypertension: analysis of its pathophysiology and clinical, laboratory and hemodynamic manifestations. *J Am Coll Cardiol* 1991; 17:492–498.

Rolando N, Philpott-Howard J, Williams R. Bacterial and fungal infection in acute liver failure. *Semin Liver Dis* 1996; 16:389–402.

Swanson KL, Wiesner RH, Krowka MJ. Natural history of hepatopulmonary syndrome: impact of liver transplantation. *Hepatology* 2005; 41:1122–1129.

Verne GN, Soldevia-Pico C, Robinson ME, et al. Autonomic dysfunction and gastroparesis in cirrhosis. *J Clin Gastroenterol* 2004; 38:72–76.

Diabetes mellitus and perioperative glucose control

Ruma R. Bose and Balachundhar Subramaniam

According to the Centers for Disease Control and Prevention, diabetes mellitus (DM) is present in 24 million people (7% of the US population; www.cdc.gov/medicalpressure/2008/r080624.htm, 2008). The prevalence of hyperglycemia in hospitalized patients is 26%, of whom 12% have previously unrecognized diabetes or hospital-related DM. A high blood glucose level predisposes patients to organ morbidity and increased mortality. Hyperglycemia in the intraoperative and perioperative settings has been seen not only in diabetics but also in nondiabetics. This condition is associated with poor outcome, increased hospital mortality, infection, sepsis, poor wound healing, and ischemic events. In the intensive care unit (ICU), hyperglycemia has been correlated with prolonged mechanical ventilation, sepsis, renal insufficiency, and neurologic deficits. Therefore, knowledge of the optimal intraoperative blood glucose level, which is still a topic of contention, is of utmost importance to the anesthesiologist.

The American Diabetes Association (ADA) Expert Committee on the Diagnosis and Classification of Diabetes Mellitus describes in-hospital hyperglycemia as follows:

- Medical history of diabetes – DM previously diagnosed and acknowledged by the patient's treating physician
- Unrecognized diabetes – hyperglycemia (fasting blood glucose $\geq$126 mg/dl or random blood glucose $\geq$200 mg/dl) occurring during hospitalization and confirmed as diabetes after hospitalization by standard diagnostic criteria, but unrecognized as diabetes by the treating physician during hospitalization
- Hospital-related hyperglycemia – hyperglycemia (fasting blood glucose $\geq$126 mg/dl or random blood glucose $\geq$200 mg/dl) occurring during hospitalization and reverting to normal after hospital discharge.

Types of diabetes mellitus

Type 1 diabetes

Different types of diabetes mellitus are listed in Fig. 9.1. Type 1 involves 5% to 10% of patients with diabetes. The β-cells of the pancreas are affected by an autoimmune process, leading to

decreased production of insulin. Patients with type 1 DM are prone to develop ketoacidosis.

Type 2 diabetes

Type 2 is present in 90% to 95% of diabetic patients. Insulin resistance is stated as the primary cause of diabetes. Hence, there is hyperglycemia despite high or normal circulating levels of insulin. This level eventually falls as a result of feedback inhibition of insulin production by the pancreas. Patients with type 2 DM are less likely to develop ketoacidosis but are prone to develop a hyperglycemic, hyperosmolar, nonketotic state.

Gestational diabetes

Gestational diabetes manifests during pregnancy and is more common in patients with a family history of diabetes. Twenty percent to 50% of patients diagnosed with gestational diabetes go on to develop type 2 diabetes within the next 5 to 10 years.

Stress-related diabetes

During stressful events such as surgery and hospitalization, hyperglycemia occurs as a result of multiple factors that lead to an increase in concentration of blood glucose, a decrease in production of insulin, and insulin resistance (Fig. 9.1). The stress of surgery leads to the production of corticosteroids and stress hormones such as glucagon, growth hormone, epinephrine, and norepinephrine. These substances cause an increase in gluconeogenesis and glycogenolysis by the liver, ultimately leading to an increase in glucose production. In addition, the catabolic hormones cause insulin resistance, which decreases glucose uptake by muscle and fat. Epinephrine and norepinephrine inhibit insulin release by their action on α-adrenergic receptors. The net result is an increase in blood glucose concentration, eventually leading to an increase in insulin secretion by β-cells of the pancreas. Normally, because it is an anabolic hormone, insulin decreases the production of glucose by inhibiting gluconeogenesis and glycogenolysis and enhances its uptake peripherally. However, in stressful situations the blood glucose level remains elevated because of the reasons mentioned earlier.

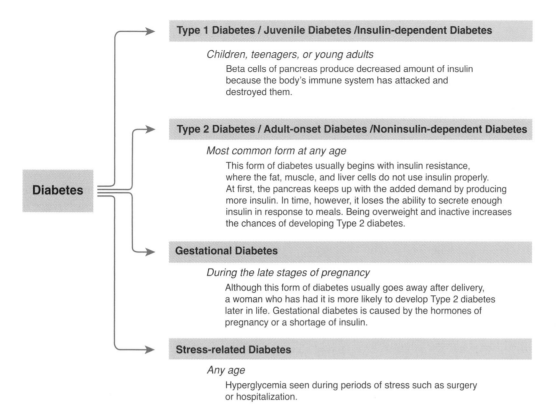

Figure 9.1. Classification of DM.

Adverse effects of hyperglycemia

Complications related to diabetes can be classified into acute and chronic. Acute complications are diabetic ketoacidosis, nonketotic hyperosmolar state, and hypoglycemia. Long-term effects are seen in virtually all the organ systems and include retinopathy, cataract, coronary artery disease, peripheral vascular disease, and renal insufficiency, to name a few.

In the perioperative setting, hyperglycemia is associated with an increase in overall hospital mortality. There is an increase in the incidence of pneumonia, wound infection, and sepsis. In acute myocardial infarction (MI), hyperglycemia is associated with increased mortality, congestive heart failure, and cardiogenic shock. In cardiac surgery patients, there is an increase in sternal wound infection, in-hospital mortality, postoperative renal failure, delayed stroke, and length of hospital stay. In ICU patients, hyperglycemia is associated with poor neurologic outcome, prolonged mechanical ventilation, sepsis, and renal failure.

Endothelial function

Hyperglycemia alters the integrity of the endothelium by inhibiting nitric oxide, which leads to an increase in cellular permeability, inflammation, angiogenesis, and thrombogenesis.

Thrombosis

Animal and human studies have demonstrated an increase in thrombosis associated with hyperglycemia, which is the result of an increase in the production of thromboxane and von Willebrand factor, coupled with the inhibition of plasminogen activator. As a result, there is platelet activation and aggregation, which in the setting of shear stress, as seen during hemodynamic fluctuations in the perioperative period, increases the incidence of thrombus formation.

Wound infection

Hyperglycemia has been associated with an increased incidence of postoperative wound infection, which may be explained by microvascular changes in the tissues that limit blood supply to the tissue. Another contributing factor is the decrease in phagocytosis and chemotaxis of the polymorphonuclear cells. A marked reduction in phagocytic and cytotoxic activity of the polymorphonuclear cells was observed in patients with poorly controlled blood glucose levels. A decrease in the incidence of sternal wound infections in diabetic patients after coronary artery bypass grafting was seen in those with a blood glucose level <200 mg/dl in the immediate postoperative period. The effect of perioperative hyperglycemia and hyperinsulinemia on monocytes was studied, and a decrease in HLA-DR expression was seen, which correlated with infectious complications and mortality.

Wound healing

Glycemic control in the perioperative period improves wound healing by increasing granulation tissue formation, fibroblast proliferation, and collagen synthesis. Hyperglycemia may cause nonenzymatic glycosylation with the production of abnormal proteins that decrease elastance and tensile strength, which are an essential part of the wound healing process. Diminishing insulin activity also decreases capillary proliferation, which worsens the tissue healing process.

Hyperglycemia and outcomes in critically ill patients

Glucose homeostasis is altered in critically ill patients, leading to increased glucose production and insulin resistance. Hyperglycemia in ICU patients has been associated with a higher incidence of MI, congestive heart failure, and cardiogenic shock. It also has been associated with a prolonged length of stay in the ICU as well as a prolonged duration of mechanical ventilation. A significant correlation has been found with stroke, neurologic injury, polyneuropathy, and renal insufficiency in these patients. In a landmark study, Van Den Berghe et al. in 2001 showed a reduction in mortality from 8% to 4.6% in ICU patients who maintained their blood glucose concentrations between 80 and 110 mg/dl. The largest reduction was seen in multiple organ failure due to sepsis. There was a decrease in in-hospital mortality, bloodstream infection rate, and acute renal failure requiring dialysis. There also was a decrease in the median number of blood transfusions, polyneuropathy, and the need for prolonged mechanical ventilation.

Neurologic injury

Supranormal blood sugar levels at the time of cerebral insult, be it traumatic head injury, subarachnoid hemorrhage, intracerebral hemorrhage, cerebrovascular accident, or stroke, are associated with a worsened neurologic outcome. Evidence suggests a profound benefit of blood glucose control in patients with global central nervous system ischemia. Glucose acts as a substrate for anaerobic metabolism, increasing lactate levels, worsening intracellular acidosis, and disrupting normal intracellular homeostasis. There is a correlation of poor functional recovery in stroke patients with hyperglycemia. The tissue most vulnerable to ischemia is the penumbra or the area surrounding the area of primary insult, and the progression of stroke depends on the viability of this region. Hyperglycemia has been associated with irreversible damage to this vulnerable region of the brain.

Myocardial infarction

Type 2 diabetes has been referred to as a "cardiovascular disease associated with hyperglycemia." Patients with diabetes tend to suffer painless MI, which makes timely detection and treatment difficult. The size of the infarct is larger and recovery is poor compared with the general population. During an MI, there is an increased production of stress hormones, which, in conjunction with preexisting insulin resistance, leads to a decrease in the utilization of glucose by the myocardium. The energy

Table 9.1. Signs and symptoms of autonomic imbalance

• Asymptomatic hypoglycemia	• Nocturnal diarrhea
• Lack of sweating	• Bladder atony
• Lack of pulse rate variability with respiration	• Erectile dysfunction
• Orthostatic hypotension	• Peripheral neuropathy
• Resting tachycardia	• Dysrhythmias
• Gastroparesis	• Asymptomatic hypoglycemia

requirements are fulfilled by fatty acid metabolism, which utilizes more oxygen, increasing the myocardial oxygen requirement and widening the demand–supply gap, thereby worsening ischemia.

Some of the other mechanisms that cause poor outcomes with hyperglycemia are worsening of ischemic preconditioning, a decrease in the formation of collateral blood supply, accelerated myocyte death, and worsening of reperfusion injury. The DIGAMI (Diabetes Mellitus Insulin-Glucose Infusion in Acute Myocardial Infarction) trial showed the beneficial effects of blood glucose control in patients with acute MI. A continuous insulin infusion was used to control blood sugar during acute MI, followed by intensive subcutaneous insulin therapy for 3 months. This regimen improved long-term survival and caused an absolute reduction in mortality by 11%. A moderate perioperative target range of 100 to 150 mg/dl in vascular surgical patients has the potential to reduce perioperative MI rates.

Autonomic imbalance

Patients with diabetes have a 10% to 50% incidence of autonomic neuropathy. Some of the signs and symptoms are listed in Table 9.1.

Patients with autonomic neuropathy lack the compensatory mechanisms to deal with hemodynamic fluctuations and hypoxia and are therefore more prone to sudden cardiac death, arrhythmias, and postoperative MI. Additionally, they are more likely to aspirate due to gastroparesis.

Ketoacidosis

Diabetic ketoacidosis usually occurs in type 1 diabetics but may also occur in type 2 diabetics. It is a life-threatening condition resulting from lack of insulin and highly elevated blood glucose levels (up to 500 mg/dl). There is accumulation of ketone bodies (acetoacetate and β-hydroxybutyrate). The resulting anion gap metabolic acidosis leads to dyspnea, nausea and vomiting, thirst (hypovolemia), abdominal pain, constant urination (diuretic effect of glucose), agitation, and confusion. If the blood glucose levels are not corrected coma may result.

Diabetic ketoacidosis is treated with aggressive hydration, insulin drip (10 units/h or 0.1 units/kg/h to decrease blood glucose levels at a rate of not more than 100 mg/dl/h), and replacement of electrolytes (especially potassium; insulin carries glucose and potassium into the cell). When the blood

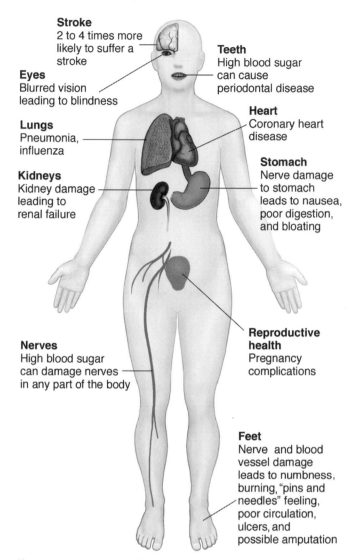

Stroke
2 to 4 times more likely to suffer a stroke

Eyes
Blurred vision leading to blindness

Lungs
Pneumonia, influenza

Kidneys
Kidney damage leading to renal failure

Teeth
High blood sugar can cause periodontal disease

Heart
Coronary heart disease

Stomach
Nerve damage to stomach leads to nausea, poor digestion, and bloating

Nerves
High blood sugar can damage nerves in any part of the body

Reproductive health
Pregnancy complications

Feet
Nerve and blood vessel damage leads to numbness, burning, "pins and needles" feeling, poor circulation, ulcers, and possible amputation

Figure 9.2. Complications of DM.

glucose reaches 250 mg/dl, an infusion of 5% dextrose in water is started to prevent hypoglycemia. Patients are actively monitored with repeated measurements of blood glucose, urine output, and vital signs.

Intraoperative blood glucose management
Preoperative evaluation

Preoperative evaluation of diabetic patients should include assessment of glycemic control; early detection and treatment of electrolyte disturbances, hypoglycemia, and ketoacidosis; and determination of the extent of end-organ disease. The American College of Cardiology/American Heart Association guidelines state that a patient's risk for cardiac complications is a function of the patient's medical history, current functional status, and the specific surgical procedure. DM is considered an intermediate risk factor for postoperative cardiac morbidity. Complications of DM are shown in Fig. 9.2.

Cardiovascular disease is the most common cause of morbidity in diabetic patients. A thorough history and physical examination should be performed and a baseline electrocardiogram (ECG) obtained in every patient. The presence of arrhythmias, Q waves, left ventricular hypertrophy, or ST changes have been correlated with increased cardiac morbidity. Noninvasive and invasive cardiac testing may be warranted in high-risk patients undergoing major or intermediate-risk surgical procedures. Asymptomatic patients with diabetes have shown significant perfusion defects during thallium testing.

Signs and symptoms of autonomic neuropathy should be elicited. The tilt test is an easy method for assessing orthostatic hypotension (a positive test is a decrease in blood pressure of approximately 30 mm Hg in the upright position). A pulse rate variability of ≤ 5 bpm during deep inspiration and expiration (normal being 15 bpm) also is an indicator of autonomic imbalance. Renal insufficiency is a common complication associated with diabetes and requires further evaluation.

The type of diabetes and its management with regard to insulin regimen or oral hypoglycemic agents should be determined. Patients should be asked about the occurrence and frequency of hypoglycemic episodes. Type 2 diabetic patients who are on oral hypoglycemics may need to be started on an insulin regimen perioperatively to ensure adequate control of blood sugar in the setting of stress, fasting, and change in nutritional regimen while in the hospital. However, well-controlled type 2 diabetic patients undergoing same-day surgery may not require insulin.

Airway examination

Patients with a history of longstanding diabetes may demonstrate the "prayer sign," which is difficulty in approximating the metacarpophalangeal joints of the two hands. These patients also may have restricted neck extension, which may cause problems during airway management. The restricted neck extension is a result of atlanto-occipital joint fusion. Patients showing the prayer sign have a greater incidence of microvascular disease.

Laboratory tests

In addition to routine laboratory tests, blood glucose, ECG, blood urea nitrogen, creatinine, and plasma electrolyte levels should be evaluated. Twenty-four-hour creatinine clearance is recommended in some patients with renal insufficiency. Urine should be checked for ketones and albumin. The hemoglobin A_{1c} level (an indicator of glycosylated hemoglobin) may be checked to determine the adequacy of blood sugar control during the previous 4 to 6 weeks.

Medications

Whenever possible, the surgery should be scheduled in the morning to minimize the catabolic state and hypoglycemia. If the patient is on metformin, some have advocated stopping it

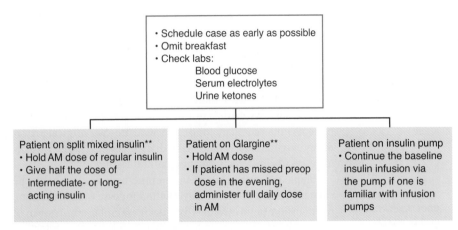

Figure 9.3. Preoperative management of blood sugar in patients with DM.

at least 24 hours before surgery because of its rare propensity to cause lactic acidosis, but this is no longer widely accepted. Sulfonylureas and thiazolidinediones may be stopped the day before surgery. Preoperative blood sugar should always be checked; the goal is to maintain an optimum glucose level and prevent hypoglycemia. One has to be cognizant of the fact that intraoperatively and immediately postoperatively, all the signs and symptoms of hypoglycemia may be masked; therefore, frequent blood sugar measurements are advised.

Insulin pumps deliver a continuous infusion of short-acting insulin, and the rate of infusion is controlled by the patient based on periodic blood sugar measurements. The insulin pump delivers baseline insulin, and it is important to maintain this infusion rate in insulin-dependent diabetics. However, some experts advocate substituting intravenous insulin infusions for the subcutaneous pump because of concerns for altered cutaneous blood flow during surgery. Rhodes and Ferrari in 2005 laid out practice guidelines for the preoperative management of pediatric patients with diabetes, and these

Table 9.2. Insulin time chart

Type of insulin	Start of action	Peak of action, h	Duration of action, h
Humalog (rapid)	15 min	1.5–2	4
Regular (short)	30 min	2–3	5
NPH (intermediate)	1–2 h	4–8	14–20
Lente (intermediate)	2–3 h	8–12	16–24
Ultralente (long)	2–4 h	8–14	18–24
Lantus (long)	1–2 h	6	18–26

may be applied to adults as well. Preoperative management of diabetic patients based on these guidelines is summarized in Figs. 9.3 and 9.4, and Tables 9.2 and 9.3.

Intraoperative management

It is universally accepted that intraoperative hyperglycemia is deleterious to patient outcome, but there is continuing debate regarding the ideal target blood glucose level. Earlier studies suggested a more generous margin for blood glucose levels; for example, Pomposelli et al. in 1998 showed a benefit in outcome if the limit was 220 mg/dl. Later studies lowered this limit to anywhere between 100 and 120 mg/dl. Van Den Berghe's study in ICU patients showed a difference in outcome when blood glucose was maintained at <110 mg/dl. The major concern with dropping the safe level of blood glucose is the risk of hypoglycemia, with its attendant life-threatening complications. The recent NICE-SUGAR (Normoglycemia in Intensive

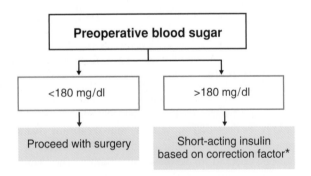

*Correction factor (CF) = 1500/ [Total daily dose (TDD) of insulin]
Example: If TDD is 50 U, CF = 1500/50 = 30 U
1 U of regular insulin will decrease the blood sugar by 30 mg/dl. Blood sugar is maintained between 100 and 150 mg/dl.

Figure 9.4. Insulin regimen to manage hyperglycemia.

Table 9.3. Insulin regimen for patients who require continuous IV infusion.

- Continuous background infusion of 10% dextrose and $\frac{1}{2}$ NS is required
- Insulin infusion is piggybacked (1U for 3g dextrose)
- Blood glucose is maintained at 100–500 mg/dl
- Subsequent dose adjustment of insulin is based on the current insulin infusion rate and the rate of decline of blood glucose levels

Source: Adapted from figure 7; Rhodes RT, Ferrari LR. Perioperative management of pediatric surgical patients with diabetes mellitus. *Anesth Analg* 2005; 101:986–999.

Care Evaluation – Survival Using Glucose Algorithm Regulation) study seriously challenged the tight glucose target range. A moderate target of 100 to 150 mg/dl seems to have more benefits than risks.

In 2004, the American College of Endocrinology set up a taskforce whose recommendation for the target blood glucose level was 110 mg/dl in ICU patients and a maximum of 180 mg/ml in non-ICU patients. The goal at our institution is to maintain the intraoperative blood glucose level between 100 and 150 mg/dl in all patients with diabetes. Blood glucose should be measured immediately preoperatively and every hour intraoperatively and during the immediate postoperative period. There are many insulin regimens for managing intraoperative hyperglycemia. A background glucose infusion is recommended to prevent hypoglycemia, ketosis, and protein breakdown, especially when using continuous insulin infusion. Potassium levels should be measured periodically. Insulin and epinephrine stimulate potassium uptake by the cells, whereas hyperosmolality and acidosis translocate potassium out of the cells.

If intraoperative blood glucose measurements warrant insulin administration, the bolus dose is calculated as follows: For insulin-dependent diabetic patients, the daily insulin requirement is divided by 24, and that is the initial dose (approximately 0.1 units/kg body weight); in patients who are insulin naïve the dose is 0.02 units/kg intravenously (IV). Repeat doses are calculated by the rapidity of change in blood glucose level and incorporation of a correction factor. If the surgery is emergent, preoperative assessment and optimization of metabolic status and adequate volume replacement should be the goal. Surgery should be delayed if possible to achieve metabolic control. If surgery cannot be delayed, adequate fluid replacement and timely correction of electrolyte imbalance, especially potassium levels, will decrease the occurrence of arrhythmias and hypotension.

Postoperative management

Postoperative management includes measurement of blood glucose levels and continuation of the IV or a subcutaneous insulin regimen until the patient can resume caloric intake. Nausea and vomiting should be treated aggressively. Adequate pain control is important to minimize the release of catabolic hormones that increase blood glucose levels. Renal dysfunction should be kept in mind when prescribing analgesics. Patients should be monitored closely for signs of hypoglycemia, respiratory depression, and hemodynamic instability. A postoperative ECG should be obtained to monitor for ischemic changes. With regard to patients receiving an insulin infusion, consideration for continuing it should be given in postoperative patients discharged from the ICU, those on corticosteroids, and those who have had an organ transplant or stroke.

Suggested readings

Alberti KG. Diabetes and surgery. *Anesthesiology* 1991; 74:209–211.

Alberti KG, Gill GV, Elliot MJ. Insulin delivery during surgery in the diabetic patient. *Diabetes Care* 1982; 5(Suppl. 1):65–67.

Furnary A, Zerr K, Grunkemeier G, Starr A. Continuous intravenous insulin infusion reduces the incidence of deep sternal wound infection in diabetic patients after cardiac surgical procedures. *Ann Thorac Surg* 1999; 67:352–362.

Furnary AP, Gao G, Grunkemeier GL, et al. Continuous insulin infusion reduces mortality in patients with diabetes undergoing coronary artery bypass grafting. *J Thorac Cardiovasc Surg* 2003; 125:1007–1021.

Gandhi GY, Nuttall GA. Intensive intraoperative insulin therapy versus conventional glucose management during cardiac surgery: a randomized trial. *Ann Intern Med* 2007; 146:233–243.

Levetan CS, Passaro M, Jablonski K, et al. Unrecognized diabetes among hospitalized patients. *Diabetes Care* 1998; 21:246–249.

NICE-SUGAR Study Investigators; Finfer S, Chittock DR, Su SY, et al. Intensive versus conventional glucose control in critically ill patients. *N Engl J Med* 2009; 360:1283–1297.

Pomposelli J, Baxter J, Babineau T, et al. Early postoperative glucose control predicts nosocomial infection rate in diabetic patients. *J Parenter Enter Nutr* 1998; 22:77–81.

Rhodes RT, Ferrari LR. Perioperative management of pediatric surgical patients with diabetes mellitus. *Anesth Analg* 2005; 101:986–999.

Subramaniam B, Panzica PJ, Novack D, et al. Continuous perioperative insulin infusion decreases major cardiovascular events in patients undergoing major vascular surgery: a prospective, randomized controlled trial. *Anesthesiology* 2009; 110: 970–977.

Umpierrez GE, Isaacs SD, Bazargan N, et al. Hyperglycemia: an independent marker of in-hospital mortality in patients with undiagnosed diabetes. *J Clin Endocrinol Metab* 2002; 87:978–982.

Van Den Berghe G, Wouters P, Weekers F, et al. Intensive insulin therapy in critically ill patients. *N Engl J Med* 2001; 345:1359–1367.

Zerr KJ, Furnary AP, Grunkemeier GL, et al. Glucose control lowers the risk of wound infection in diabetics after open heart operations. *Ann Thorac Surg* 1997; 63:356–361.

Chapter 10

Common blood disorders

Jonathan D. Bloom and Edward A. Bittner

Erythrocyte disorders

Anemia

Anemia is defined as a deficiency in the concentration of functional red blood cells (RBCs) in the circulation. It should be noted that a change in reported hemoglobin (Hb) or hematocrit (Hct) does not necessarily indicate a change in erythrocyte mass, as dehydration may falsely elevate a normal value whereas hemodilution may falsely lower it. Conversely, the Hb/Hct may be reported as normal in the setting of acute bleeding, prior to fluid resuscitation and re-equilibration.

Clinical considerations

Perioperative concerns about the anemic patient are based on the physiologic expectation that anesthesia, surgery, and the postoperative period commonly increase a patient's oxygen demand in the setting of an already limited oxygen reserve. Despite this, evidence that blood product transfusions are associated with adverse outcomes (e.g., transfusion-related acute lung injury, transfusion reactions) have altered perioperative transfusion practices, prompting the physician to weigh the benefit of the acute increase in transfused product against the risks of transfusion.

Knowledge of the clinical consequences and physiologic responses to anemia is essential for providing appropriate perioperative care. Basic compensatory responses to anemia involve central, regional, and microcirculatory alterations in blood flow, as well as a shift of the oxyhemoglobin dissociation curve to the right. Acute normovolemic anemia results in increased cardiac output resulting from both increased venous return and decreased afterload. This is further augmented by decreased blood viscosity and increased inotropy from sympathetic stimulation. Regional blood flow is altered by redistribution from nonvital to vital organs (e.g., from skeletal muscle to the heart and brain). Microcirculatory changes enable increased tissue oxygen extraction via capillary recruitment. Finally, anemia results in increased 2,3-diphosphoglycerate concentrations in RBCs, which shift the oxyhemoglobin curve to the right, favoring oxygen unloading. Oxygen delivery remains essentially unchanged until hemoglobin concentration falls below 7 g/dl.

The increase in cardiac output in response to acute normovolemic anemia differs between awake and anesthetized patients. Increased cardiac output in awake patients is the result of an increase in stroke volume and heart rate, whereas increased cardiac output in anesthetized patients primarily is the result of an increase in stroke volume alone. Consequently, tachycardia in the anesthetized patient in the setting of acute anemia most likely is a sign of hypovolemia and should be treated with crystalloids or colloids.

Causes of anemia

The three major causes for anemia are (1) blood loss, (2) decreased RBC production, and (3) increased RBC destruction. The diagnosis for most causes of anemia can be determined from a thorough history and physical examination. Symptoms of anemia are variable and depend on a patient's coexisting diseases. For example, in a healthy patient, symptoms of anemia may not develop until the Hb level decreases below 7 g/dl. Laboratory tests that may be helpful in distinguishing the cause(s) of the anemia include a peripheral smear (for erythrocyte size and shape), mean cell volume, and reticulocyte count. The reticulocyte count typically is elevated in anemia caused by RBC destruction and is inappropriately low in anemia caused by a failure of RBC production. Other tests that may be useful include serum iron and ferritin levels; vitamin B_{12}/folate levels; serum bilirubin, lactate dehydrogenase, and haptoglobin levels; and the direct antiglobulin test (direct Coombs).

Types of Anemia

Anemias can be classified into two categories, primary and secondary. The former results from a structural abnormality of the hemoglobin molecule or of the erythrocyte membrane. The second category is more common, having multiple etiologies, which are described briefly later.

Megaloblastic anemias are caused by impaired DNA synthesis and are most commonly a result of deficiency of folic acid (the most common vitamin deficiency, commonly seen in severely ill patients, alcoholics, and parturients because of dietary deficiencies) and/or vitamin B_{12}. In the general surgical population, megaloblastic anemia commonly is caused by disease or partial resection of the gastrointestinal tract. Signs and symptoms, in addition to anemia, may include glossitis, tachycardia, flow murmurs, splenomegaly, and neurologic disorders (mainly in B_{12} deficiency) such as ataxia, loss of deep tendon reflexes, loss of posterior column sensations, confabulation, dyspnea, headache, fatigue, diarrhea, and other gastrointestinal symptoms. Management, as with all causes of anemia, is focused on maintenance of adequate oxygen delivery to the tissues. Long-term exposure to nitrous oxide has been shown to produce a megaloblastic anemia with neurologic changes and may exacerbate the effects of preexisting vitamin B_{12} deficiency. Preexisting neurologic deficits should be documented and may preclude use of regional anesthetic techniques.

Iron deficiency anemia results from insufficient iron intake or a rapid turnover of cells (e.g., chronic blood loss or hemolysis). The finding of a microcytic, hypochromic anemia, together with a low serum ferritin level, is a rapid and effective method of making the diagnosis.

Anemia of chronic disease, the second most common cause of anemia after iron deficiency, occurs in patients with acute or chronic immune activation. Abnormal uptake and accumulation of iron within the cells of the reticuloendothelial system result in impaired erythropoiesis and blunted response to erythropoietin. The diagnosis is largely one of exclusion. Laboratory evaluation reveals a mild normochromic, normocytic anemia with a low reticulocyte count and normal total body iron (ferritin) stores. Treatment currently centers on managing the underlying disease.

Sickle cell disease

Sickle cell disease (SCD) is an inherited blood disorder stemming from production of the abnormal hemoglobin molecule HbS. A single amino acid substitution (glutamic acid to valine at the sixth position of the hemoglobin β-chain) results in a loss of negative charge, which allows for neighboring HbS molecules to associate and polymerize upon deoxygenation, resulting in the distorted, sickled erythrocyte shape. Even when fully oxygenated, a fraction of erythrocytes remains dense, dehydrated, and sickled, resulting in the vaso-occlusive manifestations. Injury to a sickled erythrocyte cell membrane as a result of polymerization causes adherence to vascular endothelial cells, resulting in reduced blood flow, which initiates the vicious cycle of ischemia, hypoxia, and further polymerization and sickling (Fig. 10.1).

Complications of SCD are hemolysis, anemia, aplastic crisis (sudden cessation of bone marrow activity), painful crisis, splenic atrophy (with associated increased infection risk to encapsulated bacteria), hypercoagulability, stroke, pulmonary embolism, asthma, hepatopathy, renal insufficiency/failure (from repeated infarcts), acute chest syndrome (the most common cause of death in adults with SCD), and secondary pulmonary hypertension. The various clinical manifestations of SCD are listed in Table 10.1.

Treatment of SCD consists of supportive regimens (folate, magnesium, zinc), pneumococcal vaccine, prophylactic penicillin, hydroxyurea (increases HbF levels, which interfere with HbS polymerization), anhydration agents, transfusion (for aplastic crisis or sequestration), pain therapy for painful crisis, and (rarely) bone marrow transplantation.

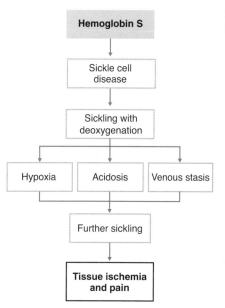

Figure 10.1. Factors precipitating sickling.

Preoperative assessment should include evaluation for infection, dehydration, vaso-occlusion, and end-organ damage. Intraoperatively, the patient should avoid sickling triggers, such as hypothermia, hypoxemia, hypovolemia, acidosis, and hypotension. In addition, fluid replacement should be selected over vasoconstrictors when possible. The use of tourniquets should be minimized, as they produce local stasis and acidosis. If a tourniquet is unavoidable, the limb should be carefully exsanguinated and the cuff duration minimized.

Perioperative prophylactic transfusion frequently is used in surgical patients with SCD, but no consensus exists regarding the best regimen. Prophylactic red blood exchange has not been shown to be superior to simple RBC transfusion in the preoperative setting. Regional techniques may be used, but epinephrine should be avoided. Acute chest syndrome, especially common the first 48 to 72 hours postoperatively, is characterized by chest pain, cough, progressive anemia, hypoxemia, and the presence of new pulmonary infiltrates on chest radiograph.

Table 10.1. Clinical manifestations of SCD

System	Complications
Neurologic	Pain crisis, stroke, retinopathy, neuropathy, chronic pain syndrome
Pulmonary	Acute chest syndrome, airway hyperreactivity, restrictive lung disease
Genitourinary	Hyposthenuria, chronic renal insufficiency, urinary tract infection, priapism, increased obstetric complications
Gastrointestinal	Cholelithiasis, liver disease, dyspepsia
Hematologic	Hemolytic anemia, acute aplastic anemia, splenic enlargement/fibrosis
Orthopedic	Osteonecrosis, osteomyelitis, dactylitis
Vascular	Leg ulcers
Immunologic	Immune dysfunction, erythrocyte auto/alloimmunization

Less common causes of anemia

Thalassemias are a group of inherited disorders characterized by decreased rates of production or failure to synthesize normal globin chains. Clinical features of thalassemia include anemia, hemolysis, and bone marrow hyperplasia. Treatment is based on the severity of the anemia. Bone marrow transplantation for patients with severe anemia may be curative. Regular transfusion may be required if the thalassemia is severe.

Hereditary spherocytosis is a rare anemia caused by an inherited RBC cytoskeletal abnormality. A defect of the spectrin protein in the cell membrane results in a more rounded and fragile RBC. Anemia typically results from splenic destruction of the abnormal cells. Cholelithiasis secondary to chronic hemolysis and elevated serum bilirubin concentrations are common. Hemolytic crises, triggered by folate deficiency or infection may worsen the anemia. Treatment of hereditary spherocytosis is splenectomy.

Glucose-6-phosphate dehydrogenase (G6PD) deficiency is the most common inherited RBC enzyme disorder, affecting 400 million people worldwide. Chronic hemolytic anemia is the most common manifestation. Drugs that form peroxides by interactions with oxyhemoglobin can trigger hemolysis in patients with G6PD deficiency. These agents include antimalarial drugs, nitrofurantoin, probenecid, phenacetin, vitamin K, quinidine, and nitroprusside. There is considerable variability in the hemolytic response to drugs. Hemolysis typically begins 2 to 5 days after the offending drug's administration. Bacterial infections also may trigger hemolytic episodes. Patients with G6PD deficiency cannot reduce methemoglobin; therefore, drugs such as nitroprusside and prilocaine should not be used in these patients. Anesthetic drugs have not been incriminated as triggering agents.

Immune hemolytic anemias are characterized by antibody formation against the RBC membrane. These antibodies may be acquired through drug exposure, disease, or erythrocyte sensitization. Immune hemolytic anemias can be divided into (1) autoimmune hemolysis, (2) drug-induced hemolysis, and (3) alloimmune hemolysis. Autoimmune hemolytic anemia includes warm and cold antibody hemolytic anemia, according to the optimal temperature at which the antibodies act to destroy RBCs. Cold hemolytic anemias are of special concern in the perioperative setting, because the cold operating room environment and hypothermia during cardiopulmonary bypass may precipitate a hemolytic crisis. Maintaining a warm environment is essential; in rare instances, plasmapheresis may be required to reduce cold antibody titer before hypothermic procedures. Of note, clinically insignificant cold-reacting RBC autoantibodies often are detected incidentally in the blood bank laboratory. Only the rare examples of cold autoantibodies that cause hemolysis in vivo require special measures in the operating room.

Several clinical entities, including neoplasia, infection, and collagen vascular diseases, may result in immune hemolytic anemias. Immune hemolytic anemias also may be drug induced from several commonly administered drugs, including acetaminophen, cephalosporins, hydralazine, and hydrochlorothiazide. Alloimmune hemolytic anemia most commonly manifests as hemolytic disease of the newborn, in which maternal antibodies against fetal RBCs with incompatible Rh or ABO blood groups are produced and cross the placenta.

Polycythemia

In contrast to the previously mentioned erythrocyte disorders, polycythemia is defined by an elevated hemoglobin concentration and increased hematocrit. It can be divided pathophysiologically into primary polycythemias (those not caused by increased erythropoietin) and secondary polycythemias (those caused by increased erythropoietin production). Polycythemia vera, the most common type of primary polycythemia, is a neoplastic stem cell disorder. Untreated polycythemia vera may result in an increased risk of thrombosis as well as hemorrhage. Possible clinical manifestations of thrombosis include myocardial infarction (MI), ischemic stroke, pulmonary embolism, peripheral arterial thrombosis, and deep venous thrombosis.

Secondary polycythemias result from increased erythropoietin production in response to chronic tissue hypoxia (e.g., as occurs with ascent to high altitude or with cardiopulmonary disease), tumors that secrete erythropoietin (e.g., kidney tumors), or inherited conditions that result in overproduction or exaggerated response of erythropoietin. The main goal in treating polycythemia is to correct the condition responsible for the increased cell mass, if possible. Phlebotomy is used to lower the hematocrit and prevent hyperviscosity while the primary condition is being corrected. Treatment of polycythemia vera additionally involves myelosuppressive drugs such as hydroxyurea.

Coagulation disorders

Coagulation is a complex process, occurring in response to an injury, in which the blood forms clot or thrombus. Injury usually occurs to the endothelial lining of the blood vessel, which initiates a coagulation cascade leading to hemostasis (cessation of blood loss from the damaged vessel).

Coagulation of blood involves two important processes, formation of a platelet plug (primary hemostasis) and formation of fibrin strands to strengthen the platelet plug (secondary hemostasis). The latter occurs via proteins known as clotting/coagulation factors. Spontaneous thrombus formation in normal endothelium is prevented by proteins and factors such as heparan proteoglycans, prostacyclin, nitric oxide, and tissue plasminogen activator. However, when the endothelium is damaged, these anticoagulant proteins are down-regulated and other proteins (procoagulants) are up-regulated.

Once the endothelial lining is damaged, it exposes collagen to which circulating platelets bind (primary hemostasis). This adhesion is facilitated by von Willebrand factor (vWF), causing the platelets to become activated. Activated platelets release

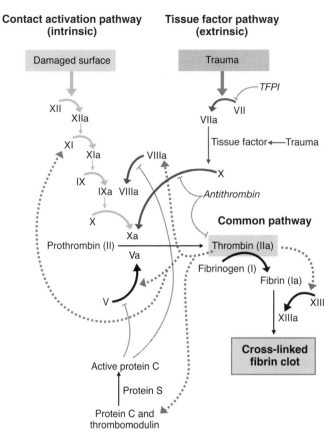

Figure 10.2. The coagulation cascade.

Table 10.2. Coagulation factors

Factor	Name	Plasma concentration, μg/ml	% of normal required for hemostasis
I	Fibrinogen	3000	30
II	Prothrombin	100	40
III	Tissue factor	–	–
IV	Calcium	–	–
V	Proaccelerin	10	10–15
VII	Proconvertin	0.5	5–10
VIII	Antihemophilic	0.1	10–40
IX	Thromboplastin	5	10–40
X	Stuart	10	10–15
XI	Prethromboplastin	5	20–30
XII	Hageman	30	0
XIII	Fibrin stabilizing	30	1–5

that includes both disorders. They are classified further by the hemostatic component involved, that is, platelet or clotting factors.

Platelet disorders

Thrombocytopenia

Platelet disorders are subdivided into disorders of platelet number and platelet function. *Thrombocytopenia* is defined

humoral factors such as adenosine diphosphate (ADP), platelet activating factor, and thromboxane, which in turn activate the platelets. Activated platelets contain an increased amount of calcium, which activates protein kinase C, which in turn modifies the membrane protein "integrin," increasing its affinity to bind fibrinogen.

Secondary hemostasis consists of the coagulation cascade, which is a series of reactions, to form fibrin. The coagulation cascade consists of two initial pathways (Fig. 10.2): the tissue factor (extrinsic) pathway and the contact activation (intrinsic) pathway. These two initial pathways converge into a common pathway leading to the formation of thrombin and fibrin.

The coagulation cascade consists of various clotting/coagulation factors, all of which are serine proteases or glycoproteins. The various coagulation factors are listed in Table 10.2. All factors, except factors III, IV, and VIII, are synthesized in the liver. Factors II, VII, IX, and X (plus proteins C and S) are vitamin K dependent for their synthesis. Proper functioning of the coagulation cascade requires cofactors such as phospholipids and vitamin K. Regulators of the coagulation cascade include protein C, antithrombin, tissue factor pathway inhibitor, plasmin, and prostacyclin. Common laboratory tests of hemostasis are listed in Table 10.3.

Coagulation disorders can be broadly divided into disorders of hemostasis or thrombosis, with an intermediate group

Table 10.3. Common laboratory tests for hemostasis

Class	Test	Normal value
Platelet function	Platelet count	100,000–400,000 cells/μl
	Bleeding time	<10 min
	Platelet function and aggregation analysis	
Coagulation studies	PT–tissue pathway	Normal, 11–14 sec; prolonged with low levels of factor I, II, V, VII, or X, or liver disease. INR standardizes results across laboratories.
	PTT–contact activation pathway	Normal, 24–35 sec; prolonged with low levels of factor I, II, V, VIII, IX, X, XI, or XII. Heparin prolongs PTT.
	Thrombin time	Normal, 22–32 sec; prolonged with low levels of factor I or II
	ACT	Normal, 80–180 sec. Monitor heparin therapy with large doses in the operating room.
	Thromboelastography	Measure of time to initial clot formation, time to clot formation, clot strength, clot lysis
Fibrinolysis tests	D-dimer levels	When plasmin cleaves cross-linked fibrin (fibrinolytic states)
	Fibrin degradation products	Excessive activity of plasmin, which degrades fibrin (DIC)

INR, international normalized ratio.

as a platelet count <150,000/μl. Major causes of thrombocytopenia include decreased production, increased destruction/consumption, sequestration, and dilution. Common causes of decreased production of platelets include drug effects, infections, chemotherapy or radiation therapy, alcohol toxicity, and certain vitamin deficiencies (B_{12}/folate). Increased platelet destruction and consumption occur in several conditions, including disseminated intravascular coagulation (DIC), drug exposure, autoimmune states (idiopathic thrombocytopenic purpura, thrombotic thrombocytopenic purpura/hemolytic uremic syndrome, antiphospholipid antibody syndrome), HELLP syndrome (hemolytic anemia, elevated liver enzymes, and low platelet count), physical destruction (cardiopulmonary bypass, giant hemangiomas, large aortic aneurysms, large tissue wounds), and adherence to grafts. Dilution typically occurs after massive resuscitation/transfusion. Splenic sequestration is found in patients with portal hypertension.

Some forms of thrombocytopenia are associated with thrombotic risk (e.g., heparin-induced thrombocytopenia and antiphospholipid syndrome) rather than bleeding. Surgical bleeding due to thrombocytopenia does not typically occur until the platelet count falls below 50,000/μl, and spontaneous bleeding is not typically seen unless the platelet count falls below 5000 to 10,000/μl. Dilutional thrombocytopenia is the most common cause of intraoperative coagulopathy. Assuming the preoperative platelet count is normal, as much as 80% of the circulating blood volume may have to be replaced before clinically significant thrombocytopenia occurs. Rapid diagnosis is important to minimize bleeding or thrombotic risk through appropriate therapy.

There are multiple causes of *qualitative platelet abnormalities*. Inherited causes stem from abnormalities of the platelet membrane (e.g., Bernard-Soulier syndrome, Glanzmann disease) or granule abnormalities. The former typically are associated with more significant bleeding than the latter. Inherited conditions are rare and usually are diagnosed in childhood. The most common causes of acquired platelet dysfunction are the various antiplatelet agents used to prevent thrombosis and decrease the risk of MI, stroke, and other thrombotic complications. Platelet transfusion may be necessary to support surgery. The major offending classes are cyclooxygenase inhibitors, phosphodiesterase inhibitors (dipyridamole), ADP receptor antagonists (ticlopidine and clopidogrel), and glycoprotein IIb/IIIa antagonists (abciximab, tirofiban, eptifibatide).

Perioperative risk of hemorrhage in patients taking antiplatelet agents varies with the agent used and the surgical procedure. In general, bleeding risk increases when a patient receives two or more agents or when the agent is combined with another anticoagulant medication. Risks of perioperative bleeding must be weighed against the risk of thrombosis by withholding agents. It is important to note that several commonly used herbal supplements, including garlic, ginkgo, ginseng, and vitamin E, also are inhibitors of platelet function and should be discontinued at least 1 week prior to surgery. Qualitative platelet disorders also may be seen in various

Table 10.4. Classification and treatment of vWD

Type	Mechanism of disease	Treatment of choice
1	Partial quantitative deficiency of vWF (and factor VIII)	Desmopressin
2	Qualitative defects of vWF	
2A	Defective platelet-dependent vWF functions, associated with lack of larger multimers	Factor VIII–vWF concentrates
2B	Heightened platelet-dependent vWF functions, associated with lack of larger multimers	Factor VIII–vWF concentrates
2M	Defective platelet-dependent vWF functions	Factor VIII–vWF concentrates
2N	Defective vWF binding to factor VIII	Factor VIII–vWF concentrates
3	Severe or complete vWF deficiency and moderately severe factor VIII deficiency, *without* alloantibodies	Factor VIII–vWF concentrates
	Severe or complete vWF deficiency and moderately severe factor VIII deficiency, *with* alloantibodies	Recombinant factor VIII

Adapted from Soliman DE, Broadman LM. Coagulation defects. *Anesthesiol Clin* 2006; 24:549–578.

systemic conditions, including uremia, liver disease, myelodysplastic syndromes, and DIC. Finally, the reversible qualitative platelet dysfunction caused by cardiopulmonary bypass is a major cause of nonsurgical bleeding in cardiac surgery.

von Willebrand disease

von Willebrand disease (vWD) deserves special attention as it is relatively common, present in 1% to 2% of the general population. vWD arises from a qualitative or quantitative deficiency of vWF. This multimeric protein acts as an adhesive link between platelets and the injured blood vessel wall, as well as a carrier for factor VIII. Acquired forms of vWD are associated with lymphoproliferative disease, tumors, autoimmune disease, hypothyroidism, cardiac and valvular defects, and medications (e.g., valproic acid). The most common symptom is mucocutaneous bleeding, such as easy bruising, epistaxis, gingival bleeding, and menorrhagia. vWD should be considered in any patient with a history of unexplained postoperative bleeding. If vWD is suspected in a patient about to undergo an elective procedure, the case should be canceled until a proper hematologic workup is obtained. The mechanisms behind the various types of vWD, as well as their treatments, are shown in Table 10.4.

Clotting disorders
Inherited coagulation disorders
Hemophilias

The most common examples of an inherited coagulation disorder are the hemophilias, characterized by a partial or complete deficiency of a coagulant factor. The two most common are deficiencies in factors VIII and IX, corresponding to hemophilia A and B, respectively. Both diseases have X-linked recessive inheritance; therefore, males are far more commonly affected than females. Up to 50% of hemophilia cases appear de novo as a result of new mutations. Female carriers may actually behave as mild cases, as some have significantly reduced coagulation factors themselves, and obstetric anesthesiologists, in particular, should be aware of these.

Preoperatively, unexplained bruising or bleeding in young males or a positive family history usually indicates referral to a hematologist. Patients with hemophilia A or B usually demonstrate an isolated prolongation of activated partial thromboplastin time (aPTT), that is, normal prothrombin time (PT), thrombin clotting time, fibrinogen level, and platelet count. However, very mild cases may actually demonstrate a normal aPTT, and direct factor level measurements become necessary for diagnosis. Bleeding may occur anywhere, but the most common sites are into joints (80%) and muscles, as well as from the gastrointestinal tract. Bleeding severity relates to the degree of factor deficiency. For example, spontaneous bleeds occur in severe cases (<1% coagulant factor), whereas patients with moderate (1%–5%) and mild (>5%) factor deficiencies may bleed excessively only after trauma or surgery.

Treatment is aimed toward replacement of the specific coagulation factor. Historically, the use of plasma-derived coagulation factor concentrates tragically caused HIV and hepatitis C virus infections among thousands of hemophilia patients. Recombinant factor replacement is now available to minimize infectious disease exposure. Moreover, all coagulation factor concentrates are now required to undergo viral inactivation steps during manufacturing. Like products such as albumin, factor concentrates currently are considered to have zero risk of viral transmission.

Up to 30% of patients with severe hemophilia A may develop alloantibody inhibitors to factor VIII. In most cases, these patients cannot be treated using factor concentrates and must be managed using "bypass" agents, such as recombinant factor VIIa. Close consultation with a hematologist is mandatory.

Acquired coagulation disorders

Acquired inhibitors of coagulant factors

Another class of closely related bleeding disorders consists of the acquired inhibitors of coagulant factors, typically associated with autoimmune disorders, drug reactions, or the postpartum period. Elective surgery should be postponed until inhibitor formation is suppressed.

Vitamin K deficiency

A more common form of acquired bleeding disorder is deficiency of vitamin K, a compound necessary for the synthesis of factors II, VII, IX, and X, as well as the anticoagulant proteins C and S. Vitamin K consists of two subunits: vitamin K_1, found in green leafy vegetables, and vitamin K_2, synthesized by intestinal bacteria. Patients therefore can acquire vitamin K deficiencies by poor diet and/or by taking antibiotics that destroy intestinal bacteria. Biliary obstruction, malabsorption, cystic fibrosis, and resection of the small intestine also may contribute to vitamin K deficiency. The PT usually is prolonged first, as factor VII typically is depleted relatively early. Urgent treatment of vitamin K deficiency requires intravenous vitamin K, administered slowly to prevent hypotension. Improvement in coagulopathy usually is apparent 6 to 8 hours after administration.

Medications

A few commonly used medications act on the coagulation cascade in a similar manner. These systemic anticoagulants are used to prevent or treat thromboembolic complications and are recommended for an increasing number of medical conditions, including mechanical heart valves, atrial fibrillation, venous thromboembolism, acute MI, and stroke. A typical example is warfarin, which works by inhibiting vitamin K epoxide reductase, preventing vitamin K synthesis. Because warfarin is a highly protein-bound compound in the plasma, unintentional increases in anticoagulation may occur when warfarin is displaced by other protein-bound drugs.

Other drug interactions occur by medications inhibiting or activating the cytochrome P-450 system, as it is metabolized almost entirely by the liver. Rapid reversal can be accomplished by administration of fresh frozen plasma (FFP) and vitamin K. In urgent cases (e.g., intracerebral hemorrhage on warfarin), the infusion of prothrombin complex concentrate (PCC) should be considered. PCCs contain factors II, VII, IX, and X, and thus provide immediate replacement of factors that are deficient from warfarin therapy.

Unfractionated heparin acts by binding reversibly to antithrombin III, accelerating its inhibition of coagulation factors XII, XI, X, IX, plasmin, and thrombin. This effect can be reversed by administering protamine, although stopping the heparin infusion usually is adequate during a short period, as the half-life of heparin is <1 hour. Low molecular weight heparin (LMWH) also acts via antithrombin III but has a greater ability to inhibit factor Xa than thrombin. The half-life, in contrast, is longer, as LMWH can be given once daily as a maintenance dose. Two additional classes of anticoagulant medications are direct thrombin inhibitors, such as argatroban, and direct factor Xa inhibitors, such as fondaparinux.

Disorders of fibrinolysis

The typical example of a disorder of fibrinolysis is DIC, a consumptive coagulopathy characterized by inappropriate and widespread systemic activation of coagulation and excessive fibrinolysis, resulting in small vessel thrombosis and generalized bleeding. DIC also is associated with thrombocytopenia, elevated fibrin split products, and elevated D-dimers. Various triggers of DIC are shown in Fig. 10.3. Treatment primarily is supportive and aimed toward correcting the underlying cause.

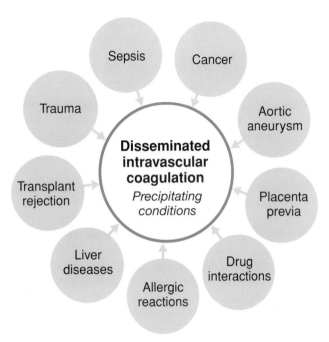

Figure 10.3. Conditions associated with DIC.

Theoretically, a key strategy to managing DIC is interruption of the coagulation process. Very rarely, the use of heparin is considered for this purpose – particularly for patients with overt thromboembolism or extensive deposition of fibrin. Treatment with FFP (to replace coagulation factors), cryoprecipitate (to replace fibrinogen), and platelet concentrates may be of value in the setting of diffuse bleeding.

Disorders of thrombosis

Most, if not all, cases of thromboembolism result from a convergence of underlying genetic predisposition and acquired precipitating events. Virchow's triad, consisting of altered blood flow (stasis), vascular endothelial injury, and altered blood constituents (inherited or acquired hypercoagulable states), provides a simplified model for venous thromboembolism.

Inherited hypercoagulable states are associated with venous rather than arterial thrombosis. These may be the result of increased prothrombotic protein activity or quantity (factor V Leiden, prothrombin gene mutation G20210A, or increased levels of factor VII, VIII, IX, or XI, or vWF) or from decreased activity or quantity of antithrombotic proteins (protein C, protein S, and antithrombin). Coagulation and anticoagulation proteins are consumed acutely during a thrombotic event, so testing should take place 2 to 3 weeks after the thrombotic event. Hypercoagulable laboratory workup typically includes a complete blood count, PT, partial thromboplastin time (PTT), fibrinogen, protein C assay, protein S antigen, anticardiolipin antibody, factor V Leiden assay, lupus anticoagulant panel, homocysteine assay, and functional antithrombin assay. Patients with suspected or documented hypercoagulable states are treated with warfarin for 6 months or until they are thrombosis-free for 2 months. Patients who develop a second thrombotic event or have other risk factors require long-term anticoagulation.

Acquired hypercoagulable states also are possible. The perioperative setting itself is associated with increased risk of thrombosis secondary to both an increased prothrombotic state and inhibition of fibrinolytic pathways. This is especially true for orthopedic, major vascular, neurosurgical, and oncologic procedures. Additional risk factors among surgical patients include age, previous thrombotic event, malignancy, thrombophilia longer surgery and immobilization times.

An additional acquired hypercoagulable state the clinician should be aware of is heparin-induced thrombocytopenia (HIT), a transient antibody-mediated, prothromboic disorder initiated by exposure to heparin. Diagnosis is made when HIT antibody formation is accompanied by an otherwise unexplained fall in platelet count (usually >50%) and/or by other clinical sequelae, such as thrombosis, skin lesions, or acute systemic reaction. Treatment for patients with suspected or confirmed HIT is cessation of heparin and initiation of non-heparin anticoagulants, such as direct thrombin inhibitors, to prevent thrombotic complications. LMWHs should be avoided, as they cross-react with HIT antibodies. Vigilance should be maintained in identifying and eliminating sources of heparin exposure, including heparin-coated lines and line and port flushes.

Autoimmune hypercoagulable states may be inherited or acquired. The two typical examples, anticardiolipin antibody and lupus anticoagulant, may result in venous or arterial thromboses, thrombocytopenia, and recurrent fetal losses. These autoantibodies usually occur in association with other autoimmune diseases but can occur independently. Patients with these disorders are at increased risk for developing ischemic and valvular heart disease, as well as recurrent cerebral infarcts, headaches, and visual disturbances. As such, these patients commonly receive chronic anticoagulation. Additional perioperative measures to decrease thrombotic risk include the use of elastic stockings and maintenance of normovolemia and normothermia. Additionally, because the autoantibodies inhibit phospholipid-dependent coagulation in vitro, heparin monitoring should be performed using whole-blood coagulation tests only (e.g., activated clotting time [ACT]).

Suggested readings

Brash PG, Cullen BF, Stoelting RK, eds. *Clinical Anesthesia.* 5th ed. Philadelphia: Lippincott Williams & Wilkins; 2006.

Firth PG. Anaesthesia for peculiar cells – a century of sickle cell disease. *Br J Anaesth* 2005; 95:287–299.

Lasne D, Jude B, Susen S. From normal to pathological hemostasis. *Can J Anesth* 2006; 53:S2–S11.

Levi M, Cate H. Disseminated intravascular coagulation. *N Engl J Med* 1999; 341:586–592.

Levy JH, Tanaka KA, Hursting MJ. Reducing thrombotic complications in the perioperative setting: an update on heparin-induced thrombocytopenia. *Anesth Analg* 2007; 105:570–580.

Madjdpour C, Spahn DR, Weiskopf RB. Anemia and perioperative red blood cell transfusion: a matter of tolerance. *Crit Care Med* 2006; 34:S102–S108.

Martlew VJ. Peri-operative management of patients with coagulation disorders. *Br J Anaesth* 2000; 85:446–455.

Oranmore-Brown C, Griffiths R. Anticoagulants and the perioperative period. *Cont Edu Anaesth Crit Care Pain* 2006; 66:156–159.

Park KW. Sickle cell disease and other hemoglobinopathies. *Int Anesthesiol Clin* 2004; 42:77–93.

Soliman DE, Broadman LM. Coagulation defects. *Anesthesiol Clin* 2006; 24:549–578.

Weiss G, Goodnough LT. Anemia of chronic disease. *N Engl J Med* 2005; 352:1011–1023.

The elderly patient

Ruma R. Bose and Sheila R. Barnett

The term *geriatric/elderly* generally is reserved for patients 65 years and older; however, this definition combines a large group of individuals with a wide range of abilities. Aging is an inevitable process producing measurable changes in the structure and function of tissues and organ systems. One of the main problems encountered by anesthesiologists when dealing with elderly patients is distinguishing the impact of age versus the effect of disease on organ function. The anesthesiologist is faced with the challenge of estimating the reserve capacity of vital organ systems and predicting the ability of the individual to deal with the stress of anesthesia and surgery.

Risk factors and the elderly

Although chronologic age per se is not a contraindication for surgery or anesthesia, elderly patients are at increased risk for adverse events following surgery. Certain factors are known to increase the risk associated with surgery in older patients. These include:

- Operative site: intra-abdominal and intrathoracic procedures are less well tolerated.
- Physical status at the time of surgery: preoperative stabilization is important. The presence of congestive heart failure, renal failure, or ischemic heart disease carries a higher risk of morbidity and mortality.
- Emergency surgery: this carries a poor prognosis.

Guidelines for treating geriatric patients

Elderly patients may be challenging to care for because of the tremendous heterogeneity within this age group. However, a few common themes arise that can help guide the care of the elderly patient:

- Clinical presentation of disease frequently is atypical, leading to delays and errors in diagnosis. This may result in a later presentation to the operating room, a more advanced disease condition, and greater likelihood of instability.
- Individuals over age 65 years have, on average, three or four medical diseases, often limiting function and increasing morbidity.

- Polypharmacy is a major issue in this population. Many older patients are on multiple medications that may affect the administration of anesthesia.
- Diminished organ reserve may be unpredictable, and even significant limitations may become apparent only during stressful events.
- The impact of extrinsic factors such as smoking, environmental factors, and socioeconomic status on physiologic age is difficult to quantify.
- Significant interindividual variability and heterogeneity exist in the aged population, making responses difficult to predict based on age alone.
- A disproportionate increase in perioperative risk may occur without adequate preoperative optimization, and adverse events are more frequent when cases are done on an emergent basis.
- Meticulous attention to detail may help avoid minor complications, which in elderly patients may rapidly escalate into major adverse events.

Aging and major organ systems
Cardiovascular system

Cardiovascular complications represent the primary source of perioperative complications in elderly patients. Preexisting cardiac conditions, such as coronary artery disease, hypertension, and abnormal left ventricular function, put the patient at risk for a postoperative cardiac event (Fig. 11.1).

The combined effects of these aging changes result in a decrease in compensatory response of the cardiovascular system to stress and hypotension. Elderly patients cannot compensate for hemodynamic fluctuations by altering heart rate, stroke volume, cardiac output, and oxygen delivery to the same extent as younger individuals, rendering them vulnerable to the side effects of anesthetic agents that alter hemodynamics and the consequences of surgery.

Pulmonary system

Perioperative pulmonary morbidity and mortality increase with age. There is a gradual decrease in pulmonary reserve, and it may be difficult to separate age-related changes from those

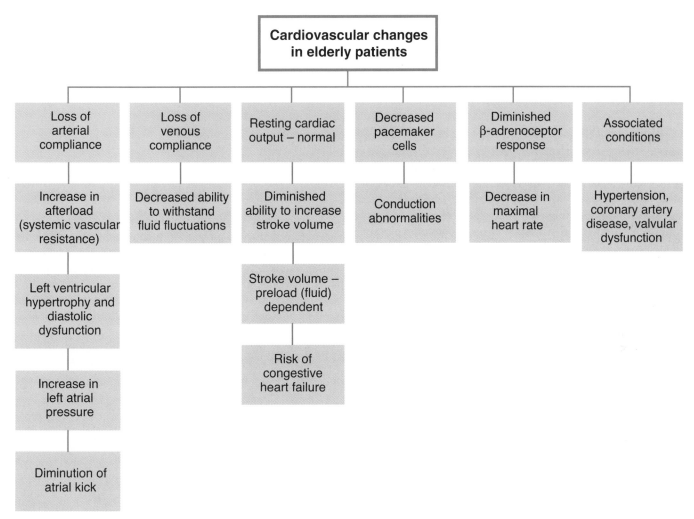

Figure 11.1. Cardiovascular (CV) changes in elderly patients. CO, cardiac output; SVR, systemic vascular resistance; SV, stroke volume; HR, heart rate; HTN, hypertension; CAD, coronary artery disease; LVH, left ventricular hypertrophy; CHF, congestive heart failure.

secondary to disease and environmental factors. The influences of prior smoking and environmental exposures are particularly difficult to distinguish from senescence (Table 11.1).

These mechanical changes are exacerbated by an aging central nervous system with diminished responsiveness to hypoxemia as well as to hypocapnia and hypercapnia. In addition, older patients exhibit increased sensitivity to opioid-induced blunting of the normal ventilatory response to hypercarbia. Residual anesthetic agents may further suppress these reflexes. Thus, older patients are more susceptible to developing hypoxia, making them unable to respond appropriately to hypoxemia and hypercarbia. In general, supplemental oxygen and close monitoring are required, especially in the immediate postoperative setting.

Central nervous system

There is continual neuronal loss with aging, which is more prominent in gray matter versus white. There is a gradual decline in cerebral metabolic rate, oxygen consumption, and cerebral blood flow. Decreases in neurotransmitter action of

Table 11.1. Changes in pulmonary functions in the elderly

FRC	↔
RV	↑
RV/total lung capacity	↑
Closing capacity	↑
Dead space	↑
Work of breathing	↑
V/Q mismatch	↑
FEV_1	↓
PaO_2	↓
$PaCO_2$	↔
HPV	↓
Thoracic wall compliance	↓
Alveolar elasticity	↓
Vital capacity	↓
Total lung capacity	↓
MBC	↓

FRC, functional residual capacity; RV, residual volume; V/Q, ventilation-perfusion; FEV_1, forced expiratory volume in the first second of expiration; HPV, hypoxic pulmonary vasoconstriction; MBC, maximal breathing capacity; ↑, increase; ↓, decrease; ↔, equivocal.

acetylcholine, dopamine, and serotonin may predispose older patients to delirium and increased sensitivity to effects of centrally acting medications. Simple pain thresholds rise with age, reflecting a reduction in end-organ pain neurons and peripheral deafferentation. However, central processing of pain and thalamic amplification probably remain normal.

Peripheral nervous system

Sensory changes occur and may lead to decreased visual acuity and increases in dark adaptation. Diminished hearing, particularly at the high frequencies above 10 kHz, has been observed. Attrition of taste buds, diminished ability to detect smell, and diminished thirst sensation have been noted and may lead to dehydration and orthostatic hypotension. Joint perception and vibration sense are compromised, contributing to an increased risk of falls. The risk of falls is exacerbated by the changes in the peripheral nervous system as well. Electrical conduction falls in both sensory and motor nerve pathways by about 2% to 3% per decade after adulthood, or approximately 0.15 m/sec/year. Peripheral neurogenic atrophy is common, resulting in decreased muscle strength and fine motor control. Aging also is accompanied by a progressive predominance of type 1 (slow-twitch) over type 2 (fast-twitch) muscle fibers.

These changes may lead to increased difficulty with balance and coordination following surgery, especially if the surgery involves a limb. Postoperatively, regional blockade may further distort the older patient's ability to balance or use crutches or walking aids. These may be important considerations when choosing the surgical setting (inpatient versus ambulatory) and the type of anesthesia (regional versus general).

Postoperative delirium, cognitive dysfunction, and stroke

Postoperative mental status changes are one of the events about which elderly patients are most concerned. Common postoperative mental status changes result from delirium, cognitive dysfunction, or perioperative stroke.

Delirium is an acute confusional state associated with fluctuating mental status and disorientation (Chapter 55). It may be accompanied by agitation or combative behavior. The incidence of postoperative delirium ranges from 5% to 50% and has been linked to numerous preexisting conditions and medications (Table 11.2). Delirium may manifest as postoperative agitation, and confusion may occur unexpectedly, usually appearing 1 to 4 days following surgery and often after an initial lucid period. Certain medications are associated with an increased incidence of delirium, including meperidine, benzodiazepines (especially lorazepam and diazepam), and medications with anticholinergic effects (diphenhydramine and atropine).

Initial management of delirium is supportive, addressing the ABCs: airway, breathing, and circulation. Once hemodynamic stability is assured, the next step is to search for an etiology. This requires a search for a physical illness, infection, or drug toxicity. Untreated pain is a common cause of agitation

Table 11.2. Causes of delirium

Advanced age
Preexisting dementia
Depression
Hypoxia, hypocarbia
Hypotension
Alcohol or sedative withdrawal
Impaired vision and hearing
Metabolic disturbances, e.g., hypo- and hypernatremia
Acute myocardial infarction
Infection
Emergency surgery

and confusion in the postoperative period and may go unrecognized in demented patients with communication problems. Opioids should be considered early in treatment, and haloperidol, in small doses, may be useful in treating acutely agitated elderly patients. Supportive measures include safety precautions such as rails and close supervision. The use of simple measures, such as provision of clocks, good daytime lighting, familiar photos, and personal objects, may help reorient older people facing a new environment and may improve their ability to cope. Postoperative delirium is associated with significant increases in length of stay, nursing home admission, and morbidity and mortality.

Postoperative cognitive dysfunction (POCD), in contrast to delirium, refers to subtle cognitive changes usually detected on neuropsychological testing after surgery. Early POCD is related to increasing age, increasing duration of anesthesia, a low level of education, a second operation, postoperative infection, and respiratory complications. Prolonged POCD (3 months) is associated only with increasing age. Patients with POCD at discharge have a higher mortality at 1 year after surgery. POCD continues to be investigated, and the role of anesthesia in the development of POCD is not yet fully understood. Potential mechanisms currently under investigation include, but are not limited to, exaggerated decline in central cholinergic function, perioperative hypoxia and hypotension, genetic predisposition, and abnormal stress response with prolonged hypercortisolemia.

Postoperative stroke is also a significant cause of altered mental status and morbidity following surgery. In general, the dramatic increase in cerebral arteriosclerosis observed with advanced age is associated with an increase in the incidence of stroke. The overall incidence of stroke is 1.5 times higher in individuals 65 to 74 years old, twice as high in patients 75 to 84 years old, and three times as high in patients aged 85 years or older compared with younger age groups. Perioperative stroke risk increases from 0.2% in patients less than 65 years of age to 3.4% in patients older than 80 years.

Renal system

As many as 30% of elderly patients have renal impairment prior to surgery, which predisposes them to acute tubular necrosis postoperatively (Table 11.3). Acute renal failure accounts for

Table 11.3. Renal changes in the elderly

Decrease in renal blood flow (mainly in cortex)
Variable decline in glomerular filtration rate
Decline in ADH response
Decrease in total body water
Decreased ability to conserve sodium
Diminished urine-concentrating ability (urine osmolarity declines from 1200 mOsm/kg at age 30 y to 900 mOsm/kg by age 80 y)
Decline in renin–aldosterone levels
Decreased thirst perception (dehydration)

ADH, antidiuretic hormone.

one-fifth of the postoperative deaths in the elderly. A steady decrease in glomerular filtration rate is accompanied by a decline in lean body mass. Thus, creatinine production declines, and seemingly normal creatinine values may not accurately reflect true renal function. Measuring creatinine clearance gives a more accurate idea of renal function.

Hepatic system

Aging is associated with a loss of functioning mass of hepatocytes. The decrease in drug metabolism parallels the loss of functional mass, but there is significant interindividual variation. Hepatic blood flow diminishes, leading to decreased clearance of drugs. Albumin production declines with age and is reduced further by malnutrition and chronic and acute diseases, which may result in an increase in the free portion of protein-bound drugs. Phase II metabolism appears to be unaltered.

Pharmacokinetic and pharmacodynamic changes

The administration of medications in the elderly is especially challenging. Older patients exhibit increased sensitivity to medications such as opioids and inhalational agents, and the effects may be prolonged because of delayed clearance and excretion (Table 11.4). In general, it is important to reduce the initial doses and increase the interval between repeated doses in older patients.

As a person ages, there is a decrease in total body water and an increase in fat reservoirs, leading to a decrease in the initial volume of distribution of water-soluble medications. A delay in intercompartmental clearance further affects the initial redistribution of drugs, potentially leading to a higher initial plasma concentration of medications such as propofol. Albumin levels tend to decrease with age; in addition, the quality of protein

Table 11.4. Elimination half-life of drugs

Drug	Young people	Older people
Fentanyl	4 h	15 h
Alfentanil	1.5 h	2 h
Diazepam	24 h	72 h
Midazolam	2.8 h	4.3 h
Vecuronium	16 min	45 min

binding deteriorates with advanced age. The decrease in plasma albumin increases the free fraction of the drugs, increasing the available concentration at the receptor site and causing a more profound effect. This becomes more important in drugs that are highly protein bound, such as barbiturates, benzodiazepines, and opioids. Reductions in liver blood flow and renal function lead to a prolonged duration of action of the drugs and their metabolites. The increase in body fat may act as a reservoir for lipid-soluble drugs, leading to prolonged duration and elimination half-life of lipophilic drugs, such as morphine.

In older patients, these changes may result in an increased potential to manifest adverse effects associated with medications. For instance, hypotension associated with propofol administration may be prolonged and increase the risk of ischemia in patients with underlying cardiac or cerebrovascular disease. Adverse events may be increased by polypharmacy, and in older patients it is advisable to minimize the number of different agents used when possible.

Anesthetic management

There is no "best" anesthetic for an elderly patient. In contrast to pediatric patients, in whom it is possible to make assumptions about anesthetic requirements based on age-specific physiologic changes, elderly patients are a heterogeneous population and chronologic age may not reflect the physiologic age. Older patients require a careful preoperative assessment for the presence of concomitant disease, medication use, and functional status, all of which will influence the choice of anesthesia.

Preoperative examination

The preoperative evaluation is critical for the safe administration of anesthesia to elderly patients. The goal of a preoperative assessment is to establish the baseline health and functional status of the patient, identify comorbid conditions, and determine whether further evaluation and optimization are required. Elderly patients have an average of three diseases after the age of 65 and are frequently on multiple medications, making the preoperative assessment especially challenging. Chronic pain, agitation, and dementia may prohibit the patient from lying still during the procedure, making a plan for deep sedation unfeasible, even if the procedure is minor. The early identification of patients requiring further investigation or those with special issues may help with advance planning and room scheduling.

The preoperative evaluation of patients with extensive medical histories may be very difficult in those with baseline dementia and memory loss, and every effort should be made to obtain prior medical records. A mental status examination should be considered for all geriatric surgical patients. Preoperative depression and alcohol abuse are relatively common and not always admitted by the patient or family, but these will increase the risk of delirium in the postoperative period. Frail older patients frequently need assistance postoperatively, and the plan for postoperative care should be discussed in advance with the patient and relevant relatives or caretakers.

As with all preoperative testing, requests for laboratory studies or further investigations should be directed by the history and a physical examination that includes a functional assessment. A baseline electrocardiogram (ECG) generally is indicated in women over the age of 55 years and men over 45 years. Further testing beyond the history and physical is determined by an assessment of the surgical procedure and the baseline comorbidities of the patient. For instance, a patient with significant cardiac morbidity about to undergo cataract surgery may not need further investigation, whereas a patient with fewer cardiac risk factors coming in for high-risk surgery will need a comprehensive cardiac evaluation.

Polypharmacy is a common occurrence in elderly patients, and a complete list of medications, including over-the-counter and alternative treatments, should be included in the preoperative assessment. It may be helpful to ask patients to bring all their medications to the preoperative clinic or on the day of surgery to lessen confusion regarding multiple prescriptions.

Intraoperative management

Premedication

A general principle when treating the geriatric patient is to avoid any unnecessary medications. Premedication should be administered carefully because of increased sensitivity to the drugs and a higher incidence of postoperative delirium. Midazolam is a popular benzodiazepine administered in the preoperative period. Older patients are more sensitive to the effects of midazolam; therefore, the starting dose may need to be reduced and the interval between supplemental doses increased. Anticholinergic agents such as diphenhydramine and scopolamine should be avoided because of increased incidence of delirium.

Induction

Profound hypotension may occur following the induction of general anesthesia in older patients. Several factors contribute to the development of hypotension, including a decreased volume of distribution for induction agents, leading to a more pronounced effect for the same dose. Hypovolemia also exaggerates this effect, especially in patients who are fasting, hypertensive, or on diuretics and those who have had bowel preparations.

Aging results in a diminished capacity to respond to hypotension because of blunting of the baroreceptor reflex, leading to a reduction in heart rate increases. This may be exacerbated by medications that further reduce the ability to respond to hypotension, such as β-blockers and angiotensin-converting enzyme inhibitors. Therefore, the dose of induction agent may need to be decreased, vasopressors should be readily available, and the interval between doses of repeated medications should be lengthened as necessary.

Drug administration

Benzodiazepines

Elderly patients exhibit increased central nervous system sensitivity to midazolam; therefore, a lower starting dose is recommended. Reduced hepatic microsomal oxidation and clearance result in an elimination half-life roughly twice that in younger patients. Longer-acting benzodiazepines, such as lorazepam and diazepam, have significantly prolonged action in the elderly and may lead to delirium and confusion; therefore, they should probably be avoided in this population.

Propofol

In the elderly, propofol has a smaller volume of distribution and initial target organ levels are higher, which may result in a greater degree of hypotension compared with other agents, because of vasodilatory effects. The initial redistribution likely also is slowed in the older patient, so dosing intervals should be increased; this is particularly true in patients with reduced cardiac output. The short duration of action and minimal side effects associated with propofol are advantageous in the older patient with baseline cognitive dysfunction and multiple comorbidities, provided the hypotension is tolerable. In general, the induction dose of propofol may need to be reduced by 25% to 50% and titrated slowly to effect.

Thiopental

Thiopental has a slower onset of action and causes a reduction in cardiac output in older patients. The dosage generally should be reduced 25% to 50% in the elderly. The elimination half-life is prolonged to almost 25 hours in older individuals, compared with 12 hours in younger patients. Thiopental should be used with caution in frail elderly patients with cardiac or renal disease.

Etomidate

Etomidate is a short-acting agent metabolized by ester hydrolysis. A rapid recovery and minimal cardiac depressant effects make it a useful agent in the elderly patient with multiple comorbidities, especially in the presence of hypovolemia. The 11-β-hydroxylase blockade caused by a single bolus of etomidate should be considered. Drug clearance is hepatic flow dependent and may be prolonged; thus the overall dose may need to be reduced.

Opioids

Aging is associated with increased sensitivity to opioid medications, resulting in a predisposition to respiratory depression and apnea. Hepatic metabolism is reduced, the volume of distribution generally is increased, and renal clearance of metabolites is reduced. As with other medications for the elderly, the dose of opioids should be reduced and the interval between doses prolonged.

Remifentanil, metabolized by plasma and tissue esterases, has an extremely short half-life. Its noncumulative nature offers advantages in the elderly patient, particularly in cases requiring sedation and in those with intense short periods of pain and stimulation. The clinician should be aware of the potential bradycardia associated with remifentanil administration, particularly in patients who already are β-blocked. Fentanyl has minimal cardiac side effects, although older patients exhibit increased sensitivity. In general, the dose should be reduced 50% and titrated slowly to effect. Morphine is longer acting, with active metabolites; thus, there may be increased risk of respiratory depression, as with all long-acting opioids.

Inhalational agents

The minimum alveolar concentration (MAC) of inhalational agents declines 4% every decade over age 40. By the age of 70 years, the MAC is reduced 20% to 30% compared with that of a younger subject. This may reflect an age-related loss of central nervous system reserve and a decrease in neurotransmitter levels. Cardiac effects of these agents, such as reduced myocardial contractility, are exaggerated in most elderly patients, especially those with already compromised cardiac function. Shorter-acting agents such as desflurane offer some advantages in the elderly, but there are no consistent data to support the use of one short-acting inhalational agent over another.

Muscle relaxants

Aging results in a decrease in muscle mass and strength, as well as a slowing in time and rate of relaxation, likely as the result of decreased rate and maximal speed of calcium uptake in the endoplasmic reticulum. The duration of action of nondepolarizing muscle relaxants is prolonged in the elderly because of slower hepatic metabolism and decreased renal clearance; however, this generally has little effect on the clinical administration of the medications. Agents that undergo Hoffman's degradation, such as atracurium and cisatracurium, are not affected by aging. Mivacurium, which is metabolized by plasma cholinesterase, can demonstrate a prolonged duration of action because of a decrease in the level of cholinesterase in frail elderly patients. The pharmacokinetics of depolarizing muscle relaxants are not affected by aging. Complete reversal of neuromuscular blockade is important to prevent adverse events associated with prolonged weakness in the recovery area. Tachycardia associated with anticholinergic medications such as glycopyrrolate may not be well tolerated in patients with underlying ischemic disease. Reducing the dosage or administration of short-acting β-blockers such as esmolol may offset the tachycardia.

Airway management

Elderly patients have diminished pharyngeal sensitivity and a loss of protective laryngeal reflexes, and are at increased risk from silent passive aspiration. Sedation and residual anesthetic drug effects may compound this risk. Establishment of an airway may be difficult in elderly patients. The factors that may complicate airway management include limited neck extension, advanced arthritis, increased vertebrobasilar insufficiency worsened by neck extension, and reduced mouth opening. Although the edentulous state can make intubation easier, it also can make mask ventilation much more difficult, and an oral airway may be required to achieve an adequate mask fit. Sympathetic response to laryngoscopy is exaggerated in elderly patients, and the resulting hypertension and tachycardia may be poorly tolerated by patients with underlying cardiac disease.

Regional anesthesia

Although anecdotal evidence suggests there may be significant advantages to spinal or epidural anesthesia over general anesthesia, there are few data to support a clear advantage in the elderly patient. Certain advantages that have been shown in patients undergoing epidural or spinal anesthesia include a reduction in the incidence of postoperative thrombosis, blood transfusion, and blood loss during orthopedic procedures. Age-related decreases in the clearance of local anesthetics and subsequent accumulation may predispose the older patient to toxicity. Lower doses of local anesthetics may be needed because nerve size and conduction are reduced with aging. The quantity of myelinated fibers is diminished in older patients, and by age 90, one third of myelinated fibers have disappeared.

Placement of regional techniques may be more difficult secondary to arthritis and calcification of spinal ligaments. Other comorbidities and chronic pain may restrict optimal positioning. Local anesthetics in the epidural and subarachnoid space ultimately are absorbed into the circulation, and the plasma concentration depends on their absorption, distribution, and elimination. With age there is a decrease in the size and compliance of the epidural space, and equivalent doses of local anesthetics may cause a higher level of sensory blockade in the elderly than in the younger individual. Elderly patients also tend to exhibit more dramatic decreases in blood pressure, and vasopressors should be immediately at hand to treat hypotension. Postdural puncture headaches are less common in elderly patients.

Positioning

Many elderly patients have characteristics that predispose them to accidental injury from seemingly benign positions. These factors include accelerated loss of subcutaneous and intramuscular fat, resulting in bony prominences requiring extra padding; demineralized long bones susceptible to fractures; atrophied skin tissues, leading to skin tears after tape and intravenous line placement; and, in general, slow healing. Vertebrobasilar insufficiency may predispose older patients to unexpected cerebral ischemia with neck extension during airway manipulation or positioning for surgery. Osteoarthritis and ankylosing spondylitis may limit optimal positioning during intubation and during placement of central neuraxial blockade.

Monitoring

Older patients need careful monitoring during and after anesthesia. The significant incidence of cardiovascular disease requires careful vigilance for ischemia and arrhythmias, and a five-lead ECG may offer more information than a basic three-lead ECG monitor. Similarly, elderly patients are at increased risk for hypoxemia, and continuous monitoring of oxygen saturation should be accompanied by end-tidal CO_2 monitoring for ventilation, even during simple monitored anesthesia cases. The ability to compensate for hemodynamic fluctuations is impaired in older patients, and an arterial line may be very useful for continuous monitoring. In general, more aggressive use of invasive monitoring should be considered.

Thermoregulation

Hypothermia is both more common and less well tolerated in the older frail patient. The normal thermoregulatory response to cold stress involves peripheral vasoconstriction, shivering, and eventual activation of brown fat metabolism. These mechanisms may be impaired in the elderly. The major age-related changes that predispose the elderly patient to hypothermia are a steady decline in basal metabolic rate, leading to reduced heat production, and a parallel increase in heat loss. Adverse effects from hypothermia include an increase in blood loss from platelet dysfunction and coagulopathies, myocardial ischemia, and poor wound healing. Active warming of the older patent should be performed both within the operating room and in the postoperative period.

Postoperative recovery

Some of the common problems facing the elderly during recovery are respiratory depression, delayed awakening from anesthesia, postoperative delirium, and inadequate pain management. Postoperative respiratory insufficiency is a common problem seen in the elderly and frequently is the result of residual effects of medications used intraoperatively. With advanced age, the respiratory response to hypoxia and hypercarbia is decreased, and this is exaggerated further by intraoperative use of opioids. Respiratory effort frequently is insufficient in frail older patients with weakened thoracic musculature, and the ability to cough and clear secretions is diminished. This predisposes patients to aspiration, atelectasis, and pneumonia. Lingering effects of anesthetics also increase postoperative respiratory insufficiency.

The accurate assessment of pain in the elderly may be difficult because of sedation, dementia, confusion, and delirium, which may result in under-treatment of pain. Regional techniques may be advantageous, minimizing the need for parenteral opioids. Nonopioid pain medications, such as the α_2-agonists (gabapentin) and acetaminophen, may be useful adjuncts and help reduce the dose of opioids. When opioids are used, careful monitoring and potentially reduced dosing should be considered. Patient-controlled analgesia offers significant advantages in the cognitively intact elderly patient. In more impaired patients, continual pain assessment and treatment are important.

Suggested readings

Ciccocioppo R, Candelli M, Di Francesco D, et al. Study of liver function in healthy elderly subjects using the 13C-methacetin breath test. *Aliment Pharmacol Ther* 2003; 17(2):271–277.

Cook DJ, Rooke GA. Priorities in perioperative geriatrics. *Anesth Analg* 2003; 96(6):1823–1836.

Dyer CB, Ashton CM, Teasdale TA. Postoperative delirium. A review of 80 primary data-collection studies. *Arch Intern Med* 1995; 155:461–465.

Fowler RD. Aging and lung function. *Age Ageing* 1985; 14(4): 209–215.

Franklin SS, Gustin WT, Wong ND, et al. Hemodynamic patterns of age-related changes in blood pressure: the Framingham Heart Study. *Circulation* 1997; 96:308–315.

Kam PCA, Calcroft RM. Peri-operative stroke in general surgical patients. *Anaesthesia* 1997; 52:879–883.

Khuri SF, Daley J, Henderson W, et al. The National Veterans Administration surgical risk study: risk adjustment for the comparative assessment of the quality of surgical care. *J Am Coll Surg* 1995; 180:519–531.

Kronenberg RS, Drage CW. Attenuation of the ventilatory and heart rate responses to hypoxia and hypercapnia with aging in normal men. *J Clin Invest* 1973; 52:1812–1819.

McDowell I, Kristjansson B, Hill GB, Hebert R. Community screening for dementia: the Mini Mental State Exam (MMSE) and Modified Mini-Mental State Exam (3MS) compared. *J Clin Epidemiol* 1997; 50:377–383.

Moller JT, Cluitmans P, Rasmussen LS, et al. Long-term postoperative cognitive dysfunction in the elderly ISPOCD1 study. ISPOCD investigators. International Study of Post-Operative Cognitive Dysfunction. *Lancet* 1998; 351(9106):857–861.

Monk TG, Weldon BC, Garvan CW, et al. Predictors of cognitive dysfunction after noncardiac surgery. *Anesthesiology* 2008; 108(1):18–30.

Muravchick S. Central nervous system. In: Craven L, ed. *Geroanesthesia: Principles for Management of the Elderly Patient.* St. Louis: Mosby; 1997:78–113.

Redfield MM, Jacobsen SJ, Borlaug BA, et al. Age- and gender-related ventricular-vascular stiffening: a community-based study. *Circulation* 2005; 112(15):2254–2262.

Schnegg M, Lauterburg BH. Quantitative liver function in the elderly assessed by galactose elimination capacity, aminopyrine demethylation and caffeine clearance. *J Hepatol* 1986; 3(2):164–171.

Seymour DG, Vaz FG. A prospective study of elderly general surgical patients: II. post-operative complications. *Age Ageing* 1989; 18:316–326.

Chapter 12

Neurologic diseases and anesthesia

Spiro G. Spanakis, John Lin, and Pankaj K. Sikka

Patients with neurologic disease require special consideration and preparation in the perioperative period. Preoperatively, the current status of the patient's disease must be assessed and optimized, if possible. Medications should be reviewed and a plan established for their administration or discontinuation in the perioperative period. Regional anesthesia may be used in patients with certain neurologic diseases, but in others it may exacerbate their disease or be contraindicated. Consent for surgery and anesthesia may need to be obtained from a health care proxy if associated cognitive impairment is present.

Intraoperatively, a plan for neuromuscular blockade for endotracheal intubation and maintenance must be established. Patients with neurologic disease may exhibit an atypical response to nondepolarizing and depolarizing muscular blockers. Outward manifestations of neurologic disease may include motor and sensory deficits, but autonomic dysfunction also may be present.

Postoperatively, patients may exhibit impaired respiratory function leading to respiratory insufficiency in the recovery room, an exacerbation of their sensory or motor symptoms, or impaired cognitive function that may interfere with recovery from anesthesia.

Cerebrovascular disease

Cerebrovascular disease is usually manifested as transient ischemic attacks (TIAs) or stroke. TIAs are defined as facial or extremity weakness and speech problems lasting <24 hours. Patients with TIAs should undergo further neurologic evaluation, because they are prone to developing stroke. Presence of a carotid bruit may or may not be associated with significant carotid disease. Following a stroke, elective surgery should be deferred for at least 2 to 3 months, to allow resolution of regional blood flow abnormalities and CO_2 responsiveness.

Preoperatively, patients with stroke should undergo detailed neurologic and cardiac evaluation. Strokes may be thrombotic, embolic, or hemorrhagic. Thrombotic strokes usually occur in elderly patients with coronary artery disease (atherosclerosis), hypertension, or diabetes mellitus. Embolic (air, calcium debris, fat, fibrin) strokes usually are associated with valvular heart surgery. Hemorrhagic strokes are the result of intracranial hemorrhage due to hypertension, cerebral aneurysm rupture, or arteriovenous malformation. Patients (except those with

hemorrhagic strokes) are usually on warfarin, aspirin, or dipyridamole therapy. These drugs may need to be stopped preoperatively.

Intraoperatively, patients with stroke should have a smooth induction with avoidance of succinylcholine, as denervation of the muscles may lead to a hyperkalemic response. Blood pressure should be maintained at a level higher than normal because of the rightward shift of cerebral autoregulation. Neuromuscular blockade should be monitored on the normal extremity, as the affected extremity may show an exaggerated response to nerve stimuli and thus an underestimation of the degree of blockade.

Use of shorter-acting anesthetic agents may be beneficial for faster recovery and assessment of neurologic function postoperatively. Adequate pain and blood pressure control and avoidance of hyperglycemia should be the goal. Risk of postoperative stroke for nonneurologic surgery is estimated to be about 0.25%. Risk of stroke is higher in patients undergoing neurologic and cardiovascular surgery and those with prolonged hypotension or hypertension. Hypotension may result in cerebral hypoperfusion, which may cause thrombosis and infarction. Sustained hypertension may disrupt the blood–brain barrier and cause intracranial hemorrhage.

Seizure disorders

Seizures are either idiopathic or the result of a central nervous system disorder. Recurrent paroxysmal seizures are termed *epilepsy*. Seizures occur because of abnormal brain electrical activity and may result from decreased inhibitory neurotransmitter activity (γ-aminobutyric acid), increased excitatory neurotransmitter activity (glutamic acid), or increased neuronal firing.

Seizure activity may be focal or generalized in the brain. Seizures may be classified as generalized (grand mal or tonic–clonic), petit mal (staring or repeated blinking of the eyes), or partial (simple or complex to varying degrees). Tonic–clonic seizures are characterized by tonic motor activity (30 seconds), followed by a clonic (jerking) phase, with or without loss of consciousness. When accompanied with loss of consciousness, they are termed *grand mal seizures*. *Status epilepticus* is defined as two consecutive tonic–clonic seizures without regaining consciousness, or seizure activity for 30 minutes or longer.

Patients presenting for surgery with a history of seizures should be asked about the type of seizures they have, medications they are taking, and the frequency of seizures. Seizures, if not idiopathic, may occur as a result of head injury, stroke, cranial tumors, metabolic abnormalities (hypoglycemia, uremia), or drug toxicity. Antiseizure medications should be continued until surgery, and may even have to be supplemented intraoperatively.

Intraoperatively, antiseizure medications decrease the duration of neuromuscular blockade. Antiseizure medications cause hepatic microsomal enzyme induction. Potentially epileptogenic medications such as enflurane, methohexital, and ketamine should be avoided. It is important to remember that atracurium is metabolized to laudanosine, and meperidine to normeperidine, which have epileptogenic potential.

Postoperatively, antiseizure medications should be restarted as soon as possible. Seizures are more likely to occur during the postoperative period. Grand mal seizures should be treated aggressively. Management includes maintaining the airway to prevent hypoxia and administering intravenous drugs such as midazolam (2–5 mg), diazepam (5–10 mg), thiopental (75–125 mg), or propofol (50–75 mg) to control the seizure. Phenytoin (500–1000 mg) is often administered for prevention of additional seizures.

Autonomic dysfunction

Autonomic dysfunction is usually seen in disorders of the central or peripheral nervous system, such as diabetes mellitus, chronic alcoholism, multiple sclerosis, syringomyelia, and spinal cord injury. Common manifestations of autonomic dysfunction are summarized in Table 12.1.

Intraoperatively, these patients manifest hypotension, which may cause coronary and cerebral hypoperfusion. Vasodilatory effects of general anesthetic agents and epidural and spinal anesthesia are poorly tolerated. Patients with severe hemodynamic instability should be observed with invasive arterial blood pressure monitoring. These patients are usually hypovolemic and tolerate blood loss poorly. Management consists of treatment of hypotension, preferably with direct-acting vasopressors; fluid administration; and maintenance of normothermia.

Alzheimer's disease

Alzheimer's disease is characterized by irreversible impairment of cognitive function, memory disturbances, and difficulty maintaining and sustaining attention. Progressive

Table 12.1. Common manifestations of autonomic dysfunction

Orthostatic hypotension
Bladder dysfunction
Gastrointestinal dysfunction
Lacrimation and salivation
Decreased sweating

degeneration of cholinergic neurons in the cortex, amygdala, and hippocampus results in marked cortical atrophy. Patients also may experience gait and motor disturbances, seizures, or myoclonus, eventually leading to apraxia and aphasia later in the disease course.

Outpatient pharmacologic therapy of the disease is aimed at slowing disease progression and delaying the onset of symptoms and apraxia. Tacrine, donepezil, and rivastigmine are cholinesterase inhibitors used to treat the disease and should be continued in the perioperative period. Tacrine induces down-regulation of postsynaptic acetylcholine receptors, and patients may exhibit altered responses to nondepolarizing blocking agents. Donepezil blocks acetylcholine hydrolysis and therefore exaggerate depolarizing blockade by succinycholine. Anticholinergics (except glycopyrrolate, which does not cross the blood–brain barrier) may exacerbate symptoms in the postoperative period, giving rise to confusion and cognitive dysfunction.

Preoperatively, patients may be disoriented and uncooperative, so a health care proxy should give consent for all procedures. Regional anesthesia may be used only if the patient can remain cooperative. Premedication should be minimized and short-acting agents used when possible for sedation and analgesia.

Recent research shows that general anesthetics induce long-lasting neurotoxicity (at the molecular level) and cognitive dysfunction in animal models. For example, desflurane increases β-amyloid production in human neuroglioma cells. β-amyloid plaques have been implicated in the pathogenesis of Alzheimer's disease; however, the implications of these studies for clinical practice have yet to be determined.

Parkinson's disease

Parkinson's disease affects individuals between the ages of 50 and 70 years and is an important cause of perioperative morbidity. Apoptosis of the dopaminergic neurons in the substantia nigra of the basal ganglia gives rise to thalamic and brainstem nuclei inhibition, resulting in suppression of the motor cortex. Excessive thalamic inhibition results in suppression of the cortical motor system, leading to akinesia, cogwheel rigidity, and tremor, whereas inhibition of brainstem locomotor areas contributes to abnormalities of posture and gait. Intellectual function is preserved early in the disease course.

Three classes of drugs are used to treat Parkinson's disease; they provide symptomatic relief because no cure exists. Dopamine agonists include bromocriptine, pergolide, ropinirole, pramipexole, and cabergoline. Levodopa (a metabolic precursor of dopamine) administered with carbidopa (which inhibits peripheral breakdown of dopamine) also is commonly used. Early use may be associated with a quicker onset of bradykinesia, so therapy sometimes is delayed in the disease course. The type B monoamine oxidase inhibitor selegiline, which prolongs the action of dopamine in the striatum, also may be used.

Autonomic instability manifesting as hypotension or hypertension may be related to treatment with levodopa or may be a result of the disease process itself. Other side effects of levodopa therapy include orthostatic hypotension, cardiac irritability, and nausea and vomiting. Dopamine agonists also may precipitate hypotension. Drug interactions with meperidine, serotonergic drugs, and catecholamines also must be considered in any patient on monoamine oxidase inhibitors. Anticholinergic drugs and antihistamines may be used during acute exacerbation of symptoms.

Preoperatively, a thorough history and physical examination should be performed, focusing on specific areas commonly affected by Parkinson's disease. A history of orthostatic hypotension, cardiac arrhythmias, hypotension, hypertension, autonomic dysfunction, and impaired temperature regulation should be identified. Existing respiratory impairment should be assessed, along with a history of pharyngeal muscle dysfunction and dysphagia and the degree of muscle rigidity. History of gastrointestinal reflux and nutritional and mental status also should be assessed (Table 12.2).

Medications should be continued until the day of surgery, but the side effects must be appreciated during the administration of anesthesia. Because the half-life of levodopa is short (1–3 hours), interruption of therapy may result in severe muscle rigidity that interferes with ventilation or in the development of parkinsonism hyperpyrexia syndrome, which is the result of an acute suppression of central dopaminergic activity. Intravenous levodopa has been used during the perioperative period, although it may result in side effects such as hypertension, hypotension, and dysrhythmias. Also, a rapid sequence induction may be indicated in patients with delayed gastric emptying, who are at increased risk for pulmonary aspiration.

Table 12.2. Assessment of the patient with Parkinson's disease

System	Assessment by history
Head and neck	Pharyngeal muscle dysfunction Dysphagia Sialorrhea Blepharospasm
Respiratory	Respiratory impairment from rigidity or bradykinesia
Cardiovascular	Orthostatic hypotension Cardiac arrhythmias Hypertension Hypovolemia Autonomic dysfunction
Gastrointestinal	Weight loss Poor nutrition Susceptibility to reflux
Urologic	Difficulty in micturition
Endocrine	Abnormal glucose metabolism (selegiline)
Central nervous system	Muscle rigidity, akinesia, tremor, confusion, depression, hallucination, speech impairment

Adapted from Rudra A, Rudra P, Chatterjee S. Parkinson's disease and anaesthesia. *Indian J Anaesth* 2007; 51(5):382–388.

Table 12.3. Neurologic disease and neuromuscular blocking agents

Disease	Depolarizing neuromuscular blockade	Nondepolarizing neuromuscular blockade
Alzheimer's disease	No disease-related contraindication	Prolonged effect in patients on donepezil receiving atracurium
Parkinson's disease	Single case report of hyperkalemia	No disease-related contraindication or altered response
Huntington's disease	Decreased plasma cholinesterase may lead to prolonged response	Increased sensitivity
ALS	Vulnerable to hyperkalemia after administration	Prolonged response
MS	Avoid if paresis or paralysis is present	Prolonged response possible
GBS	Contraindicated	Prolonged response possible
Neurofibromatosis	Increased sensitivity	Increased sensitivity

Dopamine antagonists such as metoclopramide, phenothiazines, and butyrophenones should not be given, because they may cause extrapyramidal symptoms. Because Parkinson's disease may result in autonomic insufficiency, hemodynamic instability and altered response to vasopressors sometimes are seen during anesthesia. Patients with Parkinson's disease exhibit a normal response to nondepolarizing muscle blockade. There is only an isolated report in the literature of hyperkalemia following succinylcholine administration, although other factors probably contributed to the incident. Alterations in the response to neuromuscular blocking agents in neurologic diseases are summarized in Table 12.3.

There are no reports of adverse responses to modern inhalational gases such as isoflurane, sevoflurane, and desflurane. Ketamine has been reported to potentiate sympathomimetic properties of levodopa, whereas morphine, alfentanil, and fentanyl have been reported to exacerbate muscle rigidity. Regional anesthesia may have some potential advantages over general anesthesia, such as avoidance of neuromuscular blockers and manipulation of the airway. No data from randomized controlled trials exist that can point to the best anesthetic technique. During the postoperative period, these patients are susceptible to symptom exacerbation, aspiration, respiratory failure, and mental confusion.

Huntington's disease

Huntington's disease is an autosomal dominant disease characterized by the triad of choreiform movements, progressive dementia, and personality changes, with an onset age of 35 to 40 years. The mechanism of the disease involves marked atrophy of the basal ganglia, particularly the caudate nucleus and globus pallidus.

There is no cure for the disease, and treatment is symptomatic. Haloperidol is used to decrease choreoathetoid movements by nonselectively antagonizing dopamine receptors. Fluphenazine also may relieve chorea, hallucinations, and delusions.

Preoperatively, the history and physical examination should focus on symptoms of dysphagia, because pharyngeal muscle dysfunction, common in this disease, increases the risk of aspiration in the perioperative period. Dysphagia also leads to malnutrition and cachexia.

Sodium thiopental has been implicated in prolonged apnea in afflicted patients if used at dosages >3 to 5 mg/kg. Decreased plasma cholinesterase levels may lead to a prolonged response after succinylcholine administration. These patients also may exhibit prolonged responses to nondepolarizing muscle relaxants.

Amyotrophic lateral sclerosis

Amyotrophic lateral sclerosis (ALS) is a degenerative disease of the motor ganglia in the anterior horn of the spinal cord and the spinal pyramidal tracts, resulting in upper and lower motor neuron dysfunction. Weakness and atrophy of respiratory muscles eventually result in respiratory failure and death.

Preoperatively, the severity of the disease may be assessed by spirometry. Patients with ALS exhibit reduced vital capacity with adequate gas exchange until late in the course of the disease. These effects are exacerbated further by general anesthesia. Successful epidural analgesia has been described in these patients, whereas there have been reports of neurologic sequelae in patients receiving spinal anesthesia.

Patients with ALS exhibit a prolonged response to nondepolarizing muscular blockade. Depolarizing agents induce hyperkalemia and therefore should be avoided. Bulbar involvement may occur, with resulting dysphagia and increased risk of pulmonary aspiration. Autonomic dysfunction also may be present, giving rise to orthostatic hypotension and a resting tachycardia.

Multiple sclerosis

Multiple sclerosis (MS) is an autoimmune disorder characterized by a progressive demyelination of the brain and spinal cord. Women are affected twice as often as men, with an onset of disease between the ages of 20 and 40 years. There are several categories of the disease, the most common being relapsing–remitting MS, eventually resulting in gradual neurologic deterioration.

Exacerbations of MS are characterized by paresthesias, visual problems, and motor weakness. Visual disturbances result from optic neuritis and diplopia. Only symptomatic treatment is available with a variety of drug classes, including corticosteroids, used for acute relapses. History of steroid use should be obtained in the preoperative evaluation, because patients may have received high doses for an extended period, resulting in adrenal insufficiency later. Other drugs used include interferon-β, glatiramer acetate, intravenous immunoglobulin, methotrexate, and cyclophosphamide.

Patients with MS exhibit varied responses to general anesthesia. An exacerbation of their symptoms may be expected in the postoperative period in general. When indicated, peripheral nerve blocks and epidural anesthesia may be used, spinal anesthesia is somewhat controversial, with limited evidence of either safety or harm. Autonomic dysfunction also may be present late in the disease. If paresis or paralysis is present, depolarizing muscle blockade should be avoided. Patients with MS may exhibit a prolonged response to depolarizing neuromuscular blockade and should be monitored if these drugs are administered to them. Intraoperatively, hyperthermia should be avoided because it may exacerbate symptoms.

Guillain-Barré syndrome

Guillain-Barré syndrome (GBS), an acute demyelinating polyneuropathy, usually occurs after a viral illness, resulting in ascending motor paralysis. Bulbar involvement may occur, resulting in respiratory failure requiring ventilatory support in an otherwise healthy person. GBS also may present in pregnancy.

GBS associated with pregnancy results in an increased need for ventilatory support and an increased risk of maternal mortality. Regional anesthesia has been used for labor but may exacerbate neurologic symptoms. This risk must be weighed against the risks of general anesthesia in pregnant patients.

Neurofibromatosis

Neurofibromatosis is a progressive autosomal dominant disorder involving multiple organ systems. The airway may be compromised if neurofibromas are present in the cervical, laryngeal, or mediastinal regions. Intracranial tumors may be the presenting diagnosis in the perioperative period. Intellectual function also is compromised with disease progression. The endocrine system may be involved, and patients may present with pheochromocytomas, carcinoid tumors, medullary thyroid carcinoma, or hyperparathyroidism. Spinal neurofibromas may complicate or contraindicate spinal anesthesia.

Syringomyelia

Syringomyelia is thought to occur as the result of obstruction of the cerebrospinal fluid outflow from the fourth ventricle. The increased pressure causes dilation and cavitation of the spinal cord, leading to neurologic symptoms. Most commonly, the cervical spine is affected, causing sensory and motor deficits in the upper extremities. Associated craniovertebral anomalies, including Arnold-Chiari malformation and thoracic scoliosis, are common.

These patients typically present to the operating room for decompressive procedures, including ventricular–peritoneal shunting. Respiratory function should be assessed preoperatively and any neurologic deficits documented. Patients may have increased sensitivity to neuromuscular blocking drugs because of the presence of muscle wasting.

Autonomic hyperreflexia

Autonomic hyperreflexia is a reaction caused by hyperstimulation of the autonomic nervous system. In the United States, the reported prevalence of this syndrome in individuals with spinal cord injuries at the T6 level and above is 48% to 90%. Although it commonly occurs in patients with spinal cord injuries above T6, patients with a spinal cord injury at T6 through T10 also may be susceptible. Autonomic hyperreflexia syndrome is manifested by systemic hypertension, bradycardia, sweating, and flushing of the skin. If not treated promptly, it may lead to seizures, stroke, myocardial infarction, and death.

Causes and triggering factors

The most common cause of autonomic hyperreflexia is spinal cord injury above the T6 level. Other causes include effects of cocaine and amphetamines, GBS, and severe head trauma.

Distention of a hollow viscus such as the rectum or bladder is the most common triggering stimulus (Table 12.4). However, the reflex may occur from any endogenous or exogenous stimulus occurring below the level of the cord lesion. Tactile or thermal skin stimulation, decubitus ulcers, labor contractions, and urinary tract infections also have been reported precipitants of this syndrome. Although most incidences occur in the operating room, it is important for the anesthesiologist to consider other causes in the postoperative period following recovery from regional or general anesthesia. The differential diagnosis of autonomic hyperreflexia also includes carcinoid syndrome, thyroid storm, neuroleptic malignant syndrome, pheochromocytoma. and toxemia of pregnancy.

Symptoms and signs

Autonomic hyperreflexia is seen only after resolution of spinal shock (loss of sensation and reflexes below the level of injury, flaccid paralysis) and return of spinal cord reflexes. This period of "postacute spinal cord injury" begins approximately 1 to 3 weeks after initial injury and remains for the duration of the patient's life. Symptoms of autonomic hyperreflexia often are divided between symptoms seen above versus below the level of spinal cord transection (Table 12.5).

In addition, some patients may experience difficulty breathing, changes in body temperature, and muscle spasms.

Table 12.4. Triggering factors of autonomic hyperreflexia – below the level of injury

Bladder distention (most common) – blockage of urinary catheter, infection, stones
Bowel distention – constipation, gas, digital stimulation, anal fissures
Pregnancy – labor and delivery
Miscellaneous – skin irritants, wounds, burns, appendicitis and other infections

Table 12.5. Symptoms and signs of autonomic hyperreflexia

Above the lesion	Below the lesion
Bradycardia (vagal stimulation)	Hypertension (severe)
Nasal stuffiness	Mesenteric ischemia, abdominal pain
Cutaneous flushing	Cold skin, vasoconstriction
Headache, blurred vision, seizures, aphasia	Acute renal failure
Cerebral and retinal hemorrhage	
Dysrhythmias, pulmonary edema	

Associated morbidity includes cerebral and subarachnoid hemorrhage, retinal hemorrhage, seizures, and pulmonary edema secondary to left ventricular failure. Spinal cord lesions at or above T6 generally result in intense manifestation of the syndrome, whereas lesions between T6 and T10 result in mildly elevated blood pressure with few other associated symptoms. Lesions below T10 generally do not result in hypertensive changes with compensatory reflex responses. Systolic blood pressure elevations >15 to 20 mm Hg above baseline in adults or children with spinal cord injuries may be significant enough to warrant consideration of autonomic hyperreflexia syndrome.

Pathophysiology of the reflex

Cutaneous sensory endings, as well as mucosal and muscle afferent pathways of hollow organs, ascend in the spinothalamic tracts and dorsal columns. Motor outflow reflexes occur via sympathetic inputs in the spinal cord lateral horns, which target blood vessels and viscera. In patients without spinal cord injury, this reflex is normally inhibited by outflow from higher central nervous system centers. However, in the presence of spinal cord transection, this inhibitory outflow fails to reach back to the effector organs innervated by spinal cord roots below the level of transection. Essentially, the sympathetic nervous system below the level of spinal cord injury becomes functionally isolated from all inhibiting (parasympathetic) influences of the brainstem and hypothalamus (Fig. 12.1).

Stimulation below the level of spinal cord injury elicits a vasoconstrictive response in the splanchnic sympathetic outflow (T5–L2). The carotid and aortic arch sinus baroreceptors detect this intense hypertension. As expected, a reflex bradycardia via the intact cranial nerve X (vagus) pathway ensues. In addition, the stimulation of afferent pathways (sympathetic) from these receptors to the vasomotor center in the medulla results in vasodilation (parasympathetic) above the level of cord injury. This vasodilation may help to correct the hypertension elicited by the sympathetic outflow; but in patients exhibiting autonomic hyperreflexia, this compensatory response is inadequate and systemic hypertension with associated symptoms persists.

Prevention and treatment

Preventive measurements are important considerations in managing patients with the potential for developing autonomic hyperreflexia. Application of topical anesthesia to the bladder

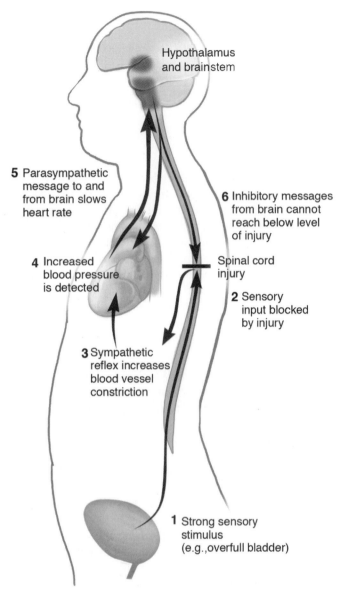

5 Parasympathetic message to and from brain slows heart rate

6 Inhibitory messages from brain cannot reach below level of injury

4 Increased blood pressure is detected

Spinal cord injury

2 Sensory input blocked by injury

3 Sympathetic reflex increases blood vessel constriction

1 Strong sensory stimulus (e.g.,overfull bladder)

Hypothalamus and brainstem

Figure 12.1. The autonomic reflex arc.

or rectal mucosa may be helpful in patients undergoing bladder or rectal instrumentation. Unfortunately, this technique is unreliable because the underlying muscular layer proprioceptors are not anesthetized. Spinal anesthesia (preferable) or epidural anesthesia is a reliable technique for preventing autonomic hyperreflexia during surgical operations of the lower abdomen, pelvis, and lower extremities. Alternatively, general anesthesia may be used if spinal or epidural anesthesia is not indicated, to prevent autonomic hyperactivity in these types of surgeries. It is important to remember that administration of succinylcholine ≥24 hours after spinal cord transection may

cause hyperkalemia. Injuries to the phrenic nerve or diaphragmatic innervation (C3–5) may require endotracheal intubation and ventilatory support. Maintenance of body temperature is of primary importance in patients with spinal cord transection. Because of immobility, patients with chronic spinal cord transection may develop muscle atrophy, decubitus ulcers, osteoporosis, deep vein thrombosis, or chronic urinary tract infections, with renal failure being the most common cause of death.

Among pregnant patients with spinal cord lesions above T6, the risk of developing autonomic hyperreflexia is about 80% to 90%, especially during labor. Autonomic hyperreflexia can be prevented in pregnant patients during childbirth by using spinal or epidural anesthesia. It is important to differentiate autonomic hyperreflexia (hypertension may occur with uterine contractions) from preeclampsia of pregnancy.

Removal of the inciting stimulus is important in terminating the reflex. This may be all that is needed for the reflex to subside. If the suspected cause is urinary blockage, the catheter should be checked for any kinks or blockage. Pharmacologic treatment of hypertension includes drugs such as sodium nitroprusside, nitroglycerin, nifedipine, hydralazine, and prazosin or clonidine for recurrent or chronic episodes. Bradycardia may be treated with anticholinergics. Men with spinal cord injuries and erectile dysfunction should be questioned about the use of sildenafil, as profound hypotension may occur with the administration of nitrates.

Suggested readings

Baraka A. Epidural meperidine for control of autonomic hyperreflexia in a paraplegic parturient. *Anesthesiology* 1985; 62:688–690.

Broecker BH, Hranowsky N, Hackler RH. Low spinal anesthesia for the prevention of autonomic dysreflexia in the spinal cord injury patient. *J Urol* 1979; 122:366.

Claydon VE, Elliott SL, Sheel AW. Cardiovascular responses to vibrostimulation for sperm retrieval in men with spinal cord injury. *J Spinal Cord Med* 2006; 29(3):207–216.

Hambly PR, Martin B. Anaesthesia for chronic spinal cord lesions. *Anaesthesia* 1998; 53(3):273–289.

Karlsson AK. Autonomic dysreflexia. *Spinal Cord* 1999; 37(6): 383–391.

Kewalramani LS. Autonomic dysreflexia in traumatic myelopathy. *Am J Phys Med* 1980; 59:1–21.

Lambart DH, Deane RS, Mazuzan JE. Anesthesia and the control of blood pressure in patients with spinal cord injury. *Anesth Analg* 1982; 61:344–348.

Naftchi NE, Richardson JS. Autonomic dysreflexia: pharmacological management of hypertensive crises in spinal cord injured patients. *J Spinal Cord Med* 1997; 20(3):355–360.

National Guideline Clearinghouse. Acute management of autonomic dysreflexia. *J Spinal Cord Med* 1997; 20(3):284–308.

Chapter 13

Anesthetic considerations in psychiatric diseases

Houman Amirfarzan and Pankaj K. Sikka

Each year, about 44 million people in the United States experience a mood or psychological disorder ranging from mild to severe mental illness. Patients on medications often present for surgery; therefore, it is important for the anesthesiologist to be aware of any drug interactions that may occur perioperatively.

Mood disorders

The *Diagnostic and Statistical Manual of Mental Disorders*, 4th edition (DSM-IV), divides mood disorders into the following categories: major depression, bipolar I, bipolar II, dysthymic, cyclothymic, disorders due to general medical conditions, those due to substance abuse, and depressive, bipolar, and mood disorders not otherwise specified.

Depression

Depression is characterized by persistent depressed mood, loss of interest, sleep disorder, fatigue, difficulty concentrating, and recurrent thoughts of death or suicide. Symptoms should cause significant impairment and not be the result of substances or bereavement. The exact mechanism of depression is not known but is believed to be the result of deficiency of catecholamines (dopamine [D_2], serotonin, or norepinephrine [NE]) in the brain. Therefore, pharmacologic treatment is directed toward increasing the concentrations of these catecholamines in the brain (Fig. 13.1). Electroconvulsive therapy (discussed in Chapter 96) is reserved for severe depression, refractory cases, or depression with suicidal ideation.

Brain catecholamine concentration may be increased by inhibiting (1) the reuptake of the catecholamines back into the cell (reuptake inhibitors) or (2) catecholamine metabolism, by inhibiting the enzyme monoamine oxidase. Commonly used drugs are the selective serotonin reuptake inhibitors (SSRIs), tricyclic antidepressants (TCAs), monoamine oxidase inhibitors (MAOIs), and miscellaneous other drugs.

The first line of treatment for major depressive disorder is a regimen consisting of antidepressant drugs, with four main categories: TCAs, MAOIs, serotonin–NE reuptake inhibitors, and one heterogenous group not otherwise classified. Mood stabilizers often are also part of the drug regimen. Because MAO is an enzyme promoting the breakdown of NE, MAOIs indirectly

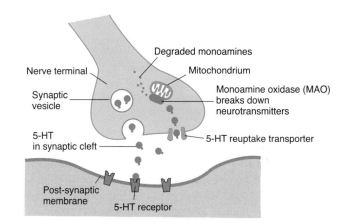

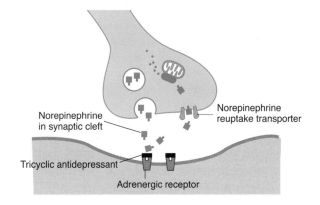

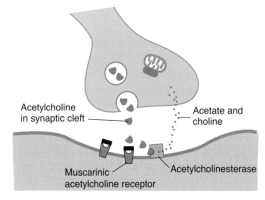

Figure 13.1. Mechanism of action of antidepressants.

Table 13.1. Side effects of SSRIs

Agitation	Anxiety, sweating
Headache	Nausea
Insomnia	Restlessness
Appetite suppression	Inhibition of cytochrome P-450

Table 13.2. Side effects of TCAs

Anticholinergic – dry mouth, blurred vision, constipation, urinary retention, tachycardia, confusion, delirium	Cardiac – prolonged PR and QT intervals, wide QRS complexes, arrhythmias, sudden cardiac death
Sedation (decreases MAC), weight gain	Postural hypotension
Hypertensive response	Sexual dysfunction

increase NE in the brain. Similarly, SSRIs indirectly increase brain serotonin levels. Mood is critically dependent on the neurotransmitters NE, D_2, and serotonin. Trials with antidepressants may take more than 3 to 4 weeks to identify the drug with the best results, but reliable predictors for its success are not available.

Selective serotonin reuptake inhibitors

Fluoxetine was the first SSRI released in the United States. Between 1987 and 1994, it was prescribed for more than 10 million people, making it the second most widely prescribed medication in the United States. SSRI agents currently available include fluoxetine (Prozac; Eli Lilly, Indianapolis, IN), paroxetine (Paxil; Pfizer, New York, NY), sertraline (Zoloft; Pfizer), citalopram (Celexa; Forest Pharmaceuticals, St. Louis, MO), and fluvoxamine (Luvox; Jazz Pharmaceuticals, Palo Alto, CA). Their relatively mild side effect profile and once-daily dosing schedule make them a safe and convenient alternative to the TCAs and MAOIs. SSRIs have low sedative and anticholinergic properties, do not cause postural hypotension or cardiac conduction defects, and have a very low risk of death from overdose compared with the TCAs. SSRIs are activating (stimulating) and therefore are taken during the day. Their side effects are listed in Table 13.1.

Fluoxetine and paroxetine may inhibit the activity of the cytochrome P-450 enzyme and so have a greater potential than other SSRIs for interaction with other drugs. Sertraline and citalopram only mildly inhibit this enzyme and hence have a lower likelihood of interactions with coadministered medications. In addition, paroxetine has a mild affinity for muscarinic receptors and may cause more anticholinergic side effects than other SSRIs (although much less than the TCAs).

Tricyclic antidepressants

TCAs are used to treat depression and chronic pain syndromes. They inhibit the reuptake of catecholamines in general, thus increasing their concentration in the nerve synapses and brain. Commonly used TCAs include amitriptyline (Elavil; AstraZeneca, Wilmington, DE, and Laroxyl; Roche, Nutley, NJ), doxepin (Sinequan; Pfizer), desipramine, nortriptyline (Aventyl; Eli Lilly), and imipramine (Tofranil; Mallinckrodt Inc., Hazelwood, MO). It is important to remember that an increase in catecholamine activity may increase the minimum alveolar concentration (MAC) of inhalation anesthetics.

The most common side effects of TCAs are anticholinergic effects, as listed in Table 13.2. Amitriptyline has the most marked anticholinergic effects, whereas doxepin has the fewest cardiac effects. The elderly are particularly susceptible to memory impairment, confusion, and hallucinations. Sedation and weight gain may result from concomitant blockade of histamine H_1 receptors, and orthostatic hypotension may occur from blockade of α_1-receptors. Atropine and glycopyrrolate have been noted to have increased muscarinic activity in the presence of TCAs.

Compared with normal patients, a decrease in intraoperative core temperature and an increased incidence of shivering have been observed in patients taking TCAs. The most important interaction between anesthetic agents and TCAs is an exaggerated response to indirect-acting vasopressors and sympathetic stimulation (hypertensive crisis). Administration of ketamine, meperidine, pancuronium, ephedrine, or epinephrine-containing local anesthetic solutions should be done with caution. Management consists of treating the hypertension emergently with a drug such as phentolamine or nitroprusside.

Monoamine oxidase inhibitors

Catecholamines are metabolized by the enzyme MAO. Hence, MAO inhibitors increase the availability of catecholamines in the nerve synapses. Two common isoforms of the MAO enzyme are the type A (selective for serotonin, NE) and type B (selective for phenylethylamine) isoforms. MAOIs often are not used for treatment because of their potential to precipitate enhanced sympathetic activity and severe hypertension (hypertensive crisis) with the concomitant ingestion of tyramine-containing foods (aged cheeses, beer, champagne, soy sauce, avocados, bananas, overripe or spoiled food, and any fermented, smoked, or aged fish or meat). The hypertensive reaction is dose-dependent and may be exacerbated if the patient is also taking a sympathomimetic drug. In the past, it was suggested that MAOIs be discontinued 2 to 3 weeks before any elective procedure involving general anesthesia. This precaution is no longer encouraged or practical for many procedures, because discontinuation of the drug may acutely place the patients at a greater risk for depression or suicide. MAOIs for clinical use include phenelzine, isocarboxazid, and tranylcypromine.

Miscellaneous drugs

Venlafaxine (Effexor; Pfizer), bupropion (Wellbutrin; Glaxo-SmithKline, Research Triangle Park, NC), and duloxetine (Cymbalta; Eli Lilly) have been shown to reduce neuropathic pain; therefore, they are preferred in treating depressed patients

Table 13.3. Potential interaction with drugs used in anesthesia

Class	Interacting drugs	Response
TCAs and MAOIs	Ephedrine, NE, epinephrine	Exaggerated pressor responses
	Halothane	Cardiac arrhythmias
	Meperidine	Hyperthermia, coma, seizures
	Atropine, scopolamine	Mental confusion
Lithium carbonate	Neuromuscular blocking drugs	Prolonged action

Table 13.4. Manifestations of lithium toxicity

System	Effects
Central nervous	Confusion, sedation (decreases MAC), muscle weakness (prolongs muscular blockade), ataxia, tremors, slurred speech, seizures
Cardiovascular	Widening of QRS complexes, AV heart block, hypotension
Endocrine	Hypothyroidism
Hematologic	Leukocytosis, aplastic anemia
Renal	Nephrogenic diabetes insipidus, tubular acidosis
Gastrointestinal	Nausea, vomiting, abdominal pain

AV, atrioventricular.

with chronic pain, to alleviate both the pain symptoms and treat the underlying depression. These drugs also are used to treat depression in patients who do not respond to typical antidepressant drugs. St. John's wort is an herbal product used for treating depression. Studies in the United States do not support its efficacy in the treatment of severe depression. The side effect profile of St. John's wort is extensive, but the main concern for anesthesiologists is the similarity this drug bears to the MAOIs in their potential for precipitating hypertension and hyperpyrexia. Concomitant use with SSRIs may lead to a form of "serotonin syndrome," characterized by agitation, hyperthermia, diaphoresis, tachycardia, and neuromuscular rigidity. In summary, detailed information on antidepressant drugs is important because they are widely prescribed and have interactions with drugs used in anesthesia. Table 13.3 shows potential interactions of antidepressant drugs with drugs used in anesthesia.

Bipolar disorder

The true prevalence of bipolar disorder (alternate periods of mania [elation] and depression) is uncertain; the diagnosis likely is missed when patients are seen for depression but are not asked specifically about symptoms suggesting prior episodes of mania or hypomania. Bipolar disorders are divided into types I and II, the former characterized by at least one manic or mixed episode, the latter by at least one hypomanic episode (lower severity than mania) and major depressive episodes. A mixed episode is defined as one that fits the criteria for both major depressive and manic episodes for 1 week. Mania is treated most effectively by administration of lithium (orally), carbamazepine (especially in lithium-refractory patients), and atypical antipsychotics.

Lithium

Despite its efficacy in the treatment of mania, lithium has a very narrow therapeutic index. The plasma level of lithium must be monitored routinely and perioperatively. A serum concentration of 0.6 to 0.8 mEq/L is considered therapeutic for the treatment of stable mania. Slightly higher levels, up to 1.2 mEq/L, are acceptable for treating acute episodes. Levels >2.0 mEq/L are considered toxic and require withdrawal of the drug and aggressive hydration with sodium-containing solutions or administration of osmotic diuretics, such as mannitol. Lithium

alters sodium transport across cell membranes by inhibiting the sodium–potassium pump, thus inhibiting the intracellular formation of cyclic adenosine monophosphate. Lithium toxicity (Table 13.4) is compounded by sodium depletion, and concurrent use of diuretics that inhibit the uptake of sodium in the renal tubule (loop diuretics and thiazides) is hazardous and should be avoided. Lithium also inhibits the action of antidiuretic hormone on the distal renal tubule, leading to nephrogenic diabetes insipidus in severe cases of lithium toxicity. Lithium can prolong the action of neuromuscular blocking agents.

Atypical antipsychotics

The term *atypical* refers to an antipsychotic medication that produces minimal extrapyramidal side effects (sustained contraction of muscle groups [neck, jaw, tongue, eyes], restlessness, agitation), has a low propensity to cause tardive dyskinesia (repetitive, purposeless involuntary movements – grimacing, tongue protrusion, lip smacking) with long-term treatment, and treats both positive and negative signs and symptoms of schizophrenia as well as bipolar disorders. A systematic review and meta-analysis found that the efficacy of atypical antipsychotics was comparable with that of mood stabilizers in treating acute mania but that a combination of antipsychotic and mood-stabilizing agents was more effective than mood stabilizers alone.

In addition to lower D_2-receptor potency and occupancy at therapeutic doses, atypical agents selectively antagonize mesolimbic D_2 receptors more than those in the nigrostriatum and prefrontal cortex. As a result, side effects attributable to nigrostriatal D_2 blockade (extrapyramidal symptoms) occur less frequently, as do side effects attributable to prefrontal D_2 blockade (neurocognitive impairment). Serotonin–D_2 antagonism is the reason atypical antipsychotics may be given in smaller doses, producing fewer extrapyramidal side effects while maintaining clinical efficacy.

Atypical agents currently available include clozapine, risperidone (Risperdal; Janssen, Titusville, NJ), olanzapine (Zyprexa; Eli Lilly), quetiapine (Seroquel; AstraZeneca), and ziprasidone (Geodon; Pfizer). Although each agent has different affinities for specific receptors, most drugs fall into one of two groups. The first group consists of clozapine, olanzapine,

Table 13.5. Side effects of antipsychotic drugs

System	Effects
Central nervous	Extrapyramidal symptoms, seizures (especially clozapine), sedation, cognitive dysfunction
Autonomic nervous	Orthostatic hypotension, anticholinergic effects (tachycardia, dry mouth, urinary retention)
Cardiovascular	Prolonged QT interval, torsades de pointes
Respiratory	Laryngospasm, dyskinesia
Hematologic	Leukopenia, pancytopenia
Endocrine	Weight gain, sexual dysfunction, galactorrhea
Gastrointestinal	Constipation, jaundice

and quetiapine, all of which demonstrate multiple receptor antagonism (α_1, H_1, and muscarinic$_1$). The second group consists of risperidone and ziprasidone, which demonstrate only α_1-adrenergic receptor antagonism.

Schizophrenia

Schizophrenia, the most common psychotic disorder, is thought to occur as the result of hyperactivity of the dopaminergic system. Symptoms include delusions, hallucinations, agitation, social incompatibility, withdrawal, and lack of hygiene. Schizophrenia may be associated with depression or mania. Commonly used antipsychotic drugs used to treat schizophrenia include phenothiazines (chlorpromazine, thioridazine), butyrophenones (haloperidol), loxapine (Loxapac; Wyeth-Ayerst, Radnor, PA), clozapine, and risperidone. Side effects of antipsychotic drugs are listed in Table 13.5.

Agitation

Safety is the first consideration with any psychiatric patient. When confronted with an agitated patient, physical restraint, including room seclusion, should be applied only as necessary to maintain the safety of the patient and staff or to avoid destruction of property.

Among the neurotransmitters, serotonin plays a major inhibitory role in aggressive behavior. Atypical antipsychotic medications, which affect both serotonin and D_2 activity, may have primary antihostility properties, which the traditional antipsychotic medications lack. Patients requiring injectable antipsychotics may be given olanzapine, ziprasidone, aripiprazole, or haloperidol. Additionally, for patients who agree to take oral medication but whose cooperation is marginal, risperidone and olanzapine are available as tablets that disintegrate in the mouth and therefore do not allow the patient to conceal a pill and surreptitiously discard it. The tablets are absorbed through the gastrointestinal tract at the same rate as standard pills (i.e., those not absorbed transmucosally). Oral and injectable preparations appear to be comparable in efficacy in acutely agitated patients.

Agitated patients also may benefit from a benzodiazepine. Lorazepam (Ativan; Pfizer) has the advantages of compatibility with antipsychotics, evidence of efficacy, and availability in oral, intramuscular, and intravenous formulations. Lorazepam, 0.5 to 2 mg, may be administered at the same time and by the same route as the antipsychotic.

Neuroleptic malignant syndrome

Perhaps the most feared complication of neuroleptics is neuroleptic malignant syndrome (NMS). NMS may be caused by antipsychotics, meperidine, or metoclopramide. Higher dosages or a rapid and large increase in dosage also may trigger the development of NMS. The first symptom to develop is usually muscular rigidity, followed by high fever and changes in cognitive functions. Other symptoms may vary but include unstable blood pressure, confusion, coma, delirium, and muscle tremors. The creatine phosphokinase plasma concentration will be elevated as a result of increased muscular activity. Patients may be hypertensive and usually have a metabolic acidosis, with mortality rates around 20% to 30%.

Treatment requires withdrawal of the offending agent, initiation of bromocriptine or dantrolene therapy, and supportive care. Anesthesia personnel must be aware of the similarity of NMS and malignant hyperthermia (MH), and especially vigilant when providing care to persons with a documented history of either. A primary defect in skeletal muscle has been suggested in view of similarities in the clinical presentations of NMS and anesthetic-induced MH, although NMS is associated with a normal muscle biopsy (unlike MH). Patients with neuroleptic-induced parkinsonism may develop intercurrent fever caused by infections or dehydration and be mistaken for cases of NMS. Although NMS has been reported before and after surgery, it appears unlikely to develop intraoperatively, in contrast to MH. Among differential diagnoses, serotonin syndrome should be mentioned because in its most severe form, which is associated with MAOIs, it presents as an NMS-like hypermetabolic state (although it usually presents with milder and more transient symptoms indicative of an agitated delirium).

Suggested readings

Allen MH, Currier GW, Carpenter D, et al. The expert consensus guideline series. Treatment of behavioral emergencies 2005. *J Psychiatr Pract* 2005; 11(Suppl 1):5.

Ely EW, Inouye SK, Bernard GR, et al. Delirium in mechanically ventilated patients: validity and reliability of the confusion assessment method for the intensive care unit (CAM-ICU). *JAMA* 2001; 286:2703–2710.

Heres S, Davis J, Maino K, et al. Why olanzapine beats risperidone, risperidone beats quetiapine, and quetiapine beats olanzapine: an exploratory analysis of head-to-head comparison studies of second-generation antipsychotics. *Am J Psychiatry* 2006; 163:185.

Inouye SK, Bogardus ST, Charpentier PA, et al. A multicomponent intervention to prevent delirium in hospitalized older patients. *N Engl J Med* 1999; 340:669–676.

Levenson JL. Neuroleptic malignant syndrome. *Am J Psychiatry* 1985; 142:1137.

Lieberman JA, Stroup TS, McEvoy JP, et al. Effectiveness of antipsychotic drugs in patients with chronic schizophrenia. *N Engl J Med* 2005; 353:1209.

Mann JJ. The medical management of depression. *N Engl J Med* 2005; 353:1819.

Milbrandt E, Deppen S, Harrison P, et al. Costs associated with delirium in mechanically ventilated patients. *Crit Care Med* 2004; 32:955–962.

Pandharipande P, Shintani A, Peterson J, et al. Lorazepam is an independent risk factor for transitioning to delirium in intensive care unit patients. *Anesthesiology* 2006; 104(1):21–26.

Shapiro BA, Warren J, Egol AB, et al. Practice parameters for intravenous analgesia and sedation for adult patients in the intensive care unit: an executive summary. Society of Critical Care Medicine. *Crit Care Med* 1995; 23:159.

Trivedi MH, Rush AJ, Wisniewski SR, et al. Evaluation of outcomes with citalopram for depression using measurement-based care in STAR*D: implications for clinical practice. *Am J Psychiatry* 2006; 163:28.

Williams JW Jr, Mulrow CD, Chiquette E, et al. A systematic review of newer pharmacotherapies for depression in adults: evidence report summary. *Ann Intern Med* 2000; 132:743.

14 Substance abuse and anesthesia

Thomas J. Graetz and Lisa R. Leffert

Recreational drugs are substances used without medical justification, causing changes in consciousness, habituation, and, in some cases, addiction (Table 14.1). The illicit use of these substances, which include alcohol, cocaine, amphetamines, marijuana, and opioids, is common; it is estimated that almost 10% of the US population >12 years of age have ingested recreational drugs in the past month. Acute and chronic substance abuse affect anesthetic care through the associated physiologic derangements and interactions with perioperative medications.

The following discussion highlights the epidemiologic, pharmacologic, and anesthetic implications of recreational drug use; in addition, the effects on pregnant women and their developing fetuses are highlighted.

Optimal care of the substance-abusing patient includes knowledge of which drugs he or she has ingested. The anesthesia consultation should contain detailed questions about the patient's use of recreational drugs, asked in a private and nonjudgmental fashion. Because patients tend to underreport their recreational drug use, it is important to recognize the relevant signs, symptoms, and comorbidities and to use drug testing when feasible. The most common specimen tested is urine (Table 14.2), although bioassays are available to test blood, hair, fetal meconium, and umbilical cord tissue.

Tobacco
General considerations

Tobacco use is common; more than 72 million Americans over 12 years of age (approximately 30% of the population) have used a tobacco product in recent months. Tobacco-containing products include cigarettes, the focus of this discussion. Other use includes chewing and pipe tobacco, snuff, and cigars.

Tobacco smoke contains more than 3000 active substances, including carbon monoxide and nicotine. Carbon monoxide decreases available oxygen for delivery to cells by avidly binding to hemoglobin to form carboxyhemoglobin and shifting the hemoglobin dissociation curve to the left. Inhaled nicotine acts on nicotinic (cholinergic) receptors in the brain and the periphery immediately upon exposure, causing sympathetic stimulation. Nicotine is metabolized by the liver to cotinine prior to being excreted in the urine.

Inhalation of tobacco smoke has diverse systemic effects, including increases in heart rate, blood pressure, and myocardial contractility. Smoking tobacco increases the rate of cardiovascular disease, and also affects the lungs, changing the quality and quantity of mucus production, decreasing mucociliary clearance, and predisposing patients to bronchitis and chronic obstructive pulmonary disease (COPD). Tobacco is addictive; cessation of smoking may lead to withdrawal symptoms including cravings, insomnia, and headaches. Some patients use nicotine replacement therapies such as gum, patches, or inhalers to facilitate cessation; the American College of Obstetricians and Gynecologists recommends they be used in pregnant patients only when nonpharmacologic interventions have failed.

Anesthetic implications

Smokers are at increased risk for perioperative complications, including pneumonia, respiratory failure, decreased wound healing, and unanticipated intensive care unit admission. Smoking cessation should be encouraged preoperatively, as oxygen delivery and exercise capacity have been shown to improve even after only a few hours. Longer duration of cessation (up to 6 months) may be required to confer additional benefits in terms of decreasing perioperative pulmonary complications.

Anesthetic management of a smoker should include a thorough investigation of frequently associated comorbidities, including cardiovascular and pulmonary disease. Of particular concern is the propensity for increased secretions, decreased ciliary motility, and impairment of gas exchange. Airway "irritability" associated with general anesthesia is thought to occur in smokers, although the published data are not entirely supportive of this concept. When feasible, neuraxial and peripheral regional techniques may be beneficial in these patients as their use can minimize airway manipulation.

Alcohol (ethanol)
General considerations

Ingestion of alcohol as beer, wine, or distilled liquor is common; 51% of Americans over 12 years of age report current drinking, whereas 23% of the population 12 years or older report binge drinking. Acute ethanol exposure places the individual at risk

Table 14.1. Recreational drugs

Substances	Drug properties	Systemic effects	Anesthetic implications
Tobacco	Nicotine – works via nicotinic cholinergic receptors in a variety of complex neurotransmitter systems, including peripheral autonomic effects. Metabolized to cotinine. Carbon monoxide – interacts with hemoglobin to form carboxyhemoglobin, which decreases the available oxygen for cells and increases the affinity of oxygen for red blood cells	Increased heart rate Increased blood pressure Increased myocardial contractility Decreased tissue oxygen levels Increased mucus production Decreased mucociliary clearance Small airway dysfunction	Increased risk for pulmonary complications Potential for airway "irritability" and bronchospasm Regional technique allows airway manipulation to potentially be avoided Cessation should be encouraged

Ethanol	Absorbed rapidly from GI tract
	Metabolized by alcohol dehydrogenase
		Acute
		  Impaired cognition
		  Increased gastric acidity
		  Hypovolemia
		Chronic
		  Hypertension
		  Anemia
		  Peripheral neuropathy
		  Cardiomyopathy
		  Liver cirrhosis
		  Pancreatitis
		  Malnutrition
		  Cancer
		  Metabolic derangements
		  Withdrawal
		  Tremor
		  Hypertension
		  Tachycardia
		  Nausea and vomiting
		  Agitation
		  Potential for delirium tremens
			Acute
			  Potential for uncooperative patient
			  Impaired airway reflexes
			  Decreased MAC
			Chronic
			  Manifestations of comorbid diseases
			  Altered drug metabolism
			  Empirically increasing anesthetic doses is *not* recommended (conflicting data)
			  Withdrawal
			  Altered hemodynamics
			  Potential for seizures

Cocaine	Reuptake inhibitor of presynaptic sympathomimetic neurotransmitters. Metabolized by serum and liver esterases	Local anesthetic properties CNS stimulation Cardiovascular complications including arrhythmias, hypertension, myocardial ischemia Seizures Proteinuria	Potentially uncooperative patient Altered pain perception Delayed gastric emptying β-Blockers may lead to unopposed alpha stimulation Resistance to ephedrine Reports of increased risk of thrombocytopenia (conflicting data)
Amphetamines	Indirect sympathomimetics that stimulate the CNS	Dose-dependent CNS stimulation Cardiovascular complications including arrhythmias, hypertension, myocardial ischemia Seizures Proteinuria	Toxic effects potentiated when combined with ethanol Potentially uncooperative patient Altered pain perception Resistance to ephedrine β-Blockers may lead to unopposed alpha stimulation
Marijuana	Smoked or ingested (slower onset)	Tachycardia Mucociliary dysfunction Elevated carboxyhemoglobin Biphasic effects Lower doses leading to increased sympathetic activity and decreased parasympathetic activity Higher doses leading to increased parasympathetic activity including bradycardia and potentially hypotension	Likely use of other drugs concomitantly Arrhythmias Potential for pulmonary complications

Opioids	Variable route of administration	Acute
		  Decreased ventilatory drive
		  Dysphoria
		  Unconsciousness
		  Miotic pupils
		Withdrawal
		  Occurs 4–6 h after opioid intake and peaks at 48–73 h
		  Agitation
			Potential for acute withdrawal syndrome if opioid antagonists or agonist–antagonists given to chronic users
			Clonidine can ameliorate some withdrawal symptoms
			To treat acute pain in chronic user:
			  Develop care plan with patient
			  Multimodal therapy (including NSAIDs, regional techniques) is recommended

(continued)

Table 14.1. (continued)

Substances	Drug properties	Systemic effects	Anesthetic implications
		Tachycardia Hypertension Insomnia Lacrimation Rhinorrhea Yawning Diarrhea	Maintain baseline opioid requirements Anticipate increased acute analgesic needs (30%–100% or more than in opioid-naïve patients)
Hallucinogens (LSD)	Complex mechanisms of action with agonist, partial agonist, and antagonist effects at various serotonin, dopaminergic, and adrenergic receptors Effects begin in 15–45 min and last 4–6 h, with metabolism by the liver	Mild sympathetic effects relative to cocaine, amphetamines, or ecstasy Euphoria Anxiety Paranoia Visual and auditory hallucinations	Agitation my be treated with benzodiazepines Supportive therapy, with resolution of symptoms usually within 12 h Avoid use of neuroleptic drugs because these may worsen symptoms Patients may have an exaggerated response to sympathomimetics
Solvents	Diverse group of substances Specific properties vary by specific substance	Euphoria, excitement, and feeling of invulnerability Sympathetic stimulation Hypotension Cardiomyopathy Renal failure	Tachyarrhythmias Hypoxia from respiratory depression, aspiration Formation of carboxy- and methemoglobin, airway edema

GI, gastrointestinal; NSAIDs, nonsteroidal anti-inflammatory drugs.

for antegrade amnesia and impaired judgment: a blood alcohol level of 50 mg/dl leads to impairment of some skilled tasks, and 80 mg/dl is the legal limit for driving in many states. Ethanol is metabolized by alcohol dehydrogenase, aldehyde dehydrogenase, and cytochrome P-450, leading to elevated levels of cellular NADH, which results in metabolic derangement.

Acute intoxication from ethanol ingestion increases gastric acidity. Chronic use may lead to myriad medical problems, including hypertension, cardiomyopathy, anemia, gastritis, hepatic cirrhosis, and/or chronic pancreatitis. Cognitive motor deficits and peripheral neuropathy also may ensue. Withdrawal from ethanol in a chronic abuser may occur 6 to 48 hours after consumption and usually manifests as tremor, hypertension, tachycardia, nausea, vomiting, and hallucinations. Benzodiazepines and α_2-agonists are the mainstays of treatment for withdrawal. Delirium tremens, with its attendant autonomic instability, is a potential complication of untreated withdrawal and may be fatal if left untreated.

Anesthetic implications

Whether or not they have eaten recently, acutely alcohol-intoxicated patients are at increased risk for aspiration because of delayed gastric emptying, increased gastric acid secretion, and impaired airway reflexes. As such, pretreatment with a nonparticulate antacid and histamine (H_2) blocker should be instituted. For general anesthesia, a rapid sequence induction should be performed unless a difficult intubation is anticipated. Intoxicated patients may be hypoglycemic or volume depleted secondary to vomiting, poor fluid intake, and/or diuresis.

Classic teaching has been that acute alcohol intoxication decreases patients' anesthetic needs, partly because of the additive effect of alcohol and other central nervous system (CNS)

depressants. The notion that chronic alcoholics have a higher anesthetic requirement than their non–alcohol-using counterparts seems based originally on an abstract published by Han in 1969, which described an alteration in mean minimum alveolar concentration (MAC) values of halothane in six chronic alcoholic patients compared to six "normal healthy adult subjects." Of note, a subsequent study showed that thiopental pharmacodynamics and pharmacokinetics were not statistically significantly different in 11 chronic alcohol users compared with nine controls. Additionally, a small study from 1993 looking at propofol induction doses in humans showed a slightly higher dose of propofol was needed at induction of general anesthesia. Given the presence of additional vulnerabilities in this patient population, such as decreased nutritional status and increased cardiac comorbidities, empirically increasing anesthetic dosing should be done with caution.

Table 14.2. Drug detection in urine

Drug	Analyte	Detection window via urine, days
Tobacco	Cotinine	2–4
Cocaine	Benzoylecgonine	~2–3
Amphetamines	Methamphetamine	~3–6
Ecstasy	MDMA	~2
Marijuana	THC	~1–2
	THCCOOH	~4
LSD	LSD	~1–2
	2-Oxo-3OH-LSD	~4
Opioids (heroin)	Morphine	~1–3

THCCOOH, 11-Nor-Δ^9-tetrahydrocannabinol-9-carboxylic acid.
Data from Haufroid and Lison 1998; Wallach 2000; Verstraete AG. Detection times of drugs of abuse in blood, urine, and oral fluid. *Ther Drug Monit* 2004; 26(2):200–205.

Peripheral and neuraxial anesthesia may be used safely in these patients in appropriate surgical circumstances, provided that (1) the patient is cooperative (benzodiazepines may be beneficial), (2) coagulopathy (due to associated liver disease) has been ruled out, (3) the patient is euvolemic, and (4) baseline neurologic deficits (e.g., peripheral neuropathy) are taken into consideration.

Cocaine
General considerations

Approximately 15% of the population over 12 years of age have used cocaine. An alkaloid derived from the *Erythroxylon coca* plant, cocaine commonly is prepared as a water-soluble hydrochloride salt that can be snorted, injected intravenously, or absorbed intrarectally or intravaginally. Cocaine also may be modified using ether and ammonia or sodium bicarbonate to form "free-base" or "crack" cocaine, respectively. Both free-base and crack can be smoked.

Cocaine has a biologic half-life of 0.5 to 1.5 hours and is metabolized primarily by plasma and liver esterases to ecgonine methyl ester and benzoylecgonine. Patients who are homozygotes for atypical plasma cholinesterase have impaired in vitro ability to metabolize cocaine in addition to succinylcholine. Acquired deficiencies in the quantity of plasma cholinesterase secondary to liver disease, pregnancy, plasmapheresis, hypothyroidism, and malnutrition also may alter cocaine metabolism, although these may or may not have a clinically significant effect. If cocaine is metabolized in the presence of ethanol, cocaethylene, which has a longer half-life than cocaine and amplified physiologic effects, is formed.

Cocaine exerts its pharmacologic action by preventing reuptake of dopamine, norepinephrine, and serotonin. Increased CNS levels of dopamine lead to feelings of euphoria and contribute to the addictive nature of cocaine. Repeated exposure to cocaine may cause dopamine depletion and anhedonia. Cocaine is unique in that it also functions as a local anesthetic with inherent vasoconstrictive properties.

Anesthetic implications

The anesthetic implications of cocaine use relate to its multi-organ system effects and to the frequent concomitant use of other recreational drugs. Cardiovascular sequelae of acute and chronically elevated catecholamine levels include hypertension, dysrhythmias, and conduction disturbances, in addition to an increased risk of developing myocardial ischemia, dilated cardiomyopathy, valvular disease, and aortic dissection.

Some authors advocate pretreatment with benzodiazepines and antihypertensive agents prior to induction of general anesthesia to attenuate the adrenergic effects of cocaine. Recommended therapy for severe cocaine-induced hypertension includes hydralazine, nitroprusside, nitroglycerin, or phentolamine. β-Blockers are relatively contraindicated because of the risk of unopposed alpha activity, leading to a further increase in blood pressure and coronary vasoconstriction. Labetalol, with its concomitant (albeit weak) alpha effects, may be less problematic. Given the variable effects of cocaine on myocyte calcium metabolism, some authors have cautioned against the use of calcium channel blockers in cocaine-intoxicated patients, although others advocate its use.

Treatment for cocaine-induced hypotension should begin with intravenous (IV) fluids and a search for underlying causes. If a vasopressor is needed, direct-acting vasoconstrictors such as phenylephrine may be advisable because ephedrine may be associated with an exaggerated or attenuated response depending on levels of circulating catecholamines. Cardiac arrhythmias should be treated according to Advanced Cardiac Life Support (ACLS) protocol, using cardioversion or defibrillation if indicated. Use of volatile anesthetics during general anesthesia, most notably halothane, may increase the risk of cardiac arrhythmias. Of note, an animal study published in 1988 by Hayashi showed that epinephrine-exposed dogs had fewer ventricular arrhythmias when exposed to isoflurane than to sevoflurane. Finally, the use of ketamine is relatively contraindicated in patients with acute cocaine intoxication as it may provoke an exaggerated hemodynamic response.

Patients who abuse cocaine also may suffer neurologic consequences including headache, agitation (may respond to benzodiazepines), depression, seizures, psychosis, stroke, and cerebral atrophy. Additionally, opioid receptor modulation secondary to chronic cocaine use may lead to breakthrough pain during spinal or epidural anesthesia as well as postoperatively, despite an adequate sensory level. The MAC of halothane has been shown to be increased during acute cocaine intoxication in animals.

Pulmonary comorbidities associated with cocaine use occur primarily in the setting of inhalation. As is the case for tobacco smokers, these patients have an increased risk of asthma, chronic cough, and diffusion abnormalities. Other related complications include pneumothorax and pulmonary edema. Because individuals who smoke cocaine are at risk for upper airway burns, extra care must be taken if intubation is planned. Snorting cocaine may lead to nasal septal injury, which precludes insertion of airway, temperature, and nasogastric devices through the nares.

Gastric emptying is delayed by cocaine ingestion, so pretreatment with a nonparticulate antacid and H_2 blocker should be instituted. For general anesthesia, a rapid sequence induction should be performed, unless a difficult intubation is anticipated.

Although cocaine has been shown to cause increased platelet activation and aggregation, the presence of cocaine-induced thrombocytopenia is both supported and refuted in the literature. If feasible, the platelet count should be checked in these patients prior to placing a regional anesthetic. In addition, for those who have end-stage liver disease, it is prudent to assess coagulation status.

Finally, patients who inject cocaine or any other illicit drugs are more likely to have infectious complications (including HIV and viral hepatitis) and difficult intravenous access.

Amphetamines

General considerations

Amphetamines cause the release of catecholamines from presynaptic nerves, leading to CNS stimulation with feelings of euphoria. Six percent of the population have used amphetamines at some point during their lives; methamphetamines are the most commonly used drugs in this class. 3,4-Methylenedioxymethamphetamine (MDMA or "ecstasy") is chemically related to methamphetamines and also has hallucinogenic properties (see Hallucinogens).

Metabolism of amphetamines is variable; up to 30% of the drug is excreted unchanged in urine. The plasma half-life varies from 5 to 30 hours, depending on urine output and pH (increased pH leading to decreased excretion). Amphetamines frequently are taken in combination with other drugs; for example, ethanol plus methamphetamines is known to provide more pleasurable sensations for the user and also to be more demanding on the cardiovascular system than either substance alone.

Anesthetic implications

The signs, symptoms, and anesthetic considerations of amphetamine intoxication are generally similar to those of cocaine, and therapy should be directed accordingly: benzodiazepines to blunt the excitatory effects of amphetamines and nitrates, hydralazine and phentolamine for treatment of severe hypertension. Hypotension in a chronic amphetamine user likely is the result of catecholamine depletion and possibly down-regulation of α- and β-adrenergic receptors; as such, phenylephrine may be a more effective corrective therapy than an indirect agent such as ephedrine.

Regional or general anesthetic techniques may be used in amphetamine-intoxicated patients, depending on the overall clinical picture. Of note, chronic use of methamphetamines is associated with severe tooth decay ("meth mouth"), which puts these patients at risk for having teeth dislodged during intubation. In addition, the results of animal studies suggest that MAC for volatile anesthetics is decreased in the setting of chronic amphetamine use and increased in the setting of acute ingestion. Because MDMA intoxication may lead to hyperpyrexia, core body temperature should be measured in these patients and active warming devices used with caution.

Marijuana (cannabis)

General considerations

Marijuana was used recreationally by about 16% of the population 18 to 25 years old and 8% of those over 12 years old in 2006. Derived from the *Cannabis sativa* or *C. indica* plant, marijuana contains over 400 different compounds, including over 60 cannabinoids. The most potent and studied cannabinoid in marijuana is Δ^9-tetrahydrocannabinol (THC). Marijuana is frequently smoked, although it can be orally ingested.

Cannabinoids, which are metabolized by the liver and eliminated in the urine, have complex effects mediated by endogenous receptors. Marijuana users experience anxiolysis, sedation, intoxication, and analgesia; dysphoria and paranoia also may occur. A biphasic effect on the autonomic nervous system occurs: low to moderate doses lead to sympathetic stimulation, tachycardia, and hypertension, whereas high doses lead to sympathetic inhibition with resultant bradycardia and hypotension. Life-threatening arrhythmias in patients without preexisting cardiac disease are rare, although ectopy may occur.

Smoking three to four cannabis cigarettes per day has been estimated to result in the same degree of bronchopulmonary damage as smoking 20 cigarettes a day. The cannabinoids are lipid-soluble substances, leading to their long elimination half-life (about 7 days). Withdrawal from chronic marijuana use reportedly is associated with headache, restlessness, tremor, and anxiety.

Anesthetic implications

Because marijuana cigarettes contain many of the compounds in tobacco (excluding nicotine), inhalation may lead to mucociliary dysfunction, bronchial irritation, and decreased tissue levels of oxygen secondary to increased carboxyhemoglobin. As is the case with tobacco, use of peripheral or neuraxial regional anesthetics may enable the anesthesiologist to avoid instrumenting the airway. Caution should be taken when administering anticholinergics and other vagolytic medications (e.g., pancuronium), as these medications may worsen the tachycardia frequently seen with marijuana. Marijuana also may potentiate the sedative effects of other medications.

Opioids

General considerations

The opioid class of medications includes "opiates" derived from the poppy plant (e.g., morphine and codeine) and other semisynthetic or synthetic formulations, such as heroin, oxycodone, and methadone. These drugs frequently are injected intravenously but also may be injected subcutaneously or ingested orally. The prevalence of heroin abuse in the population over 12 years of age is 1.5%, and that of nonmedical use of pain relievers (e.g., oxycodone) is estimated at 14%. Heroin, an acetylated morphine, is highly addictive and reaches the brain in <10 seconds when injected intravenously; it is metabolized in the liver prior to excretion by the kidneys and has an elimination half-life of 1 to 2 hours.

Oxycodone is a popular opioid of abuse because of its high oral bioavailability and potency.

Methadone is a synthetic opioid used recreationally and in medical practice as substitution therapy for heroin addicts and to treat chronic pain. Its peak concentration after oral administration occurs at 4 hours; its elimination half-life is highly variable and prolonged (15–40 hours). Opioid intoxication leads to decreased ventilatory drive and decreased airway reflexes. Withdrawal symptoms include agitation, tachycardia, hypertension, insomnia, lacrimation, rhinorrhea, and yawning.

Anesthetic implications

When caring for a patient who chronically uses opioids, it is essential to communicate effectively, to maintain the patient's baseline opioid requirements, and to anticipate acute additional analgesic needs. Tolerance to opioids and abnormal pain sensitivity in these patients make achieving optimal pain control more challenging; they are more likely to report breakthrough pain intraoperatively when regional anesthesia is used and postoperatively regardless of the mode of anesthesia. As such, multimodal therapy including nonsteroidal medications, peripheral and neuraxial techniques, and adequate doses of opioids (30%–100% above what is expected in opioid-naïve patients) is indicated. Medical therapy is enhanced when coupled with a detailed conversation outlining the care plan. Withholding necessary opioids for fear of relapse in a formerly addicted patient is not medically justified.

Patients on chronic methadone maintenance should continue receiving their baseline-dosing regimen. Opioid antagonists (e.g., naloxone) and mixed agonists–antagonists (e.g., nalbuphine) are relatively contraindicated in chronic opioid users, unless they have overdosed or are undergoing medically supervised detoxification. Withdrawal symptoms can be ameliorated by α_2-agonists (e.g., clonidine) or by careful reintroduction of opioids. IV abuse of opioids and other recreational drugs frequently is associated with subsequent difficult IV access and infectious complications including cellulitis, viral hepatitis, HIV, and endocarditis.

Hallucinogens

General considerations

Five percent of the population over the age of 12 years have used hallucinogens (e.g., lysergic acid diethylamide [LSD], phencyclidine [PCP], psilocybin, or mescaline) during their lifetime. Hallucinogens have complex mechanisms of action, including agonist, partial agonist, and antagonist effects at serotonin, dopamine, and adrenergic receptors; ingestion typically produces mind-altering CNS stimulation, including visual, auditory, and tactile hallucinations, and mild adrenergic stimulation compared with cocaine and amphetamines. These effects typically occur approximately 1 hour after ingestion and may last up to 12 hours. No specific withdrawal syndrome is associated with abrupt discontinuation of these substances, although psychological dependence frequently occurs.

Anesthetic implications

Management of the hallucinogen-intoxicated patient typically is supportive and noninterventional. As such, the choice of regional versus general anesthesia depends primarily on the clinical situation. If necessary, agitation can be treated with benzodiazepines. Neuroleptic agents should be avoided because they may potentiate the undesirable effects of these compounds. Hallucinogens may cause arrhythmias and hypertension, which can be managed in the usual fashion. As these patients may have an inadequate response to ephedrine, phenylephrine may be more effective in the treatment of hypotension.

Solvents

General principles

Solvents are popular substances of abuse because they are readily available and inexpensive. Approximately 9% of the population over 12 years of age have used inhalants during their lifetime. Solvents may be ingested orally or inhaled because they readily vaporize at room temperature. The primary effect of these recreational drugs is on the CNS, causing a "rush" of excitement and disinhibition. These effects, typically of short duration, may be prolonged by sequential inhalations. Solvent abuse may lead to irritation of mucous membranes, epistaxis, rhinorrhea, aspiration, fatal arrhythmias, burns, and accidental death. Chronic use may result in multiorgan system pathology, including renal failure, leukemia, aplastic anemia, hepatocellular carcinoma, cardiomyopathy, and brain atrophy.

Anesthetic implications

A careful neurologic examination is important in order to document preexisting sensory and motor deficits. Solvent intoxication may lead to hypoxemia as a result of suffocation and/or methemoglobinemia. The drug user's airway also may be injured by the inhalation process, leading to mucosal injury and edema. Repeated use of nitrates may lead to syncope, hypotension, and the potential for methemoglobinemia. Care should be used with epinephrine-containing medications, as the inhalational agents may sensitize the myocardium. Respiratory and neurologic abnormalities should be specifically evaluated. Additionally, electrolyte abnormalities may occur and should be identified and corrected, if present.

Pregnant patients and their developing fetuses

An estimated 17% of pregnant women smoke cigarettes. Smoking tobacco leads to in utero exposure to carcinogens and toxic metabolites of tobacco, as well as to hypoxia from placental vasoconstriction and increased levels of carboxyhemoglobin. Smoking places pregnant women at risk for complications such as intrauterine growth restriction (IUGR), placental abruption, premature rupture of membranes, low birth weight, and perinatal mortality. A negative association between smoking and preeclampsia has been reported in the literature.

Approximately 12% of pregnant women report alcohol use. Fetal alcohol syndrome (FAS) secondary to in utero ethanol exposure is the leading cause of preventable birth defects and developmental abnormalities. Key features of the diagnosis of

FAS are facial dysmorphia (smooth philtrum, thin vermilion border, and small palpebral fissure) and neurologic and developmental abnormalities. No level of alcohol exposure has been identified as "safe" for use during pregnancy.

Cocaine use may lead to placental abruption, preterm labor, spontaneous abortion, IUGR, preterm delivery, stillbirth, and neonatal abstinence syndrome. Pregnant women who abuse cocaine are at higher risk for needing cesarean delivery for fetal distress. Cocaine-exposed infants weigh less, are shorter, and have an increased incidence of infections, particularly those that are sexually transmitted. Early reports suggested that in utero cocaine exposure is associated with congenital anatomic defects, although more recent data have not supported this observation.

Amphetamine use during pregnancy has been implicated in some fetal anomalies in animal studies (e.g., cardiac abnormalities and cleft lip) as well as in IUGR. Additionally, prematurity, placental abruption, and fetal distress have been associated with amphetamine use in pregnancy.

Marijuana use during pregnancy allows the potent metabolite THC to readily cross the placenta. Although THC is not an established teratogen, chronic use may lead to IUGR, uteroplacental insufficiency, and low birth weight.

Specific concerns regarding the fetus associated with chronic opioid use include decreased birth weight, longer and more frequent hospital stays, increased fetal mortality, and neonatal abstinence syndrome (NAS). The latter is a withdrawal syndrome seen in neonates exposed to opioids in utero and is characterized by gastrointestinal, respiratory, and nervous system dysfunction manifesting as irritability, high-pitched cry, tremors, hypertonicity, vomiting, diarrhea, and tachypnea. When maternal abstinence is not feasible, methadone maintenance therapy (MMT) is used as replacement/maintenance therapy for heroin addiction. MMT has been shown to increase prenatal medical care, decrease NAS, and reduce maternal illicit drug use at delivery.

There is conflicting evidence as to whether prenatal PCP exposure has negative effects on the developing fetus. PCP use during pregnancy has been associated with smaller and more premature infants.

Solvent abuse in pregnancy has been associated with an increased incidence of IUGR, preterm labor, and prenatal death. Toluene may contribute to FAS with concomitant use of alcohol.

Suggested readings

Ashton CH. Pharmacology and effects of cannabis: a brief review. *Br J Psychiatry* 2001; 178:101–106.

Fleming JA, Byck R, Barash PG. Pharmacology and therapeutic applications of cocaine. *Anesthesiology* 1990; 73(3):518–531.

Floyd RL, O'Connor MJ, Sokol RJ, et al. Recognition and prevention of fetal alcohol syndrome. *Obstet Gynecol* 2005; 106(5 Pt 1):1059–1064.

Ghuran A, Nolan J. Recreational drug misuse: issues for the cardiologist. *Heart* 2000; 83(6):627–633.

Han YH. Why do chronic alcoholics require more anesthesia. *Anesthesiology* 1969; 30(3):341.

Hayashi Y, Sumikawa K, Tashiro C. et al. *I Anesthesiology* 1988 Jul; 69(1) 145–147. (PMID:3389556 on Pubmed.)

Jatlow P, Barash PG, Van Dyke C, et al. Cocaine and succinylcholine sensitivity: a new caution. *Anesth Analg* 1979; 58(3):235–238.

Johnston RR, Way WL, Miller RD. Alteration of anesthetic requirement by amphetamine. *Anesthesiology* 1972; 36(4):357–363.

Kuczkowski KM. Anesthetic implications of drug abuse in pregnancy. *J Clin Anesth* 2003; 15(5):382–394.

Lange RA, Hillis LD. Cardiovascular complications of cocaine use. *N Engl J Med* 2001; 345(5):351–358.

Lieber CS. Medical disorders of alcoholism. *N Engl J Med* 1995; 333(16):1058–1065.

Ludvig J, Miner B, Eisenberg MJ. Smoking cessation in patients with coronary artery disease. *Am Heart J* 2005; 149(4):565–572.

Orser B. Thrombocytopenia and cocaine abuse. *Anesthesiology* 1991; 74(1):195–196.

Reynolds EW, Bada HS. Pharmacology of drugs of abuse. *Obstet Gynecol Clin North Am* 2003; 30(3):501–522.

Verstraete AG. Detection times of drugs of abuse in blood, urine, and oral fluid. *Ther Drug Monit* 2004; 26(2):200–205.

Williams JF, Storck M. (2007). Inhalant abuse. *Pediatrics* 2007; 119(5):1009–1017.

Airway Management

William H. Rosenblatt, editor

Anatomy of the human airway

Sarah H. Wiser

Understanding the anatomy of the human airway is critical to safe and efficient airway management. The upper airway consists of the passages from the nose and mouth to the larynx. The lower airway includes structures distal to the glottis (Fig. 15.1).

Nasal cavity

The nasal cavity provides for the passage, filtration, humidification, and warming of inhaled air. Its anatomic borders are the cribriform plate superiorly, the hard palate inferiorly, and the turbinates laterally. It is divided in the midsagittal plane by the septum. From the nares anteriorly, the nasal passage extends posteriorly and slightly caudad to reach the nasopharynx.

General sensation to the mucous membranes of the nasal cavity is derived from the trigeminal nerve (Table 15.1). The anterior lateral wall and anterior septum are supplied by the anterior ethmoid nerves (V1), whereas the sphenopalatine nerves (V2) provide sensation to these structures posteriorly. The floor of the nasal cavity (or hard and soft palates) is supplied by the infraorbital and greater palatine nerves (V2) anteriorly and posteriorly, respectively. The nasal cavity has a rich and redundant blood supply from the ophthalmic, maxillary, and facial arteries.

Oral cavity

The mouth includes the dentition, anterior two-thirds of the tongue, floor of the mouth, and undersurface of the hard and soft palates. The division between the oral cavity and the oropharynx is marked by the anterior tonsillar pillars or palatoglossal folds. The tongue is attached to the mandible anteriorly and laterally; posteriorly it is attached to the stylohyoid process and the hyoid bone. The tongue continues posteriorly into the pharynx and is attached to the epiglottis by mucosa. This mucosa creates the glossoepiglottic fold (medially) and the pharyngoglottic folds (laterally). The vallecula is the fossa formed by these folds.

General sensation to the tongue is supplied by three cranial nerve branches: the lingual branch of the trigeminal nerve (anterior two-thirds), the glossopharyngeal nerve (posterior one-third), and a small component derived from the vagus nerve (Table 15.1). The primary blood supply to the oral cavity is from a branch from the external carotid artery.

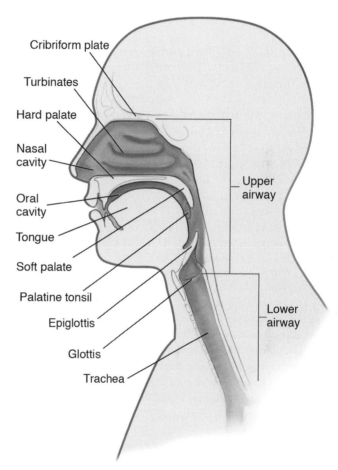

Figure 15.1. Anatomy of the upper human airway.

The mandible is the primary bony structural support of the mouth. It is a horseshoe-shaped structure with two vertical rami that articulate with the temporal bones of the cranium. The temporomandibular joint provides for two types of movement: rotation and translation. These movements allow for opening of the mouth. The space between the horizontal rami of the mandible is called the mandibular space.

Pharynx

The pharynx is a U-shaped fibromuscular tube that, anatomically and functionally, is divided into three areas: the

Table 15.1. Sensory innervation of the airway

Nerve	Sensory distribution
Trigeminal nerve (CN V)	Mucous membranes of the anterior nasal cavity
V1 anterior ethmoidal nerve	Mucous membranes of the posterior nasal cavity
V2 sphenopalatine nerves	Hard and soft palate
V2 palatine nerves	Roof of the nasopharynx
V2 pharyngeal branch	General sensation to the anterior two-thirds of the tongue
V3 lingual nerve	
Facial nerve (CN VII)	Taste to the anterior two-thirds of the tongue
Glossopharyngeal nerve (CN IX)	General sensation and taste to the posterior third of the tongue
	Nasopharynx (except the roof – supplied by V)
	Oropharynx
	Tonsils
	Laryngopharynx, pharyngeal surface of the epiglottis
Vagus nerve (CN X)	Contributes to the glossopharyngeal nerve for sensation to the oropharynx and laryngopharynx
Internal laryngeal nerve	Sensation of the pyriform recesses
Recurrent laryngeal nerve	Laryngeal surface of the epiglottis, and laryngeal structures to the vocal cords
	Sensation below the vocal cords and distal airways

CN, cranial nerve.

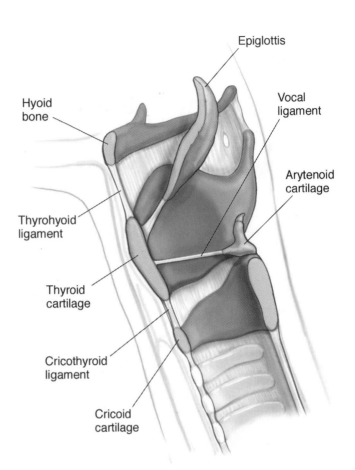

Figure 15.2. The cartilaginous skeleton of the larynx.

nasopharynx, oropharynx, and hypopharynx. The nasopharynx, as discussed earlier, is posterior to the nasal cavity and serves as an air conduit. The oropharynx is the main passage of the aerodigestive tract. The palatoglossal folds separate the oropharynx from the oral cavity anteriorly. The hypopharynx, the continuation of the aerodigestive tract, extends from the epiglottis to the lower border of the cricoid cartilage; it is contiguous with the esophagus. The larynx bulges posteriorly into the hypopharynx, thus creating lateral recesses on either side, called the pyriform recesses.

General sensation to the pharynx is supplied by the trigeminal, glossopharyngeal, and vagus nerves (Table 15.1). The trigeminal nerve supplies sensory innervation to the roof of the nasopharynx, and the glossopharyngeal nerve supplies sensory innervation to the remainder of the nasopharynx. The glossopharyngeal and vagus nerves both contribute sensory innervation of the oropharynx, including the posterior third of the tongue. The blood supply to the pharynx is derived from the external carotid artery.

Larynx

The larynx lies at the level of the third to sixth cervical vertebrae, anterior to the hypopharynx. Functionally, the larynx is the organ of phonation and the passageway for air into the trachea and lungs. The epiglottis acts to protect the lower airways from contamination from the alimentary tract. The larynx

consists of a cartilaginous skeleton bound by ligaments, membranes, and muscles.

The cartilaginous skeleton of the larynx consists of three unpaired cartilages – the epiglottis, thyroid, and cricoid, and three paired cartilages – the arytenoid, cuneiform, and corniculate (Fig. 15.2). The epiglottis is the functional division between the oropharynx and larynx. The thyroid cartilage houses the glottic opening and is attached to the hyoid bone by the thyrohyoid membrane superiorly and to the cricoid cartilage inferiorly by the cricothyroid membrane. The cricoid cartilage is signet ring–shaped and is the only complete cartilaginous ring in the airway. The cricothyroid ligament continues posteriorly behind the thyroid cartilage to form the anterior commissure and subsequently to create the true vocal cords, which attach and continue between the arytenoids medially to meet in the midline. The arytenoids are attached to the epiglottis laterally

Table 15.2. Motor innervation of the larynx

Superior laryngeal nerve (external branch) (CN X)	Cricothyroid muscle
Recurrent laryngeal nerve (CN X)	All other muscles of the larynx

CN, cranial nerve.

Table 15.3. Clinical manifestations of motor nerve injury

Nerve	Subtypes of Injury	Clinical manifestation	Cord position/appearance
Superior laryngeal nerve (external branch)	Unilateral injury		
	• Acute	Hoarseness	Aryepiglottic fold shortened on the affected side and lengthened on the normal side; affected cord appears wavy
	• Chronic	Generally has minimal effect (the other vocal cord compensates), but there may be residual dysphonia	
	Bilateral injury	Hoarseness, tiring of voice	Cords appear wavy
Recurrent laryngeal nerve	Unilateral injury	Hoarseness	Affected cord – adducted to the paramedian position
	Bilateral injury		
	• Acute	Stridor, respiratory distress	Cords nearly closed
	• Chronic	Aphonia	Cords are paramedian
Vagus nerve (prior to branching of the nerve)	Unilateral injury	Hoarseness	Affected cord – midline
	Bilateral injury	Aphonia	Midway between abduction and adduction (cadaveric position)

by the aryepiglottic ligaments and have articular facets inferiorly with the cricoid cartilage.

The branches of the vagus nerve supply all the motor and sensory innervation to the larynx (Tables 15.1 and 15.2) via its branches, the superior and recurrent laryngeal nerves. The superior laryngeal nerve divides into the internal laryngeal (sensory) and the external laryngeal (motor) nerves before entering the larynx. The internal laryngeal nerve pierces the lateral edge of the thyrohyoid membrane, inferior to the greater cornu of the hyoid bone, and travels superficially in the pyriform recess to enter the larynx. The internal laryngeal nerve supplies sensation to the base of the tongue, laryngeal surface of the epiglottis, and larynx to the vocal cords. The left recurrent laryngeal nerve loops around the aortic arch and the right loops around the right subclavian artery. Both then travel to supply sensory innervation to the vocal cords, trachea, carina, and distal airways.

The larynx is designed for phonation and protection of the airway. The muscles that perform these functions are divided into external and internal groups. The external group allows for position and movement of the entire larynx, whereas the internal group provides for delicate movements that affect glottic opening. The exception to this is the cricothyroid muscle, which lies external to the larynx and acts to provide tension to the vocal cords (adductor). The recurrent laryngeal nerve supplies all motor function to the internal laryngeal muscles (Table 15.2), whereas the cricothyroid muscle is supplied by the external branch of the superior laryngeal nerve. Laryngeal blood supply is derived from the carotid and subclavian arteries. Occasionally, a small cricothyroid artery crosses the superior portion of the cricothyroid membrane. Clinical manifestations of motor nerve injury are summarized in Table 15.3.

Trachea

The trachea is a tubular structure that begins at the inferior border of the cricoid cartilage at the level of the sixth cervical vertebra. It consists of 16 to 20 C-shaped hyaline cartilaginous rings connected posteriorly by the membranous trachea. The adult trachea is approximately 12 mm in diameter and 9 to 15 cm in length and bifurcates into the left and right mainstem bronchi at the carina. The carina is at the level of the sternal angle, which corresponds to the junction of the fourth and fifth thoracic vertebrae. The right mainstem bronchus is 1 to 2 cm in length and divides into upper, middle, and lower lobes, whereas the left mainstem bronchus is 4 to 5 cm in length and divides into upper and lower lobes. Air continues through the bronchioles to reach the alveoli, where gas exchange occurs.

Suggested readings

Gray H. *Anatomy of the Human Body*. 20th ed., thoroughly revised and reedited by Warren H. Lewis. Philadelphia: Lea & Febiger; 1918.

Krohner RG, Ramanathan S. Functional anatomy of the airway. In: Hagberg CA, ed. *Benumhof's Airway Management*. 2nd ed. Philadelphia: Mosby; 2007:3–21.

Mali M, Esch O, Lang J, et al. Magnetic resonance imaging of the upper airway: effects of propofol anesthesia and nasal continuous positive airway pressure in humans. *Anesthesiology* 1996; 84(2):273–279.

Morris IR. Functional anatomy of the upper airway. *Emerg Med Clin North Am* 1988; 6(4):639–669.

Netter FH. *Atlas of Human Anatomy*. Philadelphia: Saunders; 1989:32–75.

Rajagopal MR, Paul J. Applied anatomy and physiology of the airway and breathing. *Indian J Anaesth* 2005; 49(4):251–256.

16 Airway assessment

Rahul Koka and B. Scott Segal

The preoperative evaluation of the airway and the ability to predict difficulty in airway management are essential components of preparing the patient for surgery. American Society of Anesthesiologists (ASA) Closed Claims Project analysis of adverse outcomes associated with anesthesia reveals that the most common cause of serious injury during anesthesia is inadequate ventilation. More often than not, this is secondary to problems with laryngoscopy and/or mask ventilation, that is, the "difficult airway." Being able to predict the difficult airway is an essential tool that allows the anesthetist to select appropriate airway devices, techniques, and procedures.

Patient history

Preoperative airway management must include a focused and detailed history of diseases or symptoms related to the airway as well as a review of prior airway management events. There are recognized associations between a variety of congenital, acquired, and traumatic disease states and problems with airway management (Table 16.1). These diseases are usually associated with specific findings on physical examination that correlate with difficult laryngoscopy or ventilation.

In addition, there are other factors that may compromise airway functionality, including edema, burns, smoke inhalation, and history of oral or nasal bleeding. Tracheal/esophageal stenosis may occur after prior tracheostomy or prolonged intubation. Snoring may suggest obstructive sleep apnea, difficulty with mask ventilation, and problems during emergence and extubation.

A history of prior attempts at intubation and ventilation also should be reviewed and may be the best predictor of difficulty with future events. A history of a difficult intubation, mask ventilation, or supraglottic airway placement may be a significant warning sign of future difficulties. If an anesthetist encounters airway problems, it is important to document such information and advise the patient. To date, there is no national searchable database of difficult airway patients in the United States; however, such databases have been started in Austria and the United Kingdom.

Physical examination

Examination of the airway should start with an evaluation of issues that would present problems during mask ventilation, intubation, supraglottic device placement, or tracheostomy. These components of the physical examination are listed in Table 16.2.

Prediction of difficult airway management

Fortunately, true difficult airways are uncommon. In anesthetic practice, not only are most patients easy to ventilate and intubate, most of those who are predicted to be difficult are not.

Prediction of difficult mask ventilation

According to the ASA Task Force on Management of the Difficult Airway (2003), difficult bag–mask ventilation occurs when the anesthetist cannot provide adequate ventilation because of an inadequate mask seal, excessive gas leak, or excessive resistance to the entry or exit of gas. The incidence of this difficulty is small (only 1%–5% for difficult and 0.01%–0.14% for impossible mask ventilation). Risk factors for difficult ventilation are shown in Table 16.3.

Other risk factors suggested, but not proven, to cause difficulty include lack of teeth, limited mandibular protrusion, macroglossia, massive jaw or heavy jaw muscles, and abnormal neck anatomy. Additional factors that should be considered are facial dressings or burns, skin sensitivity, and pharyngeal pathology such as the lingual tonsil, lingual tonsillar hypertrophy, and a thyroglossal cyst.

Prediction of difficult intubation

Direct laryngoscopy with a rigid laryngoscope is the historical tool used for orotracheal intubation. In addition to patient characteristics, the most important factor in determining the success or failure of airway management is the skill of the personnel managing the airway and their ability to recognize and react to the difficult airway. If direct laryngoscopy is predicted to be difficult on preoperative assessment of the patient, other approaches should be considered.

Table 16.1. Conditions associated with difficult endotracheal intubation

Syndrome/pathology	Description/difficulty
Congenital syndromes	
Down's	Large tongue, small mouth make laryngoscopy difficult; small subglottic diameter is possible; laryngospasm is common
Klippel-Feil	Neck rigidity because of cervical vertebral fusion
Pierre Robin	Small mouth, large tongue, mandibular anomaly; awake intubation essential in neonate
Treacher Collins	Direct laryngoscopy is difficult
Turner's	High likelihood of difficult direct laryngoscopy
Acquired disease states	
Angioedema	Obstructive swelling renders ventilation and intubation difficult
Ankylosing spondylitis	Fusion of cervical spine may render direct laryngoscopy impossible
Diabetes mellitus	May have reduced mobility of atlanto-occipital joint
Hypothyroidism	Large tongue and abnormal soft tissue (myxedema) make ventilation and intubation difficult
Laryngeal edema (postintubation)	Irritable airway, narrowed laryngeal inlet
Obesity	Upper airway obstruction with loss of consciousness; tissue mass makes mask ventilation difficult
Papillomatosis	Airway obstruction
Radiation therapy	Fibrosis may distort airway or make manipulations difficult
Rheumatoid arthritis	Mandibular hypoplasia, temporomandibular joint arthritis, immobile cervical spine, laryngeal rotation, and cricoarytenoid arthritis make intubation difficult
Sarcoidosis	Airway obstruction (lymphoid tissue)
Scleroderma	Tight skin and temporomandibular joint involvement make mouth opening difficult
Soft tissue, neck injury (edema, bleeding, emphysema)	Anatomic distortion of airway, obstruction
Temporomandibular joint syndrome	Severe impairment of mouth opening
Tetanus	Trismus renders oral intubation impossible
Infection	
Abscess (submandibular, retropharyngeal, Ludwig's angina)	Distortion of airway may render mask ventilation or intubation extremely difficult
Croup, bronchitis, pneumonia (current or recent)	Airway irritability with tendency for cough, laryngospasm, bronchospasm
Epiglottitis	Laryngoscopy may worsen obstruction
Trauma	
Basilar skull fracture	Nasal intubation attempts may result in intracranial trauma
Cervical spine injury	Neck manipulation may traumatize spinal cord
Maxillary or mandibular injury	Airway obstruction, difficult mask ventilation and intubation; cricothyroidotomy may be necessary with combined injuries

Adapted from Miller RD. *Miller's Anesthesia* 2000: 5th edition; Tables 42–2 and 42–3.

Table 16.2. Components of the airway physical examination

Parameter	Factors for consideration
General appearance	Level of consciousness; evidence of respiratory distress, stridor, or cyanosis; body habitus; cervical collar or evidence of external trauma; pregnancy and body jewelry
Face	Beard or obvious facial abnormalities that might prevent adequate seal during mask ventilation
Nares	Patency, masses, evidence of trauma
Temporomandibular joint	Interincisor distance ($\geq$4 cm or 2 fingerbreadths is desirable), ability to prognath the mandibular teeth anterior to the maxillary teeth
Palate	High arched palate or a long narrow mouth may present difficulty
Tongue	Piercings or large tongue may cause difficulty
Submental space	Thyromental distance $\geq$7 cm is desirable
Dentition	Dentures, loose teeth, prominent upper incisors or canines, with or without overbite
Neck	Short thick neck is associated with difficult intubation, decreased neck mobility, or inability to sniff

Atlanto-occipital joint extension

Direct laryngoscopy typically is performed with the patient supine and the operator standing at the head of the bed. The goal of laryngoscopy is to visualize the laryngeal opening. Therefore, the operator attempts to position the patient in such a way as to create a straight line between the observer and the larynx. The three-axis alignment theory describes the airway as consisting of the oral and pharyngeal anatomic axes, leading the laryngoscopist to the opening of the laryngotracheal axes (Fig. 16.1). According to the theory, two former lines need to be in alignment for visualization of the vocal cords. Elevation of the head (about 10 cm) with pads below the occiput and the shoulders remaining on the table helps align the laryngeal and pharyngeal axes. In addition, head extension at the atlanto-occipital joint creates the shortest distance (almost a straight line) from the incisors to the glottic opening. Therefore, risk factors for difficult intubation include those that prevent alignment of this axis or anatomic structures that block direct visualization.

The "sniffing position" (Fig. 16.2), originally suggested by Magill to help align a patient's head during tracheal intubation, requires some degree of neck mobility (actually Magill suggested an "elderly gentleman sniffing the early morning air" or "draining a pint of beer"). Reduced atlanto-occipital joint

Table 16.3. Prediction of difficult mask ventilation

Body mass index >26 kg/m^2
Age >55 y
Obstructive sleep apnea or history of snoring
Presence of a beard

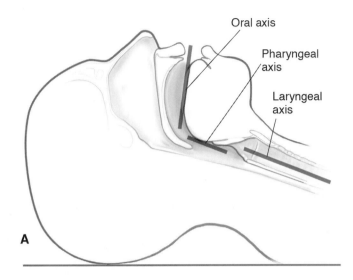

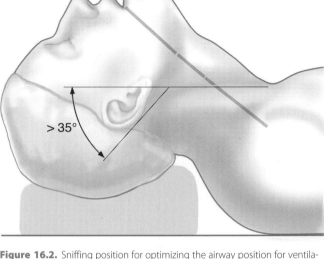

Figure 16.2. Sniffing position for optimizing the airway position for ventilation or endotracheal intubation.

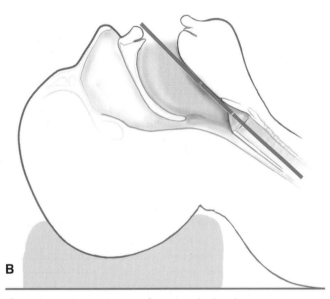

Figure 16.1. Ideal head position for endotracheal intubation.

extension is a predictor of difficult intubation based on measurements made of the cervical spine, mandible, and upper jaw in patients considered to be difficult to intubate. In general, neck extension <35° is associated with difficulty in intubation; the average neck extension is 54° to 64°. Therefore, the range of motion of the neck plays a large part in the prediction of difficult intubation.

Mallampati classification

In 1983, Mallampati suggested and tested the following hypothesis: "If the base of the tongue is disproportionately large, it overshadows the larynx, rendering exposure of the latter by direct laryngoscopy poor or difficult." From this premise, a rating system was devised comparing tongue size to pharyngeal size. The Mallampati classification system, later modified by

Samsoon and Young (1987), has since become a standard practice in airway assessment (Fig. 16.3). The test is done as the patient sits with the head in a neutral position, the mouth open, and the tongue protruding to its limit. The airway is assessed and classified according to the pharyngeal structures seen. The patient is not asked to phonate during this maneuver, as it raises the soft palate and, on average, the view of the pharynx. In addition, the test should be repeated twice to avoid false positives and negatives. The Mallampati classification is as follows:

Class I – soft palate, pharyngeal wall, entire uvula, and pillars
Class II – soft palate, pharyngeal wall, portion of uvula
Class III – soft palate, base of uvula or no uvula
Class IV – hard palate only

The Mallampati examination is the most commonly used test in airway assessment. It is relatively easy to perform, with no need for extra equipment. However, it has a sensitivity of only about 50% for predicting difficult intubation, with a high false-positive rate. The results of the test depend a great deal on patient cooperation and proper positioning, two factors that have been shown to be difficult to replicate.

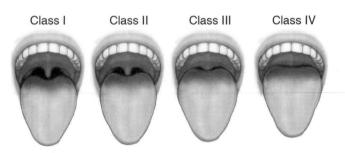

Figure 16.3. The modified Mallampati classification system.

Mouth opening and mandibular space

In addition to the Mallampati classification, other screening tests include measuring the mouth opening using interincisor distance and measuring mandibular space using the thyromental distance. The former is reflected in the Mallampati examination, and although it is assessed often, it has not been shown to be an independent predictor of difficult tracheal intubation. Normal interincisor distance is about 4 cm.

Thyromental distance is defined as the distance from the chin (mentum) to the thyroid cartilage notch with the patient's neck in an extended position. Normal distance is 6.5 to 7.0 cm. Distances of 6.0 to 6.5 cm have been associated with difficult laryngoscopy and those <6.0 cm with difficult intubation. The combination of Mallampati score and thyromental distance is one of the best overall predictors of difficult intubation.

Dentition

Although injury to a patient's teeth during intubation is unusual, it still is one of the most common complications of anesthesia. In addition, prominent teeth may hinder direct laryngoscopy by limiting the alignment of the oral and pharyngeal axis during laryngoscopy. Risk factors for dental injury and difficult laryngoscopy include prominent upper incisors or canines or an overbite. An edentulous state can help with direct laryngoscopy (oral axis alignment) but may cause hypopharyngeal obstruction by the tongue during bag–mask ventilation.

Prediction of difficult supraglottic device insertion

Supraglottic devices often are the first rescue devices used in the "cannot intubate, cannot ventilate" scenario. Placement of the laryngeal mask airway (LMA) is not always easy, and seating above the vocal cords rarely is not possible. The rate of failure to place an LMA is 0.24%, and studies correlating the ease of LMA insertion with Mallampati classification are controversial at best.

Prediction of difficult surgical airway

The emergent surgical airway is a situation of last resort for most anesthesiologists. It is a rare event, thus there are limited data on the prediction of difficult tracheostomy. Obese patients, particularly those with obstructive sleep apnea, may pose a problem because excess skin and redundant tissue may impair the operation. Tracheostomy placement also may be difficult in infants and children because of their relatively short necks.

Suggested readings

Adnet F, Borron SW, Dumas JL, et al. Study of the "sniffing position" by magnetic resonance imaging. *Anesthesiology* 2001; 94:83–86.

Bannister FB, MacBeth RG. Direct laryngoscopy and tracheal intubation. *Lancet* 1944; 2:651–654.

Benumof JL. Difficult laryngoscopy: obtaining the best view. *Can J Anaesth* 1994; 41:361–365.

Chou UC, Wu TL. Large hypopharyngeal tongue: a shared anatomic abnormality for difficult mask ventilation, difficult intubation, and obstructive sleep apnea? [letter]. *Anesthesiology* 2001; 94:936–937.

El-Ganzouri AR, McCarthy RJ, Tuman, KJ, et al. Preoperative airway assessment: predictive value of a multivariate risk index. *Anesth Analg* 1996; 82:1197–1204.

Magill IW. Endotracheal anesthesia. *Am J Surg* 1936; 34:450–455.

Mallampati RS, Gatt SP, Gugino LD. A clinical sign to predict difficult tracheal intubation: a prospective study. *Can Anaesth Soc J* 1985; 32:429.

Practice guidelines for management of the difficult airway: an updated report by the American Society of Anesthesiologists Task Force on Management of the Difficult Airway. *Anesthesiology* 2003; 98(5):1269–1277.

Samsoon GLT, Young JRB. Difficult tracheal intubation: a retrospective study. *Anaesthesia* 1987; 42:487–490.

Savva D. Prediction of difficult tracheal intubation. *Br J Anaesth* 1994; 73:149–153.

White A, Kander PL. Anatomical factors in difficult direct laryngoscopy. *Br J Anaesth* 1975; 47:468–474.

Wilson ME, Spiegelhalter D, Robertson L, Lesser P. Predicting difficult intubation. *Br J Anaesth* 1988; 61:211–216.

Perioperative airway management

Sibinka Bajic and Sarah H. Wiser

Airway management is fundamental to the practice of anesthesia. To provide safe and effective airway management, the anesthesiologist must be knowledgeable in both airway techniques and equipment. In addition, knowledge of basic airway anatomy and an understanding of the patient's characteristics will help determine the appropriate approach to the patient's airway in clinical practice.

A general approach to airway management is outlined in Fig. 17.1. This represents an effective preoperative exercise to help guide perioperative airway management and the path to be followed through the American Society of Anesthesiologists (ASA) difficult airway algorithm.

Noninvasive airway maintenance techniques

The noninvasive airway maintenance technique is suitable for procedures that allow for a local or regional anesthetic, supplemented with sedation and oxygen, when general anesthesia is not required. The patient needs to be cooperative and

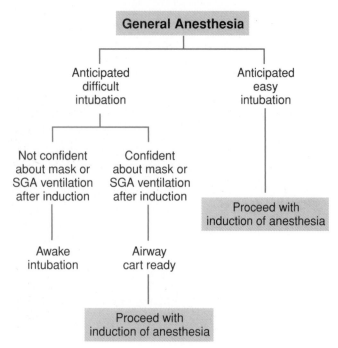

Figure 17.1. A general approach to airway management.

to understand that light sedation may not make him or her unaware of the surgical procedure. Furthermore, the patient should be informed that a general anesthetic may be necessary in the event of an inadequate block or a surgical/anesthetic complication.

Nasal cannula

Supplemental oxygen may be delivered either by nasal cannula or a simple face mask. A nasal cannula can be placed rapidly and comfortably in most patients. The continuous flow of oxygen causes nearly 80% of the gas to be wasted during expiration. During quiet respiration, the fraction of inspired oxygen content (FiO_2) increases by 1% to 2% (above 21%) per each liter of oxygen flow. The maximal level of FiO_2 that can be achieved with a nasal cannula is 40% to 50% at oxygen flows >10 L/min. Flows >5 L/min create gas jetting into the nasal cavity, with subsequent drying and crusting of the nasal mucosa, leading to patient discomfort. In situations in which a higher FiO_2 is required, a face mask is a better alternative. Pooling of oxygen beneath drapes has been a factor in operating room fires, and caution must be exercised whenever the surgical site is proximal to the airway or oxygen source.

Face masks

The nonreservoir simple face mask is suitable for patients who require a moderately increased level of oxygen therapy for short periods (e.g., during an operation, medical transport, care in the postanesthesia recovery or emergency room). The FiO_2 received depends on the mask volume, pattern of ventilation, and oxygen flow rate. At low flows, exhaled carbon dioxide is retained in the mask, resulting in rebreathing; thus the minimal flow rate should be 5 L/min. One should expect an FiO_2 of 30% to 60% with flows of 5 to 10 L/min, respectively.

Two types of reservoir masks are commonly available for use: the partial rebreathing mask and the nonrebreathing mask. The partial rebreathing mask, a simple mask with a reservoir bag, is considered a low-flow system. At flow rates of 6 to 10 L/min, the system can provide an FiO_2 of 40% to 70%. The nonrebreathing mask is similar to the partial rebreathing mask, except that it has a series of one-way valves between the bag and mask. These valves prevent exhaled air from returning to the

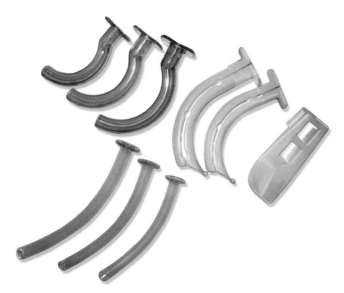

Figure 17.2. Artificial airways: oropharyngeal, Ovassapian intubating airway, and nasopharyngeal airways.

bag, thereby preventing rebreathing. Because a nonrebreathing mask coupled with high oxygen flow (15 L/min) may provide an FiO_2 of nearly 100%, it is commonly used in intensive care settings as a preoxygenation device prior to intubation.

During sedation with spontaneous respiration, the oxygen saturation, pattern of breathing, and end-tidal CO_2 should be monitored continuously. The clinician should be vigilant for potential airway compromise secondary to excessive sedation. Partial airway compromise often manifests with airway "noises." Inspiratory noises of snoring occur as a result of loss of pharyngeal muscle tone due to central nervous system depression. This loss of pharyngeal muscle tone can be corrected by airway maneuvers such as a head tilt/chin lift and/or a jaw thrust, or by placement of an artificial (nasal or oral) airway (Fig. 17.2). Inspiratory noises of stridor or "crowing" may indicate serious and impeding laryngeal obstruction or laryngospasm, which should be recognized rapidly and treated with positive pressure ventilation and/or removal of airway secretions. This may require deeper anesthesia and airway control if not resolved quickly. The total lack of respiratory noises combined with ongoing inspiratory effort (e.g., suprasternal and costal retractions) occurs in the setting of total airway collapse and must be treated immediately.

Oro- and nasopharyngeal airway

The oropharyngeal airway may be used for airway patency or as a bite block (Fig. 17.2). It is a hollow, rigid structure with a proximal flange, bite block, and curvature that mimics the contour of the airway. It is contraindicated if pharyngeal and laryngeal reflexes are intact, as it may lead to gagging with regurgitation or laryngospasm. Other potential complications include airway trauma during insertion and airway obstruction.

Alternatively, the nasopharyngeal airway is used to maintain upper airway patency and is better tolerated in sedated or

lightly anesthetized patients, even if pharyngeal and laryngeal reflexes are intact (Fig. 17.2). It is a curved cylinder made of one of several pliable materials, with a proximal flange to prevent overinsertion into the airway, and is beveled on one side to minimize mucosal trauma. Contraindications to nasopharyngeal airway use include nasal airway obstruction, nasal and basilar skull fractures, a markedly deviated septum, coagulopathy, and cerebrospinal fluid rhinorrhea. Complications include epistaxis, nasopharyngeal submucosal tunneling, and pressure sores.

Invasive airway maintenance techniques
Bag–mask ventilation

Bag–mask ventilation is minimally invasive and remains the mainstay to assist or control ventilation in the peri-induction/emergence period of a general anesthetic, for the delivery of an anesthetic, and during resuscitation. The most important aspect of effective mask ventilation is achieving a good mask seal. An adequate mask seal requires proper handling of the mask and often placement of the patient's head and neck in the "sniffing" position. The sniffing position is flexion of the neck at the lower cervical vertebrae with extension at the atlanto-axial joint. In the supine patient, the sniffing position can be achieved easily by placing a small ring or folded blanket under the patient's head to flex the neck and tilt the head backward.

There are two techniques for holding a mask, the one-handed and two-handed/two-person techniques. The one-handed technique involves placement of the mask onto the patient's face with the thumb and index fingers around the circuit connecter of the mask, down-placing the mask onto the face with concurrent upward displacement of the mandible with the remainder of the fingers, known as a "jaw thrust" (Fig. 17.3). This technique frees the other hand for delivery of positive pressure breaths by squeezing the reservoir bag. Difficulty with mask ventilation is encountered in elderly, obese, edentulous,

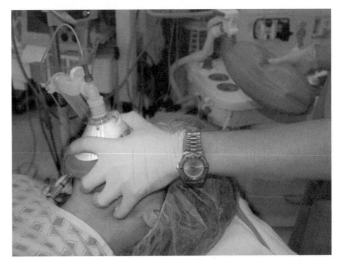

Figure 17.3. Proper finger/hand position during one-handed bag–mask ventilation.

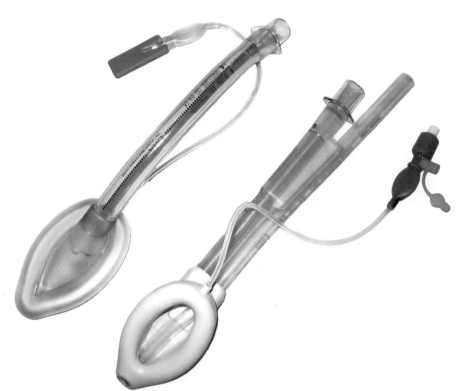

Figure 17.4. Disposable LMA (*left*) and ProSeal LMA (*right*).

or bearded patients, as well as in patients with a history of obstructive sleep apnea. In such instances, a two-handed/two-person technique may be required to deliver adequate ventilation. Here, the primary operator acts to ensure a good seal between the mask and the patient's face while performing a bilateral jaw thrust and mask seal with both hands; the second operator ventilates the patient by squeezing the reservoir bag. One should be cautious not to cause trauma to the eyes or branches of the facial and trigeminal nerves while providing mask ventilation.

Whenever mask ventilation is used, no more than 15 to 20 mm Hg of positive pressure should be required, unless pulmonary pathology or obesity is present. Applying higher pressure may lead to gastric insufflation, compromise of oxygenation, regurgitation, and/or aspiration. If greater pressure is required or difficult ventilation is present, the clinician should adjust the mask fit, try a two-handed technique, and consider placement of oro/nasopharyngeal airway devices. If initial troubleshooting is unsuccessful, more "invasive" methods should be considered.

Supraglottic devices

Supraglottic devices are designed to keep the airway patent without entering the larynx. Several types of supraglottic devices are available; the one most commonly used is the Laryngeal Mask Airway (LMA). Recently, many new supraglottic devices became available that vary by material composition, shape, and, in some instances, functionality. The Combitube has been used largely in rescue/emergency airway situations. Another device, the King laryngeal tube (King LT;

King Systems, Noblesville, IN), has been used increasingly for standard anesthetic procedures. The latter two devices are promoted as conferring some protection against aspiration, although randomized controlled trials are lacking to confirm this potential benefit. In general, supraglottic devices are indicated for nonemergent anesthetic cases, in healthy patients without the risk of aspiration, and for routine, short procedures. Outside these indications, they may be used for rescue when tracheal intubation fails or is not available.

Laryngeal Mask Airway

The LMA (Fig. 17.4) is composed of an airway tube with a standard 15-mm anesthetic connector at the proximal end and an inflatable mask at the distal end. As with cuffed endotracheal tubes (ETTs), inflation is controlled by a pilot balloon system. The opening of the airway tube is covered by two bars to prevent the epiglottis from being trapped in the airway tube, which might cause obstruction of airflow. Once inserted, the LMA sits in the hypopharynx with the opening overlying the laryngeal entrance and the tip of the mask within the upper esophageal sphincter. The LMA, an alternative to mask ventilation and tracheal intubation, is used in 35% of all general anesthetic cases in the United States. In addition, the LMA is a useful tool in the ASA difficult airway algorithm as a rescue device in patients with unexpected difficult airways or as a conduit for intubation.

When correctly placed, the LMA can seal the hypopharyngeal space and allow for spontaneous or positive pressure ventilation of up to 20 cm H_2O pressure. Although the LMA will protect the larynx from oropharyngeal secretions, it was

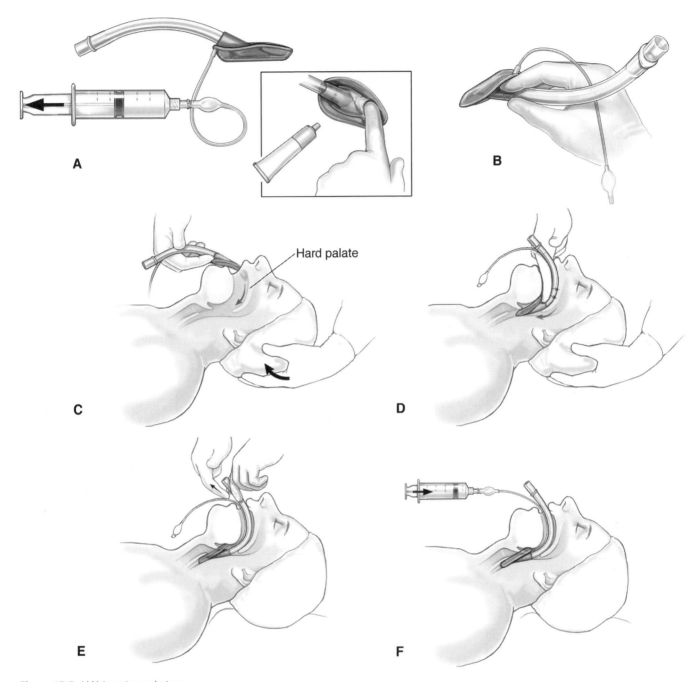

Figure 17.5. LMA insertion technique.

not designed to protect the airway from regurgitated contents. However, reports of aspiration are rare. The LMA is best suited for nonemergent, short procedures in supine ASA I or ASA II patients with no risk of aspiration. However, the LMA has been used for airway management in a wide variety of cases, including transesophageal echocardiography, cardioversions, head and neck operations, pulmonary procedures, surgery in patients in a nonsupine position, and laparoscopic cholecystectomies. Contraindications for elective LMA placement include patients who have not fasted; laboring women; and any patient with risk of pulmonary aspiration, hiatal hernia with significant positional gastroesophageal reflux disease (GERD), oropharyngeal, glottic or subglottic airway obstruction; poor pulmonary compliance; or a limited mouth opening.

Multiple techniques for placing an LMA have been described. However, to ensure proper placement of the LMA, the recommended technique is the one described by its inventor, Dr. Archie Brain (Fig. 17.5). This technique involves the following:

- Completely deflating and lubricating the mask (however, some trials have shown greater success with partial cuff inflation)

- Holding the LMA with the dominate hand, with the index finger between the airway tube and the mask
- Placing the patient's head and neck in the sniffing position and widening the oropharyngeal angle by placing the nondominant hand at the vertex of the head to open the mouth, allowing for visualization of the hard palate
- Inserting the LMA by flattening the mask against the hard palate and advancing the LMA posteriorly with the index finger while maintaining cranial pressure
- Removing the index finger of the dominant hand
- Inflating the mask, upon which the LMA lifts out by 1 to 2 cm and the cricoid cartilage moves forward. Once the LMA is inflated, the anesthesia circuit can be connected for conformation of adequate ventilation, with either spontaneous or controlled ventilation (with or without muscle relaxation).

Several LMA types and sizes are available (made by LMA Inc., San Diego, CA), including LMA Classic and its disposable version (LMA Unique); LMA ProSeal, which has a separate port used to verify its position and can accommodates a tube for gastric suctioning, and its disposable version (the LMA Supreme); LMA Fastrach, or intubating LMA, designed to facilitate blind or fiber-optically guided endotracheal intubation; and the LMA CTrach, which adds video capability to the Fastrach. A variety of adult and pediatric sizes are available, and appropriate size selection and cuff inflation is vital for a successful LMA seal (Table 17.1). With proper use, the incidence of gastric content aspiration with an LMA is equal to that of the tracheal tube.

Finally, it is important to be aware of complications of LMA insertion, including sore throat, vascular compression due to an overinflated and improperly positioned device, mucosal injury, and neurapraxias. The lingual, hypoglossal, and recurrent laryngeal nerves are the three most commonly involved in LMA-related nerve injury.

Combitube

The Combitube is a double-cuffed, double-lumen tube that allows ventilation and oxygenation with either tracheal or esophageal intubation. It is used occasionally for routine anesthesia, emergency airway control (during cardiopulmonary resuscitation), and difficult airway management (massive upper

Table 17.1. Recommended LMA size according to various patient weights

LMA size	Weight, kg
1	<5
1½	5–10
2	10–20
2½	20–30
3	30–50
4	50–70
5	70–100
6	>100

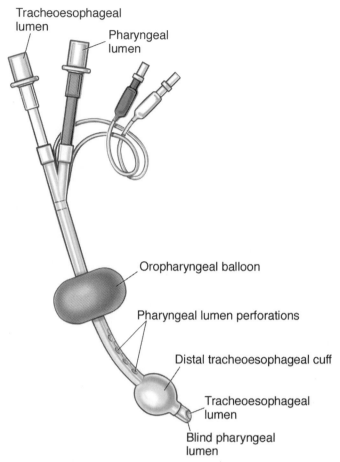

Figure 17.6. Cross-section of the Combitube.

gastrointestinal bleed, massive regurgitation, or unanticipated difficult intubations). Distally, the "pharyngeal" lumen is blind and has eight perforations at the level between the cuffs. The second lumen is "tracheoesophageal" and is open distally. The proximal balloon (oropharyngeal) is located at the middle portion of the Combitube, and the distal cuff (tracheoesophageal) is located at the distal end (Fig. 17.6). A unique tube design allows ventilation both when the Combitube is inserted into the esophagus (via the perforations of the pharyngeal lumen) and when it is inserted into the trachea, through the opened distal end of the tracheoesophageal lumen. In either case, the proximal or oropharyngeal balloon seals the oral and nasal cavity after inflation, and the distal conventional tracheal tube cuff isolates the respiratory from the gastrointestinal tract. It is important to remember that the oropharyngeal balloon is made of latex. When it is inserted, the teeth or alveolar ridge should fall between the two black rings printed on the proximal end of the double-lumen tube indicating the limit of insertion.

The Combitube is available in two sizes: 37F fits patients who are 4 to 6.5 feet tall, and 41F fits those taller than 6 feet, with some overlap. It is inserted "blindly," with 90% of Combitube placements resulting in an esophageal position, and ventilation is carried out via the perforations of the pharyngeal lumen. Advantages of the Combitube include rapid airway control and protection from aspiration, no requirement for

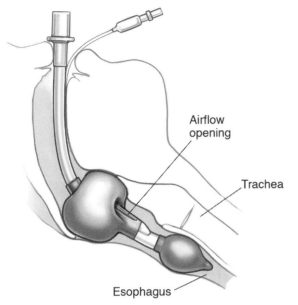

Figure 17.7. King LT in proper position. The bigger balloon is the pharyngeal balloon; the smaller one is the esophageal balloon.

visualization of the larynx, and the ability to maintain the neck in neutral position. Contraindications include the presence of esophageal obstruction or other pathology, upper airway foreign body, intact gag reflex, lower airway obstruction, patients with latex allergy, and patients <4 feet tall. Reported complications include laceration of the esophageal wall and pyriform sinus, as well as complications similar to those of the LMA.

King laryngeal tube

The King LT consists of a silicon airway tube and two (distal and proximal) low-pressure cuffs (Fig. 17.7). The airway tube is short and J-shaped (with approximately a 130° midshaft angle) and has a blind tip. The King LT has two ventilation outlets located on the ventral aspect of the tube, between the two cuffs. When the tube is inserted correctly, the proximal cuff lies in the pharynx and the distal cuff in the upper esophagus; both cuffs inflate simultaneously via a single inflation line. The King LT is designed for use during spontaneous or controlled ventilation. Spontaneous or positive pressure ventilation occurs via the midcuff openings. It is reusable (a disposable version also is available) and can be inserted "blindly" or with the aid of the laryngoscope. Inadvertent tracheal intubation occurs rarely. Six sizes are available, and size selection is based on the patient's weight (sizes 0–2) and height (sizes 3–5). The King LT is not appropriate for patients with an increased risk of aspiration, poor lung compliance, increased airway resistance, or lesions of the oropharynx or epiglottis.

Laryngeal tube suction (LTS; King Systems) is similar to the King LT but incorporates a second, posterior esophageal lumen. This esophageal lumen represents a release valve for increases in gastric pressure and permits gastric suctioning.

Endotracheal intubation

Perioperative endotracheal intubation provides a means for airway patency and protection, mechanical ventilation, and the ability to remove tracheobronchial secretions in the anesthetized patient. Primary surgical indications for endotracheal intubation are prevention of loss of the airway, complicated cases (requiring a significant proportion of time to be focused on nonairway tasks), unusual positioning for surgery, cases in which high airway pressures may occur, and those in which gas exchange is likely to be impaired. Primary patient indications for endotracheal intubation include airway protection, the need for close control of end-tidal CO_2, and postoperative intubation. A secondary need for tracheal intubation arises when surgical or anesthetic complications occur, such as high spinal, massive blood loss; malignant hyperthermia; or inadequate regional anesthesia.

Orotracheal intubation is the commonest route of intubation for general anesthesia and cardiopulmonary resuscitation (Fig. 17.8). The nasotracheal approach is reserved for surgical procedures requiring free access to the oropharynx or for patients with limited access to the oral cavity. Standard ETTs are made of polyvinyl chloride and shaped to follow the contour of the airway. However, the shape and rigidity of the ETT may be altered by inserting a stylet through the tube. It is important to note that the proximal end of the stylet should not protrude from the ETT, as it may cause trauma to the airway. ETTs usually have a lateral opening at the proximal end (Murphy's eye) to prevent occlusion. Besides the standard ETTs, wire-reinforced flexible tubes (armored) and preshaped tubes (oral and nasal) are available. Armored tubes are resistant to kinking and occlusion and therefore are preferable for use in head and neck and prone-position surgeries.

To ensure a proper seal in the trachea, cuffed ETTs are available. Cuffed ETTs consist of a balloon at the proximal end, which can be inflated via a pilot cuff. These cuffs may be high pressure (low volume) or low pressure (high volume). High-pressure cuffs may cause tracheal mucosal ischemia, especially if tracheal intubation is continued for lengthy cases. Low-pressure (high-volume) cuffs may cause sore throat (large surface area) and provide an improper seal to guard against aspiration.

Selecting the proper ETT size is important. Larger tubes provide better airway gas flow, whereas smaller ones cause less airway trauma. For an adult male, about a size 8.0 (internal diameter in millimeters) is preferable, whereas about a size 7.0 is preferred for an adult female. In children, ETT size can be calculated by the formula 4 + age/4. For example, in an 8-year-old child, one can use a 6.0 ETT. Uncuffed ETTs generally are used for children <5 years old.

Standard intubation technique utilizes direct laryngoscopy. There are many types of laryngoscopes and blades available, but the two in most widespread use are the Macintosh (curved) blade and Miller (straight) blade. Other available blades have different angles of curvature, lengths, optical components, and even movable parts.

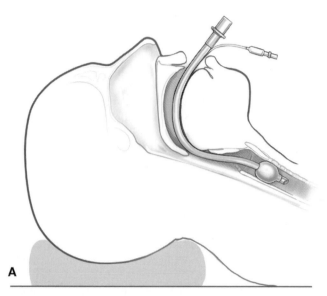

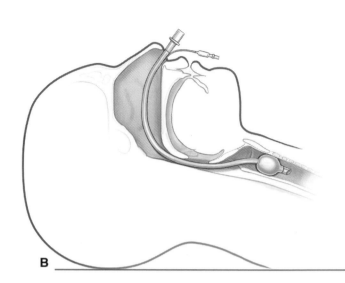

Figure 17.8. (**A**) Orotracheal intubation. (**B**) Nasotracheal intubation.

The Macintosh blade is designed to be advanced into the vallecula (space between the base of the tongue and the lingual surface of the epiglottis), and its blade displaces the tongue and soft tissues forward, exposing the larynx. Advantages of the Macintosh blade include less trauma to the teeth, more space in the oro- and hypopharynx for passage of the ETT, and less bruising and damage to the epiglottis. The Miller straight blade is designed to lift the epiglottis to expose the vocal cords. The Miller blade may produce a better view of the glottic opening compared with curved-type blades. However, its blade flattens tissue with less displacement, thus providing less space for passage of the tube. The Miller blade is more advantageous in patients with a small mandibular space, large incisors, or a large epiglottis, whereas the Macintosh blade may be better for patients with a small mouth (Fig. 17.9).

Preparation for general anesthesia and tracheal intubation should include appropriate airway equipment checked for proper function, an oxygen source, suction, and a flowing intravenous line; anesthetics and muscle relaxants of choice; proper patient positioning; and preoxygenation. The latter also is termed *denitrogenation* and involves replacement of the lung's nitrogen volume with oxygen, so an oxygen reservoir is present after the onset of apnea. Preoxygenation is performed by placing a tightly fitting face mask and delivering 100% oxygen for 5 minutes to a spontaneously breathing patient. Without preoxygenation, arterial desaturation may occur after 1.5 to 2 minutes of apnea, whereas a healthy preoxygenated patient will not develop desaturation until after about 7 or more minutes of apnea. An alternative method that is less time-consuming is to ask the patient to take eight vital capacity breaths of 100% oxygen.

Successful laryngoscopy requires proper positioning of the patient to gain adequate visualization from the lips to the glottis. The most frequently used position for intubation is the sniffing position (described earlier). This position creates maximal

alignment of the axes of the airway, allowing direct visualization of the glottis. The typical technique for laryngoscopy includes the following steps: (1) The laryngoscope is held in the left hand. (2) The mouth is opened with a scissoring motion of the right thumb and index finger on the teeth or gingiva. (3) The laryngoscope is inserted into the right side of patient's mouth and advanced toward the epiglottis while sweeping the tongue to the left. (4) With the wrist held straight, the laryngoscopist's arm and shoulder lift the tongue and pharyngeal soft tissue in an anterior and caudal direction to expose the glottic opening.

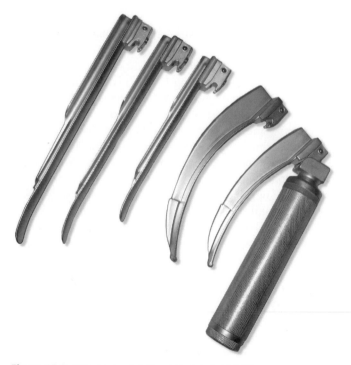

Figure 17.9. Miller blades (*left* 3) and Macintosh (*right* 2).

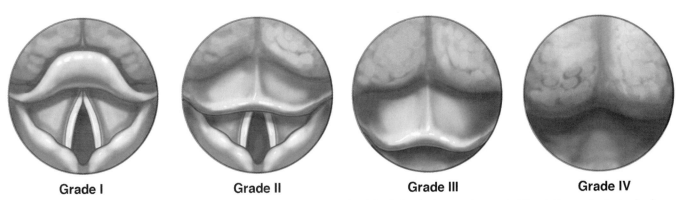

| Grade I | Grade II | Grade III | Grade IV |

Figure 17.10. View of the vocal cords. Grade I: the entire glottic opening is visualized. Grade II: only the posterior aspect of the glottic opening is visualized. Grade III: only the tip of the epiglottis is visualized. Grade IV: only the soft palate is visualized.

(5) The ETT is passed through the glottic opening from the right-hand side to avoid obstruction of the glottic view during insertion. The laryngoscopist should never use the blade as a lever, as this may cause significant damage to the teeth or gingiva.

The view of the larynx and vocal cords may be complete, partial, or impossible. Four grades of laryngeal views were described by Cormack and Lehane (Fig. 17.10).

If a good laryngeal view is not achieved during laryngoscopy, external laryngeal manipulation of the cricoid cartilage may improve the view. Furthermore, many types of intubation guides and stylets have been designed and are useful during difficult laryngoscopy. Intubation using an introducer known as a bougie is an essential adjunct to direct laryngoscopy. Many of the available bougies have a curved distal tip that allows for intubation into the trachea, even with suboptimal views (grade II or III). The bougie is "hooked" beneath the epiglottis and advanced into the trachea. A tactile click may be sensed as the tip moves over the tracheal rings; if the tactile sensation is smooth, the bougie likely has passed into the esophagus and should be repositioned. Once the bougie is in the trachea, the ETT can be placed over the bougie.

Nasotracheal intubation (Fig. 17.8b) typically is reserved for surgical procedures requiring free access to the oropharynx (e.g., maxillofacial surgery) and when there is limited access to the oral cavity. An ETT 0.5 to 1 mm smaller than that planned for oral intubation is selected. If a difficult airway is not anticipated, the naris is prepared with a vasoconstrictor (phenylephrine drops), and a lubricated ETT is passed through the nose after induction. A laryngoscope (direct, fiberoptic, or video) often is used to advance the tube under visual guidance. Manipulation of the head position, larynx, or ETT with Magill's forceps may be needed to guide the ETT into the larynx.

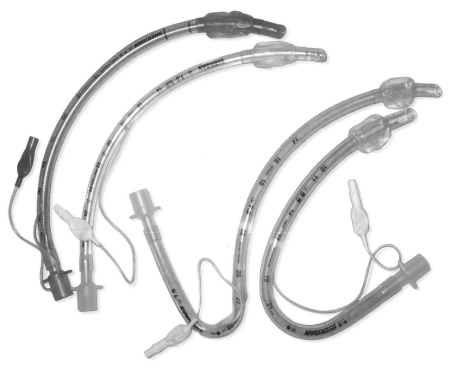

Figure 17.11. Various endotracheal tubes. From left to right: armored, regular, nasal RAE, and oral RAE tubes.

Relative contraindications of nasotracheal intubation include basal skull fractures, coagulopathy, planned systemic anticoagulation or thrombolysis, and elevated intracranial pressure. Complications include epistaxis (seen with inadequate topical vasoconstriction, large tube size, and anatomic abnormalities), retropharyngeal laceration/abscess, turbinectomy, and paranasal sinusitis (with prolonged nasotracheal intubation).

Proper placement of the ETT can be verified by a variety of methods. The gold standard techniques include visualization of the ETT passing between cords, bronchoscopy, and sustained detection of the end-tidal CO_2. Other techniques of confirmation include auscultation of both lung fields and the stomach, chest expansion, condensation in the ETT during exhalation, palpation of the cuff in the suprasternal notch, expansion of a self-inflating bulb applied to the ETT, and chest radiography. If breath sounds are heard unilaterally, a mainstem bronchial intubation should be suspected, and the ETT should be withdrawn until breath sounds are auscultated bilaterally. Additional complications of laryngoscopy and endotracheal intubation include (1) airway trauma (damage to teeth, lips, tongue, pharynx, vocal cords, arytenoid cartilages, or trachea), (2) physiologic responses to airway manipulation (hypertension, tachycardia, increase in ocular or intracranial pressure, laryngospasm), (3) tube malposition (esophageal or endobronchial placement, unintentional extubation), and (4) tube malfunction (cuff perforation, ignition, and obstruction).

Airway injury remains a common anesthetic complication. Approximately 6% of all recent anesthesia-related injury claims were for airway injury, with the most frequent sites of injury being the larynx (33%), pharynx (19%), and esophagus (18%). According to Closed Claims Project data, injuries to the esophagus and trachea were more frequently associated with difficult intubation, whereas injuries to the temporomandibular joint and larynx were more frequently associated with non-difficult intubation. The incidence of dental injuries during airway manipulation is approximately one per 2073 patients, with maxillary incisors being the most frequently injured teeth. Compared with patients with normal teeth, those with poor dentition are three times more likely to have dental injuries if they are easy to intubate and a 20 times more likely if they are moderate to difficult to intubate.

Rapid sequence induction

In the rapid sequence induction (RSI) of anesthesia, after adequate preoxygenation, intravenous administration of an induction agent is quickly followed by a rapidly acting neuromuscular blocking agent with the application of constant cricoid pressure (Sellick's maneuver, 30-40N) prior to the loss of consciousness. Cricoid pressure causes the downward displacement of the cricoid cartilage (a complete signet-shaped ring) against vertebral bodies so that the esophagus or hypopharynx lumen is compressed. Direct laryngoscopy and endotracheal intubation are performed following the onset of muscle relaxation. This technique minimizes the time between loss of consciousness and intubation and theoretically confers increased protection against pulmonary aspiration. It is indicated in patients undergoing general anesthesia with a high risk of aspiration of gastric contents (full stomach, impaired gastroesophageal sphincters, delayed gastric emptying, loss of protective airway reflexes). Patients at risk include those who are in labor, morbidly obese, or diabetic; patients with positional GERD; and those undergoing emergency procedures. However, the effectiveness of cricoid pressure has been questioned recently. MRI studies revealed that the esophagus is displaced laterally relative to the cricoid in more than 50% of normal patients without cricoid pressure and that this proportion reaches 90% when cricoid pressure is applied.

Classic RSI precludes the ability to "test" the airway with mask ventilation. In theory, a muscle-relaxed patient who cannot be intubated or mask ventilated might be encountered. If such a situation arises, the clinician should follow the ASA difficult airway algorithm emergency pathway sequence. Many leaders in the field are now questioning the necessity of not ventilating RSI patients prior to intubation. A review of the literature has shown that the reason for omitting ventilation during RSI is based on marginal, anecdotal evidence.

Extubation

The time of emergence and tracheal extubation may be a vulnerable period for patients. The ASA Task Force on Management of the Difficult Airway commented that since their publication of the original guidelines in 1993, there has been little change in extubation-related claims. During extubation, there is risk of aspiration, laryngospasm, bronchospasm, airway obstruction, vocal cord paralysis, hypertension, or hypoventilation. Extubation criteria include return of consciousness and spontaneous respiration, ability to follow simple commands, intact gag reflex, sustained head lift for 5 seconds (the resolution of neuromuscular blockade), adequate pain control, and stable vital signs. Objective extubation criteria include respiratory rate <30/min, tidal volumes >5 ml/kg, vital capacity >10 ml/kg, peak negative inspiratory force of −20 cm H_2O, dead space/tidal volume ratio of <0.6, PaO_2 >70 mm Hg, and $PaCO_2$ <55 mm Hg on an FiO_2 of 40%. The patient is asked to open his or her mouth, and secretions and/or blood are removed with a suction catheter. The ETT is removed after the cuff is deflated. Because of the risk of hypoxia due to hypoventilation and diffusion hypoxia, it is essential to have an oxygen source available at the time of extubation. Patients who presented with a difficult airway at the induction of anesthesia should be considered at risk for extubation failure. Preparation for extubation includes performance of the leak test (air escape when the ETT is cuff deflated), pre-extubation oxygenation, full neuromuscular blocking agent reversal, and verification of the patient's ability to follow commands. In cases of prolonged intubation or suspected airway edema, a leak test may be performed to detect air escape when the ETT cuff is deflated. If there is any anticipation of difficulty, advanced airway rescue equipment should be available. An airway exchange catheter (a hollow-lumen tube placed in the trachea via the ETT) may be used if there is suspicion of extubation failure. On ETT removal, the catheter may be left in place for minutes to hours and facilitates a "Seldinger-like" reintubation or is used for oxygen insufflation.

Suggested readings

American Society of Anesthesiologists Task Force on Management of the Difficult Airway. Practice guidelines for management of the difficult airway. *Anesthesiology* 2003; 98:1269–77.

Benumof JL. Preoxygenation: best method for both efficacy and efficiency [editorial]. *Anesthesiology* 1999; 91:603–605.

Cormack RS. Laryngoscopy grades. *Anaesthesia* 1999; 54(9):911–2.

Gambee AM, Hertzka RE, Fisher DM. Preoxygenation techniques: comparison on three minutes and four breaths. *Anesth Analg* 1987; 66:468–470.

Gold MI, Duarte I, Muravchick S. Arterial oxygenation in conscious patients after 5 minutes and after 30 seconds of oxygen breathing. *Anesth Analg* 1981; 60:313–315.

Hagberg CA. *Benumof's Airway Management, Principles and Practice.* 2nd ed. Philadelphia: Mosby Elsevier; 2007.

Keller C, Brimacombe J. Mucosal pressure, mechanism of seal, airway sealing pressure, and anatomic position for the disposable versus reusable laryngeal mask airways. *Anesth Analg* 1999; 88:1418–1420.

Langeron O, Masso E, Huraux C, et al. Prediction of difficult mask ventilation. *Anesthesiology* 2000; 92:1229–1236.

Rosenblatt WH. The Airway Approach Algorithm: a decision tree for organizing preoperative airway information. *J Clin Anesth* 2004; 16:312–316.

Rosenblatt WH. Airway Management. In: Barash PG, Cullen BF, Stoelting RK, eds. *Clinical Anesthesia.* 5th ed. Philadelphia: Lippincott Williams and Wilkins; 2006:595–642.

Vanner R. Cricoid pressure. *Int J Obst Anes* 2009; 18:103–105.

Chapter 18

Management of the difficult airway

Essi M. Vulli and Wariya Sukhupragarn

Management of a difficult airway is one of the more challenging tasks for an anesthesiologist. It necessitates dexterity with various airway devices and techniques as well as the ability to adapt rapidly to complex and evolving situations involving diverse patient factors and clinical scenarios. Competency in dealing with a difficult airway is expected of all anesthesiologists and is of critical importance, for it can have a profound impact on patient outcome (death, brain injury, cardiopulmonary arrest, unnecessary tracheostomy, and airway trauma). The American Society of Anesthesiologists (ASA) Closed Claims Project database demonstrates that difficult intubation is the second most frequent primary damaging event leading to anesthesia malpractice claims.

Definition

In 2003, the ASA Task Force on Management of the Difficult Airway published an updated report that defined the difficult airway as "the clinical situation in which a conventionally trained anesthesiologist experiences difficulty with face mask ventilation of the upper airway, difficulty with tracheal intubation, or both." This publication includes a revised difficult airway algorithm (DAA), which is a simple yet invaluable tool to guide the practitioner in these situations (Fig. 18.1). As stated in *Current Anaesthesia and Critical Care* journal, an alternative and often-used definition of a difficult airway is a "an intubation requiring more than three attempts at laryngoscopy or taking longer than ten minutes."

Preoperative evaluation of the airway is of paramount importance. It allows the practitioner to anticipate problems with mask ventilation and/or intubation. This evaluation includes a concise medical history, review of previous anesthesia documents when available, and a focused physical examination. Such an evaluation should be performed whenever possible prior to induction of anesthesia.

Difficult airway algorithm

A practitioner enters the DAA by first examining the airway and making a premanagement decision of awake intubation (entrance point A) or airway control after the induction of general anesthesia (entrance point B). In doing so, the practitioner either anticipates difficulty with airway manipulation or feels that no difficulty should be encountered. In this context,

"airway manipulation" should be interpreted as meaning supraglottic airway (SGA) ventilation (mask ventilation, laryngeal mask airway [LMA], or other SGA device) and/or endotracheal intubation. The importance of this distinction is to stress that it is not only anticipated intubation but also anticipated difficulty with ventilation that should drive a practitioner to proceed with caution and to perhaps choose option A.

Alternative airway devices and techniques

This section discusses the many devices and techniques available to assist the practitioner when a difficult airway is encountered. They may be of particular use in situations involving unsuccessful initial intubation attempts after induction of general anesthesia (i.e., most commonly, failed conventional direct laryngoscopy) or when conventional mask ventilation is difficult, or both.

If the clinician encounters the cannot-intubate/cannot-ventilate situation, it is imperative to consider (1) calling for help, (2) returning to spontaneous ventilation, and/or (3) awakening the patient. The following devices and techniques are helpful in these critical situations, but calling for help early is critical.

Laryngeal Mask Airway (LMA)

As discussed in Chapter 17, the LMA was developed by Archie Brain and first introduced into clinical practice in Great Britain in the mid-1980s; it was approved for use in the United States by the US Food and Drug Administration in 1991. The LMA is recognized by the ASA as a critical tool for the difficult airway patient. It appears in the 2003 iteration of the DAA as the third recommended strategy after failed "laryngoscopy/face mask ventilation." Although each of the three mentioned techniques – laryngoscopy, mask ventilation, and LMA – is expected to fail in one to three in 1,000 patients, unanticipated failure of all methods is expected to occur in fewer than one in 500,000 cases. The LMA ProSeal (LMA Inc., San Diego, CA) may add to this resuscitation potential by allowing the rescuer to empty the stomach.

The LMA Fastrach (LMA Inc.), also known as intubating LMA (ILMA), was developed by Brain and introduced into clinical practice in 1997 (Fig. 18.2). The Fastrach has been used for patients with normal and anticipated difficult airways,

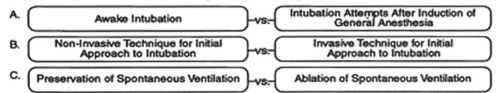

DIFFICULT AIRWAY ALGORITHM

1. Assess the likelihood and clinical impact of basic management problems:
   - A. Difficult Ventilation
   - B. Difficult Intubation
   - C. Difficulty with Patient Cooperation or Consent
   - D. Difficult Tracheostomy

2. Actively pursue opportunities to deliver supplemental oxygen throughout the process of difficult airway management

3. Consider the relative merits and feasibility of basic management choices:

   A. Awake Intubation — vs.— Intubation Attempts After Induction of General Anesthesia

   B. Non-Invasive Technique for Initial Approach to Intubation — vs.— Invasive Technique for Initial Approach to Intubation

   C. Preservation of Spontaneous Ventilation — vs.— Ablation of Spontaneous Ventilation

4. Develop primary and alternative strategies:

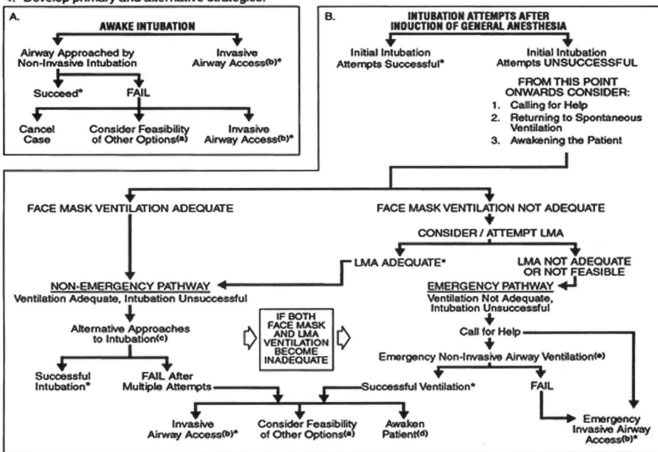

* Confirm ventilation, tracheal intubation, or LMA placement with exhaled CO_2

a. Other options include (but are not limited to): surgery utilizing face mask or LMA anesthesia, local anesthesia infiltration or regional nerve blockade. Pursuit of these options usually implies that mask ventilation will not be problematic. Therefore, these options may be of limited value if this step in the algorithm has been reached via the Emergency Pathway.

b. Invasive airway access includes surgical or percutaneous tracheostomy or cricothyrotomy.

c. Alternative non-invasive approaches to difficult intubation include (but are not limited to): use of different laryngoscope blades, LMA as an intubation conduit (with or without fiberoptic guidance), fiberoptic intubation, intubating stylet or tube changer, light wand, retrograde intubation, and blind oral or nasal intubation.

d. Consider re-preparation of the patient for awake intubation or canceling surgery.

e. Options for emergency non-invasive airway ventilation include (but are not limited to): rigid bronchoscope, esophageal-tracheal combitube ventilation, or transtracheal jet ventilation.

Figure 18.1. The difficult airway algorithm (*Anesthesiology*, Vol. 98, #5, May 2003, Page 1273).

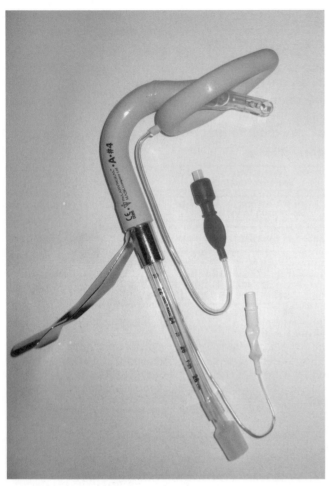

Figure 18.2. LMA Fastrach.

immobilized cervical spines, and airways distorted by tumors, surgery, or radiation therapy and for patients wearing stereotactic frames. It was designed for use as a tool for blind endotracheal intubation. It consists of an anatomically curved steel tube and handle that allows for easy insertion, following the palate (as will all laryngeal masks) without the need to insert fingers into the oral cavity or move the patient's cervical spine. Furthermore, the steel handle allows the clinician to direct the aperture of the LMA during intubating attempts. The ILMA can be used to introduce an endotracheal tube (ETT) up to 8.5 mm in diameter.

During Fastrach insertion, the head and neck are kept in the neutral position with the device handle parallel to the patient's chest. With the cuff fully deflated, the Fastrach distal tip is placed against the palate and rotated along the palate and posterior pharyngeal wall until resistance is met. The cuff is inflated to a pressure of not more than 60 cm H_2O.

Once in situ, the Fastrach is used as a ventilation device. It is advised that the operator continually support the handle during ventilation and subsequent intubation attempts. One recommended technique consists of two separate movements used to optimize both Fastrach ventilation and blind intubation. The first step involves using the handle to rotate the Fastrach in the sagittal plane until the best ventilation is obtained. The second movement involves lifting the Fastrach slightly from the posterior pharynx using the handle. These two steps allow for easy placement of the ETT through the device. Once the position has been optimized, a lubricated ETT is blindly placed via the Fastrach. If intubation fails, the up–down maneuver (whereby the Fastrach is rotated out by 6 cm and then back into the airway with the cuff inflated) reseats the epiglottis. A new-generation Fastrach, the LMA CTrach includes a handle-mounted monitor that allows the operator to view the glottis during intubation.

Once endotracheal intubation is done successfully, the next step is to remove the ILMA. This should be done with extreme caution so as not to extubate the patient. The ETT adapter is removed, and the cuff is deflated. A stylet is used to push the ETT down while gently pulling the LMA out. The adapter is then put back in the ETT, the cuff is inflated, and ventilation is checked for end-tidal CO_2 ($ETCO_2$). Some have advocated leaving both the ETT and the LMA in place, particularly when this technique has been used in a difficult airway. As with all new devices, it is strongly advised that the operator use the Fastrach and CTrach on normal patients prior to applying them to difficult airway scenarios.

Endotracheal tube guides

Numerous ETT guides are available. These devices serve as "Seldinger-like" conduits over which an ETT may be passed into the trachea and/or one endotracheal tube may be exchanged for another. One of the most commonly used tube guides is the gum elastic bougie with a coudé tip (angled up). During a direct laryngoscopy with a poor laryngeal view, the bougie is threaded under the epiglottis and passed blindly into the trachea. As the coudé tip gently moves across the anterior tracheal wall, the practitioner can appreciate the cartilaginous tracheal rings. Failure to appreciate the rings means probable esophageal placement, and the bougie is repositioned. ETT guides are capable of traumatizing and even perforating the airway or esophagus. Care should be taken not to advance the guide beyond the carina. During advancement of the ETT over the guide, the use of jaw thrust, laryngoscopy, and/or a rotating movement (90° counterclockwise) of the ETT may decrease the risk of entrapping glottic structures.

The Aintree AEC ET Guide (Cook Critical Care, Bloomington, IN) is designed to be used in conjunction with a flexible fiberoptic bronchoscope (FOB) (Fig. 18.3). This guide is a 19F hollow polyethylene tube through which a pediatric-sized FOB may be passed. It is supplied with Rapi-Fit adapters for attachment to a ventilation circuit or high-pressure oxygen source. An Aintree guide/FOB technique may be used for placing an ETT after airway rescue with an LMA or other SGA.

Lighted stylets

Lighted stylets serve to transilluminate the soft tissue structures of the anterior neck to direct the ETT into the trachea. As the

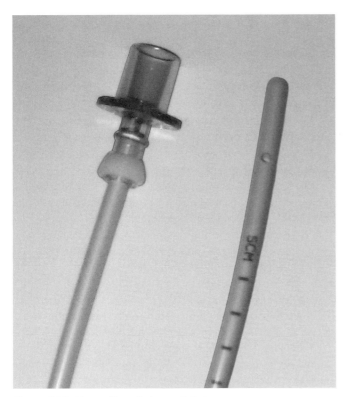

Figure 18.3. Aintree Airway Exchange Catheter.

infections/abscesses, foreign bodies, and trauma. They are relatively contraindicated in obese patients and those with limited neck extension (transillumination may prove difficult).

Indirect fiberoptic laryngoscopes

New laryngoscopic devices have all but abandoned the concept of direct laryngoscopy in favor of indirect visualization of the larynx. The earliest of these modern devices is the Bullard laryngoscope (Circon Corp., Stamford, CT; Fig. 18.5). The Bullard

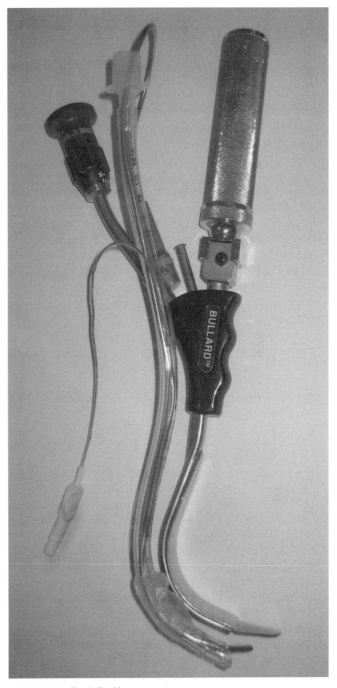

Figure 18.5. The Bullard laryngoscope.

stylet enters the glottic opening, this transillumination is seen as a distinct glow immediately below the thyroid prominence. A more diffuse glow is seen if the stylet tip is located in the esophagus. The Trachlight (Laerdal Medical Corp. Armonk, NY; Fig. 18.4) has a reusable handle, a flexible disposable wand, and a stiff retractable stylet. This device has an improved light source compared with older models. The stylet allows the ETT to be molded to a 90° angle for better transillumination and then easily advanced into the trachea as the stylet is retracted. Rigid and semirigid fiberoptic stylets are now available with or without video-assisted technology. Examples of these include the Seeing Optical Stylet (SOS; Clarus Medical, Golden Valley, MN), Bonfils Retromolar Intubation Fiberscope (Karl Storz GmbH, Tuttlingen, Germany), Weiss video-optical intubation stylet, and Nanoscope (Nanoptics, Inc., Gainesville, Florida).

Lighted stylets such as the Trachlight may be inappropriate for patients with known airway abnormalities such as tumors,

Figure 18.4. Trachlight.

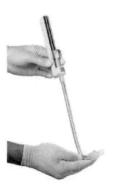

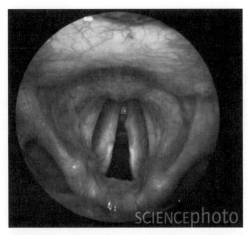

Figure 18.6. Video Macintosh intubating laryngoscope system (used with permission).

incorporates an anatomically curved blade that facilitates visualization of the larynx without the need for a wide-mouth opening or neck extension. A fiber-optic bundle runs along the posterior aspect of the blade and ends near the distal aspect. Light can be supplied from a standard battery laryngoscope handle or via a fiberoptic cable from a high-intensity light source. The eyepiece can be used directly or with a camera that transmits the image to a video screen. A working channel located on the posterior aspect of the blade can be used for suction, insufflation of oxygen, or administration of saline flush or local anesthetics. The Bullard has a detachable stylet (one stylet version is hollow for passage of an ETT exchange catheter). As with any airway device, proficiency comes only with practice in nonchallenging airway situations.

Newer video-laryngoscopes incorporate image technology into the distal aspect of the blade, eliminating the need for fragile and expensive fiberoptic bundles. The video Macintosh intubating laryngoscope system (VMS) was designed using a standard Macintosh blade and laryngoscope handle (Fig. 18.6). The GlideScope (Verathon Medical, Bothell, WA) has more acute distal angulation (60°) of the laryngoscope blade, so the operator need not displace the tongue for optimal laryngeal viewing on a remote screen. The McGrath laryngoscope includes the acute angulation blade but is highly portable, incorporating the image screen onto the laryngoscope handle itself.

Flexible fiberoptic intubation

Flexible fiberoptic bronchoscopy is arguably the most important alternative airway technique with which one must have proficiency. The flexible FOB may be used in a myriad of clinical situations; it may be used in the awake or the anesthetized patient (orally or nasally) who has or is suspected of having a difficult-to-manage airway. It is useful for the intubation of patients with upper or lower airway abnormalities and unstable or immobile cervical spines. It also may be used as a means to confirm proper ETT placement, to aid in the placement

of double-lumen tracheal tubes, or for performing pulmonary lavage or toilet.

Unlike many other tools available to the airway manager, use of the FOB requires the development of a sophisticated plan and skill set. The following are essential steps in the preparation and proper use of the bronchoscope:

- Assess the shaft of the FOB by holding the handle and allowing the objective end to hang freely. If the insertion shaft shows excessive bends or curvatures, there may be damage to the nonglass elements.
- Check proper functioning of the control lever. The distal 1 to 2 cm should move smoothly in the sagittal plane, typically 90° or more from midline.
- Ensure that the working channel is clear by attaching suction or an oxygen source. A "clogged" channel may indicate poor cleaning or damage.
- Check the fiber bundle by focusing on text a few millimeters from the lens. The inability to produce a clear image may indicate poor cleaning of the lens or moisture within the sealed elements. Note the number of black dots in the visual field. These represent individual broken fibers, and too many may make the FOB unusable. You may want to document the number of broken fibers before and after use.

When using the FOB for intubation, the following steps may improve technique:

- The handle of the FOB is held in the nondominant hand, with the thumb over the control lever and first finger positioned over the valve of the working channel. Oxygen or suction should be attached for clearing secretions and lens defogging.
- The objective end is held as close to the patient as possible; the insertion cord should always be kept straight. Turning of the objective during advancement is accomplished with both hands in a coordinated fashion.
- As one enters the airway, identifiable structures should always be visible, such as tracheal rings and the carina (Fig. 18.7). Using a device such as the Ovassapian intubating oral airway (in both awake and induced patients) facilitates the creation of a visible path and protects the scope from biting.
- Using the smallest clinically adequate tracheal tube or turning the bevel 90° counterclockwise facilitates ETT entrance into the larynx.
- Prior to anesthetic induction (after awake intubation), the operator should strive to see the tracheal carina and ETT simultaneously to confirm successful intubation.

Minimally invasive techniques

Approach to the airway via the extrathoracic trachea and larynx presents the airway manager with a completely new access to the airway. This may be vital if airway management from above has failed or is likely to fail. Unfortunately, the Closed Claims database has shown that when the anesthesiologist chooses to use an invasive technique, it may be successful but usually is done too late to affect the outcome.

The technique of *retrograde guided intubation* has historical importance for the airway manager. Prior to the advent of many of the current supraglottic and video-assisted devices, retrograde intubation was a mainstay of difficult airway teaching. The basic technique involves the retrograde passage, via a large-bore needle, of a catheter, suture, or wire through the cricothyroid membrane, up through the larynx, pharynx, and mouth or nose. The wire, suture, or catheter is recovered and is used to pass a tracheal tube in the antegrade direction through the larynx. In the opinion of the current authors, this technique may be considered useful but not "essential," and the reader is referred to other sources for details.

Transtracheal jet ventilation (TTJV) is a percutaneous emergency airway option included in the DAA. It is a relatively simple procedure, and although it may be lifesaving, it may be fraught with complications. A large-bore (12- to 16-gauge) nonkinking needle–catheter is inserted at a 90° angle to all planes in the midline of the cricothyroid membrane with the patient supine and the neck extended (unless contraindicated). The right-handed practitioner should stand to the right of the patient and use the nondominant hand to stabilize the laryngeal cartilages. A Luer-Lok syringe should be attached to the needle–catheter and continuous aspiration performed once the skin is punctured. Once air is aspirated, the needle and catheter are advanced slightly, then the catheter is advanced alone into the airway (in the direction of the carina) and the needle is removed. Several devices currently are available for jet ventilation once the catheter is in position. Low-pressure systems such as an Ambu bag or anesthesia circuit cannot provide sufficient pressure for oxygenation and ventilation during TTJV. Several nonkinking catheters are available and should be used in place of an angiocatheter (e.g., the Cook transtracheal jet ventilation catheter; Cook Critical Care).

Complications of TTJV may be life threatening (e.g., subcutaneous emphysema, pneumomediastinum, pneumothorax, esophageal puncture), and most can be avoided by using careful air aspiration during the needle placement, beginning the insufflation process with low pressure (e.g., 10–15 cm H_2O), and maintaining an open upper airway with an oral airway or SGA. It is important that a regulated oxygen injector, such as the Manujet III (VBM, Sulz, Germany), be used to prevent accidental overpressurization. Inflation pressure should be increased to a maximum of 50 cm H_2O, using chest movement as a guide. TTJV may be especially dangerous if there is outlet obstruction. In these cases, surgical cricothyrotomy may be a better choice of airway.

Cricothyrotomy and *emergency tracheostomy* are invasive, lifesaving procedures performed for the "cannot-intubate/cannot-ventilate" clinical scenario, in which awakening the patient is not an option. They are especially useful when total upper airway obstruction is known or suspected, a situation in which TTJV likely would be ineffective. Surgical cricothyrotomy and tracheostomy procedures are usually performed by an experienced surgical team. Percutaneous cricothyrotomy systems are available and may be more appropriate for the occasional user. The Melker Emergency Cricothyrotomy Kit (Cook Critical Care) uses a Seldinger catheter over-the-wire technique. A 2-cm skin incision is made over the cricothyroid membrane and a needle is inserted via the cricothyroid membrane until air is aspirated. A guidewire is passed through the needle, which is then removed. A catheter/dilator (3.4, 4, or 6 mm internal diameter) is inserted over the wire and into the airway. The catheter is available in cuffed and uncuffed versions. Complications are similar to those listed for TTJV. This technique is not recommended for children under 5 years of age. Damage to the cricoid cartilage may lead to life threatening airway collapse.

Awake intubation

If difficulty with airway management is anticipated, awake intubation (box A of the DAA) may be the most prudent choice. This is especially true if the practitioner expects difficulty with ventilation as well as intubation and/or there is a significant aspiration risk. The awake state provides several advantages over an anesthetized state: spontaneous ventilation is maintained, the size and patency of the pharynx and retropalatal spaces are increased, the tone of both the upper and lower esophageal sphincters is maintained, and important airway reflexes, including cough and gag, are preserved.

Successful awake intubation requires patience on behalf of the practitioner and methodical preparation of the patient. Adequate preparation of the patient includes not only the use of topical and intravenous medications, but also psychological guidance. The mature patient should be informed of the rationale for the decision to proceed with awake intubation and be reassured that once the airway is prepared, discomfort will be minimal. The use of medications to decrease anxiety may be considered but should be used with discretion. Benzodiazepines such as midazolam may be administered in small amounts to decrease anxiety, and opioid agonists such as fentanyl also may be used for their analgesic, sedative, and antitussive properties.

Ketamine and the α₂-agonist dexmedetomidine are becoming increasingly popular agents for sedation for awake intubation, as they have fewer respiratory depressive effects. However, the operator must be cognizant that anxiolytic agents can produce airway obstruction, especially in patients prone to obstructive sleep apnea or when multiple agents are combined, therefore leading to loss of airway control. Furthermore, an overly sedated patient may no longer be capable of cooperating with procedures or protecting his or her own airway.

An antisialagogue such as glycopyrrolate (0.2–0.4 mg intravenously/intramuscularly) is an important component of awake intubation. Antisialagogues increase the effectiveness of topical anesthetics and make the use of fiber-optic devices easier by minimizing secretions on lenses. If nasal intubation is to be performed, a vasoconstrictor such as oxymetazoline, phenylephrine, or cocaine should be applied to the nasal mucosa to prevent bleeding.

Local anesthetics may be applied topically by numerous methods or injected as part of a regional anesthetic technique. Anesthesiologists should be knowledgeable of each agent's toxicities, toxic doses, and acceptable doses. Lidocaine, an amide local anesthetic, is a commonly used agent. It is available in many different preparations (solution, viscous, ointment) and concentrations (0.5%–5%). Cocaine, available as a 4% solution, also is commonly used because it is both an effective local anesthetic and a potent vasoconstrictor; therefore it commonly is used for nasal airway preparation. Its use is contraindicated in patients with ischemic heart disease, hypertension, tachydysrhythmias, or preeclampsia or in those taking monoamine oxidase inhibitors. Other local anesthetics used for airway topicalization include tetracaine and benzocaine. Tetracaine has a relatively long duration of action but a narrow therapeutic window. Benzocaine has the advantage of rapid onset and short duration of action but may produce methemoglobinemia.

All anesthesiologists must have a thorough knowledge of the airway anatomy, including its sensory and motor innervations, to provide adequate airway anesthesia for awake airway manipulation. For practical purposes, there are three general anatomic areas of importance: the nasal cavity/nasopharynx, oropharynx, and hypopharynx/larynx/trachea.

Techniques for topicalization are as follows:

1. Non-needle technique

   · A noninvasive method of anesthetizing all three anatomic areas at once involves nebulized lidocaine and a face mask. Nebulization results in high levels of drug absorption and blunts all airway reflexes. This technique should not be used in patients at risk for aspiration of gastric contents.

   · Nasal passage/nasopharynx: Local anesthetic–soaked cotton swabs are advanced slowly into the nasal passage up toward the sphenoid bone over a period of a few minutes, or cotton pledgets may be placed with bayonet forceps.

   · Base of tongue/posterior oropharyngeal wall: Local anesthetic–soaked swabs are placed at the base of the palatoglossal arch (bilateral), where the glossopharyngeal nerve travels, and are applied for 5 minutes.

   · Hypopharynx/larynx/trachea: The tip of the patient's tongue is wrapped with unfolded gauze while the tongue is extended maximally to prevent the patient from swallowing the local anesthetic. The local anesthetic solution is dripped on the tongue base slowly via a 5-ml syringe fitted with a plastic catheter. This procedure should take 1 to 2 minutes and is accompanied by coughing as the agent is aspirated. The patient should be reassured that this spontaneous coughing is desirable.

2. Needle technique

   · Sphenopalatine nerve block may be performed by injection of local anesthetic through the greater palatine foramen, which is located between the second and third maxillary molars, 1 cm medial to the palatogingival margin. This block will cover the nasal turbinates and posterior two thirds of the nasal septum.

   · Glossopharyngeal nerve block (blocks gag reflex and decreases the hemodynamic response during laryngoscopy): There are two approaches. The landmark for the anterior approach (palatoglossal fold) is the end of the gutter between the tongue and teeth at the base of the palatoglossal arch. The posterior approach (palatopharyngeal fold) requires a tonsillar needle to inject local anesthetic from behind the palatoglossal arch at its midpoint.

   · Superior laryngeal nerve block (inhibits sensation of the larynx above the vocal cords): The external approach can be performed with three different landmarks: the hyoid cornu, thyroid cornu, and upper border of thyroid cartilage 2 cm from the thyroid notch.

   · The translaryngeal block (transtracheal technique) anesthetizes the tracheal mucosa, which is innervated by the recurrent laryngeal nerve. Local anesthetic is injected via an angiocatheter passed through the cricothyroid membrane. Coughing during injection may spread local anesthetic to the inferior and superior surfaces of the vocal cords.

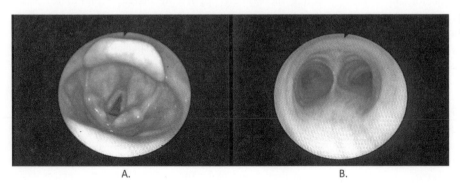

Figure 18.7. Fiber-optic view of the (**A**) vocal cords and (**B**) carina.

A. B.

Once adequate patient preparation and airway topicalization are achieved, the clinician may choose from many different methods for placing an ETT in an awake patient. For example, one may choose to use an FOB (Fig. 18.7), perform direct laryngoscopy or video-laryngoscopy, or even perform blind nasotracheal intubation. As long as the patient can cooperate and has been rendered analgesic, the operator has many options from which to choose. Awake fiberoptic intubation using a flexible bronchoscope is the most commonly used method. As soon as the ETT is advanced, the carina visualized, and $ETCO_2$ detected, anesthesia can be safely induced.

Although uncommon, there are a few contraindications to awake intubation, including patient refusal or inability to cooperate or a true allergy to local anesthetics. Patients in whom the clinician should use caution include those with ischemic heart disease, who likely would not tolerate significant cardiovascular stimulation; those with poorly controlled bronchospasm; and those in whom one wishes to avoid raising intracranial or intraocular pressures.

Suggested readings

Cook TM, Seller C, Gupta K, et al. Non-conventional uses of the Aintree Intubating Catheter in management of the difficult airway. *Anaesthesia* 2007; 62:169–174.

Cooper RM. Use of a new videolaryngoscope (Glidescope®) in the management of a difficult airway. *Can J Anesth* 2003; 50:611–613.

Current Anaesthesia & Critical Care 2001; 12:197–200.

Ferson DZ, Rosenblatt WH, Johansen MJ, et al. Use of the Intubating LMA-Fastrach in 254 patients with difficult-to-manage airways. *Anesthesiology* 2001; 95:1175–1181.

Hagberg CA, ed. *Benumof's Airway Management: Principles and Practice*. Philadelphia: Mosby; 2007.

Hooker EA, Danzl DF, O'Brien D, et al. Percutaneous transtracheal ventilation: resuscitation bags do not provide adequate ventilation. *Prehosp Disaster Med* 2006; 21:431–435.

Hudgel DW, Hendricks C. Palate and hypopharynx – sites of inspiratory narrowing of the upper airway during sleep. *Am Rev Resp Dis* 1988; 138:1542–1547.

Hung OR, Pytka S, Morris I, et al. Clinical trial of a new lightwand device (Trachlight) to intubate the trachea. *Anesthesiology* 1995; 83:509–514.

Kaplan MB, Ward DS, Berci G. A new video laryngoscope – an aid to intubation and teaching. *J Clin Anesth* 2002; 14:620–626.

Nandi PR, Charlesworth CH, Taylor SJ, et al. Effect of general anaesthesia on the pharynx. *Br J Anaesth* 1991; 66:157–162.

Peterson GN, Domino KB, Caplan RA, et al. Management of the difficult airway: a closed claims analysis. *Anesthesiology* 2005; 105:33–39.

Practice guidelines for the management of the difficult airway: an updated report by the American Society of Anesthesiologists Task Force on Management of the Difficult Airway. *Anesthesiology* 2003; 98:1269–1277.

Rosenblatt WH. The use of the LMA-proseal in airway resuscitation. *Anesth Analg* 2003; 97:1773–1775.

Rosenblatt WH, Sukhupragarn W. Airway management. In: Barash PG, Cullen BF, Stoelting RK, eds. *Clinical Anesthesia*. 6th ed. Philadelphia: Lippincott Williams & Wilkins; 2008.

Stewart RD, LaRosee A, Stoy WA, Heller MB. Use of a lighted stylet to confirm correct endotracheal tube placement. *Chest* 1987; 92:900–903.

Medical gas supply, vacuum, and scavenging

Jesse M. Ehrenfeld and Yasodananda Kumar Areti

If anything can go wrong, it will (Fig. 19.1). Although infrequent, several accidents and mishaps have been reported with the use of medical gases. Adequate safety precautions therefore must be taken to ensure that accidents are minimized and adequate backup measures are in place. In the United States, the Department of Transportation has published requirements for manufacturing, labeling, filling, transportation, storage, handling, and maintenance of medical gas cylinders and containers. The Department of Labor and the Occupational Safety and Health Administration (OSHA) regulate matters affecting the safety and health of employees in all industries.

Medical-grade gas is supplied to the operating room via two delivery mechanisms – a central supply and portable cylinders. Most anesthetizing locations have access to a central supply of the three most commonly used medical gases – oxygen, nitrous oxide (N_2O), and air. These and all other gases also may be supplied via gas cylinders – most commonly "E"-size cylinders – mounted on anesthesia machines. A waste anesthetic gas scavenging system and a medical suction system for surgical and anesthetic use also are provided centrally.

Physical principles

Medical gases are stored in cylinders either as compressed gases (oxygen, air) or liquefied gases (oxygen, N_2O, carbon dioxide). Table 19.1 depicts the relationships among gas volume, pressure, and temperature.

Pressure

Anesthesiologists make pressure measurements in both patients and machines, and hence should have a good understanding of pressure and its units of measurement. Pressure is expressed as force per unit area. Although the SI unit is the pascal, this represents a tiny pressure; therefore, the kilopascal (kPa) is used more commonly. The other units commonly used are presented in Table 19.2.

Critical temperature and critical pressure

Critical temperature is defined as the temperature above which gases cannot be liquefied by applying pressure. *Critical pressure* is the pressure at which a gas can be liquefied at its critical temperature. The critical temperature of N_2O is 36.5°C, hence

Table 19.1. Common gas laws

Law	Relationship	Formula
Boyle's	Pressure and volume	P1V1 = P2V2
Charles's	Volume and temperature	V1/T1 = V2/T2
Gay-Lussac's	Temperature and pressure	P1/T1 = P2/T2
Ideal gas	Pressure, volume, and temperature	PV = nRT

P, absolute pressure; V, volume; T, absolute temperature; n, number of moles; R, universal gas constant.

N_2O is supplied as a liquefied gas in the cylinders at room temperature. The critical temperature of oxygen is −118°C, hence at room temperature oxygen cannot be liquefied, and exists as compressed gas. Liquid oxygen (LOX) can be obtained only if the oxygen is cooled below its critical temperature and pressurized. To maintain this temperature, special insulated and refrigerated containers are required for supply of LOX.

Avogadro's hypothesis

Equal volumes of gases at the same temperature and pressure contain an equal number of molecules. This number of particles is 6.022×10^{23} and is known as Avogadro's number. One mole of any gas occupies 22.4 L at standard temperature and pressure (0°C, 1 atm) and 24 L at room temperature and pressure (RTP; 20°C, 1 atm). This principle is used to calculate the contents of a cylinder containing liquefied gas and the amount of vapor that can be generated from a given amount of volatile liquid.

Medical gases and supply

Oxygen

Medical-grade oxygen (99% pure or greater) is a necessity in any operating room. Oxygen is synthesized commercially by first

Table 19.2. Units of pressure

kPa	Kilopascal
cm H_2O	Centimeters of water
psi	Pounds per square inch
mm Hg	Millimeters of mercury
101 kPa = 760 mm Hg = 1030 cm H_2O = 14.7 psi = 1 atm at sea level	
1 kPa = 7.5 mm Hg	
1 mm Hg = 1.35 cm H_2O	

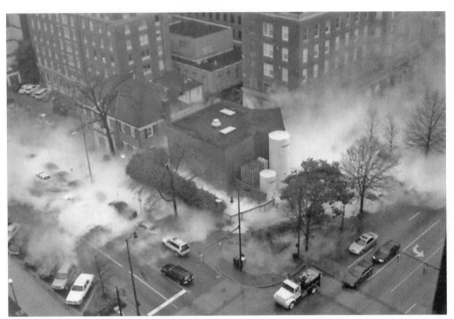

Figure 19.1. University of Alabama LOX spill. Eight thousand gallons of LOX escaped, making it temporarily impossible to assess either the primary tank or secondary reserve tank. Efficient implementation of predetermined protocol ensured that there was no adverse patient outcome despite peak use at the time of the incident. (Reproduced with permission from Schumacher SD, Brockwell RC, Andrews JJ, Ogles D. Bulk liquid oxygen supply failure. *Anesthesiology* 2004; 100:186–189.)

liquefying compressed air. Oxygen is separated from liquid air by using the difference in the boiling points of oxygen and nitrogen (fractional distillation). Nitrogen evaporates first, leaving liquid oxygen, which is then evaporated. Dried and purified oxygen is supplied as compressed gas in cylinders at ambient temperature. It also may be supplied in cryogenic containers containing liquid oxygen.

Liquid oxygen

Oxygen often is stored as a liquid, although it is used primarily as a gas. Liquid storage is less bulky and less costly than the equivalent capacity of high-pressure gaseous storage. Physical properties of oxygen are shown in Table 19.3.

Because the temperature difference between the product and the surrounding environment is substantial, even in the winter, keeping LOX insulated from the surrounding heat is essential. The product also requires special equipment for handling and storage. A typical storage system consists of a cryogenic storage tank, one or more vaporizers, a pressure control system, and piping necessary for the fill, vaporization, and supply functions. The cryogenic tank is constructed, in principle, like a thermos bottle. There is an inner vessel surrounded by an outer vessel. Between the vessels is an annular space that contains an insulating medium, from which all the air has been removed. This space keeps heat away from the LOX held in the inner vessel. Vaporizers convert the LOX into a gaseous state. A pressure control manifold then controls the pressure of the gas fed to the pipelines. A backup system may comprise another smaller-sized LOX container or manifold of oxygen cylinders. The backup system should have a separate feed line to the pipeline network to lessen the risk of interrupted supply.

Oxygen concentrator

Oxygen concentrators are devices that can be used as a primary source of oxygen to feed pipelines in remote locations. Oxygen is generated onsite using pressure swing adsorber technology. Oxygen in the atmospheric air is concentrated by adsorption of nitrogen by a molecular sieve (a zeolite). Oxygen produced by this method has a concentration of 93% ± 3%. Pressurized air passes through a bed of zeolite usually contained in two containers. As one container adsorbs nitrogen, the other is purged of adsorbed nitrogen and the zeolite is regenerated. The adsorbent has a high affinity for water; hence, the design should include adequate purges, low dead space, and heat exchangers. The beds should be sealed so that atmospheric moisture cannot seep into the zeolite. The output concentration of oxygen should be monitored carefully to ensure delivery of adequate oxygen to the pipelines. The size of the adsorption beds determines the output. They must always have a pressurized reservoir large enough to cope with peak flows. Portable oxygen concentrators also are available and are quite popular for home oxygen therapy.

Nitrous oxide

N_2O often is provided for use as an anesthetic gas. It is synthesized commercially by heating ammonium nitrate and is stored

Table 19.3. Physical properties of oxygen

- Boiling point at 1 atm: −183.0°C (90°K)
- Critical temperature: −118.4°C
- Critical pressure: 729.1 psia (49.6 atm)
- Expansion ratio, liquid to gas, boiling point to 20°C : 1:860

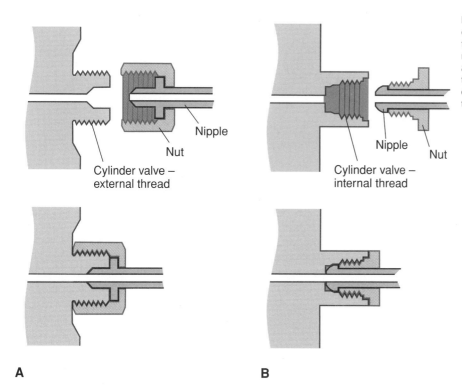

Figure 19.2. Valve outlet connections for large cylinders. The threads of the valve outlet must match those on the nut. When the nut is tightened, the nipple seats against the valve outlet. (**A**) The threads are on the outside of the cylinder valve outlet and the nut screws over the valve outlet. (**B**) The valve outlet thread is internal so that the nut screws into the outlet.

A   B

as a liquid at room temperature because the critical temperature of this gas is 36.5°C. N_2O usually is stored in large H-cylinders that are cross-connected via an auto-switching manifold. The banks usually have a smaller number of cylinders compared with an oxygen supply because of the higher content of liquefied gas and lower consumption of N_2O. As N_2O becomes vaporized from a liquid to a gas, heat is absorbed from the surrounding atmosphere, which may lead to the formation of frost on the outside of a gas cylinder.

Medical air

Air is the natural atmosphere of the earth – a nonflammable, colorless, odorless gas that consists of a mixture of gaseous elements (nitrogen, oxygen, water vapor, a small amount of carbon dioxide, and traces of many other constituents). Medical air may be provided by a manifold of cylinders or a central compressor plant. Usually two compressors are used; these may run alternately or concurrently depending on the demand. This also ensures that during servicing or repairing, the supply is not interrupted. Air from the intake to the compressors is drawn through a filter and silencer. There usually is an air cooler to cool the compressed air. The air then passes through a non-return valve into a large reservoir to maintain a constant air pressure. After leaving the reservoir, the air is cleaned by passing it through baffled separators and filters to remove particulate impurities such as oil droplets. The air is then passed through two driers containing a desiccant to remove any excess

humidity. Finally, the air is passed through a bacterial filter to ensure removal of any contaminants.

Medical gas cylinders

Medical gases are stored in metal cylinders of various sizes. Table 19.4 indicates the color codes, state in cylinders, and pressure for different medical gases. Cylinders are made of aluminum or steel alloys; each is tested by visual inspection and with a hydraulic stretch test to ensure its integrity when subjected to test pressures 1.66 times the service pressure. Each cylinder is permanently stamped on its shoulder to indicate the contents, service pressure, serial number, manufacturer's symbol, owner's symbol, test date (original test date and retest date), and mark of the testing facility.

Valves

The bulk cylinders supplying the pipelines (type H) are fitted with bullnose valves with a non-interchangeable screw-thread system (Fig. 19.2), which is different from the Diameter Index Safety System (DISS), discussed later. The type E or smaller cylinders that serve as backups on anesthesia machines are fitted with a pin-indexed valve (Fig. 19.3).

Filling

The pressure inside a cylinder may vary with ambient temperature. To prevent buildup of excessive pressure, a cylinder should not be filled above the service pressure stamped on the cylinder

Table 19.4. Medical gas cylinders

Gas	Formula	Color (US)	Color (international)	psi at 21°C	State in cylinder	E-cylinder capacity, L
Oxygen	O_2	Green	White	1900–2200	Gas	660
Carbon dioxide	CO_2	Gray	Gray	838	Gas and liquid <31°C	1590
Nitrous oxide	N_2O	Blue	Blue	745	Gas and liquid <37°C	1600
Helium	He	Brown	Brown	1600–2000	Gas	500
Nitrogen	N_2	Black	Black	1800–2200	Gas	660
Air		Yellow	White and black	1800	Gas	600

for compressed gases. The filling limit on cylinders containing liquefied gases is based on the filling ratio or filling density, which is the percent ratio of weight of a gas in the cylinder to the weight of water the cylinder would hold at 60°F. The filling density of N_2O and carbon dioxide is 68%.

Safety pressure release

Every cylinder is fitted with a safety pressure release device to vent the contents into the atmosphere if the inside pressure increases to a dangerous level. The venting orifice is closed with a disk that ruptures at a given pressure, a fusible plug (Wood's metal) that melts at high temperatures, or a spring-loaded pressure relief valve. In pin-indexed valves, this device is present just below the conical depression for the screw clamp; hence, care should be taken to prevent any inadvertent damage while mounting the cylinder on the anesthesia machine.

Devices to open or close the cylinder

Large cylinders are fitted with a "hand wheel" to open and close the valve. Small cylinders come with a spindle valve, and the spindle can be opened or closed with a wrench or handle. A wrench usually is fixed to the anesthesia machine to prevent misplacement. While using these wrenches, one must be careful not to handle the hexagonal gland nut that fixes the spindle valve to the cylinder.

Contents of the cylinder

The contents of a cylinder containing compressed gases such as oxygen can be calculated using Boyle's law, using the pressure inside the cylinder and the water capacity of the cylinder:

$$P1 \times V1 = P2 \times V2$$
$$V1 = \frac{P2 \times V2}{P1},$$

where P1 is the atmospheric pressure, V1 is the volume of oxygen available at atmospheric pressure, P2 is the pressure in the cylinder, and V2 is the water capacity of the cylinder or volume of oxygen in the compressed state.

For example, in a type E cylinder with a water capacity of 4.7 L, if the pressure gauge reads 100 atm (1470 pounds per square inch gauge [psig]), the approximate amount of oxygen available (V1) to be used at 1 atm will be

$$V1 = \frac{100 \text{ atm} \times 4.7 \text{ L}}{1 \text{ atm}} = 470 \text{ L}$$

The water capacity of a type H bulk cylinder is 47.2 L. For all practical purposes, if one learns to read the pressure in the cylinder in atmospheric pressures (the number labeled as kPa × 100), then multiplying this by 4.7 (or even with 5 for approximate values) will give an estimate of the contents of the type E cylinder for compressed gases.

The contents of a cylinder containing liquefied gases (N_2O and carbon dioxide) cannot be estimated by measuring the pressure inside the cylinder, because the pressure remains nearly constant until all the liquid is evaporated. However, they can be estimated using Avogadro's principle. The molecular weight of N_2O and carbon dioxide is the same: 44 g/mole. According to Avogadro's hypothesis, 44 g would occupy a volume of 24 L at RTP (20°C, 1 atm). Hence, a liter of N_2O weighs about 1.8 g. The actual weight of the gas in the cylinder should be estimated by the difference between the actual weight and the tare (empty) weight of the cylinder. This weight in grams divided by 1.8 (one may use 2 for approximation and ease of calculation) gives us an estimate of the contents of the cylinder. This aspect is particularly useful for laparoscopic surgeons and their teams to have an idea of the contents of carbon dioxide cylinders prior to starting the surgery.

Manifold and pipeline network

Normally, the main gas supply to the anesthesia machine is the hospital pipeline system, delivered at approximately 50 to 55

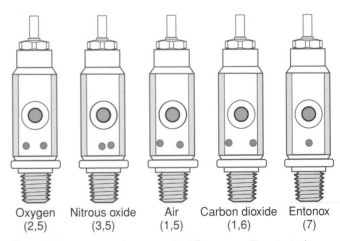

Figure 19.3. Pin-index safety system for different gases. Two pins in the hanger yoke of the anesthesia machine are aligned with two corresponding holes on the cylinder head to prevent mounting of a wrong cylinder.

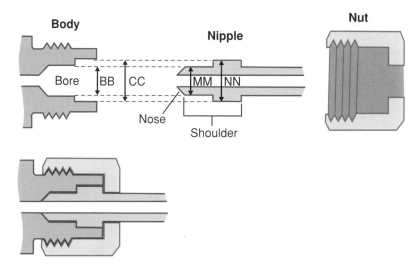

Figure 19.4. DISS – see text for details.

psig. The gas supply to the pipeline supply may be from one of the following sources:

1. Primary LOX tank with a smaller, secondary LOX tank as a backup
2. Primary LOX tank with a manifold of compressed gas cylinders as a backup
3. Two banks of compressed gas cylinders with a smaller bank of compressed gas cylinders as a backup

The capacity of the primary supply depends on the demand of the hospital. It should be more than enough for 2 days' consumption, and the backup should be enough for at least 1 day's consumption. The high-pressure source is connected to the pipeline through a two-stage pressure regulator. If a manifold of cylinders is used, only one of the two banks supplies the pipeline at any time. When this bank reaches exhaustion, the second bank automatically begins supplying gas. The status of the banks is indicated by visual indicators at the source, as well as at a manned control station, to enable a prompt change of empty cylinders.

The supply and manifolds usually are located outside the hospital. From the manifold, the gases are carried to various points of care through a network of pipelines made of copper. These networks consist of risers and branches to individual areas of the hospital. Each area should have pressure monitors and shutoff valves so that repairs and maintenance can be performed without having to shut down the entire system. The network should not result in a decrease in pressure of >5 psig from the source to the outlet. The pipelines should be clearly labeled as to the contents by letters, color-coded bands, and the direction of gas flow at periodic intervals.

Outlets

The pipelines end in terminal wall outlets with color-coded plates. These outlets may be either non-interchangeable quick-coupling outlets or DISS outlets.

Quick connectors

Quick connectors (automatic quick-coupler valves, quick connects, quick-connect fittings, quick couplers) allow apparatus (e.g., hoses, flow meters) to be connected or disconnected by a single action using one or both hands, without the use of tools or undue force. Quick connectors are more convenient than DISS fittings but tend to leak more. Each quick connector consists of a pair of gas-specific male and female components. A releasable spring mechanism locks the components together. Hoses and other equipment are prevented from being inserted into an incorrect outlet by using different shapes and different spacing of the mating portions.

The Diameter Index Safety System

The DISS was developed to provide non-interchangeable connections for medical gas lines at pressures ≤ 1380 kPa (200 psi). Each DISS connector consists of a body, nipple, and nut combination (Fig. 19.4). There are two concentric and specific bores in the body and two concentric and specific shoulders on the nipple. The small bore (BB) mates with the small shoulder (MM), and the large bore (CC) mates with the large shoulder (NN). To achieve non-interchangeability between different connectors, the two diameters on each part vary in opposite directions so that as one diameter increases, the other decreases. These dimensions are unique for each gas, and only properly mated parts will fit together and allow the threads of the nut and body of the valve to engage.

Safe use of cylinders

To prevent injury, gas cylinders must always be properly secured and stored in a cool environment protected from fire and open flame. Care should be taken to ensure that cylinders are never dropped, because damage to a pressurized cylinder may lead to the creation of a fatal projectile. The personnel handling the cylinders should be trained adequately. The cylinders should be kept closed at all times, except when they are in use. A cylinder should always be opened slowly, to prevent a rapid rise in temperature due to adiabatic expansion.

Other medical gases of interest to anesthesiologists

Entonox

Entonox (BOC, Manchester, UK) is a mixture of 50% oxygen and 50% N_2O stored in cylinders at a pressure around 2000 psig. Although the critical temperature of N_2O is 36.5°C, in a mixture of gases such as Entonox, it remains in gaseous phase. However, at a temperature below −5.5°C, a liquid phase containing 20% oxygen and 80% N_2O may form below the gas; this sometimes is referred to as pseudo-critical temperature. To prevent delivery of a hypoxic mixture, it is recommended that Entonox cylinders be stored at temperatures >10°C. Entonox is used mostly for obstetric and dental analgesia; it also is used for wound dressing changes and during transport of patients with long bone fractures but no other injuries. It usually is self-administered under the supervision of medical or paramedical personnel through a two-stage pressure regulator and a demand valve.

Nitric oxide

The role of inhaled nitric oxide (iNO) for clinical use has increased remarkably during the past decade. The discovery of iNO's role in pulmonary vascular tone led to a flood of research from basic science to large randomized clinical trials in patients of all ages, resulting in thousands of publications. In 1992, the journal *Science* named nitric oxide the "Molecule of the Year." Several researchers received a Nobel Prize in medicine and physiology for their work with nitric oxide in 1998. The only US Food and Drug Administration–approved indication for iNO is the treatment of term neonates with hypoxic respiratory failure associated with pulmonary hypertension, as a means to improve oxygenation.

Nitric oxide is supplied as a gaseous blend of nitric oxide (800 ppm) and nitrogen in a nonliquefied form at a cylinder pressure of 2000 psig at 21°C. Cylinders are constructed of an aluminum or steel alloy. Nitric oxide is administered into the ventilator breathing circuit through a monitoring unit (NOx box, NOdomo unit [Dräger, Lübeck, Germany], INOvent [INO Therapeutics, Clinton, NJ]), which operates at 55 to 60 psig. The most commonly used initial dose is 5 to 20 ppm by inhalation. Monitoring the levels of inspired nitric oxide, nitrogen dioxide, and methemoglobin is essential. Weaning should be achieved gradually in decrements of 5 ppm over 6 to 8 hours.

Heliox

Helium and oxygen mixtures (heliox) have been used for medicinal purposes since 1934. Heliox has been reported to be effective in a variety of respiratory conditions, such as upper airway obstruction, status asthmaticus, decompression sickness, post-extubation stridor, bronchiolitis, and acute respiratory distress syndrome. Helium, an inert gas, is odorless and tasteless and does not support combustion or react with biologic membranes. Helium is 86% less dense (0.179 g/L) than room air (1.293 g/L). It is seven times lighter than nitrogen and eight times less dense than oxygen. The lower density of helium reduces the Reynolds number associated with flow through the airways, favoring laminar over turbulent flow. Hence, heliox mixtures have the potential to decrease the work of breathing in patients with increased airway resistance. Heliox also increases the deposition of inhaled particles to the distal airways in patients with severe asthma.

Heliox is commercially available and supplied at the point of care as compressed medical gas cylinders in sizes H, G, and E. Helium and oxygen typically are blended to percentage concentrations of 80/20, 70/30, and 60/40. Gas regulators manufactured specifically for helium must be used to deliver the gas safely and accurately. The mixture can be administered to the patient via either an endotracheal tube or a face mask with a reservoir bag.

Vacuum

A vacuum is a volume of space that is essentially empty of matter, such that its gaseous pressure is much less than atmospheric pressure (negative pressure). Vacuums commonly are

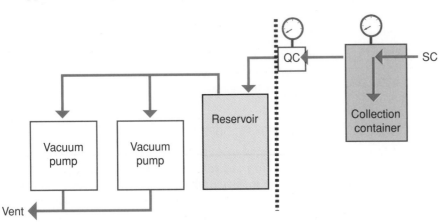

Figure 19.5. Complete suction system. Normally, liquids and solids do not move any further than the collection container. SC, suction catheter; QC, quick coupler at the wall.

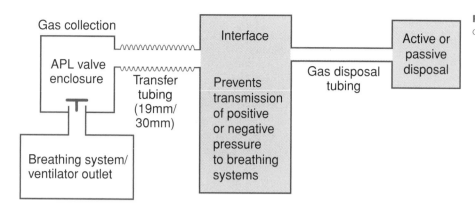

Figure 19.6. Schematic representation of the components of a scavenging system.

used to produce suction. Suctioning is an important part of anesthesia practice to remove and/or collect solids, gases, and liquids from the patient, airway devices, and the patient's environment.

The most common source of vacuum in health care facilities is the pipeline system (Fig. 19.5). The system must be capable of maintaining a vacuum of approximately 40 kPa (300 mm Hg) at the user end. The suctioning apparatus is connected to a wall inlet through a non-interchangeable coupler similar to those used for medical gas pipelines. The pipelines are connected to a central vacuum source. These pipelines are constructed of copper and are slightly larger than the medical gas pipelines. Vacuum is created by two pumps connected in parallel. These pumps are essentially air compressors mounted in reverse to create a partial vacuum. There is a reservoir between the pumps and the pipeline to even out the vacuum and collect any fluids or debris that may enter the system.

Scavenging systems

The anesthetic gases and vapors that leak into the surrounding room during medical procedures are considered waste anesthetic gases. It is estimated that more than 250,000 health care professionals in the United States who work in hospitals, operating rooms, dental offices, and veterinary clinics potentially are exposed to waste anesthetic gases. The relationship between exposure to trace concentrations of waste anesthetic gases in the operating room and the possible development of adverse health effects has concerned health care professionals for many years. Some potential effects of exposure to waste anesthetic gases are nausea, dizziness, headaches, fatigue, and irritability, as well as sterility, miscarriages, birth defects, cancer, and liver and kidney disease, among operating room staff and their spouses (in the case of miscarriages and birth defects). The reports on the effects of exposure to waste anesthetic gases are controversial. However, scavenging of waste anesthetic gases is recommended for all areas, as are work practices to reduce contamination. In addition, there should be a program for management of waste anesthetic gases, with a documented maintenance schedule for all anesthesia machines and the ventilation system in the operating room and postanesthesia care units.

Factors contributing to operating room pollution include:

1. Use of breathing systems with high-flow techniques
2. Poorly fitting masks
3. Failure to turn off gases at the end of anesthesia
4. Filling of anesthetic vaporizers without key systems
5. Liquid agent spills
6. Leaks in the machine and breathing systems
7. Improper scavenging

The components of a scavenging system are shown in Fig. 19.6. The waste gases are collected by suitable modification of adjustable pressure-limiting valves and ventilator relief valves and are transferred via special tubing to the scavenging interface. These tubes are of different sizes and appearances to prevent misconnection or direct connection to breathing systems (19 mm/30 mm; corrugated tubes used in breathing systems are 22 mm). The interface protects the breathing systems from excessive positive or negative pressure. From the interface, the gases are conducted through collapse-proof tubing to the gas disposal assembly, which eliminates excess waste gas.

There are two types of gas disposal systems:

1. *Active:* This is the most common system and uses central vacuum. It provides for high flows but only slight negative pressure.
2. *Passive:* The pressure of the waste gas itself produces flow through the system, and no vacuum is used.

Occlusion of scavenging systems may produce high levels of positive pressure in the breathing systems, leading to barotrauma. In active systems, failure of the interface may transmit excess negative pressures to the patient.

Suggested readings

Eisenkraft JB. Anesthesia delivery systems. In: Longnecker D, Brown D, Newman M, Zapol W, eds. *Anesthesiology*. New York: McGraw Hill; 2008:767–820.

Gentile MA. The role of inhaled nitric oxide and heliox in the management of acute respiratory failure. *Respir Care Clin* 2006; 12:489–500.

Pamphlet P-1. *Safe Handling of Compressed Gases in Containers*. New York: Compressed Gas Association.

Parbrook GD, Davis PD, Parbrook EO. *Basic Physics and Measurement in Anesthesia.* 2nd ed. Norwalk, CT: Appleton-Century-Crofts; 1986.

Sandberg WS, Urman RD, Ehrenfeld JM. *The MGH Textbook of Anesthetic Equipment.* 1st ed. Philadelphia: Elsevier; 2010.

Schumacher SD, Brockwell RC, Andrews JJ, Ogles D. Bulk liquid oxygen supply failure. *Anesthesiology* 2004; 100: 186–189.

Web sites

US Department of Labor, Occupational Safety & Health Administration (OSHA) web site. Available at: http://www.osha.gov/SLTC/wasteanestheticgases/solutions.html. Accessed December 28, 2008.

http://www.bocmedical.co.uk/product_information/Cylinder_data_chart.pdf. Accessed December 29, 2008.

http://www-safety.deas.harvard.edu/services/oxygen.html. Accessed December 29, 2008.

Chapter 20

Anesthesia machine

Yasodananda Kumar Areti

From Morton to Zeus

Since the first demonstration of ether anesthesia by William T. G. Morton in 1846, the apparatus to administer anesthesia evolved from a simple Morton inhaler to the present-day sophisticated anesthesia workstations care stations (Fig. 20.1). The 20th century saw anesthesia machines built around the prototype of Henry Edmund Gaskin Boyle in 1917 (1875–1941). Dräger (Telford, PA) adopted the name *Zeus* for its latest brand of anesthesia workstations. Zeus, according to Greek mythology, is the king of all gods and is all powerful. The name *Zeus* is supposed to indicate the power packed into these machines. They incorporate safe systems for target controlled inhalational anesthesia, total intravenous anesthesia, sophisticated ventilators matching intensive care unit ventilators, extensive monitoring capability, and data networking capabilities.

This chapter covers the principles of anesthesia machines used to deliver inhalational anesthesia. In the United States, the two major manufacturers of anesthesia machines are GE Datex-Ohmeda and Dräger Medical. Anesthetic mishaps due to machines are becoming a rarity thanks to the safety features incorporated in these machines, as recommended by the American Society of Testing and Materials (ASTM) International. However, one of the common reasons for adverse outcomes related to anesthesia equipment is lack of familiarity with the equipment, as well as inadequate pre-use checking. Hence, it is advisable for all users to familiarize themselves with the machine and safety documents that come with it before using any equipment.

Structure of the anesthesia machine

The machine itself can be divided into three sections (Fig. 20.2):

1. **High pressure:** This part of the machine is exposed to the high pressures in the cylinders (yoke, pressure gauge, and pressure regulators).
2. **Intermediate pressure:** This part of the machine is exposed to the pressures in the pipelines (pipeline connections, oxygen failsafe devices, oxygen flush, ventilator gas outlets, pressure gauge, and flow meter needle valves).
3. **Low pressure:** This part of the machine lies from the needle valves of the flow meters to the common gas outlet (rotameters, vaporizers, back bar, pressure-relief valve). This section should not be confused with the breathing systems, which are also referred to as low-pressure systems.

Components of the machine

Power supply

The electrical and pneumatic components of most modern machines are powered by electricity, and the master switch should be turned on before using the machines. The master switch activates the flow of gases into the intermediate-pressure pneumatic circuit of the machine. The emergency oxygen flush can be activated even when the power is off. The machines also come with a backup battery system, which keeps charging when the machine is plugged in, even if the master switch is in the off position. Once the power is turned on, there is always a "minimum assured flow" of oxygen at 200 ml/min, and the machines perform self-checks. In an emergency situation, the operator can bypass these checks. Some machines limit the number of consecutive times this bypass can be used. The machines are also equipped with visual and/or audible alarms to indicate loss of power.

Medical gas inlets

The medical gases (oxygen, nitrous oxide [N_2O], and air) are supplied through pipelines, which are connected to the machine through non-interchangeable connections (Fig. 20.3). The ASTM standards for anesthesia workstations require that every anesthesia machine have a Diameter Index Safety System (DISS) fitting for each pipeline inlet to prevent incorrect connections (DISS is discussed in Chapter 19).

All piped supplies have a backup cylinder supply (one or two E-type cylinders). The outlet port of the cylinder is aligned with the gas inlet nipple. A Bodok seal is placed between the cylinder and the yoke to ensure leak-free fitting. The assembly has a pin-indexed safety system to prevent incorrect connection of gases. The two pins on the machine should be aligned with the corresponding holes in the cylinder head. Before mounting the cylinder, it should be opened gently (cracked) to blow away any dust in the port, then closed. The cylinder is securely mounted with a screw clamp. Presence of leaks in this area can be detected

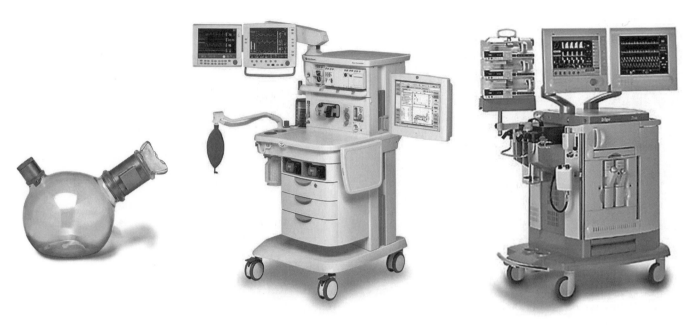

Figure 20.1. Morton inhaler; GE Aisys Carestation (courtesy GE Healthcare); Dräger Zeus workstation.

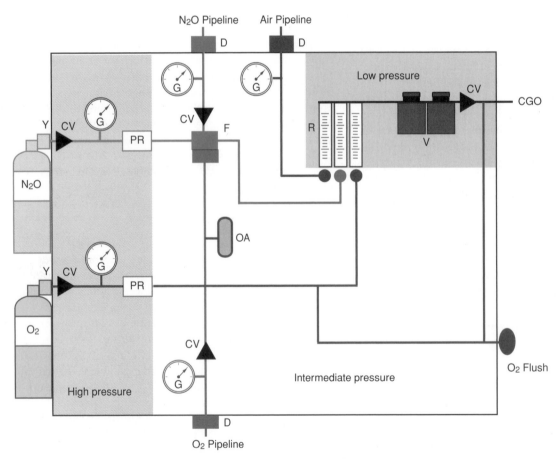

Figure 20.2. Structure of an anesthesia machine. Y, yoke; D, Diameter Index Safety System (DISS); G, pressure gauge; PR, pressure regulator; F, oxygen failsafe device; OA, oxygen alarm; R, rotameters; V, vaporizer assembly; CV, check valve.

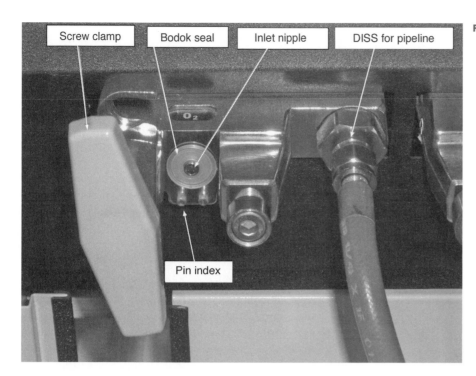

Screw clamp | Bodok seal | Inlet nipple | DISS for pipeline

Pin index

Figure 20.3. Cylinder inlet yoke and pipeline inlet.

by applying soapy water to the junction and observing for any bubble formation.

Pressure gauge

All machines are equipped with Bourdon pressure gauges (patented in 1849) to monitor the pressure in the cylinders and pipelines (Fig. 20.4). A flexible tube within this gauge straightens when exposed to gas pressure. This motion is transmitted to a pointer through a gearing mechanism. In modern machines, these gauges are located at the front panel. The dials carry two types of units of measurement of pressure (psi and kPa × 100). Monitoring the pressure will ensure an adequate gas supply at all times, and the pressure in the oxygen cylinder gives a clue as to

the quantity of oxygen backup. The gauges on the N_2O cylinder do not give any indication of the amount of N_2O in the cylinder, because N_2O exists as a liquid (see Chapter 19).

Pressure regulator

Each gas supplied from the cylinders to the machine must have a pressure regulator (Fig. 20.5). Pressure regulators not only reduce the pressure of gases from the cylinders, but also provide gases at a nearly constant reduced pressure to the flow meters, despite the changing pressures in the cylinders. Because pressure is defined as force per unit area, a high pressure acting on a small area may be balanced by a low pressure acting on a large area (large diaphragm in the regulator). A simple pressure-reducing valve constructed using this principle, however, results in decreasing reduced pressure as the cylinder contents empty. To smooth the flow and keep the reduced pressure nearly constant, a set of high-force springs was added to the modern

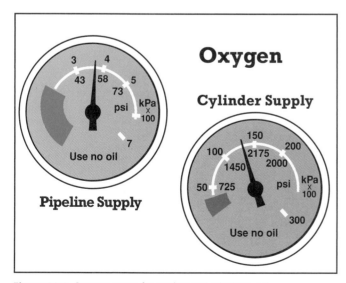

Figure 20.4. Pressure gauge for pipeline and cylinder supply.

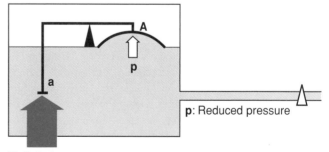

Figure 20.5. Basic principle of the pressure regulator: P × a = p × A (high pressure acting on a small area is balanced by low pressure acting on a large area diaphragm).

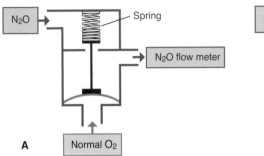

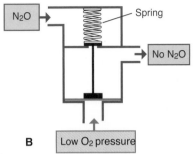

Figure 20.6. Oxygen failsafe device. (**A**) Normal function. (**B**) N_2O cut off because of oxygen pressure failure.

regulator. The pressure regulators on anesthesia machines are factory preset to reduce the high pressure in the cylinders to 300 to 350 kPa (45–50 psi). The pipeline pressures are supplied at a pressure of 350–400 kPa (50–55 psi) to ensure that the pipeline supply is used preferentially even if the cylinder is left open unintentionally. Some machines have second-stage regulators in the intermediate-pressure section before the flow meters and oxygen flush. The second regulator reduces the oxygen pressure further to approximately 20 psi gauge (psig) for oxygen and 38 psig for N_2O. This ensures lower pressure at oxygen flush; minimizes pressure fluctuation to the flow meter, thereby maintaining constant flow; and decreases the wear and tear of needle valves of the flow meters. Two-stage regulators are also used in the demand-flow Entonox (BOC, Manchester, UK) apparatus.

Check valves

Check valves are present on the yoke after the fresh gas entry port to prevent leaks during the change of cylinders and to prevent filling of the cylinders from pipelines or the second backup cylinder, even if the cylinders are inadvertently left open. These valves are also present at the entry of pipelines to prevent back-flow into the pipeline in the event pressures fall in the pipeline while the backup cylinder is being used. A check valve is also present downstream of the vaporizer bank to ensure that back pressure is not transmitted to the vaporizers, particularly when oxygen flush is activated.

Safety devices to prevent administration of a hypoxic gas mixture

A devastating complication of administering anesthesia is delivering a hypoxic gas mixture. The incorporation of ASTM-recommended standards in the anesthesia work station and its components has made this occurrence much rarer than in the past. Color coding of cylinders and pipelines, non-interchangeable threaded connections to the regulators of bulk cylinders, a pin-indexed safety system for cylinders mounted on the anesthesia machine, non-interchangeable quick couplers, and DISS for pipelines have all improved safety. Appropriate calibration and monitoring of the oxygen concentration delivered by the machine and inspired by the patient is another important advance in the standard of care. The following

devices incorporated in the anesthesia machine itself are additional measures to prevent accidental administration of hypoxic gas mixtures.

Oxygen failsafe device

In Datex-Ohmeda machines, N_2O is always connected to its flow meter through an oxygen failsafe device. This device has a spring-loaded valve (Fig. 20.6). Oxygen pressure acts against the force of the spring and keeps this valve open so that N_2O can flow to its flow meter. Once oxygen pressure drops below 30 psig (205 kPa), the unopposed force of the spring closes the valve and N_2O can no longer be administered.

In some machines, air supply also flows through a failsafe device. However, some manufacturers allow air to be delivered directly to the flow meter, which enables the anesthesiologist to administer air in the event of oxygen failure. Modern machines incorporate an electronic switch that will not allow air and N_2O to be used at the same time.

Oxygen failure protection device

The oxygen failure protection device (OFPD), used in Dräger machines, proportionately decreases the N_2O pressure based on the oxygen pressure. In oxygen failsafe devices, the flow is "all or none." In the OFPD, the flow is proportional and variable and maintains a desired level of fraction of inspired oxygen (FiO_2). Only at extremely low oxygen pressure is the N_2O flow is entirely stopped.

Proportioning systems

Newer machines are equipped with proportioning devices that ensure a minimum FiO_2 at all times.

Datex-Ohmeda Link 25

The flow meter control valves of oxygen and N_2O are mechanically linked to each other with chains. Normally, both knobs can be operated independently. Whenever the proportion of oxygen approaches 25%, the gear engages and both control knobs move simultaneously. This mechanical system is supported by a pneumatic system in which both flow meters operate at different pressures because of the differential setting in the respective second-stage pressure regulators. The resulting combination ensures a minimum FiO_2 of 0.25.

Dräger oxygen ratio monitor controller

Oxygen and N_2O are interlocked pneumatically to ensure a fresh gas oxygen concentration of at least 25% ± 3%. The pressures downstream of the flow control valves of N_2O and oxygen and upstream of the resistors before the flow meter tubes are linked through pressure transducers. This system controls the slave control valve, which controls the N_2O inlet pressure.

Oxygen low-pressure alarm

The low-pressure or oxygen supply failure alarm will sound when there is a significant increase or decrease in oxygen supply pressure. This occurs when there is a sudden loss of cylinder or pipeline pressure or when the anesthesia machine is turned on or off. A commonly used mechanism uses a pressurized canister that is filled with oxygen when the anesthesia machine is turned on. The stream of oxygen that enters the canister passes through a whistle, and a sound can be heard when the machine is turned on. If the oxygen pressure then falls below a certain value, this canister will empty and direct a reversed stream of oxygen through the whistle. This alarm may not be heard if the oxygen supply pressure drops very gradually over a long period. Some machines have a visual alarm as well. The audible alarm should be activated within a few seconds after oxygen pressure drops below 200 kPa, and has a minimum noise level of 60 dB at 1 m. The alarm can be switched off only by restoring the oxygen supply.

Flow meters

A needle valve controls the flow of individual gases into the flow meter (Fig. 20.7). A needle valve has a relatively small orifice with a long, tapered, conical seat. As the control knob is turned, the plunger is retracted and gases flow between the seat and plunger. Because it takes many turns of the fine-threaded screw to retract the plunger, precise regulation of the flow rate is possible. To avoid damage to the seat and prevent the stem from disengaging from the body, there are stops at the "off" and "maximum" flow positions. The control knobs are labeled clearly, color coded, and tactilely distinguishable. The oxygen control knob is larger and has a fluted profile. Electronic, solenoid-controlled flow devices are used in new machines.

The actual flow is measured by cylindric tubes with varying internal diameters (Thorpe tubes). The flow meters on anesthesia machines are traditionally called *rotameters* (a trade name adopted by the British Oxygen Company). They are variable-orifice, fixed–pressure difference devices. As the flow increases, the rotating bobbin rises in the flow meter and the annular orifice around the cylindric bobbin increases. The calibration is either etched on the flow meter or written immediately to the right of the tube. One reads the flow at the top of a cylindrical bobbin or the center of a spherical bobbin.

At low flows, the flow meters are calibrated in milliliters per minute (or in decimal fractions of liters per minute), whereas at high flows they are calibrated in liters per minute. To facilitate accuracy at low flows, two tubes may be used to measure

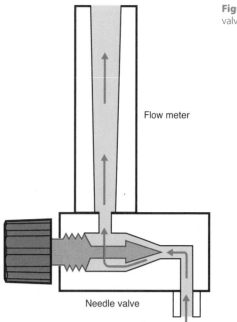

Figure 20.7. Needle valve.

Flow meter

Needle valve

flows for a single gas. One tube measures up to 1 L/min, and the higher flows are measured in the second tube. However, there is only one control knob and the flow meter tubes are connected in a series.

Flow tubes are equipped with float stops at the top and bottom of the tube. The upper stop prevents the float from ascending to the top of the tube and plugging the outlet. It also ensures that the float is visible at maximum flows instead of being hidden in the manifold. The bottom float stop provides a central foundation for the indicator when the flow control valve is turned off.

In a flow meter assembly, the oxygen flow meter joins downstream of all the flow meters to ensure oxygen flow, even if there is a leak in another flow meter. However, damage to the oxygen flow meter will result in a hypoxic mixture if N_2O is also being used (Fig. 20.8). Continuous monitoring of the inspired oxygen concentration, with associated alarms if a hypoxic mixture is being delivered, is the only option to ensure that a hypoxic mixture is not delivered to the patient.

Most modern machines use conventional flow control and an electronic flow sensor. The flow measured by the sensor is represented digitally and/or by a simulated flow meter on the anesthesia machine screen. An *auxiliary flow meter* for oxygen is incorporated in some modern machines that can deliver an oxygen flow of up to 10 L/min without the machine being turned on. This enables the anesthesiologist to deliver oxygen therapy during regional anesthesia and for emergency resuscitation.

The "back bar"

The back bar is a structure that supports the flow meter block and vaporizers. This term is used to describe these supporting components and the gaseous pathways connecting them. Many

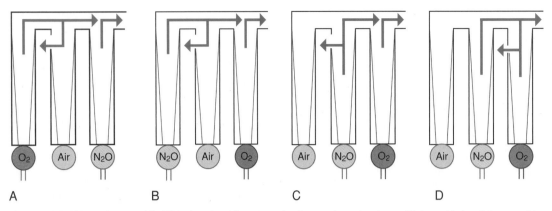

Figure 20.8. Flow meter assembly. (**A**) Leak in the airflow meter, leading to a hypoxic mixture. (**B**) Assembly in a Dräger machine. (**C**) Assembly in a Datex-Ohmeda machine. (**B and C**) A leak in the air or N_2O flow meter does not deliver a hypoxic mixture. (**D**) Regardless of the sequence of flow meters, a break in the oxygen flow meter always leads to a hypoxic mixture if N_2O is being used.

machines use a system that allows the user to add or remove specific vaporizers quickly and easily while maintaining a gas-tight system. Some machines have space for a single vaporizer only; others allow the attachment of two or more vaporizers. However, only one vaporizer can be turned on at any given time. There are two popular interlock systems to achieve this: Selectatec (Datex-Ohmeda) and the Dräger medical mounting system. Once a vaporizer is attached and turned on, gas flow is diverted from the back bar into the vaporizer to provide the required concentration of anesthetic vapor.

High pressure relief valves

Anesthesia machines are also fitted with pressure-relief valves. In the intermediate-pressure section, these valves are set to open at about 95 to 110 psig to protect against a defective pressure regulator. In the low-pressure section, they are set to open at about 40 kPa (6 psig). These relief valves protect the machine (not the patient) from high pressures. The patient should be protected from excessive pressures by relief valves within the breathing system.

Vaporizers

Vaporizers are devices used in anesthesia equipment that convert volatile anesthetic liquid into vapor and facilitate inhalational anesthesia. All modern vaporizers are precise and agent specific. Color-coded filling systems are used to ensure the vaporizers cannot be filled with the wrong agent. The currently used vaporizers are constructed to be on the machine and are not suitable for use in the breathing system after the common gas outlet (CGO). They are calibrated at sea level and are flow and back pressure compensated. Several types are used in modern machines.

Variable bypass vaporizers

Sevoflurane, isoflurane, and halothane are administered using variable bypass vaporizers (e.g., Tec 5 and Tec 7 [Ohmeda] and

Dräger Vapor). The fresh gas stream is split into two streams, a bypass stream and a stream passing through the vaporizing chamber. The ratio of the two streams (i.e., the splitting ratio) depends on the saturated vapor pressure of the specific volatile agent and is controlled by the concentration dial (Fig. 12.9).

Functional analysis of the vaporizers:

1. *Method of vaporization:* The fresh gas passing through the vaporizing chamber picks up the vapor as it flows over the liquid agent (flow over or plenum). The gases are directed to flow through a spiral of wicks soaked with liquid agent, to increase the time of contact and surface area of vaporization, thus improving efficiency. The gas exiting the vaporizing chamber is fully saturated with the vapor, and the amount of vapor up picked will depend on the atmospheric pressure (ATP) and the saturated vapor pressure (SVP) of the agent (Table 20.1) per the

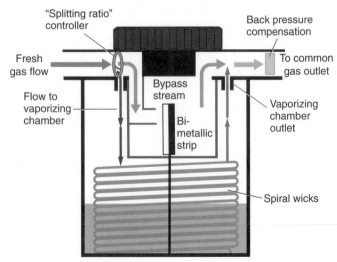

Figure 20.9. Schematic representation of the structure of a variable bypass vaporizer.

following equation:

$$Vapor\,(ml) = Fresh\,gas\,flowing\,through\,vaporizing\,chamber\,(ml)$$
$$\times \frac{SVP}{ATP - SVP}$$

This equation is useful to understand the performance of a vaporizer if it is filled with the wrong agent, or if the vaporizer is being used at a different ambient pressure. The amount of vapor picked up at sea level when a given amount of fresh gas ("x" ml) passes through the vaporizing chamber is as shown here for different agents:

$$Sevoflurane\,vapor\,(ml)\,x(ml) \times \frac{157}{760 - 157} = x(ml) \times 0.26$$

$$Isoflurane\,vapor\,(ml) = x(ml) \times \frac{238}{760 - 238}$$
$$= x(ml) \times 0.456$$

$$Halothane\,vapor\,(ml) = x(ml) \times \frac{243}{760 - 243}$$
$$= x(ml) \times 0.47$$

2. *Regulating the output concentration:* The flow through the vaporizing chamber is controlled by the control dial, which adjusts the ratio of carrier gas entering the vaporizing chamber to the gas bypassing it (splitting ratio); hence, it is termed the *variable bypass vaporizer.* As the dial is turned to give a higher concentration, the proportion of gas passing through the vaporizing chamber increases and the vapor output increases. Because the splitting ratio, which controls the output concentration, remains constant over a wide range of fresh gas flows (FGFs), fairly reliable output concentration can be obtained, even at very low FGFs.

3. *Temperature compensation:* As volatile liquid vaporizes, it consumes heat, known as latent heat of vaporization. This results in the cooling of the liquid and a consequent change in the SVP, and therefore a drop in the output concentration. This heat is supplied to some extent by the metal sink used in the construction (thermostabilization). In addition, the bypass/vaporizer flow ratio is altered by either a bimetallic strip or liquid-filled bellows so that the output remains constant, even after long usage (thermocompensation).

4. *Filling with the wrong agent:* Most present-day vaporizers are fitted with agent-specific filling systems (e.g., keyed filling system, quick-fill system, easy-fill system). However, some still use the funnel-fill system, in which it is possible to fill the vaporizer with the wrong agent. Theoretically, the ratio of different vapor outputs, as calculated from the earlier equations, can be used to estimate the output concentration of an agent administered through a different vaporizer (Table 20.1).

In the event a vaporizer is filled with the incorrect agent, in addition to the different output concentrations, one is also

Table 20.1. Approximate output concentration of an agent when administered through a different vaporizer set to deliver 1%

Agent	SVP, mm HG at 20°C	Vaporizer	Output concentration %
Sevoflurane	157	Isoflurane	0.57
Isoflurane	238	Sevoflurane	1.75
Halothane	243	Isoflurane	1.03
Isoflurane	238	Halothane	0.97

likely to face a mixture of two agents. Hence, the current recommendations state that the unit must be completely drained and all the liquid discarded. Fresh gas must be allowed to flow through the emptied unit until the wicks are dry and no vapor is detected at the outlet.

5. *Performance at different ambient pressures:* The output concentration of a vaporizer, calibrated at sea level, changes when the unit is used at a different ambient pressure. At a higher altitude, the output concentration is higher than that set on the dial; in hyperbaric conditions, the output concentration is lower than that set on the dial. The magnitude of changes is significantly less when output partial pressures are considered instead of concentrations. The effect of ambient pressure on the output concentration also depends on the changes in density at different ambient pressures. Consequently, the performance of these vaporizers at different ambient pressures is variable; hence, the ASTM anesthesia workstation standards require that the effects of changes in ambient pressure on vaporizer performance be stated in the accompanying documents.

Electronic vaporizers

Desflurane vaporizer

Because of the high SVP of desflurane, a special electronic vaporizer (Tec 6; Ohmeda) is required to administer this agent (Fig. 20.10).

Functional analysis of the vaporizers:

1. *Method of vaporization:* The desflurane vaporizer electrically heats the anesthetic in a sealed chamber to 39°C, creating a pressure of approximately 1550 mm Hg. At this temperature and pressure, desflurane exists partly as liquid and partly as vapor. The vapor is added to the fresh gases in a controlled manner. There are heaters in the gas pathway to prevent condensation of vapor.

2. *Regulating the output concentration:* The FGF inlet pressure (varies with FGF) and the agent's vapor pressure (varies with dial setting) are sensed by means of a pressure transducer (P). Based on the dial setting and FGF, the required amount of vapor is added to produce the desired output concentration. This can be considered an addition of a measured amount of vapor to the FGF. A microprocessor control achieves this through integration of a pressure regulator (R1), a variable resistor (R2), and

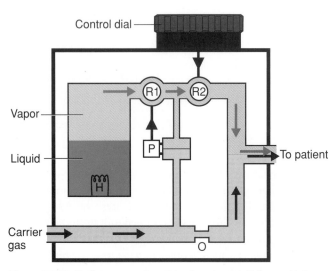

Figure 20.10. Desflurane vaporizer. H, heating element; O, flow restriction orifice; P, pressure transducer; R1: pressure regulator; R2: variable resistor.

pressure transducer (P). The saturated agent flow and FGF mix before their delivery to the CGO.

3. *Temperature compensation:* Because the liquid is heated to a constant temperature above the boiling point of desflurane and a measured amount of vapor is added to the FGF, no additional temperature compensation is required.

Aladin vaporizing system

The Aladin vaporizing system, used in Datex-Ohmeda workstations (S5/ADU and Aisys), is designed for desflurane, sevoflurane, isoflurane, enflurane, and halothane. The cassettes are magnetically coded to be recognized by the machine as they are inserted. Only one cassette can be inserted into the machine at any given time. The electronic controls and concentration dial are part of the anesthesia workstation, whereas the cassette contains the liquid anesthetic.

Functional analysis of the vaporizers:

1. *Method of vaporization:* The fresh gas passing through the vaporizing chamber picks up the vapor as it flows over the liquid agent (flow over or plenum). The fresh gas passing through the vaporizer is fully saturated with vapor because it flows between the agent-soaked wicks and baffles.

2. *Regulating the output concentration:* These vaporizers perform like variable bypass vaporizers, but with electronic controls. The FGF is split into a bypass flow in the machine and a vaporizing chamber flow in the cassette, and both flows are monitored constantly. A central processing unit (CPU) integrates the inputs from the bypass flow sensor, cassette pressure sensor, cassette flow sensor, and control dial setting to determine the ratio of bypass to vaporizing chamber flow and hence the outlet concentration, which is also monitored constantly.

3. *Temperature compensation:* Input from the cassette temperature sensor is integrated into the CPU and provides temperature compensation by adjusting the flow

through the vaporizing chamber. The metal wicks and baffles provide thermostability. If the temperature falls below 18°C, a fan is activated to facilitate heat transfer.

Direct injection of volatile agents

Technologic advances have led to innovative and reliable concepts of precise dosing of modern inhaled anesthetics. The volatile anesthetic agents are injected directly into the breathing system. When combined with a basal FGF in a circle breathing system, this technique enables rapid control of the agent concentration as well as minimal consumption of anesthetic. Direct injection of volatile agents (DIVA) has been implemented in the PhysioFlex and Zeus anesthesia machines (both from Dräger).

The DIVA unit comprises a reservoir unit, dosing chamber, and heating unit. The reservoir unit stores a quantity of liquid anesthetic in a tank and delivers it by means of an automatic injection system. The agent is vaporized in a heated vaporizing chamber, and the vapor is delivered to the breathing system via a heated pipe. The user can set the expiratory target concentration directly, independent of FGF. A closed-loop feedback mechanism is used to achieve the target concentration. A circuit flow provided by a blower located in the inspiratory limb of the breathing system provides a homogenous agent concentration.

Oxygen flush

The oxygen flush allows administration of 100% oxygen at rate of 35 to 75 L/min to the breathing system. The pressure downstream of the pressure regulator is supplied directly to the flush valve. The oxygen joins downstream of the vaporizers. There is a check valve to ensure that retrograde flow to the vaporizers is prevented when oxygen flush is activated. The flush is suitable for emergency jet ventilation in only a few models, depending on the position of the check valve; hence, it is not recommended for this purpose by the manufacturers. The flush works even if the main switch is not turned on. The valve is placed in a recessed position to prevent accidental activation. Overzealous intraoperative use may lead to patient awareness due to dilution of anesthetic agent. Accidentally sticking or activating it during inspiration may lead to pulmonary barotrauma.

Common gas outlet

The mixture of gases and vapors exits the machine via a 22-mm male/15-mm female conically tapered pipe. The connector is sometimes fixed, although some manufacturers provide a swiveling connector. The emergency oxygen flush is located close to the CGO, although this is not always the case in modern machines.

Suggested readings

ASTM Standard F 1850, 2000 (2005) *Standard Specification for Particular Requirements for Anesthesia Workstations and Their Components*. West Conshohocken, PA: ASTM International.

Brockwell RC, Andrews JJ. Inhaled anesthetic delivery systems. In: Miller RD, ed. *Miller's Anesthesia.* 6th ed. Philadelphia: Elsevier Churchill Livingstone; 2005:273–311.

Dorsch JA, Dorsch SE. *Understanding Anesthesia Equipment.* 5th ed. Philadelphia: Lippincott Williams & Wilkins; 2008.

Eisenkraft J. Anesthesia delivery system. In: Longnecker D, Brown D, Newman M, Zapol W, eds. *Anesthesiology.* New York: McGraw-Hill; 2007:767–820.

Meyer JU, Küllik G, Wruck N, et al. Advanced technologies and devices for inhalational anesthetic drug dosing. In: Schüttler J, Schwilden H, eds. *Modern Anesthetics (Handbook of Experimental Pharmacology).* Berlin: Springer-Verlag; 2008:451–470.

Web site

Schematic diagram of desflurane vaporizer. Available at: http://www.frca.co.uk/article.aspx?articleid=100151. Accessed January 17, 2009.

Chapter 21

Anesthesia ventilators

Yasodananda Kumar Areti and Edward R. Garcia

The anesthesia ventilator has undergone considerable evolution since the Cattlin bag, used with Boyle's original anesthesia machine in 1917. The earliest delivery of anesthesia, in 1846, used a simple vaporization chamber that required spontaneous ventilation by the patient to inhale air and diethyl ether. Seventy years later, Boyle's anesthesia machine incorporated a breathing circuit and reservoir bag containing the anesthetic gases, finally allowing the clinician to ventilate the patient, although this required manually squeezing the reservoir bag. Blease's eventual invention of the "pulmoflator" (a simple bellows ventilator) in 1945 enabled automatic positive pressure ventilation for patients undergoing surgery. This was followed by continued refinement with the Bird and Bennett ventilators two decades later. The contemporary anesthesia ventilators on the anesthesia workstations by Dräger, Datex-Ohmeda, and others integrate many advanced intensive care unit–type ventilation features and can provide ventilation to the most challenging patients brought to the operating room. These anesthesia ventilators have sophisticated computerized controls, have several modifications to the circle breathing system, and can provide advanced types of ventilatory support, such as synchronized intermittent mandatory ventilation (SIMV), pressure-controlled ventilation (PCV), positive end-expiratory pressure (PEEP), and pressure-support ventilation (PSV), in addition to conventional control-mechanical ventilation (CMV). To use these complicated techniques safely, it is critical for every anesthesiologist to have a basic understanding of the mechanics of these ventilators and breathing circuits.

Common modes of ventilation in anesthesia ventilators

Volume-controlled ventilation

The most commonly used mode of ventilation during anesthesia is volume-controlled ventilation (VCV), also called volume-targeted or volume-limited ventilation. In VCV, the ventilator attempts to deliver a specified tidal volume by delivering a constant inspiratory flow for the programmed inspiratory time. The airway pressure rises throughout inspiration as the lung volume steadily increases. The rate of airway pressure rise depends on the inspiratory flow rate, as well as the total compliance of the lungs and chest wall. The tidal volume is delivered despite

a decrease in total compliance, at the cost of increased airway pressure, with the potential for barotrauma. To minimize the risk of barotrauma, a pressure limit is usually set, and once this pressure is reached, the ventilator no longer delivers the set tidal volume. The traditional use of large tidal volumes during ventilation in the intensive care unit (ICU) is also linked to volutrauma, and current recommendations suggest that low-volume PCV may be superior. More challenging patients are undergoing surgery and anesthesia, and the newer options available in contemporary anesthesia workstations ensure adequate intraoperative gas exchange. Some of these ventilator options may be particularly useful for patients requiring extremes of ventilation, such as neonates with very low tidal volumes and patients with stiff or resistive lungs due to diseases such as acute respiratory distress syndrome (ARDS).

Pressure-controlled ventilation

In PCV or pressure-limited ventilation, the controlled parameter is the airway pressure during inspiration. The ventilator varies the inspiratory flow rate to generate the specified inspiratory airway pressure (Fig. 21.1), which tends to produce larger tidal volumes at lower pressures; therefore it is very useful when lung compliance is low, such as in laparoscopy, obesity, ARDS, and pregnancy. In patients with lung disease, there is some evidence that PCV may result in better matching of ventilation and perfusion.

Disadvantages

Like VCV, PCV is a time-cycled method of ventilation because the inspiration terminates at the end of the set inspiratory time (as set by respiratory rate and inspiratory/expiratory ratio). Because the inspiratory flow rate varies, the total volume delivered at the end of the inspiratory time varies depending on the overall lung and system compliance during each inspiration, which sometimes may result in wide swings of resultant tidal volumes. If the compliance of the lungs and breathing circuit is constant, the volumes delivered tend to be constant. If lung compliance decreases, as with abdominal insufflation, external pressure on the chest, or a momentary contraction of the diaphragm (as with a cough), the airway pressure will increase. The ventilator will decrease the inspiratory flow to maintain the set airway pressure; consequently, the volume delivered will

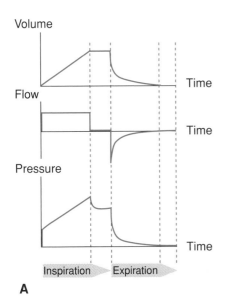
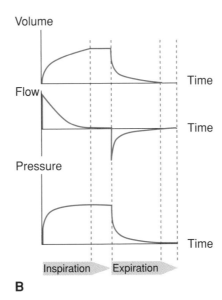

Figure 21.1. Relationship among tidal volume, flow, and pressure. (**A**) VCV and (**B**) PCV.

A

B

decrease. Conversely, when there is a sudden increase in lung compliance, such as during release of abdominal pressure at the end of laparoscopy, the subsequent tidal volume will increase significantly unless the set inspiratory pressure is immediately decreased.

Synchronized intermittent mandatory ventilation

SIMV was initially introduced as a weaning mode; however, it has become a standard mode of ventilation from initiation to weaning. The ventilator delivers a preset number of breaths and allows patients to breathe spontaneously between ventilator breaths. If a spontaneous breath is initiated before a controlled breath is due, the controlled breath is synchronized with the spontaneous breath, preventing the "stacking" of the machine-delivered breath on the patient's spontaneous breath. The total respiratory rate includes the machine breaths and spontaneous additional breaths. SIMV has found application in the operating room to facilitate emergence from anesthesia as the patient transitions from controlled to spontaneous ventilation.

Pressure-support ventilation

The use of laryngeal mask airways has led to a dramatic increase in spontaneous ventilation in the operating room. PSV is a useful adjunct to such techniques. In PSV, the ventilator supports the patient's effort by providing programmed pressure assistance throughout the breath. Low values of pressure support primarily overcome the resistance of the endotracheal tube or laryngeal mask airway and the ventilator circuit, decreasing the patient's work of breathing. The patient's own ventilatory musculature provides the remainder of the work to generate the tidal volume. The level of support can be increased to provide the desired tidal volume after each breath initiation. In strict PSV, all breaths are patient initiated. Consequently, if there is inadequate stimulus for the patient to breathe, apnea will ensue. With

many ventilators, pressure support includes a "backup" or safety mode. If the patient does not initiate a breath within a certain period, the machine defaults to a mode of controlled ventilation to ensure adequate ventilation. PSV mode allows more patients to breathe spontaneously during surgery.

Positive end-expiratory pressure

General anesthesia and positioning during surgery decrease functional residual capacity, which may lead to pulmonary atelectasis and intraoperative pulmonary shunting, resulting in hypoxemia. The magnitude of shunt is correlated with the formation of pulmonary atelectasis, which appears within minutes after induction of anesthesia in 85% to 90% of patients. Application of PEEP has an obvious advantage in such situations, instead of using a very high inspired oxygen concentration, which itself predisposes to atelectasis. In addition, PEEP is essential for patients on ventilator therapy in the ICU who are undergoing surgery and anesthesia. Application of PEEP is also known to reduce the incidence of atelectasis in obese patients undergoing general anesthesia. Application of continuous positive airway pressure (CPAP) during preoxygenation also is well tolerated and has been shown to prevent atelectasis during induction, even in morbidly obese patients. Application of CPAP to the unventilated lung also has been used to improve oxygenation during one-lung anesthesia.

Challenges specific to anesthesia ventilators
Low-flow inhalational anesthesia

Inhalational anesthesia requires administration of a known concentration of oxygen, volatile agent vapor, and air or nitrous oxide. Low flows are used to save costs and minimize pollution and necessitate the use of breathing circuits with carbon dioxide absorption techniques. Traditionally, spontaneous breathing is largely unassisted (manual assistance is done if required)

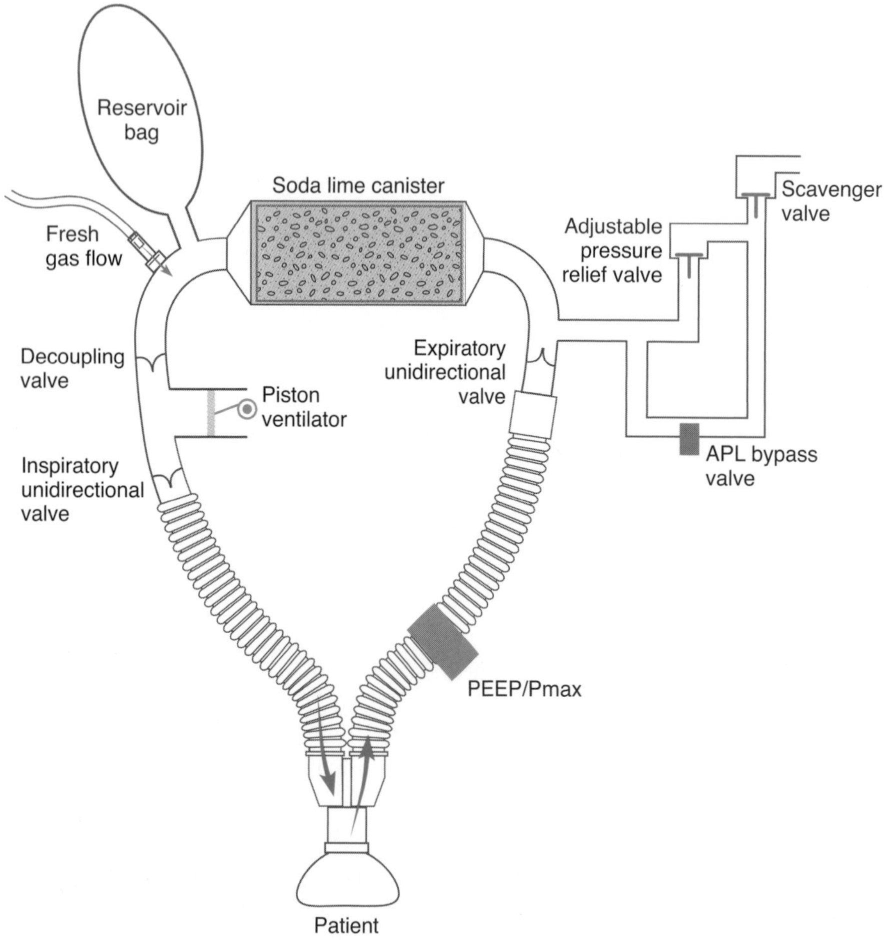

Figure 21.2. Modifications in the anesthesia breathing system using a piston ventilator to achieve fresh gas decoupling.

and controlled ventilation is achieved by partially closing the adjustable pressure limiting (APL) valve and squeezing the reservoir bag.

Traditional ventilators achieve mechanical ventilation with all the aforementioned objects by enclosing the reservoir bag (bellows replaced the reservoir bag) in a rigid box, which is pressurized intermittently, mimicking the intermittent squeezing of the reservoir bag. This results in two circuits: one with inhalational agents connected to the patient and the other in which the driving gas pressurizes the rigid box – hence the name *double-circuit technology*. These ventilators also are known as "bag-in-bottle" or "bellows-in-box" ventilators. These bellows may be hanging bellows or, more commonly, ascending bellows, based on whether the bellows descend or ascend during expiratory filling. Descending bellows have the disadvantage of creating negative pressure during expiration or filling with gases from the box if there is a leak in the bellows.

Driving the ventilator

Gas-driven ventilators

The driving gas in anesthesia ventilators may be compressed air, oxygen, or a a mixture of oxygen and air delivered by a Venturi device. If oxygen is the driving gas, one must switch to manual ventilation in the event of a failure in the pipeline supply necessitating use of oxygen from a type E cylinder.

Piston ventilators

With regard to some modern ventilators (e.g., Dräger ventilators), there has been a resurgence in the use of mechanical devices such as pistons to drive them (Fig. 21.2). These piston-type ventilators use a computer-controlled stepper motor instead of compressed drive gas to actuate gas movement in the breathing system. Instead of dual circuits, with gas for the patient in one and the drive gas in another, these systems have a single gas circuit for the patient. These ventilators are classified as piston-driven, single-circuit ventilators. The piston operates much like the plunger of a syringe to deliver the desired tidal volume or airway pressure to the patient. The major advantage of the piston ventilator is its ability to deliver tidal volume accurately to all patients under a wide variety of clinical conditions. There is no oxygen cost of driving gas, and the loss of tidal volume due to internal compliance of the bellows is eliminated. However, because these ventilators run on electricity, one must depend on limited battery backup (about 30 minutes) in the event of a power failure.

Turbo-Vent

The latest advance in anesthesia ventilation is the use of Turbo-Vent (Dräger Zeus), a revolutionary closed-system ventilator consisting of an electric-driven and – controlled compressor turbine placed in the inspiratory limb. The compressor turbine is dynamically driven by a brushless DC motor, enabling it to (i) build up the breathing pressure and deliver the corresponding flow to the patient during inspiration time and (ii) deliver the circuit flow required to mix the gas within the breathing system independently from patient inspiratory effort. This ventilator allows spontaneous respiration in all breathing modes and with virtually unlimited inspiratory flow. Turbo-Vent is suitable for all forms of ventilation, even those required in the ICU.

Effect of fresh gas flow on the delivered tidal volume

Traditionally the fresh gas flow (FGF) is delivered directly into the breathing system (circle system). This flow, which is added to the tidal volume delivered by the ventilator, is termed *fresh gas coupling* (Chapter 22, Fig. 22.4). If FGF is low, this contribution will be small; if FGF is high, it significantly contributes to ventilation. For example, if FGF is set at 6 L/min, then approximately 100 ml of fresh gas flows into the circuit every second. If the ventilator is set to deliver a tidal volume of 600 ml in 2 seconds, then 200 ml of fresh gas will be added to this volume, resulting in a total inspiratory tidal volume of 800 ml. If the FGF is low at 1 L/min, then the additional volume is only about 33 ml, a minor contribution. Fresh gas coupling might be particularly hazardous to infants and small children when FGF is altered.

Fresh gas decoupling

The aim of the contemporary anesthesia ventilator is to ensure that tidal volume is not affected by FGF. There are several approaches to dealing with the problem of fresh gas coupling. The Dräger Julian, Narkomed 6000, and Fabius GS use fresh gas decoupling, that is, fresh gas is not added to the delivered tidal volume. Thus, fresh gas decoupling helps ensure that the set and delivered tidal volumes are equal. These machines use a piston ventilator, which may be present in either the inspiratory limb (Fig. 21.2) or expiratory limb. The action of the piston closes a one-way decoupling valve, diverting the FGF to the manual breathing bag during the inspiratory cycle. A series of electronically controlled valves must work in concert with the ventilatory phase to accomplish this decoupling. In machines in which the ventilator is present in the inspiratory limb, because of this decoupling valve, there is no back pressure to close the expiratory unidirectional valve. Hence, a PEEP/maximum pressure valve is interposed between the patient and the expiratory unidirectional valve.

The visual appearance of the reservoir bag during this type of decoupling is unusual:

- The manual breathing bag, normally quiescent during mechanical ventilation, moves with each breath.
- The manual breathing bag movement is opposite the movement seen in a mechanical ventilator bellows – the manual breathing bag *inflates* during inspiration (because of FGF), and *deflates* during expiration as the contents empty into the ventilator. If the reservoir bag is removed, atmospheric air is entrained and the ventilator functions without activating any alarms; hence the anesthesiologist must be aware of this potential problem.

The second approach is fresh gas compensation, which is used in the Aestiva and S/5 Anesthesia Delivery Unit (ADU). The volume and flow sensors provide feedback, allowing the ventilator to adjust the delivered tidal volume so that it matches the set tidal volume, despite the total FGF, or if there is a change in FGF. These measurements may be done in the first few breaths, and compensation is instituted from subsequent breaths, which may result in high tidal volumes during the first few breaths.

The third approach used to minimize the effects of FGF on tidal volume is FGF interruption (Dräger Julian). With this approach, FGF is measured and reported electronically and the computer controls interrupt the flow during inspiration.

Effect of breathing system compliance and leaks on delivered tidal volume

During intermittent positive pressure ventilation, a part of the tidal volume gets compressed in the breathing system, leading to a decrease in the delivered tidal volume. This is known as the internal compliance of the breathing system, which is approximately 5 to 10 ml/cm H_2O. Traditional ventilators did not compensate for this loss, and anesthesiologists had to depend on chest expansion, spirometry, and end-tidal CO_2 to ensure that the ventilation was adequate, and they could not rely on the volume indicated on the ventilator controls. Compliance compensation is incorporated in some of the modern ventilators (e.g., Datex-Ohmeda SmartVent 7900, Dräger Fabius). During the pre-use test, the ventilator assesses the internal compliance and makes the appropriate changes to ensure that the set tidal volume is delivered. One has to repeat the self-tests if the circuit is changed between patients on the surgical list. Alternately, some machines (SmartVent) monitor the volumes and flows at both the inspiratory and expiratory limbs of the breathing system and ensure that the set tidal volume is delivered through a servo-feedback loop.

Small leaks around uncuffed endotracheal tubes or laryngeal mask airways result in a loss of tidal volume, which is not detected by pre-use check. This can be compensated only by measuring the inspiratory and expiratory flows and making the necessary adjustments to deliver the set tidal volume.

Ability to switch from mechanical to manual ventilation

During induction of anesthesia, patients are transitioned through spontaneous breathing to manual ventilation, followed by controlled mechanical ventilation. The opposite occurs during recovery. The isolation of the patient circuit from the ventilator circuit helps achieve this objective. Adjusting the pressure-relief valve helps transition from spontaneous to manual ventilation. A manual switch is incorporated in the circuit to switch between the reservoir bag and the ventilator bellows. The relief valve in the ventilator circuit is distinct from the APL valve. It relieves excess gas from the patient's breathing circuit at the end of *exhalation*, contrary to the APL valve during manual ventilation, which relieves excess patient gas during *inspiration*. The relief valve in the ventilator is kept sealed during inspiration.

Use of oxygen flush

A more significant problem with fresh gas coupling may result from activation of the oxygen flush valve during the inspiratory phase of the ventilator. As with FGF, this additional flow (35–75 L/min) adds to the inspiratory flow. This translates to >1000 ml/sec of flow, leading to buildup of excessive pressures in the circuit, possibly resulting in barotrauma. Hence, activation of the oxygen flush valve during inspiration must be avoided, except if using an anesthesia machine specifically designed to allow it.

Pediatric ventilation

The loss of tidal volume due to breathing system compliance and leaks around the uncuffed endotracheal tubes has maximal effect in pediatric patients; therefore, appropriate breathing systems are chosen for pediatric subjects. In the bellows-in-box arrangement, smaller ventilator bellows must be used to deliver small tidal volumes accurately. The new piston and turbine ventilators give the clinician flexibility in delivering a wide range of tidal volumes more accurately and obviate the need to change bellows.

Waste anesthetic gas scavenging

The exhaled gases in ICU ventilators are vented to the atmosphere. However, anesthesia ventilators should be able to vent the exhaled gases to the waste gas–scavenging systems in operating rooms to eliminate operating room pollution. Both the APL valve in the circle system and the relief valve in the ventilator are suitably modified to achieve this.

Application of positive end-expiratory pressure

Application of PEEP is a solution to counter the effects of anesthesia on the pulmonary system. In the past, PEEP valves were used for this purpose; however, because of the dangers in using them incorrectly, they no longer are recommended. Modern ventilators incorporate electronic PEEP control. In standing bellow ventilators, there normally is an end-expiratory pressure of +2.5 cm H_2O because of the PEEP effect of the ventilator relief valve. Application of PEEP might result in a loss of tidal volume set on the ventilator. The position of the PEEP valve varies in different models of anesthesia ventilators. The Datex-Ohmeda SmartVent applies PEEP at the ventilator relief valve, resulting in no loss of tidal volume. Any deviation from the tidal volume set is sensed by the inspiratory flow transducer, and a correction is made via the SmartVent compensation system.

Commonly used current models of anesthesia ventilators

Dräger Divan ventilator

The Dräger Divan is a modern ventilator offering features such as pressure-control mode, SIMV, correction for compliance losses, and integrated electronic PEEP. Its piston-driven bellows are inconspicuous and horizontally mounted. Fresh gas decoupling is achieved by diverting fresh gas to the manual breathing bag, which inflates during mechanical ventilator inspiration and deflates during expiration. A disconnect causes the manual breathing bag to lose volume gradually (in addition to activating other apnea alarms). A pressure transducer within the ventilator measures compliance losses and leaks in the total breathing circuit (absorber head and corrugated limbs), and appropriate adjustments are made by the ventilator microprocessor to ensure that the set tidal volume is delivered to the patient.

Dräger Fabius GS ventilator

The Fabius GS is an electronically controlled, electrically driven piston ventilator; it consumes no drive gas. The piston is vertical and continuously visible. This ventilator has a wide range of operating parameters to suit adult as well as pediatric patients. Fresh gas decoupling is achieved by diverting the fresh gas to a reservoir bag during inspiration. Compliance compensation is achieved by checking the circuit compliance during the pre-use check. Leaks in the reservoir bag may lead to air dilution and possible awareness.

Dräger AV-E and A-2

The Dräger AV-E and A-2 are electrically powered, double-circuit, pneumatically driven, ascending-bellows, time-cycled, electronically controlled ventilators. The tidal volume must be preset with pressure limiting. Inspiratory flow control must be set properly so that driving gas flow does not create an inspiratory pause.

Ohmeda 7000

The Ohmeda 7000 is an electrically powered, double-circuit, pneumatically driven, ascending-bellows, time-cycled, electronically controlled ventilator. It also is a minute-volume preset ventilator (unique among current ventilators). Tidal volume cannot be set directly but is calculated from settings of minute volume and respiratory rate. Inspiratory flow stops when driving gas equivalent to the set tidal volume has been delivered to the driving circuit side of the bellows chamber, or if a pressure >65 cm H_2O is attained.

Ohmeda 7900 SmartVent

The SmartVent is a pneumatic, double-circuit, ascending-bellows ventilator. A microprocessor control delivers the set tidal volume despite changes in FGF, small leaks, or losses in breathing system or bellows compliance proximal to the sensors. The flow sensors are placed between the corrugated plastic breathing circuit and the absorber head, in both limbs. These are connected to pressure transducers in the ventilator. This ventilator offers desirable features such as integrated electronic PEEP control and PCV mode. It has been reported that the sensors may be quite sensitive to humidity, causing ventilator inaccuracy or outright failure; therefore the use of a heat/moisture exchange filter is recommended.

Datex-Ohmeda S/5 ADU ventilator

The S/5 ADU is an electronically controlled, pneumatic, double-circuit, ascending-bellows ventilator with several unique features. Single-switch activation (setting the bag/vent switch to "auto") is all that is needed to start mechanical ventilation. FGF is located between the inspiratory unidirectional valve of the circle system and the patient. Delivered tidal volume is adjusted to compensate for changes in FGF and total breathing circuit compliance losses through the D-Lite sensor at the elbow. This ventilator can use either oxygen or air as the driving gas and can switch automatically from one to the other if pipeline pressure is lost. VCV, PCV, and SIMV modes are offered, along with integrated electronic PEEP.

Suggested readings

Badgwell M, Swan J, Foster AC. Volume-controlled ventilation is made possible in infants by using compliant breathing circuits with large compression volume. *Anesth Analg* 1996; 82:719–723.

Brochard L, Rua F, Lorino H, et al. Inspiratory pressure support compensates for the additional work of breathing caused by the endotracheal tube. *Anesthesiology* 1991; 75:739–745.

Eisenkraft J. Anesthesia delivery system. In: Longnecker D, Brown D, Newman M, Zapol W, eds. *Anesthesiology*. New York: McGraw-Hill; 2008.

Gajic O, Dara SI, Mendez JL, et al. Ventilator-associated lung injury in patients without acute lung injury at the onset of mechanical ventilation. *Crit Care Med* 2004; 32:1817–1824.

Gammon RB, Shin MS, Buchalter SE. Pulmonary barotrauma in mechanical ventilation: patterns and risk factors. *Chest* 1992; 102:568–572.

Klemenzson GK, Perouansky M. Contemporary anesthesia ventilators incur a significant "oxygen cost." *Can J Anesth* 2004; 51(6):616–620.

Nathan SD, Ishaaya AM, Koerner SK, Belman MJ. Prediction of minimal pressure support during weaning from mechanical ventilation. *Chest* 1993; 103:1215–1219.

Stayer SA, Bent ST, Campos CJ, et al. Comparison of NAD 6000 and Servo 900C ventilators in an infant lung model. *Anesth Analg* 2000; 90:315.

Tobin MJ. Medical progress: advances in mechanical ventilation. *N Engl J Med* 2001; 344:1986–1996.

Web sites

The Anesthesia Gas Machine. Available at: http://www.udmercy.edu/crna/agm/08.htm Dosch MP. Accessed on January 5, 2009.

Educational Animated presentation of Fabius GS anesthesia work station. Available at: http://www.simanest.org/FabiusGS.html. Accessed on January 5, 2009.

Comparison of breathing circuits of modern anesthesia machines: a transitional graphic presentation. Available at: www.apsf.org/assets/documents/circuit.ppt. Accessed on January 10, 2009.

Modern anesthesia machines offer new safety features. APSF News Letter. 2003: Summer. Available at: www.apsf.org/resource_center/newsletter/2003/summer/machines.htm. Accessed on January 10, 2009.

Chapter 22

Anesthesia breathing apparatuses

Jingping Wang and Charles A. Vacanti

Anesthesia breathing apparatuses represent very simple and logical devices that are exceedingly important for anesthesiologists to understand. We have elected to start with what we believe is the simplest example of a basic breathing apparatus. We explore its limitations and then suggest modifications that may be beneficial, depending on one's needs. For the purpose of this chapter, *anesthesia breathing apparatuses* are defined as devices that enhance the ability to breathe a desired or defined gas or vapor. The reader should note that this discussion does not include anesthesia machines by which one can effectively designate the compound to be delivered, ventilators that assist breathing but are not considered the actual breathing apparatus, or masks and other aids to breathing (such as Ambu bags, Venturi masks, and nasal prongs) not directly related to the administration of anesthesia.

Our first recollection of a very simple yet effective breathing apparatus was demonstrated in one of the early Tarzan films, in which the "ape man" eluded capture by submerging himself in a pond and harvesting a long reed, through which he was able to breathe until the natives lost interest and abandoned their pursuit (Fig. 22.1).

The reed through which he was breathing functioned similarly to a modern-day snorkel, with some important differences. A "standard" snorkel is about 50 cm long, with an internal diameter of 2 cm, resulting in a capacity, or dead space, of about 150 cm³. If Tarzan's reed had an internal diameter of 1 cm, it would have contained the same dead space at a length of approximately 7.5 feet. A smaller-diameter "breathing" tube would have significantly increased resistance to breathing (try breathing through a standard soda straw for a period of time), whereas a tube of larger diameter or length would have resulted in an unacceptably large dead space (see how long you can survive by breathing through a garden hose). Too large a dead space would have prevented Tarzan from effectively eliminating carbon dioxide (CO_2), resulting in rebreathing. Tarzan might effectively breathe through a tube with a very large dead space if he were to exhale into the water rather than back into the tube (this can be achieved easily by adding a one-way valve that directs inhaled air from the tube into the lungs, and exhaled air into the water rather than back into the breathing tube. This simple maneuver converts an open breathing system to a semi-closed apparatus.

In Tarzan's reed, or any effective breathing apparatus, the critical elements are:

1. A sufficiently large and sufficiently compliant reservoir of inhaled gas (air, in Tarzan's case) to fully expand the lungs as needed with little effort. The reservoir in the example is the virtually unlimited supply of air above the water that feeds directly into the breathing tube.
2. A conduit of sufficient diameter to conduct the gas being breathed without creating significant resistance to breathing. In the example, the reed was at least 1 cm in diameter.
3. A mechanism to effectively eliminate exhaled CO_2. In this case, breathing through a tube with a dead space <150 cm³. Alternatively, a one-way valve could be used to prevent rebreathing of CO_2 by diverting exhaled air into the water, rather than back into the breathing tube. In Tarzan's case, this would have created exhaled bubbles in the pond, revealing his location and resulting in a feast for the natives. That is precisely why Tarzan did not use a one-way valve but rather chose a reed with a dead space <150 cm³.

Based on this simple example, it becomes obvious that if one wishes to design an effective breathing device for any purpose, one must identify the objectives, evaluate the theoretical limitations of the device being developed, and make appropriate modifications to meet each successive need (Table 22.1). This is

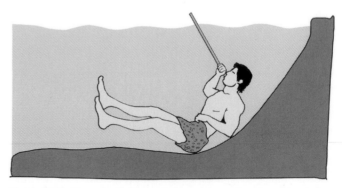

Figure 22.1. "Tarzan," with his new haircut and store-bought trunks, eluding capture by breathing through a reed while submerged in a pond.

Table 22.1. Classification of breathing systems

Type	Inhalation	Exhalation to	Reservoir	Rebreathing	Example
Open	Air + agent	Atmosphere	Nil	Nil	Open drop T-piece
Semi-open	Air + agent from machine	Atmosphere	Small	Minimal	T-piece with small reservoir
Semi-closed	From machine	Atmosphere + machine	Large	Possible	Magill attachment Mapleson systems
Closed	From machine	Machine	Large	Yes + CO_2 absorbent	Circle system

indeed what occurred historically in the development of breathing devices used in anesthesia.

If we want to deliver a known mixture of gases and vapors (in the case of anesthesia, oxygen and anesthetic agents), we refer to the gas outlet of an anesthesia machine as the *gas source*. Because the anesthesia machine itself is presented later, we schematically represent the machine and its outlet as a box with a tube (hose) protruding from it and label it *gas source*. Now let us put Tarzan to sleep. First, we fashion the infamous "reed" or basic breathing apparatus out of corrugated tubing to add flexibility and some compliance while reducing kinks. We also place the breathing apparatus over his mouth using a mask, then examine the most effective ways to connect this breathing apparatus to the gas source (Fig. 22.2).

It appears the simplest approach is to run the gas outlet hose from the machine into the inside of the larger-diameter breathing tube. This indeed may be quite effective, depending on how far into the breathing tube the gas source hose is placed (Fig. 22.3).

We now have created one of the simplest and most effective "open circuit" breathing apparatuses, called a *Bain circuit*. Although it appears to be the simplest, most logical circuit to develop and one of the most effective open circuits, it was not described until after several less effective configurations were developed (see later). The breathing apparatus we designed thus far is also referred to as a *modified Mapleson D circuit*, or even a *modified Ayre T-piece* (that was introduced in 1937 and itself was known as a modified Mapleson E circuit). These circuits were named according to the order of their historical description, rather than by a logical or intuitive nomenclature. Described and analyzed by Mapleson in 1954, all are variations of the Mapleson circuit, but in fact, they are all simple

variations of the breathing apparatus Tarzan was described as using many years earlier. The reason seemingly more complicated breathing apparatuses were developed before these simpler, more effective designs is that earlier devices were designed around a need to provide a gas source contained in a pressurized cylinder. In 1907, Barth used a reservoir bag and Clover inhaler to deliver nitrous oxide from a cylinder. A simple anesthetic delivery system known as the "Magill circuit" was introduced later.

In one variation of the aforementioned circuit, rather than run the gas source hose through the entire internal length of the breathing apparatus, the source hose can run along the breathing tube and enter the wall of the tube near the mask (Fig. 22.4e), allowing it to function in exactly the same manner. When configured in this manner, it is referred to as a Mapleson E or Ayre T-piece (the modification in which the gas source tube runs inside the breathing tube was described later, consequently being called a *modified Ayre T-piece*). A bag (with a pop-off valve on its base) can be placed on the end of the breathing tube (Fig. 22.4f) to enable assisted ventilation, which enhances CO_2 removal and reduces the need for high fresh gas flows to prevent rebreathing. This additional modification is referred to as a *Mapleson F*, or the *Jackson-Rees modification of an Ayre T-piece*.

Other modifications to this simple breathing apparatus involve the relocation of pop-off valves at various positions in the circuit in hopes of reducing rebreathing. As they largely have been abandoned from clinical use in modern anesthesiology, they are mentioned for historical significance and because knowledge of their names and configuration may be deemed

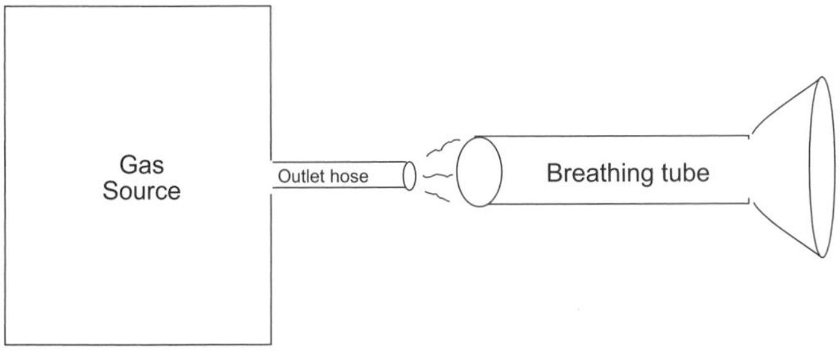

Figure 22.2. The anesthesia machine is represented by a box labeled *gas source* with an outlet hose that supplies the gas to the breathing tube. Unless the gas hose is placed well within the breathing tube, only room air will be inspired.

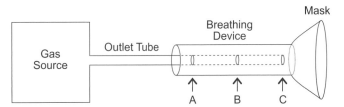

Figure 22.3. If the gas outlet hose resides only slightly within the breathing tube (to *A*), the patient will breathe exhaled air mixed with room air and very little fresh gas from the gas source hose. Advancing the gas supply hose to *B* improves the delivery of gas and if the flow is sufficient, helps remove exhaled CO_2 by blowing it out of the circuit. The optimal placement of the gas source outlet tube is as far into the breathing tube (as close to the breathing mask) as possible (*C*). When the flow of fresh gas is 1.5 to 2 times the minute ventilation, exhaled CO_2 is effectively washed out of the breathing tube, preventing rebreathing and CO_2 buildup.

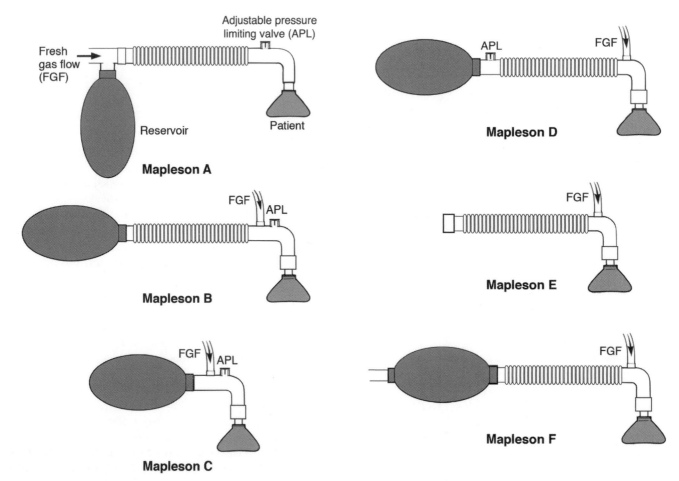

Figure 22.4. (A–D) The historical classification by Mapleson of various breathing apparatuses. **(E)** Rather than the gas outlet hose being run through the end of the breathing tube, it can run for a short distance outside the tube and then enter it closer to the mask. This will allow for the addition of a bag on the end of the tube to assist ventilation. **(F)** The gas supply hose can run external to the breathing tube and enter the tube adjacent to the mask. This is what is done in an Ayre T-piece. Again, a bag may be added to assist ventilation, making it a Mapleson F circuit or a Jackson-Rees modification to an Ayre T-piece.

important in an examination. Also analyzed by Mapleson, they are referred to as Mapleson A through D and are presented schematically in Fig. 22.4:

- Mapleson A (Magill) – The expiratory valve is near the face mask. Fresh gas enters the distal end of the tube, prior to the reservoir bag (Fig. 22.4a).
- Mapleson B – Similar to Mapleson A, but the fresh gas supply is moved near the face mask, just before the expiratory valve (Fig. 22.4b).
- Mapleson C (Ambu bag) – Same as Mapleson B, but with a much shorter conduit (Fig. 22.4c).
- Mapleson D – Identical to Mapleson B, except the expiratory valve is moved away from the mask, near the reservoir bag (Fig. 22.4d).

To–fro system

Although these circuits and modified Ayre T-piece systems are effective and efficient, a high gas flow (1.5–2 times the minute

ventilation) is necessary to prevent hypercapnia. Although this is useful in small children, in adults it necessitates fresh gas flows of 10 to 20 L/min that is expensive and inefficient and produces large amounts of waste gases to be scavenged. A simple solution to reduce gas flows and waste (called a "to–fro" system) is to add a CO_2 absorber to any of the aforementioned open circuit systems. The fresh gas inlet may be connected proximal or distal to the CO_2 absorber. An example of adding the CO_2 absorber in a line to a Mapleson F (Jackson-Rees) open system is shown in Fig. 22.5.

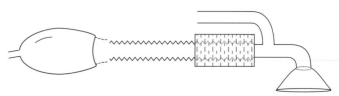

Figure 22.5. Mapleson F (Jackson-Rees) open system. In this example, the fresh gas flow enters proximal to the canister.

The first to–fro canister was developed by Waters to deliver cyclopropane. The system is quite effective but results in less than optimal mixing of fresh and expired gases when low flows are used. In addition, the distance from the mask to the CO_2 absorber is added as dead space. To reduce the dead space and improve mixing of gases, an expiratory limb with one-way valves may be added to the system. The expiratory limb and gases can then be directed back to the inspiratory limb of the system after being channeled through the CO_2 absorber by means of the one-way valves. These improvements result in a "circle system" as described in the following section.

Circle system

In 1926, Brian Sword developed a unidirectional rebreathing system, referred to as a circle system (Fig. 22.6). The circle system consists of a fresh gas inflow directed to an inspiratory limb and unidirectional valve, an expiratory limb and unidirectional valve, a CO_2 absorber, an expiratory pop-off valve, and a reservoir bag. Circle systems may be classified as semi-open, semi-closed, or closed, depending on the amount of fresh gas inflow.

During inspiration, the fresh gas, along with the CO_2 in the reservoir bag, flows through the inspiratory limb and its associated unidirectional valve to the patient. During expiration, the inspiratory unidirectional valve closes and the expired gas flows through the expiratory unidirectional valve in the expiratory limb to the soda lime canister and to the reservoir bag. The CO_2 is absorbed in the canister. The fresh gas flow from the machine continues to fill the reservoir bag. When the reservoir is full, the relief valve opens and the excess gas is vented into the atmosphere or, better still, a scavenging system. This system has the advantages of reduced fresh gas flow (as low as 250–500 ml/min of oxygen), economy of anesthetic consumption, reduction in atmospheric pollution, and conservation of heat and humidity. Disadvantages include a complex design with increased opportunity for malfunction or incorrect arrangement, slow changes in the inspired anesthetic concentration with low flows, increased resistance to breathing due to the CO_2 canister and valves in the system, and inhalation of soda lime dust.

Many classifications used in the literature are a source of confusion and inconsistency. Because it is important for an anesthesiologist to understand carbon dioxide homeostasis while using different systems, it is advisable to classify the systems based on CO_2 elimination (Table 22.2). One also should understand whether a system is efficient during spontaneous breathing, controlled ventilation, or both, and whether it can be used for pediatric patients, adults, or both.

Carbon dioxide absorption systems

Circle absorber systems have been used extensively in North America for more than 30 years. As mentioned earlier, they were developed to reduce the cost and use of expensive gases and

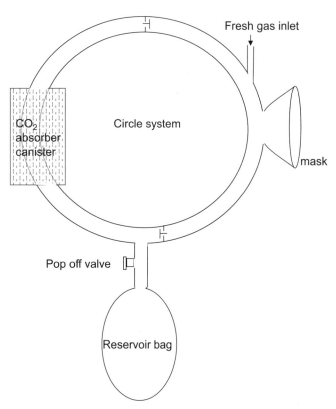

Figure 22.6. A circle system.

inhalational anesthetic agents as well as to reduce the amount of gas needing to be scavenged, and ultimately the extent of environmental pollution.

Two types of absorber are widely used: soda lime and Baralyme. Soda lime consists of 80% calcium hydroxide, 15% water, 4% sodium hydroxide, and 1% potassium hydroxide. As these pellets are fragile, small amounts of silicate are added to provide strength and prevent powdering. Baralyme, which is used more

Table 22.2. Classification based on CO_2 rebreathing (normal working condition)

No CO₂ rebreathing	CO₂ rebreathing is possible, but the CO₂ level in the patient is determined by the interaction of: Minute ventilation Fresh gas flow and Arrangement of components
Non-rebreathing valves: these separate exhaled gases from inhaled gases: Nonrebreathing circuits Self-inflating resuscitation equipment	*Mapleson systems* Efficient for spontaneous respiration: Mapleson A, Lack's Efficient for controlled ventilation: Mapleson D, Bain's Efficient for both spontaneous and controlled A-D switches Enclosed afferent reservoir system
CO₂-absorbent systems: To–fro system Circle system	*T-piece systems* Ayre, Jackson-Rees, Bain's

commonly in the United States than in other countries, consists of 80% calcium hydroxide and 20% barium hydroxide; it also may contain some potassium hydroxide. Unlike soda lime, the addition of silica to Baralyme granules is not necessary to ensure hardness. The reaction of Baralyme differs from that of soda lime because more water is liberated by a direct reaction of barium hydroxide and CO_2.

The reactions of CO_2 with absorbers are as follows: For both soda lime (containing sodium hydroxide) and Baralyme (containing barium hydroxide), the first several steps are the same, as they both involve reactions of CO_2 and water to form carbonic acid ($CO_2 + H_2O \rightarrow H_2CO_3$). In each system, the carbonic acid reacts with both calcium hydroxide and potassium hydroxide (present in each mixture) to form calcium carbonate, potassium carbonate, water, and heat. In addition, the carbonic acid also reacts very quickly with either the sodium hydroxide of soda lime, to form sodium carbonate, or to the barium hydroxide of Baralyme, to form barium carbonate, heat, and water. With Baralyme, this concludes the reaction, whereas with soda lime, the sodium carbonate then reacts with a calcium hydroxide mixture (as does the potassium bicarbonate) to form calcium carbonate as well as to reform the sodium hydroxide and potassium hydroxide found in the original mixture.

The absorbents interact with inhaled anesthetics to some extent. In some circumstances, interaction of sevoflurane with the strong bases present in soda lime or Baralyme results in the formation of compound A that has been shown to cause nephrotoxicity in animals. These circumstances include (1) low total gas flow rate (below 1 L/min), (2) higher concentration of sevoflurane, (3) the use of Baralyme rather than soda lime, (4) higher absorbent temperatures, and (5) desiccated CO_2 absorbent. Exposure of desflurane and isoflurane to soda lime and Baralyme results in formation of carbon monoxide. Factors increasing formation include (1) higher anesthetic concentration, (2) higher temperature, (3) dry absorbent, (4) the use of Baralyme rather than soda lime, and (5) the agent; the magnitude of CO production from greatest to least is: desflurane > isoflurane > halothane = sevoflurane.

Newer CO_2 absorbers (e.g., Amsorb; Armstrong Medical, Londonderry, Northern Ireland) have recently become available. They consist of calcium hydroxide with a compatible humectant (a hygroscopic substance with the affinity to form hydrogen bonds with molecules of water), namely calcium chloride. The absorbent mixture does not contain strong bases such as sodium and potassium hydroxide but does include two setting agents (calcium sulfate and polyvinylpyrrolidone) to improve hardness and porosity. New materials are designed to be effective absorbents of CO_2 while being chemically nonreactive with sevoflurane, isoflurane, and desflurane.

To be effective, the granules in the absorbing canisters must be properly configured to minimize resistance to airflow and to maximize the mixing of gases. To prevent rebreathing, the intergranular space should be greater than the patient's tidal volume. Soda lime absorbs up to 26 L of CO_2 per 100 g. Soft and crushable granules are converted to hard and noncrushable ones (calcium hydroxide changes to calcium carbonate – limestone), indicating exhausted soda lime. Different manufacturers add different indicator dyes to the absorber: some change from pink when fresh to white when exhausted; others change from white to purple. Correctly packed canisters allow absorption throughout, rather than in a columnar fashion. A larger cross-sectional diameter allows less turbulence, with reduced resistance and less dust. Baffles in the canisters reduce gas tracking down the walls, where spaces are relatively larger.

Indication of absorbent exhaustion

Methods to determine whether the absorbent is exhausted include the following:

1. Capnography: Appearance of CO_2 in the inspired gas is the best way to detect absorbent exhaustion.
2. Indicators: An indicator is an acid or base whose color depends on the pH, and the color change is indicative of absorbent exhaustion. Different manufacturers use different indicators, including phenolphthalein (white to pink), ethyl violet (white to purple), Clayton yellow (red to yellow), ethyl orange (orange to yellow), and mimosa Z (red to white). Color change may be misleading in certain circumstances, particularly those resulting in regeneration (peaking) after a rest period. Amsorb turns purple when desiccated, an additional advantage that prevents use of desiccated absorbant.
3. Temperature in the canister: Because CO_2 neutralization is an exothermic reaction, changes in the absorbent temperature occur earlier than color changes. Studies have suggested that when the temperature of the downstream canister is higher than that of the upstream one, the absorbent should be changed in both canisters.
4. Clinical signs: Clinical signs of hypercapnia, such as tachycardia, hypertension, cardiac arrhythmias, and sweating, are usually late signs and are nonspecific.

In conclusion, by understanding these few relatively simple principles, one should be able to easily evaluate the advantages and disadvantages of any breathing system with which he or she is presented, and to effectively troubleshoot problems. We strongly recommend that those interested in pursuing the principles of breathing systems in more depth refer to the web site listed below.

Suggested readings

Bain JA, Spoerel WE. A streamlined anaesthetic system. *Can Anaesth Soc J* 1972; 19:426–35.
Shankar R, Kodali B. Anesthesia breathing system. Available at http://www.capnography.com/.

Chapter 23

Electrical safety

Jesse M. Ehrenfeld, Seetharaman Hariharan, and Stephen B. Corn

Introduction

Anesthesiologists have become recognized for their commitment to safety. The specialty of anesthesiology is composed of several societies whose focus includes taking a proactive role in developing safety-enhancing approaches to patient care. For example, the Anesthesia Patient Safety Foundation (APSF) was highlighted in a *Wall Street Journal* article for providing an excellent model for identifying and controlling risk not just for the specialty of anesthesiology, but for other disciplines of medicine as well.

Just as drugs and techniques have evolved in the specialty of anesthesiology, so have technologic developments. Today the anesthesiologist is faced with an array of displays, monitors, and alarm systems. Further, with the development of embedded computer and operating systems, anesthesia equipment has gotten less intuitive in design and in many instances resembles "black boxes" with complex functions.

Although anesthesiologists can, and often do, become quite skilled at using a wide variety of anesthesia delivery systems and monitoring and imaging equipment, most do not have a formal engineering or electrical safety background, nor can they be expected to be experts in all subtleties of equipment design. Therefore, this chapter provides some basic electrical information and an overview of electrical equipment safety issues in the operating room (OR). It also supplies some simple models to enhance the clinician's understanding of OR design and devices that have been introduced to provide for electrical safety in patient care areas.

Of note, the goal of this chapter is not to give the reader the impression that he or she can or should be functioning as a clinical biomedical engineer. It is hoped that an understanding of the basic design goals and alarm devices will allow the anesthesiologist to be cognizant of a potential or real electrical safety issue so that he or she can either remedy it immediately or recognize that additional assistance is needed. Clearly, the vigilant anesthesiologist should remain focused on patient care and invoke the necessary resources.

The bird and the trolley car: a simplified approach to patient electrical isolation

A complete understanding of patient electrical safety requires familiarity with concepts such as isolated power supplies, induced current, grounded circuits, ungrounded circuits, isolation transformers, and primary and secondary power supplies. Cursory descriptions of these terms in the clinical classroom environment rarely seem to clarify the simple reason we strive to keep patients electrically isolated.

Hence, the bird and the trolley car

Electrical trolley cars get their power from high-voltage overhead lines. As the trolley travels under the high-voltage line, a "trolley pole" reaches up and makes electrical contact with the exposed wire. This contact completes an electrical circuit that allows current to flow through the trolley pole and power the motor, lights, and other critical systems of the trolley; finally, the current flows through the rails to the ground.

The power line (Fig. 23.1) to the trolley car supplies an enormous amount of electrical energy, enough to move a train at high speeds, and certainly enough to "cook" a small bird. However, birds land directly on the noninsulated power line, enjoy the sights, and fly off, without even a singed feather. They can do so because they are "isolated from ground," that is, there is no path for the electricity from the high-voltage line to go through the bird and then to a grounding source. There is no flow of current through the bird, and no harm ensues. Similarly, the goal is to electrically isolate each patient. That is to be sure to NOT provide a potential pathway for electricity to exit the patient if we were to inadvertently contact the patient with a source of electricity, such as a faulty piece of electrical equipment. (Discussions related to arcing and other electrical phenomena are

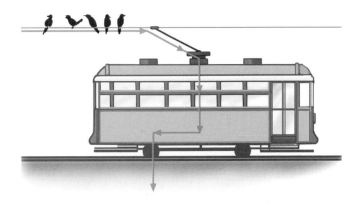

Figure 23.1. Trolley car and power line.

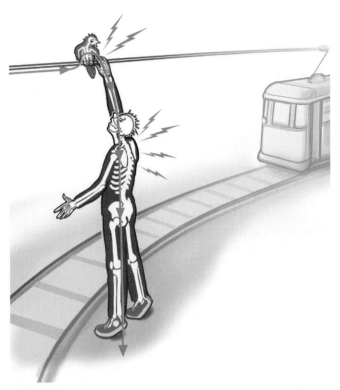

Figure 23.2. A curious individual.

beyond the scope and intent of this chapter and are left to the reader to explore further.) *Ideally*, we aim to isolate the patient from *both* the power supply line and ground.

In Fig. 23.2, the curious individual makes contact with the bird and creates a path for the electrons to flow: from the wire, through the bird, through the human, and into the ground. An electrical circuit is completed, with its associated consequences. It suffices to say that this is not a pleasant experience for either the bird or the curious person.

Now imagine the bird is a patient on an operating table. The patient may be electrically connected to one or more pieces of medical equipment. We need to be sure that we are not putting the patient in danger by creating a pathway to ground as we contact the patient and connect monitoring and therapeutic devices.

These examples are used to clarify some rather complex OR and hospital circuitry and are not intended to make light of a significant risk. The examples also should serve as reminders to clinicians who may be faced with responding to a victim of electrocution: before physically approaching or contacting any individual to be rescued, make sure the person and his or her immediate environment are no longer in contact with an active power source, as you could become part of the potentially deadly circuit.

Having discussed the importance of isolating the patient, it leads us to address the line isolation monitor (LIM). Most simply, the LIM is a device that continually monitors the impedance (resistance and capacitance) from all lines in the room in relation to ground and indicates what current *might* flow to a patient if he or she came into contact with a line conductor (i.e., defective equipment). It basically determines how much grounding is present if a power source were to be applied, as that will in part determine how much current *might* flow through the patient. An alarming LIM does *not* mean current is presently flowing through the patient – it only quantifies the grounding potential present in the room at that time.

It is understood that unlike the bird sitting on the wire, which is completely isolated from ground, the circuitry and equipment in the OR will allow some electrons to "leak" out. These small ground faults are quantified by the LIM. As long as the cumulative potential ground leak from all OR equipment remains small enough, the monitor does not alarm. However, *if* the potential ground leak is of a magnitude great enough that *if* a current were applied, significant flow *might* occur through the patient, *then* the LIM alarms.

Another device with which to be familiar is the ground fault circuit interrupter (GFCI) that is commonly found in household kitchens and bathrooms. These devices typically are not used in hospital OR environments or where lifesaving equipment is used, because when they are "tripped" or activated by a ground fault, they interrupt the power supply until they are manually reset.

It is hoped that the aforementioned models will serve to enhance the understanding of the following text, which is a more detailed discussion of some basic electrical principles in relation to equipment commonly used in hospital environments.

Basic concepts of electricity

Electricity is the flow of electrons from one point to another through a substance that is capable of conducting them. When electrons flow in a constant single direction, the current is said to be a *direct current* (DC); when the flow cyclically changes direction, it is known as an *alternating current* (AC). The frequency with which the current alternates is measured in terms of cycles per second or, equivalently, hertz (Hz).

A defibrillator delivers a short DC pulse intended to effect cardioversion. Household outlets in many countries (such as in the United States) supply a standardized AC source of 110 volts at 60 Hz to power electrical equipment. A rectifier can convert AC to DC power.

Voltage (V), the potential difference between two points of a conductor (points *A* and *B* in Fig. 23.3), is measured in *volts*. Electrons move through a conductor when a potential difference (voltage) and a conduction path exist. Current (I), the number of electrons per second flowing between the two points,

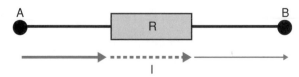

Figure 23.3. Basic principle of electricity.

is measured in amperes. Resistance (R) is a measure of how difficult it is for current to flow through the conductor. The typical unit of measure for resistance is ohms.

The simple flow of electricity through a conductor as described by voltage, current, and resistance is completely analogous to the flow of water through a garden hose connected to a spigot at point A with an open end at point B. As the tap is opened, a difference in pressure (voltage) between points A and B drives a stream of water (current) down the hose. A kink in the hose (resistance) slows the flow of water from A to B (reduces the electrical current), even though the pressure difference remains the same. If the tap is opened further, more water will flow, even though the resistance has not changed.

This somewhat intuitive relationship among voltage, current, and resistance leads to the most basic law of electrical engineering, Ohm's law. Qualitatively, the current is proportional to the voltage between two points and inversely proportional to the resistance. Thus, these three parameters are interrelated by Ohm's law:

$$I \propto V \quad \text{and} \quad I \propto 1/R$$

$$V = I \times R$$

Concept of grounding

Figure 23.4 shows the supply of electricity from a wall outlet that powers a piece of electrical equipment. Point A is the live terminal of the power source, and point B is the neutral terminal. The potential difference or voltage between points A and B alternates between +110 V and −110 V at a frequency of 60 Hz (in the United States) so that together they constitute an alternating current source. When an electrical device is plugged into an outlet, it contacts both points A and B and completes an electrical circuit between them. Current then flows between the two points – through the equipment – providing power for lights, gauges, pumps, computers, and other equipment.

The neutral terminal of an electrical outlet is connected to a very large conductor capable of receiving an infinite amount of electrical charge. This large conductor is the earth, which provides the most common and accessible voltage reference for electrical circuits and equipment. An electrical connection to the earth typically is referred to as earth or ground, and things

that are thus connected are said to be grounded. A conductor that is grounded loses its charge and assumes a neutral potential relative to the earth. This is the concept of grounding that is the basic principle of electrical safety.

When someone plugs a piece of household electrical equipment into an outlet, he or she also is connected to the earth ground either directly or capacitively through his or her environment. Because both the person and the neutral outlet terminal are grounded, they are at the same voltage and the person could touch that terminal without issue. The live terminal, however, has an alternating voltage relative to the earth, and touching that terminal would drive current through the person to ground – resulting in an electrical shock.

Modern outlets have added a third terminal, the ground terminal, illustrated as point C in Fig. 23.4. This terminal provides a backup safety path to ground to avoid electrical shock or arcing in cases in which the electrical equipment is somehow compromised. Typically, external metallic cases of electrical equipment are connected directly to the ground terminal of the outlet – reducing the potential for a person to contact a nongrounded surface.

The outlet described earlier is quite sufficient for most household uses. However, in areas likely to come in contact with water, such as kitchens, bathrooms, and outdoor areas, safety is supplemented through the use of GFCIs. These devices are set to trip, or turn off the current source, whenever they detect a difference in current flowing in the live and neutral wires; the assumption is that the current difference represents current flowing from the live wire through an individual to ground. GFCIs work very well in most homes, where shutting down a piece of equipment is unlikely to have severe consequences. However, they are not used in ORs because of the risk of interrupting power to a piece of lifesaving equipment.

In the modern OR, two other electrical devices are commonly used to reduce the possibility of electrical shock: line isolation transformers (LITs) and LIMs. An LIT serves to isolate the circuitry providing power to OR equipment from the base power supply of the hospital that is connected to an earth ground. Creating an isolated (or floating) power supply separates the alternating current source that powers the equipment from earth ground completely. This protects clinical workers and patients by reducing the possibility of a shock due to an electrical short or ground fault within the equipment. A perfectly isolated power supply does not allow any current to flow from either terminal to earth ground. Therefore, a *single* short between earth ground and either of the isolated power supply's terminals will *not* result in arcing or shock. The floating power supply will simply "float" to the new potential and continue to operate. This has obvious advantages over GFCI protection as it allows OR equipment to operate continuously, even in the case of an earth ground fault.

It should be noted that an isolated power supply that is shorted to the earth-based power supply reverts to earth-based power supply behavior. That is, a *second fault* would lead to a short circuit that may result in arcing, shock, and/or loss of

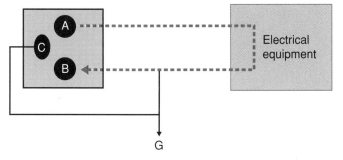

Figure 23.4. Concept of grounding.

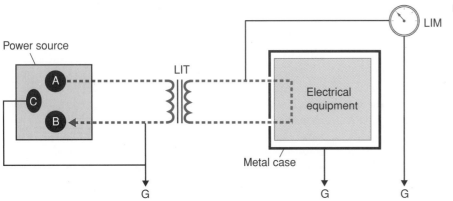

Figure 23.5. Line isolation.

power due to a circuit breaker. Of note, isolated power supplies are sometimes referred to as *ungrounded*. This term has become part of the nomenclature, but it can be somewhat confusing. In the strictest sense, the isolated power supply still has a circuit ground – generally taken to be one of the power terminals. The distinction is simply that this is not an earth ground but rather a *floating ground*. Hence, the term *unearthed* may be more appropriate than *ungrounded*.

Working in conjunction with an LIT is an LIM (Fig. 23.5). As discussed earlier, the LIM constantly monitors the isolated power supply and determines the current that *could* flow to earth ground if either of the isolated terminals *were* to be shorted to ground. The LIM alarms when the current that *could* flow in that case, reaches a preset limit. Although a ground fault may lead to an LIM alarm, a more likely cause of a LIM alarm is the buildup of small current "leakages" from all the equipment connected to the isolated power supply and from the LIT itself. When these small leakages add up to a current sizeable enough to harm the patient, the LIM alarms.

It should be noted that *microshocks*, discussed later, may be a result of currents well below the sensitivity of a typical LIM and the LIM does NOT protect against microshock.

Interestingly, there is not universal agreement regarding the installation and use of isolated OR power supplies and devices as such as LIMs. Some argue that the incidence of medical device failures that result in patient or caregiver harm is not well quantified and that evidence should be provided to justify the cost and maintenance of these systems. It should be noted further that these complicated electrical safety systems are not without their own issues. For example, it has been reported that LIMs have produced spike-like electrocardiographic (ECG) interference.

Presently, OR design is guided by the National Fire Protection Association 99 (NFPA 99) Standard for Health Care Facilities, 2005. The scope of this document is to establish criteria to minimize the hazards of fire, explosion, and electricity in health care facilities providing services to humans.

ECRI, formerly the Emergency Care Research Institute (www.ECRI.org), is a nonprofit organization with the mission of bringing the discipline of applied scientific research to health care to uncover the best approaches to improving patient care.

The 2010 NFPA 99 document is pending at the time of this writing. This proposed standard is worded to require that isolated power, or other protective mechanisms, be included in ORs by default, and may be omitted only when a risk assessment indicates it is not needed. ECRI has submitted commentary to the NFPA because ECRI does not believe that isolated power offers significant electrical safety benefits for most ORs. The evidence demonstrating adverse incidents is lacking. Of note, there may be exceptions, such as rooms in which large amounts of fluids are routinely present on the floor; in these cases, isolated power is advisable. However, ECRI believes it is reasonable for most ORs not to have isolated power, and that this can be decided for specific rooms or facilities on an individual basis when there are special concerns (personal communication).

Electrical hazards in the operating room environment

Electric shock

An electric shock occurs when the human body contacts any source of voltage high enough to cause sufficient current through the tissues.

Static electricity

In earlier days, when highly flammable volatile anesthetic agents such as diethyl ether were used, most anesthetic equipment (including the anesthesiologist's shoes) was required to be "antistatic" to prevent discharge of static electricity. Static electricity is produced by surface contact that builds up an electrical charge that gets discharged when the surface comes into contact with a conductor. This discharge is sufficient to produce a spark that may cause a fire in the presence of highly flammable anesthetics.

Macroshock

Macroshock is caused by large voltages or currents applied to the skin or tissues. The effects of the current passing through human tissue depend on the strength of the current (Table 23.1). Electrical burns usually are caused by high-density current if the strength is >100 mA/cm^2.

Table 23.1 Effects of 60-Hz AC on an average human for a 1-second duration of contact

Current	Effect
Macroshock	
1 mA (0.001 A)	Threshold of perception
5 mA (0.005 A)	Threshold of pain and accepted as maximum harmless current intensity
10–20 mA	"Let-go" current before sustained muscle contraction
50 mA	Pain, possible fainting, mechanical injury; heart and respiratory functions continue
100–300 mA	Ventricular fibrillation will start, but respiratory center remains intact
6000 mA	Sustained myocardial contractions, followed by normal heart rhythm; temporary respiratory paralysis; burns if current density is high
Microshock	
100 μA (0.1 mA)	Ventricular fibrillation
10 μA (0.01 mA)	Recommended maximum allowable 60-Hz leakage current

Reproduced with permission from Ehrenwerth J. Electrical safety. In: Ehrenwerth J, Eisenkraft JB, eds. *Anesthesia Equipment Principles and Applications.* St. Louis: Mosby-Year Book Inc.; 1993.

Microshock

Microshock is caused by small voltages or currents applied directly or in close proximity to the heart. Microshock may be applied intentionally, as in pacemaker electrodes; however, when it occurs inadvertently, it may lead to life-threatening cardiac dysrhythmias such as ventricular fibrillation. Saline-filled central venous catheters and arterial lines are potential sources of microshock if the electrodes of the transducers come in contact with an electrical source. The present design of pressure transducers is such that they are connected to the monitors by means of telephone cables using very small voltages, thus they are relatively safer than older models.

Surface ECG electrodes are relatively safe with regard to producing microshock. With the increasing use of monitored anesthesia care for interventional radiologic procedures, and given the number of indwelling catheters filled with electrolyte solution, the potential for the electrical hazard of microshock exists and needs to be thoroughly understood by the anesthesiologist and all members of the team.

The American National Standards Institute has set 10 μA as the maximum allowable current leakage level in the connections of catheters and electrodes contacting the heart. LIMs cannot detect this small leakage because 2 mA (i.e., 2000 times larger) is the level at which LIMs warn of leakage.

Electrical hazards from surgical diathermy

Electrically operated surgical electrocautery units discharge high-intensity currents through a pointed tip to a small surface area of high resistance. This generates intense heat in the area, causing tissue coagulation and cutting. The electrocautery units discharge currents at very high frequency levels, in the range of 300 kHz to 2 MHz. Because excitable tissues cannot respond to such high frequencies, frequency electrocautery currents do not cause ventricular fibrillation.

Two types of electrosurgical electrocautery units are commonly used by surgeons: unipolar and bipolar. In unipolar electrocautery, the more commonly used modality, the current is passed through the tip of the pencil point equipment (active electrode), which passes through the tissues of the patient, and the circuit is completed by the passage of current through the dispersive electrode pad or return pad (sometimes incorrectly referred to as the grounding pad). The return pad is often applied to the patient's body surface. This pad should be applied to a wide surface area well coated with conducting gel, and as far from the heart as possible. Burns may occur if the area is dry of gel, or if the contact of the dispersive electrode pad is poor if, for example, it is applied to very hairy skin. Similarly, when a patient becomes wet, which commonly happens during surgery, the electrocautery current may take different routes other than the return electrode. ECG electrodes may become the alternate route for completion of the circuit and may cause electrical burns if the return electrode contact is defective.

Bipolar electrocautery is commonly used by neurosurgeons and vascular surgeons. In this mode, the cauterization is done by an appliance resembling forceps with two prongs. The current is discharged by one prong and passes through the tissue and then through the other prong back to the console of the electrosurgical unit.

Another, newer modality, known as the argon beam coagulator, is also a type of electrocautery; anesthesiologists should not confuse it with argon beam lasers. A jet of ionized argon gas carries electrical charge from a probe to tissue. This system also utilizes a return electrode from the patient, as in conventional electrocautery.

Many concerns with electrical safety in the OR arise from the use of electrosurgical units, because they can cause electric shock, burns, explosions, arrhythmias, and disturbances in pacemakers. In patients who have cardiac pacemakers, electrocautery units may cause interference with the pacemaker's discharge of cardiac impulses. Unipolar units may be more hazardous than bipolar ones in patients with implanted pacemakers. Hence, for these patients, bipolar electrocautery is advised whenever possible. If unipolar electrocautery is used, the return electrode pad should be placed so that the path of the current from the operative site to the return electrode does not cross the pacemaker. Backup plans with appropriate pacemaker magnets and pharmacologic support should always be available. Though beyond the scope of this chapter, one must exercise extreme caution when utilizing electrical equipment in the presence of oxygen sources.

In summary, to prevent electrical hazards in the OR environment, the following points are noteworthy:

- Anesthesiologists should be aware of the concepts of electricity in general and know specifically about the circuitry in their particular hospital.

- They also should have a thorough knowledge of the operating principles of anesthetic and electrosurgical equipment.
- Proper maintenance of electrical equipment such as monitors, anesthetic machines, modern vaporizers, and electrocautery units is paramount for electrical safety. All equipment should be checked at regular intervals for electrical leakage and other malfunctions.
- Meticulous efforts should be undertaken to prevent macro- and microshock.
- There should be interaction among all the OR personnel with respect to the application and use of electrical equipment such as electrosurgical units.
- In special situations, such as patients with cardiac pacemakers, anesthesiologists should be well prepared to prevent patient morbidity due to the use of electrical equipment.

Acknowledgments

The authors thank Martin D. Wells, Ph.D., cofounder of Granite Peak Technology, Newton, MA, for his review of the manuscript.

Suggested readings

Antony A, Zhang C, Austen W. Operating Room Electrical, Fire,Laser, and Radiation Safety. In: Sandberg WS, Urman RD, Ehrenfeld JM, eds. *MGH Clinical Essentials of Anesthesia Equipment*, 1st ed. New York: Elsevier Press; 2010: Chapter 29.

Bernstein MS. Isolated power and line isolation monitors. *Biomed Instrum Technol* 1990; 24:221–223.

Buczko GB, McKay WP. Electrical safety in the operating room. *Can J Anesth* 1987; 34:315–322.

Day FJ. Electrical safety revisited: a new wrinkle. *Anesthesiology* 1994; 80:220–221.

Hallinan J. Heal thyself once seen as risky. One group of doctors changes its ways. Anesthesiologists now offer model of how to improve safety, lower premiums. Surgeons are following suit. *Wall Street Journal* June 21, 2005:A1.

Kerr DR, Malhotra IV. Electrical design and safety in the operating room and intensive care unit. *Int Anesthesiol Clin* 1981; 19:27–48.

Litt L. Electrical safety in the operating room. In: Miller RD, ed. *Miller's Anesthesia*. 6th ed. Philadelphia: Churchill Livingstone; 2005;3139–3148.

Litt L, Ehrenwerth J. Electrical safety in the operating room: important old wine, disguised new bottles. *Anesth Analg* 1994; 78:417–419.

National Fire Protection Association (NFPA 99) Standard for Health Care Facilities. NFPA 99; 2005.

Hemodynamic patient monitoring

Amit Asopa, Theodore E. Dushane, and Swaminathan Karthik

Anesthesiologists have many and varied perioperative roles. Clearly, one of the most important roles is serving as the ever-vigilant set of "eyes" to ensure patient safety. Despite the introduction of new methods to monitor the anesthetized patient, hemodynamic monitoring and the analysis of these well-known parameters remain central to assessing patient well-being.

Standards for basic anesthetic monitoring

In an effort to ensure patient safety, the American Society of Anesthesiologists (ASA) has created "Standards for Basic Anesthetic Monitoring" (approved by the ASA House of Delegates on October 21, 1986 and last affirmed on October 25, 2005).

In general:

These standards apply to all anesthesia care although, in emergency circumstances, appropriate life support measures take precedence. These standards may be exceeded at any time based on the judgment of the responsible anesthesiologist. They are intended to encourage quality patient care, but observing them cannot guarantee any specific patient outcome. They are subject to revision from time to time, as warranted by the evolution of technology and practice. They apply to all general anesthetics, regional anesthetics, and monitored anesthesia care. This set of standards addresses only the issue of basic anesthetic monitoring, which is one component of anesthesia care. In certain rare or unusual circumstances 1) some of these methods of monitoring may be clinically impractical and 2) appropriate use of the described monitoring methods may fail to detect untoward clinical developments. Brief interruptions of continual[†] monitoring may be unavoidable. These standards are not intended for application to the care of the obstetrical patient in labor or in the conduct of pain management.

STANDARD I states, "Qualified anesthesia personnel shall be present in the room throughout the conduct of all general anesthetics, regional anesthetics and monitored anesthesia care."

STANDARD II states, "During all anesthetics, the patient's oxygenation, ventilation, circulation and temperature shall be continually evaluated."

Standard II includes specific recommendations with regard to hemodynamic evaluation.

Specifically, Standard II aims to "ensure the adequacy of the patient's circulatory function during all anesthetics":

1. Every patient receiving anesthesia shall have the electrocardiogram continuously displayed from the beginning of anesthesia until preparing to leave the anesthetizing location.[*]
2. Every patient receiving anesthesia shall have arterial blood pressure and heart rate determined and evaluated at least every five minutes.[*]
3. Every patient receiving general anesthesia shall have, in addition to the above, circulatory function continually evaluated by at least one of the following: palpation of a pulse, auscultation of heart sounds, monitoring of a tracing of intra-arterial pressure, ultrasound peripheral pulse monitoring, or pulse plethysmography or oximetry.

The need for real-time invasive hemodynamic data versus noninvasive assessment of cardiovascular function is determined by several factors, including the ASA physical status, type of surgery, anticipated blood loss, and likelihood for hemodynamic instability during surgery. The ACC/AHA 2007 guidelines on perioperative cardiovascular evaluation and care for noncardiac surgery can be used as a risk assessment tool.

Of note, "These guidelines are intended for physicians and nonphysician caregivers who are involved in the preoperative, operative, and postoperative care of patients undergoing noncardiac surgery. They provide a framework for considering cardiac risk of noncardiac surgery in a variety of patient and surgical situations."

Hemodynamic monitoring is an essential part of every anesthetic and includes directly or indirectly monitoring pressure, flow, and resistance in the arterial and venous systems of every patient. The ASA standards of basic anesthetic monitoring require assessment of adequate circulatory function during all anesthetics, including measurement of arterial blood pressure (ABP) and heart rate at least every 5 minutes and continuously monitoring the electrocardiogram (ECG). Other clinical signs, such as skin and mucosal color, palpation of a peripheral pulse, and auscultation of heart sounds, may aid in the assessment of the cardiovascular system. An adequate signal from a pulse

---

[†] Note that "continual" is defined as "repeated regularly and frequently in steady rapid succession," whereas "continuous" means "prolonged without any interruption at any time."

[*] Under extenuating circumstances, the responsible anesthesiologist may waive the requirements marked with an asterisk (*); it is recommended that when this is done, it should be so stated (including the reasons) in a note in the patient's medical record.

Table 24.1. Methods for NIBP measurement

Auscultatory	• 1st Korotkoff sound at systolic pressure
	• Disappearance of sounds at diastolic pressure
	• Mean pressure may be estimated as diastolic pressure + 1/3 pulse pressure
Oscillatory	• Uses the oscillation of the mercury column to determine the mean arterial pressure
	• The basis of automated sphygmomanometers
	• Pressure at maximal oscillations closely estimates mean arterial pressure
	• Pressures at 50% of maximal oscillation on either side of the mean pressure yield estimates of the systolic and diastolic pressures
	• **Cannot be used in the presence of nonpulsatile flow, such as during cardiopulmonary bypass or when an LVAD is in place**
Palpation	• Appearance of a distal pulse at systolic pressure
	• Cannot determine diastolic or mean pressure
Ultrasound	• Similar to palpation
Arterial tonometry	• Uses the principle of photoplethysmography
	• Blood flow detected by reflectance of infrared light
	• Dynamic pressure applied by cuff to determine real-time pressures
	• Might potentially work during cardiopulmonary bypass

LVAD, left ventricular assist device

Table 24.2. Complications of NIBP monitoring

- Bruising and petechiae formation
- Neuropathy
- Measurement errors
- Limb ischemia

oximeter or the presence of expired CO_2 on capnography may be a gross indicator of circulation.

The need for real-time invasive hemodynamic data versus continual noninvasive assessment of cardiovascular function is determined by the acuity of the patient, type of surgery, and physiologic reserve of the patient.

Noninvasive arterial blood pressure monitoring

Noninvasive arterial blood pressure (NIBP) monitoring may involve direct palpation, use of a Doppler probe, auscultation, arterial tonometry, or more commonly, oscillometry. Several methods of NIBP estimation are described in Table 24.1.

Automated NIBP machines frequently use the oscillometric method. Blood pressure cuff oscillations are sensed by a transducer. The lowest cuff pressure with the greatest average oscillation amplitude is sensed as the mean arterial pressure (MAP). Systolic and diastolic blood pressures are determined by identifying the cuff pressures where the amplitudes of oscillations are specific ratios of the maximum oscillation amplitude.

Here are some important points to consider:

- Cuff width influences the accuracy of blood pressure measurements. A narrow cuff may overestimate blood pressure, whereas a wide cuff may underestimate the pressure. This is because the pressure necessary to occlude

the artery is greater with a narrow cuff and less with a wide one. Importantly, a narrow cuff more greatly *overestimates* the systolic blood pressure than a wide cuff *underestimates* the systolic blood pressure.
- Patient movement during oscillometric measurement, including shivering, may cause artifact and can result in inaccurate measurement.
- Counter-intuitively, more peripheral arterial measurements result in an exaggeration of the systolic and pulse pressures as the result of changes in the waveform morphology. For example, the dorsalis pedis artery pressure reading may be higher than the aortic root pressure. It should also be noted that changes in vascular resistance, such as from hypothermic cardiopulmonary bypass and vasodilating drugs, can further affect relative differences in pressure measurements recorded from site to site.
- Korotkoff described five sounds heard when taking blood pressure measurements with the auscultatory method. Typically, systolic blood pressure is measured as the pressure at which the first Korotkoff sound is first heard, whereas diastolic blood pressure measured as the pressure at which the fourth Korotkoff sound is just audible. Interestingly, the mechanism by which Korotkoff sounds are generated has not been well understood and many theories exist.
- The auscultatory gap is the period during which sounds indicating true systolic pressure fade away and reappear at a lower pressure point. Failure to recognize this gap can result in not indentifying hypertensive patients.

Potential complications of NIBP monitoring are listed in Table 24.2.

Invasive pressure monitoring
Principles of invasive pressure monitoring

Placing a hollow cannula in a vessel of the cardiovascular system connecting to calibrated transducers with a fluid-filled high-pressure tubing system allows for accurate invasive pressure measurements (Table 24.3). Cannulas may be placed in

Table 24.3. Checklist for invasive monitoring

- Intravascular cannula (arterial line/CVC/PAC)
- Infusion and tubing
- Transducer
- Display screen
- Mechanism for zeroing and calibration

virtually any portion of the cardiovascular system. Commonly, they are placed in central or peripheral arteries for arterial pressure, the superior vena cava or right atrium for central venous pressure (CVP), and the pulmonary artery for pulmonary artery pressure and pulmonary artery wedge pressure (PAWP).

Electronic transducer

The cannula is connected to high-pressure tubing that is filled with saline. This acts as a continuous column of fluid that transmits intraluminal pressure changes to the transducer diaphragm that oscillates in response to the pressure waveform. The movement is converted to an electrical signal by a transducer. The transducer accomplishes this by acting as part of a capacitor, inductor, or, most commonly, a strain gauge.

The strain gauge uses variable resistors, the electrical resistance of which increases with increasing length. The diaphragm of the transducer moves a small plate connected to four strain gauges. With any one movement, two gauges are compressed and the other two stretched. All four strain gauges form part of a Wheatstone bridge, increasing the sensitivity.

Calibration

Calibration is the process of validating a measurement technique or equipment. It was an important consideration for older electronic transducers. The standard calibration is a 50 microvolt change in potential per 10 mm Hg. Modern systems typically do not require external calibration because they are manufactured in a standardized manner to tight standards.

Zeroing

Zeroing removes the effect of atmospheric pressure on transmural pressure of the tubing system by exposing the transducer system to ambient atmospheric pressure. Zeroing is performed by opening the transducer to atmospheric pressure and electronically setting this atmospheric pressure to zero. Occasionally, this zero baseline may drift and should be checked frequently, because even a 5 mm Hg drift can represent a significant difference in low-pressure systems such as CVP.

Leveling

Leveling refers to the placement of an *already zeroed* transducer at a particular height where the pressures are sought to be measured (a reference point). The electrical transducer needs to be aligned to the superior aspect of the right atrium to measure the pressure at the level of the heart. This eliminates errors of measurement that might occur from the hydrostatic pressure exerted by the column of blood above or below the point of reference to be measured. A 10 cm change in height will increase or decrease the pressure reading by 7.5 mm Hg.

To standardize measurements, the position of the right atrium is assumed to be along the mid axillary line. For intracranial procedures, in which the pressure in the circle of Willis is important, the transducer may be leveled to the tragus.

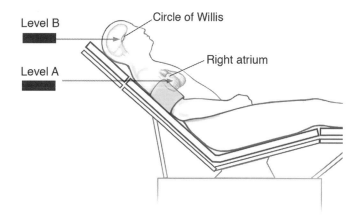

Figure 24.1. Influence of hydrostatic pressure on monitoring arterial blood pressure.

Invasive blood pressure monitoring devices measure blood pressure at the *level of transducer* and are not affected by level of the insertion point in the extremity as long as the *transducer* is maintained level to the heart. NIBP measurement devices measure pressure at the level of peripheral artery. Therefore, if the NIBP measurements are made above or below the level of heart, then a correction for hydrostatic pressure should be made before extrapolating the pressure at the level of heart (Fig. 24.1).

Resonance and damping

The arterial pressure waveform can be represented as a sum of sine waves (using Fourier analysis). Transducer systems have their own natural oscillatory frequency, or resonant frequency, and if the resonant frequency of the transducer system coincides with one of the frequencies making a substantial contribution to the arterial waveform, resonance and subsequent distortion of the signal will occur. Arterial pressure monitoring is designed to keep its natural frequency above 40 Hz, which is above any of the frequencies making up the arterial waveform, thus minimizing resonance. Venous waveforms generally do not require high-frequency response systems because they do not have steep waves or high-frequency components of significant amplitude. Simply, the natural frequency of the *monitoring system* needs to exceed the natural frequency of the *arterial system*.

Damping is an effect that reduces the amplitude of oscillations in an oscillatory system. It acts to slow the rate of a change in signal. The amount of damping in a system is indicated by the damping coefficient (Fig. 24.2, Fig. 24.3), which describes how rapidly an oscillating system comes to rest.

Resonance is the tendency of a system to oscillate with larger amplitude at some frequencies than at others.

- Optimally damped: The system responds rapidly to a change in signal by allowing a small amount of overshoot (damping coefficient 0.7).
- Critically damped: No overshooting occurs, but the system may be too slow (damping coefficient 1.0).

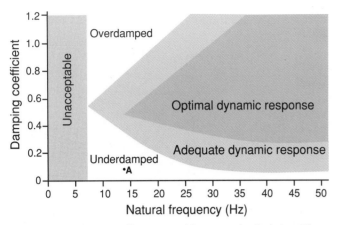

Figure 24.2. Damping coefficient–natural frequency plot displaying different areas into which pressure monitoring systems fall. (Modified from Mark JB. *Atlas of Cardiovascular Monitoring.*)

- Underdamped: Resonance occurs, causing the signal to oscillate and overshoot (damping coefficient <0.7).
- Overdamped: The signal takes a long time to reach equilibrium but will not overshoot. It may not reach equilibrium in time for a true reading to be given (damping coefficient >1.0). This may be the result of soft tubing, an air bubble, a blood clot, or a constriction.

Factors affecting errors in invasive monitoring

1. Zeroing error
2. Leveling error
3. Simultaneous infusion of fluids and drugs

   · Rapid administration of fluid in the CVP catheter will alter measurements

4. Variation with respiration

   · Variations occur in all pressure measurements with spontaneous and positive pressure ventilation
   · Considerable variations may occur in CVP and pulmonary artery pressures during both spontaneous ventilation and positive pressure ventilation
   · Variations may be the result of changes in intrapleural pressure during the respiratory cycle
   · All CVP/pulmonary artery measurements should be performed at end expiration, when intrapleural pressure is zero
   · Arterial pressure waveform variation with respiration may be suggestive of hypovolemia or other conditions, such as cardiac tamponade

5. Excessive positive end-expiratory pressure (PEEP)

   · Measured CVP is the intraluminal pressure
   · True filling pressure is the transmural pressure in the right atrium, which is equal to the right atrial pressure (RAP) minus the sum of intrathoracic pressure and intrapericardial pressure

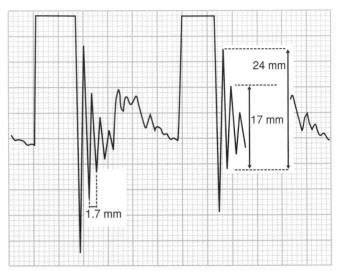

Figure 24.3. Fast flush method to calculate natural frequency and damping coefficient of a pressure monitoring system as described by Gardner. The graph is at tracing speed of 25 mm/sec and shows the arterial pressure waveform and two *square wave* flush. Natural frequency is determined by measuring the period of one cycle between adjacent oscillation peaks (1.7 mm) and the recording speed (25 mm/sec). The natural frequency is 25 mm/sec × 1 cycle/1.7 mm = 14.7 Hz. The damping coefficient is determined by measuring the height of adjacent oscillation peaks (17 and 24 mm), calculating the ratio $(A_2/A_1)(17/24 = 0.71)$, and using the formula derived by Gardner: $D = LN\{(A_2/A_1)/[\Pi^2 + ln(A_2/A_1)\}^2]^{1/2}\}$ to arrive at damping coefficient (D) of 0.11. (Modified from Mark JB. *Atlas of Cardiovascular Monitoring.*)

· As transmural pressure varies throughout the ventilatory cycle, there is a corresponding variation in venous return
· Application of PEEP increases intrathoracic pressure throughout the respiratory cycle
· Compliant lungs tend to transmit this pressure to the right atrium and impede venous return

Arterial pressure

Arterial pressure waveform

The systemic arterial blood pressure (ABP) waveform is generated when the blood is ejected from the left ventricle into the aorta during systole, followed by peripheral arterial runoff of this stroke volume during diastole (Fig. 24.4 and Fig. 24.5).

The morphology of ABP waveform changes as the wave travels from the aorta to the periphery. Compared with aortic pressures, peripheral arterial waveforms have a higher systolic pressure, a lower diastolic pressure, and thus a wider pulse pressure. The pulse arrives at the peripheral site after some delay, and this is seen in the waveform display. Pressure wave reflection off the tapering arterial tree is the predominant factor that influences the shape of the arterial blood pressure waveform. Patients with reduced arterial compliance (e.g., atherosclerosis, advancing age) have an increased pulse pressure, late systolic pressure peak, and disappearance of the diastolic pressure wave (Fig. 24.6), which is the result of an early return of the reflected pressure wave.

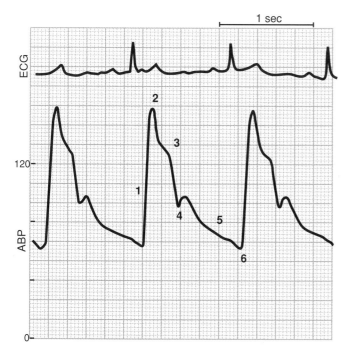

Figure 24.4. The systolic components following the R wave on ECG consist of (1) steep pressure upstroke, peak; (2) systolic peak pressure; and (3) decline, which correspond to the period of left ventricular systole. The down-slope is interrupted by the (4) dicrotic notch, which reflects aortic valve closure at end systole. The remaining decay of waveform, (5) diastolic runoff, occurs during diastole following the ECG T wave and reaches its nadir at end diastole, (6) end-diastolic pressure. (Modified from Mark JB. *Atlas of Cardiovascular Monitoring.*)

Indications for invasive arterial pressure monitoring include the following:

1. The need for real-time blood pressure monitoring
2. The need for repeated arterial blood gas sampling

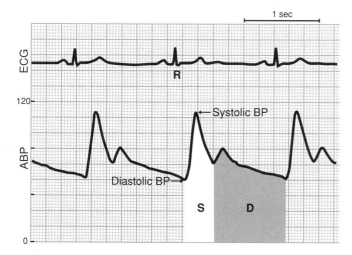

Figure 24.5. Systolic (S) and diastolic (D) pressures are shown with *arrows.* Mean arterial pressure (MAP) is represented by the area beneath the arterial pressure curve divided by the beat period, and it incorporates the S and D portions of the cardiac cycle. (Modified from Mark JB. *Atlas of Cardiovascular Monitoring.*)

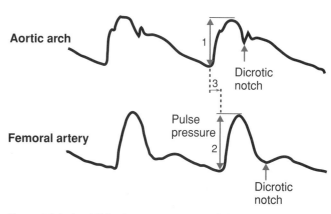

Figure 24.6. Arterial blood pressure waves recorded simultaneously from the aortic arch and femoral artery have different morphologies. In this example, the femoral artery waveform has a wider pulse pressure (1 and 2); a delayed upstroke (3); a delayed, slurred dicrotic notch (*arrows*); and a more prominent diastolic wave following the dicrotic notch. (Modified from Mark JB. *Atlas of Cardiovascular Monitoring.*)

3. Unreliable noninvasive blood pressure; for example, during cardiopulmonary bypass, severe shock, extreme peripheral vasoconstriction, arrhythmias, severe burns, morbid obesity, or patients with an LVAD
4. Dynamic monitoring of fluid resuscitation: systolic pressure variation, mean pressure variation, or pulse pressure variation may be used as an indicator of volume status

Arterial line placement

The most common site for arterial line cannulation is the radial artery, given its superficial location and the presence of good collateral circulation. Other sites include the femoral, axillary, brachial, ulnar, dorsalis pedis, and posterior tibial arteries (Table 24.4).

Table 24.4.	Sites of insertion of arterial lines
Radial	• Most commonly performed; technically easy
	• Allen's test not shown to be predictive of ischemic sequelae
Ulnar	• Not recommended if multiple cannulation attempts were made on the ipsilateral radial artery
	• Primary source of hand blood flow
Brachial	• Risk of median nerve damage
	• Anatomic end artery
Axillary	• Risk of nerve injury
	• Good collateral circulation
	• Hematomas may be difficult to tamponade
	• Higher risk of air or atherosclerotic emboli into cerebral vessels
Femoral	• Risk of retroperitoneal hemorrhage
	• Large artery – ease of placement in emergencies
	• Risk of atherosclerotic emboli to lower extremity
	• **Rarely used in pediatrics because of the high risk of thrombosis**
Dorsalis pedis	• Overestimates systolic pressure
Posterior tibial	• Avoid in peripheral vascular disease

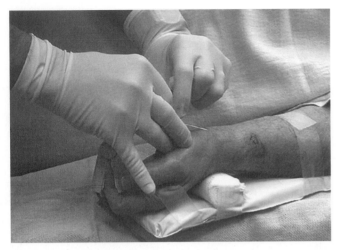

Figure 24.7 Positioning the wrist.

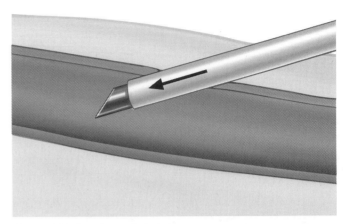

Figure 24.8. Over-the-needle technique.

The Allen's test is used to demonstrate collateral circulation in a hand prior to cannulating the radial artery. After elevating the patient's hand and having the patient make a fist for 30 seconds, pressure is applied over the ulnar and radial arteries to occlude them. The hand is opened and ulnar pressure is released. If color does not return or returns after 7–10 seconds, then the ulnar arterial supply to the hand is considered not sufficient and the radial artery cannot be safely cannulated.

Utility of the test, however, is questionable as there are case reports of ischemic complications despite a normal Allen's test. Specifics of the surgery and the patient's characteristics often influence the site and side of arterial cannulation.

Several techniques of insertion of the arterial line are used, including direct arterial puncture, the Seldinger technique, and the transfixion–withdrawal technique. Ultrasound guidance can be of value in arterial line placement.

Technique

The wrist is placed in the supine position and dorsiflexed on a roll of gauze, thus stabilizing the artery and making it more superficial. A soft board and tape may be used to secure and position the wrist (Fig. 24.7). The radial artery is palpated between the bony head of the distal radius and the flexor carpi radialis tendon. The radial nerve is usually found lateral to the artery. Infiltration of local anesthetic around this area may prevent arterial spasm and also makes the procedure more tolerable for an awake patient.

Catheter over needle

A soft catheter mounted on a sharp metallic needle (or an intravenous catheter) is introduced at about a 45° angle. Once the pulsatile flash of blood is seen at the hub, the angle of the catheter is lowered to about 10° to 15°. The catheter-over-needle assembly is advanced a few millimeters to ensure that the tip of catheter is in the artery. The catheter is then advanced over the needle into the artery (Fig. 24.8).

Catheter over wire (Seldinger technique)

A metallic hollow cannula is used to access the artery (with or without a syringe at the end of the needle). When pulsatile flow is seen, a guidewire is inserted through the cannula into the artery. Then, the hollow cannula is removed and a soft arterial catheter is advanced over the wire into the artery (Fig. 24.9).

Transfixation

Transfixation is a modification of the catheter-over-wire technique. Following entry of the cannula into the artery, the needle is advanced through the posterior wall of the artery. The cannula is then withdrawn slowly until pulsatile blood flow is seen. The guidewire is then advanced into the artery through the cannula. Then, the cannula is removed, and the soft arterial catheter is advanced over the wire into the artery.

Ultrasound or Doppler guidance may sometimes be required in cases of difficulty with blind techniques.

Ultrasound for arterial cannulation

Ultrasound may be used as an aid in the placement of arterial cannulas. All the techniques described previously can be used under ultrasound guidance. Improved success and decreased

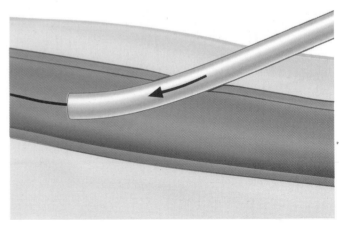

Figure 24.9. Over-the-wire technique.

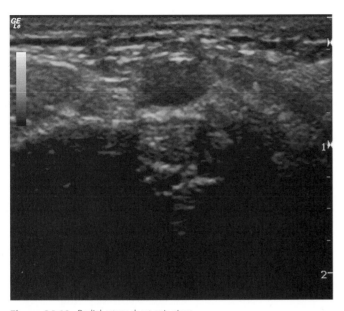

Figure 24.10. Radial artery short-axis view.

complications are some of the advantages of using ultrasound guidance. However, these benefits have not yet been shown consistently. Both short-axis (Fig. 24.10) and long-axis (Fig. 24.11) approaches may be used for cannulation.

Complications

Major complications are extremely rare in the absence of other contributing factors, such as previous arterial injury, protracted shock, high-dose vasopressor administration, prolonged cannulation, and severe atherosclerosis (Table 24.5).

Central venous and pulmonary artery pressure monitoring
Physiology

Blood returns to the right atrium and generates a pressure that is referred to as right atrial pressure (RAP) or central venous

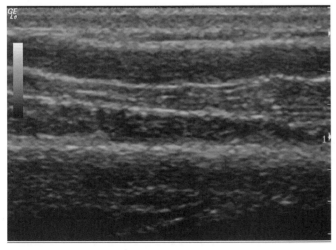

Figure 24.11. Radial artery long-axis view.

Table 24.5. Complications of arterial catheterization

Mechanical complications	• Hematoma
	• Bleeding
	• Vasospasm
	• Pseudoaneurysm
	• Nerve damage
	• Atrioventricular fistula
Thromboembolic	• Arterial thrombosis
	• Air or thromboembolism
Infectious	• Bacteremia
	• Cellulitis
	• Compartment syndrome
Management errors	• Interpretation errors
	• Measurement errors
	• Unintentional intra-arterial drug injection

pressure (CVP). The terms *right atrial pressure* and *central venous pressure* generally can be used interchangeably. Direct left atrial pressure (LAP) measurement is far less common than RAP measurement because of the inherent dangers in its measurement, most notably arterial air embolus and cardiac tamponade.

Cardiac *preload* is defined as the resting end-diastolic length of myofibrils and is clinically represented by end-diastolic right ventricular volume.

Pressure–volume dynamics

The relationship between change in volume and change in pressure yields a compliance curve. Pressure can be measured using a central venous catheter (CVC), whereas volume measurement is more difficult, requiring calculation. Therefore, this relationship between pressure and volume is used to extrapolate right ventricular end-diastolic volume from measured filling pressure or CVP. This pressure–volume compliance curve is not constant and varies among individuals and also under different physiologic conditions, even within the same patient. Thus, assessment of volume status from CVP is fraught with error. The reader is referred to elsewhere in the textbook for further discussion of the limitations of CVP in reflecting patient volume status.

Compliance = change in volume/change in pressure

In normal hearts, CVP also reflects the preload of the left ventricle. In patients with ventricular dysfunction or pulmonary vascular disease, this relationship is lost and a PAWP will be more reflective of LAP and left ventricular end diastolic volume.

CVP waveform

A tracing of the CVP yields three positive waves – a, c, and v – and two negative descents – x and y. These are described further in Table 24.6. Both the atria and the ventricles have systolic and diastolic phases. For clarity, the ventricular phases of the cardiac cycle are used to describe the timing of various events. Therefore, *systole* refers to ventricular systole. These phases can be identified most accurately if an ECG tracing is also used

Table 24.6. CVP/RAP waves

Component wave	Atrial phase	Ventricular phase	ECG phase	Causative event	Normal pressures, mm Hg
a wave	Systole	End diastole	P wave	Atrial contraction	2–7
c wave	Diastole	Isovolumic ventricular contraction	After R wave	Tricuspid valve motion toward the atrium	
x descent	Diastole	Late systole	S-T segment	Atrial relaxation and geometric changes due to ventricular systole	
v wave	Diastole	Late systole to isovolumic ventricular relaxation Early diastole	After T wave	Pressure produced when the blood filling the atrium comes up against a closed tricuspid valve	2–7
y descent	Diastole	Early diastolic filling		Atrial emptying into ventricle on opening of tricuspid valve	

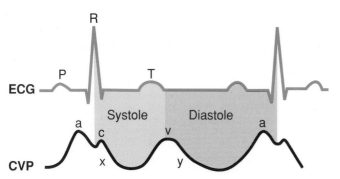
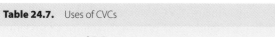

Figure 24.12. CVP waves synchronized to ECG. (From Mark JB. *Atlas of Cardiovascular Monitoring.*)

Table 24.7. Uses of CVCs

- Measurement of CVP
- Administration of vasoactive/inotropic drugs
- Administration of hypertonic solutions and parenteral nutrition
- Administration of chemotherapy, antibiotics, and immunosuppressants
- Hemodialysis and hemofiltration
- Diagnosis of dysrhythmias, particularly nodal rhythms

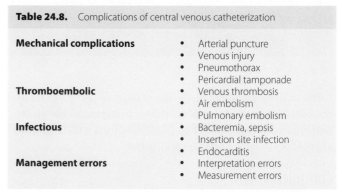

Table 24.8. Complications of central venous catheterization

Mechanical complications	• Arterial puncture
	• Venous injury
	• Pneumothorax
	• Pericardial tamponade
Thromboembolic	• Venous thrombosis
	• Air embolism
	• Pulmonary embolism
Infectious	• Bacteremia, sepsis
	• Insertion site infection
	• Endocarditis
Management errors	• Interpretation errors
	• Measurement errors

From Mark JB, Slaughter TF. *Miller's Anesthesia.* 6th ed. New York: Churchill Livingstone; 2004:1265–1362.

(Fig. 24.12). Electrical activity always precedes mechanical activity; there is usually a very short delay of less than 0.1 second before pressure changes are noted on the CVP waveform. Alterations in the ECG rhythm often are reflected in the CVP waveform, as explained later in this chapter.

Mean CVP is measured as the mean a-wave pressure and normally ranges from 2 to 6 mm Hg. It can be approximated by averaging the a wave pressure and the trough of the y descent. (See also Tables 24.7 and 24.8.)

Abnormal CVP waves

Atrial arrhythmias

Because a coordinated atrial contraction does not occur in atrial flutter/fibrillation, an a wave will be absent from the CVP tracing. Occasional flutter waves may be discernable instead of a single a wave (Fig. 24.13).

Junctional rhythm and complete heart block

Atrial contraction is usually normally timed to coincide with ventricular diastole, thus allowing the tricuspid valve to open

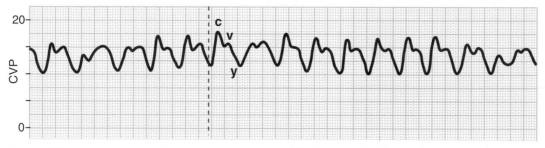

Figure 24.13. Absent a wave as well as a larger c wave seen in atrial fibrillation. (Modified from Mark JB. *Atlas of Cardiovascular Monitoring.*)

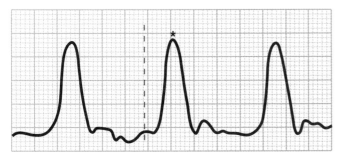

Figure 24.14. Tall cannon a waves are the result of atrial contraction against a closed tricuspid valve.* denotes an example of a cannon wave. (Modified from Mark JB. *Atlas of Cardiovascular Monitoring*.)

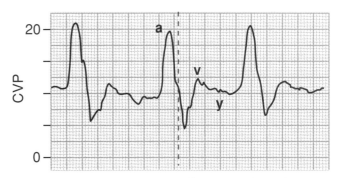

Figure 24.16. Tricuspid stenosis, with a tall a wave and a blunted y descent. (Modified from Mark JB. *Atlas of Cardiovascular Monitoring*.)

and allow blood flow. In cases of altered rhythms such as junctional rhythms, reentrant supraventricular tachycardia, or complete heart block, atrial contraction occurs during ventricular systole. Atrial contraction during tricuspid closure results in tall "cannon" a waves (Fig. 24.14). False cannon a waves can be produced when a transduced port passes through the mitral valve and detects right ventricular pressures.

a-c Wave

In cases in which the PR interval is shortened, the a and c waves may temporally appear to have merged, resulting in an a-c wave. In the case of tachycardia, diastolic shortening may result in v and a waves appearing fused.

Tricuspid regurgitation and decreased right ventricular compliance

Tricuspid regurgitation is a ventricular systolic event resulting in a rise in atrial pressure due to transmission of ventricular systolic pressure to the atrium. This coincides with the v wave of the atrium, resulting in a tall systolic c-v wave and an obliteration of the x descent (Fig. 24.15). Differential diagnosis includes conditions in which right atrial compliance is decreased, because this also may lead to a large v wave. Note that the common clinical sign of acute tricuspid regurgitation is an enlarged y-descent, whereas the common clinical sign of acute mitral regurgitation is a large v wave. This occurs because the compliance of the pulmonary veins is much lower than the compliance of the central venous system, so the regurgitant volume produces a larger pressure increase (v wave) in the left side compared with the right.

Tricuspid stenosis

In tricuspid stenosis, the higher pressure gradient required for flow across the tricuspid valve results in atrial hypertrophy as well as impedance of passive emptying of the atrium. Thus, a tall a wave and attenuated y wave are seen (Fig. 24.16). Decreased right ventricular compliance also may result in a tall a wave. Because right ventricular diastolic pressure is elevated when compliance is poor, a higher atrial pressure is required to fill the ventricle. This is achieved by more forceful contraction of the atrium.

Pericardial tamponade

Fluid in the pericardium results in decreased ventricular compliance, resulting in impairment of diastolic filling. Because the y wave occurs as the result of early diastolic filling, y-descent attenuation is seen in tamponade (Fig. 24.17). The x descent occurs during ventricular systole, which is unaffected by fluid in the pericardium.

Pericardial constriction

Chronic constrictive pericarditis results in similar hemodynamic alterations to that of pericardial tamponade restrictive. Diastolic filling of the ventricles is restricted, reducing stroke volume and cardiac output. As in tamponade, the x descent is unchanged but the y descent is prominent because of rapid initial filling of the ventricle, which is abruptly terminated by pericardial restraint. This is often described as the *M* or *W configuration*. Following the deep y descent, a mid-diastolic plateau is often seen, which is called the *dip and plateau* or the *square root sign* (Fig. 24.18).

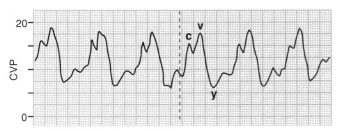

Figure 24.15. Tricuspid regurgitation showing tall c-v waves is shown with a lack of a well-defined x descent. (Modified from Mark JB. *Atlas of Cardiovascular Monitoring*.)

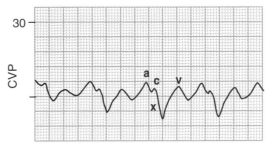

Figure 24.17. Pericardial tamponade showing a dampened y descent. (Modified from Mark JB. *Atlas of Cardiovascular Monitoring*.)

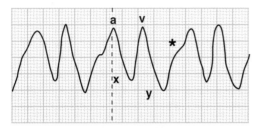

Figure 24.18. Pericardial constriction showing deep x and y descents as well as a flatter curve after the y descent marked by an *asterisk* (*). (Modified from Mark JB. *Atlas of Cardiovascular Monitoring.*)

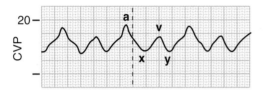

Figure 24.19. The CVP pattern for right ventricular ischemia can mimic that seen in pericardial restriction or restrictive cardiomyopathy with pronounced x and y descents. (Modified from Mark JB. *Atlas of Cardiovascular Monitoring.*)

Right ventricular ischemia

Right ventricular ischemia depresses ventricular systole as well as diastole. Diastolic impairment results in a tall a wave. Systolic impairment may result in tricuspid regurgitation, causing a tall v wave, which may be accompanied by a deep x and y descent (Fig. 24.19). This may appear similar to the tracing seen in pericardial constriction.

Central venous cannulation

Seldinger's technique of using a guidewire to insert central lines has become the standard method. An additional finder needle is often used in internal jugular venous access to decrease the incidence of carotid puncture with a large-bore needle. This step is typically omitted at other sites.

Ultrasound guidance may increase safety and is typically used at two stages: first, to surface-mark the anatomy of the

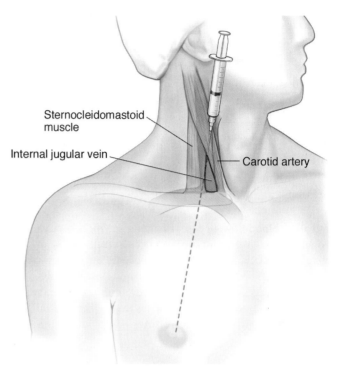

Figure 24.20. Landmarks and position for internal jugular venous cannulation.

target vessel, and second, to access the vein as well as visualize intraluminal placement of the guidewire in real time.

A number of sites for central venous cannulation are available (Table 24.9).

Internal jugular vein cannulation

For internal jugular vein (IJV) cannulation, the patient is placed in Trendelenburg position, which helps distend the vein. The IJV lies deep to the sternocleidomastoid muscle and follows a course from just anterior to the mastoid process to behind the sternoclavicular joint (Fig. 24.20). The IJV may be cannulated at different sites along the course, using landmarks or

Table 24.9. Insertion sites for central venous cannulation

Site	Location	Advantages	Disadvantages
Internal jugular	Central	• Ease of access to the neck for the anesthesiologist • Ease of floating PACs	• Risk of stroke from carotid punctures • Difficult to place in patients with unstable cervical spine
External jugular	Central	• Visible superficially • Lower risk of carotid puncture	• Difficult threading of catheter under clavicle
Subclavian	Central	• Consistent landmarks • Good site for tunneled catheters	• Highest risk of pneumothorax • Arterial puncture • Chest retractors can dampen waveforms or even occlude catheters • Floating PAC via right SCV can be difficult • Tip needs to be supradiaphragmatic to read true CVP
Femoral	Central	• Ease of placement • No risk of pneumothorax	• Highest risk of infection • Venous thrombosis
Basilic	Peripheral	• Can be used for longer durations	• Needs to be positioned in the central veins or right atrium to read CVP

From Clutton-Brock TH, Hutton P. *Monitoring in Anaesthesia and Intensive Care* 1st ed. Edited by Hutton P. Philadelphia, PA: W.B. Saunders; 1994:145–155.

ultrasound guidance. A finder needle is invariably used in landmark-guided IJV cannulation to decrease the incidence of carotid punctures.

Anterior (high) approach

The IJV is cannulated at the level of the larynx. The needle is inserted along the medial border of the sternocleidomastoid, angled at 30° to the skin, and directed toward the ipsilateral nipple.

Middle approach

The cannula is inserted at the apex of the triangle formed by the two heads of the sternocleidomastoid muscle. This landmark is more reliable when carotid pulsation is weak or absent (as in cardiac arrest).

Posterior approach

The cannula is inserted along the lateral border of the sterno-cleidomastoid muscle at the level of the external jugular vein.

Subclavian vein cannulation

The subclavian vein is the continuation of the axillary vein and arises at the lateral border of the first rib. It passes over the first rib anterior to the subclavian artery, separated from it by the scalenus anterior, to join the IJV at the medial end of the clavicle (Fig. 24.21).

The insertion point is at the junction of medial third and middle third of the clavicle. This point is also marked by a notch that can be felt on the undersurface of the clavicle. The needle is introduced while aspirating under the clavicle at this point and is directed toward the sternal notch. When the vein has

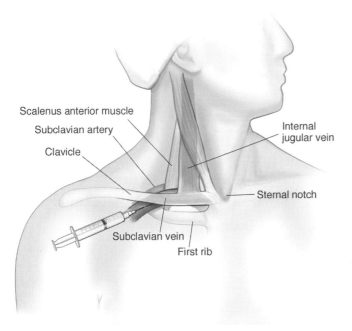

Figure 24.21. Landmarks and position for subclavian vein cannulation.

been cannulated, the Seldinger technique is used to introduce the catheter over the wire. The subclavian vein cannot be compressed with direct pressure – therefore, this route is contraindicated in patients with a coagulopathy (Table 24.10).

It should be noted that there is a risk, in any patient, of inadvertent cannulation and even laceration of the subclavian artery. This can cause a large uncontrolled hemorrhage into the thoracic cavity. For this reason, many centers do not attempt percutaneous subclavian access without the personnel and equipment immediately available to accommodate this rare, but potentially catastrophic, complication.

Ultrasound for central venous cannulation

Vascular access by the landmark technique depends on the anatomic landmarks; however, anatomic variations often are encountered. In addition, vessels may be diminutive, thrombosed, or even absent in certain circumstances. Ultrasound offers the advantage of real-time visualization of the vessels, demonstrates patency and flow, and differentiates arteries from veins using color Doppler or pulse wave Doppler. B-mode ultrasound provides two-dimensional (2-D) images that can be used to examine structures in the transverse and longitudinal planes. For differentiation, arteries are pulsatile and difficult to compress with the ultrasound probe while veins are nonpulsatile and collapse or distend, depending on probe pressure, patient position, and respiration.

Ultrasound is becoming increasingly popular for CVC insertion because it has been shown to reduce the complication rate and allows for cost saving. The use of ultrasound has increased catheterization success rates, reduced the number of needle passes required for success, and decreased the incidence of complications compared with traditional landmark techniques. The Agency for Healthcare Research and Quality recommends the use of ultrasound guidance for placing CVCs to improve patient care and patient safety.

The *Guidance on the Use of Ultrasound Locating Devices for Placing Central Venous Catheters* from the National Institute for Clinical Excellence provides the following major recommendations:

- 2-D imaging ultrasound guidance is the preferred method for insertion of CVCs into the IJV in adults and children in elective situations.
- The use of 2-D imaging ultrasound guidance should be considered in most clinical circumstances in which CVC insertion is indicated.
- Everyone involved in placing CVCs using 2-D imaging ultrasound guidance should undertake appropriate training to achieve competence.
- Audio-guided Doppler ultrasound guidance is not recommended for CVC insertion.

The American College of Surgeons supports the uniform use of real-time ultrasound guidance for the placement of CVCs in all patients.

Table 24.10. Derived parameters

Derived parameter	Formula	Normal value
Cardiac index	CO/BSA	2.6–4.2 L/min/m^2
Systemic vascular resistance	(MAP − CVP)/CO × 80	900–1300 dyn ∗ s/cm^5
Pulmonary vascular resistance	(MPAP − PAWP)/CO − 80	40–180 dyn ∗ s/cm^5
Left ventricular stroke work	SV × (MAP − PAWP) × 0.0136	58–104 gm-m/beat
Right ventricular stroke work	SV − (MPAP − PAWP) × 0.0136	8–16 gm-m/beat
Stroke volume (SV)	CO/HR × 1000	60–100 ml/beat
Coronary artery perfusion pressure	Diastolic BP − PAWP	60–80 mm Hg
Arterial oxygen content (CaO$_2$)	(0.0138 × Hb × SaO$_2$) + (0.0031 × PaO$_2$)	17–20 ml/dl
Venous oxygen content (CvO$_2$)	(0.0138 × Hb × SvO$_2$) + (0.0031 × PaO2)	12–15 ml/dl
A-V oxygen content difference [C(a-v)O$_2$]	CaO$_2$ − CvO$_2$	4–6 ml/dl
Oxygen delivery	CaO$_2$ × CO × 10	950–1150 ml/min
Oxygen consumption	[C(a − v)O$_2$] × CO × 10	200–250 ml/min

A-V, arteriovenous; BP, blood pressure; BSA, body surface area; gm-m, gram-meter; Hb, hemoglobin; HR, heart rate; MAP, mean arterial pressure; MPAP, mean pulmonary artery pressure; SaO$_2$, arterial oxygen saturation; SvO$_2$, venous oxygen saturation.

However, ultrasound guidance does not eliminate all adverse outcomes. For example, difficulty in visualizing the tip of the inserted needle and the related potential for injury is driving the development of advanced ultrasound machines. Incorporating embedded sensors in both the needle and ultrasound probe, these new ultrasound machines are capable of tracking the tip of the needle in real time.

Performing real-time ultrasound-guided vessel cannulation

Ultrasound can be used to assist with venous cannulation of internal jugular or femoral veins at their usual locations. The subclavian vein is accessed at the level of the axillary vein. Asepsis is maintained by using sterile gel and a sterile sheath to cover the probe and cable. The vessels may be visualized in long-axis (Fig. 24.22) or short-axis (Fig. 24.23) views. Both views have

their advantages and disadvantages. The short-axis view of the vessel allows for simultaneous visualization of the artery, but the needle appears as a pinpoint. This may lead to confusion as to the exact location of the needle tip. Long-axis allows for visualization of the entire needle at all times but, depending on the patient and location, may or may not allow for simultaneous visualization of the artery. This may lead to inadvertent cannulation of the artery if care is not taken.

The image of the vessel to be cannulated should be kept in the middle of the screen while the needle is introduced. It is important to minimize pressure on the transducer, particularly for the internal jugular approach, as excessive pressure will distort the anatomy visualized, often compressing the internal jugular vein, making the placement of the needle more difficult. The needle is usually visible, but often its initial presence is seen as a distortion of local tissues. As the needle tip approaches the

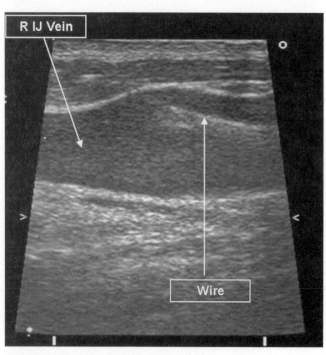

Figure 24.22. IJV with the guidewire visualized in long-axis view.

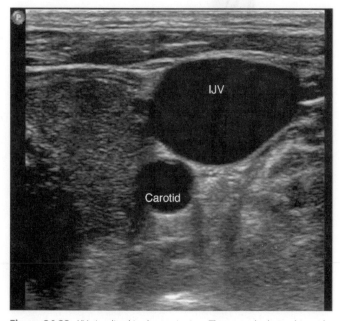

Figure 24.23. IJV visualized in short-axis view. The normal relationship with the carotid artery also is seen in this view.

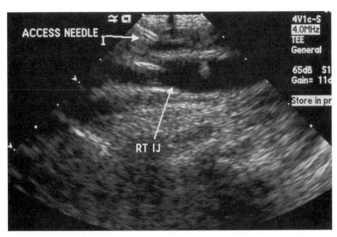

Figure 24.24. Access needle seen within the lumen of the IJV on real-time ultrasound.

anterior wall, an indentation is seen until a "give-way" sensation is felt and the vein re-expands. The needle tip should then be visible within the lumen (Fig. 24.24). The probe is temporarily set aside on a sterile drape and the guidewire passed in the usual way. The probe then may be used to confirm that the guidewire is within the lumen. Visualization of the guidewire in the correct vessel may not imply that the tip of the wire is in the vein or the right side of the heart; thus, it may still be necessary to use manometry or echocardiography to confirm venous access.

Pulmonary artery catheters

Pulmonary artery catheters (PACs) play a vital role in the hemodynamic monitoring of critically ill patients. However, there has been considerable debate about their use.

In 1993, the ASA published practice guidelines looking at the evidence supporting the clinical effectiveness of PACs; these guidelines were updated in 2003. The guidelines suggest that PAC monitoring may reduce perioperative complications if critical hemodynamic data obtained from an "appropriately" placed PAC are "accurately" interpreted and "appropriate" treatment is initiated.

"Assessment of the clinical effectiveness of Pulmonary Artery Catheters in Management of patients in intensive care (PAC-Man): a randomized controlled trial concluded that there is no clear evidence of benefit or harm in managing critically ill patients with a PAC. The decision to use PAC must be taken considering risks and benefits on a case by case basis."

Measured and derived parameters

Measured parameters include the following:

- Intracardiac pressures (normal values mentioned)
  - CVP/RAP: 2 to 6 mm Hg
  - Pulmonary artery systolic pressure (PASP): 15 to 25 mm Hg
  - Pulmonary artery diastolic pressure (PADP): 8 to 15 mm Hg
  - Mean pulmonary artery pressure (MPAP): approximated by PASP + (2 × PADP)]/3 = 10 to 20 mm Hg
  - PAWP: 6–12 mm Hg
- Thermodilution cardiac output (CO)
- Mixed venous oxygen saturation
- Calculation of shunt fractions and gradients
- PCWP may be used to indirectly assess left ventricular preload. This relationship is based on the assumption:

$$PCWP \cong LAP \cong LVEDP \cong LVEDV$$

Derived parameters are listed in Table 24.10.

Invasive methods to measure cardiac output
Fick principle

The Fick principle, developed by Adolf Eugen Fick, is based on the conservation of mass and states that the amount of a substance taken up by an organ (or whole body) per unit time is equal to the arterial minus venous concentration of the substance multiplied by blood flow.

This principle can be used to measure the blood flow through any organ that adds substances to, or removes substances from, the blood. The heart does not do either of these, but the CO equals the pulmonary blood flow and the lungs add oxygen to the blood and remove carbon dioxide from it. CO is a function of VO_2, CaO_2, and CvO_2, where:

- VO_2, oxygen consumption, can be measured from the difference in oxygen concentration between expired and inspired gas
- CVO_2 – venous oxygen content of blood
- CaO_2 – arterial oxygen content of blood

$$CO = VO_2/CaO_2 - CvO_2$$

Substituting normal values, $CO = (250 \text{ ml/min})/5 \text{ml dl}^{-1} = 50 \text{ dl/min} = 5 \text{ L/min}$

The Fick method is accurate and can be calculated using a PAC. Several variants of the basic method have been devised, but their accuracy usually is not validated.

Dilution techniques
Dye dilution technique

A known amount of dye is injected into the pulmonary artery, and its concentration is measured peripherally. A curve is generated and is graphed semi-logarithmically to correct for recirculation of the dye. CO is calculated from the injected dose, the area under the curve (AUC), and its duration (Fig. 24.25).

Thermodilution technique

A known volume of cold saline is injected through the port of a PAC. A distal thermistor measures temperature changes. The degree of change in the temperature is inversely proportional to the CO. A plot of temperature change against time gives a curve

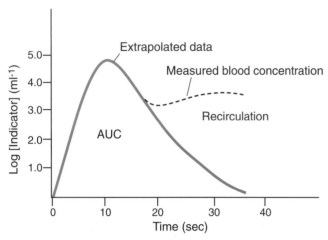

Figure 24.25. CO is derived from the area under curve. Note that the curve is made by extrapolation. (From Allsager CM, Swanevelder J. Measuring cardiac output. *Br J Anaesth CEPD Rev* 2003; 3(1):15–19.)

similar to the dye curve (but without the second peak). CO is calculated using the Stewart-Hamilton equation. This makes certain assumptions:

1. Complete mixing of blood and indicator
2. No loss of indicator between the injection site and detection site and constant blood flow

$$\dot{Q} = \frac{n}{\int c\, dt} = \frac{k(T_{core} - T_{indicator})\, V_{indicator}}{\int_{t_1}^{t_2} -\Delta T\, dt}$$

$$\dot{Q} = \frac{n}{\int c\, dt} = \frac{k(T_{core} - T_{indicator})\, V_{indicator}}{\int_{t_1}^{t_2} -\Delta T\, dt}$$

The amount of indicator (n) is related to its mean concentration (c), CO (Q), and the time for which it is detected ($t_2 - t_1$).

Some newer catheters allow for continuous measurement by using a thermal filament. However, the accuracy of the thermodilution technique may be influenced by various factors:

1. Right and left ventricular output may differ in the presence of a cardiac shunt.
2. Tricuspid or pulmonary valve regurgitation may cause underestimation or overestimation of CO.
3. Core blood temperatures may vary.
4. Positive pressure ventilation produces beat-to-beat variations in right ventricular stroke volume during the respiratory cycle; measured CO will depend on the timing of the bolus injection.
5. Volume of injectate: even small errors in injectate volume may result in errors of CO measurement.
6. Speed of injection: duration of injection should be brief (<3 seconds) and consistent across measurements.

7. Errors in measurement can be created by simultaneous administration of fluids at a significant rate, even if administered via a peripheral IV site.

Pulmonary artery catheter flotation

The PAC may be inserted in any of the large central veins. The right IJV is the preferred route, as it offers the straightest course to the right heart. When an RAP waveform is seen, approximately 20 cm from the right IJV (see CVP waveform section), the balloon is gently inflated with 1.0 to 1.5 ml of air and then advanced until it crosses the tricuspid valve.

The position of the PAC in the heart is recognized by different waveforms (Fig. 24.26). Right ventricular pressure is characterized by a marked increase in systolic pressure (systolic rise). The PAC then enters the right ventricular outflow tract and floats across the pulmonic valve into the main pulmonary artery. Often, this may be complicated by arrhythmias, as the catheter irritates the right ventricular infundibulum. The pulmonary arterial waveform is characterized by an increase in diastolic pressure (Fig. 24.27). On reaching wedge position, the waveform resembles an LAP waveform, with a, c, and v waves as described earlier. At this point, the balloon occludes the blood flow and creates a static column of blood between the catheter tip and the left atrium (Fig. 24.28). As a surrogate for LAP, the PAWP waveform shares many **of its** morphologic features: a and v waves and x and y descents are usually identifiable (Fig. 24.29). However, PAWP is a representation of LAP that is delayed by about 160 ms.

Guidelines for catheter placement

Guidelines for catheter placement are as follows:

1. Prior to insertion, proper assembly and functioning should be confirmed (Table 24.11).
2. A defibrillator and a transcutaneous pacemaker should be available.
3. As the balloon fills with air, it tends to float to nondependent regions; certain maneuvers help in flotation:

   · Head down aids flotation past the tricuspid valve.
   · Right tilt and/or head up aids flotation out of the right ventricle.
   · Head up may reduce the frequency of arrhythmias.
   · Valsalva maneuver and release during spontaneous ventilation increase right heart venous return and may help flotation.
   · Continuous positive airway pressure of 30 to 40 cm H_2O and release during mechanical ventilation increase right heart venous return and may help flotation.

4. Transesophageal echocardiography may be used to visualize the catheter position during flotation.
5. Typical distances observed when placing a PAC from the RIJ insertion site are mentioned in Table 24.12.

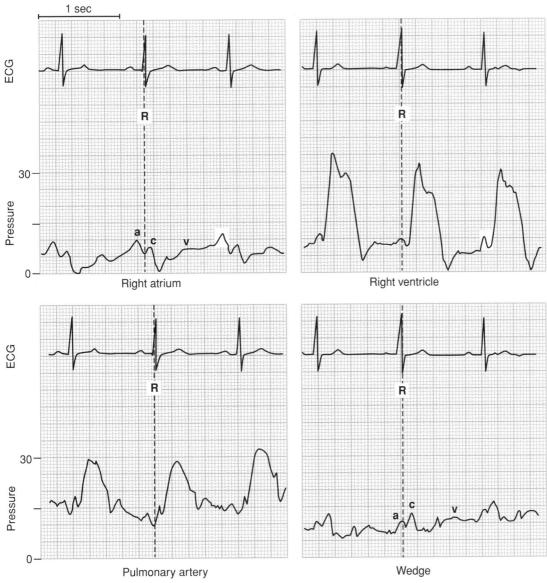

Figure 24.26. Pressure waveforms recorded from a PAC as it passes through the heart. (Modified from Mark JB. *Atlas of Cardiovascular Monitoring.*)

Complications of pulmonary artery catheterization are listed in Table 24.13.

Minimally invasive hemodynamic monitors

- **Esophageal Doppler:** The esophageal Doppler monitor measures blood flow velocity in the descending thoracic aorta using a flexible ultrasound probe. This is then combined with estimated aortic cross-sectional area to give stroke volume and cardiac output measurements. Disadvantages include that the aortic cross-sectional area is typically taken from stored normograms, which limits accuracy. Erroneous readings may also result from suboptimal probe positioning. Advantages include that the device is simple to use and does not require access to the circulation. There are many clinical studies proving its utility. Further, it can calculate corrected flow time (FTc) as

a measure of cardiac preload and thus be used to monitor volume responsiveness in goal-directed therapy. Of note, the ultrasound CO monitor (USCOM) is a completely noninvasive Doppler device that measures CO from a suprasternal Doppler probe.

- **Lithium dilution device:** Lithium chloride is injected into either a peripheral or a central vein, and lithium concentration decay is then measured with a lithium-sensitive electrode attached to an arterial line. Cardiac output is then calculated by integrating the area under the curve of concentration versus time. Disadvantages include that the system requires access to the circulation with repetitive blood draws and that nondepolarizing neuromuscular antagonists interfere with the sensor and can give erroneous results. Advantages include ease of setup and continuous CO measurement

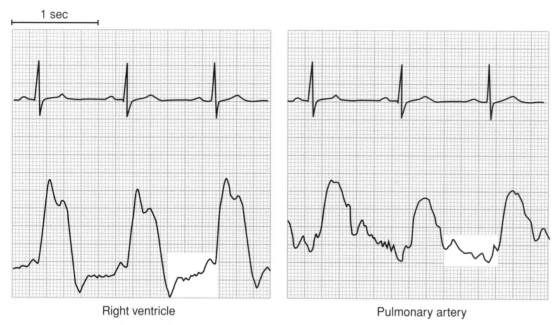

Figure 24.27. The diastolic contour helps distinguish right ventricular from pulmonary artery pressure. (Modified from Mark JB. *Atlas of Cardiovascular Monitoring*.)

with just one arterial line. Further, it can be used to measure stroke volume and stroke volume variation for use in goal directed therapy.

- **Partial nonrebreathing systems:** These systems use the Fick method for determining CO. Disadvntages include many technical difficulties, including that changes in dead space or V/Q matching affect CO measurement. The device also measures only CO and is not useful for evaluating intravascular volume and fluid responsiveness. Advantages include that the device is easy to set up, it does not require access to the circulation, and it provides for continuous CO determination.

- **Arterial pulse contour analysis:** The origin of the pulse contour method for estimation of beat-to-beat stroke volume is based on the Windkessel (air chamber) model described by Otto Frank in 1899. The Windkessel effect is the distension of the aorta when blood is ejected from the left ventricle. Advanced statistical principles are applied to the arterial pressure tracing to calculate cardiac output. Disadvantages of this method include requirement for access to the circulation and the need for a high-fidelity arterial waveform. Initial systems required calibration, although a newly released device requires no calibration with an intravascular indicator and does not need to be

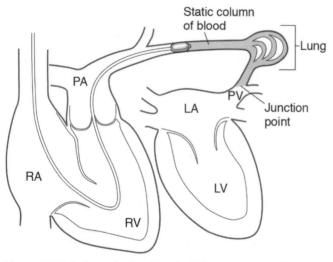

Figure 24.28. In the wedged position, the PAC creates a static column of blood connecting the catheter tip to a junction point, where flow resumes in the pulmonary veins (PV) near the left atrium (LA). (Modified from Mark JB. *Atlas of Cardiovascular Monitoring*.)

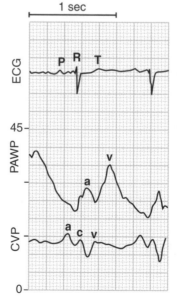

Figure 24.29. The PAWP waveform generally displays two pressure peaks (a and v waves) compared with the CVP tracing, which displays three pressure peaks (a, c, and v waves). Note that the a and v waves of the PAWP trace are delayed relative to the CVP trace, both because the right ventricle normally contracts before the left ventricle and because of the timing delays in the propagation of left atrial waves to an occluded pulmonary artery (Modified from Mark JB. *Atlas of Cardiovascular Monitoring*.)

Table 24.11. Components of a typical PAC

Component	Function
Proximal lumen	• Measures RAP • Injects fluid for thermodilution CO
Distal lumen	• Measures pressures as catheter is advanced • When appropriately positioned, measures PASP, PADP, and PCWP
Balloon	• When inflated, directs catheter forward with blood flow • Occludes a branch of pulmonary artery to create a continuous, static column of blood that connects the pulmonary artery, via a segment of the pulmonary vasculature, to the left atrium
Thermistor	• Located just proximal to distal port and balloon • Helps calculate CO by thermodilution
Additional features	• Additional lumen for drug infusion • Lumen for pacing wire • Atrial and ventricular pacing electrodes • Fiberoptic bundles that allow continuous determination of mixed venous oxygen saturation • Ability to perform continuous CO monitoring using a thermal filament • Rapid-response thermistor to measure right ventricular ejection fraction

Table 24.13. Complications of pulmonary artery catheterization

During insertion	• Arrhythmias/fibrillation • Right bundle branch block • Complete heart block in patient with prior left bundle branch block
Mechanical	• Placement in incorrect locations • Pulmonary artery rupture • Catheter knots • Pulmonary artery pseudoaneurysm • Endocardial injury • Cardiac valves damage • Catheter migration
Infectious	• Endocarditis • Sepsis
Thromboembolic	• Mural thrombus • Pulmonary infarction • Venous thrombosis
Management errors	• Interpretation errors • Measurement errors

recalibrated during hemodynamic instability. Advantages include its ease of use, the need for only an arterial line (no central line), continuous CO measurements are provided, and stroke volume and stroke volume variation can be measured.

- **Transpulmonary thermodilution technique (TTT):** The TTT system uses a central line to calculate CO by transpulmonary thermodilution and an arterial line (femoral, axillary or brachial, but *not* radial) as a pulse contour device to measure CO. Disadvantages include the requirement of a central line *and* arterial catheter placed in a major artery. As such, the technology is not truly minimally invasive. Advantages include the provision of continuous CO measurements, estimation of extravascular fluid, and use in goal-directed therapy. Further, the system can be used with in-situ arterial and central lines.

- **Thoracic electrical bioimpedance (TEB):** TEB is based on the assumption that thoracic impedence is dependent on the blood flow within thoracic cavity. High-frequency low-amplitude current is transmitted from electrodes and the impedance to the current flow is measured with

another set of electrodes. Disadvantages include that the system relies on numerous mathematical assumptions and is prone to errors from hemodynamic instability, arrhythmias, changes in venous blood and lung water, ventilation, electrocautery, and surgical manipulation. Although the device is completely noninvasive, current iterations of the technology do not suggest that the device will become a routine modality for measuring CO.

In a well-written recent study, Harvey et al. note that of the available minimally invasive CO monitors, the esophageal Doppler and arterial pulse contour devices have the best likelihood of replacing the PAC for CO measurement. Further, both the esophageal Doppler and the arterial pulse contour devices have been shown to reduce postoperative morbidity when used with an intraoperative goal-directed fluid strategy.

Suggested readings

ACC/AHA 2007 Guidelines on Perioperative Cardiovascular Evaluation and Care for Noncardiac Surgery: A Report of the American College of Cardiology/American Heart Association Task Force on Practice Guidelines. *J Am Coll Cardiol* 2007 50: e159–242.

Allsager CM, Swanevelder J. Measuring cardiac output. *Br J Anaesth CEPD Rev* 2003; 3(1):15–19.

American College of Surgeons. [ST-60] Statement on recommendations for uniform use of real-time ultrasound guidance for placement of central venous catheters. Available at: http://www.facs.org/fellows_info/statements/st-60.html.

American Society of Anesthesiologists Task Force on Pulmonary Artery Catheterization. Practice guidelines for pulmonary artery catheterization: an updated report by the American Society of Anesthesiologists Task Force on Pulmonary Artery Catheterization. *Anesthesiology* 2003, 99(4):988–1014.

Blaivas M, Adhikari S. An unseen danger: frequency of posterior vessel wall penetration by needles during attempts to place internal jugular vein central catheters using ultrasound guidance. *Crit Care Med* 2009; 37(8):2345–2349.

Clutton-Brock TH, Hutton P. *Monitoring in Anaesthesia and Intensive Care.* 1st ed. Edited by Hutton P. Philadelphia, PA: W.B. Saunders; 1994; 145–155.

Table 24.12. Distances for PAC placement from right internal jugular cannulation site

Puncture site	Destination	Distance, *cm*
Right internal jugular vein	Right atrium Right ventricle Pulmonary artery Pulmonary artery wedge	20 30–35 40–45 50

Dinardo JA. *Anesthesia for Cardiac Surgery.* 2nd ed. Stamford, CT: Appleton & Lange; 1998:62–70.

Funk DJ, Moretti EW, Gan TJ. Minimally invasive cardiac output monitoring in the perioperative setting. *Anesth Analg* 2009; 108:887–897.

Galloway S, Bodenham A. Ultrasound imaging of the axillary vein – anatomical basis for central venous access. *Br J Anaesth* 2003; 90(5):589–595.

Ganesh A, Kaye R, Cahill AM, et al. Evaluation of ultrasound-guided radial artery cannulation in children. *Pediatr Crit Care Med* 2009; 10(1):45–48.

Hatfield A, Bodenham A. Ultrasound for central venous access: continuing education in anaesthesia. *Crit Care Pain* 2005; 5(6):187–190.

Harvey S, Harrison DA, Singer M, Ashcroft J, Jones CM, Elbourne D, Brampton W, Williams D, Young D, Rowan K: Assessment of the clinical effectiveness of pulmonary artery catheters in management of patients in intensive care (PAC-Man): a randomized controlled trial. *Lancet* 2005; 366:472–477.

Hind D, Calvert N, McWilliams R, et al. Ultrasonic locating devices for central venous cannulation: meta-analysis. *BMJ* 2003; 327: 361.

Langton JA, Stoker M. Principles of pressure transducers, resonance, damping & frequency response. *Anaesth Intensive Care Med* 2001; 2:186–190.

Levin PD, Sheinin O, Gozal Y. Use of ultrasound guidance in the insertion of radial artery catheters. *Crit Care Med* 2003, 31(2):481–484.

Levitov AB, Aziz S, Slonim AD. Before we go too far: ultrasound-guided central catheter placement. *Crit Care Med* 2009; 37(8):2473–2474.

Mark JB. *Atlas of Cardiovascular Monitoring.* 1st ed. New York: Churchill Livingstone; 1998.

Mark JB, Slaughter TF. *Miller's Anesthesia.* 6th ed. New York: Churchill Livingstone; 2004; 1265–1362.

National Institute for Clinical Excellence. *Guidance on the Use of Ultrasound Locating Devices for Placing Central Venous Catheters.* London: National Institute for Clinical Excellence (NICE); 2002. Technology appraisal guidance no. 49.

Otto CW. *Monitoring in Anesthesia and Critical Care Medicine.* 3rd ed. Edited by Blitt CD et al. New York: Churchill Livingstone; 1994; 173–212.

Phillips R, Lichtenthal P, Sloniger J, Burstow D, West M, Copeland J. Noninvasive cardiac output measurement in heart failure subjects on circulatory support. *Anesth Analg* 2009; 108:881–886.

Randolph AG, Cook DJ, Gonzales CA, Pribble CG. Ultrasound guidance for placement of central venous catheters: a meta-analysis of the literature. *Crit Care Med* 1996; 24:2053–2058.

Rothschild JM. Ultrasound guidance of central vein catheterization. In: *On Making Health Care Safer: A Critical Analysis of Patient Safety Practices.* Rockville, MD: AHRQPublications; 2001;245–255. Also available at: http://www.ahrq.gov/clinic/ptsafety/chap21.htm.

Spiess BD, Gomez MN. *Principles and Practice of Anesthesiology.* 2nd ed. St. Louis, MO: Longnecker; 1998; 802–828.

Ward W, Langton JA. Blood pressure measurement. *Br J Anaesth CEPD Rev* 2007; 7(4):122–126.

Web sites

http://www.asahq.org/publicationsAndServices/standards/02.pdf.

Chapter 25

The electrocardiogram and approach to diagnosis of common abnormalities

Usha B. Tedrow

In 1924, William Einthoven received the Nobel Prize in Medicine for his description of the electrical waves coming from the heart measured at the body surface. He named the components of the waves, which are discussed later, and identified many disease states of the heart associated with abnormalities of these waves. The electrocardiogram (ECG), as we use it today, is an essential tool for the management of patients. It represents a variety of vectors from each of the body surface electrodes placed in standard fashion. The information gleaned from these vectors can give information about heart rhythm disorders, presence of ischemic heart disease, cardiomyopathy, and even some extracardiac processes.

The ECG is printed on standard paper with single square millimeter boxes and heavier 5-mm increments. These heavier increments are further demarcated into 25-mm square boxes. The standard paper speed is 25 mm/sec, so the 25-mm squares each represent 1 second of time, the 5-mm increments represent 200 ms, and the 1-mm boxes represent 40 ms. The amplitude of the signals is determined by the standardization signal at the upper left of the ECG, indicating the number of boxes for a 1-mV signal. A normal standardization shows 10 mm for a 1-mV signal (Fig. 25.1), although in patients with hypertrophy, standardization may be only 5 mm.

ECG leads

There are two types of leads represented on the surface ECG: limb leads and precordial leads. The limb leads are the result of vectors between electrodes placed on the right arm, left arm, right leg, and left leg. The standard precordial leads are derived from electrodes placed on the anterior chest wall from the sternum to the midaxillary line.

Limb leads

Limb lead I has the negative electrode on the right arm and the positive electrode on the left arm, and points at 0° in the cardiac frontal plane (Fig. 25.2). Therefore, right-sided cardiac impulses create a positive deflection in lead I, and left-sided cardiac impulses create a negative deflection in lead I. Limb lead II has the negative electrode on the right arm and the positive electrode on the left leg and points at 60° in the frontal plane. Limb lead III has the negative electrode on the left arm and the positive electrode on the left leg, and points at 120° in the frontal

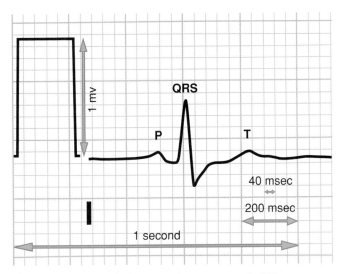

Figure 25.1. Grid, standardization, and measurements for ECG.

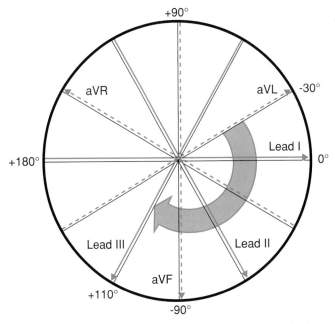

Figure 25.2. Frontal plane axis. The standard and augmented limb leads are shown on a plot of the frontal plane axis. The *curved arrow* indicates the range of normal axis, from −30° to 110°.

plane. Leads II and III, along with lead aVF (described later) are the "inferior" leads. Impulses initiating from high to low in the heart inscribe a positive deflection on these leads, whereas an impulse from near the diaphragmatic surface heading in a more superior direction would inscribe a negative deflection.

The augmented limb leads are aVL, aVR, and aVF. The augmented vector left (aVL) has a positive electrode on the left arm and a shared negative electrode on the right arm and left leg, and it points at $-30°$ (Fig. 25.2). This lead gives left–right information similar to lead I. The augmented vector right (aVR) points at $-150°$ and has a positive electrode on the right arm and a shared negative electrode on the left arm and left leg. It is sometimes termed an *intracavitary* lead because it can give vector information about the direction of endocardial activation of the left ventricle. Last, lead aVF, the augmented vector foot, is formed by the positive electrode on the left leg and the combined negative electrode on the right and left arms. This lead points at $90°$ and is one of the inferior leads.

Precordial leads

The standard precordial leads in adults are placed across the left chest. They are unipolar leads, unlike the limb leads discussed earlier. Their negative electrode is a shared common ground for the whole ECG system, called the Wilson's central terminal. The positive electrode for V_1 is placed to the right of the sternum at the fourth intercostal space. The electrode for V_2 is placed opposite, to the left of the sternum at the fourth intercostal space. V_4 is placed at the midclavicular line in the fifth intercostal space, and V_3 is placed between V_2 and V_4. V_6 is placed at the midaxillary line, and V_5 is placed between V_4 and V_6. The precordial leads give a horizontal depiction of the cardiac activation, in contrast to the limb leads, which give a depiction of the vertical axis. Leads V_1 and V_2 give an idea of the direction of ventricular basal septal activation, and V_5 and V_6 give an idea of apical left ventricular activation.

Electrical events in the heart

The normal heartbeat originates from the sinoatrial node, a structure located on the outside (epicardial) surface of the junction between the superior vena cava and the right atrium. The signal from these pacemaker cells propagates through the atrium to the atrioventricular (AV) node, located at the junction between the atria and the ventricles at the septum. The atrial depolarization is from high to low and therefore produces a positive P-wave deflection in the inferior ECG leads (II, III, and aVF).

The AV node has slow conduction relative to the rest of the myocardium and acts mainly to delay impulses traveling from atrium to ventricle, producing the isoelectric component of the PR interval. The AV node consists of a compact portion and two or three lobes that join with the His bundle, the beginning of the His–Purkinje system, located at the anterior aspect of the ventricular side of the tricuspid annulus. In contrast to the AV node, the His–Purkinje system, consisting of the right and left

bundle branches, has very rapid conduction relative to the rest of the myocardium; therefore, conduction spreads rapidly down the bundle branches, with subsequent activation from apex to base. The left bundle branch is activated slightly before the right, producing the initial upward deflection in V_1 in normal hearts and the physiologic septal Q waves in V_6. Ventricular depolarization proceeds from endocardium to epicardium, inscribing the rest of the QRS complex (Fig. 25.1). Ventricular repolarization then produces the ST segment and T wave.

A place to start

As is the case for chest radiography or other diagnostic tests, it is important to have a system for assessing the ECG, so that both important and subtle ECG abnormalities are discovered. One proposed sequence for looking at the ECG is to evaluate the rate, rhythm axis, and intervals and then turn to chamber enlargement, bundle branch blocks, and ST-T–wave abnormalities.

Rate

A normal adult heart rate is between 60 and 100 bpm; slower rates are considered bradycardia and faster ones tachycardia. The heart rate can be estimated by taking the number of milliseconds between heartbeats and dividing it into 60,000 ms/min. For example, if there are 10 1-mm boxes between QRS complexes, each representing 40 ms, or a total of 400 ms/beat, this would yield a heart rate of 150 bpm (60,000 ms/min divided by 400 ms/ = 150 bpm). For irregular rhythms, the number of QRS complexes on a rhythm strip in 3 seconds multiplied by 20 can give an estimate of the average heart rate.

Rhythm

The assessment of heart rhythm is more challenging. First, is there a P wave in front of each QRS complex? Does the P wave look like a sinus rhythm P wave (positive in the inferior leads)? Is the rhythm regular or irregular? Are there more P waves than QRS complexes, such as in atrial flutter, or are there more QRS complexes than P waves, as in ventricular tachycardia? Is pacing present?

Bradycardia

If bradycardia is identified, typically defined as a heart rate leas than 60 bpm, it requires further assessment for the etiology. Young, healthy athletes may have asymptomatic sinus bradycardia and even sinus pauses nocturnally due to vagal tone. However, older patients with age-related sinus node dysfunction also may have sinus bradycardia or even junctional rhythm. Sinus bradycardia has a P wave in front of each QRS complex with a fixed PR interval. If the P waves are regular, the PR interval prolongs with each successive beat, and ultimately there are blocked P waves with no accompanying QRS complex, this is considered second-degree heart block, Mobitz type I (Fig. 25.3). This suggests an AV conduction problem at the level of the AV node. If the P waves are regular and the PR interval is fixed with blocked

Sinus Bradycardia

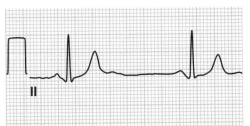

Mobitz I Block

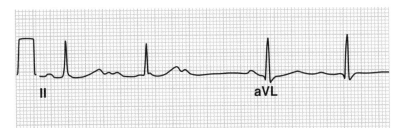

Mobitz II Block

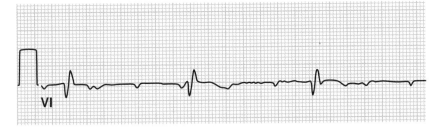

Complete Heart Block

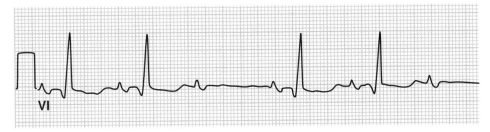

Figure 25.3. Bradycardia.

P waves, this is a second-degree Mobitz type II block. Mobitz II is more serious than Mobitz I in that Mobitz II suggests a diseased infranodal conduction system and potentially unreliable ventricular rhythm. Even more serious is complete heart block, in which the P waves are regular and normal to bradycardic in rate, the QRS complexes are regular, there is AV dissociation, and the ventricular rate is slower than the atrial rate. Whereas complete heart block may occur paroxysmally related to delay in the AV node, complete AV block often is an unstable rhythm associated with a severely diseased distal conduction system and an unreliable ventricular escape.

Tachycardia

Patients with tachycardia also warrant close inspection of the ECG to determine the etiology. Sinus tachycardia – a heart rate >100 bpm and P waves positive in the inferior leads, similar to normal sinus rhythm – is most common. Etiologies include pain, hypovolemia, and hyperadrenergic states such as hyperthyroidism. More rarely, sinus tachycardia may be an intrinsic state (inappropriate sinus tachycardia) or even the consequence of sinus node reentry.

Narrow complex (QRS < 120 ms) or supraventricular tachycardias (SVTs) are divided into regular and irregular categories (Fig. 25.4). Regular tachycardias include several entities. Atrial tachycardia, in which the P wave is different from that of sinus rhythm, has an RP that is longer than the PR interval. AV node reentrant tachycardia is the result of a reentrant circuit involving the tissue of the AV node and most typically has an RP that is exceedingly short, because the atria and ventricles are activated nearly simultaneously. AV-reciprocating tachycardia is a circuit involving an accessory pathway for the retrograde limb; it also has a short RP, but the retrograde conduction times are slightly longer than for AV node reentrant tachycardia. Common atrial flutter is a regular tachycardia caused by a large macroreentrant circuit with a wave front revolving around the tricuspid annulus. In typical counterclockwise atrial flutter, the wave front proceeds up the atrial septum and down the right atrial free wall, inscribing negative P waves in the inferior leads. Patients in

Atrial Tachycardia

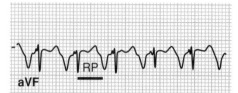

Multifocal Atrial Tachycardia

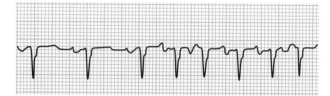

AV Node Reentrant Tachycardia

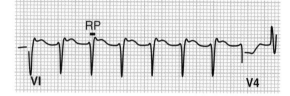

Atrial Flutter

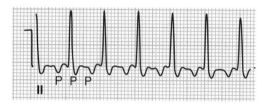

AV Reciprocating Tachycardia

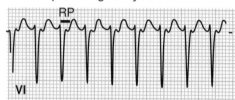

Atrial Fibrillation

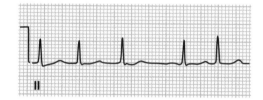

Figure 25.4. Narrow tachycardia.

typical atrial flutter may present with variable heart rates but often present with a heart rate near 150 bpm with P waves at twice the ventricular rate (Fig. 25.4). Regular narrow complex tachycardias, including junctional ectopic tachycardia and junctional reciprocating tachycardia, are rarer in adults but more common in the pediatric population.

Irregular narrow complex rhythms include multifocal atrial tachycardia (Fig. 25.4), in which there are P waves in front of each QRS complex, but they are of differing morphologies. A minimum of three different P waves is required to diagnose multifocal atrial tachycardia. The arrhythmia is commonly secondary to an active pulmonary process. In contrast, atrial fibrillation is irregularly irregular, with no clear P waves seen.

Wide complex rhythms (QRS duration >120 ms) are more challenging. They may result from a supraventricular rhythm with bundle branch block (see later). Ventricular tachycardia is marked by evidence of AV dissociation, sometimes with fusion or capture beats interrupting the rhythm. These beats represent AV conduction capturing the ventricle during AV dissociation, and one is marked C in Fig. 25.5. Ventricular pacing also may produce a wide complex. More rarely, an accessory pathway acting as the antegrade limb for SVT also may produce a wide complex rhythm.

Special scenario: accessory pathways and Wolff–Parkinson–White syndrome

When the normal His–Purkinje system is bypassed by a band of myocardial tissue connecting the atrium and ventricle, this is termed an *atrioventricular bypass tract*. Bypass tracts or accessory pathways allow antegrade-only, retrograde-only, or bidirectional conduction. Antegrade-only conducting accessory pathways are rare, occur most commonly on the right ride of the heart, and connect atrial tissue to portions of the right bundle branch. Because they insert directly into Purkinje tissue, these are called *atriofascicular fibers*, also known as *Mahaim fibers*. In contrast, retrograde-only AV accessory pathways are called *concealed* because their existence is not apparent on the surface ECG; however, the pathway can still support orthodromic AV reentry. Wolff–Parkinson–White (WPW) syndrome is defined as occurring in the setting of a bidirectional conduction accessory pathway.

WPW syndrome is a common cause of SVT and atrial fibrillation, and may be a cause of sudden cardiac death. In sinus rhythm, the ECG demonstrates a delta wave: fusion of conduction down the normal His–Purkinje system and the accessory pathway producing a slurred upstroke to the QRS complex and a shortened PR interval (Fig. 25.6). During AV reentry

Ventricular Tachycardia with Capture Beat

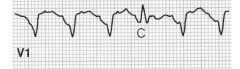

Ventricular Pacing

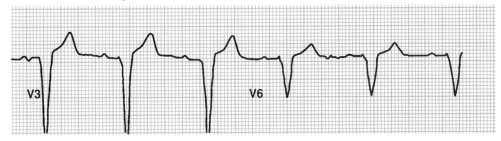

Atrial Pacing with Bundle Branch Block

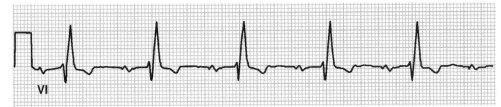

Figure 25.5. Wide complex.

tachycardia (AVRT), the arrhythmia may be orthodromic with conduction down the normal AV node and His–Purkinje system and retrograde conduction up the pathway. In this setting, the QRS complex is narrow in tachycardia and no delta wave is seen, because the accessory pathway is being used for the retrograde limb of the tachycardia (as seen in Fig. 25.4).

Less commonly, the AVRT circuit also may proceed in the opposite direction, with conduction down the accessory pathway and retrograde up the AV node, termed *antidromic AVRT*. The tachycardia in this case is a regular wide complex tachycardia that at times is difficult to distinguish from

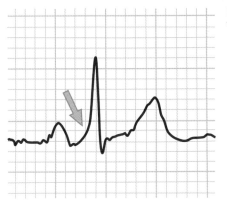

Figure 25.6. Delta wave.

ventricular tachycardia. In WPW syndrome, the accessory pathway refractory period may be exceedingly short, allowing for rapid conduction to the ventricles not possible via the AV node. The presence of the accessory pathway itself also predisposes to atrial fibrillation. The danger of sudden cardiac death in WPW syndrome comes in the setting of atrial fibrillation when the accessory pathway refractory period is short. In this situation, conduction through the pathway may be exceedingly rapid (Fig. 25.7), producing a rapid, irregular, wide complex rhythm. Because of the rapid ventricular conduction, degeneration to ventricular fibrillation is possible.

Axis

The normal frontal plane axis ranges from −30° to 110° (Fig. 25.2). More negative axes are termed *left axis deviation* and more positive ones are known as *right axis deviation*. If leads I and II are completely positive, the frontal place axis is normal. If lead I is positive and leads II and III are negative, there is left axis deviation. If lead I is positive, lead III is negative, and lead II is indeterminate, this is a leftward but physiologic axis (Fig. 25.8). Conversely, if lead I is negative, there is right axis deviation, usually accompanied by positive deflections in the inferior leads.

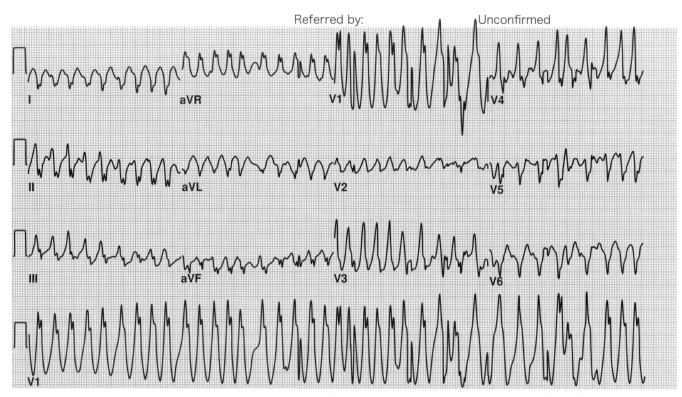

Figure 25.7. Preexcited atrial fibrillation in WPW syndrome.

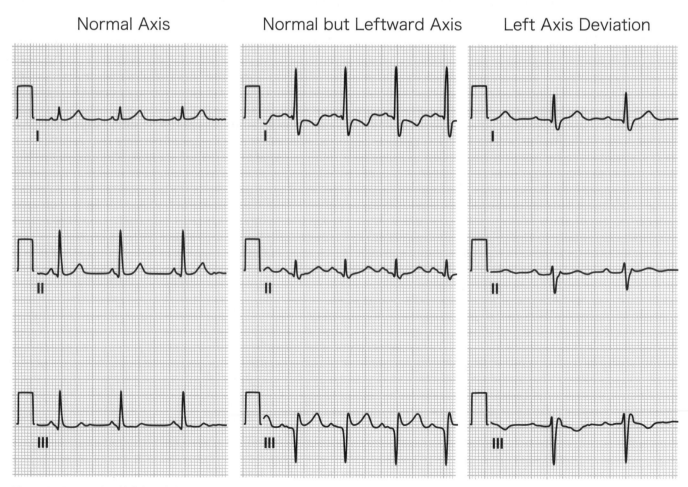

Figure 25.8. Normal and left frontal plane axis.

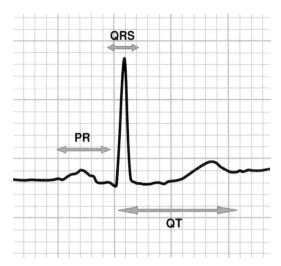

Figure 25.9. ECG intervals.

When thinking about the axis, it is important to consider the causes of an abnormal axis. Common causes of left axis deviation include left ventricular hypertrophy (LVH), left anterior hemiblock, elevated hemidiaphragm, and posterior pathway preexcitation in WPW syndrome. Causes of right axis deviation may include mechanical shifts due to emphysema or pneumothorax, right ventricular hypertrophy, left posterior hemiblock, anterior pathway preexcitation in WPW, and dextrocardia.

Intervals

The normal intervals on surface ECG should be assessed from the limb leads only, and from the lead that gives the longest measurement. The upper limit of the PR interval (Fig. 25.9) is 200 ms, or five 40-ms 1-mm boxes. Prolongation of the PR interval suggests so-called first-degree AV block. The upper limit of normal QRS duration is 120 ms, or three 1-mm boxes. Prolongation suggests ventricular myocardial conduction delay, in the form of a bundle branch block, preexcitation, ectopic ventricular beats, or ventricular pacing.

The QT interval is heart-rate-dependent and is normally shorter at faster heart rates and longer at slower ones. Thus, an instantaneous measurement of the QT should be corrected to the QTc using Bazett's formula to account for the heart rate dependence. The QTc is equal to the measured QT divided by the square root of the RR interval in seconds. For a heart rate of 60 bpm, the QTc is equal to the measured QT. A normal QTc ranges from 300 to 450 ms. Prolongation of the QT may be congenital, as in congenital long QT syndrome. (See Fig. 25.10.)

Perhaps more importantly, however, QT prolongation may be drug induced. Antiarrhythmic drugs, methadone, phenothiazines, and macrolide antibiotics are frequent causative agents (www.Qtdrugs.org). Dramatic QT prolongation is associated with sudden cardiac arrest due to torsades de pointes and therefore is very important to recognize. Drug-induced torsades de pointes is typically induced by a short-long–short interval sequence with a characteristic undulating disorganized ventricular arrhythmia that follows (Fig. 25.11).

Chamber enlargement

P-wave morphology can help determine whether there is atrial enlargement or abnormality. Leads II and V$_1$ give the best assessment of atrial enlargement. If the P wave is more than 2.5 1-mm boxes wide (100 ms) in lead II (Fig. 25.12), this suggests left atrial enlargement. Supporting evidence is that the larger component of the P wave in V$_1$ is downgoing and at least a 1-mm square in size. Conversely, right atrial enlargement is suggested by a P wave that is more than 2.5 1-mm boxes in height.

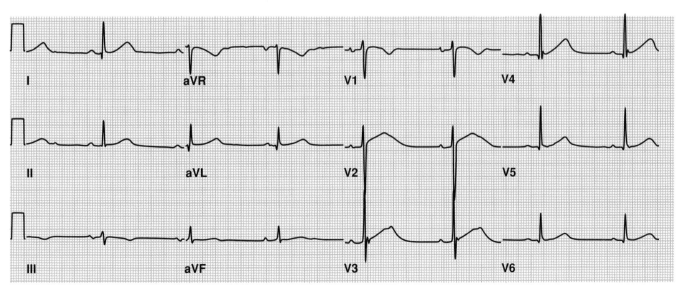

Figure 25.10. ECG with QT prolongation.

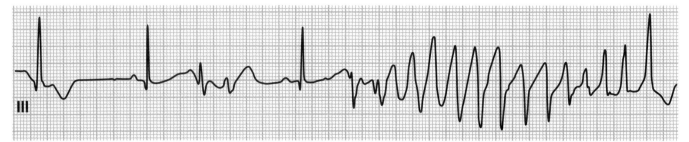

Figure 25.11. Torsades de pointes.

An upgoing component to the P wave in lead V_1 is also supportive of right atrial enlargement.

The QRS morphology can give evidence of LVH. The following assumes a normal QRS duration. A simple criterion for LVH is an R wave in aVL >11 mm, as seen in Fig. 25.13. An S wave in lead V_2 or V_3 plus an R wave in V_5 >35 mm also suggest LVH. A leftward axis (as in Fig. 25.8) or frank left axis deviation may accompany LVH. Additionally, repolarization abnormalities consequent to strain are often seen in the lateral and apical leads in this setting.

Bundle branch blocks

Bundle branch blocks occur when there is disease of the His–Purkinje system causing more delay in one of the bundle branches relative to the other. Bundle branch block may be caused by ischemia or infarction of the heart, cardiomyopathy, or age-related calcification. Because the His–Purkinje tissue has more rapid conduction than the surrounding myocardium, when the bundle branches are functioning normally, the QRS complex is narrow. When one of the bundle branches is diseased, conduction proceeds rapidly down the unaffected bundle branch, then propagates more slowly through the myocardium on the affected side. The result is lengthening of the QRS duration beyond 120 ms (three 1-mm boxes). Additionally, when the QRS is prolonged, the normal axis of the T wave (repolarization) is opposite the main axis of the QRS, also known as appropriate T-wave discordance.

Left Atrial Enlargement   Right Atrial Enlargement

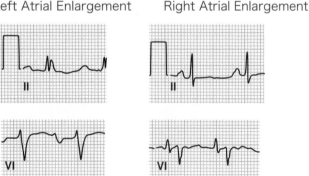

Figure 25.12. Atrial enlargement.

Left bundle branch block

In the case of left bundle branch block, the complex is mainly downgoing in lead V_1 with a QS wave or rS wave in lead V_1 and a monotonic R wave in leads I and V_6. The example in Fig. 25.14 shows an rS in lead V_1 (small R wave, large S wave). It also is notable in the example that where the QRS is downgoing (leads V_1–V_3), the T wave is upgoing. Conversely, where the QRS is upgoing (e.g., in leads II, III, and aVF), the T wave is downgoing. Left bundle branch block does not completely preclude the diagnosis of ischemia or infarction in patients with chest pain. ST-segment or T-wave changes from a baseline ECG may indicate ischemia or infarction. Normally, T-wave changes are in the direction opposite the major QRS deflection. Certain findings are highly suggestive of acute infarction, including ST elevation ≥1 mm in same direction as the major deflection of the QRS complex, ST depression >1 mm in V_1 through V_3, and ST elevation >5 mm in the opposite direction of the major deflection of QRS.

Fascicular blocks or hemiblocks

The left bundle has two fascicles: anterior and posterior. Block of only one of these results in a hemiblock, also known as a fascicular block. Left anterior hemiblock manifests as left axis deviation without a discernable cause, whereas left posterior hemiblock presents as marked right axis deviation. The QRS duration typically is between 100 and 120 ms. The left axis deviation seen in Fig. 25.8 is an example of left anterior hemiblock.

Right bundle branch block

In right bundle branch block, the complex in V_1 is mainly positive with a terminal R wave. The complex may have an rSR′ pattern, as shown in Fig. 25.15, but a qR or an R wave also is acceptable. There also should be a slurred S wave in leads I and V_6, which is seen best in lead I in our example. Interestingly, in right bundle branch block, some leads are wide and others are narrow. In the narrow leads (e.g., I, V_5, and V_6), the T wave is the same direction as the QRS complex. In the wide leads (e.g., III and V_1–V_3), the T wave again exhibits normal T-wave discordance, with the T wave opposite the main axis of the QRS. These are all part of the normal repolarization pattern in right bundle branch block. Ischemia and infarction are identified more readily in right bundle branch block and have similar criteria to those described in the following section.

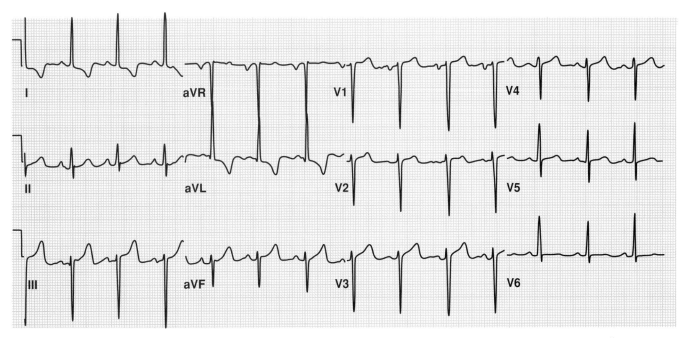

Figure 25.13. Left ventricular hypertrophy.

ST and T waves

Ischemia and infarction

An important application of the ECG and the analysis of ST segments and T waves is the diagnosis of ischemia and infarction. Acute infarction is the result of a coronary artery occlusion. Early phases of infarction may display tall-peaked T waves on the surface ECG, called *hyperacute T waves*. As early as minutes into the infarction, ST-segment elevation (Fig. 25.16) is seen in characteristic leads. Infarction of a small territory can also manifest as ST-segment depression or T-wave inversion in some patients. Injury usually is not reversible without prompt restoration of blood flow to the myocardium. In contrast, ischemia is caused by an insufficient blood supply to meet the demands of the myocardium. Ischemia usually is a combination of fixed coronary narrowing and increased myocardial demand (e.g., hypertension, tachycardia, anemia, metabolic stress) and can be controlled in most settings by decreasing myocardial demand with medication. The ECG in ischemia most typically shows ST-segment depression but also may show T-wave inversion.

The coronary arteries usually supply stereotypic areas of the heart, reflected in particular leads on the surface ECG. The left anterior descending coronary artery supplies the anterior

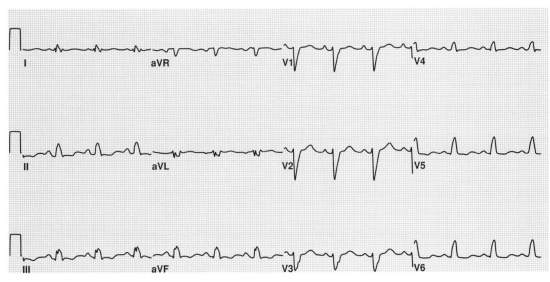

Figure 25.14. Left bundle branch block.

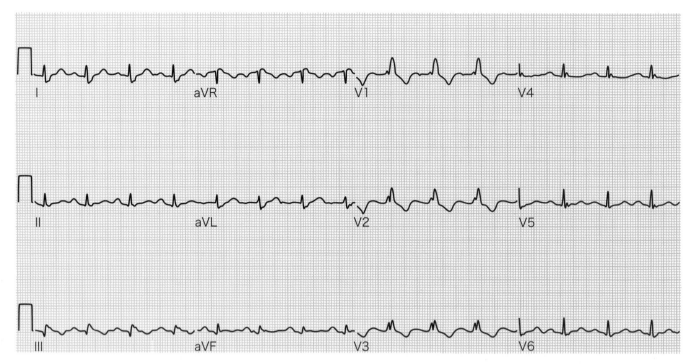

Figure 25.15. Right bundle branch block.

wall, the anteroseptum, and the anteroapex of the left ventricle. Leads V_1 and V_2 represent the septum, V_3 and V_4 represent the midanterior wall, and V_5 and V_6 represent the anteroapex. The left anterior descending coronary artery usually has diagonal branches supplying the lateral wall, represented by leads I and aVL. The right coronary artery supplies the inferior wall of the left ventricle in most patients and is represented on the surface ECG by leads II, III, and aVF, the inferior leads. The left circumflex supplies the posterior wall in most patients, and depending on the size of the artery, it also may supply some

of the inferior and even lateral territory. The posterior wall is least well seen on surface ECG, but acute injury can manifest as ST-segment depression in V_1 and V_2 (opposite that seen in the anterior wall). Right ventricular infarction also may be difficult to discern on surface ECG, but if a right-sided precordial rV_4 lead is placed (at the right midclavicular line at the fifth intercostal space), ST-segment elevation can confirm right ventricular infarction.

If coronary blood flow is not restored quickly after an acute infarction, Q waves will develop in the infarcted zones.

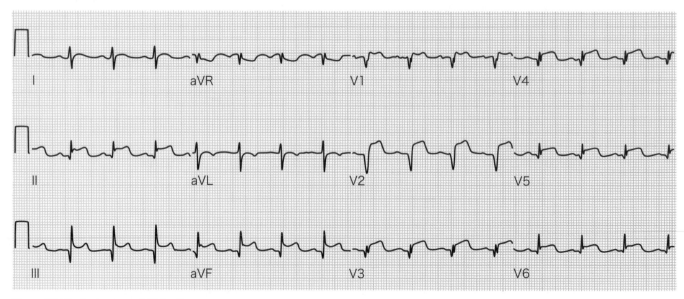

Figure 25.16. Acute myocardial infarction.

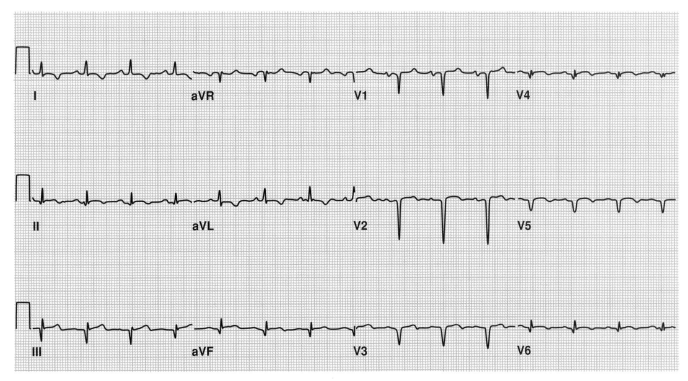

Figure 25.17. Old myocardial infarction.

Pathologic Q waves generally are defined as those lasting 40 ms (one 1-mm box) or with an amplitude 25% of the QRS complex. T-wave inversions appear next and may persist for weeks; if they persist beyond 6 weeks, this suggests development of an aneurysm.

Figure 25.16 shows an acute anterior infarction due to occlusion of a large left anterior descending coronary artery. This artery was large enough to "wrap around" some of the inferior wall and produce the ST-segment elevation in the inferior leads. Fig. 25.17 shows the same patient weeks later, with resolution of most of the ST-segment elevation and repolarization change. Large pathologic Q waves are present in leads V_1 through V_5 as well as leads III and aVF.

It is important to mention that other entities can mimic myocardial ischemia and infarction. Repolarization abnormalities with strain in LVH can produce T-wave inversion and ST-segment depression. Early repolarization and rare entities such as Brugada syndrome may produce ST-segment elevation. WPW syndrome can produce Q waves similar to those seen in old infarction because of preexcitation of the ventricle via an accessory pathway. Pericarditis and electrolyte abnormalities such as hyperkalemia also can mimic acute ischemia and infarction.

Electrolyte abnormalities

Many electrolyte abnormalities can produce characteristic changes on the surface ECG. Hyperkalemia causes dramatic prolongation of the cardiac action potential. Signs of hyperkalemia on ECG include tall-peaked T waves, which sometimes are confused with the early stages of acute myocardial infarction (hyperacute T waves). The QRS complex may become prolonged in a pattern often uncharacteristic of a typical bundle branch block pattern (Fig. 25.18), and the heart rate may be slowed. P waves may be reduced in amplitude or may be absent. The PR interval may be prolonged, and AV dissociation may be present. When hyperkalemia is severe (e.g., >7.0 mmol/L), both bradyarrhythmias and ventricular tachycardia may occur. Pacemaker systems also may fail to capture the myocardium in this setting despite good positioning of the leads and other connections. Hypokalemia, in contrast, can produce an ECG similar to that seen in hypocalcemia (discussed later). There may be flattening of the T waves or even ST depression or T-wave inversion; a prominent U wave may be seen as well.

In hypercalcemia, the action potential repolarization is accelerated, which can produce tall-peaking T waves with a slightly shortened QT interval. When hypercalcemia is severe, the QRS may become broadened, in a pattern very similar to that seen in hyperkalemia. In the setting of hypocalcemia (Fig. 25.18), the QT interval is prolonged consequent to delayed action potential repolarization. The T waves are characteristically flattened, sometimes with a prominent U wave. The QRS typically is narrow. The PR interval may be shortened, and the ST segment may be slightly depressed.

Digitalis effect and toxicity

Digitalis (or digoxin) blocks the sodium–potassium adenosine triphosphatase-mediated exchanger in myocardial cells and also has modest vagolytic properties. The normal effect of

Hyperkalemia

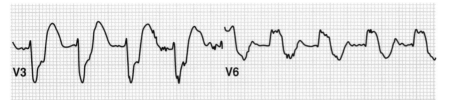

Figure 25.18. Common electrolyte abnormalities.

Hypocalcemia

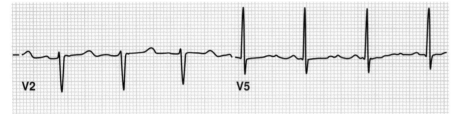

Figure 25.19. Digitalis effect/toxicity.

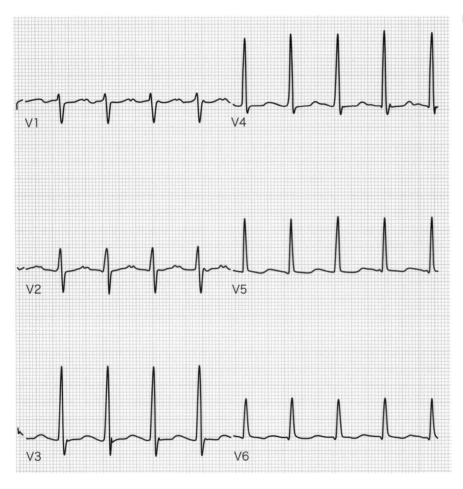

digoxin compounds is to slow the heart rate without lowering blood pressure, although this effect is limited in the setting of high sympathetic tone. Digoxin also mildly increases contractility, although an important effect in outcomes of heart failure populations has not been consistently demonstrated. At normal levels, slight depression of the ST segment is often seen, predominantly in V_3 through V_6, and is termed *digitalis effect*; it is not evidence of toxicity. At higher doses, toxicity may be present. It is important to remember that digitalis toxicity is a continuum and that despite a "normal" digoxin level, a susceptible patient may have toxicity if his or her clinical syndrome is characteristic. The classic arrhythmia seen in early digitalis toxicity is paroxysmal atrial tachycardia with block. The patient in Fig. 25.19 has classic signs of digitalis effect, seen in leads V_5 and V_6, but also has an oddly slow atrial tachycardia with prolonged PR interval, suggesting digitalis toxicity. As the degree of toxicity worsens, bradyarrhythmias and ventricular tachycardia may be present. To reverse toxicity in this setting, use of the antidote compound Digibind (GlaxoSmith-Kline, Research Triangle Park, NC), a purified Fab fragment of a digoxin-specific antibody raised in sheep, should be considered. Ventricular arrhythmias, when present, are best treated with the sodium channel blocker phenytoin or lidocaine, and temporary pacing should be considered to bridge the patient through bradyarrhythmias.

Summary

Overall, when approaching the surface ECG, it is important to have an organized system for looking at the large amount of information contained therein. Suggested in this chapter is a system for looking at the rate, rhythm, axis, and intervals. This is followed by assessment of chamber enlargement and bundle branch blocks. Last, ST and T waves are examined carefully for evidence of ischemia and infarction or metabolic derangement. Although not exhaustive, this system may give the reader a starting point for learning more about the surface ECG and its implications.

Suggested readings

Braat SH, Brugada P, den Dulk E, et al. Value of lead V4R for recognition of the infarct related artery in acute inferior myocardial infarction. *Am J Cardiol* 1984; 53:1538–1541.

Braunwald E, Morrow AG. Sequence of ventricular contraction in human bundle branch block; a study based on simultaneous catheterization of both ventricles. *Am J Med* 1957; 23(2):205–211.

Delacretaz E. Clinical practice. Supraventricular tachycardia. *N Eng J Med* 2006; 354(10):1039–1051.

de Lemos JA, Braunwald E. ST segment resolution as a tool for assessing efficacy of reperfusion therapy. *J Am Coll Cardiol* 2001; 38:1283–1294.

Einthoven W. The different forms of the human electrocardiogram and their signification. *Lancet* 1912; (1):853–861.

Epstein AE, DeMarco J, Ellenbogen KA, et al. ACC/AHA/HRS 2008 Guidelines for Device-Based Therapy of Cardiac Rhythm Abnormalities: a report of the American College of Cardiology/American Heart Association Task Force on Practice Guidelines. *Circulation* 2008; 117(21):e350–e408.

Josephson ME, Kastor JA, Morganroth J. Electrocardiographic left atrial enlargement. Electrophysiologic, echocardiographic and hemodynamic correlates. *Am J Cardiol* 1977; 39(7):967–971.

Sokolow M, Lyon TP. The ventricular complex in left ventricular hypertrophy as obtained by unipolar precordial and limb leads. *Am Heart J* 1949; 37:161.

Surawicz B. Electrocardiographic diagnosis of chamber enlargement. *J Am Coll Cardiol* 1986; 61:1089–1101.

Chapter 26

Pulse oximetry and capnography

Zhiling Xiong and Bhavani S. Kodali

Pulse oximetry

Pulse oximetry (oximeter) is a standard of care for monitoring oxygen during anesthesia. It is a noninvasive method of measuring oxygen saturation of hemoglobin (SpO_2) on a continuous basis to detect hypoxia. The device displays digital numbers for oxygen saturation and pulse rate, in addition to a continuous display of perfusion waveform (plethysmography).

Principles of pulse oximetry

The general principle of pulse oximetry is based on the Beer-Lambert law. It is a measurement of the transmission of red (600- to 750-nm wavelength) and infrared (850- to 1000-nm) light through the pulsatile tissue beds, which subsequently determines the light absorption characteristics of oxygenated and deoxygenated hemoglobin (Hb). According to the Beer-Lambert law, the intensity of transmitted light decreases exponentially as both the concentration of the substance (due to absorption) and the distance traveled through the substance increase. Oxygenated Hb absorbs more infrared light and allows more red light to pass through, thus appearing bright red to the naked eye. In contrast, deoxygenated (or reduced) Hb absorbs more red light and allows more infrared light to pass through, thus appearing blue or cyanotic (Fig. 26.1).

Sensing the pulsatile arterial flow is required for pulse oximetry to work. At the measuring site, many constant light absorbers are always present. These include the skin, soft tissue, bone, as well as venous, capillary, and nonpulsatile components of arterial blood, all constituting baseline absorption of the light. The pulsatile expansion of the arteriolar bed increases the light path length and further increases light absorbency over the baseline (Beer-Lambert law; see earlier). This change in light absorption during arterial pulsation is the basis of oximetry determinations. The variation in the absorbability of light during pulsatile flow compared with baseline is displayed as the arterial waveform (plethysmography).

Pulse oximetry sensor

The pulse oximetry sensor consists of a pair of small red (R; 660-nm) and infrared (IR; 940-nm) light-emitting diodes (LEDs) and a single silicone photodetector mounted inside a rigid

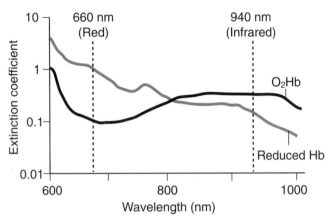

Figure 26.1. Hemoglobin light spectrum absorption curve. The *black curve* denotes the oxygenated hemoglobin (O_2Hb), and the *blue curve* denotes the deoxygenated (reduced) hemoglobin. The two *vertical dotted lines* represent wavelengths in the red (660-nm) and infrared (940-nm) parts of the spectrum used by the LEDs of pulse oximeters.

spring-loaded clip, a flexible probe, or an adhesive wrap. The sensor is placed on a translucent site of the patient's body such as a fingertip, toe, earlobe, nose, lip, or even the foot or palm (for an infant).

There are two modes of sending light through the measuring site: transmittance and reflectance. In the transmittance sensor (Fig. 26.2), the LEDs and photodetector are opposite each other, with the measuring site between them. The light passes through the site. In the reflectance mode, the LEDs and photodetector are mounted side by side on top of the measuring site, and the light bounces from the LEDs to the detector across the site. The transmittance mode is the more commonly used type.

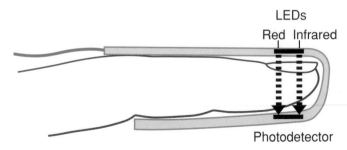

Figure 26.2. Fingertip pulse oximetry sensor.

The absorption ratio of R/IR is calculated by a microprocessor and is compared with a "lookup" table (based on experimental studies in healthy human volunteers) that converts the ratio to an SpO_2 value. For example, an R/IR ratio of 0.5 equates to approximately 100% SpO_2, 1.0 to approximately 85% SpO_2, and 2.0 to 0% SpO_2.

Functional versus fractional hemoglobin saturations

It should be noted that the SpO_2 measured by pulse oximetry differs from the arterial oxygen saturation (SaO_2) measured by a laboratory carbon monoxide (CO) oximeter. Pulse oximetry measures the functional Hb SaO_2, which is defined as Hb capable of carrying oxygen. It is the ratio of oxyhemoglobin (O_2Hb) to O_2Hb plus reduced Hb:

Functional $SaO_2 = O_2Hb/(O_2Hb + $ reduced Hb).

Laboratory CO-oximeters measure the fractional Hb SaO_2, which is defined as the ratio of O_2Hb to total Hb, which includes nonfunctional Hb such as methemoglobin (MetHb) and carboxyhemoglobin (COHb; incapable of carrying oxygen):

Fractional $SaO_2 = O_2Hb/(O_2Hb + $ reduced Hb + MetHb $+ $ COHb).

Therefore, the SpO_2 number measured by pulse oximetry (functional SaO_2) should be higher than the SaO_2 reported by the laboratory blood gas. In the usual clinical circumstances, however, patients' concentrations of MetHb and COHb are so low that the values of both functional and fractional saturations are nearly identical.

Calibration and practical limitations

Pulse oximeters are calibrated during manufacture, and their internal circuits are automatically checked when they are switched on; they cannot be altered by users. They are accurate in the range of oxygen saturations from 70% to 100%, with a standard error of $\pm$ 2%, but less accurate in the range of 70% to 50% ($\pm$ 3%).

Pulse oximeters have been used widely for monitoring patients' oxygenation and pulse rates in a variety of clinical settings, including perioperative, intensive care unit, and intravenous (IV) conscious sedation cases. Their use has improved the margin of safety for patients. However, pulse oximetry provides no indication of the adequacy of ventilation because of lack of information about CO_2 level. In addition, several factors and clinical situations limit the effectiveness and accuracy of pulse oximetry, including:

1. Nonfunctional hemoglobins (COHb and MetHb). The light absorption of COHb and O_2Hb at 660 nm is identical, meaning the COHb is red and "detected" by pulse oximetry as O_2Hb; therefore, in the presence of a large amount of COHb (e.g., in patients with CO poisoning or heavy tobacco smokers), the pulse oximetries read the sum of O_2Hb and COHb, registering a falsely high SpO_2 reading. In this situation, CO oximetry is required to measure the COHb level. In contrast, MetHb has the same absorption at 660-nm and 940-nm wavelengths. This 1:1 absorption ratio is interpreted by pulse oximetry as 85% of SpO_2 regardless of the true saturation.

2. A reduction in peripheral pulsatile blood flow due to vasoconstriction, hypovolemia, severe hypotension, hypothermia, or shock.

3. Surgical dyes such as methylene blue, indocyanine green, and indigo carmine. These transiently decrease pulse oximetry readings and absorb light in the region of 660 nm.

4. Excessive ambient lights, such as the high-intensity overhead lights in operating rooms or some IR heat lamps. These may interfere with photodetector signal sensing.

5. Artifacts due to motion, shivering, and radiofrequency diathermy apparatus.

6. Nail polish, especially black, blue, and green.

In summary, pulse oximetry is a mandatory monitor for patients receiving anesthesia, and it plays an important role in early detection of hypoxia. Although it rarely may cause local tissue injury due to the heat (from the light source) and sensor pressure, there are no contraindications for its use. "New-generation" pulse oximetry with advanced technology has demonstrated significant improvement in the ability to read through motion and low perfusion states, thus making this medical device more reliable.

Capnography

Capnography is the continuous monitoring of instantaneous CO_2 concentration using a graphic display (waveform) in respired gas. This CO_2 waveform is also called a *capnogram*, and a device that generates the CO_2 waveform is called a *capnograph*. Use of capnographic monitoring can reliably and quantitatively provide vital respiratory information of intubated patients. Alterations in cardiac output, distribution of pulmonary blood flow, and metabolic activity may also be reflected by the change of CO_2 concentration in expired gases. The American Society of Anesthesiologists mandates the use of capnography in all patients undergoing anesthesia. Many intensive care units use capnography as an adjunct to ensure patient safety and the adequacy of ventilation.

Principles of capnography

Whereas a variety of techniques may be used for CO_2 measurement, such as mass spectrometry, Raman scattering, and photoacoustic measurement, by far the most widely used method is IR absorption spectrometry. The principle of this technique is based on the fact that CO_2 is a polyatomic gas that absorbs IR radiation of a specific wavelength. CO_2 shows strong absorption in the far IR light at 4.3 μm, which lies way beyond the visible

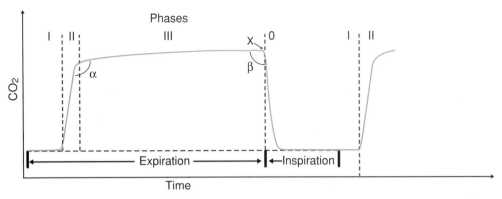

Figure 26.3. Normal capnogram with three phases of expiration: phase I, dead space; phase II, mixture of dead space and alveolar gas; phase III, alveolar gas plateau. Point X delineates the PETCO$_2$, which is the best reflection of the alveolar CO$_2$ tension.

wavelength (0.4–0.8 μm). The basic elements of IR spectrometry include an IR light source, a sample chamber, and an IR detector. The absorption of the IR light also is governed by the Beer-Lambert law, that is, the absorption is proportional to the concentration of the absorbing gas in the sample chamber.

Types of capnographs

Depending on the location of the CO$_2$ sensor, capnographs can be divided into two types: sidestream (aspiration) and mainstream (flow-through) capnographs. In sidestream capnographs, the gas sample is continuously aspirated by a fine tube from the breathing circuit (usually located at the T-piece); it then passes to a measuring unit containing the CO$_2$ sensor. The CO$_2$ concentration is determined by comparing the IR light absorption in the sample cell with a chamber free of CO$_2$. A unique advantage of sidestream capnography is that it allows monitoring of spontaneously breathing nonintubated patients, as a sample of the expired gas can be obtained from the face mask or nasal cannula. In mainstream capnographs, a cuvette containing a CO$_2$ sensor with an IR source and detector is inserted between the breathing circuit and the endotracheal tube, so CO$_2$ is measured within the breathing circuit. Compared with sidestream capnography, the advantages of mainstream capnography are that the response time is faster, no gas is subtracted from the breathing circuit, and there is no need for sampling pumps. Disadvantages include the relatively heavy measuring adapter with an electrical cord (which may lead to an endotracheal tube kinking), added dead space, and the high cost of maintenance and repair. Needless to say, the newer-generation mainstream sensors are remarkably lighter and smaller.

Calibration

Capnographs must be calibrated at specific intervals based on manufacturer recommendations, but usually at least daily. Modern instruments use a self-calibration process and maintain a satisfactory degree of accuracy, usually about ± 0.1% in the range of 0% to 10% CO$_2$ (0–76 mm Hg). They are fairly accurate, even in the extended range up to 100 mm Hg,

which is useful in rare cases of hypoventilation or malignant hyperthermia.

Normal capnogram

A capnogram may be displayed as CO$_2$ versus time (time capnogram) or versus volume (volume capnogram). The time capnogram is the method most commonly used in anesthesia and other clinical practices, because the volume capnogram needs elaborated equipment for plotting the trace. Thus, all capnograms mentioned in this chapter are time capnograms unless indicated otherwise.

A standard nomenclature has been assigned for delineating various phases of a capnogram. A capnogram may be considered as having two segments, an inspiratory and an expiratory segment, and two angles, an alpha and a beta angle. The inspiratory segment is also designated phase 0. The expiratory segment is divided further into phases I, II, and III, and occasionally phase IV, which represents the terminal rise in CO$_2$ concentration (Fig. 26.3). Phase I represents the initial stage of expiration; there is no rise in expired CO$_2$ as anatomic and apparatus dead space gases are exhaled. As expiration continues, there is a sharply rising upstroke (phase II) due to the mixing of dead space gas with CO$_2$-containing alveolar gas, followed by a plateau phase (phase III). The CO$_2$ concentration at the end of the plateau is referred to as end-tidal CO$_2$ (PETCO$_2$). PETCO$_2$ is the best reflection of alveolar CO$_2$ (PACO$_2$), and normally the arterial CO$_2$ (PaCO$_2$)–PETCO$_2$ difference is about 5 mm Hg because of the dead space. It is important to note that the expiratory plateau is not an isocapnic trace; rather it progresses with a very slight and steady increase in PCO$_2$ as the alveolar fraction is expelled from the lungs. As the patient begins to inspire, fresh gas is entrained and there is a steep downstroke back to the baseline (phase 0). The angle between phases II and III, called the alpha angle, increases as the slope of phase III increases; normally it is about 100° to 110°. Airway obstruction increases the angle because of the increasing slope. The response time of the capnograph, the sweep speed, and the respiratory cycle time also affect the angle. The angle between phases III and 0, called the beta angle, normally is about 90°.

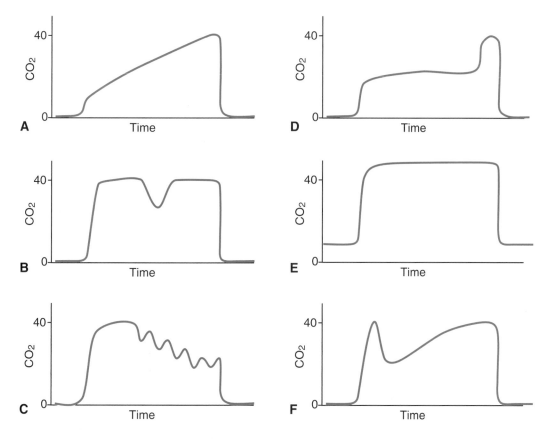

Figure 26.4. Abnormal capnograms. (**A**) Capnogram from a patient with severe obstructive pulmonary disease or another cause leading to increased airway resistance, such as asthma, endobronchial intubation, or endotracheal tube kinking. No plateau is reached before the next inspiration. The gradient between $PETCO_2$ and arterial CO_2 is increased. (**B**) Downward wave during the plateau phase, indicating spontaneous respiratory effort. (**C**) Cardiogenic oscillations appearing as small regular, tooth-like "humps" at the latter part of the expiratory phase. The rate of the humps is identical to the patient's heart rate. (**D**) A leak in the sampling line during positive pressure ventilation. (**E**) Failure of inspired CO_2 to return to zero because of an incompetent expiratory valve or exhausted CO_2 absorbent. (**F**) Bifid waveform of expired CO_2 in a patient with emphysema undergoing elective surgery after unilateral lung transplantation. The initial upstroke represents gas from the normal (transplanted) lung, which is followed by gas exhaled from the remaining (emphysematous) lung.

During rebreathing, this angle increases. Occasionally, an upward blip or spike, known as phase IV, may occur toward the end of phase III; this is akin to phase IV of the single-breath nitrogen curve. This terminal elevation represents the emptying of alveoli with long-time constants containing a higher CO_2 concentration.

Abnormal capnograms and clinical considerations

In analyzing an abnormal capnogram, five characteristics should be evaluated: size (height), shape, frequency, rhythm, and baseline. For example, in patients with an obstructed airway (e.g., those with emphysema or asthma), the capnogram shows a slow rate of rise of phase II (upstroke) and the increased slope of phase III (plateau). In an unrecognized esophageal intubation, the capnograms are flat or may have occasional baseline blips. However, after attempted face mask ventilation (driving some expired gas into the esophagus and stomach) or in patients who have recently consumed carbonate beverages, some CO_2 waves may be observed as the result of gastric CO_2 returning

to the breathing system. However, such a CO_2 tracing has a peak effect only with a progressively decreasing amplitude, and it does not resemble the usual end-tidal plateau. The CO_2 concentration decreases to zero after about five breaths of ventilation. Fig. 26.4 shows several capnograms in a variety of clinical scenarios.

The $PETCO_2$ concentration measured from the capnogram provides important clinical information about a patient's ventilatory status. Because the measurement of $PETCO_2$ is an estimate of $PaCO_2$, the characteristic abnormal CO_2 waveforms and concentrations may help in the diagnosis of many clinical and technical abnormalities. Table 26.1 summarizes the common causes that may be reflected by $PETCO_2$ changes during anesthesia care, including alterations in metabolism, circulation, ventilation, airway, or breathing. Abnormal CO_2 measurements also may occur as a result of a malfunction in sampling or measurement of CO_2.

Although it is believed that capnograms predominantly identify respiratory abnormalities, they also can forewarn of major impending depression of the cardiovascular system, such

Table 26.1. Factors that may change PETCO$_2$ during anesthesia

Increase in PETCO$_2$	Decrease in PETCO$_2$
Due to an increase in CO$_2$ production	Due to a decrease in CO$_2$ production
Increases in metabolic rate	Decreases in metabolic rate
Sepsis	Hypothermia
Malignant hyperthermia	Hypothyroidism
Shivering/seizure	Due to an increase in CO$_2$ elimination
Hyperthyroidism	Hyperventilation
Due to a decrease in CO$_2$ elimination	Due to a decrease in alveolar CO$_2$ delivery
Hypoventilation	Hypoperfusion
Rebreathing	Pulmonary embolism
CO$_2$ absorber exhaustion	Due to artifact
Due to artifact	Gas sampling tube leak or loose connection
Malfunction of CO$_2$ measuring system	Malfunction of CO$_2$ measuring system

as hypotension associated with massive blood loss, impending circulatory arrest, or pulmonary embolism.

In summary, capnography has become an important, integral part of monitoring in anesthesia. The proper use and understanding of it not only can help in the correct placement of endotracheal tubes, but can also rapidly facilitate a differential diagnosis of hypoxia, impending hypoxia, or equipment malfunction so that corrective action can be implemented before the patient suffers irreversible, life-threatening injury.

Suggested readings

Barash PG, Cullen BF, Stoelting RK, eds. *Clinical Anesthesia*. 5th ed. Philadelphia: Lippincott Williams & Wilkins; 2006.

D'Mello J, Butani M. Capnography. *Indian J Anaesth* 2002; 46(4):269–278.

Kodali BS. Capnography.com Web site. Available at: www.capnography.com. Accessed May 2010.

Kodali BS, Kumar AY, Mosely H, Hallsworth RA. Terminology and the current limitations of time capnography. *J Clin Monit* 1995; 11:175–182.

Mendelson Y. Pulse oximetry: theory and applications for noninvasive monitoring. *Clin Chem* 1992; 38(9):1601–1607.

Miller RD. *Miller's Anesthesia*. Vol. 1, 5th ed. New York: Churchill Livingstone; 2000.

Chapter 27

Monitoring of neuromuscular blockade

Kai Matthes and Neelakantan Sunder

Introduction

Muscle paralysis commonly is desired during general anesthesia to facilitate endotracheal intubation and to blunt responses to surgical stimuli. Endotracheal intubation without the use of muscle relaxation is possible but requires profound anesthesia, and intubation conditions are less optimal compared with complete neuromuscular blockade. Improving intubation conditions decreases postoperative hoarseness, vocal cord damage, and patient discomfort. Neuromuscular reversal of muscle relaxation and return of respiratory function must be achieved before the trachea is extubated. Neuromuscular blockade can improve surgical conditions and is most beneficial in abdominal surgery. Muscle relaxation also may be used to prevent patient movement with lighter anesthesia or in procedures such as intracranial or complex eye surgery, in which even slight movement may result in major complications. Muscle paralysis occurs over a narrow range of receptor occupancy. There is no detectable block until 75% to 85% of receptors are occupied, and paralysis is complete at 90% to 95% receptor occupancy. Therefore, adequate muscle relaxation corresponds to a narrow range of 85% to 90% receptor occupancy, requiring an adjustment to the individual patient as there is considerable variation in individual responses.

To monitor muscle relaxation, a peripheral nerve is stimulated electrically by a battery-powered device that delivers a depolarizing current via two electrodes. The response of the corresponding muscle is assessed and depends on the current applied, the duration of the current, and the position of the electrodes. A current in the range of 60 to 80 mA is usually chosen. Durations of 0.1 to 0.2 ms are acceptable. The threshold current is the lowest current required to depolarize the most sensitive fibers in a given nerve bundle to elicit a detectable muscle response. Supramaximal current is approximately 10% to 20% higher than the current required to depolarize all fibers of the nerve bundle, generally a current two to three times higher than the threshold current.

Electrocardiogram electrodes placed on the skin are used to apply the current on the appropriate nerve. Subcutaneous needles deliver the impulse in the immediate vicinity of the nerve and have the advantage of bypassing the tissue impedance. Disadvantages include local irritation, infection, nerve damage, and diathermy burns. Thus, surface electrodes are commonly preferred over needle electrodes. The first electrode should be placed on the skin overlying the nerve to be stimulated. The second electrode is positioned proximally or distally along the stimulated nerve, avoiding stimulation of neighboring nerves. Practically, no differentiation between positive and negative electrodes is considered for proximal or distal placement along the nerve. In theory, if the negative electrode is placed directly on the nerve in the proximal location, the threshold to supramaximal stimulation is less than for the positive electrode.

Monitoring modalities

Recording the response

The electrical stimulation of a peripheral nerve can be assessed by visual and tactile evaluation of the twitch response of the corresponding muscle (Table 27.1). Using the train-of-four (TOF), four successive stimuli are delivered at 2 Hz (every 0.5 seconds). Immediately available stores of acetylcholine are depleted with each current, and the amount released by the nerve decreases with each successive stimulus until it levels off. In the presence of a nondepolarizing block, the twitches progressively fade starting with the fourth, and one by one eventually disappear with increasing degrees of block. The ratio of the height of the fourth response to the first has been defined as the TOF ratio (T4/T1). It has been shown that a TOF ratio >0.9 at the adductor pollicis is necessary to achieve adequate airway protection to avoid postoperative atelectasis or pneumonia. At TOF ratios < 0.9, a significantly reduced upper esophageal sphincter resting tone and reduced muscle coordination have been demonstrated (Table 27.2).

The assessment of TOF is prone to subjective assessment errors, as the quantitative determination of the TOF ratio is difficult to make during recovery and depends on the experience of the observer. TOF ratios as low as 0.3 may remain undetected, but with double-burst stimulation, fade can be detected reliably in the range of 0.5 to 0.6.

High-frequency stimulation ($\geq$50 Hz) results in sustained or tetanic contraction of the muscle during normal neuromuscular transmission despite a decrement in acetylcholine release. During tetanus, progressive depletion of acetylcholine output is balanced by increased synthesis and transfer of transmitter from its mobilization stores. The presence of nondepolarizing

Table 27.1. Indications for and specifics of various nerve simulation techniques

Technique	Indication	Frequency/time/interval	Location/muscle	Limitations
Single twitch	Assessment of onset of muscular blockade	Single square wave stimuli lasting 0.2 ms are applied at intervals of >10 sec Usually supramaximal current is applied Amplitude may be varied in increments up to 80 mA	Central muscles (facial nerve) to assess readiness for intubation is preferred over peripheral muscles (adductor pollicis)	Response must be compared to control preblockade twitch. Difficult to assess magnitude of response over time.
TOF	Monitoring of muscle relaxation during surgery or readiness for reversal of muscular blockade	Four 2-Hz square wave stimuli each lasting 0.2 ms Observation of degree of fade between fourth and first stimulus: interpretation as a fraction of 1 (TOF ratio) Intervals of 12–15 sec between measurements Surgical relaxation: TOF 0.15–0.25 TOF >0.9 is sufficient recovery for extubation	Central muscles (facial nerve) to monitor adequate surgical relaxation (proximity to diaphragm) Peripheral muscles (adductor pollicis) to detect residual paralysis before extubation	Does not require preblockade control measurement Difficult to evaluate by visual or tactile means Not ideal for determining residual paralysis before extubation because of subjective difficulty determining residual block if TOF ≥0.4
Tetanus	Assessment of residual muscular blockade Sensitivity for detecting residual block >single twitch or TOF	5-sec stimulus with a frequency >30 Hz Observation of fade (more fade is seen with 100 Hz than with 50 Hz) Intervals of 1–2 min between measurements	Preferably peripheral muscles (adductor pollicis) to detect residual paralysis before extubation	Does not require preblockade control measurement Difficult to evaluate by visual or tactile means At 100 Hz, fade may be seen even in the absence of neuromuscular blockade Posttetanic facilitation depends on frequency and duration of stimulation
PTC	Assessment of profound neuromuscular blockade if there is no response to the other modalities	50-Hz tetanus for 5 sec followed by a 3-sec pause and then stimulation at 1 Hz Count of visible twitches correlates inversely with time required to return of single twitch or TOF (PTC of 1 to reappearance of first twitch is 10–20 min, PTC of 10 indicates immediate reappearance of first twitch) Intervals of 1–2 min between measurements	Central muscles (facial nerve) to detect recovery from profound muscular blockade Peripheral muscles (adductor pollicis) to detect residual paralysis before extubation	Does not require preblockade control measurement Commonly used to detect profound muscular blockade
Double-burst stimulation	Assessment of residual muscular blockade Sensitivity for detecting residual block >single twitch or TOF	Three 0.2-ms impulses at 50 Hz separated by 750 ms Fade ratio correlates closely with TOF ratio but is easier to detect manually Intervals of 12–15 sec between measurements	Preferably peripheral muscles (adductor pollicis) to detect residual paralysis before extubation	Does not require preblockade control measurement Fade can be detected reliably up to TOF ratios of 0.5–0.6

muscle relaxants impairs the mobilization of acetylcholine within the nerve terminal, thereby contributing to the fade in response to tetanic and TOF stimulation. This perhaps is the most painful method of monitoring the neuromuscular junction and therefore is not suitable for patients being lightly anesthetized. Tetanic stimulation facilitates the neuromuscular response during and after its application, artificially shifting all subsequent neuromuscular events toward normality. Because it provides only one point on the continuum of neuromuscular response, it is less useful than TOF. With 100-Hz tetanic stimulation, fade might be detected at TOF ratios of 0.8 to 1.0 but also may be seen in individuals with no neuromuscular block.

During profound neuromuscular blockade, quantification of neuromuscular blockade can be done using the posttetanic count (PTC), based on the principle of posttetanic facilitation. Mobilization and enhanced synthesis of acetylcholine continue during and after cessation of tetanic stimulation. Following the end of tetanus, there is an increase in the immediately available store of acetylcholine and the quantal content. Thus after tetanus, there is an increase in the amount of transmitter released in response to nerve stimulation, and a single twitch evoked after cessation of tetanus may be stronger than the pretetanic control. The number of evoked posttetanic twitches detected is referred to as the PTC. The number of posttetanic twitches correlates inversely with the time

Table 27.3. Objective assessment of neuromuscular blockade

Assessment tool	Technique	Advantages/disadvantages
Mechanomyography	Mechanomyographic device objectively quantifies the force of isometric contraction of adductor pollicis muscle in response to ulnar nerve stimulation. The force is translated into an electrical signal that can be displayed on an interfaced pressure monitor and then recorded. Balloon pressure methods may be used to monitor the larynx or corrugator supercilii. Measurement of force indirectly by change of pressure exerted onto the balloon compressed by movement of the thumb or contraction of the corrugator supercilii. A constant amount of baseline muscle tension (preload) should be applied to the monitored muscle, which serves to align the contractile elements (actin and myosin filaments).	Gold standard of muscle relaxation monitoring. Requires most stringent preparations and precautions (e.g., placement of arm in a molded cast to prevent changes of position). Mechanomyographic devices are awkward and bulky to prepare. Drift may be a problem, implying that the response does not return to the control amplitude. Slight movement of the hand may lead to a change in amplitude of the evoked potential.
Electromyography	Measurement of electrical response of muscle after evoked stimulation of a motor nerve; interpretation as an integrated EMG response. The latency of the compound MAP is the interval between stimulus artifact and evolved muscle response. The amplitude of the compound MAP is proportional to the number of muscle units within the designated time interval (epoch). This correlates with the evoked mechanical responses. Mostly for experimental studies.	May be used at various muscle sites (larynx, diaphragm, adductor pollicis; with restrictions, corrugator supercilii and ocularis oculi). Smaller muscles create a smaller action potential and therefore are more difficult to monitor. Monitoring of the diaphragm is possible (measuring the pressure induced within the esophagus). May underestimate the degree of paralysis. Drift over time may arise (failure to descend completely in fully relaxed muscles). Interference with other electronic devices may occur.
Accelerometry	A miniature piezoelectric transducer is used to determine the rate of angular acceleration of the thumb (adductor pollicis). The principle is based on the constant relationship between force (F) and acceleration (a), as long as mass (m) is constant (Newton's second law: $F = ma$). One requirement for accelerometry is that the muscle must be able to move freely. The piezoelectric crystal is distorted by the movement of the crystal inlaid transducer applied to the finger, and an electric current is produced with an output voltage proportional to the deformation of the crystal. Interpretation is from a digital readout. Elastic preload to the thumb has been shown to decrease TOF variability.	Easy to use, practical, versatile, and inexpensive; may be applied to various muscles. Good correlation with mechanomyography and electromyography. Has been shown to reduce the incidence of residual paralysis. Difficult to use with muscles that do not create a distinct movement (e.g., corrugator supercilii). Cannot be used at the larynx or diaphragm.
Kinemyography	Measurement of the movement of the end organ (e.g., thumb) by a piezoelectric transducer. Use of a molded plastic device with the contour of the outstretched thumb and index finger.	Slight clinical differences from mechanomyography in studies. Accuracy is not superior to that of acceleromyography. Careful hand positioning is necessary to avoid artifact. Monitoring of recovery may be misleading.
Phonomyography	Contracting muscle emits low-frequency sounds, which are recorded with special microphones. Interpretation of fade of TOF.	Easy to apply at various muscles. Promising agreement with mechanomyography. Change in contact with the skin surface may change the signal amplitude. Currently, no commercial devices are available.

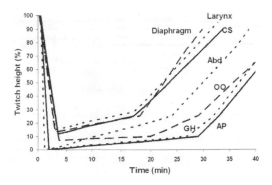

Legend:
CS: M. corrugator supercilii
Abd: Abdominal muscles
OO: M. orbicularis oculi
GH: M. geniohyoid (upper airway)
AP: M. adductor pollicis

Figure 27.1. Approximate time course of twitch height after administration of rocuronium, 0.6 mg/kg, to different muscles. (Modified with permission from Barash PG, Cullen BF, Stoelting RK. *Clinical Anesthesia*. 5th ed. Philadelphia: Lippincott Williams & Wilkins; 2006.)

Table 27.2. Relationship between receptor occupancy, T1, T4, T4/T1 ratio, and tetanus during nondepolarizing muscular blockade

Percentage blocked	T1, % *normal*	T4, % *normal*	T4/T1, % *normal*	Tetanus
100				
95			T1–T4 lost	
90	10		T2–T4 lost	
85	20		T3–T4 lost	
80	25		T4 lost	Onset of fade at 30 Hz
	80–90	55–65	TOF 0.6–0.7	
	95	70	TOF 0.7–0.75	
75	100	75–100	TOF 0.75–1	
70			TOF 0.9–1	Onset of fade at 50 Hz
50				Onset of fade at 100 Hz
30				Onset of fade at 200 Hz

for spontaneous recovery. PTC is a prejunctional event; the response may vary with the nondepolarizing muscle relaxant used.

Following intense neuromuscular blockade by vecuronium, the first detectable twitch of the TOF will appear an average of 8.5 minutes (6–15 minutes) after a PTC of 1. A PTC of 8 to 9 indicates imminent return of TOF. The recovery of atracurium is similar to that of vecuronium; the interval is larger for pancuronium. It takes approximately 38 minutes after the first post-tetanic twitch for the reappearance of the first response to TOF stimulation. A PTC of 9 to 11 predicts imminent return of TOF response. Children have a shorter interval between PTC 1 and onset of T1. The PTC may be useful for cases in which profound muscle relaxation is required (e.g., ophthalmic surgery) or for the continuous infusion of intermediate nondepolarizing muscle relaxants.

Because of the unreliability of visual/tactile assessment of neuromuscular function, there has been an emerging interest in the development of quantitative devices for the assessment of neuromuscular blockade (Table 27.3). These devices measure either the compound muscle action potential (MAP) or the evoked contractile response. The compound MAP is the cumulative electrical signal generated by the individual action potentials of individual muscle fibers.

For research purposes, mechanomyography is the gold standard for objective muscle relaxation monitoring. The most versatile method in the clinical setting is acceleromyography because it can be applied at various muscles and has a long track record of clinical utility.

Choice of muscle

Muscles differ in terms of onset, offset, and peak effect of neuromuscular blockade. There is a variation in responses of individual muscles to electric stimulation, which serve different purposes or indications. Possible causes for the varying responses of different muscle groups are the differences in the

margin of safety of the neuromuscular junction of differ muscle groups, fiber composition, innervation ratio (numbe neuromuscular junctions), blood flow, and muscular temp ture (Fig. 27.1).

Important means of providing optimal relaxation sho consider monitoring muscles of the surgical site or, alte tively, muscles that adequately reflect neuromuscular bl ade at the surgical site (Table 27.4). Complete neuromusc blockade at the adductor pollicis does not necessarily r complete relaxation of the diaphragm. Monitoring the corr tor supercilii better reflects the degree of relaxation at the gical site during thoracic surgery. In general, for surgery upper or lower extremities, monitoring of the adductor cis, or any other hand muscle, is preferable. For surgery v the chest or abdomen in which relaxation of the diaph is necessary, monitoring of the corrugator supercilii be used.

Current evidence shows that monitoring of the co tor supercilii should be used to establish the earliest tir optimal conditions for tracheal intubation, as it reflects geal relaxation better than monitoring of the adductor p Recovery of neuromuscular transmission is best monit the adductor pollicis because, in general, this is the last group to recover from neuromuscular blockade. TOF st tion with a ratio >0.9 indicates sufficient recovery of neu cular transmission for awakening the patient and ensuri tracheal extubation.

Factors affecting the monitoring of neuromuscular blockade

Many drugs interfere with neuromuscular function. clinical settings make the interpretation of monito neuromuscular blockade difficult. Neuromuscular blo prolonged if the patient is hypothermic due to a de metabolism of the blocking drug.

Overestimation of neuromuscular blockade may a cold extremity without central hypothermia. Unde tion of neuromuscular blockade is seen in the setting o hypothermia. Central and peripheral nerve damage le resistance to nondepolarizing muscle relaxants at the site (e.g., hemiplegia) presumably as a result of an ex tional expression of acetylcholine receptors on the par A misinterpretation of the relaxation of the patient ca potential of overdosing muscle relaxants because of a d response to the monitoring methods. Central and pe nerve damage can be based on nerve trauma, cord tra or stroke.

Maintenance of neuromuscular blocka

The goal of muscle relaxation is to maintain the n depth of block required for surgery. Adequate relax abdominal surgery can be achieved with >80% twitc sion, which correlates with one or two twitches prese TOF. The diaphragm is relatively resistant and require

Table 27.4. Comparison of various monitoring sites

M. adductor pollicis (ulnar nerve)	Stimulation of ulnar nerve: first electrode on proximal wrist on the radial side of flexor carpi ulnaris muscle, second electrode 2 cm proximal on volar forearm or over the olecranon grove Relatively sensitive to nondepolarizing neuromuscular blocking drugs During recovery, more blocked than respiratory muscles
First dorsal interosseous muscle (ulnar nerve)	Preferably used for electromyography Electrodes are relatively undisturbed by hand movement Sensitivity of this muscle correlates with M. adductor pollicis
M. abductor digit quiniti (ulnar nerve)	Less sensitive than M. adductor pollicis to muscle relaxants May overestimate recovery from blockade Prone to stimulus artifact
Muscles surrounding the eye (facial nerve)	Stimulation of facial nerve 2–3 cm posterior to the lateral border of the orbit; use less current (20–30 mA) M. orbicularis oculi: covers eyelid movement Monitoring the onset of neuromuscular blockade at the orbicularis oculi can predict good intubation conditions M. corrugator supercilii: small muscle around the eyebrow, responsible for vertical frowning Movement of eyebrow is similar to that of laryngeal adductors Onset of blockade is more rapid and recovery occurs sooner vs. adductor pollicis Accurately reflects the response of laryngeal muscles or diaphragm Acceleromyography is difficult to perform because of the small size of the muscle
Vastus medialis (femoral nerve)	The vastus medialis muscle has been used as an alternative monitoring site Stimulation of muscular branches of the femoral nerve Onset and recovery from neuromuscular blockade are faster vs. the adductor pollicis
Muscles of the foot (tibial nerve)	Stimulation of posterior tibial nerve behind the internal malleolus to produce flexion of the big toe by contraction of the flexor hallucis Response is better vs the adductor pollicis but with inconsistent results, limiting usability Stimulation of external peroneal nerve produces dorsiflexion Sensitivity of muscles has not been measured
Laryngeal muscles (recurrent laryngeal nerve)	Neuromuscular blockade at the larynx is less intense vs. the adductor pollicis, with more rapid onset and offset Monitoring of the larynx is based on mechanomyography, electromyography, or phonomyography Placement of the endotracheal cuff between the vocal cords allows measurement of the force of the adducting laryngeal muscles via the degree of pressure changes within the cuff A special endotracheal tube with incorporated electrodes may be used for electromyography; alternatively, small microphones may be placed at the larynx to monitor the laryngeal muscles This technique obviates the risk of endotracheal tube dislodgement, as associated with techniques requiring tube positioning Transcutaneous stimulation of the recurrent laryngeal nerve may be accomplished medially, between the jugular notch and the thyroid cartilage or lateral to the sternocleidomastoid muscle in the tracheoesophageal groove
Diaphragm (phrenic nerve)	Neuromuscular blockade at the diaphragm is less intense vs. adductor pollicis, with more rapid onset and offset Monitoring of the diaphragm is possible with electromyography and mechanomyography using transcutaneous needles or superficial skin electrodes The seventh or eighth intercostal space, between the anterior axillary and midclavicular line, may be used to record the signal Mechanomyography may be used indirectly by inserting a balloon in the esophagus to record pleural pressure and another in the stomach to record abdominal pressure. The balloons are connected to air-filled catheters to identical transducers. Transdiaphragmatic pressure = gastric (intra-abdominal) pressure – esophageal (intrathoracic) pressure. However, this technique is more invasive and difficult to apply. It cannot be used in open abdominal or laparoscopic cases.

plasma concentration of nondepolarizing muscle relaxants. When paralysis of the diaphragm is required, the administration of neuromuscular blockade is titrated to paralysis of the corrugator supercilii muscle, whose recovery profile is similar to that of the diaphragm.

Detecting reversible block

Airway patency and adequate ventilation require more than an intact diaphragm. Therefore, it is important to assess the degree of block at a muscle that does not overestimate the rate of recovery of muscles maintaining the airway. The increased sensitivity and slower time course of the adductor pollicis muscle make this site preferable for monitoring recovery. PTC may be used when no twitch response is attainable. The time to recovery of twitch response is inversely proportional to the number of PTC. In the absence of objective monitoring devices, double-burst stimulation may be preferable to TOF to reliably detect a fade. Atracurium-, vecuronium-, and pancuronium-induced neuromuscular blockade is antagonized by neostigmine in 30 minutes when the single twitch height is ≥10% of control or just prior to emergence of the second twitch of the TOF count and in 10 minutes, when all four responses to TOF stimulation are present. When zero twitches are present in the TOF, the block is considered not antagonizable.

Table 27.5. Clinical tests to assess recovery from neuromuscular blockade

Both legs lifted off the bed	TOF 0.6 Probably not sufficient to ensure protection of airway
Head lift >5 sec	TOF 0.6 Probably not sufficient to ensure protection of airway
Normal hand grip strength	TOF 0.7
Teeth clenched to prevent removal of wooden spatula (masseter muscle strength)	TOF 0.86 Most sensitive test to ensure adequate recovery, but not all patients may be able to demonstrate

Clinical tests to evaluate residual muscular blockade

Aside from peripheral nerve stimulation, a variety of clinical tests are used in clinical practice to assess for adequate recovery from neuromuscular blockade. Subjective evaluation consists of the assessment of residual paralysis based on the patient's ability to perform certain tasks. These tests depend on the degree of consciousness and cooperation of the patient (Table 27.5).

Ensuring adequate neuromuscular function before extubation

Safe extubation from the trachea can be performed only after adequate restoration of neuromuscular function. A TOF ratio >0.75 at the thumb correlates with restoration of strength of the muscles of respiration and airway protection, vital capacity, maximum expiratory force, peak expiratory flow rate, hand grip, and 5-second head lift. Historically, a TOF ratio of 0.7 was used as an indication of adequate recovery from neuromuscular blockade. Current evidence, however, indicates that a TOF ratio of 0.9 rather than 0.7 is required to ensure recovery. A residual block (TOF < 0.9) is associated with functional impairment of the pharynx and upper esophagus, likely predisposing to regurgitation and aspiration.

Postoperative residual curarization (PORC) might occur because of administration of excess neuromuscular blocking agents, early administration of reversal, or an abnormal response of the patient. PORC continues to be a common problem in postanesthesia care units. Given that PORC is a potentially preventable patient safety problem, it is important to find ways to reduce the incidence. PORC is a major risk factor for many critical events in the immediate postoperative period, such as ventilatory insufficiency, hypoxemia, and pulmonary infections.

Subjective evaluation of the evoked muscular response to TOF stimulation is extremely inaccurate. In addition, many practitioners are unclear about the current standards that define adequate recovery from neuromuscular blockade. Also, there is conflicting evidence regarding the utility of conventional peripheral nerve stimulators in preventing PORC. The incidence of PORC was found to be significantly lower after the use of intermediate neuromuscular blocking drugs.

Not all clinicians believe PORC is a clinical problem that may affect their patients. Disinclination to use peripheral nerve stimulator devices suggests that many practitioners do not accept the premise that these devices are helpful. Thus, four decades after the first battery-operated nerve stimulators were described, unacceptable levels of residual paresis in postanesthesia care units continue to be reported. It should be emphasized that objective monitoring of neuromuscular blockade may provide enhanced safety to prevent PORC.

Suggested readings

Baillard C, Clec'h C, Catineau J, et al. Postoperative residual neuromuscular block: a survey of management. *Br J Anaesth* 2005; 95:622–626.

Baurain MJ, Hennart DA, Godschalx A, et al. Visual evaluation of residual curarization in anesthetized patients using one hundred-hertz, five-second tetanic stimulation at the adductor pollicis muscle. *Anesth Analg* 1998; 87:185–189.

Berg H, Roed J, Viby-Mogensen J, et al. Residual neuromuscular block is a risk factor for postoperative pulmonary complications. A prospective, randomised, and blinded study of postoperative pulmonary complications after atracurium, vecuronium and pancuronium. *Acta Anaesthesiol Scand* 1997; 41:1095–1103.

Debaene B, Beaussier M, Meistelman C, et al. Monitoring the onset of neuromuscular block at the orbicularis oculi can predict good intubating conditions during atracurium-induced neuromuscular block. *Anesth Analg* 1995; 80:360–363.

Dhonneur G, Kirov K, Motamed C, et al. Post-tetanic count at adductor pollicis is a better indicator of early diaphragmatic recovery than train-of-four count at corrugator supercilii. *Br J Anaesth* 2007; 99:376–379.

Donati F, Plaud B, Meistelman C. A method to measure elicited contraction of laryngeal adductor muscles during anesthesia. *Anesthesiology* 1991; 74:827–832.

Drenck NE, Ueda N, Olsen NV, et al. Manual evaluation of residual curarization using double burst stimulation: a comparison with train-of-four. *Anesthesiology* 1989; 70:578–581.

Dupuis JY, Martin R, Tessonnier JM, Tetrault JP. Clinical assessment of the muscular response to tetanic nerve stimulation. *Can J Anaesth* 1990; 37:397–400.

Eriksson LI, Lennmarken C, Staun P, Viby-Mogensen J. Use of post-tetanic count in assessment of a repetitive vecuronium-induced neuromuscular block. *Br J Anaesth* 1990; 65:487–493.

Eriksson LI, Sundman E, Olsson R, et al. Functional assessment of the pharynx at rest and during swallowing in partially paralyzed humans: simultaneous videomanometry and mechanomyography of awake human volunteers. *Anesthesiology* 1997; 87:1035–1043.

Hemmerling TM, Donati F. Neuromuscular blockade at the larynx, the diaphragm and the corrugator supercilii muscle: a review. *Can J Anaesth* 2003; 50:779–794.

Katz RL. Clinical neuromuscular pharmacology of pancuronium. *Anesthesiology* 1971; 34:550–556.

Kopman AF, Yee PS, Neuman GG. Relationship of the train-of-four fade ratio to clinical signs and symptoms of residual paralysis in awake volunteers. *Anesthesiology* 1997; 86:765–771.

Lee C, Katz RL. Fade of neurally evoked compound electromyogram during neuromuscular block by d-tubocurarine. *Anesth Analg* 1977; 56:271–275.

Lieutaud T, Billard V, Khalaf H, Debaene B. Muscle relaxation and increasing doses of propofol improve intubating conditions. *Can J Anaesth* 2003; 50:121–126.

Mencke T, Echternach M, Kleinschmidt S, et al. Laryngeal morbidity and quality of tracheal intubation: a randomized controlled trial. *Anesthesiology* 2003; 98:1049–1056.

Moorthy SS, Hilgenberg JC. Resistance to non-depolarizing muscle relaxants in paretic upper extremities of patients with residual hemiplegia. *Anesth Analg* 1980; 59:624–627.

Naguib M, Kopman AF, Ensor JE. Neuromuscular monitoring and postoperative residual curarisation: a meta-analysis. *Br J Anaesth* 2007; 98:302–316.

Williams MT, Rice I, Ewen SP, Elliott SM. A comparison of the effect of two anaesthetic techniques on surgical conditions during gynaecological laparoscopy. *Anaesthesia* 2003; 58:574–578.

Thermoregulation and temperature monitoring

Matthias Stopfkuchen-Evans, Elliott S. Farber, and Francis X. Vacanti

Introduction

Control of body temperature is mediated via behavioral and autonomic mechanisms to maintain effective enzymatic activity and normal bodily functions. Behavioral mechanisms are far more powerful than autonomic thermoregulatory defenses in allowing humans to survive in diverse environments. Once anesthetized, the patient loses all behavioral means to self-regulate temperature.

Thermoregulation

Under normal conditions, the hypothalamus seeks to establish an equilibrium of heat generation and dissipation to maintain core temperatures in a very narrow range. Core temperature consists of the well-perfused tissues, and this compartment maintains a warmer and more uniform state. Sensory information is gathered primarily from the transient receptor potential (TRP) family of ion channels and conveyed by unmyelinated C and myelinated A-δ fibers. Thermal inputs from the skin surface, deep abdominal and thoracic tissues, the spinal cord, and nonhypothalamic regions in the brain contribute equally and are further integrated on several levels within the brain and spinal cord, before the information gets relayed to the anterior hypothalamus, the dominant thermoregulatory controller. The thresholds for increasing or decreasing core temperature lie within approximately 0.2°C of the hypothalamic thermoregulatory set point; however, there is a nearly 1°C sinusoidal circadian variation around the set point temperature, with the maximum occurring midafternoon and the minimum occurring 12 hours later. The primary autonomic response to heat consists of sweating and active capillary vasodilation, whereas the primary autonomic response to cold results in shivering and vasoconstriction.

Heat production

The energy lost in the biochemical conversion of glucose to adenosine triphosphate (ATP) and in the expenditure of ATP appears as heat. Human activity is such that ATP utilization varies immensely, and the human body must be able to deal with significant swings in endogenous heat production. Humans handle the heat load of varying activities such as sleeping with an energy expenditure of approximately 0.7 metabolic

equivalents (MET) to vigorous activity of 10 to 12 MET, where 1 MET is defined as the caloric consumption of 1 kcal/kg/h. Anesthetic agents, opioids, and sedatives incapacitate or alter some mechanisms of heat production (shivering to generate heat). Infants are capable of increased heat production via nonshivering thermogenesis from the metabolism of brown fat. This fat is loaded with mitochondria and is found close to the large blood vessels and intrascapular space. When sympathetically activated, it can increase the production of heat by as much as 100%.

Mechanisms of heat loss: transfer of thermal energy

The transfer of thermal energy from humans (i.e., heat loss) occurs through four mechanisms:

- Conduction
- Convection
- Radiation
- Evaporation

Conduction resulting in heat loss occurs via direct contact with surrounding substances (e.g., air, water, intravenous [IV] fluids, operating room [OR] table, laryngoscope blades) and is related to the area of contact and differences in temperature. Convection is related to conduction, as contact with a substance is required; however, convection differs in that continued renewed contact with that substance (i.e., a breeze or a current of water) occurs. However, *most* heat is lost in the form of infrared electromagnetic waves via radiation. All objects above absolute zero emit electromagnetic radiation, and the rate of heat loss by this mechanism is related to the temperature of the object. The human body radiates energy in the infrared portion of the electromagnetic spectrum, as do the surrounding walls and other objects. It is usually the case that the temperature of the surrounding objects is lower than that of the human body, and there is a net loss of heat from the body to the environment. The body loses 0.58 kcal of heat with each gram of water that evaporates from its surfaces. Approximately 20% of the total heat loss normally is the result of evaporation, but this can increase markedly under thermal stress, and evaporation then becomes the major means of heat loss. Evaporation is the only mechanism whereby heat energy is transferred to a warmer

Table 28.1. Intraoperative phases of heat redistribution and loss

Phase	I	II	III
Temperature	↓ core temperature by 1–2°C during first hour	Gradual decline over 3–4 h Heat loss exceeds heat production	Equilibrium at around 33°C T_{core} Heat production equals loss
Characteristics	Heat redistribution from abdomen and thorax to extremities	Linear reduction	Core-to-peripheral temperature gradient is restored
Mechanisms	Inhibition of tonic thermoregulatory vasoconstriction	Radiation, 60%; convection, 30%; conduction, 5%; evaporation, 5%	Peripheral vasoconstriction
Heat loss	No net heat loss	Net heat loss	No net heat loss
Prophylaxis	Preemptive skin warming before surgery (decrease core-to-peripheral temperature gradient)	Active warming measures intraoperatively	Active warming to maintain core temperature plateau at or above 36°C

environment. Sympathetic cholinergic neurons activate sweat glands to excrete sweat, which is then evaporated from the skin surface.

Altered regulation and environmental response under anesthesia

Table 28.1 summarizes the three phases of intraoperative core temperature changes. The ability to self-regulate temperature is greatly affected under anesthesia. Anesthetics alter the range of normal adaptive response to temperature changes by some 20-fold, such that mechanisms for heat production and dissipation may not be triggered until detrimental effects of hypo- or hyperthermia are already present. In the normal awake state, heat is unevenly distributed throughout the body as a result of tonic thermoregulatory vasoconstriction. Redistribution of body heat, however, occurs from the alteration of this vasoconstriction by various anesthetics and is responsible for the initial decrease in core temperature that follows induction (Fig. 28.1). The magnitude of redistributory heat loss is inversely proportional to the percentage of body fat and the weight-to-surface area ratio. Following this redistribution, temperature changes happen at a slower rate. This nearly linear decrease in temperature is a result of heat loss dominating over metabolic heat production. Again, the magnitude of the core cooling rate during the second phase is inversely proportional to the weight-to-surface ratio. The mechanisms for increased heat generation, heat conservation, and heat dissipation remain intact; however, trigger responses for these mechanisms are blunted and response curves are shifted such that wider temperature ranges will occur. Fig. 28.2 shows changes in thermoregulatory thresholds seen with various anesthetic agents.

Phase 3 is characterized by reaching a thermal steady state at which heat loss equals metabolic heat production and no heat is lost. This stage may be reached either by effective warming efforts, thus reaching a passive thermal steady state, or by allowing sufficient hypothermia to occur, which leads to the reactivation of thermoregulatory vasoconstriction and therefore to the reestablishment of the normal core-to-peripheral temperature gradient. This, of course, is attained at significantly lower core temperature levels, as outlined in Fig. 28.3.

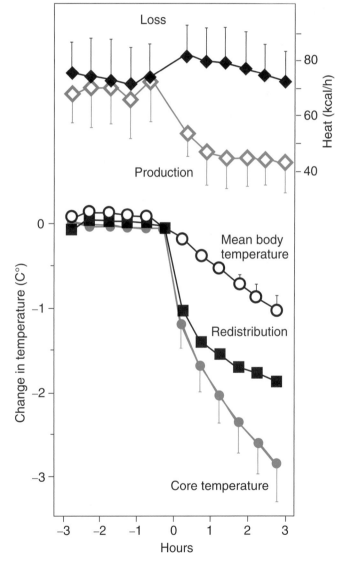

Figure 28.1. Changes in heat content and distribution of heat in the body before and after the induction of general anesthesia; mean (±SD) changes in thermoregulatory thresholds associated with anesthetics. (Modified from Kurz A. Physiology of thermoregulation. *Best Pract Res Clin Anaesthesiol* 2008;2:627–644.)

Table 28.2. Organ system effects of hypothermia

- Cardiovascular
  - Bradycardia → Osborne J waves → conduction slowing → atrial fibrillation → ventricular irritability → ventricular fibrillation
  - Altered oxygen supply and demand → increased blood viscosity → reduced microcirculatory flow → increased systemic vascular resistance → cardiac output reduction
- CNS
  - Ataxia → delirium → stupor → coma
  - EEG slowing → ↓ EEG amplitude → EEG isoelectricity (maximum decrease in CMRO$_2$)
  - ↓ CMRO$_2$ → ↓ Decreased cerebral blood flow
  - Respiratory
  - ↑ Breathing rate → ↓ PaCO$_2$ → ↓ peripheral O$_2$ unloading
  - ↓ HPV
  - ↑ PVR
- Renal
  - Renal vasoconstriction → ↓ ADH release → diuresis
  - ↓ Renal blood flow → ↓ GFR → ↓ renal tubular function → ↓ urine-concentrating ability
  - ↓ Renal oxygen consumption
- Hepatic
  - ↓ Drug metabolism
  - Platelet sequestration
- Endocrine
  - ↑ Hypothalamic thyrotropin-releasing hormone → ↑ T$_3$/T$_4$ → ↑ metabolic rate
  - ↑ Adrenocortical and medullary hormones (norepinephrine and epinephrine) → ↑ blood glucose
- Coagulation system
  - ↓ Platelet function
  - Platelet sequestration
  - ↓ Activity of clotting cascade

ADH, antidiuretic hormone; CMRO$_2$; EEG, electroencephalogram; GFR, glomerular filtration rate; HPV; PVR.
Adapted from Stoelting RK, Hillier SC. *Pharmacology and Physiology of Anesthetic Practice*. 4th ed. Philadelphia: Lippincott Williams & Wilkins; 2005.

Table 28.3. Common causes of hyperthermia

- Disorders associated with excessive heat production
  - Malignant hyperthermia
  - Neuroleptic malignant syndrome
  - Thyrotoxicosis
  - Delirium tremens
  - Pheochromocytoma
  - Salicylate intoxication
  - Drug abuse (cocaine, amphetamines)
  - Status epilepticus
  - Exertional heat stroke
- Disorders associated with decreased heat loss
  - Autonomic nervous system dysfunction
  - Anticholinergics
  - Dehydration
  - Occlusive dressings
  - Heat stroke
- Disorders associated with dysfunction of the hypothalamus
  - Trauma
  - Cerebrovascular accident
  - Encephalitis
  - Neuroleptic malignant syndrome

Adapted from Stoelting RK, Hillier SC. *Pharmacology and Physiology of Anesthetic Practice*. 4th ed. Philadelphia: Lippincott Williams & Wilkins; 2005.

to developing surgical wound infections. Table 28.2 summarizes the effects of hypothermia on various organ systems.

Shivering is a complex response to hypothermia that often is perceived as particularly uncomfortable and increases postoperative pain sensation. It may double or triple oxygen consumption and carbon dioxide production and double metabolic heat production. It is absent in newborns and infants and is rarely seen in elderly patients because of impaired thermoregulatory control. Pharmacologic interventions to decrease shivering in the postoperative care unit may consist of central α_2-adrenergic agonists or small doses of meperidine, which decreases the shivering threshold temperature significantly more than the vasoconstriction threshold.

Untoward effects of hyper- and hypothermia

Hypothermia

Hypothermia exists when core temperature is <36°C. At increased risk of perioperative hypothermia are elderly patients, neonates, and those with cachexia, burns, or paraplegia because of their already-existent altered heat conservation. Despite the demonstrated benefits in some clinical scenarios (severe traumatic brain injury with Glasgow Coma Score < or = 8, comatose patients after an out-of-hospital cardiac arrest, potentially after acute ischemic stroke), the untoward effects of hypothermia generally outweigh the ischemic protection benefits. Untoward effects of hypothermia include impaired coagulation from decreased activation of the coagulation cascade and inhibited platelet function, increased oxygen and metabolic demand from postoperative shivering, and slowed drug metabolism, contributing to a delayed recovery from anesthesia. In addition, hypothermic patients have impaired resistance

Hyperthermia

Hyperthermia exists when core temperature is >38°C and is different from fever in that it is in excess of the hypothalamic set point. For comparable deviation from normothermia, hyperthermia is more detrimental to the body than hypothermia, with the brain and central nervous system (CNS) being most sensitive. Hyperthermia increases the release of excitatory neurotransmitters and has been shown to worsen neurologic injury following ischemic events and status epilepticus. Under anesthesia, most cases of hyperthermia result from excessive intraoperative warming techniques; however, excessive metabolic production of heat in the setting of impaired heat dissipation also is possible. Common causes of hyperthermia are listed in Table 28.3.

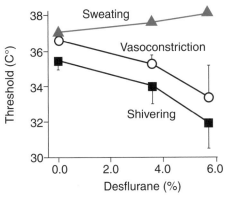

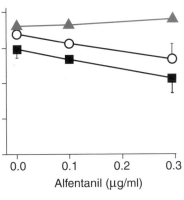

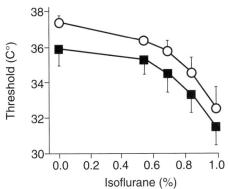

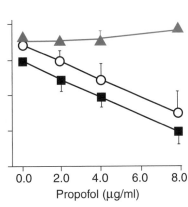

Figure 28.2. Anesthetic-induced inhibition of thermoregulatory control usually is the major factor determining perioperative core temperature. Concentration-dependent thermoregulatory inhibition by desflurane, isoflurane (halogenated volatile anesthetics), alfentanil (a μ-agonist opioid), and propofol (an intravenous anesthetic). The sweating (*triangles*), vasoconstriction (*circles*), and shivering (*squares*) thresholds are expressed in terms of core temperature at a designated mean skin temperature of 34°C. Anesthesia linearly, but slightly, increases the sweating threshold. In contrast, anesthesia produces substantial and comparable linear or nonlinear decreases in the vasoconstriction and shivering thresholds. Typical anesthetic concentrations thus increase the interthreshold range (difference between the sweating and vasoconstriction thresholds) approximately 20-fold from its normal value near 0.2°C. Patients do not activate autonomic thermoregulatory defenses unless body temperature exceeds the interthreshold range; surgical patients thus are poikilothermic over a 3°C–5°C range of core temperatures.

Accuracy and reliability of temperature monitoring

The gold standard for temperature monitoring is a thermistor within the pulmonary artery, as it most accurately reflects core temperature in a continuous manner. Its invasiveness, however, lends to other monitoring techniques. The nasopharynx and tympanic membrane are close to the blood flow to the brain and thus reliably reflect core temperature. Continuous tympanic membrane monitoring is possible; however, it requires that a transducer be placed in contact with the tympanic membrane, which may be technically undesirable. An esophageal probe positioned above the hard palate allows continuous monitoring of the nasopharynx. Rectal temperature may be confounded by heat-producing bacteria; fecal insulation of the temperature probe, delaying responsiveness; or blood return from the lower extremities. Bladder temperature closely approximates core temperature but can be affected by an open abdomen and is subject to the same delayed responsiveness as rectal monitoring in settings of reduced urinary output. An appropriately placed temperature probe in the distal esophagus accurately reflects core temperature. When the site is not distal enough, readings may be affected by inhaled gases. Table 28.4 shows possible sites for temperature measurement.

Techniques for maintaining normothermia

Because patients under anesthesia are more susceptible to the temperature influences of their environment and the standard OR environment is cold, active techniques must be employed to maintain normothermia. Patient covering is extremely effective because as much as 80% of heat loss is from radiation and convection. This is most effective when a patient is covered prior to the induction of anesthesia, especially with prewarming of the skin to minimize early intraoperative hypothermia. Forced-air convection blankets are extremely effective when covering >25% of the body surface area and require continuous temperature monitoring to prevent hyperthermia. Table 28.5 outlines various techniques to prevent perioperative heat loss and maintain normothermia.

Table 28.4. Sites for temperature monitoring

- Core temperature monitoring sites
  - Pulmonary artery (gold standard)
  - Nasopharynx
  - Tympanic membrane
  - Distal esophagus
- Transitional zone monitoring sites
  - Axillary
  - Rectum
  - Bladder
- Peripheral temperature monitoring
  - Skin

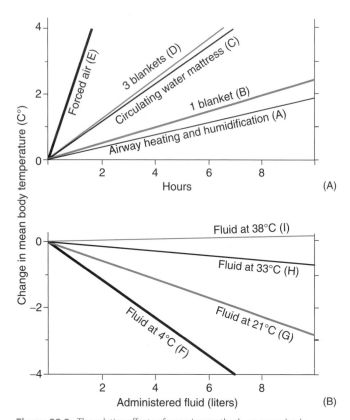

Figure 28.3. The relative effects of warming methods on mean body temperature. Figure 28.3 (A) shows the change in mean body temperature according to the time elapsed since the start of treatment; (B) shows the change in mean body temperature according to the quantity of fluid administered. Mean body temperature is the average temperature of body tissue and is usually somewhat lower than core temperature. The calculations are for a hypothetical, undressed patient weighing 70 kg, with a metabolic rate of 80 kcal/h, in thermal steady state in a typical OR (ambient temperature, 21°C). *Line A* indicates the change in mean body temperature in a patient inspiring warmed humidified gas. *Line B* indicates the change in a patient with all skin below the neck covered by a warmed or unwarmed blanket. *Line D* indicates the change in mean body temperature in a patient similarly covered with three blankets. (Similar amounts of heat loss are prevented by one or three layers of other passive insulators.) *Line C* indicates the change in a patient on a full-length circulating-water mattress and *line E* the change in mean body temperature in a patient covered with a full-length forced-air blanket. *Lines F, G, H, and I* indicate the change in mean body temperature per liter of administered blood or crystalloid at various fluid temperatures.

Postoperatively, these devices may be less effective in the presence of peripheral vasoconstriction, as this might limit heat transfer. Concerns regarding increased airborne bacterial wound contamination with the use of these devices have not been confirmed by studies. Radiant heat lamps are more effective for use with infants because of their greater surface

Table 28.5. Measures to prevent heat loss and reverse hypothermia

Use blankets during transport from the scene
Increase trauma room and OR temperatures >80°F
Minimize duration of exposure to cold environment
Use warming devices for all infusions in the trauma room and OR
Cover patient's head and other parts of the body with warming devices (Bair Hugger[a])
Irrigate nasogastric and thoracostomy tubes with warm saline
Irrigate open body cavities with warm saline
Consider extracorporeal warming

[a] Registered trademark of Arizant, Eden Prairie, MN.

area–volume ratio compared with adults. Radiant heat lamps also are more effective in terminating postoperative shivering than the application of warm blankets. Thermal mattresses have been more effective in the infant than in the adult population. Warming is hampered by decreased tissue perfusion from compressive contact with these devices. Heat loss from ventilation represents 8% to 10% of the total caloric expenditure of the infant. Active heating and humidification of inhaled gases can minimize damage to respiratory cilia. Fluid and blood warming help minimize intraoperative heat loss, especially when large volume resuscitation is required, as each liter of IV fluid at ambient temperature that is infused into adult patients decreases mean core body temperature by about 0.25°C. Fig. 28.3 shows the relative effects of warming methods on mean body temperature.

Suggested readings

Faust RJ, Cucchiara RF, Rose SH, Spackman TN, Wedel DJ, Wass CT, eds. *Anesthesiology Review*, 3rd ed. Philadelphia: Churchill Livingstone; 2001: 91–93.

Insler SR, Sessler DI. Perioperative thermoregulation and temperature monitoring. *Anesthesiol Clin* 2006; 24:823–837.

Lake CL, Hines RL, Blitt CD. *Clinical Monitoring: Practical Applications for Anesthesia and Critical Care*. Philadelphia, 2001.

Ryan JF, Vacanti FX. Temperature regulation. In: Ryan JF, Todres ID, Cote CJ, Goudsouzian NG, eds. *A Practice of Anesthesia for Infants and Children*. New York and Orlando FL: Grune & Stratton; 1986:19–23.

Sessler DI. Mild perioperative hypothermia. *N Engl J Med* 1997; 336(24):1730–1737.

Stoelting RK, Hillier SC. *Pharmacology & Physiology in Anesthetic Practice*, 4th ed. Philadelphia, Lippincott Williams & Wilkins; 2005.

Wilson WC, Grande CM, Hoyt DB. *Trauma: Emergency Resuscitation, Perioperative Anesthesia, Surgical Management*. New York: Informa; 2007.

Neurophysiologic monitoring

Kai Matthes and Mary Ellen McCann

Introduction

The assessment of neurologic function during surgery can be challenging because many general anesthetics depress the central nervous system (CNS). Fortunately, a variety of neuromonitoring techniques have been devised to monitor the integrity of the CNS, which may be compromised by ischemia, hypothermia, hypotension, or direct structural damage. Electroencephalography and evoked potentials are used to assess ischemia, surgical injury, and anesthetic depth. Monitoring of intracranial hypertension is utilized primarily in the intensive care unit and occasionally in the operating room. Methods to assess cerebral blood flow (CBF) and oxygen saturations also have been developed to aid in the detection of intraoperative ischemia.

Electroencephalography

Electroencephalographic (EEG) monitoring analyzes the spontaneous electrical potentials generated by pyramidal cells of the granular cortex via scalp electrodes, which are interpreted as waveforms on a monitor. EEG waveforms are interpreted by pattern recognition and quantification, which involves measuring frequency and amplitude. Frequency is measured in hertz (Hz) and is defined as the number of times per second the wave crosses the zero voltage line. Amplitude is measured in microvolts (μV) and represents the electrical height of the wave. Commonly, EEG is a plot of voltage versus time using 16 channels. The scalp EEG oscillations have characteristic frequency ranges which are divided into different bands that are associated with different states of brain functioning (Table 29.1).

Certain EEG changes are observed during anesthesia. During induction of anesthesia, a decrease in alpha activity and an increase in beta activity are observed. With a more profound depth of anesthesia, theta and delta activity is predominant. By further deepening of anesthesia, a burst suppression pattern may be observed as a depression of cerebral metabolic activity. Isoelectricity is the maximum degree of suppression achievable with anesthetic agents, which is the goal when inducing barbiturate coma.

The primary use of intraoperative EEG is to monitor for cerebral ischemia and hypoxia during carotid endarterectomy, cerebral aneurysms, arteriovenous malformations, and cardiopulmonary bypass procedures. Other indications for EEG monitoring include the assessment of barbiturate-induced burst suppression, CBF during deliberate hypotension, coma and death states, and diagnosis and treatment of epilepsy (Table 29.2).

The major advantage of intraoperative EEG monitoring is that it allows early detection of cerebral hypoxia and ischemia, because inadequate PaO_2 or insufficient CBF is reflected within seconds in the EEG.

Electrocorticography

Electrocorticography (ECoG) is the localization of epileptic foci by the placement of electrodes directly on the exposed surface of the cortex to record electrical activity. In cooperative patients, ECoG can be performed in the operating room while the craniotomy is accomplished with light sedation and local anesthesia. Agents used for this light anesthesia include nitrous oxide,

Table 29.1. EEG frequency ranges

Delta rhythm (0–3 Hz)	Deep sleep Deep anesthesia Pathologic states: brain tumors, hypoxia, metabolic encephalopathy
Theta rhythm (4–7 Hz)	Sleep and anesthesia in adults Hyperventilation in awake children and young adults
Alpha rhythm (8–13 Hz)	Resting, awake adult with eyes closed; predominantly in occipital leads
Beta rhythm (>13 Hz)	Mental activity Light anesthesia

Table 29.2. Factors affecting the EEG

PaO_2	Hypoxia initially may produce EEG activation, followed by slowing or electrical silence
$PaCO_2$	Hypocarbia: EEG slowing Mild hypercarbia: increased frequency Severe hypercarbia: decreased frequency and amplitude
Temperature	Hypothermia: progressive slowing Electrical silence at 15°C–20°C
Sensory stimulation	EEG activation

opioids, and low-dose isoflurane (maximum 0.25% end-tidal concentration). Seizure activity is provoked with agents or techniques that lower the seizure threshold (methohexital, alfentanil, hyperventilation).

In noncooperative patients and children, likely areas of epileptic foci are identified prior to the craniotomy. "Grids and strips" of electrodes embedded in a matrix are implanted into the cortex, and ECoG is performed after the surgery.

Although ECoG is the "gold standard" used to define epileptogenic zones, newer technologies using structural MRI and scalp EEG to integrate information and define first principal vectors have proven to be a promising noninvasive approach to locating epileptogenic zones.

Evoked potentials

Somatosensory evoked potentials

Somatosensory evoked potentials (SSEPs) monitor the integrity of the sensory pathways of the spinal cord. The waves of evoked potentials are thought to represent potentials from specific neural generators. A peripheral stimulus is applied to a distal nerve – usually the median or posterior tibial nerve – and the cephalad progression of the stimulus is monitored along the popliteal fossa, lumbar spine, cervical spine, and cortex. The amplitude of the cortical responses is very small ($0.1–20\ \mu V$) and difficult to discern from background bioelectrical activity (EEG, electrocardiogram, muscle activity) and extraneous electrical activity in the room, such as infusion pumps and blood warmers. However, this background noise is eliminated by the averaging process.

The individual peaks in the waveform of sensory evoked potentials are described by:

- Polarity (negative, positive)
- Poststimulus latency (ms)
- Peak-to-peak amplitude (μV or nV)
- Distance separating neural generators and recording electrodes (near-field, far-field)

Compromise or injury to a neurologic pathway is manifested by an increase in latency and/or decrease in amplitude of evoked potential waveforms. In general, it must be stressed that because most anesthetics affect evoked potential monitoring, it is very important to maintain constant anesthetic drug levels so that changes seen in the monitoring can be seen as a reflection of possible neurologic damage. Specifically, bolus administration of intravenous agents and step changes in inspired agent concentration should be avoided, especially during parts of the surgery when neurologic injury might occur. High concentrations of end-tidal inhalational agents essentially eliminate cortical evoked potentials (SSEPs or visual evoked potentials [VEPs]). Newer inhalational agents, such as desflurane and sevoflurane, may permit higher inhaled concentrations during electrophysiologic monitoring than older agents. In general, volatile agents cause a dose-dependent increase in latency and a decrease in amplitude of cortical SSEPs or VEPs.

Many intravenous agents, such as narcotic infusions, propofol, ketamine, dexmedetomidine, and methohexital alter SSEPs less than volatile anesthetics or nitrous oxide.

Motor evoked potentials

Motor evoked potentials (MEPs) may be produced by direct (epidural) or indirect (transosseous) stimulation of the brain or spinal cord. Following transcranial stimulation, the signal descends through motor pathways located in the corticospinal tract of the spinal cord. The signal is localized primarily in the pyramidal tracts and can be recorded from the spinal cord, peripheral nerves, and muscle using conventional electromyographic (EMG) and evoked potential techniques. Stimulation of the motor cortex elicits contralateral peripheral nerve signals, EMG signals, or limb movements. Transosseous activation of motor neurons is accomplished by either electrical or magnetic stimulation. Transcranial electrical stimulation is achieved by delivering brief high-voltage pulses through scalp electrodes. Transcranial magnetic stimulation is produced by placing a magnetic coil over the motor cortex. With either electrical or magnetic stimulation, it is possible for repetitive stimulation to induce epileptic activity, neural damage, and cognitive or memory dysfunction. In patients with seizures, skull fractures, implanted metallic devices, or pulmonary artery catheters, this technique should be used with caution.

In addition, it is very important to make sure that a soft bite block is in place orally to prevent injury to the patient's tongue and teeth during MEP stimulation. MEPs are particularly useful in monitoring for surgically induced damage during scoliosis surgery or resection of cerebral tumors. Myogenic MEP monitoring can detect ventral horn ischemia during aortic reconstruction (Tables 29.3 and 29.4).

Physiologic changes in systemic blood pressure, PaO_2, $PaCO_2$, and temperature may alter evoked potentials. Systemic hypotension below levels of cerebral autoregulation produces progressive decreases in amplitude of evoked potentials.

Wake-up test

The purpose of the wake-up test is to monitor voluntary motor function of the lower extremities once the vertebrae have been distracted during scoliosis surgery. This test was frequently used in scoliosis surgery but now is generally reserved for cases in which there is a decrease or loss of evoked potentials after excessive retraction during surgery. The wake-up test involves gradually lightening the anesthetic depth while maintaining adequate analgesia, to the point at which the patient can respond to verbal commands such as "squeeze my hands" or "wiggle your toes." The patient needs to be educated about the wake-up test prior to surgery, including reassurance about not feeling any pain during the test and very small likelihood of intraoperative awareness.

During the actual wake-up test, it is important to remember that patients with idiopathic scoliosis generally are young, healthy, and strong. Therefore, some anesthesiologists

Table 29.3. Evoked potentials monitoring

Monitoring	Technique	Anesthetic considerations
SSEPs	Evaluation of functional integrity of ascending sensory pathways by somatosensory stimulation	A significant change of SSEPs is considered if the amplitude is reduced by 50% from baseline in response to surgical manipulation. TIVA may be preferred over inhalational agent anesthesia. End-tidal concentrations of 0.6 MAC of volatile agent are compatible with satisfactory readings. Nitrous oxide in combination with a volatile anesthetic produces profound depression unless total MAC < 1.0.
VEPs	Evaluation of functional integrity of ascending sensory pathways by visual stimulation	TIVA may be preferred over inhalational agent anesthesia. End-tidal concentrations of 0.5 MAC of volatile agent are compatible with satisfactory readings. VEPs tend to be more sensitive than SSEPs to the effect of inhalational anesthetics. Nitrous oxide in combination with a volatile anesthetic produces profound depression.
BAEPs	Evaluation of functional integrity of ascending sensory pathways by auditory stimulation at the brainstem	BAEPs are less vulnerable than SSEPs or VEPs to anesthetic influences. Most anesthetic regimens are compatible. Increase of latency with minimal amplitude effects. An increase in latency of >1 ms is considered clinically significant. Large step of inhalational agent increases (>0.5 MAC) should be avoided during critical periods.
MEPs	Evaluation of functional integrity of descending motor pathways	MEPs are extremely sensitive to volatile agents, but less so to nitrous oxide. Benzodiazepines, barbiturates, and propofol produce marked depression of myogenic MEPs. Fentanyl, etomidate, and ketamine have little or no effect. Muscle relaxants affect the recorded EMG response by depressing myoneural transmission but may be used as a continuous infusion maintaining 1 or 2 twitches.

BAEPs, brainstem auditory evoked potentials; MAC, minimum alveolar concentration; TIVA, total intravenous anesthesia.

administer a small dose of nondepolarizing muscle relaxant (i.e., 0.015 mg/kg of vecuronium) just before the test to mildly weaken the patient. It is important to inform the neurophysiologist if any muscle relaxants are given. It is advisable to have an assistant, in addition to the anesthesiologist, at the head of the bed just before the test and to have an additional assistant under the drapes viewing the patient's feet. In general, volatile agents should be discontinued 20 minutes before the test and nitrous oxide discontinued 1 to 3 minutes before the test. If an infusion of methohexital or propofol was used, then it needs to be discontinued for a sufficient period. After the test is accomplished, the anesthesiologist can reanesthetize the patient with a small dose of an induction agent and/or midazolam. The induction agent must be given carefully considering that the patient might demonstrate hemodynamic changes such as hypotension in the setting of hypovolemia. In most cases, only a small amount of induction agent is needed to reinitiate general anesthesia. The anesthesiologist then must reassess the patient's positioning and padding because some patients move more than their hands and feet.

It is very important that the wake-up test is performed by an experienced anesthesiologist, because an uncontrolled wake-up test may lead to inadvertent extubation of the trachea as well as disconnection of arterial and venous catheters and patient injury.

Table 29.4. Effect of intravenous agents on evoked potentials

Agent	Effect
Propofol	Increases latency and decreases amplitude of SSEPs; decreases amplitude of VEPs
Etomidate	Increases latency and amplitude of cortical SSEPs; increases latency of VEPs
Thiopental	Induction dose may increase latency and decrease amplitude of SSEPs; increases latency and decreases amplitude of VEPs Increasing doses result in dose-dependent increase in latency and decrease in amplitude of cortical SSEPs and progressive increases in latency in BAEPs
Pentobarbital	Increases latency and decreases amplitude of SSEPs and VEPs
Ketamine	Increases latency and amplitude of SSEPs; increases latency and decreases amplitude of VEPs
Midazolam	No change or increase in latency and decrease of amplitude of SSEPs
Diazepam	No change or increase in latency and decrease of amplitude of SSEPs; decreases amplitude of VEPs
Opioids	Minimal change in SSEP waveforms

BAEPs, brainstem auditory evoked potentials.

Table 29.5. ICP monitoring techniques

Method	Technique	Advantages	Disadvantages
Intraventricular catheters (standard)	Small scalp incision Small burr hole through skull Insertion of a soft nonreactive plastic catheter into the lateral ventricle, connection to transducer	Relatively reliable measurement of ICP Allows CSF drainage and compliance measurement	Occlusion of tubing may obliterate recording Ventricle is difficult to locate in the setting of brain swelling Brain injury is possible during passage of catheter Risk of hematoma and infection of catheter
Subdural–subarachnoid bolts or catheters	Hollow screw fixed into the skull with the tip passing through the incised dura	No brain tissue penetration or knowledge of ventricular position May be placed in any skull location with avoidance of venous sinuses	Occlusion of tubing may obliterate recording Brain tissue may obstruct the tip of the bolt Risk of infection, epidural bleeding, or focal seizures if bolt is positioned too deeply
Epidural transducers	Placement of epidural catheter with a pressure-sensitive membrane or a Numoto pressure switch (Ladd transducer)	Lower risk of brain infection because of extradural placement	Difficult placement in potential space Risk of bleeding No possibility for compliance testing or CSF drainage
Intraparenchymal fiber-optic devices	Fiber-optic catheter introduced within cortical gray matter	Direct measurement of brain tissue pressure Easy insertion Small diameter Less disruptive of brain tissue Lower risk of infection (no fluid column) New fiber-optic ICP monitors allow measurement of local CBF, PO_2, PO_2, PCO_2, pH, and other metabolic markers	No possibility of calibration in situ No possibility of compliance testing or CSF drainage

CSF, cerebrospinal fluid.

Cranial nerve monitoring

Potential injury to the cranial nerves may occur during posterior fossa and lower brainstem procedures. The integrity of these cranial nerves can be preserved by monitoring the EMG potential of cranial nerves with motor components (CN V, VII, IX, X, XI, and XII). Both spontaneous and triggered muscle activity can be recorded. With accidental surgical contact, spontaneous neural activity changes into phasic "bursts" or "train" activity, which allows the surgeon to realize that he or she is in danger of damaging the cranial nerve. It is recommended that muscle relaxants not be administered during cranial nerve monitoring.

Intracranial pressure monitoring

Continuous intracranial pressure (ICP) monitoring has been used to guide the perioperative management of patients with head injury, large brain tumors, ruptured intracranial aneurysms, cerebrovascular occlusive disease, and hydrocephalus (Table 29.5). With continuous ICP monitoring, one can optimize cerebral perfusion pressure, which is critical in the treatment of brain hemorrhage, swelling, and herniation. Another important indication for ICP monitoring is to detect intracranial hypertension during neurosurgical procedures.

Transcranial Doppler ultrasound

Transcranial Doppler ultrasound (TCD), used for clinical imaging of intracranial vasculature, uses a 2-MHz range-gated probe. This probe is placed over low-density bone regions of the skull, and the beam is focused on the appropriate vessel, usually between the junction of the middle cerebral artery and the anterior cerebral artery. The blood flow of the vessel produces a Doppler shift proportional to the blood velocity, and thus a continuous assessment of systolic, diastolic, and mean flow velocities is possible. TCD primarily is a technique to measure relative changes in blood flow rather than a method to determine the actual blood flow. TCD can be used to measure CO_2 reactivity and autoregulation and to estimate cerebral perfusion pressures by using the pulsatile index: systolic velocity – diastolic velocity/mean velocity. TCD is used to identify patients with vasospasm, hyperemia, emboli, stenosis, abnormal collateral flow, and inadequate CBF.

Cerebral oxygenation metabolism

Several monitoring modalities are available to prevent ischemia by measuring the cerebral oxygen saturation during cardiac and vascular surgery (Table 29.6).

Table 29.6. Cerebral oxygen/metabolism monitoring techniques

Monitoring method	Technique	Anesthetic considerations
Brain tissue oxygenation	A multiparameter sensor is available for measuring brain tissue PO_2, PCO_2, pH, and temperature using a combined electrode-fiber-optic system	The placement of the sensor requires insertion into the cortex tissue under direct visualization.
Jugular bulb venous oximetry	Measurement of $SjVO_2$ through a percutaneous retrograde cannulation of the internal jugular vein using a catheter with embedded optical fibers. Normal $SjVO_2$ is 60%–70%.	Increases in $SjVO_2$ indicate relative hyperemia as a result of reduced metabolic requirement (comatose or brain-dead patient) or excessive flow (severe hypercapnia). A value <50% reflects increased oxygen extraction and potential risk of ischemic injury. This also may be caused by increased metabolic demand (fever, seizure) or by an absolute reduction in flow. A major limitation is the inability to detect focal ischemia.
Transcranial oximetry	NIRS is a noninvasive optical method for monitoring cerebral regional oxygenation. It reflects off oxy- and deoxyhemoglobin and allows quantitative assessment of those based on the absorption of light at several wavelengths. It is used as a monitor during carotid endarterectomy, head injury, and subarachnoid hemorrhage.	Major limitations include intersubject variability, variable optical path length, potential contamination from extracranial blood, and lack of a definable threshold. It can be used only as a trend monitor. As a bilateral monitor, it is useful to detect regional ischemia during carotid endarterectomy and temporary clip application during intracranial aneurysm surgery.

Cerebral oximetry

Near-infrared spectroscopy (NIRS) provides a noninvasive assessment of the cerebral intravascular oxyhemoglobin, deoxyhemoglobin, and mitochondrial cytochrome aa3 oxygen levels by measuring the ability of these chromophores to absorb near-infrared light. The pathway of light photons in mammalian tissue is characterized by light attenuation as photons are absorbed by tissues and by scattering of the pathways as the photons are deflected from the different types of tissues. NIRS technology takes advantage of this by having the light emitter and detector on the same plane and measuring light that takes an elliptical pathway. In experimental settings, NIRS has been used along with other monitoring modalities to assess O_2 delivery and extraction, cerebral blood volume, CBF, and the redox state of the brain.

Most medical uses of NIRS center on its ability to measure relative changes in oxygen extraction in the total blood volume in a small brain area. Approximately 75% of the blood volume in the brain is venous, thus measures of the oxyhemoglobin content of this blood volume gives an estimate of venous oxygen saturation and thus extraction. This modality is called *regional cerebral oximetry* (rSO2; INVOS, Somanetics Corporation, Troy, MI), and it is currently being used in cardiac and neurosurgical as well as pediatric critical care units.

Brain tissue oxygen monitors

Brain tissue oxygen monitors are catheters inserted through an intracranial bolt that measures O_2, brain tissue temperature, and ICP. The interstitial partial pressure of oxygen in brain tissue ($P_{bt}O_2$) depends on the CBF and arteriovenous difference in oxygen tension, thus these types of monitors may be a more sensitive tool in assessing cerebral hypoxia. Intensivists can individualize the care of a patient with traumatic brain injury (TBI) because the $P_{bt}O_2$ is dependent not only on CBF but also on hemoglobin and lung function.

Jugular venous bulb oximetry

Continuous jugular venous bulb oximetry ($Sjvo_2$) provides a means to indirectly assess the brain's ability to extract and metabolize oxygen. Cerebral oxygen delivery depends on CBF and arterial oxygen content. In healthy patients, the extraction ratio between arterial and venous blood remains constant because CBF increases when cerebral oxygen requirements increase. However, >50% of patients with TBI exhibit evidence of cerebral dysautoregulation and thus are at risk for localized or generalized cerebral hypoxia. A study comparing brain tissue oxygen Pao_2 levels with $Sjvo_2$ found that both monitoring methods provided complementary information and that neither method alone identified all episodes of ischemia. Brain tissue monitors are capable of monitoring only a local area, whereas $SjVO_2$ monitors give a broader picture of the overall oxygen extraction. Because of difficulties in positioning the probe in a retrograde fashion from the internal jugular vein, these probes are used rarely in a clinical operating room setting.

Summary

Neuromonitoring during anesthesia and critical care allows for more insightful therapeutic management of patients who have had nonsurgical brain injury or who are at risk for neurologic injury during neurosurgical and back procedures. More studies are needed to determine which monitoring modalities or which combinations of monitoring modalities lead to optimal outcomes during the perioperative and critical care periods. It is possible that in the future, some of these techniques will become standard of care, but it also is important for outcome studies to demonstrate a therapeutic advantage before they are adopted as standard of care.

Suggested readings

Banoub M, Tetzlaff JE, Schubert A. Pharmacologic and physiologic influences affecting sensory evoked potentials: implications for perioperative monitoring. *Anesthesiology* 2003; 99:716–737.

Botes K, Le Roux DA, Van Marle J. Cerebral monitoring during carotid endarterectomy – a comparison between electroencephalography, transcranial cerebral oximetry and carotid stump pressure. *S Afr J Surg* 2007; 45:43–46.

Cheng MA, Theard MA, Tempelhoff R. Anesthesia for carotid endarterectomy: a survey. *J Neurosurg Anesthesiol* 1997; 9:211–216.

Cortinez LI, Delfino AE, Fuentes R, Munoz HR. Performance of the cerebral state index during increasing levels of propofol anesthesia: a comparison with the bispectral index. *Anesth Analg* 2007; 104:605–610.

Cuadra SA, Zwerling JS, Feuerman M, et al. Cerebral oximetry monitoring during carotid endarterectomy: effect of carotid clamping and shunting. *Vasc Endovasc Surg* 2003; 37:407–413.

Debatisse D, Pralong E, Dehdashti AR, Regli L. Simultaneous multilobar electrocorticography (mEcoG) and scalp electroencephalography (scalp EEG) during intracranial vascular surgery: a new approach in neuromonitoring. *Clin Neurophysiol* 2005; 116:2734–2740.

Edmonds HL Jr, Ganzel BL, Austin EH 3rd. Cerebral oximetry for cardiac and vascular surgery. *Semin Cardiothorac Vasc Anesth* 2004; 8:147–166.

Edmonds HL Jr, Paloheimo M. Computerized monitoring of the EMG and EEG during anesthesia. An evaluation of the anesthesia and brain activity monitor (ABM). *Int J Clin Monit Comput* 1985; 1:201–210.

Edmonds HL Jr, Rodriguez RA, Audenaert SM, Austin EH 3rd, et al. The role of neuromonitoring in cardiovascular surgery. *J Cardiothorac Vasc Anesth* 1996; 10:15–23.

Florence G, Guerit JM, Gueguen B. Electroencephalography (EEG) and somatosensory evoked potentials (SEP) to prevent cerebral ischaemia in the operating room. *Neurophysiol Clin* 2004; 34:17–32.

Gopinath SP, Valadka AB, Uzura M, Robertson CS. Comparison of jugular venous oxygen saturation and brain tissue Po2 as monitors of cerebral ischemia after head injury. *Crit Care Med* 1999; 27:2337–2345.

Lotto ML, Banoub M, Schubert A. Effects of anesthetic agents and physiologic changes on intraoperative motor evoked potentials. *J Neurosurg Anesthesiol* 2004; 16:32–42.

McGrath BJ, Matjasko MJ. Anesthesia and head trauma. *New Horiz* 1995; 3:523–533.

Moehle DA. Neuromonitoring in the cardiopulmonary bypass surgical patient: clinical applications. *J Extra Corpor Technol* 2001; 33:126–134.

Murkin JM. Perioperative detection of brain oxygenation and clinical outcomes in cardiac surgery. *Semin Cardiothorac Vasc Anesth* 2004; 8:13–14.

Niparko JK, Kileny PR, Kemink JL, et al. Neurophysiologic intraoperative monitoring: II. Facial nerve function. *Am J Otol* 1989; 10:55–61.

Peterson DO, Drummond JC, Todd MM. Effects of halothane, enflurane, isoflurane, and nitrous oxide on somatosensory evoked potentials in humans. *Anesthesiology* 1986; 65:35–40.

Rosenthal G, Hemphill JC, Sorani M, et al. The role of lung function in brain tissue oxygenation following traumatic brain injury. *J Neurosurg* 2008; 108:59–65.

Samra SK, Dy EA, Welch K, et al. Evaluation of a cerebral oximeter as a monitor of cerebral ischemia during carotid endarterectomy. *Anesthesiology* 2000; 93:964–970.

Schaffranietz L, Heinke W. The effect of different ventilation regimes on jugular venous oxygen saturation in elective neurosurgical patients. *Neurol Res* 1998; 20(Suppl 1):S66–S70.

Smith MJ, Stiefel MF, Magge S, et al. Packed red blood cell transfusion increases local cerebral oxygenation. *Crit Care Med* 2005; 33:1104–1108.

Soriano SG, McCann ME, Laussen PC. Neuroanesthesia. Innovative techniques and monitoring. *Anesthesiol Clin North Am* 2002; 20:137–151.

Vets P, ten Broecke P, Adriaensen H, et al. Cerebral oximetry in patients undergoing carotid endarterectomy: preliminary results. *Acta Anaesthesiol Belg* 2004; 55:215–220.

Williams IM, Vohra R, Farrell A, et al. Cerebral oxygen saturation, transcranial Doppler ultrasonography and stump pressure in carotid surgery. *Br J Surg* 1994; 81:960–964.

Chapter 30

Intraoperative awareness

Scott D. Kelley

One of the fundamental goals in providing general anesthesia is to render the patient unconscious and oblivious to the events of the surgical procedure. If the anesthetic state becomes inadequate, a patient may regain consciousness and potentially form memories of the intraoperative period. This complication of anesthesia – intraoperative awareness with recall – has been recognized for decades, and it recently has become the focus of concerted efforts to reduce its frequency. Anesthesia strategies can be developed to minimize the occurrence and consequences of intraoperative awareness.

Incidence and etiology

Several prospective investigations documented the prevalence of intraoperative awareness with recall at approximately 0.1% to 0.2%; that is, it occurs in one in 500 to 1000 patients undergoing general anesthesia. These incidence measures have used a specific and simple structured interview to determine whether intraoperative memories have been formed. Patient recall of intraoperative events may be delayed; consequently, several interviews during the first 7 days will detect a greater occurrence of awareness. Initial interviews in the postanesthesia care unit likely detect only two-thirds of awareness episodes. The incidence of awareness determined using a patient interview approach may be substantially lower than the frequency of spontaneous patient complaints of awareness. In one survey of a large anesthesia practice, a quality assessment survey detected a much lower incidence of awareness based on patient feedback.

Based on clinical experience and investigation, the incidence of intraoperative awareness is greater in a recognized spectrum of patient types, surgical procedures, and anesthetic techniques (Table 30.1). In some of these clinical situations, such as emergency trauma surgery or a patient's cardiovascular status may preclude the administration of an adequate anesthetic dose to produce unconsciousness and suppress memory formation, and can increase the risk of awareness tenfold, up to 1%. Intravenous anesthesia may lead to a higher incidence of awareness due to the inability to monitor anesthetic drug levels with the equivalent of end-tidal agent analysis. General anesthesia provided solely by the combination of nitrous oxide and opioid administration has a higher incidence of awareness. Administration of neuromuscular blocking agents is associated with an increased risk of awareness, presumably because these

Table 30.1. Potential risk factors for awareness

Surgical procedures	Cardiac, trauma, emergency surgical procedures; emergent cesarean section
Patient characteristics	Substance use or abuse Chronic pain patients on high doses of opioids ASA physical status 4 or 5 Limited hemodynamic reserve
Anesthetic history	Anticipated or history of difficult intubation Previous episode of awareness Total intravenous anesthesia Nitrous oxide–opioid anesthesia
Anesthetic management	Planned use of neuromuscular blocking agents during maintenance phase Reduced anesthetic doses during paralysis

agents mask somatic signs of inadequate anesthesia. The early period of a general anesthetic, particularly in cases involving endotracheal intubation, is a high-risk period for intraoperative awareness. During management of anticipated or unexpected difficult intubation, the focus and attention of securing the airway may allow the anesthetic level to decrease and permit consciousness and recall. Similarly, the acute increase in anesthetic requirement with surgical incision represents another high-risk period for the occurrence of awareness.

By definition, intraoperative awareness occurs when an inadequate anesthetic effect permits a patient to regain consciousness, permitting memory formation. Inadequate anesthesia may result from an inadequate dose selected by the clinician, a failure (mechanical and/or human error) of the anesthetic delivery system to deliver the intended dose of anesthesia, or potentially, unrecognized resistance to anesthetic agents. The last etiology has been particularly difficult to characterize. To date, no genetic link to anesthetic requirement has been identified. In contrast, however, a patient's medication and substance use may alter the anesthetic dose required to maintain consciousness.

Consequences of intraoperative awareness

The consequences of intraoperative awareness are quite varied, ranging from tragic and horrific patient experiences to episodes that appear to have no sequelae. In one large prospective investigation, the occurrence of awareness was the greatest risk factor for patient dissatisfaction with anesthesia care. In addition, a detailed follow-up of patients who experienced intraoperative awareness demonstrated that awareness may result in substantial psychological injury. During the period of intraoperative awareness, a patient may experience varying degrees of sensation (e.g., audible, tactile, pain, paralytic) as well as acute psychological symptoms (e.g., fear, panic, helplessness). The variety of these experiences and the duration of the awareness episodes likely are factors that contribute to the severity of psychological injury following awareness. The psychological injury may be transient and minor but also has been documented to result in substantial permanent long-term psychological disturbance, classified as posttraumatic stress disorder.

The occurrence of intraoperative awareness may be the basis for medicolegal action against the anesthesia professional who cared for the patient. The American Society of Anesthesiologists (ASA) Closed Claims Project has examined the settlement history for awareness claims in the database. In the most recent report, claims involving anesthesia awareness accounted for approximately 3% of cases. Payment was made in 46% of claims, and the median payment was $41,210 (range, $3960–$1,016,470). Although the *frequency* of payments is similar to that of other general anesthesia claims, the *median* payment is

significantly less than that for other anesthesia claims. Several experts believe the recent focus on intraoperative awareness may increase the likelihood of medicolegal claims; however, it will be several years before this concern is reflected in the Closed Claims Project.

Preventing intraoperative awareness

The continued occurrence of awareness in modern anesthesia practice – in both high-risk and routine cases – has prompted efforts to develop practice strategies to prevent awareness. In the past 5 years, several anesthesia professional societies around the world, including the ASA, issued guidelines for their members regarding awareness. In addition, the Joint Commission for Accreditation of Healthcare Organizations (JCAHO) issued a Sentinel Event Alert to hospitals encouraging them to develop policies to prevent and manage intraoperative awareness. Common themes from these approaches include appropriate patient assessment and risk stratification, intraoperative use of routine clinical monitoring techniques, specific consideration of brain function and anesthetic agent monitoring in select cases, and postoperative assessment of patients to detect and manage awareness, if it occurred (Fig. 30.1).

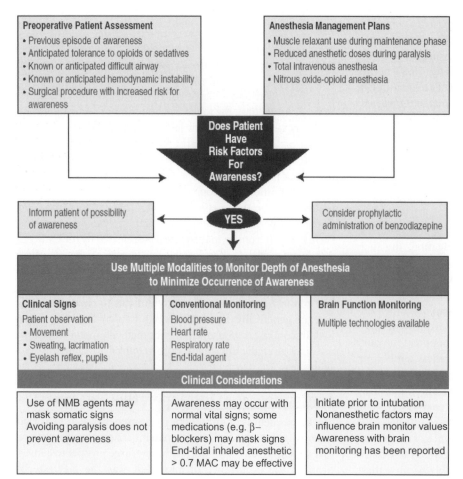

Figure 30.1. Approach to avoiding awareness.

Preoperative period

Preoperative patient assessment should include identification of patient and procedural factors known to increase the risk of awareness. If a patient is at higher risk for awareness, this should be communicated during the informed consent process. Preoperative administration of benzodiazepine – despite its known amnestic effect – should not be considered protection against intraoperative awareness. In addition, preanesthesia checkout of the anesthetic machine and other drug delivery devices is essential to ensure the delivery of the intended anesthetic dose.

Clinical monitoring techniques

The routine clinical monitoring of the patient's vital signs and responses is important to assess the adequacy of the anesthetic state. However, intraoperative awareness may be particularly difficult to recognize based on routine clinical monitoring. A common assumption is that other indicators of inadequate anesthesia will alert the anesthesia clinician to a patient regaining consciousness. However, based on detailed reviews of anesthesia records from cases of intraoperative awareness, most patients did not exhibit hemodynamic signs of hypertension or tachycardia that would indicate inadequate anesthesia. As described earlier, neuromuscular blocking agents can prevent a patient from exhibiting somatic movement as a sign of inadequate anesthesia.

Brain function monitoring

Brain function monitoring devices provide anesthesia clinicians with another method to assess anesthetic effect. These devices use the patient's electroencephalogram (EEG) and/or auditory evoked responses as biological signals of anesthetic effect. To improve the utility of these devices, the manufacturers developed signal processing techniques and algorithms to translate raw EEG waveforms into numeric indicators of anesthetic effect. Typically, these devices scale anesthetic depth from a dimensionless score of 100, indicating the "awake" state, to 0, indicating maximal anesthetic effect on the EEG. As a class, these devices are very accurate in distinguishing an awake patient from an "unconscious" one. Consequently, the utility of this monitoring modality has been investigated as a measure to minimize intraoperative awareness.

Although other devices are available, only the bispectral index (BIS) monitor has been used in prospective trials to date. Two large trials studied the incidence of awareness when BIS monitoring was added as an adjunct to routine patient care and management. In a prospective investigation of 4945 patients undergoing routine anesthesia including neuromuscular blocking administration, addition of BIS monitoring led to a 78% reduction in the incidence of awareness compared with a historical cohort of 7826 patients. In a more rigorous prospective randomized controlled trial enrolling 2463 patients at high risk for awareness, the addition of BIS monitoring resulted in an 82% reduction in the incidence of awareness.

Anesthetic agent monitoring

The broad availability of end-tidal anesthetic agent analysis allows anesthesia clinicians to accurately measure the effective dose of delivered volatile anesthetic. In addition, the well-appreciated concept of volatile anesthetic potency, measured by minimum alveolar concentration (MAC), offers the ability to determine anesthetic requirements such as MAC_{awake}. A recent prospective trial measured the incidence of awareness in 1941 high-risk patients randomly assigned to undergo a BIS-guided anesthesia protocol (maintaining BIS between 40 and 60) or an end-tidal anesthetic-guided protocol (maintain 0.7–1.3 MAC). There were two cases of awareness in each treatment group, substantially less than would be expected in high-risk patients. This study did not find a difference in the incidence of awareness between the BIS-guided and MAC-guided anesthetic requirement techniques. However, the study may have been underpowered to detect a difference between the interventions.

Currently, anesthetic agent monitoring is available only for volatile anesthetic agents and nitrous oxide. Real-time measurement of intravenous anesthetic concentration is not available. There are no data available comparing the effectiveness of target-controlled infusions of propofol as a method to reduce awareness with that of conventional propofol infusion regimens. During anesthesia involving total intravenous anesthesia, brain function monitoring may provide additional confirmation of anesthetic delivery and effect.

Postoperative assessment and management

Early detection of awareness may minimize patient consequences. Although the Joint Commission recommends that all patients be assessed to detect the occurrence of awareness, other organizations suggest that only patients at increased risk need to be assessed. If intraoperative conditions (e.g., mechanical failure of anesthetic delivery, prolonged cessation of anesthetic agent administration due to hypotension) suggest an increased likelihood of awareness, the patient should be assessed as soon as possible. A structured approach modified from Brice is the easiest to use: What is the last thing you remember before you went to sleep? What is the first thing you remember when you woke up? Do you remember anything in between? Did you have any dreams? All patients who report intraoperative awareness should be followed up by the anesthesia team. It is important to express empathy with the patient's experience and concerns. The anesthesia team is in the best position to determine whether a patient's report of awareness represents intraoperative recall or perhaps recall during emergence, during extubation, or at a later time point. A discussion of the possible etiology or risk factors for awareness should be presented. Because of the potential for psychological injury, additional consultations should be obtained regarding the best course of counseling and other follow-up. Awareness cases should be discussed at departmental quality assurance meetings to increase efforts to avoid them in the future.

Suggested readings

Avidan MS, Zhang L, Burnside BA, et al. Anesthesia awareness and the bispectral index. *N Engl J Med* 2008; 358:1097–1108.

Ekman A, Lindholm M, Lennmarken C, Sandin R. Reduction in the incidence of awareness using BIS monitoring. *Acta Anaesthesiol Scand* 2004; 48:20–26.

Ghoneim MM. Awareness during anesthesia. *Anesthesiology* 2000; 92:597–602.

Kent C, Domino K. Awareness: practice, standards, and the law. *Best Pract Res Clin Anaesthesiol* 2007; 21:369–383.

Lennmarken C, Bildfors K, Enlund G, et al. Victims of awareness. *Acta Anaesthesiol Scand* 2002; 46:229–231.

Myles P, Leslie K, McNeil J, et al. Bispectral index monitoring to prevent awareness during anaesthesia: the B-Aware randomised controlled trial. *Lancet* 2004; 363:1757–1763.

Myles PS, Williams DL, Hendrata M, et al. Patient satisfaction after anaesthesia and surgery: results of a prospective survey of 10,811 patients. *Brit J Anaesth* 2000; 84:6–10.

Practice advisory for intraoperative awareness and brain function monitoring: a report by the American Society of Anesthesiologists Task Force on Intraoperative Awareness. *Anesthesiology* 2006; 104:847–864.

Preventing, and managing the impact of, anesthesia awareness. *Sentinel Event Alert* 2004; 1–3.

Sandin RH, Enlund G, Samuelsson P, Lennmarken C. Awareness during anaesthesia: a prospective case study. *Lancet* 2000; 355:707–711.

Sebel P, Bowdle T, Ghoneim M, et al. The incidence of awareness during anesthesia: a multicenter United States study. *Anesth Analg* 2004; 99:833–839.

Part 5

Inhalation Anesthetics

James H. Philip, editor

Chapter

31 Inhalation anesthetics

Matthias Stopfkuchen-Evans, Lina M. Bolanos-Diaz, Alimorad G. Djalali, and Beverly K. Philip

The term *inhalation anesthetic* refers to anesthetics administered in a gaseous form. These include nitrous oxide (N_2O), a gas at room temperature, and the volatile anesthetics, which are nonflammable liquids at room temperature. Inhalation anesthetics are the most common drugs used for maintenance of general anesthesia because of their ease of administration and the ability to reliably monitor their effects with clinical signs and end-tidal concentration. This chapter presents the clinical pharmacology of commonly used and future inhaled anesthetics (Table 31.1).

Halothane
Physical properties

Halothane (2-bromo-2-chloro-1,1,1-trifluoroethane) is a halogenated alkane compound. It is colorless and pleasant smelling but unstable in light; therefore, it is packaged in amber bottles with thymol preservative. Halothane became popular as a nonflammable general anesthetic, replacing older, flammable volatile anesthetics such as diethyl ether and cyclopropane. Halothane is a potent bronchodilator and is the least expensive volatile anesthetic. Although it is still used in developing countries, especially for the inhalation induction of anesthesia in children, it is no longer available in the United States.

Biotransformation and toxicity

The MAC (minimum alveolar concentration; see Chapter 33) for halothane is 0.75%, and its blood/gas partition coefficient ($\lambda_{b/g}$) is 2.4. Approximately 25% of administered halothane is metabolized to trifluoroacetic acid (TFA), chloride, and bromide. The major metabolite in humans is TFA, formed from oxidative metabolism primarily by CYP2E1. The TFA metabolite also reacts with tissue proteins to form trifluoroacetylated protein adducts (discussed later in the chapter).

Nitrous oxide
Physical properties

N_2O is a colorless, odorless, nonflammable gas. Although nonflammable, N_2O will support combustion. The MAC is 105%; therefore, N_2O is frequently used in combination with other anesthetic agents. The blood/gas partition coefficient ($\lambda_{b/g}$) is

0.47, and with its lower solubility, N_2O has a very rapid uptake and elimination. N_2O also is analgesic and is commonly used for dental sedation/analgesia.

N_2O increases the volume of air-filled cavities, air bubbles in blood, and air-containing intestines. All air-filled spaces contain nitrogen, which has a very low blood/gas partition coefficient (0.014). Compared with nitrogen, N_2O is much more soluble and much more diffusible. When N_2O enters an air-filled cavity down a partial pressure gradient, nitrogen cannot leave the cavity as quickly as N_2O enters. Hence, the volume of, of the gas pressure in, the cavity increases until its N_2O partial pressure equals that in the blood that is perfusing it. There are several clincial scenarios when this effect is particularly undesirable. N_2O should not be used when a pneumothorax is suspected. N_2O added to trapped air in the skull after head trauma may lead to brain damage. An air embolus becomes more dangerous when N_2O is in the bloodstream. The common presence of intravascular air during cardiopulmonary bypass makes N_2O an undesirable agent for cardiac surgery. In abdominal procedures, N_2O may cause an increase in the volume of the gas-filled intestine, depending on the concentration and duration of N_2O administration and the composition of the bowel gas. If an ileus is present, the volume change may cause bowel ischemia and difficulty closing the abdomen. Breathing 70% to 80% N_2O and air may double the volume of the intestinal gas in approximately two hours. For elective abdominal surgery, this change may not be of any significance. Because diffusion coefficients of CO_2 and N_2O are similar, N_2O may be used during laparoscopic procedures using CO_2 for insufflation.

Biotransformation and toxicity

N_2O is minimally metabolized (0.004%), and during emergence almost all is eliminated by exhalation. It has a very low short-term toxicity. Long-term, intensive care unit use of N_2O has been associated with clinical sequelae of inhibition of methionine synthase. N_2O irreversibly oxidizes cobalamin, a cofactor (along with folic acid) for methionine synthase, thus impairing DNA synthesis and causing hyperhomocysteinemia. Bone marrow depression may occur after prolonged exposure. Symptoms of vitamin B_{12} deficiency, including sensory neuropathy, myelopathy, and encephalopathy, may develop after several days of exposure to N_2O anesthesia. Patients with heterozygous

Table 31.1.   Properties of inhalation agents

Parameter	Nitrous oxide	Isoflurane	Sevoflurane	Desflurane	Halothane
MAC	104	1.15	2.05	6.0	0.75
Vapor pressure[a]	39,000	240	160	664	244
Blood/gas pc	0.47	1.46	0.69	0.42	2.54
Brain/blood pc	1.1	1.6	1.7	1.3	1.9
Muscle/blood pc	1.2	2.9	3.1	2	3.4
Fat/blood pc	2.3	45	47.5	27	51
CO_2 absorbent stability	Yes	CO formation when dry	Compound A formation, heat production	CO formation when dry	CO formation when dry
Pungency	No	Yes	No	Yes	No

[a] vapor pressure in mm Hg at 20°C.
pc, partition coefficient; CO, carbon monoxide.

mutations in the gene encoding for methionine synthase or with vitamin B_{12} deficiency are at risk for acute hyperhomocysteinemia and neuropathy, even after a single exposure to N_2O for as few as 80 minutes.

Isoflurane
Physical properties

Isoflurane (2-chloro-2-[difluoromethoxy]-1,1,1-trifluoroethane) is a halogenated ether with a moderately high pungency that can irritate the respiratory system.

Biotransformation and toxicity

The MAC of isoflurane is 1.17%, and its blood/gas partition coefficient ($\lambda_{b/g}$) is 1.4. There has been controversy regarding the use of isoflurane in patients with coronary artery disease because of the possibility of "coronary steal," which is diversion of blood from areas of myocardium with inadequate perfusion to myocardium with more adequate perfusion. However, this has not been shown to be any clinical significance. Isoflurane exposure has been demonstrated to induce cognitive decline in mice. Exposure of cultured human cells to isoflurane has been reported to induce apoptosis as well as accumulation and aggregation of amyloid beta protein. However, no link between clinical exposure to isoflurane and cognitive decline or dementia in humans has been established.

Sevoflurane
Physical properties

Sevoflurane (2,2,2-trifluoro-1-[trifluoromethyl]ethyl fluoromethyl ether) is a sweet-smelling drug used for induction and maintenance of general anesthesia. Sevoflurane is the preferred agent for mask (inhalational) induction because of its low airway irritation; it also is a potent bronchodilator.

Biotransformation and toxicity

The MAC of sevoflurane is 2.05%, and its blood/gas partition coefficient ($\lambda_{b/g}$) is 0.65. Sevoflurane metabolites include fluoride (F^-), which has the potential to cause high-output renal failure. However, because of sevoflurane's low blood/gas solubility and its rapid elimination, fluoride concentrations fall very quickly after surgery and renal toxicity from fluoride does not occur. The interaction of sevoflurane with dry carbon dioxide absorbents produces a chemical toxic to rats called "*compound A.*"

Desflurane
Physical properties

Desflurane (2-[difluoromethoxy]-1,1,1,2-tetrafluoroethane) is structurally similar to isoflurane but differs in its substitution of a fluoride for isoflurane's single chloride atom. This change results in (1) low solubility in blood and tissues, allowing tissue levels to follow inhaled levels closely; (2) a decrease in potency; and (3) high vapor pressure. Desflurane boils at 22.8°C, which is near room temperature, requiring a unique anesthetic administration device that heats the desflurane liquid to 39°C (and <2 atm) to deliver desflurane as a vapor (Chapter 20).

Biotransformation and toxicity

Desflurane's MAC is 6.0%, and its blood/gas coefficient ($\lambda_{b/g}$) is 0.42. It is minimally metabolized. The interaction of desflurane with dry CO_2 absorbents produces carbon monoxide (possibly resulting in increased levels of blood carboxyhemoglobin). The major clinical drawbacks of desflurane are its airway pungency and cardiovascular reactivity.

Xenon

Xenon is a nonflammable, colorless, and odorless gas that does not irritate the respiratory tract. Xenon is a trace gas in atmospheric air, unlike all other inhaled anesthetics, and is not an environmental pollutant. Xenon has a low blood/gas partition coefficient (0.14), allowing rapid uptake and elimination. The MAC is 60% to 70%, which prohibits the use of overpressure as an induction technique.

Xenon is well tolerated for inhalation induction, producing unconsciousness with analgesia, a degree of muscle relaxation, and respiratory depression. It has minimal cardio-vascular effects. Xenon is not metabolized in the body and is eliminated rapidly via the lungs. It is nontoxic, not associated with allergic reactions, and stable in storage, with no interaction with alkali CO_2 absorbents. Xenon should not be used with rubber anesthesia circuits as there is a high loss through the rubber. The high price of xenon has prevented its use in clinical anesthetic practice. Xenon, therefore, needs to be delivered in a closed circuit. The accumulation of nitrogen is a significant problem within the closed circuit and necessitates flushing, which in turn increases gas expenditure.

Clinical effects of inhalational anesthetics

Central nervous system

Volatile inhalation agents produce general anesthesia, which comprises a lack of awareness and lack of physical and physiologic response to surgical stimulation as primary therapeutic effects. All volatile inhalation agents produce a dose-dependent increase in cerebral blood flow through vasodilation, increased intracranial pressure (ICP), and decreased cerebral metabolic rate of oxygen (CMR_{O_2}). Below 1 MAC, the decrease in CMR_{O_2} effect dominates; above 1 MAC, the cerebral vasodilatory effect dominates. Hypocapnia, opioids, and barbiturates can attenuate the increase in ICP if needed in patients with intracranial lesions or head injuries. Because of their vasodilator properties, volatile anesthetics diminish cerebral blood flow autoregulation. Halothane is the most potent cerebral vasodilator, and isoflurane is the least potent. Volatile anesthetics cause predictable EEG changes. During induction, volatile anesthetics increase the frequency and amplitude of EEG, which may relate to the excitement phase (stage II). As 1 MAC is reached, the EEG begins to slow, and then becomes isoelectric at 1.5 to 2 MAC. Volatile anesthetics also affect evoked potentials, increasing latency and decreasing amplitude.

Cardiovascular system

Volatile anesthetics cause a concentration-dependent decrease in mean arterial blood pressure by a variety of mechanisms. All volatile anesthetics decrease systemic vascular resistance (SVR), with halothane having the least effect on SVR. Halothane decreases blood pressure mainly by decreasing cardiac contractility, more so than do isoflurane, desflurane, or sevoflurane. In contrast, isoflurane, sevoflurane, and desflurane decrease blood pressure primarily by decreasing SVR. Volatile anesthetics have a protective effect on the myocardium called *anesthetic preconditioning*.

Volatile anesthetics increase heart rate as a compensatory response to the decrease in blood pressure, except for halothane, which blunts the baroreceptor reflex. With desflurane, a rapid increase in inspired concentration may lead to a rapid increase in heart rate and/or blood pressure, likely as a result of sympathetic stimulation. This effect may be attenuated by the prior administration of a β-blocker or moderate doses of opioid. All inhaled anesthetics, especially isoflurane and desflurane, prolong the QT interval.

N_2O is a mild negative inotrope, slightly reducing contractility by inhibiting transsarcolemmal Ca^{+2} flux. It does not change heart rate, it maintains SVR by increasing sympathetic tone, and it causes vasoconstriction of epicardial coronary arteries. N_2O further increases pulmonary vascular resistance in patients with preexisting pulmonary hypertension. Unlike other agents, halothane sensitizes the heart to the arrhythmogenic effects of epinephrine, predisposing to arrhythmias. Combined use of halothane with local anesthetics containing epinephrine should be limited to epinephrine doses <1.5 μg/kg. Beta-blockers and calcium channel blockers may exacerbate the myocardial depression induced by halothane. Halothane also slows sinoatrial conduction, which may result in junctional rhythms; adults are more susceptible than children.

Respiratory system

Inhaled anesthetics produce concentration-dependent depression of respiratory drive via depression of the ventilatory centers in the medulla and reduction of intercostal muscle function. The result is a rapid, shallow breathing pattern, even in the absence of surgical stimulation, with decreased tidal volume and a compensatory increase in respiratory rate. However, this compensation may be insufficient to maintain adequate minute ventilation. Resting $PaCO_2$ is elevated, as is the apneic threshold. Ventilatory responses to arterial hypoxemia and hypercapnia are diminished by inhaled anesthetics. Desflurane, more than isoflurane, can cause airway irritation during induction, resulting in coughing, breath holding, laryngospasm, and salivation. Among the other volatile anesthetics, the order of airway irritation is isoflurane > halothane > sevoflurane. Halothane, sevoflurane, and isoflurane are potent bronchodilators, while desflurane may cause bronchoconstriction, especially in smokers and persons with asthma.

Hepatic system

Ether-based anesthetics (isoflurane, sevoflurane, desflurane) decrease portal vein blood flow but increase hepatic artery blood flow, thus maintaining total hepatic blood flow and oxygen delivery. This is in contrast to halothane anesthesia, in which decreases in portal vein blood flow are not compensated by increases in hepatic blood flow. Postoperative liver dysfunction has been associated most commonly with halothane use, although there are reports after isoflurane and, rarely, desflurane use. There are two major types of hepatotoxicity, type I and type II.

Type I hepatotoxicity

Type I hepatotoxicity is benign and self-limiting. It occurs in 25% to 30% of those who receive halothane. Signs are mild transient increases in serum transaminase, nausea, fever, but usually not jaundice.

Type II hepatotoxicity

Type II hepatotoxicity (also called "halothane hepatitis") has been reported in one per 35,000 cases of halothane administration. It is immune-mediated and believed to result from the metabolism of halothane to TFA via oxidative reactions in the liver. Clinical signs of liver injury include fever, eosinophilia, jaundice, and grossly elevated serum transaminase levels, with positive IgG against TFA. Severe cases are associated with massive centrilobular liver necrosis that may lead to fulminant liver failure, with a mortality rate of 50%. Risk factors for halothane hepatitis include (1) multiple exposures, especially at intervals of < 6 weeks – reexposure at short intervals is the single greatest risk factor for halothane hepatitis; (2) a history of postanesthetic fever or jaundice, which may indicate previous subclinical disease; (3) obesity; (4) female sex; and (5) age > 50 years. There also may be a genetic predisposition.

The incidence of liver injury caused by fluorinated inhaled anesthetics follows the order of halothane > isoflurane > desflurane, and it correlates with the extent of their oxidative metabolism, which is halothane (20%), isoflurane (0.2%), and desflurane (0.02%). Because all these inhaled anesthetics appear to form protein adducts that are identical or related in structure to those produced by halothane, it seems probable that they cause liver injury by a similar mechanism. The reduced incidence of injury from the other inhalational anesthetics compared with halothane appears to result from the lower levels of potentially immunogenic protein adducts formed when they are oxidatively metabolized by CYP2E1. Sevoflurane does not produce TFA, so it does not cause hepatotoxicity.

Renal system

Volatile anesthetics produce a concentration-dependent reduction in renal blood flow, glomerular filtration rate, and urinary output due to decreases in blood pressure and cardiac output. These may be attenuated by adequate perioperative hydration. Inorganic fluorides are released by the oxidation of halogenated anesthetics. Fluoride levels of >50 μmol/L may cause renal injury, consisting of polyuria hypernatremia, the inability to concentrate urine, and increased serum osmolality. Methoxyflurane is the only agent known to cause clinical fluoride-induced toxicity by this mechanism.

Sevoflurane in contact with the soda lime in a CO_2 absorber forms several degradation products, including *compound A*. Larger amounts of breakdown products are produced at lower fresh gas flows, as a result of increased temperature of the soda lime, and when the soda lime is desiccated. Compound A causes serious injury to kidneys in rats but is not proven to cause the same in humans. It is hypothesized that the difference is the result of different levels of renal cysteine conjugate β-lyase enzymes, which catalyze the conversion of compound A into thiol, which may cause toxicity. However, β-lyase is eight to 30 times less active in humans.

Neuromuscular system

Volatile anesthetics produce skeletal muscle relaxation and potentiate the effect of neuromuscular blocking drugs (both nondepolarizing and depolarizing). Sevoflurane can produce adequate muscle relaxation for intubation of children and adults, at sufficient depth.

Malignant hyperthermia

Malignant hyperthermia (MH) is a pharmacogenetic disorder of skeletal muscle triggered in susceptible individuals by all volatile inhalation anesthetics (desflurane, halothane, isoflurane, and sevoflurane). In addition to volatile agents, depolarizing skeletal muscle relaxants (e.g., succinylcholine) can also trigger MH. This syndrome has been linked to a missense mutation in the type 1 ryanodine receptor (RyR1) in more than 50% of cases studied to date. Signs of MH include tachycardia, increased expired CO_2, muscle rigidity, and increased temperature, and are related to increased metabolism (hypermetabolic state).

The treatment of MH is dantrolene (see Chapter 110). Dantrolene markedly attenuates the loss of calcium from sarcoplasmic reticulum, restoring the metabolism to normal and reversing the signs of metabolic stimulation.

Inhalational induction technique

Since Morton's demonstration of the inhalation of ether in 1846, inhalation induction has been a useful technique to produce unconsciousness. Subsequently, chloroform, cyclopropane, N_2O, and halothane became popular agents for inhalational induction. Halothane was administered to millions of adult and pediatric patients worldwide for more than 30 years, but because of its cardiac depressive effect, arrhythmogenicity, and potential for hepatic dysfunction, it has been replaced by newer and safer agents, such as sevoflurane.

Sevoflurane is a sweet-smelling agent, having a nonirritant odor and a low blood/gas partition coefficient. It can be rapidly and conveniently administered without discomfort, and its low solubility facilitates precise control over the depth of anesthesia. This agent's low solubility, clinically useful overpressure capability, and high airway and cardiovascular tolerability combine to produce a rapid and smooth induction of general anesthesia.

Inhalation induction is widely used in the pediatric population and is a great alternative for adult patients with difficult intravenous access or an aversion to needles. Among the advantages of inhalation induction is the avoidance of the discomfort of a painful injection (propofol) and the "hangover" associated with intravenous agents (thiopental). Anesthesia "masks" have improved in the past several years and now are clear and more comfortable. They can be flavored with fruit essence or mint to make the induction a more pleasant experience.

Several clinical trials have evaluated and described mask inhalation induction techniques with sevoflurane, including:

- Gradual technique: The gradual technique consists of increasing the sevoflurane concentration by 1% every two breaths. This technique may be initiated with 66% N_2O before introducing sevoflurane, because N_2O is odorless and has a pleasant effect.
- Vital capacity single-breath technique: The anesthesia circuit is primed with 8% sevoflurane and up to 75% N_2O in O_2 at 4 L/min (3:1) for at least 1 minute. The patient exhales to residual volume, then inhales to vital capacity and attempts to hold his or her breath as long as tolerated or until unconsciousness.

Studies have shown that there is little statistical or clinical difference between the two induction techniques, or between the vital capacity technique and intravenous induction with propofol.

Suggested readings

Bito H, Ikeda K. Closed-circuit anesthesia with sevoflurane in humans. Effects on renal and hepatic function and concentrations of breakdown products with soda lime in the circuit. *Anesthesiology* 1994; 80:71.

Doi M, Ikeda K. Airway irritation produced by volatile anesthetics during brief inhalation: comparison of halothane, enflurane, isoflurane, and sevoflurane. *Can J Anaesth* 1993; 40:122.

Epstein RH, Mendel HG, Guarnieri KM, et al. Sevoflurane versus halothane for general anesthesia in pediatric patients: a comparative study of vital signs, induction, and emergence. *J Clin Anesth* 1995; 7(3):237–244.

Epstein RH, Stein AL, Marr AT, Lessin JB. High concentration versus incremental induction of anesthesia with sevoflurane in children: a comparison of induction times, vital signs, and complications. *J Clin Anesth* 1998; 10(1):41–45.

Fernandez M, Lejus C, Rivault O, et al. Single-breath vital capacity rapid inhalation induction with sevoflurane: feasibility in children. *Pediatr Anaesth* 2005; 15(4):307–313.

Iyer RA, Anders MW. Cysteine conjugate beta-lyase-dependent biotransformation of the cysteine S-conjugates of the sevoflurane degradation product compound A in human, nonhuman primate, and rat kidney cytosol and mitochondria. *Anesthesiology* 1996; 85:1454–1461.

Kenna JG. Immunoallergic drug-induced hepatitis: lessons from halothane. *J Hepatol* 1997; 26(Suppl 1):5–12.

Philip BK, Lombard LL, Philip JH. Vital capacity induction with sevoflurane in adult surgical patients. *J Clin Anesth* 1996; 8: 426.

Philip BK, Lombard LL, Roaf ER, et al. Comparison of vital capacity induction with sevoflurane to intravenous induction with propofol for adult ambulatory anesthesia. *Anesth Analg* 1999; 89(3):623–627.

Stoelting RK. *Pharmacology and Physiology in Anesthetic Practice.* 3rd ed. Philadelphia: Lippincott Williams & Wilkins; 1999.

Yang T, Riehl J, Steve E, et al. Pharmacologic and functional characterization of malignant hyperthermia in the R163C RyR1 knock-in mouse. *Anesthesiology* 2006; 105(6):1164–1175.

Yurino M, Kimura H. Vital capacity breath technique for rapid anesthetic induction: comparison of sevoflurane and isoflurane. *Anaesthesia* 1992, 47:946–949.

Yurino M, Kimura H. Induction of anesthesia with sevoflurane, nitrous oxide, and oxygen: a comparison of spontaneous ventilation and vital capacity rapid inhalation induction (VCRII) techniques. *Anesth Analg* 1993; 76:598–601.

Yurino M, Kimura H. Vital capacity rapid inhalation induction technique: comparison of sevoflurane and halothane. *Can J Anesth* 1993; 40:440–443.

32

Pharmacokinetics of inhalational agents

James H. Philip

The kinetics of inhaled anesthetics is fundamental to the clinical practice of anesthesia. This subject is often called the *uptake and distribution of anesthetics*. It explains the time course of anesthetic movement from the delivery system to the site of action, which is the patient's central nervous system. Although the site of action of inhaled anesthetic agents includes the brain and spinal cord, the word *brain* is used alone in the remainder of this chapter. See Chapter 35 for further discussion of anesthesia site of action.

Inhaled agents are either gases or vapors, depending on their physical state at room temperature and pressure. Nitrous oxide and xenon are gases. For these agents, the anesthetic source is a flow controller with flow meter. Halothane, isoflurane, sevoflurane, and desflurane are vapors. In this chapter, the agent source for all these is called a *vaporizer*. The physical properties of some of these agents are listed in Table 32.1.

Definitions

The measure of anesthetic concentration in a compartment or location is the partial pressure. Partial pressure is also called tension. *Tension* is a generic term that applies to variables that equalize in connected locations. Examples are hydrostatic tension (water height) and electrical tension (voltage). The interchangeable terms *high-tension wires* and *high-voltage wires* are familiar examples of this.

Anesthetic partial pressure or tension could be expressed in common pressure units such as mm Hg, Pa, or kPa. However, the most commonly used unit for anesthetic partial pressure is % atm (percent of one sea level atmosphere). One percent partial pressure represents $1\% \times 760$ mm Hg $= 7.6$ mm Hg. The anesthetic tension is then said to be 1%. Commercial vaporizers state their delivered tension as a percentage and thus are consistent with this description.

Equilibrium is achieved when the tensions in compartments are equal. The locations or compartments of interest for inhaled agents are breathing circuit (inspired gas), lungs (alveolar gas), arterial blood, and the idealized body compartments: the vessel-rich group (VRG; brain, heart, liver, and kidneys), muscle, fat, and venous blood. Fig. 32.1 displays the Gas Man model (registered trademark of the author), showing the compartments and their partial pressures. The model has been validated for induction and emergence of anesthesia

and has been used to elucidate fine points of inhalation kinetics.

Although equilibrium is achieved when the anesthetic tensions in compartments are equal, anesthetic concentrations in connected compartments differ at this equilibrium according to agent solubility in each location. For blood and gas in equilibrium, the ratio of concentration in blood to concentration in gas is the blood/gas solubility ratio or blood/gas solubility. The following example explains this.

A 10-ml syringe is filled with 5 ml blood and 5 ml air. A small amount of liquid or vapor anesthetic is added to the syringe, which is then capped and shaken. In the syringe, the tension of anesthetic in the blood and gas compartments equalizes while the concentrations equilibrate. At equilibrium, the ratio of concentration in the blood to concentration in the gas is the blood/gas solubility ratio or blood/gas solubility. The ratio of drug quantity in these two equal-size compartments also equals the blood/gas solubility. When the term *solubility* is used by itself, it usually refers to blood/gas solubility or blood/gas solubility ratio.

Movement of anesthetic

As blood passes through the capillaries of the lungs, anesthetic equilibrium is achieved across the alveolar–capillary membrane. Thus, arterial tension equals alveolar tension. The concentration of anesthetic in blood is equal to the product of the partial pressure and the solubility.

Arterial blood perfuses each tissue, and tissue tension rises toward arterial tension. During this period, anesthetic tension in venous blood leaving the tissue equals that in each tissue itself. Eventually, anesthetic tension in the tissue equals that in arterial blood. At this time, venous tension equals arterial tension and there is no longer anesthetic uptake into that tissue. The tissue is in equilibrium with blood. All tissues, fast and slow, eventually reach equilibrium, some after many hours. When this final equilibrium is reached, anesthetic tensions in all gas, liquid, and tissue compartments are equal.

The alveolar tension curve

To understand the kinetics of inhaled agents, we analyze the time course of anesthetic tension in the patient's lungs or alveoli

Table 32.1. Physical and kinetic properties of anesthetic agents

	Units	Halothane	Isoflurane	Sevoflurane	Desflurane	N$_2$O	Xenon
MAC	%	0.8	1.1	2.1	6.0	110	70
Blood/gas solubility		2.47	1.30	0.65	0.42	0.47	0.13
VRG/blood solubility		1.94	1.62	1.69	1.29	0.89	1.30
Muscle/blood solubility		4.01	3.46	3.69	2.31	1.15	2.00
Fat/blood solubility		60.7	53.8	52.3	31.0	2.30	10.0
Alveolar plateau height		0.24	0.38	0.55	0.66	0.63	0.86
VRG = brain	Tau	Minutes	3.1	2.6	2.7	2.0	1.4	2.1
Muscle	Tau	Hours	2.4	2.1	2.3	1.4	0.7	1.2
Fat	Tau	Hours	49	43	42	25	2	8

(P$_A$) in response to a step change in inspired tension (P$_I$), as described by Kety in 1950. This is called the *alveolar step response* or, sometimes, the *alveolar tension curve*. The alveolar tension curve describes the time course of alveolar tension (P$_A$) in response to a step change in inspired tension (P$_I$).

Initial rise of the alveolar tension curve

The alveolar tension curve has the same general shape for all inhaled agents because they share the same physiology of drug delivery and removal. The alveolar tension curve components are called the *initial rise*, *plateau*, *knee*, and *tail*, as described by Kety. The alveolar tension curve for isoflurane is shown in Fig. 32.2.

The first portion of the curve is called the initial rise (Fig. 32.3). This is what the shape would look like if there were no removal of anesthetic from the alveoli by blood. This would happen in the following imaginary situations: if cardiac output

were zero, if the lungs were not connected to the cardiovascular system, or if the agent's solubility in blood were zero. The initial portion of the alveolar tension curve follows this shape for all inhaled agents whose inspired tension rises in the shape of a step. The curve shape of the initial rise is an exponential curve, shown in Fig. 32.3 and expressed mathematically as

$$\frac{P_A}{P_I} = 1 - e^{-\frac{t}{\tau}} \qquad \text{(Eqn. 1)}$$

where τ (Greek letter tau) is called the *time constant*. The time constant can be computed as the ratio of volume to flow in the alveolar compartment. The volume (V) is the functional residual capacity (FRC), or resting volume, of the lung and the flow (F) is the alveolar ventilation (VA), equal to the effective average minute ventilation of the alveoli:

$$\tau = \frac{V}{F} = \frac{FRC}{VA} \qquad \text{(Eqn. 2)}$$

For the average adult, FRC = 2 L and VA = 4 L/min, so

$$\tau = \frac{FRC}{VA} = \frac{2L}{4 \text{ L/min}} = 0.5 \text{ min} \qquad \text{(Eqn. 3)}$$

The shape of the exponential curve of Eqn. 1, shown in Fig. 32.3, can be understood as follows. Initially, t = 0 and e^0 = 1, like any number raised to the zero power. Thus, P$_A$/P$_I$ = 0 initially.

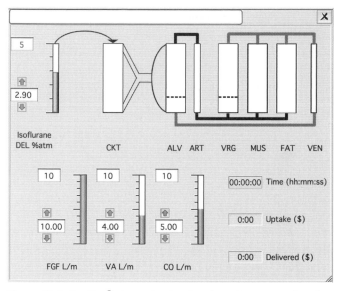

Figure 32.1. Gas Man® picture showing the schematic representation of the model for inhalation kinetics. The upper half shows compartments in which anesthetic partial pressure will rise from left to right. The lower half shows the flows that link the compartments, FGF, alveolar ventilation (VA), and cardiac output (CO). With permission of the owner, James H. Philip, and the licensee, Med Man Simulations, Inc. (www.gasmanweb.com), a nonprofit charitable organization, PO Box 67160, Chestnut Hill MA 02467. (Gas Man is a registered trademark of James H. Philip and Med Man Simulations, inc., a nonprofit charitable organization.)

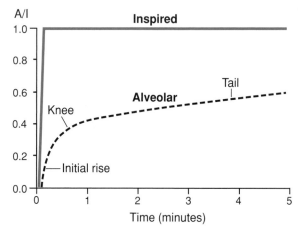

Figure 32.2. Alveolar tension curve for isoflurane. The *vertical axis labeled A/I* reflects the alveolar over inspired ratio of concentration, fraction, partial pressure, or tension. The curve shows the characteristic initial rise, knee, and tail described in the text.

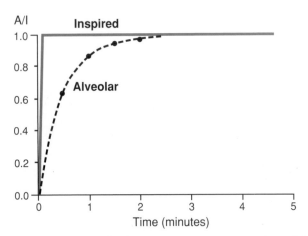

Figure 32.3. Rise in alveolar tension in response to a step change in inspired tension in the absence of uptake into blood. *Small circles* represent values at 1, 2, 3, and 4 time constants, which occur at 0.5, 1.0, 1.5, and 2.0 minutes.

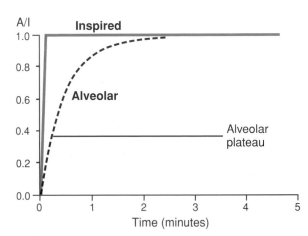

Figure 32.4. The alveolar plateau is formed as alveolar ventilation delivers agent to the alveoli while blood flow removes it. The removal rate equals cardiac output times blood/gas solubility.

As time passes, t eventually reaches the value of τ. This is at 0.5 minute in the example. At this time, the exponent of e is -1 and $e^{-1} = 1/e = 1/2.72718 \sim 0.37$. One minus this value is 0.63. Thus, when $t = \tau$, $P_A/P_I = 0.63$. After a second time constant has passed ($2 \times 0.5 = 1$ minute in this example), P_A/P_I has reached 0.63 of the remainder or 0.84 of the total. The value at $3 \times \tau = 0.92$ and at $4 \times \tau = 0.98$. Thus, at the end of four time constants, the curve has reached 0.98 on its way toward 1. It will reach 1.0 only after infinite time has elapsed.

An exponential curve depicts the input–output relationship for any fully mixed single compartment subjected to a step change in the tension entering it. This applies to tissue compartments as well. For a tissue compartment, the effective volume is the actual volume times the tissue/gas solubility. The effective flow is the actual blood flow times the blood/gas solubility. Solubilities of successive areas relate to each other such that tissue/gas solubility ($\lambda_{t/g}$) equals tissue/blood solubility ($\lambda_{t/b}$) times blood/gas solubility ($\lambda_{b/g}$).

$$\lambda_{t/g} = \lambda_{t/b} \times \lambda_{b/g} \qquad \text{(Eqn. 4)}$$

Plateau of the alveolar tension curve

The next portion of the alveolar tension curve is called the alveolar plateau. It reflects the added effect of removal of anesthetic by the blood (Fig. 32.4). This portion of the alveolar tension curve is created by the balance between delivery of anesthetic by alveolar ventilation (VA) and the removal of anesthetic by the product of cardiac output (CO) and blood/gas solubility ($\lambda_{b/g}$). The alveolar plateau height is computed as:

$$\frac{P_A}{P_I}_{\text{plateau}} = \frac{1}{1 + \dfrac{CO \times \lambda}{VA}} \qquad \text{(Eqn. 5)}$$

The equation and plateau height can be understood as follows. Imagine a drug with solubility = 1 and call it *unithane*. Further, consider the patient whose cardiac output equals his

or her alveolar ventilation. In this situation, $CO \times \lambda/VA = 1$ and the alveolar plateau height is calculated to equal $\frac{1}{1+1} = 0.5 = 1/2$. Thus, the height of the plateau tension is half the height of inspired tension. This shows the balance of delivery exactly offset by removal, establishing equilibrium where alveolar tension is halfway between zero and inspired tension. If ventilation is higher, the plateau is higher. If cardiac output or solubility is higher, the plateau is lower.

The presence in the plateau equation of the mathematical term $CO \times \lambda/VA$ is clinically very significant. A change in any one of these parameters is offset by a proportional or inverse change in another term. Thus, halving the ventilation is the same as doubling the solubility. Moreover, doubling the ventilation is the same as halving the solubility, and tripling the ventilation is the same as reducing the solubility by a factor of three. This is important in that desflurane, sevoflurane, and isoflurane have relative solubilities of 1, 2, and 3. Table 32.1 shows solubilities and plateau heights, and Fig. 32.5 shows the plateaus.

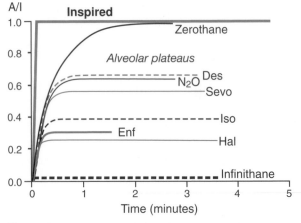

Figure 32.5. Alveolar plateaus for real anesthetics and the imaginary zerothane (solubility zero) and infinithane (solubility infinity) anesthetics.

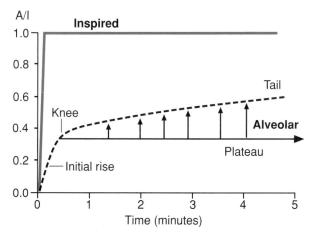

Figure 32.6. Tail of the alveolar tension curve. The rise in alveolar tension that transforms the plateau into a knee is produced by venous return of anesthetic-laden blood to the lungs.

Knee and tail of the alveolar tension curve

The final portion of the alveolar tension curve is called the tail. It is formed as a result of venous blood from tissues returning anesthetic to the alveoli; this causes alveolar tension to rise. Because arterial blood anesthetic tension follows alveolar tension closely, arterial tension also rises. As anesthetic tension from fast tissues (VRG) rises in the first few minutes after the inspired step, the flat plateau is transformed into an upgoing knee and the name of this portion of the curve changes (Fig. 32.6). The plateau exists in theory, whereas the knee and tail exist in reality. The first portion of the tail is formed by anesthetic-laden blood from VRG, the next portion by anesthetic-laden blood from muscle (a few hours later), and the final portion by anesthetic-laden blood from fat (more than 10 hours later). The alveolar tension curve for many agents is shown in Fig. 32.7 along with lines depicting the plateau heights. Actual plateau heights and values are shown in Table 32.1.

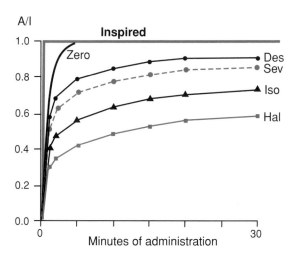

Figure 32.7. Alveolar tension curves of several anesthetics. *Graphs* are redrawn from the data of Yasuda, Eger et al., *Anesth Analg* 1991; 72:316–324.

Fine points of end-tidal, alveolar, and arterial tension

Lung shunt

Arterial blood anesthetic tension follows alveolar gas tension closely. Blood that passes through alveolar capillaries attains an anesthetic tension identical to that in alveolar gas. However, some blood flow does not pass through alveolar capillaries equilibrating with alveolar gas. This blood is called *lung shunt*. Lung shunt adds mixed venous blood with its lower anesthetic tension to the perfect alveolar-equilibrated blood. Thus, arterial tension is slightly lower than alveolar tension during deepening and higher than alveolar tension during lightening of anesthesia.

Alveolar dead space

Agent monitors measure end-expired gas tension. In reality, this "end-expired" gas comprises alveolar gas plus a small amount of inspired gas. The fraction of inspired gas mixed into the expired gas is the alveolar dead space fraction. This is usually around 10%.

End-expired gas monitor errors

The end-tidal agent tension measured by agent monitors differs from arterial blood tension by two errors: alveolar shunt and alveolar dead space. The total error with isoflurane is approximately 20%. Stated differently, $P_{art}/P_{ET} = 0.8$.

End-expired gas misinterpretations that ignore brain delay

At all times during anesthesia, anesthetic tension in the brain lags behind that in the arterial blood. The brain is a compartment perfused by blood and takes time to equilibrate with it. Based on brain/blood solubilities all being approximately 1.5 (Table 32.1), the brain time constant is between 1.5 and 3 minutes for all anesthetic agents.

Clinical kinetics: control of anesthetic depth

The goal of administering inhaled anesthetics is to bring the anesthetic tension in the brain to the desired level, manipulate it as clinical conditions dictate, and reduce the brain level to as close to zero as possible at the end of anesthesia. During anesthesia, brain tension is held somewhere near 1 MAC with pure inhalation anesthesia and < 1 MAC when other agents form a significant part of the patient's anesthetic. Even if inspired agent tension could be controlled accurately, alveolar and VRG tension would be lower and delayed according to the alveolar tension curve described earlier.

In clinical care, the vaporizer dial is set and fresh gas flow (FGF) with the delivered tension enters the breathing circuit. The FGF mixes with the patient's exhaled gas flow, producing an inspired tension that is an average of exhaled and delivered tensions, each weighted by its relative flow and possibly affected by uneven mixing. Dilution of the delivered tension occurs unless FGF greatly exceeds ventilation. This occurs rarely in clinical practice, in which such excess is considered wasteful. The limit of low FGF is closed circuit anesthesia, in which FGF is set to exactly match the patient's uptake of oxygen and inhaled anesthetic agent. Closed circuit anesthesia is not addressed in this chapter.

Careful adjustment of the vaporizer setting combined with consideration of FGF, ventilation, cardiac output, and blood/gas solubility of the chosen anesthetic are required to achieve and maintain the desired brain anesthetic tension. FGF, vaporizer setting, inspired tension, and expired tension should all be observed for good control and understanding of brain anesthetic tension. This is important because changing FGF and patient ventilation often requires changes in the vaporizer setting, and these changes might not otherwise be appreciated if only expired tension is observed and recorded.

Emergence from anesthesia

Emergence from anesthesia of very long duration is the inverse of anesthesia induction. The alveolar tension curve is inverted. The shape could be described as comprising the initial fall, the knee, and the tail of the curve.

The level of anesthesia in the VRG at which 50% of patients follow commands is termed MAC_{awake}. For all agents, MAC_{awake} is approximately 0.33 MAC. Other benchmark levels of anesthesia are 0.75 MAC, 0.5 MAC, 0.2 MAC, and 0.1 MAC. Figure 32.8 shows a graph of emergence after very long anesthesia created by inverting the anesthesia induction curves of Fig. 32.7. It can be seen that for most agents, even in the context of a very long anesthetic at 1.0 MAC, the 0.75 MAC level is reached immediately and the 0.5 MAC level is attained in just a few minutes. The time to reach one-half the steady-state initial value is called

the *half-time*. This value is commonly used as a benchmark for drugs. More sensitive differentiation among drugs is achieved by observing 0.67, 0.80, and 0.90 reduction (shown as dotted lines in Fig. 32.8).

Emergence is faster after short anesthetics than after long anesthetics. This is because very slow body compartments, such as fat, remain empty enough to remove anesthetic *from* blood. The effect of the muscle compartment changes within clinical durations of anesthesia. As muscle fills with anesthetic, it is transformed from a compartment that augments awakening to one that retards it. Any compartment with a tension lower than that in the blood helps emergence, whereas any compartment with a tension above that in blood hinders it.

Subtle kinetic effects
The concentration effect

The concentration effect and second gas effect describe the effect of gas uptake on the gas volume and the concentration that remains in the alveolar compartment. The concentration effect describes the kinetic impact of breathing a gas in a high concentration or fraction. When a high concentration is breathed, most of the gas taken up from the lung is that gas. When alveolar volume is reduced by uptake into blood during one breath, inspired tidal volume is increased in the next breath to offset the missing volume.

This phenomenon increases alveolar ventilation during the period of rapid uptake into blood. The high-concentration effect is usually described regarding nitrous oxide, because currently it is the only agent safe to breathe in a high concentration. Fig. 32.5 shows that the plateau height for nitrous oxide is lower than that for desflurane. In Fig. 32.5, the line is drawn as if nitrous oxide were breathed in a low concentration like the other gases. To avoid confusion, Fig. 32.7 omits the curve for nitrous oxide because in the actual experiment depicted, nitrous oxide was breathed in a high concentration (65%–70%) and the concentration effect displaced the nitrous oxide curve above that of desflurane. Figure 32.9 demonstrates the

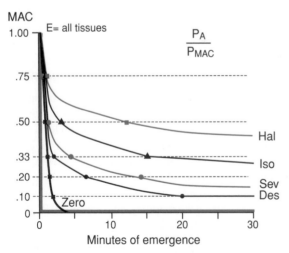

Figure 32.8. Alveolar tension fall for various anesthetic agents after an infinitely long anesthetic. These curves are created by inverting the curves of Fig 32.7. *Dotted lines* are shown at reduction from 1 MAC to 0.75, 0.50, 0.33, 0.20, and 0.10 MAC, reflecting fractional reductions of 0.25, 0.50, 0.67, 0.80, and 0.90 MAC.

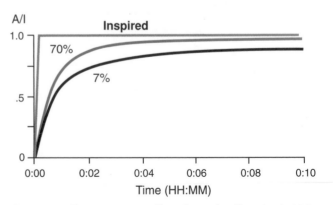

Figure 32.9. The concentration effect refers to the effect whereby high-concentration (70%) nitrous oxide increases the rise of alveolar nitrous oxide compared with a low concentration of nitrous oxide (7%). The figure was created using Gas Man.

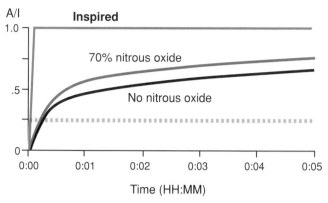

Figure 32.10. Second gas effect shows the higher alveolar tension curve for isoflurane combined with 70% nitrous oxide compared with the curve for isoflurane alone. The figure was created using Gas Man.

impact of concentration by overlaying simulated alveolar tension curves when breathing high-concentration (70%) and low-c-oncentration (7%) nitrous oxide.

The second gas effect describes the impact of the presence of a high-concentration first gas such as nitrous oxide on the alveolar tension curve for a second, lower-concentration gas, such as isoflurane (Fig. 32.10). The absorption of the high-concentration high-volume nitrous oxide concentrates the isoflurane remaining in the alveoli. This absorption also augments all ventilation into the lungs by the increased inspired ventilation from the concentration effect. Because the alveolar isoflurane concentration is low compared with the inspired concentration, the alveolar concentration of the second gas can be raised by the presence of the first gas. For the less soluble drugs sevoflurane and desflurane, the second gas effect has less clinical impact.

The effect of tissue solubilities and blood flows

The clinical impact of tissue/blood solubility and the shape of the tail of the alveolar tension curve are subtle. Simulation provides insights. When anesthetic tension in a tissue compartment exceeds MAC_{awake} or any other specified threshold, that tissue compartment delays blood and brain tension from reaching the threshold level. Early in the course of anesthesia, low muscle and fat anesthetic tensions will speed emergence, whereas later, high anesthetic tensions will delay it. The subtleties of tissue solubility and unknown tissue volume and blood flow make this even more complex.

Summary

Inhalation anesthesia kinetics is important. The alveolar tension curve in response to a step change in inspired tension unveils the kinetic relationship created by the interconnection of the inspired gas with the alveolar gas, blood, and key body compartments.

Suggested readings

Bouillon T, Shafer S. Editorial – hot air or full steam ahead? An empirical pharmacokinetic model of potent inhaled agents. *Brit J Anaesth* 2000; 84:429–431.

Eger EI 2nd. *Anesthetic Uptake and Action.* Baltimore: Williams & Wilkins; 1974.

Eger EI, Shafer SL. Context-sensitive decrement times for inhaled anesthetics [tutorial]. *Anesth Analg* 2005; 101:688–696.

Frei FJ, Zbinden AM, Thomson DA, Reider HU. Is the end-tidal partial pressure of isoflurane a good predictor of its arterial partial pressure? *Brit J Anaesth* 1991; 66:331–339.

Kety SS. The physiological and physical factors governing the uptake of anesthetic gases by the body. *Anesthesiology* 1950; 11: 517.

Philip JH. *GAS MAN® – Understanding Anesthesia Uptake and Distribution.* 5th ed. www.gsmanweb.com. Chestnut Hill: Med Man Simulations; 2008.

Yasuda M, Lockhart SL, Eger EI, et al. Comparison of kinetics of sevoflurane and isoflurane in humans. *Anesth Analg* 1991; 72:316–324.

Chapter 33

Pharmacodynamics of inhalational agents

Jan Boublik and Richard D. Urman

The minimum alveolar concentration (MAC) of an inhaled anesthetic is the concentration at 1 atm that prevents visible skeletal muscle movement in response to skin incision in 50% of patients. MAC is the inhaled anesthetic equivalent to the 50% effective dose (ED_{50}) of other medications. Several basic assumptions form the foundation of the concept of MAC.

First, alveolar concentration is an assessment of blood level. The brain is perfused by this blood, but the effect on the brain occurs several minutes after it appears in end-tidal gas, which we use to estimate alveolar gas. MAC equals the partial pressure of anesthetic at the anesthetic site of action. This is based on the assumption that the alveolar partial pressure is transmitted without change to arterial blood and that, given sufficient time for equilibration, the partial pressure at the site of action equals the partial pressure in arterial blood. The time constant for the brain and spinal cord is approximately 3 minutes for all inhaled agents. Thus, alveolar level to assess brain level can be applied only when anesthetic level is constant for several brain time constants. In research studies, end-expired anesthetic level is held constant for 15 minutes before measures of anesthesia depth are made.

The second assumption is that alveolar and end-tidal concentrations are equal. This is true only when there is no alveolar dead space and no alveolar shunt. Otherwise, dead space and shunt cause end-tidal and arterial concentrations to differ. Third, when the term *concentration* is used, it applies only at sea level. For the term to apply universally, *partial pressure* must replace *concentration* in the definition. (Chapter 32 explores this concept further.) The final assumption is that it is possible to elicit an all-or-nothing response to skin incision.

Mechanism of immobility

The immobility produced, as measured by MAC, is primarily mediated by the effects of volatile anesthetics on the spinal cord, with only a minor cerebral component. For example, decerebration of animals does not change MAC, whereas delivery of inhaled anesthetics only to the brain increases the MAC more than 2.5-fold and selective delivery to the spinal cord decreases MAC by a third.

The effects of volatile anesthetics on the spinal cord represent a diverse combination of drug-induced depression of excitement as well as enhancement of inhibition. Inhaled anesthetics inhibit excitatory α-amino-3 adenosine monophosphate-hydroxy-5-methyl-4-isoxazolepropionic acid (AMPA) and N-methyl-D-aspartate (NMDA) receptor currents independently of γ-aminobutyric acid A ($GABA_A$) and glycine receptor activity. Sodium, but not potassium, ion channels also may be important in producing immobility. Cholinergic receptors do not seem to be involved in producing immobility at the spinal cord level. Opioids and α_2-adrenoreceptor stimulation decrease MAC, but it is unlikely that the immobility produced by volatile anesthetics is mediated via these receptors. In summary, immobility cannot be explained by action of volatile anesthetics on a single group of receptors, nor does immobility seem to be the effect of concurrent action on several receptors.

Significance of MAC

The value of the MAC concept lies in the fact that it establishes a common measure of potency (partial pressure at steady state) for inhaled anesthetic with relatively small (10%–20%) variation among individuals (Table 33.1). The concept serves as a guide for several important clinical issues.

MAC provides a means for uniform dosage comparison of inhaled anesthetics. It establishes relative amounts of inhaled anesthetics to reach set clinical end points (described later). MAC serves as a guide to elucidate potential mechanisms of inhaled anesthetic/anesthetic action, and the use of MAC as a benchmark allows examination of the effect of equally potent doses (at spinal level) on other organ systems.

It is of crucial importance to understand that MAC represents only one point on the dose–response curves of the inhaled anesthetics. A modest increase to 1.3 MAC abolishes movement in at least 95% of patients as a result of the steep dose–response curves. This is why in clinical practice in which the inhalational

Table 33.1. Comparative MACs at sea level for adults aged 30 to 55 years

Agent	MAC, %
Nitrous oxide	104
Isoflurane	1.15
Sevoflurane	2.05
Desflurane	6.0
Halothane	0.75
Xenon	70

Table 33.2. Factors affecting MAC

Factor	Effect on MAC	Mechanism
Age	Young age (6 mo): increase Increasing age: decrease	Brain development and neuron formation before and loss of neurons after age 6 mo
Red hair	Increase	? Increased pheomelanin concentrations caused by melanocortin-1 receptor gene mutations, antagonism with opioid receptors, or influence on nociception
Body temperature	Hyperthermia: increase Hypothermia: decrease	Intrinsic properties in the brain
Blood pressure (MAP)	< 40 mm Hg: decrease	? Possibly impaired brain perfusion
Postpartum	Decrease by 30% immediately postpartum	Cardiovascular and hormonal changes of postpartum period
Oxygenation	$PaO_2 < 38$ mm Hg: decrease	Attenuation of glutamate excitotoxicity
Cardiopulmonary bypass surgery	Decrease	Not known
Length of surgery	Constant or decrease	Not known
Sodium	Hypernatremia: increase Hyponatremia: decrease	Inhaled anesthetics inhibit synaptosomal sodium channels; amount of sodium in the body affects level of inhibition
Cyclosporine	Increase	Pharmacodynamic interaction seems to be likely, perhaps consequent to an effect of cyclosporine on ligand-gated sodium channels
Opioids	Decrease	Indirect (modulating) role but not a direct (mediating) role; provide analgesia and thus decrease MAC
Benzodiazepines	Decrease	Modulation by inhibition of GABA receptor
Ketamine	Decrease	NMDA receptor antagonism decreases temporal summation of pain stimuli
Lithium	Decrease	Not known
Lidocaine	Decrease	Modulating effect by providing analgesia
Alcohol	Acute: decrease Chronic: increase	Acute alcohol ingestion: synergistic with inhaled anesthetics Chronic alcoholism causes tolerance (?) by alteration of cytochrome P-450 system

agent is the sole anesthetic, >1 MAC often is needed to prevent the patient from moving in response to surgical stimulation. Several other "MACs" are of clinical relevance, as discussed below.

Various MAC parameters

MAC_{awake} represents the point on the volatile anesthetic concentration curve that defines the return of response to verbal command during emergence from anesthesia. For most agents, MAC_{awake} is 0.33 MAC. Interestingly, the transition from awake to unconscious requires 0.4 to 0.5 MAC.

$MAC_{intubation}$ is the concentration of volatile anesthetic at which no movement or cough occurs during endotracheal intubation. Its value is approximately 2.0 MAC.

MAC_{BAR} is the concentration at which we observe blocked autonomic response (no blood pressure, heart rate, or catecholamine release) to an incision. Its value is 1.6 to 1.7 MAC.

The ratios among $MAC_{(skin)}$, MAC_{BAR}, $MAC_{intubation}$, and MAC_{awake} are constant for the respective inhaled anesthetics.

Factors affecting MAC

MAC lends itself to the analysis of physiologic and pharmacologic factors that may or may not affect inhalational anesthetic requirements in humans (Tables 33.2 and 33.3, respectively) as a result of the remarkable homogeneity of inhaled anesthetic requirements in humans.

Physiologic variables

Several factors may significantly alter MAC requirements. Maximum MAC requirement is achieved at 6 months after birth. Age accounts for a 6% average decrease in MAC per decade of life for all inhaled anesthetics. This is attributed to brain development and formation (increase MAC) and degeneration of neurons (decrease MAC) in the human brain.

Hyperthermia increases MAC, whereas hypothermia decreases it. In the early postpartum period, MAC is decreased by nearly 30% and returns to normal within 12 to 72 hours as a result of postpartum hormonal and cardiovascular changes.

Table 33.3. Factors not affecting MAC

Gender (except for xenon)
Duration of anesthesia (see Table 33.2)
Anesthetic metabolism
Thyroid gland dysfunction
Hypo-/hyperkalemia
PaO_2 variation if > 38 mm Hg
Hypertension
Hypotension

Although gender does not affect MAC, women with naturally red hair have a 20% increase in MAC, stemming from increased pheomelanin concentrations caused by melanocortin-1 receptor gene mutations. Most sources describe MAC as time independent, but there is some evidence to suggest that the MAC for isoflurane decreases with length of surgery as well as cardiopulmonary bypass use. Hypoxia with a $PaO_2 < 38$ mm Hg decreases MAC by attenuating glutamate excitotoxicity. Changes in the sodium concentration in the blood alter MAC requirements by affecting synaptosomal sodium channels, whereas changes in potassium levels have no effect.

Pharmacologic variables

MAC values for different inhaled anesthetics are additive, meaning that 0.5 MAC each of two anesthetics provides the same effect as 1 MAC of either agent alone. Nitrous oxide cannot be used as the sole inhaled anesthetic in young patients, as its MAC surpasses safe concentrations. Opioids at clinical doses can reduce MAC by up to 50% in a modulating, indirect fashion when they provide profound analgesia. Comparatively smaller effects on MAC are observed with benzodiazepines and ketamine through $GABA_A$ inhibition and NMDA antagonism (causing decreased temporal summation of nociceptive stimuli). Whereas acute alcohol ingestion decreases MAC, chronic alcohol use increases it. Table 33.2 summarizes the various factors affecting MAC.

Limitations of MAC

Although the MAC concept is undoubtedly useful in discussing the potency of volatile anesthetics and the depth of anesthesia, it also has several inherent limitations. MAC determination requires a constant alveolar concentration to be maintained for 15 minutes to allow for equilibration of the vessel-rich group and blood. The best use of MAC is in interpreting the end-tidal anesthetic agent concentration in the recent past to predict the level of anesthetic in the brain at present. Lung shunt and alveolar dead space cause differences between end-tidal and arterial anesthetic tension.

It is important to remember that MAC is a measure of ED50 established in clinical trials, not ED100 on a population level. The required concentration to prevent movement in response to skin incision therefore differs slightly from patient to patient. MAC measures somatic response, not lack of awareness. It applies only to inhaled not intravenous anesthetics, thereby limiting the ability to compare the two classes of drugs. MAC always depends on a specific clinical end point, and different values have to be elucidated for each end point (e.g., skin incision, awake).

Suggested readings

Barash PG, Cullen BF, Stoelting RK. *Clinical Anesthesia*, 5th ed. Philadelphia: Lippincott Williams and Wilkins; 2006.

Eger EI. Age, minimum alveolar anesthetic concentration, and minimum anesthetic concentration-awake. *Anesth Analg* 2001; 93:947–953.

Eger EI, Laster MJ, Gregory GA, et al. Women appear to have the same alveolar concentration as men. A retrospective study. *Anesthesiology* 2003; 99:1059–1061.

Gross JB, Alexander CM. Awakening concentrations of isoflurane are not affected by analgesic doses of morphine. *Anesth Analg* 1988; 67(1):27–30.

Katoh T, Suguro Y, Kimura T, Ikeda K. Cerebral awakening concentration of sevoflurane and isoflurane predicted during slow and fast alveolar washout. *Anesth Analg* 1993 77(5):1012–1017.

Liem EB, Lin C-M, Suleman MI, et al. Anesthetic requirement is increased in redheads. *Anesthesiology* 2004; 101:279–283.

Niemann CLI, Stabernack C, Serkova N, et al. Cyclosporine can increase isoflurane MAC. *Anesth Analg* 2002; 95:930–934.

Petersen-Felix S, Zbinder AM, Fischer M, Thomson DA. Isoflurane minimum alveolar concentration decreases during anesthesia and surgery. *Anesthesiology* 1993; 79:959–965.

Sebel PS, Glass PS, Fletcher JE, et al. Reduction of MAC of desflurane with fentanyl. *Anesthesiology* 1992; 76:52–59.

Sonner JM, Antognini IE, Dutton RC, et al. Inhaled anesthetics and immobility: mechanisms, mysteries and minimum alveolar concentration. *Anesth Analg* 2003; 97:718–740.

Zhou HH, Norman P, DeLima LG, et al. The minimum alveolar concentration of patients undergoing bilateral tubal ligation in the postpartum period. *Anesthesiology* 1995; 82:1364–1368.

Chapter

34

Intravenous induction agents

Aakash Agarwala and Mark Dershwitz

Sedative–hypnotic agents such as barbiturates, benzodiazepines, etomidate, and propofol, as well as medications such as ketamine, all may be used to induce general anesthesia and are therefore classified as induction agents. They also may be used for maintenance of sedation or general anesthesia, either via intermittent bolus injection or constant intravenous (IV) infusion. When administered in large doses, as during the induction of general anesthesia, they may cause significant cardiovascular and ventilatory effects. These effects, as well as the adverse effects specific to each agent, are discussed in this chapter. The choice of medications used for induction should be tailored to each patient based on his or her medical history and the pharmacologic effects of each drug. The choice may consist of an induction agent alone or may include the use of opioids, muscle relaxants, inhalational agents, and/or vasoactive medications to maximize patient safety and comfort and provide optimal surgical conditions.

Overview

Benzodiazepines, barbiturates, etomidate, and propofol function primarily through their interaction with the γ-aminobutyric acid (GABA) neurotransmitter system. Through different mechanisms, they augment the function of this inhibitory system. GABA receptor activation results in the influx of chloride ions into neurons, causing hyperpolarization and inhibition of the neuron by increasing the potential difference that must be overcome to generate an action potential (see Chapter 35).

Ketamine, in contrast to the other induction agents, acts primarily by antagonizing the N-methyl-D-aspartate (NMDA) receptor, although it also inhibits neuronal nicotinic acetylcholine receptors (see Chapter 35). Through its interaction with NMDA receptors, it causes a simultaneous depression of the thalamocortical system and stimulation of the limbic system, resulting in what is called "dissociative anesthesia."

During induction, a rapid onset of action is generally desired to minimize the time the patient is in the excitatory stage of anesthesia. Characteristics of these drugs that favor a more rapid onset include high lipid solubility and greater fraction of drug in the nonionized form. Following administration, these drugs distribute rapidly to the central nervous system

(CNS) because of the large fraction of cardiac output received by the CNS as well as their lipophilic nature.

The effects of opioids and IV induction agents are synergistic, and the use of opioids prior to induction generally reduces the dose of induction agent required to produce unconsciousness. In addition, opioids typically potentiate the cardiovascular and ventilatory effects of the IV induction agents.

Elderly patients usually require lower doses of most agents used for induction because of decreased CNS sensitivity, decreased metabolic and renal clearance, and decreased plasma protein concentration that results in an increased fraction of "free" drug within the circulation. Elderly hypovolemic patients who have been pretreated with opioids and/or benzodiazepines may have more cardiovascular instability with a given dose of an induction agent; thus, a lower dose of induction agent and concomitant administration of vasoactive medications should be considered in these patients.

Induction agents

Barbiturates

Thiopental and methohexital are the shortest-acting of the barbiturates and are used for induction of general anesthesia. Through rapid redistribution, they produce a loss of consciousness, followed by prompt awakening following the usual induction doses (Table 34.1). Thiopental is prepared as a 2.5% solution that is relatively painless when injected intravenously. Allergies to barbiturates are rare, estimated at one in 30,000, and barbiturates are contraindicated in patients with porphyria. Thiopental may cause hyperalgesia in sedative doses.

CNS effects

Thiopental decreases the cerebral metabolic rate of oxygen consumption ($CMRO_2$), cerebral blood flow (CBF), and intracranial pressure (ICP) (Table 34.2). By decreasing cerebral metabolism, the administration of thiopental protects the brain against ischemic injury during periods of decreased oxygen delivery. This neuroprotective effect may be advantageous for patients undergoing surgery for intracranial aneurysms or arteriovenous malformations. Although thiopental also causes decreases in mean arterial pressure, reductions in ICP may be greater, favoring increased cerebral perfusion in these patients.

Table 34.1.   Pharmacokinetic characteristics of IV anesthetic agents

Drug	Induction dose, *mg/kg*	Onset, *sec*	Duration, *min*	Redistribution half-life, *min*	Terminal half-life, *h*
Thiopental	4–7	< 30	5–10	2–4	6–12
Methohexital	1–3	< 30	5–10	5–6	2–5
Propofol	1–3	< 30	3–8	1–2	4–6
Etomidate	0.2–0.3	< 30	5–10	2–4	2–5
Diazepam	0.3–0.6	45–60	15–30	10–15	20–40
Lorazepam	0.03–0.06	60–120	60–120	3–10	10–20
Midazolam	0.2–0.4	30–60	15–30	7–15	2–4
Ketamine	1–2	45–60	10–20	11–17	2–3

Adapted with permission from Dershwitz M, Rosow CE. Intravenous anesthetics. In: Longnecker DE, Brown D, Newman M, Zapol WM, eds. *Anesthesiology.* 3rd ed. New York: McGraw-Hill; 2008.

The neuroprotective effect of thiopental occurs only if administered prior to an anticipated reduction of cerebral perfusion. No benefit has been found if thiopental is given following the onset of cerebral ischemia.

Progressively increasing doses of thiopental result in changes in the electroencephalogram (EEG) from alpha and beta waves to delta waves that are characteristic of surgical anesthesia. At higher doses, an isoelectric EEG may be attained, a state characterized by significant decreases in cerebral oxygen metabolism and blood flow. Thiopental's anticonvulsant properties make it useful in the treatment of status epilepticus, although the cardiovascular and ventilatory effects may necessitate mechanical ventilation and the use of vasopressors.

Methohexital, in contrast to thiopental, has some epileptogenic activity at lower doses, which makes its use less desirable in patients with seizure disorders. This property is of benefit, however, when trying to isolate epileptic foci in the brain during surgical ablation. It is often used to induce anesthesia in patients undergoing electroconvulsive therapy.

Cardiovascular effects

Induction doses of thiopental (4–7 mg/kg) may cause hypotension, although to a lesser degree than following induction with propofol. Decreases in blood pressure and cardiac output occur primarily though preload reduction due to venodilation and secondarily through decreases in myocardial contractility

(Table 34.3). Decreases in blood pressure are usually accompanied by reflex tachycardia. The hypotension may be exaggerated in the elderly, in hypovolemic patients, or in those who have been pretreated with opioids, benzodiazepines, or antihypertensive medications. Thiopental also causes nonimmunologic histamine release that also contributes to hypotension, but histamine levels return to normal soon after thiopental administration.

Ventilatory effects

Apnea is common following an induction dose of thiopental. Lower doses cause ventilatory depression with decreases in rate, tidal volume, and carbon dioxide responsiveness. Airway responsiveness is increased more than with propofol. Bronchospasm and laryngospasm resulting from airway stimulation occur more frequently because barbiturates do not depress laryngeal or cough reflexes as much as propofol does.

Metabolism and elimination

The short period of unconsciousness following an induction dose of thiopental is the result of redistribution. Repeated bolus doses or a continuous infusion results in accumulation and a longer period of unconsciousness following the last dose or termination of the infusion.

Table 34.2.   CNS effects of IV anesthetic agents

Drug	CMRO$_2$	CBF	CPP	ICP
Thiopental	– –	– –	±	– –
Methohexital	– –	– –	±	– –
Propofol	– –	– –	–	–
Etomidate	– –	– –	+	– –
Benzodiazepines	–	±	0	–
Ketamine	+	+ +	±	+

CMRO$_2$, cerebral metabolic rate for oxygen; CBF, cerebral blood flow; CPP, cerebral perfusion pressure; ICP, intracranial pressure.

Adapted with permission from Dershwitz M, Rosow CE. Intravenous anesthetics. In: Longnecker DE, Brown D, Newman M, Zapol WM, eds. *Anesthesiology.* 3rd ed. New York: McGraw-Hill; 2008.

Table 34.3.   Cardiovascular effects of IV anesthetic agents

Drug	MAP	HR	CO	Contractility dP/dt	SVR	Venous dilation
Thiopental	–	+	–		±	+ +
Methohexital	–	+ +	–	–	±	+
Propofol	– –	–	–		– –	+ +
Etomidate	0	0	0	0	0	0
Diazepam	0/–	±	0	0	–/0	+
Midazolam	0/–	±	0/–	0	–/0	+
Ketamine	+ +	+ +	+	±	±^{a}	0

^{a} Change depends on concurrent sympathetic tone.

dP/dt, delta pressure/delta time; MAP, mean arterial pressure; HR, heart rate; CO, cardiac output; SVR, systemic vascular resistance.

Adapted with permission from Dershwitz M, Rosow CE. Intravenous anesthetics. In: Longnecker DE, Brown D, Newman M, Zapol WM, eds. *Anesthesiology.* 3rd ed. New York: McGraw-Hill; 2008.

Thiopental is oxidatively metabolized by cytochrome P450 (CYP) to several metabolites. One of these metabolites results from replacing the sulfur atom in the barbituric acid ring with an oxygen atom, yielding the active metabolite pentobarbital. Because pentobarbital has a longer duration of action than thiopental, its presence as an active metabolite causes thiopental to appear longer acting than it actually is. These characteristics make thiopental less ideal for maintenance of anesthesia or sedation; therefore, it rarely is given by repeated bolus dosing or by infusion.

Patients with liver disease generally maintain normal total clearance of thiopental. This observation may be explained by the opposing effects of decreased hepatic clearance and decreased protein binding due to hypoalbuminemia. All barbiturates induce δ-aminolevulinic acid (ALA) synthase, the initial enzyme in heme biosynthesis. Patients with certain types of porphyria (acute intermittent porphyria, hereditary coproporphyria, variegate porphyria) are deficient in enzymes downstream from ALA synthase in the heme biosynthesis pathway. Administration of barbiturates to such patients may result in accumulation of ALA, which is neurotoxic. Barbiturates thus are contraindicated in patients with these types of porphyria.

Thiopental and methohexital are supplied as sodium salts in powdered form and are mixed with sterile water prior to administration. Barbiturates may precipitate when dissolved in an acidic solution such as lactated Ringer's. If thiopental is accidentally given by intraarterial injection, vasospasm, thrombosis, and tissue necrosis may occur. Treatment includes vasodilator therapy with papaverine or nitroglycerin and anticoagulation with heparin.

Propofol

Propofol is the most commonly used induction agent because its use is characterized by rapid return of consciousness with minimal residual CNS effects (Table 34.1). It also has antiemetic and amnestic properties at subhypnotic doses.

CNS effects

Like thiopental, propofol decreases $CMRO_2$, CBF, and ICP (Table 34.2). It has an anticonvulsant effect and may be used for treatment of status epilepticus. Although it has not been studied as extensively as thiopental for neuroprotection, it appears to have a similar profile. Relative to thiopental, however, the decreases in systemic blood pressure may be more significant than decreases in ICP, potentially resulting in a greater reduction in cerebral perfusion pressure.

Cardiovascular effects

Propofol causes a greater decrease in systemic vascular resistance than does thiopental, but it causes a similar decrease in cardiac contractility (Table 34.3). By virtue of its inhibition of the barostatic reflex and vagal stimulation, there is a smaller increase in heart rate for a given decrease in blood pressure, thereby exaggerating the hypotensive effect as compared with thiopental. Elderly persons, patients with hypovolemia, and patients with ventricular dysfunction are more likely to become hypotensive.

Ventilatory effects

Compared with thiopental, propofol causes diminished airway reactivity, decreasing the incidence of coughing or laryngospasm. Induction doses result in apnea, and lower doses cause decreases in tidal volume, minute ventilation, and carbon dioxide responsiveness. Pretreatment with benzodiazepines or opioids may augment the ventilatory depressant effect. Propofol does not cause histamine release.

Metabolism and elimination

Propofol is short acting following an induction dose because of its rapid redistribution. Compared with thiopental, it is metabolized more rapidly, not only by the liver, but by the kidney as well. Even in the presence of liver and kidney disease, propofol clearance is usually not significantly decreased. Propofol therefore is often given by infusion, and recovery is typically predictable (see Chapter 36). Propofol is approximately 98% bound to plasma protein. Unlike thiopental, propofol is safe in patients with porphyria.

In the United States, propofol is available as a 1% emulsion containing soybean oil, glycerol, and lecithin. Depending on the manufacturer, the bacteriostatic agent is EDTA, metabisulfite, or benzyl alcohol. Different lipid preparations are available in other countries, and some of them cause less pain on injection. Aseptic technique is important when withdrawing and administering propofol, and vials or syringes that have been exposed to air should be discarded 6 hours after exposure.

True allergy to propofol, if it exists, is exceedingly rare. Although the emulsion contains soybean oil and egg lecithin, it contains no soy protein or egg albumin. Therefore, persons allergic to soy or egg protein can be given propofol safely. IV administration of propofol often causes pain during the injection, especially if it is given via a small vein. The pain may be minimized by choosing a larger vein for IV placement. Alternatively, placing a tourniquet proximal to the IV catheter and then preceding the administration of propofol with an IV injection of lidocaine (0.5 mg/kg) may be effective in reducing this discomfort. Accidental arterial administration of propofol may be very painful but generally does not cause the potentially severe consequences of thrombosis and tissue necrosis that often occur with intraarterial injection of thiopental.

Etomidate

Etomidate, an imidazole derivative, is structurally different from other induction agents. However, like thiopental and propofol, it increases GABA activity. Induction doses result in both rapid onset of anesthesia and rapid emergence

(Table 34.1). In contrast to thiopental and propofol, it produces only minimal changes in blood pressure and cardiac output.

CNS effects

Etomidate produces CNS effects similar to those of propofol and thiopental. Etomidate decreases $CMRO_2$, CBF, and ICP (Table 34.2). Because etomidate reduces ICP while having little effect on mean arterial pressure, it typically produces an increase in cerebral perfusion pressure. Etomidate is an anticonvulsant and may be used in treating status epilepticus. It also may increase EEG activity in epileptogenic areas, a property that makes it useful in locating seizure foci during brain mapping surgery. Unlike other induction agents, which depress somatosensory evoked potentials (SSEPs), etomidate increases both the amplitude and latency of SSEPs. Following induction of anesthesia with etomidate, there is increased incidence of myoclonic jerking compared with thiopental or propofol.

Cardiovascular effects

Perhaps the greatest pharmacologic advantage of etomidate is the hemodynamic stability that follows its administration. Induction of anesthesia with etomidate, in contrast to propofol or thiopental, results in minimal changes in blood pressure, heart rate, or cardiac output because it has minimal effect on cardiac contractility and vascular tone (Table 34.3). Etomidate therefore may be the induction agent of choice in patients with hypovolemia or significant ventricular dysfunction.

Ventilatory effects

Etomidate causes less ventilatory depression than propofol and thiopental, but transient apnea still occurs with induction doses. Opioids often are given in conjunction with etomidate to minimize the sympathetic response to intubation.

Metabolism and elimination

Etomidate inhibits 11β-hydroxylase, the mitochondrial isozyme of CYP responsible for the final reaction in the biosynthesis of cortisol. Following a typical induction dose, cortisol release from the adrenal gland is suppressed for about 12 hours. Whether the short-term adrenal suppression that occurs with a single dose of etomidate is of clinical significance remains controversial. However, the adrenal suppression that occurs with continuous infusions of etomidate may have significant adverse consequences. Etomidate infusions given for several days have been associated with increased mortality in critically ill patients.

Etomidate is metabolized primarily via ester hydrolysis in the liver to a water-soluble metabolite excreted in the urine. Compared with thiopental and propofol, a slightly smaller fraction of etomidate is bound to plasma proteins. Because etomidate has a high hepatic extraction ratio of about 0.7, decreased hepatic blood flow will decrease its clearance. Because etomidate induces ALA synthase in rats, it should be used with caution in patients with porphyria.

Etomidate is supplied as a 0.2% solution in 35% propylene glycol at neutral pH. Intravenous injection may be painful,

Table 34.4. Comparative clinical effects of IV anesthetic agents

Drug	Advantages	Disadvantages
Thiopental	Rapid onset, rapid recovery No pain on injection ↓ CMRO₂, CBF, ICP	↑ Airway responsiveness ↓ BP, CO ↓ Ventilatory drive
Propofol	Rapid onset, rapid recovery ↓ Airway resistance ↓ CMRO₂, CBF, ICP ↓ Nausea and vomiting	Pain on injection ↓ BP, CO ↓ Ventilatory drive
Etomidate	Minimal changes in BP, CO Rapid onset, rapid recovery ↓ CMRO₂, CBF, ICP	Adrenal suppression Pain on injection ↑ Nausea and vomiting ↓ Ventilatory drive
Midazolam	Anxiolysis, amnesia Minimal changes in BP, CO Minimal ventilatory depression Effects reversible with flumazenil ↓ CMRO₂, CBF, ICP Effective by IM route	Longer duration than other agents
Ketamine	Minimal ventilatory depression Preservation of airway reflexes ↑ HR, BP, CO Effective by IM route	Emergence delirium Longer duration than other agents ↑ Ischemia risk in CAD

BP, blood pressure; CAD, coronary artery disease; CO, cardiac output; HR, heart rate.

although much less than with propofol. Etomidate is the most emetogenic of the intravenous induction agents. The combination of etomidate and an opioid may further promote its emetogenic effects. Therefore, antiemetic therapy is advisable with its use. See Table 34.4 for more details.

Benzodiazepines

Diazepam, lorazepam, and midazolam have properties that differentiate them from other induction agents. They are used most commonly for premedication to produce sedation, anxiolysis, and anterograde amnesia, accompanied by minimal ventilatory depression, prior to induction. Although they act primarily by augmenting the inhibitory effects of GABA, they do so via a mechanism distinct from that of other induction agents. They bind to a specific benzodiazepine receptor located near the GABA receptor and increase the affinity of the GABA receptor for GABA. Midazolam and diazepam occasionally are used for induction of anesthesia because of their rapid onset following IV administration; however, emergence is delayed compared with that following thiopental, propofol, or etomidate administration (Table 34.1).

CNS effects

Benzodiazepines decrease $CMRO_2$, CBF, and ICP, although more modestly than thiopental, propofol, or etomidate (Table 34.2). Benzodiazepines are excellent anticonvulsants and may be used to treat status epilepticus. Even following very large doses, benzodiazepines do not cause burst suppression on the

EEG, and cannot cause an isoelectric EEG. Benzodiazepines produce anterograde amnesia at doses that may be only minimally sedating. In most patients, this is a desirable effect. They also cause skeletal muscle relaxation, an effect probably mediated by agonism at the glycine receptor.

Many patients take benzodiazepines chronically for management of anxiety disorders. Such patients develop tolerance with continued use, that may result in cross-tolerance to thiopental, propofol, or etomidate. The development of cross-tolerance leads to an increased dose requirement for these induction agents, as well as to benzodiazepines, administered in the perioperative period.

Cardiovascular effects

Benzodiazepines produce minimal depression of the cardiovascular system in normovolemic patients. They cause a mild decrease in blood pressure secondary to decreased systemic vascular resistance (Table 34.3). Myocardial contractility is relatively unaffected. The decrease in preload and afterload resulting from induction with a benzodiazepine makes them reasonable choices for induction in patients with heart failure. Benzodiazepines may cause a significant decrease in blood pressure in patients with hypertension due to anxiety.

Ventilatory effects

When used alone in sedating doses, benzodiazepines cause minimal ventilatory depression. However, when given in combination with opioids, benzodiazepines act synergistically to produce sedation and ventilatory depression. When used in higher doses (e.g., for induction of anesthesia), benzodiazepines may cause transient apnea.

Metabolism and elimination

Allergy to benzodiazepines is rare. They also generally do not cause nausea or vomiting. In contrast to diazepam and lorazepam, which cause pain on injection because of their propylene glycol solvent, midazolam is relatively painless when given intravenously owing to its water solubility. Benzodiazepines may be given orally, although the extensive first-pass metabolism of midazolam requires that high doses be given. Midazolam (along with ketamine) is one of the few induction agents that may be given intramuscularly, resulting in reliable absorption into the circulation.

Midazolam, diazepam, and lorazepam are metabolized by the liver. Because a high fraction of diazepam and lorazepam is bound to protein, these agents are cleared by the liver more slowly. Metabolism of midazolam results in a metabolite with only minimal activity, and it is rapidly conjugated to glucuronic acid and excreted. Lorazepam is metabolized to an inactive metabolite. Diazepam is metabolized to several active metabolites, including nordazepam that has a long half-life (100 hours), and oxazepam. Unless these medications are given by multiple repeated bolus doses or by a prolonged infusion, termination of the drug effect is the result of redistribution. When given by infusion, midazolam has a longer context-sensitive half-time

than thiopental or propofol (see Chapter 36). Patients with porphyria generally should avoid benzodiazepines, as some of these agents were found to induce ALA synthase in rats.

Benzodiazepines are the only induction agents for which there is a specific antagonist: flumazenil. Therefore, it is possible, although not always advisable, to reverse the CNS effects of a benzodiazepine by administering flumazenil. Flumazenil is an antagonist at the benzodiazepine receptor. The relative concentrations of benzodiazepine and flumazenil determine the overall level of pharmacologic effect. Some studies found flumazenil to have inverse agonist activity, meaning it produces an effect opposite that of the agonist. Thus, flumazenil may cause anxiety and panic if given alone. Patients on chronic benzodiazepine therapy who are given flumazenil may have symptoms and signs of acute withdrawal, including seizures.

Reversal of benzodiazepine effects with flumazenil should be done with caution, not only because of the adverse effects that may occur, but because flumazenil is much shorter acting than the benzodiazepines whose effects it may be used to reverse. Thus, repeated dosing may be necessary to maintain benzodiazepine antagonism. Flumazenil does not reliably reverse the ventilatory depression caused by benzodiazepines, and ventilatory support may be required in patients receiving flumazenil to treat a large overdose of benzodiazepine. If opioids also were administered with the benzodiazepine, then naloxone may be needed to reverse the ventilatory depression.

Ketamine

Ketamine, unlike other induction agents, acts primarily by NMDA receptor antagonism as opposed to GABA potentiation. It is structurally related to phencyclidine. It is supplied as a racemic mixture, and the S-isomer produces more analgesia, less delirium, and shorter emergence times than the R-isomer.

Anesthesia with ketamine is markedly different from that of other agents. It produces a cataleptic state, often termed "dissociative anesthesia," typically characterized by signs consistent with continued consciousness. Patients given ketamine may have open eyes and nystagmus; they may move and vocalize, yet they do not respond to stimuli, cannot communicate, and have no recollection of events. They may report vivid dreams, hallucinations, or dysphoria postoperatively. These effects may be mitigated by the concurrent administration of propofol or a benzodiazepine.

Ketamine produces profound analgesia that typically persists into the postoperative period. Its ability to produce amnesia and analgesia in the presence of minimal ventilatory depression makes it a useful analgesic when trying to maintain spontaneous ventilation while managing pain.

CNS effects

In contrast to the other induction agents, ketamine increases $CMRO_2$, CBF, and ICP (Table 34.2). Thus, ketamine generally is not used in patients with increased ICP, intracranial lesions, or recent head trauma. The EEG changes caused by ketamine are quite different from those of the other induction agents. Therefore, monitors of anesthesia depth that rely on processing the EEG signal, such as the bispectral index (BIS) monitor, do reliably indicate the depth of ketamine-induced anesthesia. Like etomidate, ketamine is associated with a high risk of postoperative nausea and vomiting.

Cardiovascular effects

Ketamine is the only induction agent that causes cardiovascular stimulation through centrally mediated increased sympathetic tone and increased release of adrenal catecholamines. Patients experience a transient increase in heart rate, systemic vascular resistance, pulmonary artery pressure, and cardiac output (Table 34.3). These effects may be beneficial in maintaining hemodynamic stability in a hypovolemic patient or in a patient with reduced ventricular function. These same properties make ketamine a poor choice in patients with coronary artery disease or poorly controlled hypertension, because the increase in myocardial oxygen demand may exceed the increase in oxygen delivery, causing ischemia. Although the cardiovascular effects of ketamine are indirect, ketamine may cause direct myocardial depression in patients whose sympathetic tone is maximal.

Ventilatory effects

Ketamine does not cause significant ventilatory depression when given to healthy patients or those with chronic obstructive pulmonary disease. Ketamine causes bronchodilation, making it useful for induction in patients prone to bronchospasm. However, it depresses airway reflexes to a lesser degree than other induction agents. Nevertheless, aspiration is still a risk in patients anesthetized with ketamine and not intubated. Laryngospasm may occur during light anesthesia with ketamine as it causes an increase in salivary, tracheal, and bronchial secretions. Pretreatment with an antisialagogue (e.g., glycopyrrolate) is generally recommended.

Metabolism and elimination

Ketamine may be given intravenously or intramuscularly. Like midazolam, it is reliably absorbed following intramuscular injection. Ketamine undergoes high first-pass metabolism following oral administration, although it is sometimes given orally in children.

In contrast to induction of general anesthesia with thiopental, propofol, or etomidate, unconsciousness following IV induction with ketamine may last up to a half hour, and it may take much longer for the patient to become fully oriented (Table 34.1). Upon emergence from anesthesia following ketamine administration, patients may experience "emergence delirium," characterized by confusion, impaired short-term memory, auditory and visual hallucinations, or even nightmares. Concurrent administration of propofol or a benzodiazepine may decrease the incidence and severity of these adverse effects.

The prolonged effect of ketamine is partly a result of its metabolism by CYP to norketamine, an active metabolite with approximately one-fourth the potency of ketamine. After norketamine is hydroxylated and conjugated, forming a water-soluble metabolite, it is renally excreted. Because ketamine has a high hepatic extraction ratio of about 0.8, decreased hepatic blood flow will decrease its clearance. Ketamine is generally considered safe in patients with porphyria.

Suggested readings

Brain Resuscitation Clinical Trial I Study Group. Randomized clinical study of thiopental loading in comatose survivors of cardiac arrest. *N Eng J Med* 1986; 314:397–403.

DeBalli P. The use of propofol as an antiemetic. *Int Anesthesiol Clin* 2003; 41:67–77.

Dershwitz M, Rosow CE. Intravenous anesthetics. In: Longnecker DE, Brown D, Newman M, Zapol WM, eds. *Anesthesiology.* 3rd ed. New York: McGraw-Hill; 2008.

Eames WO, Rooke GA, Wu RS, et al. Comparison of the effects of etomidate, propofol, and thiopental on respiratory resistance after tracheal intubation. *Anesthesiology* 1996; 84:1307–1311.

Fragen RJ, Shanks CA, Molteni A, et al. Effects of etomidate on hormonal responses to surgical stress. *Anesthesiology* 1984; 61:652–656.

Gooding JM, Weng, JT, Smith RA, et al. Cardiovascular and pulmonary response following etomidate induction of anesthesia in patients with demonstrated cardiac disease. *Anesth Analg* 1979; 58:40–41.

Grounds RM, Twigley AJ, Carli F. The haemodynamic effects of intravenous induction. Comparison of the effects of thiopentone and propofol. *Anaesthesia* 1985; 40:735–740.

Hiraoka H, Yamamoto K, Miyoshi S, et al. Kidneys contribute to the extrahepatic clearance of propofol in humans, but not lungs and brain. *Br J Clin Pharmacol* 2005; 60:176–182.

Hudson RJ, Stanski DR, Burch PG. Pharmacokinetics of methohexital and thiopental in surgical patients. *Anesthesiology* 1983; 59:215–219.

Hudson RJ, Stanski DR, Saidman LJ, et al. A model for studying depth of anesthesia and acute tolerance to thiopental. *Anesthesiology* 1983; 59:301–308.

Picard P, Tramèr MR. Prevention of pain on injection with propofol: a quantitative systematic review. *Anesth Analg* 2000; 90:963–969.

Russo H, Bressolle F. Pharmacodynamics and pharmacokinetics of thiopental. *Clin Pharmacokinet* 1998; 35:95–134.

Sato M, Tanaka M, Umehara S, et al. Baroreflex control of heart rate during and after propofol infusion in humans. *Br J Anaesth* 2005; 94:577–581.

Servin F, Cockshott ID, Farinotti R, et al. Pharmacokinetics of propofol infusions in patients with cirrhosis. *Br J Anaesth* 1990; 65:177–183.

Veselis RA, Reinsel RA, Feshchenko VA, et al. The comparative amnestic effects of midazolam, propofol, thiopental, and fentanyl at equisedative concentrations. *Anesthesiology* 1997; 87:749–764.

Watt I, Ledingham IM. Mortality amongst multiple trauma patients admitted to an intensive therapy unit. *Anaesthesia* 1984; 39:973–981.

White PF, Way WL, Trevor AJ. Ketamine: its pharmacology and therapeutic uses. *Anesthesiology* 1982; 56:119–136.

Chapter 35

Mechanisms of anesthetic actions

Ken Solt and Douglas E. Raines

General anesthetics are structurally diverse (Fig. 35.1). Drugs with anesthetic activity include noble gases, alkanes, alcohols, ethers, and other structurally unrelated compounds. To account for this diversity, early theories regarding general anesthetic action were heavily influenced by the notion that all anesthetics act by a common mechanism.

Lipid theories of anesthetic action

At the end of the 19th century, Meyer and Overton independently reported a strong correlation between the potencies of general anesthetics and their lipid solubilities (Fig. 35.2a). Their observations suggested that all anesthetics produce their behavioral effects in the same manner, by interacting nonspecifically with lipid components of neuronal cell membranes. Although the details were vague regarding how these interactions led to specific anesthetic effects, the Meyer-Overton correlation and lipid theories of anesthetic mechanisms dominated thinking in the field for many years.

Evidence has accumulated over the past several decades, however, that argues against lipids as anesthetic targets. *First*, anesthetic-induced changes in lipid properties (i.e., fluidity) are mimicked by small changes in temperature that do not alter behavior in animals. *Second*, anesthetics act stereoselectively to produce anesthesia, a characteristic generally associated with specific interactions with protein targets. For example, the R-$^+$ enantiomer of etomidate is more than an order of magnitude more potent than the S-enantiomer. Similarly, optical isomers of isoflurane possess different anesthetic potencies, although the magnitude of this difference is relatively small. *Third*, there is a "cutoff" in anesthetic potency in homologous anesthetic compounds. Anesthetic cutoff is the phenomenon in which the anesthetic potencies of homologous compounds increase with anesthetic size until a cutoff point is reached, after which anesthetic activity either no longer increases or disappears completely. This is best illustrated with straight-chain alcohols (e.g., methanol, ethanol, n-propanol, n-butanol) in which anesthetic potency increases with alkyl chain length up to n-dodecanol, but longer alcohols are devoid of anesthetic activity. *Fourth*, some volatile compounds (e.g., di-[2,2,2,-trifluoroethyl]ether) possess no anesthetic activity even though they are highly lipid soluble and therefore are predicted by the Meyer-Overton correlation to be potent anesthetics.

These compounds, termed *nonimmobilizers*, typically produce convulsions when given at partial pressures predicted to produce anesthesia.

A series of experiments by Franks and Lieb in the 1980s demonstrated that anesthetic inhibition of firefly luciferase, a water-soluble protein in a lipid-free system, obeys the Meyer-Overton correlation (Fig. 35.2b). This work led most researchers to abandon lipid theories and agree that proteins are the likely targets of general anesthetics. Recent work has focused largely on identifying the specific proteins involved in producing anesthetic effects.

Ion channels in the central nervous system

Anesthetics have been shown to bind to a diverse range of proteins, but ion channels in the central nervous system (CNS)

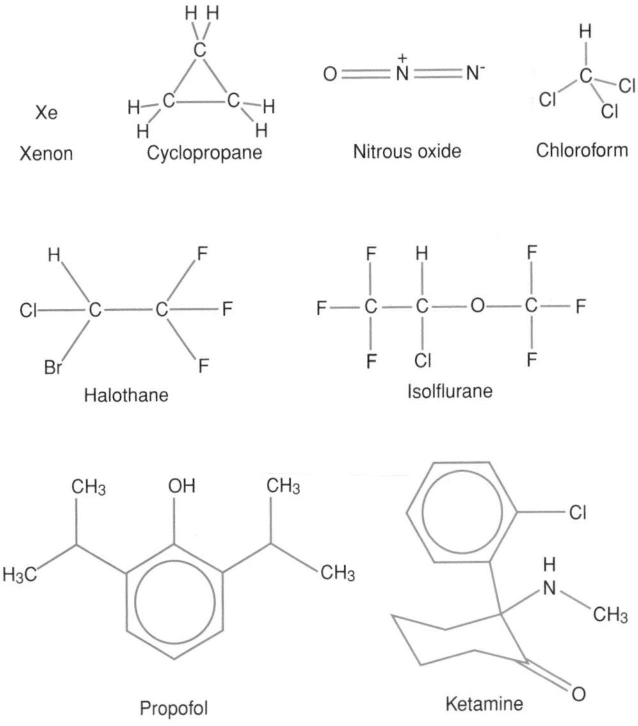

Figure 35.1. The structural diversity of general anesthetics. Although the pharmacologic profiles of these drugs vastly differ, all of them are capable of producing amnesia and immobility in response to noxious stimuli.

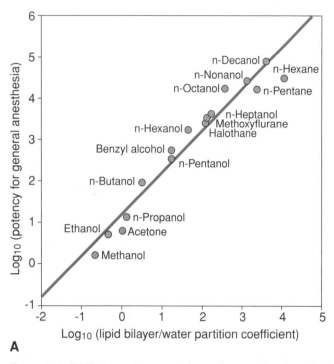

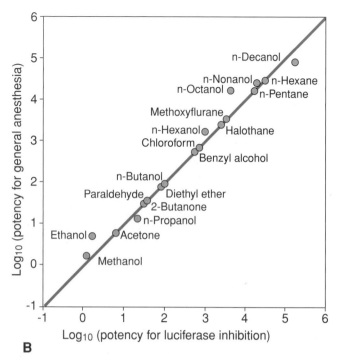

Figure 35.2. (**A**) The Meyer-Overton correlation, illustrating the relationship between anesthetic potency and lipid solubility. (**B**) The strong correlation between anesthetic potency and potency for luciferase inhibition demonstrates that a protein target can account for the observations of Meyer and Overton. (Modified from Figure 3 in Franks NP. Molecular targets underlying general anesthesia. *Br J Pharmacol* 2006; 147:S72–S81.)

are considered to be among the most likely targets that mediate the behavioral effects of these drugs. In particular, neurotransmitter-gated ion channels that regulate synaptic transmission are thought to play important roles; among these, γ-aminobutyric acid (GABA) receptors have been studied most extensively.

The GABA type A (GABA$_A$) receptor belongs to a family of neurotransmitter-gated ion channels that include the nicotinic acetylcholine, serotonin type 3 (5-HT$_3$), and glycine receptors. GABA$_A$ receptors are the most abundantly expressed inhibitory receptors in the brain. Binding of GABA to these receptors causes opening of a chloride-selective ion channel and hyperpolarization of the neuronal membrane. Many inhaled and intravenous anesthetics have been shown to enhance the activity of GABA$_A$ receptors, leading to an increase in inhibitory neurotransmission in the CNS.

Propofol and etomidate

Although many anesthetic-sensitive ion channels, such as GABA$_A$ receptors have been identified, it is difficult to prove from in vitro data whether a specific target is responsible for a drug's behavioral effects. Recent advances in genetic engineering have provided a powerful new tool for testing the relevance of putative anesthetic targets, and genetic approaches have been particularly successful in elucidating the mechanisms underlying the actions of propofol and etomidate.

Electrophysiologic studies have demonstrated that a single amino acid substitution in the β$_3$ subunit of the GABA$_A$

receptor renders the entire receptor insensitive to the enhancing effects of propofol and etomidate. When this point mutation was introduced in mice to produce "knock-in" animals, the mutants were highly resistant to the hypnosis, immobility, and respiratory depression produced by these anesthetics. This result indicates that GABA$_A$ receptors containing β$_3$ subunits play a critical role in mediating important CNS effects of propofol and etomidate.

Ketamine, nitrous oxide, cyclopropane, and xenon

Unlike propofol and etomidate, ketamine, nitrous oxide, cyclopropane and xenon have little or no effect on GABA$_A$ receptors. However all these drugs are potent inhibitors of N-methyl-D-aspartate (NMDA) receptors. NMDA receptors are a subtype of glutamate receptors, which are the most widely expressed excitatory receptors in the brain. Unlike inhibitory GABA$_A$ receptors, glutamate receptors cause neuronal depolarization upon glutamate binding. NMDA receptors have received the most attention among the glutamate receptor subtypes, as they play important roles in learning and memory as well as nociception. Anesthetic-induced inhibition of NMDA receptors may produce behavioral effects by decreasing excitatory neurotransmission in the CNS.

In addition to inhibiting glutamate receptors, ketamine and nitrous oxide inhibit neuronal nicotinic acetylcholine receptors, which are also important excitatory receptors in the CNS. TREK-1, a tandem-pore K$^+$ channel widely expressed in the CNS, also is activated by nitrous oxide, xenon, and cyclopropane, leading to neuronal hyperpolarization. Although ketamine, nitrous oxide, cyclopropane, and xenon all appear to produce their behavioral effects by similar mechanisms, the relevance of their proposed targets has yet to be elucidated.

Halogenated volatile anesthetics

Halogenated alkanes (e.g., chloroform, halothane) and ethers (e.g., isoflurane, sevoflurane, desflurane) exhibit the least selectivity for putative anesthetic target proteins. Targets sensitive to halogenated volatile anesthetics include $GABA_A$ receptors, glutamate receptors, tandem-pore K^+ channels, neuronal nicotinic acetylcholine receptors, $5\text{-}HT_3$ receptors, mitochondrial adenosine triphosphate–sensitive K^+ channels, and HCN (hyperpolarization-activated cyclic nucleotide-gated) channels, among others. Effects on some targets may be important in mediating anesthetic side effects such as nausea and vomiting, whereas others may lead to potentially beneficial effects, such as ischemic preconditioning. So far, genetic methods to identify targets relevant to immobility have produced only modest results for these anesthetics, suggesting that many molecular targets may contribute to their behavioral effects.

Anatomic sites of anesthetic actions

General anesthetics have myriad reversible effects on the CNS, including sedation, excitation, confusion, amnesia, euphoria, hypnosis, and immobility. Although most scientists had assumed that the brain was responsible for mediating all the CNS effects of general anesthetics, a series of animal studies conclusively demonstrated that anesthetic-induced immobility in response to noxious stimuli is the result of of an effect on the spinal cord, not the brain. Therefore, even a single anatomic site cannot account for all the CNS effects of general anesthetics.

Summary

Although early theories focused on a single, lipid-based mechanism of anesthetic action, it has become evident that multiple sites and mechanisms likely are responsible for the behavioral effects of general anesthetics. Furthermore, the sites and mechanisms likely are different depending on the anesthetic. As we continue to learn more about how general anesthetics act to produce their desirable and undesirable effects, the design of safer drugs with improved therapeutic indices may be attainable.

Suggested readings

Campagna JA, Miller KW, Forman SA. Mechanisms of actions of inhaled anesthetics. *N Engl J Med* 2003; 348:2110–2124.

Franks NP. Molecular targets underlying general anesthesia. *Br J Pharmacol* 2006; 147:S72–S81.

Jurd R, Arras M, Lambert S, et al. General anesthetic actions in vivo strongly attenuated by a point mutation in the GABA(A) receptor beta3 subunit. *FASEB J* 2003; 17:250–252.

Koblin DD. Mechanisms of action. In: Miller RD, ed. *Miller's Anesthesia*. 6th ed. Philadelphia: Elsevier; 2004:105–130.

Solt K, Forman SA. Correlating the clinical actions and molecular mechanisms of general anesthetics. *Curr Opin Anaesthesiol* 2007; 20:300–306.

Pharmacokinetics of intravenous agents

Lisbeth Lopez Pappas and Mark Dershwitz

Pharmacokinetics is the study of "what the body does to the drug," whereas pharmacodynamics is the study of "what the drug does to the body." This chapter considers the pharmacokinetics of anesthetic drugs given by the intravenous route. Age and certain diseases (e.g., heart failure, liver failure, renal failure) may require adjustments from the typical doses of a drug. An understanding of pharmacokinetic parameters, which may be altered by certain disease states, provides a rational approach to drug and dosage selection. These parameters include the volume of distribution (V_d), drug clearance (CL), and drug half-life ($t_{1/2}$).

Pharmacokinetic parameters

Drug distribution

The injection of a medication intravenously provides complete absorption, with a rapid and predictable rise in the drug concentration in the plasma. From the systemic circulation, drugs rapidly distribute to highly perfused organs such as the brain, heart, lungs, liver, and kidneys. This vessel-rich group accounts for about 10% of total body mass, yet it receives about 75% of the cardiac output. Factors that influence drug distribution and tissue uptake include lipid solubility, ionization, and protein binding.

For drugs that are lipid soluble, nonionized, and unbound to protein, the concentration gradient will dictate the degree and direction of transfer. A tissue's capacity to function as a drug reservoir depends greatly on the drug's solubility in that tissue, its binding to macromolecules, and tissue pH. Saturation of these stores, as may occur with repeated or large initial doses of the drug, results in a prolonged duration of action. This effect might convert an apparently "short-acting" drug such as thiopental or fentanyl into one that actually has a long duration of action. As the drug's concentration in the circulation falls with respect to that in highly perfused tissues (e.g., brain), redistribution of drug to less perfused tissues (e.g., muscle, fat) occurs. This process accounts for the "short" duration of action of medications such as propofol and sufentanil.

Ionization

The degree of ionization is determined by the drug's pK_a (dissociation constant) and the pH of the liquid in which it is dissolved. The pK_a is the pH at which 50% of the drug exists in the ionized form and 50% in the nonionized form. Small variations in pH may have significant effects on the ratio of ionized to nonionized drug. Nonionized molecules typically have greater lipid solubility. Most clinically used medications are either weak acids or weak bases and therefore exist in both ionized and nonionized forms. At a low (acidic) pH, weak acids (e.g., barbiturates) become uncharged and more lipid soluble whereas weak bases (e.g., local anesthetics, opioids) become charged and more water soluble.

Protein binding

Drug disposition is significantly affected by the degree of protein binding. Factors that determine the extent of protein binding include the concentrations of both the drug and the protein to which it binds, the affinity of the drug for the protein, and the number of available protein binding sites. In general, the binding of drugs to proteins is reversible and involves hydrophobic or ionic interactions. The ability of a drug to bind to proteins in the circulation or within a tissue affects the drug concentration in that compartment. In general, drugs with high lipid solubility also have greater protein binding.

In the circulation, acidic drugs (e.g., barbiturates) tend to bind to albumin, whereas basic drugs (e.g., opioids) tend to bind to α_1-acid glycoprotein (AAG), an acute-phase reactant that increases with physiologic stresses such as surgery and trauma. It is the free (i.e., unbound) fraction of a drug that largely contributes to the pharmacologic effect. For drugs with negligible protein binding (i.e., free fraction $\approx$ 1), there is no relationship between changes in protein concentration and changes in the free fraction of drug. However, for drugs that approach 100% protein binding (i.e., free fraction $\approx$ 0), there is an inverse relationship between the change in protein concentration and the change in the free fraction of drug in the plasma. For example, a small decrease in the binding capacity (e.g., from 98% to 96%) of diazepam, a highly protein-bound drug, doubles the free fraction of drug in the circulation.

Factors that affect protein binding include age, liver disease, kidney disease, and physiologic stress or trauma. Both kidney and liver disease can produce a quantitative as well as qualitative change in the binding of drugs to proteins. Protein binding also may be altered by changes in tissue pH (e.g., acidosis, alkalosis) and the presence of other drugs or endogenous compounds (e.g., bilirubin) that can compete for protein binding sites. Only unbound drug equilibrates between the circulation and tissues and ultimately undergoes metabolism and elimination. With reduced protein binding (e.g., hypoalbuminemia), the increased free fraction of drug produces a larger gradient between the circulation and peripheral tissues; as a result, equilibrium is achieved at a lower drug concentration in the circulation. In addition, the concentration of drug at the site of action increases (i.e., increased apparent potency), which translates to a lower required dose.

Elimination

Elimination includes the processes of metabolism and excretion. The primary organ involved in drug metabolism is the liver via hepatic microsomal enzymes (e.g., cytochrome P450 [CYP]). Microsomal enzymes are induced by many drugs (e.g., barbiturates, rifampin, phenytoin) and inhibited by others (e.g., cimetidine, azole antifungal agents, macrolide antibiotics, antiretroviral protease inhibitors). The biotransformation of drugs involves phase I and/or phase II reactions. Phase I reactions include oxidation, reduction, and hydrolysis, whereas phase II reactions involve conjugation to moieties such as glucuronic acid or sulfate. The overall effect is to convert lipid-soluble drugs to water-soluble metabolites that are more easily excreted in urine and bile.

Factors that affect hepatic drug metabolism include hepatic blood flow and the intrinsic capacity of the liver to metabolize the drug. The fraction of unbound drug cleared by the liver is known as the hepatic extraction ratio (ER). Hepatic clearance is calculated by the following equation:

$$CL = Q \times ER,$$

where Q is the hepatic blood flow.

For drugs that have a high hepatic extraction ratio (ER > 0.9), drug clearance is affected primarily by hepatic blood flow (perfusion-dependent metabolism), whereas drugs that have a low extraction ratio (ER < 0.2) are minimally affected by hepatic blood flow and greatly affected by the metabolic capacity of the liver (capacity-dependent elimination). For example, propofol (ER ≈ 1), shows a linear relationship between drug clearance and hepatic blood flow, whereas alfentanil (ER ≈ 0.1) demonstrates a linear relationship between drug clearance and the intrinsic metabolic capacity of the liver. Alfentanil therefore is much more likely than propofol to participate in drug interactions due to induction or inhibition of CYP.

In general, biotransformation of drugs by the liver results in metabolites that are less pharmacologically active. There are exceptions, however, such as codeine and morphine, and variations in the extent of hepatic metabolism may cause clinically significant differences in the drug's effects. For example, codeine is metabolized to morphine by CYP2D6, which exhibits a greater degree of genetic polymorphism than any other isozyme of CYP. Morphine is metabolized further to

morphine-6-glucuronide, an active metabolite with greater potency than morphine. These metabolites are responsible for the analgesic effects of codeine. Patients with nonfunctional versions of CYP2D6 (about 10% of persons of western European descent) experience no analgesic effect from codeine, whereas patients with CYP2D6 gene duplication or amplification demonstrate ultrarapid codeine metabolism and an exaggerated opioid effect.

Some drugs undergo extrahepatic metabolism. For example, certain tissues are rich in esterases, and several important medications undergo extrahepatic hydrolysis, including succinylcholine (plasma), remifentanil (skeletal muscle), and esmolol (red blood cells). The overall clearance of propofol significantly exceeds hepatic blood flow because of substantial metabolism in the kidney. In addition, other drugs (e.g., atracurium, cisatracurium) undergo nonenzymatic Michael (occasionally referred to as Hofmann) elimination in the circulation at physiologic pH and temperature. This reaction is independent of disease or genetic variations.

The clearance of water-soluble metabolites or drugs that do not undergo metabolism occurs primarily in the kidney, and the clearance is correlated with creatinine concentration or creatinine clearance. Excretion of drugs by the kidney involves both glomerular filtration and tubular secretion. The glomerular filtration rate, protein binding, lipid solubility, and urine pH can influence the rate and extent of renal clearance. Alkalinization of the urine can enhance the renal excretion of weak acids such as glucuronides by shifting the fraction of drug in the ionized form so that tubular reabsorption occurs to a lesser degree.

Pharmacokinetic models

The first fundamental pharmacokinetic parameter, the volume of distribution (V_d), represents the volume into which a drug *appears to be* diluted. It is calculated by the following formula:

$$V_d = \frac{Dose}{Concentration}.$$

The classic yet simplest one-compartment pharmacokinetic model has served as the basis for calculating dosage regimens (Fig. 36.1). Applying this model to the lipid-soluble drugs used in anesthesia (e.g., hypnotics, opioids) results in huge deviations from physiologic behavior. A multicompartmental model involves more complex mathematic equations but is better suited to predicting the behavior of most anesthetic medications.

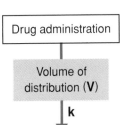

Figure 36.1. The one-compartment pharmacokinetic model. Clearance equals $k \times V$. (Redrawn with permission from Figure 52-13 in Shafer SL. Principles of pharmacokinetics and pharmacodynamics. In *Principles and Practice of Anesthesiology*. 2nd ed. St. Louis: Mosby; 1998.

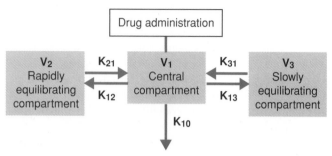

Figure 36.2. The three-compartment pharmacokinetic model. Drug is administered into a central compartment from which it is cleared by metabolism and/or elimination. Drug rapidly distributes into a peripheral compartment, and this compartment reaches equilibrium with the central compartment quickly. Drug distributes more slowly into a third compartment. The volume of distribution at steady state, V_d, equals $V_1 + V_2 + V_3$. Redrawn with permission from Figure 52-16 in Shafer SL. Principles of pharmacokinetics and pharmacodynamics. In *Principles and Practice of Anesthesiology*. 2nd ed. St. Louis: Mosby; 1998.

The three-compartment pharmacokinetic model divides the body into theoretic volumes from which pharmacokinetic parameters are derived (Fig. 36.2). The initial volume into which a drug is introduced is referred to as the central volume of distribution, V_1, and represents some fraction of the circulating volume. Two peripheral compartments, one representing rapidly equilibrating tissues (V_2) and the other the slowly equilibrating tissues (V_3), are linked to the central compartment. Drug transfer from one compartment to another is known as intercompartmental clearance and is represented by a rate constant, k. Drug transfer directly out of the central compartment is known as central clearance, k_{10}. The distribution of drug throughout the body results in the ultimate equilibrium of drug throughout all body tissues, also known as steady state. In this situation, the volume of distribution at steady state, $V_{d_{ss}}$, includes the central as well as the peripheral compartments and can be calculated as follows:

$$V_{d_{ss}} = V_1 + V_2 + V_3 = \frac{X}{C},$$

where X is the dose of drug administered and C is the drug concentration in the plasma at steady state.

Anesthetic drug distribution is typically extensive and reflects the properties of the drug (e.g., solubility, protein binding) as well as the composition of a given compartment (e.g., protein vs. fat, water content). In general, drugs that are lipid soluble undergo extensive distribution out of the central compartment and have large volumes of distribution (e.g., propofol, diazepam). Conversely, drugs that are water soluble tend to distribute to body water and thus have smaller volumes of distribution (e.g., vecuronium, epinephrine). The volume of distribution of lipid-soluble drugs often greatly exceeds the total volume of the body and thus cannot be correlated with actual anatomic volumes (e.g., V_d for propofol $\approx$ 5000 L).

The second fundamental pharmacokinetic parameter is clearance (CL). It refers to the portion of the volume of distribution from which a drug *appears* to be removed during a

Table 36.1. Drug concentration as a function of half-lives

Elapsed half-lives, n	Original concentration remaining, %
1	50
2	25
3	12.5
4	6.25
5	3.125
6	1.5625

given period. From the one-compartment model, the relationship between clearance and volume of distribution is:

$$CL = k \times V_d,$$

where k is the rate constant.

In the one-compartment model, the half-life ($t_{1/2}$) is defined as the time it takes drug concentration to decrease by 50%. The half-life is related to the rate constant, k, according to the following equation:

$$t_{1/2} = \frac{\ln 2}{k} = \frac{0.693}{k}.$$

As each half-life elapses, the drug concentration decreases to 50% of its previous value. Thus, the decrease in drug concentration as a function of the number of half-lives that have elapsed is shown in Table 36.1.

The rate at which the central compartment drug concentration decreases depends on clearance (primarily hepatic metabolism) as well as on the distribution of drug out of the central compartment into the peripheral compartments, also known as the intercompartmental clearances. The intercompartmental clearances reflect blood flow to the peripheral tissues as well as the properties of the drug itself (e.g., lipid solubility).

The three-compartment model is necessary to approximate the pharmacokinetic behavior of the lipid-soluble intravenous anesthetic agents. A graphic depiction of drug concentration as a function of time following an intravenous bolus injection of 10 mg of morphine is shown in Fig. 36.3. The shape of the curve is characterized by three phases. The first phase lasts about 6 minutes and has a half-life of 1 minute. It is characterized by a steep decrease in the plasma concentration of morphine, primarily as a result of drug distribution from the central compartment to the rapidly equilibrating compartment. The second phase lasts about 50 minutes and has a half-life of 8 minutes. It is characterized by a more gradual decrease in the plasma drug concentration and results primarily from drug distribution into the slowly equilibrating compartment. The third, or terminal, phase has a half-life of 96 minutes, is characterized by a much slower decrease in plasma drug concentration, and results from the metabolism and renal elimination of morphine as well as the return of morphine from both peripheral compartments to the central compartment.

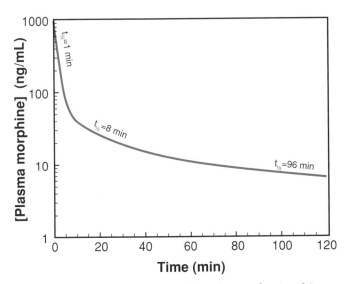

Figure 36.3. The plasma concentration of morphine as a function of time following a 10-mg bolus dose. The three phases of the disappearance curve have half-lives of 1 minute, 8 minutes, and 96 minutes, respectively. Redrawn with permission from Figure 5 in Dershwitz M, Walsh JL, Morishige RJ, et al. Pharmacokinetics and pharmacodynamics of inhaled versus intravenous morphine in healthy volunteers. *Anesthesiology* 2000; 93:619–628.

The plasma drug concentration as a function of time following the administration of the intravenous bolus, Conc(t), can be calculated as follows:

$$\text{Conc}(t) = Ae^{-\alpha t} + Be^{-\beta t} + Ce^{-\gamma t},$$

where t is the time following the bolus; A, B, and C are fractional coefficients; and α, β, and γ are rate constants. The first, second, and third exponential terms in the equation correspond to the rapid, intermediate, and slow phases of the disappearance curve shown in Fig. 36.3, respectively. The fractional coefficients describe the importance of each of the three phases in the overall disappearance of the drug.

The rate constants used in the three-compartment model are related to the half-lives of each of the three phases:

$$t_{1/2\alpha} = \frac{\ln 2}{\alpha} \quad t_{1/2\beta} = \frac{\ln 2}{\beta} \quad t_{1/2\gamma} = \frac{\ln 2}{\gamma}.$$

For all practical purposes, a pharmacokinetic process may be considered complete after five half-lives have elapsed (although it should be apparent that such a process is *never* complete in a mathematic sense).

The use of half-lives as the basis for drug dosing may be misleading. Although the terminal half-lives of most of the commonly used intravenous anesthetics are quite long (e.g., propofol $\approx$ 5 hours, sufentanil $\approx$ 9 hours), recovery from a bolus dose of a lipophilic drug can occur in minutes because of its rapid redistribution. When intravenous anesthetics are administered by infusion, redistribution continues to play a significant role in the termination of the drug's effect.

Intravenous anesthetics have become widely used in the practice of anesthesia. It is intuitive that when a volatile agent is

used for maintenance of general anesthesia, the longer the duration of administration the longer it will take to eliminate the agent to permit the patient to awaken. Analogously, the longer the duration of intravenous drug infusion, the longer the time required for emergence from anesthesia. However, the terminal half-life cannot be used to predict the decline in drug concentration in the central compartment.

Although intravenous anesthetics have been in clinical use since the 1940s, it was not until the 1990s that quantitative methods were introduced to permit the clinician to predict accurately the amount of time required for emergence following the intravenous infusion of an anesthetic drug. This concept, called the *context-sensitive half-time* (CSHT), describes the time required for the central compartment drug concentration to fall by 50% as a function of the duration of the infusion. The term *context* refers to the duration of an infusion designed to maintain a constant central compartment drug concentration. It has been demonstrated that the CSHTs of commonly used anesthetic drugs are substantially shorter than their respective terminal half-lives.

As expected, the time to recovery (i.e., awakening) after the termination of a continuous intravenous infusion depends on the drug concentration in the central and peripheral compartments at the time the infusion is discontinued. At the end of a short infusion, there remains a large concentration gradient between the central and peripheral compartments, and the drug concentration in the central compartment will decrease rapidly. In contrast, at the end of a long infusion, both the rapidly and the slowly equilibrating compartments may approach steady state with the central compartment; therefore, the decline in the central compartment drug concentration will occur more slowly.

The CSHTs for five common intravenous anesthetics as a function of infusion duration are illustrated in Fig. 36.4. From

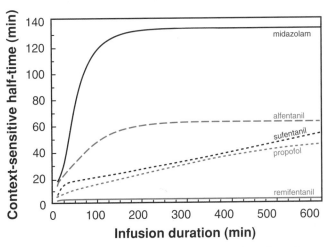

Figure 36.4. The context-sensitive half-times for midazolam, alfentanil, sufentanil, propofol, and remifentanil as a function of infusion duration. The simulations were performed using the program RECOV, written by Steven Shafer.

this graph, it is apparent that the choice of anesthetic to be given by a continuous intravenous infusion can be made based on the anticipated duration of the surgical procedure. As shown in the figure, midazolam has a CSHT of about 120 minutes after a 2-hour infusion; thus, it would not be a good choice for a hypnotic agent when rapid emergence is desired. Alfentanil, an opioid with a short terminal half-life that often is used in brief procedures, is not short acting when given by a continuous infusion. Although alfentanil has shorter distribution and terminal half-lives than sufentanil, recovery following a sufentanil infusion is much more rapid than that with alfentanil for infusions less than 9 hours. Sufentanil and propofol display similar curves, suggesting that these anesthetic agents may be discontinued simultaneously in the course of an anesthetic. The CSHT of remifentanil remains constant at about 4 minutes, regardless of the duration of the infusion. This is because metabolic clearance of remifentanil is so much greater than its intercompartmental clearances that accumulation of remifentanil does not occur, even after prolonged infusions. Because there is no accumulation, a remifentanil infusion may be discontinued at the very end of surgery.

Effects of coexisting diseases
Effects of hepatic disease

Hepatic drug clearance involves numerous metabolic pathways and liver disease effects, each to a different degree. Typically liver disease affects hepatic phase I reactions to a greater degree than hepatic phase II reactions. Currently, there is no clinically available laboratory test that predicts the degree of impairment of metabolic reactions (although such tests are commonly used in research protocols).

In chronic liver disease (e.g., cirrhosis), decreased hepatic blood flow, altered enzyme activity, and reduced protein synthesis may coexist and result in altered pharmacokinetic behavior and drug disposition. The severity of disease, as well as drug characteristics (e.g., protein binding, hepatic extraction ratio), will affect the pharmacokinetic alterations.

Metabolism of drugs with a low hepatic extraction ratio (e.g., alfentanil) depends on liver function and not on hepatic blood flow. Clearance of these drugs may be severely impaired in the setting of end-stage liver disease, in which the enzyme capacity of the liver is limited. In contrast, decreased hepatic blood flow (e.g., shock, congestive heart failure) may impair the metabolism of drugs with a high extraction ratio (e.g., fentanyl). Overall, reduced drug clearance results in an increased plasma drug concentration and a prolonged terminal half-life.

Advanced liver disease alters protein binding as a result of decreased protein synthesis. A common finding in advanced liver disease is a low serum albumin concentration, which results in an increased free fraction of drugs bound to albumin. Clinically significant changes in protein binding generally are seen with drugs that are highly bound to albumin (e.g.,

warfarin) such that a small decrease in plasma protein concentration produces a significant rise in the circulating free drug concentration. Drug binding to AAG does not appear to be affected by liver disease.

Effects of renal disease

The most useful indicator of renal function is creatinine clearance. Significant renal dysfunction primarily affects the clearance of water-soluble drugs (e.g., pancuronium) and metabolites (e.g., normeperidine, morphine-6-glucuronide). In the setting of renal failure, such drugs or metabolites may accumulate significantly and result in an increased pharmacologic effect as well as a prolonged duration of action. In addition, increased drug effects also may be expected in patients with uremia as a result of decreased protein binding. Repeated dosing or infusions of long duration may cause significant drug accumulation.

Individual pharmacokinetic variability

In addition to the genetic polymorphisms previously discussed, there also may be pharmacokinetic differences due to age. The effects of aging include a loss of nephrons and changes in the volumes of distribution and protein binding. In the older patient population, total body water decreases while the percentage of body fat increases, resulting in a smaller central compartment V_d. Renal clearance is decreased because of the decrease in the number of nephrons. Protein binding capacity is decreased as a result of reduced albumin levels. These effects result in increased drug sensitivity as a result of increased plasma drug concentrations and the potential for drug accumulation.

The concurrent administration of multiple drugs may result in drug–drug interactions and account for multiple and diverse variations in pharmacokinetic behavior. As discussed earlier, there are numerous drugs that can cause inhibition or induction of CYP and alter the metabolism of other drugs (see Chapter 35).

Suggested readings

Alston TA. Hofmann, Schmofmann: atracurium undergoes Michael elimination. *Anesthesiology* 2001; 95:273.

Dershwitz M, Walsh JL, Morishige RJ, et al. Pharmacokinetics and pharmacodynamics of inhaled versus intravenous morphine in healthy volunteers. *Anesthesiology* 2000; 93:619–628.

Grandison MK, Boudinot FD. Age-related changes in protein binding of drugs. *Clin Pharmocokinet* 2000; 38:271–290.

Hiraoka H, Yamamoto K, Miyoshi S, et al. Kidneys contribute to the extrahepatic clearance of propofol in humans, but not lungs and brain. *Br J Clin Pharmacol* 2005; 60:176–182.

Hudson RJ, Henthorn TK. Basic principles of clinical pharmacology. In Barash PG, Cullen BF, Stoelting RK, eds. *Clinical Anesthesia*. 5th ed. Philadelphia: Lippincott Williams & Wilkins; 2006:247–263.

Hughes MA, Glass PSA, Jacobs JR. Context-sensitive half-time in multicompartment pharmacokinetic models for intravenous anesthetic drugs. *Anesthesiology* 1992; 76:334–341.

Rodighiero V. Effects of liver disease on pharmacokinetics. *Clin Pharmacokinet* 1999; 37:399–431.

Shafer SL. Principles of pharmacokinetics and pharmacodynamics. In: *Principles and Practice of Anesthesiology*. 2nd ed. St. Louis: Mosby; 1998:1159–1209.

Shafer SL, Varvel JR. Pharmacokinetics, pharmacodynamics, and rational opioid selection. *Anesthesiology* 1991; 74:53–63.

Opioids

Darin J. Correll and Carl E. Rosow

Opioids are the oldest known anesthetic and analgesic agents, with documented use as early as 6000 B.C. by the Sumerians, Babylonians, and Egyptians. Opium is derived from the exudate of the seed pod of *Papaver somniferum*. An opioid is any substance – natural or synthetic, endogenous or exogenous – with activity at opioid receptors. An opiate is an alkaloid derived naturally from opium, such as morphine or codeine. *Narcotic* is not a medical term but rather a legal term in the United States applied to any substance with abuse potential.

Mechanism of action

Opioids bind to G protein–coupled receptors located in the central nervous system (CNS; e.g., cortex, midbrain, thalamus, spinal cord), peripheral nervous system (e.g., mesenteric plexus of the gastrointestinal tract, primary afferent neuron), and peripheral tissues (e.g., joints and lung). The receptors are both presynaptic (inhibitory and excitatory) and postsynaptic (inhibitory). Opioid binding to presynaptic receptors inhibits voltage-sensitive calcium channels, decreases adenylyl cyclase activity, and decreases the release of various neurotransmitters (e.g., substance P, glutamate, acetylcholine, norepinephrine, and serotonin). Opioid binding to postsynaptic receptors increases outward potassium conductance, which results in hyperpolarization and a reduction of neural transmission.

Opioid receptors

Four distinct opioid receptors have been identified and cloned: μ, κ, δ, and nociceptin-orphanin FQ. These are sometimes abbreviated MOP, KOP, DOP, and NOP respectively. Most opioids used in clinical anesthesia are agonists that are relatively selective for μ-opioid receptors, and they produce a similar group of clinical effects. There are multiple human μ-opioid receptor subtypes, and their expression differs between tissues and among individuals. Each opioid has different efficacies after binding to the various μ-opioid receptor subtypes, and this may help explain why some patients respond better to a particular drug. Different subtypes also may account for the fact that tolerance to one μ-opioid agonist does not produce complete cross-tolerance to all other μ-opioid agonists. κ-Opioid and δ-opioid receptors mediate analgesia and also may contribute to the analgesic effect when high doses of μ-opioids are administered. A few κ-opioid agonists are used clinically, and κ-opioid actions probably account for the dysphoria and hallucinations occasionally reported with these drugs. There are no selective δ-opioid or NOP agonists available for clinical use.

Endogenous opioids

The body produces five different classes of opioid peptides that act throughout the CNS and peripheral nervous system to affect nociception, thermoregulation, hormone release, gastrointestinal function, and cardiovascular control.

- The enkephalins are pentapeptides derived from proenkephalin A. They are moderately selective for δ-opioid receptors and probably act within the spinal cord and brainstem.
- The dynorphins (A and B) are polypeptides derived from prodynorphin (also called proenkephalin B). They are agonists at the κ-opioid receptor.
- β-Endorphin, derived from proopiomelanocortin, is the most important of the humoral endogenous opioids, and an important endogenous ligand at μ-opioid receptors.
- Orphanin FQ (also called nociceptin), derived from proorphanin, binds the NOP receptor. Orphanin FQ is found in the hippocampus and sensory cortex. It has a supraspinal *antianalgesic* effect while producing spinal analgesia. It may have roles in pain modulation, learning, and drug reward.
- The endomorphins are tetrapeptides with high affinity for the μ-opioid receptor. No precursor molecule has been identified yet. In vivo studies suggest that endomorphin-1 acts via stimulation of μ-opioid receptors. Endomorphin-2 is less specific, acting at both μ-opioid and κ-opioid receptors.

Pharmacokinetics

Because all the commonly used opioids produce similar effects, the choice of opioid generally is based on pharmacokinetics, that is, the speed of onset, the duration of action, or the desired route of administration (Table 37.1). The lipid solubility of opioids is most commonly expressed as an octanol/water partition coefficient (Table 37.2). The partition coefficient is adjusted for

Table 37.1. Equianalgesic opioid doses, time to peak effect, and duration of analgesia

Agent	Dose, mg[a]	Peak effect, min	Duration of effect, h[b]
Morphine	10	>30	3–4
Hydromorphone	1.5	10–20	2–3
Methadone	10	15–20	3–4
Meperidine	80	5–7	2–3
Fentanyl	0.1	3–5	0.5–1
Sufentanil	0.01	3–5	0.5–1
Alfentanil	0.75	1.5–2	0.2–0.3
Remifentanil	0.1	1.5–2	0.1–0.2

[a] Approximately equianalgesic doses. Data for fentanyl derivatives are derived from intraoperative studies, the remainder from postoperative pain studies.
[b] Typical duration of initial dose.

the amount ionized at pH 7.4, because only uncharged species will partition between aqueous and lipid environments. Opioids are weak bases, and most have a dissociation constant (pK_a) > 7.4; therefore, they are predominately ionized at body pH.

Distribution

After intravenous (IV) bolus injection, a relatively lipophilic opioid (e.g., fentanyl) undergoes rapid distribution into highly perfused tissues such as brain, lung, heart, and viscera. After a single bolus dose, the effects of such a drug usually appear rapidly and then disappear rapidly as the opioid is redistributed into muscle and fat. More hydrophilic opioids, such as morphine, hydromorphone, and oxymorphone, have a slower onset and offset. It must be emphasized that lipid solubility is only one factor determining the rate of equilibration with receptor sites in the brain. Alfentanil is less lipophilic than sufentanil, yet its $t_{1/2}k_{e0}$ (equilibration half-time) is shorter. This may be a result of its lower pK_a (more uncharged drug) as well as a smaller cerebral volume of distribution. Opioids undergo variable amounts of protein binding in tissues and plasma. In plasma, opioids usually bind to α_1-acid glycoprotein, an acute-phase reactant that changes concentration in many disease states. Drug that is protein bound in plasma will not diffuse across membranes, may not be metabolized in the liver, and will not be filtered by the kidney.

Table 37.2. Lipid solubility, pK_a, and protein binding of opioid agonists

Drug	Octanol/water partition coefficient at pH 7.4	pK_a	Protein binding, %
Morphine	1.42	7.9/9.4	30–35
Hydromorphone	1.28	8.1	8–19
Methadone	117	8.25	85–90
Meperidine	38.8	8.5	64
Fentanyl	860	8.4	80–85
Sufentanil	1757	8.0	93
Alfentanil	128	6.5	92
Remifentanil	17.9	7.07	70

Clearance

The offset of opioid effects after a bolus dose initially is the result of rapid redistribution. All opioids, except remifentanil, then undergo hepatic metabolism with renal excretion of active or inactive metabolites. The biotransformation pathways include oxidative metabolism by various cytochrome P-450 (CYP) isozymes as well as glucuronidation. The polar opioid metabolites are then eliminated in urine and bile.

Pharmacokinetics of commonly used opioids

Morphine

Morphine has a relatively slow onset of action. It is rapidly distributed and eliminated from the circulation. More than 90% of morphine is metabolized and excreted within 24 hours. The drug is metabolized to the 3- and 6-glucuronides, as well as to normorphine. The metabolites are then excreted in the urine (90%) and bile (10%). Morphine-6-glucuronide (M6G), which represents about 15% of the total metabolites, has significant agonist activity. M6G probably has little effect after a single morphine dose, but it accumulates with repeated dosing and then contributes substantially to the overall opioid effect. The blood concentration of M6G may reach high values in patients with renal insufficiency and result in adverse effects such as sedation and ventilatory depression.

Hydromorphone

Compared with morphine, hydromorphone has a slightly faster onset of action and a slightly shorter duration of action. Hydromorphone is rapidly metabolized to inactive compounds. Its water solubility allows it to be formulated in a high-concentration solution useful for patients who are opioid tolerant.

Methadone

Methadone is much more lipophilic than morphine and has high oral bioavailability. The commercial preparation is a racemic mixture with all opioid activity residing in the *l*-isomer. There is huge interindividual variability in the metabolic clearance of both isomers, and clearance is subject to many drug interactions. Because the terminal half-life is about 35 hours, repeated doses may result in substantial accumulation, with subsequent doses lasting much longer than the initial dose. Methadone undergoes metabolism in both the liver and gastrointestinal mucosa, primarily via *N*-demethylation. The metabolite is then excreted mostly by the kidneys, and some also in bile.

Meperidine

Compared with morphine, meperidine has a faster onset of effect and a shorter duration of action. Meperidine has a very high rate of hepatic clearance and is primarily *N*-demethylated in the liver to form normeperidine, which is then renally excreted. Normeperidine is an active metabolite that may cause

CNS excitation, manifested as restlessness, tremors, myoclonus, seizures, and occasionally death. It has a long terminal half-life of about 21 hours and repeated doses of meperidine may cause normeperidine to accumulate in persons with renal failure, leading to significant toxicity.

Fentanyl

Fentanyl is extremely lipophilic and is readily absorbed through intact skin and mucous membranes. After IV injection, it has a rapid onset and relatively short duration of action. It is rapidly distributed to the brain, heart, and other highly perfused tissues. Termination of effect occurs when fentanyl rapidly redistributes away from the CNS. Elimination is much slower (terminal half-life, 4–5 hours) due to the slow return of drug from peripheral tissues to the bloodstream. Fentanyl is metabolized in the liver and gastrointestinal mucosa to inactive metabolites excreted by the kidneys (90%) and in the bile (10%).

Sufentanil

Sufentanil is even more lipophilic than fentanyl, and its pharmacokinetic profile is similar, with a slightly shorter duration of action. Despite a terminal half-life of about 9 hours, sufentanil has a relatively short context-sensitive half-time (see Chapter 36). Its duration of action remains relatively short when administered by infusion for up to about 12 hours. Sufentanil is metabolized in the liver and the gastrointestinal mucosa, and the metabolites are excreted in urine and bile.

Alfentanil

Alfentanil has an extremely rapid onset and relatively short duration of effect after a bolus dose. Alfentanil is less likely than fentanyl to produce cumulative effects after repeated doses. Despite its short terminal half-life of 90 minutes, it has a longer context-sensitive half-time than sufentanil when given by infusion for up to about 12 hours (see Chapter 36). Alfentanil is metabolized in the liver, primarily by CYP3A4, and inhibitors of this isozyme (e.g., erythromycin) can greatly reduce its clearance.

Remifentanil

Remifentanil is an ester hydrolyzed by nonspecific esterases, primarily in skeletal muscle. The onset of effect is extremely rapid and similar to that of alfentanil. A bolus dose lasts only a few minutes, so the drug generally is administered by continuous infusion. Its high clearance gives the drug a context-sensitive half-time of about 4 minutes, irrespective of the duration of infusion. Redistribution of remifentanil occurs, but it plays a minor role in termination of the drug effect. Remifentanil is not a substrate for pseudocholinesterase; therefore, the dose does not need to be altered in persons with pseudocholinesterase deficiency.

Clearance is unchanged in patients with hepatic or renal failure, and the dose does not need to be adjusted in such patients. Extremes of age and body weight may influence clearance, but

recovery is still very rapid. The primary remifentanil metabolite has very weak opioid activity, but significant amounts do not accumulate with typical clinical dosing. The ultra-short duration of this analgesic may be a drawback in patients who are expected to have significant postoperative pain. These patients should receive a longer-acting opioid prior to stopping the remifentanil infusion.

Pharmacodynamics

Nervous system

Analgesia

The analgesic effects of opioids are the result of actions at many locations. In the brain, opioids activate various endogenous descending inhibitory (antinociceptive) pathways via action in the periaqueductal gray matter, locus ceruleus, and raphe nuclei. Opioids also act at receptors in the limbic system to alter the emotional response to a noxious stimulus. Opioid analgesia sometimes leads to feelings of euphoria – a possible etiology of the abuse potential of opioids – but dysphoria also may occur. In the spinal cord, opioids act both pre- and postsynaptically on the nociceptive neurons in the dorsal horn. In the periphery, opioids reduce activity in the primary nociceptor during states of inflammation.

The relative potencies of the older opioid agonists are derived from studies of acute pain, whereas the fentanyl analogues primarily have been studied in intraoperative settings. These data have been used to estimate equianalgesic doses (Table 37.1). However, there is large interindividual variability, and doses necessary for a given intensity of effect may vary as much as tenfold between patients.

The opioids listed in Table 37.1 are all considered full μ-opioid agonists, and all are capable of producing intense analgesia and complete cessation of breathing in opioid-naïve patients. Some animal data suggest that higher-potency opioids (e.g., fentanyl derivatives) may be more effective analgesics in patients with a high degree of opioid tolerance. Tolerance involves down-regulation of a portion of the available receptor population, and higher-potency opioids exert a full effect with lower levels of receptor availability (i.e., they have more "spare receptors").

Sedation

All opioids produce sedation, even at moderately analgesic doses, and the effect varies greatly among patients. When opioids are used concomitantly with other CNS depressants (especially benzodiazepines), the sedative effects may be marked. Sleep disturbances and even hallucinations may occur during opioid use. Intraoperatively, opioids should not be used as the primary agents to produce hypnosis or amnesia.

Miosis

Pupillary constriction occurs as the result of stimulation of the Edinger-Westphal nucleus, the accessory parasympathetic nucleus of cranial nerve III (oculomotor nerve). A maximal miotic effect may occur in tolerant individuals, even after relatively low doses of μ-opioid agonists, so this is not a reliable end point for analgesia. However, absence of miosis suggests absence of opioid effect. In cases of opioid overdose, mydriasis may occur if the patient becomes hypoxemic.

Antitussive effect

Opioids depress the cough reflex, at least partly, by action at a putative medullary cough center. The effect is mediated by a receptor mechanism different from that of analgesia; low-potency analgesics (e.g., codeine) and analgesically inactive stereoisomers (e.g., dextromethorphan) are effective antitussives.

Pruritus

Itching may be generalized but often is limited to the area around the nose. The etiology is activation of μ-opioid receptors in the rostral medulla, although some animal data suggest a peripheral component as well. The itching is specifically antagonized by low doses of naloxone or nalbuphine, but these μ-opioid antagonists often reverse some analgesia. Opioid-induced itching rarely involves histamine, so the small amount of relief produced by diphenhydramine is probably a result of its sedative properties.

Nausea and vomiting

Opioids stimulate the chemoreceptor trigger zone on the floor of the fourth ventricle, which then activates the emetic center in the pontine lateral reticular formation. The emetic effect is increased by input from the vestibular apparatus in the inner ear. Thus, patients may not be nauseated while lying still but may become so when they are moved or sat upright. Any of the various antiemetics may be used, but none has been proven to be specific for opioid-induced nausea. In theory, an antiemetic with strong anticholinergic effects (e.g., scopolamine or promethazine) should be effective if the problem is triggered by motion. The various opioid analgesics appear to cause a similar incidence of nausea and vomiting, and despite numerous assertions to the contrary, there are no data that reproducibly indicate an advantage or disadvantage for one opioid. In animals, high doses of opioids directly depress the emetic center, and it is possible that this effect may occur during some high-dose intraoperative use.

Ventilatory depression

Opioids produce a dose-dependent depression of ventilation by decreasing medullary sensitivity to hypercarbia. This results in a rightward shift and a decrease in the slope of the carbon dioxide response curve. Tidal volume initially is preserved, but minute ventilation falls because of a decrease in respiratory rate. When a patient falls asleep, ventilation is depressed further and the degree of hypercarbia and hypoxemia will increase. Other patient-related risk factors for increased ventilatory depression include advanced age, a history of obstructive sleep apnea, morbid obesity, and the concomitant use of other CNS depressants.

Opioids also decrease hypoxic ventilatory drive and may cause a periodic or Cheyne-Stokes breathing pattern. Sufficient opioid will cause apnea, but the patient may still be arousable and will often breathe if told to do so. All the opioids produce equivalent amounts of ventilatory depression at equianalgesic doses. Treatment depends on the degree of depression and ranges from supplemental oxygen administration to assisted ventilation, with slow naloxone titration.

Muscle rigidity

Generalized hypertonus of skeletal muscle may occur during induction with moderate to large doses of opioids, which can make ventilation extremely difficult. The etiology is a μ-opioid receptor–mediated inhibition of GABAergic neurons in the striatum. For many years, this has been characterized as "chest wall" or "truncal" rigidity. Although there undeniably is a loss of compliance in the chest wall and abdomen, difficulty in ventilation probably is caused by constriction of the laryngeal and pharyngeal musculature. This upper airway obstruction can mimic laryngospasm and may be severe enough to require treatment with a skeletal muscle relaxant. The effect also may be reversed with naloxone, although this is usually undesirable during induction.

Cerebral blood flow/intracranial pressure

Opioids do not directly affect cerebral blood flow, but intracranial pressure (ICP) may be elevated if ventilatory depression is allowed to produce hypercarbia and cerebral vasodilatation. During anesthesia induction, however, the opioids are excellent adjuncts for patients with increased ICP. In this circumstance, ventilation can be controlled, and the opioid will help blunt the increased ICP due to laryngoscopy and intubation.

Tolerance

Tolerance is a physiologic phenomenon in which the response to a drug's effect diminishes over time. To maintain the same effect, the dose needs to be increased as the result of both receptor uncoupling and down-regulation. There are two types of tolerance to opioid action: *acute* tolerance, which occurs immediately after a single large dose, and *chronic* tolerance, which occurs when opioids are administered frequently over longer periods of time.

In general, tolerance develops to all the depressant effects described earlier but not to the stimulant effects, such as constipation and miosis. In addition, when tolerance to an opioid occurs, there is simultaneous development of *cross-tolerance* to all other opioid agonists, although this cross-tolerance is often incomplete (perhaps because of the heterogeneity of μ-opioid receptor subtypes). Thus, a patient who is tolerant to one opioid often can get additional relief by switching to another – a process known as "opioid rotation."

The precise mechanisms of both acute and chronic tolerance are still unclear, although down-regulation of adenylyl cyclase and other second-messenger mechanisms play a role. A current area of active investigation suggests that chronic opioid administration may actually cause hyperalgesia, and this may be mediated by activation of the glutamate N-methyl-D-aspartate (NMDA) receptor. Inhibitors of NMDA can reduce tolerance development in animals, but the data are inconsistent in humans.

Dependence

Physical dependence is a physiologic state defined by the occurrence of a specific withdrawal syndrome when the drug is stopped abruptly, the dose is reduced dramatically, or an antagonist is given. The symptoms of withdrawal can be terminated rapidly with small doses of IV opioids. The presence of physical dependence (and tolerance) is not the same as psychological dependence or *addiction*, which is a chronic, multifactorial neurobiological disease manifested by drug-seeking behavior, impaired control over drug use, and continued use despite negative social and physiologic consequences. Epidemiologic studies have shown that the risk of addiction from *appropriate* medical use of opioids is very low.

Other CNS effects

High doses of opioids may cause myoclonic activity, but without evidence of seizure activity on the cortical electroencephalogram (EEG). As stated previously, chronic administration of meperidine may cause accumulation of its metabolite, normeperidine, which is a true convulsant. Unlike with propofol or volatile anesthetics, even high doses of opioids will not produce EEG suppression.

Cardiovascular system

Vasomotor tone

Opioids produce peripheral vasodilation by depressing vasomotor centers in the medulla, causing a reduction in sympathetic activity. Unlike volatile anesthetics or propofol, they do not block high- or low-pressure baroreflex responses. There is little effect on blood pressure in the awake, normovolemic patient, although analgesic doses can sometimes cause orthostatic hypotension. More significant hemodynamic effects may be seen when higher doses are used or when opioids are combined with other sedative medications (e.g., benzodiazepines). Opioids are most likely to cause hypotension in patients relying on a high sympathetic tone to maintain their blood pressure (e.g., hypovolemia, congestive heart failure).

Heart rate

Opioids produce a dose-dependent reduction in heart rate by stimulating the central vagal nuclei. Bradycardia is most likely to occur when large doses of opioids are administered rapidly.

It may be prevented or reversed by atropine, pancuronium, or other vagolytic drugs.

Contractility and excitability

Opioids do not produce significant direct myocardial depression, and they do not sensitize the myocardium to the effects of catecholamines.

Smooth muscle effects

Gastrointestinal

Through both central (brain and spinal cord) and peripheral (enteric muscle and nerve) effects, opioids cause a reduction in propulsion throughout the entire length of the gastrointestinal system. Therefore, there can be delayed gastric emptying and the development of ileus or constipation. With extended use of opioids, constipation is common, so prophylactic use of stool softeners and stimulant laxatives is recommended. New quaternary opioid antagonists (see "Antagonists") appear to antagonize the constipating effects without influencing analgesia.

Biliary

Opioids increase smooth muscle tone throughout the biliary tree and sphincter of Oddi. This effect may be less with the agonist–antagonist opioids. The increase in biliary pressure occasionally may lead to epigastric distress or frank biliary colic. Opioid-induced biliary spasm can be relieved specifically with naloxone or nonspecifically with smooth muscle relaxants such as nitroglycerin. The latter is important because biliary pain can sometimes be hard to distinguish from the pain of myocardial ischemia.

Urinary

Urinary retention may result from decreased contraction of the detrusor muscle and an increase in tone of the involuntary sphincter. The patient also may become inattentive to the stimulus of a full bladder. The effect is more prevalent in males and often occurs after neuraxial opioid administration. A part of the effect appears to be peripheral, because it can be reversed by the quaternary antagonist N-methylnaltrexone.

Opioid effects not mediated by opioid receptors

Histamine release

Morphine and meperidine can cause dose-dependent histamine release from tissue mast cells and circulating basophils. This cannot be prevented by administration of an opioid antagonist, thus it is not mediated through opioid receptors. The effect often is manifested as a short-lived wheal-and-flare reaction near the site of an IV cannula. After larger doses of morphine, sufficient histamine may be released to cause flushing and transient hypotension. It must be emphasized that this reaction is the result of a nonspecific displacement of the amine from mast cells and does not involve an immunologic mechanism. True allergy to any of the opioids is extremely rare.

Inhibition of serotonin reuptake

Meperidine (and probably normeperidine) and tramadol appear to inhibit the presynaptic serotonin transporter. This effect may form the basis for the well-described and potentially fatal interaction between meperidine and monoamine oxidase inhibitors (MAOIs). Patients chronically taking MAOIs (isocarboxazid, phenelzine, tranylcypromine, or selegiline) who are given meperidine or tramadol may suffer a serotoninergic crisis, manifested as clonus, agitation, hyperreflexia, hyperthermia, and occasionally death.

Inhibition of shivering

Subanalgesic doses of meperidine (12.5–25 mg IV) are effective for treating shivering from a variety of causes (e.g., general or regional anesthesia, bacteremia, transfusion reactions). The mechanism partly may be a result of the serotonin mechanism mentioned earlier, because serotonin is an important neurotransmitter in the posterior hypothalamus. Meperidine also is known to be an agonist at α_{2B}-adrenoceptors, so it may work in a manner similar to that of dexmedetomidine.

NMDA antagonism

Methadone is available commercially as a racemic mixture containing the *l*-isomer (a μ-opioid agonist and noncompetitive NMDA antagonist) and the *d*-isomer (a noncompetitive NMDA antagonist). NMDA antagonism has led some to propose that methadone may have advantages over other opioids in reversing or attenuating the development of opioid tolerance and possibly in treating hyperalgesia or neuropathic pain. The data supporting these advantages are inconsistent at best. Methadone is capable of producing substantial tolerance with chronic dosing, which is why addicts on methadone maintenance have such high opioid requirements.

Perioperative opioid uses

Opioids are used for premedication, IV sedation, balanced general anesthesia, total IV anesthesia (TIVA), and postoperative analgesia. There is little reason to give opioids prior to transfer to the operating room unless the patient is already in pain. Opioid use for premedication makes most sense when sedation is accompanied by the need for analgesia (e.g., during painful procedures like line placement or the performance of regional blocks). The use of small doses of opioids immediately prior to induction might properly be considered part of the anesthetic technique.

Intraoperatively, opioids produce a concentration-dependent suppression of the hemodynamic responses to painful stimuli. The effective concentration varies widely among individuals, although the transition from inadequate to adequate analgesia occurs over a small range for each patient

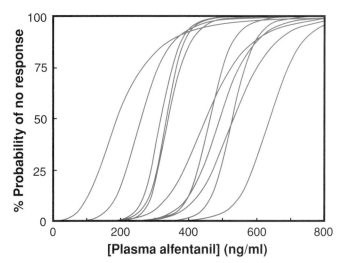

Figure 37.1. Alfentanil plasma concentrations versus effect curves for each patient during the intra-abdominal part of upper abdominal surgery. (Patients also were receiving 66% nitrous oxide in oxygen.) The plasma concentration for 50% probability of response Cp₅₀ and slope (γ) of these curves were defined from the quantal responses of the individual patients to the stimulus using logistic regression. (Redrawn with permission from Ausems ME, Hug CC Jr, Stanski DR, Burm AG. Plasma concentrations of alfentanil required to supplement nitrous oxide anesthesia for general surgery. *Anesthesiology* 1986; 65:362–373.)

(Fig. 37.1). Increasing doses of opioids reduce the requirements for other intravenous and inhaled anesthetics. For example, low plasma concentrations of fentanyl (2–3 ng/ml) or remifentanil (3 ng/ml) can reduce the amount of propofol necessary to prevent the movement response to pain by about 75%. The opioid agonists all reduce minimum alveolar concentration (MAC) for various volatile anesthetics by a maximum of about 70%. Recent data suggest that there is less of an effect in lowering MAC_awake.

Opioids are not reliable hypnotics. They do not consistently produce amnesia or unconsciousness or suppress movement by themselves, so they should not be considered anesthetics. The use of high opioid doses (e.g., 50–150 μg/kg fentanyl) with only oxygen was popular for a time, particularly in cardiac anesthesia, because it was thought to produce stable hemodynamics. Unfortunately, many patients given fentanyl–oxygen "anesthesia" still had wide fluctuations in blood pressure, some remembered intraoperative events, and all required prolonged postoperative ventilation. Currently, almost all intraoperative opioid use is in combination with true hypnotics, such as propofol (i.e., TIVA), or with volatile agents.

Individualization of doses

The range of effective concentrations (therapeutic window) is narrow for each patient but varies widely among patients. The clear implication is that "cookbook" analgesia likely is inadequate or excessive much of the time. With this caveat, Table 37.3 presents some "typical" intraoperative doses for various opioids. It is intended only as a reasonable place to start titration.

Table 37.3. Typical IV opioid dosages

Agonist	Adjunct to induction	Bolus for maintenance	Infusion for maintenance
Morphine	0.1–0.25 mg/kg	0.02–0.05 mg/kg	NA[a]
Hydromorphone	0.015–0.04 mg/kg	0.003–0.0075 mg/kg	NA[a]
Methadone	Patients who are on methadone chronically may require very large opioid doses intraoperatively. A reasonable starting dose is to administer intravenously the same daily oral dose on which the patient is maintained.	–	NA[a]
Fentanyl	1.5–5 µg/kg	0.4–1.5 µg/kg	0.01–0.1 µg/kg/min
Sufentanil	0.2–0.5 µg/kg	0.1–0.2 µg/kg	0.002–0.01 µg/kg/min
Alfentanil	10–75 µg/kg	3–15 µg/kg	0.1–2 µg/kg/min
Remifentanil	0.5–1 µg/kg	0.1–0.3 µg/kg	0.025–1 µg/kg/min

[a] Rarely given intraoperatively via infusion.
NA, not applicable.

The choice of doses will depend on factors unique to the patient and to the procedure:

- Lower starting or maintenance doses are advisable in some circumstances. Elderly patients, for example, may be sensitive, but some elderly patients may require substantial doses. (Undertreatment of pain in the elderly is a significant problem.)
- Lower doses also should be considered in patients who are hypovolemic, debilitated, hypothyroid, or treated with other CNS depressants.
- Patients with obstructive sleep apnea may need normal doses but require more intensive postoperative monitoring for ventilatory depression.
- Patients with hepatic or renal insufficiency may become excessively sedated or experience ventilatory depression from accumulation of the parent drug or metabolites.
- Higher starting or maintenance doses should be considered in some cases – for example, a thoracotomy in which intense postoperative pain is anticipated. However, multimodal analgesia, including epidural analgesia, often is a better choice in cases such as these.
- A patient with obvious opioid tolerance or a history of recent, consistent opioid use may require a substantial amount of opioid. In many cases, intraoperative dosing can be guided by the response (or lack of response) to opioids given preoperatively. One should not hesitate to give adequate doses to patients who have become highly tolerant. Checking intraoperatively for spontaneous ventilation may be reassuring in such cases. If the patient will breathe during general anesthesia, there is a high likelihood that ventilation will continue in the postoperative period.

Agonist–Antagonists

The clinically available agonist–antagonists bind to both µ-opioid and κ-opioid receptors, but they have different intrinsic activities at each site (Table 37.4). Equipotent IV doses for analgesia also are listed in Table 37.4. All the agonist–antagonists behave as partial agonists, with lower efficacy than that of the pure agonists; thus, there is a ceiling for both the analgesic and ventilatory-depressant effects. These agents offer no major benefits compared with the pure agonists for use during balanced anesthesia. Even extremely large doses will not produce the intensity of analgesia produced by fentanyl or morphine, and they are less effective in reducing MAC of the volatile anesthetics.

The subjective effects of buprenorphine are similar to morphine. The κ-opioid agonists nalbuphine and butorphanol have been described as producing "apathetic sedation," and patients generally do not experience mood elevation like that seen with morphine. After analgesic doses, patients often appear extremely sedated, yet they are able to carry on conversations. The lack of euphoric effects makes these analgesics much less desired by opioid addicts, which is thought to be a key factor in their lower abuse liability. Butorphanol may be used as a premedicant because it produces sedative effects in doses lower than those routinely used for analgesia. Unlike the benzodiazepines, it produces very little anterograde amnesia.

Table 37.4. Agonist–antagonist opioid receptor effects and equianalgesic doses

Drug	µ-Opioid receptor	κ-Opioid receptor	Analgesic dose, mg[a]
Buprenorphine	Partial agonist	Antagonist	0.3
Butorphanol	Antagonist	Partial agonist	2
Nalbuphine	Antagonist	Partial agonist	10

[a] Equivalent to morphine, 10 mg.

Because these opioids are partial agonists, the ventilatory-depressant effects are limited in intensity, reaching a maximum after about 30 mg of nalbuphine or about 4 mg of butorphanol. Severe ventilatory depression still is possible in sensitive individuals, such as those with concomitant CNS or pulmonary disease or those receiving other depressant drugs. Buprenorphine has limited ability to cause ventilatory depression. This is important because it has high affinity for μ-opioid receptors, and complete reversal using naloxone may be difficult. Reversal cannot be achieved with another agonist–antagonist.

Nalbuphine and butorphanol do not cause significant elevation of intrabiliary pressure, whereas buprenorphine may cause mild biliary effects. The agonist–antagonists appear to have small effects on smooth muscle in the intestine and bladder, and they cause less constipation than the pure agonists. The cardiovascular effects of buprenorphine and nalbuphine are similar to those of morphine. Butorphanol also may increase pulmonary artery pressure, but heart rate and blood pressure usually decrease slightly.

Nalbuphine and buprenorphine are strong μ-opioid antagonists, and they may be used for this purpose. Reversal of agonist effects with an agonist–antagonist has never been demonstrated to be safer or more reliable than reversal with a pure antagonist such as naloxone. Administration of an opioid antagonist to an opioid-dependent patient will precipitate withdrawal; therefore, agonist–antagonist agents should be avoided in such patients.

Antagonists

Naloxone

Naloxone acts as a competitive antagonist at all opioid receptors, but it has greatest affinity for μ-opioid receptors. Small doses of naloxone reliably reverse or prevent the effects of pure opioid agonists and most mixed agonist–antagonists. The block is reversible, so it can be overcome by additional agonist. Given by itself to an opioid-naïve person, naloxone is nearly devoid of clinically demonstrable effects.

Naloxone is widely distributed and rapidly achieves effective concentrations in the CNS. Plasma and brain concentrations decrease rapidly because of redistribution. The drug is cleared rapidly by hepatic biotransformation. The terminal half-life is 1 to 2 hours. The onset of antagonist effect is extremely rapid, but the duration of action is quite brief. A total IV dose of 0.4 mg will usually antagonize morphine for less than 1 hour, and increasing the dose does not increase the duration appreciably. With the exception of remifentanil, the duration of naloxone is shorter than the opioids it is used to antagonize.

The presence of excessive opioid effects is a common problem in the postoperative setting. Small doses of naloxone (0.04 mg in an adult, repeated every few minutes) can be given intravenously, usually with dramatic improvement. In many cases, there is partial reversal of analgesia as well, but careful dosing can minimize this effect. Patients who receive naloxone need continued observation, and possibly repeated doses. Postoperative ventilatory compromise is frequently caused by a combination of factors, and therapy with naloxone does not eliminate the need to search for and treat conditions such as residual paralysis, bronchospasm, and airway edema.

Opioid reversal may sometimes have important hemodynamic consequences. Increases in systemic pressure, heart rate, and plasma levels of catecholamines may occur. This may be because of the sudden onset of pain, but these effects have been reproduced experimentally in the absence of painful stimuli. There have been several case reports of fulminant pulmonary edema, dysrhythmias, and even death in young, previously healthy individuals given naloxone. In one case, the dose of naloxone was only 0.1 mg. The etiology of this is not known.

Naltrexone

Naltrexone is available for oral administration or as a depot injection given monthly. The main clinical use of naltrexone is in the treatment of opioid addiction and alcoholism. Naltrexone blocks the euphoriant effects of opioids and decreases drug craving, thus helping prevent relapse. In the event a patient on naltrexone requires opioid treatment for acute pain, naltrexone antagonism is competitive and may be overcome with high doses of morphine or fentanyl.

N-methylnaltrexone

N-methylnaltrexone (MNTX) is a new quaternary analogue of naltrexone. The permanently charged molecule does not cross the blood–brain barrier and achieve significant concentrations in the CNS. It is given subcutaneously as a treatment for opioid-induced bowel dysfunction (OBD). In healthy volunteers and patients given morphine, IV MNTX reversed depression of gastric emptying and intestinal motility but did not interfere with analgesia.

Alvimopan

Alvimopan is another permanently charged new opioid antagonist that does not achieve significant concentrations in the CNS. It is poorly absorbed after oral administration and does not reverse opioid analgesia. Alvimopan is given orally for the treatment of postoperative ileus.

Suggested readings

Ausems ME, Hug CC Jr, Stanski DR, Burm AG. Plasma concentrations of alfentanil required to supplement nitrous oxide anesthesia for general surgery. *Anesthesiology* 1986; 65:362–373.

Davies G, Kingswood C, Street M. Pharmacokinetics of opioids in renal dysfunction. *Clin Pharmacokinet* 1996; 31: 410–422.

Dershwitz M, Randel GI, Rosow CE, et al. Initial clinical experience with remifentanil, a new opioid metabolized by esterases. *Anesth Analg* 1995; 81:619–623.

Fukuda K. Intravenous opioid anesthetics. In: Miller R, ed. *Miller's Anesthesia*. 6th ed. New York: Elsevier; 2005.

McClain DA, Hug CC Jr. Intravenous fentanyl kinetics. *Clin Pharmacol Ther* 1980; 28:106–114.

Philbin DM, Rosow CE, Schneider RC, et al. Fentanyl and sufentanil anesthesia revisited: how much is enough? *Anesthesiology* 1990; 73:5–11.

Rosow CE, Dershwitz M. Opioid analgesics. In: Longnecker DE, Brown D, Newman M, Zapol WM, eds. *Anesthesiology*. 3rd ed. New York: McGraw-Hill; 2008.

Chapter 38

Muscle relaxants

Torin D. Shear and J. A. Jeevendra Martyn

Neuromuscular block (NMB) refers to the interference with nerve signal transmission at the neuromuscular junction (NMJ) resulting in skeletal muscle paralysis. Several pharmacologic agents are clinically available to produce this paralysis and are collectively known as muscle relaxants. These relaxants block the action of the neurotransmitter acetylcholine (ACh), which initiates muscle contraction. Muscle relaxants are conveniently subdivided into two categories according to the mechanism of action at the NMJ: *depolarizing neuromuscular blockers* and *nondepolarizing neuromuscular blockers*. Both classes of drug block the action of ACh at the nicotinic ACh receptor on skeletal muscle.

Clinically, neuromuscular blocking drugs (NMBDs) facilitate tracheal intubation, mechanical ventilation, and optimization of surgical conditions by producing skeletal muscle paralysis. The pharmacologic effect of NMBDs can be monitored using electrical stimulation of peripheral nerves and assessment of the evoked twitch response. Neuromuscular paralysis can be reversed with the careful titration of anticholinesterase drugs and, more recently, by direct binding of the drug.

Neuromuscular junction

The NMJ comprises a presynaptic motor nerve terminal and a postsynaptic skeletal muscle membrane (Fig. 38.1). Between the presynaptic nerve terminal and the postsynaptic membrane is the synaptic cleft. ACh is stored in the nerve terminal in special organelles called vesicles. ACh receptors (AChRs) cluster in the highly folded motor endplate opposite the nerve terminal.

In the adult NMJ, there are approximately 5 million AChRs. These are nicotinic cholinergic receptors that form transmembrane ion channels permeable to sodium and calcium (into the cell) and potassium (out of the cell). The AChRs are formed by a five-subunit glycoprotein weighing about 250,000 Da. This pentameric protein consists of two α subunits and one each of β, δ, and ε subunits in the adult NMJ. Also located on the postsynaptic membrane is acetylcholinesterase.

Alterations in the conventional AChR subunits have been described in denervated muscle, leading to increased membrane permeability associated with hyperkalemic cardiac arrest following administration of depolarizing NMBDs. These immature receptors are expressed in extrajunctional areas of the skeletal muscle membrane in response to many pathologic states, including muscle denervation. More recently, another isoform, the α_7 AChR, consisting of five α_7 subunits, has been described following denervation.

Normal muscle contraction occurs in a predictable manner. In response to nerve stimulation, an action potential is generated, causing voltage-dependent N-type calcium channels, which are located in the nerve terminal, to open. The ensuing rapid influx of calcium generates an increase in the intracellular calcium concentration in the nerve terminal. This causes ACh-filled synaptic vesicles to fuse with the cell membrane, releasing ACh into the synaptic cleft. ACh molecules bind to nicotinic AChRs on the motor endplate, thereby changing membrane permeability to sodium, calcium, and potassium. This causes an increase in the transmembrane potential from -90 mV to -45 mV. The motor endplate action potential is then propagated throughout the skeletal muscle via sodium channels, leading to muscle contraction.

Neuromuscular blockers

All NMBDs bind to the AChR and antagonize the action of ACh. The NMBDs are quaternary ammonium compounds and, like ACh, bind to the α subunit of AChRs. Nondepolarizing NMBDs can be subdivided based on duration of action or structure (steroid vs. benzylisoquinoline). The evoked twitch response to depolarizing and nondepolarizing NMB differs. Depolarizing block is characterized by a dose-dependent decrease in twitch height without fade during repetitive stimulation. Nondepolarizing block is characterized by fade during repetitive stimulation, the inability to maintain tetanus, and by posttetanic potentiation.

Depolarizing NMBDs

Depolarizing NMBDs are agonists at the nicotinic AChR. They mimic the action of ACh by binding to the AChR and causing skeletal muscle contraction through depolarization of the motor endplate. Persistent endplate depolarization prevents further muscle contraction. Succinylcholine (SCh) is currently the only depolarizing NMBD in clinical use. SCh structurally consists of two ACh molecules linked by methyl groups. It is unique in its rapid onset and short duration. The dose of SCh

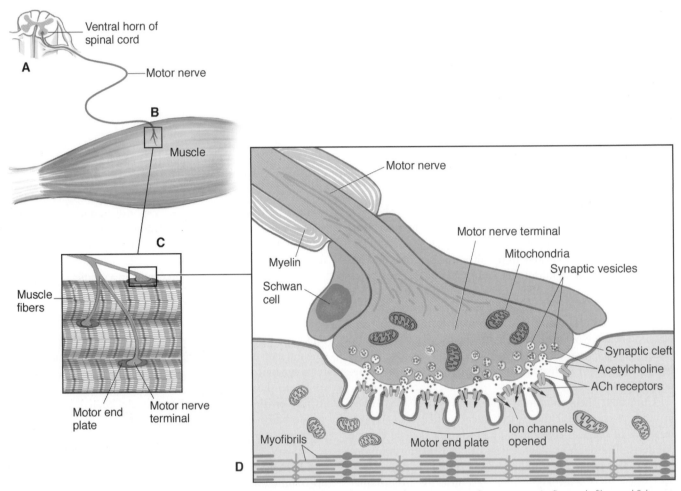

Figure 38.1. Structure of the adult NMJ with the three structures that constitute the synapse: the motor neuron (i.e., nerve terminal), muscle fiber, and Schwann cell. (**A**) The motor nerve originates in the ventral horn of the spinal cord or brainstem. (**B**) As the nerve approaches its muscle fibers, it divides into branches that innervate many individual muscle fibers. (**C**) Each muscle receives only one synapse. (**D**) The nerve terminal, covered by a Schwann cell, has vesicles clustered about the membrane thickenings as well as mitochondria and microtubules. A synaptic cleft separates the nerve from the muscle. The muscle surface is corrugated, and dense areas on the shoulders of each fold contain ACh receptors. Acetylcholinesterase, proteins, and proteoglycans that stabilize the NMJ are present in the synaptic clefts.

has been extensively studied during its long history of clinical use, and ranges from 0.6–1.5 mg/kg. Although studies demonstrate adequate intubating conditions with doses as low as 0.6 mg/kg, a dose of 1 mg/kg is most commonly used.

Rapid onset of skeletal muscle paralysis occurs in 30 to 60 seconds, and paralysis lasts 5 to 10 minutes. With an initial bolus dose of SCh (e.g., 1 mg/kg), phase I neuromuscular block occurs. Higher bolus doses or a prolonged infusion will cause phase II block. Phase I block is the typical depolarizing block and is manifested as a decrease in twitch height without fade in response to peripheral nerve stimulation. As the block resolves, there is an increase in twitch height. During phase II block, the evoked twitch response is similar to that seen during nondepolarizing block in that fade occurs (Fig. 38.2).

SCh is metabolized by plasma butyrylcholinesterase (also known as pseudocholinesterase or plasma cholinesterase), and the NMB produced by SCh is prolonged in patients with plasma butyrylcholinesterase deficiency. A history of prolonged paralysis after general anesthesia or family history of such should raise concern. Butyrylcholinesterase activity can decrease in states such as burns and liver disease. Genetic variations of butyrylcholinesterase also occur. Normal plasma butyrylcholinesterase can be inhibited by the local anesthetic dibucaine. An in vitro assay using dibucaine measures the atypical genetic variations. In normal patients, dibucaine will inhibit 80% of enzyme activity with the corresponding *dibucaine number* of 80. Heterozygous atypical plasma butyrylcholinesterase occurs in about 4% of the population with the corresponding dibucaine number between 30 and 65. Homozygous atypical plasma butyrylcholinesterase occurs in about 0.04% of the general population and corresponds to a dibucaine number of 20. That is, atypical genetic variant plasma butyrylcholinesterase, that does not metabolize SCh, is inhibited less effectively by dibucaine.

Other genetic variants have been described. In addition, plasma butyrylcholinesterase may be inhibited by exogenous compounds such as organophosphates (e.g., insecticides, chemical warfare agents, and echothiophate, a drug used topically

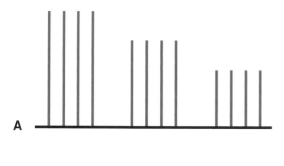

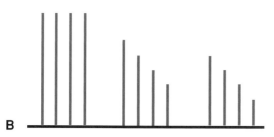

Figure 38.2. Illustration of train-of-four stimuli following administration of neuromuscular blockers. (**A**) With incremental doses of SCh, the twitch height decreases. All four twitches are decreased by the same height. (**B**) During nondepolarizing relaxation, increasing doses result in a decrease of twitch height and a lower second, third, and fourth twitch compared with the first (the twitch amplitude fades during train-of-four stimulation).

in the eye to treat glaucoma), anticholinesterase agents (e.g., neostigmine, pyridostigmine, edrophonium), and monoamine oxidase inhibitors.

Since its introduction in 1951, the pharmacodynamic advantages of SCh have been invaluable in facilitating intubation in and out of the operating room. Its desirable properties allow rapid muscle relaxation of short duration. In contrast, SCh has many undesirable and occasionally lethal adverse effects.

Myalgias secondary to skeletal muscle depolarization are more pronounced in young, muscular individuals. Many clinical trials have evaluated pharmacologic therapies to prevent and or treat this adverse effect. Pretreatment with a nonsteroidal anti-inflammatory agent or a small dose of a nondepolarizing NMBD may be effective.

Hyperkalemia may occur after the administration of SCh. Normal patients typically experience a 0.5 to 1 mEq/L increase in plasma potassium concentration after SCh. Patients at risk for developing life-threatening hyperkalemia after SCh are listed in Table 38.1. Up-regulation and spread of the immature isoform as well as proliferation of the α_7 AChR throughout the muscle membrane plays a role in hyperkalemia following SCh administration. These isoform changes are seen in pathologic states listed in Table 38.1.

Dysrhythmias induced by SCh include sinus bradycardia, junctional rhythm, and, more commonly in children, sinus arrest. Sinus arrest in children can be prevented by pretreatment with atropine. These cardiac effects are secondary to the agonistic action of SCh at parasympathetic nerves.

Table 38.1. Risk factors for the development of hyperkalemia after the administration of depolarizing NMBDs

Upper or lower motor neuron defect
Prolonged chemical denervation (e.g., muscle relaxants, magnesium, clostridial toxins)
Direct muscle trauma, tumor, or inflammation
Thermal trauma
Disuse atrophy
Severe infection

SCh may also can produce other adverse effects, including elevated intracranial pressure and increased intraocular pressure. Both these effects may be mitigated by a higher dose of an intravenous induction agent and pretreatment with a small dose of a nondepolarizing NMBD.

Nondepolarizing NMBDs

Nondepolarizing NMBDs are often subdivided based on their duration of action (short, intermediate, or long acting) or chemical structure (benzylisoquinoline or steroid). NMBDs from the two different chemical classes will act synergistically and prolong the duration of action compared with either drug alone. Drugs from the same chemical class will act in an additive manner. Pancuronium, vecuronium, and rocuronium are steroids. Atracurium, cisatracurium, and mivacurium are benzylisoquinolines. Nondepolarizing NMBDs are competitive antagonists of ACh at the NMJ and bind to the α subunits of the AChR. Unlike SCh, nondepolarizing drugs do not cause depolarization of the postsynaptic muscle membrane.

Long-acting NMBDs

Pancuronium, a steroid, is the longest-acting NMBD available clinically. Its prolonged effect is a result of the action of the parent compound and its active metabolite, 3-hydroxypancuronium, produced in the liver. Pancuronium and its metabolite are eliminated equally in the urine and bile. The initial dose is 0.06 to 0.1 mg/kg, with a maintenance dose of 0.01 mg/kg every 25 to 60 minutes after the initial dose. The time to 25% twitch recovery is 80 to 100 minutes. Hepatic disease can double the terminal half-life and prolong neuromuscular recovery time. Because of its vagolytic properties, tachycardia, increased cardiac output, and hypertension may occur.

Because of pancuronium's prolonged neuromuscular effect, residual paresis may occur in the postanesthesia care unit. Studies comparing the incidence of postoperative residual paresis between long-acting NMBDs and intermediate-acting agents show a decreased risk of residual paresis when shorter-acting relaxants are used. For this reason, the use of pancuronium may be more appropriate when postoperative intubation is planned.

Intermediate-acting NMBDs

Most NMBDs currently in use fit into the intermediate-acting class. Vecuronium, rocuronium, atracurium, and cisatracurium are the intermediate-acting agents.

Table 38.2. Onset and duration of action of rocuronium on laryngeal adductors at varying doses

Dose, mg/kg	Onset at laryngeal adductor muscles, sec	Duration (T1 + 25%), min
0.4	92 ± 29	NA
0.8	96 ± 29	25 ± 9
1.2	54 ± 30	43 ± 13

Data from Wright PM, Caldwell JE, Miller RD. Onset and duration of rocuronium and succinylcholine at the adductor pollicis and laryngeal adductor muscles in anesthetized humans. *Anesthesiology* 1994; 81:1110–1115.

Vecuronium

Vecuronium is an intermediate-acting steroid NMBD used for both intubation and surgical muscle relaxation. The intubating dose is 0.1 mg/kg, with good intubating conditions within 2 to 3 minutes. Maintenance doses of 0.01 to 0.015 mg/kg may be given 25 to 40 minutes after the initial dose. If SCh is used for intubation, a lower initial dose of 0.04 to 0.06 mg/kg is adequate. The time to 25% twitch recovery is approximately 25 to 30 minutes, with a half-life of 51 to 80 minutes. Vecuronium undergoes both renal and hepatic elimination, with 80% excretion in the bile. The active metabolite, 3-desacetyl vecuronium, has half the potency of the parent compound. During prolonged administration, as in the intensive care setting, metabolite accumulation may cause prolonged recovery from paralysis, especially in the presence of renal failure. Vecuronium has little effect on the cardiovascular system.

Rocuronium

Rocuronium is an intermediate-acting steroidal NMBD whose rate of onset is directly related to the dose. Therefore, with larger initial doses (e.g., 1.2 mg/kg), intubating conditions can be achieved within 60 seconds (Table 38.2). It can be used as an alternative to SCh for rapid-sequence intubation. When compared with SCh, the onset of rocuronium at the adductor pollicis, in doses >1 mg/kg, is similar. Larger doses of rocuronium also significantly increase the duration of action. Repeat dosing for maintenance of paralysis is 0.1 to 0.2 mg/kg. Metabolism occurs in the liver to 17-desacetyl rocuronium, which has 5% to 10% of the activity of the parent compound. The terminal half-life is 60 to 70 minutes. More than 70% of the elimination occurs via the liver, with 30% eliminated renally.

Sugammadex is a novel investigational selective relaxant binding agent. It is a modified γ-cyclodextrin derivative that causes chemical encapsulation of rocuronium as well as vecuronium. Published data show that increasing doses of sugammadex reduced the mean recovery time of rocuronium from 122 minutes (spontaneous recovery) to less than 2 minutes in a dose-dependent manner. Signs of recurrence of paralysis did not occur. It has failed to achieve US Food and Drug Administration approval because of concerns regarding the incidence of hypersensitivity reactions.

Atracurium

Atracurium is an intermediate-acting benzylisoquinoline NMBD. It has four chiral centers, and there are theoretically 16 isomers. The clinical preparation is a mixture of 10 of these isomers. The intubating dose is 0.4 to 0.5 mg/kg, with good intubating conditions achieved in 2 to 3 minutes. However, it causes histamine release when given rapidly, thereby resulting in hypotension. It undergoes both Michael elimination (commonly referred to as Hofmann elimination) and ester hydrolysis, with a time to 25% recovery of 25 to 30 minutes. The metabolite laudanosine can cross the blood–brain barrier and has central nervous system–stimulating properties (convulsions). It is cleared both by the liver and kidneys. Adverse clinical effects of this metabolite are uncommon.

Cisatracurium

Cisatracurium is an intermediate-acting benzylisoquinoline NMBD. It is one of the isomers of atracurium and is the isomer with the largest ratio of NMB activity to histamine-releasing activity. It is approximately two to three times more potent than atracurium. Adequate conditions for intubation are achieved in 3 to 5 min with an intubating dose of 0.15 to 0.2 mg/kg. Cisatracurium undergoes Michael elimination to laudanosine, although the levels of laudanosine are less than those seen in atracurium. Its action and metabolism are not affected by renal or hepatic disease. The terminal half-life is 26 to 28 minutes, and the time to 25% recovery is 50 to 60 minutes.

Factors altering NMBD pharmacology

Various medications potentiate the clinical pharmacologic effects of NMBDs (Table 38.3). In addition, various disease states antagonize or potentiate the effects of NMBDs (Table 38.4).

Renal disease

In the presence of impaired renal function, renal clearance will be reduced. Prolonged recovery is not typically seen after a single bolus dose, because redistribution terminates the drug effect. However, after multiple bolus doses or a continuous

Table 38.3. Effect of various medications on the neuromuscular junction

Decreases synthesis of ACh	Impairs release of ACh by block of presynaptic calcium channels	Postsynaptic block of the AChR (by allosteric binding)
Furosemide	Volatile anesthetics	Volatile anesthetics
	Magnesium	Aminoglycoside antibiotics
	Calcium channel blockers	Quinidine
	Aminoglycoside antibiotics	Tricyclic antidepressants
		Ketamine
		Midazolam
		Barbiturates

Table 38.4. Pathologic states affecting neuromuscular block

Conditions that antagonize NMB	Conditions that potentiate NMB
Alkalosis	Hyponatremia
Hypercalcemia	Hypocalcemia
Demyelinating lesions	Hypokalemia
Peripheral neuropathies	Hypermagnesemia
Denervation states	Certain neuromuscular diseases
Infection	Acidosis
Immobilization	Acute intermittent porphyria
Muscle trauma	Eaton-Lambert syndrome
	Myasthenia gravis
	Renal failure
	Hepatic failure

infusion, the relaxant effect of drugs cleared by the kidney (especially pancuronium) will be prolonged. Atracurium and cisatracurium do not undergo renal clearance; thus, their duration of action is largely independent of renal function. In the presence of decreased metabolism of SCh (e.g., homozygous butyrylcholinesterase deficiency), the termination of its effect depends on renal elimination.

Hepatic disease

Following multiple bolus doses or a continuous infusion of rocuronium, vecuronium, or pancuronium, prolonged paralysis will occur in patients with significant hepatic dysfunction. However, because liver failure is often associated with fluid retention and/or ascites, a larger volume of distribution may be present. This larger volume of distribution may increase the initial dose needed to achieve the desired clinical effect. The duration of a single bolus dose is typically unchanged, because redistribution terminates the drug effect. A decreased synthesis of plasma butyrylcholinesterase may occur with decreased liver function, potentially prolonging the duration of SCh.

Diseases of the neuromuscular junction

Myasthenia gravis is an autoimmune disorder resulting in a decrease in the number of AChRs at the NMJ. This decrease in receptor number causes an increased sensitivity to nondepolarizing NMBDs. In addition, the decreased number of receptors requires an increased dose of SCh to effectively depolarize skeletal muscle. Eaton-Lambert syndrome is a paraneoplastic disorder in which antibodies bind to presynaptic voltage-gated calcium channels. This decreases ACh release at the NMJ, causing increased sensitivity to both nondepolarizing and depolarizing NMBDs.

Infection

Severe infection and immobilization in the intensive care unit can cause resistance to nondepolarizing NMBDs and a hyperkalemic response to SCh. This is secondary to up-regulation of AChRs. Infection with *Clostridium botulinum*, or administration of a large therapeutic dose of botulinum toxin, may lead

to a denervated state, resulting in a hyperkalemic response to SCh. Therapeutic exposure to botulinum toxin, in which only a single area or muscle is injected (i.e., forehead or for torticollis or blepharospasm), does not increase the risk of hyperkalemia. Animal data indicate that clostridial infection may lead to increased sensitivity to nondepolarizing NMBDs. This is an exception to the usual response, where resistance to nondepolarizing NMBDs is usually seen when AChRs are increased.

Drug interactions

Drugs that alter liver cytochrome P450 (CYP) will alter the pharmacokinetics of NMBDs cleared by the liver, specifically the steroidal NMBDs. Several studies have demonstrated increased elimination of vecuronium with the concomitant use of anticonvulsants (phenytoin, phenobarbital, carbamazepine) secondary to induction of CYP. In contrast, vecuronium activity was prolonged after inhibition of CYP by cimetidine. Other medications interact with muscle relaxants at the level of the NMJ by decreasing ACh synthesis, impairing the release of ACh or binding the α subunit of the AChR, and/or blocking the ion channel (see Table 38.3).

Data regarding the use of anti-inflammatory glucocorticoids and their interaction with NMBDs are contradictory. One study in humans found a prolonged effect of vecuronium in patients given concomitant glucocorticoids, whereas another study found no effect of acute glucocorticoid therapy on nondepolarizing muscle relaxants. Given this contradiction, care should be taken when administering NMBDs to patients on chronic glucocorticoid therapy.

Suggested readings

Alston TA. Hofmann, Schmofmann: atracurium undergoes Michael elimination. *Anesthesiology* 2001; 95:273.

Brown MM, Parr MJ, Manara AR. The effect of suxamethonium on intracranial pressure and cerebral perfusion pressure in patients with severe head injuries following blunt trauma. *Eur J Anaesthesiol* 1996; 13:474–477.

de Boer HD, Dreissen JJ, Marcus MA, et al. Reversal of rocuronium-induced (1.2 mg/kg) profound neuromuscular block by sugammadex: a multicenter, dose-finding and safety study. *Anesthesiology* 2007; 107:239–244.

Fiekers, JF. Sites and mechanisms of antibiotic-induced neuromuscular block: a pharmacological analysis using quantal content, voltage clamped end-plate currents and single channel analysis. *Acta Physiol Pharmacol Ther Latinoam* 1999; 49: 242–250.

Frick C, Richtsfeld M, Sahani N, et al. Long-term effects of botulinum toxin on neuromuscular function. *Anesthesiology* 2007; 106:1139–1146.

Ghoneim MM, Long JP. The interaction between magnesium and other neuromuscular blocking agents. *Anesthesiology* 1970; 32:23–27.

Martyn JA, Richtsfeld M. Succinylcholine-induced hyperkalemia in acquired pathologic states: etiologic factors and molecular mechanisms. *Anesthesiology* 2006; 104:158–169.

McCarthy G, Mirakhur RK, Elliott P, Wright J. Effect of H2-receptor antagonist pretreatment on vecuronium and atracurium induced neuromuscular block. *Br J Anaesth* 1991; 66:713–715.

Miller R, ed. *Miller's Anesthesia*. 6th ed. New York: Elsevier, Churchill-Livingstone; 2010.

Murphy GS. Residual neuromuscular blockade: incidence, assessment, and relevance in the postoperative period. *Minerva Anestesiol* 2006; 72:97–109.

Scheller M, Bufler J, Schneck H, et al. Isoflurane and sevoflurane interact with the nicotinic acetylcholine receptor channels in micromolar concentrations. *Anesthesiology* 1997; 86: 118–127.

Schreibe J, Lysakowski C, Fuchs-Buder T, Tramer M. Prevention of succinylcholine-induced fasciculation and myalgia: a meta-analysis of randomized trials. *Anesthesiology* 2005; 103:877–884.

Schwartz AE, Matteo RS, Ornstein E, Silverberg PA. Acute steroid therapy does not alter nondepolarizing muscle relaxant effects in humans. *Anesthesiology* 1986; 65:326–327.

Soriano SG, Sullivan LJ, Venkatakrishnan K, et al. Pharmacokinetics and pharmacodynamics of vecuronium in children receiving phenytoin and carbamazepine for chronic anticonvulsant therapy. *Br J Anaesth* 2001; 86:223–229.

Vachon CA, Warner DO, Bacon DR. Succinylcholine and the open globe. *Anesthesiology* 2003; 99:220–223.

Zimmerman AA, Funk KJ, Tidwell JL. Propofol and alfentanil prevent the increase in intraocular pressure caused by succinylcholine and endotracheal intubation during a rapid sequence induction of anesthesia. *Anesth Analg* 1996; 83:814–817.

Chapter 39

Reversal of neuromuscular blockade

Thor C. Milland and Neelakantan Sunder

When the need for muscular relaxation has passed, one may either await spontaneous return or administer one of several agents to hasten the return of neuromuscular function. Adequate muscle strength is a prerequisite for protective airway reflexes to prevent aspiration, as well as to maintain adequate spontaneous ventilation to prevent hypoxemia and hypercarbia. If mechanical ventilation is to be continued postoperatively for longer than the duration of action of the neuromuscular blocking agents used, reversal is most often omitted.

Depolarizing neuromuscular blockers

Succinylcholine, a depolarizing neuromuscular blocker, has the most rapid metabolism of any neuromuscular blocking drug. Most of this agent is metabolized by the circulating enzyme plasma butyrylcholinesterase (also known as pseudo-cholinesterase or plasma cholinesterase), even before it reaches the neuromuscular junction (NMJ). If this enzyme is phenotypically normal, the duration of neuromuscular blockade is short, with full spontaneous recovery within 4 to 10 minutes. Several medications can decrease butyrylcholinesterase activity, including metoclopramide, oral contraceptives, esmolol, some cytotoxic drugs, anticholinesterase agents, monoamine oxidase inhibitors, and echothiophate (a glaucoma agent). Individuals heterozygous or homozygous for a range of mutations in the butyrylcholinesterase gene may have increased duration of blockade, ranging from modest prolongation to up to 4 to 8 hours. There is no medication that increases the rate of recovery from succinylcholine neuromuscular blockade.

Nondepolarizing neuromuscular blockers

The neuromuscular blockers that are typically reversed are the nondepolarizing agents. These neuromuscular blockers are competitive antagonists of acetylcholine (ACh) at the NMJ. The return of normal transmission of excitation–contraction coupling at the NMJ depends on the reestablishment of the ability of ACh to bind to its receptor. Several factors either prolong or decrease the duration of neuromuscular blockade.

The major factors that influence the reversal of neuromuscular blockade are (1) concentration of ACh in the synapse, (2) concentration of neuromuscular blocker at the ACh receptor, (3) removal of the neuromuscular blocker from the synapse,

and (4) metabolism and/or excretion of the neuromuscular blocker from the body. Numerous factors can potentiate neuromuscular blockade, including volatile anesthetics, acidosis, hypothermia, and drugs such as aminoglycosides and polypeptide antibiotics. Electrolytes also have an influence on neuromuscular blockade, with hypokalemia and hypermagnesemia prolonging it and hypercalcemia antagonizing it.

Removal of neuromuscular blockers from the synapse occurs primarily by diffusion away from the synapse to the interstitial fluid, and then to the bloodstream. For most, hepatic metabolism ensures that a gradient favorable to their diffusion away from the synapse will be maintained. Cisatracurium is a notable exception, most of it being degraded by Michael (commonly referred to as Hofmann) elimination, and therefore largely independent of organ function. The primary route of elimination of neuromuscular blockers is via hepatic metabolism and/or renal excretion.

Assessment of neuromuscular blockade

The degree of neuromuscular blockade present, as well as its assessment, is of crucial importance in determining reversal strategy. There is a nonlinear relationship between the time to return of muscular function and depth of neuromuscular blockade when reversal agents are administered. Peripheral nerve twitch monitoring with the train-of-four (TOF) pattern of stimulation is used most commonly. Either the number of twitches observed or the ratio of the amplitude of the first twitch to the fourth twitch (TOF ratio) indicate the degree of neuromuscular blockade present. When TOF is used, the simplest method to assess neuromuscular blockade is visual or tactile assessment of the number of twitches present.

Without a quantitative measurement of twitch amplitude, TOF is inherently an inaccurate method. A single twitch remaining on the TOF represents approximately 90% blockade. If four twitches are visible, the degree of blockade is about ≤ 25%. TOF monitoring without accurate quantization of twitch amplitude should not be used to assess the degree of spontaneous recovery or the success of reversal, as there may be a clinically significant neuromuscular blockade in the absence of a manual or visually perceptible difference between the first and fourth twitches.

The preferred method to assess the degree of recovery or the success of reversal is to use the double-burst pattern of stimulation. The double-burst consists of a series of two short 50-Hz tetanic stimuli separated by 0.75 seconds. A difference in the ratio of the first and second responses is determined more easily visually or with the palpating finger. However, lack of apparent difference following a double-burst stimulus is still no guarantee that the patient has a clinically insignificant degree of NMB.

Another method to assess degree of recovery or the success of reversal is to elicit sustained tetanus for 5 seconds at 100 Hz without fade in degree of muscular contraction (in anesthetized patients, because it is painful) or eliciting a sustained head lift for 5 seconds (in awake patients). Following administration of tetanus, there will be posttetanic potentiation of the TOF and double-burst, so these methods of assessment then become less accurate. Other clinical methods include leg lift, grip strength, response to verbal communication, and adequate ventilatory parameters (tidal volume 3–5 ml/kg, maximum inspiratory force −20 mm Hg).

Monitoring site

To assess the degree of neuromuscular blockade, the twitch-monitoring site is important. The larynx, diaphragm, and other central muscles are more rapidly affected by neuromuscular blockers and also have a quicker recovery. Stimulation of the facial nerve with observation of the orbicularis oculi muscle is closely correlated with laryngeal adductor paralysis, and is a good indicator of intubating conditions. However, it is often difficult to differentiate between direct versus evoked responses when the facial nerve is used. For recovery from neuromuscular blockade, the ulnar nerve and adductor pollicis muscle provide the best correlation with the tone of the muscles involved in protective airway reflexes. Furthermore, when adduction of the thumb is used as the response, there is no interference from direct stimulation.

Although spontaneous movement and respiratory activity are also measures of return of neuromuscular function, they are inherently inaccurate, and a twitch monitor should be used whenever possible. It is important to remember that in hemiplegic patients, peripheral nerve twitch monitoring should be done on the normal side, as monitoring on the weak side may lead to an overdose of neuromuscular blockers because of an exaggerated response on the weaker side due to the presence of extrajunctional receptors.

When to reverse

When considering reversal of neuromuscular blockade with an inhibitor of acetylcholinesterase, two important factors should be considered: (1) the time elapsed since the last dose of the neuromuscular blocker and (2) the dose of neuromuscular blocker administered. Although administration of neostigmine during profound neuromuscular blockade will indeed result in shortening of the interval before a TOF ratio of 0.9 is achieved, waiting until the TOF ratio is > 0.1 will result in a far speedier

reversal. If reversal is attempted at a deeper degree of block, residual blockade is likely. A good practice is to reverse the neuromuscular blockade when at least two twitches (TOF) are detectable.

Spontaneous recovery

If the route of spontaneous recovery of neuromuscular blockade is chosen, it is important to allow sufficient time for recovery to occur. Even then, it is important to realize that despite apparent adequate muscular tone, as gauged by nonquantitative methods of measurement such as sustained head lift for 5 seconds, leg lift, or grip strength, a significant amount of residual paralysis may still be present. This subclinical paralysis may cause a significant compromise of protective airway reflexes. In addition, these clinical signs are subject to significant interobserver variability, which significantly decreases their reliability. Even when a TOF ratio of 0.9 is set as the limit of adequate reversal of neuromuscular blockade, 13% of patients will still have pharyngeal dysfunction. Given this evidence, many anesthesiologists feel it is prudent to reverse neuromuscular blockade prior to extubation in all patients who have received nondepolarizing neuromuscular blockers.

Agents for neuromuscular blockade reversal

Various pharmacologic agents are available to reverse neuromuscular blockade. These agents produce their effect by increasing the amount of ACh available to compete with the NMB at the NMJ by inhibiting acetylcholinesterase, the enzyme that degrades ACh. This mechanism for reversal will be effective as long as there is not such a surplus of neuromuscular blocker at the synapse that it is impossible to overcome the blockade by the levels of ACh achieved. In overdose, acetylcholinesterase inhibitors can themselves cause paradoxic weakness due to the production of a depolarizing block from the excess of ACh present at the NMJ. Acetylcholinesterase inhibitors also prolong the effect of succinylcholine by inhibition of butyrylcholinesterase.

Neostigmine, edrophonium, pyridostigmine

Anticholinesterase agents available for clinical use at present are neostigmine, edrophonium, and pyridostigmine. Neostigmine is the most potent and widely used neuromuscular blockade reversal agent because its pharmacokinetics closely matches that of the commonly used neuromuscular blockers. Its onset is within 5 minutes, and its duration is about 1 to 2 hours.

Pyridostigmine is slower in onset and longer in duration compared with neostigmine. It is sometimes used in the reversal of deep neuromuscular blockade. Edrophonium is more rapid in onset than neostigmine (approximately 2 minutes) and shorter in duration (≪1 hour). Because of its short duration, there is the possibility of reparalysis, especially with longer-acting neuromuscular blockers.

All anticholinesterase drugs are metabolized in the liver and excreted in the urine. However, in the presence of hepatic or renal disease, their doses usually do not need to be adjusted, because the neuromuscular blockers are also metabolized hepatically or excreted renally.

Although the aforementioned anticholinesterase agents are quaternary ammonium compounds, physostigmine, also an anticholinesterase agent, is a tertiary ammonium compound and is lipid soluble. It is the only anticholinesterase agent that can cross the blood–brain barrier into the central nervous system (CNS). Therefore, CNS symptoms of anticholinergic toxicity (due to scopolamine or atropine) can be reversed with physostigmine.

Adverse effects of acetylcholinesterase inhibitors

When neuromuscular blockade is reversed by acetylcholinesterase inhibitors at the NMJ, the acetylcholinesterase enzyme is inhibited at all cholinergic synapses, resulting in increased ACh at both nicotinic and muscarinic receptors. Although the nicotinic receptor at the NMJ is the targeted receptor, ACh is also the neurotransmitter at the nicotinic receptors in autonomic ganglia as well as at the muscarinic receptors at parasympathetically innervated organs. The increase in ACh leads to bradycardia, hypersalivation, and bronchoconstriction. Severe parasympathetic overstimulation may lead to the so-called SLUDGE (salivation, lacrimation, urination, defecation, gastrointestinal upset, emesis) or cholinergic syndrome. These effects are seen least following the use of edrophonium.

Anticholinergics

To offset the aforementioned cholinergic effects, a muscarinic antagonist (vagolytic/anticholinergic) is usually given in combination with the anticholinesterase agent (Table 39.1). The three commonly used anticholinergic drugs are scopolamine, atropine, and glycopyrrolate, of which the latter two are used in neuromuscular blockade reversal. Scopolamine and atropine are tertiary amines and can cross the blood–brain barrier, whereas glycopyrrolate is a quaternary amine and does not cross the blood–brain barrier. The anticholinergic drugs competitively block the effect of ACh at the muscarinic receptors.

Glycopyrrolate has a longer duration (1–2 hours) and a slower onset of action compared with atropine This makes it well suited for use in conjunction with neostigmine. Atropine occasionally may cause a paradoxic bradycardia in lower doses

Table 39.1. Typical combinations of acetylcholinesterase inhibitors and vagolytic agents

Combination	Dose, *mg/kg*
Neostigmine/glycopyrrolate	Neostigmine: 0.04–0.07 Glycopyrrolate: 0.005–0.01
Edrophonium/atropine	Edrophonium: 0.5–1 Atropine: 0.01
Pyridostigmine/glycopyrrolate	Pyridostigmine: 0.2–0.35 Glycopyrrolate: 0.005–0.01

Table 39.2. Effects of anticholinergic agents on various organ systems

Antisialagogue effect	Drying of secretions, rise in body temperature
Cardiovascular[a]	Tachycardia, shortening of PR interval
CNS[b]	Sedation, amnesia, stimulation/depression
Respiratory	Inhibition of secretion of respiratory mucosa, bronchodilation
Gastrointestinal	Decreased intestinal motility, increased risk of aspiration as lower esophageal sphincter tone is decreased
Renal	Urinary retention
Ophthalmic	Pupillary dilation and cycloplegia[c]

[a] Atropine produces the highest cardiovascular effects and scopolamine the least.
[b] Glycopyrrolate does not cross the blood–brain barrier and does not produce CNS effects. Scopolamine produces the most CNS effects.
[c] Cycloplegia is the inability to accommodate to near vision.

(<0.5 mg). All muscarinic antagonists are antisialagogues and inhibit perspiration (Table 39.2), both of which are desirable characteristics in the setting of imminent extubation and hypothermia, often the case at the end of an operative procedure. Heart transplant patients, despite having a theoretic parasympathetic denervation of the transplanted organ, may suffer pronounced bradycardia or asystole if an acetylcholinesterase inhibitor is administered, regardless of the concurrent administration of a vagolytic agent.

Administration of a centrally acting anticholinergic agent such as scopolamine may lead to the so-called central anticholinergic syndrome characterized by excitation, delirium, and hyperpyrexia. Physostigmine, a cholinesterase inhibitor, may be used to treat the central anticholinergic syndrome.

Sugammadex

Sugammadex, formerly known as Org 25969, is a cyclodextrin whose mechanism of reversal is by encapsulation of rocuronium or vecuronium. (It is much less active against pancuronium.) As acetylcholinesterase inhibitors and antimuscarinic agents are not administered, the adverse effects attributable to these agents are absent. Sugammadex possesses several unique characteristics that may drastically change the practice of neuromuscular blockade and its reversal.

Return of a TOF ratio of 0.9 within 1 minute of intravenous administration of sugammadex (8 mg/kg) has been demonstrated. In addition, although a higher dose is required for reversal with increasing depth of neuromuscular blockade, this agent can be used immediately after the blockade is established. The adverse effect profile is benign; the most noteworthy effect was signs of insufficient depth of anesthesia after sugammadex administration in 20% of patients in a dose-finding study. The therapeutic range is wide, with up to a 10-fold overdose being tolerated without incident. The ability to rapidly reverse profound neuromuscular blockade may offer an alternative to succinylcholine and may be beneficial for rescue in a certain subset of patients in a "can't ventilate, can't intubate" scenario.

Although approved for use in Europe, sugammadex has failed to achieve US Food and Drug Administration approval due to concerns regarding the incidence of hypersensitivity reactions.

Suggested readings

Alston T. Hofmann, Schmofmann: atracurium undergoes Michael elimination. *Anesthesiology* 2001; 95:273.

Beecher HK, Todd DP. A study of the deaths associated with anesthesia and surgery: based on a study of 599, 548 anesthesias in ten institutions 1948-1952, inclusive. *Ann Surg* 1954; 140: 2–35.

Debaene B, Plaud B, Dilly MP, Donati F. Residual paralysis in the PACU after a single intubating dose of nondepolarizing muscle relaxant with an intermediate duration of action. *Anesthesiology* 2003; 98:1024–1047.

Eriksson NW. Videoradiographical computerized manometry in assessment of pharyngeal function in partially paralyzed humans. *Anesthesiology* 1995; A886.

Katz RL. Clinical neuromuscular pharmacology of pancuronium. *Anesthesiology* 1971; 34:550–556.

Molina AL, de Boer HD, Klimek M, et al. Reversal of rocuronium-induced (1.2 mg/kg) profound neuromuscular block by accidental high dose sugammadex. *Br J Anaesth* 2007; 98:624–627.

Sparr HJ, Vermeyen KM, Beaufort AM, et al. Early reversal of profound rocuronium-induced neuromuscular blockade by sugammadex in a randomized multicenter study: efficacy, safety, and pharmacokinetics. *Anesthesiology* 2007; 106:935–943.

Tramèr MR, Fuchs-Buder T. Omitting antagonism of neuromuscular block: effect on postoperative nausea and vomiting and risk of residual paralysis. A systematic review. *Br J Anaesth* 1999; 82:379–386.

Chapter 40

Perioperative pulmonary aspiration prophylaxis

John P. Broadnax and B. Scott Segal

Pulmonary aspiration of gastric contents is a complication that causes significant trepidation among anesthesia providers. Indeed, the first clearly anesthesia-related death was probably the result of aspiration. Pulmonary aspiration involves the regurgitation of gastric contents and their subsequent entrance into the respiratory tract, which may lead to acute lung injury mediated by particulate matter and the acidic nature of gastric contents. Aspirated particulate matter may lead to a focal inflammatory and foreign body reaction. The low pH of gastric contents causes diffuse acid-mediated damage. Animal models suggest that aspiration of material with pH < 2.5 is associated with pulmonary morbidity, whereas more alkaline material causes little or no injury. The volume required to cause injury is controversial. Early data suggesting 0.4 ml/kg (or approximately 25 ml in a 70-kg adult) was sufficient probably overestimated the risk; more recent, larger studies suggest 1 ml/kg in the lung (not merely in the stomach) is required.

Together, the twin insults of acid and particulate matter can act synergistically, leading to increased pulmonary damage. Acutely, pulmonary aspiration may lead to aspiration pneumonitis. After the initial insult, pulmonary aspiration may later evolve into aspiration pneumonia, respiratory failure, or acute respiratory distress syndrome.

The overall risk of pulmonary aspiration of gastric contents during general anesthesia is actually quite low, on the order of one to five in 10,000 anesthetic procedures. In the setting of modern pulmonary care, the aspiration of gastric contents is fortunately associated with minimal morbidity and negligible mortality. The incidence of aspiration is slightly greater in the obstetric and pediatric patient populations, but overall morbidity and mortality are not increased. Studies in trauma patients indicate a much higher incidence of aspiration.

The first step in preventing pulmonary aspiration is to identify patients who are at an increased risk for this complication. Several risk factors for pulmonary aspiration have been identified: increased gastric pressure, increased gastric regurgitation, and laryngeal incompetence. The specific entities that predispose patients to these conditions are outlined in Table 40.1.

Traditionally, pregnancy and obesity have been thought to be associated with an increased risk of aspiration due to associated decreased gastric emptying. However, these assumptions appear to be untrue in both the obese and the nonlaboring parturient.

To minimize the risk associated with pulmonary aspiration, surgical patients are required to be nil per os (NPO) prior to undergoing general anesthesia. The current American Society of Anesthesiologists (ASA) NPO guidelines recommend patient fasting of 2 hours after clear fluids, 4 hours after breast milk for neonates and infants, and 6 hours after infant formula, nonhuman milk, or a light meal (ASA 1999). Many anesthesiologists favor a more conservative fast of 8 hours, or NPO after midnight the day of surgery.

Several anesthetic techniques have been proposed to reduce the risk of pulmonary aspiration in high-risk patients. Rapid sequence intubation and the application of cricoid pressure are widely used in anesthetic practice. Neither, however, has been shown to reduce the incidence of aspiration or affect the morbidity or mortality from pulmonary aspiration. Nonetheless, most anesthesiologists consider such techniques to be the standard of care for patients known to have elevated risk of pulmonary aspiration.

Pharmacologic approaches to reducing the risk of aspiration include the preoperative administration of nonparticulate antacids, histamine H_2 antagonists, proton pump inhibitors (PPIs), and prokinetic agents. Table 40.2 summarizes suggested aspiration prophylaxis drugs, doses, and routes of administration.

Table 40.1. Risk factors for perioperative pulmonary aspiration

Increased gastric volume	Increased gastric regurgitation	Decreased laryngeal competence
Delayed gastric emptying	Gastroesophageal reflux disease	General anesthesia
Diabetic gastroparesis	Decreased lower esophageal sphincter tone	Depressed level of consciousness
Labor	Esophageal obstruction	Head injury
Pain/stress	Zenker's diverticulum	Stroke
Gastric hypersecretion	Achalasia	Neuromuscular disorders
Overfeeding	Extremes of age	Muscular dystrophies
Recent meal	Esophageal/upper abdominal surgery	
	Esophagectomy	
	Increased intra-abdominal pressure	

Table 40.2. Suggested aspiration prophylaxis drugs, doses, and routes of administration

Drug	Dose	Route of administration
Citric acid/sodium citrate	30 ml	PO
Metoclopramide	5–15 mg	PO/IV/IM
Rabeprazole	20 mg	PO/IV
Omeprazole	20–40 mg	PO/IV
Pantoprazole	40–120 mg	PO/IV
Lansoprazole	15–30 mg	PO/IV
Esomeprazole	20–40 mg	PO/IV
Nizatidine	150–300 mg	PO/IV/IM
Famotidine	20–40 mg	PO/IV/IM
Cimetidine	400–800 mg	PO/IV/IM
Ranitidine	75–150 mg	PO/IV/IM

IM, intramuscular; IV, intravenous; PO, oral.

Nonparticulate antacids administered immediately preoperatively significantly raise gastric pH. The most commonly used solution is sodium citrate or a citrate/citric acid buffer. These agents have a very rapid onset of action but a relatively short-lived gastric acid–neutralizing effect.

Histamine H_2 antagonists and PPIs have been used to increase gastric pH. Both pharmacologic classes act by limiting parietal cell acid secretion in the stomach. Histamine H_2 antagonists exert their effect by antagonizing the action of histamine on gastric parietal cells via competitive inhibition. PPIs bind to and block the action of the H^+,K^+-ATPase pump on parietal cells. Both methods effectively increase gastric pH when administered appropriately preoperatively. Their onset of action is slower but they last considerably longer than antacids.

Metoclopramide is a dopamine receptor antagonist with prokinetic properties due to peripheral cholinergic agonism. Its effects include increased gastric contractions, relaxation of the pyloric sphincter, and increased small bowel peristalsis. Metoclopramide is administered preoperatively to increase gastric emptying, thereby theoretically reducing the risk of perioperative aspiration because of decreased gastric volume. Its onset time after intravenous administration is approximately 20 minutes. In emergency settings, it may help reduce the risk of aspiration at extubation, even if it has no effect at induction.

Although each of these agents has proven to be effective in achieving the goals of reducing gastric volume and increasing gastric pH, none has been shown to affect the morbidity or mortality from perioperative pulmonary aspiration. In large part, this may be the result of insufficient power given the rare incidence of perioperative pulmonary aspiration and associated morbidity and mortality. Therefore, routine prophylaxis with these agents for all patients is not recommended. Despite the paucity of outcome data, however, these agents likely are useful in patients at high risk for pulmonary aspiration or in whom the consequences of such an event would be poorly tolerated.

Suggested readings

American Society of Anesthesiologists Task Force on Preoperative Fasting. Practice guidelines for preoperative fasting and the use of pharmacological agents for the prevention of pulmonary aspiration: application to healthy patients undergoing elective procedures. *Anesthesiology* 1999; 90:896–905.

Blitt CD, Gutman HL, Cohen DD, et al. 'Silent' regurgitation and aspiration during general anesthesia. *Anesth Analg* 1970; 49:707–713.

Cohen MM, Duncan PG, Pope WDP, Wolkenstein C. A survey of 112,000 anaesthetics at one teaching hospital (1975–83). *Can Anaesth Soc J* 1986; 33:22–31.

Coriat P, Labrousse J, Vilde F, et al. Diffuse interstitial pneumonitis due to aspiration of gastric contents. *Anaesthesia* 1984; 39:703–705.

Engelhardt T, Webster NR. Pulmonary aspiration of gastric contents in anaesthesia. *Br J Anaesth* 1999; 83:453–460.

Ezri T, Szmuk P, Stein A, et al. Peripartum general anaesthesia without tracheal intubation: incidence of aspiration pneumonia. *Anaesthesia* 2000; 55:421–426.

Harkness GA, Bentley DW, Roghmann KJ. Risk factors for nosocomial pneumonia in the elderly. *Am J Med* 1990; 89:457–463.

Harrison GG. Death attributable to anaesthesia. A ten year survey (1967–1976). *Br J Anaesth* 1978; 50:1041–1046.

Hovi-Viander M. Death associated with anaesthesia in Finland. *Br J Anaesth* 1980; 52:483–489.

Ishihara H, Singh H, Giesecke AH. Relationship between diabetic autonomic neuropathy and gastric contents. *Anesth Analg* 1994; 78:943–947.

Knight PR, Rutter T, Tait AR, et al. Pathogenesis of gastric particulate lung injury: a comparison and interaction with acidic pneumonitis. *Anesth Analg* 1993; 77:745–760.

Kulkarni PN, Batra YK, Wig J. Effects of different combinations of H2 receptor antagonist with gastrokinetic drugs on gastric fluid pH and volume in children – a comparative study. *Int J Pharmacol Ther* 1997; 35:561–564.

La Rosa M, Piva L, Ravanelli A, et al. Aspiration syndrome in cesarean section. Our experience from 1980 to 1990. *Minerva Anestesiol* 1992; 58:1213–1220.

Leigh JM, Tytler JA. Admissions to the intensive care unit after complications of anaesthetic techniques over 10 years. *Anaesthesia* 1990; 45:814–820.

Manchikanti L, Colliver JA, Marrero TC, Roush JR. Assessment of age-related acid aspiration risk factors in pediatric, adult, and geriatric patients. *Anesth Analg* 1985; 64:11–17.

Ng A, Smith G. Gastroesophageal reflux and aspiration of gastric contents in anesthetic practice. *Anesth Analg* 2001; 93:494–513.

Nishina K, Mikawa K, Takao Y, et al. A comparison of rabeprazole, lansoprazole and ranitidine for improving preoperative gastric fluid property in adults undergoing elective surgery. *Anesth Analg* 2000; 90:717–721.

Olsson GL, Hallen B, Hambraeus-Jonzon K. Aspiration during anaesthesia: a computer-aided study of 185–358 anaesthetics. *Acta Anaesthesiol Scand* 1986; 30:84–92.

Phillips S, Daborn AK, Hatch DJ. Preoperative fasting for paediatric anaesthesia. *Br J Anaesth* 1994; 73:529–536.

Tiret L, Hatton F. Complications associated with anaesthesia – a prospective survey in France. *Can Anaesth Soc J* 1986; 33: 336–344.

Warner MA, Warner ME, Weber JG. Clinical significance of pulmonary aspiration during the perioperative period. *Anesthesiology* 1993; 78:56–62.

Wong CA, McCarthy RJ, Fitzgerald PC, et al. Gastric emptying of water in obese pregnant women at term. *Anesth Analg* 2007; 105:751–755.

Perioperative antiemetic therapies

John P. Broadnax and B. Scott Segal

Introduction

Postoperative nausea and vomiting (PONV) has been a perpetual problem since the introduction of ether anesthesia. It has often been referred to as the "big little problem" (Kapur 1991). Although this condition rarely results in significant mortality, the morbidity has a significant effect on the patient's perioperative experience and perception. PONV may lead to incisional suture dehiscence, aspiration, and delayed postoperative patient discharge. In several studies, patients identified their primary perioperative concern as PONV, even greater than pain. Over the past few decades, a substantial amount of research has been dedicated to this topic, leading to better mechanistic understanding and development of rational solutions. This chapter reviews the pharmacology of antiemetic drugs. The assessment of PONV risk and strategies for rational use of these drugs are discussed in Chapter 54.

Physiology of PONV

Nausea and vomiting are the results of a complex integration of inputs from various physiologic systems (Fig. 41.1). It is the manifestation of the stimulation of the salivary center, respiratory center, and pharyngeal, gastrointestinal (GI), and abdominal muscles. These centers receive their stimulatory input from the central vomiting center, which has been classically postulated to be located in the lateral reticular formation of the medulla. More recent evidence suggests it is not a single anatomic center but a group of closely integrated areas in the brainstem. This central vomiting center is responsible for integrating and coordinating the complex processes involved in vomiting. The vomiting center receives input from the chemoreceptor trigger zone (CTZ), the vestibular apparatus, the cerebral cortex, and the visceral afferent nerves from the GI tract. The CTZ, also located in the brainstem (in the area postrema at the floor of the fourth ventricle) lies outside the blood–brain barrier and thus is uniquely positioned to receive blood-borne chemical emetogenic stimuli. The stimulation of dopamine, opioid, histamine, acetylcholine, neurokinin-1, or serotonin type-3 receptors in these centers initiates the cascade that leads to emesis. These receptors are the targets of the various antiemetic therapies, and it is through them that they enact their antiemetic effects.

Rational administration of antiemetic therapy

The preoperative identification of independent risk factors followed by the use of a risk-dependent stratification management model should form the foundation of a rational, evidence-based approach to the prophylaxis and treatment of established nausea and vomiting in the postoperative setting. Please refer to Chapter 54 for a detailed discussion of this topic.

Number needed to treat and number needed to harm

Comparison of the efficacy and side effects of antiemetic drugs is complex, and few head-to-head comparisons are available. Instead, it is common to compare a given drug with placebo. The apparent effect of the tested drug depends on its effectiveness or harmfulness as well as the incidence of PONV or side effects in the placebo-treated group. A common way to standardize this comparison across studies and drugs is to compute the number needed to treat (NNT) or number needed to harm (NNH). This number is simply the reciprocal of the absolute difference in risk in the treatment and placebo groups. For example, if 25% of the drug-treated group experiences PONV, compared with 50% of the placebo-treated patients, then the absolute risk reduction is 25%, and the NNT is $1/(0.5 - 0.25) = 4$.

Pharmacology of antiemetic drugs
Anticholinergics

Anticholinergics presumably produce their antiemetic effects via inhibition of postganglionic muscarinic receptors in the central nervous system. They prevent cholinergic transmission from the vestibular nuclei and reticular formation to the central vomiting center. The most effective antiemetic in this drug class is scopolamine. As a tertiary amine, scopolamine crosses the blood–brain barrier to exert its central anticholinergic effects. Scopolamine is available as either a parenteral solution or a transdermal patch delivery system. Transdermal scopolamine premedication has been shown to decrease the incidence of vomiting following general anesthesia when applied the evening before surgery or 4 hours before the end of anesthesia. Early

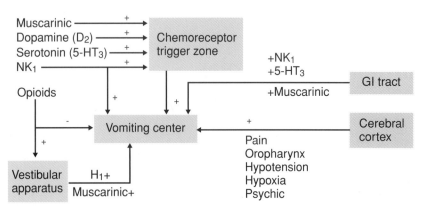

Figure 41.1. The neurobiology of PONV.

application of the patch is necessary because of its 2- to 4-hour delay in onset of an antiemetic effect. Conversely, a single patch may provide up to 72 hours of antiemetic treatment.

A meta-analysis of randomized studies (Kranke et al. 2002) found the NNT with scopolamine to prevent postoperative vomiting was 5.9 patients. Transdermal scopolamine also has been shown to decrease nausea and vomiting caused by epidural and intrathecal morphine. It may find particular benefit in outpatient surgery, because its anti–motion sickness effect is prominent. Side effects are mild but common; the NNH is 5.6 for visual disturbances such as blurry vision and 12.5 for dry mouth. Other common side effects include sedation, memory disturbance, confusion, constipation, and urinary retention. Table 41.1 shows currently used PONV prophylaxis drugs, as well as their suggested doses and time of administration.

Serotonin-3 antagonists

The antiemetic properties of many classic antiemetics initially were attributed solely to dopaminergic antagonism (see later), but serotonin receptor antagonism later was discovered to also partially play a role in this effect. This discovery led to the research and eventual development of the serotonin-3 (5-HT$_3$) antagonists. These drugs act via antagonism of 5-HT$_3$ receptors in the CTZ and the vagal afferents in the GI tract. They have been shown to be effective in both the prophylaxis and treatment of PONV. The first 5-HT$_3$ antagonist to be marketed in the United States and the most studied drug in the class is ondansetron. Its efficacy has been documented in numerous randomized placebo-controlled trials (Tramer et al. 1997). The NNT for prevention of nausea is 6 to 7, compared with 5 for prophylaxis against vomiting, indicative of the class's superiority in preventing vomiting over nausea. The optimal timing of administration is at the end of surgery (Sun et al. 1997).

Other 5-HT$_3$ antagonists include dolasetron, granisetron, tropisetron, and ramosetron (the latter two are not available in the U.S.). When used in equipotent doses, 5-HT$_3$ receptor antagonists are equally effective in the prevention of PONV (Naguib et al. 1996).

The side effect profile of the 5-HT$_3$ antagonists includes constipation, with an NNH of 23; headache, with an NNH of 36; elevated liver enzymes, with an NNH of 31; and more rarely, dizziness, electrocardiogram abnormalities, and flushing. The lack of sedation with drugs of this class makes them particularly suitable for use in ambulatory surgery. Recently, the FDA withdrew approval of intravenous dolasetron for chemotherapy-induced nausea and vomiting because of the risk of dose-dependent QT interval prolongation. All 5-HT$_3$ antagonists prolong the QT interval to some extent, but the risk with dolasetron seems to be highest. Because the dose for PONV is so much lower than that for chemotherapy patients, the risk in the perioperative period is still relatively small. Another part of the new FDA warning is that dolasetron should not be given to patients with congenital long QT syndrome or with hypokalemia or hypomagnesemia.

Table 41.1. Suggested PONV prophylaxis drugs, doses, and times of administration

Drug	Dose	Time of administration[a]
Dexamethasone	4–5 mg IV	Induction of anesthesia
Dimenhydrinate	1 mg/kg IV, 25–50 mg PO	Undetermined
Dolasetron	12.5 mg IV	End of surgery
Droperidol	0.625–1.25 mg IV	End of surgery
Granisetron	0.35–1.5 mg IV	End of surgery
Haloperidol	0.5–2 mg IM/IV	? / End of surgery
Prochlorperazine	5–10 mg IM/IV	End of surgery
Promethazine	6.25–25 mg IV	Induction of anesthesia
Ondansetron	4 mg IV	End of surgery
Scopolamine	Transdermal patch	Preoperatively
Aprepitant	40 mg PO	Preoperatively

[a] The stated times of administration are based on the best currently available evidence; however, significant controversy remains regarding the optimal timing of perioperative antiemetic administration.
IM, intramuscularly; IV, intravenously; PO, orally.
Data from Gan T, Meyers T, Apfel C. Consensus guidelines for managing postoperative nausea and vomiting. *Anesth Analg* 2003; 97:62–71.

Glucocorticoids

Dexamethasone is the most extensively evaluated and frequently used glucocorticoid in the prophylaxis and treatment of PONV. The mechanism by which glucocorticoids exert their antiemetic effect is unknown. Dexamethasone has been shown to be effective for both the immediate and late onset of PONV. Its effects on late-onset PONV appear to be more pronounced. The NNT for early-onset PONV is 7.1, compared with 3.8 for later-onset PONV (Henzi et al. 2000). To provide prophylaxis for both early- and late-onset PONV, dexamethasone should be administered relatively early in the immediate perioperative period. For example, dexamethasone was demonstrated to be more effective at preventing PONV during the first 2 hours following surgery when given before induction of anesthesia, as opposed to at the end of surgery; however, administration at either time was effective in preventing late-onset symptoms from 2 to 24 hours postoperatively (Wang et al. 2000). Most studies on dexamethasone have focused on doses of 8 to 10 mg, but some data suggest that lower doses of 2.5 to 5 mg may be effective as well. Given the short duration of therapy for PONV, long-term adverse effects of glucocorticoids, such as reduction in bone mineral density, diabetes, and cataracts, have not been reported (Henzi et al. 2000).

Dopaminergic antagonists

The butyrophenones most often used as antiemetics are droperidol and haloperidol. These drugs act via antagonism of the dopamine D_2 receptor in the CTZ and in the postremal area. Although both drugs have shown efficacy in PONV, droperidol is more frequently used in anesthetic practice. Droperidol doses as low as 0.625 mg have been shown to be effective in the prophylaxis of PONV (Henzi et al. 2000a). Doses <1 mg are more effective for the prevention of nausea than of vomiting; however, doses between 1 and 2.5 mg improve antiemetic efficacy. Droperidol's efficacy is similar to that of ondansetron for PONV prophylaxis, with an NNT of approximately 5 (Tramer 2001).

On November 26, 2001, the US Food and Drug Administration (FDA) issued a "black box" warning for droperidol regarding the potential for QT interval prolongation and cardiac arrhythmias that may result in torsades de pointes and sudden cardiac death. Continuous cardiac rhythm monitoring for 2 to 3 hours is recommended for any patient receiving droperidol at the approved (labeled) dose of ≥2.5 mg. Although the aforementioned cardiac morbidity is a well-documented effect seen with high doses of droperidol, questions have been raised regarding its relevance at the lower doses (0.625–1.25 mg) used for PONV prophylaxis and treatment.

Of the numerous cases reported to the FDA involving droperidol-associated QT prolongation, arrhythmia, or cardiac death, only 10 cases involved droperidol administered at a dose of ≤1.25 mg. Droperidol was not conclusively found to be causally related to the deaths in any of the reported cases. Because of the lack of submitted data, the FDA has declined to comment on the efficacy or safety of droperidol at these lower doses. Also of note, the FDA has reiterated the importance of off-label drug use in medical practice and neither restricts physicians' discretionary use of approved drugs nor regulates the off-label use of approved drugs (Ludwin et al. 2008; Rappaport 2008).

The second class of antiemetic dopaminergic antagonists is the phenothiazines. Their antiemetic effects are primarily via antagonism of the dopamine D_2 receptor in the CTZ.

Phenothiazines also antagonize histamine H_1 receptors. Prochlorperazine, an agent in this class of medications, has been shown to be an effective antiemetic when administered at the end of surgical procedures. Caution should be taken when using prochlorperazine in the perioperative period because of its profound antagonism of α-adrenoceptors.

Antihistamines

Antihistamines exert their antiemetic effects via antagonism of the histamine H_1 and muscarinic receptors in the vestibular system. The most effective antiemetic antihistamines used frequently in anesthetic practice are members of the ethanolamine, piperazine, and phenothiazine families.

Dimenhydrinate, an ethanolamine, appears to have antiemetic efficacy similar to that of the 5-HT$_3$ receptor antagonists, dexamethasone and droperidol. A meta-analysis of randomized controlled trials showed the NNT for nausea and vomiting prophylaxis to be approximately 5 within 48 hours after surgery. The optimal timing and dose response for administration could not be calculated because of insufficient data (Kranke et al. 2002). Also of note, dimenhydrinate is pharmacologically similar to diphenhydramine, as it is composed of the salts of diphenhydramine and 8-chlorotheophylline.

The most used antiemetic antihistamines in the piperazine family are cyclizine and hydroxyzine. Hydroxyzine also has been found to be a favorable option because of its other properties, including anxiolysis and potentiation of opioid analgesia.

Another commonly used antiemetic with significant antihistamine activity is promethazine. Promethazine is chemically a phenothiazine; however, it does not block dopamine receptors at the usual clinical doses. Promethazine therefore exerts most of its antiemetic effects via histamine H_1 and muscarinic receptor antagonism.

Antihistamines share a similar side effect profile, which tends to be the limiting factor in their perioperative use. These side effects include sedation, dry mouth, constipation, confusion, blurred vision, delirium, urinary retention, and tachycardia. In particular, sedation limits their popularity for outpatient surgery.

Neurokinin-1 receptor antagonists

Substance P has been implicated in the pathogenesis of PONV via both central and peripheral mechanisms. Substrate P is a ligand of the neurokinin-1 (NK$_1$) receptor, which may be found centrally in the CTZ and vomiting center, as well as peripherally in the vagal afferents of the GI tract. The first NK$_1$ receptor agonist approved for clinical use by the FDA in the United States was aprepitant. This drug was shown to be superior to ondansetron in preventing vomiting up to 48 hours postoperatively and equivalent in reducing the incidence of nausea and need for rescue antiemetics in the first 24 hours (Gan et al.

2007). Aprepitant should be given within 3 hours prior to induction of anesthesia.

Other antiemetics

The current available data suggest that several drugs traditionally used for PONV prophylaxis are relatively ineffective for that purpose. Metoclopramide, at least at the standard clinical dose of 10 mg, has no antinausea effect and is only minimally effective in prophylaxis against vomiting (Henzi et al. 1999). Other agents that have shown poor clinical efficacy for PONV include ginger root and the cannabinoids.

Nonpharmacologic strategies

Nonpharmacologic approaches to PONV prophylaxis have been explored as inexpensive and noninvasive alternatives and adjuncts to traditional treatments. These therapies also confer the additional benefit of allowing patients to avoid the numerous side effects involved with pharmacologic treatments. Therapies such as acupuncture, transcutaneous electrical nerve stimulation, acupoint stimulation, and acupressure have shown some antiemetic efficacy when used prior to surgical procedures. The NNT for these procedures has been estimated to be approximately 5 (Lee and Done 1999). Other nonpharmacologic therapies shown to be effective in at least limited settings include intravenous hydration, high supplemental inspired fractional oxygen content, and inhalation of isopropyl alcohol vapor.

Conclusion

Although significant advances have been made in antiemetic therapy, PONV continues to be a problem for patients and anesthesiologists alike. There likely is no "magic bullet" that will eliminate PONV, the most common anesthetic side effect. The keys to overcoming it are to continue to refine methods for identifying high-risk patients, to continue to find ways to reduce baseline risk factors, to optimize multimodal prophylactic combination regimens, and to continue the research and development of novel antiemetic agents and strategies.

Suggested readings

Bailey PL, Streisand JB, Pace NL, et al. Transdermal scopolamine reduces nausea and vomiting after outpatient laparoscopy. *Anesthesiology* 1990; 72:977–980.

Chang NS, Simone AF, Schultheis LW. From the FDA: what's in a label? A guide for the anesthesia practitioner. *Anesthesiology* 2005; 103(1):179–185.

Chen JJ, Frame DG, White TJ. Efficacy of ondansetron and prochlorperazine for the prevention of postoperative nausea and vomiting after total hip replacement or total knee replacement procedures: a randomized, double-blind, comparative trial. *Arch Intern Med* 1998; 158:2124–2128.

Diemunsch P, Schoeffler P, Bryssine B, et al. Antiemetic activity of the NK1 receptor antagonist GR205171 in the treatment of established postoperative nausea and vomiting after major gynaecological surgery. *Br J Anaesth* 1999; 82:274–276.

Domino KB, Anderson EA, Polissar NL, Posner KL. Comparative efficacy and safety of ondansetron, droperidol, and metoclopramide for preventing postoperative nausea and vomiting: a meta-analysis. *Anesth Analg* 1999; 88:1370–1379.

Ernst E, Pittler MH. Efficacy of ginger for nausea and vomiting: a systematic review of randomized clinical trials. *Br J Anaesth* 2000; 84:367–371.

Fortney JT, Gan TJ, Graczyk S, et al. A comparison of the efficacy, safety, and patient satisfaction of ondansetron versus droperidol as antiemetics for elective outpatient surgical procedures: S3A-409 and S3A-410 Study Groups. *Anesth Analg* 1998; 86: 731–738.

Gan TJ, Apfel C, Kovac A, et al. Aprepitant-PONV Study Group. A randomized, double-blind comparison of the NK1 antagonist, aprepitant versus ondansetron for the prevention of postoperative nausea and vomiting. *Anesth Analg* 2007; 104:1082–1089.

Gan T, Meyers T, Apfel C. Consensus guidelines for managing postoperative nausea and vomiting. *Anesth Analg* 2003; 97:62–71.

Gesztesi Z, Scuderi PE, White PF, et al. Substance P (Neurokinin-1) antagonist prevents postoperative vomiting after abdominal hysterectomy procedures. *Anesthesiology* 2000; 93:931–937.

Goll V, Ozan A, Greif R, et al. Ondansetron is no more effective than supplemental intraoperative oxygen for prevention of postoperative nausea and vomiting. *Anesth Analg* 2001; 92:112–117.

Greif R, Laciny S, Rapf B, et al. Supplemental oxygen reduces the incidence of postoperative nausea and vomiting. *Anesthesiology* 1999; 91:1246–1252.

Harnett MJ, O'Rourke N, Walsh M, et al. Transdermal scopolamine for prevention of intrathecal morphine-induced nausea and vomiting after cesarean delivery. *Anesth Analg* 2007; 105:764–769.

Henzi I, Walder B, Tramer MR. Dexamethasone for the prevention of postoperative nausea and vomiting: a quantitative systematic review. *Anesth Analg* 2000; 90:186–194.

Henzi I, Sonderegger J, Tramer MR. Systematic review: efficacy, dose-response, and adverse effects of droperidol for prevention of postoperative nausea and vomiting. *Can J Anaesth* 2000a; 47:537–551.

Henzi J, Walder B, Tramer MR. Metoclopramide in the prevention of postoperative nausea and vomiting: a quantitative systematic review of randomized placebo-controlled studies. *Br J Anaesth* 1999; 83:761–771.

Kapur PA. The big "little problem." *Anesth Analg* 1991; 73:243–245.

Khalil S, Philbrook L, Rabb M, et al. Ondansetron/promethazine combination or promethazine alone reduces nausea and vomiting after middle ear surgery. *J Clin Anesth* 1999; 11:596–600.

Kotelko DM, Rottman RL, Wright WC, et al. Transdermal scopolamine decreases nausea and vomiting following cesarean section in patients receiving epidural morphine. *Anesthesiology* 1989; 71:675–678.

Kranke P, Morin AM, Roewer N, et al. The efficacy and safety of transdermal scopolamine for the prevention of postoperative nausea and vomiting: a quantitative systematic review. *Anesth Analg* 2002a; 95:133–143.

Kranke P, Morin AM, Roewer N, Eberhart LH. Dimenhydrinate for prophylaxis of postoperative nausea and vomiting: a metaanalysis of randomized controlled trials. *Acta Anaesthesiol Scand* 2002b; 46:238–244.

Kreisler NS, Spiekermann BF, Ascari CM, et al. Small-dose droperidol effectively reduces nausea in a general surgical adult patient population. *Anesth Analg* 2000; 91:1256–1261.

Lee A, Done ML. The use of nonpharmacologic techniques to prevent postoperative nausea and vomiting: a meta-analysis. *Anesth Analg* 1999; 88:1362–1369.

Lewis IH, Campbell DN, Barrowcliffe MP. Effect of Nabilone on nausea and vomiting after total abdominal hysterectomy. *Br J Anaesth* 1994; 73:244–246.

Liu K, Hsu CC, Chia YY. The effective dose of dexamethasone for antiemesis after major gynecological surgery. *Anesth Analg* 1999; 89:1316–1318.

Loper KA, Ready LB, Dorman BH. Prophylactic transdermal scopolamine patches reduce nausea in postoperative patients receiving epidural morphine. *Anesth Analg* 1989; 68:144–146.

Lorhan PH. Cyclizine lactate (marezine) for post operative control of nausea and vomiting after cataract surgery. *Anesth Analg* 1958; 37:247–248.

Ludwin DB, Shafer SL. Con: the black box warning on droperidol should not be removed (but should be clarified!). *Anesth Analg* 2008; 106(5):1418–1420.

McKenzie R, Wadhwa RK, Uy NT, et al. Antiemetic effectiveness of intramuscular hydroxyzine compared with intramuscular droperidol. *Anesth Analg* 1981; 60:783–788.

Merrit BA, Okyere CP, Jasinski DM. Isopropyl alcohol inhalation: alternative treatment of postoperative nausea and vomiting. *Nurs Res* 2002; 51:125–128.

Morin AM, Betz O, Kranke P, et al. Is ginger a relevant antiemetic for postoperative nausea and vomiting? *Anasthesiol Intensivmed Notfallmed Schmerzther* 2004; 39:281–285.

Naguib M, el Bakry AK, Khoshim MH, et al. Prophylactic antiemetic therapy with ondansetron, tropisetron, granisetron and metoclopramide in patients undergoing laparoscopic cholecystectomy: a randomized, double-blind comparison with placebo. *Can J Anaesth* 1996; 43:226–231.

Rappaport BA. FDA response to droperidol black box warning editorials. *Anesth Analg* 2008; 106(5):1585.

Sun R, Klein KW, White PF. The effect of timing of ondansetron administration in outpatients undergoing otolaryngologic surgery. *Anesth Analg* 1997; 84:331–336.

Tramer MR. A rational approach to the control of postoperative nausea and vomiting: evidence from systemic reviews. I. Efficacy and harm of antiemetic interventions, and methodological issues. *Acta Anaesthesiol Scand* 2001; 45:4–13.

Tramer MR, Reynolds DJM, Moore RA, McQuay HJ. Efficacy, dose-response, and safety of ondansetron in prevention of postoperative nausea and vomiting: a qualitative systematic review of randomized placebo-controlled trials. *Anesthesiology* 1997; 87:1277–1289.

Wang JJ, Ho ST, Lee SC, et al. The use of dexamethasone for preventing postoperative nausea and vomiting in females undergoing thyroidectomy: a dose-ranging study. *Anesth Analg* 2000a; 91:1404–1407.

Wang JJ, Ho ST, Tzeng JI, Tang CS. The effect of timing of dexamethasone administration on its efficacy as a prophylactic antiemetic for postoperative nausea and vomiting. *Anesth Analg* 2000b; 91:136–139.

Wilhelm SM, Dehoorne-Smith ML, Kale-Pradhan PB. Prevention of postoperative nausea and vomiting. *Ann Pharmacother* 2007; 41:68–78.

Yogendran S, Asokumar B, Cheng DC, Chung F. A prospective randomized double-blinded study of the effect of intravenous fluid therapy on adverse outcomes on outpatient surgery. *Anesth Analg* 1995; 80:682–686.

COX inhibitors and α_2-adrenoceptor agonists

Benjamin Parish and Mark Dershwitz

Cyclooxygenase (COX) inhibitors are nonopioid drugs that reduce pain (analgesic) and fever (antipyretic). All except acetaminophen also reduce inflammation. Commonly used COX inhibitors include aspirin, acetaminophen, ibuprofen, ketorolac, and celecoxib. A major advantage of COX inhibitors over opioids is that COX inhibitors do not produce sedation, ventilatory depression, or tolerance. Adverse effects, however, limit their use. The following section considers the pharmacology of the parenteral COX inhibitor ketorolac.

Ketorolac

Indications

In 1990, ketorolac was the first parenteral COX inhibitor approved for use for postoperative pain. It is used for short-term management (<5 days in adults) of moderate to severe acute pain. It is not indicated for use in children (<17 years) or for chronic pain conditions.

Mechanism of action

Ketorolac's primary mechanism of action is thought to be competitive and reversible inhibition of the enzyme COX, resulting in the inhibition of prostaglandin synthesis, as shown in Fig. 42.1. There are two isozymes of COX: COX-1 is a constitutive enzyme that participates in the protection of the gastrointestinal (GI) mucosa from acid damage, in the activation of platelets, and in the regulation of renal blood flow; COX-2 is an inducible enzyme that participates in the mediation of inflammation, pain, and fever. Ketorolac is a racemic mixture of the "S" active form and the "R" inactive form. The active form inhibits both COX-1 and COX-2 (as do aspirin and ibuprofen). Selective COX-2 inhibitors, such as celecoxib, are selective for the COX-2 isozyme. The therapeutic effects of these medications are additive, as are their adverse effects (except that celecoxib has little effect on the GI mucosa and on platelets).

Pharmacokinetics

Ketorolac can be administered orally, intramuscularly (IM), or intravenously (IV). Its bioavailability is 100% following oral administration. The recommended dosage for postoperative pain management is 30 mg IM or IV every 6 hours, with a maximum daily dose of 120 mg. The dose should be halved in persons over 65 years of age, in persons with renal insufficiency, or in adults weighing <50 kg. The onset of analgesia is slow, occurring about 30 minutes following IV and in about 60 minutes following IM administration. Oral ketorolac may be given at 10 mg every 6 hours. The duration of therapy should not exceed 5 days.

Ketorolac is metabolized by the liver, and the metabolites are excreted primarily in the urine. About 40% of an administered dose is metabolized, whereas the remainder is excreted unchanged.

The comparative doses of ketorolac and other COX inhibitors are shown in Table 42.1.

Alternative to opioids

Although potency ratios are difficult to measure, a 30-mg dose of ketorolac is approximately equipotent to 4 mg of morphine. Using ketorolac as an alternative to opioids avoids the adverse effects of sedation and ventilatory depression. Most patients also will experience less nausea and vomiting. For these reasons, ketorolac has become particularly popular in ambulatory surgery, in which its use may permit shorter patient discharge times. When given in combination with opioids, the opioid requirement likely will be lower. The adverse effect profile of ketorolac is summarized in Table 42.2.

Table 42.1. Doses of COX inhibitors

Drug	Dose, mg	Interval, h	Maximum daily dose, mg
Ketorolac	30 IV/IM	6	120
	10 PO	6	40
Acetaminophen	500–1000	4–6	4000
Aspirin	500–1000	4–6	4000
Ibuprofen	200–800	4–6	2400
Naproxen	500 initially, then 250	6–8	1500
Celecoxib	200–400 initially, then 100–200	12–24	400

PO, orally.

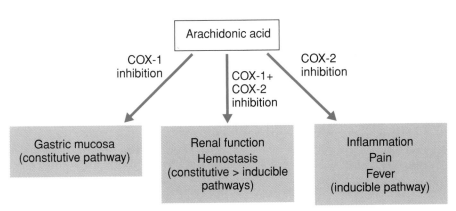

Figure 42.1. Mechanism of action of the COX inhibitors. Ketorolac, aspirin, and ibuprofen inhibit both COX-1 and COX-2, whereas celecoxib is a selective COX-2 inhibitor.

Special populations

Elderly patients

The dose of ketorolac should be halved in persons over 65 years of age. Such patients are also at higher risk for experiencing adverse effects, especially GI ulceration.

Pediatric population

Ketorolac is contraindicated in children <17 years of age.

Pregnancy

Ketorolac is contraindicated during labor and delivery and for nursing mothers. Inhibiting prostaglandin synthesis may decrease uterine blood flow and contractions. Ketorolac is excreted in breast milk.

Drug interactions

Because the effects of ketorolac are additive with other COX inhibitors, their concurrent administration is not recommended. Ketorolac may reduce the natriuretic effect of furosemide and thiazide diuretics in some patients, leading to increased edema. Administration of ketorolac with angiotensin-converting enzyme inhibitors may cause renal impairment, especially in volume-depleted patients. The effects of ketorolac on GI bleeding are synergistic with warfarin and

heparin; therefore, ketorolac should not be used in the presence of coagulation disorders or in patients on anticoagulant therapy.

α_2-Adrenoceptor agonists

Currently, there are two α_2-adrenoceptor agonists used in clinical practice. Dexmedetomidine is a useful adjunct in anesthesiology and critical care medicine. Clonidine, although not used by anesthesiologists as often as dexmedetomidine, has profound effects in anesthetic management.

The primary effect of the α_2-adrenoceptor agonists is to decrease sympathetic outflow from the central nervous system (CNS), leading to a decrease in heart rate and blood pressure. There is a significant sedative effect that is not accompanied by ventilatory depression. Analgesia and a decreased requirement for opioid analgesics also occur.

Although these medications cannot produce general anesthesia, they may be useful as anesthetic adjuvants. Dexmedetomidine decreases the minimal alveolar concentration of halothane by 95% in animals, whereas clonidine does so by up to 50%. In contrast to benzodiazepines, α_2-adrenoceptor agonists do not produce reliable amnesia.

Ventilatory effects

At doses used to provide sedation, there is a minimal reduction in minute ventilation secondary to decreased tidal volumes.

Table 42.2. Adverse effects of ketorolac

System	Effect	Patient restrictions	Notes
Renal	Renal papillary necrosis	Elderly patients, preexisting renal disease, hypovolemia	
Hematologic	Inhibition of platelet aggregation	Coagulation disorders, use of anticoagulants	Unlike aspirin, platelet inhibition disappears 24–48 h after discontinuation
GI	Ulceration	Peptic ulcer disease, bleeding or perforation	
Respiratory	Bronchospasm	Aspirin-sensitive asthma cross-reactivity	Indirect stimulation of leukotriene pathway
Cardiovascular	Inhibition of platelet aggregation	Myocardial infarction, thrombotic events, stroke	Contraindicated following cardiac surgery
Hepatic	Liver necrosis, hepatitis	Impaired hepatic function	
Reproductive	Decreased uterine contractions	Pregnant women	Also decreases uterine blood flow

However, the ventilatory response to carbon dioxide remains intact.

Cardiovascular effects

Through its centrally acting sympatholytic effects, there are frequent decreases in heart rate, blood pressure, and cardiac output. If the initial bolus of dexmedetomidine is given too rapidly, there may be a paradoxic increase in blood pressure. This is thought to be a result of agonist effects at vascular α_1-adrenoceptors.

CNS effects

As mentioned previously, α_2-adrenoceptor agonists produce sedation and analgesia. When given in combination with opioids, the requirement for opioid is lessened. Their amnestic effect is much less reliable than with benzodiazepines.

Clonidine has been used in nerve blocks with varying results. Some studies have suggested improved onset and quality of the block, whereas others have documented prolongation of the block. The mechanism of action is unknown.

Use of dexmedetomidine

Dexmedetomidine is approved for sedation in the intensive care unit and for procedural sedation, including for awake fiberoptic intubation. The usual loading dose is 1 μg/kg given over 10 minutes. Maintenance doses are typically 0.1 to 1 μg/kg/h.

Suggested readings

American Pain Society. *Principles of Analgesic Use in the Treatment of Acute Pain and Cancer Pain*. 5th ed. Glenview, IL: American Pain Society; 2003.

Barash PG, Cullen BF, Stoelting RK, eds. *Clinical Anesthesia*. 5th ed. Philadelphia: Lippincott Williams & Wilkins; 2006.

Ding Y, White PF. Comparative effects of ketorolac, dezocine, and fentanyl as adjuvants during outpatient anesthesia. *Anesth Analg* 1992; 75:566–571.

Morgan GE, Mikhail MS, Murray MJ. *Clinical Anesthesiology*. 4th ed. New York: Lange Medical Books; 2006.

Tollison CD, Satterthwaite J. *Practical Pain Management*. 3rd ed. Philadelphia: Lippincott Williams & Wilkins; 2002.

Watcha MF, Issioui T, Klein KW, White PF. Costs and effectiveness of rofecoxib, celecoxib, and acetaminophen for preventing pain after ambulatory otolaryngologic surgery. *Anesth Analg* 2003; 96: 987.

Diuretics

Edward R. Garcia

The therapeutic goal of diuretics is to reduce edema by decreasing total body water. Diuretics may also be used to alter electrolyte or osmotic levels. Essentially all diuretics interfere with sodium ion (Na^+) reabsorption in some way at various segments of the nephron. They achieve this by increasing sodium chloride (NaCl) output, which results in a net NaCl loss and, therefore, water loss along with it. Fig. 43.1 shows sites of diuretic action along the nephron.

Proximal convoluted tubule diuretics

The proximal convoluted tubule is the primary site for Na^+ reabsorption and seems a likely site for effective diuretic action. However, the number of downstream reabsorption sites limits the effectiveness of any diuretic targeting this region. Carbonic anhydrase inhibitors are the only commonly used diuretics that particularly target this region, although they are rarely used primarily as diuretics. They work by blocking the enzyme carbonic anhydrase, which acts to help reabsorb bicarbonate in the proximal tubule. The net effect is reduction of bicarbonate ion (HCO_3^-) reabsorption, which instead remains in the filtrate (metabolic acidosis). To maintain electrochemical neutrality, Na^+ (the most abundant cation) accompanies HCO_3^- out of the proximal tubule. The thick ascending limb (TAL) of the loop of Henle is capable of reabsorbing increased loads of NaCl. As a result, a large amount of the Na^+ is reabsorbed there, accounting for the relatively weak diuretic effect of acetazolamide. In the distal tubule, Na^+ is exchanged for potassium (K^+), with a net result of a small increase in the excretion of HCO_3^-, K^+, and water.

Acetazolamide occasionally is used for the treatment of glaucoma, as it inhibits the production of aqueous humor by the ciliary body, resulting in lowered intraocular pressure. It also is used for the treatment of acute mountain sickness (AMS). Its precise mechanism of action in ameliorating the symptoms of AMS is unclear, although it is presumed to counter the hyperventilation-induced respiratory alkalosis that results from exposure to the hypoxia of high altitude. Acetazolamide is contraindicated in patients with sickle cell anemia, sulfonamide allergy, or diabetes.

Osmotic diuretics

Osmotic diuretics act primarily at the loop of Henle. Examples of osmotic diuretics include mannitol, glycerin, and, occasionally, glucose. Mannitol and glycerin are freely filtered into the tubular fluid but are inert, and are not reabsorbed from the filtrate. In the proximal tubule, Na^+ is reabsorbed, resulting in an increase of filtrate osmolality due to the increasing concentration of mannitol. The increased oncotic pressure opposes water reabsorption from the filtrate and results in increased excretion of water as well as Na^+. Osmotic diuretics also increase the serum osmolarity following their administration, which results in net water extraction from the extravascular to the intravascular compartment. This effect is commonly observed when osmotic diuretics are administered to decrease intracranial volume/pressure. Although the increase in intravascular volume is transient, it may cause congestive cardiac failure in a minority of patients. Mannitol is the most rapidly acting and commonly used osmotic diuretic. There is some evidence that mannitol may have some renal protective activity (increases renal vasodilation), although the evidence is mixed. Glucose is also freely filtered, but it undergoes significant reabsorption by proximal tubular sodium-glucose transport proteins. Excess glucose due to severe hyperglycemia (above the capacity of proximal tubular reabsorption) also may result in an osmotic diuresis (dehydration in diabetics).

Loop diuretics

Loop diuretics act by blocking the Type 2 Na-K-Cl cotransporter (NKCC2) in the thick ascending limb of the loop of Henle. Inhibition of this cotransporter decreases reabsorption and results in increased luminal Na^+ and Cl^-. Additionally, the active Na^+ uptake in the TAL is responsible for establishing and maintaining the medullary osmolarity gradient critical for filtrate concentration. By these effects, loop diuretics decrease maximal urine concentration. This class of diuretics is the most potent and causes excretion of up to 20% of the filtered Na^+. The loop of Henle is also the primary site for reabsorption of Ca^{++} and Mg^{++}, whose reabsorption is inhibited by excess luminal

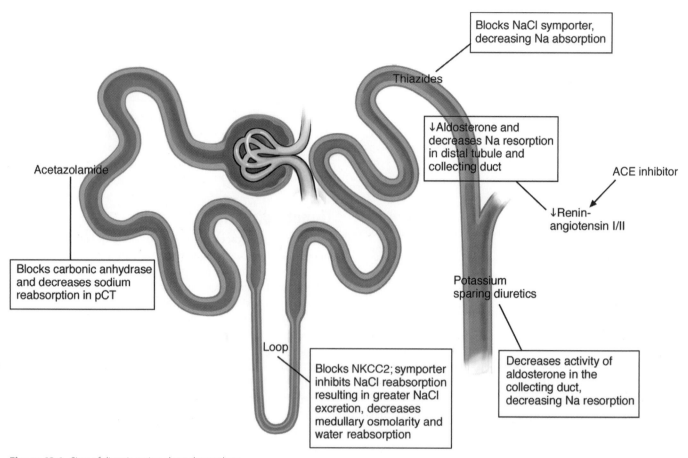

Figure 43.1. Sites of diuretic action along the nephron.

Na$^+$. Therefore, Ca^{++} (as in the treatment of hypercalcemia) and Mg^{++} are excreted along with Na$^+$, K$^+$, and water.

Because of their potency, loop diuretics may cause significant electrolyte loss, consequently hypokalemia and other electrolyte deficiencies are common with their use. Loop diuretics are often used in neurosurgical settings as a means to lower intracranial pressure. Used together with mannitol, their effect in lowering intracranial volume is synergistic. The likely mechanism for this may be their diuretic effect, but some component also may result from their vasodilatory effect, particularly in the splanchnic circulation. Dilutional hyponatremia (or syndrome of inappropriate antidiuretic hormone hypersecretion [SIADH]) can be corrected with furosemide, as excess water excretion increases the sodium plasma concentration. A small dose of furosemide may be given intravenously to differentiate prerenal from renal failure, as in the former it will lead to an increase in urine output.

Furosemide, bumetanide, and ethacrynic acid are commonly used loop diuretics. Dosages may need to be increased in the presence of reduced renal blood flow so that these agents can reach their target site. Adverse effects of loop diuretics include electrolyte loss, hyperuricemia (gout), dyslipidemia,

dehydration and metabolic alkalosis, postural hypotension, syncope, and ototoxicity (tinnitus, vertigo, or deafness).

Ascending limb and distal convoluted tubule diuretics

The thiazide and thiazide-like diuretics act at the cortical TAL and distal convoluted tubule (DCT) to inhibit Na$^+$ and Cl$^-$ transport. Only 5% to 7% of sodium is normally reabsorbed here, so inhibition in this region provides a less overall diuretic effect. Additionally, if the glomerular filtration rate (GFR) is already diminished (e.g., in renal insufficiency), less fluid will reach the distal tubule, so inhibition may have minimal effect. Diuretics such as the loop diuretics, which act more proximally in the tubule, can result in a compensatory increase of reabsorption in the distal tubule. Thiazide diuretics can block this compensatory response and therefore can be coupled with loop diuretics to provide potent diuresis. In the United States, thiazides are recommended as a first-line treatment for hypertension. They reduce the plasma volume (diuresis), decrease cardiac output, and cause peripheral vasodilation. Thiazide diuretics also inhibit the enzyme carbonic anhydrase to some extent. Adverse effects include dehydration and metabolic alkalosis, hypokalemia, hypocalcemia, hyperuricemia (gout), hyperlipidemia, impaired glucose tolerance (diabetes), and impotence.

Metolazone, a thiazide-like diuretic, is the diuretic usually selected for combination therapy with loop diuretics. It is a quinazoline diuretic with the same mechanism of action, but much greater affinity for the DCT Na^+ channel. Metolazone is generally the only DCT diuretic effective in severe renal insufficiency. In addition, metolazone also has an antihypertensive effect, the exact mechanism of which is not clear.

Collecting duct diuretics

Diuretics that act at the collecting duct generally are called *potassium-sparing diuretics*, because they tend to avoid the potassium wasting that characterizes the loop and thiazide diuretics. These agents include the aldosterone antagonist spironolactone and the distal tubule Na^+ channel antagonists amiloride and triamterene. Blockade of these pathways results in decreased Na^+ uptake in exchange for K^+ and H^+. These are generally weak diuretic agents, because more than 90% of the filtered load is reabsorbed prior to the distal tubule and only a small amount of Na^+ is reabsorbed in the terminal distal tubule and collecting duct.

Spironolactone competes with aldosterone for its receptors. It is commonly used orally to treat ascites and heart failure and has an antiandrogen effect that may result in gynecomastia and menstrual irregularities. Some studies have shown that its potassium-sparing effect can delay the development of Alzheimer's disease. In contrast to spironolactone, amiloride and triamterene are noncompetitive inhibitors of aldosterone. They inhibit Na^+ reabsorption and K^+ secretion by closing sodium channels. With all three drugs, hyperkalemia and metabolic acidosis may result in patients with renal insufficiency or in those on angiotensin-converting enzyme inhibitors.

Another diuretic that acts at the collecting duct (in addition to other locations) is atrial natriuretic peptide (ANP). ANP is released from atrial myocardial cells in response to increased intravascular volume. It is a direct vasodilator that also binds to receptors in the medullary collecting duct and increases intracellular cyclic guanosine monophosphate cGMP, which in turn decreases Na^+ channel activity. There is some evidence that ANP may also bind to receptors in the proximal convoluted tubule and inhibit Na^+ reabsorption. The net result is decreased Na^+ reabsorption and increased solute excretion accompanied by water excretion, with little effect on K^+ excretion. ANP also inhibits renin secretion and increases GFR by decreasing afferent and increasing efferent glomerular constriction. ANP appears to be a relatively weak diuretic, able to achieve only moderate diuresis. Its activity is inhibited by lowered arterial pressure or increased afferent arteriolar constriction. Brain natriuretic peptide is a similar molecule released from brain and myocardial tissue. Its levels (normally less than 20% of the natriuretic peptide fraction) are significantly increased in congestive heart failure and can be useful in differentiating between edema due to heart failure versus other etiologies. ANP levels are not significantly altered under anesthesia.

Suggested readings

Barthelmebs M, Stephan D, Fontaine C, et al. Vascular effects of loop diuretics: an in vivo and in vitro study in the rat. *Naunyn Schmiedebergs Arch Pharmacol* 1994; 349(2):209–216.

Brater DC, Pressley RH, Anderson SA. Mechanisms of the synergistic combination of metolazone and bumetanide. *J Pharmacol Exp Ther* 1985; 233(1):70–74.

Ellison DH. The physiologic basis of diuretic synergism: its role in treating diuretic resistance. *Ann Intern Med* 1991; 1/4(10):886–894.

Goetz KL. Physiology and pathophysiology of atrial peptides. *Am J Physiol* 1988; 254(1):E1–15.

Hardman JG, Limbird LE, Gilman AG, eds. *Goodman and Gilman's The Pharmacologic Basis of Therapeutics*. 11th ed. New York: McGraw-Hill; 2005.

Ip-yam PC, Murphy S, Baines M, et al. Renal function and proteinuria after cardiopulmonary bypass; the effects of temperature and mannitol. *Anesth Analg* 1994; 78:842–847.

Leaf DE, Goldfard DS. Mechanisms of action of acetazolamide in the prophylaxis and treatment of acute mountain sickness. *J Appl Physiol* 2007; 102:1313–1322.

Mathisen O, Raeder M, Kiil F. Mechanism of osmotic diuresis. *Kidney Int* 1981; 19:431–437.

Stanton B, Kaissling B. Adaptation of distal tubule and collecting duct to increased sodium delivery. II. Sodium and potassium transport. *Am J Physiol* 1988; 255:F1269–F1275.

Thenuwara K, Todd M, Brian J. Effect of mannitol and furosemide on plasma osmolality and brain water. *Anesthesiology* 2002; 96(2):416–421.

Drug interactions

Martha Cordoba-Amorocho and Jie Zhou

Anesthesiology involves the administration of multiple drugs. The goal of combining medications is to produce the best therapeutic effects with the fewest adverse effects. Anesthesiologists also care for patients with multiple underlying conditions for which they are taking medications, sometimes as part of complex therapeutic regimens. Drug combinations are a useful and unavoidable part of anesthetic practice; however, they may be a source of significant morbidity.

Drug interactions result when the effect of one drug is altered by the concurrent administration of another. To minimize unexpected or dangerous effects, it is important to know the way drugs interact with each other. The mechanisms of drug interactions may be one of three types: *pharmaceutical*, *pharmacokinetic*, or *pharmacodynamic*.

Pharmaceutical interactions

A pharmaceutical interaction is a chemical or physical interaction between drugs that occurs before they are administered or absorbed systemically. Some examples of pharmaceutical interactions include the following:

- The precipitate that forms when thiopental (a weak acid) mixes with succinylcholine (a weak base), either in a syringe or within intravenous tubing
- The precipitate that forms when thiopental mixes with vecuronium
- The precipitation of bupivacaine when bicarbonate is added
- The inactivation of catecholamine solutions (e.g., norepinephrine, epinephrine) when alkalinized by sodium bicarbonate; this situation may occur during resuscitation of a patient
- The interaction of desflurane with dry soda lime or Baralyme® to produce carbon monoxide; this situation may occur when oxygen is left flowing through the absorber canister overnight

Pharmacokinetic interactions

Pharmacokinetic interactions are a much more common source of adverse effects in anesthesia. A pharmacokinetic interaction occurs when one drug alters the absorption, distribution, metabolism, or elimination of another.

Absorption

An alteration in absorption may occur because of the direct chemical interaction between drugs in the body or because one drug affects the physiology of the absorption of another drug. Examples of drug-induced alterations in the absorption of another drug include:

- The chelation by tetracycline of the polyvalent cations (calcium, magnesium, or aluminum) contained in antacids
- The delay in gastric emptying produced by opioids and anticholinergics, thereby reducing the absorption of orally administered medications because the primary site for the absorption of most medications is the small intestine
- The increase in the speed of gastric emptying produced by metoclopramide that may increase the rate of diazepam absorption
- The decrease in the rate of absorption, and the increase in the duration of action, of local anesthetics produced by epinephrine
- The rapid uptake of nitrous oxide that may increase the alveolar concentration of a second volatile anesthetic (the "second gas effect")
- The administration of medications that increase the gastric pH (e.g., antacids, histamine H_2 antagonists, proton pump inhibitors) that may reduce the absorption of medications that are weak acids (e.g., aspirin)

Distribution

An alteration in distribution may occur because of a variation in hemodynamics, drug ionization/lipid solubility, or plasma protein binding. Some examples of drug-induced alterations in the distribution of another drug include:

- The decrease in cardiac output caused by intravenous and volatile anesthetics that increases the concentration and the effects of other drugs in the cardiovascular system and central nervous system (CNS).
- The decrease in cardiac output that also increases the end-tidal concentration of volatile anesthetics.
- The diffusion of some medications (e.g., fentanyl, meperidine) back into the stomach from the bloodstream. The medications then become ionized and trapped in the

gastric acid and are reabsorbed when the environment becomes alkaline in the small bowel. This process may produce a secondary increase in their blood concentrations.

- The occurrence of hypoproteinemia in cases of hepatic cirrhosis or nephrotic syndrome that decreases the amount of drug bound to circulating proteins. Conversely, surgery, burns, myocardial infarction, trauma, and malignancies increase α_1-acid glycoprotein. Many drugs that are weak bases (e.g., bupivacaine, lidocaine, and meperidine) bind to α_1-acid glycoprotein.
- The displacement of highly protein bound drugs (e.g., warfarin, phenytoin) by other drugs (e.g., a cyclooxygenase [COX] inhibitor).

Metabolism

Drugs are eliminated from the body by several processes. Many drugs increase or decrease the metabolism of others by the liver or other organs. Some examples of drug-induced alterations in the metabolism of another drug include:

- The inhibition of plasma butyrylcholinesterase (also known as pseudocholinesterase) by inhibitors of acetylcholinesterase (e.g., neostigmine, edrophonium, pyridostigmine) that may prolong the effect of succinylcholine.
- The inhibition of plasma butyrylcholinesterase that may also increase the toxicity of ester local anesthetics by decreasing their rate of metabolism in the circulation.
- The potentiation of indirect-acting sympathomimetics (e.g., ephedrine, amphetamine) by monoamine oxidase inhibitors (MAOIs; e.g., phenelzine, tranylcypromine, isocarboxazid, selegiline). MAOIs increase the amount of presynaptic transmitter available to be released. A typical clinical dose of ephedrine may then produce a severe hypertensive crisis.
- The production of serotonin syndrome (excitation, hyperpyrexia, hypertension, profuse sweating, rigidity) by the interaction of an MAOI and a medication that has serotonin reuptake–inhibiting activity (e.g., meperidine, methadone, dextromethorphan).

Many anesthetic drugs undergo oxidative metabolism by one of the isoforms of cytochrome P450 (CYP). A wide range of chemical compounds may interact with CYP, resulting in either an increase or decrease in activity.

Based on the fraction of a drug metabolized in a single pass through the liver, drugs may be classified as "high extraction" or "low extraction." The metabolism of high-extraction drugs (e.g., morphine, fentanyl, sufentanil, lidocaine) is decreased by drugs or maneuvers that decrease cardiac output and/or hepatic blood flow (e.g., β–blockade, vasoconstrictors, halothane, hypotension, upper abdominal surgery). The metabolism of low-extraction drugs (e.g., alfentanil, diazepam) is affected by medications that induce or inhibit drug metabolism.

Some examples of inducers of CYP are phenobarbital, phenytoin, rifampin, carbamazepine, ethanol, and the polycyclic aromatic hydrocarbons present in cigarette smoke and charred meat. In contrast, some examples of drugs than inhibit CYP are cimetidine, antifungal agents (e.g., fluconazole, ketoconazole, itraconazole), macrolide antibiotics (e.g., erythromycin, clarithromycin, but not azithromycin), antiretroviral protease inhibitors (e.g., ritonavir, indinavir), verapamil, and grapefruit juice.

The list of potential drug interactions due to the induction or inhibition of CYP is enormous. An excellent and frequently updated list of clinically relevant drug interactions as a result of these mechanisms may be found at http://www.drug-interactions.com.

Elimination

Alteration in drug elimination may involve changes in renal clearance or in pulmonary excretion. For certain cellular barriers, such as in the stomach, placenta, or renal tubules, the pH on either side of the barrier is very different. Many drugs are weak acids or bases that are partially ionized at physiologic pH. Because it is only the un-ionized fraction that diffuses across such barriers, small alterations in pH may have a large effect on the degree of ionization and therefore the rate of transport as a result of of diffusion. For example, an increase in urinary pH may cause phenobarbital or aspirin to become trapped in the urine because its rate of tubular reabsorption decreases.

Organic anions and cations are actively secreted by different transporters in the renal tubules. Various anions or cations may compete for their respective transporter systems. Examples of drugs eliminated by the anion system are aspirin, β-lactam antibiotics (penicillins, cephalosporins), and many diuretics. Probenecid is an inhibitor of the anion transporter and may decrease the rate of elimination of drugs dependent on that transporter for their elimination. The cation system transports atropine, isoproterenol, neostigmine, and meperidine.

Pharmacodynamic interactions

A pharmacodynamic interaction occurs when one drug alters the sensitivity of a target receptor or tissue to the effect of another drug. These interactions can be classified as *additive*, *antagonistic*, or *synergistic*.

Additive interactions occur when drugs with the same mechanism of action are administered concurrently. Examples of such additive interactions include:

- Rocuronium and vecuronium, two aminosteroid nondepolarizing muscle relaxants
- Two volatile anesthetics, or nitrous oxide with a volatile anesthetic
- The additive CNS toxicity produced by lidocaine and tetracaine

Table 44.1. Claimed effects and potential toxic effects of herbal preparations

Name	Common use	Potential toxicity
Ephedra	Energy building, weight loss, antitussive, bacteriostatic	Hypertension, tachycardia, dysrhythmias; stroke, seizure. Effects potentiated by agents with MAOI activity
Echinacea	Respiratory and urinary infections, promote wound and burn healing	Hepatotoxicity Decreased glucocorticoid effects Macrophage and natural killer cell activation
Garlic	Hyperlipidemia, hypertension, antiplatelet, antioxidant, and antibiotic effects	Increased risk of perioperative bleeding, potentiation of anticoagulant effects; risk of interactions with cardiovascular medications, MAOIs, hypoglycemics
Ginger	Antinausea, antispasmodic; respiratory ailments; motion sickness	Increased risk of perioperative bleeding, potentiation of anticoagulant effects; hyperglycemia
Ginkgo	Circulatory stimulant; dementia, Alzheimer's disease; asthma, angina	Increased risk of perioperative bleeding, potentiation of anticoagulant effects; neurotoxicity, decreased seizure threshold, decreased efficacy of anticonvulsants; interaction with MAOIs
Ginseng	Energy building	Elevates digoxin concentration by 75%; interaction with MAOIs
Goldenseal	Diuretic, antiinflammatory, laxative, hemostatic	Oxytocic, paralysis, edema, hypertension
Kava	Anxiolytic	Hepatotoxicity; potentiates barbiturate and benzodiazepine effects
Licorice	Peptic ulcer disease, respiratory infections	Hypertension, hypokalemia, edema; reduction in ADH, aldosterone and plasma renin activity
St. John's wort	Depression, anxiety, insomnia	Decreased digoxin concentrations; prolonged general anesthesia, sedation; induction of CYP and P-glycoprotein (i.e., numerous drug interactions)
Valerian	Sedative, anxiolytic	Potentiates barbiturate and benzodiazepine effects
Vitamin E	Antiaging; prevention of stroke, blood clots, and atherosclerosis; promotes wound healing	Increased risk of perioperative bleeding, potentiation of anticoagulant effects

ADH, antidiuretic hormone.

There are multiple mechanisms that produce antagonistic drug reactions. Examples of antagonistic drug interactions include:

- Two medications with opposite physiologic effects administered concurrently (e.g., phenylephrine and nitroglycerin)
- A partial agonist or a competitive antagonist given concurrently with a full agonist that decreases the effect of the full agonist (e.g., the partial μ-opioid agonist buprenorphine concurrently with the full agonist fentanyl)
- A medication that increases agonist concentration overcoming the action of a competitive antagonist (e.g., using neostigmine to reverse the effect of vecuronium)

Synergistic drug interactions are very important clinically when small doses of two or more drugs produce greater than additive effects. Some examples of synergistic drug interactions include:

- The concurrent administration of an aminosteroid and a benzylisoquinoline muscle relaxant (e.g., vecuronium and cisatracurium)
- The potentiation of opioid analgesia by COX inhibitors (e.g., morphine and celecoxib)
- The potentiation of nondepolarizing muscle relaxants by volatile anesthetics (e.g., vecuronium and isoflurane)
- The potentiation of nondepolarizing muscle relaxants by aminoglycoside antibiotics (e.g., vecuronium and gentamicin)

- The potentiation of the ventilatory depressant effect when an opioid is administered concurrently with a benzodiazepine (e.g., fentanyl and midazolam)
- The decrease in the minimum alveolar concentration of a volatile anesthetic when an opioid is administered concurrently (e.g., isoflurane and fentanyl)
- The decrease in the required dose of a hypnotic when an opioid or a benzodiazepine is given preoperatively (e.g., propofol and fentanyl)
- The potentiation of the effects of an opioid or a benzodiazepine by a centrally acting α_2-adrenoceptor agonist (e.g., fentanyl and dexmedetomidine)

Cardiovascular medications and drug interactions

Some patient are particularly prone to experiencing drug interactions. Patients who are chronically ill and/or elderly are at high risk because of the number of medications they consume. The severity of the underlying disease state(s) may also place these patients at higher risk.

Most cardiovascular medications should not be discontinued prior to surgery, so it becomes important to predict how they will interact with the medications administered during anesthesia. Fortunately, most of the interactions with cardiovascular medications are simply extensions of the known pharmacologic effect of these agents:

- α-Adrenoceptor antagonists: hypotension, vasodilation, reflex tachycardia

- β-Adrenoceptor antagonists: hypotension, decreased contractility, bradycardia, atrioventricular (AV) block
- Calcium channel antagonists: hypotension, vasodilation; with verapamil only: decreased contractility, bradycardia, AV block
- Vasodilators: hypotension, vasodilation, reflex tachycardia
- Angiotensin-converting enzyme inhibitors and angiotensin antagonists: hypotension, vasodilation, hyperkalemia
- Diuretics: hypovolemia, hypokalemia, vasodilation

Herbal preparations and drug interactions

An increasing number of patients are taking herbal preparations, vitamins, or other over-the-counter preparations in addition to their medications. Although these preparations may have some benefits, adverse effects are often associated with their use. Unfortunately, some patients may not report the use of these alternative medications. During the preoperative assessment, anesthesiologists should specifically ask patients about their use of these agents.

Herbal preparations are classified as dietary supplements and are exempt from the safety and efficacy requirements that prescription and over-the-counter medications must fulfill. Different brands or even batches of the same herbal preparation may not contain the same amount of the active compound, or any active compound at all. Some of the claimed efficacious effects and potential toxic effects of herbal preparations are listed in Table 44.1. Herbal medications with the greatest impact on hemostasis are garlic, ginkgo, and ginseng. However, presently, mandatory discontinuation of the herbals is not recommended before surgery or anesthesia.

Anesthesiologists should also be aware of medications with narrow therapeutic indices. Such medications are risky in overdose, and drug interactions that increase their concentrations or effects are particularly hazardous. Table 44.2 lists some commonly used medications with a narrow therapeutic index. Additional topics related to alternative medicine and anesthesia are covered in Chapter 177.

Suggested readings

American Society of Anesthesologists. What you should know about herbal and dietary supplement use and anesthesia. Available at: http://www.asahq.org/patientEducation/herbPatient.pdf. Accessed May 1, 2008.

Table 44.2. Commonly used medications with a narrow therapeutic index

Aminoglycoside antibiotics (e.g., gentamicin, tobramycin, amikacin)
Anticoagulants (e.g., warfarin, heparin)
Antidysrhythmics (e.g., procainamide, quinidine)
Carbamazepine
Cyclosporine
Digoxin
Hypoglycemic agents (e.g., glyburide, metformin)
Lithium
Phenytoin
Theophylline
Thyroid hormone
Tricyclic antidepressants (amitriptyline, imipramine, doxepin)
Valproic acid

Bovill JG. Adverse drug interactions in anesthesia. *J Clin Anesth* 1997; 9:3S.
Brown CH. Overview of drug interactions. Available at: http://www.uspharmacist.com. Accessed on January 1, 2011.
Cheng B, Hung CT, Chiu W. Herbal medicine and anesthesia. *Hong Kong J Med J Med* 2002; 8:123.
Hodges PJ, Kam PCA. The peri-operative implications of herbal medicines. *Anesthesia* 2002; 57:889.
Horlocker TT, Wedel DJ, Rowlingson JC, et al. Regional anesthesia in the patient receiving antithrombotic or thrombolytic therapy: American Society of Regional Anesthesia and Pain Medicine Evidence-Based Guidelines (3rd edition). *Reg Anesth Pain Med.* 2010 Jan-Feb; 35(1):64–101.
Ingelmo PM, Ferri F, Fumagalli R. Interactions between general and regional anesthesia. *Minerva Anesthesiol* 2006; 72:437.
Kam PCA, Chang GWM. Selective serotonin reuptake inhibitors. *Anesthesia* 1997; 52:982.
Kam PCA, Liew S. Traditional Chinese herbal medicine and anesthesia. *Anesthesia* 2002; 57:1083.
Kissin I. Anesthetic interactions following bolus injections. *J Clin Anesth* 1997; 9:14S.
Peter SA, Glass MB, Gan TJ, et al. Drug interactions: volatile anesthetics and opioids. *J Clin Anesth* 1997; 9:18S.
Roig RJ, Orfila GM, Masanes RJ. Manejo perioperatorio de la medicacion cronica no relacionada con la cirugia. *An Med Interna (Madrid)* 2004; 21:291.
Rosow C, Levine W, Barash P. Drug interactions. In: Barash P, Cullen B, Stoelting R, eds. *Clinical Anesthesia.* 5th ed. Philadelphia: Lippincott Williams & Wilkins; 2006.
Rosow CE. Anesthetic drug interaction: an overview. *J Clin Anesth* 1997; 9:27S.
Sweeney BP, Bromilow J. Liver enzyme induction and inhibition: implications for anesthesia. *Anesthesia* 2006; 61:159.
Vuyk J. Pharmacokinetic and pharmacodynamic interactions between opioids and propofol. *J Clin Anesth* 1997; 9:23S.

Allergic reactions

Karan Madan and David L. Hepner

An allergic or hypersensitivity reaction is an immunologic response to stimulation by an antigen. Anesthesiologists frequently encounter allergic reactions while managing patients in the perioperative period. Patients are exposed to multiple medications, including antibiotics, anesthetic agents, sedatives and hypnotics, neuromuscular blocking (NMB) agents, polymers such as protamine, blood products, and environmental agents such as latex. All of the aforementioned agents can cause mild to severe (anaphylactic) allergic reactions. The incidence of life-threatening reactions has been reported to be approximately one in 3500 to 13,000 anesthetics. Although anaphylaxis is a rare intraoperative event, most drugs used during the perioperative period have been associated with severe allergic reactions. Muscle relaxants and latex are the most common agents that may lead to anaphylaxis, and prevention is the most important component to decrease the incidence of anaphylaxis.

Pathophysiology

When an individual is exposed to an allergen for the first time, sensitization takes place. This process involves a fixation of IgE to human mast cells and basophils, preparing these cells for activation on reexposure to the allergen. IgE-mediated activation of human mast cells leads to the solubilization and swelling of the secretory granules, as well as fusion of multiple granules and their membranes with the plasmalemma. This initiates a signal transduction cascade that culminates in the increase of intracellular calcium and the release of preformed mediators such as histamine, proteases (tryptases), proteoglycans, and platelet-activating factor.

Phospholipid metabolism, the main component of the lipid mediator pathway, then leads to the generation of potent inflammatory leukotrienes (LTC_4, LTD_4, LTE_4, and LTB_4) and prostaglandins (PGD_2) (Fig. 45.1). Histamine, PGD_2, and LTC_4 are potent vasoactive mediators implicated in vascular permeability changes, flushing, urticaria, angioedema, hypotension, and bronchoconstriction. Leukotriene B_4 mediates leukocyte–endothelial cell adhesion and chemotaxis. In addition, there is generation and release of cytokines involved in the perpetuation of the reaction, including tumor necrosis factor-α (TNF-α), interleukin (IL)-4, IL-5, IL-6, IL-13, and granulocyte macrophage colony-stimulating factor (GM-CSF).

The immunologic pathways, as a result of mast cell activation, are summarized in Fig. 45.2. Mediator release leads to several responses, including adherence and chemotactic leukocyte responses, proliferation of fibroblast and collagen production, activation of the coagulation cascade, and changes in venous and capillary permeability, including constriction and dilatation.

Types of hypersensitivity reactions

Immune-mediated allergic reactions are classified according to their mechanism (Table 45.1). Whereas anaphylaxis is a type I IgE-mediated hypersensitivity reaction involving mast cells and basophils, contact dermatitis is a type IV T-lymphocyte cell–mediated delayed-type hypersensitivity reaction. Other immune-mediated reactions include type II reactions, in which IgG, IgM, and complement mediate cytotoxicity, and type III reactions, in which immune complex formation and deposition lead to tissue damage. Anaphylactoid reactions (i.e., non-allergic anaphylaxis) occur through a direct non–immune-mediated release of mediators from mast cells or basophils or as a result of direct complement activation. However, they present with clinical symptoms similar to those of anaphylaxis.

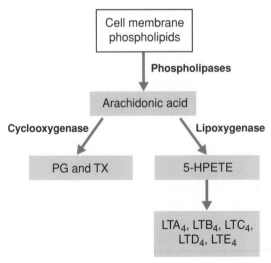

Figure 45.1. Lipid mediator generation. PG, prostaglandin; TX, thromboxane; LT, leukotriene; HPETE, hydroperoxyeicosatetraenoic acid.

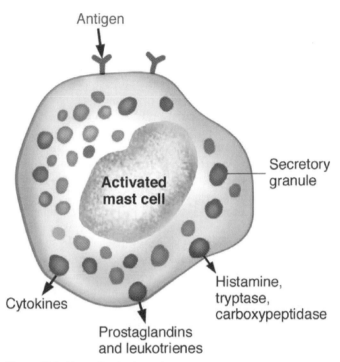

Figure 45.2. Mast cell activation and responses.

Table 45.1. Types of hypersensitivity reactions (Gell and Coombs classification)

Type	Description
I (immediate)	Atopy, urticaria, anaphylaxis
II (cytotoxic)	Autoimmune hemolytic anemia, heparin-induced thrombocytopenia, hemolytic transfusion reactions
III (immune complex mediated)	Serum sickness, Arthus reaction, acute hypersensitivity pneumonitis
IV (delayed cell mediated)	Contact dermatitis, tuberculin-type hypersensitivity, chronic hypersensitivity pneumonitis

Clinical presentation

The onset of anaphylaxis may be delayed by a few minutes to 2 to 3 hours, depending on the route of exposure. After parenteral administration, the onset of anaphylaxis is usually immediate. Dermatologic manifestations include urticaria, itching over the skin and eyes, rash, warmth, and swelling of the face. Conscious patients may complain of dizziness, chest tightness, difficulty breathing, and coughing. In addition, wheezing, tachypnea, laryngeal stridor, and cyanosis may be observed, with the potential to progress to glottic, epiglottic, and pharyngeal edema accompanied by acute respiratory distress. In an anesthetized patient, the first sign of an anaphylactic reaction may be respiratory (bronchospasm) or cardiovascular collapse (sudden massive hypotension). This is the result of the end-organ response to vasoactive mediators leading to bronchospasm, laryngeal edema, reduced effective intravascular volume, and decreased systemic vascular resistance, resulting in shock.

In the latest epidemiologic survey of anaphylactic and anaphylactoid reactions occurring during anesthesia in France and published in the English literature (January 1999–December 2000), anaphylactic reactions were diagnosed in 518 cases (66%), whereas 271 cases (34%) were attributed to anaphylactoid reactions. The most common causes of anaphylaxis were NMB agents (59%), latex (17%), and antibiotics (15%). Anaphylactic reactions to colloids (4%), hypnotics (3%), opioids (1%), and other agents (1%) also were reported. These incidences are illustrated in Fig. 45.3.

Muscle relaxants

Muscle relaxants are the most common agents responsible for intraoperative anaphylaxis. Because environmental contact with cosmetics and disinfectants may lead to sensitization to NMB, anaphylactic reactions to NMB may occur without previous exposure. Females are more likely than males to develop an allergic reaction to NMB agents. Rocuronium (43%) and succinylcholine (23%) were the most frequently incriminated NMB agents. Cross-reactivity between NMB agents was observed in 75% of cases of anaphylaxis; antibodies to NMB agents seem to persist for years. Therefore, cross-reactivity with other NMB agents should be assessed through skin tests in order to propose a safe alternative for further procedures when anaphylaxis to a definite NMB agent has been documented. Rocuronium and vecuronium account for 80% of the sales of nondepolarizing muscle relaxants in the United States. An analysis done in 2005 revealed that in the United States, there was no difference in the incidence of anaphylaxis between the two drugs. However, reports from abroad have found a higher incidence of anaphylaxis with rocuronium.

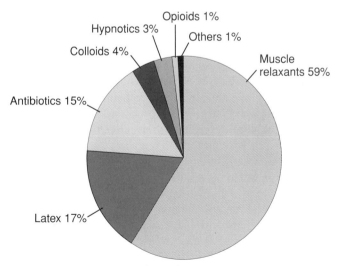

Figure 45.3. Incidence of allergic reactions by agent.

Latex allergy

Allergy to latex was first recognized in 1979 as a result of the use of "universal precautions" promoted by the Centers for Disease Control and Prevention to decrease the spread of HIV and hepatitis B and C viruses. This effort resulted in a 25-fold increase in the use of latex-containing surgical gloves, causing it to emerge as the second most common cause of anaphylaxis in surgical suites (17% of cases) over the following two decades. Health care workers, who come in contact with latex in the form of gloves or other latex-containing medical equipment, may become sensitized to latex. Other high-risk groups include non–health care workers with occupational exposure to latex, patients with an atopic background, and children with spina bifida or genitourinary abnormalities who have undergone multiple surgeries. In addition, some fruits, such as bananas, avocados, and kiwis, contain proteins that cross-react with latex.

Latex-mediated reactions include irritant contact dermatitis (most common reaction), allergic contact dermatitis (type IV), and type I IgE-mediated hypersensitivity reactions (anaphylaxis). Whereas *latex sensitization* is the presence of IgE antibodies to latex without clinical manifestations, *latex allergy* refers to any immune-mediated reaction associated with clinical symptoms that may include urticaria, rhinitis, and conjunctivitis. Latex-specific IgE can be detected in the patient's serum by radioallergosorbent test (RAST) or enzyme allergosorbent test. No standardized antigens for skin testing are commercially available in the United States. Most health care facilities have institutional guidelines for precautions used during management of patients with known latex allergy that must include the use of non–latex-containing gloves and other medical equipment, particularly in patients with IgE-mediated hypersensitivity reactions. There are no data that support the use of pharmacologic prophylaxis (i.e., histamine H_1 and/or H_2 antagonists and/or steroids) prior to a surgical procedure.

Antibiotics

Prevention of postoperative surgical infections has increased preoperative antibiotic use. In the general population, antibiotics, particularly the β-lactams, are the most common drugs causing anaphylaxis, accounting for about 75% of anaphylaxis-related deaths in the United States. Antibiotics that share the β-lactam ring include penicillins, cephalosporins, carbapenems, and monobactams. Although cross-reactivity between cephalosporins and penicillins has been reported, with an incidence between 8% and 10%, recent data suggest the actual incidence is lower. Taking a detailed history of the reaction to penicillin will remove most of the questionable cases of penicillin allergy, which usually are related to nonimmunologic adverse effects. In addition, most of the reported reactions of cross-sensitivity between cephalosporins and penicillins consist of rashes that are not immunologic in origin. Furthermore, earlier generations of cephalosporins contained trace amounts of penicillin; therefore, patients with an allergy to penicillin were more likely to experience an anaphylactic reaction. It is also important to understand that patients who have a definite allergic reaction to a specific antibiotic are more likely to develop anaphylaxis upon exposure to any other antibiotic. More recently, side chain structure attached to the beta-lactam ring has been identified as an important component in determining the allergenicity of the molecule. Because first-generation cephalosporins and cefamandole share a similar side chain with penicillin and amoxicillin, a higher incidence of allergic reactions to first generation cephalosporins and cefamandole is likely to occur in those with a history of penicillin allergy. In contrast, second- and third-generation cephalosporins have different side chains from penicillin and amoxicillin and are unlikely to cross-react with penicillin. There is an increasing trend toward using cephalosporins in patients without a convincing history of penicillin allergy.

It is important to distinguish between a chemically mediated response that may be prevented upon further exposure, such as red man syndrome due to a too-rapid administration of vancomycin, and a true allergic or anaphylactic reaction. Allergic reactions to antibiotics may present as urticaria, pruritus, erythema, angioedema, rhinitis, bronchospasm, hypotension, cardiac arrhythmias, or full-blown anaphylaxis.

Colloids

Albumin, dextran, hetastarch, and gelatin are colloids commonly used in the operating room. Gelatin is the colloid most likely to cause an allergic reaction (although gelatin-based intravenous fluids are not available in the United States). Gelatins and dextrans are more likely than albumin or hetastarch to cause an allergic reaction, with the latter being the colloid least likely to cause an allergic reaction. IgE-mediated anaphylaxis has been proven by demonstrating IgE antibodies and positive intradermal tests against gelatins. Increased circulating IgG dextran-reactive antibodies are found in most adults with dextran anaphylaxis. Enzyme-linked immunosorbent assay (ELISA) is used for detecting hetastarch- and dextran-reactive antibodies (IgG and IgM) in human sera. Although there is no known cross-reactivity among the different groups of colloids, those that belong to the same group, such as Haemaccel (Piramal, Mumbai, India) and Gelofusine (B. Braun, Bella Vista, NSW, Australia), which are both gelatins, have been shown to have cross-reactivity.

Individuals with prior drug allergies are more likely to develop anaphylaxis, with males more likely than females to develop an allergic reaction. Egg allergy does not appear to be a contraindication to the use of albumin, because the principal egg protein, ovalbumin (45 kDa), is different from human serum albumin (67 kDa).

Hypnotics

Cases of propofol-induced bronchoconstriction and allergy have been reported. Although large doses of propofol inhibit histamine-induced contraction in isolated human airway smooth muscle, some reports have suggested that propofol may cause histamine release in healthy and atopic patients and may induce bronchospasm. Propofol is currently formulated in a lipid emulsion vehicle containing 10% soybean oil, 1.2% egg lecithin, and 2.25% glycerol. True allergic reactions to propofol likely are secondary to the two isopropyl groups. Most cases of drug allergy to propofol are IgE mediated, and specific IgE-RIA and intradermal skin tests have been reported. The egg lecithin component of the lipid vehicle is highly purified egg yolk. Ovalbumin, the principal protein of eggs, is present in the egg white. Current evidence suggests that patients allergic to eggs likely will not develop anaphylaxis when exposed to propofol.

An anaphylactoid reaction to thiopental is seen in one in 30,000 anesthetics. Although some of these reactions may be a result of the release of histamine, others are true IgE-mediated anaphylactic reactions.

Opioids

The incidence of allergic reactions to opioids is one in every 100,000 to 200,000 anesthetics. Some opioids (e.g., morphine, meperidine) cause the direct release of histamine, leading to dermatologic manifestations such as urticaria, itching, and vasodilation. Large doses of morphine used during cardiac anesthesia did not show any increased incidence of bronchospasm or angioedema. Anaphylactoid reactions to codeine and morphine have been reported; however, skin tests were negative when affected patients were tested.

Local anesthetics

Although allergy to local anesthetics is frequently reported by patients and there are case reports of such reactions, it is extremely rare to encounter a true IgE-mediated allergic reaction to local anesthetics, especially in the amide class. The most common immune-mediated reaction to local anesthetics is a delayed hypersensitivity (type IV) reaction or contact dermatitis. The metabolism of amide local anesthetics primarily is in the liver, whereas that of esters is via plasma cholinesterases. Para-aminobenzoic acid (PABA) is the main metabolite of ester local anesthetics implicated in causing allergic reactions. Preservatives such as methylparaben, propylparaben (both metabolized to PABA), and metabisulfite are often added to multiple-dose vials of local anesthetics. Many reactions attributed to local anesthetics are actually a result of reactions to PABA. It is also important to distinguish an allergic reaction from more common reactions due to anxiety or epinephrine, as are seen frequently preoperatively and in dentists' offices. Cross-reactivity exists among the ester local anesthetics and is unusual among amides. There is no cross-reactivity between amide and ester local anesthetics. Skin and antigen-challenge testing may be used to identify local anesthetics that are safe for a particular patient, but it should be done with preservative-free solutions.

Blood products

Urticarial reactions are seen in 0.5% of all transfusions with frozen plasma. Because there is a small amount of plasma in all blood products, allergic reactions to plasma contained in units of red blood cells and platelets may occur as well. The reaction may present as itching, swelling, or a rash. These symptoms can be avoided by pretreating patients with previous severe urticarial reactions with diphenhydramine. In addition, it is recommended that such patients be transfused with saline-washed red cells. The prophylactic use of acetaminophen prior to transfusion is controversial, because it has potential toxicity and studies have not shown that it prevents transfusion reactions.

True anaphylactic reactions to blood products are infrequent, except in patients with IgA deficiency, who may have been previously sensitized by either a transfusion or a prior pregnancy.

Radiocontrast agents

Most reactions to nonionic contrast agents are minor events such as flushing or skin rashes and are not immune in origin. The incidence of anaphylactoid reactions is 1% to 2% during infusion of radiocontrast agents, and these reactions occur as a result of nonspecific histamine release. The incidence of repeat reactions on reexposure to radiocontrast material is 17% to 35%, and the severity of these reactions may be reduced by premedication with antihistamines and glucocorticoids. Premedication has not been proven to prevent these reactions.

Protamine

Protamine, a histone derived from salmon sperm, is used to reverse the effects of heparin. Exposed patients may develop an allergic reaction to protamine in 0.4% to 0.8% of cases, with the risk increased in patients previously exposed to protamine. Some forms of insulin, such as NPH and protamine zinc insulin, contain protamine; therefore, diabetic patients exposed to them may have an increased risk for a protamine reaction. Although antigenic crossover is possible in patients with fish allergies, and some vasectomized men have IgG antibodies to protamine, recent reports have failed to demonstrate an association between protamine allergy and vasectomy, infertility, or fish allergy.

Protamine reactions include IgE- and IgG-mediated hypersensitivity, complement activation, nonimmunologic histamine release, and augmentation of thromboxane, which may lead to urticaria, systemic hypotension, and an elevation in pulmonary artery pressure with pulmonary vasoconstriction. Although cutaneous testing will identify IgE-mediated sensitivity, protamine-specific IgE and IgG antibodies can be measured by solid-phase immunoassay, ELISA, and RAST.

Treatment of allergic reactions

The first step in treating an anaphylactic reaction (Table 45.2) consists of withdrawing the drug likely to be the cause of the reaction, interrupting the effects of the preformed mediators, and preventing more mediator release. An immediate assessment of airway, breathing, and circulation (ABC), in addition to early administration of epinephrine, is mandatory

Table 45.2. Treatment of anaphylaxis

Withdrawal of agent
Assessment of airway, breathing, circulation
Early administration of epinephrine
Oxygen supplementation
Intravenous fluids
Histamine H_1 and H_2 antagonists, bronchodilators, hydrocortisone

to avoid airway compromise and cardiovascular collapse. Epinephrine, in doses of 5 to 10 μg IV (0.2 μg/kg), is used in the treatment of mild to moderate hypotension, and is titrated to effect. Doses of 0.1 to 0.5 mg IV are used in the presence of cardiovascular collapse. In addition, it is important to decrease or discontinue anesthetic agents likely to cause vasodilation, such as inhalational agents, as well as any medications with negative inotropic effects. Recently, the concept of anaphylactic shock refractory to epinephrine has been introduced. If incremental doses of epinephrine fail to restore the cardiovascular collapse associated with severe cases of anaphylaxis, norepinephrine, metaraminol, arginine vasopressin or glucagon for patients taking β-blockers should be utilized.

Other important steps in the treatment of anaphylaxis include airway support with 100% oxygen to compensate for the increased oxygen consumption, IV crystalloid replacement (2–4 L) to compensate for the peripheral vasodilatation, histamine H_1 antagonists (diphenhydramine, 0.5–1 mg/kg), histamine H_2 antagonists (ranitidine, 150 mg, or cimetidine 400 mg IV), bronchodilators (nebulized albuterol and/or ipratropium bromide), and glucocorticoids (hydrocortisone) to decrease airway swelling and prevent recurrence of symptoms.

There are no randomized controlled trials that address the treatment of anaphylaxis, and clinical treatment protocols for anaphylaxis are based on our understanding of its cellular mechanism, animal experiments, and clinical presentation. Immediate discontinuation of the offending agent and administration of epinephrine are the cornerstones of treating anaphylaxis.

Suggested readings

Apter AJ, Kinman JL, Bilker WB, et al. Is there cross-reactivity between penicillins and cephalosporins? *Am J Med* 2006; 119:354.e11–20.

Dewachter P, Mouton-Faivre C, Emala CW. Anaphylaxis and anesthesia: controversies and new insights. *Anesthesiology* 2009; 111:1141–1150.

Fisher MM, Baldo BA. The incidence and clinical features of anaphylactic reactions during anesthesia in Australia. *Ann Fr Anesth Reanim* 1993; 12:97–104.

Harper NJ, Dixon T, Dugué P, et al. Suspected anaphylactic reactions associated with anaesthesia. *Anaesthesia* 2009; 64:199–211.

Hepner DL, Castells MC. Latex allergy: an update. *Anesth Analg* 2003; 96:1219–1229.

Hepner DL, Castells MC. Anaphylaxis during the perioperative period. *Anesth Analg* 2003; 97:1381–1395.

Joint Task Force on Practice Parameters; American Academy of Allergy, Asthma and Immunology; American College of Allergy, Asthma and Immunology; Joint Council of Allergy, Asthma and Immunology. The diagnosis and management of anaphylaxis practice parameter: 2010 update. *J Allergy Clin Immunol* 2010; Aug 6. Epub ahead of print.

Kroigaard M, Garvey LH, Gillberg L, et al. Scandinavian Clinical Practice Guidelines on the diagnosis, management and follow-up of anaphylaxis during anaesthesia. *Acta Anaesthesiol Scand* 2007; 51: 655–670.

Lieberman P. Anaphylactic reactions during surgical and medical procedures. *J Allergy Clin Immunol* 2002; 110: S64–S69.

Lieberman P, Nicklas RA, Oppenheimer J, et al. The diagnosis and management of anaphylaxis practice parameter: 2010 update. *J Allergy Clin Immunol* 2010; 126:477–80.

Mertes PM, Laxenaire MC. Allergic reactions occurring during anesthesia. *Eur J Anaesthesiol* 2002; 19:240–262.

Mertes PM, Laxenaire MC. Adverse reactions to neuromuscular blocking agents. *Curr Allergy Asthma Rep* 2004; 4:7–16.

Mertes PM, Laxenaire MC, Alla F; Groupe d'Etudes des Réactions Anaphylactoïdes Peranesthésiques. Anaphylactic and anaphylactoid reactions occurring during anesthesia in France in 1999–2000. *Anesthesiology* 2003; 99:536–545.

Mertes PM, Laxenaire MC, Lienhart A, et al. Working Group for the SFAR; ENDA; EAACI Interest Group on Drug Hypersensitivity. Reducing the risk of anaphylaxis during anaesthesia: guidelines for clinical practice. *J Investig Allergol Clin Immunol* 2005; 15: 91–101.

Pichichero ME, Casey JR. Safe use of selected cephalosporins in penicillin-allergic patients: a meta-analysis. *Otolaryngol Head Neck Surg* 2007; 136: 340–347.

Vervloet D, Magnan A, Birnbaum J, Pradal M. Allergic emergencies seen in surgical suites. *Clin Rev Allergy Immunol* 1999; 17: 459–467.

Strom BL, Schinnar R, Apter AJ, et al. Absence of cross-reactivity between sulfonamide antibiotics and sulfonamide nonantibiotics. *N Engl J Med* 2003; 349:1628–35.

Pharmacology of Local Anesthetics

Pradeep Dinakar and Gary R. Strichartz, editors

Mechanism of action and pharmacokinetics

Peter Gerner and Pradeep Dinakar

Overview

Local anesthesia is defined as the temporary or permanent loss of sensation in localized areas of the body by either chemical or physical modalities. The chemical modalities include the use of local anesthetic agents, which reversibly inhibit the generation and propagation of nerve impulses in excitable tissues, producing a transient loss of sensory, motor, and autonomic functions.

Chronology of discovery of local anesthetics

In 1860 Neimann isolated and described the chemical structure of cocaine. Koller introduced cocaine as the first local anesthetic clinically in 1884, but the development of dependence and addiction with prolonged use and local irritant properties paved the way for development of newer and related drugs that were less toxic and less addictive. Procaine was the first clinically relevant local anesthetic, introduced in 1905, which formed the prototype of the modern local anesthetics. Changes in the benzoic acid moiety resulted in chloroprocaine and tetracaine initially. This was followed by a change in the linkage from ester to amide, resulting in the introduction of lidocaine in 1948. Lidocaine was soon succeeded by the introduction of bupivacaine, levobupivacaine, mepivacaine, and ropivacaine. The chronology of introduction of local anesthetics into clinical practice and the intermediate chain type, which formed the basis of local anesthetic classification, is shown in Table 46.1.

Chemical structure of local anesthetics

Local anesthetics have a lipophilic benzene ring, a hydrophilic tertiary amine separated by an ester or amide linked intermediate chain. The link which contains either the ester or amide linkages formed the basis of the local anesthetic classification into amino-ester-linked or amino-amide-linked local anesthetics (Table 46.2). The amino-amide local anesthetics were far superior to the early amino-ester local anesthetics in that chemically they were more stable in solution and at higher temperatures. Structural variations in the amino-ester linkage further classified the amino-ester local anesthetics into aminoacyl and aminoalkyl amides. The newer aminoacyl-amide local anesthetics also had the advantages of being longer acting among all anesthetics, associated with fewer allergic reactions compared

to the ester anesthetics, and exibiting stereo selectivity, which reduced cardiac side effects.

Pharmacodynamics of local anesthetics
Type of nerve fibers affected

Axons differ in their size and structure. The larger the diameter of an axon, the faster is the speed of propagation of the action potential along that axon. A greater degree of myelination also yields faster transmission of electrical impulses by insulating the axon membrane and allowing the "action current" to move more efficiently to the subsequent, uninsulated regions called nodes of Ranvier. Thus, based on the fiber size and myelination, the nerve fibers are classified into type A, B, or C (Fig. 46.1a). This process by which depolarization travels rapidly from one uninsulated region to another along the axon is called *saltatory conduction* (Fig. 46.1b). Sensitivity to blockade is determined by axonal diameter, degree of myelination, and various other physiologic factors as described below (Table 46.3).

Role of sodium ion channel conformational states on blockade

The generation and propagation of impulses in nerve axons that carry afferent (sensory) and efferent (motor, sympathetic) information require the flow of specific ionic currents through channels in the plasma membrane. Many of these channels open and close depending on the electrical potential across the cell membrane. The major determinant of depolarization and

Table 46.1. Chronology of clinical use of local anesthetics

Anesthetic agent	Type of linkage	Year of introduction
Cocaine	Ester	1884
Procaine	Ester	1905
Tetracaine	Ester	1933
Lidocaine	Amide	1948
Chlorprocaine	Ester	1955
Mepivacaine	Amide	1956
Prilocaine	Amide	1960
Bupivacaine	Amide	1963
Ropivacaine	Amide	1997
Levobupivacaine	Amide	1999

Table 46.2. Classification of local anesthetics based on linkages

Anesthetic agent	Type of linkage
General local anesthetic structure	Aromatic portion — Ester or amide — Amine portion
Aminoacyl-Ester local anesthetic (e.g. Lidocaine)	
Aminoalkyl-Ester local anesthetic (e.g. Dibucaine)	
Amino-Amide local anesthetic (e.g. Procaine)	

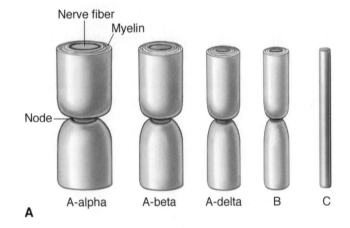

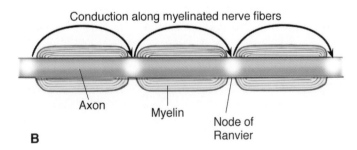

Figure 46.1. (**A**) Diameters of various types of nerve fibers. Only the C-fibers are unmyelinated. (**B**) Impulse conduction includes simultaneous active depolarization of several nodes of Ranvier in myelinated nerve fibers, with active inward (Na^+) currents occurring only at the nodes.

Table 46.3. Properties of different nerve fibers

Property	A-α	A-β	A-δ, A-γ	B	C
			Nerve fiber		
Diameter, μm	12–20	5–12	2–5	<3	0.4–1.2
Speed, m/sec	70–120	30–70	4–30	3–15	0.5–3
Sensitivity to block	++	++	+++	++++	++++
Myelination	+++	+++	++	+	–
Function	Motor, proprioception	Touch, pressure, proprioception	Pain, Temperature, Touch, Motor	Autonomic	Pain, Temperature, Touch

impulse propagation is the influx of sodium (Na$^+$) ions through specific voltage gated sodium channels located in the nerve axons. Local anesthetic agents reversibly bind to and block these sodium channels and reduce the sodium currents across the channels (see Fig. 46.2), thereby preventing the initiation and propagation of action potentials.

The sodium ion conformational state, which depends on the depolarization–repolarization cycle, could be in a resting, open, or inactivated state. The local anesthetics have a minimal effect on the resting states and have the greatest affinity to the open state followed by the inactivated state. Thus local anesthetics create a "state dependent block" by showing greatest affinity to the open Na$^+$ channels (Fig. 46.3).

Although local anesthetics may interfere with other channels (K$^+$ and Ca^{2+}), their interaction with sodium channels is clinically most relevant. Additional mechanisms of local anesthetic action include the nonspecific expansion of the neuronal lipid membrane to compress and thus affect the function of various ion channels and alteration of neuronal membrane surface charge. Also, local anesthetic drugs directly interact with specific neuronal membrane receptors (nicotinic acetylcholine-activated receptors, the substance P receptor, and many of the G protein–coupled receptors). These alternative actions may contribute to local anesthesia actions, particularly at synapses in the spinal cord and also play a role in local anesthetic toxicity.

Differential blockade

Local anesthetics differ in their ability to block autonomic, sensory, and motor action potentials on nerves in different parts of

the body. The reason for this differential blockade is unclear and many theories exist with some clinical correlation. Fiber size, which was thought to play a role in differential blockade, has not been shown to play a significant role in a clinical setting. C fibers (unmyelinated) are the most sensitive to the local anesthetic action and A fibers (myelinated) the least sensitive. This is the reason for analgesia seen prior to the loss of pressure and touch sensations. Other theories on efficacy of the local anesthetics relating to the anatomical arrangement and location of the nerve fibers, vasodilating properties of the individual local anesthetics, and differential effects on other ion channels have been proposed as some of the causes. Bupivacaine has the most favorable sensory-to-motor differential blockade and is widely used in obstetric analgesia and chronic pain procedures, where preservation of motor function is essential. If the local anesthetic concentration is increased to a sufficiently high level, all local anesthetics will cause complete blockage of all modalities.

Systemic actions of local anesthetic agents

Various chronic pain syndromes, including neuropathic pain syndromes and fibromyalgia, show a favorable response to the systemic administration of local anesthetics. Intravenous lidocaine infusion is an approved pain treatment modality in refractory pain conditions, and the mechanism of its systemic action is unclear. Presumed sites of action are the activated sodium channels on the central and peripheral nervous system, the dorsal root ganglia, and the sympathetic nervous system.

Pharmacokinetics of local anesthetics
Absorption of local anesthetics

Local anesthetics are rapidly absorbed from mucous membranes (conjunctiva), whereas absorption from intact skin requires time and increased dosage. Local anesthetics are frequently applied directly on or near their target via the injection techniques of regional anesthesia, where their pharmacodynamic effects are directly related to tissue concentrations in the immediate vicinity of injection. Plasma levels of local anesthetic rarely bear a relationship to their desired effects; however, plasma levels are directly related to systemic toxicity. Peak plasma levels of local anesthetic reach the highest concentrations after direct intravenous or intra-arterial injection and are lowest after subcutaneous injection (intravenous > tracheal >

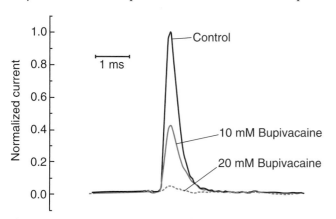

Figure 46.2. Decrease in amplitude of Na$^+$ currents by local anesthetic drugs (bupivacaine).

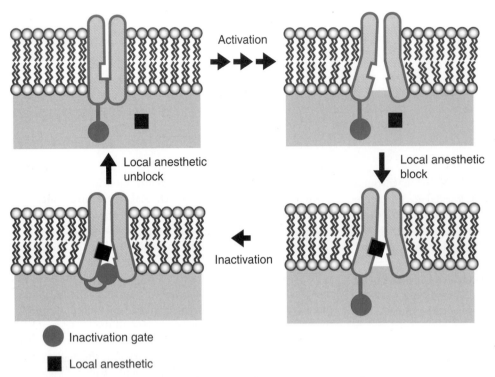

Figure 46.3. Conformational change of Na$^+$ ion channel from active to inactive and resting state. LA, local anesthetic.

intercostal > caudal > epidural > brachial plexus > sciatic > subcutaneous). Following injection, local anesthetics absorbed into the circulation are taken up first by the highly perfused organs (brain, heart, liver, kidney, lung), and then by less well-perfused tissues (muscle and fat).

Metabolism and clearance

Metabolism and clearance of amide-type local anesthetics (Table 46.4) depend on liver function (hydroxylation and *N*-dealkylation by microsomal cytochrome P-450) and may be limited in any disease state that reduces hepatic blood flow or liver function (e.g., liver disease, congestive heart failure). An increase of α_1-acid glycoprotein and other plasma proteins (e.g., due to cancer, trauma, inflammatory disease) may lead to slower hepatic metabolism and slower clearance, as more drug is bound to proteins. However, dissociation rates from plasma proteins are relatively rapid compared with clearance rates and have only modest effects on overall biotransformation. Metabolites of prilocaine and benzocaine can cause methemoglobinemia.

Ester-type local anesthetics are hydrolyzed by plasma pseudocholinesterase enzymes to an alkylamine and para-aminobenzoic acid (PABA). Thus, patients with genetically abnormal pseudocholinesterase levels are at increased risk for toxic side effects. In addition, PABA may cause allergic reactions in some patients; allergy to ester-type local anesthetics is far more common than allergy to amide local anesthetics. Benzocaine, a local anesthetic commonly used to produce topical anesthesia in the upper airway, exists only in the uncharged form. It passes rapidly through the skin and is rapidly hydrolyzed in plasma, leading to potentially high levels of PABA. To a limited degree, the liver also extracts and metabolizes ester-type compounds (especially cocaine). Termination of action of intrathecally administered ester-type local anesthetics (tetracaine) is by systemic absorption into the blood, as cerebrospinal fluid lacks the esterase enzymes. Renal disease has little effect on the pharmacokinetics of local anesthetics.

Role of pH

Local anesthetics are weak bases that pass through the phospholipid membrane into the cell when they are in their uncharged

Table 46.4. Pharmacokinetics of local anesthetics most often used clinically

Anesthetic agent	VD, L/kg	CL, L/kg/h	T$_{1/2}$, h	Relative potency[a]
Amides				
Lidocaine	1.3	0.85	1.6	1
Prilocaine	2.73	2.03	1.6	1
Mepivacaine	1.2	0.67	1.9	1
Ropivacaine	0.84	0.63	1.9	4
Bupivacaine	1.02	0.41	3.5	4
Esters				
Chloroprocaine	0.5	2.96	0.11	0.5
Procaine	0.93	5.62	0.14	Data not available

[a] Measured after epidural administration.
VD, volume of distribution at steady state; CL, total plasma clearance; T$_{1/2}$, terminal half-time.

Table 46.5. pK$_a$ and pH of commonly formulated local anesthetics

Drug	pK$_a$[a]	pH of solution in vial
2-Chloroprocaine	9.1	2.5–4
Procaine	8.9	5.5–6
Lidocaine	7.7	5.6 (without epinephrine)
		3.5–5.5 (with epinephrine)
Levobupivacaine	8.1	4.0–6.5 (without epinephrine)
Bupivacaine	8.1	4.5–5.5 (without epinephrine)
		3.5–5.5 (with epinephrine)
Mepivacaine	7.7	5.5

[a] Depends on temperature and ionic condition.

Table 46.6. Advantages of adding epinephrine to local anesthetic drugs

Prolongs the duration of nerve block
Increases the intensity of nerve block
Decreases systemic absorption and reduces blood levels of LAD
Decreases surgical blood loss
May be used as a test dose to identify intravascular injection of LAD
Has weak local anesthetic property of its own

LAD, local anesthetic drug.

lipid-soluble form. However, once inside the cell, they are rapidly converted to the charged form, which more effectively blocks the sodium channel. The Henderson-Hasselbach equation relates the pH to the dissociation constant (pK$_a$) and the relative concentrations of uncharged base (B) and charged base (BH$^+$). Given the reaction, $B + H^+ \leftrightarrow BH^+$, the pH determines the ratio of B and BH$^+$.

$$pH = pK_a + \log_{10}[B]/[BH^+].$$

pK$_a$ is the pH at which 50% of the local anesthetic is uncharged ([B] = [BH$^+$]). As shown in Table 46.5, the pK$_a$ values for commonly used local anesthetics lie within the range between about 8 and 9. For amide local anesthetics, the pK$_a$ usually correlates with the speed of onset. In general, it is thought that drugs with a pK$_a$ closer to the pH in the tissue surrounding the nerve (physiologic pH) have faster block onset, as there are more local anesthetic molecules available in the neutral (uncharged) form, which is largely responsible for traversing the membranes that ensheath the nerve.

Sodium bicarbonate is often added to increase the pH of these local anesthetic solutions, thus increasing the concentration of nonionized lipophilic free-base. This increases the rate of membrane permeation of the drug and its speed of onset. Clinically, the addition of 1 mEq of sodium bicarbonate to each 10 ml of commercially prepared 1.5% to 2% lidocaine solution (0.1 mEq to each 10 ml bupivacaine) produces a significantly faster onset of anesthesia and more rapid spread of sensory block. Excessive alkalinization, particularly of more concentrated local anesthetic solutions, will cause the local anesthetic to precipitate from solution.

Effect of lipid solubility

Lipid solubility is also an important factor in determining the speed of onset of action. Although higher lipid solubility would be expected to promote drug entry into membranes by increasing the diffusion rate, very high lipophilicity results in a dominant absorption of the drug into the membrane, with concomitantly slow dissociation and net transport across the membrane. Very lipid-soluble drugs, such as etidocaine, have both a slow onset of action and an extraordinarily long duration. Lipid solubility is directly proportional to potency of the drug, because of hydrophobic binding to the Na$^+$ channel.

Role of additives

Commonly used additives to local anesthetic drugs include opioids and vasoconstrictors. Opioids such as fentanyl are added to supplement analgesia. Epinephrine (5 µg/ml, or 1:200,000) is the vasoconstrictor most commonly added to local anesthetic drugs. Advantages of adding epinephrine are listed in Table 46.6. Addition of epinephrine in patients with coronary artery disease and hypertension should be done with caution, as direct intravascular injection will produce tachycardia and hypertension. Epinephrine should not be added to local anesthetic drugs when peripheral nerve blocks are performed in tissues with inadequate collateral blood circulation (wrist, ankle, digits, penis) or when intravenous regional anesthesia is administered.

47

Clinical applications of local anesthetics

Pradeep Dinakar and Peter Gerner

Overview

The clinical application of local anesthetic agents depends on the type of local anesthetic, stereoselectivity, clinical potency, and the side effect profile. Local anesthetic potency is based on a multitude of factors including time of onset of action, duration of action, and type of regional anesthetic block.

Clinical characteristics of local anesthetics

Type of local anesthetics

Clinically used local anesthetics, as described in Chapter 46, may be classified as amino-amides (lidocaine, mepivacaine, prilocaine, bupivacaine, levobupivacaine, and ropivacaine), or amino-esters (procaine, chloroprocaine, tetracaine, and cocaine). This classification is based on the type of linkage, which is either an amide or an ester, that links the lipophilic benzene ring with the hydrophobic tertiary amine (see Table 46.2).

Amide and ester local anesthetics differ in their chemical stability, metabolism, and allergic potential. Amides are extremely stable, whereas esters are relatively unstable, particularly in neutral or alkaline solution. Amide compounds undergo enzymatic degradation in the liver, whereas the ester compounds are hydrolyzed in plasma by the pseudocholinesterase enzymes. Cocaine, an ester, is an exception, as it is metabolized predominantly by the liver. The metabolites of esters include para-aminobenzoic acid (PABA), which can occasionally induce allergic-type reactions. Allergies to amides are extremely rare.

Stereochemistry

Local anesthetics are available as individual enantiomers and racemic mixtures. An *enantiomer* is one of two stereoisomers of a given molecule that cannot be superimposed. Enantiomers differ only in their ability to rotate the plane of polarized light, and thus are named for the direction of that polarization, levorotatory (left) or dextrorotatory (right). A *racemic mixture* contains equal amounts of the two enantiomers. The two enantiomers can have significantly different chemical and physiologic properties that are of clinical importance.

Potency of local anesthetics

Local anesthetics differ in their potency based on onset of action, duration of action, lipid solubility, vasodilating property, and the type of regional block.

The uncharged form of a local anesthetic is more likely to cross the cell membrane than the charged (protonated) form, thus the proportion of the local anesthetic that is in the uncharged form will significantly impact the speed of onset of action. Local anesthetics (bases) are poorly soluble in water but can be dissolved in hydrophobic organic solvents. Therefore, most local anesthetics are commercially formulated as the more soluble hydrochloride salts, accounting for their low (acidic) pH (see Table 46.5). Hence, speed of onset of local anesthetics depends on their pKa and the pH of the anesthetic solution which influences the ratio of the unprotonated and protonated forms. Low pKa of an agent and high pH of the solvent are most favorable for rapid onset of action. Other favorable factors include high lipid solubility, low vasodilating property, and higher dose of local anesthetic (Table 47.1).

Table 47.1. Maximum recommended doses of local anesthetics[a]

Drug	Onset[b]	Maximum dose for plain solution, mg/kg	Maximum dose with epinephrine, mg/kg[c]
Lidocaine	Rapid	5	7
Mepivacaine	Rapid	5	7
Chloroprocaine	Rapid	10	15
Prilocaine	Rapid	7[d]	8[d]
Ropivacaine	Slow	3	3
Bupivacaine	Slow	2.0	2.5
Levobupivacaine	Slow	2.5	3
Procaine	Slow	8	10

[a] The maximal recommended dose of local anesthetics is influenced by various factors (see text) and should be adjusted for each injection site.
[b] Onset times vary significantly with the injection site – for example, all the above commonly used local anesthetics have fast onset when used for infiltration anesthesia, but most are very slow topical anesthetics.
[c] The maximal adult recommended dose of epinephrine is 250 μg per dose; for children, 3 μg/kg per dose.
[d] The maximal recommended adult dose of prilocaine is 600 mg because of clinically significant methemoglobinemia.

Table 47.2. Tissue infiltration[a]

Drug	Volume for 70-kg person, *ml*	Usual duration, *min*
Lidocaine 0.5%–1%, plain	70–35	30–60
Lidocaine 0.5%–1%, with epinephrine (1:200,000–1:400,000)[b]	100–50	60–120
Mepivacaine 0.5%–1%, plain	70–35	45–90
Mepivacaine 0.5%–1%, with epinephrine (1:200,000–1:400,000)[b]	100–50	120
Bupivacaine 0.25%–0.5%, plain	56–28	180
Bupivacaine 0.25%–0.5%, with epinephrine (1:200,000–1:400,000)[b]	70–35	180
Levobupivacaine 0.25%–0.5%	70–35	120
Levobupivacaine 0.25%–0.5%, with epinephrine (1:200,000–1:400,000)[b]	84–42	120
Ropivacaine 0.2%–0.5%	105–42	120

[a] Do not exceed the maximum dosage listed in Table 47.1.
[b] Caution: The maximal *adult* recommended dose of epinephrine is 250 μg per dose; for children, the maximum dose is 3 μg/kg per dose.

The duration of action varies for each local anesthetic agent. Bupivacaine, levobupivacaine, and ropivacaine have one of the longest durations of anesthesia. This is followed by lidocaine, mepivacaine, and prilocaine. Procaine and chloroprocaine have the shortest durations (Table 47.2).

The duration and onset of action are also affected by the type of regional block. Peripheral nerve/plexus blocks have a slow onset of action but last the longest given their relative tissue

Table 47.3. Minor nerve blocks[a,b]

Drug	Volume, *ml*	Usual duration, *min*
Lidocaine 1%–2%, plain	5–10	60–120
Lidocaine 1%–2%, with epinephrine (1:200,000–1:400,000)[c]	5–10	120–180
Chloroprocaine 2%–3%, plain	5–10	15–30
Chloroprocaine 2%–3%, with epinephrine (1:200,000–1:400,000)[c]	5–10	30–60
Mepivacaine 1%–1.5%, plain	5–10	60–120
Mepivacaine 1%–1.5%, with epinephrine (1:200,000–1:400,000)[c]	5–10	120–360
Bupivacaine 0.25%–0.5%, plain	5–10	180–480
Bupivacaine 0.25%–0.5%, with epinephrine (1:200,000–1:400,000)[c]	5–10	240–960
Levobupivacaine 0.25%–0.5%	5–10	180–480
Levobupivacaine 0.25%–0.5%, with epinephrine (1:200,000–1:400,000)[c]	5–10	240–960
Ropivacaine 0.2%–0.5%	5–10	120–480

[a] Single nerve, such as ulnar or radial, and blocks below the knee.
[b] Of note, most minor nerve blocks are performed without the addition of epinephrine. Epinephrine is contraindicated in blocks of the digits or penis, as is plain cocaine, because tissue ischemia may result. Also, do not exceed maximum dosage listed when blocking several nerves simultaneously.
[c] Caution: The maximal *adult* recommended dose of epinephrine is 250 μg per dose; for children, the maximum dose is 3 μg/kg per dose.

Table 47.4. Major nerve blocks[a,b]

Drug	Volume, *ml*	Usual duration, *min*
Lidocaine 1%–2%, plain	50–30	60–180
Lidocaine 1%–2%, with epinephrine (1:200,000–1:400,000)[c]	50–30	120–240
Mepivacaine 1%–1.5%, plain	50–30	60–180
Mepivacaine 1%–1.5%, with epinephrine (1:200,000–1:400,000)[c]	50–30	180–300
Levobupivacaine 0.25%–0.5%, plain	50–30	180–270
Levobupivacaine 0.25%–0.5%, with epinephrine (1:200,000–1:400,000)[c]	50–30	360–1440
Ropivacaine 0.5%–0.75%, plain or with epinephrine (1:200,000–1:400,000)[c]	50–30	360–720

[a] Several nerves or a plexus.
[b] Do not exceed maximum dosage listed in Table 47.1.
[c] Caution: The maximal *adult* recommended dose of epinephrine is 250 μg per dose; for children, the maximum dose is 3 μg/kg per dose.

avascularity and large block volume required (Table 47.3 and Table 47.4). Intrathecal, epidural, and subcutaneous blocks have a much faster onset of action but have a much shorter duration of action (Table 47.5 and Table 47.6).

Local anesthetic toxicity

Local anesthetics are the mainstay of regional anesthesia and pain management; however, their toxicity is a major limitation to their use. Because of the constant concern about systemic or local neurotoxicity, clinicians have to use the lowest concentrations/dosages of local anesthetics possible, thereby effectively limiting the full potential of these agents, lowering the success rate, and shortening the duration of block.

Table 47.5. Epidural anesthesia[a]

Drug	Volume, *ml*	Usual duration, *min*
Chloroprocaine 2%–3%, plain or with epinephrine (1:200,000)	30–15	30–60
Lidocaine 1%–2%, plain	25–15	45–60
Lidocaine 1%–2%, with epinephrine (1:200,000)	25–15	60–75
Mepivacaine 1%–2%, plain	25–15	45–75
Mepivacaine 1%–2%, with epinephrine (1:200,000)	25–15	60–180
Bupivacaine 0.25%–0.75%, plain	20–10	90–240
Bupivacaine 0.25%–0.75%, with epinephrine (1:200,000)	25–10	120–300
Levobupivacaine 0.25%–0.75%,	25–10	Same as plain
Levobupivacaine 0.25%–0.75%, with epinephrine (1:200,000)	30–10	bupivacaine
Ropivacaine 0.2%–1.0%, plain or with epinephrine (1:200,000)	20–10	90–300

[a] Do not exceed the maximum recommended dose listed in Table 47.1. Administration in fractionated doses of 3–5 ml is recommended.

Table 47.6. Spinal anesthesia: commonly used agents/doses

Drug	Dose, *mg*	Usual duration, *min*
Procaine 5%–10%	80–160	30–75
Lidocaine 1%–2%	20–100	30–90
Mepivacaine 1.5%–4%	20–80	30–90
Bupivacaine 0.5%–0.75%	5–18	75–300
Levobupivacaine	Same as bupivacaine	
Ropivacaine 0.5%–1%	8–18	75–300

Direct local toxicity (direct neurotoxicity and nerve degeneration) may occur at clinically used concentrations and cause permanent nerve lesions. This is particularly disabling, as its frequency is greater in the spinal cord than in peripheral nerves, potentially causing damage to the nerves of the cauda equina (cauda equina syndrome, which manifests with varying neurologic deficits depending on the nerves affected, including incontinence, impotence, and paresthesia in the buttocks, perineal area, and legs), and even paraplegia. *Transient neurologic symptoms* (TNS) have been reported after spinal anesthesia with almost every local anesthetic agent, especially lidocaine. The cause is thought to be direct irritation of one or more spinal nerves, characterized by burning pain in the lower extremities and the buttocks. Symptoms usually resolve over 3 to 5 days (Table 47.7).

Systemic toxicity may occur as a result of vascular absorption or accidental intravascular injection of local anesthetics. Systemic toxicity usually is heralded by restlessness, twitching, metallic taste, and seizures. Severe systemic toxicity manifests as generalized seizures and cardiac arrhythmias, which can progress to ventricular tachycardia and asystole at higher blood levels. Usually, much higher blood levels of local anesthetic (about three times) are required to cause cardiotoxicity than to cause neurotoxicity. Lidocaine and bupivacaine (approved by the US Food and Drug Administration in 1947 and 1963, respectively) are still the two most widely used local anesthetic agents. Bupivacaine is more cardiotoxic than lidocaine, in part

because it binds to and dissociates more slowly from sodium channels than lidocaine. Two homologues of bupivacaine, ropivacaine (less lipid soluble) and levobupivacaine (stereoisomer of bupivacaine), are believed to be less toxic than racemic bupivacaine. However, neither is dramatically less toxic, as evidenced by similar dosage guidelines and recurring case reports of their toxicity, including fatalities.

In recent years, the administration of intravenous intralipid solution, termed *lipid rescue,* has shown some promise of reducing systemic local anesthetic toxicity. Specifically, the intravenous administration of a 20% intralipid solution in a dose of 1.5 ml/kg as an initial bolus, followed by 0.25 ml/kg/min for 30 to 60 minutes has been shown to improve the survival of animals with bupivacaine-induced asystole.

Currently, there is no therapy for permanent nerve damage from local anesthetics, either in the spinal cord or the peripheral nervous system. Minor reactions to local anesthetic agents may resolve spontaneously, probably by repair of neuronal damage. The best approach is to adopt practices that minimize the risk of systemic local anesthetic toxicity. Administering local anesthetic in small, incremental doses while frequently assessing the patient for signs or symptoms of toxicity is prudent. If the restlessness, twitching, metallic taste or seizures appear, further administration of any local anesthetic should be halted and oxygen/airway management provided immediately. Seizures are most often transient, but persistent seizures can be treated with thiopental, propofol, or midazolam. In the event of cardiac arrest, cardiopulmonary resuscitation and standard treatment of any apparent arrhythmias, including direct cardiac defibrillation should be instituted. Lipid rescue should be considered if standard resuscitation measures fail. Prompt efforts to institute cardiopulmonary bypass can be life-saving.

Clinically used local anesthetics
Amino-amide local anesthetics
Lidocaine

Lidocaine, the first widely used local anesthetic, is available for infiltration as well as peripheral (including intravenous regional anesthesia of Bier block), spinal, and epidural blocks. It has a rapid onset of action, moderate duration of action limited by its vasodilating properties, and a favorable side effect profile. Its use for spinal anesthesia has declined because of concerns about neurotoxicity and transient neurologic symptoms. It can be applied topically as an ointment or jelly, or nebulized as an aerosol to anesthetize the upper airway. Intravenous injection of lidocaine to achieve low plasma levels (<5 μg/ml) results in systemic analgesia; this is due to lidocaine's action in the central nervous system (CNS) as well as its effect on peripheral nerves or cutaneous nerve endings. Clinically, lidocaine has been administered as an infusion to treat chronic neuropathic pain and can predict the efficacy of oral sodium channel blocking drugs, such as mexiletine.

Table 47.7. Symptoms and signs of local anesthetic toxicity

Central nervous system	Transient neurologic symptoms, cauda equina syndrome, dizziness, perioral and tongue numbness, blurred vision, tinnitus, restlessness, agitation, slurred speech, seizures, unconsciousness
Respiratory system	Decreased ventilatory drive to hypoxia, apnea, depression of respiratory center in the medulla
Cardiovascular system	Decreased myocardial automaticity, contractility–bradycardia, ventricular arrhythmias, heart block, hypotension, cardiac arrest
Hematologic system	Decreased platelet aggregation, increased fibrinolysis, deceased embolic events
Prolonged action of	Muscle relaxants, opioids
Action prolonged by	Propranolol, cimetidine – decreased hepatic blood flow

Lidocaine causes vasodilation at most concentrations. Thus, the addition of epinephrine can significantly reduce the absorption of lidocaine by nearby vasculature, allowing more of the initially administered dose to rapidly enter the neural compartment, thereby prolonging the duration of action by as much as 50%. Experimentally, intravenous lidocaine profoundly suppresses both increased peripheral neuronal "firing" induced by injury and inflammation and central sensitization of wide dynamic range neurons in the dorsal horn of the spinal cord.

Prilocaine

Prilocaine has a clinical profile similar to that of lidocaine and is used for infiltration, peripheral nerve blocks, and spinal and epidural anesthesia. Because prilocaine causes significantly less vasodilation than lidocaine, addition of epinephrine is not necessary to prolong the duration of action. This may be advantageous when epinephrine is contraindicated. Prilocaine shows the least systemic toxicity of all the amide local anesthetics; therefore, it is useful for intravenous regional anesthesia. However, because it causes methemoglobinemia (>500 mg dose) because of its metabolite, *o*-toluidine, it largely has been abandoned for regional anesthetic use.

Mepivacaine

The anesthetic profile of mepivacaine is also similar to that of lidocaine, but its duration of action is slightly longer. However, it is not as effective when applied topically. Although toxicity appears to be less than that with lidocaine, the metabolism of mepivacaine is prolonged in the fetus and newborn. Consequently, mepivacaine is not used for obstetric anesthesia. Vasodilation is mild, but adding epinephrine can attain significant prolongation of action.

Bupivacaine

Bupivacaine provides prolonged and intense sensory analgesia, often outlasting the motor block. For epidural analgesia and anesthesia, bupivacaine usually is used at concentrations from 0.25% to 0.5%, with a 2- to 5-hour duration of action. Peripheral nerve blocks are also performed with these concentrations, depending on the amount of motor block sought. The block may last for 12 to 24 hours. Intrathecal use provides approximately 2 to 3 hours of anesthesia and 4 to 6 hours of analgesia. Other clinical uses include tissue infiltration with 0.25% concentration, useful in "trigger point" injections for treating myofascial pain. Epinephrine is sometimes added as a marker for intravascular injection and to prolong the duration of action because of its decreased vascular absorption. However, as vasoconstriction has less impact on the duration of more hydrophobic agents, epinephrine is more commonly added to agents that are more hydrophilic, such as lidocaine.

Many reports of sudden cardiac arrest with bupivacaine injection were associated with considerable morbidity and mortality. This agent's high affinity for the local anesthetic receptor protein and its high lipid solubility may be the main causes. By consensus, the 0.75% concentration of bupivacaine is not used in obstetrics because of the associated mortality/toxicity.

Levobupivacaine

Levobupivacaine is the *S*-enantiomer of bupivacaine, which is a racemic mixture containing equal amounts of the *R* and *S* enantiomers. Compared with bupivacaine, the CNS and cardiovascular toxicity of levobupivacaine is considerably reduced, allowing a larger dose to be given. The clinical profile and potency of levobupivacaine appear similar to those of bupivacaine. Levobupivacaine is particularly useful when large doses are required, as for plexus blocks.

Ropivacaine

Concerns about the cardiotoxicity of bupivacaine led to the development of ropivacaine. Ropivacaine can be administered in larger doses than bupivacaine before early signs of toxicity develop. The clinical profile of ropivacaine is similar to that of bupivacaine, but ropivacaine is less lipid soluble and less potent than bupivacaine. Epidural application may allow for even greater sensory block without significant motor block. An intrinsic vasoconstricting effect (also true for levobupivacaine) may augment the duration of action and reduce the incidence of cardiotoxicity.

Amino-ester local anesthetics

Procaine

Procaine was used mainly for infiltration and spinal blocks in the last century, before lidocaine use became popular (Table 46.2). Low potency, slow onset (probably a result of its high dissociation constant [pK$_a$]), and short duration of action all limit the use of procaine. Allergic reactions are possible because of the production of the metabolite PABA (see Figure 47.1).

Chloroprocaine

Because of its relatively low potency and extremely low toxicity, relatively high concentrations of chloroprocaine can be used. This agent also has an extremely short plasma half-life because it is metabolized very rapidly by cholinesterase. Reports of CNS

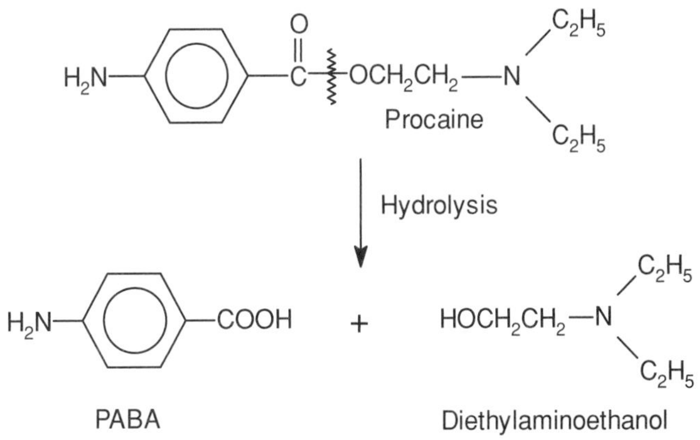

Figure 47.1. Metabolism of a typical ester local anesthetic.

toxicity are extremely unusual. Chloroprocaine is thought to have the lowest CNS and cardiovascular toxicity rates of all agents in current use. Chloroprocaine is used commonly for epidural anesthesia. It also is used for peripheral blocks in combination with other long-acting, slow-onset local anesthetics, for the combined effect of rapid onset and prolonged duration. In obstetrics, epidural chloroprocaine, with or without bicarbonate, is used to rapidly attain surgical levels of anesthesia in preparation for cesarean section. Another advantage in obstetrics is that there is virtually no transmission of chloroprocaine to the fetus. Epidurally administered chloroprocaine may, however, interfere with the action of epidurally administered amide anesthetics or opioids.

There is controversy regarding the use of chloroprocaine related to reports of persistent, serious neurologic deficits associated with accidental massive subarachnoid injection. Initially, the agent itself was thought to be implicated. Subsequent evaluation suggests that the preservative, antioxidant bisulfite, may by itself produce the phenomenon. However, after elimination of bisulfite, several reports of back pain appeared. Moreover, renewed interest led to a report suggesting that bisulfite actually may have been neuroprotective in an animal model.

Tetracaine

Tetracaine is a slow-onset, potent, intermediate- to long-acting ester-type local anesthetic. Even longer duration of action can be achieved when it is administered with a vasoconstrictor such as epinephrine; however, it is quite toxic. Animal studies suggest that tetracaine might cause neurotoxicity at high doses and may cause cauda equina syndrome with repeated spinal dosing. It is used mainly topically or sometimes for spinal anesthesia. Tetracaine is highly lipid soluble, and a significant amount may get absorbed when used on mucous membranes or wounded skin.

Cocaine

Cocaine, the only naturally occurring local anesthetic used clinically, is also the only local anesthetic that causes intense vasoconstriction. Thus, it is used as a topical anesthetic, such as in anesthetizing the cornea or the nasal airway before endotracheal intubation. Cocaine inhibits the neuronal reuptake of catecholamines and therefore may cause hypertension, tachycardia, dysrhythmias, and other serious cardiac effects.

Benzocaine

Benzocaine has a slow onset and short duration of action and is both minimally potent and minimally toxic. Its clinical use is limited to topical anesthesia to anesthetize mucous membranes – for example, to anesthetize the oral and pharyngeal mucosa before fiberoptic endotracheal intubation. Excessive use of benzocaine is associated with methemoglobinemia.

Mixture of local anesthetics

The rationale for mixing local anesthetics is an attempt to benefit from their respective pharmacokinetics: a quick onset with the short-acting drug while prolonging anesthesia with the long-acting drug. However, the beneficial effects of local anesthetic agent mixtures may be overstated. For example, bupivacaine provides a clinically acceptable onset of action as well as prolonged anesthesia. In addition, catheter techniques for many forms of regional anesthesia make it possible to extend the duration of action of rapid- and short-acting agents such as chloroprocaine and lidocaine. Most importantly, one should be cautioned against the use of maximum doses of two local anesthetics. Toxicities of these agents are independent; the toxicities should be presumed to be additive, or even synergistic/supra-additive.

Topical local anesthetics

Eutectic mixture of local anesthetic

Eutectic mixture of local anesthetic (EMLA) cream is a mixture of lidocaine and prilocaine, each at a concentration of 2.5%. It is a eutectic mixture because it has a melting point below room temperature and therefore exists as a viscous liquid rather than a solid powder. EMLA should be applied to intact skin surfaces, because application to breached skin surfaces may lead to unpredictably rapid absorption. It provides dermal analgesia by the release of the lidocaine and prilocaine from the cream into the skin, which leads to blockade of pain transmission originating from the free nerve endings. The onset, quality, and duration of dermal analgesia depend primarily on the duration of skin application. Although there is considerable interpatient variation, EMLA cream should be applied under an occlusive dressing for about 1 hour to provide adequate analgesia for insertion of an intravenous catheter. The maximum recommended duration of exposure is 4 hours, although exposures of up to 24 hours have not led to toxic plasma levels of local anesthetics.

For intravenous catheter placement or the drawing of blood, roughly 2.5 g of the cream should be applied over a 25-cm^2 area of skin, about 1 hour before the procedure. Caution must be taken in children or very small adults, as plasma levels of lidocaine and prilocaine depend on patient size and the rate of systemic drug elimination. A large application area, a long duration of application, and impaired elimination may result in high blood values of the local anesthetics.

Lidocaine patch (5%)

The lidocaine patch (Lidoderm; Endo Pharmaceuticals, Newark, DE) was approved by the US Food and Drug Administration in 1999 for the treatment of pain associated with postherpetic neuralgia, a chronic neuropathic pain condition. The patch is a topical delivery system intended to deliver low doses of lidocaine to superficially damaged or dysfunctional cutaneous nociceptors in an amount sufficient to produce analgesia but not mechanosensory block. Its recommended dosing is an application of up to three patches to intact painful skin areas for 12 hours per day.

Pharmacokinetic studies have demonstrated that clinically insignificant plasma levels are achieved with this formulation. The levels are one tenth of those required to produce cardiac activity and 1/32 of those required to produce toxicity. However, patients often report pain relief even during the 12 hours between patch applications, although lidocaine plasma half-life is much shorter. This suggests that some cumulative benefit results from prolonged delivery of the drug.

Suggested readings

Ferrante FM, Paggioli J, Cherukuri S, Arthur GR. The analgesic response to intravenous lidocaine in the treatment of neuropathic pain. *Anesth Analg* 1996; 82(1):91–97.

Hampl KF, Schneider MC, Ummenhofer W, Drewe J. Transient neurologic symptoms after spinal anesthesia. *Anesth Analg* 1995; 81(6):1148–1153.

Heavner JE. Pharmacology of Local Anesthetics. *Longnecker's Anesthesiology*. McGraw-Hill; 2008: 954–971.

Rowbotham MC, Davies PS, Verkempinck C, Galer BS. Lidocaine patch: double-blind controlled study of a new treatment method for post-herpetic neuralgia. *Pain* 1996; 65(1):39–44.

Strichartz GR, Berde CB. Local anesthetics. In: Miller RD, ed. *Miller's Anesthesia*. 6 ed. New York: Churchill Livingstone; 2004:573–603.

Stymne B, Lillieborg S. Plasma concentrations of lignocaine and prilocaine after a 24-h application of analgesic cream (EMLA) to leg ulcers. *Br J Dermatol* 2001; 145(4):530–534.

Throm MJ, Stevens MD, Hansen C. Benzocaine-induced methemoglobinemia in two patients: interdisciplinary collaboration, management, and near misses. *Pharmacotherapy* 2007; 27(8):1206–1214.

Tucker GT, Mather LE. Properties, absorption, and disposition of local anesthetic agents. In: Cousin MJ, Bridenbaugh PO, eds. *Neural Blockade in Clinical Anesthesia and Management of Pain*. 3 ed. Philadelphia: Lippincott Williams & Wilkins; 1998:55–95.

Woolf CJ. Windup and central sensitization are not equivalent [editorial]. *Pain* 1996; 66(2–3):105–108.

Woolf CJ, Thompson SW. The induction and maintenance of central sensitization is dependent on N-methyl-D-aspartic acid receptor activation; implications for the treatment of post-injury pain hypersensitivity states. *Pain* 1991; 44(3):293–299.

Anesthesia Techniques

Sascha S. Beutler, editor

Administration of general anesthesia

Francis X. Dillon and Rana Badr

Introduction

The primary goal of anesthesia is to provide patient comfort and safety during surgery or to facilitate the surgical procedure itself. Anesthesia can be general, regional, and local, depending on the needs of the patient and surgeon. In this chapter, we will discuss general anesthesia.

General anesthesia is a reversible drug-induced state of unconsciousness with hypnosis, amnesia, analgesia, and elimination of the patient response to the painful stimuli, sometimes accompanied by paralysis.

Preoperative preparation

Preoperative evaluation

Preparation for administration of general anesthesia is affected by whether the surgery is elective or emergency, the extent of the procedure, and the patient's comorbidities. Table 48.1 summarizes the steps usually involved in preoperative preparation.

For elective procedures, a preoperative visit to the hospital's pre-admitting test center several days before surgery can have tremendous value. This is an opportunity to evaluate the patient for comorbidities, perform necessary tests and consults, discuss the anesthesia plan with the patient, and address the patient's concerns. Anesthesia information leaflets provided preoperatively have been shown to have a significant effect on patient satisfaction and are a way to evaluate comorbidities, decrease patient anxiety, and prevent an unnecessary cancellation of surgery.

Decisions regarding specific preoperative tests and procedures should be individualized and depend on information obtained from patient's medical record, history and physical examination, and the type and invasiveness of the planned procedure. For example, a patient with renal failure may need dialysis before the procedure, a patient with an implantable cardioverter–defibrillator may need the device turned off, or a hypovolemic patient may need fluid resuscitation before induction to minimize hemodynamic instability. Of course, in an emergency situation, time for preparation is scarce. The most important aspects of the preoperative evaluation include a problem and medication list, allergies, NPO (nothing by mouth) status, chest examination, and airway evaluation.

Preparing anesthesia equipment

There are basic steps that need to be addressed before each anesthesia case, including anesthesia machine checkout, preparation of appropriate equipment for intubation, basic ASA (American Society of Anesthesiologists) monitors, and medications. In trauma centers, it is necessary to have a dedicated trauma room available at all times for emergent cases. This room should be checked on a daily basis and contain medications, intravenous (IV) fluids, a rapid infusion device, and other equipment ready to be used. Obstetric centers should have a dedicated emergency cesarean section room.

Preparing the patient

Discussion of the anesthetic plan with the patient or guardian will help address his or her concerns and help ease the patient's anxiety. An informed consent should also be obtained at this time, although it may not always be possible in emergent cases. In such a situation, the attempt to obtain informed consent and the reasons for proceeding without it should be clearly documented in the chart before the surgical procedure is undertaken. The anesthesiologist should also become familiar with the surgical plan.

Table 48.1. Preoperative preparation

Preoperative preparation step	Considerations
Evaluating the patient	History and physical Laboratory tests NPO status Airway evaluation Anesthetic plan
Preparing anesthesia equipment	Anesthesia machine Monitors Fluid warmer Emergency medications
Preparing the patient	Discussion of anesthetic plan Obtaining consent Preoperative medication Line placement
Assessing need for blood products	Type and screen, cross-match, contact blood bank

IV access

Adequate and reliable IV access is an important part of preparation for anesthesia and surgery. In surgeries with significant risk of bleeding or fluid loss, at least two large-bore IV lines (≥16-gauge) are necessary. If a reliable peripheral IV line is not available, central line placement should be considered. When obtaining access, it is important to pay attention to patient-specific factors, such as history of radical mastectomy or previous arteriovenous fistula.

Premedication

Relief of anxiety and pain is an important aspect of premedication. Reassurance and appropriate interaction with the patient are effective ways to relieve patient anxiety. One may use a benzodiazepine or an opioid premedication, with midazolam and fentanyl being the most commonly used agents for this purpose. Occasionally, clonidine and other medications are used as well. In the case of an emergency surgery or underlying gastroesophageal reflux, H_2-receptor blockers and metoclopramide may be given by slow intravenous infusion. Metaclopramide is a useful tool to promote gastric emptying, but it must be administered slowly, over 3 to 4 minutes. If given as a rapid bolus injection, it often results in severe anxiety or panic attack. If an awake fiber-optic intubation is part of the anesthetic plan, glycopyrrolate may be used to decrease airway secretions, and airway topicalization with local anesthetic and phenylephrine or oxymetazoline spray, if the nasotracheal route is planned, may be performed. Sometimes β-blockers are administered preoperatively to control heart rate, especially in patients with ischemic heart disease.

Blood products

Blood product availability is important any time there is possibility of significant bleeding. Before surgery is begun, there should be clear documentation that the blood or blood products previously requested to be put on reserve are indeed available. There should be clear communication with the blood bank whenever the emergency release of blood products is necessary.

Monitoring plan

The decision for additional monitoring is usually made during the preoperative evaluation and sometimes may evolve during surgery. In addition to basic ASA monitoring required for all patients undergoing general anesthesia, the following may be necessary:

Arterial line: Indications include significant blood loss and fluid shifts, as well as underlying comorbidities that can result in hemodynamic instability. An indwelling arterial line is a convenient way to draw arterial blood gases. An arterial line is also indicated when the surgery itself is associated with rapid changes in blood pressure, for example, resection of a pheochromocytoma or clipping of an intracranial aneurysm.

Central venous pressure line and *pulmonary artery catheter:* Indications may include patients with significant cardiac or renal disease undergoing major surgery, large fluid shifts and blood loss, and the possibility of significant change in peripheral vascular resistance and cardiac output. With the advent of portable ultrasound devices to aid in insertion of a central venous catheter, these devices should be used whenever possible to decrease the incidence of inadvertent carotid artery puncture or cannulation.

Transesophageal echocardiogram (TEE): TEE may be used in cardiovascular surgery or in patients with reduced cardiac function undergoing major surgery. It is increasingly being used instead of a pulmonary artery catheter in cardiac surgery. An evaluation by TEE may be required to obtain the most precise information to guide surgical interventions (e.g., myocardial revascularization, valvular competence, and repair of congenital heart defects), pharmacologic support, or fluid administration in the perioperative period.

Esophageal Doppler monitor (EDM): The EDM is a promising noninvasive technique to estimate left ventricular preload and cardiac output. An esophageal probe is inserted into the lower esophagus. Blood flow in the descending aorta is calculated from the area under the velocity–time curve and the aortic cross-sectional area.

Foley catheter: Urine output monitoring is necessary whenever there is a risk of significant bleeding, fluid shifts, long surgical time, or preexisting renal impairment. A Foley catheter is also employed for abdominal hysterectomy and other major gynecologic procedures to monitor urine output in case a ureter is inadvertantly transected during the procedure. If suspected, the surgeon will ask the anesthetist to administer methylene blue, which appears in the Foley bag within minutes. If irrigation fluid in the surgical field turns blue after the methylene blue is given, it indicates that a ureter or the bladder may have been lacerated.

Bispectral index (BIS) monitor (or other depth-of-anesthesia monitors): This monitor has become popular with increasing scientific and media attention about awareness under anesthesia. The utility of electroencephalogram monitoring remains controversial. Patients at high risk for awareness under anesthesia include those undergoing cardiac surgery, trauma surgery, or obstetric surgery under general anesthesia, and those with unusually high anesthetic requirements.

Induction of anesthesia

Application of appropriate monitoring, measuring of preinduction vital signs, and preoxygenation should precede induction of anesthesia. In emergency and trauma cases, additional preinduction considerations may include full-stomach precautions, possibility of alcohol and drug intoxication, and cervical spine and hemodynamic instability. Table 48.2 outlines common induction-related issues and considerations.

Table 48.2. Induction of anesthesia

Induction-related issue	Considerations
Choice of anesthetic agent	Intravenous Intramuscular Inhalational
Stages of anesthesia	Guedel's stages of anesthesia (Table 48.3)
Airway management	Endotracheal tube Laryngeal mask airway Fiberoptic intubation Management of a difficult intubation
Positioning	Nerve and soft tissue injury Hemodynamic changes

Choice of anesthetic agents

Inhalation induction, using only inhalational agents, is often chosen for induction of general anesthesia in children and occasionally in adults when IV access is difficult to obtain prior to induction. An inhalational induction is also used, with an IV in place, when the airway is compromised and the goal is to maintain spontaneous respiration throughout the induction until the airway can be secured with an endotracheal tube. Most commonly, sevoflurane is used as it is thought to be relatively non-irritating to the airway, although other agents, such as isoflurane and halothane also have been used successfully. Table 48.3 outlines Guedel's four stages of general anesthesia. Guedel's stages were formulated around the time of World War II to aid medical corps and nursing personnel in administering ether because it was the only induction agent used at the time. When using the newer inhalational agents, it is more difficult to appreciate the stages, especially when an IV induction agent, such as propofol, is used along with them.

IV induction agents are considered the principal route of anesthetic induction, especially in adults and in emergency cases. In emergency cases, induction is usually performed in rapid sequence (see later) and with in-line neck stabilization in trauma cases. In hemodynamically unstable patients, etomidate or ketamine may be a better choice. Muscle relaxants are used to improve intubating conditions. With the exception of rapid-sequence induction, the ability to ventilate the lungs is usually assessed prior to the administration of a muscle relaxant.

Rapid-sequence induction refers to induction in which the IV injection of a drug to produce unconsciousness is followed immediately by a neuromuscular blocking drug that produces a rapid onset of skeletal muscle paralysis (e.g., succinylcholine). Mask ventilation is traditionally avoided until the patient's airway is secured with an endotracheal tube. In addition, cricoid pressure may be applied from the beginning of induction until the correct placement of the endotracheal tube is confirmed. The goal of these maneuvers is to reduce the risk of aspiration during induction. Therefore, rapid-sequence induction is typically performed in patients with significant reflux disease, bowel obstruction, or a full stomach, and in trauma patients and pregnant patients. All are considered a high risk for aspiration.

Intramuscular induction agents, mainly ketamine, occasionally are used in combative, mentally challenged patients. Detailed information about different induction agents can be found in Chapter 34.

Airway management and anesthetic techniques

The decision to use mask ventilation, laryngeal mask airway, or an endotracheal tube (orotracheal vs. nasotracheal) depends on the risk of aspiration, necessity of muscle relaxation, length of surgery, and patient positioning. Regardless of the primary plan of airway management, anesthesiologists must always be prepared for the need to perform an endotracheal intubation. This requires precise preoperative evaluation of the airway and readiness to deal with potentially difficult intubations. A difficult intubation cart should be readily available. Discussion regarding management of a difficult intubation is presented elsewhere in the text. Hemodynamic effects of laryngoscopy may be significant and severe degrees of arterial oxygen desaturation may occur if the anesthesiologist is unable to insert quickly an endotracheal tube. It is always advisable to preoxygenate before attempting endotracheal intubation, especially when a difficult airway is suspected or encountered.

Table 48.3. Guedel's stages of general anesthesia with ether as the sole agent

Stage	General description	Guedel's clinical criteria, simplified				
		Respiratory pattern	Eyeball activity	Pupil size	Eyelid reflex	Risk of vomiting, laryngospasm
I	Analgesia	Slow, regular	Baseline	Baseline	Present	
II	Delirium Excitement Unconsciousness	Irregular	Markedly increased	Reactive to light, may be dilated	Present, starts to disappear	Increased
III	Surgical anesthesia	Regular, then progresses to complete paralysis	Decreases progressively, then ceases	Gradual dilation	None	
IV	Respiratory paralysis Cardiovascular collapse	Complete paralysis	None	Complete dilation	None	

Positioning

Proper patient positioning requires particular attention from the anesthesia team to avoid pressure on the peripheral nerves and soft tissues. This is especially important in the prone, lateral, and lithotomy positions. Hemodynamic effects of positioning may be significant as well. In a patient with an arteriovenous fistula, it is important to avoid excessive pressure and to confirm its patency.

Maintenance

Maintenance of anesthesia is achieved with either IV or inhalational agents, or a combination thereof. Close attention to the patient's vital signs, ventilation, the surgical field, and blood loss is an important aspect of care during this time. Communication with the surgical team also is important. For example, excessive pressure on the diaphragm might be the reason for bradycardia, or if it is challenging to catch up with blood loss, the surgeon may be able to temporarily stop the procedure and prevent ongoing bleeding by applying direct pressure on the vessels.

The total IV anesthesia (TIVA) technique uses only IV drugs for the induction and maintenance of anesthesia. Drugs used for this technique may include hypnotics such as propofol, opioids such as fentanyl and remifentanil, and sometimes a muscle relaxant. No inhalational agents are used for this type of anesthesia. TIVA is the main route of administration of anesthesia in patients susceptible to malignant hyperthermia (MH). This mode of anesthesia may be associated with less postoperative nausea and vomiting. A detailed description of this technique is discussed in Chapter 49.

Inhalational anesthetic techniques are widely used and are an alternative to TIVA. These agents, except for nitrous oxide (N_2O), are not safe to use in MH-susceptible patients. Desflurane is a potential airway irritant, and caution is advised when using it in patients with reactive airway disease.

Opioids and N_2O (65%–75%) are safe agents in MH-susceptible patients. The likelihood of intraoperative awareness with the pure opioid/N_2O method is greater than with other general anesthetic techniques. Use of depth-of-anesthesia monitoring is advised along with a propofol by infusion or intermittent boluses to help ensure an adequate anesthetic depth. A bispectral anesthesia depth monitor is of particular value in such situations. N_2O is contraindicated in surgery for bowel obstruction, pneumothorax, or in pneumoencephalograms due to its tendency to diffuse into closed air spaces, and is relatively contraindicated in patients with severe pulmonary hypertension.

Fluid management

In calculating fluid requirements under anesthesia, one needs to consider the fluid deficit from NPO status, maintenance fluid requirements, additional fluid requirements secondary to blood and other fluid loss, and metabolic state. Other fluid losses include evaporative loss (depending on the size of the incision),

losses through the gastrointestinal and respiratory systems, and third space loss. The maintenance fluid requirement is calculated based on weight: 4 ml/kg/h for the first 10 kg of weight, 2 ml/kg/h for >10 kg up to 20 kg of weight, and 1 ml/kg/h thereafter. For example, the maintenance fluid requirement for a 70-kg man is 110 ml/h. Fluid deficit is calculated based on the maintenance fluid requirement times the number of hours the patient has been NPO. Replacement of blood by crystalloid is roughly calculated by a ratio of 1:3 and for colloid by the ratio of 1:1. This means that every milliliter of blood loss should be replaced with 3 ml of crystalloid or 1 ml of colloid. When the decision is made to replace blood with packed red blood cells (PRBC), the ratio is 1:2 because the hematocrit of PRBC is twice that of whole blood. Crystalloid versus colloid replacement of fluid loss has long been debated. There is no consensus regarding the current outcome data, as each method has its advantages and disadvantages.

Blood components may be necessary during surgery if blood loss exceeds the allowable amount or if there is continuous loss and the patient remains unstable. With rapid blood loss, measured hematocrit may not be accurate. The threshold for blood transfusion also depends on the patient's age and coexisting diseases. In the case of massive transfusion, the administration of platelets and fresh frozen plasma may be necessary. Detailed information about transfusion and fluid management may be found in Sections XI and XII of this textbook.

Pain management

The ASA practice guidelines recommend using two analgesic agents that have a single route but act by different mechanisms, allowing better analgesic response with equal or fewer adverse effects. Examples include the administration of epidural opioids with local anesthetics or clonidine, or administration of IV opioids in combination with ketorolac or ketamine. Multimodal pain management is a growing trend in acute postoperative pain management. It has been shown that nociceptive neurons are involved primarily in the attraction of opioid-containing leukocytes during early stages of inflammation. Compared with patient-controlled IV analgesia, epidural analgesia may result in significantly decreased migration of β-endorphin–containing leukocytes to the injured site 24 hours after surgery. Regional anesthesia such as epidural, peripheral nerve block, single dose, or continuous nerve block may improve postoperative pain control and reduce the inflammatory response. Acupuncture also has been shown to reduce the analgesic requirement by up to 21%. Clonidine has been used for postoperative pain control, with dose-dependent side effects of hypotension and sedation. Nonsteroidal anti-inflammatory drugs, opioids, ketamine, and clonidine all have been used in multimodal pain management.

Intraoperative problems

Airway difficulties, hypotension, arrhythmias, anaphylaxis, and emergence have been shown to cause the most serious intraoperative anesthesia problems. A trained anesthesiologist will have an armamentarium of "mental algorithms" to quickly approach these serious problems and also to resolve less serious but common intraoperative problems.

Table 48.4 provides an overview of common intraoperative problems that may occur during anesthesia. Table 48.5 is a more elaborate algorithmic approach to intraoperative hypoxemia. Neither of these tables represents an exhaustive presentation of the topics.

In the following sections, selected intraoperative problems are discussed.

Hypotension

Hypotension is very common during induction. Anesthetics cause a dose-dependent decrease in blood pressure as a result of pharmacologically induced myocardial depression, decreased systemic vascular resistance (SVR) from lowered sympathetic outflow, or both. Compounding this hypotensive tendency is the possibility that the patient may be dehydrated and may have reduced preload.

The usual, initial approach to dealing with intraoperative hypotension is to treat it immediately with a single dose of a short-acting pressor such as phenylephrine, 40 to 80 μg IV, ephedrine, 5 to 10 mg IV, to lighten the anesthesia if feasible; and to infuse fluid boluses.

The use of pressors and fluids is often the only temporizing measure until the source of hypotension is identified and resolved. Besides the anesthetic, other causes include surgical procedure itself (e.g., bleeding, retractors compressing the inferior vena cava), the patient's medical condition necessitating the surgical procedure (e.g., septic shock, ruptured aortic aneurysm, trauma), or co-morbidities (e.g., heart failure).

It is also important to recognize that spinal or epidural anesthesia should not be used in patients with hemorrhagic hypotension from acute blood loss, such as a gunshot wound to the lower extremity. In such patients, the onset of a sympathetic block from the regional anesthetic may cause pooling of blood in the lower extremities, thereby decreasing venous return to the heart (preload) and exacerbating the hypotension. In extreme cases, pulseless electrical activity and death can result.

Hypertension

Hypertension also is commonly encountered. Most brief hypertensive episodes are benign and are related to a sudden increase in surgical stimulation. Thus, the best first option is simply to deepen anesthesia with an IV bolus of propofol and to increase the concentration of a volatile inhaled anesthetic. Administration of an opioid medication such as fentanyl also may be appropriate.

If inadequate anesthetic depth likely is not the contributor to hypertension, practitioners generally consider the use of short-acting antihypertensive medication (e.g., nitroglycerin, 40 μg IV bolus), especially when the hypertensive episode may be catastrophic (e.g., bleeding intracranial aneurysm).

Infusion of a short-acting antihypertensive drug (e.g., nitroglycerin, nitroprusside, or esmolol) may be needed to control blood pressure throughout the surgical procedure. The agent should be infused via a stopcock near the hub of the venous intracatheter. That way, the dead space of the IV line is low, meaning changes in medication infusion rates will reach the patient quickly. Nitroprusside administration requires the use of intra-arterial monitoring because reduction of systolic pressure occurs so rapidly that severe hypotension can result within 2 to 3 minutes, and if undetected could be dangerous.

If it becomes evident that the hypertension will persist well into the postoperative period, longer-acting antihypertensive medications (e.g., hydralazine IV, labetalol IV) may be considered. However, there is a tendency to overtreat hypertension until the cumulative overdosage is evident and the patient is hypotensive.

Hypoxemia

Hypoxemia deserves special emphasis. When it occurs during anesthesia, diagnosis and therapy must be done expeditiously. Uncorrected hypoxemia leads to anaerobic metabolism and metabolic acidosis from lactic acid. This adversely affects the biochemistry of the cell and may indeed be irreversible, leading to organ damage or death. See Table 48.5 for a good approach to intraoperative hypoxemia. The brain is at extreme risk from severe hypoxia lasting longer than 4 to 8 minutes, the reason being that cerebral neuronal function is almost entirely dependant on the aerobic metabolism of glucose. Sustained periods of anoxia carry a high probability of irreversible brain damage.

Failure to ventilate

Failure to ventilate may occur at any stage during an anesthetic. At induction, it can occur when the anesthetist is unable to ventilate by mask or to insert an endotracheal tube during a rapid intubation for a full stomach. In severe cases, insertion of a laryngeal mask airway may restore the ability to ventilate. In any such event, the ASA Difficult Airway Algorithm should be familiar to every anesthesiologist and followed in such situations. During the anesthetic itself, after an airway is established, ventilation can be lost because of a disconnection, a leak in the circuit or tube or from an obstruction, or the endotracheal tube itself becoming dislodged. This constitutes an emergency and immediate threat to the patient. The surgical team should be informed immediately; they may be able to help quickly by reconnecting the circuit if it is in the surgical field.

The commonest site of disconnection is where the 15-mm polyethylene adapter connects to the tracheal tube or the circuit. If the ventilator or capnography alarm indicates failure to ventilate, the entire length of the circuit and tube should be inspected or palpated. The connections from the machine to the circuit's inspiratory and expiratory limbs (called 22-mm adapters) should be checked; they also are common sites of disconnection.

Table 48.4. Common intraoperative problems and differential diagnoses

Problem	Differential diagnosis	Remarks
Hypotension	Hypovolemia	The most common cause is blood loss or preoperative fasting and dehydration.
	Vasodilatation from medication	Any opioid, sedative, or anesthetic may reduce central sympathetic outflow and cause vasodilation.
		Virtually every anesthetic induction or heavy sedation will be accompanied by this finding.
	Sepsis or SIRS	During surgery for an infectious process, sudden decreases in blood pressure are often from sepsis or SIRS.
	Low cardiac output	Many anesthetics decrease cardiac output; congestive heart failure or myocardial infarction may do this also.
	Severe bradycardia	This may cause low cardiac output, resulting in hypotension.
	Severe tachycardia	If atrial fibrillation or flutter conduction to the ventricle becomes too fast, hypotension may result.
	Pneumothorax	This is uncommon but may spontaneously arise during positive pressure ventilation with or without anesthesia.
Hypertension	Pain or surgical stimulus	The first thing to consider if blood pressure rises: "light" or insufficient anesthetic depth.
	Essential hypertension	Such patients may be adequately anesthetized but still markedly hypertensive.
	Tourniquet or cuff	A surgical tourniquet on an extremity produces a hard, recalcitrant kind of hypertension called "cuff hypertension."
	Lightening anesthesia	Has blood loss, an empty vaporizer or medication infusor, or rapid drug clearance made the patient "light"?
	Preeclampsia	Perhaps the most common cause of acute peripartum hypertension. May be accompanied by seizures, proteinuria, acute renal injury, acute liver failure, thrombocytopenia, or coagulopathy.
	Hypervolemia	In the setting of hypertension, it is possible to overfill or overtransfuse and predispose to pulmonary edema and congestive heart failure acutely.
	Pheochromocytoma	Patients have been known to have an occult tumor secreting epinephrine or norepinephrine, but this is rare.
	Hyperadrenocorticalism	Patients who are cushingoid, hypertensive, or hypokalemic may have this.
Hypoxemia	Low FiO_2	Increase FiO_2 immediately while searching for the cause.
	Hypoventilation	May be the result of opioids, benzodiazepines, muscle relaxants, or inhalation agents, which decrease respiratory drive and/or muscle strength.
	Disconnection of circuit	The commonest cause of serious hypoxemic accidents
	Atelectasis	A result of patients being intubated and receiving positive pressure ventilation. Consider gentle recruitment maneuvers.
	Mucus plugging	Suction and recruitment maneuvers.
	Right main stem intubation	Maximum depth for tracheal tubes measured from teeth (on average): females, 21 cm; males, 23 cm. May visualize with bronchoscope.
	Pulmonary thromboembolism	Significant pulmonary embolism leads to sudden drop in end-tidal CO_2, and hypoxemia that does not improve on 100% FiO_2, accompanied by tachycardia and hypotension.
	Pulmonary edema	May be secondary to fluid overload, diastolic dysfunction, systolic dysfunction, or myocardial infarction.
	Venous air embolism	Also causes drop in end-tidal CO_2, and an increase in end-tidal N_2.
Failure to ventilate	Kinked tube	Most likely during ENT anesthetics or in prone position if no armored endotracheal tube is used.
	Biting on tube	Especially during "light" anesthesia or emergence.
	Disconnection of tube from circuit or adapter	Still the commonest cause of severe hypoxia during general anesthesia.
	Complete obstruction from mucus or tissue	May occur very rapidly in infants and children whose endotracheal tubes are narrow; worse when no humidification is used. May need to replace tube very quickly. Encountered more often in the ICU setting.
	Hole in tube or punctured cuff	Laser airway surgery and tracheostomies are particularly common settings for this problem. Beware of the risk of airway fire in tracheostomy and laser airway surgery!
High peak airway pressures	Kinked tube	May require the use of an armored (metal spring–reinforced) tube to prevent kinking.
	Biting on tube	May require the use of a bite block or mouth gag, or the emergent use of a neuromuscular blocking drug.
	Bronchospasm	First approach usually is to deepen anesthesia, then consider neuromuscular blockade; administer β-agonists, inhaled or IV corticosteroids, and methylxanthines (e.g., aminophylline) occasionally.
	Mucus plugging (smaller tubes, copious mucus production, and nonhumidified gases predispose)	Patients with COPD, asthma, cystic fibrosis, tracheostomy, pneumonia, or otherwise excessive secretions may have plugging of significance. It may require replacement of the endotracheal tube but usually improves with suctioning and humidification of anesthetic gases.
	Pneumothorax (although this may happen in any anesthetic, predisposing surgeries include thyroidectomy, mastectomy, tracheal procedures, nephrectomy, and the use of high PEEP)	This causes increased peak airway pressures if the pneumothorax is extreme. Likewise, a complete inability to ventilate may be caused by a pneumomediastinum or a pneumothorax.
High mean airway pressures	Bronchospasm	May be severe enough to prevent ventilation.
	Stacking or auto-PEEP of mechanical breaths	This happens when the expiratory phase is not long enough to allow exhalation. Slow the respiratory rate.

Table 48.4 (continued)

Problem	Differential diagnosis	Remarks
	Dynamic airway obstruction	May be from airway neoplasm or mediastinal mass.
	Pneumothorax	Other things would be observable first: hypotension, hypoxia.
	Obesity or chest wall restriction of excursion	Fairly common and may be difficult to treat.
	ARDS	Common cause of high mean pressures in ICU patient with respiratory failure.
Hypocarbia	Hypothermia	Most evident in severe hypothermia.
	Massive pulmonary embolus	A sudden drop in expired CO_2 should make one think of this.
	Hyperventilation	Patients who are anxious (awake) or mechanically hyperventilated (anesthetized) may have this.
	Leak in CO_2 sampling tubing	This also may cause an abnormal shape of the capnograph waveform or envelope.
Hypercarbia	Hyperthermia	Metabolic rate increases 15% for every 1°C.
	Malignant hyperthermia	Uncoupling of calcium metabolism in mitochondria from a rare (1:15,000) genetic defect in the ryanodine receptor of the calcium channel.
	Hypoventilation	May be from opioid medication, residual neuromuscular blocking drug, or weakness from a variety of reasons.
	Increased "dead space"	From a variety of causes: long endotracheal tube, lung disease, etc.
	Increased diffusion gradient in lung	From COPD, interstitial lung disease, ARDS, pulmonary edema, or previous chemotherapy.
	Increased metabolic rate from feedings	Feeding patients with COPD often makes it difficult to liberate (wean) them from mechanical ventilation in the ICU.
Hypothermia	Administration of unwarmed fluid or blood products	Ideally, all fluids should be warmed by an FDA-approved device. No microwave or ad hoc fluid heating methods are safe!
	Anesthetic effects on hypothalamus	Every general anesthetic causes impaired central thermoregulation due to its effect on the hypothalamus.
	Conductive, radiative, evaporative losses	Wet drapes or sheets; exposed skin or body cavities, or nonheated breathing circuits.
	Massive blood loss	Very difficult to keep patients warm after 1 blood volume has been lost. Use FDA approved warming devices only!
	TURP or other irrigation with unwarmed fluid	Surprisingly few urology suites use warmed TURP/TURBT irrigation. Hypothermia is common after TURP/TURBT.
Hyperthermia	Malignant hyperthermia	Specific therapy for MH: dantrolene IV plus other measures. If MH is suspected, call for help and consult.
	Fever from SIRS, sepsis, or transfusion reaction	Use acetaminophen or ibuprofen in addition to a cooling blanket.
	Stroke	Sudden extreme hyperthermia (> 105°F) may be from a stroke to the hypothalamus.
	Neuroleptic malignant syndrome	Relatively uncommon side effect that may develop after use of an antipsychotic medication, e.g., chlorpromazine, haloperidol, olanzapine, escitalopram.
	Excessive warming	Use the air-warming blanket at room temperature setting to cool the patient.
Bradycardia	Increased vagal tone	Spinal anesthesia causes sympathectomy and may lead to profound bradycardia or even asystole. Surgical stimulus on the gut or bladder (or other organs) may feed back and cause vagal tone to increase.
	Hypoxia	Occurs with severe hypoxia and is a bad prognosticator. Correct hypoxia immediately if possible.
	Increased SVR with intact baroreceptor reflex	In patients with an intact baroreceptor reflex, increased systemic vascular resistance causes increased blood pressure, which in turn causes reflex bradycardia. Phenylephrine may induce this, especially in young patients.
	β-Blockers	A common cause.
	Degenerative fibrosis of nodal tissue	This is actually considered the most common cause of bradyarrhythmias; it occurs in all settings, not just the operating room.
	Calcium channel blockers	Diltiazem is most likely to cause heart rate decreases and is used for this purpose in atrial fibrillation and flutter.
	Reversal of neuromuscular blockade with cholinesterase inhibitors such as edrophonium or neostigmine	Usually, coadministration of an anticholinergic medication such as atropine or glycopyrrolate is standard practice, so this happens rarely. However, edrophonium may be used alone to try to convert SVT or slow heart rate, or in a common test for myasthenia gravis (Tensilon test).
	Sick sinus syndrome	May require temporary or permanent pacemaker.
	Myocardial infarction	Especially if the right coronary artery and sinus node are involved in the infarction
	Third-degree heart block	The ECG rhythm strip will provide the diagnosis.
Sinus tachycardia	Pressors or inotropes	Ephedrine, epinephrine, norepinephrine, isoproterenol.
	Increased pain or surgical stimulus	The commonest cause at the start of the surgical procedure; suggests insufficient anesthesia.
	Myocardial infarction	The commonest dysrhythmia associated with MI.
	Malignant hyperthermia	Tachycardia in MH follows an observed increase in CO_2 production, and it precedes hyperthermia.
	Atropine, scopolamine, or glycopyrrolate given	These are given for drying (antisialagogues), heart rate control (vagolytics) or nausea control (antiemetics).
	β-Adrenergic agonists	Bronchodilators, tocolytics, decongestant medications, and anorexigenics (diet medications) may do this.

Note and disclaimer: Any table such as this one must necessarily be incomplete and imperfect.
ARDS, acute respiratory distress syndrome; COPD, chronic obstructive pulmonary disease; ECG, electrocardiogram; ENT, ear, nose, throat; FiO_2, fraction of inspired oxygen; FDA, US Food and Drug Administration; MI, myocardial infarction; PEEP, positive end-expiratory pressure; SIRS, systemic inflammatory response syndrome; SVT, supraventricular tachycardia; TURBT, transurethral resection of bladder tumor ; TURP, transurethral resection of the prostate .

301

Table 48.5. Steps to consider immediately and a few minutes after sudden hypoxemia in the operating room

Immediately	In a minute or so	In 3–5 minutes
Inform all caretakers Ventilate by hand; assess compliance and chest excursion Ensure 100% FiO_2 delivery. Look for disconnection: circuit, tube, 15-mm connector. Check expired gases for $ETCO_2$. Examine capnograph waveform Inspect the tube and circuit for kinking, biting, obstruction Inspect tube for excessively deep insertion: 21 cm (females); 23 cm (males). Palpate the cuff in the sternal notch while inflating and deflating it. Withdraw it if it is in too far.	Suction the tracheal tube with a thin catheter to remove secretions and assess patency or obstruction Perform direct laryngoscopy to verify tube placement in the trachea Reassess compliance and chest excursion If in doubt, replace tracheal tube under direct laryngoscopy Try bronchodilator inhaler empirically Apply recruitment maneuvers to open alveoli	Perform bronchoscopy through the tube Apply PEEP Obtain arterial blood gases Try alternate means of obtaining SaO_2 Obtain chest radiograph to rule out atelectasis or pneumothorax Consider TTE or TEE

$ETCO_2$; end-tidal CO_2; FiO_2, fraction of inspired oxygen; PEEP, positive end-expiratory pressure; SaO_2 – arterial oxygen saturation; TEE, transesophageal echocardiography; TTE, transthoracic echocardiography.

Removable plastic plugs, sampling tube fittings, cracks, and holes also should be checked for leaks, and the circuit should be checked for manufacturing defects. Next, the large rubber seals of any carbon dioxide (CO_2)-absorbent canister fittings on the anesthesia machine should be assessed, because these may become dislodged slightly when the canisters are replaced, resulting in a leak. Another source of a gross leak in the anesthesia circuit is the insertion point of the CO_2 sensor. Typically, the hole at the machine where the sensor inserts has a width of several centimeters. If the sensor falls out, it will result in an enormous leak with inability to ventilate. Although uncommon, this can generally be avoided by a thorough leak check of the anesthesia circuit prior to induction and by making certain that the sensor is firmly plugged in.

After these measures have been used and the leak diagnosed and corrected, the anesthesiologist should verify that the patient is receiving adequate ventilation. Checking the CO_2 trace may be insufficient to ensure that ventilation is optimal. The anesthesiologist should auscultate the breath sounds while giving breaths by hand and restoring mechanical ventilation. This gives valuable information as to inspiratory pressures required and the presence of rales or wheezing. The inspiratory pressure valve should also be viewed to quantitate the pressures required to ventilate. A bag–valve oxygen supply (e.g., Ambu bag) should be available on each anesthesia machine to connect to the endotracheal tube or mask in the event of circuit or machine failure that is not immediately repairable.

Obstruction of the circuit or tracheal tube or a sudden increase in airway peak pressure

One cause of obstruction of the circuit or tracheal tube or a sudden increase in airway peak pressure is concretions of dried mucus that can accumulate and, over time, completely obstruct a large adult-size tracheal tube. This phenomenon is even more common in pediatric patients, whose tracheal tubes are smaller. Humidification may reduce the risk of obstruction, but

may not prevent it entirely. When it does happen, replacement of the tracheal tube with a new one may be the only way to restore patency if suctioning with a catheter down the tube is insufficient.

More common is biting on or kinking the tracheal tube. To prevent kinking, use of an armored (embedded metallic spring) tube at the beginning of the procedure is effective. Armored tubes are especially valuable in prone and sitting cases where the endotracheal tube may be subject to torsion. A patient biting on the tube during maintenance of anesthesia usually is a sign of light anesthesia and should be treated quickly by deepening anesthesia, inserting (gently) a bite block, and/or giving a dose of neuromuscular blocking drug (10 to 20 mg of succinylcholine is sufficient to relax the jaw within 30 to 60 seconds in such a situation).

Other, less likely causes of sudden obstruction to ventilation are severe, sudden coughing or bronchospasm, pneumomediastinum causing tracheal obstruction, and tension pneumothorax. Bronchospasm is treated with bronchodilators, whereas coughing can be decreased with muscle relaxants and deeper anesthesia. Tension pneumothorax and pneumomediastinum are likely to be accompanied by severe hypotension. Needle or tube thoracocentesis is the first, emergent step for these complications.

Arrhythmias

Studies have demonstrated that approximately 50% of serious intraoperative arrhythmias are anesthesia related. The majority consist of extreme bradycardia or asystole, often resulting from spinal anesthesia with a high level, widespread sympathetic block and overriding vagal tone. Such an event usually responds to atropine (1 mg IV), IV ephedrine, and even a brief period of external cardiac massage to get the drug circulating in the event of asystole. Laparoscopy can result in sudden severe bradycardia or even asystole when the trochar pierces the peritoneum, causing an intense vagal stimulus. Again, atropine 0.2-1 mg IV (depending on severity of bradycardia) is usually effective in this situation and typically restores heart rate to 60 or greater within 45 to 90 seconds. Sudden onset of sinus tachycardia with hypertension commonly is a sign of insufficient depth of anesthesia (see earlier). Sudden onset of tachycardia with hypotension may be an ominous sign indicating an immediate life-threatening event, such as venous air embolus (e.g., intracranial surgery), pulmonary embolus (e.g., patient with known deep vein thrombosis), or myocardial ischemia with a sudden drop in cardiac output. Please refer to Chapter 155 on arrhythmias Part 28 and to the Advanced Cardiac Life Support algorithms (Chapter 153) to review the differential diagnosis of arrhythmias in detail.

Allergy problems

Severe anaphylactoid or anaphylactic reactions occur in a small but significant percentage of cases. Often, the adverse allergic reaction to a specific drug is not known prior to the anesthetic. One study demonstrated that a severe allergic reaction to neuromuscular blocking drugs occurred in one in 3000 cases of general anesthesia. If the allergy is unknown, prevention is difficult, but early diagnosis and prompt and aggressive treatment may prevent morbidity. An anaphylactic reaction is a life-threatening event, calling for immediate vigorous fluid administration to combat cardiovascular collapse, IV epinephrine, H_2-blockers, and corticosteroids.

Emergence and extubation

Preparation for emergence includes reversal of muscle relaxants and discontinuation of inhalational and IV anesthetics. The patient should meet the criteria for extubation before the endotracheal tube is removed. The decision to extubate depends on the patient's ability to ventilate and oxygenate, the provider's ability to mask ventilate or reintubate if necessary upon extubation, and the impact on the patient if the extubation fails. Tracheal extubation may be complicated by laryngospasm, aspiration, hypoventilation, or negative pressure pulmonary edema. The premature removal of an endotracheal tube during the second stage of anesthesia may be particularly dangerous.

Criteria for extubation include stable vital signs, adequate ventilation and adequate reversal of muscle relaxant (4/4 twitches on the train-of-four and sustained 100 Hz tetanus), and an awake and cooperative patient. A good clinical measure of adequate reversal of neuromuscular blockade is the patient's ability to perform a sustained head lift for 5 to 10 seconds. Occasionally, the anesthesiologist may choose "deep" extubation to prevent coughing and bucking during emergence. This technique is particularly useful in a patient with significant reactive airway disease, but may not be advisable in a patient with difficult intubation.

Common problems during emergence from general anesthesia include residual neuromuscular blockade and delayed emergence (see Chapter 52).

Residual neuromuscular blockade may be demonstrated by the use of the transcutaneous peripheral nerve stimulator, which will show posttetanic fade or significant blockade on train-of-four stimulation (see section immediately above). If maximal anticholinesterase medication has been given, the proper treatment is conservative: passive or forced-air warming, correction of metabolic acidosis, and ensuring amnesia as recovery of muscle strength occurs. Mechanical ventilation with varying degrees of support is needed in the postanesthesia care unit (PACU) or intensive care unit (ICU). Great care must be taken in such situations to ensure that the patient is adequately ventilated and not experiencing dyspnea. Dyspnea from inability to breathe adequately or spontaneously is a frightening sensation and, if possible, the patient should be asked if he or she feels that he or she is "getting enough air while being mechanically ventilated." In such cases, additional sedation may be indicated along with careful settings on the ventilator to ensure adequate ventilation.

Delayed emergence, that is, delayed regaining of consciousness following the end of an anesthetic administration, is almost always from residual anesthetic effect and is longer if surgery lasts longer. The patient is supported with mechanical ventilation, and reassuring the family (and other caretakers) is key. Drugs such as scopolamine may cause delayed emergence and distort the pupil examination. Of course, CT scanning frequently is done to reassure caretakers that no intracranial event has occurred. Neurologic consultation usually is not necessary, but patience is. Pressure points should be padded carefully, and the eyes and airway cuff should be cared for as if a prolonged anesthetic were taking place.

Agitation occasionally occurs in patients on emergence and is more common in young patients who have received general anesthesia with an inhalational agent. The anesthesiologist should rule out physiologic causes of agitation, including hypoxia, hypercarbia, a full bladder, and pain. Clonidine has been used to reduce the incidence of emergence agitation in children, but it also may delay awakening from anesthesia.

Mortality and morbidity

Overall mortality from general anesthesia is approximately one in 200,000. Morbidity related to anesthesia includes dental injury, soft tissue and nerve injury, awareness under anesthesia, and postanesthesia respiratory and cardiac complications. Administration of anesthesia has become far safer during the past 30 years, owing to improved monitoring techniques and the widespread adoption of safety standards modeled after those in the airline industry. Claims for death and brain damage decreased between 1975 and 2000. From 1986 to 2000, adverse respiratory events decreased, whereas adverse cardiovascular events increased. By 1992, respiratory- and cardiovascular-damaging events occurred in approximately the same proportion (28%), a trend that continued through 2000. The overall downward trend did not seem to be affected by the use of pulse oximetry and end-tidal carbon dioxide monitoring, which began in 1986.

There is emerging evidence that the choice of anesthetic technique may influence patients' long-term outcome, especially following surgery for certain types of cancer. The perioperative inflammatory response to surgical stress, but also to anesthetics, appears to influence particularly the cell-mediated immune response, which plays a pivotal role in scavenging cancer cells spilled into the circulation during surgery. Two small retrospective studies suggest less frequent cancer recurrence after removal of the primary tumor when regional anesthesia was used for analgesia rather than systemic opioids. Currently, larger prospective trials are under way to further explore the potentially significant impact anesthesia might have on long-term patient outcome.

Transport

The decision to transport to the PACU versus ICU depends on the need to keep the patient intubated after surgery, hemodynamic stability, significant comorbidities, and the need for frequent checks. Transfer with or without supplemental oxygen to the PACU depends on the type and length of surgery and anesthesia, as well as the patient's comorbidities. Monitoring for transport depends on the patient's stability and the length of travel. If oxygen is to be administered during transport, it is essential that the tank be checked prior to leaving the operating room. An "E" tank, most commonly used for transport, holds 660 liters when fully pressurized at 2000 p.s.i. At a 6L/min flow, a full tank will last 110 minutes; that is, just under two hours. The reserve times are directly proportional to the gauge pressure; that is, 1000 p.s.i. allows 55 minutes at 6L/min. This is of great importance when a patient is taken to the PACU or SICU (surgical intensive care unit) at the end of the anesthetic. An E-cylinder with 250 p.s.i. will only last about 15 minutes at 6L/min. This can be disastrous if an elevator is caught between floors during transit to the SICU.

Reporting to the accepting team either in the PACU or ICU by the anesthesia team is an important component of perioperative care. This report should include the patient's medical history, preoperative and intraoperative medications, ease of intubation, any problems in the operating room, intraoperative blood loss, and fluid management. A postoperative visit is a standard of practice, if feasible, in order to elicit any postoperative complications and patient satisfaction.

Suggested readings

Capuzzo M, Gilli G, Paparella L. Factors predictive of patient satisfaction with anesthesia. *Anesth Analg* 2007; 105: 435–442.

Cheney FW, Posner KL, Lee LA, et al. Trends in anesthesia-related death and brain damage: a Closed Claims analysis. *Anesthesiology* 2006; 105(6):1081–1108.

Clinical Anesthesia Procedures of the Massachusetts General Hospital. 7th ed. Philadelphia: Lippincott Williams and Wilkins; 2007.

Ead H. Post-anesthesia tracheal extubation. *Dynamics* 2004; 15:20–25.

Elicitation of expert knowledge about the post-anesthesia extubation decision. *Anesthesiology* 2001; 95:A1187.

Fasting S, Gisvold SE. Serious intraoperative problems. *Can J Anesthesiol* 2002; 49(6):545–553.

Miller RD, ed. *Miller's Anesthesia.* 7th ed. Philadelphia: Elsevier Churchill Livingstone; 2009.

Practice advisory for preanesthesia evaluation: a report by the American Society of Anesthesiologists Task Force on Preanesthesia Evaluation. *Anesthesiology* 2002; 96:485–496

Practice guidelines for acute pain management in the perioperative setting: an updated report by the American Society of Anesthesiologists Task Force on Acute Pain Management. *Anesthesiology* 2004; 100:1573–1581.

Standards for postanesthesia care. Approved by the ASA House of Delegates on October 12, 1998 and last amended on October 27, 2004. Available at http://www.asahq.org.

Statement on Transesophageal Echocardiography. Approved by House of Delegates, American Society of Anesthesiologists on October 17, 2001 and last amended on October 18, 2006. Available at http://www.asahq.org.

Chapter 49

Total intravenous anesthesia (TIVA)

Amit Gupta and J. Lance Lichtor

Introduction

Total intravenous anesthesia (TIVA) may be defined as a technique of general anesthesia using a combination of agents given solely by the intravenous (IV) route and in the absence of all inhalational agents, including nitrous oxide.

The IV route has been used to administer drugs for hundreds of years. The administration of anesthesia solely by the IV route using chloral hydrate was documented as early as the 1870s. In 1934, thiopental was introduced into clinical practice, and IV induction of anesthesia became popular. However, only in more recent years has TIVA become possible and practical; there are two reasons for this. First, only drugs with a rapid onset and shorter recovery profiles, such as propofol and the newer synthetic, short-acting opioids, are suitable for maintenance of anesthesia with IV infusion. Second, advances in computer technology have allowed the development of easier-to-use infusion delivery systems.

Indications and advantages

TIVA is indicated for any general anesthetic provided a well-functioning IV is in place. With TIVA, there is no operating room pollution by nitrous oxide or potent inhalation agents. After TIVA, patients have been shown to feel better and report a more pleasant anesthetic experience, in part because of less postoperative nausea and vomiting (PONV). In an ambulatory setting, these patients may be able to leave the recovery room earlier, reducing costs of stay. However, it has also been noted that the combination of certain IV drug infusions (e.g., propofol and dexmedetomidine) without the use of a depth-of-anesthesia monitor, may result in gross overdose and delayed awakening. Initial reports also showed that postoperatively, patients experience less pain with TIVA compared with maintenance with isoflurane.

For individuals with a personal or family history of malignant hyperthermia TIVA is frequently chosen because the use of inhalational agents is generally contraindicated for this disorder (Chapter 110).

Intravenous hypnotic drugs

Modern hypnotic drugs suitable for TIVA include propofol, midazolam, ketamine, etomidate, and dexmedetomidine. Most commonly, a hypnotic drug is combined with an opioid.

Table 49.1 provides suggested dosages for hypnotic agents used in TIVA.

Propofol has become the hypnotic drug of choice for the TIVA technique. It has a short context-sensitive half-time that is prolonged only to a minor extent as the infusion duration increases (Fig. 49.1). This allows for fast awakening, even after several hours of continuous administration. It should be noted that the time to recovery also depends on other factors (see Chapter 36). Propofol can be used by itself, with no other drugs. It causes a decrease in peripheral vascular resistance and mean arterial blood pressure (30%), but these hemodynamic side effects can be attenuated with slow injection and careful titration to effect. When used for maintenance of anesthesia, propofol is associated with less PONV than inhalation anesthesia. For example, in a study of 5161 patients, propofol reduced nausea and vomiting by 19% compared with a volatile anesthetic (Fig. 49.2).

In contrast to propofol, the context-sensitive half-time of thiopental increases rapidly following all but the shortest infusions owing to cumulation (Fig. 49.1). This property renders it unsuitable for maintenance of anesthesia. Midazolam is also rarely used as a maintenance infusion since significant and prolonged psychomotor impairment often occurs following the administration of larger doses.

Etomidate has many unfavorable side effects, such as PONV, phlebitis, excitatory movements, venous irritation, and adrenal cortical suppression, limiting its use in TIVA. When dexmedetomidine is included as an adjunct to propofol and an opioid, PONV is decreased as a result of a decreased use of intraoperative opioids. In addition, dexmedetomidine can help reduce central sympathetic outflow, a property that

Table 49.1. Suggested dosages for anesthetic agents used in general anesthesia

Agent	Loading dose, mg/kg	Maintenance infusion rate
Midazolam	0.15–0.35	–
Propofol	1–3	50–200 µg/kg/min
Thiopental	3–6	–
Etomidate	0.2–0.4	–
Ketamine	1–2	5–10 µg/kg/min
Dexmedetomidine	1 µg/kg	0.2–1.0 µg/kg/h

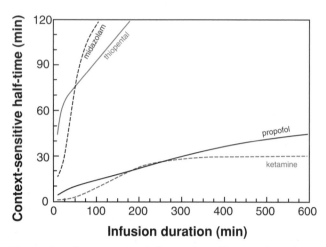

Figure 49.1. Context-sensitive half-time values of hypnotic drugs, shown as a function of infusion duration. Adapted from Figure 36.4.

enhances sedation, analgesia, anxiolysis, and amnesia, reducing the requirements and associated side effects of other drugs.

Analgesics for TIVA

Analgesia during IV anesthesia may be provided by opioids, ketamine, or local anesthetics.

The opioid analgesic chosen for TIVA must have a fast onset and be easily titratable. Fentanyl is the most commonly used opioid. It can be administered by intermittent boluses or as an infusion, and provides good postoperative pain control. However, the context-sensitive half-time of fentanyl

Table 49.2. Suggested opioid dosages for TIVA

Agent	Loading dose, μg/kg	Maintenance infusion rate	Additional boluses
Alfentanil	25–100	0.5–2 μg/kg/min	5–10 μg/kg
Sufentanil	0.25–2	0.005–0.025 μg/kg/min	2.5–10 μg
Fentanyl	4–20	0.03–0.17 μg/kg/min	25–100 μg
Remifentanil	1–2	0.025–1 μg/kg/min	0.1–1.0 μg/kg

increases markedly with prolonged infusion owing to cumulation at higher dosages. This effect may result in delayed recovery after prolonged administration. Other opioids suitable for TIVA include alfentanil and sufentanil. Remifentanil has gained popularity for the administration of TIVA because it has a short onset time, high metabolic clearance, and short context-sensitive half-time, which is independent of the duration of infusion. This desirable property is a function of its rapid enzymatic degradation in all patients, regardless of ethnicity or coexisting hepatic or renal impairment. When postoperative analgesia is desired, a longer-acting analgesic such as fentanyl or morphine should be administered.

Ketamine is a dissociative anesthetic with sedative, hypnotic, and analgesic properties. Ketamine can be used with continuous infusions of propofol as an adjunct to help reduce the opioid requirement.

Approximate opioid bolus doses, maintenance infusion rates, and additional maintenance doses are listed in Table 49.2.

Drug interactions and TIVA

In recent years, advances in computer technology and pharmacokinetic modeling have allowed us to gain a better understanding of individual drugs as well as the interactions between drugs when administered by the IV route. The context-sensitive half-times of the intravenous opioids given by infusion are shown in Figure 49.3.

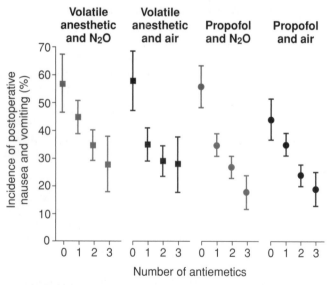

Figure 49.2. Postoperative nausea and vomiting (PONV). PONV occurs least after a propofol anesthetic with either air or nitrous oxide that also includes one or more antiemetics. Illustrated is the incidence of PONV when different anesthetics and different numbers of prophylactic antiemetic treatments are administered.

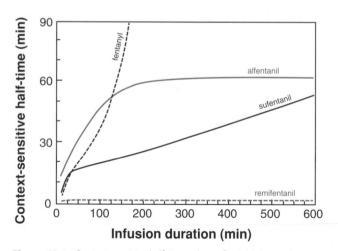

Figure 49.3. Context-sensitive half-time values of opioid drugs, shown as a function of infusion duration. Among the opioids, remifentanil is associated with the most rapid return to consciousness. Adapted from Figure 36.4.

Infusion delivery systems: manual-controlled infusion and target-controlled infusion

Two types of infusion devices can be distinguished: manual-controlled infusion (MCI) and target-controlled infusion (TCI) systems.

MCI is a continuous IV infusion with a syringe pump programmed for use with any drug used for TIVA; the anesthesiologist sets the pump's rate. These systems are widely used in operating rooms and intensive care units across the United States to administer various drugs as continuous infusions. These infusion systems are commonly referred to as *infusion pumps*.

TCI devices are now available worldwide, except in the United States. This worldwide availability primarily reflects the widespread approval of the Diprifusor (AstraZeneca, Wilmington, DE) for the administration of propofol. The anesthesiologist enters the patient's age and weight and sets the initial target blood concentration. He or she also estimates the target drug concentration based on the patient's physiologic state. The device then achieves and maintains the target concentration, with no further intervention required by the anesthesiologist. If signs of inappropriate anesthetic depth are manifested, the anesthesiologist has to adjust the set point up or down to achieve the appropriate depth of anesthesia.

Randomized trials have explored the differences in quality of anesthesia, adverse event rate, and drug cost between the two types of delivery systems (TCI vs. MCI) when administering propofol. The comparative effectiveness of the two systems remains controversial. A recent systematic review by the Cochrane Collaboration comparing the two systems did not demonstrate an advantage of either delivery system in clinical practice. The authors therefore concluded that there is not sufficient evidence to recommend the use of TCI versus MCI in clinical anesthetic practice.

This may be not surprising if one considers that the described TCI systems do not take into account many factors that influence the optimal IV dose, such as the type of operation (superficial, intra-abdominal), preexisting diseases (hepatic, renal, cardiac), and intraoperative interventions (laryngoscopy, skin incision). Anesthesiologists are very well aware that the appropriate depth of anesthesia remains a moving target that requires constant adjustments – a challenge that has not been resolved by the TCI systems on the market.

Open-loop versus closed-loop control systems

Currently, all TCI devices on the market are "open-loop" control systems, meaning that the anesthesiologist must recognize changes in the required depth of anesthesia and then adjust the target concentration appropriately (as described earlier).

"Closed-loop" control systems are in development. These systems will measure feedback signals from the patient, such as evoked potential and/or bispectral index (BIS). Based on the feedback signals, these systems will automatically adjust the target concentration, without the intervention of the anesthesiologist. These closed-loop control systems are purely investigational at this time but most likely will be part of the future technological advances in the field of anesthesia.

Limitations of TIVA

Although there is some controversy concerning TIVA and intraoperative awareness, the incidence of awareness with TIVA probably is no different than that of inhalation anesthesia. During TIVA, direct drug concentration measurements are not available and the relationships between infusion rates and adequate effect-site concentrations are not easy to establish. However, in one study, 11,785 patients were questioned for explicit recall on three occasions after anesthesia. Although TIVA was used for only about 3% of all patients, no patients who received TIVA reported recall. In that study, all the patients who did report unpleasant effects during or after wakefulness had been paralyzed. In another study of 1000 patients who specifically received TIVA with propofol, alfentanil, and paralysis, the incidence of recall (0.2%) was similar to that found in other studies. Depth-of-anesthesia monitors have been shown to reduce, but not eliminate, the incidence of recall (Chapter 30). Another study showed that intraoperative recall is possible even with a BIS value below 60. The most common reasons for intraoperative awareness are related to technical problems such as infusion pump malfunctions or disconnections. Other potential limitations of the TIVA technique include significant cumulation of the infused drugs after prolonged infusions, leading to delayed awakening, and the side effects of propofol administration, including pain on injection and postoperative fatigue and confusion. Finally, prolonged infusion of propofol may result in significant expense.

Suggested readings

Apfel CC, Korttila K, Abdalla M, et al. A factorial trial of six interventions for the prevention of postoperative nausea and vomiting. *N Engl J Med* 2004; 350:2441–2451.

Bulow NM, Barbosa NV, Rocha JB. Opioid consumption in total intravenous anesthesia is reduced with dexmedetomidine: a comparative study with remifentanil in gynecologic videolaparoscopic surgery. *J Clin Anesth* 2007; 19;280–285.

Cheng SS, Yeh J, Flood P. Anesthesia matters: patients anesthetized with propofol have less postoperative pain than those anesthetized with isoflurane. *Anesth Analg* 2008; 106;264–269.

Leslie K, Clavisi O, Hargrove J. Target-controlled infusion versus manually-controlled infusion of propofol for general anaesthesia or sedation in adults. *Cochrane Database Syst Rev* 2008; CD006059.

Nordstrom O, Engstrom AM, Persson S, Sandin R. Incidence of awareness in total i.v. anaesthesia based on propofol, alfentanil and neuromuscular blockade. *Acta Anaesthesiol Scand* 1997; 41:978–984.

Ramsay MA, Luterman DL. Dexmedetomidine as a total intravenous anesthetic agent. *Anesthesiology* 2004; 101;787–790.

Sandin RH, Enlund G, Samuelsson P, Lennmarken C. Awareness during anaesthesia: a prospective case study. *Lancet* 2000; 355:707–711.

Visser K, Hassink EA, Bonsel GJ, et al. Randomized controlled trial of total intravenous anesthesia with propofol versus inhalation anesthesia with isoflurane-nitrous oxide: postoperative nausea with vomiting and economic analysis. *Anesthesiology* 2001; 95:616–626.

Vuyk J, Mertens MJ, Olofsen E, et al. Propofol anesthesia and rational opioid selection: determination of optimal EC50-EC95 propofol-opioid concentrations that assure adequate anesthesia and a rapid return of consciousness. *Anesthesiology* 1997; 87:1549–1562.

Shubjeet Kaur

Introduction

The use of monitored anesthesia care (MAC) as an anesthetic technique for the care of patients both in the operating room and in a procedural setting continues to increase. Currently, MAC is the first choice in an estimated 10% to 30% of all surgical procedures in the operating room.

Monitored anesthesia care

The American Society of Anesthesiologists (ASA) defines MAC as a "specific anesthesia service for a diagnostic or therapeutic procedure." The standards of anesthesia care are no different from those of general or regional anesthesia. MAC includes a preprocedure assessment, intraprocedure care, and postprocedure anesthesia management. The anesthesiologist either provides the anesthesia himself or herself or supervises another anesthesia care provider (resident, nurse anesthetist).

During MAC, an anesthesiologist may administer medications that produce analgesia, anxiolysis, amnesia, or hypnosis. The anesthesiologist is always responsible for monitoring the patient's vital functions. Often, analgesia is provided by the surgeon via local anesthesia or nerve blocks on the surgical field. Sometimes the anesthesiologist may not need to administer any medications at all.

An important component of successful MAC is that the anesthesiologist providing this service is responsible for anticipating, diagnosing, and treating any medical problems that may arise during the procedure. MAC may need to be converted to a general anesthetic at a moment's notice. Therefore, the anesthesia care provider must be able to ensure adequate airway support and ventilation.

Moderate sedation/analgesia (formerly known as "conscious sedation") by nonanesthesiologists

It is important to have a clear understanding of the differences between MAC and moderate sedation/analgesia: MAC is provided by a fully trained anesthesia care provider and adheres to the same standard as any other choice of anesthetic (as outlined earlier). Therefore, during MAC cases, at least two independently functioning healthcare providers are present: the health care provider performing the procedure and the anesthesiologist/nurse anesthetist. This is in contrast to moderate sedation/analgesia cases, in which the physician performing the procedure is also directing and supervising the provider administering the sedation.

Although anesthesiologists have specific training to provide sedation and analgesia, in most institutions these services often are provided by nonanesthesiologists for various reasons, including scheduling issues, convenience, lack of availability of anesthesiologists, and cost.

To improve patient safety, most institutions have developed policies and procedures for moderate sedation/analgesia with the help of the anesthesiologists. An ASA task force has published practice guidelines for sedation and analgesia by nonanesthesiologists to assist anesthesiologists in the process of developing these institutional policies. The ASA practice guidelines define four levels of sedation that represent a continuum (Table 50.1). At one end of the spectrum is "minimal sedation," which may progress to "moderate sedation/analgesia (conscious sedation)" to "deep sedation/analgesia," and finally to "general anesthesia."

Moderate sedation/analgesia (formerly known as "conscious sedation") is defined as a medically controlled state of depressed consciousness that allows protective reflexes to be maintained, retaining the patient's ability to maintain a patent airway and to respond to verbal and physical stimulation. A "conscious sedation" case therefore should never exceed the level of moderate sedation. Sedation beyond moderate sedation may lead to airway compromise and the immediate need for airway intervention to avoid adverse patient outcome.

Most institutions exclude high-risk patient groups from undergoing moderate sedation/analgesia (e.g., patients with morbid obesity, chronic pain issues, sleep apnea, severe cardiac, pulmonary, hepatic, renal, central nervous system disease) and require anesthesiologists to provide MAC or general anesthesia for these patient groups.

Sedation with propofol is classified as deep sedation by the ASA practice guidelines. Therefore, most institutions exclude propofol and sometimes other medications from being used by nonanesthesiologists in an attempt to avoid adverse patient outcomes. In addition, institutions often require nonanesthesiologists to undergo training in monitoring, resuscitation skills, and

Table 50.1. Continuum of depth-of-sedation definitions

Parameter	Minimal sedation (anxiolysis)	Moderate sedation/analgesia (conscious sedation)	Deep sedation/analgesia	General anesthesia
Responsiveness	Normal response to verbal stimulation	Purposeful response to verbal or tactile stimulation[a]	Purposeful response following repeated or painful stimulation[a]	Unarousable even with painful stimulus
Airway	Unaffected	No intervention required	Intervention may be required	Intervention often required
Spontaneous ventilation	Unaffected	Adequate	May be inadequate	Frequently inadequate
Cardiovascular function	Unaffected	Usually maintained	Usually maintained	May be impaired

[a] Reflex withdrawal from a painful stimulus is *not* considered a purposeful response.
From ASA. Continuum of Depth of Sedation Definition of General Anesthesia and Levels of Sedation/Analgesia. (Approved by ASA House of Delegates on October 13, 1999 and amended on October 27, 2004.)

medication knowledge before they are given privileges to provide moderate sedation/analgesia.

Indications for MAC

Choosing MAC as the anesthetic technique over regional techniques or general anesthesia depends on various considerations, such as the type of procedure; the patient's medical condition, including the patient's mental status; specific positioning requirements during the procedure; and the surgeon's and patient's preference. Examples of procedures that are usually well tolerated under MAC are breast biopsy, indwelling central venous catheter placement, eye operations, minor plastic surgery, diagnostic cystoscopy, hysteroscopy, dilatation and curettage (D&C), creation of AV fistula for dialysis access, insertion of pacemaker or ICD, many interventional radiology cases, and upper and lower gastrointestinal endoscopic procedures.

Communication with the surgeon and the patient about the advantages and limitations of MAC prior to the start of the procedure facilitates the successful conduct of a MAC anesthetic.

Preprocedure evaluation

A thorough preprocedure evaluation must be completed, an anesthetic plan formulated, and informed consent obtained for every patient scheduled for MAC. The patient must be informed that although a MAC anesthetic is planned, there is always a possibility that it may get converted to a general anesthetic in order to complete the procedure safely. A detailed medical history and focused physical examination with emphasis on airway evaluation must be performed, along with a review of current medications and any drug allergies. The patient's medical condition should be optimized prior to the planned procedure, and the indicated laboratory workup and diagnostic studies should be ordered. ASA fasting guidelines should be used and are the same as those for a general anesthetic.

Monitoring

The standards for basic monitoring apply to all patients under the care of an anesthesiologist, regardless of whether the anesthetic is general, regional, or MAC.

The continuous presence of a qualified anesthesia provider (an anesthesiologist or, in the case of medical direction, a certified registered nurse anesthetist/anesthesia resident) is a requirement for the conduct of MAC (monitoring standard I as defined by the ASA). There is no substitute for a vigilant anesthesia caregiver. Continuous observation of the patient, along with verbal communication, provides a wealth of information in a dynamic clinical situation. In addition, every patient must have the following parameters continually monitored: oxygenation, ventilation, circulation, and body temperature (basic anesthetic monitoring standard II as defined by the ASA).

Techniques for MAC

Patient safety and operating conditions that facilitate timely and satisfactory completion of the procedure are the key goals from the provider's perspective. Generally, the following end points must be met: analgesia, sedation/comfort, anxiolysis, and early discharge/return to baseline function. In addition to verbal reassurance and preemptive communication with the patient, a variety of medications may be used to achieve the aforementioned end points. The surgeon will commonly inject local anesthetic to provide analgesia. The anesthesiologist is in a position to advise the surgeon about the maximum allowable dose to prevent local anesthetic toxicity and be constantly vigilant for symptoms and signs of toxicity. The anesthesia provider must be prepared to manage this potential complication immediately.

Systemic agents used for MAC

The ideal drug used during MAC should have a quick onset of action, minimal side effects, a high therapeutic index, short duration of action, and rapid elimination (noncumulative). The aim is to have a rapid return to baseline status and to facilitate early discharge. Some key pharmacologic concepts with which the anesthesiologist should be familiar are ESET (effect site equilibration time), therapeutic index, and context-sensitive half-time (see Part 6 in this book). Drugs may have a synergistic or additive effect, and there may be considerable interpatient variability. Various techniques ranging from intermittent boluses to multiple concurrent continuous infusions of drugs

Table 50.2. Commonly used intravenous agents in MAC

Desired end point	Drug group	Commonly used agents
Sedation	Benzodiazepines α₂-Agonists	Midazolam Dexmedetomidine
Hypnosis	Hypnotics	Propofol
Analgesia	Opioids	Fentanyl Alfentanil Remifentanil
	Nonopioids	Ketamine
Amnesia	Benzodiazepines	Midazolam

Table 50.4. Benzodiazepine and opioid antagonists

Factor	Flumazenil	Naloxone
Antagonist	Benzodiazepines	Opioids
Dose	0.2 mg IV Repeat 0.2 mg every 1 min maximum 1 mg IV	40 μg IV Repeat to effect every 1–2 min
Duration of action	30–60 min	30–45 min
Side effects	Seizures Agitation/confusion Acute anxiety Sweating or shivering Blurred vision Headache	Reversal of analgesia Nausea and vomiting[1] Hypertension, tachycardia, ventricular dysrhythmias Pulmonary edema

[1] Dependent upon the prior dose of opioid and the dose of naloxone; an antagonist like naloxone might be very effective in treating opioid-induced nausea and vomiting.

to achieve the goals of providing sedation and analgesia have been described. Table 50.2 provides a summary of common intravenous (IV) agents used to achieve the different end points of MAC; Table 50.3 provides examples of dosing regimens of these drugs.

The most important pharmacologic principle in this setting is "titration to effect." To help prevent overdosing, titration involves ensuring that the drug administered into the IV tubing is actually being delivered into the patient's circulation, and also waiting for the peak effect prior to redosing. Heightened caution is especially important in the elderly and in patients who have multiple comorbid conditions. The changing level of stimulation and the concurrent use of multiple drugs may result in undesirable end points in spite of using a conservative approach. The anesthesiologist may have to temporarily support the patient's airway and ensure adequate ventilation.

Benzodiazepine and opioid antagonists

Sometimes pharmacologic agents may have to be given to reverse the unintended side effects of administered drugs such as benzodiazepines and opioids. Flumazenil is a specific competitive benzodiazepine antagonist that can reverse the sedation as well the ventilatory depression produced by benzodiazepines. It can be titrated in increments of 0.2 mg IV at 60-second intervals (total dose of 1 mg IV) until the desired level of consciousness is achieved. Naloxone is an opioid antagonist that reverses all opioid effects, including ventilatory depression and analgesia. It is titrated in 20- to 40-μg IV increments. It produces peak effects in 1 to 2 minutes, and titration is essential to avoid severe pain in patients. Sudden, complete

antagonism of opioid effects may cause hypertension, tachycardia, ventricular dysrhythmias, and pulmonary edema. Table 50.4 lists these two antagonist agents and provides a brief summary of the key pharmacologic features.

Discharge criteria

Postprocedure, a patient who has undergone MAC has to be monitored under the care of a registered nurse who has the clinical skills and core competencies required in a postanesthesia care unit (PACU) until discharge criteria are fulfilled. The anesthesiologist should be immediately available to address any patient management issues during the recovery phase. Return to baseline mental status, minimal pain, vital signs within 20% of preprocedure values, and control of nausea and vomiting must be achieved prior to discharge. A responsible adult must be available to escort the patient home and observe the patient for any unexpected events in the postprocedure period. A patient who has undergone MAC must be provided the same standard of postprocedure care given to patients who underwent a regional or general anesthetic.

Outcomes and safety of MAC

MAC sometimes is requested for patients who are considered "too sick" to have a general anesthetic. In addition, anesthesiologists are being asked to provide this care in settings remote from the operating room with greater frequency. Some of the factors that contribute to adverse outcomes are the use of multiple drugs, inadequate monitoring, and lack of timely resuscitation efforts. Combining a benzodiazepine with an opioid may result in frequent episodes of hypoxemia and apnea. Administering propofol with opioids produces a synergistic or additive effect and diminishes the ventilatory response to hypercarbia. A recently published Closed Claims analysis revealed that "respiratory depression after absolute or relative overdose of a combination of sedative and/or opioid drugs was the most common specific damaging event in claims

Table 50.3. Typical dosing regimens for MAC

Drug	Induction bolus dose	Maintenance infusion rate, μg/kg/min	Maintenance intermittent boluses
Midazolam	0.5–5 mg	–	0.5–2 mg
Propofol	10–80 mg	10–75	10–50 mg
Fentanyl	25–50 μg	0.01–0.03	25–50 μg
Alfentanil	20–50 μg	0.25–1	20–50 μg
Remifentanil	10–25 μg	0.025–0.1	10–25 μg
Ketamine	10–50 mg	2–10	10–50 mg
Dexmedetomidine	1.0 μg/kg over 10–20 min	0.2–1.0 μg/kg/h	10–30 μg

associated with Monitored Anesthesia Care." In addition, "nearly half of these claims were judged preventable by better monitoring, including capnography, improved vigilance, or audible alarms." In this claims analysis, although death or permanent brain damage was present with similar frequency whether the claim was filed for a MAC or general anesthetic, patients undergoing MAC were found to be sicker and older than those who had a general anesthetic. The authors concluded that the use of capnography as a monitor for ventilation may enhance patient safety. Current ASA practice guidelines state that "continual monitoring for the presence of expired carbon dioxide shall be performed unless invalidated by the nature of the patient, procedure or equipment."

Conclusion

MAC is a safe anesthetic technique when it is chosen for the right procedure in a patient who has been medically optimized. It allows the anesthesiologist an opportunity to provide a more intimate level of care and reassurance to patients than can be given during most general anesthetics. Patients undergoing MAC deserve the same level of vigilance and care before, during, and after the procedure. One might say that MAC should stand for *maximum anesthesia caution*, not *minimal anesthesiology care*.

Suggested readings

Bhananker SM, Posner KL, Cheney FW, et al. Injury and liability associated with monitored anesthesia care. *Anesthesiology* 2006; 104:228–234.

Burton JH, Harrah JD, Germann CA, Dillon DC. Does end-tidal carbon dioxide monitoring detect respiratory events prior to current sedation monitoring practices? *Acad Emerg Med* 2006; 13(5):500–504.

Definitions of monitored anesthesia care. *ASA Newsletter* 2004; 68:6.

Distinguishing Monitored Anesthesia Care ("MAC") from Moderate Sedation/Analgesia (Conscious Sedation). (Approved by ASA House of Delegates on October 27, 2004 and last updated on September 2, 2008.) Available at: http://www.asahq.org.

Position on Monitored Anesthesia Care (approved by the House of Delegates on October 21, 1986, and last amended on October 25, 2005 and last updated on September 2, 2008). Available at: http://www.asahq.org.

Soto RG, Fu ES, Vila Jr, H Miguel RV. Capnography accurately detects apnea during monitored anesthesia care. *Anesth Analg* 2004; 99:379–382.

Chapter 51

Patient positioning and common nerve injuries

Christian D. Gonzalez

Introduction

Although monitoring vital signs is an important part of the anesthesiologist's responsibility perioperatively, it is far from being the sole task. As advocates of patient safety, anesthesiologists are also involved in setting and monitoring the patient's position during surgery.

Because nerve injuries resulting from patient malpositioning may lead to serious morbidity, the American Society of Anesthesiologists (ASA) published a practice advisory for the prevention of peripheral neuropathies associated with positioning in the perioperative period. Furthermore, a task force was created aiming at practice improvement based on limited available scientific data. In this chapter, we discuss the most common patient positions during surgery; explore how patient positioning may lead to adverse outcomes, particularly nerve injuries; and review the current guidelines for preventing nerve injuries due to malpositioning.

Preparation

Planning the intraoperative patient position begins in the preoperative visit. At this time, the anesthesiologist should have an understanding of the procedure and the patient's expected position during surgery. This knowledge helps determine which structures are at high risk of injury. Any existing nerve injury should be documented carefully, with emphasis on focal motor or sensory deficits. Examples include a history of hand numbness, radicular pain in the extremities, and chronic back pain. There are other aspects of the medical history that are important risk factors associated with adverse outcomes due to positioning. The ASA task force enumerated six risk factors:

    Preexisting neurologic symptoms
    Body habitus
    Diabetes mellitus
    Peripheral vascular disease
    Alcohol dependency
    Arthritis

Thus, a thorough knowledge of the patient's medical history is vital in assessing the risk of nerve injury due to positioning. In addition, during the preoperative visit, the practitioner should discuss with the patient any potential risks of nerve injury. The patient's position during surgery is a joint decision between the surgeon seeking to facilitate surgery and the anesthesiologist assessing for risk of injury. After induction of anesthesia and once a sterile field has been created, the patient's position is final.

Monitoring

After the patient has been positioned in the operating room, the anesthesiologist must make one final position check before the sterile field is created: All pressure points must be cushioned and vulnerable joints well supported. The patient under general anesthesia should look as if sleeping comfortably.

There are many instances during surgery in which patient movement or change in position might occur, potentially leading to adverse outcomes. For example, the surgeon might lean on the patient's arm or face, the Trendelenburg position might be too steep, or the patient's arm might fall off the arm board. Constant monitoring, quick assessment, and possible correction of these changes are of the utmost importance in preventing adverse outcomes. General preparation and monitoring of the patient's position are indeed essential to prevent nerve injury. However, specific knowledge of different surgical positions, and the risks associated with them, is equally important.

Common positions and their related injuries

Supine position

The supine position is the most common position during surgery (Fig. 51.1). The arms may be abducted or adducted

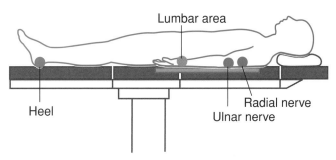

Supine

Figure 51.1. Supine position.

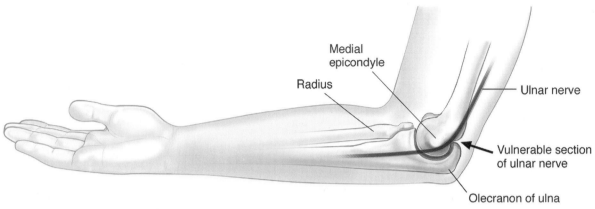

Figure 51.2. Arm positioning: olecranon, ulnar nerve, and surrounding structures.

depending on the type of surgery and the surgeon's preference. When the arm is in the *abducted* position, the ASA task force recommends that the angle be ≤90°. In fact, multiple studies have demonstrated that arm abduction beyond 90° is associated with brachial plexus injury. In the abducted position, the ASA recommends placing the forearm so that the olecranon process rests on the padded board, minimizing pressure on the ulnar nerve (Fig. 51.2). However, for some patients this position may be uncomfortable. Furthermore, upper-extremity supination may cause brachial plexus stretching. The decision to pronate or supinate often is made by the anesthesiologist based on the patient's comfort, before induction of anesthesia. The ASA task force generally advises that the forearm be supinated or placed in a neutral position. When the *adducted* position is selected, care must be taken to avoid arm compression by any external device (e.g., metal side rails) and to ensure appropriate padding. The forearm should be placed in a neutral position.

The most common nerve injury following surgery is ulnar neuropathy. There is evidence that placement of the arm in a nonsupinated position may contribute to the development of ulnar neuropathy. Although classically this injury was believed to always be the result of compression of the ulnar nerve at the level of the elbow, more recent nerve conduction studies have proved this belief incorrect. Current data indicate that the patient's susceptibility to injury, in the form of preexisting illness or other risk factors, may play a more important role. It is important to note that 40% of the general, asymptomatic population has anatomic variations of the ulnar nerve at the elbow. For this reason, it is important to pad generously around the medial epicondyle.

Although less common, other nerve injuries may occur in the supine position. Relaxation of the paravertebral spine muscles secondary to anesthesia may cause the loss of normal lumbar lordosis. If the patient has chronic low back pain secondary to herniated disks, listhesis, or other abnormalities of the spine, there is a likelihood that the patient may suffer from nerve root compression or radiculopathy. Radial nerve injury also may occur, most often as a result of external pressure on the nerve as it traverses the spiral groove of the humerus in the lower third of the arm. At this point, it is most sensitive to injury

secondary to pressure. Caution should be exercised to avoid any external pressure on the patient's arms, especially in the presence of metal side frames. Finally, focal alopecia also has been documented with the supine position. It can be prevented by moving the patient's head every 2 hours or using a foam pad.

Prone position

Potential pressure points in the prone position (Fig. 51.3) include the cheek, ear, acromion process, breasts (women), genitalia (men), patella, and toes. In the prone position, the head may be tilted to one side; however, this may worsen any pre-existing cervical spine pathology. It is recommended that for any patient with cervical spine pain or cerebral vascular disease placed in the prone position, specialized padding be used to keep the head in the neutral position. However, care must be taken not to cause pressure buildup on the face, especially the eyes, as this may lead to retinal ischemia. The arms may be placed at the patient's sides or flexed at the elbow and shoulder and placed on arm boards alongside the patient's head. Pads or rolled towels may be used to support areas of the arms suspended. A pillow usually is placed under the lower legs to alleviate pressure on the toes and feet. If the arms are to be placed above the patient's head, a preoperative examination should rule out thoracic outlet syndrome, which might lead to brachial plexus injury. If the arms are to be placed alongside the patient's body, attention must be given to placing the padding above the elbow to prevent equipment or personnel-related pressure over

Prone

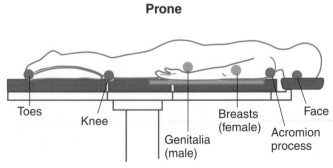

Toes · Knee · Genitalia (male) · Breasts (female) · Acromion process · Face

Figure 51.3. Prone position.

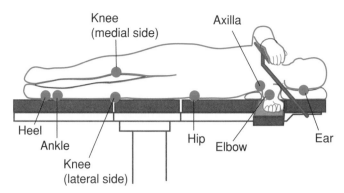

Figure 51.4. Lateral decubitus position.

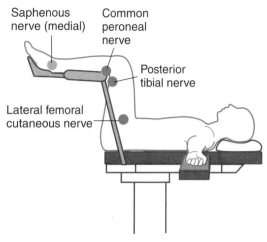

Figure 51.5. Lithotomy position.

the ulnar nerve. The patient may require a chest roll to allow for diaphragmatic excursion.

Lateral decubitus position

Potential pressure points in the lateral decubitus position include the ear, acromion process, ribs, ilium, greater trochanter, medial and lateral condyles, and malleolus (Fig. 51.4). The lateral decubitus position also places the patient at an increased risk for brachial plexus injury. Typically, the bottom arm is placed in an arm board and the top arm is supported by a pillow or other supporting devices parallel to the lower arm. An axillary roll helps prevent damage to the brachial plexus. However, if the axillary roll is displaced or misplaced, pressure over the head of the humerus may result in a brachial plexus injury secondary to compression. Stretching of the brachial plexus of the nondependent upper extremity can be limited by aligning the cervical and thoracic spine and keeping the head in the neutral position. Care must be taken to avoid pressure over the axilla, which may cause compression of the brachial plexus and nerve damage. Proper head support also prevents straining of the spinal facet joints. The patient's head can be supported by a pillow, keeping the head in normal anatomic alignment with the rest of the body. The patient's bottom leg should be flexed, and a pillow should be placed between the legs.

Lithotomy position

The use of the lithotomy position is associated with multiple peripheral nerve injuries (Fig. 51.5). The nerves at increased risk for injury are the femoral, common peroneal, sciatic, saphenous, and obturator nerves. Reducing the risk of injury to these nerves is accomplished by proper padding over susceptible areas. These vulnerable nerve sites should be clear of hard surfaces or metal braces.

If shoulder braces are used, the patient is at a higher risk for injury. The use of these braces has become more controversial, and there is now evidence that they are associated with brachial plexus injury, likely as a result of the weight of the torso compressing the plexus. A patient with a history of lumbosacral spine pathology also is at an increased risk for worsening symptoms. The best way to prevent further injury is

to have the patient try the position while awake and report any discomfort.

Trendelenburg position

The Trendelenburg (or "head-down") position (Fig. 51.6) is common, especially during laparoscopic surgery. In this position, the patient may be at a high risk for brachial plexus injury, especially if pressure is placed on the shoulders to prevent the patient from sliding in the cephalad direction.

Sitting position

Potential pressure points in the sitting position include the scapulae, ischial tuberosities, back of the knees, and calcaneus. Common nerve complications of the sitting position include excessive neck flexion leading to spinal cord ischemia, and sciatic nerve injury from excessive lower-extremity extension.

Subsequent care of nerve injury

Intraoperative positional nerve injuries manifest immediately when the patient wakes from surgery. A delayed diagnosis is not uncommon, however, and may be secondary to the postoperative patient being intubated, sedated, casted, or not ambulatory. The deficit is usually most severe immediately after surgery

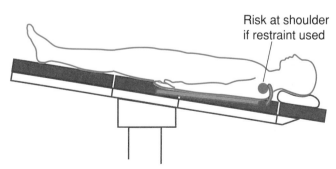

Figure 51.6. Trendelenburg position.

and often improves with time. The anesthesiologist should be informed as soon as possible of any adverse outcomes in the perioperative period. In case of suspected nerve damage, a detailed history should be taken and a focused physical examination performed. Sensory or motor changes should be noted and compared with the preoperative assessment.

If nerve injury is suspected after the initial assessment, a neurology consultation should be obtained for further examination and testing. The hiatus for a neurology consult should be within the first 2 weeks postinjury. Testing within this time-frame is important to determine the temporal nature of the nerve injury. Electromyography (EMG) may show no changes within the 2-week time period if the injury is acute. If the injury is chronic (preexisting), the EMG may be abnormal within that period. If testing is done beyond that, EMG may be positive for both acute and chronic injuries. Thus, the combination of initial testing within the first 2 weeks and repeated testing after this period will allow determination of whether the nerve injury occurred during surgery or was preexisting. The operative position used should be reviewed carefully by the surgeon and anesthesiologist. Any erythema or other skin changes indicative of prolonged pressure should be documented. The alternative diagnosis of an inflammatory (noncompressive) neuritis can be ruled out if the neurologic deficit is present immediately after surgery, because neuritis often takes several days to develop. Some practitioners also test the opposite limb to determine whether there are any unrecognized abnormalities that might predispose the patient to injury.

If a diagnosis of acute peripheral neuropathy is made, the patient should be reassured that most symptoms resolve within the first 6 weeks. Symptoms will resolve faster if the nerve injury causes only a sensorial deficit. Studies show that up to 80% of patients have no residual symptoms 6 months after the injury. Persisting pain can then resolve within the year. However, after

1 year, only a minority will get better within 24 months and after that the symptoms will more than likely be permanent. If the symptoms do not improve within 6 weeks, or if there is disruption of daily living activities, the patient should be referred to a pain management specialist. Although interventions such as nerve blocks will not hasten overall recovery, pain relief can allow more aggressive physical therapy. This is particularly important because physical therapy decreases the incidence and severity of complex regional pain syndrome and allows faster recovery of function.

Suggested readings

Coppieters MW. Shoulder restraints as a potential cause for stretch neuropathies: biomechanical support for the impact of shoulder girdle depression and arm abduction on nerve strain. *Anesthesiology* 2006; 104(6):1351–1352.

Coppieters MW, Van de Velde M, Stappaert KH. Positioning in anesthesiology: toward a better understanding of stretch-induced perioperative neuropathies. *Anesthesiology* 2002; 97(1):75–81.

Prielipp RC, Morell RC, Butterworht J. Ulnar nerve injury and perioperative arm positioning. *Anesthesiol Clin North Am* 2002; 20(3):589–603.

Rupp-Montpetit K, Moody ML. Visual loss as a complication of nonophthalmologic surgery: a review of the literature. *AANA J* 2004; 72(4):285–293.

Stambough JL, Dolan D, Werner R, Godfrey E. Ophthalmologic complications associated with prone positioning in spine surgery. *J Am Acad Orthop Surg* 2007; 15(3):156–165.

Warner MA, Blitt CD, Butterworth JR, et al. Practice advisory for the prevention of perioperative peripheral neuropathies. *Anesthesiology* 2000; 92(4):1168–1182.

Warner MA, Warner DO, Harper CM, et al. Lower extremity neuropathies associated with lithotomy positions. *Anesthesiology* 2000; 93(4):938–942.

Warner MA, Warner ME, Matin JT. Ulnar neuropathy. Incidence, outcome, and risk factors in sedated or anesthetized patients. *Anesthesiology* 1994; 81(6):1332–1340.

Emergence from anesthesia

Michael P. Storey and Richard D. Urman

Emergence from anesthesia is a critical time for the patient and the anesthesia provider. As surgery comes to a close, a patient emerging from anesthesia requires the full attention and focus of the anesthesia provider. At the end of anesthesia and surgery, the patient should typically be awake or easily arousable, be able to protect the airway, maintain adequate ventilation, and have his or her pain adequately controlled. Time to emergence from anesthesia varies, depending on many patient factors as well as the type and length of surgery and the type of anesthetic administered.

Delayed emergence

Delayed emergence or awakening is common after prolonged surgery and anesthesia. Although no specific definition of delayed awakening exists, it is commonly described as the case in which a patient takes longer to awaken from a specific circumstance than a clinician would expect. The causes of delayed awakening from anesthesia are listed in Table 52.1.

Residual drug effects

Most often, delayed awakening may be attributed to the residual effects of drugs. The speed of emergence from a volatile anesthetic primarily depends on the patient's alveolar ventilation and the anesthetic's blood/gas solubility. Less soluble agents, such as nitrous oxide and desflurane, are eliminated faster than more soluble agents, such as isoflurane. In addition, hypoventilation will result in prolonged emergence. Finally, as a case lengthens, the anesthesia provider must factor in the anesthetic agent's total tissue uptake that is related to the drug's solubility, the concentration being delivered, and duration of administration. End-tidal gas monitoring is now used routinely, and it is important to ascertain that it is working properly. Using a bispectral index monitor may provide an estimate of the level of consciousness if an unexpected delay is encountered.

Table 52.1. Causes of delayed awakening from anesthesia

Residual drug effects
Respiratory failure (hypercarbia and reduced oxygen delivery)
Cardiovascular complications
Metabolic derangements
Neurologic complications

The anesthesia provider should always suspect a drug overdose or error, as well as the possibility of an increased sensitivity to a particular drug. This may be particularly true of elderly and chronically ill patients and patients with impaired drug metabolism because of underlying liver, kidney, or enzymatic deficiency. It is important to assess for the possibility of an overdose of the commonly used medications, such as benzodiazepines, opioids, and neuromuscular blockers.

For intravenous (IV) anesthetic agents, immediate recovery generally depends on redistribution from the brain to less vascular organs, muscle, and fat. Propofol is rapidly metabolized in the liver, with a short terminal half-life and minimal accumulation over time. Thiopental, a formerly popular induction agent, is metabolized at a slower rate and has a longer terminal half-life than propofol. As a result, it may demonstrate cumulative effects following higher doses.

Respiratory failure

Respiratory failure may lead to delayed emergence. Hypoventilation may lead to hypercarbia that can cause sedation and even unconsciousness (i.e., carbon dioxide [CO_2] narcosis) when profound. Respiratory failure may be a result of a preexisting condition such as chronic obstructive pulmonary disease but also may be the result of persistent paralysis from neuromuscular blockers, respiratory depression following opioids, or airway obstruction. In this case, a blood gas measurement may be helpful.

Cardiovascular complications

Cardiovascular causes of delayed emergence, such as heart failure, cardiac arrhythmias, or hypotension, may result in inadequate delivery of blood and oxygen to the brain. The hypotension should be reversed (by IV fluids or blood products and/or vasopressors, as appropriate) and the underlying rhythm and contractility issues treated appropriately.

Metabolic causes

Hypoglycemia may occur in patients taking insulin or oral hypoglycemics. It is more common in infants and in patients with liver failure. Hyperglycemia may occur in diabetic patients, possibly leading to diabetic ketoacidosis or diabetic coma.

Table 52.2. Stages of anesthesia

Stage	Description
I	Amnesia, induction of anesthesia to loss of consciousness
II	Delirium, excitation, potential for vomiting, laryngeal spasm, hypertension, tachycardia, uncontrolled nonpurposeful movements, dilated pupils
III	Surgical anesthesia, constricted pupils, regular respiration, adequate anesthetic depth, prevention of hypotension and tachycardia, absence of movement
IV	Overdosage; shallow or no respiration; dilated, nonreactive pupils; hypotension

Table 52.3. Effects of anesthesia at different stages

Stage	Pupil	Pulse	Blood pressure	Respiration
I (induction)		Fast	Baseline	Normal
II (excitement)		Fast	High	Automatic and regular
III (surgical)		Slow	Baseline	Intercostal muscle paralysis
IV (overdose)		Weak, thready	Low	Diaphragmatic paralysis

Serum glucose should be checked if an abnormal glucose level is suspected. Serum electrolytes should be checked to detect a sodium, potassium, calcium, or magnesium imbalance.

Severe hypothermia may lead to reduced consciousness. Body temperature in the low 30°C range may lead to respiratory depression, potentiate the central nervous system effects of anesthetic drugs, reduce the minimum alveolar concentration of inhalational anesthetics, potentiate muscle relaxants, and slow metabolism of other drugs.

Neurologic complications

It also is important to rule out neurologic causes of delayed awakening, such as increased intracranial pressure, cerebral hemorrhage, and air or fat embolism. If a neurologic cause is suspected, a neurologic consultation should be ordered and the patient should remain intubated until all the potential causes are explored.

Extubation

Near the end of emergence, the anesthesia provider must decide when to remove the airway device – generally an endotracheal tube (ETT) or a laryngeal mask airway (LMA). If the ETT or LMA is removed too early, the patient may not adequately breathe or protect the airway. If the patient is still in stage II of anesthesia (see Tables 52.2 and 52.3), the patient may develop laryngospasm or not be able to support his or her airway. However, if the ETT or LMA is in place when the patient is fully conscious, it may cause severe discomfort to the patient.

Extubation criteria

Extubation criteria are listed in Table 52.4. Ideally, the patient should be able to perform simple actions on command, such as eye opening, hand grasping, or holding his or her head off the operating table for at least 5 seconds. Additionally, the anesthesia provider should assess for other useful extubation criteria, such as a regular respiratory pattern, a respiratory rate of <30 breaths per minute, tidal volumes of at least 5 ml/kg, positive end-expiratory pressure (PEEP) requirements ≤ 5 cm H_2O, and a negative inspiratory force > -20 cm H_2O. It is also important to ensure that the patient is not hypoxic or hypercarbic (end-tidal $CO_2 < 50$ mm Hg). A vital capacity > 10 ml/kg indicates

that the patient's coughing should be able to clear secretions and help maintain airway patency.

For extubation to be attempted, the patient should be breathing 100% oxygen with a high flow rate. The increased flow rate will help expedite the removal of residual anesthetic gases from the patient and the anesthesia circuit. If the anesthesia provider believes extubation can be performed successfully, the patient's oropharynx should be gently suctioned to remove any secretions from above the cuff of the ETT. After suctioning, the ETT cuff should be fully deflated, the reservoir bag squeezed, and the breathing tube gently removed from the trachea. The purpose of squeezing the reservoir bag is to create a positive pressure, thereby helping to blow any remaining secretions above the ETT cuff upward, instead of allowing them to fall onto the vocal cords. The anesthesia mask should then be attached to the anesthesia circuit and placed on the patient to ensure he or she is breathing adequately after extubation. After it has been determined that the patient can maintain a patent airway and adequate oxygenation while breathing spontaneously, supplemental oxygen may be delivered via a simple face mask or nasal cannula may be used during transport to the postanesthesia care unit (PACU).

Airway complications during emergence
Upper airway obstruction

Upper airway obstruction in a patient emerging from anesthesia may occur for a variety of reasons. Possible causes include

Table 52.4. Extubation criteria

Negative inspiratory force > -20 cm H_2O
Tidal volume > 5 ml/kg
PaO_2 65–70 mm Hg on $FiO_2 < 40\%$
Respiratory rate < 30/min
Vital capacity > 10 ml/kg
$PaCO_2 < 50$ mm Hg
PEEP < 6 cm H_2O

secretions, glottic edema, and foreign bodies such as teeth or dentures, secretions, blood, or vomit. The most common cause of upper airway obstruction is the tongue. Airflow is blocked when the tongue falls back into a position that occludes the pharynx, resulting in a partial or total obstruction. Common signs and symptoms of upper airway obstruction include snoring, intercostal and suprasternal retractions, paradoxic respirations, and use of the accessory muscles of respiration. To relieve an upper airway obstruction, a patent airway must be established. This can often be accomplished simply by stimulating the patient, repositioning the head, or using the "head tilt, chin lift" technique or a jaw thrust. At times, an airway adjunct such as a nasal or oral airway may be needed.

Laryngospasm

Laryngospasm is a true life-threatening emergency. Laryngospasm occurs with stimulation of the superior laryngeal nerve, when the vocal cords spontaneously close and remain closed. This may be the result of light anesthesia, irritating gas in the airway, or a mechanical cause such as instrumentation in the airway or secretions falling onto the vocal cords. Signs and symptoms of laryngospasm include the inability to ventilate the patient, acute respiratory distress, absent breath sounds, severe agitation, and oxygen desaturation.

Laryngospasm must be treated immediately. Suctioning of the oropharynx and positive pressure ventilation with 100% oxygen should be initiated at once. Maintaining PEEP may be helpful. Performing a jaw thrust while applying positive pressure with a tight-fitting anesthesia mask and inserting an oral or nasal airway also may be helpful. These maneuvers often are enough to break intermittent or complete laryngospasms. However, if they fail, 10 to 20 mg of IV succinylcholine may be administered to aid in breaking the laryngospasm.

Laryngeal edema may cause swollen vocal cords to approximate and, as a result, allow little air to pass; it is characterized by a high-pitched inspiratory noise. Laryngeal stridor is often confused with a partial airway obstruction. Initially, treatment should include suctioning the oropharynx or performing a "head tilt, chin lift" or jaw thrust. If the patient still remains stridorous, additional options include placing an oral or nasal airway and, finally, attempting continuous positive airway pressure (CPAP) with a tight-fitting anesthesia mask. If stridor still does not resolve, it most likely is laryngeal in nature. Treatment in this case consists of racemic epinephrine (0.5 ml in 2 ml normal saline) via a nebulizer. These measures are usually adequate. However, if the patient is still struggling to breathe, heliox with a maximum fraction of inspired oxygen content (FiO$_2$) of 35% may be instituted. When heliox is administered, an FiO$_2$ > 35% may be ineffective because of the increasing density of the gas mixture with increasing FiO$_2$. In addition to heliox, mild sedation and anxiolysis may be beneficial.

Bronchospasm

Bronchospasm is caused by increased bronchial smooth muscle tone. A bronchospastic patient experiences closure of the small airways, resulting in "tight" breathing. Patients with reactive airway disease and smokers are at greater risk than others for bronchospasm. These patients may be treated prior to induction and emergence with a β$_2$-agonist bronchodilator such as albuterol. Bronchospasm also may be the result of aspiration, secretions, airway instrumentation, or reaction to medications. Any mechanical triggers of bronchospasm, such as oropharyngeal secretions, should be removed or alleviated. Patients are then usually treated with β$_2$-agonists via a nebulizer or inhaler. If the bronchospasm is life threatening, epinephrine may be administered endotracheally or IV.

Pulmonary aspiration

Aspiration during emergence may result in severe hypoxemia and morbidity. An actively vomiting patient should be vigorously suctioned in a head-down tilt. Aspiration of gastric contents may lead to adult respiratory distress syndrome, hypoxia, atelectasis, bronchospasm, infection, or chemical pneumonitis. Aspiration is treated by alleviating the hypoxemia, maintaining airway patency, and supporting hemodynamic status. Antibiotics should be given only in response to culture-proven pneumonia. Some patients who have aspirated gastric contents may need to remain intubated postoperatively to prevent hypoxemia.

Pulmonary edema

Pulmonary edema is characterized by engorgement of the perivascular and peribronchial interstitial tissues and by alveolar edema. During emergence, it is often the result of one of two causes.

Negative pressure pulmonary edema occurs when a patient creates a strong negative pressure within the chest. This often results from an attempt to take a large-volume breath through a small ETT or to breathe against a closed glottis. Negative pressure pulmonary edema may result in severe hypoxemia. Supportive treatment, including reintubation, is often necessary.

Pulmonary edema that is cardiac in nature may occur during emergence and extubation. Treatment of cardiogenic pulmonary edema also begins with supplemental oxygen therapy. Occasionally patients may need to be reintubated or placed on CPAP to maintain oxygenation. Therapy such as furosemide diuretics and fluid restriction also may be beneficial to the patient postoperatively.

Hypoventilation

Hypoventilation is a common finding after general anesthesia, especially if opioids have been given. Depression of respiratory drive, inadequate reversal of paralytics, pain from surgery, and neuromuscular disease also may result in hypoventilation. Hypoventilation is often defined as a PaCO$_2$ > 45 mm Hg, although it often is clinically apparent only when the PaCO$_2$ rises above 60 mm Hg and the arterial pH is < 7.25. A prominent sign of hypoventilation is a decreased respiratory rate and tidal volume. There may or may not be a concurrent decrease in

Table 52.5. Common causes of emergence delirium

Physiologic		Pharmacologic
Hypoxemia	Gastric dilation	Ketamine
Hypercapnia	Bladder distention	
Electrolyte imbalance	Pain	Benzodiazepines
Alcohol withdrawal	Hypothermia	Metoclopramide
Intracranial injury	Sensory overload	Atropine, scopolamine
Sepsis	Sensory deprivation	Inhalational anesthetics

oxygen saturation, especially if the patient had been ventilated with a high concentration of oxygen. Treatment should be aimed at the underlying cause, such as treating opioid overdosage with naloxone in titrated doses and fully reversing neuromuscular blocking drugs. Adequate ventilation should be assured either by assisting the patient's respirations or through positive pressure ventilation.

Emergence delirium

Emergence delirium or agitation may be caused by a variety of factors, both physiologic and pharmacologic (Table 52.5). It often occurs in very young or in elderly patients. Emergence delirium is characterized by severe disturbances in attention, orientation, perception, arousal, and intellectual function. It is often associated with fear and agitation, occasionally requiring the use of restraints to prevent injury to the patient or care providers. Periods of excitement or agitation may be followed by periods of lethargy and inappropriate behavior.

Arterial hypoxemia or hypercapnia should be ruled out as a cause of agitation, as should possible pharmacologic or physiologic causes. Benzodiazepines may be useful for sedating and calming patients. Other useful agents include physostigmine, haloperidol, analgesics, and α_2-agonists (e.g., dexmedetomidine). Fortunately, most incidences of emergence delirium are time limited and resolve prior to the patient's discharge from the PACU.

Suggested readings

Burns SM. Delirium during emergence from anesthesia: a case study. *Crit Care Nurs* 2003; 23: 66–69.

Forman S. Administration of general anesthesia. In: Hurford WE, ed. *Clinical Anesthesia Procedures of the Massachusetts General Hospital.* 6th ed. New York: Lippincott Williams & Wilkins; 2002:210–213.

Lepouse C, Lautner CA, Liu L, et al. Emergence delirium in adults in the post-anaesthesia care unit. *Br J Anaesth* 2006; 96(6):747–753.

Miller KA, Harkin CP, Bailey PL. Postoperative tracheal extubation. *Anesth Analg* 1995; 80:149–172.

Pavlin EG, Holle RH, Schoene RB. Recovery of airway protection compared with ventilation in humans after paralysis with curare. *Anesthesiology* 1989; 70:381–385.

West JB. *Pulmonary Physiology and Pathophysiology: An Integrated Case-Based Approach.* New York: Lippincott Williams & Wilkins; 2001:102.

Chapter 53

Postoperative complications in the PACU

Ala Nozari and Edward A. Bittner

Patients are often admitted to a postanesthesia care unit (PACU) for recovery after procedures that require anesthesia or sedation. It is essential that specially trained personnel are immediately available to supervise the postprocedural care of these patients, particularly if they have complicating medical problems or have undergone challenging surgical procedures. Complications in the PACU are common (Fig. 53.1). Anticipation, identification, and timely management of postoperative problems lead to decreased perioperative morbidity and mortality, improve the overall care, and enhance patient satisfaction.

The American Society of Anesthesiologists (ASA) has published standards for postoperative care (Table 53.1). These standards provide five general principles intended to ensure safe postoperative recovery.

Patients admitted to the PACU should be monitored and assessed as follows:

- Respiratory: respiratory rate, oxygen saturation, airway patency
- Cardiovascular: heart rate, blood pressure, electrocardiogram (ECG)
- Neuromuscular strength
- Pain
- Mental status
- Nausea or nausea/vomiting (see Chapters 41 and 54)
- Temperature
- Urine output
- Surgical site bleeding or drainage

Airway obstruction

Complete or partial airway obstruction is among the most common perioperative complications and without treatment, it may lead rapidly to life-threatening hypoxemia. Pharyngeal obstruction caused by posterior tongue displacement or soft tissue collapse can be managed successfully with simple maneuvers such as a chin lift, jaw thrust, and lateral decubitus positioning. Nasopharyngeal or oropharyngeal airways may be helpful but are not always tolerated by awake patients. Laryngeal or subglottic edema is often treated with head-up positioning and nebulized epinephrine and steroids, but it may require emergency reintubation or tracheostomy.

Laryngospasm may be precipitated by the presence of an airway irritant such as blood or secretions, or by the insertion of an oropharyngeal airway or other foreign bodies. Unrelieved laryngospasm may lead to the development of negative pressure pulmonary edema. Jaw thrust and positive pressure ventilation may be helpful, but occasionally a small dose of succinylcholine or intravenous (IV) anesthetic may be required to relieve the spasm.

Other common postoperative complications that may result in complete or incomplete airway obstruction include direct laryngeal trauma, extrinsic airway compression from an expanding neck hematoma, and vocal cord paralysis caused by recurrent laryngeal nerve injury. Unilateral vocal cord paralysis results in hoarseness, with the ipsilateral vocal cord fixed in a paramedian position, whereas bilateral paralysis results in airway occlusion and requires emergent intubation or a surgical airway.

Exacerbation of obstructive lung disease is frequent in the postoperative course of patients with preexisting disease and may require treatment for bronchospasm and airway inflammation, as well as correction of hypoxemia and hypercapnia.

Hypoxemia

Common causes of hypoxemia ($PaO_2 < 60$ mm Hg) in the early postoperative period include hypoventilation and atelectasis. Hypoventilation may be caused by respiratory muscle weakness, decreased ventilatory drive, or exacerbation of chronic pulmonary disease. Incomplete reversal of neuromuscular blockade, more commonly observed in patients who receive long-acting muscle relaxants such as pancuronium, may result in generalized weakness with uncoordinated movements, shallow breathing, atelectasis, and hypoxemia.

Inadequate analgesia, gastric distention, restrictive surgical dressings, and obesity may increase the work of breathing and contribute to the development of respiratory failure and hypoxemia. Residual anesthetics and ventilatory depression from opioids and benzodiazepines also may cause significant hypoventilation with carbon dioxide retention, respiratory acidosis, and hypoxemia.

A cerebrovascular accident should be ruled out in a patient with hypoventilation and altered mental status.

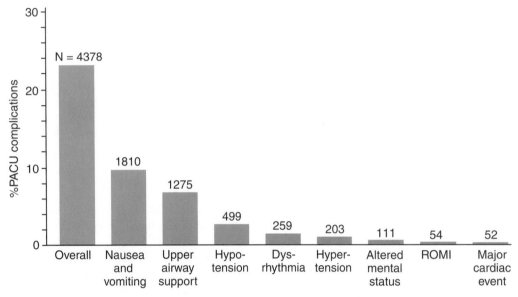

Figure 53.1. Major PACU complications by percentage of occurrence, from a prospective study of 18,473 patients. Reproduced with permission. (From Hines R, et al. Complications occurring in the postoperative care unit: a survey. *Anesth Analg* 1992; 74:503–509.) ROMI, rule out myocardial infarction.

Aspiration is an infrequent cause of perioperative hypoxemia but may result in severe morbidity. Inhalation of sterile acidic gastric contents may cause aspiration pneumonitis, whereas contents colonized with pathogenic bacteria may cause pneumonia. Symptoms depend on the type and volume of the material aspirated and include bronchospasm, tachypnea, hypoxemia, tachycardia, and hypotension. Aspiration of large volumes may require bronchoscopy to remove particulate matter from the tracheobronchial tree, administration of bronchodilators, and mechanical ventilation for correction of hypoxemia and hypercapnia. Empiric antibiotic treatment is not recommended. Steroids have not been shown to be beneficial.

Pulmonary edema caused by left ventricular dysfunction or mitral valve disease (cardiogenic pulmonary edema) or

increased pulmonary capillary permeability (noncardiac pulmonary edema) may hinder gas exchange and lead to significant hypoxemia. Supplemental oxygen, diuretics, and vasodilators may reverse the course of the disease, but mechanical ventilation with positive end-expiratory pressure may be required in some cases. A cardiology evaluation may be indicated if myocardial ischemia or valvular disease is a contributing factor.

Pulmonary embolism is another cause of hypoxemia. It is associated with significant perioperative morbidity and mortality. The most common cause of pulmonary embolism is a venous thrombosis, usually originating in a leg or pelvic vein. Thrombosis is triggered by venous stasis, hypercoagulability, and inflammation of the vascular wall.

Other common materials that can form emboli include fat that escapes into the blood from a long bone fracture or mobilized during orthopedic surgery, and amniotic fluid embolized into the pelvic veins during a tumultuous childbirth.

Symptoms of pulmonary embolism include dyspnea, pleuritic pain, hypoxemia, and, in severe cases, cardiovascular compromise or collapse. As thrombolysis and aggressive anticoagulation often are contraindicated in the early postoperative period, treatment generally is only supportive. However, an inferior vena cava filter may be beneficial in preventing further embolism.

Pneumothorax should always be considered in patients with respiratory distress or hypoxemia, particularly after thoracic or upper abdominal procedures, tracheostomy, or central line placement. Auscultation of the lungs will reveal decreased or absent breath sounds over the affected lung, but chest radiography often is required to confirm the diagnosis.

Tension pneumothorax causes rapid deterioration in gas exchange and marked hemodynamic instability and requires immediate decompression.

Table 53.1. ASA standards for postoperative care

I	All patients who have received general anesthesia, regional anesthesia, or monitored anesthesia care shall receive appropriate postanesthesia management.
II	A patient transported to the PACU shall be accompanied by a member of the anesthesia team who is knowledgeable about the patient's condition. The patient shall be continually evaluated and treated during transport with monitoring and support appropriate to the patient's condition.
III	Upon arrival to the PACU, the patient shall be reevaluated and a verbal report provided to the responsible PACU nurse by the member of the anesthesia care team who accompanies the patient.
IV	The patient's condition shall be evaluated continually in the PACU.
V	A physician is responsible for discharge of the patient from the PACU.

From the ASA Standards for Postanesthesia Care. Available at: http://www.asahq.org/publicationsAndServices/standards/36.pdf. Accessed August 2008.

Hypotension

Hypotension is a common postoperative complication, and hypotension may result from intravascular volume depletion or decreased cardiac output or vascular tone. Perioperative hemorrhage, inadequate fluid replacement, and fluid sequestration are common causes of intravascular volume depletion, and assessment requires consideration of the patient's preoperative volume status, type and duration of surgery, and intraoperative blood loss and fluid replacement. Administration of a fluid bolus is considered a safe maneuver for the initial assessment of a patient's intravascular volume status. Nevertheless, echocardiography may be required if hypotension persists despite seemingly adequate fluid replacement.

Myocardial ischemia and infarction and dysrhythmias are common causes of decreased cardiac output and should always be considered in the hypotensive patient. If present, they should be treated immediately. Systemic vasodilation due to rewarming, systemic inflammation and sepsis, neuraxial blockade, or residual anesthesia also may cause systemic hypotension by decreasing vascular tone and impairing venous return. Diagnosis of the specific etiology is crucial, although vasoconstrictors such as phenylephrine or norepinephrine may be used for symptomatic treatment.

Cardiac dysrhythmia

Cardiac dysrhythmias, common causes of decreased cardiac output and hypotension in the postoperative period, are most likely to occur in patients with underlying structural heart disease. However, sinus tachycardia, the most common cardiac dysrhythmia in the immediate postoperative period, is usually benign and resolves when its underlying etiology, such as pain, anxiety, anemia, hypovolemia, or hypoxia, is treated. Nevertheless, in patients at risk for myocardial ischemia, the rate should be controlled by correcting the underlying cause. Pharmacological management of tachycardia (e.g., with β-blockers or calcium channel blockers) should not be attempted until the aforementioned treatable etiologies are excluded.

Atrial fibrillation, a common dysrhythmia, has the potential for serious consequences in the postoperative period. Unstable patients with a rapid ventricular rate require urgent cardioversion, whereas rate control can be achieved in stable patients with β-blockers, calcium channel blockers, or amiodarone.

Bradycardia without hypotension is benign and requires no treatment. In a patient with symptomatic bradycardia, anticholinergics may improve atrioventricular nodal conduction, but epinephrine, isoproterenol, or ventricular pacing may be required to increase the ventricular rate. Electrolyte imbalances, acid–base abnormalities, hypoxia, and pharmacologic effects of drugs such as digoxin should be ruled out. Complete heart block may develop in patients with preexisting conduction disease and often will result in hypotension and inadequate organ perfusion. A cardiologist should be consulted to assist in the management of patients with dysrhythmias associated with hemodynamic compromise.

Myocardial ischemia

ECG changes are common after anesthesia and surgery, resulting from the effects of anesthetics and other administered drugs, increased sympathetic tone, hypothermia, and electrolyte imbalances. Changes in P- or T-wave morphology, intraventricular conduction, or ST segments may occur in the absence of a cardiac abnormality or ischemia. Perioperative myocardial ischemia and infarction often occur within the first 2 days following surgery and may be difficult to diagnose in the PACU, as residual anesthesia and analgesia may mask chest pain, and pain perception may be altered because of the competing stimulus of surgical pain.

ECG and serial markers of myocardial injury should be examined if myocardial ischemia is suspected, and measures to enhance the myocardial oxygen supply/demand ratio (oxygen administration, rate control, aspirin, and nitrates) should be implemented immediately. Early consultation with a cardiologist should be considered, particularly in a hemodynamically unstable patient or a patient with evidence of ongoing myocardial ischemia who may require invasive monitoring and reperfusion therapy (e.g., thrombolysis, percutaneous angioplasty).

Pacemaker and implantable cardioverter–defibrillator dysfunction

Permanent pacemakers and implanted cardiac defibrillators (ICDs) deserve special consideration in the perioperative period. The patient's medical history and pacemaker dependency and possible perioperative complications should be discussed with the operating room team and the patient's cardiologist. Electrocautery used during surgery may increase the pacing rate or inhibit the pacing function, convert a pacemaker to "noise reversion" mode, or damage the lead–tissue interface or the pacemaker or ICD circuitry. ECG monitoring is essential in the postoperative setting, and all patients with a pacemaker or ICD should remain in a monitored setting postoperatively until the device is interrogated to confirm proper functioning.

Hypertension

Hypertension, a common postoperative problem, frequently is observed in patients who did not receive their regular antihypertensive medications preoperatively and is more commonly present after neurosurgical, vascular, and cardiac procedures. If uncontrolled, postoperative hypertension can potentially precipitate surgical bleeding and lead to end-organ damage, including myocardial ischemia and dysrhythmias, congestive heart failure, cerebral bleeding, and edema.

Reversible causes of hypertension, such as pain, anxiety, hypoxemia, and hypercarbia, should be treated before antihypertensive treatment is initiated. The decision to treat hypertension should take into consideration the patient's baseline blood pressure, coexisting diseases, and perceived risk of complications. Short-term treatment in the PACU is achieved using IV agents such as β-blockers (e.g., esmolol, metoprolol), vasodilators (e.g., hydralazine), or labetalol (that is both a β-blocker and vasodilator). For persistent or refractory hypertension, continuous infusion of a vasodilator such as nitroglycerin or nitroprusside may be needed.

Oliguria and urinary retention

Oliguria, defined as urine output < 0.5 ml/kg/h, may be a sign of acute renal failure, with the risk for significant perioperative morbidity and mortality. Acute renal failure may be broadly categorized as prerenal, renal, or postrenal.

Prerenal failure is the result of reduced renal perfusion, usually related to hypovolemia or hypotension. In prerenal failure, renal function is impaired, but there is no parenchymal damage. Administration of an IV fluid bolus may be helpful in the assessment of the fluid status, but more extensive workup, including echocardiography, may also be required.

Postrenal failure is caused by an obstruction to urine flow. Assessing the urinary catheter for kinking or obstruction (by irrigation) or catheter migration is important to exclude those causes, but obstruction of the bilateral urinary tracts also may cause postrenal failure and may require diagnosis with ultrasound or CT imaging of the kidneys.

Acute tubular necrosis refers to necrosis of kidney tubules and is used to describe the clinical syndrome of reversible acute intrinsic renal failure that follows an episode of renal ischemia or exposure to nephrotoxins such as organic solvents, aminoglycoside antibiotics, radiologic contrast media, and myoglobin. Analysis of urine and plasma osmolality and electrolytes, acid–base status, and urine microscopy is helpful in the assessment of the etiology, but an ultrasound scan of the kidneys, urography, or renal biopsy may be required for definitive diagnosis. Consultation with a nephrologist may be indicated.

Delirium

Postoperative delirium, the most commonly encountered serious mental disturbance in the postoperative period, may present as reduced awareness, apathy, or drowsiness, although restlessness, hyperactivity, and agitation are more commonly associated signs. Elderly patients and those with a history of organic brain disease or mental disorders are at particular risk. Ruling out physiologic causes of delirium, such as hypoxemia, hypotension, and hypoglycemia, should be the first priority in management.

Other common causes include postoperative pain, bladder distention, and electrolyte and acid–base disturbances. Anticholinergics, opioids, and benzodiazepines are medications commonly associated with postoperative delirium. Physostigmine may be helpful if centrally acting anticholinergic drugs are the suspected cause. The catatonic effect of droperidol or haloperidol may be beneficial by protecting the patient from physical harm, although it does not improve the disordered thinking of delirium.

Pain

Most patients experience pain in the PACU, with approximately 20% describing the pain as severe. Adequate postoperative analgesia should always begin in the operating room and continue into the PACU (see Chapter 144). Opioids remain the mainstay of postoperative analgesia, with patient-controlled analgesia being preferred over intermittent boluses (see Chapter 37). Intravenous patient-controlled analgesia results in greater patient satisfaction compared with intermittent analgesia administered by nursing staff and should be promptly initiated in the PACU when indicated..

COX inhibitors are effective complements but have potential side effects, such as nephrotoxicity, decreased platelet aggregation, and gastrointestinal bleeding (see Chapter 42). Regional or peripheral sensory blockade is an effective alternative for patients in whom opioids are contraindicated.

Temperature abnormalities

Hypothermia remains a common problem in the postoperative period, despite an increasing body of evidence supporting intraoperative temperature control and advances in warming technology. Even mild hypothermia is associated with adverse postoperative complications, including myocardial ischemia, arrhythmias, coagulopathy, and wound infection. Warm blankets usually are sufficient therapy for patients with mild hypothermia, although forced-air warming devices are more efficient. Pharmacologic control of shivering may sometimes be achieved with a small dose of meperidine (e.g., 12.5–25 mg).

Significant hyperthermia is relatively uncommon in the immediate postoperative period. Mild elevation in body temperature, however, is not infrequently associated with the inflammatory response that accompanies surgery. Although infection is always a concern in the postoperative patient with hyperthermia, it is less likely than other etiologies to be the cause, unless bacteremia is provoked by the procedure or the patient had a preexisting infection. Febrile reaction to a medication or blood product should always be considered. Less common causes of postoperative hyperthermia include hyperthyroidism, malignant hyperthermia, and neuroleptic malignant syndrome. Treatment should be targeted toward the most likely etiology, although symptomatic treatment with acetaminophen may be helpful for patient comfort and to minimize the metabolic demands of fever.

Fluid administration in PACU

The use of colloid solutions or crystalloids for perioperative fluid resuscitation continues to generate significant debate. A possible advantage of colloids is related to their potential for effective and prolonged intravascular volume expansion. Regardless of the type of fluid administered, goal-directed perioperative fluid management has been shown to have a positive impact on outcome and to shorten the hospital stay.

Similar to the controversy over the ideal perioperative fluid management, the blood transfusion threshold for patients has been extensively debated in the literature. Recent reports that blood transfusion may adversely affect outcomes in critically ill patients support the application of a more conservative perioperative transfusion policy. Hence, it is recommended that clinicians consider the risk and benefit for each patient when deciding whether to use a volume replacement strategy that may involve blood component therapy.

Hemorrhage

Postoperative bleeding requires rapid evaluation to differentiate poor surgical hemostasis, potentially requiring an immediate reoperation, from a diffuse coagulopathy. Surgical and nonsurgical bleeding often coexist. Ongoing hemorrhage in the postoperative patient is an emergency requiring immediate treatment. Risk factors for postoperative hemorrhage, such as anticoagulation therapy and surgical complications, should prompt close monitoring in the postoperative period.

Saturated dressings, increased drain output, decrease in hemoglobin level, hypotension, tachycardia, or decreased urine output can guide the clinician in assessing the bleeding patient, but internal bleeding is not always obvious and may not be identified until the patient is severely compromised. Coordination among the surgical and anesthesia teams, the operating room staff, and the blood bank is essential.

Adequate IV access should be established immediately and the availability of appropriate blood products ensured. Thrombocytopenia, hypothermia, and loss of coagulation factors are common causes of coagulopathy in these patients, but preexisting medical conditions, such as liver failure and bone marrow suppression, and specific surgical or nonsurgical complications, such as disseminated intravascular coagulation and consumption coagulopathy, also should be considered.

Suggested readings

Adesanya AO, De Lemos JA, Greilich NB, Whitten CW. Management of perioperative myocardial infarction in noncardiac surgical patients. *Chest* 2006; 130:584–596.

Badner NH, Knill RL, Brown JE, et al. Myocardial infarction after noncardiac surgery. *Anesthesiology* 1998; 88:572–578.

Bittner EA, Grecu L, George E. Postoperative complications. In: DE Longnecker et al., eds. *Anesthesiology*. New York: McMcGraw-Hill; 2008.

Cheney FW. The American Society of Anesthesiologists Closed Claims Project: what have we learned, how has it affected practice, and how will it affect practice in the future? *Anesthesiology* 1999; 91:552–556.

Cheney FW, Domino KB, Caplan RA, Posner KL. Nerve injury associated with anesthesia: a closed claims analysis. *Anesthesiology* 1999; 90:1062–1069.

Dagi TF. The management of postoperative bleeding. *Surg Clin N Am* 2005; 85:1191–1213.

Domino KB. Office-based anesthesia: lessons learned from the Closed Claims Project. *ASA Newsletter* 2001; 65(6):9–11, 15.

Gan TJ, Meyer T, Apfel CC, et al. Consensus guidelines for managing postoperative nausea and vomiting. *Anesth Analg* 2003; 97:62–71.

Grecu L, Bittner EA, George E. Recovery of the healthy patient. In: DE Longnecker et al., eds. *Anesthesiology*. New York: McGraw-Hill; 2008.

Grocott MPW, MG Mythen, Gan TJ. Perioperative fluid management and clinical outcomes in adults. *Anesth Analg* 2005; 100: 1093–1106.

Lee LA. Postoperative visual loss data gathered and analyzed. *ASA Newsletter* 2000; 64(9):25–27.

Lepouse C, Lautner CA, Liu L, et al. Emergence delirium in adults in the post-anaesthesia care unit. *Br J Anaesth* 2006; 96:747–753.

Noble DW. Hypoxia following surgery – an unnecessary cause of morbidity and mortality? *Minerva Anestesiol* 2003; 69:447–450.

Practice guidelines for acute pain management in the perioperative setting. An updated report by the American Society of Anesthesiologists Task Force on Acute Pain Management. *Anesthesiology* 2004; 100:1573–1581.

Chapter 54

Management of postoperative nausea and vomiting

Robert M. Knapp

Introduction

Postoperative nausea and vomiting (PONV) is common following anesthesia; the overall occurrence rate is 20% to 30%. Much of the variability reflects the fact that some patients are more prone to PONV than others and that some anesthetic agents are more prone to inducing PONV than others. Identifying patients with PONV-related traits, as well as those who receive PONV-inducing agents, allows identification of subgroups of patients whose PONV risk runs as high as 70%.

Patients dislike PONV; however, this does not mean that they all dislike it equally or that they all fear it as the worst possible postoperative experience. Attempts to quantify how much patients dislike PONV have mostly involved measuring how much they claim to be willing to pay to avoid having it after surgery. The numbers are not entirely reliable, however. The dollar values given by individual patients cover enormous spreads, and the group median values vary widely from study to study. Also, it turns out that the values change when the study population is broken down into subgroups based on factors such as age, sex, level of preoperative anxiety, or household income.

Furthermore, even though preoperative questionnaires tend to rank PONV as the postoperative event most concerning to patients, those who actually experienced both pain *and* PONV felt otherwise. For example, adults who experienced postoperative pain increased the dollar value they had previously placed on pain relief. They did *not*, however, change the value they placed on PONV treatment after having PONV. Similarly, children who experienced PONV were more likely to view pain as their primary concern, even if better pain control meant a higher risk of vomiting.

Definition of PONV

PONV refers to both nausea and vomiting. Strictly speaking, the two are different. Nausea is a conscious sensation of an urge to vomit, whereas vomiting is a reflexive expulsion of gastric contents. The two symptoms seem to be intimately related, however, and the same measures generally are used to relieve both. For this reason, PONV is usually referred to and treated as a single entity.

For treatment purposes, PONV is classified as either early or late. Early PONV occurs up to 6 hours after surgery. Late PONV generally occurs up to 24 hours following surgery, although some studies expand this definition to 48 hours. Differentiating between 24 and 48 hours generally reflects an attempt to differentiate the treatment effects of different drugs.

Mechanisms of PONV

PONV is often described as multifactorial, because the list of neurotransmitters known or at least suspected to influence PONV includes histamine, opioid, acetylcholine, muscarine, neurokinin-1, serotonin, and dopamine. Stimulation of several specific nerves, particularly the vestibular-cochlear, vagus, and glossopharyngeal nerves, also may play a role. Because of the multiple possible neurotransmitters involved, the optimal management of PONV may require drugs that interact with multiple receptors.

How is PONV managed?

The management of PONV involves three steps. First, the patient's risk of having PONV is estimated preoperatively. Second, appropriate drugs are given intraoperatively to reduce this risk. Finally, those who experience PONV nonetheless are treated in the postanesthesia care unit (PACU). Occasionally, the anesthetic regimen itself is adjusted to affect PONV risk.

Estimating the risk

A given patient's risk of having PONV is increased by each "risk factor" that can be applied. Risk factors are certain traits or exposures that predispose some people toward having PONV. The four most prominent risk factors in use today are (1) a previous history of PONV, (2) a history of not smoking, (3) female gender, and (4) use of perioperative opioids. Increasing duration of surgery and certain types of surgery are also associated with elevated risk. In addition, the act of having anesthesia of any kind introduces risk, with some agents producing somewhat more risk than others.

In the most popular risk estimation algorithm in use today, the following is an approximate guide to estimating overall PONV risk: The simple fact of having any sort of anesthesia introduces its own small degree of risk, approximately 10%. (This approximately doubles with the use of a volatile agent with nitrous oxide [N_2O]). Next, the four primary risk factors each add approximately 10–20% to the risk level. The mean overall risk with one, two, three and four risk factors is approximately 20%, 40%, 60%, and 80%, with less precision in the estimates of the highest risk group (see the studies by Apfel et al. for more detail). In practice, the precise estimates are less important than the overall classification of risk to low (0–1 risk factors), moderate (2 factors), and high (3–4 factors). In addition, if the operation itself has a known association with PONV, or the duration seems significant, many anesthesiologists would consider the patient to be at least at moderate risk.

Reducing the risk

Reducing the risk of PONV is almost entirely a matter of giving medications that are known to reduce the baseline risk. It is important to remember that risk reduction, rather than risk elimination, is the expected result. Also, the results from any one drug are only modest under the best of circumstances – no medication is a complete preventive. In fact, the most effective medications stop or prevent one patient in four or five *at best* from having PONV. Given this, the primary strategy for reducing the incidence of PONV is to give the number and combination of drugs that obtain the most effective decrease in baseline risk. To maximize effectiveness, the medications selected should provide some degree of relief beyond the immediate recovery period and should also address the fact that PONV can be triggered from many different sites. The medications given should reflect a spread of durations as well as a spread of mechanisms of action.

Numerous regimens have been studied for the prophylaxis of PONV. Direct comparisons between them are complicated by differences in the studied patient population and therefore baseline risk. Moreover, many trials have focused on newer agents in preference to older drugs (which may be far less expensive but also less likely to attract funding for large studies). Several algorithms have been suggested based on the estimated PONV risk and most share a common framework. For the lowest risk patients, no prophylaxis is recommended. For those of low to moderate risk, one or two drug regimens are suggested. The most popular such regimens are a serotonin antagonist alone, or the combination of dexamethasone and a serotonin antagonist. Although the data supporting timing of administration are sparse, most authorities recommend steroids be given early in the case, and anti-serotonin agents just prior to emergence. As noted earlier, there are likely other regimens of similar efficacy, although none has been studied as extensively nor compared head-to-head with this combination. For high-risk patients, a three- or four-drug regimen (with drugs from different classes) is commonly recommended. In addition, efforts to reduce anesthetic-related factors contributing to PONV risk are indicated (see "Adjusting the anesthetic regimen"). Reasonable alternatives to dexamethasone include scopolamine patches and perhaps the neurokinin-1 receptor antagonists, though the latter are very expensive. Low-dose butyrophenones (droperidol, haloperidol) are very effective alternatives or supplements

to serotonin antagonists and likely do not significantly increase the risk of dangerous dysrhythmias such as torsades de pointes. Metoclopramide is likely effective only in higher doses and not as effective as serotonin antagonists.

Treating PONV in the PACU

Comparatively little research has been directed at the treatment of established PONV. Treating PONV in the PACU is partly an extension of prophylactic regimens and partly an extension of older regimens passed on by oral tradition. The medications used in current prophylactic regimens also may be used as treatments for PONV. The most important caveat is that if they already were given as prophylaxis, the medications are unlikely to have much treatment effect if repeated in the PACU. However, medications such as low-dose butyrophenones droperidol 0.625 mg intravenously (IV); and haloperidol, 1 mg IV, may be overlooked as prophylactics so are then available for PACU therapy. Some medications, such as dexamethasone and transdermal scopolamine, are not well suited for PACU therapy because of their prolonged time to onset.

Medications that block the histamine H_1 receptor, such as promethazine and hydroxyzine, are commonly used as antiemetics. Promethazine has been studied and found to be more efficacious than a repeat dose of ondansetron given for PONV in the PACU. The dose most commonly given is 6.25 mg IV, which has shown the same efficacy as doses of 12.5 and 25 mg. If serotonin antagonists have not been used for prophylaxis, very low doses (e.g., ondansetron 1 mg) may be effective.

Principles for PACU treatment are as follows:

1. Do not repeat drugs already given for prophylaxis.
2. Consider drugs with good antiemetic properties that have not already been given, such as a low-dose butyrophenone.
3. When implementing a prophylactic regimen, and if considering a 5-hydroxytryptamine 3 (5-HT$_3$) antagonist such as ondansetron, consider reserving it for rescue.
4. Older drugs given on the basis of tradition, such as promethazine, 6.25 mg IV, may have a significant antiemetic effect.

Adjusting the anesthetic regimen

In any patient with elevated risk of PONV, it is prudent to minimize the contribution of the anesthetic to this risk.

Volatile agents/N$_2$O

Both volatile agents and N_2O are widely thought to increase the incidence of PONV. However, determining the effect of omitting N_2O is complicated by the requirement to substitute another agent, sometimes potent volatile anesthetics, which may themselves contribute to PONV risk. A meta-analysis of 24 trials found that omitting N_2O reduced the risk by 27% overall, with an NNT of 13. However, the effect was highly dependent on the baseline risk of PONV. In studies in patients with lower than average risk, the effect of omitting N_2O was not statistically significant; in those with above average baseline risk the effect was stronger and the NNT was 5. The authors also cautioned that the NNT for intraoperative awareness was 46 compared to anesthetics in which N_2O was used, limiting the overall benefit of its omission. In separate meta-analyses of trials comparing propofol, with or without N_2O, to inhaled anesthetics with or without N_2O, little benefit was found in substituting propofol for N_2O. The NNT was 9 when propofol was used for induction only, and 6 when used for maintenance, relative to other techniques. The early prevention (0–6 hr after surgery) of nausea was the strongest effect of propofol. TIVA (with propofol) had a NNT of 6 when compared to general anesthesia, including N_2O. General anesthesia with both volatile anesthetics and N_2O produced more PONV than the other techniques.

Propofol

Propofol is often described as being protective against PONV. There are three clinical contexts in which this claim is made: propofol infused as a general anesthetic, propofol used as a bolus induction agent, and propofol given in small amounts as a rescue drug used to treat PONV in the PACU.

In the general anesthetic context, propofol is almost universally said to protect against PONV, and by a significant amount. However, the preceding analysis of PONV risk with volatile/N_2O anesthesia shows that the difference between volatile and propofol techniques is not very great. The second context, propofol used as a bolus induction agent was shown by meta-analysis to cause nearly no significant reduction in PONV. Only in patients with a relatively high baseline risk of PONV was there any discernable effect, and the NNT was 9.

Finally, propofol given in subhypnotic doses, 20 mg every 5 minutes as needed according to one study, appears to have a good antiemetic effect, although the duration is uncertain.

Neostigmine

The effects of neostigmine on PONV are somewhat controversial. One meta-analysis found that neostigmine at dosages over 2 mg was associated with an increased risk. However, a later review found no association between neostigmine and PONV at any dose.

Clinical summary for providing PONV prophylaxis

A reasonable strategy for PONV prophylaxis is as follows:

1. Estimate the risk. Get a sense of whether the patient appears to be at low or medium to high risk for PONV. The presence of only one of the common risk factors establishes a low sense of risk, unless there are additional considerations, such as the likelihood that the patient will receive a significant amount of postoperative opioids or is undergoing a surgery associated with a high PONV rate. The risk should then be considered at least moderate. Two risk factors establish a moderate sense of risk, particularly

in the presence of a volatile-based general anesthetic or for a surgical procedure that either is associated with PONV or is of longer duration. More than two risk factors should by themselves indicate a moderate to high risk.

2. Give prophylaxis according to the sense of risk. A low sense may merit a wait-and-see approach (no drugs) or baseline prophylaxis (two drugs). A moderate to high sense merits full prophylaxis (three or four drugs).

3. Use dexamethasone as the foundation drug (unless it is inappropriate for the patient). Dexamethasone works well with others and has a relatively long duration. Transdermal scopolamine is a cost-effective alternative; aprepitant is a very costly one.

4. When using a serotonin antagonist, combine it with a longer acting drug, generally give it near the end of surgery, and consider giving it in the PACU. Once it is given, there is no effect from a second dose. Finally, when PONV rescue is needed in the PACU, ondansetron is an excellent choice.

Suggested readings

Apfel CC, Korttila D, Abdalla M, et al. A factorial trial of six interventions of the prevention of postoperative nausea and vomiting. *N Engl J Med* 2004; 350:2441–2451.

Apfel CC, Uiara E, Koivuranta M, et al. A simplified risk score for predicting postoperative nausea and vomiting. *Anesthesiology* 1999; 91:693–700.

Cheng C, Sessler DI, Apfel CC. Does neostigmine administration produce a clinically important increase in postoperative nausea and vomiting? *Anesth Analg* 2005; 101:1349–1355.

Dolin SJ, Cashman JN. Tolerability of acute postoperative pain management: nausea, vomiting, sedation, pruritus, and urinary retention. Evidence from published data. *Br J Anaesth* 2005; 95:584–591.

Fortney JT, Gan TJ, Graczyk S, et al. A comparison of the efficacy, safety, and patient satisfaction of ondansetron versus droperidol as antiemetics for elective outpatient surgical procedures. *Anesth Analg* 1998; 86:731–738.

Gan TJ. Risk factors for postoperative nausea and vomiting. *Anesth Analg* 2006; 102:1884–1889.

Gan TJ, Meyer TA, Apfel CC, et al. Society for ambulatory anesthesia guidelines for the management of postoperative nausea and vomiting. *Anesth Analg* 2007; 105:1615–1628.

Henzi I, Walder B, Tramer MR. Dexamethasone for the prevention of postoperative nausea and vomiting: a quantitative systematic review. *Anesth Analg* 2000; 90:186–194.

Kovac AL, Jense HG, O'Conner TA, et al. Efficacy of repeat intravenous dosing of ondansetron in controlling postoperative nausea and vomiting: a randomized, double-blind, placebo-controlled multicenter trial. *J Clin Anesth* 1999; 11:453–459.

Parlak I, Erdur B, Parlak M, et al. Midazolam vs. diphenhydramine for the treatment of metoclopramide-induced akathisia: a randomized controlled trial. *Acad Emerg Med* 2007; 14: 715–721.

Scuderi PE, James RL, Harris L, Mims GR. Antiemetic prophylaxis does not improve outcomes after outpatient surgery when compared to symptomatic treatment. *Anesthesiology* 1999; 90:360–371.

Tang J, Wang B, White, PF, et al. The effect of timing of ondansetron administration on its efficacy, cost-effectiveness, and cost-benefit as a prophylactic antiemetic in the ambulatory setting. *Anesthesia Analgesia* 1998; 86:274–282.

Tramer M, Moore A, McQuay H. Omitting nitrous oxide in general anaesthesia: meta-analysis of intraoperative awareness and postoperative emesis in randomized controlled trials. *Br J Anaesth* 1996; 76:186–193.

Tramer M, Moore A, McQuay H. Propofol anaesthesia and postoperative nausea and vomiting: quantitative systematic review of randomized controlled studies. *Br J Anaesth* 1997; 78:247–255.

Van Den Bosch JE, Bonsel GJ, Moons KG, Kalkman CJ. Effect of postoperative experiences on willingness to pay to avoid postoperative pain, nausea, and vomiting. *Anesthesiology* 2006; 104:1033–1039.

Wallenborn J, Gelbrich G, Bulst D, et al. Prevention of postoperative nausea and vomiting by metoclopramide combined with dexamethasone: randomized double blind multicentre trial. *BMJ* 2006; 333:324.

Chapter 55

Cognitive changes after surgery and anesthesia

Joshua C. Vacanti, Gregory J. Crosby, and Deborah J. Culley

It has long been recognized that patients subjected to the stress of surgery are at risk for the development of a host of neurologic impairments postoperatively. These may result from well-known metabolic or physiologic derangements that occur intraoperatively. Conversely, patients who undergo seemingly uneventful surgery routinely develop cognitive dysfunction that cannot easily be attributed to any clear operative event. In the acute phase, cognitive dysfunction presenting as transient confusion is commonly referred to as *postoperative delirium*. It is typified by an acute fluctuating course that may begin at emergence from anesthesia, during recovery in the postanesthesia care unit, or more typically after discharge to the floor. More concerning is the fact that a small subset of patients appear to suffer from long-term cognitive changes following surgery; this constellation of changes in a patient's cognitive function is generally referred to as *postoperative cognitive dysfunction*.

Although postoperative changes in cognition have not yet been as thoroughly researched as other areas in anesthesia, such as postoperative nausea and vomiting, the significance of these pathologies in terms of physical, emotional, and monetary cost may be enormous. The postoperative patient who suffers from delirium also suffers from an increased risk of self-injury, extended hospital stays, and a higher incidence of placement in long-term care facilities, all of which increase the cost of health care. These additional costs add to the financial burden of the US health care system by adding billions of dollars in payments per year. The potential impact of long-term postoperative cognitive dysfunction on society extends well beyond the health care industry, and the societal contributions are likely to be even more burdensome.

Postoperative delirium

Delirium is the most common form of cognitive impairment in hospitalized patients. Although delirium may occur at any age, it is especially common in hospitalized elders; 40% of elderly medical patients and 10% to 40% of elderly surgical patients become delirious during their hospital stay. In fact, delirium is the most common perioperative morbidity in elders. Delirium is an acute transient organic brain syndrome characterized by disturbances of consciousness and cognition that develop over a relatively short period (hours to days) and wax and wane over the course of the day. The *Diagnostic and Statistical Manual of Mental Disorders* (DSM-IV) criteria for delirium include a disturbance of consciousness with altered awareness of the environment, inability to sustain or shift attention, and a change in cognition or development of perceptual disturbances that are not better explained by preexisting, established, or evolving dementia. The Confusion Assessment Method (CAM) and its variant for intubated, nonverbal patients in the intensive care unit, the CAM-ICU, are widely used at the bedside to diagnose delirium. They both have the benefits of ease, speed, reliability, and validity (Table 55.1).

Delirium is generally divided into three types: hyperactive, hypoactive, and mixed. Agitation, irritability, restlessness, and aggression characterize the hyperactive form, whereas hypoactive delirium is typified by somnolence and psychomotor

Table 55.1. Confusion Assessment Method[a]

CAM diagnostic algorithm – the diagnosis of delirium requires the presence of features 1 and 2 *and* the presence of feature 3 or 4

Feature 1: acute or fluctuating course
This feature is usually obtained from a family member or nurse and is shown by positive responses to the following questions: Is there evidence of an acute change in mental status from the patient's baseline? Did the (abnormal) behavior fluctuate during the day, i.e., did it tend to come and go, or increase and decrease in severity?

Feature 2: inattention
This feature is shown by a positive response to the following question: Did the patient have difficulty focusing attention, e.g., was he or she easily distractible or did he or she have difficulty keeping track of what was being said?

Feature 3: disorganized thinking
This feature is shown by a positive response to the following question: Was the patient disorganized or incoherent, e.g., did he or she engage in rambling or irrelevant conversation, an unclear or illogical flow of ideas, or unpredictable switching from subject to subject?

Feature 4: altered level of consciousness
This feature is shown by any answer other than "alert" to the following question: Overall, how would you rate this patient's level of consciousness? (Alert [normal], vigilant [hyperalert], lethargic [drowsy, easily aroused], stuporous [difficult to arouse], comatose [unarousable].)

[a] The CAM diagnostic algorithm is a short test used by clinicians to differentiate delirium from other cognitive impairments. Through correlation with DSM-IV criteria for delirium, the CAM diagnostic algorithm has a reported sensitivity of 94% to 100% and a specificity of 90% to 95%. From Inouye SK, van Dyck CH, Alessi CA, et al. Clarifying confusion: The confusion assessment method. A new method for detection of delirium. *Ann Intern Med* 1990; 113:041–8.

Table 55.2. Risk factors for delirium[a]

Nonmodifiable factors	Modifiable factors
Age > 70 y	Metabolic/physiologic derangements
Preexisting cognitive impairment	Hypoxemia
History of delirium	Hypercarbia
History of depression	Hypoglycemia
Multiple comorbidities	Hypoalbuminemia[b]
Poor functional status	Perioperative anemia[b]
Genetic factors – apo E4	Electrolyte disturbances
Type of surgery	Hypothermia
Major orthopedic	Occult infection
Cardiac	Occult cerebrovascular event
Thoracic	Iatrogenic causes[c]
Vascular	Pain
Emergency	Acute systemic disturbances
	Urinary retention, fecal impaction

[a] Patients with any of the nonmodifiable factors demonstrate an increased risk for the development of delirium postoperatively and should be identified during the preoperative assessment. Patients who develop delirium after surgery should be evaluated for any of the modifiable factors and treated accordingly.

[b] Linked to the development of postoperative delirium, although perioperative correction has not been demonstrated to improve the clinical course of delirium.

[c] Anticholinergics (with the exception of glycopyrrolate), benzodiazepines, and antidopaminergic agents are the most commonly implicated agents.

slowing. Because delirious patients who are hypoactive look sedated and are not bothersome to hospital staff, the delirium frequently goes undetected. A common misconception is that delirium is transient and harmless. In fact, delirium may last days to weeks. It is associated with a longer hospital stay (and cost) and a greater chance of requiring discharge to a post-acute care nursing facility; and patients with delirium have a higher 1-year mortality than those who do not develop it in the hospital.

Conditions contributing to delirium can be divided into nonmodifiable and modifiable factors (Table 55.2).

Age greater than 70 years, preexisting cognitive impairment, a history of delirium, depression, multiple comorbidities, poor functional status, and the apolipoprotein (apo) E4 genotype are important predictors. The type of surgery is also important, with major orthopedic, cardiac, thoracic, vascular, and emergency surgery carrying the greatest risk. Among the modifiable factors, metabolic and physiologic derangements are common causes of confusion. Hypoxemia, hypercarbia, and hypoglycemia are readily identifiable and potentially life-threatening causes of postoperative delirium and should be treated without delay. There is also evidence that low serum albumin concentration or hematocrit values are associated with development of postoperative confusion, but it is not established that correction of these abnormalities alters the clinical course of the delirium. The role of intraoperative hypotension in development of delirium is unclear, with some studies indicating elders maintained at a mean arterial blood pressure of 45 to 55 mm Hg are no more likely to develop postoperative delirium than those whose

mean arterial pressure is maintained between 55 and 70 mm Hg. Electrolyte disturbances, mild hypothermia, subclinical infection, and an occult neurologic event such as a stroke should also be considered.

Anesthetic agents and drugs used in conjunction with surgical anesthesia have been implicated in postoperative delirium. Anticholinergic agents may be best avoided in elders. The aged brain has a relative cholinergic deficiency, and these drugs, with the exception of glycopyrrolate, which does not cross the blood–brain barrier, increase the risk of postoperative delirium, presumably by further reducing cholinergic neurotransmission. In susceptible elderly patients, even small dosages of drugs with anticholinergic effects may produce symptoms of confusion, agitation, and disorientation. If these symptoms occur, physostigmine, a centrally active acetylcholinesterase inhibitor, may be useful in partially reversing the symptoms.

Benzodiazepines are also problematic. They have prolonged effects in the elderly and sometimes produce paradoxic disinhibition and agitation.

Antihistamines given for their antiemetic effects, such as diphenhydramine, hydroxyzine, and promethazine, all have significant central anticholinergic effects. Antagonism of dopamine may exacerbate symptoms in patients at risk for postoperative delirium.

What is curious and surprising is that the type of anesthesia used does not seem to affect delirium risk. Specifically, there is no benefit of spinal or epidural anesthesia in elders in terms of the risk of developing delirium perioperatively and no indication that delirium is more likely with the use of nitrous oxide or a particular volatile agent.

Pain is an important and underrecognized contributor to delirium in the postoperative period. Elderly, cognitively intact patients with inadequately treated postoperative pain are nine times more likely to develop delirium than those whose pain is controlled. The specifics of pain treatment are less important than the quality of pain control. Indeed, in the postoperative period, low but not high opioid use is a factor in the development of delirium. This is relevant because studies show that cognitively impaired patients receive only 30% to 50% as much opioid as cognitively intact patients. This suggests that suboptimal pain management in demented and delirious patients may contribute further to their cognitive deterioration. Meperidine is an exception to this rule and should probably be avoided in geriatric patients. It has been associated with the development of postoperative delirium, presumably because of accumulation of toxic metabolites or its anticholinergic activity.

The key to managing postoperative delirium is to avoid it by identifying patients at greatest risk, correcting metabolic or physiologic abnormalities that may contribute, and selecting anesthetic adjuvants carefully and using them sparingly and deliberately. There is also evidence that a preoperative geriatric consultation and perioperative use of visual aids, environments, and cognitive and physical activities designed specifically for at-risk patients may reduce the incidence of delirium significantly. Once delirium occurs, it is important to look aggressively for treatable causes (e.g., hypoxia, electrolyte disturbances, drug effects, infection) and to correct them before embarking on pharmacotherapy. Pharmacologic treatment of delirium is controversial, and one should resort to it only after treating remediable medical conditions. Haloperidol remains the mainstay of pharmacologic treatment of agitated delirium but may produce extrapyramidal side effects. Sedating a delirious patient with lorazepam or another benzodiazepine is inadvisable because these agents have themselves been implicated in development of delirium and may produce a paradoxic reaction of agitation and disinhibition in elders. Thus, whenever pharmacologic treatment of delirium is considered, it is wise to abide by the geriatrician's adage: "start low, and go slow."

Postoperative cognitive dysfunction

Postoperative cognitive dysfunction (POCD) is operationally defined as a subtle and long-lasting impairment in cognitive function after surgery and anesthesia. First described more than 50 years ago, it has only recently been accepted as a legitimate and common perioperative morbidity, especially in the elderly. POCD is present in 25% to 40% of elderly patients in the first week after noncardiac, nonneurologic surgery and even in 10% to 14% 3 months postoperatively. In contrast, only about 3% of age-matched controls (not hospitalized, no surgery) decline over the same interval. Postoperative cognitive impairment is not unique to the elderly. The incidence is similar in young, middle-aged, and aged patients during the first postoperative week, but it persists only in elders. Besides advanced age, important patient- or procedure-specific risk factors include low educational level, history of a previous stroke, the type of surgery (lower incidence with minor ambulatory surgery), duration of anesthesia, prolonged hospital stay, and postoperative infectious and respiratory complications (Table 55.3). Genetic predisposition may play a role, but the only study thus far looked at apo E4, a susceptibility gene for Alzheimer's disease, and no association with POCD was found.

Unlike delirium, which is a clinical diagnosis, POCD is defined by performance on various neuropsychological tests. One problem this creates is that not all studies adhere to the same test batteries and statistical criteria, leading to variability in the reported incidence of POCD. In fact, standardization of the definition of POCD and improvement in conventional methods for identifying it are needed for the field to advance. Another issue is that although patients with preexisting cognitive impairment or dementia would seem more likely to be at risk for POCD, these patients have been excluded from studies to date – so the true incidence of POCD may be higher.

The cognitive domains most often affected are memory and/or executive function. Particularly in those with dysfunction in both of these domains, POCD is associated with limitations in activities of daily living. Moreover, POCD at the time of hospital discharge and 3 months later is associated with higher 1-year mortality. Thus, POCD occurs in at least one third of patients in the first week after surgery, lasts 3 months or more in some elderly persons, and is associated with functional limitations and greater 1-year mortality. The encouraging news is that patients seem to recover completely within 1 to 2 years or less, but this optimism is based on follow-up of only a small subgroup.

The key question is, what causes POCD? The answer is that no one is certain. Surprisingly, intraoperative hypotension (mean arterial pressure $< 60\%$ for ≥ 30 minutes) and hypoxemia (oxygen saturation of hemoglobin ≤ 80 for > 2 minutes) are not predictors of cognitive decline 3 months postoperatively in elders. Surgery and/or general anesthesia may, however, contribute to POCD by more subtle and insidious means. Surgery induces a robust peripheral inflammatory response, and there is an associated inflammatory response in the cerebrospinal fluid (CSF) and brain. Because inflammatory cytokines interfere with neural events involved in memory and, in high concentrations, produce neurotoxicity and neurodegeneration, surgery may impair cognition and contribute to POCD via inflammation. General anesthesia also may be involved. Of course, the most profound change in cognition in the perioperative period occurs during general anesthesia, and evidence from animal studies shows that general anesthesia without surgery caused impaired spatial learning for days to weeks in aged rats. These data imply either that the neurobiological machinery of memory is altered in an enduring way by anesthesia itself or that damage occurs. There is some support for both concepts, with reports that general anesthesia leads to persistent changes in gene expression in the brain of old animals and that common volatile anesthetics promote formation and/or reduce clearance of amyloid β, a protein implicated in the pathogenesis of Alzheimer's disease, and change its physical properties to augment its neurotoxic qualities. The roles of inflammation and anesthesia in POCD remain unclear, however, because inflammatory markers in the CSF return to normal within days of surgery. Clinical studies find no difference between regional and general anesthesia regarding the risk of prolonged POCD and do not identify previous general anesthesia as a risk factor for development of Alzheimer's disease. This issue has garnered considerable attention recently, but more work is necessary

Table 55.3. Risk factors for POCD[a]

Age > 70 y
Low educational level
History of cognitive impairment
Type of surgery
Duration of anesthesia
Prolonged hospital course
Postoperative infection
Postoperative respiratory complications
? Genetic predisposition[b]

[a] Patients with any of these risk factors demonstrate an increased incidence of POCD.
[b] Currently under investigation.

before the etiology, neurobiology, and clinical significance of POCD are fully understood.

The uncertainty about the mechanisms of POCD makes it difficult to recommend specific prevention or treatment strategies. Other than recognizing that elders are often cognitively fragile and treating them accordingly, there presently is no scientific basis for recommending (or avoiding) a particular anesthetic agent or technique on the basis of concerns about POCD. This may change quickly with ongoing research.

The aged brain is different from the young brain in many respects, making elders more vulnerable to perioperative cognitive complications such as delirium and persistent POCD. These perioperative cognitive morbidities are a major challenge for the anesthesiologist and perioperative physician because they may lead to prolonged hospital stay and poor postsurgical functioning, and appear to be associated with increased 1-year mortality. The specific features of hospitalization, surgery, and anesthesia that contribute to these cognitive morbidities are not well defined, making prevention and treatment difficult. With the population aging, the challenge for the decades ahead is to better understand the role of surgery and anesthesia in causation of these complications so that perioperative physicians can tailor care for the elderly patient with the aged brain in mind.

Suggested readings

Adunsky A, Levy R, Mizrahi E, Arad M. Exposure to opioid analgesia in cognitively impaired and delirious elderly hip fracture patients. *Arch Gerontol Geriatr* 2002; 35:245–251.

Carnes M, Howell T, Rosenberg M, et al. Physicians vary in approaches to the clinical management of delirium. *J Am Geriatr Soc* 2003; 51:234–239.

Culley DJ, Yukhananov RY, Xie Z, et al. Altered hippocampal gene expression 2 days after general anesthesia in rats. *Eur J Pharmacol* 2006 549:71–78.

Dyer CB, Ashton CM, Teasdale TA. Postoperative delirium. A review of 80 primary data-collection studies. *Arch Intern Med* 1995; 155:461–465.

Johnson T, Monk T, Rasmussen LS, et al. Postoperative cognitive dysfunction in middle-aged patients. *Anesthesiology* 2002; 96:1351–1357.

Lynch EP, Lazor MA, Gellis JE, et al. The impact of postoperative pain on the development of postoperative delirium. *Anesth Analg* 1998; 86:781–785.

Marcantonio ER, Flacker JM, Wright RJ, Resnick NM. Reducing delirium after hip fracture: a randomized trial. *J Am Geriatr Soc* 2001; 49:516–522.

Newman S, Stygall J, Hirani S, et al. Postoperative cognitive dysfunction after noncardiac surgery: a systematic review. *Anesthesiology* 2007; 106:572–590.

Price CC, Garvan CW, Monk TG. Type and severity of cognitive decline in older adults after noncardiac surgery. *Anesthesiology* 2008; 108:8–17.

Sandberg O, Gustafson Y, Brannstrom B, Bucht G. Clinical profile of delirium in older patients. *J Am Geriatr Soc* 1999; 47:1300–1306.

Williams-Russo P, Sharrock NE, Mattis S, et al. Cognitive effects after epidural vs general anesthesia in older adults. A randomized trial [see comments]. *JAMA* 1995; 274:44–50.

Xie Z, Tanzi RE. Alzheimer's disease and post-operative cognitive dysfunction. *Exp Gerontol* 2006; 41:346–359.

Anatomy of the vertebral column and spinal cord

Assia Valovska

Osseous anatomy

The spinal column consists of both the vertebral column and the spinal cord. It comprises 33 vertebrae (Table 56.1) and has characteristic curves in the lumbar and thoracic regions, which give it a "double S" shape (Fig. 56.1). A lordosis is an anteriorly convex curve, seen in the cervical and lumbar region, and kyphosis is a posteriorly convex curve, seen in the thoracic and sacral sections of the spinal column. The natural curves of the spinal column may influence the spread of medications injected in the subarachnoid space. The bony vertebral column fulfills several functions (Table 56.2).

Vertebral arch and body

Each vertebra has an anterior part or body and a posterior part or vertebral arch (Fig. 56.2). The vertebral arch has two pedicles and two laminae, and together they enclose a foramen, the *vertebral foramen*. All the vertebral foramina constitute the spinal canal, which houses the spinal cord and nerve roots. Each vertebral arch supports seven processes:

- One spinous process, a midline structure arising between the two laminae, a place for attachment of muscles and ligaments.
- Two transverse processes, laterally at the junction of the laminae and the pedicles.
- Four articular processes – two superior, projecting upward, and two inferior, projecting downward – that participate in each zygapophyseal joint above and below. The pedicles of two adjacent vertebrae form the intervertebral foramina on each side, through which nerve roots exit the spinal column.

Cervical vertebrae

The vertebral bodies of the cervical spine are the smallest and have horizontal spinous processes, permitting an easy midline approach for performing neuraxial blockade. Each transverse process has a foramen. The first six foramina transversaria give passage to the vertebral artery and vein and a plexus of sympathetic nerves.

The atlas (the first cervical vertebra [C1]) lacks a body and spinous process and consists of an anterior and posterior arch

Table 56.1. Vertebral groups according to region

Cervical	7 vertebrae in the neck (C1–7)
Thoracic	12 vertebrae in the upper back corresponding to each pair of ribs (T1–12)
Lumbar	5 vertebrae in the lower back (L1–5)
Sacral	5 vertebrae fused together, forming the sacrum (S1–5)
Coccygeal	4 vertebrae fused together to form the coccyx

and two lateral masses containing the facets. The ring of the atlas is divided by the transverse atlantal ligament into a small anterior part receiving the odontoid process of the axis, and a larger posterior part housing the spinal cord. Inflammatory and arthritic changes in this ligament in patients with rheumatoid arthritis, diabetes mellitus, or trisomy 21 may lead to overt or occult subluxation of the two vertebral bodies and present a challenge at intubation. The axis (C2) has a distinct process, the odontoid (or dens axis) that represents the fusion of the bodies of the atlas and the axis. It rises perpendicularly toward the atlas and forms the pivot on which the C1 rotates to enable head rotation. The spinous process is short and bifid. The seventh vertebra (C7) has a prominent spinous process.

Thoracic vertebrae

The thoracic vertebrae are intermediate in size and increase in size from cephalad to caudad. All transverse processes, except the 11th and 12th vertebrae, have facets for articulation with the tubercles of the ribs. The laminae are thick and overlap the subjacent vertebrae like tiles on a roof. The facet joints are nearly horizontal. The spinous processes are very long, are steeply inferiorly directed, and overlap from the fifth to the eighth vertebrae. The paramedian approach to neuraxial anesthesia may be preferred to avoid the slanted spinous process.

Table 56.2. Functions of the vertebral column

Protection	Encloses the spinal cord and nerve roots
Base	Attachment place for ligaments, tendons, muscles
Structural support	Supports the head, shoulders, chest; connects the upper and lower body
Mobility	Ensures flexibility of the upper body by enabling flexion, extension, rotation

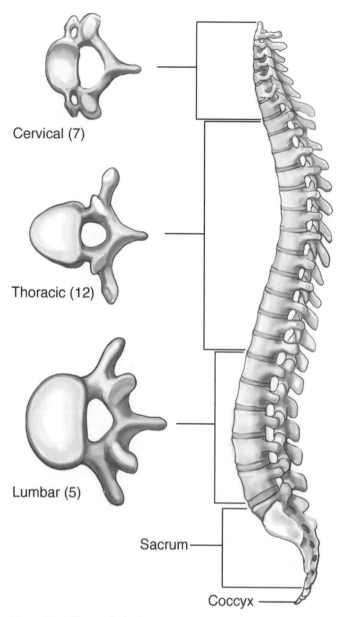

Figure 56.1. The vertebral column.

Cervical (7)

Thoracic (12)

Lumbar (5)

Sacrum

Coccyx

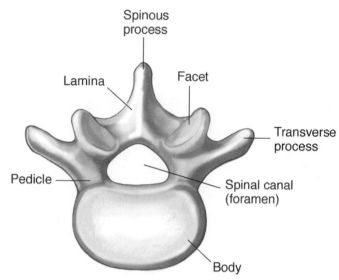

Figure 56.2. A typical lumbar vertebra.

Spinous process

Lamina

Facet

Transverse process

Pedicle

Spinal canal (foramen)

Body

Lumbar vertebrae

The vertebrae in the lumbar region have longer and wider pedicles and horizontal spinous processes. The vertebral bodies are thick and almost square. The lowest lumbar vertebra, L5, articulates with the sacrum.

Sacral vertebrae

The sacrum comprises five bones fused together in a triangular shape. The spinal canal extends into the sacrum, and the sacral nerves exit the canal through bony foramina. The lamina of S5, and partially that of S4, normally does not fuse and comprises the sacral hiatus. The coccyx is made up of four or five vertebrae fused together. All the segments lack pedicles, laminae, and spinous processes.

Intervertebral discs

The intervertebral discs are structures composed of three main components: a strong avascular annulus fibrosus, that encloses the soft nucleus pulposus, and a cartilaginous endplate (Fig. 56.3). The outer layer is richly innervated by multiple nerves and is a source of some chronic back pain.

Joints

Each vertebra joins the ones above and below it with several different types of joints. The atlanto-occipital joint is a condyloid joint between the atlas of the vertebral column and the occipital bone of the skull. The atlantoaxial articulation is a pivot joint between the atlas and the odontoid process of the axis.

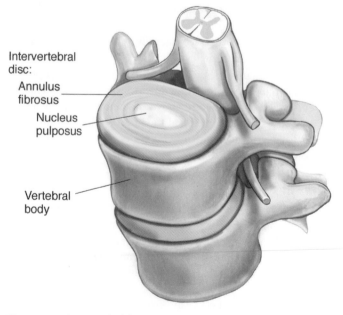

Intervertebral disc:

Annulus fibrosus

Nucleus pulposus

Vertebral body

Figure 56.3. Intervertebral disc in relation to vertebral body.

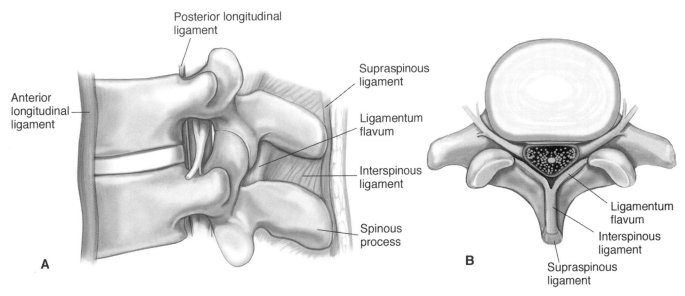

Figure 56.4. Ligaments of the spinal column. (**A**) Lateral view. (**B**) Transverse view.

The uncovertebral joints (Luschka's joints) articulate each cervical vertebral body to the one immediately below it. The costovertebral and costotransverse joints are articulations between the ribs and the vertebral bodies or transverse processes of the thoracic spine. The facet or zygapophyseal joints are formed by the inferior and superior processes of adjacent vertebral bodies.

Ligaments

The ligaments of the spine provide stability and protection from injury while allowing flexion, extension, and rotation. They are typically traversed during neuraxial anesthesia techniques. There are five main ligamentous structures seen throughout the spine (Fig. 56.4).

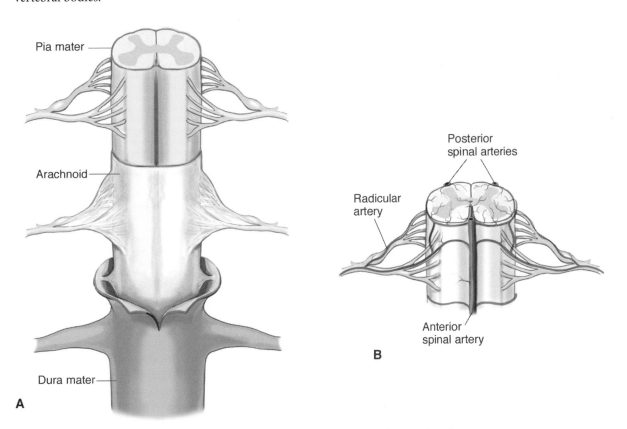

Figure 56.5. Spinal cord anatomy. (**A**) Coverings of the spinal cord. (**B**) Arterial supply of the spinal cord.

The anterior longitudinal ligament extends throughout the whole length of the spine and adheres to the anterior surface of the vertebral body and annulus fibrosus. The posterior longitudinal ligament runs along the posterior surface of the vertebral bodies and adheres to the annulus fibrosus but not to the vertebra. The supraspinous ligament connects the tips, and the interspinous ligament connects the bases of the spinous processes.

The ligamentum flavum defines the dorsolateral margins of the spinal canal from the base of the skull to the pelvis and classically is portrayed as a single ligament. In reality, there are two ligamenta flava, that join in the middle, forming an acute angle with a ventral opening. The distance from skin to ligamentum flavum ranges from 3–8 cm in most patients. The thickness of the ligament differs at different vertebral levels, ranging from 1.5 mm at the cervical level to 6.0 mm in the lumbar area. Penetration of the ligamentum flavum with the tip of an epidural needle is thought to be the cause of loss of resistance in identifying the epidural space. However, investigations have demonstrated that the ligament frequently exhibits incomplete fusion, with gaps being more frequent at cervical and thoracic levels and less frequent at lumbar levels.

Spinal cord anatomy

The spinal cord is located in the vertebral canal and extends from the foramen magnum caudad to the first or second lumbar vertebra. The spinal cord gives rise to the eight cervical, 12 thoracic, five lumbar, and five sacral nerves and one coccygeal spinal nerve. The spinal nerves comprise the sensory nerve roots that enter the spinal cord at each level, and the motor roots that emerge from the cord at each level. C1–7 nerves emerge above their respective vertebrae. C8 emerges between the C7 and T1 vertebrae. The remaining nerves emerge below their respective vertebrae.

The spinal cord terminates with the conus medullaris that is attached to the coccyx by the filum terminale. This is surrounded by the cauda equina (lumbar and sacral nerve roots). The dural sac ends at the S2 level, whereas the spinal cord ends at L1 in adults and L3 in children. Performing spinal anesthesia below these levels is necessary to avoid needle trauma to the cord.

The spinal cord is covered by three membranes known as meninges (Fig. 56.5). The outermost layer is the dura mater, a tough fibrous sheath closely applied to the inner layer of bone surrounding the spinal canal. The epidural space is a potential space between the dura and the bone (see Chapter 58 for details).

Beneath the dura mater is a thin and delicate membrane called the arachnoid mater. Normally, the arachnoid mater is closely applied to the dura, but between them exists a potential space, the subdural space, that is the result of separation within the meninges. Beneath the arachnoid mater and intimately applied to the spinal cord is the pia mater. Cerebrospinal fluid is contained between the arachnoid mater and the pia

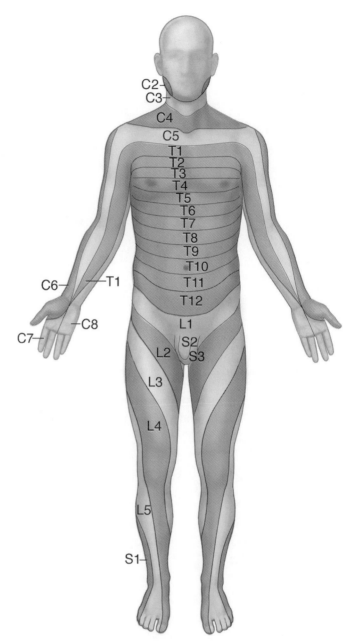

Figure 56.6. Dermatomes of human body.

mater in the subarachnoid space. The pia mater continues caudally as the filum terminale through the dural sac and attaches to the coccyx.

Arterial supply and venous drainage

The spinal cord is supplied by a single anterior spinal artery and two posterior spinal arteries. The anterior spinal artery enters the anterior median fissure of the spinal cord and supplies the anterior two-thirds of the cord. The posterior spinal arteries supply the posterior one-third of the spinal cord. The blood to the roots, as well as the cord, is segmentally supplied by radicular arteries. Usually, a few large segmental radiculospinal

Table 56.3. Important dermatome levels

C6–median nerve	1st digit (thumb)	T6–7	Xyphoid process
C7–radial nerve	2nd and 3rd digits	T10	Umbilical level
C8–ulnar nerve	4th and 5th digit	T12	Pubic symphysis
T4	Nipple level	L1	Inguinal ligament
T5	Inframammary fold	L4	Knee level

arteries are noted, including the artery of Adamkiewicz (or artery of the lumbar enlargement), that is larger than the others. In 75% of cases, it originates between T9 and T12, almost always on the left, and supplies the lower one-third of the cord. Injury to this artery may result in anterior spinal artery syndrome. This is also referred to as *Beck's syndrome* and consists of weakness, urinary and fecal incontinence, and loss of temperature and pain sensation below the level of injury with relative sparing of position and vibratory sensation.

Veins draining the spinal cord have a distribution similar to that of the arteries. The internal vertebral venous plexus (Batson plexus) is in the epidural space and consists of four interconnecting longitudinal vessels, two anterior and two posterior. Increased intra-abdominal pressure or obstruction of the inferior vena cava distends the epidural venous plexus. The epidural veins engorge during pregnancy and with uterine contraction and pushing efforts. Epidural veins connect to the azygous vein, potentially delivering local anesthetic inadvertently injected intravascularly directly to the heart.

Dermatomes and myotomes

A dermatome is an area of skin associated with a pair of dorsal roots from the spinal cord. Dermatomal maps (Fig. 56.6) portray sensory distributions for each level and provide information about the spread of a neuraxial block. The term *myotome* is used to describe the muscles served by a single spinal nerve. It is the motor equivalent of a dermatome. Table 56.3 shows important dermatome levels frequently used in assessing neuraxial blocks.

Suggested readings

Hogan QH. Lumbar epidural anatomy. A new look by cryomicrotome section. *Anesthesiology* 1991; 75(5):767–775.

Hogan QH. Epidural anatomy examined by cryomicrotome section. Influence of age, vertebral level, and disease. *Reg Anesth* 1996; 21:395–406.

Lirk P, Kolbitsch C, Putz G, et al. Cervical and high thoracic ligamentum flavum frequently fails to fuse in the midline. *Anesthesiology* 2003; 99(6):1387–1390.

Meijenhorst GC. Computed tomography of the lumbar epidural veins. *Radiology* 1982; 145:687–691.

Spinal anesthesia

Ivan T. Valovski and Assia Valovska

Spinal anesthesia is produced by injection of a local anesthetic drug into the subarachnoid space creating a conduction blockade of the spinal nerves and resulting in a rapid, dense, and predictable state of anesthesia.

Indications

Spinal anesthesia is an ideal choice for surgeries below the level of the umbilicus. Examples include low abdominal, inguinal, genitourinary, gynecologic, rectal, and lower-extremity surgeries. Spinal anesthesia is not widely used for upper abdominal procedures because of the need for a very high level of block that may increase the risk of cardiovascular and respiratory complications. A low spinal anesthetic or "saddle block" can be used for perineal or perianal surgery (Table 57.1).

Contraindications

Contraindications to spinal anesthesia are absolute and relative (Table 57.2). Patient refusal is the only absolute contraindication. Spinal anesthesia may be discussed with the reluctant patient and the surgeon and the risks and benefits of the procedure fully understood by the patient. However, patients should not be coerced into accepting the technique.

The presence of active infection at the site of needle insertion may predispose the patient to spread of the infection into the epidural and subarachnoid spaces. Fever alone is not an absolute contraindication, provided appropriate antibiotic therapy is initiated before dural puncture and the patient has shown a response to therapy. Spinal anesthesia, especially higher thoracic levels, will block multiple preganglionic sympathetic nerve fibers, and if the patient is hypovolemic, this may result in severe hypotension; therefore, correction of preoperative hypovolemia is advised.

The major concern regarding full anticoagulation is the development of spinal bleeding leading to hematoma formation. In patients with severe cardiac disease (especially severe stenotic defects) a high thoracic block may result in refractory hypotension and cardiac arrest because of an inability to increase cardiac output. Neuraxial anesthesia may be considered as an option in these patients if a lower level of blockade is adequate for the surgery. There is little evidence that

Table 57.1. Level of spinal anesthesia required for common surgical procedures

Spinal level required	Surgical procedure
T4–5 (nipple)	Upper abdominal surgery, cesarean section
T6–8 (xiphoid)	Lower abdominal surgery, appendectomy, gynecologic surgery, ureteral surgery
T10 (umbilicus)	TURP, vaginal delivery
L1 (inguinal ligament)	Thigh surgery, lower limb surgery
L2–3 (knee and below)	Foot surgery
S2–5 (perineal)	Perineal surgery, hemorrhoidectomy

TURP, transurethral resection of the prostate.

spinal anesthesia may worsen preexisting neurologic disease, but some anesthesiologists avoid it because of medicolegal considerations. Advantages and disadvantages of spinal anesthesia are summarized in Table 57.3.

Physiologic responses to spinal anesthesia

Injection of local anesthetic into the subarachnoid space produces a multitude of physiologic responses that depend on the patient's preexisting medical conditions, height of the block, and the medications and doses used (see Chapter 47).

Neural blockade

Small-diameter C-fibers (conducting pain impulses) are located to a greater extent in spinal nerve roots and the periphery of

Table 57.2. Contraindications to spinal anesthesia

Absolute	Relative	Controversial
Patient refusal	Bacteremia	Chronic back pain
	Preexisting neurologic deficit	Severe headache
	Stenotic valvular lesions	Back surgery with instrumentation
	Spinal column deformities	Complex or prolonged surgery
	Anticoagulation or coagulopathy	
	Hemorrhagic diathesis	
	Elevated intracranial pressure	

Table 57.3. Advantages and disadvantages of spinal anesthesia

Advantages	Disadvantages
Cost-effectiveness	Difficult needle placement
High patient satisfaction	Inability to obtain CSF
Preserved protective reflexes	Hypotension
Decreased risk of aspiration	PDPH
Less bleeding	Urinary retention
Rapid return of bowel function	Infection
Decreased incidence of DVT	Possible conversion to general
Less incidence of nausea	anesthesia
Decreased postoperative pain	Failed spinal
Lower incidence of cognitive impairment	

DVT, deep vein thrombosis; PDPH, postdural puncture headache.

the spinal cord; thus, they are more easily accessible to the local anesthetic. This might explain why sensory anesthesia occurs more rapidly than motor blockade (block from first to last: sympathetic > temperature > sensory > motor). Classically, the level of sympathectomy is said to be about two levels above the sensory loss level, but more recent data suggest the degree of sympathetic blockade may be at, below, or above the level of sensory loss.

Cardiovascular response

Sympathetic outflow from the spinal cord originates from T1 to L2, whereas the parasympathetic outflow is primarily craniosacral. Sympathetic fibers from T1–4 (cardioaccelerator fibers) increase the cardiac rate. Blocking these fibers causes cardiac sympathetic denervation and a decrease in heart rate, as well as a decrease in cardiac contractility and cardiac output. Systemic effects of spinal anesthesia include dilatation of arteries and venous capacitance vessels, leading to decreased systemic vascular resistance; decreased venous return; decreased cardiac output; and ultimately, hypotension. Spinal blockade at lower levels produces less hemodynamic change and is better tolerated by hypovolemic patients, elderly patients, or those with cardiac disease.

Respiratory response

In healthy patients, spinal anesthesia has no major effects on ventilation, even with a high spinal block. This is because spinal anesthesia does not alter the ventilatory response to carbon dioxide. In addition, phrenic nerve function is usually preserved. Spinal anesthesia may cause paralysis of intercostal and abdominal muscles that may affect patients with preexisting pulmonary disease and decrease their ability to cough. A high spinal level may not be a good choice for patients with severe pulmonary disease.

Gastrointestinal response

Spinal anesthesia may cause nausea and vomiting in a significant number of patients because of unopposed parasympathetic visceral activity. Consequently, parasympatholytics (e.g., atropine, glycopyrrolate) and sympathomimetics (e.g., ephedrine, phenylephrine) may be helpful in treating these symptoms. In addition, spinal anesthesia may cause a decrease in hepatic blood flow proportional to the decrease in mean arterial blood pressure.

Renal response

Spinal anesthesia tends to decrease renal blood flow as a result of arterial hypotension. However, the kidneys autoregulate to maintain renal blood flow.

Neuroendocrine response

The body's response to surgical trauma includes localized production of inflammatory mediators and activation of somatic and visceral afferent nerve fibers. These responses lead to an increase in the activity of adrenocorticotropic hormone, cortisol, epinephrine, norepinephrine, vasopressin, and the renin–angiotensin–aldosterone system. Spinal anesthesia suppresses part of this neuroendocrine response to a greater degree than general anesthesia.

Thermoregulation

Spinal anesthesia inhibits normal thermoregulation. There is loss of heat due to peripheral vasodilation as a result of sympathectomy.

Spinal anesthetic agents

The most common local anesthetics used for spinal anesthesia are lidocaine, tetracaine, and bupivacaine (Table 57.4). Mepivacaine and ropivacaine, though more commonly used in peripheral nerve blocks or epidural anesthesia, may be used for spinal anesthesia, although this is not a labeled use in the United States. Since procaine is associated with a slow onset and short duration of spinal anesthesia, it is rarely used. Chloroprocaine is not approved for spinal anesthesia and formerly was felt to be neurotoxic, although it has been used successfully in some studies.

The usual doses, onset time, and duration of action of various local anesthetics are shown in Table 57.4. Lidocaine once was the most popular local anesthetic for spinal anesthesia, but its use has declined significantly because of its association with transient neurologic symptoms. Bupivacaine and tetracaine are popular choices for longer surgery. While epinephrine has minimal effects on the duration of bupivacaine, epinephrine or phenylephrine significantly prolong the duration of tetracaine anesthesia.

Preparation for spinal anesthesia

Informed consent is an absolutely necessary part of patient preparation. It involves discussing the risks and benefits of

Table 57.4. Drugs used for spinal anesthesia

Drug and concentration	Dose, *mg*	Onset, *min*	Duration (plain drug[a]), *h*	Duration (drug + epinephrine, 0.2 mg[b]), *h*
Procaine (5%)	100–150	3–5	<1	<1.5
Lidocaine (1.5% with dextrose 7.5%, 2% plain[c])	50–100	3–5	1–2	1.5–2.5
Bupivacaine (0.75% with dextrose 8.25%, 0.5% plain[c])	8–15	5–10	1.5–3	2–4
Tetracaine (0.5%)	6–16	5–10	1.5–3.5	3–5

[a] Times are approximate; dextrose-containing solutions spread over more dermatomes and thus a given dose will provide shorter duration of anesthesia than plain solutions.
[b] Motor block is extended more than sensory block, particularly for dextrose-containing solutions.
[c] Plain lidocaine and bupivacaine solutions are not approved in the United States for spinal anesthesia.

the procedure as well as alternative techniques to spinal anesthesia.

Physical examination

Routine physical examination, including airway examination, is performed prior to administering spinal anesthesia. Patients should be questioned about a history of bleeding problems. The lumbar spine should be examined, and rash, infection, prior lumbar surgery, or severe spine deformities should be documented if present. In addition, any history of a neurologic condition or existing neurologic deficit should be documented.

Laboratory tests

Specific tests that should be considered prior to administering spinal anesthesia are usually determined by the patient's history and physical examination. If the patient reports a history of coagulopathy or easy bleeding and bruising, then prothrombin time (PT), partial thromboplastin time (PTT), and platelet count may be useful.

Premedication

Midazolam, 1 to 2 mg intravenously IV immediately, or diazepam, 5 to 10 mg orally 1 hour prior to administering spinal anesthesia, may be used to allay the patient's anxiety. An opioid may be used to help relieve pain during patient positioning.

Intravenous preloading

Patients receiving spinal anesthesia must have an IV cannula placed. Anesthesiologists commonly infuse 500 to 1000 mL of crystalloid fluid immediately before the spinal anesthetic, to mitigate the effects of sympathectomy.

Monitoring

Blood pressure may fall precipitously following induction of spinal anesthesia. Therefore, spinal anesthesia must be administered in an environment in which the ASA monitoring standards are achieved (see Chapter 24). Warning signs of falling blood pressure include pallor, sweating, nausea, and feeling generally unwell.

Equipment

Spinal needles generally fall into two categories: those that cut the dura and those designed to spread the dural fibers (Fig. 57.1).

The Whitacre and Sprotte needles have a rounded or pencil-point tip, no cutting edges, and a side hole proximal to the tip. The Quincke–Babcock needle is the "traditional" needle design. It is a cutting–type needle with sharp edges, medium bevel length, sharp point, and an end hole located on the cut bevel.

Needle size and tip design have been shown to correlate with the incidence of postdural puncture headache (PDPH). Smaller-gauge needles (25–27 G) have a lower incidence of PDPH than larger-gauge needles (22 G). Pencil-point needles (e.g., Whitacre, Sprotte) have a lower incidence of PDPH compared with cutting-type needles (e.g., Quincke) of similar or even smaller diameter.

Techniques
Landmarks

The iliac crests are palpated, and if a line is drawn at this level perpendicular to the spinal column it will generally intersect the L4–5 interspace or the L4 body. However, imaging studies

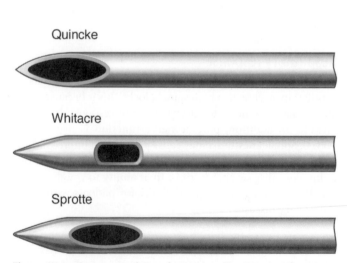

Figure 57.1. Common tip designs for spinal needles: Quincke, Whitacre, and Sprotte needles.

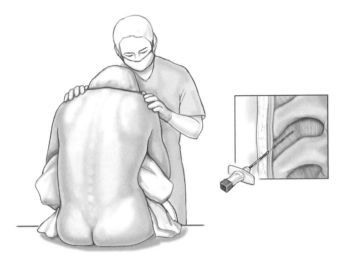

Figure 57.2. Neuraxial anesthesia in the sitting position. The patient sits on the edge of the bed and is supported by an assistant or a specially designed stand. Note the direction of the needle, shown on the right.

indicate poor correlation between anesthesiologists' landmark-predicted interspace and the anatomically verified interspace. The injection site is then prepared with a skin antiseptic and draped. If accidentally introduced into the spinal space, antiseptic solutions may cause chemical meningitis. The skin is anesthetized at the level chosen using 1% lidocaine, and the spinal needle is then inserted directly (Quincke needle), or through a larger introducer needle (Whitacre or Sprotte needle).

Positioning

Spinal anesthesia can be administered in the sitting (Fig. 57.2), lateral decubitus (Fig. 57.3), or prone positions. The lateral decubitus and sitting positions are most commonly used. Oxygen by face mask or nasal cannula may be administered, especially if a sedative has been given.

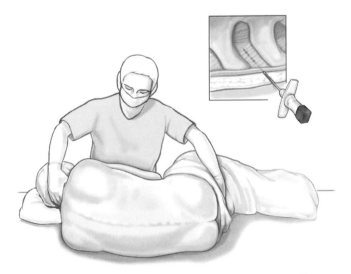

Figure 57.3. Neuraxial anesthesia in the lateral decubitus position. The patient lies on his or her side with the back slightly rounded and the knees flexed toward the abdomen. An assistant holds the patient at the neck and behind the knees. Note the direction of the needle, shown on the right.

Sitting position

The sitting position is a popular position for spinal anesthesia, and is also chosen when low lumbar or sacral levels of anesthesia are needed. This position allows easier identification of lumbar structures, especially in obese patients or patients with scoliosis. The patient is positioned at the edge of the bed with the legs hanging or supported by a foot rest. He or she is asked to bend forward and arch the lower back posteriorly (reversing the lumbar lordosis); assuming this position allows "opening" of the interspaces and easier access to the subarachnoid space. An assistant or a specially designed support device then supports the patient. Once the spinal injection is performed, the patient is positioned for surgery. If a hyperbaric solution is used, spread of the local anesthetic solution can be facilitated by tilting the operating table to the side as needed, or to a Trendelenburg (head-down) position to increase cephalad spread of the local anesthetic.

Lateral decubitus position

The lateral decubitus position allows administration of more sedation and is less dependent than the sitting position on a well-trained assistant. The patient is placed close to the edge of the table in a comfortable position with a pillow underneath the head and sometimes between the knees. The hips and knees are flexed and knees drawn up to the chest. The neck is flexed toward the knees to provide maximum anterior flexion of the spinal column. The hips and shoulders should be perpendicular to the surface of the table. If a hyperbaric solution is used, the surgical site is often placed dependently if the planned surgery is unilateral. If the surgical site is placed nondependently, then a hypobaric or isobaric anesthetic solution may be used.

Prone position

The prone position (Fig. 57.4) is usually reserved for patients undergoing rectal, perineal, or lumbar surgery. The patient is placed in the desired position, often with jackknife modification, and this position is maintained during surgery. Most often, the operative site is caudad to the level of injection; therefore, the prone position is well suited to the use of hypobaric anesthetic solutions. An isobaric solution will also provide satisfactory sacral anesthesia.

Approach

Lumbar puncture can be performed using either a midline or a paramedian approach.

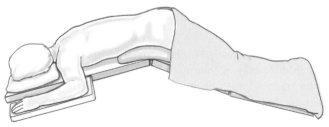

Figure 57.4. Patient position for neuraxial anesthesia in the prone position.

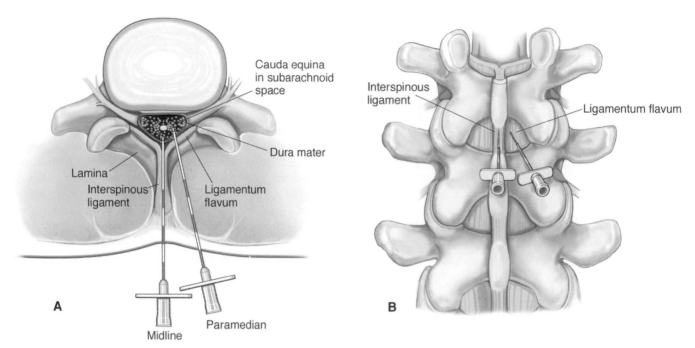

Figure 57.5. Spinal anesthesia via the midline and paramedian approaches. (**A**) Transverse view. (**B**) Posterior view.

Midline approach

In the midline approach, the spinal needle is inserted and advanced between the upper and lower spinal processes in the midline, taking into account the minimal cephalad angulation of the spinal processes in the lumbar area (Fig. 57.5). If the needle is angled and advanced correctly, it will pierce through the supraspinous and interspinous ligaments, and then the ligamentum flavum. After entering the epidural space, it pierces the dura to reach the subarachnoid space. At any time, bone may be encountered, and this should be used as an indication as to where in the interspace the needle could be. Superficial contact with bone usually indicates spinal process, whereas deeper contact implies contact with the lamina. When the ligamentum flavum is encountered, there is an increase in needle resistance, followed by decreased resistance ("pop") when the subarachnoid space is entered. The stylet is then removed. Correct position in the subarachnoid space is confirmed by spinal fluid flowing through the needle hub.

Paramedian approach

In some patients with difficult anatomy, such as kyphoscoliosis or severe arthritis, the paramedian approach (Fig. 57.5) may be the technique of choice. In the presence of severe scoliosis, the approach should be from the concave rather than the convex side of the curvature. With this technique, the needle insertion point is approximately 1–1.5 cm lateral and 1–1.5 cm caudal to the inferior edge of the superior spinal process of the chosen interspace. A longer needle may be needed for this approach. The needle is advanced with an angle of 10° to 15° off the sagittal plane and 45° cephalad. If the lamina is contacted, the needle is redirected and "walked off" the lamina in a slight medial and cephalad direction. With this approach, the interspinous ligament has been bypassed and the needle encounters the ligamentum flavum before entering the spinal space.

Taylor approach

The lumbosacral approach is useful in patients who have had lumbar spine fusions. The point of needle insertion is about 1 cm caudal and 1 cm medial from the posterior superior iliac spine. In this technique, a 5-inch spinal needle is directed upward, medially, and anteriorly at an angle that approximates the angle of the dorsal aspect of the sacrum. The needle is then advanced so that its point enters the lumbosacral space between the sacrum and the last lumbar vertebra at the L5–S1 interspace.

Factors affecting spinal block

In the past, numerous factors were thought to affect the spread of spinal local anesthetic, including the patient's body habitus, technique of injection, characteristics of the spinal fluid, and the anesthetic solution. In clinical practice, only baricity, patient posture, and perhaps total dose of anesthetic have any important effects.

The *baricity* of a local anesthetic solution refers to the density of the solution compared with the density of human CSF. Hyperbaric solutions contain glucose and have a specific gravity greater than 1.008 and therefore tend to migrate toward dependant areas. Hypobaric anesthetic solutions have a specific gravity less than 1.003 and are prepared by mixing local anesthetic with preservative-free water. Hypobaric anesthetic solutions tend to move opposite the dependant areas. Isobaric anesthetic solutions (specific gravity same or close to CSF) will stay near the site of injection, with minimal spread.

Despite a long tradition of calculating spinal anesthetic dose based on desired level of anesthesia and patient height, there is little direct evidence for the influence of either parameter, except at the extremes. Most adult patients will achieve a midthoracic level with any reasonable dose of hyperbaric solution (unless the patient remains in the sitting position while the block "sets"), and an upper lumbar or low thoracic level with an isobaric solution. The curves of the spine in the supine position make the midthoracic spine the most dependent point, thus solutions denser than CSF (hyperbaric) will reach these levels. The position of this curve is independent of height, so the latter rarely is a clinically significant determinant of anesthetic level. At extremes of height, the level may vary modestly, although this may be the result of altered spinal curves rather than height per se. Controlling the position of the most dependent point in the spine by patient positioning or tilting the bed can influence this distribution.

It may seem logical that a greater dose or volume of solution would block more spinal segments, but there is little evidence that this is true. The effect of baricity so overwhelms other effects, including dose, that the small effect that may be caused by the drug dose is clinically meaningless. Isobaric injections may show some modest dose or volume dependency, and any block will be more intense and last longer when a larger dose is used.

Adverse effects of spinal anesthesia
Cardiovascular effects

The most common cardiovascular effects after spinal anesthesia are hypotension and bradycardia. Cardiac arrest (asystole) is a rare but more serious complication.

Hypotension, the most common complication of spinal anesthesia, is the result of venous and arterial vasodilation from sympathectomy, resulting in reduced venous return, cardiac output, and systemic vascular resistance. The incidence of hypotension following spinal anesthesia is estimated to be about 10%–40%. Hypotension, if severe, should be treated with appropriate administration of IV fluids and careful administration of vasoactive drugs, such as ephedrine (5–10 mg IV bolus) or phenylephrine (40–80 µg IV bolus).

Bradycardia is caused by widespread sympathetic blockade, leading to unopposed vagal tone. Risk factors for bradycardia during spinal anesthesia include a baseline heart rate less than 60 bpm, age younger than 50 years, American Society of Anesthesiologists status I, use of β-blockers, a high spinal level, and a prolonged PR interval. Bradycardia during spinal anesthesia may be associated with hypotension and hypoxemia, but also may occur independently. It may be related to surgical manipulations, peritoneal traction and decreased venous return, or reflex bradycardia (Bezold-Jarisch reflex). In cases of severe bradycardia that compromise myocardial oxygen supply, further deterioration may follow. Consequently, severe or symptomatic bradycardia should be treated aggressively with glycopyrrolate, atropine, or ephedrine. Epinephrine should be used if other agents are not effective.

Neurologic effects

The incidence of serious neurologic complications is reported to be 0.5 per 10,000 spinal anesthetics. The most common neurologic complications are described in the following text.

Aseptic meningitis is usually benign and presents within 24 hours of spinal anesthesia. Clinically, nuchal rigidity and photophobia may be present, accompanied by a fever. CSF cultures are negative for bacteria but may show abundant polymorphonuclear leukocytes. Infectious meningitis should always be in the list of differential diagnoses and needs to be ruled out, especially if fever is present. Aseptic meningitis requires only symptomatic treatment and usually resolves within a few days.

Postdural puncture headache (PDPH) is thought to be caused by persistent CSF leak through the dural puncture site. Age (young > older), gender (female > male), the size and type of the needle, orientation of the bevel (parallel > perpendicular to the long axis of the body for cutting needles), and pregnancy all are risk factors for developing PDPH. Management of PDPH is discussed in Chapter 58.

Transient neurologic symptoms (TNS) were first described in 1993 and originally termed transient radicular irritation. It presents with pain in the lower back, limbs, buttocks, thighs, or calves after uncomplicated spinal anesthesia. The pain may last for 5 to 10 days. There are no associated motor or sensory deficits with TNS. Somatosensory evoked potential, electromyography, and nerve conduction studies do not show any abnormalities. TNS is more common after the lithotomy position, in obese patients, and in outpatient operations. Although TNS may develop after injection of any local anesthetic, the highest incidence has been found after administration of lidocaine. There is no association of TNS with gender, age, needle type, difficulty with block placement, or paresthesia during needle placement. The first line of therapy is patient reassurance and analgesics such as COX inhibitors if the pain is severe.

Nerve damage is a rare complication of spinal anesthesia, with an incidence of fewer than one in 10,000 cases. Spinal nerve roots may be damaged directly from the needle contact, and this is usually preceded by paresthesias or pain during placement. Under no circumstances should the needle be advanced or injection continued if the patient complains of pain or paresthesia.

Meningitis may rarely follow spinal anesthesia, particularly if there is a breach of sterile technique or if the patient has severe untreated bacteremia. The incidence is estimated to be approximately one in 50,000. Oral commensal organisms have been isolated in some cases, implying the source may be the anesthesiologist's mouth. Careful attention to sterile precautions, including universal use of a mask and sterile gloves, pretreatment of patients with suspected bacteremia with appropriate antibiotics, and vigilance for signs of meningitis followed by aggressive treatment, can help minimize morbidity.

Table 57.A1. Anticoagulation Guidelines of ASRA

Drug Class	Drug(s)	Recommendations
Thrombolytics	Urokinase, streptokinase, alteplase, releptase	Timing of neuraxial blockade at least 10 d after or 10 d before thrombolytic therapy Avoid neuraxial blocks, except for highly unusual situations If thrombolytics are given at or near the time of neuraxial block, continue neurologic monitoring for an appropriate interval If thrombolytics are administered while neuraxial catheter is in place, minimize sensory and motor block to allow for monitoring of neurologic function No recommendation for removal of neuraxial catheters can be made; consider measuring fibrinogen levels, and monitor neurologic function
Unfractionated Heparin	Subcutaneous heparin	No contraindication for neuraxial techniques Time of insertion of needle or removal of catheter: 4 h after last dose, 24 h before next dose Consider platelet count check in patients receiving subcutaneous heparin for >4 d
	Intraoperative anticoagulation with IV heparin for vascular surgery	Avoid neuraxial technique in patients with other coagulopathies Delay heparin dose for 1 h after needle placement Remove catheter after evaluation of coagulation status, 1 h before any subsequent dose and 2–4 h after last dose Consider postoperative neurologic monitoring every 2 h and use of weak local anesthetic concentrations
	Prolonged therapeutic heparinization	Neuraxial technique should be avoided If systemic anticoagulation is begun with catheter in place, delay catheter removal for 2–4 h after discontinuation of heparin. Evaluate coagulation status prior to removal of catheter.
Low Molecular Weight Heparin (LMWH)	*High-dose LMWH (therapeutic dosing)* Enoxaparin, 1 mg/kg every 12 h or 1.5 mg/kg/d; Dalteparin, 120 U/kg every 12 h; Tinzaparin, 175 U/kg/d	Start first dose > 24 h after neuraxial block, > 2 h after catheter removal Remove catheter before initiating therapy
	Low-dose LMWH (prophylactic dosing)	*Twice-daily dosing:* Avoid neuraxial technique if LMWH is given within 2 h prior to planned block First dose > 24 h after neuraxial block Remove indwelling catheters > 2 h before first dose *Once-daily dosing (European dosing):* First dose 68 h postoperatively Second dose no sooner than 24 h after first dose Catheter removal > 10–12 h after last LMWH dose; subsequent LMWH at least 2 h after removal
Oral anticoagulants	Warfarin	Discontinue chronic oral anticoagulation 4–5 d prior to neuraxial block Measure PT/INR prior to performing neuraxial block: only normal PT/INR reflects adequate levels of factors II, VII, IX, X Check PT/INR prior to performing neuraxial block if initial dose was given > 24 h earlier or if second dose of warfarin was given Monitor PT/INR daily for patients on low-dose warfarin (5 mg) receiving epidural analgesia. PT/INR should be < 1.5 before removing catheter. Neurologic testing of sensory and motor function should continue until at least 24 h after catheter removal Withhold or reduce warfarin dose if INR > 3 Consider reducing warfarin dose for patients likely to have enhanced response to the drug
	Antiplatelet agents	NSAIDS alone do not interfere with performance of neuraxial blocks. COX-2 inhibitors should be considered in patients on anticoagulation who require anti-inflammatory therapy. Discontinue ticlopidine 14 d prior to neuraxial block Discontinue clopidogrel 7 d prior to neuraxial block
GP IIb/IIIa receptor inhibitors		Avoid neuraxial blockade until platelet function has recovered: Abciximab: 24–48 h Eptifibatide, tirofiban : 48 h If GP IIb/IIIa receptor inhibitors are administered in the postoperative period, monitor the patient carefully
Herbal therapy		Herbal medications alone do not interfere with performance of neuraxial blocks
Fondaparinux		The actual risk of spinal/epidural hematoma with fondaparinux is unknown. If neuraxial block is planned, seek alternative method of prophylaxis.

COX, cyclooxygenase; GP, glycoprotein; LMWH, low molecular weight heparin; PT/INR, prothrombin time/international normalized ratio. Adapted from Horlocker TT, et al., Reg Anesth Pain Medicine 2010; **35**:64–101.

Spinal hematoma is a potentially devastating complication that if left untreated, may result in a partial or permanent neurologic deficit. The most common site is the epidural space, however subdural and subarachnoid hematomas are also documented. The actual incidence of spinal hematoma is unknown, however based on the incidence cited in the literature, it is estimated to be 1 in 220,000 for spinal anesthesia and 1 in 150,000 for epidural anesthesia. Known or suspected risk factors include therapeutic anticoagulation or coagulopathy, multiple attempts, and traumatic needle placement. (See the Appendix at the end of this chapter.) The clinical presentation of the spinal hematoma may vary from persistent back pain with or without distinctive motor or sensory deficits to frank paraplegia. Close postoperative neurologic monitoring for signs consistent with hematoma formation is essential for early diagnosis and treatment. An unresolving spinal block in the recovery room should be appropriately investigated. If there is suspicion of a spinal hematoma, an MRI is the gold standard for confirming the diagnosis. Early surgical decompression and evacuation usually are indicated within 6 to 8 hours. If surgery is postponed, recovery is unlikely after 8 to 12 hours.

High spinal or total spinal anesthesia is a serious anesthetic complication caused by depression of cervical spinal cord and brainstem function due to high cephalad spread of local anesthetic. It has a variable presentation and may present with tingling of the fingers, indicating spread of local anesthetic to the C7–T1 level. The patient may complain of nausea, followed by hypotension, bradycardia, difficulty breathing, and respiratory depression. If the anesthetic spreads to C3–5, apnea may occur as a result of blockade of the phrenic nerve (diaphragm). Treatment is supportive, involving IV fluids and pressors to maintain the blood pressure and heart rate, and adequate oxygenation (face mask or tracheal intubation) for respiratory support.

Respiratory effects

Dyspnea is described as an unpleasant sensation of difficulty breathing. This complication has been seen frequently after spinal anesthesia. It results from loss of intercostal muscle proprioception and the inability of patients to sense chest wall movements. Motor blockade of the abdominal and intercostal muscles may have a negative impact on coughing. Patents with preexisting pulmonary problems such as chronic obstructive pulmonary disease are more severely affected. Reassurance and confirmation of adequate ventilation are essential. Apnea may result from a high spinal and direct blockade of C3–5 (phrenic nerve) or severe hypotension. Hypotension may lead to impaired medullary blood flow and hypoxemia of the ventilatory center and may be perceived as chest heaviness.

Other effects

Backache may occur in up to 40% of patients after a lumbar puncture and may last for 1 to 2 weeks. The pain may be related to periosteal trauma from multiple attempts or stretching of the muscles or ligaments associated with muscle relaxation, TNS, or a spinal hematoma. It is important to remember that the backache may not be related to the spinal injection. Usually, the pain is not severe or debilitating. Application of heat, rest, and massage therapy are usually sufficient.

Urinary retention is common after spinal anesthesia and is caused by blockade of the sacral nerve roots S2–4. The loss of bladder tone may lead to bladder distention. Considering that sacral autonomic fibers are among the last to recover following a spinal anesthetic, bladder distention may be significant, and catheterization may be needed. If a longer spinal anesthetic is planned, it might be prudent to insert a bladder catheter to avoid problems with bladder distention. Bladder distention, if not recognized postoperatively, may be associated with hemodynamic changes such as hypertension and tachycardia or bradycardia. Blockade of higher sympathetic efferent fibers (T5–L1) may result in an increase in sphincter tone, again producing urinary retention.

Nausea and vomiting may occur after a spinal anesthetic as a result of hypotension, administration of opioid in the spinal solution or IV, sympathectomy itself (leading to unopposed vagal tone), or surgical stress. Hypotension should be treated, and antiemetics such as ondansetron may be administered.

Appendix: anticoagulation guidelines of the American Society of Regional Anesthesia

Although preoperative screening is not indicated for healthy patients undergoing neuraxial anesthesia, coagulation studies and platelet count should be checked if the clinical history suggests the possibility of a bleeding diathesis. The decision to perform neuraxial anesthesia in the anticoagulated patient should be made after weighing the risks of bleeding and development of spinal hematoma or other complications versus the benefits of the procedure. Guidelines for specific anticoagulant medications are given in Table 57.A1.

Suggested readings

Auroy Y, Narchi P, Messiah A, et al. Serious complications related to regional anesthesia: results of a prospective survey in France. *Anesthesiology* 1997; 87:479–486.

Carp H, Bailey S. The association between meningitis and dural puncture in bacteremic rats. *Anesthesiology* 1992; 76: 739.

Carpenter RL, Caplan RA, Brown DL, et al. Incidence and risk factors for site effects of spinal anesthesia. *Anesthesiology* 1992; 76: 906.

Freund FG, Bonica JJ, Ward RJ, et al. Ventilatory reserve and level of motor block during high spinal and epidural anesthesia. *Anesthesiology* 1967; 28:834.

Horlocker TT, et al. Regional anesthesia in the patient receiving antithrombotic or thrombolytic therapy: American Society of Regional Anesthesia and Pain Medicine evidence-based guidelines (third edition). *Reg Anesth Pain Medicine* 2010; 35:64–101.

Horlocker TT, Wedel DJ, Benzon H, et al. Regional anesthesia in the anticoagulated patient: defining the risks (the second ASRA

Consensus Conference on Neuraxial Anesthesia and Anticoagulation). *Reg Anesth Pain Med* 2003; 28(3):172–197.

Mackey DC. Physiological effects of regional block. In: Brown DL, ed. *Regional Anesthesia and Analgesia*. Philadelphia: WB Saunders; 1996:397–422.

Mulroy MF. Spinal headaches: management and avoidance. In: Brown DL, ed. *Problems in Anesthesia: Regional Anesthesia at the Virginia Mason Medical Center: A Critical Perspective*. vol. 1, no 4. Philadelphia: Lippincott; 1987.

Pollock JE. Transient neurologic symptoms: etiology, risk factors, and management. *Reg Anesth Pain Med* 2002; 27(6):581–586.

Ravin MB. Comparison of spinal and general anesthesia for low abdominal surgery in patients with chronic obstructive pulmonary disease. *Anesthesiology* 1971; 35:319.

Schnider M, Ettlin T, Kaufmann M, et al. Transient neurologic toxicity after hyperbaric subarachnoid anesthesia with 5% lidocaine. *Anesth Analg* 1993; 76:1154–1157.

Tryba M. Epidural regional anesthesia and low molecular weight heparin: pro [in German]. *Anesthesiol Intensivmed Notfallmed Schmertzthe* 1993; 28:179.

Vandam LD, Dripps RD. Long-term follow-up of patients who received 10,098 spinal anesthetics: III. Syndrome of decreased intracranial pressure (headache and ocular and auditory difficulties). *JAMA* 1956; 161:586.

Vandermeulen EP, Van Aken H, Vermylen J. Anticoagulants and spinal-epidural anesthesia. *Anesth and Analg* 1994; 79:1165.

Wedel DJ, Horlocker TT. Regional anesthesia in the infected patient. *Reg Anesth Pain Med* 2006; 31:324–333.

Epidural anesthesia

Richard S. Field and B. Scott Segal

Introduction

Neuraxial anesthesia is the term used to describe both intrathecal (spinal) and epidural nerve blocks. Drugs delivered into the epidural space do not behave as drugs in the intrathecal space. Understanding the differences allows the anesthesiologist to choose which space to deliver a drug based on the benefits of each (Table 58.1). The epidural space is located within the spinal canal but lies outside the dural sac. Anesthetics delivered into this space may provide regional surgical anesthesia, prolonged postoperative analgesia, or treat chronic pain syndromes. Successful epidural anesthesia depends on proper patient selection, knowledge of the surgery, its location and duration, excellent three-dimensional appreciation of the neuraxial anatomy, and appropriate choice of anesthetic agent. This chapter focuses on these factors and also describes the complications associated with epidural anesthesia.

Anatomy

Appreciation of the bony spinal anatomy, the ligaments connecting these bones, and the contents and borders of the epidural space itself is important for the safe and expeditious performance of epidural blocks. For a detailed description of the spinal bony and ligamentous anatomy, please refer to Chapter 56.

Anatomy of the epidural space

The anatomy of the epidural space is as follows:

- Space inside the vertebral foramen but outside the dural sac
- Enclosed cranially by the foramina magnum and caudally by the sacrococcygeal ligament
- Discontinuous space divided into anterior, posterior, and lateral compartments

  - The lateral compartment is filled with spinal nerves, epidural fat, and blood vessels; communicates with the paravertebral space
  - The anterior compartment is a thin space that also includes the valveless veins of Batson's plexus
  - The posterior epidural compartment is the widest part of the epidural space; it is filled with epidural fat and some minute vessels

Table 58.1. Comparison of spinal and epidural anesthesia

Benefits of spinal anesthesia	Benefits of epidural anesthesia	Benefits of an epidural catheter
Smaller total dose of drug	Less respiratory depression	Ability to titrate a drug to effective level of sensory block
Fewer systemic side effects	Lower incidence of high block	Outlasts a single-shot block
Quicker onset time	Less hemodynamic instability	Can use the catheter for days after surgery
	Use of catheter	Helps reduce chronic pain levels

The dura often touches but does not attach to the periosteum of the spinal canal, unless inflammation has occurred. This results in separate compartments of epidural space, interspersed with areas of potential epidural space. These areas can be opened up, or epidural space created by, injection of a bolus of air or liquid. Epidural fat is abundant in the posterior but also in the lateral compartment. This fat can affect the flow of epidural solutions and act as a sink in sequestering lipid-soluble opioids and local anesthetics.

Performing epidural anesthesia

Increasing evidence supports the use of neuraxial techniques to lower perioperative morbidity and mortality (Table 58.2). Contraindications to epidural anesthesia are the same as for spinal anesthesia (see Chapter 57). The only absolute contraindication

Table 58.2. Beneficial effects of neuraxial anesthesia in the perioperative period

Reduced stress response to surgery
Less intraoperative blood loss (and lower transfusion requirements)
Fewer thromboembolic events (deep vein thrombosis, pulmonary embolism, graft occlusions)
Fewer postoperative pulmonary complications
Increased regional blood flow
Earlier return of gastrointestinal function
Earlier ambulation
Earlier hospital discharge for some surgeries
Less perioperative mortality

to epidural anesthesia is patient refusal. Relative contraindications include bacteremia, coagulopathy, and hypovolemia.

Preparation

Preparation for placement of an epidural block initially includes taking a patient history, examining the patient, reviewing the patient's records and results of relevant laboratory and imaging investigations, and obtaining written informed consent. Once completed, the preparation for the procedure can begin. This includes checking the equipment, placing the monitors on the patient, and correctly positioning the patient. Surface landmarks help identify the vertebral level at which the block will be performed (see Chapter 57 and Table 57.1), but these are imprecise and studies demonstrate that blocks are often undertaken one to three levels from the intended interspace.

Equipment

The most commonly used epidural needle used in the United States is the 17-gauge 3.5 inch Tuohy needle (with the addition of lateral wings it is known as the Weiss needle). Needles used for epidural blocks are larger gauge than spinal needles to facilitate the loss of resistance technique and to pass a 19- or 20-gauge catheter through the needles. The Weiss needle has a blunt, curved tip (similar to Tuohy) that facilitates threading of the catheter. The blunt tip transmits tactile information to the clinician as the needle is advanced through the "gritty" interspinous and "tough" ligamentum flavum (Fig. 58.1).

The needles also are supplied with stylets to prevent superficial tissue from becoming embedded within the needle lumen during insertion. Centimeter markings are displayed on the outside of the epidural needle to determine the distance from skin to epidural space. These markings facilitate placement of specific lengths of catheter within the epidural space. The plastic catheters themselves typically have markings every centimeter for the distal 20 cm. By measuring the catheter marking at the skin (after the needle has been removed) and subtracting from this the distance from the skin to the epidural space (measured on the epidural needle), the practitioner can determine the length of catheter left in the epidural space (commonly 3–5 cm). The catheters may be single- or multi-orifice. Some evidence points to fewer patchy and one-sided blocks with multi-orifice catheters. The tip of the catheter is dark colored to ensure that the entire length of the catheter has been removed from the patient at the conclusion of the anesthetic. Epidural catheters also vary in their stiffness. Less stiff catheters are believed to result in fewer paresthesias on insertion and intravascular placements. Stiffer catheters are easier to thread longer distances into the epidural space.

Syringes for loss of resistance are also present in the epidural kits. Often a glass syringe is used after lubricating the interior walls with saline to reduce friction on the plunger; plastic loss-of–resistance (LOR) syringes are also available and do not require such lubrication but have a distinctly different feel to most operators. In addition to the equipment necessary to perform epidural anesthesia, emergency equipment should be available, including a source of oxygen, suction, bag–valve–mask resuscitator (Ambu bag), equipment to secure an airway, and resuscitation drugs. All patients should have vascular access established, and a "safety pause" should be performed prior to starting the procedure.

Monitoring

The patient's mental status should be continually monitored by verbal communication. Hemoglobin saturation (SpO_2), heart rate and rhythm, and blood pressure should also be monitored throughout the procedure.

Positioning

The sitting, lateral decubitus, or (less commonly) prone position can be used (see Chapter 57 and Figs. 57.2, 57.3, 57.4). Specialized stands that facilitate proper patient positioning have been developed. A trained attendant who can maintain communication and reassure the patient may optimize establishment and maintenance of appropriate patient position.

Lumbar technique

The spinal cord terminates at L1 in most adults and L3 in most children. Therefore, there is less risk of damage to the spinal cord by placing an epidural block in the lumbar region. After adequate preparation and positioning of the patient, an antiseptic solution is used to clean the back. Sterile drapes are placed, and the surface anatomy is identified. Local anesthetic is used to raise a skin wheal and is then injected deeper to the level of the interspinous ligament. A midline or paramedian approach is then used to introduce the epidural needle and stylet into the subcutaneous tissue. The needle is advanced until the interspinous ligament is identified by its "gritty" texture. A glass or plastic syringe is filled with 2–4 ml of air or saline, or both, and attached to the needle. Several techniques for hand positioning have been described for advancing the epidural needle (Fig. 58.2). Constant or intermittent pressure on the syringe plunger is applied during advancement. As the ligamentum flavum is reached, increased resistance to pressure on the plunger is felt. As the epidural space is reached, a loss of resistance is felt and the contents of the syringe freely enter the space. At this point,

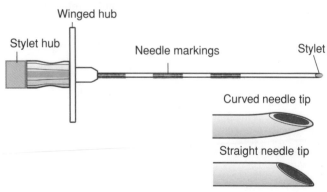

Figure 58.1. Epidural needle design.

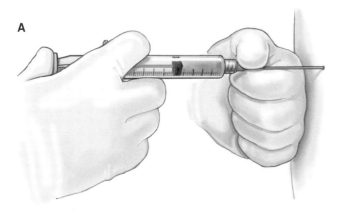

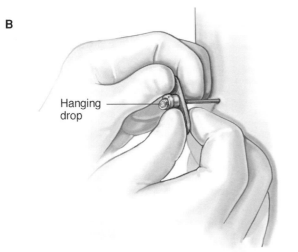

Hanging drop

Figure 58.2. Epidural techniques. **(A)** LOR technique (continuous pressure variant). **(B)** Hanging drop technique.

pressure on the plunger should be released to prevent injection of all the air or saline in the syringe. A "single shot" of anesthetic may then be administered, or a catheter may be advanced and the needle withdrawn.

An alternate method of identifying needle entry into the epidural space is the hanging drop technique. This technique uses the negative pressure formed in the epidural space (as the advancing needle "tents" the dura) to suck in a drop of liquid that purposely hangs off the hub of the needle. Immediately on noticing this, the clinician stops advancing the needle. This technique has lost favor in the lumbar and thoracic regions, but is still used in cervical epidural anesthesia.

Test dose

Commonly, 3 ml of 1.5% lidocaine with 1:200,000 epinephrine (5 µg/ml) is injected as a *test dose*. Intrathecal (spinal) administration of this dose of local anesthetic (lidocaine 45 mg) will rapidly result in a spinal block with motor weakness. Intravascular administration of 15 µg of epinephrine will typically result in an increase in heart rate of 30 bpm within 45 seconds, in a patient not taking β-blockers.

Thoracic, cervical, and caudal epidural anesthesia

Thoracic epidural anesthesia is most often used, in addition to general anesthesia, for procedures in the thoracic and high abdominal regions. Beneficial effects include less postoperative respiratory compromise from improved postoperative pain control, earlier ambulation, and shortened ileus after intestinal or aortic surgery. More recently, some evidence has suggested better immune function postoperatively with epidural analgesia. Performing the technique in this region is more challenging because of the presence of the spinal cord and a smaller distance from skin to epidural space, in addition to a smaller epidural space. The cervical spine also is used to perform epidural analgesia but mainly in the treatment of chronic pain.

An alternative approach to the epidural space for procedures in the rectal, perineal, genital, inguinal, and lower abdominal region is the caudal approach. A single-shot epidural anesthetic or a catheter to provide continuous infusion may be used. This technique is used more commonly in children, because the sacral hiatus is more often patent in children than in adults. The sacral hiatus is identified by palpating the sacral cornua that lie on either side of the hiatus at the top of the buttock crease or at the most caudal point of an equilateral triangle formed between the hiatus and the posterior superior iliac spines (Fig. 58.3). An epidural needle is advanced through the hiatus at an angle of about 45°. Once the "pop" of the needle passing through the sacrococcygeal ligament is felt, the angle of needle entry is reduced to advance the needle along the sacral canal. The needle is advanced 1–2 cm further. The dural sac ends at about S1 in adults and S3 in infants. Although advancing the epidural needle only 1–2 cm into the caudal canal should ensure epidural rather than intrathecal placement, it is prudent to check for CSF prior to injecting or advancing an epidural catheter.

Combined spinal–epidural anesthesia

Spinal anesthesia offers certain advantages over epidural infusion, including quicker onset, a denser motor and sensory block, and reduced total drug dose. The advantages of epidural anesthesia over an intrathecal delivery include the ability to provide a prolonged, titratable level of anesthesia. Disadvantages of subarachnoid anesthetic include anesthesia wearing off too early, an inadequate level of anesthesia, and adverse cardiovascular effects of a high spinal. The disadvantages associated with an epidural anesthetic that may be avoided by combined spinal–epidural anesthesia include slow onset time, a patchy block with inadequate motor paralysis, and an intravascular injection with subsequent CNS and cardiovascular toxicity. Combining the two techniques offers the advantages of both while minimizing the disadvantages.

The procedure is performed at the lumbar level. A standard 17-gauge 3.5 inch Weiss needle or a specifically designed epidural needle with an additional exit eye near the tip may be used (Fig. 58.4). The spinal needle used is a longer, 4.5–5 inch 24–27 gauge needle. The spinal needle should easily slide through the epidural needle and extend 12–15 mm beyond the curved tip

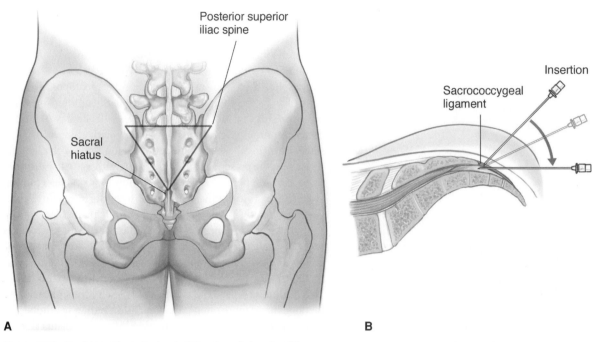

Figure 58.3. Caudal anesthesia landmarks **(A)** and needle insertion **(B)**.

of the epidural needle. After local anesthetic solution has been injected at the puncture site, the epidural needle is advanced as described for epidural anesthesia. Once in the interspinous ligament, the stylet is removed. An LOR syringe is attached, and the epidural space is identified by the loss of resistance. Once the epidural space has been found, the spinal needle is advanced through the epidural needle. As the spinal needle is advanced, a "pop" indicates puncture of the dura. Removing the stylet from the needle should result in returning CSF that will confirm intrathecal placement. The spinal drug should then be injected through the spinal needle, and this needle is then withdrawn. An epidural catheter may then be inserted, the needle removed, and the catheter secured.

A long spinal needle can be passed through the lumen of a standard epidural needle, although the needle will be slightly

deflected. Specially designed epidural needles with an additional hole for the spinal needle are available, although they may not affect block success significantly.

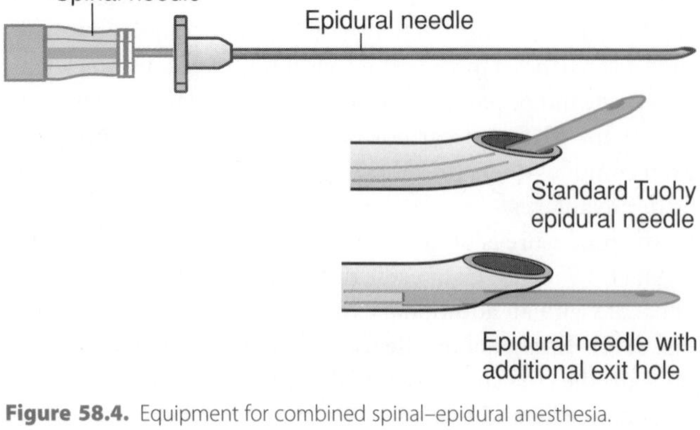

When surgical anesthesia is obtained by the spinal injection, a test dose or epidural infusion should not be started until the effect of intrathecal anesthesia starts to wear off. Although the catheter is assumed to be in the epidural space, it must be remembered that it can still be intrathecal or intravascular. Administering a bolus of local anesthetic through an epidural catheter that may have migrated into the subarachnoid space, after a full subarachnoid dose of drug has been given, may result in a high or total spinal. Once the level of intrathecal anesthesia has regressed, aspiration of the catheter may be followed by injection of a test dose. Some authorities believe it is safe to begin an epidural infusion immediately if dilute local anesthetic is used, particularly in obstetrics (see Chapter 121).

Determinants of epidural spread, onset, and duration of action

To optimize the use of epidural drug delivery, the clinician must have an understanding of what affects spread of the drug in the epidural space, the speed of onset, and the duration of anesthesia and analgesia.

Determinants of epidural spread

The site of injection of local anesthetic is the most important variable in determining segmental anesthetic coverage. Local anesthetic spreads in both cephalad and caudal directions in the epidural space. There is slightly more cephalad than caudal spread. However, it may be that it is simply easier to block the

Figure 58.4. Equipment for combined spinal–epidural anesthesia.

Spinal needle

Epidural needle

Standard Tuohy epidural needle

Epidural needle with additional exit hole

Table 58.3. Local anesthetic agents for epidural anesthesia: approximate two-segment regression time and dosing intervals for lumbar (L2–4) epidural anesthesia

Local anesthetic	Dose, mg	Peak cephalad block height	Time to two-segment regression (1 SD or range), min[a]	Recommended dose interval, min[b]
Chloroprocaine 2%–3% + 1:200,000 epinephrine	600	T5	80 (15)	45
Lidocaine 1.5%–2% + 1:200,000 epinephrine	300–400	T4	100 (50–60)	60
Mepivacaine 1.5%–2% + 1:200,000 epinephrine	300–400	T4	110–120 (40–50)	60
Bupivacaine 0.5%–0.75% (plain)	100–150	T5	150–190 (60–80)	120
Ropivacaine 1% (plain) age 30 (18–40)[c]	150	T8[d]	143 (45–298)	120
Ropivacaine 1% (plain) age 51 (41–59)[c]	150	T6[d]	190 (100–340)	120
Ropivacaine 1% (plain) age 71 (61–82)[c]	150	T4[d]	203 (105–378)	120

[a] Mean (1 SD or range).
[b] Dosing intervals are approximate guidelines. In awake and cooperative patients, clinical monitoring for signs and symptoms (increase in blood pressure and heart rate or objective evaluation of dermatomal level of block) of dermatomal regression will indicate the need for a top-up dose.
[c] Ages expressed as mean (range).
[d] Note for ropivacaine the significant difference in peak block height between the youngest and oldest age groups.
From Wong C. *Spinal and Epidural Anesthesia*. New York: McGraw-Hill; 2007.

smaller, more cranial nerve roots. Local anesthetic uptake may be slower in the more caudal regions because the caudal nerve roots are larger and more length is present in the epidural space.

Dose, volume, and concentration

Whereas the total volume injected determines the spread within the epidural space, the concentration of the drug affects the density of the block. A general guideline for the volume of drug to use is 1–2 ml of local anesthetic per dermatome to be blocked. If motor blockade is desired, the highest available concentration of local anesthetic should be used.

Age

Increasing age has been shown to affect the spread of local anesthetic in the epidural space. Older patients have increased caudal and cephalad spread of local anesthetic within the space. Anatomic changes that may account for this include a more compliant epidural space with reduced epidural fat content and a narrowing of the intervertebral neuroforamen through which the local anesthetic may escape.

Pregnancy

There is conflicting evidence in studies examining longitudinal epidural spread in pregnancy. Studies are limited because there is no practical or reliable quantitative measure of spread of the solution in the epidural space. There is some evidence to support increased local anesthetic sensitivity of nerves in pregnancy that may augment the blocks for a given dose of drug.

Onset of epidural anesthesia

The speed with which epidural anesthesia renders a patient ready for surgical incision is a characteristic of the drug used. Anesthesia is first noticed along the dermatomes nearest the site of injection within a few minutes. Onset of action of local anesthetics is determined by the fraction of the drug in the nonionized forms and the concentration of the local anesthetic solution injected.

Duration

The duration of action of local anesthetics in the epidural space depends on several factors. Time to two-segment regression from a single epidural shot of local anesthetic is summarized in Table 58.3 and include the drug itself, the dose of drug, and the presence of an adrenergic agonist. Local anesthetic duration correlates with the drug's protein-binding ability and its lipid solubility. Sequestration of the local anesthetic into epidural fat can prolong its action by acting as a depot of the drug. The use of adrenergic agonists such as epinephrine (1:200,000) is thought to prolong the block by causing local vessel vasoconstriction. This is believed to prolong the effects of epidural local anesthetics by decreasing clearance of the drug from the epidural space.

Drugs used in the epidural space

Local anesthetics, opioids, and adrenergic agonists have all been used independently and in combinations. Local anesthetics are the most frequently used epidural agents and act at the spinal cord, dorsal and ventral nerve roots, and the exiting spinal nerve itself. The most important sites of action are the lateral dural cuff regions of the dorsal and ventral nerve roots. Here, exposed arachnoid granulations facilitate local anesthetic transport into the CSF.

Opioids also may be used in the epidural space as either a bolus or an infusion. They provide analgesia by binding to pre- and postsynaptic opioid receptors in the substantia gelatinosa of the dorsal horn of the spinal cord as well as to opioid receptors located in the brainstem. Binding of opioids to these pre- and postsynaptic receptors inhibits the transmission of pain signals mediated by neurotransmitters such as substance P. Epidural opioids reach the spinal cord by diffusing across the dura. They reach the brainstem either by vascular uptake in the epidural space or by cephalad spread of hydrophilic opioids within the CSF. Adverse effects of epidural opioids include nausea, vomiting, urinary retention, pruritus, and respiratory depression. Early and late respiratory depression may result. Early respiratory depression from μ_2-opioid receptor activation may occur. Late respiratory depression occurs up to 24 hours after administration from slow cephalad CSF diffusion of hydrophilic opioids.

Adrenergic receptor agonists are also delivered into the epidural space. Clonidine is a specific α_2-adrenergic agonist with an analgesic and sedative effect. Although α_2-adrenergic receptors are found throughout the body, the analgesic activity of clonidine is believed to result from activation of receptors in the dorsal horn. Activation of these receptors mimics the descending inhibitory pain pathways that use norepinephrine in their signal transmission.

Adverse effects

Major complications from neuraxial anesthesia are uncommon events. In a large multicenter prospective study in France, complications from spinal anesthesia were found to occur significantly more often than from epidural anesthesia. Of 40,640 spinal and 30,413 epidural procedures, cardiac arrest occurred in 26 and three cases, respectively. A more recent study found a similar pattern of uncommon complications. Of 41,079 spinal and 35,293 epidural anesthetics performed at multiple centers in France, 31 serious events were reported in the spinal group and seven in the epidural group. Although serious complications from epidural anesthesia are uncommon, minor complications and adverse effects do occur more frequently. Back pain, urinary retention, pruritus, and nausea and vomiting are often seen as a result. More serious complications discussed here include intravascular injections, complications related to the inadvertent puncture of the dura, infections, and finally, epidural hematomas.

Intravascular injection

Blood vessels are located primarily in the lateral and anterior epidural space. These vessels may become engorged during pregnancy, which increases the risk of intravascular injections. Preventive measures may reduce the risk of this complication and include the use of soft-tipped catheters, restricting the length of catheter inserted to less than 5 cm, aspirating prior to any epidural injection, use of an epinephrine-containing test dose, and fractionation of doses to no more than 3-5 ml at a time. Local anesthetics injected intravascularly in the epidural space may cause CNS toxicity followed by cardiovascular toxicity and collapse.

Dural puncture

Inadvertent puncture of the dura during epidural needle placement may occur and is partly related to the skill of the practitioner. Returning CSF is a definitive sign of a "wet tap." If this occurs, the practitioner must decide whether to abandon the procedure, try again at a different level, or convert the anesthetic to a continuous spinal. Penetrating the dura either with the large-gauge epidural needle or by a catheter

that has migrated into the subarachnoid space may result in a total spinal or a postdural puncture headache (PDPH). A large epidural dose of local anesthetic unintentionally administered into the subarachnoid compartment can migrate to cervical and even intracranial levels, resulting in bradycardia, hypotension, difficulty swallowing and phonating, dyspnea, and loss of consciousness. It is termed a *high* or *total spinal*. Hypoperfusion of the brainstem may affect the higher respiratory centers and result in apnea. Treatment consists of head-down positioning to improve preload and brainstem perfusion, oxygen, airway management, and circulatory support with vasoconstrictors, inotropes, and chronotropes. Subdural anesthesia is a similar complication from unintentional dural puncture but often is less dramatic. The subdural region is a potential space lying between the closely opposed dura mater and arachnoid mater. Injection into this space by a needle positioned here or from a catheter that may have migrated into the space occurs with an estimated frequency of one in 2000 cases. Signs suggestive of a subdural block include a higher than intended level, a patchy block, Horner's syndrome (miosis, ptosis, enophthalmus, and anhidrosis), and signs of a total spinal.

Postdural puncture headache

Dural puncture, whether intended or unintended, may result in a severe bilateral fronto-occipital headache that occurs 12 to 48 hours after the procedure. Characteristically, the pain is related to position. Lying flat often relieves the pain, whereas sitting or standing increases the intensity. The pain is thought to occur following CSF leak through the dural puncture that leads to decreased intracranial cushioning effect of the CSF. This may cause increased traction on intracranial structures and result in the sensation of pain in areas innervated by compressed or stretched intracranial nerves. PDPH often resolves within 3 to 7 days but rarely may persist. Conservative management should be started upon presentation and includes reassurance, bed rest, oral or intravenous (IV) hydration, administration of caffeine or theophylline, and analgesics.

If conservative management has failed and the pain is not improving, more invasive measures may be attempted. An epidural blood patch provides rapid and complete improvement in 70%–98% of cases. The procedure involves injecting 15–25 ml of autologous blood, under sterile conditions, into the epidural space at or one interspace below the dural puncture. The procedure is believed to compress and block the defect in the dura while squeezing CSF cephalad and into the intracranial compartment.

Infection

Rarely, bacterial contaminants may cause meningitis, arachnoiditis, or an epidural abscess. Organisms responsible for such infections include skin flora such as *Staphylococcus aureus* and *Staphylococcus epidermidis* but also oral commensals such as *Streptococcus viridans*. A suspected epidural abscess should be confirmed by MRI. Treatment includes IV antibiotics and surgical incision, drainage, and decompression. Replacing or removing epidural catheters within 5 days of placement may reduce the incidence of this rare complication.

Epidural hematoma

Epidural hematomas may occur spontaneously or secondary to epidural blood vessel trauma from a needle or from insertion or removal of an epidural catheter. The incidence of epidural hematomas has been estimated to be between one in 150,000 cases for epidural anesthesia and one in 220,000 for spinal anesthesia. The increasing frequency of perioperative anticoagulation may be responsible for an increase in the incidence of this complication. Guidelines have been revised by the American Society of Regional Anesthesia and Pain Medicine (see Appendix to Chapter 57). These revised guidelines reflect the changing practice of perioperative anticoagulation. As with epidural abscess formation, early detection of the space-occupying hematoma within the epidural space is critical. Early signs of back pain and lower-extremity numbness or weakness may be masked by epidural anesthesia. However, these signs, in the setting of bowel or bladder incontinence should alert the physician to the possibility of a developing hematoma. An MRI and neurosurgical consult should be obtained immediately, because delays of more than 8 hours

before surgical decompression have been implicated in poorer outcomes.

Suggested readings

Auroy Y, Benhamou D, Bargues L, et al. Major complications of Regional Anesthesia in France: the SOS Regional Anesthesia Hotline Service. *Anesthesiology* 2002; 97:1274.

Auroy Y, Narchi P, Messiah A, et al. Serious complications related to regional anesthesia: results of a prospective survey in France. *Anesthesiology* 1997; 87:479.

Brill S, Gurman GM, Fisher A. A history of neuraxial administration of local analgesics and opioids. *Eur J Anaesthesiol* 2003; 20:682–689.

Corning JL. Spinal anesthesia and local medication of the cord. *N Y Med J* 1885; 42:483–485.

Hogan Q. Distribution of solution in the epidural space: examination by cryomicrotome section. *Reg Anesth Pain Med* 2002; 27(2):150–156.

Horlocker T, Wedel D, Benzon H, et al. Regional anesthesia in the anticoagulated patient: defining the risks (the second ASRA Consensus Conference on Neuraxial Anesthesia and Anticoagulation). *Reg Anesth Pain Med* 2003; 28:172–197.

Moen V, Dahlgren N, Irestedt L. Severe neurological complications after central neuraxial blockade in Sweden, 1990–1999. *Anesthesiology* 2004; 101:950–959.

Mandabach MG. The history of epidural anesthesia: Pages, Dogliotti, Guieterrez and Ruiz. ASA Meeting Abstract. San Francisco, CA; February 2004.

Principles of ultrasound-guided nerve blocks

Tanja S. Frey and Adam B. Collins

Ultrasound use is rapidly expanding in numerous fields of medicine. This trend is likely to continue as ultrasound image quality improves and equipment becomes less expensive and more portable. High-resolution ultrasound facilitates direct visualization of nerves, adjacent structures, block needle, and local anesthetic distribution. The ability to select an optimal needle path, guide its insertion with great precision, and obtain real-time feedback on the spread of local anesthetic is attracting substantial interest in the regional anesthesia community. A growing body of evidence demonstrates that ultrasound guidance increases the success rate and decreases morbidity compared to traditional nerve stimulator–based techniques for several peripheral nerve blocks.

Ultrasound-related physics

The transducer emits sound waves into the tissue and receives sound that is reflected or scattered back to the receiver. Ultrasound waves are high-frequency sound waves above 20 kHz that are not audible to the human ear (audible range is 20 Hz–20 kHz). Frequencies useful in regional anesthesia are in the 4–17 MHz range. Tissues with different acoustic impedance interact with incident sound waves, causing attenuation, reflection, refraction, and scattering. What is reflected back to the transducer is transformed into an electrical signal that is processed by the ultrasound machine to generate an image on the screen. The greater the echogenicity of a particular tissue, the brighter it is depicted on the sonogram. The time it takes for the sound to be received after emission is used to calculate depth, based on the assumed speed of sound in tissue, which is 1540 m/sec. Anatomic structures can appear hypoechoic, hyperechoic or isoechoic, as summarized below:

- Structures with high water content, such as blood vessels, appear *hypoechoic* (dark or black) because the ultrasound waves are transmitted through these structures easily with little reflection.
- Structures with low water content, such as bone and tendons, appear *hyperechoic* (bright) because the transmission of ultrasound waves is blocked, and the strong signal returned to the transducer gives these structures a white appearance.

- Structures of intermediate density and acoustic impedance appear gray on the screen and are called *isoechoic*.

Transducer selection

In general, linear transducers provide a rectangular image, and sector view transducers produce a pie-shaped image with a small footprint. Because frequency determines the depth of tissue penetration, the depth of the target organ/tissue in an individual patient dictates the frequency range that is most useful. *Deep* structures (>4 cm) require low-frequency transducers in the 3–7 MHz range that penetrate well but at the expense of axial resolution. *Superficial* structures (0.5–4 cm) benefit from high-frequency transducers in the 10–15 MHz range that provide high axial resolution at the expense of penetration. Advanced, high-frequency transducers in particular demonstrate the characteristic fascicular appearance of nerves and the fibrillar appearance of tendons, and differentiate them from surrounding structures. Modern ultrasound equipment offers various enhancements to make high-quality nerve imaging simpler and more consistently achieved.

Imaging plane

Nerves can be viewed in short or long axis. *Short-axis (transverse) imaging* cuts through cylindrical structures in cross-section, producing a circular image on the screen (Fig. 59.1a). This orientation generally provides the most stable and recognizable image of nerves and surrounding structures, even with moderate transducer movement during block performance.

Long-axis imaging shows the same object longitudinally and depicts the course of cylindrical objects as linear (Fig. 59.1b). It is of limited use in ultrasound-guided regional anesthesia but can help confirm catheter placement for continuous nerve block techniques along a selected nerve.

In the *out-of-plane* (OOP) technique, the needle is introduced from outside the plane of imaging and crosses the scan plane so that the needle tip or shaft is shown as an *echogenic dot* (Fig. 59.2). This technique relies on observing tissue displacement caused by the advancing needle, as well as seeking the needle tip by adjusting the transducer position and angle. Aligning the structure of interest in the center of the

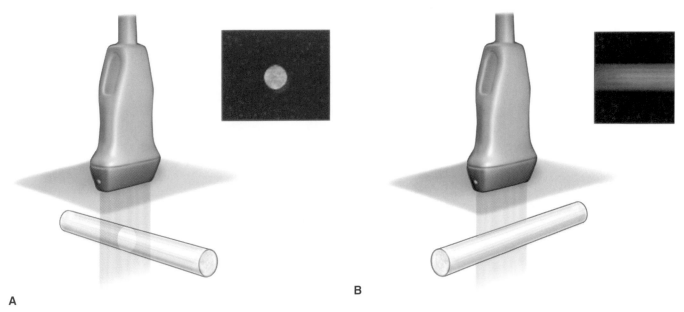

Figure 59.1. Short- or transverse-axis **(A)** and long-axis imaging planes **(B)**.

image and then inserting the needle on the centerline of the transducer helps ensure relatively accurate needle placement. A 45° insertion angle from the skin is a good starting point. The needle tip is usually sufficiently hyperechoic that it stands out from muscle and fat, but the shaft may be harder to visualize directly and may be appreciated only by the shadow it casts.

The *in-plane* (IP) technique uses a needle introduced within the plane of imaging and shows the needle as an *echogenic*

line (Fig. 59.3). Only the portion of the needle that lies within this very thin scan plane can be seen, making it possible to advance the needle further than intended when the tip strays from the scan plane. The needle tip has a stepped appearance, whereas the shaft shows reverberation artifact (Fig. 59.4). Special echogenic needles are available that produce a brighter needle image over a broader range of insertion angles. All needles show a decrement in signal intensity when they are inserted at a steeper angle relative to the active face of the transducer.

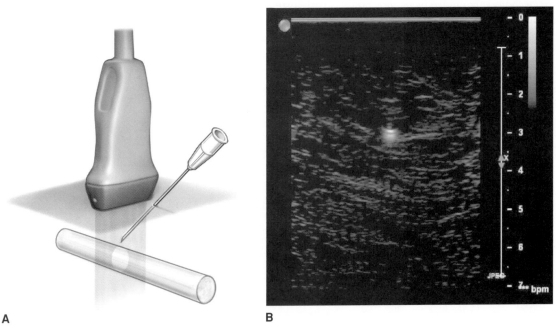

Figure 59.2. Short- or transverse-axis OOP technique **(A)** and needle tip appearance on ultrasound **(B)**.

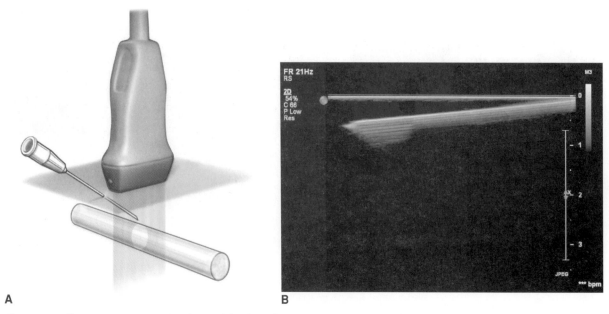

A

B

Figure 59.3. Short- or transverse-axis IP technique **(A)** and needle appearance on ultrasound **(B)**.

The IP approach requires a needle that is a few centimeters longer than the width of the transducer, to allow the needle to reach structures imaged on the side opposite the point of needle insertion.

Sonographic appearance of nerves

Nerves in ultrasound images usually have a *fascicular echotexture* that corresponds to the cross-sectional nerve structure seen on light microscopy, but with fewer fascicles resolved. The nerve fascicles appear hypoechoic, surrounded by hyperechoic epineurium and perineurium. Nerves also change shape and echotexture along their course. For example, proximal nerves, such as the roots and trunks of the brachial plexus, appear hypoechoic and monofascicular but become hyperechoic and polyfascicular as they course into the periphery (Fig. 59.5).

General considerations for ultrasound-guided nerve blocks

As with non–ultrasound-guided techniques, the patient should receive sedation, supplemental oxygen and have standard monitoring. A clean transducer with acoustic coupling gel is covered with a sterile occlusive dressing or special sterile probe cover. Air trapped between the transducer and the sterile cover will result in shadowing because of the poor impedance of air for

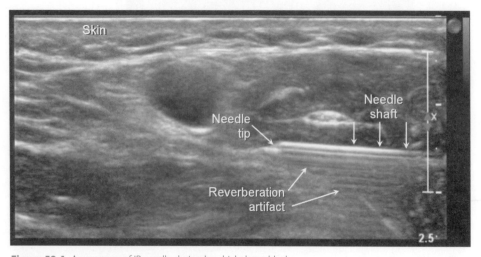

Figure 59.4. Appearance of IP needle during brachial plexus block.

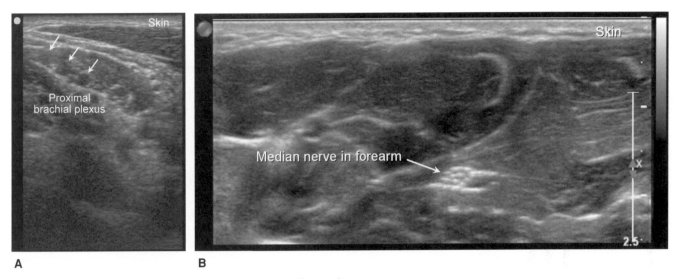

Figure 59.5. Proximal **(A)** and peripheral **(B)** nerve appearance on ultrasound.

ultrasound waves. Sterile acoustic gel is also required on the outside of the sterile cover and the patient's skin.

Touching one side of the active face confirms the *orientation* of the ultrasound transducer (Fig. 59.6). The orientation of the ultrasound transducer notch is by convention either cranial in longitudinal views or to the patient's right in transverse views. The ultrasound screen has an orientation marker that corresponds to the physical marker on the transducer.

Surface anatomy landmarks used in conventional, non–image-guided techniques can be used to guide the initial placement of the ultrasound transducer. Further adjustments are performed according to the ultrasound image to achieve the best nerve imaging. An optimal needle path is selected, and

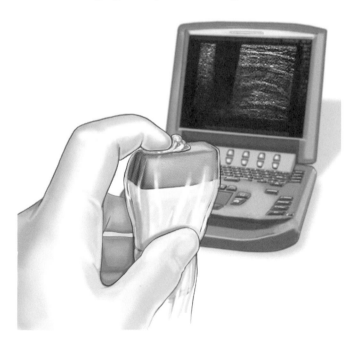

Figure 59.6. Confirmation of transducer orientation.

the puncture site is infiltrated with a local anesthetic such as lidocaine 1% via a small-gauge needle. The larger block needle is inserted through the skin wheal. It is important to respect the proximity of surrounding structures, especially the lung, arteries, veins, and spinal cord. One should avoid blind needle insertion deeper than expected by the sonogram or if the target structure or needle (tip) is poorly visualized. Nerve stimulation can confirm needle position but does not appear to improve block success rate; moreover, it adds to the complexity of the procedure.

Injection of the local anesthetic for neural blockade is made incrementally, often in multiple sites, with continuous assessment of local anesthetic distribution. Circumferential spread around nerves produces rapid and complete conduction block (Fig. 59.7). If the solution does not appear to surround all components of the target structure, the needle position is adjusted before further injections are made. Injections should be made slowly with frequent aspiration and maintaining low injection pressures (< 20 psi). If local anesthetic distribution cannot be visualized after a test dose of 1 to 2 ml, the injection should be stopped. One should aspirate and reassess needle tip placement to rule out intravascular injection. Air bubbles not removed from the syringe or tubing are highly echogenic and markedly degrade image quality after inadvertent injection (Fig. 59.7). Bicarbonate-containing solutions also may obscure imaging because of their carbon dioxide content.

All blocks can be performed either as a single-shot or continuous technique. The continuous technique is similar to the single shot, but instead of a 20- or 22-gauge short-bevel needle, a 17- or 18-gauge Tuohy needle is used. Once the needle is in optimal position, a small amount of local anesthetic is injected to facilitate passage of the catheter that is then inserted to the desired depth and secured in place. This technique can provide excellent postoperative pain control over several days that may facilitate early rehabilitation.

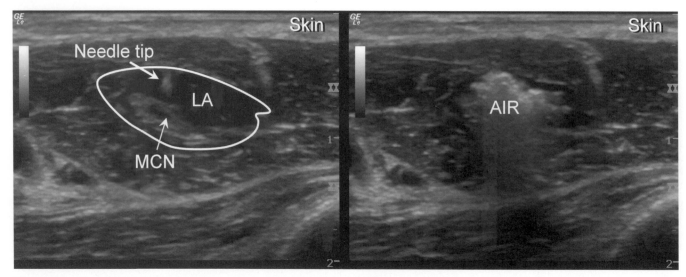

Figure 59.7. Air seen on injection while performing a musculocutaneous nerve block. MCN, musculocutaneous nerve; LA, local anesthetic.

Suggested readings

Abrahams MS, Aziz MF, Fu RF, Horn JL. Ultrasound guidance compared with electrical neurostimulation for peripheral nerve block: a systematic review and meta-analysis of randomized controlled trials. *Br J Anaesth* 2009; 102:408–17.

Adler R, Sofka C. Percutaneous ultrasound-guided injections in the musculoskeletal system. *Ultrasound Q* 2003; 19:3–12.

Gray A. Ultrasound-guided regional anesthesia – current state of the art. *Anesthesiology* 2006; 104:368–373.

Kossoff G. Basic physics and imaging characteristics of ultrasound. *World J Surg* 2000; 24:134–142.

Marhofer P, Greher M, Kapral S. Ultrasound guidance in regional anesthesia. *Br J Anesth* 2005; 94:7–17.

Peer S, Bodner G. *High-Resolution Sonography of the Peripheral Nervous System.* Berlin: Springer Verlag; 2003:3–4.

Schafhalter-Zoppoth I, McCulloch C, Gray A. Ultrasound visibility of needles used for regional nerve block: an in vitro study. *Reg Anesthesia Pain Med* 2004; 29;480–488.

Silvestri E, Martinoli C, Derchi LE, et al. Echotexture of peripheral nerves: correlation between ultrasound and histologic findings and criteria to differentiate tendons. *Radiology* 1995; 197: 291–296.

Chapter 60

Upper extremity nerve blocks

Eddy M. Feliz, Tanja S. Frey, Adam B. Collins, and Abdel-Kader Mehio

Introduction

Performing upper extremity nerve blocks requires detailed knowledge of anatomy, understanding of local anesthetic pharmacology, familiarity with the equipment, and preparation for possible complications. Upper extremity blocks are useful for a broad range of surgical procedures, ranging from the shoulder to the distal phalanges. The techniques used for nerve blocks have improved over time. Landmark-based approaches using paresthesias and nerves stimulation have largely been supplanted by ultrasound-guidance. Today ultrasound guidance is considered to be superior to older modalities in terms of maximizing success and minimizing morbidity.

Anatomy

The brachial plexus is formed by the ventral division of the cervical nerve roots of C5 through C8 and T1, with variable contribution from C4 and T2 (Fig. 60.1). These anterior divisions unite, forming trunks, divisions, cords, and terminal nerves. With the exception of the skin over the medial aspect of the arms (innervated by the intercostobrachial branch of T2) and the skin over the anterior portion of the shoulders (innervated by the cervical plexus, C1–4), the brachial plexus supplies all the motor and sensory innervation of the upper extremities.

Trunks

Nerve roots exit the spinal canal through the intervertebral foramina. In the space between the anterior and middle scalene muscles, the anterior divisions of these roots fuse together to form three trunks, the superior, middle, and inferior. The superior trunk receives fibers from C5 and C6, the middle trunk from C7, and the inferior trunk from C8 and T1. At this level, the phrenic nerve (C3–5) lies over the anterior scalene muscle. This explains its vulnerability to blockade during the interscalene approach, causing unilateral diaphragmatic paralysis.

Divisions

At the lateral border of the first rib, just behind the midpoint of the clavicle and posterior to the insertion of the anterior scalene muscle, each trunk forms an anterior and a posterior division to enter the axilla. Eventually, anterior divisions supply flexor muscles and posterior divisions supply extensor muscles.

Cords

The anterior and posterior divisions recombine to create three cords. These are named according to their relationship to the axillary artery. The lateral cord is derived from the anterior division of the superior and middle trunks. The medial cord is a continuation of the anterior division of the inferior trunk and the posterior cord originates from the fusion of the posterior divisions of all three trunks. These cords then divide into terminal branches at the lateral border of the pectoralis minor muscle.

Branches

The lateral cord gives rise to the musculocutaneous nerve and the lateral root of the median nerve. The medial cord contributes to the formation of the median nerve (medial aspect), the ulnar nerve, the medial cutaneous nerve of the forearm, and the medial cutaneous nerve of the arm. The posterior cord divides into the radial nerve and the axillary nerve.

Understanding the anatomic structure of the brachial plexus and the dermatomal innervation of each nerve root will increase the efficacy of the block while minimizing complications (Fig. 60.2). This knowledge allows one to choose the best approach to block the brachial plexus for the intended surgical procedure.

Brachial plexus blockade

Interscalene approach

The interscalene block targets the roots and trunks of the brachial plexus and is useful for surgical anesthesia and postoperative analgesia in the shoulder and arm. The patient is positioned semi-sitting or supine, with the arms adducted and the head turned to the contralateral side. Neck flexion against gravity demonstrates the sternocleidomastoid muscle, which lies just anterior to the interscalene groove. The interscalene groove is formed by the anterior and middle scalene muscles as they course toward their insertion in the first rib.

After patient preparation, a high-frequency linear transducer (10–15 MHz) is applied in the short axis. The carotid artery and internal jugular vein are identified and differentiated

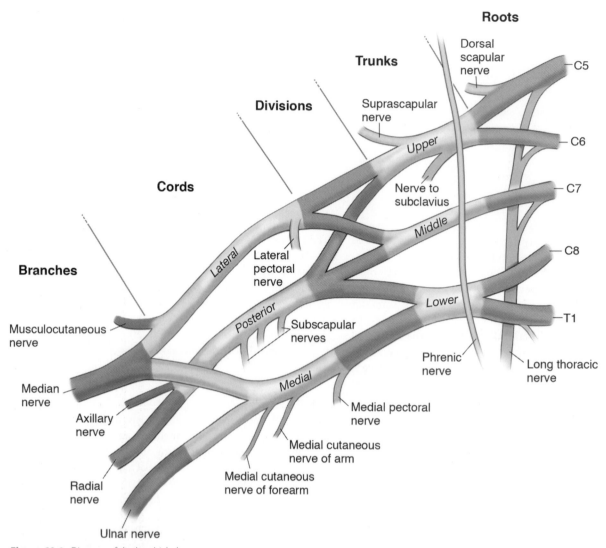

Figure 60.1. Diagram of the brachial plexus.

by compressing with the transducer. The internal jugular vein is collapsible under the pressure, whereas the carotid artery should show distinct pulsations. Sliding the transducer laterally, the roots and trunks of the brachial plexus can be visualized as round, hypoechoic structures coursing between the anterior and middle scalene muscles (Figs. 60.3 and 60.4).

The brachial plexus is usually found 0.5 to 1.5 cm beneath the skin surface. It can be approached with the needle in or out of plane, depending on what appears to be the safest needle trajectory in a given patient. The puncture site is infiltrated with 1% lidocaine via a small-gauge needle. The out-of-plane (OOP) approach uses a 22-gauge short-bevel 1–2 inch needle inserted from outside the plane of imaging either cranial to caudal (Fig. 60.3) or lateral to medial. This may result in unconventional needle approaches that have the potential to cause complications, especially those resulting from the proximity of the lung, carotid, and vertebral arteries, as well as the spinal cord. Hence, it is important to image the needle tip while it is still superficial and to avoid blind passes.

The in-plane (IP) approach (Fig. 60.4) requires a longer needle, depending on the width of the transducer and depth of the target structures. A 22-gauge 2–3 inch needle is advanced slowly into the plane of imaging under real-time visualization. The needle trajectory can be either posterior to anterior, as shown in Fig. 60.4, or anterior to posterior. The IP approach may afford a greater degree of safety as long as the needle is imaged well throughout the procedure. When using the IP approach it is safer to insert the needle lateral to the ultrasound probe. Inserting the needle medial or anterior to the ultrasound probe may result in injury to the phrenic nerve. It is common to see physical separation of the roots of the brachial plexus in the interscalene groove (Fig. 60.4). An injection of 25 to 30 ml of local anesthetic solution is made incrementally, targeting the deeper roots (C8, T1) first so that the mass of local anesthetic does not drive these nerves deeper and make them less accessible later in the procedure. If spread around the more superficial roots is incomplete, the anesthetic should be reserved and the needle repositioned to obtain spread around the entire brachial plexus.

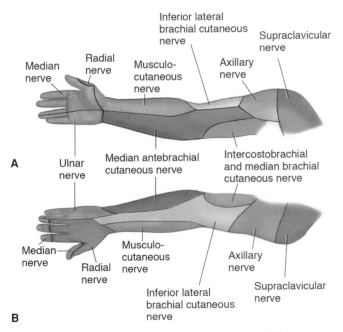

Figure 60.2. Cutaneous innervation of the upper extremity. **(A)** Arm supinated. **(B)** Arm prone.

Adverse effects and complications

Neural injury secondary to direct needle trauma can occur, but it is uncommon and self-limited. Ipsilateral phrenic nerve blockade leading to hemiparesis of the diaphragm occurs in almost 100% of patients and can result in up to 30% reduction in pulmonary function. Bilateral interscalene brachial plexus

blockade should be avoided. Frequent aspiration should be done during injection of local anesthetics, even though it does not exclude an intravascular injection. Pneumothorax is a rare complication but is more likely if the needle is directed too caudad (>45°). Recurrent laryngeal, vagus, and cervical sympathetic nerve blockade have also been described. Epidural and intrathecal injection can be avoided if the needle orientation is maintained slightly caudad.

Supraclavicular approach

For a supraclavicular block, the patient is positioned in a semi-sitting, upright, or supine position with the arms adducted and the head turned to the opposite side. The clavicle and lateral border of the clavicular head of the sternocleidomastoid muscle provide a reference for where to place the high-frequency linear transducer. After patient preparation, the transducer is applied in the short axis. At this height, the trunks or divisions of the brachial plexus are typically visualized. The ultrasound picture is usually described as hypoechoic clusters of grapes between the anterior and middle scalene muscles, just cephalad to the subclavian artery (Fig. 60.5b). The lung or pleura can be seen deep to the first rib. Careful attention must be paid to the proximity of the lung and subclavian artery when performing a supraclavicular block, because this block carries a higher risk of inadvertent vascular puncture and pneumothorax.

For the OOP approach, the needle can be advanced in a cranial-to-caudal direction similar to the classical approach, the point of needle insertion being 2–3 cm above the

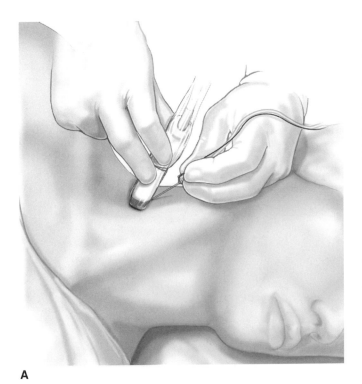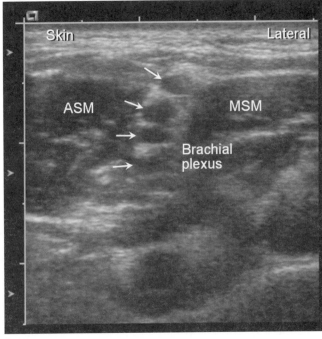

Figure 60.3. Interscalene block OOP approach. ASM, anterior scalene muscle; MSM, middle scalene muscle.

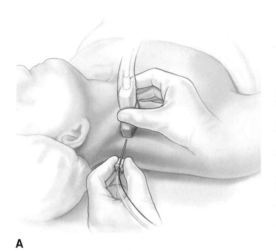

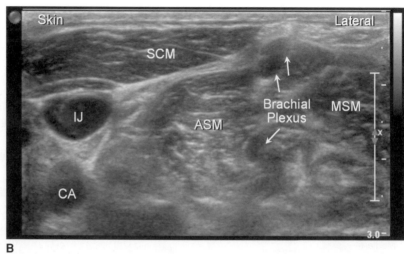

Figure 60.4. Interscalene block IP approach. CA, carotid artery; IJ, internal jugular vein; SCM, sternocleidomastoid muscle; ASM, anterior scalene muscle; MSM, middle scalene muscle.

mid-clavicle, optimally in a 30° angle (Fig. 60.5). Often, there is little working room between the transducer and the neck, and given the potential for pneumothorax, it is preferable to use the lateral-to-medial IP approach. Here, the ultrasound transducer can be placed immediately superior and parallel to the clavicle.

Shadowing artifact may be caused by the bone in this position. The needle is inserted lateral to the transducer and carefully advanced from lateral to medial under real-time visualization (Fig. 60.6). Another approach places the ultrasound transducer at a 90° angle to the clavicle. Here, the needle is inserted near

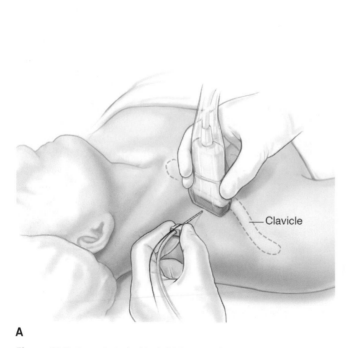

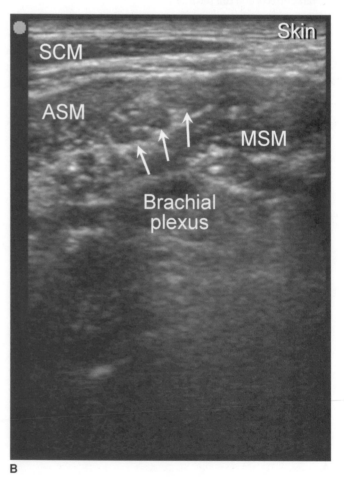

Figure 60.5. Supraclavicular block OOP approach (ASM = anterior scalene muscle, MSM = middle scalene muscle, SCM = sternocleidomastoid muscle).

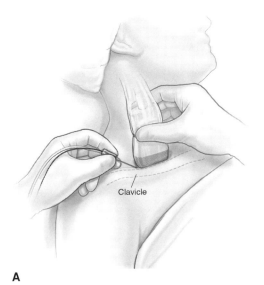
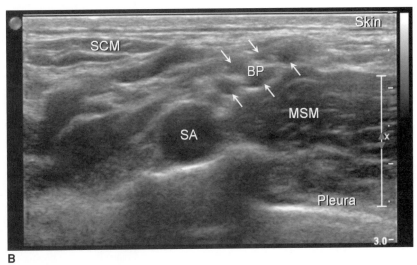

A   **B**

Figure 60.6. Supraclavicular block IP approach, lateral to medial. SA, subclavian artery; BP, brachial plexus; ASM, anterior scalene muscle; MSM, middle scalene muscle; SCM, sternocleidomastoid muscle.

the clavicular head of the sternocleidomastoid muscle, which resembles the "plumb-bob" approach, and advanced from the anterior-to-posterior direction. The transducer position and angle should be adjusted to image the advancing needle tip. Incremental injections of 25 to 30 ml of local anesthetic solution is made until the brachial plexus shows circumferential spread.

Adverse effects and complications

The most important complication associated with supraclavicular brachial plexus blockade is pneumothorax. Its incidence (0.5%–6%) is reduced with experience and the use of ultrasound to visualize the first rib and the lung while guiding the needle. However, this block should be avoided in patients with poor pulmonary reserve, and it is relatively contraindicated in outpatients if ultrasound is not available. Bilateral supraclavicular brachial plexus blocks should be avoided. Blockade of the phrenic (50%–60%), recurrent laryngeal, and cervical sympathetic plexus have also been described with this approach. Intravascular injection is possible, and frequent aspiration is advised during injection of the local anesthetic. Neural injury is rare and usually transient.

Infraclavicular approach

The patient is positioned supine, with the ipsilateral arm abducted and externally rotated. If this is impossible – for example, secondary to pain with movement – the arm also can be kept in a neutral or adducted position. This, however, may make it slightly more difficult to identify the subclavian/axillary artery. After sterile skin preparation and draping, a linear transducer (5–10 MHz) is placed immediately medial to the coracoid process in the short axis.

The subclavian/axillary artery underneath the pectoralis major and minor muscle is identified (Fig. 60.7b). Often, this is accomplished most easily by keeping the transducer very close to the inferior edge of the clavicle. One should be aware that the

close proximity to bone can cause a shadowing artifact that may reduce image quality. Adding Doppler function to the sonogram may be helpful in distinguishing the subclavian artery and vein, both of which are almost incompressible at this location. The cords may appear hyper- or hypoechoic at this level and take a lateral, medial, and posterior position with respect to the artery.

The puncture site and pectoralis muscles are infiltrated with 1% lidocaine via a small-gauge needle. Using the OOP approach, a 20- or 22-gauge short-bevel 3–4 inch needle is inserted at a 45° angle, or steeper. The needle is slowly advanced under real-time imaging from medial to lateral at this angle toward the subclavian artery and its surrounding cords (Fig. 60.7B). The medial cord may sometimes be difficult to find between the subclavian artery and vein.

For the IP approach, one can choose between the vertical paracoracoid (i.e., lateral; Fig. 60.8) or the classic approach. For the lateral approach, the transducer is placed immediately medial to the coracoid process in a parasagittal plane. If the arm is in the abducted position, the needle entry is approximately 2 cm medial and 2 cm caudal to the most prominent aspect of the coracoid process. A 22-gauge 3–4 inch needle is advanced from cranial to caudal toward the cords that surround the subclavian/axillary artery.

Alternatively, for the classic approach the transducer is applied at the middle of the clavicle in the parasagittal plane. The needle is introduced between the clavicle and the transducer and is advanced in a caudad and lateral direction within the imaging plane.

For a successful block, a total of 30 to 40 ml of local anesthetic should be injected in two locations: lateral (for the lateral and posterior cord) and medial (for the medial cord) from the artery (Fig. 60.7). Overlying muscle attenuates ultrasound waves, and the nerves deep to these muscles are often difficult to resolve well. This block is usually performed in a fairly

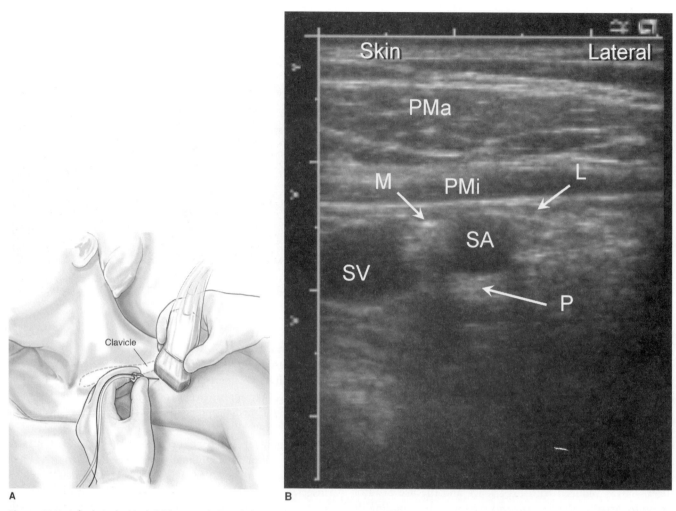

A

B

Figure 60.7. Infraclavicular block OOP approach. SA, subclavian artery; SV, subclavian vein; M, medial cord; L, lateral cord; P, posterior cord; PMi, pectoralis minor muscle; PMa, pectoralis major muscle.

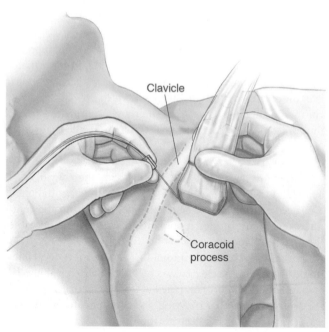

Figure 60.8. Infraclavicular block IP, lateral approach.

lateral location that makes pneumothorax less common but still possible.

This location also is preferred for a continuous brachial plexus catheter technique to provide postoperative pain control. It has the advantage of an immobile insertion point that limits the risk of dislodgement.

Adverse effects and complications

Hematoma, nerve injury, chylothorax (following left-sided block), and infection are theoretically possible. Again, the risk of intravascular injection is minimized by careful aspiration before injection. If the needle is directed too medially, pneumothorax is also a possibility.

Axillary approach

The axillary block provides safe and effective conduction block of the terminal branches of the brachial plexus for procedures on the elbow, forearm, and hand. The patient is positioned supine, with the arm abducted approximately 90° and externally rotated (Fig. 60.9). Padding under the wrist to reduce extension

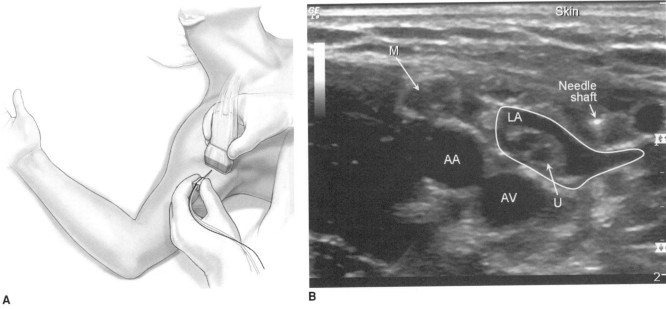

Figure 60.9. Axillary block OOP approach. AA, axillary artery; AV, axillary vein; M, median nerve; U, ulnar nerve; LA, local anesthetic.

and external rotation can make patients more comfortable while not compromising access to the brachial plexus. Surface landmarks include the pulse of the axillary artery, the coracobrachialis, and the pectoralis major muscle.

After patient preparation, a linear high-frequency transducer (10–15 MHz) is placed high in the axilla to image the nerves and vessels in short axis. The axillary artery is visualized easily with one or more nearby veins, and the median, ulnar, and radial nerves lie immediately adjacent to it. These structures usually lie 1 to 2 cm beneath the skin. The musculocutaneous nerve is outside the neurovascular bundle at this level and pierces the coracobrachialis muscle just lateral to the axillary artery.

For the OOP approach, a 22-gauge short-bevel 1–2 inch needle is inserted at a 45° angle to the skin and advanced distally to proximally crossing the plane of imaging. Local anesthetic

solution is deposited incrementally within the axillary sheath and around each accessible nerve, including the musculocutaneous nerve (Fig. 60.9b).

The IP approach requires a 22-gauge 2–4 inch needle that is advanced laterally to medially, starting at the edge of the transducer or going through the distal pectoralis major muscle (Fig. 60.10). The local anesthetic solution injection should surround each identified nerve and also spread in the axillary sheath (see Fig. 60.9b). It is usually best to perform the deep injections (the radial nerve) first so that superficial structures remain superficial and are not pushed deeper by the injected local anesthetic.

About 30 ml of local anesthetic solution is injected around the axillary artery and visible nerves or in at least two locations (anterior for the median and ulnar nerve and posterior to the axillary artery for the radial nerve; Fig. 60.11). About 5 mL of local anesthetic solution is injected around the

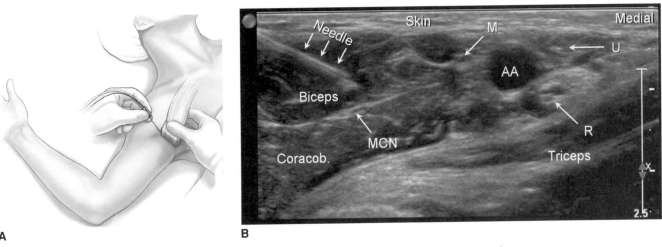

Figure 60.10. Axillary block IP approach. AA, axillary artery; M, median nerve; U, ulnar nerve; R, radial nerve; MCN, musculocutaneous nerve.

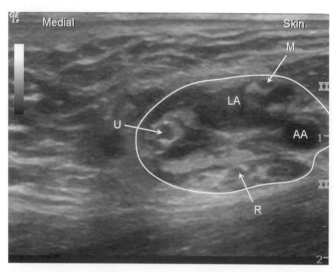

Figure 60.11. Axillary block postinjection. AA, axillary artery; U, ulnar nerve; R, radial nerve; M, medial nerve; LA, local anesthetic.

musculocutaneous nerve, seeking to fill the fascial plane in which it travels. Another 5-ml subcutaneous injection superficial to these structures blocks the intercostobrachial and medial brachial cutaneous nerves. This provides anesthesia to the medial arm and improves tourniquet tolerance.

Adverse effects and complications

Pneumothorax is not a complication of brachial plexus blockade at the axillary level. Arterial puncture can on rare occasions lead to hematoma is a possibility. Systemic toxicity and neural injury are the most significant complications associated with this approach. The risk of intravascular injection can be decreased by careful aspiration and incremental injection of the local anesthetic solution.

Distal nerve blocks of the upper extremity

Distal nerve blocks of the upper extremity can be useful after an incomplete brachial plexus block and in situations in which contraindications to the brachial plexus block exist. For example, such blocks may be useful when there is infection at the needle insertion site for a brachial plexus block and in patients in whom complications associated with brachial plexus block could be detrimental, such as bleeding diathesis, bilateral procedures and patients with limited pulmonary reserves.

Musculocutaneous nerve block

The musculocutaneous nerve provides the sensory innervation to the lateral aspect of the forearm from the elbow to the radio-carpal joint. This nerve can be blocked by injecting 3 to 5 ml of local anesthetic solution subcutaneously 1 cm proximal to the intercondylar line and 1 to 2 cm lateral to the biceps tendon.

Radial nerve block

The radial nerve provides sensory innervation to the posterior aspect of the forearm, the lateral aspect of the dorsum of the

hand, and the proximal portion of the dorsum of the thumb, index, middle, and radial side of the ring fingers. At the elbow, the radial nerve can be blocked by injecting 3 to 5 ml of local anesthetic solution in a fanlike manner, approximately 2 cm lateral to the biceps tendon on the intercondylar crease. If paresthesia is obtained or periosteum is contacted, the needle should be withdrawn 0.5 to 1 cm before injecting. At the wrist, the radial nerve is blocked by injecting 2 to 3 ml of local anesthetic solution lateral to the radial artery. In addition, a subcutaneous wheal should be raised on the lateral and dorsal aspect of the wrist.

Intravenous regional anesthesia (Bier block)

The upper extremity can be blocked for short procedures by intravenous regional anesthesia, first demonstrated by August Bier in 1908. An intravenous cannula is placed distally in the operative limb, and the limb is elevated and exsanguinated with a tight elastic wrap. A proximal tourniquet is then inflated well above arterial blood pressure (typically two adjacent cuffs are used). Local anesthetic solution is then injected via the intravenous cannula, typically 50 ml of 0.5% lidocaine without epinephrine (Fig. 60.12). Onset of anesthesia distal to the

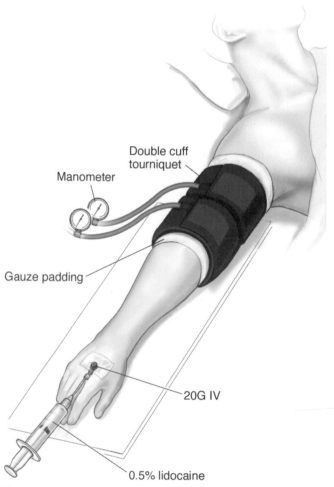

Figure 60.12. Intravenous regional anesthesia (Bier block).

cuff occurs within 5 to 10 minutes, making this technique suitable for brief procedures below the elbow. If tourniquet pain develops, the distal cuff can be inflated (over anesthetized skin) and the proximal cuff deflated. The block is usually used for no more than 60 to 90 minutes, although reinjection has been described. Most authorities recommend deflation of the cuff no sooner than 20 minutes after injection to minimize the chance of systemic local anesthetic toxicity. Some recommend deflation and rapid reinflation, followed by deflation 1 to 2 minutes later to divide the absorption of drug. The principal risk of the procedure is systemic toxicity that can be minimized by following a careful technique. The simplicity and reliability of the block makes it popular for simple upper extremity procedures.

Suggested readings

Boezaart AP. Continuous Infraclavicular Nerve Block (Brachial Plexus Cord Block). Department of Anesthesia, University of Iowa, Iowa City, IA: NYSORA meeting NY: Dec. 2006.

Brown DL. *wInterscalene block*. In: Brown DL, ed. *Atlas of Regional Anesthesia*. Philadelphia: WB Saunders; 1992:23–30.

Chan VWS, Perlas A, Rawson R, Odukoya O. Ultrasound guided supraclavicular brachial plexus block. *Anesth Analg* 2003; 97:1514–1517.

Chelly JE. *Peripheral Nerve Blocks: A Color Atlas*. Philadelphia: Lippincott Williams & Wilkins; 1999.

Fouch RA, Abram SE, Hogan QH. Neural blockade for upper-extremity pain. *Hand Clin*. 1996; 12(4):791–800.

Gerancher JC. Upper extremity nerve blocks. *Anesthesiol Clin North Am* 2000; 18(2):297–317.

Long TR, Wass CT, Burkle CM. Perioperative interscalene blockade: an overview of its history and current clinical use. *J Clin Anesth* 2002; 14:546–556.

Neal JM, Hebl JR, Gerancher JC, Hogan QH. Brachial plexus anesthesia: essentials of our current understanding. *Reg Anesth Pain Med* 2002; 27:402–428.

Ootaki C, Hayashi H, Amano M. Ultrasound guided infraclavicular brachial plexus block: an alternative technique to anatomical landmark-guided approaches. *Reg Anesth Pain Med* 2000; 25: 600–604.

Perlas A, Chan VWS. Ultrasound guided interscalene brachial plexus block. *Tech Reg Anesth Pain Management* 2004; 8:143–148.

Retzl G, Kapral S, Greher M, et al. Ultrasonographic findings of the axillary part of the brachial plexus. *Anesth Analg* 2001; 92:1271–1275.

Sandhu NS, Capan LM. Ultrasound guided infraclavicular brachial plexus block. *Br J Anaesth* 2002; 89(2):254–259.

Schroeder LE, Horlocker TT, Schroeder DR. The efficacy of axillary block for surgical procedures above the elbow. *Anesth Analg* 1996: 83:747.

Williams SR, Chouinard P, Arcand G, et al. Ultrasound guidance speeds the execution and improves the quality of supraclavicular block. *Anesth Analg* 2003; 97:1518–1523.

Chapter 61

Lower extremity nerve blocks

Mônica M. Sá Rêgo and Adam B. Collins

This chapter presents an overview of the anatomy and describes the most commonly used techniques for performance of lower extremity nerve blocks.

Lumbar plexus

The lumbar plexus (Fig. 61.1) is formed by the anterior rami of the first four lumbar spinal nerves (L1–4) with occasional contributions from T12 and L5. Lower-extremity nerves originating from the lumbar plexus include the femoral nerve (L2–4), obturator nerve (L2–4), and lateral femoral cutaneus nerve (L2–3).

Femoral nerve block

Anatomy

The femoral nerve originates from L2–4 and is the largest nerve of the lumbar plexus. It emerges from the psoas muscle, descending in the groove between the psoas and the iliacus. On its course to the thigh, it remains deep to the fascia lata and fascia iliaca, where the femoral vessels lie in a plane between these two fascial layers. At the level of the inguinal ligament, it lies anterior to the iliopsoas muscle and lateral to the femoral artery. At the level of the inguinal crease, the femoral nerve is wider and more superficial than at the level of the inguinal ligament. After passing under the inguinal ligament, the femoral nerve divides into anterior and posterior branches. The femoral nerve supplies the sartorius, pectineus, and quadriceps muscles; the knee joint; the skin of the anterior and medial thigh; and the medial aspect of the leg (Fig. 61.2). The surface landmarks for a femoral nerve block are the anterior superior iliac spine, pubic tubercle, inguinal ligament, inguinal crease, and femoral artery pulse (Fig. 61.3).

The femoral nerve is closely associated with the femoral artery and vein but is not located in the same anatomic compartment. These vessels travel in the femoral sheath, but the femoral nerve lies over the iliopsoas muscle and is physically separated from the vessels by the fascia iliaca. This position prevents local anesthetic spread around the nerve if injected on the side of the vascular bundle. The mnemonic *VAN*, which describes the relationship of the femoral vein, artery, and nerve medially to laterally, should be remembered (Fig. 61.4).

Technique

The patient should be supine with the leg to be blocked positioned in slight abduction. After sterile skin preparation and draping, the skin is infiltrated with 1% lidocaine. A 22-gauge short-bevel insulated stimulating needle is inserted at a 45° angle cephalad, 1 cm lateral to the femoral artery pulse just below the inguinal crease. The peripheral nerve stimulator is set at 1.5 to 2.0 mA. The needle is advanced slowly until upward movement of the patella is observed. The current output is decreased and the needle advanced until the patellar movement is seen with a stimulation of 0.3 to 0.5 mA. After negative aspiration, 20 ml of local anesthetic is injected in small increments.

The femoral nerve also may be blocked as part of the fascia iliaca compartment block. A short-bevel needle is introduced below the junction of the medial and lateral thirds of the inguinal ligament and slowly advanced until two losses of resistance are felt (fascia lata and fascia iliaca), then 20 to 30 ml of the local anesthetic is injected.

If using ultrasound technology, a linear high-frequency transducer (10–15 MHz) is applied in the short axis just inferior to the inguinal ligament (that extends from the anterior superior iliac spine to the pubic tubercle; Fig. 61.4). After identifying the femoral vessels, the artery and vein can be distinguished by compression with the transducer. The femoral vein is collapsible under the pressure, whereas the femoral artery has pulsations. At this level, the femoral nerve has a flattened triangular shape, is usually hyperechoic, and may show small fascicles (Fig. 61.5). It lies at an angle at the junction between the hyperechoic subcutaneous tissue and hypoechoic iliopsoas muscle.

Using the out-of plane (OOP) approach, a 22-gauge short-bevel 2–3 inch needle is inserted caudal to the transducer at a 45° cephalad inclination, aiming for the lateral edge of the femoral nerve (Fig. 61.4). Two fascial pops can be appreciated by palpation and sonogram. The first is the needle traversing the fascia lata and the second, the fascia iliaca.

For the IP approach, a longer, 22-gauge 3.5–4 inch needle is advanced laterally to medially under real-time visualization (Fig. 61.5). Efforts should be made to image the tip of the needle, not only the shaft, to avoid vascular puncture that may result from advancing the needle too far. Short-bevel needles tend to deform fascia and then produce significant recoil as they pierce

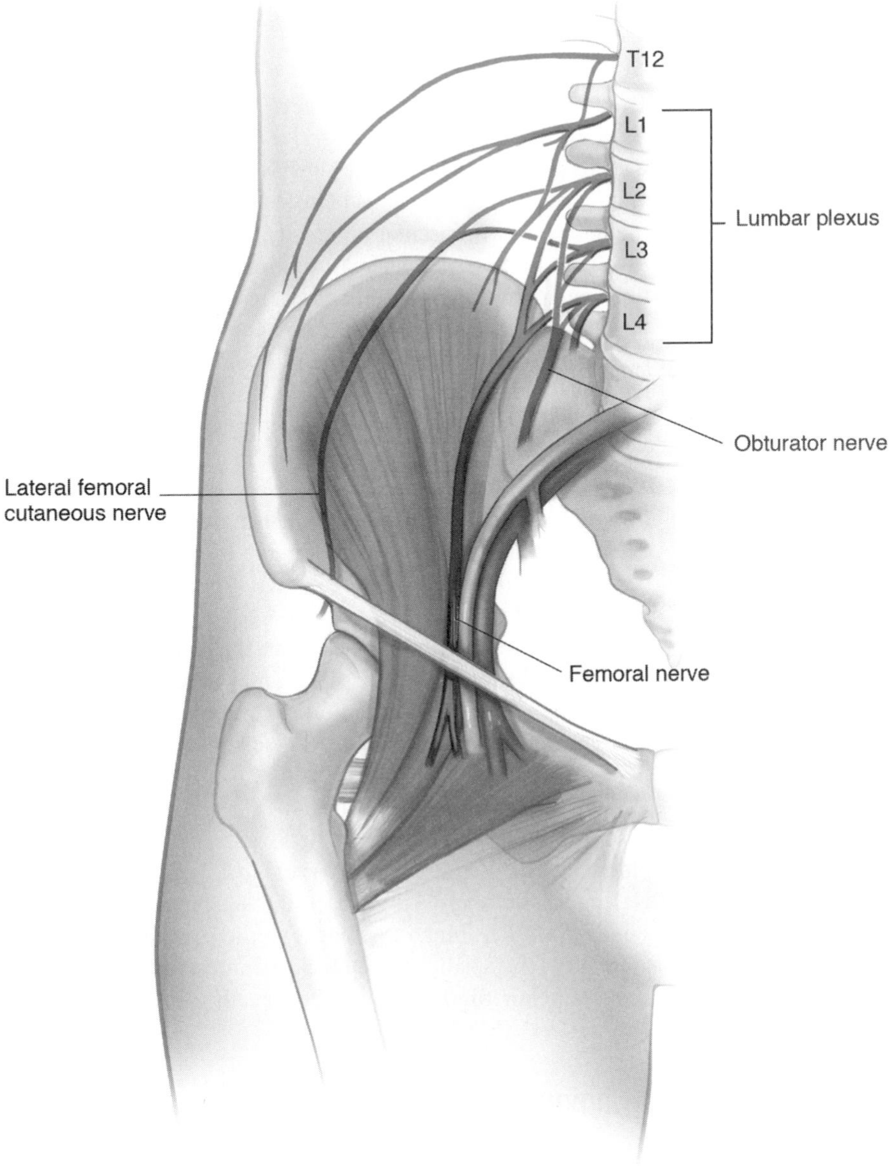

Figure 61.1. The lumbar plexus.

fascial planes, requiring some redirection to achieve optimal needle position.

After negative aspiration, 20 to 30 ml of local anesthetic solution is injected incrementally with real-time monitoring of the distribution of the solution (Fig. 61.6). Needle position may have to be adjusted to produce circumferential spread.

Lateral femoral cutaneous nerve block

Lateral femoral cutaneous nerve block is used for the diagnosis and treatment of meralgia paresthetica, and is combined with femoral and/or sciatic nerve blocks to allow the use of a thigh tourniquet. It also may be done to provide anesthesia on the lateral aspect of the thigh for skin procedures.

Anatomy

The lateral femoral cutaneous (L2–3) nerve emerges along the lateral border of the psoas muscle caudad to the ilioinguinal nerve. It courses deep to the iliac fascia to emerge from the fascia immediately inferior and medial to the anterior superior iliac spine. It divides into anterior and posterior branches below the inguinal ligament.

Technique

A short-bevel 22-gauge needle is inserted 2 cm medial and 2 cm caudal to the anterior superior iliac spine. The needle is advanced until a pop and loss of resistance are felt as the needle passes the fascia lata. About 10 ml of local anesthetic solution is injected in a fanlike fashion above and below the fascia lata.

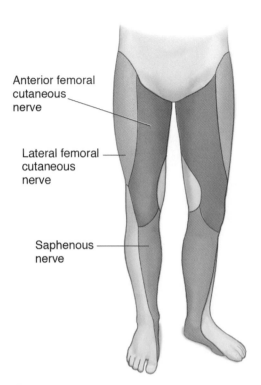

Figure 61.2. Cutaneous distribution of the femoral nerve.

Obturator nerve block

The obturator nerve block is more often combined with the femoral, sciatic, and lateral femoral cutaneous blocks for surgeries on the lower extremities. It can be used as a single nerve block in urologic surgery to suppress the obturator reflex during transurethral resection of lateral bladder wall, or to relieve adductor muscle spasm.

Anatomy

The obturator nerve (L2–4) emerges medially to the psoas muscle at the pelvic brim. It runs caudad in the retroperitoneum to the obturator canal, where it divides into anterior and posterior branches. These provide sensory innervation of the medial thigh and hip joint and motor supply to the thigh adductors. The landmarks for this block are the anterior and superior iliac spines, pubic tubercle, inguinal ligament, femoral artery, and tendon of the long abductor muscle.

Technique

The block is performed at the inguinal level to facilitate its performance and make it less uncomfortable for patients. The inguinal fold is identified, and a line is drawn from the femoral artery pulse to the tendon of the long adductor muscle (identified during leg abduction). A 22-gauge needle connected to a nerve stimulator is inserted at the midpoint of the line at a 30° angle and directed anteriorly/posteriorly and cephalad. The needle is advanced slowly and slightly laterally until a response at 0.3 to 0.5 mA from the major adductor muscle is obtained. About 10 to 15 ml of local anesthetic solution is then injected after negative aspiration.

Sciatic nerve block
Anatomy

The sciatic nerve, the largest nerve in the body, originates from L4–S3 in the pelvis on the anterior surface of the piriformis muscle (Fig. 61.7). It exits the pelvis through the greater sciatic foramen, then descends between the greater trochanter of the femur and the ischial tuberosity. It runs along the posterior thigh to the lower part of the femur, where it splits into the tibial and common peroneal nerves (usually 5–12 cm proximal to the popliteal fossa crease). In the popliteal fossa, the sciatic nerve runs slightly lateral to the midpoint between the biceps femoris (lateral) and the semitendinosus tendons (medial), where it lies lateral and superficial in relation to the popliteal vessels.

The common peroneal nerve descends along the head and neck of the fibula. Its terminal branches are the superficial and deep peroneal nerves. The tibial nerve is larger and descends vertically through the popliteal fossa. Its terminal branches are the medial and lateral plantar nerves. Because the tibial nerve has a more defined sheath, an injection of a large volume of local anesthetic in its sheath may have a higher success rate compared with injection in the common peroneal sheath. The cutaneous distribution of the sciatic nerve is shown in Fig. 61.8.

Several approaches to block the sciatic nerve have been described since Victor Pauchet first presented the sciatic nerve block in 1920. The sciatic nerve block can be performed via the classic approach (Labat), the subgluteal approach (di Benedetto), the Franco approach, or the popliteal fossa distal approach. The sciatic nerve block is indicated for major procedures below the knee, and it is usually combined with the femoral nerve block.

Technique
Classical approach

The landmarks used for the classical approach are the greater trochanter and the posterior superior iliac spine (Fig. 61.9a). The patient should be in the lateral position, slightly rotated forward, with the dependent leg extended and the leg to be blocked flexed. The landmarks are marked and a line is drawn between them. A perpendicular line is then drawn distal to the midpoint of the above line. The needle insertion site is 4 cm distal to the midpoint (Fig. 61.9b). After sterile skin preparation and draping, the skin is infiltrated with 1% lidocaine. A 4–6 inch needle is inserted perpendicular to all planes. The nerve stimulator is set at 1.5 to 2.0 mA, and the needle is advanced slowly and the current gradually reduced until twitches of the foot are seen at 0.3 to 0.5 mA (Fig. 61.10). The sciatic nerve is usually located at a depth of 5 to 8 cm with this approach. After negative aspiration, 20 to 25 ml of local anesthetic solution is injected slowly. If the aforementioned approach fails to elicit twitches, the needle is redirected in a slightly caudal or cephalad direction.

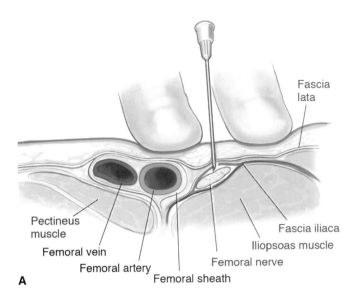

Fascia
lata

Pectineus
muscle

Femoral vein

Femoral artery

Femoral sheath

Femoral nerve

Fascia iliaca

Iliopsoas muscle

A

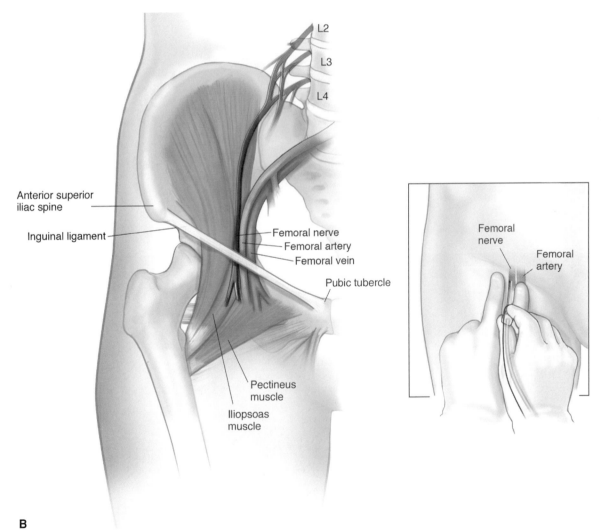

L2

L3

L4

Anterior superior
iliac spine

Inguinal ligament

Femoral nerve
Femoral artery
Femoral vein

Pubic tubercle

Pectineus
muscle

Iliopsoas
muscle

Femoral
nerve

Femoral
artery

B

Figure 61.3. Surface landmarks and technique for blockade of the femoral nerve. **(A)** Anatomic position of the femoral nerve. **(B)** Landmarks and needle insertion point for femoral nerve block.

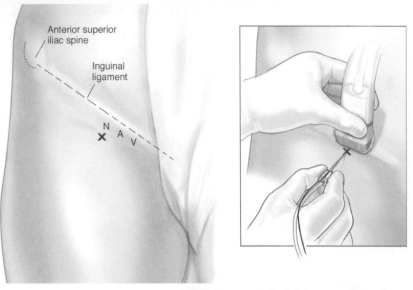

Figure 61.4. Femoral block OOP approach. VAN, femoral vein, artery, and nerve; X, needle insertion site.

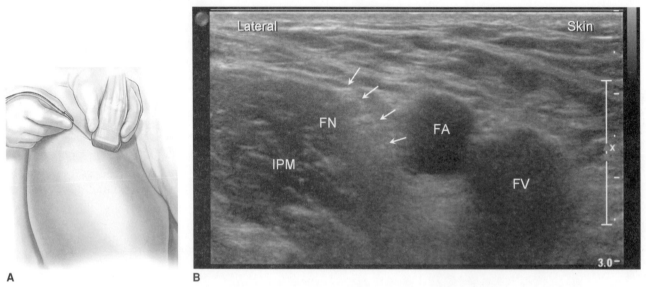

A　　　　　　**B**

Figure 61.5. Femoral block IP approach. FA, femoral artery; FV, femoral vein; FN, femoral nerve; IPM, iliopsoas muscle.

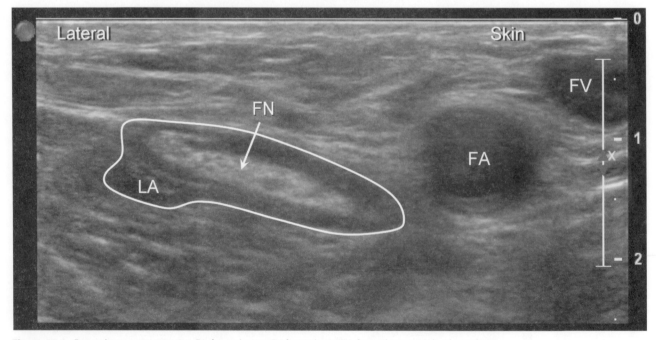

Figure 61.6. Femoral nerve post injection. FA, femoral artery; FV, femoral vein; FN, femoral nerve; LA, local anesthetic.

Subgluteal approach

The subgluteal approach has the potential to decrease the discomfort usually seen with the classical posterior approach. The patient is placed at the same position as for the classical approach. The landmarks are the greater trochanter of the femur and the ischial tuberosity. A line is drawn between the two, with the midpoint marked. The needle insertion point will be 4 cm caudad to the midpoint marked. The needle should be inserted perpendicular to all planes and foot twitches noticed, as described earlier (Fig. 61.11).

Franco approach

The Franco approach is based on the concept that the relation of the sciatic nerve to the pelvis is similar in all adults and that the posterior projection of the ischial tuberosity is located at approximately the same distance from the midline. The landmark for this approach is the intergluteal sulcus (midline). A point 10 cm lateral to the midline is marked, and the needle is inserted at this point. This approach can be performed with the patient in the lateral or prone position. The rest of the technique is similar to the classical approach.

Popliteal fossa approach (posterior and lateral)

The popliteal fossa block is used primarily for foot and ankle surgery and postoperative pain control. The analgesia provided by popliteal fossa blocks lasts longer than that of ankle blocks. The popliteal fossa block can be performed through a posterior or lateral approach, and it can be done as a single injection or continuous technique. Both approaches are discussed below.

Posterior approach

The patient should be in the prone position, and the foot to be blocked should be either protruding from the end of the bed

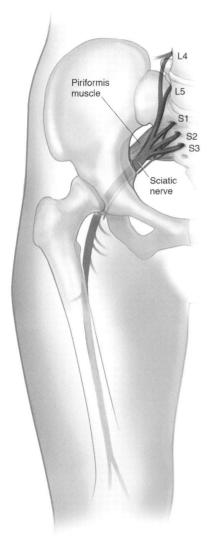

Figure 61.7. The sciatic nerve.

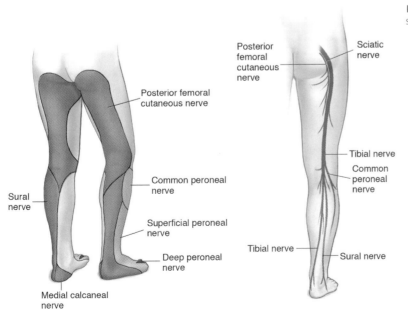

Figure 61.8. Cutaneous distribution of the branches of the sciatic nerve.

375

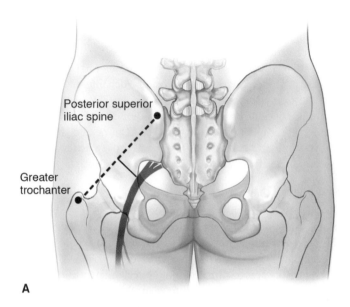

A

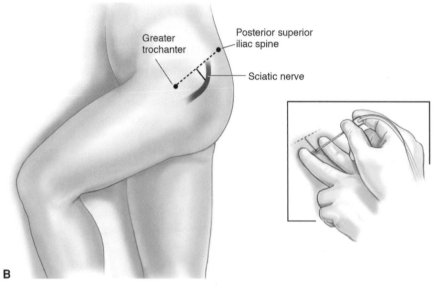

B

Figure 61.9. Posterior (classical Labat) approach to sciatic nerve block. **(A)** Landmarks. **(B)** Point of needle insertion.

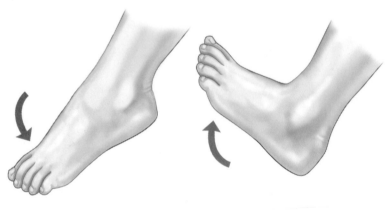
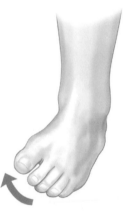
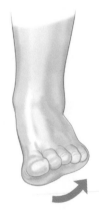

Plantar flexion – tibial nerve

Dorsiflexion – deep peroneal nerve

Inversion – tibial and deep peroneal nerves

Eversion – superficial peroneal nerve

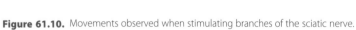

Figure 61.10. Movements observed when stimulating branches of the sciatic nerve.

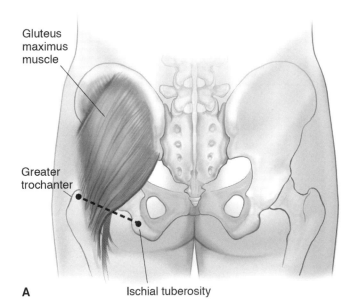

Gluteus maximus muscle

Greater trochanter

Ischial tuberosity

A

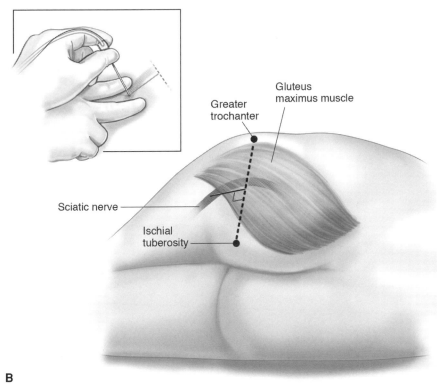

Greater trochanter

Gluteus maximus muscle

Sciatic nerve

Ischial tuberosity

B

Figure 61.11. Subgluteal approach to sciatic nerve block. **(A)** Landmarks. **(B)** Point of needle insertion.

or slightly elevated, to allow for observation of foot movement. The landmarks are the popliteal fossa crease, the tendon of the biceps femoris laterally, and the tendons of the semitendinosus and semimembranosus medially. The patient is asked to flex the knee to facilitate visualization of the tendons. The point of needle insertion is marked at 7 to 9 cm above the popliteal fossa crease, at the midpoint between the tendons (Fig. 61.12).

Under sterile technique and skin infiltration with 1% lidocaine, a 22-gauge stimulating needle is inserted and directed proximally at a 45° angle. This should not result in local muscular twitches. The stimulating current is decreased from 1.5 to 2.0 mA until foot twitches are observed at 0.3 to 0.5 mA, usually at 3 to 5 cm from the skin (Fig 61.10b). After negative aspiration, 30 ml of local anesthetic is injected. Injection of local anesthetic after stimulation of the tibial nerve is preferred, because it may result in a higher success rate.

The continuous popliteal block technique is similar to the aforementioned technique, but a 17-gauge Touhy type needle is used to allow insertion of a catheter. The catheter should be inserted 5 to 10 cm beyond the skin. Popliteal catheters

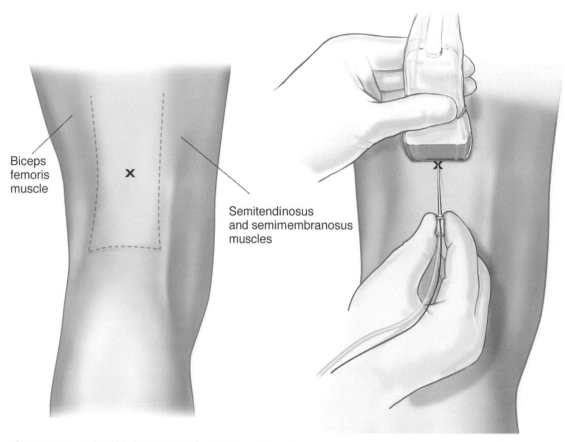

Figure 61.12. Popliteal block OOP approach. X, needle insertion site.

Biceps femoris muscle

Semitendinosus and semimembranosus muscles

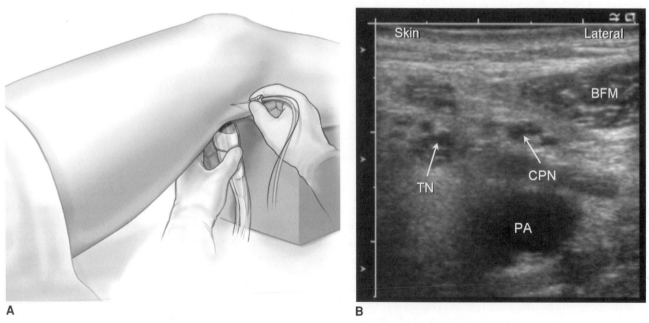

A

B

Figure 61.13. Popliteal block IP approach. PA, popliteal artery; TN, tibial nerve; CPN, common peroneal nerve; BFM, biceps femoris muscle.

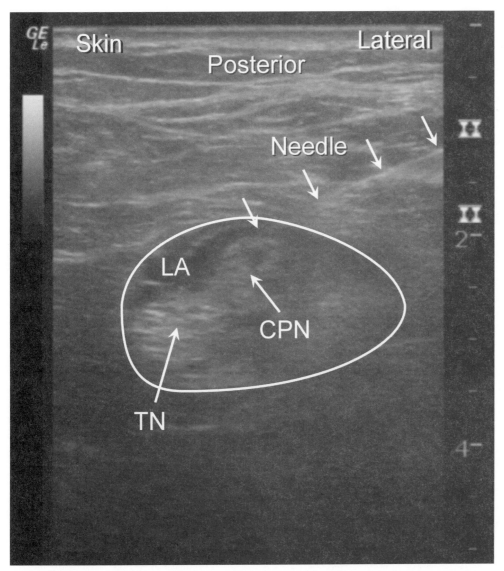

Figure 61.14. Popliteal block post injection. TN, tibial nerve; CPN, common peroneal nerve; LA, local anesthetic.

have been used successfully to manage postoperative pain after lower-extremity orthopedic procedures.

When this block is performed with the use of ultrasound imaging, the patient is positioned prone, as described above, for the OOP approach. After patient preparation, a linear high-frequency transducer (10–15 MHz) is applied in short axis slightly above the popliteal crease (Fig. 61.13). Once the popliteal artery is identified, the tibial nerve usually lies just superficial and can be traced retrograde until it joins with the common peroneal nerve, at the point of the bifurcation of the sciatic nerve (Fig. 61.13). Sliding and tilting the transducer tend to make the bifurcation more evident, as the operator can see one structure becoming two. This is usually the best location to perform a successful conduction block, because the proximal sciatic nerve is usually deeper and more encased in muscle, making it harder to image well. A 22-gauge short-bevel 2–3 inch needle is inserted with a 45° cephalad angulation and slowly

advanced as the transducer is manipulated to seek the needle tip position.

Lateral approach

The lateral approach usually is used when the patient cannot be placed in the prone position. The patient should be in the supine position with the foot to be blocked elevated to allow visualization of foot movement. The landmarks for this approach are the popliteal fossa crease, the vastus lateralis muscle, and the biceps femoris muscle. Under sterile technique, the needle is inserted in the groove between the vastus lateralis and biceps femoris muscle, about 10 cm above the popliteal crease. The needle is advanced perpendicular to skin until it contacts the femur, then it is withdrawn and redirected at a 30° angle posteriorly until foot twitches (depth of 5–7 cm) are observed, as with the posterior approach. The IP approach with the use of ultrasound imaging has the advantage of allowing the patient to remain

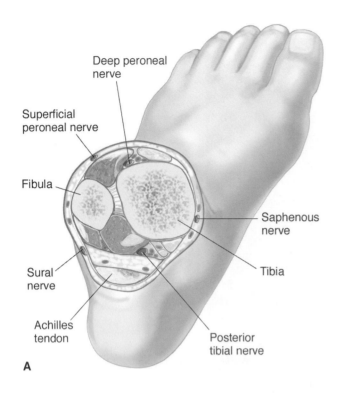

A

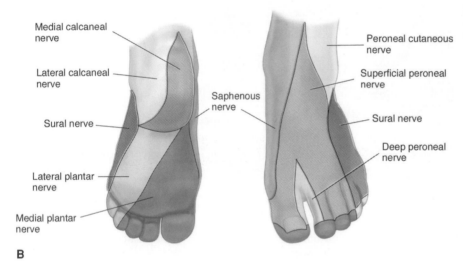

B

Figure 61.15. Innervation of the foot. **(A)** Anatomy of the five nerves innervating the foot. **(B)** Cutaneous distribution of the nerves of the foot.

supine. The ipsilateral leg is elevated on a lift or suspended by a sling to allow enough space beneath the thigh for the ultrasound probe. A 20- or 22-gauge 3–4 inch needle is introduced using landmarks as described above (Fig. 61.13). The needle is advanced under real-time visualization, adjusting the angle and position of the transducer to image the needle shaft and tip. Either the entire sciatic nerve or the tibial and common peroneal components should show local anesthetic spreading circumferentially, with approximately 30 ml of solution (Fig. 61.13 and Fig. 61.14).

The popliteal nerve block, in combination with a saphenous nerve block, provides anesthesia and postoperative analgesia for foot and ankle procedures. The saphenous nerve can be blocked just above or below the anterior and medial aspect of the knee or by performing a femoral nerve block.

Ankle block

The ankle block is indicated for distal foot surgery, the most common being surgery for the diabetic foot and for bunion surgery. It is commonly done with landmarks alone, but ultrasound can help identify many of the nerves and improve success rates.

Anatomy

There are five peripheral nerves that innervate the foot (Fig. 61.15). The saphenous nerve is a branch of the femoral nerve

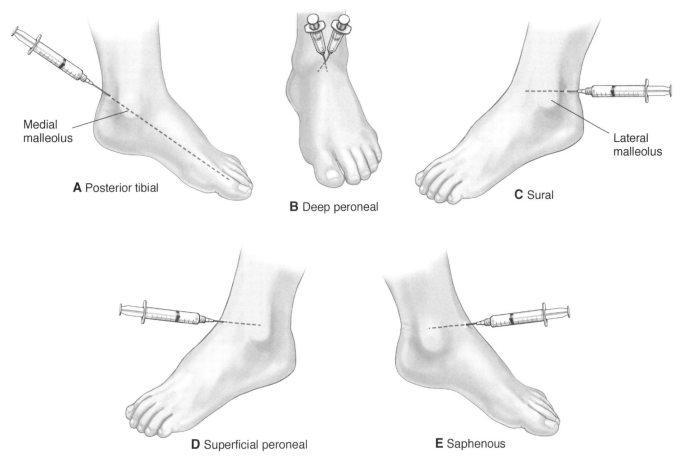

Figure 61.16. Injection sites for ankle block.

and supplies the medial aspect of the foot and ankle. The other four nerves are branches of the sciatic nerve. The sural nerve originates from the tibial nerve and the communicating superficial peroneal branches, and innervates the lateral aspect of the foot. The deep peroneal and superficial peroneal nerves are branches of the common peroneal nerve and innervate the area between the first and second toes and the dorsal aspect of the foot, respectively. The posterior tibial nerve supplies the lower and posterior surface of the heel and the plantar aspect of the foot.

Technique

The block is most easily performed with the patient supine, with the foot to be blocked elevated on a support (Fig. 61.16). The landmarks are the medial and lateral malleoli, the Achilles tendon, the extensor hallucis longus tendon, and the tibial and dorsalis pedis pulses.

The tibial nerve is blocked posterior to the medial malleolus. A 22-gauge needle is inserted posterior to the posterior tibial artery pulse, and 5 ml of local anesthetic solution is injected. The deep peroneal nerve is blocked with an injection of 5 ml of local anesthetic solution immediately lateral to

the extensor hallucis longus tendon (have the patient extend the great toe) deep to the retinaculum. The saphenous, sural, and superficial peroneal nerves are blocked at the level of the malleoli with a subcutaneous injection of 10 to 15 ml of local anesthetic solution in a circumferential line between the two malleoli.

It is advisable to block all five nerves, as there are variations in the dermatomal nerve supply. Epinephrine should not be used with the local anesthetic for ankle blocks because of the risk of causing ischemia in the foot.

Suggested readings

Boezaart AP. Anesthesia and Orthopedic Surgery. New York: McGraw-Hill; 2006.

Capdevila X, Barthelet Y, Biboulet P, et al. Effects of perioperative analgesic technique on the surgical outcome and duration of rehabilitation after major knee surgery. *Anesthesiology* 1999; 91:8–15.

Chelly JE, Greger J, Casati A. Continuous lateral sciatic blocks for acute postoperative pain management after major ankle and foot surgery. *Foot Ankle Int* 2002; 23:749–752.

Choquet O, Nazarian S, Manelli H. Bloc obturateur au pli inguinal: Etude anatomique. *Ann Fr Anesth Reanim* 2001; 20:131s.

Di Benedetto P, Bertini L, Casati A, et al. A new posterior approach to the sciatic nerve block: a prospective, randomized comparison with the classic posterior approach. *Anesth Analg* 2001; 93:1040–1044.

Franco CD. Posterior approach to the sciatic nerve in adults: is Euclidean geometry still necessary? *Anesthesiology* 2003; 98:723–728.

Gruber H, Peer S, Kovacs P, et al. The ultrasonographic appearance of the femoral nerve and cases of iatrogenic impairment. *J Ultrasound Med* 2003; 22:163–172.

Hadzic A. *Textbook of Regional Anesthesia and Acute Pain Management*. New York: McGraw-Hill; 2007.

Ilfeld BM, Morey TE, Wang DR, Enneking FK. Continuous popliteal sciatic nerve block for postoperative pain control at home: a randomized, double-blinded, placebo-controlled study. *Anesthesiology* 2002; 97:959–965.

Lee LA, Posner KL, Domino KB, et al. Injuries associated with regional anesthesia in the 1980s and 1990s: a closed claims analysis. *Anesthesiology* 2004; 101:141–152.

Marhofer P, Schrogendorfer K, Koining H, et al. Ultrasonographic guidance improves sensory block and onset time of three-in-one blocks. *Anesth Analg* 1997; 85:854–857.

McLeod DH, Wong DH, Claridge RJ, Merrick PM. Lateral popliteal sciatic nerve block compared with subcutaneous infiltration for analgesia following foot surgery. *Can J Anaesth* 1994; 41:673–676.

Singelyn F, Deyaert M, Joris D, et al. Effects of intravenous patient-controlled analgesia with morphine, continuous epidural analgesia, and continuous "3-in-1" block on postoperative pain and knee rehabilitation after unilateral total knee arthroplasty. *Anesth Analg* 1998; 87:88–92.

Singelyn F, Ebongo F, Symens B, et al. Influence of the analgesic technique on postoperative rehabilitation after total hip replacement. *Reg Anesth Pain Med* 2001; 26:39.

Vloka JD, Hadzic A, Lesser JB, et al. A common epineural sheath for the nerves in the popliteal fossa and its possible implications for sciatic nerve block. *Anesth Analg* 1997; 84: 387–390.

Fluid and Electrolyte Balance

Selwyn O. Rogers Jr., editor

Fluid replacement

Silvia Pivi and Lorenzo Berra

Despite the fact that fluid replacement therapy is one of the most fundamental elements of the anesthetic and critical care of patients, it remains one of the most difficult. Because of a lack of clear data there are no precise rules for the amount, timing, or type (crystalloid vs. colloid or which type of either) of fluid replacement, nor for the hematocrit target for RBC replacement. To further complicate the issue it is not clear on which monitoring parameter the volume given should be based, especially if invasive monitoring is not used.

Fluid compartments

Understanding the general composition of the fluid compartment is the first step in the optimal management of fluids, electrolytes, and acid–base status in the operative and critically ill patient. The multiple fluid compartments are separated by semipermeable membranes through which water can move freely. The total body water (TBW) ranges from 50% (females) to 60% (males) of body mass, is distributed differentially among body tissues (Table 62.1), and is divided into the following compartments:

- Intracellular water is approximately 66% of the TBW (40% of the body mass)
- Extracellular water is approximately 34% of the TBW (20% of the body mass) and can be further divided:

  · Intravascular water is made up of plasma and is approximately 8% of TBW (5% of the body mass)

Table 62.1. Content of water in various organs of the human body

Organ	Distribution, %
Vessel-rich organs	
Heart	79
Brain	75
Lungs	79
Liver	68
Kidney	83
Vessel intermediate-rich organ/tissue	
Muscle	75
Skin	72
Vessel-poor organ/tissue	
Adipose tissue	10

· Extravascular water is composed of lymph, interstitial fluid, bone fluid, fluids of the various body cavities, and mucosal secretory fluids, and represents approximately 25% of TBW (15% of the body mass)

Movement of water is determined by osmotic and hydrostatic pressure differences. The movement of water directly from tissue into the vasculature and the control of the flux by the relative hydrostatic and osmotic pressures in the two compartments was originally hypothesized by Ernest Starling in 1896 and is referred to as the Starling principle:

$$Q_f = K_f[(P_c - P_i) - \sigma(\pi_c - \pi_i)],$$

where Q_f = fluid flux across the capillary membrane; K_f = a constant; $P_c - P_i$ = the difference between the hydrostatic pressures in the capillary and in the interstitium; $\pi_c - \pi_i$ = the difference between the osmotic pressures in the capillary and in the interstitium; and σ = the reflection coefficient, which describes the permeability of a substance through a specific capillary membrane. Values range from 0 (completely permeable) to 1 (impermeable) in healthy tissue; reflection coefficients typically approximate 0.7.

Oncotic pressure (osmotic pressure in the intravascular compartment) is the result of negatively charged intravascular proteins to which vascular membranes are impermeable or positive ions that are associated with the negatively charged proteins. Albumin is the protein mainly responsible for the oncotic pressure (two-thirds of the total).

Clinical evaluation of fluid status

One goal of the evaluation is to determine the presence of hypovolemia or hypervolemia before the surgical procedure begins. Patients presenting in septic shock, those who may have undergone a bowel preparation preoperatively, or those who are otherwise physiologically deranged may be hypovolemic. Both hypovolemia and hypervolemia are associated with significant risks. Signs of hypo- and hypervolemia are summarized in Tables 62.2 and 62.3.

In addition, certain laboratory values, while very nonspecific, may help in assessment of volume status. For example, a high hematocrit, or plasma $[Na^+]$ may indicate a total body water deficit. A high blood urea nitrogen, a base deficit, a low mixed venous PO_2, or urine output may indicate an inadequate

Table 62.2. Signs and symptoms of hypovolemia

Signs	Fluid loss (percentage of body weight)		
	5%	10%	15%
Mucous membrane	Dry	Very dry	Parched
Sensorium	Normal	Lethargic	Obtunded
Orthostatic changes Heart rate Blood pressure	None	Present	Marked >15 bpm ↑ >10 mm Hg ↓
Urinary flow rate	Mildly decreased	Decreased	Markedly decreased
Pulse rate	Normal or increased	Increased > 100 bpm	Markedly increased > 120 bpm
Blood pressure	Normal	Mildly decreased with respiratory variation	Decreased

cardiac output. A low central venous or pulmonary artery pressure, and a high pulse rate suggest inadequate intravascular volume. In addition, indirect signs, such as the response of blood pressure to changes in patient positioning or positive-pressure ventilation, the change in stroke volume to positive-pressure ventilation or the vasodilating or negative inotropic effects of anesthetics, may aid in the assessment of volume status. Although it is true that all the above signs may be helpful in the aggregate and when combined with other findings, it must be remembered that they are nonspecific and are altered by drugs used in the perioperative period and the physiologic effects of surgical stress.

Fluid therapy

Perioperative fluid therapy includes the replacement of:

- Preexisting fluid deficits
- Normal losses (maintenance requirements)
- Surgical wound losses (including blood losses)

Evaluation of preexisting fluid deficit

The constitutive daily losses of water and electrolytes are usually replaced by a maintenance fluid intake, calculated according to the data listed in Tables 62.4 and 62.5. Calculation of estimated hourly fluid needs is shown in Table 62.6. Preoperative fluid deficits should also take into account fluid deficits due to the conditions listed in Table 62.7.

Electrolytes are usually replaced by administration of salt solutions. Although intraoperative glucose replacement is not routinely recommended, the protein-sparing effect of parenteral glucose is one of the goals of basic glucose intravenous

Table 62.3. Signs and symptoms of hypervolemia

Early signs	Late signs
Pitting edema – presacral in the bedridden patient or pretibial in the ambulatory patient	Tachycardia
Increased urinary flow	Pulmonary crackles, wheezing, cyanosis, and pink, frothy pulmonary secretions

Table 62.4. Daily water loss

Insensible water losses
Normal losses by skin and lungs: 600–800 ml/d
Sensible water losses
From kidney and gastrointestinal tract: 1700 ml/d

Table 62.5. Daily requirements of electrolyte and glucose

Electrolyte and glucose	Daily requirement
Na^+	1–2 mEq/kg/day
Cl^-	1–1.5 mEq/kg/day
K^+	1–1.5 mEq/kg/day
Glucose	100–200 mg/kg/h

Table 62.6. Hourly maintenance fluid replacement (based on body weight)

Body weight	Fluid
0–10 kg	4 ml/kg/h
For the next 11–20 kg	Add 2 ml/kg/h
For each kg above 20 kg	Add 1 ml/kg/h for each kg above 20 kg

therapy in critically ill patients. Administration of at least 100 g/d of glucose reduces protein loss by more than one half. As a caloric source supplement, glucose intake should range from 100 to 200 mg/kg/h.

Table 62.7. Fluid losses in various clinical situations

Abnormal fluid losses
  Preoperative bleeding
  Vomiting
  Diuresis
Occult losses
  Traumatized tissues
  Infected tissues
  Ascites
Increased insensible losses due to
  Hyperventilation
  Fever
  Sweating

Table 62.8. Classical procedural classification of redistribution and evaporative surgical fluid

Scale of surgery	Additional fluid requirement
Minimal (herniorrhaphy)	1–2 ml/kg
Moderate (appendectomy)	2–4 ml/kg
Severe (colectomy)	4–8 ml/kg

Maintenance requirements

Patients often present for surgery after an overnight fast without any fluid intake. This does not reduce blood volume. The presumed fluid deficit is proportional to the duration of the fast. This deficit can be estimated by multiplying the normal maintenance rate as shown in Table 62.6 by the length of the fasting period.

For example, for the average 70-kg person fasting for 8 hours, this amounts to (40 + 20 + 50) ml/h × 8 hours, or 880 ml. (In reality, this deficit will be significantly less as a result of normal renal conservation, though replacement of this amount is routine in practice.) Ideally, all deficits should be replaced preoperatively in all patients. The fluids used should be similar in composition to the fluids lost. With fever, each degree above 98.6°F (37°C) requires one to add 2.5 ml/kg/d for an increase in insensible losses. It should be realized, however, that crystalloids are physiologically distributed over the entire extracellular space. This implies that up to 80% of the fluid administered will leave the intravascular compartment (over a time course on the order of 30 minutes). However, the final distribution of the fluids will depend somewhat on the state of intravascular volume when it was given.

Surgical fluid losses
Evaporative and redistributive losses

Intraoperative fluid losses are mainly the result of evaporation and internal redistribution of body fluids. Evaporative losses classically have been assumed to be directly proportional to the surface area of the exposed surgical wound and the duration of the surgical procedure, leading to gross overestimation of intraoperative fluid requirements and overhydration. Experiments using humidity chambers indicate that evaporative losses

in adults undergoing extensive abdominal procedures merely increase to about 1 ml/kg/h.

Redistribution appears to be related to the extent of surgical trauma (Table 62.8). Internal redistribution of fluids is often called "third spacing" because large amounts of fluid are sequestered into the interstitial space or translocated into anatomic spaces, such as the bowel lumen. This occurs with burns, extensive injuries, surgical dissections, or peritonitis but is also directly proportional to the amount of fluids infused. Lastly, significant losses of lymphatic fluid may occur during extensive retroperitoneal dissections.

Blood loss

Monitoring and estimating blood loss (Table 62.9) is important for guiding fluid therapy and blood product transfusions. Selection of the type of intravenous solution depends on the surgical procedure and the expected blood loss:

- Minimal blood loss and fluid shifts: maintenance solutions
- All other procedures: lactated Ringer's solution

Fluid replacement therapy

Fluid replacement therapy should optimize cardiac preload and ensure adequate tissue oxygenation. It may consist of infusions of crystalloids, colloids, or a combination of both. The correct choice of fluid replacement therapy depends on the source and type of fluid that has been lost. In practice it is not known where the losses come from or their composition. Therefore, typically half-normal solutions are sometimes preferred for replacement of insensible losses and isotonic fluids (normal saline, lactated Ringer's or colloids) are preferred for all other deficits.

Crystalloid solutions

Crystalloid solutions are electrolyte solutions of low molecular weight ions (salts) dissolved in water, with or without glucose (Table 62.10). These solutions may be isotonic, hypotonic, or hypertonic. Crystalloid solutions are very inexpensive. They rapidly equilibrate with and distribute in the extracellular fluid space, expanding the interstitial space more than the intravascular volume.

Table 62.9. Methods for estimating blood losses

Empiric measurements	Laboratory
Measurement of blood in the surgical suction container (adjusted to account for the volume of irrigating solutions)	Serial hematocrit or hemoglobin may be useful during long procedures or when estimates are difficult (their concentrations reflect the ratio of blood cells to plasma, not necessarily blood loss; rapid fluid shifts and intravenous replacement affect measurements)
Visual estimation of the blood on surgical sponges and laparotomy pads ("laps"): Fully soaked sponge (4 × 4) holds 10 ml of blood. Soaked "lap" holds 100–150 ml of blood (the size of laparotomy pads may vary considerable among institutions)	
More accurate estimates are possible if sponges and laparotomy pads are weighed before and after use. This is especially important when large numbers are used or, for example, in pediatric patients.	

Table 62.10. Types and composition of crystalloid solutions

Solution	Na, *mEq/L*	Cl, *mEq/L*	K, *mEq/L*	Ca, *mEq/L*	Other	Osmolarity
D5W	0	0	0	0	Glucose 5 g/L	253
D5 0.45% NaCl	77	77	0	0	Glucose 5 g/L	432
0.9% NaCl	154	154	0	0		308
7.5% NaCl	1283	1283	0	0		1786
Lactated Ringer's	130	109	4	3	Lactate 28 mEq/L	273
Plasma-lyte	140	98	5	0	Acetate 27 mEq/L	294
					Gluconate 23 mEq/L	
					Mg 3 mEq/L	

D5W, 5% dextrose in water.

Crystalloids are used for maintenance and usually for the initial resuscitation fluid in the operative setting. Because administration of large amounts of saline often leads to a metabolic acidosis due to hyperchloremia, lactated Ringer's is the most common choice. In selecting between lactated Ringer's and saline, the patient's sodium-to-chloride ratio and the acid–base balance should be considered. Lactated Ringer's solution contains potassium and should be used with caution in patients with hyperkalemia or renal failure. Because they contain calcium, Ringer's solutions should not be used to dilute citrated blood products.

Colloid solutions

Colloid solutions contain high molecular weight substances, such as proteins and large glucose polymers dissolved in a solute (Table 62.11). Most colloid solutions are dissolved in isotonic saline but are available also as isotonic glucose and nonglucose solutions, as well as hypertonic saline solutions. For the most part, in healthy patients they remain intravascular and help maintain the oncotic pressure. Although the intravascular half-life of a crystalloid solution is 30 minute to 1.5 hours, most colloid solutions have intravascular half-lives of 4 to 6 hours. Colloid solutions should be used cautiously in patients with bleeding disorders, congestive heart failure, or renal disease with oliguria or anuria. The primary difference between Hetastarch and Pentastarch is that the latter has less variability in molecular size in addition to having a smaller average molecular size. The larger molecules contained in Hetastarch, of several million daltons and higher, are taken up by phagocytes in the reticuloendothelial system and are never metabolized or excreted. That is why the limit of units of Hetastarch is a lifetime limit. A reasonable molecular analogy is asbestos. Despite theoretical advantages and some demonstrated physiologic benefits in a few small studies, several large, multicenter randomized and observational cohort trials have failed to demonstrate any outcome advantage from colloid solutions over crystalloids.

Moreover, the substantial cost of colloids ($44 for 250 ml of 5% albumin and $21 for 500 ml of 6% hetastarch, versus $1.10 for 1000 ml of normal saline and lactated Ringer's solution and $1.75 for 5% dextrose in water and 5% glucose) and occasional complications (rare but severe allergic reactions, alteration in the anticoagulative pattern) associated with colloids tend to limit their use (Table 62.12).

Several types of colloid solutions are available for clinical use, including:

- Blood-derived colloids: albumin (5% and 25% solutions) and plasma protein fraction (5%). (Plasma protein fraction

Table 62.11. Types of colloids

Dextrose starches (dextran) – improves blood flow in the microcirculation by decreasing blood viscosity

Dextran 70 (Macrodex; Pharmacia, Piscataway, NJ) – average molecular weight of 70,000

Dextran 40 (Rheomacrodex; Pharmacia) – average molecular weight of 40,000
   Dose: shock – 10 ml/kg infused rapidly; 20 ml/kg maximum 1st 24 h; 10 ml/kg maximum beyond 24 h

First-generation HES: hetastarch – 6% solution with an average molecular weight of 450,000 Da, molar substitution 0.7, C_2/C_6 ratio 6:1
   Dose: volume expansion – 500–1000 ml (1500 ml/d maximum, 20 ml/kg/h rate)

Second-generation HES: pentastarch – 6% solution with average molecular weight of 264,000 Da, molar substitution 0.45, C_2/C_6 ratio 5:1
   Dose: volume expansion: 500–2000 ml (2000 ml/d maximum, 20 ml/kg/h rate)

HES 130/0.4 (Voluven; Fresenius Kabi, Bad Hmburg, Germany): 6% solution with mean molecular weight 130,000 Da, molar substitution 0.4, C_2/C_6 ratio 9:1
   Dose: volume expansion: 500–2000 ml (3500 ml/d maximum, 20 ml/kg/h rate)

HES, hydroxyethyl starch.

Table 62.12. Adverse effects associated with colloids

Colloid	Adverse effects
Dextran	Antiplatelet effect (decreased aggregation), prolonged bleeding time, interference with blood typing, allergic reactions, renal failure
Hetastarch	High doses (>1 L) may cause coagulation abnormalities (reduction in factor VIII and vWF, prolonged PTT) Newer formulations – i.e. third-generation HES 130/0.4 (Voluven; Fresenius Kabi, Bad Homburg, Germany) show improved safety profiles due to lower molecular size
Albumin	Expensive; relatively short intravenous half-life

HES, hydroxyethyl starch; PTT, partial thromboplastin time; vWF, von Willebrand factor.

contains α- and β-globulins in addition to albumin and may lead to allergic, hypotensive reactions.)

- Synthetic colloids: dextrose starches and gelatins (Table 62.11). Gelatins are associated with histamine-mediated allergic reactions and are not available in the United States.

Although isotonic saline and colloid-containing solutions both have been used to replace extracellular fluid deficits, controversy exists regarding the use of colloid versus crystalloid fluids for fluid resuscitation. There are two possible theoretical advantages of a colloid-containing solution over fluid repletion with saline:

- More rapid plasma volume expansion, because the colloid solution remains in the vascular space (replacing an intravascular volume deficit with crystalloids generally requires three to four times the volume needed when compared with colloids)
- Less risk of pulmonary edema, because dilutional hypoalbuminemia will not occur

However, as noted earlier, randomized controlled trials and systematic meta-analyses have failed to demonstrate any advantage in terms of pulmonary complications or survival for using colloid-containing solutions. Crystalloid (usually lactated Ringer's if large volumes are given quickly) solutions are therefore generally preferred. The solutions seem to be at least as safe and effective as colloid-containing solutions while costing much less. At the same time, it is important to keep in mind that rapid administration of large amounts of crystalloids (>4–5 L) is associated with significant tissue edema. Marked tissue edema may impair oxygen transport, tissue healing, and return of bowel function following major surgery.

Blood replacement therapy

Blood loss should be replaced with crystalloid or colloid solutions to maintain intravascular volume (normovolemia) until the danger of anemia outweighs the risks of transfusion. Transfusion therapy is discussed in Chapters 66, 67, and 68.

Suggested readings

Alam HB, Rhee P. New developments in fluid resuscitation. *Surg Clin N Am* 2007; 87: 55–72.

Barron ME, Wilkes MM, Navickis RJ. A systematic review of the comparative safety of colloids. *Arch Surg* 2004; 139: 552–563.

Bickell WH, Wall, MJ Jr, Pepe PE, et al. Immediate versus delayed fluid resuscitation for patients with penetrating torso injuries. *N Engl J Med* 1994; 331:1105.

Choi PT, Yip G, Quinonez LG, et al. Crystalloids vs colloids in fluid resuscitation: a systematic review. *Crit Care Med* 1999; 27: 200–210.

Finfer S, Bellomo R, Boyce N, et al. A comparison of albumin and saline for fluid resuscitation in the intensive care unit. *N Engl J Med* 2004; 350:2247.

Gold MS. Perioperative fluid management. *Crit Care Clin* 1992; 8:409–421.

Grocott MP, Mythen MG, Gan TJ. Perioperative fluid management and clinical outcomes in adults. *Anesth Analg* 2005; 100: 1093–1106.

Hayes MA, Timmins AC, Yau EHS, et al. Elevation of systemic oxygen delivery in the treatment of critically ill patients. *N Engl J Med* 1994; 330:1717.

Mange K, Matsuura D, Cizman B, et al. Language guiding therapy: the case of dehydration versus volume depletion. *Ann Intern Med* 1997; 127:848.

Mitra B, Mori A, Cameron A. Massive blood transfusion and trauma resuscitation. *Injury* 2007, 8:1023–1029.

Rather LE, Smith GW. Intraoperative fluid management. *Surg Clin North Am* 1993; 73:229–241.

Roberts I, Alderson P, Bunn F, et al. Colloids versus crystalloids for fluid resuscitation in critically ill patients. *Cochrane Database Syst Rev* 2004: CD000567.

Rosenthal MH. Intraoperative fluid management – what and how much? *Chest* 1999; 115:106S–112S.

Chapter 63

Acid–base balance in anesthesia and intensive care medicine

George P. Topulos

Despite the fact that they are both common and important in the perioperative period and in intensive care, acid–base disorders are a source of considerable confusion. The imbalance itself is usually only important as a sign that something is wrong. It is the nature of the underlying *cause* of the acid–base imbalance that principally determines the patient's prognosis and the nature of appropriate therapy. This chapter focuses on the primary causes of acid–base abnormalities, not on the abnormal $[H^+]^a$ or pH. Imagine two patients, one with an acidemia due to hyperchloremia, another with the same degree of acidemia due to shock-induced lactic acidosis. The first patient is much more likely to do well than the second, and they will need very different therapies. Determining the underlying *cause* of the acid–base imbalance is the key to successful care of the patient. Although it is true that if an acid–base disorder results in a large-enough change in $[H^+]$ or pH (pH < 7.2 or >7.6) it can cause secondary problems due to protein dysfunction (cardiac arrhythmias, vasoconstriction, or dilation), these secondary problems are uncommon (Adrogue 1998a and b).

Respiratory acid–base disturbances are easy to understand and treat. High partial pressure of carbon dioxide (PCO_2) is caused by inadequate alveolar ventilation and results in an acidosis. Low PCO_2 is caused by excessive alveolar ventilation and results in an alkalosis. Short-term therapy is directed at restoring alveolar ventilation toward normal and ensuring adequate oxygenation, often with the use of mechanical ventilation and/or supplemental oxygen. Long-term therapy is directed toward correcting the underlying problem.

It is more difficult to determine the cause and magnitude of nonrespiratory (metabolic) acid–base disturbances. The most important causes of nonrespiratory acid–base disturbances are electrolyte disturbances (Na, Cl), increased organic acids (lactic acid, keto acids), ingested toxins (methanol, ethylene glycol, aspirin), and renal failure (sulfates and phosphates). The most commonly taught methods of acid–base analysis have been the bicarbonate/anion gap (AG) approach, and the base excess/base deficit (BE) approach. More recently, Stewart applied basic physical–chemical principles to acid–base analysis (Stewart 1978, 1981, 1983). Practical clinical applications of Stewart's findings were developed first by Fencl and colleagues (Fencl

2000, 1993) and later by others (Kellum 2000, 1998, 1995). The Stewart-Fencl method is finding increasing use, especially in anesthesiology, surgery, and critical care. In medicine, considerable debate continues among members of the different schools, but in other scientific fields physical–chemical methods are used without debate (Kleypas 2006). The author believes the Stewart-Fencl method is the most effective, as well as the easiest to understand and implement, and is emphasized here. As the chapter proceeds, we also note how the AG and BE methods could be applied.

We begin by listing the components of normal plasma important in acid–base physiology and their concentrations (Fig. 63.1). This representation is called a *gamblegram*, and it is a useful tool for understanding nonrespiratory acid–base

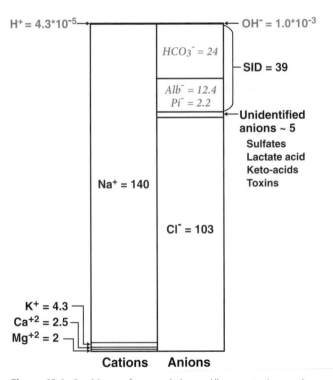

Figure 63.1. Gamblegram for normal plasma. All concentrations are in milliequivalents per liter. Weak ions are in blue italics, strong ions are in black, and water dissociation products are in bolded blue. The height of individual rectangles is proportional to the concentration of the substances within it. Because all solutions must be electrically neutral, the total height of the right and left columns must be equal.

---

a Throughout the chapter, brackets indicate concentrations, that is [x] = the concentration of x, in milliequivalents per liter unless otherwise noted.

balance. Anions are shown on the right and cations on the left. Throughout the chapter, all ion concentrations are in milliequivalents per liter to account for the valence of all ions, and to make the relative concentrations clear. The height of individual rectangles is proportional to the concentration of the substances within them. Because all solutions must be *electrically neutral*, the total height of the right and left columns must be equal (Σ all cations $= \Sigma$ all anions). Not shown in the diagram is water, which is present in a very high concentration [H_2O] = $5.55*10^4$ mEq/L, more than seven orders of magnitude greater than that of either [H^+] or [OH^-].

We then group the components into weak ions, strong ions, and water and its dissociation products.

Weak ions (shown in blue italics in Fig. 63.1) are incompletely dissociated at physiologic pH. They include the dissociation products of the CO_2 – H_2O system [HCO_3^-] = 24 mEq/L and [CO_3^{-2}] = $3.7*10^{-2}$ mEq/L, charges on albumin [Alb^-] = 12.7 mEq/L, and inorganic phosphate [Pi^-] = 2.2 mEq/L. The degree of dissociation of each weak ion depends on the net pH of the solution and the dissociation constant for that weak ion. Importantly, the net pH of the solution is determined by other independent factors, discussed later. The Henderson–Hasselbalch equation describes the dissociation of carbonic acid into bicarbonate and a hydrogen ion:

$$pH = pK + \log \frac{[HCO_3^-]}{S * PCO_2},$$

where K is the dissociation constant for carbonic acid, and S is the solubility of CO_2.

The equation's name honors the seminal contributions of Henderson and Hasselbalch. Similar equations describe the dissociation of bicarbonate into carbonate, albumin to [Alb^-], and inorganic phosphate to [P_i^-]. It is important to note that the Henderson–Hasselbalch equation *describes* the pH-dependent dissociation of carbonic acid into bicarbonate. That is, if we know the values of any two of the three variables (pH, [HCO_3^-], PCO_2) we can use the equation to calculate the third value. However, the Henderson–Hasselbalch equation alone cannot demonstrate the cause of acid–base imbalance because other factors to be discussed later, which are not present in the dissociation equations, play a key role. We must be careful not to confuse a descriptive equation with one that demonstrates causality.

We might ask ourselves, "What are the dissociation equations for NaCl, or lactic acid or keto acids, equivalent to those just discussed?" We do not need to calculate the degree of dissociation of these and other species in the second group, the *strong ions* (shown in black in Fig. 63.1), because they are completely dissociated (>99.9%) at all physiologic pH levels. The normal concentrations[b] of the strong ions [Na^+] = 140, [K^+] = 4.3, [Ca^{+2}] = 2.5, [Mg^{+2}] = 2, and [Cl^-] = 103 (all mEq/L), the electrolytes, are all commonly measured in patients. The concentrations of the strong ions lactic acid, keto acids, and sulfate are each normally less than 1 mEq/L, and their concentrations are often unmeasured; ingested toxins (e.g., methanol, ethylene

glycol, aspirin) also generate strong ions. The organic acids and toxins are often referred to as *unknown anions* (UA), a group that also includes species that are truly unknown.

Because for acid–base calculations all strong ions have the same effect, their concentrations are summarized as the *strong ion difference*, [SID] = Σ [strong cations] – Σ [strong anions]. Note that the concentrations of strong ions may be changed by adding or removing the ion or by adding or removing water. The SID is the same as the "buffer base" of Singer and Hastings. The change in the SID from its normal value of about 39 mEq/L is numerically equivalent to the base excess (normal BE = 0 mEq/L), the amount of strong acid or base in milliequivalents per liter that would be required to titrate the pH of a sample of blood to 7.40 while the PCO_2 is held at 40 mm Hg and the temperature at 37°C. Because base excess is measured with the PCO_2 held at its normal value of 40 mm Hg, it reflects the sum of all nonrespiratory acid–base disturbances.

Water and its dissociation products (shown in bolded blue in Fig. 63.1) are the third group. Water is present in a very high concentration ([H_2O] = $5.55*10^4$ mEq/L) and only very slightly dissociated, [H^+] = $4*10^{-5}$ and [OH^-] = $1.1*10^{-3}$ mEq/L.[c] However, although they are small, the concentrations of water's dissociation products ([H^+] and [OH^-]) are critically important. Because the [H_2O] is more than seven orders of magnitude greater than that of either [H^+] or [OH^-], it may be considered a constant, and the dissociation equation may be simplified to [H^+]*[OH^-] = K'_w, where K'_w is a temperature-dependent constant. Because at a fixed temperature, [H^+]*[OH^-] = a constant, if the concentration of one increases the other must decrease.

The complete development of Stewart's ideas is beyond the scope of this chapter; detailed reviews are presented elsewhere (Fencl 2000, 1993, Stewart 1981, 1983). Here, we present the principles on which the analysis is based and its major conclusions. We have just described the constituents of plasma important in acid–base physiology. To this system, Stewart applied three rules: (1) Conservation of mass, that is, the total amount of Na, H, albumin, or other entity is fixed unless some is added to or removed from the system. Note that although the total amount of H is fixed, it may exist in the form of H_2O, HCO_3^-, H^+, and so on. Similarly, the total amount of albumin is fixed, but the amount ionized, Alb^-, will vary. (2) All solutions must be electrically neutral, that is, the sum of all the positively charged ions must equal the sum of all the negatively charged ions. (3) The dissociation equilibria, described earlier, of all weak ions, and water, must be met simultaneously and at all times.

Stewart's analysis (not presented here) showed that three independent variables (i.e., causative factors) determine acid–base balance:

1. PCO_2
2. Total concentration (ionized + nonionized) of weak anions [A_{tot}], which in plasma is made up of albumin [Alb_{tot}] and inorganic phosphate [Pi_{tot}]

---

[b] Units and normal values vary according to institution.

[c] [$H+$] = $4*10^{-5}$ mEq/L = $4*10^{-8}$ Eq/L, the –log of which yields the familiar plasma pH = 7.40.

3. Strong ion difference ($[SID] = \Sigma$ [strong cations] – Σ [strong anions])

All the other acid–base variables (pH, [H+], [OH$^-$], [HCO$_3$$^-$], [CO$_3$$^{--}$], [Alb$^-$], [Pi$^-$], etc.) are dependent variables (things that change with but do not cause acid–base disturbances), the values of which depend on the values of the three independent variables.

To summarize all the preceding information: We care about the underlying causes of acid–base abnormalities; abnormal [H$^+$] or pH is merely a sign that something is wrong. All acid–base abnormalities must be the result of an abnormal value of one or more of the three independent variables: PCO$_2$, strong ion difference, and total weak anion (albumin and phosphate) concentration. Abnormalities of dependent variables are signs, not causes, of acid–base disturbances. If we want to change the acid–base status, we must change one or more of the independent variables. Next, we describe how to use the gamblegram as a tool, then examine each of the three independent causes of acid–base abnormalities; we conclude the chapter with a straightforward method for implementing this analysis in practice.

We use the gamblegram (Fig. 63.1) whenever we consider nonrespiratory (metabolic) acid–base balance – that is, the total concentration of weak anions and SID. Because the components of plasma important in acid–base physiology are represented in the diagram, it serves to remind us of all the factors we need to evaluate. In addition, it allows us a straightforward *qualitative* understanding of which dependent variables will change and in what direction after a change in an independent variable. Recall the following to make maximum use of the gamblegram:

1. Electrical neutrality requires that the sum of *all* cations equal the sum of *all* anions. The total height of the left and right columns must be the equal. However, remember that the sum of *strong* cations does *not* equal the sum of *strong* anions. In fact, normally the strong ion difference = ([Na$^+$] + [K$^+$] + [Ca^{++}] + [Mg^{++}]) – ([UA$^-$] + [Cl$^-$]) $\approx$ 39 mEq/L. The independent variable [SID] is determined by the concentration of strong ions. The [SID] is "filled in by" (but not determined by) the weak ions [HCO$_3$$^-$] + [Alb$^-$] + [Pi$^-$], which change their ionized fractions to maintain electrical neutrality. That is, the sum of the weak anions [HCO$_3$$^-$] + [Alb$^-$] + [Pi$^-$] must equal the true SID.[d] We use this fact later to estimate the concentration of unknown ions, which cannot be measured directly.

2. Clinically, we measure and control the total [Pi$_{tot}$] and [Alb$_{tot}$] (independent variables), but only the charged [Pi$^-$] and [Alb$^-$] (dependent variables) appear in the gamblegram. The values of [Pi$^-$] and [Alb$^-$] depend strongly on [Pi$_{tot}$] and [Alb$_{tot}$] and their dissociation constants, but only weakly on the net pH of the system.

Therefore, for clinical purposes, the concentrations [Pi$^-$] and [Alb$^-$] are taken to be proportional to [Pi$_{tot}$] and [Alb$_{tot}$], respectively (Fencl 2000) (see Appendix 1).

3. As the PCO$_2$ increases, [H$^+$] and [HCO$_3$$^-$] also increase. Surprisingly, as PCO$_2$ increases, the [CO$_3$$^{-2}$] falls.

4. Because at constant temperature, [H$^+$]*[OH$^-$] = constant, if one goes up the other must go down. At concentrations of [H$^+$] = 4*10^{-5} and [OH$^-$] = 1.1*10^{-3} mEq/L, neither can increase or decrease enough to make significant contributions to maintaining electrical neutrality. The same is true of carbonate.

Examples using the gamblegram

Example 1: an isolated increase in [Na$^+$]

The left column has gotten taller and so must the right column (Fig. 63.2a). Neither the concentrations of unidentified strong ions [UA$^-$] nor those of [Cl$^-$] can increase, because we have not added them (conservation of mass). So, the only way for the right column to grow to match the increased height of the left is through an increase in dissociation of all the weak anions, especially [HCO$_3$$^-$], [OH$^-$], [Alb$^-$], and [Pi$^-$]. If [OH$^-$] increases, then [H$^+$] must fall. Hence, an increase in [Na$^+$] causes an alkalosis. The same is true for anything that increases SID, such as a decrease in [Cl$^-$].

Example 2: an isolated increase in [Cl$^-$] by 4 mEq/L

If the right column grew taller by 4 mEq/L, then the left column would need to as well (Fig. 63.2b). The concentrations of [Na$^+$], [K$^+$], [Ca^{+2}], and [Mg^{+2}] cannot increase because we have not added them (conservation of mass). The only other way the left column could grow 4 mEq/L would be for the [H$^+$] to increase by 4 mEq/L (to a pH < 2.4), but [H$^+$] never exceeds even 10^{-4} mEq/L. When [Cl$^-$] increases by 4 mEq/L, the [H$^+$] does increase, but by only a tiny amount. The two columns stay the same height because other parts of the right column shrink to balance the increased [Cl$^-$]. The unidentified strong ions [UA$^-$] cannot decrease if we do not remove any of them (conservation of mass). Electrical neutrality is maintained through decreased dissociation of all the weak anions, [OH$^-$], [CO$_3$$^{-2}$], [HCO$_3$$^-$], [Alb$^-$], and [Pi$^-$]. [H$^+$] increases and [OH$^-$] decreases; an increase in [Cl$^-$] causes an acidosis. The same is true for anything that decreases SID, such as a decrease in [Na$^+$] or an increase in [UA$^-$], as in lactic acidosis or ketoacidosis.

Example 3: an isolated decrease in [Alb$_{tot}$] by 2 g/dl

If [Alb$_{tot}$] decreases, then so will the amount ionized, [Alb$^-$], by about 5 mEq/L (Fig. 63.2c). If the right column gets shorter, then so must the left column. However, the concentrations of the strong cations [Na$^+$], [K$^+$], [Ca^{+2}], and [Mg^{+2}] cannot decrease if we do not remove any of them (conservation of

---

[d] For these calculations, the [CO$_3$$^{-2}$], [OH$^-$], and [H$^+$] are so small they can be ignored.

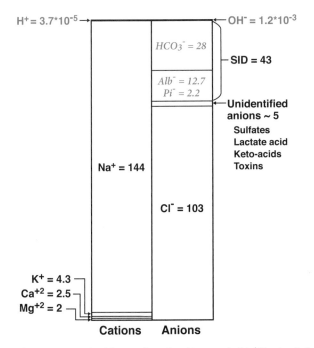

Figure 63.2A. Gamblegram for isolated increase in $[Na^+]$ by 4 mEq/L. Increase in $[Na^+]$ without change in other strong ions, so [SID] increased to 43 mEq/L. This change in SID, an independent variable, *causes* a metabolic alkalosis (pH = 7.43). No other strong ions were added or removed so their concentrations do not change. In order to maintain electrical neutrality in the face of an increased SID, the degree of ionization of all weak anions – dependent variables (principally $[HCO_3^-]$) – increases to "fill in" the gap.

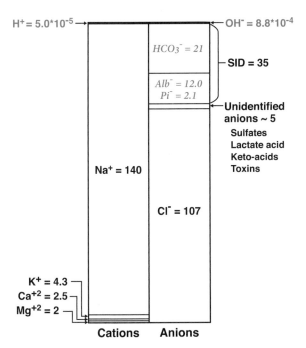

Figure 63.2B. Gamblegram for isolated increase in $[Cl^-]$ by 4 mEq/L. Increase in $[Cl^-]$ without change in other strong ions, so [SID] decreased to 35 mEq/L. This change in SID, an independent variable, *causes* a metabolic acidosis (pH = 7.30). No other strong ions were added or removed so their concentrations do not change. In order to maintain electrical neutrality with a decreased SID, the degree of ionization of all weak anions (principally $[HCO3^-]$) decreases.

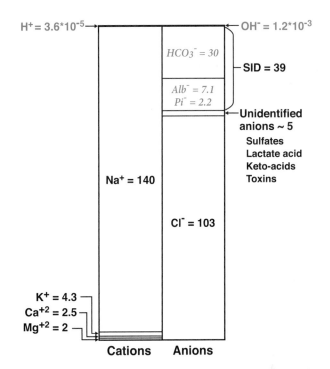

Figure 63.2C. Gamblegram for isolated decrease in $[Alb_{tot}]$ by 2 g/dL. Decreased $[Alb_{tot}]$ results in decreased $[A_{tot}]$, an independent variable *causing* a metabolic alkalosis (pH = 7.45). No strong ions were added or removed so the SID cannot change. In order for electrical neutrality to be maintained with a decreased $[A_{tot}]$, the degree of ionization of weak anions (principally $[HCO_3^-]$) increases. The $[Alb^-]$ falls as a direct consequence of the decreased $[Alb_{tot}]$ even though the ionized fraction increases somewhat. Note it is the independent variable $[Alb_{tot}]$ that we can control and which decreased by 2 g/dL, but it does not appear in the gamblegram. The dependent variable ionized albumin $[Alb^-]$ is shown.

mass). The $[H^+]$ will fall, but because it is orders of magnitude smaller than $[Alb^-]$, it cannot fall nearly enough to maintain electrical neutrality. Neither the concentrations of unidentified strong anions $[UA^-]$ nor those of $[Cl^-]$ can decrease if we do not remove any of them (conservation of mass). Electrical neutrality must be maintained through increased dissociation of the other weak anions, especially $[HCO_3^-]$ and $[Pi^-]$. $[H^+]$ decreases and $[OH^-]$ increases; a decrease in $[Alb_{tot}]$ causes an alkalosis. Conversely, an increase in $[Alb_{tot}]$ or $[Pi_{tot}]$ causes an acidosis.

Causes of acid–base disturbances

Table 63.1 summarizes all the causes of acid–base disturbances described by Stewart and Fencl. Following, we examine each of the three independent causes of acid–base abnormalities in more detail.

PCO₂ respiratory acid–base disturbances

PCO_2 respiratory acid–base disturbances are easy to understand and treat. High PCO_2 is caused by inadequate alveolar ventilation and results in an acidosis. Low PCO_2 is caused by excessive alveolar ventilation and results in an alkalosis.

Table 63.1. Summary of all causes of acid–base disturbances as described by Stewart and Fencl

	Acidosis	Alkalosis
Respiratory	↑ PCO_2	↓ PCO_2
Nonrespiratory (metabolic)	↓ [SID] or ↑ [A_{tot}]	↑ [SID] or ↓ [A_{tot}]
[SID]: [Na^+] or [H_2O]	↓ [Na^+]	↑ [Na^+]
[SID]: [Cl^-]	↑ [Cl^-]	↓ [Cl^-]
[SID]: unidentified anions	↑ [UA^-] lactic acid, keto acids, toxins	–
Total albumin	↑ [Albumin] rare	↓ [Albumin] common in critical illness
Total Pi	↑ [Pi] renal failure or acute tissue destruction	–

Table 63.3. Major causes of increase in [Cl^-] relative to [Na^+] – decrease SID acidosis.

Lose Na in excess of Cl	Gain Cl in excess of Na
Renal	
Renal tubular acidosis	Normal saline
Acetazolamide	Hyperalimentation (when cations are given
Nephrotoxic drugs	as chlorides rather than acetates)
Gastrointestinal[a]	KCl
Biliary (T-tube) drainage	
Diarrhea	

[a] Gastric fluid has very low SID because of a high [Cl^-]. Pancreatic, bile, and colonic fluids have a very high SID because of a high [Na^+].

Total concentration of weak anions, albumin [Alb_{tot}], and inorganic phosphate [Pi_{tot}]

Increases in [Alb_{tot}] or [Pi_{tot}] cause acidosis, and decreases cause alkalosis. Because the normal [Pi_{tot}] is so small, low values cannot cause significant acid–base problems. High [Pi_{tot}] is seen in chronic renal failure and, because phosphate is present in high concentrations within most cells, in acute tissue destruction. High [Alb_{tot}] is uncommon but is seen in cases of severe water loss. Low [Alb_{tot}] is very common in critically ill patients. The alkalosis caused by hypoalbuminemia is not in and of itself of great importance. However, unrecognized, the alkalosis of hypoalbuminemia can mask the presence of concurrent acidosis due to increased unmeasured anions such as lactic or keto acids. A patient with an acidosis due to a lactate of 6 mEq/L and an alkalosis due to a [Alb_{tot}] of 2 mg/dl would have a normal pH. It is primarily for this reason that measuring albumin is important in acid–base analysis. Although the [Alb_{tot}] strongly influences acid–base balance, it is regulated for reasons that are unrelated to acid–base homeostasis, mainly to regulate osmotic pressure.

Strong ion difference, [SID] = Σ[strong cations] − Σ[strong anions]

An increase in SID causes an alkalosis, and a decrease in SID causes an acidosis. The concentrations of [K^+], [Ca^{+2}], and [Mg^{+2}] each are low and cannot fall individually enough to cause a significant decrease SID. Their concentrations are

Table 63.2. Major causes of decrease in [Cl^-] relative to [Na^+] – increase SID alkalosis

Lose Cl in excess of Na	Gain Na in excess of Cl
Renal	Na HCO_3
Diuretics	
Gastrointestinal[a]	Hyperalimentation (when cations are given
Vomiting	as acetates rather than chlorides)
Nasogastric tube	
drainage	

[a] Gastric fluid has very low SID because of a high [Cl^-]. Pancreatic, bile, and colonic fluids have very high SID because of a high [Na^+].

tightly controlled for reasons unrelated to acid–base balance, and if they increase, they cause life-threatening electrophysiologic problems before causing significant acid–base problems. They are not shown in Table 63.1.

Because of their high concentrations, [Na^+] and [Cl^-] are the dominant strong ions in plasma. Because it is the strong ion *difference* that controls acid–base balance, it is the relative [Na^+] and [Cl^-] that matters, not their individual values. Note that high [Na^+] may be caused by a sodium excess *or* a water deficit, and vice versa in the case of a low [Na^+]. The distinction must be made on clinical grounds. The [Na^+] is regulated to control total body water, not for acid–base homeostasis. The causes of increased and decreased [Cl^-], relative to [Na^+], are shown in Tables 63.2 and 63.3. They are also discussed in chapters on fluids and electrolytes, and on hyperalimentation.

The normal [UA^-] ≈ 5 mEq/L is the sum of several organic anions, each normally present at a low concentration; they cannot fall enough to significantly increase SID. Strong unknown anions are a problem when their concentrations are high, such as with increased organic acids (lactic acid, keto acids) and ingested toxins (methanol, ethylene glycol, aspirin) and in renal failure, in which sulfates, Cl^-, and other unknown anions of renal failure are increased (in addition to the weak ion phosphate). Because we cannot measure their values directly, we estimate [UA^-] as described later.

Proponents of the bicarbonate anion gap approach would describe all nonrespiratory acid–base abnormalities in terms of the changes in the dependent variable [HCO_3^-], with or without an increased anion gap. The AG = [Na^+] + [K^+] − [HCO_3^-] − [Cl^-] with a normal value = 16 mEq/L. It is evident from the gamblegram that to maintain electrical neutrality, the "gap" must be filled by anions other than [HCO_3^-] and [Cl^-], namely [UA^-], [Alb^-], and [Pi^-]. The idea is that in the presence of a metabolic acidosis caused by increased UA, the anion gap will be elevated.

Proponents of the base excess approach would describe all nonrespiratory acid–base abnormalities in terms of the calculated BE. In the presence of a metabolic acidosis, the BE should be negative (base deficit); in the presence of a metabolic alkalosis, the BE should be positive. Both the AG and BE methods assume a normal [Alb_{tot}] and are inaccurate in its absence.

Methods for correcting the AG and BE for hypoalbuminemia are given in Appendix 1. Fencl and colleagues have shown that without correction, both the AG and BE methods often fail to detect important acid–base disturbances in critically ill patients (Fencl 2000, 1993, Figge 1998).

We conclude the chapter by describing two ways to implement the Stewart approach, both developed by Fencl and colleagues. Both methods quantify the qualitative information described earlier using the gamblegram and in Tables 63.1 and 63.2. The first (Fencl and Leith, personal communications 1982–1985; later a modified version was published by others (Gilfix 1993)) is easy to apply at the bedside; the only calculations necessary are done easily by hand. Initial measurements needed are as follows:

From arterial blood gas	From chemistry
$PaCO_2$, mm Hg	$[Na^+]$, mEq/L
pH	$[Cl^-]$, mEq/L
BE, mEq/L	Total [albumin], mg/dl

Step 1, determine whether the patient has an acidemia (low pH) or alkalemia (high pH); the net pH of the blood is the sum of all concurrent acidoses and alkaloses.

If there is a single primary disturbance and a secondary compensation, the direction of the primary disturbance will be given by the pH. In simple cases, a primary disturbance in SID will usually result in a respiratory compensation returning the pH toward (but not to) normal. A primary respiratory acid–base disturbance usually results in a nonrespiratory compensation (renal modulation of plasma $[Cl^-]$), returning the pH toward (but not to) normal. Respiratory compensation happens quickly, in minutes to hours. Renal compensations are not complete for several days. However, in patients, the normal compensations often are not seen because they are overwhelmed by our clinical interventions, namely intravenous fluid therapy, drugs, and mechanical ventilation. In addition, critically ill patients often have multiple concurrent independent acid–base problems, such as acidosis due to high $[Cl^-]$, alkalosis due to low $[Alb_{tot}]$, and acidosis due to increased inorganic acids (UA). Using the expected levels of compensation to differentiate the multiple causes of complex acid–base disorders in critically ill patients is ineffective.

Step 2, examine the $PaCO_2$. If it is high, there is a respiratory acidosis, if low a respiratory alkalosis.

Step 3, use the BE as a measure of the change in SID from its normal value, and determine quantitatively what nonrespiratory factors are responsible for the observed BE. Real changes in SID may be a result of changes in $[Na^+]$ or $[H_2O]$, $[Cl^-]$, or increased $[UA^-]$. In addition, although albumin is a weak ion, abnormal albumin concentrations cause an error in the measured BE, which must be accounted for. Calculate the magnitude of change in the BE due to $[Na^+]$ or $[H_2O]$, $[Cl^-]$, and $[Alb_{tot}]$, as shown in the following table. Any remaining BE must be the result of increased $[UA^-]$, which we cannot measure directly.

Factors that change BE	Magnitude of change in mEq/L
Abnormal $[H_2O]$ or $[Na^+]$	$= 0.3\,(Na-140)$
Abnormal $[Cl^-]$	$= 103-(Cl^*(140/Na))$
Abnormal $[Albtot]$	$= 3.7\,(4.5 - \text{albumin})$
Increased [UA]	$=$ Observed BE−sum of 3 terms above

where 140 and 103 are the normal $[Na^+]$ and $[Cl^-]$ in milliequivalents per liter, respectively; derivation of the factor 0.3 for abnormal $[H_2O]$ or $[Na^+]$ is shown in Appendix 1; (140/Na) is a factor to correct the measured $[Cl^-]$ for abnormal $[H_2O]$ or $[Na^+]$; 4.5 is the normal $[Alb_{tot}]$ in grams per deciliter; and 3.7 is an empiric factor to correct the BE for abnormal $[Alb_{tot}]$. The magnitude of change for each factor is the expected BE (mEq/L) if the abnormality in that row were the sole abnormality. Note the magnitude of change calculated for each variable is zero if its concentration is normal.

Step 4, if "unmeasured anions" are suspected based on the preceding information, then measure phosphate, lactate, ketone bodies, salicylates, and so on, as indicated by the patient's history. Measuring the $[K^+]$, $[Ca^{+2}]$, and $[Mg^{+2}]$ can help identify additional causes of acidosis, as they often are all low, resulting in a decreased SID.

Consider a patient with the following laboratory results:

From arterial blood gas	From chemistry
$PaCO_2$, 29 mm Hg	$[Na^+]$, 154 mEq/L
pH, 7.32	$[Cl^-]$, 123 mEq/L
BE, −10 mEq/L	$[Alb_{tot}]$, 2.9 mg/dl

Calculate the expected BE for each abnormality. The number in the last column is the expected BE (mEq/L) if the abnormality in that row were the sole abnormality.

Factors that change BE	Magnitude of change	mEq/L
Abnormal $[H_2O]$ or $[Na^+]$	$0.3\,(Na - 140) =$	4.2
Abnormal $[Cl^-]$	$103 - (Cl^*(140/Na)) =$	−8.8
Abnormal $[Alb_{tot}]$	$3.7\,(4.5 - \text{albumin}) =$	5.9
Measured BE	From laboratory tests	−10
BE due to UA $=$	$=$ observed BE − sum of 3 terms above $-10 - (4.2 - 8.8 + 5.9) =$	−11.3

The patient has:

An acidemia, a low pH

A respiratory alkalosis, a low PCO_2, probably in response to the nonrespiratory acidosis

A high Na, increasing SID, alkalosis

A high Cl (corrected for the high Na, Cl = 112), decreasing SID, acidosis

A low albumin, low weak anions, alkalosis

A measured BE of −10, and so a BE due to UA $= (-10) - (4.2 - 8.8 + 5.9) = -11.3$

We must now look to the patient's history to determine the likely explanations for the BE due to UA of −11.3, and which laboratory studies we might order next. The patient presented with hypotension and an acute abdomen, and renal failure (creatinine = 6.5 mg/dl), making high sulfates and phosphates, and the other anions of renal failure, likely in addition to the known high chloride. The blood sugar is normal and the patient has no history of diabetes mellitus, so ketoacidosis is unlikely. The next steps would be to measure phosphate because of the renal failure, lactate because of the history of hypotension and an acute abdomen, and potassium, calcium, and magnesium. In addition, dialysis will help correct much of the problem while causes and therapy for the acute abdomen are pursued.

The second implementation of the Stewart method, detailed in several highly recommended papers by Fencl, Figge, and colleagues (Fencl 2000, 1993, Figge 1991, 1992) is outlined here only briefly. It is more rigorous, but requires a calculator or, even better, a computer. Recall from Fig. 63.1 and the previous discussion that the true $[SID] = ([Na^+] + [K^+] + [Ca^{++}] + [Mg^{++}]) - ([UA^-] + [Cl^-])$ and to maintain electrical neutrality, it must $= [HCO_3^-] + [Alb^-] + [Pi^-]$. If we define a new quantity, the measured or apparent SID $[SIDapp] = ([Na^+] + [K^+] + [Ca^{++}] + [Mg^{++}] - [Cl^-])$, then $[UA^-]$ is estimated as: $[UA^-] = [SIDapp] - ([HCO_3^-] + [Alb^-] + [Pi^-])$. $[Na^+]$, $[K^+]$, $[Ca^{++}]$, $[Mg^{++}]$, $[Cl^-]$, and $[HCO_3^-]$ are all routinely measured. $[Alb^-]$ and $[Pi^-]$ can be estimated from measured $[Alb_{tot}]$ and $[Pi_{tot}]$, respectively, as described by Figge and Fencl, and in Appendix 1. $[UA^-]$ is then calculated $= [SIDapp] - ([HCO_3^-] + [Alb^-] + [Pi^-])$, and lactate, ketone bodies, salicylates, and so on are measured as indicated by the patient's history. It often is the case that all sources of unknown anions will not be discovered, because, as mentioned earlier, the category contains species that are still truly unknown, as is the case in shock.

Suggested readings

Adrogue HJ, Madias NE. Management of life-threatening acid-base disorders. First of two parts. *N Engl J Med* 1998; 338:26–34.

Adrogue HJ, Madias NE. Management of life-threatening acid-base disorders. Second of two parts. *N Engl J Med* 1998; 338: 107–111.

Bunker JP. The great trans-Atlantic acid-base debate. *Anesthesiology* 1965; 26:591–594.

Fencl V, Jabor A, Kazda A, Figge J. Diagnosis of metabolic acid-base disturbances in critically ill patients. *Am J Respir Crit Care Med* 2000; 162:2246–2251.

Fencl V, Leith DE. Stewart's quantitative acid-base chemistry: applications in biology and medicine. *Respir Physiol* 1993; 91:1–16.

Figge J, Jabor A, Kazda A, Fencl V. Anion gap and hypoalbuminemia. *Crit Care Med* 1998; 26:1807–1810.

Figge J, Mydosh T, Fencl V. Serum proteins and acid-base equilibria: a follow-up. *J Lab Clin Med* 1992; 120:713–719.

Figge J, Rossing TH, Fencl V. The role of serum proteins in acid-base equilibria. *J Lab Clin Med* 1991; 117:453–467.

Gamble JL. *Chemical Anatomy, Physiology and Pathology of Extracellular Fluid.* Cambridge, MA: Harvard University Press; 1949.

Gilfix BM, Bique M, Magder S. A physical chemical approach to the analysis of acid-base balance in the clinical setting. *J Crit Care* 1993, 8:187–197.

Kellum JA. Determinants of blood pH in health and disease. 2000; *Crit Care* 4:6–14.

Kellum JA. Metabolic acidosis in the critically ill: lessons from physical chemistry. *Kidney Int Suppl* 1998; 66:S81–S86.

Kellum JA, Kramer DJ, Pinsky MR. Strong ion gap: a methodology for exploring unexplained anions. *J Crit Care* 1995; 10:51–55.

Kleypas JA, Feely RA, Fabry VJ, et al. Impacts of Ocean Acidification on Coral Reefs and Other Marine Calcifiers: A Guide for Future Research, report of a workshop held 18–20 April 2005, St. Petersburg, FL, sponsored by NSF, NOAA, and the US Geological Survey. Available at: http://www.ucar.edu/communications/Final_acidification.pdf.

McAuliffe JJ, Lind LJ, Leith DE, Fencl V. Hypoproteinemic alkalosis. *Am J Med* 1986; 81:86–90.

Severinghaus JW. Siggaard-Andersen and the "Great Trans-Atlantic Acid-Base Debate." *Scand J Clin Lab Invest Suppl* 1993; 214:99–104.

Siggaard-Andersen O, Fogh-Andersen N. Base excess or buffer base (strong ion difference) as measure of a non-respiratory acid-base disturbance. *Acta Anaesthesiol Scand Suppl* 1995; 107:123–128.

Singer RB, Hastings AB. An improved clinical method for the estimation of disturbances of the acid-base balance of human blood. *Medicine (Baltimore)* 1948; 27:223–242.

Stewart PA. *How to Understand Acid-Base: A Quantitative Acid-Base Primer for Biology and Medicine.* New York: Elsevier; 1981.

Stewart PA. Independent and dependent variables of acid-base control. *Respir Physiol* 1978; 33:9–26.

Stewart PA. Modern quantitative acid-base chemistry. *Can J Physiol Pharmacol* 1983; 61:1444–1461.

Appendix 1:

I. Calculation of $[Alb^-]$ from $[Alb_{tot}]$ and $[Pi^-]$ from $[Pi_{tot}]$, as described by Fencl et al. (Fencl 2000):

$[Alb^-]$ mEq/L $= [Alb_{tot}]$ (g/dL)$^*(1.23^*(pH - 0.631))$, which for clinical purposes may be approximated by $[Alb^-]$ mEq/L $\approx 2.8^*[Alb_{tot}]$ (g/dL)

$[Pi^-]$ mEq/L $= [Pi_{tot}]$ (mmol/L)$^*(0.309^*(pH - 0.469))$, which for clinical purposes may be approximated by $[Pi^-]$ mEq/L $\approx 1.8^*[Pi_{tot}]$ (mmol/L) or $[Pi^-]$ mEq/L $\approx 0.6^*[Pi_{tot}]$ (mg/dl)

II. Correcting the AG and BE, both mEq/L, for abnormal $[Alb_{tot}]$ g/dL, as described by Figge et al. (Figge 1998) and McAuliffe et al. (McAuliffe 1986):

$AG_{corr} = AG_{observed} + 2.5^*([\text{normal albumin}] - [\text{observed albumin}])$

$BE_{corr} = BE_{observed} + 3.7^*([\text{normal albumin}] - [\text{observed albumin}])$

III. Derivation of magnitude of change in BE due to abnormal $[H_2O]$ or $[Na^+] = 0.3(Na - 140)$

For 140 is the normal $[Na^+]$ and 42 is the normal [SID], both in mEq/L

Fractional change in Na (or H_2O) $= (Na - 140)/140$

Change in SID due to Na (or H_2O) = $42*(Na - 140)/140$
and $42/140 = 0.3$, then
Magnitude of change in BE due to abnormal $[H_2O]$ or $[Na^+] = 0.3(Na - 140)$

Appendix 2: simplified "classical" blood gas analysis

Analysis of blood gases is sometimes presented in a vastly simplified manner, in which one considers only the pH, PCO_2, and HCO_3. As discussed earlier, this approach is incomplete and sometimes misleading in the presence of abnormalities of albumin or in mixed or complex acid–base disorders, which characterize many critically ill patients. Only in patients with a single disorder will this approach give a satisfactory interpretation, so it is presented here for completeness with this caveat.

The simplified approach for patients with one primary acid-base disorder proceeds by following an ordered series of questions. The primary disorder may be metabolic, respiratory, or both and can be determined by assessing $PaCO_2$ and HCO_3.

1. What is the pH? Is it an acidosis or alkalosis?
2. Is the change in $PaCO_2$ consistent with a respiratory component?
3. If the change in $PaCO_2$ does not explain the change in arterial pH, does the change in HCO_3 indicate a metabolic component?

With these questions answered, an initial diagnosis of the underlying primary disorder can be made; then, one can determine whether there is a compensation (see the list at the end of this paragraph). These compensation rules were determined empirically from animal experiments in which a single derangement was induced. If the compensatory response is more or less than expected, a mixed acid–base disorder exists. Measurement of electrolytes provides additional data to determine whether there is an anion gap in the case of metabolic acidosis. In the case of metabolic alkalosis, the urinary chloride concentration is measured. If the urinary $Cl^- < 10$ mmol/L, the metabolic alkalosis is chloride sensitive and can be corrected with NaCl. Examples include gastric and intestinal losses and diuretic therapy. If the urinary $Cl^- > 10$ mmol/L, the metabolic alkalosis is chloride resistant. Examples include renal artery stenosis, Cushing's syndrome, primary aldosteronism, and exogenous mineralocorticoids.

Empirically observed compensatory responses to acid-base disturbances:

Metabolic acidosis: $1 \downarrow HCO_3 \geq 1 \downarrow PCO_2$
Metabolic alkalosis: $10 \uparrow HCO_3 \geq 7 \uparrow PCO_2$
Acute respiratory acidosis: $10 \uparrow PCO_2 = 1 \uparrow HCO_3$
Chronic respiratory acidosis: $10 \uparrow PCO_2 = 4 \uparrow HCO_3$
Acute respiratory alkalosis: $10 \downarrow PCO_2 \geq 2 \downarrow HCO_3$
Chronic respiratory alkalosis: $10 \downarrow PCO_2 \geq 5 \downarrow HCO_3$

Following are a few examples of arterial blood gases in which the reader can follow the aforementioned steps to diagnose the disturbance.

Example 1

pH, 7.25
PCO_2, 60
HCO_3, 26

Given the pH of 7.25, there is an acidosis. With a PCO_2 of 60, there is a 20−mm Hg elevation of the PCO_2. Given the 2-mEq/L increase in HCO_3, this example represents an acute respiratory acidosis.

Example 2

pH, 7.35
PCO_2, 60
HCO_3, 32

The pH of 7.35 indicates an acidosis. With the elevated PCO_2 of 60, it is a respiratory acidosis. Given the 8-mEq/L increase in HCO_3, this is a compensated chronic respiratory acidosis.

Example 3

pH, 7.31
PCO_2, 30
HCO_3, 15
Na, 138
Cl, 112
Anion gap, $138 - (112 + 15) = 11$

There is an acidosis. The change in PCO_2 is not consistent with a respiratory component; hence, it is a metabolic acidosis. The HCO_3 decrease is proportionate to the CO_2 decrease. With an anion gap that is normal, this points to a non−anion gap metabolic acidosis.

Chapter 64

Ion balance

Tommaso Mauri and Lorenzo Berra

In this chapter, we discuss sodium, potassium, calcium, magnesium, and phosphorus ion balance. The normal concentrations of each of those electrolytes in the various body compartments are summarized in Table 64.1. Sodium is the most abundant extracellular ion, whereas potassium is the most abundant intracellular ion.

Basic definitions

Basic definitions are as follows:

- The *osmolarity* of a solution is the number of osmotically active particles (osmoles) per liter of solvent.
- The *osmolality* of a solution is the number of osmotically active particles per kilogram of solvent.
- *Tonicity* is the effective osmolality of a solution. It refers to the capacity to exert an osmotic force across a membrane. Hypertonic solutions decrease cell volume, hypotonic solutions increase cell volume, and isotonic solutions have no effect on cell volume.

$$\text{Osmolality (mOsm/kg)} = [\text{Na}^+] \times 2 + \frac{\text{glucose}}{18} + \frac{\text{BUN}}{2.8}$$

(Normal plasma osmolality = 280–290 mOsm/kg)

Sodium

Sodium is critical in regulating extracellular and intravascular fluid volumes. Consequently, total body sodium usually determines clinical volume status, as sodium draws water wherever it is concentrated. Sodium is also essential for generation of action potentials in various tissues of the body. Sodium is regulated mainly by aldosterone, antidiuretic hormone, and atrial natriuretic peptide. The normal range of plasma sodium is 135 to 145 mEq/L, and the adult requirement of daily sodium is 1 to 2 mEq/kg/day.

Hypernatremia (plasma sodium > 145 mEq/L)

Hypernatremia has a relatively high prevalence in the intensive care unit (ICU), usually due to the use of diuretics. About 9% of medical ICU patients have a sodium level > 150 mEq/L

at admission, and an additional 6% develop hypernatremia during the ICU stay. Hypernatremia is always associated with hypertonicity. It can be classified according to the underlying mechanism and the resulting volume status of the patient. Table 64.2 lists common differential diagnoses based on the total body water (TBW) status.

Clinical manifestations

The primary symptoms of hypernatremia are caused by the loss of cell volume. Symptoms include irritability, spasticity, and tremulousness. A decrease in brain volume causes lethargy, weakness, and headache. If sodium levels rise above 158 mEq/L, severe symptoms may emerge, such as seizures, coma, and eventually death. Symptoms are more likely to occur when there are rapid changes in sodium concentration.

Treatment

The aim is to treat the underlying cause (e.g., hypernatremia secondary to drugs, hormonal derangements or central and nephrogenic diabetes insipidus, diabetic ketoacidosis, acute tubular necrosis, chronic renal failure, fever). Treatment may be guided by defining the type of hypernatremia (hypovolemic, euvolemic, or hypervolemic).

- *Hypovolemic hypernatremia*: isotonic saline initially for volume repletion in symptomatic patients with orthostasis, hypotension, or prerenal azotemia, followed by hypotonic crystalloid solutions, such as 0.45% normal saline.
- *Euvolemic hypernatremia*: replacement of free water.

Table 64.1. Fluid electrolyte composition of body compartments

Ions		Plasma, mEq/L	Interstitial, mEq/L	Intracellular, mEq/L
Cations	Sodium	142	145	10
	Potassium	4	4	159
	Calcium	5	5	<1
	Magnesium	2	2	40
Anions	Chloride	104	117	3
	Bicarbonate	24	27	7
	Proteins	16	<0.1	45
	Others	9	9	154

Table 64.2. Causes of hypernatremia

Hypovolemic	TBW loss > sodium loss	Renal loss (urine [Na$^+$] >20 mmol/L): osmotic or loop diuretic, postobstructive diuresis, recovery phase of acute tubular necrosis Extrarenal loss (urine [Na$^+$] <20 mmol/l): excessive sweating, diarrhea, burns, fistulae
Euvolemic	TBW loss	Renal losses: diabetes insipidus Hypodipsia, insensible losses
Hypervolemic	TBW increase < total sodium increase	Infusions of hypertonic sodium bicarbonate or hypertonic saline, hypertonic dialysate, overdose of salt tablets, Cushing's syndrome, primary hyperaldosteronism

- *Hypervolemic hypernatremia*: removal of the excess sodium (e.g., thiazide or loop diuretics) while replacing water. Intravenous infusions should be hypotonic compared with the urine.

Free water deficit can be calculated as:

$$\text{Free water deficit} \approx \text{Total body water} \times \{1 - (140/[\text{Na}^+])\}.$$

One-half of the calculated water deficit can be administered either enterally or parenterally during the first 24 hours and the rest over the following 1 to 2 days. Sodium can be safely lowered by 10 mEq/L in the first day of therapy, but patients with acute increases in sodium can safely be corrected at 1 mEq/L/h. It is important to remember that if sodium is lowered too quickly, cerebral edema may occur.

Hyponatremia (plasma sodium < 135 mEq/L)

Hyponatremia, the most common electrolyte derangement occurring in hospitalized patients, is usually accompanied by hypo-osmolality but in rare circumstances may be associated with iso-osmolality or hyperosmolality (Table 64.3). Hypo-osmolar hyponatremia may further be classified as hypovolemic, isovolemic, or hypervolemic hyponatremia.

Clinical manifestations

Symptoms seen in hyponatremia are largely neurologic and increase in severity with lower sodium levels. Symptoms are often vague and nonspecific and include malaise, nausea, confusion, and lethargy. Symptoms that are more dangerous follow when [Na$^+$] falls below 120 mEq/L (e.g., headache, obtundation, seizures, coma, and death).

Treatment

A plasma sodium level < 130 mmol/L should result in initiation of treatment, and the cause of hyponatremia should be identified and addressed. Water restriction should be started if appropriate. Symptomatic patients with plasma sodium levels < 120 to 125 mmol/L generally need more aggressive management. However, rapidly restoring normal osmolality may cause the plasma to be relatively hypertonic to the cells, resulting in

Table 64.3. Causes of hyponatremia

Isotonic hyponatremia (pseudohyponatremia)	Asymptomatic: hypertriglyceridemia, hyperproteinemia (i.e., multiple myeloma) Symptomatic: glycine absorption
Hypertonic hyponatremia	Hyperglycemia, mannitol therapy, radiocontrast
Hypotonic hyponatremia	Hypovolemic hypotonic hyponatremia: renal loss (diuretic therapy or salt-wasting nephropathy), gastrointestinal loss (vomiting, diarrhea, tube drainage), skin loss (sweating, burns, cystic fibrosis), peritonitis Isovolemic hypotonic hyponatremia: antidiuretic hormone excess (SIADH, thiazide diuretics or oral hypoglycemic agents), pain, postoperative status (transurethral prostatic resection syndrome), cortisol deficiency, hypothyroidism, decreased solute intake, psychogenic polydipsia Hypervolemic hypotonic hyponatremia (TBW excess): congestive heart failure, cirrhosis of liver, nephrotic syndrome, renal failure

SIADH, syndrome of inappropriate antidiuretic hormone secretion.

the osmotic movement of water out of the cells. In the central nervous system, this may cause a condition called central pontine myelinolysis or osmotic demyelination syndrome, which results in severe morbidity or death. Therefore, in acute, symptomatic hyponatremia, sodium may be raised more rapidly, initially 1 to 2 mmol/h, but not to exceed 8 to 10 mEq/L in the first 24 hours. Even in patients with seizures and hyponatremia, a correction of 1 to 6 mmol usually leads to a resolution of symptoms. Chronic asymptomatic hyponatremia is well tolerated and should be treated conservatively.

- *Isotonic hyponatremia*, also known as pseudohyponatremia, requires no therapy.
- *Hypertonic hyponatremia* is the result of the increased osmotic pressure (e.g., glucose, mannitol) that moves the water from the intracellular space to the extracellular compartment. Hyperglycemia, for example, decreases plasma sodium concentration by approximately 1.6 mEq/L for each 100 mg/dl of blood glucose. The goals of therapy are to remove the osmotically active substance and to restore euvolemia.
- *Hypotonic hyponatremia*, the most common form of hyponatremia, is subdivided according to the extracellular fluid volume status:
  1. *Hypovolemic hypotonic hyponatremia*: Sodium is lost in greater proportion than water. Therapy should focus on replacement of extracellular volume with isotonic sodium solution.
  2. *Isovolemic hypotonic hyponatremia*: Usually, therapy is focused on water restriction. See Table 64.4.
  3. *Hypervolemic hypotonic hyponatremia*: The goal of therapy depends on the primary cause of hyponatremia. However, fluid and salt restriction and the use of proximal and loop diuretics are usually acceptable.

Table 64.4. Calculation of desired negative TBW balance

Estimated TBW: percentage of body weight in kilograms, 60% in children and men, 50% in women and elderly men, 45% in elderly women

TBW (excess) $\approx$ (actual plasma Na^+/desired plasma Na^+) $\times$ (Normal) $\times$ (TBW)

TBW (excess) represents **the amount of negative water balance needed to increase plasma Na^+ to desired level**

Potassium

The human body contains 50 mEq/kg of potassium, more than 95% of which is intracellular. Plasma potassium concentration is kept in a narrow range via two main regulating mechanisms: potassium shift between intracellular and extracellular compartments and modulation of renal potassium excretion. In addition, potassium is regulated by aldosterone, insulin, hydrogen ion concentration, and epinephrine. The electrocardiogram (ECG) is useful for the diagnosis of true potassium imbalance, because cardiovascular effects are usually noted early. The level of polarization of an excitable cell and the ability for repolarization are determined by the extracellular and intracellular potassium concentration. Average daily intake of potassium is approximately 1 to 1.5 mEq/kg/d.

Hyperkalemia (plasma potassium > 5.5 mEq/L)

Hyperkalemia usually develops in patients with advanced renal dysfunction (Table 64.5). Succinylcholine may transiently raise the plasma potassium level by 0.5 to 1.0 mEq/L in normal patients. Succinylcholine should not be used in paraplegic or burn patients because it may result in excessive potassium release. Many cases of hyperkalemia are associated with metabolic acidosis. Elective surgery should not be undertaken in the presence of significant hyperkalemia.

Clinical manifestations

Muscle weakness and, rarely, flaccid paralysis, abdominal distention, and diarrhea may occur. With the worsening of hyperkalemia, ECG changes may occur and include atrial and ventricular ectopy, decreased QT interval, peaked T waves, loss

Table 64.5. Causes of hyperkalemia

Decreased renal excretion	Acute and chronic renal failure, drugs (potassium-sparing diuretics, ACE inhibitors, COX inhibitors, decreased mineralocorticoid activity (HIV)
Redistribution	Trauma, burns, rhabdomyolysis, severe infections, acidosis, hyperosmolar states, vigorous exercise
Increased intake	Salt substitutes, blood transfusions, potassium salts of antibiotics
Pseudohyperkalemia	Hemolysis, leukocytosis (WBCs > 50,000/mm³), thrombocytosis (PLT > 1,000,000/mm³)

ACE, angiotensin-converting enzyme; PLT, platelets; COX inhibitors, nonsteroidal anti-inflammatory drugs; WBCs, white blood cells.

of P waves, widening of the QRS complex, and merging of the widened QRS complexes with the T wave, leading to ventricular fibrillation and possibly to cardiac arrest.

Treatment

One must first confirm that the elevated level of plasma K^+ is genuine. Continuous monitoring of the ECG is indicated. Renal dysfunction should be ruled out. The following measures can temporarily reduce the plasma K^+ level via redistribution to other compartments, or mitigate its effects:

- Calcium chloride (10 ml of 10% solution) intravenously (IV) to stabilize the cellular membrane
- Insulin with glucose (1 U of IV insulin for 2 g of dextrose) is administered to shift the extracellular potassium intracellularly and to stabilize the cellular membrane
- Sodium bicarbonate (50–100 mEq) to shift the potassium intracellularly

The following measures will reduce the plasma K^+ level by increasing its excretion:

- Loop diuretics (e.g., furosemide) to reduce total body potassium, although patients in renal failure may not respond to diuretics.
- Exchange resins (e.g., sodium polystyrene sulfonate) administered orally may reduce total body potassium in about 1 to 3 hours.
- One or two standard doses of nebulized albuterol can reduce plasma K^+ within 30 minutes after administration in dialysis patients.
- Hemodialysis, if other measures fail.

Hypokalemia (plasma potassium < 3.5 mEq/L)

Severe hypokalemia may induce dangerous arrhythmias and even rhabdomyolysis (Table 64.6). It is important to remember that the plasma potassium concentration correlates poorly with the total body potassium deficit. Nevertheless, plasma concentration may be used as a rough guide to total body levels, and in the steady state 1-mEq/L change in plasma potassium reflects about a 100- to 200-mEq change in total body

Table 64.6. Causes of hypokalemia

Potassium shift into the cell	Insulin, alkalosis, trauma, barium ingestion, β₂-adrenergic agonists, hypothermia
Renal potassium loss	Primary and secondary hyperaldosteronism, renovascular hypertension, ACTH and renin-producing tumor, congenital abnormality of steroid metabolism, diuretics, salt-wasting nephropathy, hypomagnesemia
Extrarenal potassium loss	Vomiting, diarrhea, laxatives, NG tube suctioning
Inadequate intake	Usually not a single cause of hypokalemia, because of very effective decrease of renal potassium excretion

ACTH, adrenocorticotropic hormone; NG, nasogastric.

potassium. Usually, mild and asymptomatic hypokalemia (K^+ > 3.0 mEq/L) does not warrant cancellation or delay of surgery, especially if it is chronic. Acute hypokalemia is less well tolerated than mild chronic hypokalemia. As a general rule, patients with clinical signs of hypokalemia and/or ECG changes might require correction prior to proceeding with elective surgery. Patients on digoxin are at a higher risk of developing side effects when hypokalemic. Glucose-free infusion solutions should be used in hypokalemic patients, because glucose supports potassium shift into the cell, further reducing the plasma concentration.

Clinical manifestations

Muscular weakness, fatigue, and muscle cramps are frequent in mild to moderate hypokalemia. Flaccid paralysis, hyporeflexia, hypercapnia, tetany, rhabdomyolysis, and arrhythmias may be seen with severe hypokalemia (<2.5 mEq/L). ECG changes that may occur consist of widening of the QRS complex with plasma potassium levels around 3 mEq/L. Furthermore, the ST segments become depressed, and the T waves begin to flatten (inversion). U waves become more prominent. The tendency for ventricular ectopy increases and puts the patient at risk for ventricular fibrillation.

Treatment

Mild to moderate potassium deficiency is safely treated with oral potassium. In the setting of abnormal renal function and mild to moderate diuretic dosage, 20 mEq/d of oral potassium is generally sufficient to prevent hypokalemia, whereas 40 to 100 mEq/d is needed to treat hypokalemia if it occurs. Intravenous potassium replacement is indicated for patients with severe hypokalemia and for those who cannot take oral supplementation. For severe deficiency, potassium may be given through a peripheral IV line in a concentration that should not exceed 40 mEq/L at rates of up to 10 mEq/h because of its local and systemic toxicity. When a central line is present, it should be the route of choice to administer IV potassium. Rates of 10 to 20 mEq/h require continuous ECG monitoring. Daily potassium replacement should not exceed 240 mEq.

Calcium

The normal total plasma (or plasma) calcium concentration is 8.5 to 10.5 mg/dl. Ionized calcium (4.4–5.3 mg/dl; the normal range may vary slightly from laboratory to laboratory) is the physiologically active calcium. Calcium is necessary for almost every function in the human body, including muscle contraction, nerve function, and blood coagulation. Calcium is regulated primarily by parathyroid hormone and vitamin D. Albumin levels do not affect ionized calcium levels, although total calcium increases or decreases with a decrease or an increase in albumin levels, respectively. An albumin level decrease of 1 g/dl increases the calcium level by 0.8 mg/dl. It is also important to remember that metabolic acidosis increases ionized calcium levels.

Table 64.7. Causes of hypercalcemia

Increased intake	Excess vitamin D, vitamin A, or calcium intake
Cancer	Multiple myeloma
Endocrine disorders	Primary hyperparathyroidism, adrenal gland insufficiency
Other	Thiazide diuretics, sarcoidosis, Paget's disease of bone, immobilization

Hypercalcemia (plasma calcium > 10.5 mg/dl)

Tumor production of parathyroid hormone–related protein accounts for most cases of hypercalcemia (Table 64.7). The neoplasm is clinically apparent in nearly all cases when the hypercalcemia is detected, and the prognosis is often poor from the underlying malignancy.

Clinical manifestations

Mild hypercalcemia is often asymptomatic. Symptoms usually occur if the plasma calcium is > 12 mg/dl. Typical symptoms are constipation, polyuria, nausea and vomiting, muscle weakness, ataxia, and confusion. ECG shows a shortened QT interval.

Treatment

Until the primary disease is controlled, renal excretion of calcium with a resultant decrease in plasma calcium concentration should be promoted. Hypercalcemia should be considered a medical emergency, and elective surgeries should not be performed until the calcium level is corrected. Serial measurements of potassium and magnesium should also be done while the calcium is being corrected.

- Saline (250–500 ml/h) with furosemide (20–40 mg every 2 hours) is the treatment of choice.
- Bisphosphonates (pamidronate) or calcitonin is the mainstay of treatment of hypercalcemia of malignancy.

Hypocalcemia (plasma calcium < 8.5 mg/dl)

Development of true hypocalcemia (decreased ionized calcium) implies an insufficient level or impaired action of parathyroid hormone or active vitamin D (Table 64.8).

Table 64.8. Causes of hypocalcemia

Decreased intake or absorption	Malabsorption, small bowel bypass, vitamin D deficit
Increased loss	Alcoholism, chronic renal insufficiency, diuretics, chelation of calcium by citrate ions when large volume of blood is administered
Endocrine disease	Hypoparathyroidism, sepsis, medullary carcinoma of the thyroid
Physiologic	Hyperphosphatemia, aminoglycoside antibiotics

Clinical manifestations

Extensive spasm of skeletal muscle may cause weakness, cramps, tetany, and eventually, laryngospasm with stridor. Seizure, paresthesias of the lips and extremities, and abdominal pain may occur. Carpopedal spasm (Trousseau's sign) or masseter muscle spasm (Chvostek's sign) may be seen. The ECG shows prolongation of the QT interval (due to lengthened ST segment), which predisposes the patient to developing hypotension and ventricular arrhythmias.

Treatment

In the presence of tetany, arrhythmias, or seizures, calcium gluconate 10% (10–20 ml), administered IV over 10 to 15 minutes, is indicated. Its duration of action is short; therefore, an infusion is usually required to maintain the plasma calcium level at 7 to 8.5 mg/dl. ECG monitoring is recommended. Asymptomatic hypocalcemia can be treated with oral calcium and vitamin D.

Magnesium

Normal plasma magnesium ranges between 1.5 and 2.5 mEq/L. Mg^{2+} promotes enzyme reactions within the cell during metabolism, helps in the production of adenosine triphosphate (ATP), participates in protein synthesis, and plays a role in coagulation, platelet aggregation, and neuromuscular activity. Magnesium slows atrioventricular conduction and potentiates the action of both depolarizing and nondepolarizing neuromuscular blocking agents. About two-thirds of magnesium is stored in the bone.

Hypermagnesemia (plasma magnesium > 2.5 mEq/L)

Increased intake, mainly as a result of magnesium-containing antacids and laxatives, may commonly lead to hypermagnesemia (Table 64.9).

Clinical manifestations

Skeletal muscle weakness, hyporeflexia, sedation, vasodilation, bradycardia, hypotension, and impaired breathing may occur.

Treatment

Treatment includes immediate cessation of Mg^{2+} administration/intake, administration of calcium gluconate, increased urinary excretion (diuretic), and dialysis in patients with renal failure.

Table 64.9. Causes of hypermagnesemia

Reduced excretion and/or increased intake	Magnesium-containing antacid or laxative intake, acute and chronic renal failure, clinically induced hypermagnesemia state with preeclampsia treatment
Uncommon causes	Addison's disease, acute diabetic ketoacidosis, hypothyroidism, pituitary dwarfism, lithium therapy, viral hepatitis, milk-alkali syndrome

Table 64.10. Causes of hypomagnesemia

Gastrointestinal	Decreased intake, reduced absorption (chronic diabetes, diarrhea, emesis, steatorrhea, short bowel syndrome, pancreatitis)
Renal excretion	Loop and thiazide diuretics, hypercalcemia, removal of parathyroid tumor, diabetic ketoacidosis, hypersecretion of aldosterone, thyroid hormones or ADH, nephrotoxins, chronic ethanol ingestion
Acute intracellular shift	Refeeding syndromes, glucose infusions, amino acid infusions, insulin, catecholamines, metabolic acidosis

Hypomagnesemia (plasma magnesium < 1.5 mEq/L)

Hypomagnesemia is commonly seen in ICU patients. Common causes of hypomagnesemia are listed in Table 64.10.

Clinical manifestations

Increased neuromuscular irritability, hyperreflexia, confusion, and seizures may occur. Hypomagnesemia is commonly associated with hypocalcemia and hypokalemia and, hence, with their associated manifestations. ECG changes seen with magnesium deficiencies include prolonged PR and QT intervals, widened QRS complexes, depression of ST segments, and inversion of T waves. Atrial fibrillation may be associated with hypomagnesemia.

Treatment

Patients with mild/moderate Mg^{2+} deficiency may require 50 mEq of oral Mg^{2+} per day (i.e., about twice the amount of the estimated deficit in patients with intact renal function, because about 50% of the administered Mg^{2+} is excreted in urine). Serious manifestations of hypomagnesemia (seizures) should be corrected by IV replacement (2- to 4-g infusion over 30–60 min). It is prudent to avoid an IV bolus of magnesium sulfate, as it may cause cardiac arrhythmias.

Phosphorus

In plasma, phosphate is present mainly as a very small inorganic fraction (PO_4, normal range 2.5–4.5 mg/dl). About 85% of phosphorus is stored in the bone. It is used to form ATP, nucleic acids, 2,3-diphosphoglycerate (off-loading oxygen from hemoglobin), and cyclic adenosine monophosphate.

Hyperphosphatemia (plasma phosphate > 4.5 mg/dl)

Clinical manifestations

Clinical signs of hyperphosphatemia are related primarily to the development of hypocalcemia and ectopic calcification. Because renal failure is the most common cause of hyperphosphatemia, other signs and symptoms of renal failure may also be associated with it (Table 64.11).

Table 64.11. Causes of hyperphosphatemia

Increased intake	Intravenous infusion, oral supplementation, vitamin D intoxication, phosphate-containing enemas, acute phosphorus poisoning
Increased production	Tumor lysis syndrome, rhabdomyolysis, bowel infarction, malignant hyperthermia, hemolysis, acid–base disorders
Reduced loss	Acute and chronic renal insufficiency, hypoparathyroidism, acromegaly, tumoral calcinosis, magnesium deficiency, multiple myeloma

Treatment

In renal failure, dialysis will reduce plasma phosphate. Absorption of phosphate can be reduced by administration of aluminum hydroxide/carbonate, which binds phosphates. Diuresis can be induced with acetazolamide.

Hypophosphatemia (plasma phosphate < 2.5 mg/dl)

Hypophosphatemia may occur in the presence of normal phosphate stores. Serious depletion of body phosphate stores may exist even with normal or high phosphorus in plasma.

Clinical manifestations

In the presence of severe hypophosphatemia ($PO_4 < 1$ mg/dl), decreased levels of 2-3 DPG will result in an increased affinity of hemoglobin for oxygen, which impairs tissue oxygenation and thus cellular metabolism. Muscle weakness or even rhabdomyolysis, paresthesias, encephalopathy (e.g., irritability, confusion, or seizures), platelet dysfunction, leukocyte dysfunction, respiratory failure, and myocardial dysfunction may occur.

Treatment

The best treatment is prophylaxis, by including phosphate in repletion and maintenance fluids (total parenteral nutrition). When possible, oral replacement of phosphate is preferable, as rapid correction may cause hypocalcemia. For severe, symptomatic hypophosphatemia, an infusion should provide 279 to 310 mg (9–10 mmol)/12 h until the plasma phosphorus exceeds 1 mg/dl; the patient can then be switched to oral therapy.

Suggested readings

Adrogue HJ, Madias NE. Hypernatremia. *N Eng J Med* 2000; 342:1493–1499.

Alfonzo AVM, Isles C, Geddes C, Deighan C. Potassium disorders – clinical spectrum and emergency management. *Resuscitation* 2006; 70(1):10–25.

Desmeules S, Bergeron MJ, Isenring P. Acute phosphate nephropathy and renal failure. *N Engl J Med* 2003; 349: 1006–1007.

Gennari FJ. Hypokalemia. *N Eng J Med* 1998; 339:451–458.

Gums JG. Magnesium in cardiovascular and other disorders. *Am J Health Syst Pharm* 2004; 61(15):1569–1576.

Hall JB, Schmidt GA, Wood LDH. *Principles of Critical Care.* 3rd ed. New York: McGraw-Hill; 2005.

Nolan CR, Qunibi WY. Treatment of hyperphosphatemia in patients with chronic kidney disease on maintenance hemodialysis. *Kidney Int Suppl* 2005; 95:S13–S20.

Offenstadt G, Das V. Hyponatremia, hypernatremia: a physiological approach. *Minerva Anestesiol* 2006; 72(6):353–356.

Schlingmann KP, Konrad M, Jeck N, et al. Salt wasting and deafness resulting from mutations in two chloride channels. *N Engl J Med* 2004; 350:1314–1319.

Sterns RH, Silver SM. Brain volume regulation in response to hypo-osmolality and its correction. *Am J Med* 2006; 119:S12–S16.

Weisinger JR, Bellorin-Font E. Magnesium and phosphorous. *Lancet* 1998; 352:391–396.

Chapter 65

Total parenteral nutrition

Mallory Williams and Gyorgy Frendl

Total parenteral nutrition (TPN) is intravenous (IV) administration of nutrients for the purposes of metabolic support. TPN
can be used in various clinical settings, almost always as an alternate approach to nutrition when nourishment of the patient via
the enteral route is not feasible.

The objectives of nutrition therapy are to supply the patients'
caloric needs and to provide the appropriate proportions of protein, carbohydrate, and fat to support the metabolic needs of the
patient. Enteral nutrition, if possible, should always be the preferred route of nutrient administration. Multiple studies comparing enteral nutrition with TPN in critically ill medical and
surgical patients have found that enteral nutrition is safer than
TPN, is less expensive, and results in at least similar and sometimes superior clinical outcomes.

Initiation of nutrition therapy

The management of nourishment begins with a nutritional
assessment of the patient. It should be acknowledged that nutritional assessments in critically ill patients are often inaccurate.
Simple measurements, such as weight, cannot be used because
of edema, ascites, and overall fluid overload states that often
accompany the postoperative or critical care state. Well-known
nutritional parameter levels are affected by underlying disease,
inflammatory states, and medications.

Malnutrition in hospitalized patients often goes unrecognized; its prevalence may be 30% to 50%, with 40% of these
patients being malnourished at the time of admission. The subjective global assessment (SGA) is a clinical method to evaluate the nutritional status of a patient. The components of this
assessment are history taking and physical examination, determination of any effects of malnutrition on end-organ function,
and a determination of how the patient's overall disease process affects nutrient requirements. The SGA has been found to
be reproducible among blinded observers assessing the same
patient, with 80% interrater reliability. It is also a good predictor of complications in general surgery patients. Components
of the SGA are described in Table 65.1.

The next step for patients requiring nutritional support is
to determine whether they are candidates for enteral nutrition.
TPN is not indicated in patients who have a gastrointestinal
tract capable of adequate nutrient absorption. For patients who

cannot tolerate enteral nutrition (Table 65.2), TPN may be an
option.

Nutrition as pharmacotherapy

The role of nutrition has progressed from maintaining a positive
nitrogen balance to using specific nutrients to modulate organ
function.

Branched-chain amino acids

Branched-chain amino acids (BCAAs), including leucine,
isoleucine, and valine, undergo very little metabolism by the
liver and remain intact until they reach the skeletal muscle.
Leucine in skeletal muscle increases protein synthesis by 50%
and decreases protein degradation by 25%. This increased protein synthesis reaches physiologic significance during stress or
injury states. Increased concentration of BCAAs in TPN may
increase prealbumin and retinol-binding protein, leading to
lower mortality.

Table 65.1. Subjective global assessment

Medical history	Physical examination
Weight Change	***Muscle Wasting***
No Change Change	Biceps
	Triceps
% Weight Loss	Quadriceps
<5% 5–10% >10%	Temple
Weight change in past 2 weeks	***Subcutaneous Fat Wasting***
Increase No change Decrease	Eyes
Dietary intake	Perioral
Reduction	Palmar
Unintentional	
Intentional	
Overall Change	***Edema***
Change	Upper Extremities
No change	Sacral
Increase or Decrease	Lower Extremities
Gastrointestinal Symptoms	
None Nausea Diarrhea Vomiting	
Dysphagia Anorexia	
Functional Impairment	
Overall Impairment	
None Mild Severe	
Duration	
Days Weeks Months	

Table 65.2. Contraindications to enteral nutrition

Intractable emesis
Bowel obstruction
Malabsorption
Inflammation of gastrointestinal tract
Acute pancreatitis
Postoperative ileus
Pseudo-obstruction
Mechanical obstruction
Short bowel syndrome
Inflammatory bowel disease
Severe diarrhea – sprue
Radiation enteritis
Diverticulitis
Appendicitis
Cholecystitis
Esophagitis
Gastroenteritis
Mucositis – radiation induced or graft-versus-host disease

Glutamine

Glutamine is synthesized and stored in skeletal muscle. Catabolism induced by surgery, sepsis, burns, or major injury results in increased release of glutamine from skeletal muscle to the plasma. Patients receiving L-glutamine supplementation have a better nitrogen balance (−1.4 g/d vs. −4.2 g/d) and a lower incidence of infection.

Omega-3 fatty acids

The omega-3 fatty acids are potential immuno*stimulants*. Infections, length of intensive care unit (ICU) stay, and nitrogen balance (−2.2 g/d vs. −6.6 g/d) are better in patients receiving fish oil. Whereas omega-3 fatty acids are present in enteral formulas, the only commercially available IV emulsions in the United States are long-chain triglycerides with omega-6 fatty acids, which are potential immuno*suppressants*. High intake of omega-6 fatty acids (linoleic acid) is associated with increased synthesis of prostaglandin E_2, which inhibits the immune system.

However, omega-3 fatty acid-rich infusion during parenteral nutrition was recently reported in a prospective open label study and found to reduce both ICU and hospital length of stay and improve mortality in critically ill patients after major abdominal surgery, or who were experiencing peritonitis and abdominal sepsis, non-abdominal sepsis, multi-trauma, and severe head injury (reference listed in recommended readings). This study was not controlled or blinded and variations in dose of omega-3-fatty acids occurred in the trial. These interesting findings need confirmation in randomized controlled trials before they can be considered cost effective.

Route of TPN administration

TPN can be delivered via centrally or peripherally placed venous access catheter port. TPN solutions contain glucose, amino acids, and lipids. Lipid solutions of 10–20% can be given peripherally, whereas lipid concentrations of 30% are prescribed in the admixture and are administered centrally. Glucose-amino acid solutions of greater than 10% glucose are damaging to peripheral veins and can cause thrombophlebitis. It is very important that the tip of the central venous catheter be evaluated for its presence in the superior vena cava. The tonicity of hypertonic nutrient solutions (>1900 mOsm/L) is so great that thrombophlebitis and venous sclerosis are potential complications of peripheral administration. Superior vena cava placement allows for rapid dilution of this nutrient-rich solution.

The port used for TPN administration should be a dedicated port. Medications, blood draws, or administration of other fluids is not preferred because of an increase in infection risk. In addition, initial placement of a central venous catheter that will be used for TPN should follow the full barrier precautions and nursing checklist protocol. No catheters placed for emergency use should be used to administer TPN. Catheters should never be advanced into patients post placement. Lines need to be secured to patients using a dermal stitch with three-point fixation of the catheter. Clear dressings are used so the line site can be monitored daily.

Occasionally, there are patients in whom percutaneous central venous access is difficult to achieve. These patients are candidates for peripheral IV central catheter (so-called PICC) lines. These lines are placed centrally from peripheral veins using wires (most often by designated IV services). As with central venous catheters, the central venous position of the tip should be confirmed on a regular basis. The administration of TPN through a femoral line is not optimal because of increased risk of infection. If options are confined to femoral line administration, time periods should be limited. However, burn units present unique challenges that at times may call for administration of TPN through a femoral line. Clear documentation as to the risks and benefits of the therapy and the overall lack of IV access in the patient may provide a rationale for administering TPN through a femoral catheter.

The traditional preferred site for TPN infusion is through the subclavian vein due to low infection rates. In general quoted infection rates for subclavian catheters are approximatedly 3.5–6 per 1000 catheter days versus 6–10 per 1000 catheter days for internal jugular catheters in ICUs. Femoral catheter sites have infection rates that range from 12–16 per 1000 catheter days in ICUs. Peripherally inserted central catheters (PICC) have similar infection rates to centrally venous catheters but sustain a longer duration of treatment before infection. Tunneled catheters can also serve as a long term source for treatment without infection. In general, peripherally placed intravenous catheters and central venous catheters are short-term access sites. PICC are considered midterm access sites, and tunneled catheters are long-term access sites (see Table 65.3).

Nutrient composition of the TPN mixture

The existing body cell mass is the major determinant of total caloric requirement, which is either estimated or measured

Table 65.3. Suggested fluid concentrations, duration of use, and common complications associated with catheters used for TPN administration

Catheter Site	Concentration of IV Fluids (mOsm/L)	Complications
Peripheral IV catheter	<500	Infection Phlebitis
Femoral Vein	>900	Infection Bleeding DVT
Centrally Placed Catheters		
SubclavianVein /Internal Jugular Vein	>900	Pneumothorax Injury to heart Retained guidewire
Peripherally Inserted Central Catheter Tunneled Catheters or Ports		Infection, bleeding, DVT

directly. There is controversy regarding whether strict calculation and matching of energy expenditure with energy input improve clinical outcomes. Promotion of anabolic functions and avoidance of overfeeding are the goals, meaning that a 25-kcal/kg ideal body weight is usually sufficient. The American College of Chest Physicians consensus statement recommendations are listed in Table 65.4.

In general, 1 ml is required to administer 1 kcal of nutrients. Therefore, a volume of 2 to 2.5 L/d will provide the patient with 2000 to 2500 kcal of energy. This caloric load is sufficient for 90% of surgical patients. The base solution is commonly 500 ml of 10% amino acids and 500 ml of 50% dextrose (Table 65.5). Fluid, electrolytes, vitamins, and trace elements are added to this solution. The final volume is usually 2 to 2.5 L/d. Providing a fat emulsion (500 ml, 20%) 1 d/wk to patients will meet their essential fatty acid requirements.

Modulating the fat content of the mixture is important in specific patient populations. For example, it has been shown that administration of excessive calories to patients on the ventilator elevates CO_2 production due to excessive carbohydrate intake and prolongs efforts at discontinuation of mechanical ventilation. However, in patients with severe COPD, Steiner et al. demonstrated that carbohydrate supplementation improved pulmonary rehabilitation in well-nourished patients.

All three major nutrients may be mixed in a 3-L bag (triple mix or three-in-one). Sodium and potassium are added as chlorides or acetates, with the ratio of acetates to chlorides increasing in patients with hyperchloremia or acidosis. Sodium bicarbonate is incompatible with the nutrient solution; therefore, acetate is used. Phosphate is given as a potassium or sodium salt. Commercially available solutions of vitamins, minerals,

and trace elements are added to the nutrient mix for daily administration. Vitamin K, proton pump inhibitors or histamine H_2-receptor blockers, and insulin also may be included in the nutrient mix. Iron should be avoided in patients with sepsis. Slightly hypertonic (600–900 mOsm/L) solutions can be made for peripheral administration. These low–caloric density solutions include 5% amino acids, 10% dextrose, and 20% fat emulsion and are administered in a large volume of fluid.

There are studies suggesting that immunomodulation is possible via parenteral and enteral diets. Arginine, glutamine, and omega-3 fatty acids all have been shown to be immunomodulatory when given as a component of the diet. Patients who are septic seem to benefit from the administration of BCAAs.

Metabolic monitoring

All patients receiving parenteral nutritional support should receive accurate daily weights, and data on their fluid balance should be recorded rigorously. Serum glucose should be measured regularly, and euglycemia (serum glucose, 110–150 g/dl) should be maintained. Most alterations of patient weight in the ICU are reflective of excess fluid. However, if the patient's weight decreases and this is persistent, additional calories (500–1000 kcal/d) should be added to maintain lean body mass. The metabolic rate can be calculated and the energy input then

Table 65.4. TPN mixture recommendations

Glucose, 30%–70% of total calories
Fat, 15%–30% of total calories
Protein, 5%–20% of total calories
Micronutrient repletion

Table 65.5. Various additives/properties of a TPN mixture

Property	Standard solution	Triple mix
Volume, *ml*		
Amino acids 10%	500	1000
Dextrose 50%	500	1000
Fat emulsion 20%	–	250
Contents, *g*		
Amino acids	50	100
Dextrose	250	500
Total nitrogen	8.4	16.8
Total calories	1050	2600
Caloric density, *kcal/ml*	1.0	1.15
Osmolality, *mOsm/L*	1970	1900

matched to this figure:

$$\text{Metabolic rate (kcal/day)} = VO_2 \text{ (ml/min)} \times 60 \text{ min/h}$$
$$\times 1 \text{ L/1000 ml} \times 4.83 \text{ (kcal/L)} \times 24\text{h/d},$$

where VO_2 is the amount of oxygen consumed per minute.

In patients not on ventilators, metabolic carts offer bedside estimates of oxygen uptake for calculation of metabolic rate. In patients with pulmonary artery catheters, oxygen consumption is calculated using cardiac output data:

$$Vo_2\text{(ml/min)} = \text{cardiac output (L/min)}$$
$$\times CaO_2 \text{ (ml/L)}$$
$$- CmvO_2 \text{ (ml/L)} \times 1\text{L/10 dl},$$

where CaO_2 is arterial oxygen content and $CmvO_2$ is mixed venous oxygen content.

Finally, maintenance of lean body mass should be reflected by a positive nitrogen balance, which can be measured as follows: The urine urea nitrogen (UUN) concentration is multiplied by the total volume of urine in a 24-hour period. This represents only 80% of the total nitrogen excreted. An additional 20% must be added. Also, an additional 2 g is added to account for stool and integumentary losses.

$$\text{Total nitrogen loss (g/d)} \approx \text{24-hour UUN (g/d)}$$
$$+ 0.2 \text{ (24-hour UUN g/day)} + 2\text{g/d}.$$

Complications of TPN

The most common complication of TPN administration is hyperglycemia. Maintaining euglycemia is the standard of care. Insulin protocols with close monitoring of serum glucose have made this practice possible, with a corresponding reduction in mortality and morbidity. There are complications associated with central venous access, which may be mechanical or infectious. Pneumothorax, arterial puncture, and hematomas are all detectable at the time of catheter placement. Infectious complications often occur in a delayed manner. Coagulase-negative staphylococci are the most common pathogens in catheter-related bloodstream infections, followed by enterococcus. Signs of catheter infection, such as fever, leukocytosis, erythema at the puncture site, and positive blood cultures, should prompt catheter removal. A new bag of TPN should be initiated when a new, appropriately positioned central venous catheter is available.

Perioperative and periprocedural management of TPN

Once TPN is initiated, unless otherwise indicated by the procedure, it is recommended that the infusion of TPN should continue during the procedure and in the operating room to maximize the nutritional benefits for critically ill patients.

However, when TPN is discontinued, it is particularly important to be vigilant about the risk of hypoglycemia. This may happen as TPN runs out and the new supply is not yet available, or when TPN infusion is discontinued (e.g., because of the removal of the central venous catheter or travel of the patient). When TPN is discontinued, it is imperative to regularly measure serum/blood glucose levels (every 30 minutes or every hour, but even more frequently when the measured values are < 60 mg/dl). The administration of 50% dextrose solution is also recommended when blood glucose levels fall below 45 to 60 mg/dl (these levels are determined by institutional guidelines for hypoglycemia). To prevent this scenario, if the TPN needs to be discontinued, the patient should be placed on 10% dextrose infusion at the same rate the TPN was infused, with regular blood glucose measurements.

Refeeding syndrome

Malnourished patients suffer from the depletion of total body phosphorus. In an attempt to maintain homeostasis, phosphorus is redistributed from the intracellular space. Once nutrition is initiated, the delivery of a large amount of glucose causes an insulin surge that initiates cellular glucose uptake, as well as uptake of potassium and phosphate from the extracellular space. The body also begins to retain fluid. Under these conditions, the serum concentration of potassium and phosphorus falls rapidly. The cardiac effects of this are increased cardiac workload, increased stroke work, and increased oxygen consumption with a resultant increase in the respiratory quotient and minute ventilation. Patients may have tachypnea, dysrhythmias, seizures, coma, or respiratory or cardiac failure.

Prevention of refeeding syndrome is best accomplished by a gradual increase in calories per day when nutrition is initiated combined with monitoring and replacement of electrolytes, particularly magnesium, phosphate, and potassium. Refeeding syndrome may occur in any patient who is malnourished or has been subjected to a significant period of starvation prior to the administration of nutrients.

Suggested readings

Baker JP, Detsky AS, Wesson DE, et al. Nutritional assessment: a comparison of clinical judgement and objective measurement. *N Engl J Med* 1982; 306:969–972.

Beattie AH, Prach AT, Baxter JP, et al. A randomized control trial evaluating the use of enteral nutritional supplements postoperatively in malnourished surgical patients. *Gut* 2000; 46:813–818.

Brennan MF, Cerra F, Daly JM, et al. Report of a research workshop: branched chain amino acids in stress or injury. *J Parenter Enteral Nutr* 1986; 10:446–452.

Cerra FB, Benitez MR, Blackburn GL, et al. Applied nutrition in ICU patients. A consensus statement of the American College of Chest Physicians. *Chest* 1997; 111:769–778.

Daly JM, Lieberman MD, Goldfine J, et al. Enteral nutrition with supplemental arginine, RNA, and omega-3 fatty acids in patients after operation: immunologic, metabolic, and clinical outcome. *Surgery* 1992; 112:56.

Dudrick SJ, Wilmore DW, Vars HM, Rhoads JE. Long-term total parenteral nutrition and growth, development and positive nitrogen balance. *Surgery* 1968; 64:134–142.

Furst P, Albers S, Stehle P. Stress-induced intracellular glutamine depletion. *Ther Clin Nutr* 1987; 17:117.

Garcia-de-Lorenzo A, Ortiz-Leyba C, Planas M, et al. Patenteral administration of different amounts of branched chain amino acids in septic patients: clinical and metabolic aspects. *Crit Care Med* 1997; 25:418.

Heller AR, Rossler S, Litz RJ, et al. Omega-3 fatty acides improve the diagnosis-related clinical outcome. *Crit Care Med* 2006; 34:97.

Heyland DK. Enteral and parenteral nutrition in the seriously ill, hospitalized patient: a critical review of the evidence. *J Nutr Health Aging* 2000; 1:31–41.

McWhirter JP, Pennington CR. The incidence and recognition of malnutrition in the hospital. *BMJ* 1994; 308:945–948.

Muller J, Brenner U, Dienst C, et al. Preoperative parenteral feeding in patients with gastrointestinal carcinoma. *Lancet* 1982; 1: 68–71.

Torosian MH. Perioperative nutrition support for patients undergoing gastrointestinal surgery: critical analysis and recommendations. *World J Surg* 1999; 23:565–569.

Transfusion Medicine

Richard M. Kaufman, editor

Blood products

Edward R. Garcia

Blood component administration carries a significant risk of infectious, toxic, and immunologic complications. All clinicians must be familiar with indications and alternatives to decrease the risks of this therapy (Table 66.1).

Red blood cells

Red blood cells (RBCs) are given to improve oxygen (O_2)-carrying capacity and do not contain viable platelets or significant amounts of coagulation factors or neutrophils. All RBC transfusions must be ABO compatible. RBC units are stored at 1° to 6°C to decrease metabolism and inhibit bacterial growth.

A unit of RBCs (often referred to as "packed" red cells) is prepared from whole blood using a closed sterile system. First, approximately 450 ml of whole blood is collected from a screened volunteer donor into a bag containing 63 ml of a citrate-phosphate-dextrose (CPD) anticoagulant preservative. The donated whole blood unit may then be processed to produce one RBC unit, one platelet concentrate, and one unit of fresh frozen plasma (FFP). To generate a unit of RBCs, a whole-blood unit is centrifuged to separate the RBCs from the plasma. Most of the plasma is then expressed from the unit, leaving about 180 (160–275) ml of RBCs, 30 ml of residual plasma, and 30 ml of CPD solution. Such a CPD RBC unit has a volume of about 250 ml and a hematocrit (Hct) of 70% to 80%, and may be stored for up to 21 days. Typically, an additive solution is added to CPD RBC units to extend the allowable storage time to up to 42 days (below).

The solutions used in manufacturing RBC units are:

- CPD is the basic anticoagulant preservative solution used to collect whole blood. Citrate acts as an anticoagulant by binding calcium, and dextrose serves as an energy source for the RBCs. CPD units may be stored for up to 21 days at 1° to 6°C.
- CPDA-1 is identical in composition to CPD, except for the addition of 17.3 mg of adenine. Adenine provides a substrate for the production of adenosine triphosphate. CPDA-1 RBC units may be stored for up to 35 days at 1° to 6°C.
- Additive solutions are crystalloid solutions that include dextrose, adenine, and other components in varying concentrations. Currently licensed additive solutions are

AS-1 (Adsol; Baxter, Round Lake, IL), AS-3 (Nutricel; Miles Inc, Elkhart, IN), and AS-5 (Optisol; Oxonica, Bucks, UK). Typically, 100 ml of an additive solution is added to a CPD RBC unit, resulting in a final product of about 310 ml with an Hct of 55% to 65%. Additive solutions contain monobasic sodium phosphate (AS-3) or mannitol (AS-1 and AS-5) to limit cell lysis. The additive solutions serve to extend RBC survival, increasing the unit's shelf-life to 42 days. Also, by lowering the product's viscosity, additive solutions yield excellent flow characteristics.

Recently, there has been some discussion regarding a possible link between "older" blood (still within the 42-day shelf life) and increased morbidity and mortality in transfused patients. At this point, currently available evidence does not indicate a clear linkage, although some large randomized trials (e.g., Red Cell Storage Duration study, Age of Blood Evaluation trial) are currently investigating this question.

Leucocyte-reduced red blood cells

Patients who have a history of febrile nonhemolytic transfusion reactions, require cytomegalovirus-negative blood, are at risk for HLA alloimmunization, or are receiving an exchange transfusion should receive leukocyte-depleted RBCs. These RBC units are prepared with special filters that remove $\geq$ 99.99% of white blood cells (WBCs) prior to storage. Leukoreduction is usually effective in preventing febrile nonhemolytic transfusion reactions and also has been shown to be effective in decreasing platelet alloimmunization and cytomegalovirus transmission. The filtration system used will remove some portion of the other cellular components present but the RBC unit should still have a therapeutic efficacy equal to at least 85% of the original component. Leukoreduction does not prevent graft-versus-host disease (GVHD). Cryoprecipitate and FFP do not contain significant numbers of viable leukocytes, so leukoreduction is unnecessary.

Washed red blood cells

Patients who have a history of severe reaction to transfusion, such as anaphylactoid reactions, should receive washed RBCs. RBCs are washed using 0.9% sodium chloride to remove almost all IgA (99%) and other plasma proteins and WBCs. This may not be sufficient to prevent hypersensitivity reactions, so blood collected from an IgA-deficient donor may be needed to support an IgA-immunized patient. Because units are typically washed using an open system, washed products must be transfused within 4 hours of preparation. The wash process reduces RBC content by approximately 20%.

Frozen red blood cells

RBC units with rare antigen combinations and other requirements for extended storage can be frozen with the addition of glycerol as a cytoprotective agent. Expired units that are rare can be "rejuvenated" by washing in a biochemical solution, and can then be glycerolized and frozen. These units are stored at $\leq -65°C$ for up to 10 years. They must be washed with successively lower concentrations of sodium chloride to remove the glycerol prior to transfusion. These units contain at least 80% of the RBCs present in the original unit and have the same expected posttransfusion survival.

Platelets

Platelet transfusions are indicated to prevent or treat bleeding in patients with qualitative or quantitative platelet deficiencies. Platelet concentrates ("random donor platelets") are derived from donated whole blood. First, a whole blood unit is gently centrifuged ("soft spin") to produce a bag of platelet-rich plasma (PRP) plus one unit of RBCs (see earlier). The PRP is centrifuged a second time ("hard spin") to produce a platelet concentrate plus one unit of plasma. The platelet concentrate is resuspended in 40 to 70 ml of plasma and should contain a minimum of 5.5×10^{11} platelets. Platelet concentrates are stored at room temperature $(20°–24°C)$ with continuous gentle agitation for up to 5 days. Platelet metabolic activity continues during storage; agitation of platelet units facilitates gas exchange and helps preserve the pH of the unit. Because platelets are stored at room temperature, bacterial growth may occur during storage. Rarely, septic transfusion reactions are observed, particularly in immunocompromised recipients.

A single platelet concentrate is expected to increase the platelet count of a 70-kg adult by 5 to 10,000/μl. Platelet concentrates are usually pooled into packs of four to six units of platelets for transfusion in adults. Pooling requires entry into the sterile units, so platelet concentrates are required to be transfused within 4 hours of pooling. Low numbers of RBCs are present in platelet concentrates. Rarely, Rh sensitization may be induced if an Rh-positive platelet unit is transfused to an Rh-negative recipient, but sensitization can be prevented by administering Rh immune globulin.

Most platelet units used in the United States are actually obtained via plateletpheresis, in which a therapeutic adult dose can be harvested from a single donor (hence, "single-donor platelets"). In plateletpheresis, whole blood is withdrawn and centrifuged by an automated device, and the red cells, leukocytes, and most plasma are returned to the donor. Apheresis platelet units contain the equivalent of four to eight whole-blood–derived platelet concentrates (at least 3×10^{11} platelets per unit in a volume of about 300 ml). Most apheresis platelets contain $<1 \times 10^6$ leukocytes and can be labeled *leukocyte reduced*. Apheresis platelet units contain very low numbers of contaminating RBCs, typically <0.1 ml.

Blood banks strive to provide ABO-compatible platelet units; however, transfusing ABO-compatible platelets is not required. In rare cases, hemolytic transfusion reactions have been seen as a result of high-titer isoagglutinins (e.g., anti–A antibody) present in the donor plasma in the platelet unit.

Lower-than-expected posttransfusion platelet count increments may represent a refractory state. Nonimmune factors that can cause refractoriness to platelets include fever, sepsis, medications, disseminated intravascular coagulation (DIC), bleeding, splenomegaly, hepatic veno-occlusive disease, and GVHD. In a subset of cases, refractoriness to platelets is immune mediated, which is generally the result of class I anti-HLA antibodies in the recipient. These patients may respond to HLA-matched platelets or crossmatched platelet units. Although platelets express class I HLA antigens, transfusion recipients are usually stimulated to make anti-HLA antibody not by the platelets themselves, but rather by HLA-expressing leukocytes present in the unit. Providing leukoreduced blood products has been demonstrated to be highly effective in preventing HLA alloimmunization.

Fresh frozen plasma

FFP is prepared by centrifuging a unit of whole blood. One unit of FFP has a volume of approximately 225 ml (200–250 ml) and contains all clotting factors in normal concentrations (1 IU/ml), as well as fibrinogen. FFP is frozen within 8 hours of collection to avoid degradation of coagulation factors (particularly the labile factors V and VIII). ABO-compatible FFP is generally used, but transfusing ABO-compatible FFP is not required. FFP is the primary source of replacement coagulation factors for patients with multiple factor deficiencies, and is the component most prone to inappropriate use.

Indications for the use of FFP include correction of bleeding due to factor deficiencies (when specific factor concentrates are not available) and states in which multiple factor deficiencies must be corrected (e.g., massive hemorrhage and transfusion, DIC, hepatic failure, acute reversal of warfarin therapy). These deficiencies should be demonstrated by abnormal coagulation studies (prothrombin time [PT] or activated partial thromboplastin time. Minor prolongations of the PT and aPTT ($<1.5 \times$ the mean of normal range), volume expansion, and nutritional support are not indications for FFP transfusion. Reversal of warfarin should be treated with vitamin K rather than FFP, unless more urgent correction is required (e.g., for ongoing hemorrhage). There are advantages and disadvantages to using Vitamin K versus FFP. The latter has the associated transfusion risks, but its action is essentially instantaneous and it permits the easy reestablishment of anticoagulation with warfarin. With Vitamin K, there is no transfusion risk; however, its action

Table 66.1. Summary of blood components

Blood component	Contents	Expected increment	Time to receive product, *min*	Volume, *ml*	Shelf life
RBCs	RBCs with ~25 ml of plasma; 100 ml of saline; additive solution (adenine, mannitol); Hct 60%	Hct, 3%	10 (if T&S complete)	340	42 d at 4°C
Pooled platelet concentrates	Platelets; includes some WBCs; 50 ml of plasma, a few RBCs	5000–10,000 plt/μl/unit (30,000–60,000 for 6-pack)	30	50 ml/concentrate; 300 ml/pool	5 d at 20°C
Apheresis platelets	Platelets; includes some WBCs; 300 ml of plasma; a few RBCs	30,000-60,000 plt/μl	15	300	5 d at 20°C
FFP	Plasma proteins; all coagulation factors; complement	Factor levels 3%/unit FFP	30	225	1 y at −18°C
Cryoprecipitate	200 mg of fibrinogen, at least 80 units of factor VIII, von Willebrand factor, factor XIII, fibronectin	Fibrinogen: 70 mg/dl (pool of 10 units)	45	15 ml	1 y at −18°C

requires hours to be manifest. In addition, a patient given Vitamin K becomes temporarily very resistant to warfarin, and this resistance decreases gradually over a period of weeks. Therefore, it becomes very difficult to establish a constant anticoagulant effect with warfarin for weeks following a dose of Vitamin K.

One milliliter of FFP per kilogram of patient weight will raise most clotting factors by approximately 1%, so one unit of FFP will raise factor levels in a 70-kg adult by about 3%. In clinically significant coagulopathy, one to two units of FFP likely is inadequate. The amount of FFP needed depends on the patient's clotting factor levels, levels needed to achieve a therapeutic effect, whether or not the patient is bleeding, and the patient's blood volume. FFP should be used as soon as possible after (and always within 24 hours of) thawing.

Cryoprecipitate

Cryoprecipitate is a concentrate prepared by thawing FFP at 1° to 6°C and isolating and refreezing the cold-insoluble precipitate that forms. Each unit of cryoprecipitate contains about 80 units each of factor VIII and von Willebrand factor and about 200 mg of fibrinogen, as well as lesser quantities of fibronectin and factor XIII. When needed, the unit is thawed, suspended in normal saline, and often pooled for administration. It must be used within 6 hours of thawing or, if pooled, within 4 hours. Compatibility testing is not needed, nor is ABO or Rh type specificity, although in infants, specificity is often observed if trace amounts of A or B isoagglutinins are present (because of their small blood volume).

Historically, cryoprecipitate was used for hemophilia and von Willebrand's disease, although now virus-inactivated factor concentrates are preferred. It is primarily used for control of bleeding with hypofibrinogenemia, such as acute DIC with bleeding. Each unit should raise the fibrinogen level in an adult by 0.1 mg/kg/dl. It is often pooled so that 10 units provide approximately enough fibrinogen to raise the fibrinogen 60 to 70 mg/dl in a 70-kg adult. Cryoprecipitate also is used for the treatment of uremic bleeding, obstetric emergencies such as abruptio placentae, and HELLP (*h*emolysis, *e*levated *l*iver enzymes, and *l*ow *p*latelet count) syndrome, and rare factor XIII deficiency. In general, it should not be used for other indications.

Irradiated blood products

Viable transfused lymphocytes present in RBC or platelet units can potentially respond to host antigens and cause transfusion-associated GVHD (TA-GVHD). Most cases have been observed in immunocompromised recipients, as infused lymphocytes are normally eradicated by a recipient's immune system. TA-GVHD is usually fatal. No effective therapy exists, but TA-GVHD can be prevented by blood product irradiation. Irradiated products must receive a minimum of 25 Gy of gamma radiation at the center of the unit. Cryoprecipitate and FFP have not been associated with TA-GVHD and do not require irradiation. RBC units that have been irradiated have a shortened shelf-life of 28 days.

Absolute indications for irradiated components include bone marrow transplant recipients (allogeneic, autologous), T-cell immunodeficiency, intrauterine transfusions, transfusions from any family member, or HLA-matched platelet transfusions. Hematologic malignancies, lymphomas, and some solid tumors (neuroblastoma and glioblastoma) are also indications for irradiated products. Patients with solid tumors of most types, those receiving chemotherapy, and those on other routine immunosuppressive (chronic steroids or solid organ transplant recipients) drugs do not typically require irradiated products. However, TA-GVHD has occurred in patients on fludarabine; therefore, patients on this agent should also receive irradiated products. Because there is no effective treatment for TA-GVHD, and because the list of indications for irradiation has expanded over time, some institutions are moving toward "universal" irradiation of blood products.

Pretransfusion testing and time to receipt of blood components

The time required to receive blood when it is ordered depends on the amount of pretransfusion testing required and laboratory processing requirements. Pretransfusion testing can reduce or eliminate the risk of hemolytic reactions and other types of transfusion reactions. Standards for testing are established by the American Association of Blood Banks, as well as local and national regulations.

ABO/Rh type

Once an adequate specimen arrives in the blood bank, pre-transfusion testing begins with determination of blood type. This phase takes about 10 minutes and involves determining what ABO antigens are present on the patient's RBCs (forward typing) by mixing the RBCs with commercial antibody preparations of anti-A and anti-B antibodies. RhD antigen determination is also performed. The blood bank also tests for the presence of expected ABO antibodies in the patient's sera (reverse typing).

Antibody screen

The patient's serum is tested for the presence of unexpected RBC antibodies to clinically significant red cell antigens. The patient's serum or plasma is mixed with commercially available reagent type O RBCs that express the 20 or so antigens most commonly associated with hemolytic transfusion reactions. The various stages of incubation conditions designed to elicit agglutination or hemolysis require about 45 minutes. If unexpected antibodies are discovered, the identification and location of appropriate antigen-negative units may require several hours or, in rare cases, days.

Crossmatch

Compatibility between a unit of RBCs and the patient's serum is assured via the crossmatch. If no antibodies are detected on the antibody screen, the unit may be crossmatched by the "immediate spin" method. Donor RBCs are mixed with recipient plasma at room temperature, and the presence or absence of agglutination is noted. This test is done simply as a final check to rule out ABO incompatibility. If a validated information system is in use in the blood bank, an electronic crossmatch can replace the immediate spin crossmatch procedure. If unexpected RBC antibodies are identified on the screen, serologic crossmatching must be performed.

If a patient has a current type and screen without unexpected antibodies, RBCs can be made available in about 10 minutes. If antibodies are present and unknown, finding crossmatch-compatible units may take considerable time. If the antibodies have been characterized, a serologic crossmatch requiring 30 minutes must be performed.

In an emergency, un-crossmatched type O or type-specific blood may be given. The risk of hemolytic reaction is low in young patients (0.1% in patients < 30 years old) but rises with a history of transfusion, age, and female sex. In patients who have received prior transfusions, the risk rises to 2% to 5% because of the presence of abnormal antibodies to RBC antigens other than A or B. A negative antibody screen decreases the risk of a hemolytic transfusion reaction to 0.06%.

Fresh frozen plasma

FFP requires 20 to 30 minutes to thaw in a 37°C water bath. No compatibility testing is required.

Platelets

Apheresis platelets are ready immediately; pooling whole-blood–derived platelet concentrates takes about 30 minutes. No compatibility testing is required.

Cryoprecipitate

Cryoprecipitate requires 45 minutes to thaw and pool. No compatibility testing is required.

Blood substitutes

Blood substitutes using hemoglobin-based O_2 carriers or inert chemicals to deliver O_2 to tissues are currently under investigation. Perfluorocarbon solutions, which are chemically inert but carry O_2 in solution, are undergoing phase II and III clinical trials in the United States and Europe. Hemoglobin-based O_2 carrier solutions (chemically modified human or bovine hemoglobin that carries O_2 in solution) are undergoing or have completed phase III clinical trials in the United States. Polyheme (Northfield Labs, Evanston, IL), a hemoglobin-based carrier, is the only blood substitute to complete phase III clinical trials, but was not approved for use by the FDA and is no longer manufactured. Both perfluorocarbons and hemoglobin-based O_2 carriers have short plasma half-lives, and none currently is licensed for use in North America.

Suggested readings

Baróti Tóth C, Kramer J, Pinter J, et al. IgA content of washed red blood cell concentrates. *Vox Sanguinis* 1998; 74:13–14.

Blood transfusion practice. In: Brecher ME, ed. *Technical Manual.* 15th ed. Bethesda, Md: AABB; 2005.

Fung MK, Downes KA, Shulman IA. Transfusion of platelets containing ABO-incompatible plasma: a survey of 3156 North American laboratories. *Arch Pathol Lab Med* 2007; 131:909–916.

Goodnough LT, Brecher ME, Kanter MH, AuBuchon JP. Transfusion medicine. I. Blood transfusion. *N Engl J Med* 1999; 340:438–447.

Goodnough LT, Brecher ME, Kanter MH, AuBuchon JP. Transfusion medicine. II. Blood conservation. *N Engl J Med* 1999; 340:525–533.

Heal JM, Rowe JM, McMican A, et al. The role of ABO matching in platelet transfusion. *Eur J Haematol* 1993; 50(2):110–117.

Lelubre C, Piagnerelli M, Vincent JL. Association between duration of storage of transfused red blood cells and morbidity and mortality in adult patients: myth or reality? *Transfusion* 2009; 49:1384–1394.

Miripol JE. ADSOL Preservation Solution – A New Additive for the Extended Storage of Red Blood Cells. Deerfield, IL: Fenwall Laboratories; 1986.

Natanson C, Kern S, Lurie P, Banks S, Wolfe S. Cell-free hemoglobin based blood substitutes and risk of myocardial infarction and death: a meta-analysis. *JAMA* 2008; 299(19): 2304–2312.

Pierce RN, Reich LM, Mayer K. Hemolysis following platelet transfusions from ABO-incompatible donors. *Transfusion* 1985; 25:60–62.

Chapter 67

Blood transfusion

Jonathan E. Charnin

Introduction

Perioperative blood transfusions comprise about two-thirds of all transfusions in the United States. All anesthesiologists must have expertise with transfusion and maintain open lines of communication with their colleagues in transfusion medicine.

Current practices in blood transfusion utilize blood component therapy. Whole blood is separated by centrifugation into red blood cell (RBC) units, platelet concentrates, and plasma. Plasma derivatives such as cryoprecipitate, albumin, pooled clotting factors, and immunoglobulins may later be generated from the separated plasma. Component therapy allows the targeted treatment of anemia, thrombocytopenia, and coagulopathy with the appropriate fraction of whole blood: RBCs, platelets, or plasma, respectively. Component therapy also facilitates storage of blood components, screening for transmissible pathogens, and management of the blood supply. The most commonly transfused blood components are RBC units (sometimes called *packed RBCs* or *PRBCs*) and fresh frozen plasma (FFP).

Blood product transfusion is a medical intervention. Whenever possible, informed consent must be obtained from the patient before transfusion. It is mandatory to discuss preoperatively the likelihood of blood transfusion and its attendant risks with patients undergoing surgery. Patients who refuse to receive blood products may present additional anesthetic challenges.

Blood compatibility testing

RBCs express a variety of surface antigens that limit the compatibility of blood for transfusion between individuals. A collection of RBC antigens produced by a single genetic locus is called a *blood group*. The ABO system is the most important blood group (Table 67.1). The *ABO* gene on chromosome 9 encodes a glycosyltransferase enzyme. An individual's ABO type – A, B, AB, or O – is dictated by which allelic forms of the *ABO* gene are inherited. The gene product of the A allele adds a terminal *N*-acetylgalactosamine (GalNAc) residue to specific RBC surface carbohydrates, forming the A carbohydrate antigen. The gene product of the B allele instead adds a galactose residue to the exact same substrates. The O allele encodes a truncated, nonfunctional protein – neither A nor B antigen is generated on the RBC surface.

An ABO-incompatible RBC transfusion may cause an immediate, life-threatening hemolytic transfusion reaction. Continuous exposure to ubiquitous environmental antigens that are structurally similar to the ABO antigens ensures that all recipients have circulating preformed antibodies against the ABO antigens their own RBCs lack. For instance, individuals who are type B always form potent, complement-fixing anti-A antibody – without ever having been exposed to type A RBCs through transfusion or pregnancy. Patterns of compatibility between recipients of a known blood type and donor blood products are worth committing to memory (Table 67.2). When transfusing RBCs, the preformed anti-ABO antibodies in the recipient are the limiting factor for transfusion. Because type O blood lacks A and B antigen, it is the "universal donor" RBC type. When transfusing plasma products (FFP and platelets), preformed anti-ABO antibodies in the donor plasma are the limiting factor for transfusion, so type AB plasma is the "universal donor" plasma type.

To determine a patient's blood type, the patient's RBCs are mixed with anti-A and anti-B reagent antibodies to provoke visible agglutination (antibody-mediated clumping). RBCs expressing A or B antigens will agglutinate when mixed with the appropriate antibody. This process is called "forward" blood typing. To confirm the forward typing results, the blood bank also tests for the expected presence of the appropriate anti-ABO antibodies in the recipient's plasma. This is called "back typing." Both forward typing and back typing are used to determine a patient's blood type.

There are many blood group antigens outside the ABO system. In most cases, these antigens represent immunogenic

Table 67.1. Blood type frequencies by percentage and skin color

ABO	Whites	Blacks
O	45	49
A	40	27
B	11	20
AB	4	4

Adapted from American Association of Blood Banks. (2005). *Technical manual* (15th ed.). Bethesda, MD: American Association of Blood Banks. Table 13–1, p. 290.

Table 67.2. ABO compatibilities for transfusion of PRBCs and FFP

Recipient blood type	ABO–compatible PRBC donor blood types	ABO–compatible FFP donor blood types
O	O	AB, A, B, O
A	A, O	A, AB
B	B, O	B, AB
AB	AB, A, B, O	AB
Rh+	Rh+, Rh−	Rh+
Rh−	Rh−	Rh+, Rh−

epitopes present on the extracellular portions of RBC membrane proteins. Most of these antigens are created by single nucleotide polymorphisms in the genome. Unlike the case with ABO antigens, prior exposure through blood transfusion or pregnancy is usually necessary for a patient to form antibodies to these antigens. Five blood group systems account for most of the clinically significant transfusion reactions that occur: the Rh blood group system, the Kell system, the Duffy system, the Kidd system, and the MNS system. After ABO, the Rh system is the most important blood group. Rh antigens are expressed on proteins encoded by two closely linked genes on chromosome 1. The *RhD* gene encodes the D antigen; the *RhCE* gene encodes the C, c, E and e antigens. The D antigen is extraordinarily immunogenic: approximately 80% of D-negative individuals will form anti-D antibody following a single D-positive RBC transfusion. For this reason, transfusion recipients are routinely matched for RhD in addition to ABO. Individuals whose RBCs express the D antigen are referred to as "Rh positive"; those lacking the D antigen are called "Rh negative." Other clinically important RBC antigens include the K antigen (Kell system), Fy^a and Fy^b (Duffy system), Jk^a and Jk^b (Kidd system), and S (MNS system).

When a patient is exposed to a foreign RBC antigen through transfusion or pregnancy, the patient may form an alloantibody to that antigen – for example, anti-K or anti-E. This primary sensitization is almost never associated with any clinical consequences. However, upon reexposure to the same antigen, a vigorous secondary immune response may occur. If reexposure to the antigen is via blood transfusion, the transfused, antigen-positive units may be cleared rapidly from the circulation of the recipient, resulting in an acute or delayed hemolytic reaction (see later). If reexposure to antigen occurs via fetomaternal hemorrhage during pregnancy, hemolytic disease of the newborn may be caused by these antigens when the mother transfers to the fetus maternal antibodies that recognize and cause hemolysis of the fetal red cells that carry other blood group antigens inherited from the father.

Prior to transfusion, a patient in need of a blood transfusion should have a sample of his or her blood sent to the blood bank. The blood bank first determines the patient's ABO type as described earlier. The patient's RhD status (positive or negative) is determined simultaneously. Next, an antibody screen is performed to test the patient's plasma for "unexpected"

anti-RBC antibodies (antibodies against non-ABO RBC antigens). The antibody screen is an example of an indirect antiglobulin test (i.e., indirect Coomb's test). In the antibody screen, patient plasma is incubated with two or three different type O reagent RBCs that have been phenotyped for the 20 or so RBC antigens that cause the vast majority of non–ABO-related hemolytic reactions. The reagent RBCs are chosen so that at least one example of each of the most important RBC antigens from the Rh, Kell, Duffy, Kidd, and other blood group systems is present. During the incubation step, anti-RBC antibodies in the patient's plasma will bind to the cognate antigens on the reagent RBCs. These antibodies, if present, are usually IgG, so they will not agglutinate the reagent RBCs directly. Therefore, to detect the antibodies, antihuman globulin (AHG, or Coomb's reagent) must be added. AHG is antibody directed against human IgG. AHG will crosslink the reagent RBCs if they have been coated with recipient antibody, causing visible agglutination. If no agglutination is observed with AHG, the antibody screen is reported as negative. If agglutination is seen, however, the blood bank must perform further testing to determine the specificity of the patient's RBC antibody (or antibodies). It is important to be aware that this testing may take several hours to days, depending on the antibodies present. If it is determined the patient has clinically significant RBC antibodies (capable of causing decreased RBC survival), RBC units lacking the appropriate antigens are selected for transfusion. The final step in pretransfusion compatibility testing is the crossmatch. If the patient's antibody screen is negative, an "immediate spin" crossmatch is done: recipient plasma is mixed with an aliquot of the RBCs intended for transfusion, and the sample is checked for agglutination. This test will detect only IgM antibody, so it essentially just serves as a last-minute confirmation that the patient's plasma and donor RBCs are ABO compatible (i.e., no ABO error has been made). At many institutions, the "immediate spin" crossmatch is actually omitted. An "electronic crossmatch" is performed instead – a validated computer system ensures that ABO-compatible units are being issued. If a patient does have a positive antibody screen, a more sensitive AHG crossmatch ("Coomb's crossmatch" or "full crossmatch") must be performed to ensure RBC compatibility.

Life-threatening hemorrhage will occasionally not wait for blood typing and crossmatching. In the most emergent circumstances in which no delay is appropriate, type O negative PRBCs can be used as universal donor blood without waiting for blood typing or crossmatching. Only for male patients is it permissible to transfuse O positive PRBCs for emergency use. In urgent situations in which transfusion can be delayed by 5 to 15 minutes, it is preferable to have the patient's blood sample sent to the blood bank for blood typing. Once the patient's blood type is known, un-crossmatched PRBCs of the same type with an appropriate Rh status, or type-specific blood, can be used to meet the needs of emergency transfusion. When the need for transfusion is not immediate, fully crossmatched PRBCs should be used. In emergency situations, universal donor FFP, which comes from type AB donors, can be used. Because it takes 30 to 45 minutes to thaw FFP, and blood typing can be performed rapidly, it is unusual to require universal donor FFP.

Platelets express ABO antigens, but they may be given without an ABO match. ABO-incompatible platelet transfusions have a reduced survival time in comparison with ABO-matched platelets, but this may not be of clinical importance in some settings.

Reactions and complications of blood transfusion

Blood component transfusions may be lifesaving, but they may also produce life-threatening complications. Anesthesiologists should focus on preventing complications of blood transfusion by transfusing blood components only when indicated and scrupulously attending to good transfusion techniques. Some immediate complications of transfusion can be recognized before the transfusion is complete, and it may be possible to limit the morbidity of a transfusion reaction by interrupting the transfusion. Transfusion reactions may be difficult to identify in patients who are anesthetized. Therefore, it is important to be mindful of adverse events and complications during transfusions, especially when transfusing emergency-released blood products when the donor blood has not been fully crossmatched with the recipient's blood.

Acute hemolytic transfusion reaction

ABO-incompatible red cell or FFP transfusions cause an immediate hemolytic transfusion reaction. Hemolytic transfusion reactions also may occur with some of the other blood group antigens, when red cells with particular antigens are transfused to a patient who has already been sensitized to those antigens. During a hemolytic transfusion reaction, a recipient may report pain at the infusion site, chest pain, dyspnea, and flank pain. He or she also may experience fever, rigors, and hypotension. Red urine, colored by free hemoglobin, and coagulopathy manifesting as diffuse bleeding at the surgical site may be observed. Acute hemolytic transfusion reactions produce red cell lysis by anti–red cell antibodies provoking both intravascular agglutination of red cells and fixing the complement system to the red cell. These reactions are life threatening and require discontinuation of the transfusion and prompt measures to support the patient. (See Table 67.3 on management of hemolytic transfusion reaction.)

Delayed hemolytic transfusion reactions

Delayed hemolytic transfusion reactions usually happen 3 or more days after PRBC transfusion. In these reactions, the recipient has an undetected antibody that coats the donor red cells and leads to hemolysis, usually in the reticuloendothelial system. These reactions may be asymptomatic or may produce anemia and jaundice a few days after a blood transfusion. Investigating delayed (and acute) hemolytic reactions by the blood bank is done by (1) rechecking identification of the patient

Table 67.3. Management of a suspected acute hemolytic transfusion reaction

Stop the transfusion, save the remaining blood product for testing

Check for an obvious error in patient identity or blood product match

Support the patient's circulation, treat hypovolemia and hypotension

If immediate transfusion is needed, give type O negative blood and AB $^+$ FFP if needed

Send a new blood sample for crossmatch to the blood bank, along with the remainder of the suspect unit for testing

Support the patient's renal function with fluids and diuretics, starting with furosemide and then mannitol if needed

Monitor the coagulation system for signs or laboratory values suggestive of disseminated intravascular coagulation, and treat if needed

Send the patient's blood for a direct antiglobulin test, free hemoglobin, and haptoglobin; send urine for free hemoglobin

Modified from Table 34–2 in *Clinical Anesthesia Procedures of the Massachusetts General Hospital*, 7th ed., 2007, p. 612.

and transfused units, (2) checking for visual hemolysis (pink or red discoloration) of the recipient plasma, and (3) performing a direct antiglobulin test (DAT, or "direct Coomb's test"). AHG is added to the recipient's sample; if recipient IgG antibody has coated the transfused RBCs, the DAT will be positive. The absence of visual hemolysis and a negative DAT essentially exclude a hemolytic transfusion reaction.

Allergic reaction

Allergic reactions may occur when a recipient has a reaction to an allergen in transfused blood products. Urticarial reactions may complicate up to 3% of transfusions. Anaphylactic, anaphylactoid, or delayed allergic rashes are possible but rare. A potential allergen is donor IgA antibodies when a recipient has a congenital IgA deficiency. Allergic transfusion reactions are not typically accompanied by fever. If an allergic reaction to transfusion is suspected, the transfusion should be stopped. If the reaction is limited to a rash, the transfusion may be restarted after an antihistamine is given. Supportive care and treatment of anaphylaxis should be given promptly if anaphylaxis is suspected. In some cases, it may be difficult to distinguish an anaphylactic reaction to transfusion from an ABO-incompatible transfusion or transfusion-related acute lung injury (TRALI). Patients with a history of IgA deficiency or allergic reactions to blood transfusion may benefit from having RBCs washed by the blood bank in saline before administration.

Febrile nonhemolytic transfusion reaction

Fever is associated with several serious transfusion reactions, including acute hemolytic transfusion reactions and transfusion of blood products infected with bacteria and is noted in about one in 300 red cell transfusions. When fever is associated with transfusion, prompt attention and evaluation are indicated. If there is no evidence of a serious complication, the reaction is called a *febrile nonhemolytic transfusion reaction*

(FNHTR). Fevers associated with transfusion are defined as a rise of > 1°C without any other explanation. FNHTR may complicate 0.5% to 6% of transfusions of non–leukocyte-reduced red cells. Recipients with prior exposures either through transfusions or gestations are at greater risk for having FNHTRs. Treatment with acetaminophen is indicated. Meperidine injection may help with rigors. For patients with a history of FNHTR, use of leukocyte-reduced blood products may prevent future reactions.

Transfusion-related acute lung injury

TRALI is a syndrome of dyspnea, hypoxia, and bilateral chest radiograph abnormalities within 6 hours of blood product transfusion. Multiple mechanisms appear to contribute to TRALI, and it is one of the leading causes of transfusion-related mortality. Most cases of TRALI appear to be caused by donor antileukocyte or anti-HLA antibodies that recognize recipient leukocytes or recipient HLA cell surface markers and then activate an inflammatory response. The occurrence of TRALI usually involves donor antibodies and therefore is related to donor plasma. Although the small amount of donor plasma transfused with PRBCs or cryoprecipitate may cause TRALI, it is about 12 times more common with FFP and eight times more common with platelet transfusions than with PRBCs. Blood product donors who have been exposed to foreign HLA through prior transfusion or prior pregnancy are more likely to have the antibodies that cause TRALI. For this reason, there is interest in using only male donor plasma for FFP transfusion.

Transfusion-associated circulatory overload

Blood product transfusion expands the intravascular space. Transfusion of blood products in sufficient quantity may induce congestive heart failure, especially in patients prone to it. This condition is referred to as *transfusion-associated circulatory overload* (TACO). When congestive heart failure manifests as respiratory distress, it may be difficult to differentiate TRALI from TACO without an assessment of the cardiac filling pressures.

Hypotensive response to transfusion with angiotensin-converting enzyme inhibitor use

Patients who take angiotensin-converting enzyme inhibitors (ACE-Is) are at risk for hypotensive reactions during PRBC transfusions. ACE-Is block the metabolism of bradykinin in addition to blocking the conversion of angiotensin. Bradykinin is a vasodilatory nonapeptide. Leukocytes in cellular blood products elaborate bradykinin that is infused with the blood product. The use of bedside leukocyte reduction filters increases bradykinin production and incidence of hypotensive reactions. Because these patients cannot metabolize bradykinin because

of the actions of ACE-Is, they experience hypotension that may be profound.

Stopping the transfusion and supporting the blood pressure are the first priorities if this reaction is observed. ACE-I cessation prevents recurrence of the reaction.

Hyperkalemia

PRBCs in storage experience a leak of intracellular potassium to plasma and the storage solution packaged with the red cells. Because the volume of plasma and storage solution packaged with the red cells is small, the potassium concentration in the fluid may be very high, ≥30 mEq/L, and its magnitude relates to the duration of red cell storage. Because the volume of the plasma is low, the total potassium given with a transfusion of red cells does not usually produce clinical hyperkalemia. Hyperkalemia is more worrisome when transfusions are given quickly or when the recipient is an infant or small child. During blood transfusion, the acute widening of the QRS complex on electrocardiography is concerning for hyperkalemia. Prompt administration of calcium chloride may be necessary while other measures to control the hyperkalemia are undertaken.

Patients who are at risk of experiencing hyperkalemia with transfusion may benefit from having RBCs washed in saline by the blood bank before administration.

Citrate toxicity

Citrate is used as an anticoagulant to prevent clotting during the storage of blood products. Citrate's anticoagulant action is mediated by chelation of the extracellular calcium required for coagulation. Typically, the citrate contained in blood products is quickly metabolized by the liver and, to a lesser degree, by many other organs. Calcium stores in the body also may be mobilized to restore blood calcium levels. During rapid transfusion, massive transfusion, liver transplantation, or hypothermia, or in patients already experiencing hypocalcemia, an accumulation of citrate may cause a profound decrease in ionized calcium that may produce muscle spasms, arrhythmias, or cardiac dysfunction. Intravenous injection of calcium chloride and correction of volume status and body temperature are recommended to treat the symptomatic decrease in ionized calcium due to citrate intoxication. Calcium gluconate requires the metabolism of the gluconate before the calcium is available and therefore may not be effective in treating citrate toxicity.

Air embolus

Rapid administration of blood product, especially when using positive pressure devices, has been associated with a life-threatening iatrogenic venous air embolism. This should be considered when hypotension complicates blood transfusions infused with positive pressure. Care should be taken when spiking blood product bags to minimize the volume of air in the plastic bags.

Table 67.4. Current risks of infection from test-negative blood

Components	Risk
HIV-1	1 in 1,525,000–2,135,000
Hepatitis C virus	1 in 1,935 000
Hepatitis B virus	1 in 205,000–488,000
West Nile virus	Approaching zero

Adapted from Stramer SL. Infectious risk from blood transfusion. *Arch Pathol Lab Med* 2007; 131:703.

Infectious complications

Blood product transfusions may transmit life-threatening infections. Transmission of viral and bacterial infections is of particular concern to physicians and patients. Transmission of blood-borne parasitic diseases such as malaria or prions such as those that cause Creutzfeldt-Jakob disease has been reported but is exceedingly rare. Testing for viral illnesses has substantially reduced the risk of transfusion-related viral transmission, especially since the introduction of nucleic acid amplification testing in 1999.

Bacterial contamination of blood products is not common, but it may produce an immediate septic reaction during transfusion. Platelets stored at room temperature are more commonly infected than other blood products, in which the rate of septic transfusion is one in 33,000 units transfused.

Screening blood donors and testing donated blood for viral contamination reduce but do not eliminate the transmission of viral illness. Some viruses, such as cytomegalovirus, may be transmitted less frequently through leukoreduced blood products. See Table 67.4 for rates of transmission.

Transfusion-associated graft-versus-host disease

Transfusion-associated graft-versus-host disease (TA-GVHD) is caused by donor lymphocytes engrafting in the recipient and attacking his or her tissues. This is a very rare but often fatal complication that is seen more commonly in immunosuppressed recipients. Leukocyte reduction filters do not eliminate the risk of TA-GVHD, but pretreatment of blood products with radiation is preventive.

Transfusion-related immunomodulation

Red cell transfusions modulate the immune response, particularly the innate immunity. The mechanisms of immunosuppression are still unclear. The deleterious effects of this immunosuppression may contribute to increased rates of hospital-acquired infections in trauma patients, as well as increased rates of cancer recurrence after surgical resection. The work by Carson and his colleagues suggests that there is a dose–response relationship between perioperative transfusion and postoperative infectious complications in patients undergoing hip fracture repair.

Transfusion triggers

Morbidity and mortality are associated both with unnecessary transfusion and uncorrected critical anemia. The desire is to transfuse when the benefits are thought to outweigh the risks. Debate continues about what degrees of anemia, coagulopathy, and thrombocytopenia should prompt a transfusion. It appears there is no one laboratory value, or transfusion trigger, that is an appropriate guide to transfuse for all patients. Few data from randomized prospective trials are available to guide the transfusion decision. Often, a clinician must consider the comorbid illnesses of the patient, the patient's vital signs, the potential for hemorrhage, and data from physiologic studies when deciding when to transfuse.

RBCs and their hemoglobin are the vehicles for oxygen transport in the body. During anemia, blood viscosity decreases and the ability of blood to transport oxygen may increase. Optimization of oxygen-carrying capacity with respect to hemoglobin concentration and viscosity appears to occur in healthy subjects when the hemoglobin is 10 g/dl. Outdated transfusion dogma suggested treating anemia with blood transfusion to keep the hemoglobin > 10 g/dl. Most patients tolerate hemoglobin levels between 7 and 9 g/dl without additional morbidity or mortality. Observational studies and small prospective trials have not demonstrated benefit for using transfusion triggers above 9 g/dl, with the exception of patients who are experiencing an ST elevation myocardial infarction. Transfusions of PRBCs are rarely indicated when the hemoglobin is >10 g/dl.

Healthy volunteers can survive profound normovolemic anemia without lasting harm, but their cognition is impaired when the hemoglobin reaches 5 g/dl. Observations of patients who experienced perioperative anemia and refused blood transfusion suggests that postoperative mortality increases when hemoglobin concentrations are <6 g/dl. To prevent this anemia-related mortality, transfusion of PRBCs is indicated when a patient's hemoglobin is below 7 g/dl. During active hemorrhage, it may be difficult to achieve a hemoglobin target. A transfusion trigger of 8 g/dl during active hemorrhage is a reasonable target to provide red cell margin during ongoing hemorrhage.

Hebert and his colleagues published the largest prospective trial evaluating red cell transfusion triggers. They randomly assigned 838 euvolemic intensive care unit patients with hemoglobin levels < 9 g/dl to a restrictive or a liberal transfusion strategy. The restrictive group had hemoglobin levels maintained by transfusion in a range of 7 to 9 g/dl, whereas the liberal group had their hemoglobin maintained in a range of 10 to 12 g/dl. The primary end point of 30-day mortality showed no statistical difference in mortality between the groups. The patients in the restrictive strategy group received 53% fewer red cell transfusions than patients in the liberal strategy group. Subgroup analyses suggest there may be additional survival benefit from restrictive transfusion in patients with less severe illness. However, because of possible selection bias, the results

Table 67.5. Cryopreciptate dosing formula

Milligrams of fibrinogen needed = [weight (kg) × 70 ml of blood/kg × (1 – hematocrit) × (desired fibrinogen in mg/dl – starting fibrinogen in mg/dl)/100 ml/dl])

Bags of cryoprecipitate needed = milligrams of fibrinogen needed/250 mg of fibrinogen per bag of cryoprecipitate

Modified from American Association of Blood Banks. (2005). *Technical Manual* (15th ed.). Bethesda, MD: American Association of Blood Banks, p. 501.

of this trial may not be applicable to patients with active coronary ischemia.

Acute coagulopathy may require both administration of clotting factors and platelet transfusion to correct thrombocytopenia. Clotting factor deficiencies and reversal of warfarin anticoagulation are commonly treated with transfusion of FFP; 10 to 15 ml of FFP per kilogram of body weight can be transfused to rapidly correct anticoagulation with warfarin. Hemostasis is usually normal when coagulation factors remain above 30% of their normal level. The clotting factor fibrinogen requires about 50% of its normal 200 to 400 mg/dl level to produce normal clot formation. Intraoperatively, transfusion of FFP likely will produce no benefit until the prothrombin time or activated partial thromboplastin timetime is prolonged to >1.5 times reference values, or when blood loss exceeds one blood volume. During active hemorrhage, many anesthesiologists begin to transfuse FFP when 4 or 6 U of PRBCs have been transfused. When clotting factors are depleted and massive transfusion is ongoing, FFP is often transfused in a 2:1 ratio of PRBCs to FFP. Some authors advocate earlier transfusion of FFP and PRBCs-to-FFP ratios of 3:2 or 1:1 during the resuscitation of hemorrhage from major trauma.

Cryoprecipitate contains the concentrated clotting factors VIII, XIII, von Willebrand, and fibrinogen that precipitate out when FFP is thawed at a temperature of 4°C. Currently, cryoprecipitate is commonly used for the treatment of hypofibrinogenemia, and the dose required to correct the fibrinogen can be estimated using a formula (Table 67.5). Cryoprecipitate may also be used to treat hemorrhage due to hemophilia A or von Willebrand disease, but commercially available factor concentrates are better therapies for these coagulopathies.

Sufficient platelet number and adequate platelet function are both important in forming an effective clot. Platelet transfusion can be undertaken to treat thrombocytopenia. The effectiveness of treating platelet dysfunction with transfusion depends on the cause of the platelet dysfunction, but it is often more effective to treat the cause of the platelet dysfunction. In the surgical setting, thrombocytopenia without platelet dysfunction should affect hemostasis only when the platelet count is $< 50,000/mm^3$. Perioperative platelet transfusion is indicated to keep the platelet count $> 50,000/mm^3$. Neurosurgical or ophthalmologic operations, in which small bleeding may create a poor outcome, may merit a platelet transfusion threshold of 80,000 or 100,000 platelets/mm^3.

Suggested Readings

American Association of Blood Banks. *Technical Manual* (15th ed.). Bethesda, MD: American Association of Blood Banks; 2005:501.

Carson JL, Altman DG, Duff A, et al. Risk of bacterial infection associated with allogenic blood transfusion among patients undergoing hip fracture repair. *Transfusion* 1999; 39(7):694–700.

Carson JL, Noveck H, Berlin JA, Gould SA. Mortality and morbidity in patients with very low postoperative hb levels who decline blood transfusion. *Transfusion* 2002; 42(7): 812–818.

Crosby ET. Perioperative haemotherapy: I. Indications for blood component transfusion. *Can J Anaesth* 1992; 39(7):695–707.

Cyr M, Eastlund T, Blais C, Jr, Rouleau JL, Adam A. Bradykinin metabolism and hypotensive transfusion reactions. *Transfusion* 2001; 41(1):136–150.

Dunn PF, Alston TA, Massachusetts General Hospital Dept. of Anesthesia and Critical Care. *Clinical Anesthesia Procedures of the Massachusetts General Hospital* (7th ed.). Philadelphia: Lippincott Williams & Wilkins; 2007.

Eder AF, Herron R, Strupp A, et al. Transfusion-related acute lung injury surveillance (2003–2005) and the potential impact of the selective use of plasma from male donors in the American Red Cross. *Transfusion* 2007; 47(4): 599–607.

Gonzalez EA, Moore FA, Holcomb JB, et al. Fresh frozen plasma should be given earlier to patients requiring massive transfusion. *Trauma-Injury Infect Crit Care* 2007; 62(1):112–119.

Hebert PC, Wells G, Blajchman MA, et al. A multicenter, randomized, controlled clinical trial of transfusion requirements in critical care. transfusion requirements in critical care investigators, Canadian critical care trials group. *N Eng Med* 1999; 340(6):409–417.

Klein HG, Spahn DR, Carson JL. Red blood cell transfusion in clinical practice. *Lancet* 2007; 370(9585):415–426.

Miller RD. *Miller's Anesthesia* (6th ed.). Philadelphia: Elsevier Churchill Livingstone.

Quillen K. Hypotensive transfusion reactions in patients taking angiotensin-converting-enzyme inhibitors. *N Eng J Med* 2000; 343(19):1422–1423.

Spiess BD, Spence RK, Shander A. *Perioperative transfusion medicine* (2nd ed.). Philadelphia: Lippincott Williams & Wilkins; 2006.

Stramer SL. Current risks of transfusion-transmitted agents: a review. *Arch Pathol Lab Med* 2007; 131(5):702–707.

68

Massive transfusion

Amy J. Ortman and Susan Vassallo

Massive transfusion is a relatively infrequent event, although the precise incidence is unknown, perhaps in part because of the variable definitions for *massive blood loss* and *transfusion*. Some authors arbitrarily define *massive transfusion* as the administration of at least 8 to 10 units (U) of blood transfused within a 12-hour period. Other definitions are the replacement of one blood volume within 24 hours, or the replacement of half of a patient's blood volume in 3 hours. Yet another, more dynamic, definition is the transfusion of ≥4 U of packed red cells within 1 hour when there is a high likelihood of ongoing need for further transfusion.

Regardless of the definition used, massive hemorrhage and the requisite massive transfusion comprise a clinical situation that presents a unique challenge to anesthesiologists. Although there is no substitute for prompt and appropriate surgical management to limit blood loss, anesthesiologists must be prepared to direct a large-volume resuscitation and have a ready, working knowledge of the issues involved.

Epidemiology and clinical context

Elective surgeries

Within hospitals, the most common cause of massive blood loss and transfusion are surgical procedures. Populations particularly at risk include those undergoing cardiopulmonary or vascular procedures, liver transplantation or resection, major orthopedic procedures, or emergency obstetric surgery. In the elective setting, resuscitation frequently begins with crystalloids, and then quickly shifts to blood products as the blood loss increases. Despite the volume of literature on the subject of transfusion, there are no precise guidelines outlining the appropriate time to transition from crystalloid resuscitation to blood product transfusion. Clinicians determine the timing by incorporating factors such as the patient's comorbidities, clinical evidence of perfusion, oxygenation and clotting ability, and anticipation of ongoing surgical losses.

Trauma

Trauma patients comprise a significant portion of patients who receive massive transfusions. Hemorrhage is the second leading cause of death following severe injury, and mortality among patients who have acute massive blood loss and transfusion

within the first 24 hours of presentation may be as high as 70%. Although the percentage of trauma patients who require a massive transfusion is relatively small, this population accounts for most blood products transfused at a trauma center. In one retrospective study linking blood bank use to trauma admissions, only 9% of all trauma admissions received blood products and of those, about 30% had a massive transfusion. Despite representing a small fraction of the total trauma admissions, the patients who received massive transfusions accounted for more than 72% of all the red blood cells (RBCs) used in the trauma center.

In the setting of trauma, massive transfusion within the first 24 hours is correlated with increased severity of injury, failure to control hemorrhage, and lower Glasgow coma scores, all of which contribute to the ongoing blood requirement and a greater mortality. Further complicating the clinical picture are the comorbidities that are frequently present when trauma patients arrive: hypothermia, hemorrhagic shock, acidosis, and coagulopathy.

Table 68.1 outlines some of the differences in massive transfusion between elective surgery and trauma situations.

Coagulopathy

Coagulation is a complex process of clot formation following vascular injury involving platelets and clotting factors, and results in hemostasis. Abnormal coagulation may occur because

Table 68.1. Differences in massive transfusion between elective surgery and trauma situations

	Elective surgery	Trauma
Tissue trauma	Controlled	Extensive and uncontrolled
Volume status	Normovolemic	Hypovolemic shock common
Temperature	Normothermic	Hypothermia common
Laboratory studies	Drawn regularly and frequently	Drawn late
Initiation of massive transfusion	Little or no delay in initiation of transfusion following hemorrhage	Transfusion may be significantly delayed following hemorrhage
Coagulopathy	Usually dilutional	Disseminated intravascular coagulopathy, dilutional, or coagulopathy of trauma

of inherited or acquired factor deficiencies, medications, hypothermia, acidosis, dilution and consumption of clotting factors, the use of fractionated blood products, or disseminated intravascular coagulation (DIC). When patients receive a massive transfusion, anticipation, recognition, and prompt intervention are essential to prevent development of a coagulopathy, further blood loss, and the resultant complications.

Hemodilution

Both trauma patients and patients undergoing elective surgery are at risk for the development of a dilutional coagulopathy. Although there is tremendous reserve and clotting factors may be decreased to approximately 30% of normal without clinical consequence, initial and ongoing resuscitation with crystalloids, colloids, or RBCs may lead to a deficiency of factors necessary for normal coagulation. Additionally, some synthetic colloid solutions may also act via platelet inhibition to further compromise coagulation.

Another important consideration is the role RBCs play in hemostasis. Erythrocytes help activate platelets by release of adenosine diphosphate and activation of platelet cyclooxygenase. RBCs also contribute to the margination of platelets against the vessel wall and thus affect their ability to act at the site of a vascular lesion. Experimental evidence suggests that in patients receiving massive transfusions, relatively high hematocrits – as high as 35% – may be required to sustain hemostasis.

Administration of fractionated blood products

Historically, administration of whole blood or modified whole blood was common and dilutional coagulopathies were rarely reported. Since then, whole blood therapy has been replaced by component therapy, largely because of storage impediments to the former and more efficient use of the components. Although component therapy is effective, massive resuscitation with fractionated blood products predisposes patients to hemodilution and development of a dilutional coagulopathy. When packed RBCs (PRBCs), fresh frozen plasma (FFP), and leukoreduced platelets are separated from whole blood, half of the platelets are lost, and the cells and clotting factors are diluted by anticoagulant and RBC nutrient solutions. Mixing the components at the classic 1:1 ratio essentially makes a reconstituted whole blood with a hematocrit of 29%, a platelet count of 88,000, and clotting factor activity of 62%.

Hypothermia

The coagulation cascade is largely a series of enzymatic reactions. Hypothermia slows the activity of the enzymatic process, reduces the synthesis of coagulation factors, increases fibrinolysis, and affects platelet function. The contribution of hypothermia to coagulopathy may be underestimated in routine testing because the laboratory studies are usually performed at a temperature of 37°C. Hypothermia, which is typically defined as a core temperature of <35°C, is a significant problem in the trauma population; Ferrara et al. reported that

hypothermia occurred in 80% of nonsurvivors and 36% of survivors in a series of 45 trauma patients. Further, hypothermia combined with trauma is associated with a worse prognosis than either insult alone.

Acidosis

Massive blood loss and resuscitation occur in patients who may also be in hemorrhagic shock. Hemorrhagic shock predisposes patients to hypoxia, anaerobic metabolism, and acidosis. Although the mechanism is not clear, the evidence is that a pH < 7.10 is associated with significant coagulopathy.

Disseminated intravascular coagulation and coagulopathy of trauma

By definition, DIC is an acquired, inappropriate, systemic activation of thrombin and deposition of fibrin with consumption of platelets and coagulation factors. In the setting of elective surgery, DIC accompanying massive transfusion is relatively uncommon. However, trauma patients are at risk for the development of a consumptive coagulopathy for three reasons. The first relates to tissue trauma such as central nervous system injuries or bone fractures with embolization of tissue; these microembolic events lead to consumption of tissue factor and inappropriate initiation of the coagulation cascade. Traumatic brain injuries also cause release of tissue thromboplastin into the circulation, rapidly resulting in activation of the extrinsic coagulation pathway. Last, significant soft tissue trauma also leads to consumption of platelets and thrombocytopenia. In each case, intravascular consumption of coagulation factors results in the development of a coagulopathy, and more specifically DIC.

Within the trauma literature, a second form of coagulopathy is described. The coagulopathy of trauma is a syndrome of nonsurgical bleeding associated with serious injury, hypothermia, acidosis, hemodilution, and occasionally DIC. Coagulopathy of trauma may occur in the setting of depleted coagulation factors, or in the setting of normal levels but dysfunctional coagulation factors. In a recent series review of 58 trauma patients without major brain injury or preexisting coagulopathy who required massive transfusion, four risk factors for the development of coagulopathy were identified using multiple logistic regression analysis. They are, in order of importance, pH < 7.10 (relative risk [RR], 12.3), core temperature <34°C (RR, 8.7), mean injury severity score >25 (RR, 7.7) and a systolic blood pressure <70 mm Hg (RR, 5.8). Patients without any risk factors had a 1% risk of coagulopathy, a single risk factor was associated with a 10% to 40% risk, and a combination of all four was associated with a 98% risk of coagulopathy.

Prevention of coagulopathy

The basic tenets of a massive transfusion and resuscitation require that one pay attention to the factors that contribute to or exacerbate a coagulopathy. Anesthesiologists should strive for normovolemic resuscitation, and regularly send studies to evaluate oxygen delivery, hemoglobin, acid–base status, and coagulation status. Failure to normalize these parameters may result in inappropriate activation of the clotting cascade and subsequent hemorrhage. It is also important to remember that even when these parameters are controlled, activation of the clotting cascade may still occur from tissue trauma alone.

Management

The basic goals of the management of massive transfusion are maintenance of tissue perfusion and oxygenation by preservation of blood volume and hemoglobin; judicious use of blood component therapy; avoidance of acidosis, hypothermia, and coagulopathy; and surgical control of the bleeding.

The essential equipment and components necessary for massive transfusion will vary depending on the clinical situation, patient comorbidities, and practice style, but should include the following:

1. Adequate intravenous (IV) access (large-bore peripheral IV line, rapid-infusion catheter, and/or central venous introducer)
2. Standard American Society of Anesthesiologists (ASA) monitors and arterial line (for invasive hemodynamic monitoring and lab draws), with or without a central line (for invasive hemodynamic monitoring, infusions, and/or medication administration)
3. Warming blankets
4. Fluid warmers and/or a rapid-infusion device
5. Adequate blood products (PRBCs, FFP, cryoprecipitate, platelets)
6. Ready access to laboratory results

Resuscitation for elective surgery

The ASA has published guidelines on perioperative blood transfusions. Although these recommendations do not specifically address massive transfusions, they are useful to review, particularly those regarding blood loss and transfusion in the setting of elective surgery. The members of the guideline committee agreed that RBCs should usually be given when the hemoglobin is <6 g/dl and are usually not necessary when the hemoglobin is >10 g/dl, and that between the two values, clinical judgment should be applied to determine the need for a transfusion. The guidelines suggest that platelets be administered when the platelet count is <50,000/dl. The committee recommends checking coagulation studies, if possible, prior to the transfusion of FFP. FFP transfusion is indicated for a prothrombin time (PT) > 1.5 times normal or for an activated partial thromboplastin time (aPTT) > 2 times normal and should be given in doses calculated to achieve a minimum of 30% of plasma factor concentrations. Last, the ASA's recommendations regarding cryoprecipitate are to administer it when the fibrinogen level is <80 to 100 mg/dl.

In the setting of elective surgery, tissue trauma is controlled and thus less extensive; blood loss is usually more predictable,

and patients are kept normothermic and normovolemic. Resuscitation is initially started with crystalloids and colloids to maintain normovolemia. As the blood loss becomes more significant, PRBCs are administered, followed by FFP and platelets – typically as guided by laboratory studies. Thus, coagulopathy is less common, and if it occurs, it is usually dilutional in origin. In a study of elective surgical patients, when normovolemia and a normal hemoglobin were maintained, abnormalities of the PT and the aPTT were found to occur after the transfusion of 12 U of PRBCs, and thrombocytopenia did not occur until after transfusion of 20 U. Similarly, in a study of ASA I and ASA II patients undergoing elective surgical procedures and resuscitated with plasma-poor RBC concentrates, critical hemostatic levels of fibrinogen and platelets were calculated to occur at losses of 1.42 and > 2 calculated blood volumes, respectively.

Resuscitation for trauma

As noted previously, massive blood loss and transfusion in a trauma patient is different from that in a patient undergoing an elective surgical procedure, for the following reasons: The initial resuscitation may be significantly delayed and is frequently complicated by hypothermia, acidosis, hypovolemic shock, and a predisposition to DIC. Prior to arrival at the hospital, patients typically receive only crystalloids, and even after arrival, the administration of RBCs may be delayed while blood typing is performed. The delay will be even greater for FFP and platelets because of the length of time required to thaw, prepare, and issue type-compatible products.

Traditionally, trauma transfusion protocols have called for 4 to 6 U of RBCs prior to administration of FFP. These empiric guidelines are based on washout equations and models that assume a stable circulating volume, which is almost never present in severely injured trauma patients who receive massive transfusions. Additionally, many of the initial studies and protocols were developed when whole blood or modified whole blood products were the standard of care. More recently, the medical literature on massive transfusion in trauma suggests that coagulopathy is common and, once present, is difficult to correct. Early and intensive therapy with plasma and platelets appears to be associated with better patient outcomes. A reasonable goal is to keep the international normalized ratio (INR) < 1.7, recognizing that in the setting of massive transfusion, the INR is unlikely to be normal.

Hirshberg et al. developed a mathematical model that captures the interactions among bleeding, hemodynamics, hemodilution, and replacement as they happen during massive hemorrhage. They investigated the time interval to the subhemostatic values of coagulation studies for a range of replacement strategies. Their model demonstrates that the sentinel event for the development of coagulopathy is the prolongation of the PT (to >1.8 times normal) and it occurs early in the resuscitation. To prevent coagulopathy, the optimal replacement ratios are 2 U of FFP for every 3 U of PRBCs, or concurrent transfusion of FFP and PRBCs. In a retrospective review of trauma patients who received a massive transfusion within the first 24 hours of admission to the intensive care unit (ICU) of a single hospital, transfusion with a traditional protocol (6 U of RBCs prior to FFP administration) before ICU admission was associated with coagulopathy and the severity of the coagulopathy was correlated with mortality. Following ICU admission and initiation of resuscitation using a 1:1 ratio of FFP to RBCs, the coagulopathy improved. The authors concluded that more aggressive early intervention to correct coagulopathy might be effective in decreasing blood requirements and improving outcomes. Similarly, Malone et al. suggested that the prevention of coagulopathy is superior to its treatment, and in trauma patients at risk for massive transfusion, a ratio of 1:1:1 (RBCs to FFP to platelets) appears to be associated with improved outcome. While provocative, these and similar studies are limited by their retrospective nature. Currently, it remains unclear whether patients survived because they received more plasma, or whether the patients who were less ill after trauma simply lived long enough for plasma to be thawed, and thus happened to receive a higher ratio of FFP to RBCs. Prospective studies in this area are badly needed.

Medical therapy
Recombinant activated factor VII

Recombinant activated factor VII (rFVIIa) was licensed for the treatment of bleeding associated with hemophilia in patients who have antibodies inactivating factor VIII and IX. It is believed to act by binding to tissue factor at the site of injury, generating thrombin, and activating platelets. Use of rFVIIa has been expanded in an attempt to minimize bleeding complications and transfusion requirements associated with major surgery and trauma. Trials investigating these indications for rFVIIa have had variable results. In a small randomized trial of rFVIIa versus placebo in patients undergoing transabdominal prostatectomy, administration of rFVIIa was associated with a 50% reduction in blood loss and elimination of transfusion of blood products, whereas 60% of patients randomly assigned to the placebo arm required transfusion. Conversely, studies in patients undergoing liver transplantation or liver resection, showed little benefit in patients who received rFVIIa versus placebo. Moreover, in two separate randomized controlled studies of patients undergoing cardiopulmonary bypass, administration of rFVIIa reduced the need for blood products, although in one of the trials, rFVIIa was associated with an increased incidence of acute renal failure. In a multicenter, randomized, controlled trial of rFVIIa in patients with blunt or penetrating trauma, administration of rFVIIa resulted in a reduction of blood transfusions in those with severe blunt trauma. In patients with penetrating trauma, there was a trend toward a reduced transfusion requirement, but the difference failed to reach clinical significance. A statistically significant difference in survival was not demonstrated. In summary, use of rFVIIa in trauma patients is controversial, and rFVIIa is not approved for this patient population.

There are trials under way investigating these issues, but until further data are available, use of rFVIIa in trauma patients should be individualized and this agent should be used with caution.

Complications
Citrate toxicity

Citrate, which binds calcium, is used as an anticoagulant in stored blood products, and FFP and platelets are the major sources of citrate. Following transfusion, citrate is rapidly metabolized by the liver and, as such, usually has little effect on plasma ionized calcium levels. However, in patients with hypothermia, massive transfusion, diminished liver perfusion, or hepatic dysfunction, and in those undergoing liver transplantation (i.e., during the anhepatic phase), citrate toxicity and the resultant decrease in ionized calcium with associated hypotension and decreased myocardial contractility may become clinically important.

In the setting of massive transfusion, ionized calcium levels should be followed at regular intervals. Ionized calcium levels are preferred because the total plasma calcium level will include the portion bound by citrate and thus may not accurately reflect the free plasma calcium. Hypocalcemia should be treated with calcium chloride rather than calcium gluconate because with the latter, liver metabolism of gluconate is required for the release of calcium.

Hyperkalemia

Over time, potassium leaks out of stored RBCs into the extracellular storage fluid because of impaired membrane integrity and diminished Na^+/K^+ adenosine triphosphatase function. With transfusion, this abnormality is rapidly reversed; consequently, hyperkalemia from massive transfusion is very uncommon. More common causes of hyperkalemia in this patient population include significant soft tissue damage from trauma or renal impairment. Regardless of the etiology, treatment includes calcium chloride administration, glucose and insulin, and bicarbonate as appropriate.

Acid–base disturbances

The pH of stored blood products is significantly acidotic owing to two factors: the acidity of the storage media and the accumulation of cell metabolites over time. Following transfusion, the metabolites (CO_2 and lactic acid) are rapidly cleared and the RBCs' buffering capacity is restored. Anecdotally, some have observed a transient metabolic alkalosis following transfusion, which some have is attributed to citrate metabolism by the liver into bicarbonate. Thus, even in the setting of massive transfusion, acidosis from transfusion itself is uncommon. Persistent acidosis in the setting of transfusion should prompt a careful evaluation for more likely causes, particularly inadequate tissue perfusion and hypovolemia, rather than empiric treatment with bicarbonate.

Suggested readings

Balldin BC, McKinley BA. Fresh frozen plasma should be given earlier to patients requiring massive transfusion. *J Trauma* 2007; 62:112–119.

Boffard KD, Riou B, Warren B, et al. Recombinant factor VIIa as adjunctive therapy for bleeding control in severely injured trauma patients: two parallel randomized, placebo-controlled, double-blind clinical trials. *J Trauma* 2005; 59:8–18.

Cosgriff N, Moore EE, Sauaia A, Kenny-Moynihan M, Burch JM, Galloway B. Predicting life-threatening coagulopathy in the massively transfused trauma patient: hypothermia and acidosis revisited. *J Trauma* 1997; 42:857–861.

Ferrara A, MacArthur JD, Wright HK, et al. Hypothermia and acidosis worsen coagulopathy in the patient requiring massive transfusion. *Am J Surg* 1990; 160: 515–518.

Friederich PW, Henny CP, Messelink EJ, et al. Effect of recombinant activated factor VII on perioperative blood loss in patients undergoing retropubic prostatectomy: double-blind placebo-controlled randomized trial. *Lancet* 2003; 361:1138.

Gonzalez EA, Moore FA, Holcomb JB, et al. Fresh frozen plasma should be given earlier to patients requiring massive transfusion. *J Trauma* 2007; 62:112–119.

Hardy JF, de Moerloose P, Samama CM. The coagulopathy of massive transfusion. *Vox Sanguinis* 2005; 89:123–127.

Hess JR, Zimrin AB. Massive blood transfusion for trauma. *Curr Opin Hematol* 2005; 12:488–492.

Hess JR, Lawson JH. The coagulopathy of trauma versus disseminated intravascular coagulation. *J Trauma* 2006; 60:S12–S19.

Hiipala ST, Myllyla GJ, Vahtera EM. Hemostatic factors and replacement of major blood loss with plasma-poor red cell concentrates. *Anesth Analg* 1995; 81:360–365.

Hirshberg A, Dugas M, Banes EI, Scott BG, Wall MJ, Mattox KL. Minimizing dilutional coagulopathy in exsanguinating hemorrhage: a computer simulation. *J Trauma* 2003; 54: 454–463.

MacIntyre AL, Hebert PC. Can we safely restrict transfusion in trauma patients? *Curr Opin Crit Care* 2006; 12:575–583.

Malone DL, Hess JR, Fingerhut A. Massive transfusion practices around the globe and a suggestion for a common massive transfusion protocol. *J Trauma* 2006; 60:S91–S96.

Mannucci PM, Levi M. Prevention and treatment of major blood loss. *N Engl J Med* 2007; 356:2301–2311.

Practice guidelines for perioperative blood transfusion and adjuvant therapies: an updated report by the American Society of Anesthesiologists Task Force on Perioperative Blood Transfusion and Adjuvant Therapies. *Anesthesiology* 2006; 105:198–208.

Wojciechowski PJ, Samol N, Walker J. Coagulopathy in massive transfusion. *Int Anesthesiol Clin* 2005; 43:1–20.

Chapter 69

Normovolemic hemodilution, perioperative blood salvage, and autologous blood donation

Thomas J. Graetz

Normovolemic hemodilution, preoperative autologous blood donation, and perioperative blood salvage are techniques that may limit the need for allogeneic blood transfusions. These are all forms of autologous transfusion, and some may even be acceptable to Jehovah's Witnesses because the blood is able to stay in continuity with the body. By limiting allogeneic blood transfusions, these techniques can conserve blood resources and limit the complications associated with them. Allogeneic transfusions should be used judiciously because they may cause alloimmunization, immunomodulation, bacterial and/or viral infection, transfusion reactions (e.g., febrile, hemolytic), and transfusion-related acute lung injury (TRALI). These techniques may all be used as part of an integrated approach to reduce the use of allogeneic blood. They may play an even larger role in patients who refuse allogeneic blood transfusions (Jehovah's Witnesses) or have rare blood phenotypes (Bombay), antibodies to common red cell antigens (anti-Kp[b], anti-Js[b]), or multiple alloantibodies (anti-c, -Fya, -S), making crossmatch difficult.

Acute normovolemic hemodilution (intraoperative autologous donation)

Acute normovolemic hemodilution (ANH) is a technique described in the 1950s. Relative anemia is iatrogenically induced by harvesting a patient's whole blood and returning an acellular substitute (e.g., crystalloid) to maintain normovolemia. A large portion of the patient's red cell mass is harvested and stored in anticoagulant-filled blood storage bags prior to major blood loss occurring in the surgical field. When surgical bleeding occurs, the patient loses lower-hematocrit (Hct) blood, thus reducing actual red cell loss. The harvested blood is reinfused after the major blood loss has occurred, or sooner if necessary to maintain the target hemoglobin level. Appropriate patient selection for preoperative hemodilution is an important issue. Some criteria have been developed by Kreimeier (Table 69.1). These are guidelines and are not a universally accepted standard. Each patient's comorbidities and clinical picture must be addressed individually by the clinician. The benefits of normovolemic hemodilution are greatest when the starting hemoglobin is high, the target hemoglobin is low, and the blood loss is high. Kreimeier proposed using an estimated blood loss of 30% of the total blood volume; however, a more recent analysis suggests the

estimated blood loss may need to be closer to 70% of the average patient blood volume to save 1 U of red cells.

One essential component of normovolemic hemodilution is calculation of the amount of blood to be removed. A commonly used integrative equation was described by Bourke et al. as blood loss = estimated blood volume (EBV) × natural log of the ratio of initial to final Hct. This logarithmic equation may be approximated by blood loss = EBV × (change in Hct) × (3 − average Hct). A more recent iterative model has been described by Meier and accounts for some factors potentially leading to an overestimation of blood loss by 15% to 20% (homogeneous distribution of red cells in large and small vessels, continuous and simultaneous substitution of the blood, and constancy of blood volume during dilution process). Crystalloid, colloid, or both are used to replace the intravascular volume. The blood volume is frequently replaced 3:1 with crystalloid or 1:1 with colloid. The replacement ratio at steady state using crystalloid may actually be closer to 5:1. The blood is harvested from an arterial catheter or large-bore venous cannula draining to gravity. The harvesting may start before the induction of anesthesia or after, but harvest should be complete prior to major blood loss. Blood is collected in standard blood collection bags, which can be kept at room temperature for up to 8 hours or refrigerated at 1° to 6°C for up to 24 hours. Blood is reinfused in the reverse order of its harvest. The blood may contain drugs circulating from when it was harvested (e.g., opioids and muscle relaxants).

ANH decreases the blood's oxygen-carrying capacity as hemoglobin is removed. The body maintains adequate oxygen delivery to the tissues by compensatory mechanisms, including an increase in cardiac output and oxygen extraction, as shown in Fig. 69.1. The decrease in blood viscosity allows venous

Table 69.1. Selection criteria for acute normovolemic hemodilution

Estimated blood loss is 1500 ml (30% of blood volume)
Preoperative hemoglobin concentration above 12 mg/dl after correction of normovolemia
Normal electrocardiogram and myocardial function
Absence of restrictive or obstructive lung disease
Absence of renal disease
Absence of liver cirrhosis
Absence of untreated hypertension
Absence of coagulation abnormalities
Absence of infection

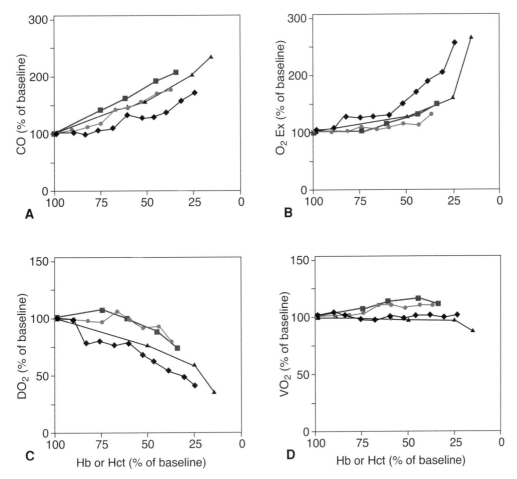

Figure 69.1. Relative changes in (**A**) cardiac output (CO, % of baseline), (**B**) O_2 extraction (O_2-Ex, % of baseline), (**C**) O_2 delivery (DO_2, % of baseline), and (**D**) O_2 consumption (VO_2, % of baseline) during progressive ANH in pigs (■), dogs (■), baboons (▲), and humans (●). Note that the combined increases of CO and O_2 extraction allow maintenance of VO_2, even at very low hemoglobin levels. Reprinted with permission from Jamnicki M, Kocian R, van der Linden P, Zaugg M. Spahn D. Acute normovolemic hemodilution: physiology, limitations, and clinical use. *J Cardiothor Vasc Anesth* 2003; 17(6):747–754.

return to increase, increasing cardiac output as well as central venous pressure. The increased cardiac output occurs through an increase in stroke volume and myocardial contractility with little change in heart rate. The increase in oxygen extraction coupled with the increase in cardiac output allows the oxygen delivery to decrease, whereas the tissue oxygen consumption does not change until a critical hemoglobin level is reached. The critical level of hemoglobin in humans is not known.

ANH is a "point-of-care" technique that eliminates blood wastage, because all collected blood is given back to the patient; it is convenient for patients and has decreased administrative costs associated with testing and collecting of allogeneic blood. Problems with the technique include the additional time and mental energy directed from other aspects of patient care. Additional assays are ordered to monitor the current hemoglobin concentration during dilution and during the operation to guide management. The literature regarding the clinical benefits of the technique is mixed with poor reporting of complications from trials. A recent meta-analysis of all trials was inconclusive; it showed a reduced likelihood of allogeneic transfusion, but there was a substantial amount of heterogeneity among trials,

many of which did not have a well-defined transfusion protocol. The ones with a protocol did not show a benefit with ANH. A recent trial with well-defined triggers showed sparing of allogeneic transfusion in patients undergoing liver resection randomly assigned to undergo hemodilution. ANH is a technique that is not part of routine practice but is supported by transfusion guidelines for specific procedures. Some, although not all, Jehovah's Witness patients will accept ANH, as long as the harvested blood bags are continuously connected with the patient.

Intraoperative blood salvage (cell saver) and postoperative blood salvage

Perioperative blood salvage includes both intra- and postoperative blood salvage as techniques used to recover and transfuse blood lost during an operation. Intraoperative blood salvage (IOBS) had its origins in the 1960s with the first attempts to salvage and re-infuse shed blood by Klebanoff using the Bentley device. In the 1970s the first acceptable surgical blood salvage system was introduced as Cell Saver (Haemonetics, Braintree, MA). The term *cell saver* is now frequently used to describe the strategy of IOBS. During IOBS, an aspiration wand draws blood from the operative field to a reservoir for the aspirated blood. The wand contains dual-chamber tubing that mixes anticoagulant with the aspirated blood. Blood is then taken from the reservoir and added to the centrifuge bowl, where it is spun and washed with normal saline. At least three times the bowl volume is used before the cell washing is considered finished; larger wash volumes lead to removal of more contaminants. The liquid wash is discarded. The washed packed cells are transferred to a bag for transfusion back to the patient. The blood should be filtered through a standard 170-μm filter prior to transfusion. The bowl fill rate and size determine the hematocrit and volume of the washed blood, but a bowl of 250 ml is commonly employed and requires 500 to 750 ml of salvaged blood to properly wash the cells. It delivers cells at a hematocrit of approximately 50% to 70%. Postoperative blood salvage is a technique whereby the contents of wound drains are either infused directly or washed prior to transfusion. The use of unwashed wound blood is falling out of favor for many because of the cell mediators, debris, and other substances that may be present and the ability to wash shed drain blood prior to transfusion. Others continue to practice the transfusion of unwashed wound blood. Those who advocate unwashed wound blood frequently limit the volumes to 500 to 1000 ml because of concerns regarding the non–red cell constituents of the wound blood.

IOBS is applied to a variety of operative domains, including trauma, vascular, cardiac, orthopedic, transplantation, urologic, and gynecologic surgery. Cell saver also has been used in surgical oncology, obstetrics, and bowel operations, but these are areas of some controversy and disagreement. If IOBS is used in these settings, two suction wands are used, one for contaminants and the other for salvaged blood. Previously, contraindications had included obstetric procedures because of the risk of amniotic fluid contamination potentially leading to amniotic fluid embolus. A small but growing body of literature describes the use of IOBS after removal of the placenta, although none of the reports has been large enough to document complete safety from this uncommon albeit potentially fatal event. Similarly, oncologic and bowel procedures (potentially including trauma) have been considered contraindications, although clinical data show its use in these circumstances. Although these data exist, it would not be considered standard practice to use IOBS for oncologic procedures or open bowel.

Autologous blood donation

Autologous donation of blood (preoperative blood donation) is a technique originally described in 1921, but the practice did not spread until subsequent publications in the 1970s. The technique is available to patients undergoing elective procedures that have a high likelihood of transfusion (e.g., redo total joints, multilevel spine cases, or major vascular procedures). Parturients who are at increased risk of peripartum hemorrhage (as in placenta previa) or who have multiple antibodies or rare blood types may also be candidates for this technique. Preoperative

Table 69.2. Contraindications to autologous blood donation

Active bacterial infection or evidence of infection

Significant aortic stenosis

Unstable angina

High-grade left main coronary artery disease

Myocardial infarction or stroke within 6 mo prior to donation

Cyanotic heart disease

Uncontrolled hypertension

Prolonged fainting episode during prior blood donation or history of epilepsy

Impaired placental blood flow (e.g., preeclampsia, diabetes, intrauterine growth retardation)

Other significant disease that has not yet been optimized preoperatively

blood should not be collected if the likelihood of transfusion is low because of the small but real risks of blood donation and the increased risk of blood transfusion if autologous blood is collected, thereby predisposing to perioperative anemia. An additional problem is the wastage of a collected but untransfused unit, thus increasing the overall expense of autologous blood.

Autologous donation requires an order from a physician. This is a decision the anesthesiologist and surgeon make based on a variety of factors that affect the eligibility of the patient for preoperative blood donation. Factors that have an impact on this decision include the likelihood of transfusion for a particular procedure, the surgeon's operative experience, the patient's medical comorbidities, and the patient's motivation to donate preoperatively. Additionally, the patient should meet certain criteria at the time of donation: Hemoglobin must be ≥ 11 g/dl, all donations are to occur more than 72 hours prior to the anticipated surgery, and a donation may not be made if the patient is at risk for bacteremia. Some contraindications to autologous donation are shown in Table 69.2, but others may disagree with some of these, having shown safe donation can occur in patients undergoing various cardiac procedures. Additional consideration should be given to patients with congestive heart failure and cerebrovascular disease. The ultimate decisions rest with the responsible clinicians and patient, weighing the risks, benefits, and alternatives for each patient with special emphasis on whether the risks of allogeneic blood transfusion outweigh the risks of donation.

Oral iron supplementation should be started prior to initial unit donation and continue afterward to mitigate iron-limited erythropoiesis; care should also be taken to limit the side effects of oral iron supplementation. Erythropoietin may be used in autologous donation programs to increase red cell production during autologous donation, although this currently is an off-label use in the United States. The effectiveness of this technique varies based on the dose used in the treatment regimen, the route of administration (intravenous vs. subcutaneous), and the degree and underlying cause of the anemia. Autologous units are generally donated at 1-week intervals, and the last unit is generally donated at least 1 week prior to the scheduled procedure. The total number of collected units is at the discretion of the ordering physician and the director of the transfusion service. An essential part of this technique is the ability of the patient to produce enough new red blood cells to replace the harvested cells, thereby reaching the goal number of units. The factors limiting harvest of additional units are frequently an inadequate hemoglobin level and the limited time frame available to collect blood units because of expiration dates of previously collected units. One possible approach, infrequently used, is freezing previously donated units of blood. This can prolong blood's shelf life, but also leads to some cell lysis during the freeze/thaw process; it also is time-consuming and expensive. The blood units are collected in standard collection bags and preservative solutions. If a unit is collected and stored as whole blood, it can be refrigerated for 35 days. The blood can be separated into its constituent components (with red cell shelf life possibly being extended to 42 days using AS-1 or another additive solution) but is frequently kept as whole blood. Autologous blood is not allowed to enter the general pool of allogeneic blood under most circumstances.

As outlined in Table 69.3, transfusion of autologous blood is not without risk. One risk is the potential for volume overloading the patient, a risk that is smaller if whole blood is used rather than packed cells. The same criteria or "trigger" (a topic outside the scope of this chapter) should be used for both allogeneic and autologous blood when deciding whether to transfuse blood, because the greatest risk to the patient is administrative in nature. If a patient who has autologous blood available is going to be transfused, great care should be taken to transfuse the autologous unit prior to the allogeneic blood. The oldest unit of blood should generally be transfused first to prolong the fixed shelf life of each collected autologous unit.

Perioperative collection of blood components including platelets is an area some have found beneficial, but it is not a routine practice and is currently not recommended for blood conservation for cardiac procedures involving cardiac bypass. Blood component collection can be performed with a standard cell salvage machine by altering the specifics of the centrifugation to optimize the collection of the components being collected. Blood is aspirated into the centrifuge bowl through a large venous access site (e.g., an introducer side port) and then separated into its components in the centrifuge bowl. The various components can then be given back to the patient as indicated during the procedure. All components are returned at the end of the procedure.

Normovolemic hemodilution, preoperative autologous blood donation, and perioperative blood salvage can all reduce the use of allogeneic blood. Nevertheless, how to best use these techniques remains controversial and merits further investigation.

Suggested readings

AABB Standards for Blood Banks and Transfusion Services. 21st ed. American Association of Blood Banks; 2002: Chapter 5.

Adrianus FCM, Moonen NT, Knoors JJ, et al. Pilot retransfusion of filtered shed blood in primary total hip and knee arthroplasty: a prospective randomized clinical trial. *Transfusion* 2007; 47(3):379–384.

Bryson GL, et al. Does acute normovolemic hemodilution reduce perioperative allogeneic transfusion? A meta-analysis. *Anesth Analg* 1998; 86:9–15.

Bourke DL, Smith TC. Estimating allowable hemodilution. *Anesthesiology* 1974; 41:609–612.

Christenson JT, et al. Plateletpheresis before redo CABG diminishes excessive blood transfusion. *Ann Thorac Surg* 1996; 62:1373–1379.

Dietrich W, et al. Autologous blood donation in cardiac surgery: reduction of allogeneic blood transfusion and cost-effectiveness. *J Cardiothor Vasc Anesth* 2005;19:589–596.

Fontana JL. Oxygen consumption and cardiovascular function in children during profound intraoperative normovolemic hemodilution. *Anesth Analg* 1995; 80:219–225.

Goodnough LT, et al. Increased preoperative collection of autologous blood with recombinant human erythropoietin therapy. *N Eng J Med* 1989; 321:1163–1168.

Goodnough LT, et al. Erythropoietin therapy. *N Engl J Med* 1997; 336:933–938.

Goodnough LT, et al. Transfusion medicine. *N Engl J Med* 1999; 340:438–447; 525–533.

Goodnough LT, et al. A randomized trial comparing acute normovolemic hemodilution and preoperative autologous blood donation in total hip arthroplasty. *Transfusion* 2000; 40:1054–1057.

Grant FC. Auto transfusion. *Ann Surg* 1921; 74:253–254.

Guyton AC, Richardson TQ. Effect of hematocrit on venous return. *Circ Res* 1961; 9:157.

Habler OP. The effect of acute normovolemic hemodilution on myocardial contractility in anesthetized dogs. *Anesth Analg* 1996; 83:451–458.

Hansen E, Pawlik M. Reasons against the retransfusion of unwashed wounds blood. *Transfusion* 2004; 44:45S–53S.

Jamnicki M, et al. Acute normovolemic hemodilution: physiology, limitations, and clinical use. *J Cardiothor Vasc Anesthesia* 2003; 17:747–754.

Kanter MH, et al. Preoperative autologous blood donations before elective hysterectomy. *JAMA* 1996; 276:798–801.

Kreimeier U. Hemodilution in clinical surgery: state of the art 1996. *World J Surg* 1996; 9:1208–1217.

Linden JV, et al. Transfusion errors in New York State: an analysis of 10 years' experience. *Transfusion* 2000; 40:1207–1213.

Table 69.3. Autologous blood donation

Advantages	Disadvantages
Prevents transfusion-transmitted disease	Does not eliminate risk of bacterial contamination
Prevents red cell alloimmunization	Does not eliminate risk of ABO incompatibility error
Supplements the blood supply	Is more costly than allogeneic blood
Provides compatible blood for patients with alloantibodies	Results in wastage of blood that is not transfused
Prevents some adverse transfusion reactions	Subjects patients to perioperative anemia and increased likelihood of transfusion
Provides reassurance to patients concerned about blood risks	

Matot I, et al. Effectiveness of acute normovolemic hemodilution to minimize allogeneic blood transfusion in major liver resections. *Anesthesiology* 2002; 97:794–800.

Meier J, et al. New mathematical model for the correct prediction of the exchangeable blood volume during acute normovolemic hemodilution. *Acta Anaesthesiol Scand* 2003; 47:37–45.

Monk TG, et al. A prospective randomized comparison of three blood conservation stragegies for radical prostatectomy. *Anesthesiology* 1999; 91:24–33.

Newman MM, Hamstra R, Block M. Use of banked autologous blood in elective surgery. *JAMA* 1971; 218:861–863.

Nieder AM, Manoharan M, Yang Y, Soloway MS. Intraoperative cell salvage during radical cystectomy does not affect long-term survival. *Urology* 2007; 69:881–884.

Ozmen V, McSwain NE, Nichols RL, et al. Autotransfusion of potentially culture-positive blood in abdominal trauma: preliminary data from a prospective study. *J Trauma* 1992; 32:36–39.

Perioperative blood transfusion and blood conservation in cardiac surgery: the Society of Thoracic Surgeons and the Society of Cardiovascular Anesthesiologists Clinical Practice Guideline. *Ann Thorac Surg* 2007; 83:S27–S86.

Potter P. Perioperative apheresis. *Transfusion* 2004; 44:54S–57S.

Practice guidelines for perioperative blood transfusion and adjuvant therapies: an updated report by the American Society of Anesthesiologists Task Force on Perioperative Blood Transfusion and Adjuvant Therapies. *Anesthesiology* 2006; 105(1): 198–208.

Reeder GD. Autotransfusion theory of operation: a review of the physics and hematology. *Transfusion* 2004; 44:35S–39S.

Shippy CR, Appel PL, Shoemaker WC. Reliability of clinical monitoring to assess blood volume in critically ill patients. *Crit Care Med* 1984; 12:107.

Thomas MJ, Gillon J, Desmond MJ. Consensus conference on autologous transfusion. Preoperative autologous donation. *Transfusion* 1996; 36:633–639.

Waters JH. Indications and contraindications of cell salvage. *Transfusion* 2004; 44:40S–44S.

Weiskopf RB. Efficacy of acute normovolemic hemodilution assessed as a function of fraction of blood volume lost. *Anesthesiology* 2001; 94:439–446.

Yamanda T, Mori H, Ueki M. Autologous blood transfusion in patients with placenta previa. *Acta Obstet Gynecol Scand* 2005; 84(3):255–259.

Cardiac Anesthesia

Stanton K. Shernan, editor

Cardiac physiology

Nelson L. Thaemert and Rena Beckerly

Introduction

A thorough understanding of cardiovascular physiology is essential for the practice of anesthesia. Heart rate (HR), blood pressure, cardiac rhythm, systemic tone, electrolytic balance, and myocardial oxygen consumption are all examples of variables to be considered part of an anesthetic, and understanding their role in cardiac physiology is important to the cerebral, scientific aspects of anesthesia and to its safe and practical delivery to patients.

The heart and circulatory blood vessels comprise the cardiovascular system, and function to provide oxygen and nutrients to the body and remove carbon dioxide and byproducts of metabolism. The heart can be considered two pumps that exist in series, separated by both the pulmonary and systemic circulatory vascular beds. As blood is perfused through the pulmonary circulation, oxygen is taken up and carbon dioxide is eliminated across the alveolar–capillary membrane. In the systemic circulation, oxygen and nutrients are delivered to perfused tissues, and carbon dioxide and metabolic wastes are removed.

Anatomy of the heart

Chambers

Anatomically, the heart is composed of four chambers, two atria and two ventricles; functionally, it is divided into two separate circulatory pumps. One pump delivers deoxygenated blood from the venous system to the pulmonary circulation, and the other delivers oxygenated blood from the lungs to the systemic circulation. Each pump consists of an atrium, which serves as a filling chamber and priming pump, and a ventricle, which serves as a pulsatile pumping chamber. Four valves exist to ensure forward flow of blood as the heart contracts. Myocardial contraction and pulsatile ejection of blood occur through a series of complex electrical and mechanical events. Understanding these concepts is essential to developing an appreciation of cardiac physiology.

Coronary blood supply

Blood is supplied to myocardium through the coronary arteries. The right and left coronary arteries arise from the aortic root and run on the surface of the heart, giving branches that supply the myocardium. Blood flows from the epicardium to the endocardial vessels to meet the metabolic demands of the heart. Thereafter, blood drains into the coronary sinus and the small anterior cardiac veins, where it empties into the right atrium. In addition, a small amount of blood drains directly into the right ventricle via the thebesian veins. Approximately 85% of coronary venous blood is returned to the right atrium through the coronary sinus.

The coronary anatomy of the heart is depicted in Fig. 70.1. The right coronary artery (RCA) exits from the aortic root and travels in the atrioventricular (AV) groove between the right atrium and ventricle. It supplies blood to the right atrium and right ventricle, and in 70% of people becomes the posterior descending artery (PDA). This anatomic configuration is known is a "right dominant" circulation. In 10% of people, the PDA arises as a branch of the left circumflex artery and is referred to as "left dominant." Finally, in about 20% of people, the PDA is supplied by both the RCA and circumflex artery and is classified as "codominant." The PDA travels in the posterior interventricular groove on the back wall of the heart between the right and left ventricles, and supplies blood to the inferior wall of the left ventricle.

The left main coronary artery exits from the aortic root and shortly divides into the left anterior descending (LAD) artery and the circumflex artery. The LAD artery travels in the anterior interventricular groove between the right and left ventricles, giving rise to the diagonal branches (D1 and D2). It supplies blood to the anterior wall of the left ventricle and the interventricular septum. The circumflex artery wraps around the left side of the heart in the AV groove between the left atrium and ventricle, giving rise to the obtuse marginal arteries (OM1 and OM2). It supplies blood to the lateral wall of the left ventricle. In some patients, a third branch called the ramus originates between the LAD and circumflex arteries. Blood supply to a large portion of the left ventricle is dependent on blood supply from the left main coronary artery. In hearts with left dominant circulation, in which the PDA circulation arises from the circumflex, all the left ventricular (LV) blood supply is dependent on a patent left main coronary artery. Fig. 70.2 depicts the typical blood supply to the different walls of the left ventricle.

Blood supply to the conduction system is variable. The sinoatrial (SA) node is perfused by the RCA in 60% of people,

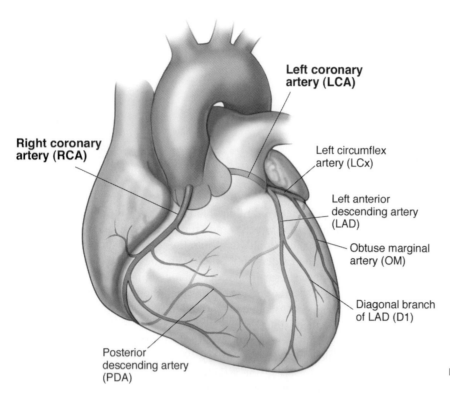

Figure 70.1. Coronary anatomy of the heart.

and the LAD in the remaining 40%. The arterial supply to the AV node is generally determined by the dominance of the circulation. The AV nodal artery arises from the RCA in right dominant hearts, from the left circulation in left dominant hearts, and from the RCA in 75% of codominant hearts. The bundle of His has a dual blood supply from the PDA and LAD.

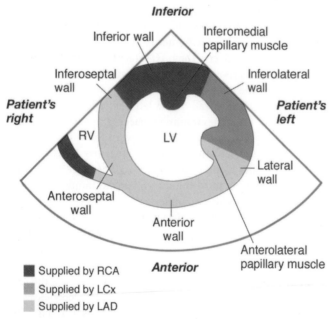

Figure 70.2. Transesophageal echocardiographic view of ventricular walls and coronary blood supply in a right dominant heart.

Blood supply to the papillary muscles tends to correlate with their anatomic location within the ventricles. The anterolateral papillary muscle, which attaches to both the anterior and lateral walls of the left ventricle, has a dual blood supply from both the LAD and circumflex arteries. The posteromedial papillary muscle is attached to the inferior wall of the left ventricle and receives its blood supply exclusively from the PDA. This solitary blood supply makes the posteromedial papillary muscle more susceptible to ischemic dysfunction and postinfarct rupture.

Cellular anatomy and electrical physiology

The heart consists of a specialized striated muscle that exists around a skeleton of connective tissue. Cardiac muscle can be divided into several different types of tissue, including atrial, ventricular, and specialized pacemaker cells. Pacemaker cells exist in various parts of the conduction system, including the SA node, AV node, bundle of His, and Purkinje network, and contain self-excitatory properties that can independently stimulate electrical activity. Low-resistance connections between individual myocardial cells allow the efficient propagation of electrical activity to adjacent cells within the atria or ventricles. Normally, no direct electrical communication exists between the atrial cells and the ventricles. Instead, specialized conductive pathways allow for the rapid and organized propagation of electrical activity from the atria to the ventricles, leading to an efficient filling of the ventricles, followed by a synchronized, pulsatile ejection of blood to the circulation.

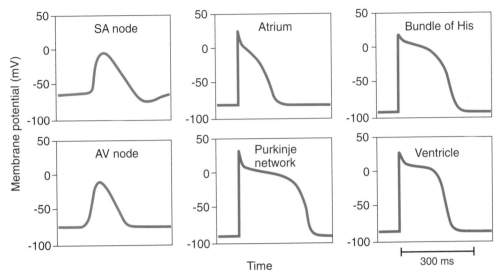

Figure 70.3. Cardiac action potential in various fibers of the heart.

Action potentials

Like other conductive cells, myocardial cell membranes are relatively impermeable to ions and maintain a membrane resting potential through the activity of Na^+/K^+–adenosine triphosphatase (ATPase). This ionic exchange serves to keep a normal voltage gradient of −80 to −90 mV. When the cell membrane becomes less negative and reaches a threshold value, a characteristic action potential is generated, which raises the membrane potential of the myocardial cell to +20 mV. This depolarizing change in voltage is a result of the opening of both fast-acting sodium channels and slower-acting calcium channels, and results in a rapid spike in action potential followed by a prolonged plateau phase of 0.2 to 0.3 seconds. Electrical balance is then restored through the action of potassium channels, which are responsible for repolarizing the myocardial cell. Following depolarization, the cells are refractory to subsequent depolarizing stimuli for a period of time.

Action potentials may be triggered by electrical impulses or occur spontaneously. Because of differences in the composition of atrial, ventricular, pacemaker, and conductive myocardial cells, the characteristics of action potentials vary with different excitatory tissues throughout the heart (Fig. 70.3). Note the prolonged plateau phases in the ventricle, bundle of His, and Purkinje network, in contrast to the rapid repolarization in the SA and AV nodes. In addition, note the unstable resting membrane potential and spontaneous depolarization in the cells of the SA node.

Cardiac impulse initiation and electrical propagation

Each cardiac cycle is initiated by generation of an action potential in the SA node, located at the posterior junction of the right atrium and the superior vena cava. Pacemaker cells of the SA node differ from other typical myocardial cells because of their relatively leaky cell membrane, permitting a slow influx of sodium and regular spontaneous depolarization, which occurs at a rate of 70 to 80 per minute, thus setting the resting HR.

The electrical impulse generated at the SA node is propagated locally through atrial myocardial cells, culminates in simultaneous atrial contraction, and is ultimately transmitted to the AV node. The AV node, located on the septal wall of the right atrium between the ostium of the coronary sinus and the septal leaflet of the tricuspid valve, serves as a gatekeeper for the fast conduction system to the ventricles. It has an intrinsic spontaneous depolarization rate of 40 to 60 per minute, allowing the faster SA node to set the HR under normal circumstances. Impulses reaching the AV node are delayed by 100 ms, allowing ventricular filling, and are then conducted to the bundle of His. This specialized group of fibers passes into the interventricular septum and divides into the right and left branches to form the Purkinje network that serves to rapidly depolarize both ventricles. The His–Purkinje fibers have the most rapid conduction velocities of any cells in the heart, allowing nearly simultaneous depolarization of the myocardium of both ventricles. The total amount of time for a depolarization to travel from the SA node to the entire ventricle is approximately 200 ms.

Electrocardiogram correlation

The appearance of electrical activity on an electrocardiogram correlates well with the electrical signal propagation described earlier. Once an electrical impulse leaves the SA node to travel across the atrium, it becomes visible as a P wave. The time to conduct across the atria is reflected in the duration of the P wave, and the normal delay within the AV node can be appreciated in the length of the P-R interval. The rapid depolarization of the ventricles is evident in the QRS complex. Any conduction delays within either the right or left Purkinje bundles can be appreciated with proper analysis. Ventricular repolarization is represented by the T wave. The relationship

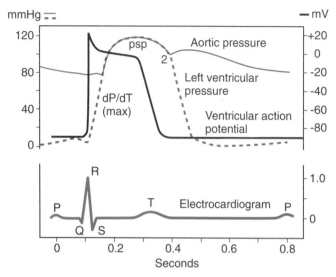

Figure 70.4. Ventricular action potential in relation to other cardiac parameters.

Mechanism of contraction

Myocardial cells contract as a result of the interaction of actin and myosin, two overlapping contractile proteins. Actin is attached to the cell membrane, or sarcolemma, via dystrophin and when allowed to interact with myosin, produces cell shortening. Normally, this interaction is prevented by two regulatory proteins, troponin and tropomyosin, which serve to cover the active binding site on actin. During depolarization, an influx of calcium from the sarcoplasmic reticulum within the cell interacts with troponin, producing a conformational change in these regulatory molecules and exposing the actin-active site to myosin. Through interactions that require ATP, a series of attachments and reengagements between actin and myosin occur, shortening the protein structure within the cell. Returning calcium to the sarcoplasmic reticulum during repolarization allows the troponin–tropomyosin complex to revert to its original confirmation, covering the actin-active site and preventing further interaction between the actin and myosin proteins.

The intracellular calcium change that occurs during the plateau phase of depolarization is insufficient to produce cellular contraction by itself. Instead, the action potential depolarizes the T tubules via dihydropyridine Ca^{2+} channels, which produce an even greater inflow of calcium from the sarcoplasmic reticulum into the cell. Upon the initiation of repolariza-

tion, calcium is pumped back into the sarcoplasmic reticulum and is also extruded extracellularly.

The force of the contraction is directly dependent on the magnitude of the calcium influx from the sarcoplasmic reticulum. The amount of calcium delivered, its rate of delivery, and its rate of removal all directly determine the amount of muscular tension developed, the rate of contraction, and the rate of relaxation. The intracellular second-messenger cyclic adenosine monophosphate (cAMP) directly affects the number of open calcium channels from the sarcoplasmic reticulum. β_1-Adrenergic stimulation results in increased cAMP via stimulatory G proteins, leading to larger intracellular calcium concentrations and more vigorous muscle contractions. Likewise, inhibited breakdown of cAMP from phosphodiesterase inhibitors such as milrinone and theophylline augment the action of calcium. Conversely, acetylcholine produces increased concentrations of cyclic guanosine monophosphate via inhibitory G proteins, leading to inhibition of the generation of cAMP. Other agents affecting strength of contraction include digoxin, which leads to larger Ca^{2+} influx after altering Na^+/K^+-ATPase; glucagon, which increases cAMP via a nonadrenergic receptor; volatile anesthetics, which depress contractility by decreasing entry of Ca^{2+} into cells during depolarization and altering kinetics of its release from sarcoplasmic reticulum; and acidosis, which affects the slow calcium channels of the plateau phase, unfavorably altering intracellular calcium action.

between the ventricular action potential, ventricular ejection, and the electrocardiogram is depicted in Fig. 70.4. Junctional rhythms, atrial and ventricular arrhythmias, varying degrees of AV block, detection of bundle branch blocks, and significance of ventricular escape beats are discussed elsewhere, but can all be appreciated when considering the conduction system and electrocardiograms.

Innervation

Although the nervous system does not directly initiate myocardial beats, it does regulate rhythm and contractility. Central control of the heart originates in the medulla and consists of the cardio-acceleratory and cardio-inhibitory centers. The cardio-acceleratory center sends signals via the sympathetic nerve fibers via T1–4 to the SA and AV nodes, in addition to widely innervating the myocardium. The sympathetic activation from norepinephrine leads to increased chronotropy (faster rate), dromotropy (faster AV conduction), and inotropy (stronger contraction) through increased β_1-adrenergic stimulation and elevations in intracellular cAMP. Additional adrenergic stimulation from circulating epinephrine produces similar effects on the myocardium. Both have additional systemic effects on the vasculature.

The cardio-inhibitory center signals the heart via the vagus nerve to the SA and AV nodes, conducting system, and selected areas of the atrium. Acetylcholine works through muscarinic receptors to produce negative chronotropic, dromotropic, and inotropic effects. Muscarinic effects of acetylcholine include increased conductance for potassium, suppressing the pacemaker current and hyperpolarizing the SA node in phase 4, increasing the time until threshold voltage is reached to initiate a new action potential. Vagal effects tend to have a fast onset and offset, whereas sympathetic influences are more gradual and take longer to reverse.

Cardiac cycle

The rhythmic nature of the heart can be characterized by two energy-requiring phases: systole, during which ventricular contraction occurs, and diastole, when ventricular relaxation occurs. Understanding the relationship of these phases to filling, ejecting, and heart valve mechanics is paramount to understanding cardiac physiology.

The entire systolic and diastolic cardiac cycle can be divided into four distinct phases: isovolumetric contraction, systolic ejection, isovolumetric relaxation, and diastolic filling. At the end of diastole, the ventricle has finished filling and the pressure in the left ventricle and left atrium have equilibrated. At the onset of systole, the ventricle depolarizes, generating a QRS complex; myocardial contraction begins; and the pressure in the left ventricle exceeds the atrial pressure, closing the mitral valve. Isovolumetric contraction continues until the pressure in the ventricle exceeds the diastolic aortic blood pressure, driving open the aortic valve. During systolic ejection of blood, the stroke volume (SV) is pumped from the left ventricle, and the peak pressure generated at this time is the systolic blood pressure. As the ventricle concludes contracting, the pressure in the aorta exceeds the pressure in the left ventricle, closing the aortic valve. The small vascular rebound that occurs here is visible as the dicrotic notch, marking the end of systole and the onset of diastole.

Isovolumetric relaxation is marked by a period of myocyte repolarization and T-wave formation. The ventricle undergoes isovolumetric relaxation until its pressure is less than the left atrial pressure, at which time the mitral valve opens and blood passively starts filling the ventricle. Diastolic filling continues in a passive manner, rapidly at first, then more slowly as the pressures equilibrate, until an atrial contraction is generated, thus actively filling the ventricle. Atrial contraction contributes up to 30% of the filled volume of the ventricle. These events are logically followed in Fig. 70.5.

The cardiac cycle can be represented in different ways – for example, as pressure and volume versus time, as shown in Fig. 70.5, or as pressure versus volume, as indicated in Fig. 70.6.

Several physiologic variables can be appreciated by studying Fig. 70.6. The volume of the left ventricle at the end of diastole is the *end-diastolic volume* (EDV), which has a corresponding *end-diastolic pressure* (EDP). The difference between the end-diastolic volume and the end-systolic volume (ESV) is the SV:

$$SV = EDV - ESV$$

Likewise, the ejection fraction (EF) is the percentage of the EDV ejected with each systolic beat:

$$EF = (EDV - ESV)/EDV = SV/EDV$$

Other variables, including aortic systolic and diastolic pressures, can also be appreciated on a pressure-versus-volume loop.

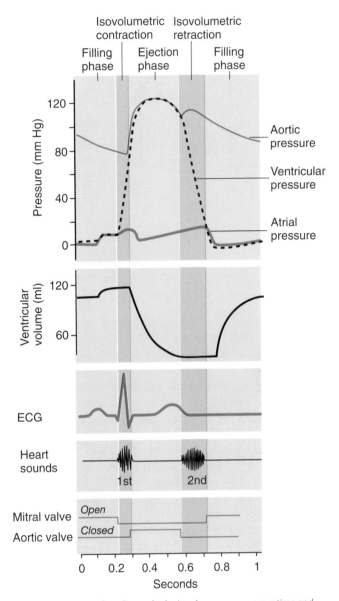

Figure 70.5. Normal cardiac cycle depicted as pressure versus time and volume versus time.

Atrial filling and emptying

Atrial filling occurs in two phases, systole and diastole; atrial emptying also occurs in two phases, passive and active. During systolic ventricular contraction, the atria fill from the venous system. Systole concludes, diastole begins, and once isovolumetric relaxation has allowed the ventricular pressure to decrease sufficiently, the mitral and tricuspid valves open and blood flows passively into the ventricles. However, even as the atria empty into the ventricles, they continue to fill to replace some of the volume passively lost. With the initiation of atrial contraction, the atria empty into the ventricle and no further atrial filling occurs from the veins. Upon initiation of systole, the mitral and tricuspid valves close, ventricular systolic ejection occurs, and atrial filling resumes.

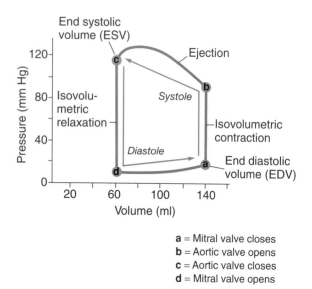

Figure 70.6. Normal cardiac cycle depicted as pressure versus volume.

a = Mitral valve closes
b = Aortic valve opens
c = Aortic valve closes
d = Mitral valve opens

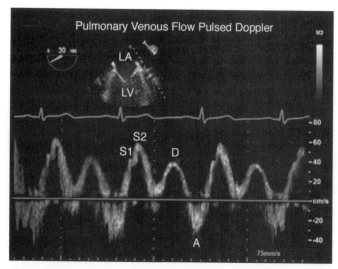

Figure 70.8. Doppler echocardiography of the pulmonary veins.

These elements can be seen on central venous pressure (CVP) tracing (Fig. 70.7). The "a" wave represents atrial contraction with active ventricular filling. Diastole ends and systole begins at the "c" wave, marked by tricuspid valve closure. As the ventricle contracts, the tricuspid annulus is slightly pulled into the ventricle, decreasing the pressure in the atrium, marked by the "x" descent. As the ventricle continues to contract, atrial filling is reflected in the "v" wave. Finally, as the tricuspid valve opens, passive emptying of the atrium into the ventricle occurs, as shown by the "y" descent. This is immediately followed by another a wave as the cycle repeats.

When studied by Doppler echocardiography, this cycle is seen in a slightly different form (Fig. 70.8). Here, the Doppler beam is measuring flow in the pulmonary vein either toward or away from the left atrium. During systole, the prominent up-spike and the much smaller phase represent two phases of systole, S1 and S2, when the atrium is filling from the pulmonary veins toward the Doppler probe near the left atrium. The second prominent hump, the D wave, indicates further forward filling of the atrium during early diastole, when the ventricle is passively being filled through the mitral valve. The down-spike is the A wave, representing a brief reversal in pulmonary venous blood during atrial contraction, when the ventricle is undergoing active filling from a contracted atrium.

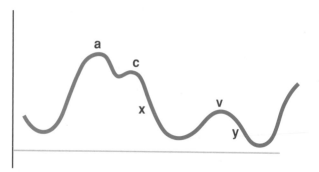

Figure 70.7. Central venous pressure waveform.

Several pathologic conditions can be detected on assessment of a CVP waveform. Large a waves occur during diastole when a pressure gradient exists during atrial contraction. This can be seen when the atrium is contracting against a closed tricuspid valve, such as during premature ventricular systole, or when tricuspid valvular stenosis is present. Prominent v waves may occur during systole when part of the ventricular ejection pressure is communicated through the tricuspid valve, such as during tricuspid regurgitation. Other pathognomonic conditions exist as well, such as a "steep x and y descent," in which the atrial pressure is very elevated and the ventricle is dangerously underfilled, such as in pericardial tamponade.

Ventricular performance

The cardiac cycle represents a unique coordination of both electrical and mechanical events, culminating in ventricular systole (contraction) and diastole (relaxation). The synchronized function of both ventricles is crucial, and factors affecting one side will invariably affect the other.

Systolic function involves ventricular ejection and primarily focuses on the left ventricle. It is often measured by the cardiac output (CO), which is the SV multiplied by HR:

$$CO = SV \times HR.$$

Average SV and HR are approximately 70 ml and 75 bpm, with a cardiac output of 4 to 6 L/min. Thus, the body's entire blood volume circulates through the heart every minute. Because changes in body size require different cardiac outputs to meet basal requirements, the cardiac index is used to account for these differences. The cardiac index is expressed as the cardiac output divided by the body surface area, with a normal range of 2.5 to 4 L/min/m^2.

In addition to cardiac output, other measures of adequacy of function include assessing for appropriate change in cardiac output with exercise and measurement of mixed venous oxygen saturation. A large amount of variability exists in baseline

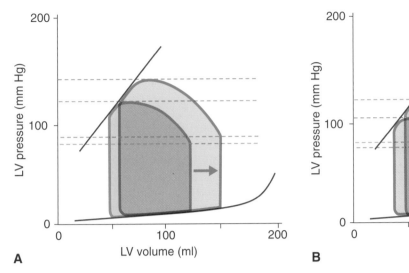

Figure 70.9. Increasing and decreasing preload.

cardiac output, and an abnormal cardiac output is not seen until gross abnormalities exist. However, failure to keep up with higher metabolic demands with exercise can be seen by a lack of an increase in cardiac output when stressed. Similarly, a falling mixed venous oxygen saturation, in which greater proportions of oxygen are extracted from the systemic blood to make up for a lack in rise of cardiac output, is indicative of inadequate ventricular performance.

Heart rate

HR is a major determinant of ventricular function and is affected by autonomic, humoral, and local factors. The intrinsic rate of the SA node is normally set at 70 to 80 bpm. It is influenced by sympathetic and parasympathetic tone, circulating inflammatory mediators, drugs, hormones, and conduction abnormalities. At normal HRs, systolic time occupies approximately one third of the entire cardiac cycle, with diastolic time occupying the remaining two thirds. However, as HR increases, this ratio changes and a lower percentage of time is spent in diastole.

Stroke volume

There are three main determinants of SV: preload, afterload, and contractility. All three variables are subject to a variety of influences, including circulating volume, ventricular compliance, systemic circulatory tone, and autonomic influences, in addition to geometric alterations in the chambers and the presence of valvular dysfunction.

Preload

Preload represents the EDV of the left ventricle and depends on ventricular filling. Starling's law describes the direct proportional relationship between cardiac output and the final volume in the ventricle prior to contraction, LV EDV. As LV EDV increases and the HR is held constant, SV increases until the

muscle fibers become maximally distended. Any further stretch compromises the heart's ability to eject that volume, and no further increase in SV is achieved. In fact, overdistention may lead to a decrease in cardiac output. Clinically, in addition to diminishing cardiac myocyte stretch, this can produce cardiac valvular incompetence.

Preload for both the left and right ventricles depends on ventricular filling, which is most heavily influenced by venous return. Circulating volume, changes in blood volume (position, intrathoracic pressure, pericardial pressure, venous tone), cardiac rhythm, and HR all influence venous return. Although the presence of other pathologic factors, such as severe mitral stenosis or aortic regurgitation, may also play a role in ventricular filling, venous tone and circulating intravascular volume have the greatest role in normal circumstances. For example, increases in venous tone from ephedrine administration or decreases in venous tone from a regional anesthetic can alter LV EDV. Likewise, hypovolemia or fluid resuscitation can also alter LV EDV.

The pressure–volume relationship of the ventricle during diastole is a nonlinear curve that depends on ventricular compliance and is not affected simply by altering the preload. Instead, this diastolic relationship holds true over a variety of filling conditions and describes the corresponding filling pressure required at any given filling volume (Fig. 70.9). Until the point at which maximum stretch is reached, a larger LV EDV produces an increased SV and increased cardiac output at a higher systemic blood pressure.

Ventricular preload is also sensitive to changes in rhythm and HR. As HR increases, diastolic time is reduced and ventricular filling is slightly impaired. Likewise, deviation from a normal sinus rhythm can adversely affect ventricular filling. Perturbation in sinus activity becomes especially crucial in patients with impaired ventricular compliance, which is discussed later.

Clinical assessment of preload may present several challenges. The most important determinant of right ventricular

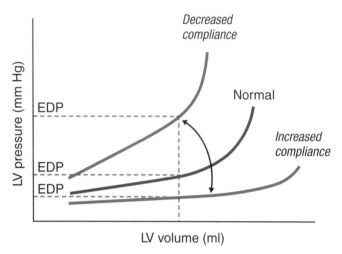

Figure 70.10. Compliance changes altering the EDP–EDV relationship.

filling is venous return, and in the absence of significant pulmonary hypertension, right heart dysfunction, or mitral valvular disease, venous return is also the most important determinant of LV filling. Trends in central venous filling *pressure* can be used to approximate LV filling *volume*. Pulmonary capillary wedge pressure (PCWP) can be used to estimate LV EDP, which with normal ventricular compliance, serves as a good surrogate measurement of LV EDV. However, this requires several assumptions, including insignificant intrathoracic positive end-expiratory pressure and absence of mitral stenosis. Other methods to try to assess the adequacy of ventricular filling include echocardiography, radionuclide imaging, and ventriculography.

Diastolic compliance determines what sort of ventricular filling pressure is generated at any given filling volume. The nonlinear curve describing the diastolic pressure–volume relationship is influenced by factors such as presence of ventricular hypertrophy, ischemia, or pericardial compression (Fig. 70.10).

"Diastolic dysfunction," a concept poorly understood by many, can be explained by examining an EDP–EDV relationship curve. The presence of factors impairing the heart's ability to relax and fill during diastole will shift this curve up and left from normal. The clinical implication is that significantly higher filling pressures may be required to achieve an adequate LV EDV. This may leave patients closer to being in pulmonary edema at what appears to be normal heart sizes. Conversely, in the event the heart deviates from a sinus rhythm, LV EDV may be significantly impaired from the loss of a higher-pressure "atrial kick."

Hearts with pathologically increased compliance are generally those that have been dilated for a long period, allowing for adaptation. Patients with dilated cardiomyopathy or chronic severe aortic insufficiency may have dramatically increased LV EDV with normal filling pressures.

Ventricular EDP–EDV relationships may be difficult to measure, but the presence of impaired relaxation and restricted filling can be assessed with echocardiography by examining inflows across the mitral valve and pulmonary veins, although

that discussion is beyond the scope of this text. However, it is important to note that conditions such as LV hypertrophy and aortic stenosis exist that shift the compliance curve up and to the left, thus requiring active atrial filling. In these situations, assessing CVP, PCWP, or LV EDP may not provide an accurate surrogate for the LV EDV.

Afterload

Afterload represents the tension the ventricle must generate during systole that is sufficient to produce contraction. In normal circumstances, this is influenced by the arterial impedance, but in the presence of aortic stenosis, it is also affected by the additional gradient across the valve. The wall tension the ventricle generates is the force required to reduce its chamber size against a given pressure. For a spherical object, the wall tension is determined by the law of Laplace:

$$\text{Wall tension} = P \times R/2h,$$

where P is the pressure in the chamber, R is the radius of the chamber, and h is the wall thickness. Therefore, hearts ejecting against higher pressures, with larger chambers, generate a higher wall tension. Having a larger wall thickness decreases wall tension but comes at a price of higher oxygen consumption and impaired oxygen delivery, which is discussed later.

In normal circumstances, the pressure the heart must develop wall tension against is determined by the arterial tone, or systemic vascular resistance (SVR). Drawing from Ohm's law, remember that voltage (V) = I (current) × R (resistance), or put another way, the pressure change across a bed of resistance is determined by the current, or flow, multiplied by the resistance:

$$\Delta P = Q \times R \; or \; R = \Delta P/Q,$$

where ΔP is the pressure change, Q is flow, and R is resistance. Therefore:

$$SVR = 80 \times (MAP - CVP)/CO,$$

where MAP is the mean arterial pressure and CVP is the central venous pressure. ΔP, or (MAP − CVP), is simply the pressure change across the vascular bed in question, in this case the systemic circulation, and 80 is a conversion factor to leave the answer in appropriate units. Normal SVR is 900 to 1500 dyne sec/cm^{-5}.

Similarly, the pulmonary vascular resistance (PVR) can be calculated applying the same concepts to the pulmonary vascular bed:

$$PVR = 80 \times (PA \; mean - LAP)/CO,$$

where PA mean is the mean pulmonary arterial pressure and LAP is the left atrial pressure. In normal circumstances, PCWP is substituted for LAP. Normal PVR is 50 to 150 dyne sec/cm^{-5}.

Increases in afterload can *decrease* the cardiac output but may be difficult to conceptualize until analyzing a pressure–volume loop (Fig. 70.11). Increases in afterload do not alter

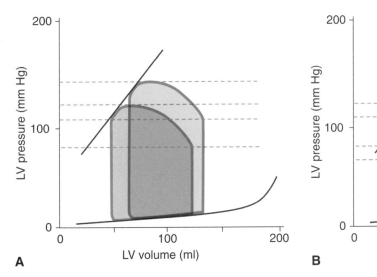

Figure 70.11. Increasing and decreasing afterload.

either the nonlinear EDP–EDV curve, which was previously discussed, or the linear end systolic pressure volume (ESP-ESV) curve, which represents the pressure–volume relationship at which the aortic valve closes at the end of systole. Instead, changes in afterload influence how SV falls between these two curves.

An increase in afterload leads to a higher systemic blood pressure but an earlier closure of the aortic valve, and thus a smaller SV for any given preload. A small amount of physiologic compensation is indicated by a subtle change in preload. The net effect is a higher systemic blood pressure, but with a lower cardiac output. Conversely, a decrease in afterload leads to a lower systemic blood pressure and a larger SV. Clinical examples of extremes of this spectrum include aortic stenosis, in which the ventricular preload must remain very high to have an adequate SV against a very high afterload, and septic shock, in which dilated systemic vascular tone leads to a high cardiac output state despite a low systemic blood pressure.

Contractility

Contractility represents the strength of ventricular contraction and is related to the rate of myocardial muscle shortening during systole. It is an intrinsic property of the muscle and is independent of preload and afterload. Myocardial contractility is influenced by neural, humoral, and pharmacologic factors. In addition, adequate intracellular calcium concentrations can improve myocardial contractility (Table 70.1).

On a pressure–volume loop, contractility is represented by the slope of the linear ESP-ESV relationship. Greater contractility shifts this curve up and to the left, whereas depressed contractility shifts it down and to the right (Fig. 70.12).

Agents that increase contractility lead to a higher systemic blood pressure, a larger SV, and a greater ejection fraction. Agents that decrease contractility lead to a lower systemic blood pressure, a smaller SV, and a decreased ejection fraction.

Changes during exercise

Several changes occur as a normal physiologic response to exercise, including increased HR, SV, and contractility, all to achieve an increase in cardiac output. Hearts that are not capable of mounting a response to this increase in physiologic demand leave the patient with an inability to tolerate the increase in exertion (Fig. 70.13). Changes in preload are still reflected as Starling curves, but the course and shape of the curves are determined by the contractile state of the heart.

Wall motion abnormalities

Regional wall motion abnormalities may lead to a decrease in SV generated under otherwise normal preload and afterload conditions. These abnormalities may be the result of ischemia, old infarction, or intraventricular conduction delays leading to asynchronous contraction. All serve to impair the ability of the ventricle to produce an SV. Normal or enhanced contractility in other regions of the ventricle may be insufficient to compensate

Table 70.1. Factors affecting myocardial contractility

Increase contractility	Decrease contractility
Sympathetic (innervate atria, ventricle, nodes)	Parasympathetic stimulation – minimal
Epinephrine and norepinephrine	Hypoxia, acidosis, hypercapnia
Hypercalcemia	Depletion of catecholamine stores in the heart (as seen in congestive heart failure, chronic hypertension, and elderly patients)
Digitalis	
Glucagon	
	Loss of functioning muscle mass with ischemia/infarction Anesthetics, especially potent inhalational agents, propofol, and thiopental
	Electrolytes: hyperkalemia, hypocalcemia
	Antiarrhythmic agents, including β-blockers and calcium blockers

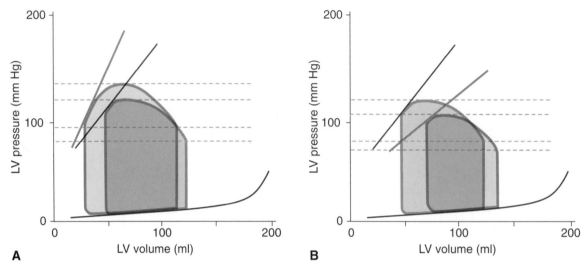

Figure 70.12. Increasing and decreasing contractility.

for hypokinetic or akinetic regional wall segments. It is through this process that patients with ischemic heart disease develop a decrease in SV and ejection fraction.

Valvular abnormalities

The presence of valvular abnormalities may further compromise the ability of the heart to fill and empty in a forward fashion. Any of the four valves may be stenotic or regurgitant. Although valvular disease is discussed in detail elsewhere, it is useful to point out some brief key concepts here and correlate them with pressure–volume loops of the heart.

Aortic stenosis produces a pressure gradient that exists between the left ventricle and aorta. Although *afterload* normally refers to SVR, here it also applies to the additional resistance the ventricle must work against by ejecting against a stenotic valve. Once the stenosis becomes critical, the afterload is dramatically increased. The only way to achieve an adequate SV is to ensure that the ventricle, which has developed worsening compliance, is adequately full. These patients are thus very sensitive to hypovolemia and arrhythmias, and can quickly decompensate or even die with loss of a sinus rhythm. The

very high wall tension generated also leads to greatly increased myocardial oxygen consumption.

Aortic regurgitation leads to diastolic retrograde filling of the left ventricle from the aorta. With time, the ventricle becomes grossly dilated and has an increase in its compliance. Forward flow to the body becomes a function of the difference between the total stroke volume and the diastolic regurgitant fraction. Physiologic conditions that worsen the regurgitation, such as higher aortic pressures and longer diastolic times, will impair forward flow. In addition, if severe, the aortic regurgitation may interfere with ventricular filling from the atrium by prematurely forcing the mitral valve shut once the pressure in the ventricle exceeds that in the atrium.

Mitral stenosis produces a pressure gradient between the left atrium and ventricle. These patients have normal systolic and diastolic pressure–volume relationships, but the ventricle is chronically underfilled. Patients may appear systemically hypovolemic with small SVs and low blood pressures even though they may present with symptoms of heart failure. Maximizing diastolic filling time and maintaining a sinus rhythm allow for optimum ventricular filling. Temporizing patients with inotropes may be an alternative if the ventricle remains grossly underfilled.

Mitral regurgitation leads to retrograde filling of the atrium during systole. Functional forward flow is the difference between the total SV and the systolic regurgitant volume. Higher atrial pressures may predispose patients to pulmonary edema, and higher ventricular systolic pressures will worsen the regurgitant fraction.

Myocardial oxygen supply and demand

Consideration of cardiac physiology, with its variables – including HR, wall tension, and contractility – requires an understanding of myocardial oxygen supply and demand. Myocardial oxygen is delivered via the coronary arteries branching off the aortic root. In contrast to other organs, perfusion to the

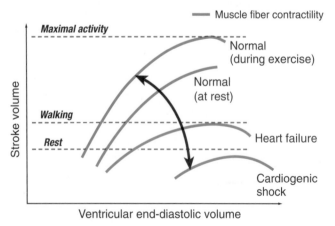

Figure 70.13. Changes in SV and LVEDP with exercise.

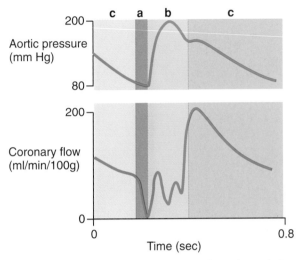

Figure 70.14. LV coronary blood flow during the cardiac cycle Note: a, isovolumetric contraction; b, systolic ejection; and c, diastole.

myocardium occurs intermittently and is timed to the cardiac cycle. Within the LV wall, the pressure generated is similar to the aortic systolic pressure, which can transiently occlude the myocardial perforating arteries. Not until diastole, when the intramyocardial pressure is low, does coronary pressure to the left ventricle occur (Fig. 70.14). The coronary perfusion pressure (CPP) to the left heart is the difference between the aortic diastolic blood pressure (AoDBP) and the LV end diastolic pressure (LVEDP):

$$CPP = AoDBP - LVEDP$$

LVEDP is generally between 10 and 20 mm Hg, so the magnitude of the coronary perfusion gradient to the left ventricle depends greatly on changes in systemic diastolic blood pressure. Conditions that decrease systemic diastolic blood pressure or increase LV end diastolic pressure may lead to decreased coronary perfusion. LV hypertrophy, which decreases overall ventricular wall tension due to increased wall thickness, impairs coronary perfusion by changing compliance and increasing LV end diastolic pressure. In addition, higher intramural pressures and compression of perforating arteries make the ventricle susceptible to subendocardial ischemia.

Perfusion to the right ventricle differs somewhat from that to the left ventricle. Because the intramyocardial pressures within the right ventricle are significantly less than those of the left ventricle, right ventricular myocardial perfusion can occur during both systole and diastole. For this reason, the coronary perfusion gradient to the right ventricle depends more on the systemic mean arterial pressure than the systemic diastolic blood pressure.

Autoregulation of coronary blood flow

In the absence of a blockage in the coronary arteries, coronary blood flow matches myocardial oxygen demand.

Autoregulation of blood flow between perfusion pressures of 50 and 120 mm Hg ensures optimum matching under most normal physiologic conditions. Changes in myocardial oxygen demand produce several effects through autonomic, humoral, and local mechanisms. Sympathetic stimulation produces both α_1- and β_2-adrenergic effects – α_1-induced vasoconstriction affects large-bore arteries, but β_2-induced vasodilation occurs in smaller intramyocardial vessels. The overall effect is for increased myocardial blood flow with sympathetic stimulation, mostly through β_2 stimulation. Likewise, local tissue hypoxia releases adenosine, leading to coronary vasodilation. All these effects help match myocardial oxygen supply to demand.

Myocardial oxygen demand

Myocardial oxygen consumption is influenced by several factors, including basal tissue oxygen consumption, generation of electrical activity, generation of wall tension under varying loading volumes and against varying pressures, and rate of systolic ejections. Hearts that beat faster, have higher filling volumes, and eject against higher pressures consume more oxygen. In addition, hearts that beat faster have less time in diastole. Therefore, increases in HR and diastolic pressure increase consumption and decrease delivery.

Myocardial tissue very efficiently extracts oxygen from arterial blood – typical blood in the coronary sinus has saturations near 30%, compared with 75% for the rest of the body. Any increase in oxygen consumption must be matched by an increase in oxygen delivery through increased coronary blood flow. For patients with a coronary blockage who cannot deliver an increase in coronary blood flow, strategies to minimize increases in myocardial oxygen demand and maximize delivery of oxygen until the blockage can be corrected are a mainstay of treatment.

Conclusion

Understanding cardiac physiology is essential to the perioperative care of patients who present for a variety of procedures. Core concepts of cardiac electrical physiology, systolic and diastolic function, ventricular filling and ejection, and myocardial oxygen supply and demand apply to almost all patients presenting for surgery, regardless of the status of their health. Developing a solid foundation of principles is essential when studying normal cardiac physiology before applying those same principles to patients with a variety of pathologic cardiovascular disorders. Conditions ranging from coronary disease to valvular disorders and hemodynamic changes from interventions such as fluid and drug administration can be explained by building on a strong understanding of cardiac physiology. The reader is advised to revisit these principles as these conditions are elaborated upon in the following chapters.

Cardiovascular pharmacology

Arti Ori and Douglas C. Shook

Introduction

Cardiovascular drugs are used to alter cardiac performance and end-organ blood flow, with the goal of maintaining adequate tissue perfusion and oxygen delivery. The choice of drug depends on the complex interrelationship among preload, contractility, afterload, and the rate and rhythm of the heart. If the patient's hemoglobin level and oxygen saturation are adequate, the cardiac output (CO) becomes an important determinant in oxygen delivery and systemic vascular resistance (SVR) for permitting optimal tissue perfusion. An understanding of these important concepts is integral to choosing among the variety of cardiovascular drugs available.

The central role of calcium

Intracellular calcium levels have a dominant effect on myocardial contractility and smooth muscle vascular tone. During the cardiac action potential, extracellular calcium enters the cell via L-type (slow) calcium channels. Calcium entry triggers calcium release from the sarcoplasmic reticulum (calcium-induced calcium release). The increased free intracellular calcium binds to the cardiac myofilament protein troponin C, which then allows actin to form cross-bridges with myosin and for contraction to occur. For myocardial relaxation, calcium must be removed from troponin C. This is accomplished by decreasing intracellular calcium levels, primarily by reuptake of calcium into the sarcoplasmic reticulum by an energy-dependent process. Calcium is also removed from the cell by ion transport channels in the cell membrane to keep the overall intracellular calcium unchanged with each contraction–relaxation cycle.

This transient increase and decrease of intracellular calcium is central to myocardial contractility. In normal hearts, only about 25% of the cardiac myofilaments are saturated with calcium. This reserve may be activated by drugs that either increase the amount of calcium in the myocyte or sensitize the myofilaments to the calcium already present. Several conditions change the sensitivity of calcium to cardiac myofilaments, and thus the effectiveness of inotropic and vasoactive drugs (Table 71.1).

Calmodulin in vascular smooth muscle modulates the interaction of actin and myosin, leading to vasoconstriction in the presence of intracellular calcium. Thus, in both vascular smooth muscle cells and cardiac myocytes, an increase in intracellular calcium promotes greater contraction, leading to increased vasoconstriction and increased contractility, respectively. All the drugs used to manage myocardial contractility and smooth muscle tone act by altering intracellular calcium.

The most common inotropic drugs augment intracellular calcium by either cyclic adenosine monophosphate (cAMP)-dependent or cAMP-independent mechanisms. β-Adrenergic agonists act via G_s proteins that activate adenylate cyclase, increasing the synthesis of cAMP. Acting as a second messenger, cAMP activates protein kinase A, which phosphorylates a variety of intracellular targets, increasing intracellular calcium for contraction (inotropy) and enhancing its reuptake, promoting relaxation (lusitropy). α-Adrenergic agonists may also increase intracellular calcium, but by a different mechanism. The clinical significance of this mechanism for myocardial contractility is uncertain, but its clinical significance in promoting vasoconstriction in vascular smooth muscle is well known. Phosphodiesterase inhibitors act by inhibiting the breakdown of cAMP, thereby increasing intracellular calcium and contractility (Fig. 71.1).

α-Adrenergic stimulation (catecholamines) and phosphodiesterase III inhibition increase cAMP, which acts via protein kinase A to phosphorylate calcium channel protein, phospholamban, and troponin I. Phosphorylation of calcium channel protein enhances sarcolemmal inward movement of Ca^{2+}, which subsequently increases Ca^{2+} movement from the sarcoplasmic reticulum (SR) through the calcium release channel (ryanodine receptor type 2) to the cytosol (calcium-induced Ca^{2+} release). Digoxin increases cytosolic Ca^{2+} by

Table 71.1. Cardiac myofilament sensitivity to calcium

Decreased sensitivity to calcium	Increased sensitivity to calcium
Acidosis	α-Receptor stimulation
Hypothermia	Myofilament calcium sensitizers
Increased phosphate	Stretching of the myofilaments (preload)
Sepsis	
Ischemia–reperfusion injury	
Myocardial stunning	
Congestive heart failure	

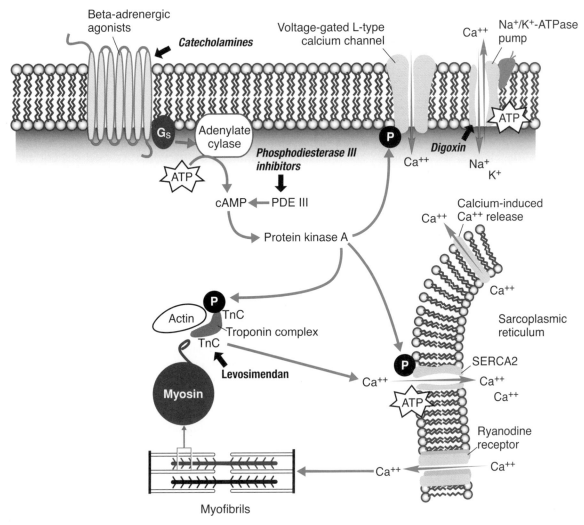

Figure 71.1. Effect of inotropic drugs on intracellular calcium.

inhibition of sarcolemmal Na–K–adenosine triphosphatase and Na–Ca^{2+} exchange. Cytosolic Ca^{2+} binds to troponin C (TnC) and initiates contraction (inotropic effect). Phosphorylation of phospholamban enhances relaxation by increased reuptake of Ca^{2+} back into the SR by the SR Ca^{2+} adenosine triphosphatase isoform 2 (SERCA2; lusitropic effect). Phosphorylation of troponin I enhances the rate of relaxation by decreasing the sensitivity of myofilaments to Ca^{2+}. Levosimendan binds to troponin C during systole and thereby increases the sensitivity of myofilaments to Ca^{2+} without alteration of Ca^{2+} levels.

In the vascular smooth muscle, cAMP and cyclic guanosine monophosphate (cGMP) have the opposite effect on intracellular calcium by promoting its reuptake into the SR, thereby decreasing its availability for contraction. Thus, drugs that increase cAMP, such as β-agonists or phosphodiesterase inhibitors, will promote vasodilation. Nitroglycerin and nitroprusside act by producing nitric oxide, which stimulates the production of intracellular cGMP, promoting vasodilation.

Inotropic drugs

In most patients with depressed CO, taking advantage of Starling's curve by increasing preload will increase stroke volume and CO. If the patient does not respond to preload management, then adding drugs that increase contractility may improve CO and tissue perfusion. Positive inotropic drugs increase cardiac contractility, stroke volume, heart rate, and CO.

The most commonly used inotropic drugs increase CO by increasing the amount of cAMP produced in the cardiac myocyte or inhibiting its breakdown. More cAMP in the cardiac myocyte promotes greater calcium interaction with troponin C, increasing contractility.

The difference among the cAMP-dependent agents is in their effect on the peripheral vasculature. Some are inoconstrictors (increase contractility and increase vasoconstriction), some are inodilators (increase contractility and promote vasodilation), and some have mixed effects on the peripheral vasculature. The choice of inotropic agent depends on the desired "side effect" on the vasculature to promote better tissue perfusion. cAMP-independent inotropes also have effects on the peripheral vasculature that must be anticipated to determine their effect on blood pressure and tissue perfusion. The most commonly used inotropic agents are listed in the following text and summarized in Table 71.2.

Epinephrine (mixed inotrope) is a naturally occurring catecholamine that directly binds to β_1-, β_2-, α_1-, and α_2-receptors, with β effects predominating at lower doses and α effects predominating at higher doses. Therefore, it is an inodilator at lower doses, in which β_1- and β_2-receptors dominate, and an inoconstrictor at higher doses, in which α-receptor stimulation becomes stronger. At higher doses, stroke volume and CO may decrease because of the intense α-receptor stimulation.

Dopamine (mixed inotrope) is another naturally occurring catecholamine, whose effects are dose dependent. Dopamine acts by directly stimulating dopaminergic receptors, as well as β_1-, β_2-, and α_1-receptors, and inducing the release of stored norepinephrine. As with epinephrine, lower doses produce increased contractility and vasodilation, which transitions to α-receptor–mediated vasoconstriction at higher doses. At higher doses, stroke volume and CO may decrease because of the intense α-receptor stimulation.

Dobutamine (inodilator) is a synthetic catecholamine with a strong affinity for β_1-receptors and weaker affinity for β_2-receptors. Its overall effect is to increase contractility and heart rate with mild vasodilation (β_2 effects).

Milrinone (inodilator) is a phosphodiesterase III inhibitor that increases myocyte and vascular smooth muscle cell cAMP by inhibiting its breakdown. Milrinone produces positive inotropy and improved diastolic relaxation (lusitropy). It may induce less tachycardia compared with catecholamine inotropes. It is a potent vasodilator affecting both venous and arterial vascular beds. Loading milrinone may cause hypotension in patients who do not have adequate preload, because of the arterial and venous dilation caused by the drug. It has a longer half-life than a catecholamine drug, which may make it harder to titrate. Milrinone is usually chosen when catecholamine drugs do not produce the desired increase in CO or the clinician wants to take advantage of its vascular dilating properties. It may also have advantages in patients with reduced available β-receptors due to chronic sympathetic stimulation (i.e., congestive heart failure) or blocked by β-receptor antagonists, and may have synergistic inotropic effects when combined with inotropes that act directly through β-receptor activation.

Glucagon (inodilator) binds to the glucagon receptor and causes an increase in intracellular cAMP. This increase in cAMP in cardiac myocytes enhances cardiac contractility. It is rarely used, however, because of its multiple side effects (nausea, vomiting, hyperglycemia, hypokalemia, and anaphylaxis).

Calcium chloride (inoconstrictor) provides a source of free calcium ions and acts as an inotrope if free ionized calcium concentrations are low within the patient. If free ionized calcium concentrations are normal, fewer inotropic effects will be noticed. Calcium chloride is also a potent vasoconstrictor and

likely will have negative effects on cardiac diastolic function. The administration of calcium *immediately* after reperfusion of the myocardium after cardiopulmonary bypass should be performed cautiously, because it may be associated with exacerbating reperfusion injury and worsening diastolic function of the heart.

Vasoconstrictors

Vasocontrictors induce contraction of vascular smooth muscle. Arterial vasoconstriction results in increased SVR, leading to increased mean arterial pressure (MAP = CO × SVR). Constriction of venous capacitance vessels results in increased preload and increased CO. When using vasoconstrictors, end-organ perfusion must be monitored closely. Vasoconstrictors may be used to temporize hypotension due to decreased preload, but should not replace adequate volume resuscitation. Table 71.3 describes the different vasocontrictors or vasopressors commonly used in the operating room.

Phenylephrine is a direct-acting α_1-agonist that causes primarily peripheral arterial vasoconstriction, with minimal venous effects. It has a short duration of action (minutes). Phenylephrine is commonly used to treat hypotension due to decreased vascular resistance by increasing afterload. It usually does not affect heart rate or contractility, but may cause a reflex bradycardia.

Ephedrine is a sympathomimetic drug that acts by indirectly releasing norepinephrine from stores in the nerve terminal. It also has mild direct α, β_1, and β_2 effects. The mild β effects will increase heart rate and contractility. Repeat dosing may lead to tachyphylaxis, with less norepinephrine being released from the nerve terminal than with the initial dose.

Norepinephrine is a direct-acting α_1-, α_2-, and β_1-agonist. The α effects dominate, causing intense α-receptor vasoconstriction throughout the dosing range. It is useful in hypotension refractory to phenylephrine (α_1 only) and has the added effect of increasing cardiac contractility.

Vasopressin is an antidiuretic hormone that at higher doses stimulates smooth muscle vasopressin receptors to cause vasoconstriction. Vasopressin does not affect α- or β-receptors. It is used in a variety of low SVR states and as a second-line agent when norepinephrine fails to adequately increase SVR (persistent vasoplegia). Vasopressin may be effective for treating angiotensin-converting enzyme inhibitor– or angiotensin receptor blocker–mediated hypotension during general anesthesia.

Methylene blue has a complex mechanism of action, and there are only a limited number of clinical trials available. It inhibits the nitric oxide/cGMP pathway by inhibiting nitric oxide synthase. Methylene blue has been used effectively in nitric oxide–mediated vasoplegic syndrome, in which patients with profound vasodilation do not respond to conventional vasopressors.

Vasodilators produce vascular smooth muscle relaxation, resulting in decreased SVR. Their primary indications are

Table 71.2. Inotropic drugs

Agent	Action	HR	Con	Preload	SVR/PVR	BP	CO	Indications	Use
Levosimendan (inodilator) (not available currently in the United States) – a calcium-sensitizing agent that acts as an inodilator. It exerts its inotropic effect by sensitizing calcium to troponin C, thereby enhancing the calcium sensitivity of the cardiac myofilaments. It does not increase intracellular calcium. It also causes vascular dilation by opening potassium-ATPase channels on vascular smooth muscle cell membranes. Levosimendan mildly inhibits phosphodiesteraseIII activity.									
Epinephrine	α_1, α_2, β_1, β_2-agonist Dose-dependent action 1–3 µg/min = β 3–10 µg/min = β > α 10+ µg/min = α > β	 ↑↑ ↑↑	 ↑↑↑	 ↑	 –/↓ –/↑ ↑↑	 ↑	 ↑ –/↓ –/↓	Reduced CO Hypotension Cardiac arrest Anaphylaxis Cardiogenic shock Bronchospasm	2–10 µg IV bolus Infusion 2–20 mcg/min (Central line) Arrest: 0.5–1.0 mg IV bolus Monitor end-organ perfusion closely Short half-life (minutes)
Dopamine	α_1, β_1, β_2, D_1-agonist Indirect NE release 1–3 µg/kg/min = D_1 3–10 = β_1, β_2 > D_1 10+ = α_1 > β_1, D_1	 – ↑↑ ↑↑	 ↑↑ ↑↑ ↑↑	 ↑ ↑ ↑	 → –/↑ ↑↑	Variable ↑ ↑	 ↑ ↑ ↑/–/↓	Low CO Low SVR Renal insufficiency (low dose)	Infusion 2–20 µg/kg/min (central line) Monitor end-organ perfusion (especially > 10 µg/kg/min) Short half-life (minutes)
Dobutamine	Strong β_1 > β_2 Weak α_1	↑/↑↑	↑↑	–	–/↓ ↑ (in β-blocked patients)	Variable	↑↑	Low CO (especially with ↑SVR/PVR) Right heart failure Stress echocardiography	Infusion: 2–30 µg/kg/min Short half-life (minutes)
Milrinone	Inhibits phosphodiesterase III Increases cAMP Does not act at β receptors	–/↑	↑↑	↓	↓/↓↓	Variable	↑↑	Low CO (especially with ↑SVR/PVR) Right heart failure Synergistic with β-agonists	25–75 µg/kg load over 10 min (beware ↓BP, esp. with ↓preload) Infusion: 0.375–0.75 µg/kg/min Longer half-life (2.4h)
Glucagon	Increases intracellular cAMP	↑	↑↑	–/↓	–/↓	↑	↑	Hypoglycemia β-Blocker toxicity Low CO Refractory CHF	Bolus: 1–5 mg IV slowly Infusion: 25–75µg/min Rarely used because of multiple side effects (Nausea, emesis, tachycardia, hyperglycemia, hypokalemia, anaphylaxis)
Calcium chloride	Free Ca^{+2} ion	–/↓	↑	–	↑	↑	↑/↓	Hypocalcemia Hyperkalemia Hypotension from hypocalcemia Calcium channel blockade Counteracts hypermagnesemia	10% calcium chloride 100mg/ml 200–1000 mg slow IVP (prefer central line) Causes vein inflammation Do not use immediately after reperfusion
Levosimendan	Calcium-sensitizing agent cAMP-independent Vascular dilation via K^+-ATPase channels	–/↑	↑↑	↓	→	Variable	↑↑	Low CO Right heart failure Supplement β-agonists Possible reduced proarrhythmic effect	Bolus: 6–24 µg/kg (10–20 min) Infusion: 0.05–0.4 µg/kg/min (up to 24 h) Active metabolite with 80-h half-life Effects last 24–48 h after infusion stopped

ATPase, adenosine triphosphatase; IV, intravenous; HR, heart rate; Con, contractility; SVR, systemic vascular resistance; PVR, pulmonary vascular resistance; BP, blood pressure; CO, cardiac output; CHF, congestive heart failure; IVP, IV push.

Table 71.3. Vasoconstrictors

Drug	Action	HR	Contractility	Preload	SVR/PVR	BP	CO	Indication	Use
Phenylephrine	α_1-agonist	−/↓ (reflex)	−	−	↑↑	↑	−/↓	Peripheral vasodilation; Low SVR; SVT (reflex vagal stimulation); TET spell	40–80 μg IV bolus; Infusion: 20–200 μg/min; Short half-life (minutes)
Ephedrine	Indirect NE release; Mild direct α, β_1, β_2; Acts like small-dose epinephrine	↑	↑	↑↑	↑	↑	↑	Low SVR (especially if HR low); Low CO (especially if HR low); Transient cardiac depression	5–10 mg IV bolus; 25–50 mg IM; Tachyphylaxis with repeat dosing; Slightly longer duration of action
Norepinephrine	α_1-, α_2-, β_1-agonist; Intense α_1 and α_2 constriction throughout dosing range	Variable	↑	↑↑	↑↑↑	↑	−/↓	Peripheral vascular collapse; Shock, vasoplegia, ↓SVR; Need ↑SVR with some ↑Con; Phenylephrine is not working	2–10 μg IV bolus (never more unless extremis); Infusion 2–20 μg/min (central line); Monitor end-organ perfusion closely; Short half-life (minutes)
Vasopressin	Direct vasoconstriction via V_1-receptors; No action at β- or α-receptors	−/↓	−	−	↑↑ (possible PVR sparing at lower doses)	↑	Variable	Second-line agent: shock, vasoplegia, sepsis, ↓SVR; Pulmonary HTN with ↓SVR? Use with milrinone to counteract ↓SVR; ACE-I/ARB–refractory hypotension	Infusion: 0.01–0.04 U/min (physiologic); Lower incidence of end-organ hypoperfusion; Infusion: 0.04–0.1 U/min (pharm dose); Monitor end-organ perfusion closely; Half-life 10–35 min
Methylene blue	Complex mechanism; Inhibits NO/cGMP; Inhibits NO synthase	−	−	−	↑↑	↑	−	Not a first-line agent; Limited clinical trials and case reports; ↓SVR, persistent vasoplegia	Bolus: 1.5–2.0 mg/kg over 15–30 min; Effect of bolus lasts 2–3 h; Infusion: 0.25–1.0 mg/kg/h; Monitor end-organ perfusion

NE, norepinephrine; NO, nitric oxide; HR, heart rate; SVR, systemic vascular resistance; PVR, pulmonary vascular resistance; BP, blood pressure; CO, cardiac output; SVT, supraventricular tachycardia; TET, tetralogy of Fallot; HTN, hypertension; ACE-I, angiotensin-converting enzyme inhibitor; ARB, angiotensin receptor blocker; IV, intravenous; IM, intramuscular.

for elevated SVR and myocardial ischemia and failure. Table 71.4 lists the most commonly used vasodilators in anesthesia.

Nitroglycerin is a direct smooth muscle vasodilator metabolized in the body to nitric oxide. This results in increased vascular smooth muscle cell cGMP, which causes vascular smooth muscle relaxation. Nitroglycerin primarily causes venous dilatation, decreasing cardiac preload, with some arterial dilation at higher doses. Coronary arterial blood vessels are dilated throughout the dosing range. Nitroglycerin may be used to control hypertensive episodes, but other agents are more effective. Nitroglycerin is also effective in treating myocardial ischemia by decreasing preload and myocardial wall tension and improving coronary blood flow to ischemic areas of myocardium, as long as perfusion pressure is maintained. Tolerance to infusions may occur after 24 hours. It is less toxic than nitroprusside, although methemoglobinemia is possible after prolonged infusions at high doses.

Nitroprusside is a direct vasodilator that acts by producing nitric oxide. It causes profound vasodilation of both arteries and veins, with arterial dilation predominating at lower doses. It is used to control systemic hypertension. Nitroprusside needs to be protected from light. Continuous blood pressure monitoring via an arterial line is recommended because of its potency. Nitroprusside may cause both cyanide and thiocyanate toxicity. Cyanide production results from nitroprusside metabolism. Cyanide inhibits oxidative phosphorylation, drastically reducing adenosine triphosphate (ATP) production in cells. Signs of toxicity include tachyphylaxis, elevated mixed venous oxygenation (cells unable to use oxygen), and metabolic acidosis. In patients receiving prolonged (>24 hours) or high-dose (>8 μg/kg/min) infusions or in those with end-organ dysfunction (liver or kidney), it is advisable to check cyanide levels. The kidneys eliminate thiocyanate, a product of cyanide metabolism by the body. Toxic levels of thiocyanate may exist in patients with renal dysfunction or after prolonged infusions, resulting in central nervous system dysfunction.

Fenoldopam is a selective peripheral dopamine receptor (DA1) agonist, rapidly lowering blood pressure by causing dilation of arteries. It also induces diuresis. It does not have toxic metabolites.

Hydralazine, a direct vasodilator, acts via the cGMP pathway. It causes more arterial than venous dilation, with little effect on preload. Its onset of action is the slowest of the drugs on this list, taking up to 20 minutes to achieve peak effect. Hydralazine is not an effective drug for acute hypertensive crisis because of its slow onset. However, it can be used to reduce doses of other, faster-acting drugs (e.g., nitroprusside).

Nicardipine is a dihydropyridine calcium channel blocker that has an intravenous formulation used to treat hypertension. It primarily causes arterial dilation with minimal venous (preload) and cardiac (contractility, heat rate) effects. It has a longer half-life than vasodilator infusions so bolusing is needed to achieve therapeutic levels.

β-Blocking drugs

β-Blocking drugs bind to β-receptors, antagonizing their effects. β-Blockers decrease heart rate and contractility and affect cardiac conduction (atrioventricular [AV] nodal conduction, refractory period). Each β-blocker has different receptor affinities (β_1, β_2, α), although selectivity for a particular receptor likely decreases as dosages of the medication are increased. Metabolism and half-life are different for each β-blocker. In patients with chronic obstructive lung disease or asthma, a selective β_1-blocker is less likely to exacerbate symptoms. Table 71.5 lists examples of selective and nonselective β-blockers commonly used in the operating room. The following bulleted list includes β-blocker indications, complications, and treatment of toxicity.

Indications:

- Hypertension
- Arrhythmias (especially supraventricular)
- Myocardial ischemia and infarction
- Dynamic ventricular outflow tract obstruction
- Perioperative cardiac morbidity and mortality

Monitor for:

- Severe bradyarrhythmias
- Heart block
- Bronchospasm (use a selective β_1-blocker in susceptible patients)
- Congestive heart failure (especially in patients with low ejection fractions)
- Withdrawal syndrome with abrupt discontinuation of β-blockers (hypertension and tachycardia)

Treatment of toxicity:

- β-Agonists (may need large doses to overcome blockade)
- Cardiac pacing
- Calcium, milrinone, glucagon, thyroid hormone (the mechanism of action of these agents does not involve β-receptors)

Hemodynamic effects:

- Decreased heart rate
- Decreased contractility
- Decreased blood pressure
- Decreased CO
- Decreased AV node conduction
- Increased refractory period

Calcium channel blockers

Calcium channel blockers interact with L-type calcium channels, blocking calcium entry into the cell. Calcium entry into the myocardial cell not only is part of the cardiac action potential but also induces calcium release from the SR, dramatically increasing calcium in the cytoplasm, thereby increasing contractility of the myocardium and increasing smooth muscle

Table 71.4. Vasodilators

Drug	Action	HR	Contractility	Preload	SVR/PVR	BP	CO	Indication	Use
Nitroglycerin	Direct vasodilator ↑cGMP production Venous > arterial Excellent coronary effects	↑ (reflex)	–	↓↓	↓	↓	↑/↓	Myocardial ischemia Increased coronary perfusion Relief of coronary spasm HTN Pulmonary HTN CHF	40–80 μg IV bolus Infusion: 10–200 μg/min At infusions higher than 200 μg/min, switch to SNP or another agent Tolerance if infused for long periods
Nitroprusside	Direct vasodilator ↑cGMP production Arterial = venous	↑ (reflex)	–	↓	↓↓	↓	↑/↓	HTN, ↑SVR Controlled hypotension	Infusion 0.1–2.0 μg/kg/min Max infusion 10 μg/kg/min (short periods only) Avoid prolonged doses > 2.0 μg/kg/min (toxicity) Protect from light Continuous BP monitoring (A-line) Use with caution in liver or kidney dysfunction
Hydralazine	Direct vasodilator Arterial ≫ venous	↑ (reflex)	–	–	↓↓	↓	–/↑	HTN, ↑SVR	2.5–5 mg IV bolus every 15 min (max. 20–40 mg) 20 min to peak effect
Fenoldopam	Synthetic dopamine receptor agonist Rapid-acting arterial dilator Maintains renal perfusion	↑ (reflex)	–	–	↓↓	↓	↑	Severe hypertension in patients with impaired renal function	IV infusion 0.01–1.6 mcg/kg/min Readjust dose every 15–20 min for effect
Nicardipine	Dihydropyridine calcium channel blocker Arterial ≫ venous	↑ (reflex)	–	–	↓↓	↓	–/↑	HTN To improve lusitropy in cardiac ischemia Coronary vasospasm	Infusion 1–4 μg/kg/min Titrate to BP May cause phlebitis in peripheral IV (if infused for > 12 h)

HR, heart rate; SVR, systemic vascular resistance; PVR, pulmonary vascular resistance; BP, blood pressure; CO, cardiac output; HTN, hypertension; CHF, congestive heart failure; IV, intravenous; SNP, sodium nitroprusside.

Table 71.5. β-Blockers

Drug	Action	Onset	β Half-life, *h*	Elimination	IV dose
Propranolol	β_1-, β_2-antagonist	2–5 min	3.5–4.0	Hepatic	0.5–1.0 mg prn
Labetalol	β_1-, β_2-, α_1-antagonist	2–5 min	3–5	Hepatic	10–40 mg prn
	Ratio of α-to-β blockade is 1:7				(max. 300 mg)
Metoprolol	Selective β_1-antagonist	5 min (peak 20 min)	3–4	Hepatic	1–5 mg prn
					(max, 15 mg)
Esmolol	Selective β_1-antagonist	Rapid	9 min	Red blood cell and plasma esterases	0.25–0.5 mg/kg prn
					Infusion: 50–300 µg/kg/min

IV, intravenous; prn, as needed.

tone in arterial vessels. By blocking the L-type calcium channel, contractility and heart rate are decreased. Calcium channel blockers are arterial vasodilators with minimal venous dilation. Verapamil and diltiazem affect the myocardium and produce arterial vasodilation. Nicardipine only produces arterial vasodilation. Table 71.6 gives examples of calcium channel blockers commonly used in the operating room. Following are the hemodynamic effects, indications, and treatment of calcium channel blocker overdose.

Hemodynamic effects:

- Prolong AV nodal refractory period (verapamil > diltiazem)
- Decrease heart rate by affecting the sinoatrial node (verapamil > diltiazem, possible reflex increase with nicardipine)
- Cause no change in preload
- Decrease SVR
- Decrease blood pressure
- Decrease CO (verapamil, diltiazem, possible increase with nicardipine)
- Depress myocardial contractility (verapamil > diltiazem, not nicardipine)

Indications:

- Hypertension
- Supraventricular arrhythmias (verapamil, diltiazem)
- Arterial and coronary vasospasm
- Myocardial ischemia (not as well established as β-blockers)

Monitor for:

- Hypotension (negative inotropic effects and vasodilation)
- Severe bradyarrhythmias
- Heart block
- Congestive heart failure (especially in patients with low ejection fractions)
- Beware of additive effects in patients on β-blockers

Toxicity: Give calcium chloride, β-agonists, α-agonists, or milrinone, or consider cardiac pacing.

Choice of inotrope or vasoactive drug

The most commonly used inotropes and vasoconstrictors are adrenergic receptor agonists (epinephrine, norepinephrine, dopamine, dobutamine, phenylephrine). They have been around for a long time, with well-documented effects on the cardiac myocyte and peripheral vasculature. Other inotropes and vasoconstrictors work via other mechanisms noted in

Table 71.6. Calcium channel blockers

Drug	Action	Onset	β Half-life	IV Dose	Comments
Verapamil	Strong myocardial effects Arterial dilation	3–5 min	3–10 h Hepatic	1–2 mg prn (low dose, especially during anesthesia)	Myocardial depression > peripheral *arterial* vasodilation Use low doses in GA, unstable patients, or patients with reduced EF Rx: SVT, HTN, vasospasm, ischemia
Diltiazem	Weaker myocardial effects Arterial dilation	2–5 min	3–5 h Hepatic and renal	20 mg bolus, then 5–15 mg/h infusion Lower doses with hemodynamic instability	Less myocardial depression compared with verapamil Causes selective coronary artery vasodilation Rx: SVT, HTN, vasospasm, angina
Nicardipine (see vasodilators)	No myocardial effects Arterial dilation	Minutes	14 min Hepatic	1–4 µg/kg/min	Titrate to blood pressure May cause phlebitis in peripheral IV if infused for > 12 h

IV, intravenous; prn, as needed; GA, general anesthesia; EF, ejection fraction; SVT, supraventricular tachycardia; HTN, hypertension.

the previous lists (milrinone, levosimendan, vasopressin, methylene blue). Each inotrope and vasoactive drug has different advantages, disadvantages, and side effect profiles. The nonadrenergic drugs often are used when adrenergic receptor agonists either cause unwanted side effects (dysrhythmias, tachycardia, changes in vascular tone) or fail to treat the cardiovascular problem (persistent vasoplegia, continued myocardial depression). In addition, the combination of an adrenergic receptor agonist (epinephrine) with a nonadrenergic inotrope (milrinone) may result in an increased, synergistic response (contractility), because both agents work to increase cAMP via different mechanisms.

Understanding the complexity of calcium modulation in cardiac myocytes and vascular smooth muscle cells is an important factor in deciding the appropriate inotrope and/or vasoactive drug needed to maintain adequate tissue perfusion and oxygen delivery. There is no gold standard for choosing an inotrope, vasoconstrictor, or vasodilator. The ideal drug would have a singular effect, such as increasing contractility, and have no effect on heart rate, rhythm, or vascular tone. Such drugs do not exist, as each has different effects or side effects. Catecholamines affect not only inotropy and chronotropy, but also vascular smooth muscle tone. Milrinone increases contractility in the cardiac myocyte by increasing cAMP, but increased cAMP also causes vasodilation. The choice of inotrope or vasoactive drug has as much to do with its intended effect as its side effects.

Suggested readings

Balser JR, Butterworth JF, Larach DR. Cardiovascular drugs. In: Frederick A, Hensley J, Martin DE, Gravlee GP, eds. *A Practical Appproach to Cardiac Anesthesia*. 4th ed. Philadelphia: Lippincott Williams & Wilkins; 2008:33–103.

Bayram M, De Luca L, Massie MB, Gheorghiade M. Reassessment of dobutamine, dopamine, and milrinone in the management of acute heart failure syndromes. *Am J Cardiol* 2005; 96:47G–58G.

Bers DM. Cardiac excitation-contraction coupling. *Nature* 2002; 415:198–205.

Groban L, Butterworth J. Perioperative management of chronic heart failure. *Anesth Analg* 2006; 103:557–575.

Holmes CL, Patel BM, Russell JA, Walley KR. Physiology of vasopressin relevant to management of septic shock. *Chest* 2001; 120:989–1002.

Kirov MY, Evgenov OV, Evgenov NV, et al. Infusion of methylene blue in human septic shock: a pilot, randomized, controlled study. *Crit Care Med* 2001; 29:1860–1867.

Levy JH, Tanaka KA, Bailey JM. Cardiac surgical pharmacology. In: Cohn LH, ed. *Cardiac Surgery in the Adult*. 3rd ed. New York: McGraw-Hill; 2008:77–110.

McGowan FX, Steven JM. Cardiac physiology and pharmacology. In: Cote CJ, Todres ID, Ryan JF, Goudsouzian NG, eds. *A Practice of Anesthesia for Infants and Children*. 3rd ed. Philadelphia: W.B. Saunders; 2001:353–390.

Notterman DA. Inotropic agents. Catecholamines, digoxin, amrinone. *Crit Care Clin* 1991; 7:583–613.

Royster RL, Butterworth J, Groban L, et al. Cardiovascular pharmacology. In: Kaplan JA, Reich DL, Lake CL, Konstadt SN, eds. *Kaplan's Cardiac Anesthesia*. 5th ed. Philadelphia: Elsevier Saunders; 2006:213–279.

Shanmugam G. Vasoplegic syndrome – the role of methylene blue. *Eur J Cardiothorac Surg* 2005; 28:705–710.

Toller WG, Stranz C. Levosimendan, a new inotropic and vasodilator agent. *Anesthesiology* 2006; 104:556–569.

Zaugg M, Schaub MC. Cellular mechanisms in sympatho-modulation of the heart. *Br J Anaesth* 2004; 93:34–52.

Although cardiovascular drugs that have a direct impact on cardiac performance are important, it is also essential to understand the mechanism, side effects, and utility of adjunct drugs that are used for controlled anticoagulation and its reversal and to minimize perioperative bleeding.

Heparin

Heparin is a naturally occurring, negatively charged mucopolysaccharide with a molecular weight that varies from 10,000 to 30,000 Da. It is derived from either bovine lung or porcine intestine. The anticoagulant effect of heparin occurs via binding of a specific pentasaccharide sequence within the heparin molecule to antithrombin, also known as antithrombin III. Antithrombin functions in the normal coagulation cascade to limit the effect of thrombin. Binding of the heparin molecule increases the activity of antithrombin by 1000- to 4000-fold. Antithrombin also regulates the activity of factors Xa, IXa, XIa, and XIIa.

Heparin has been used in clinical medicine for decades to treat acute thrombotic events, to prevent deep vein thrombosis (DVT), and for anticoagulation to facilitate cardiopulmonary bypass. The anticoagulant effect of heparin is most often measured by activated partial thromboplastin time (aPTT) or activated clotting time (ACT). Serial monitoring of anticoagulation and titrated heparin dosing is essential because of the variable and unpredictable effect of heparin in vivo. The anticoagulant effect of heparin depends on multiple factors. The size of the heparin molecule delivered is highly variable, with smaller molecules having a greater anticoagulant effect. The underlying health of the patient, the amount of circulating antithrombin, and preexisting liver disease or coagulopathy all affect heparin dosing.

Adverse effects of heparin, in addition to bleeding complications, are well described. The most important is that the drug has a narrow therapeutic window. The goal is to provide adequate anticoagulation without inducing bleeding. Given the variable response to heparin dosing, this requires frequent measurement of aPTT or ACT. As a derivative of either bovine or porcine tissues, heparin may cause allergic reaction. Additionally, heparin is known to induce osteoclast activity and therefore may lead to bone demineralization. Finally, heparin may induce thrombocytopenia.

Heparin-induced thrombocytopenia

Heparin-induced thrombocytopenia (HIT) may be the most frequent cause of drug-induced thrombocytopenia, with an estimated incidence between 10% and 20% of patients exposed to heparin. HIT describes two distinct clinical scenarios. HIT type 1 is the result of direct antiplatelet effects of heparin and produces a mild transient thrombocytopenia that is usually asymptomatic and rarely requires treatment. HIT type 2 is the result of naturally occurring IgG antibody-binding complexes within the plasma formed by heparin and platelet factor IV (PF4). HIT type 2 is much more serious and carries a significant mortality risk if not identified and promptly treated. The remainder of this discussion focuses on HIT type 2.

HIT is a clinical syndrome that may occur in any patient exposed to heparin. Risk factors include the use of unfractionated heparin, long-term exposure, a large dose, the postsurgical setting, and repeat exposure. Common findings include thrombocytopenia (platelet count decrease of 50%), occurring approximately 4 to 10 days after exposure; signs of thrombosis; and skin lesions at the site of heparin injection. In patients exposed to heparin within the preceding 90 days, HIT may develop as soon as 10 hours because of the presence of residual HIT antibodies.

Thrombotic events more commonly are venous, but may be arterial and present as venous outflow obstruction, myocardial infarction, mesenteric ischemia, cerebral vascular accident, pulmonary embolism, or upper- or lower-extremity DVT. HIT most commonly occurs in the setting of DVT prophylaxis or in patients receiving long-term therapeutic anticoagulation; however, cases have been reported after catheter flushes with doses as small as 250 IU, and in patients whose only exposure is heparin-coated central venous catheters.

HIT occurs when naturally occurring IgG antibodies bind the heparin/PF4 complex. This heparin/PF4/antibody complex binds other platelets, causing increased release of PF4 and prothrombotic particles. PF4 released from platelets binds additional heparin and IgG heparin-dependant antibodies, forming more complexes in a positive-feedback manner. Additionally, this heparin–platelet complexes and prothrombotic particles form aggregations at sites of endothelial injury. These aggregations are responsible for the two most common clinical findings in HIT, thrombocytopenia due to consumption of platelets, and thrombus formation.

A presumptive diagnosis of HIT is based on an otherwise unexplained thrombocytopenia in a patient exposed to heparin. The gold standard for diagnostic evaluation is the serotonin release assay. This test is cumbersome, time consuming, expensive, and unavailable in many laboratories. However, its sensitivity and specificity both are very high. It is performed by radiolabeling normal donor platelets with C^{14}-serotonin. These labeled platelets are then washed and exposed to patient serum with low-dose heparin (0.1 U/ml). A positive test occurs when the patient's heparin/PF4/antibody complexes bind donor platelets and cause release of the labeled serotonin.

More commonly, an enzyme-linked immunosorbent assay (ELISA) is performed to identify heparin-dependant IgG antibodies in a patient's plasma. The sensitivity of this assay is 97%, suggesting that a negative test makes the diagnosis of HIT very unlikely; however, the specificity is only 74% to 87%, making a positive test result less useful in the clinical setting. Because many patients with heparin-dependant antibodies by ELISA do not develop HIT, the clinician must carefully consider pretest probability and interpret results accordingly. In many institutions, ELISA is used as a screening test; in the case of positive results and a high pretest probability, the serotonin release assay is used to confirm the diagnosis. Treatment of HIT is focused on the removal of all heparin, including heparin-coated central lines and, in the setting of thrombosis, initiating anticoagulation.

Anticoagulation in the setting of HIT

Anticoagulation may be required for the treatment of thrombosis associated with HIT or in the event of an emergent vascular or cardiac event. Common clinical scenarios involve a patient with either acute HIT or a recent history of HIT who develops myocardial infarction or pulmonary embolism or requires anticoagulation for cardiac or vascular surgery. Therapeutic anticoagulation may be accomplished with any of the direct thrombin inhibitors, including lepirudin, bivalirudin, argatroban, and danaparoid. It should be noted that danaparoid is not available in the United States, and that ideal dosing strategies and monitor systems have not been fully developed for any of the aforementioned agents. Low molecular weight heparin, although it is less likely to trigger heparin-dependant antibody formation, has nearly 100% cross-reactivity with heparin-dependant antibodies; therefore, it cannot be used in the treatment of HIT.

Direct thrombin inhibitors

Lepirudin was the first direct thrombin inhibitor approved for the treatment of HIT in the United States. It is a recombinant form of hirudin, a naturally occurring protein found in the saliva of the medicinal leech *Hirudo medicinalis*. Metabolized and excreted by the kidney, massive overdose is possible in the setting of undiagnosed renal failure.

Bivalirudin is a synthetic drug designed from lepirudin. It also is approved for the treatment of HIT and has been approved for use in percutaneous coronary intervention (PCI). Metabolism occurs in the circulation by the action of plasma proteases; however, there is a renal component to metabolism and its effective half-life is prolonged in the setting of renal failure.

Argatroban is another direct thrombin inhibitor that has been approved for treatment of HIT and for PCI. It is metabolized primarily by the liver and may be a safer agent in the setting of renal failure.

Danaparoid has been approved for the treatment of HIT in many countries, including the European Union, Canada, and Australia. It is currently unavailable in the United States. It has approximately 17% cross-reactivity with heparin-dependant antibodies and therefore may trigger HIT.

Unlike the anticoagulant effect of heparin, which can be reversed with protamine and monitored with aPTT and ACT, the effects of direct thrombin inhibitors are irreversible and difficult to monitor. Bleeding time, aPTT, international normalized ratio, and ACT all show increased values with the direct thrombin inhibitors, but none has proven to be an ideal measure of adequate coagulation. When using direct thrombin inhibitors, the clinician must work with available laboratory resources to find the most suitable measure of anticoagulation.

Anticoagulation in a patient with HIT

None of the direct thrombin inhibitors has been approved for use in coronary bypass procedures; therefore, the following description describes off-label uses. The use of heparin for prophylaxis of DVT or treatment of acute thrombotic events continues to increase. The incidence of HIT is reportedly 0.3% to 2% of patients exposed to heparin. Therefore, the clinician is likely to encounter a patient needing anticoagulation in the setting of HIT. The choice of direct thrombin inhibitor must be based on the patient's medical history, with a focus on renal and hepatic function, and the familiarity of the anesthesiologist, surgeon, and perfusionist with the available drugs. Additionally, adequate laboratory services and monitoring equipment must be confirmed.

The American College of Chest Physicians (ACCP) published guidelines describing the approach to anticoagulation in a patient with HIT. The guidelines separate patients into three categories (Table 72.1). Those with a history of HIT and with negative heparin-dependant antibodies, those with acute HIT and positive antibodies, and those with subacute HIT whose platelet counts have normalized but who have positive heparin-dependant antibodies.

A starting reference for appropriate dosing regimens is listed in Table 72.2. These doses are not meant to be absolute recommendations. Actual dosing will depend on the type of monitoring device used, the need for bypass, and the specific underlying medical condition.

Table 72.1. Approach to anticoagulation in a patient with HIT

History of HIT, negative antibodies	Use unfractionated heparin Can use familiar drug and monitoring Avoid any heparin exposure before or after coronary bypass Safety is provided by the fact that heparin-dependant antibodies require 4–5 d to appear
Acute HIT, positive antibodies	Consider waiting until antibody negative Consider all available agents Review patient's medical history Lepirudin: renal metabolism Bivalirudin: metabolized by plasma proteases Some renal metabolism Argatroban: hepatic metabolism Consider familiarity of team with available agents and monitoring equipment
Subacute HIT, positive antibodies	Consider waiting until antibody negative If unable to wait, proceed as in the situation of acute HIT

Protamine

Protamine is the only widely available agent for the reversal of heparin. Protamine is a polycationic compound derived from salmon milt. The mechanism of action involves the formation of ionic bonds with free circulating heparin, which prevents the binding of antithrombin. It is unclear what if any effect protamine has on heparin that has already bound to thrombin. Protamine is usually dosed at 1 mg/100 U of heparin to be reversed. Caution must be used in the administration of protamine. If rapidly infused (>50 mg/10 min), hypotension may result from histamine released from mast cells. Additionally, protamine has been implicated in both allergic and anaphylactoid reactions.

IgE-mediated allergic reactions may occur in any patient who previously received protamine. IgG-mediated anaphylactoid reactions may be life threatening, leading to vasoconstriction, pulmonary hypertension, and possible right heart failure. If typical clinical manifestations of protamine reaction occur, including hypotension, urticaria, flushing, bronchospasm, pulmonary edema, or right heart failure, the initial treatment is to immediately stop the protamine infusion and institute supportive therapy.

Hypotension may be treated with volume expansion and an α-agonist such as phenylephrine or norepinephrine. Epinephrine may be required to support right ventricular function, and nitrates may be used in the setting of pulmonary hypertension. After hypotension related to histamine release is treated with fluids and pressor agents, protamine can usually be restarted and slowly infused. However, in the case of allergic or anaphylactoid reaction, protamine may be contraindicated. This has led to increasing research into agents that may be used to reverse heparin. Presently researched alternatives to protamine include heparinase, recombinant PF4, hexadimethrine, and dialysis-like heparin removal devices.

Antifibrinolytics

There are several drugs commonly in use that inhibit fibrinolysis. Aprotinin, a nonspecific protease inhibitor, and the lysine analogues tranexamic acid and aminocaproic acid are discussed in this chapter.

Aprotinin is a serine protease inhibitor that has intrinsic procoagulant effects as well as antifibrinolytic and anti-inflammatory effects mediated via its actions on thrombin, kallikrein, plasmin, and other chemical mediators. It is derived from bovine lung tissue and has been implicated in anaphylaxis and anaphylactoid reactions that have led to mortality. Exposure may lead to formation of IgG antibodies, and repeat exposure within 12 months is relatively contraindicated. It is administered most often for cardiac surgery in patients with increased risk of bleeding. Facilities should always be in place to treat precipitous hypotension, anaphylaxis, and circulatory collapse prior to administering aprotinin. It is recommended that a 1-ml test dose be given 10 minutes before additional dosing. Standard dosing varies between 1,000,000 to 2,000,000 kallikrein-inhibiting units (KIU) over 20 to 30 minutes, followed by an infusion of 250,000 to 500,000 KIU/h for the duration of surgery. Aprotinin has been associated with an increased incidence of perioperative renal failure and mortality; consequently, its current availability is exceptionally limited.

The two commonly used lysine analogues are aminocaproic acid (5-g loading dose over an hour, then 1 g/h up to 8 hours) and tranexamic acid, which share a common mechanism of

Table 72.2. Dosing regimens of alternate drugs

Drug	Half-life	Elimination	Dose	Notes
Argatroban	39–51 min	Hepatic	PCI 2–3 µg/kg/min CPB 5–10 µg/kg/min	
Danaparoid	~25 h	Renal	Not clearly defined	Unavailable in US Ab cross-reactivity
Lepirudin	~80 min	Renal	Bolus, 0.25 mg/kg Infusion, 0.5 mg/min	
Bivalirudin	25 min	Plasma proteases	Bolus, 1.5 mg/kg Infusion, 2.5 mg/kg/h	

Ab, antibody; CPB, cardio pulmonary bypass; PCI, percutaneous intervention.

action. Most often given in the setting of cardiac surgery, or in the treatment of bleeding following oral or urologic surgery, lysine analogues are competitive inhibitors of lysine binding sites located on plasminogen and fibrinogen. They inhibit the formation of plasmin and inhibit fibrinolysis. Caution should be used in the setting of renal disease; dose reduction may be considered. Lysine analogues have been known to cause transient hypotension with rapid intravenous administration.

Suggested readings

Di Nisio M, Middlethorp S, Buller HR. Direct thrombin inhibitors. *N Engl J Med* 2005; 353:1028–1040.

Kaplan KL, Francis CW. Direct thrombin inhibitors. *Semin Hematol* 2002; 39:187–196.

Mangano DT, Tudor IC, Dietzel C. The risk associated with aprotinin in cardiac surgery. *N Engl J Med* 2006; 354(4):353–365.

Miller RD, Nyhan D, Rogers JA. *Miller's Anesthesia*. 6th ed. Philadelphia: Elsevier, Churchill, Livingstone; 2005.

Murphy GS, Marymount JH. Alternative anticoagulation management strategies for the patient with heparin-induced thrombocytopenia undergoing cardiac surgery. *J Cardiothorac Vasc Anesth* 2007; 21:113–126.

Sedrakyan A, Treasure T, Elefteriades JA. Effect of aprotinin on clinical outcomes in coronary artery bypass graft surgery: a systematic review and meta-analysis of randomized clinical trials. *J Thorac Cardiovasc Surg* 2004; 128(3):442–448.

Warkentin TE, Greinacher A. Heparin-induced thrombocytopenia: recognition, treatment, and prevention: the Seventh ACCP Conference on Antithrombotic and Thrombolytic Therapy. *Chest* 2004; 126:311S.

Chapter 73

Coronary artery bypass grafting utilizing cardiopulmonary bypass

Theresa S. Chang and John A. Fox

Introduction

The introduction of cardiopulmonary bypass (CPB) techniques in the 1950s helped facilitate surgical treatment of congenital and valvular heart disease. Surgical treatment of coronary artery disease using the heart–lung machine was pioneered in the 1960s when surgeons bypassed obstructive coronary artery lesions using saphenous veins or left internal mammary arteries as conduits. In the recent decade, technologic advances in surgical instrumentation have paved the way for surgeons to employ novel techniques to graft obstructed coronary lesions, ranging from robotic and port access surgery, in which small insertions are placed in the chest, to avoiding use of the heart–lung machine entirely in so-called off-pump coronary artery bypass graft (CABG) surgery or by transmyocardial laser revascularization. However, because surgical treatment of coronary artery disease in most patients still requires use of the heart–lung machine, this chapter focuses on the anesthetic management of CABG while on CPB. In addition to CABG procedures, CPB has been used for surgical procedures such as cardiac valve repair or replacement; repair of congenital heart defects, aneurysms, septal defects; and heart transplantation.

The American College of Cardiology and the American Heart Association reviewed the literature on studies related to CABG and put together guidelines outlining the indications for the procedure. These include (1) significant left main coronary artery disease; (2) left main equivalent, defined as 70% stenosis of both the proximal left anterior descending artery (LAD) and proximal left circumflex artery (LCA); and (3) multivessel disease (with a greater survival benefit in those with normal left ventricular function, defined as a measured left ventricular ejection fraction > 50%). For those with stable angina, indications for surgery are broadened to include (1) two-vessel disease with significant proximal LAD obstruction, (2) one- to two-vessel coronary artery disease without proximal LAD stenosis but with a large area of viable myocardium at risk; and (3) severe, incapacitating angina despite maximal medical therapy.

Coronary artery anatomy

To understand coronary revascularization, one must first understand coronary artery anatomy (Fig. 73.1). The left main coronary artery (LMCA) and the right coronary artery (RCA)

originate from the aortic root. The LMCA divides into the left anterior descending coronary artery (LAD) and left circumflex coronary artery (LCA). The LAD divides further to the diagonal and septal branches, providing blood to the anterolateral portion of the heart, the interventricular groove, and the His–Purkinje system. The obtuse marginal branches coming off of the LCA, supply blood to the lateral free wall of the left ventricle. The RCA splits off into the acute marginal branches, which perfuse the anterior wall of the right ventricle. In most patients, the RCA gives rise to the posterior descending artery (PDA), providing blood to the posterior portion of the left ventricle. These patients are considered to have a right dominant system. In the remaining patients, the PDA comes off the LCA and therefore is classified as having a left dominant system. Rarely, the PDA can arise from both the LCA and RCA and be classified as a codominant system.

Myocardial oxygen supply and demand

Cardiac function depends on maintaining a balance between oxygen supply and demand. Increasing myocardial contractility, heart rate, or myocardial wall tension increases the oxygen demand of the heart, whereas myocardial oxygen supply is decreased by decreasing coronary artery blood flow, arterial oxygen content, or oxygen extraction. Heart rate and end-diastolic pressure are on both sides of the supply–demand equation. Thus, any increase in heart rate and end-diastolic pressure (volume) decreases myocardial oxygen supply while increasing myocardial oxygen demand.

Monitoring

In addition to the standard American Society of Anesthesiologists monitors, specialized monitors are used in CABG patients to help guide perioperative management. A Foley catheter measures urine output throughout the procedure. Five-lead electrocardiographic (ECG) monitoring allows for the discernment of arrhythmias, as well as the detection of more than 90% of all ischemic events if leads II and V5 are used. Arterial blood pressure monitoring permits assessment of beat-to-beat perfusion and provides a port for frequent arterial blood gas (ABG) and other laboratory measurements. Central line placement provides available ports for vasoactive medication

Figure 73.1. Coronary artery anatomy

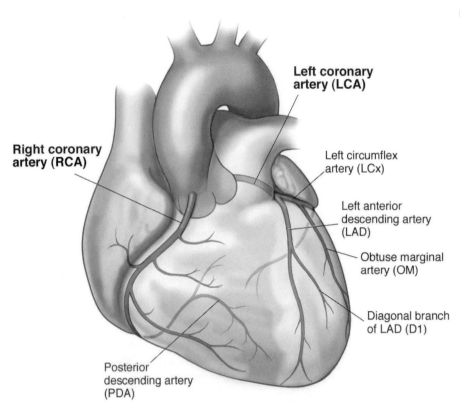

administration; the transduction of a central venous pressure waveform can provide an assessment of volume status. In more complex patients with cardiac failure or pulmonary hypertension, a pulmonary artery catheter may be placed to evaluate ventricular filling pressures, pulmonary vascular resistance, cardiac output, core temperature, and mixed venous oxygen saturation. It may also be used for transvenous pacing. Although a transesophageal echocardiogram (TEE) is not essential in all patients undergoing a CABG, in those with baseline ventricular dysfunction (left ventricular ejection fraction <40%) or valvular disease, it may be a useful tool to detect new wall motion abnormalities, areas of ischemia, or changes in valve function. The electroencephalogram or cerebral saturation may be used to monitor the well-being of the brain, and both have been used in situations in which deep hypothermic circulatory arrest is warranted to place a graft on a diseased aorta.

Perioperative management

Induction of anesthesia

Debate on the proper type of anesthetic agent to induce a patient undergoing CPB surgery has steadily evolved throughout the years. Early in the advent of cardiac surgery, barbiturates and inhalational agents were commonly used, in the first cardiac surgical patients of Gibbon and Lillihei in the 1950s. As monitoring techniques became more advanced, the need for achieving hemodynamic stability and preventing myocardial depression became recognized.

As time passed, observations were made that sedating post–cardiac surgical patients in the intensive care unit on a morphine regimen of 0.5 to 3 mg/kg provided little derangement in hemodynamic measurements. In 1969, Lowenstein et al. published hemodynamic observations based on patients undergoing cardiac surgery who were induced with 1 mg/kg of morphine, which validated the relative safety of its use, ushering in the era of a high-dose narcotic technique for these patients. This type of anesthetic was not optimal, however, because patients still had inadequate anesthesia and hypotension, likely related to the histamine effects of morphine, and required large volumes of fluid and blood perioperatively.

In the late 1970s, a fentanyl-based anesthetic was used by Stanley and Webster for inducing cardiac surgical patients and gradually supplanted the use of morphine for an opioid-based induction agent. When first used as a total anesthetic with a relaxant and a benzodiazepine, doses of up to 100 to 150 μg/kg of fentanyl comprised the total anesthetic. This technique produced hemodynamic stability and allowed a prolonged recovery time so that the heart could recuperate from the effects of CPB and achieve homeostasis. Rarely were these patients extubated the day of surgery. In the past decades, however, studies have suggested that heavy postoperative sedation does not change outcomes. It was soon appreciated that patients in the younger age range with normal ventricles who underwent an uncomplicated operation could be extubated sooner (with a potential increase in patient satisfaction and decrease in resource uti-'lization). Thus, "fast-track" anesthesia was synonymous with the goal of having patients extubated and recuperated early,

Table 73.1. Effects of anesthetics on hemodynamics

	Contractility	Rate	Afterload (SVR)	Blood pressure	Comments
Intravenous induction agents					
Propofol	↓	↑	↓	↓	Dose-dependent BP decrease, mostly secondary to decrease in contractility and SVR
Thiopental	↓	↑	↓	↓	Decreased SVR leads to venous pooling and preload with reflex tachycardia
Etomidate	–	–	↓	↓	Decline in MAP and SVR minimal compared with other agents
Ketamine	↑	↑	↑	↑	Not typically used unless tamponade is an issue
Benzodiazepines	–	↑	↓	↓	Hypotensive effect is dose-dependent, slow onset time
Fentanyl	↓/-	↓	–	↓	Previously used in large doses to achieve hemodynamic stability
Volatile agents					
Desflurane	↓/-	↑	↓	↓	Potential myocardial protection with desflurane use
Isoflurane	↓/-	↑	↓	↓	Theories of coronary steal unproven
Sevoflurane	↓/-	↑	↓	↓	Useful for inhalation induction

BP, blood pressure; MAP, mean arterial pressure.

which was advocated for CABG patients without complications. In some institutions, all patients are administered a fast-track cardiac anesthetic protocol and the decision to ventilate a patient overnight is based on the surgery or the postoperative course. An anesthetic technique using 10 to 15 μg/kg of fentanyl combined with etomidate or thiopental for induction and an inhalational agent for maintenance is used in many institutions. Recently, anesthetics such as propofol, remifentanil, sufentanil, dexmedetomidine, and desflurane have been used to allow extubation within the first few hours post cardiac surgery. Multimodal approaches with intrathecal opioids or thoracic epidural analgesia also may be used in the CABG patient, but only after discussion with the surgical and intensive care unit teams.

Any technique can (and has) been used safely and successfully in caring for cardiac surgical patients; therefore, whatever anesthetic is chosen, one must first understand the pathophysiology of the disease process for which the patient requires surgery and must treat the hemodynamic consequences accordingly. The hemodynamic effects of intravenous agents and selected inhalational agents are summarized in Table 73.1.

Effects of anesthetics on hemodynamics

A thorough understanding of the effects of anesthetic agents is crucial, because the anesthesiologist must anticipate the physiologic consequences of the medications administered to prevent imbalances in the myocardial oxygen supply–demand ratio.

Anesthetic management prior to CPB

After the induction of anesthesia, the anesthesiologist must be aware of the sequence of events leading up to a patient being safely placed on CPB. After prophylactic antibiotics are administered, antifibrinolytics are administered to prevent the onset of primary fibrinolysis triggered by CPB. Aminocaproic acid is given at a bolus of 5 to 10 g followed by an infusion at

1 g/h. If tranexamic acid is used, then a bolus of 10 mg/kg is given, followed by an infusion at 1 mg/kg/h. Aprotinin is an antifibrinolytic that previously was popular for its effectiveness in decreasing perioperative blood loss and transfusion requirements (especially for those at high risk for perioperative bleeding). In the past few years, however, its use has fallen out of favor because of the potential increased risk of renal failure, myocardial infarction, and stroke, as well as the increased mortality rates compared with the other lysine analogues.

During the maintenance of anesthesia, one must be able to anticipate the times high levels of stimulation are about to take place versus the times low levels of stimulation will occur. Periods of high sympathetic stimulation (incision, sternal split/spread, aortic cannulation) must be foreseen and managed so that tachycardia, dysrhythmias, hypertension, and heart failure can be prevented, because these alterations ultimately increase the myocardial oxygen demand and decrease the myocardial oxygen supply. In particular, during aortic cannulation, most surgeons prefer that the systolic blood pressure be dropped to below 100 mm Hg to prevent an aortic dissection or excessive bleeding during cannulation. At this time, a sufficient level of anesthetic must be achieved. If this is not enough to blunt the sympathetic response, then the administration of β-blocking agents or other blood pressure–lowering agents (venodilators such as nitroglycerin or nitroprusside) may be warranted. Doses of at least 20 μg/kg of fentanyl are commonly given preemptively to blunt the response. The patient's hemodynamic status should be thoroughly monitored with arterial pressures, central venous pressures, pulmonary artery pressures, mixed venous oxygen saturations (if applicable), and TEE. During times of low-level stimulation (saphenous vein graft/internal mammary harvesting), the pressure may decrease, and perfusion to the coronaries might be compromised, with resultant signs of ischemia. In this situation, one may add back sympathetic tone with phenylephrine or ephedrine or simply increase intravascular volume to bring the blood pressure to the desired level. Should ischemia occur persistently despite optimal anesthetic and hemodynamic management at any time before bypass, the surgical team should be informed and a discussion should take place regarding whether to initiate bypass or place an intra-aortic balloon pump. Should this need arise, it is essential that communication regarding the level of heparinization take place prior to cannulation. If a retrograde cardioplegia cannula is placed in the coronary sinus, the blood pressure should be watched vigilantly for sudden declines due to manipulation of the heart. If sudden hypotension occurs after securing the cannula, the differential diagnosis includes blood loss, compression of the heart, dysrhythmias, systemic embolization of clot/air, and aortic dissection. After the retrograde catheter is placed, the waveform should be transduced to assure proper placement and for pressure monitoring during bypass. Oftentimes, if a TEE is placed, the retrograde cannula placement can be confirmed by echoing the coronary sinus.

For repeat CABG operations, blood should be immediately available in case there is inadvertent damage to the right ventricle or grafts adherent to the sternum. In many of these patients, cannulation of the femoral vessels might be performed prior to the sternotomy, so that the patient can be placed on partial CPB. Oftentimes, this will allow the empty heart to fall away from the sternum, facilitating a safer sternotomy. Again, a proper level of heparinization should be confirmed with an intraoperative coagulation measurement.

Heparin is administered for anticoagulation prior to CPB to prevent clot formation in the CPB circuit and is monitored by checking either the activated clotting time (ACT) or heparin levels (depending on the bedside device used at each institution). An ACT level of at least 300 seconds is required before initiating CPB if the circuits are coated with a heparin/anticoagulation surface or from 400 to 480 seconds if no anticoagulation coating is used. Different institutions have different target levels. Cannulation and institution of CPB must not be performed unless adequate anticoagulation is confirmed. Anticoagulation is checked at regular intervals during CPB, and additional heparin is administered if necessary. If resistance to heparin becomes an issue, then the patient most likely has an antithrombin III deficiency. If antithrombin III is low, there is not enough of this serine protease, which irreversibly inactivates thrombin and other factors, to bind to heparin and cause adequate anticoagulation. Patients with this deficiency must then be administered fresh frozen plasma, antithrombin III concentrate, synthetic antithrombin III, or a recombinant form of the molecule. However, if the patient has a history of heparin-induced thrombocytopenia, then alternate anticoagulants such as hirudin, bivalirudin, or argatroban can be administered, because exposure to heparin might cause thrombocytopenia, with a potential for thromboembolism.

After adequate anticoagulation is achieved and the patient is cannulated, one may review the pre-CPB checklist to ensure that a patient is ready to go on CPB (Table 73.2).

Table 73.2. Pre-CPB checklist

A	Anticoagulation: Is it adequate (ACT > 300 s); anesthetic depth: Is it appropriate? (Need for hypnotic, neuromuscular blocker? Good MAC of volatile anesthetic?)
B	Blood: What was the most recent Hct? Should packed RBCs be included in the pump prime?
C	Cannulas: Are they working appropriately? Catheters: Are the monitors in place, functioning well? Pulmonary artery catheter should be pulled back a couple of centimeters to prevent a pulmonary artery rupture? Are transducers zeroed?
D	Drips: are they off?
E	Eyes: Note baseline pupil size for comparison, rule out neurologic complications, edema
F	Foley: Is the bag emptied (to ensure good urine volume while on CPB)?
G	Glucose: What is the most recent level? Should insulin be started?

Hct, hematocrit; MAC, minimum alveolar concentration; RBCs, red blood cells

CPB

The CPB circuit and heart–lung machine are complex tools used in cardiac surgery to give the surgeon a quiet (nonbeating) bloodless heart so that an efficient and effective operation may be performed. The heart–lung machine mechanically maintains systemic circulation, oxygenates the blood, and allows for carbon dioxide elimination. In addition, it provides for the rapid cooling and rewarming of blood.

The CPB machine has the following components (Fig. 73.2):

1. Venous reservoir: Venous blood is drained either by gravity or by suction from the right heart. Venous blood enters the CPB circuit via a cannula placed in the right atrium, superior vena cava (SVC), inferior vena cava (IVC), or femoral vein, and travels to the reservoir, where other fluids and medications can be mixed. *Total CPB* occurs when all the venous return goes to the venous reservoir. This occurs only when tourniquets are placed around the SVC and IVC. *Partial CPB* occurs when only a portion of blood bypasses the heart, but the rest is allowed to enter the pulmonary circulation.

2. Oxygenator: Blood is pumped from the venous reservoir to an artificial membrane that allows the diffusion of oxygen and anesthetic agents to the blood, and elimination of carbon dioxide.

3. Heat exchanger: A heat exchanger allows cooling and warming of the blood.

4. Arterial filter: It is used to prevent air and unwanted debris from being returned to the patient, and is the last device placed in the circuit before blood returns to the patient.

5. Venous blood pump (arterial pump head): This pump forces venous blood through the membrane oxygenator and then to the patient's aortic root or arterial system. The venous blood pump is the "heart" of the heart–lung machine.

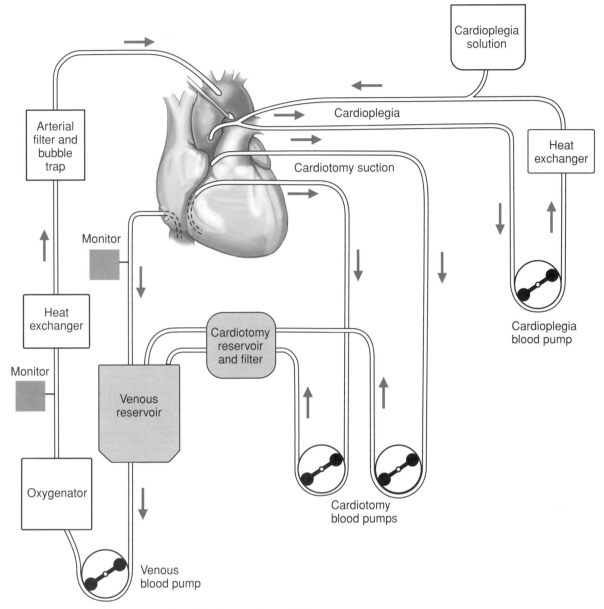

Figure 73.2. Essential components of a cardiopulmonary ciruit.

6. Cardiotomy pump: This separate device in the pump allows blood to be returned to the heart–lung machine instead of being placed in the disposal reservoir. There are usually two cardiotomy or "waste" pumps in a heart–lung machine.

7. Cardioplegia: This separate pump head is used to deliver solutions (usually high potassium) to arrest the heart during aortic cross-clamping.

8. Monitors: The perfusionist is trained to set up several pressure monitors within the circuit, level detectors on the venous reservoir that provide a feedback loop to lower the flow if the reservoir decreases and to calibrate saturation or blood gas monitors within the circuit.

9. Tubing: The tubing and connectors through which blood flows may be coated with a heparin-like material or they may be plain polyvinyl chloride.

An understanding of the physiologic effects of CPB allows for optimal perioperative management of patients undergoing cardiac surgery. The physiologic effects of CPB are shown in Fig. 70.3.

1. Change in blood flow: Systemic blood flow is dialed by the machine. Generally, blood flow is maintained at 2.5 L/min/m^2 to meet the metabolic needs of an anesthetized patient. Maximal flow is limited by the venous return, which is a function of the patient's venous capacity, or in

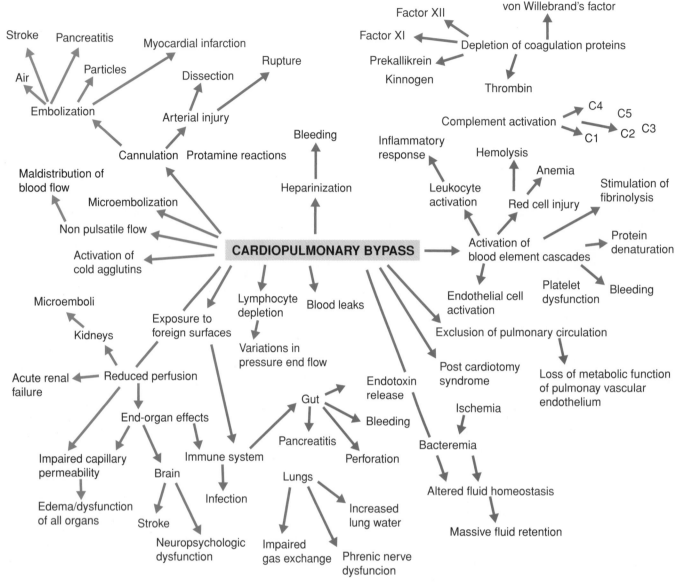

Figure 73.3. Physiologic effects of CPB.

institutions where gravity drains the right heart, can be determined by the difference in height between the operating room table and the bypass reservoir. Resistance of the venous and arterial cannulas, extracorporeal circuit, and vasculature also plays a role.

2. Change in pulsatility: When transitioning from the systemic circulation to the CPB machine, pulsatile flow stops. Potential advantages of persistent pulsatility include enhanced lymphatic flow and tissue perfusion, as well as a decreased neuroendocrine response. Although theoretically it would be better to maintain flow in the extracorporeal circulation nearly physiologic, there is still controversy over whether the proposed benefits really make a difference in outcomes. For this reason, and because methods of producing pulsatile flow are complex

and expensive, focus has turned away from achieving pulsatile flow during bypass in many centers.

3. Interaction between blood and nonphysiologic surfaces compounded by shear stresses: Initiation of CPB triggers many potential causes of adverse hematologic and inflammatory responses. An increase in shear stress causes red blood cells to become stiffer and more vulnerable to hemolysis. Neutrophil concentrations initially decrease while a patient is on the heart–lung machine, but then may rebound during rewarming. Complement is activated, and the production of anaphylatoxins from ischemia reperfusion injury causes a systemic inflammatory response. As a result, there is a decrease in systemic vascular resistance and increased capillary permeability.

Platelets are activated, degranulated, and basically rendered nonfunctional by the heart–lung machine.

4. Exaggerated stress response: Because CPB is not a natural phenomenon for the body, high concentrations of catecholamines such as epinephrine, norepinephrine, and adrenocorticotropic hormone are secreted into the circulation. Not only does this affect end-organ blood flow patterns, it also causes increased metabolic requirements and potential tissue breakdown. Hyperglycemia is common in both diabetics and nondiabetics. Thus, strict glucose monitoring and control become necessary.

5. Temperature change: Hypothermia (both systemic and myocardial) decreases myocardial oxygen consumption. Myocardial hypothermia is achieved by the administration of cold cardioplegia in the aortic root (i.e., antegrade cardioplegia) while the aorta is clamped, or in the coronary sinus (known as retrograde cardioplegia). Placing chilled saline or ice directly on the heart may allow topical cooling. Systemic cooling can be achieved with the blood heater/cooler device in the machine. Lower oxygen consumption from hypothermia should result in a lower mixed venous O_2 saturation on CPB.

6. Hyperkalemia: Cardioplegia high in potassium concentrations is used to achieve cardiac arrest. Although such high levels are anticipated during CPB, if high potassium levels persist after the patient is taken off CPB, treatment with calcium chloride or glucose and insulin may be helpful. Potassium also may be shifted into cells by hyperventilation or bicarbonate administration.

7. Hypotension: This results from several factors at the initiation of CPB that cause a decrease in systemic vascular resistance:

   · The administration of priming fluid (usually 800–1500 ml of crystalloid) decreases blood viscosity by hemodilution. Normally, the hematocrit during CPB is between 20% and 25%.
   · Dilution of systemic catecholamines
   · Temporary hypoxemia from asanguinous fluid
   · Fluid that has a low pH, and low levels of calcium and magnesium

Management of patients on CPB

Once CPB has been initiated, the cardiac output is determined by the pump flow rate, which is controlled by the perfusionist. Because all respiratory functions are also controlled by the machine, ventilation of the lungs is stopped, allowing a quiet operating field for the surgeon.

ACT is frequently monitored to ensure adequate anticoagulation while on CPB. Arterial blood gases should be checked every 30 to 60 minutes to monitor for appropriate oxygen and CO_2 levels. Electrolytes, hemoglobin, and blood glucose levels should also be monitored and treated accordingly. Although a degree of hyperkalemia is typical secondary to cardioplegia administration, potassium levels should be normalized by the time a patient is ready to be weaned from CPB.

Inhalational agents may be administered via the bypass circuit, and intravenous anesthetics may be given via an infusion. Monitoring of neurologic function may be helpful in assessing anesthetic depth.

Urine output should be monitored, and if oliguria occurs, increasing the flow rate or administration of an osmotic (mannitol) or loop diuretic (furosemide) may be considered. Temperature should be checked regularly from different sites. The core temperature monitors organs that are well perfused (bladder, nasopharyngeal probes); rectal and skeletal muscle sensors measure the shell temperatures, which may lag behind core temperature changes secondary to hypothermia-induced vasoconstriction. The pulmonary artery catheter temperature cannot be used while on CPB because of lack of blood flow through the heart. The esophageal temperature readings also may not be accurate because of the addition of ice or cold saline to the thoracic cavity during CPB.

Circulatory arrest

Circulatory arrest is used during surgery that may involve the cerebral vessels originating from the aorta, or when a severely diseased aorta cannot be cross-clamped. During circulatory arrest, the patient's systemic temperature is decreased to 15°C to 18°C. This degree of hypothermia is crucial for decreasing the cerebral metabolic rate while flow to the body is stopped. Some clinicians advocate topical hypothermia by wrapping a towel around the head and then icing the head. Additionally, some clinicians administer medications such as sodium thiopental to achieve electroencephalographic suppression), steroids (methylprednisolone, 30 mg/kg) for cerebral protection, and mannitol (25g/kg) for end-organ and renal preservation. However, few data support the benefits of these aforementioned medications, whereas the consensus is that only profound hypothermia and the shortest possible time while in circulatory arrest are actually known to prevent ischemic organ damage. During ascending and aortic arch surgery, some surgeons give antegrade cerebral perfusion to provide intermittent cerebral flow and oxygenation, thus prolonging the allowable time for repair. Other surgeons may prefer the use of retrograde cerebral perfusion through the SVC.

ABG monitoring

When monitoring ABGs, clinicians must understand the basic principles of temperature correction. Because there usually is a difference in temperature between the ABG machine and the patient, the results may vary. This is based on the idea that as the temperature of blood decreases, oxygen and carbon dioxide become more soluble. As a result, the partial pressure of the two gases decreases. Another consequence is that less water is dissociated into OH^- and H^+, causing an elevation in the pH. During analysis of the blood sample, however, the temperature of the ABG machine is higher compared with that of blood. This

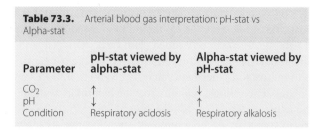

Table 73.3. Arterial blood gas interpretation: pH-stat vs Alpha-stat

Parameter	pH-stat viewed by alpha-stat	Alpha-stat viewed by pH-stat
CO_2	↑	↓
pH	↓	↑
Condition	Respiratory acidosis	Respiratory alkalosis

elevated temperature decreases the solubility of gas in the blood, causing the sample to have falsely elevated partial pressures of CO_2 and O_2. The pH also is falsely lowered, because more H^+ dissociation occurs with the higher temperature. Temperature correction takes the machine's values and corrects them to what the patient is actually experiencing in vivo. Two methods have been executed to manage patients undergoing CPB. In the pH-stat approach, CO_2 is added to the inspired gases to keep the *corrected* CO_2 level at 40 mm Hg. This in turn normalizes the pH. In the alpha-stat approach, nothing is added. It is thought that at the low in vivo temperature, although there is less dissociation of H^+, there is an equally decreased amount of OH^- dissociation. Electrochemical neutrality is thus maintained. In this method, the constant charge (of the amino acids in proteins) is preserved and homeostasis is kept. This allows the patient's *uncorrected* $PaCO_2$ and pH to be kept at normal levels. Table 73.3 shows the perspective of each method when viewed by the alternative approach.

It has been theorized that alpha-stat management might be preferential in patients undergoing CPB. This is based on the suspicion that cerebral blood flow, and therefore the risk of embolization, would increase with the addition of CO_2 in pH-stat management, because CO_2 causes cerebral vasodilation. With alpha-stat management, however, cerebral autoregulation is preserved. Because infants with congenital heart disease undergoing CPB with deep hypothermic circulatory arrest do not have atherosclerosis, the risk of embolization is extremely low. pH-stat is commonly used in this population because increased cerebral perfusion becomes the primary concern. However, studies have not shown improved long-term neurologic outcomes with either strategy.

Rewarming

Adequate time for rewarming is necessary when preparing for weaning from CPB. If the rewarming process is too fast, there is a risk of creating temperature gradients between the well-perfused organs and those that are vasoconstricted. The administration of vasodilators (e.g., nitroglycerin) can circumvent this and helps speed up the rewarming process. Rapid rewarming also may cause the formation of gas bubbles, as gas solubility decreases with increasing temperatures. During this time, because the patient's metabolic activities also escalate, intravenous medication (opioids, benzodiazepines, or muscle relaxants) is administered to provide additional anesthesia, because

the risk for recall is greatest then, unless an intravenous anesthetic was instituted at the start of CPB. As the patient's temperature rises and the aortic cross-clamp is removed, the heart's electrical activity resumes as the heart is filled with blood. A TEE may be used to evaluate for air, new valvular disease, or change in myocardial function. The ECG is assessed for ST-segment abnormalities, especially the right coronary artery – leads II, III, aVF – because it is positioned at the superior aspect of the heart and is thus vulnerable to air entrainment. If ventricular tachycardia or fibrillation is seen, the heart should immediately be defibrillated with internal paddles. A pacemaker may be used to assist with cardiac output if the heart rate is low or if the rhythm is irregular. Communication with the perfusionist about vasopressor requirements on CPB may indicate the need for intravenous support while coming off bypass. Ventilation is resumed once blood flow is permitted through the respiratory circulation.

Management of patients during the post-CPB period

Weaning from CPB is a gradual process in which 100% of the mechanical work is transitioned from the CPB machine to the patient's own heart. Assessment of whether the patient can tolerate weaning from CPB is crucial. The patient's physiologic variables must be analyzed and optimized quickly. Core temperatures should be at least 36°C. A vasodilator should also be available in case hypertension develops or new ECG changes ensue. Laboratory values should be adequate (without anemia, acid–base, or electrolyte abnormalities), and a stable rhythm should be present. A heart rate of 80 to 100 bpm is usually necessary to ensure adequate cardiac output (paced or otherwise), because otherwise there is a decreased ability to increase stroke volume post CPB. Coronary arteries that are grafted have a more favorable oxygen supply/demand ratio, so ischemia should not be an issue at higher rates. If the heart rate is > 120 bpm, however, the etiology should be identified and treated quickly, because too high a heart rate may prevent left ventricular filling. If ST changes occur, nitroglycerin should be initiated and the surgeon informed. If hemodynamic compromise is anticipated because of either poor ventricular function preoperatively or an inability to obtain complete revascularization, inotropic or vasopressor support may be started. Central filling pressure monitoring and TEE assessment can determine the need for volume or pharmacologic support. TEE monitoring is especially useful in evaluating for new regional wall motion abnormalities indicative of ischemia. If the cardiac function is insufficient despite the infusion of inotropes, the surgeon may reexamine the grafts either on or off CPB. If the grafts are patent but the patient is still showing signs of ventricular failure, then a discussion of initiating intra-aortic balloon pump (IABP) or other mechanical devices should be considered.

If, however, all the aforementioned criteria have been met, the following sequence of events will occur:

1. Prevention of venous flow back to the pump
   - The venous line is partially occluded by the surgeon or perfusionist.
   - Blood flow from the right atrium to the right ventricle increases.
   - Partial bypass is attained because some of the blood goes to the CPB machine and some goes to the heart.
   - Assessment is made about optimal preload (either by TEE or by central venous and pulmonary capillary wedge pressures).

2. Decrease of pump flow into the aorta
   - The perfusionist gradually reduces the pump flow rate as the patient's own heart is able to maintain its own cardiac output.

3. Termination of bypass
   - The CPB pump is stopped when the heart can maintain adequate systolic pressures at acceptable preloads.

After the termination of CPB, blood from the pump is usually administered in 50- to 100-ml increments to increase preload. The blood pressure and filling pressures need to be monitored closely. Volume is given slowly to avoid overdistention of the heart and to prevent inadvertent emptying of the venous reservoir. Slow volume administration should increase the cardiac output in the best circumstances. If this is not the case, one should consider investigating for the following: (1) ongoing blood loss, (2) vasodilatory effects from rewarming or systemic inflammatory response, or (3) a change in ventricular compliance. To assess that the cardiac performance is adequate, a cardiac output should be obtained and/or the TEE reviewed. Review of the physiologic variables helps determine which adjustments need to be made in the inotrope/vasopressor infusions and/or volume administration. Once it is safe to proceed, the venous and aortic cannulas can be removed. The aortic cannula can be removed when approximately half the protamine dose has been given.

Protamine administration

Protamine is given to reverse anticoagulation. Post-CPB ACT and heparin levels are evaluated to verify adequate reversal. Protamine is a large negatively charged protein from salmon known as a histone binding the DNA in the salmon sperm. It gets its negative charge from high numbers of the amino acid arginine, and hence will bind the positively charged heparin molecule. Once the heparin–protamine complex is formed, it is thought that the reticuloendothelial system removes this complex.

The protamine dosage varies from practice to practice, with a standard dose of 1 mg/100 U of heparin given for initial heparinization. Some practices use an automated heparin–protamine titration system (used to calculate heparin dosage to specific ACT by applying patient volume algorithms). This helps determine the amount of circulating heparin present at the end of bypass and hence the amount of protamine needed to bring the heparin levels back to zero. Use of this system usually results in less protamine being administered.

Adverse reactions to protamine are usually divided into three groups as a result of several different mechanisms. The first is defined as a nonimmunologic reaction known as an anaphylactoid reaction. Because the protamine molecule is a large heterogenous protein, its rapid infusion may cause a decrease in blood pressure by either vasodilation or a direct decrease in myocardial contractility and is the reason some practices advocate that protamine be given slowly over a 5- to 10-minute period. This reaction can mimic a true anaphylactic reaction.

Anaphylactic reactions to protamine imply that they are IgE mediated and therefore require the patient to have seen the molecule previously. True anaphylactic reactions to protamine in the patient after weaning from the heart–lung machine are characterized by arterial hypotension, low central venous pressure, and low left atrial pressure. Histamine levels in these patients are noted to be elevated. Patients considered at risk for a protamine reaction have included diabetics on NPH insulin (which contains protamine) and patients who have had prior catheterizations, fish allergies, or vasectomies. The evidence that patients with these risk factors will have a protamine reaction is very poor, but most clinicians believe the group at highest risk is diabetic patients. For this rare event, it has been advocated that a small test dose be given prior to administering the full dose.

The last adverse protamine reaction is a catastrophic pulmonary vasoconstriction. In this group of patients, it was noted after protamine administration that the arterial blood pressures and left atrial pressures were low and the central venous pressures were elevated. Unlike the patients who experienced anaphylactic reactions, the histamine levels drawn from these select patients were low. An animal model of this reaction noted that the large heparin–protamine complexes activated complement. This in turn induced pulmonary macrophages to produce thromboxane, ultimately causing pulmonary artery vasoconstriction and right ventricular failure.

Treatment of protamine reactions immediately post bypass depends on the severity. Protamine administration needs to be stopped, supportive therapy (epinephrine with histamine blockers) instituted, and a return to cardiopulmonary bypass (after reheparinization) considered. If bypass is reinstituted, an attempt to reverse the heparin with another protamine dose can be done after treatment with histamine H_1 and H_2 blockers and steroids. If another protamine reaction occurs, heparin reversal should be avoided and the bleeding patient should be supported with factors until the heparin is metabolized.

Fortunately, protamine reactions are rare, and because they are rare, pretreatment is not advocated in all patients who undergo cardiopulmonary bypass.

Laboratory assessment post CPB

ABGs should be monitored to ensure adequate ventilation/oxygenation and to be aware of any acid–base or electrolyte abnormalities. A hemoglobin level is also checked to estimate the need for cell saver or red blood cell administration. A complete blood count, chemistry panel, and coagulation studies are sent for analysis. If nonsurgical bleeding occurs even if thrombocytopenia is not evident, platelets may be administered because platelet dysfunction is the most prevalent cause of hemostatic abnormalities after CPB. If the coagulation panels are abnormal and there is clinical evidence of a significant coagulopathy, fresh frozen plasma and/or cryoprecipitate may be given to treat factor deficiencies or low fibrinogen.

Failure to wean off CPB

A need for inotropic support during separation from CPB may be anticipated if a patient presents with the following risk factors: a combined CABG/MV repair or MV replacement, a left ventricular ejection fraction <35%, a reoperation, moderate to severe mitral regurgitation, and a long aortic cross-clamp time. If after the administration of fluids/blood and pharmacologic support the patient still has left or right ventricular failure, then a differential diagnosis must quickly be reviewed and managed appropriately. Common causes of failure to wean off CPB are listed below.

Contractility Left or right ventricle	• Insufficient cardioplegia/ischemic injury leading to myocardial stunning/diastolic dysfunction
	• Embolic (air/atheroma)
	• Thrombotic (early graft occlusion)
	• Graft kinking
	• Prolonged aortic cross-clamp
	• Reperfusion injury
Rate	• Bradycardia, causing decreased cardiac output
	• Tachycardia, preventing adequate filling, perfusion
Rhythm	• Bradyarrhythmias
	• Tachydysrhythmias
Afterload	• Vasodilatory shock secondary to systemic inflammatory response, drug reaction (protamine)
	• Anaphylaxis
Preload	• Intraoperative, perioperative blood loss secondary to coagulopathy, surgical bleeding
	• Inadequate fluid administration
	• Excess preload, leading to overdistention of the heart
Valve failure	• During valve procedures, the prosthesis can have a leak, mechanical obstruction
	• Acute ischemic mitral regurgitation (papillary muscle rupture)

After evaluation of the patient's blood pressure, filling pressures, and TEE, if any of the above are thought to occur, the etiology of hypotension should be treated accordingly with more aggressive pharmacologic support (inotropes, pressors, or vasodilatory agents if ischemia is suspected) or fluids if necessary. If a surgical cause of the cardiovascular derangement is thought to occur or if no etiology can be determined after 3 to 5 minutes after coming off bypass, then a discussion about returning to CPB should be made. This decision should not be made lightly, considering the risk of inadequate heparinization after protamine administration and hemolysis. If the decision is made to proceed back onto CPB, then a full dose of heparin should be given based on the last ACT measurement. If the issue is nonsurgical and the patient is refractory to

medical management even after the aggressive administration of inotropes and/or pressors, one may also consider the placement of an IABP. Occasionally, the placement of a ventricular assist device may be necessary to help the myocardium recover after the period of "stunning" or to serve as a bridge to heart transplantation.

Suggested readings

Bellinger DC, et al. Developmental and neurologic effects of alpha-stat versus pH-stat strategies for deep hypothermic cardiopulmonary bypass in infants. *J Thorac Cardiovasc Surg* 2001; 121(2):374–383.

Buckberg GD. Update on current techniques of myocardial protection. *Ann Thorac Surg* 1995; 60:805–814.

Dahlbacka S, et al. Effects of pH management during selective antegrade cerebral perfusion on cerebral microcirculation and metabolism: alpha-stat vs. pH-stat. *Ann Thorac Surg* 2007; 84:847–856.

Du Plessis AJ, et al. Perioperative effects of alpha-stat versus pH-stat strategies for deep hypothermic cardiopulmonary bypass in infants. *J Thorac Cardiovasc Surg* 1997; 114(6):991–1000.

Elefteriades JA. Mini-CABG: a step forward or backward? The "pro" point of view. *J Cardiothorac Vasc Anesth* 1997; 11(5):661–668.

Fergusson D, et al. A comparison of aprotinin and lysine analogues in high-risk cardiac *N Engl J Med* 2008; 358:2319–2331.

Hagl C, et al. Hypothermic circulatory arrest during ascending and aortic arch surgery: the theoretical impact of different cerebral perfusion techniques and other methods of cerebral protection. *Eur J Cardiothorac Surg* 2003; 24(2003):371–378.

Hessel EA. Evolution of cardiac anesthesia and surgery. In: *Kaplan's Cardiac Anesthesia*. 5th ed. Philadelphia: Saunders; 2006.

Mangano D, et al. The risk associated with aprotinin in cardiac surgery. *N Engl J Med* 2006; 354:353–365.

McKinlay KH, et al. Predictors of inotrope use during separation from cardiopulmonary bypass. *J Cardiothorac Vasc Anesth* 2004; 18:404–408.

Nauphal M, et al. Effect of alpha-stat vs. pH-stat strategies on cerebral oximetry during moderate hypothermic cardiopulmonary bypass. *Eur J Anaesth* 2007; 24:15–19.

Lowenstein E. The birth of opioid anesthesia. *Anesthesiology* 2004; 100:1013–1015.

Lowenstein E, Hallowell P, Levine F, et al. Cardiovascular response to large doses of intravenous morphine in man. *N Engl J Med* 1969; 281:1389–1393.

Lowenstein E, Johnston WE, Lappas DG, et al. Catastrophic pulmonary vasoconstriction associated with protamine reversal of heparin. *Anesthesiology* 1983; 59:470.

Patel RL, et al. Alpha-stat acid-base regulation during cardiopulmonary bypass improves neuropsychologic outcome in patients undergoing coronary artery bypass grafting. *J Thorac Cardiovasc Surg* 1996; 111(6):1267–1279.

Speiss BD, Horrow J, Kaplan JA. Transfusion medicine and coagulopathyulation disorders. In: *Kaplan's Cardiac Anesthesia*. 5th ed. Philadelphia: Saunders; 2006.

Stanley TH, Webster LR: Anesthetic requirements and cardiovascular effects of fentanyl-oxygen and fentanyl-diazepam-oxygen anesthesia in man. *Anesth Analg* 1979; 57:411.

Off-pump coronary artery bypass

Theresa S. Chang and John A. Fox

Experimentation with off-pump coronary artery bypass (OPCAB) surgery began in the 1960s. Since then, its practice evolved from grafting single-vessel disease to multivessel disease with the technologic development of mechanical coronary artery stabilizers (Fig. 74.1). Although the technique is more technically demanding for the surgeon, it theoretically avoids the side effects and potential complications associated with cardiopulmonary bypass (CPB), including the development of a systemic inflammatory response, which is thought to be responsible for multiple organ dysfunction. Nonpulsatile flow achieved during CPB potentially affects the microcirculation, which also may cause end-organ damage. Avoiding aortic manipulation by avoiding aortic cannulation and cross-clamping should decrease atheroma embolization and potentially decrease stroke rate and neurocognitive impairment. With these theoretic advantages to avoiding use of the heart–lung machine, it is anticipated that the recovery time, hospital stay, and costs are reduced.

Patient characteristics

Since the advent of myocardial positioning and stabilizing devices, OPCAB surgery has been performed in patients needing myocardial revascularization on multiple coronary lesions and not just in a single area on the left anterior descending artery. As OPCAB techniques have developed, indications for this operation have expanded, from patients who initially were young and without many comorbidities to those with more

Table 74.1. Contraindications to OPCAB

Absolute contraindications	Relative contraindications
Hemodynamic instability	Cardiomegaly/congestive heart failure
Poor-quality target vessels including:	Critical left main disease
Intramyocardial vessels	Small distal targets
Diffusely diseased vessels	Recent or current acute MI
Calcified coronary vessels	Cardiogenic shock
	Poor left ventricular function (LVEF <35%)

MI, myocardial infarction; LVEF, left ventricular ejection fraction.

critical conditions, who theoretically would benefit most. Contraindications to the procedure are shown in Table 74.1.

Surgical principles

To optimize surgical conditions for OPCAB, several goals must be met:

1. The heart must be positioned appropriately to allow good surgical exposure. Many of these devices use suction to pull the heart up by its anatomic attachments (apical and nonapical).
2. The tissues surrounding the area of focus during coronary arteriotomy must be stabilized to allow the surgeon to place vascular sutures. This also is done with suction devices or by direct local compression so that certain areas of the heart can be immobilized.

The mechanical manipulation required during OPCAB surgery makes the heart vulnerable to cardiac arrhythmias.

In addition to hemodynamic changes from mechanical cardiac stabilization, temporary target vascular occlusion may contribute to regional myocardial ischemia during the anastomosis. To allow for myocardial protection, occasionally intraluminal shunts are placed to allow perfusion of the distal vessel during graft placement. Passive coronary perfusion also may be performed, allowing blood to flow from the aorta or femoral artery to the distal coronary target vessels. Another likely superior option is active coronary perfusion, in which an inline pump increases flow to the distal vessel.

Implications for anesthetic management

The placement of monitors is similar to that in coronary artery bypass graft surgery using the heart–lung machine. Standard American Society of Anesthesiologists monitors are placed prior to induction. Large-bore peripheral intravenous access is essential to allow for the rapid infusion of volume and blood products if needed. An arterial catheter helps guide intraoperative hemodynamic challenges, provides for beat-to-beat monitoring, and allows for frequent arterial blood gas/laboratory measurements. A central line facilitates the administration of pressors and inotropes in case of hemodynamic compromise, whereas a pulmonary artery catheter enables the measurement

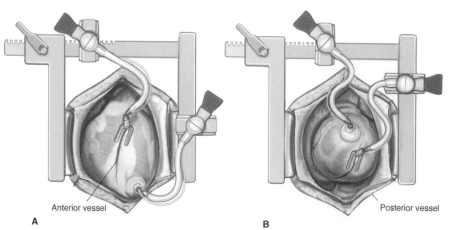

Figure 74.1. OPCAB technology in use. (A) The Medtronic (Minneapolis, MN) Octopus4 tissue stabilizer with Starfish2 heart positioner isolates and exposes the left anterior descending (LAD) coronary artery. (B) An intraluminal shunt is shown inserted and positioned across the LAD arteriotomy. The Medtronic Starfish2 heart positioner lifts the heart and exposes the posterior vessels, whereas the Octopus4 tissue stabilizer immobilizes a segment of the posterior descending artery.

of mixed venous oxygen saturation and monitoring for changes in oxygen consumption during heart manipulation, along with changes in central pressures. Transesophageal echocardiography can provide the earliest detailed information regarding myocardial ischemia, as long as images are well visualized (i.e., the heart is not malpositioned during grafting). Temperature monitoring and techniques to avoid hypothermia in the operating room must be employed.

Induction techniques are the same for those undergoing myocardial revascularization using CPB. A thorough understanding of the hemodynamic consequences of anesthetic agents as they relate to myocardial oxygen supply–demand balance is essential. "Fast-track" cardiac anesthesia is administered using a limited dose of short-acting narcotics to aid in early (1–4 hours) extubation postoperatively. Some small studies have shown that anesthetic regimens including thoracic epidural analgesia provide good results, with improved hemodynamic stability and postoperative pain control. The risk for potential epidural hematoma is still unknown, especially because some level of anticoagulation is still required in OPCAB surgery. Heparin is administered and the ACT is checked regularly to ensure adequate anticoagulation, which may vary depending on the institution, because some institutions require full heparinization as if preparing to initiate CPB, whereas other institutions use smaller doses. Toward the end of the procedure, protamine is not given, or may be given in smaller incremental doses, because acute reversal is not required. Because the heart–lung machine, with its triggering fibrinolytic processes, is not used, antifibrinolytic agents generally are not administered.

Anesthesiologists must be prepared to manage the patient promptly when surgical consequences cause sudden physiologic changes. Ensuring adequate anesthetic depth is important at the time of incision and sternotomy, when sympathetic stress is greatest. After that period, however, anesthesiologists need to prepare for immediate hypotension, preemptively giving fluids to prevent the deleterious effects from lifting and rotating the heart, reacting with inotropic support as necessary. Defibrillation pads must be on the patient, and paddles must be ready

in case arrhythmias become problematic. The surgeon must be notified immediately to stop manipulating the heart. If myocardial ischemia occurs, the patient should be managed medically until the surgical anastomosis is completed. At all times, everyone in the OPCAB room should be ready to institute CPB if the patient becomes refractory to hemodynamic manipulations. This implies that a dose of heparin to institute CPB is available and that a member of the perfusion team is present and ready to operate the heart–lung machine.

After uncomplicated OPCAB procedures, patients may be extubated immediately in the operating room if they are normothermic, are hemodynamically stable, and have no evidence of significant bleeding. Otherwise, the anesthetic technique should allow for extubation within 1 to 2 hours in the intensive care unit if extubation is not performed in the operating room.

Outcomes

Theoretic benefits of OPCAB surgery sparked a resurgence of its use in recent years. Initial studies supported a benefit of OPCAB techniques, citing decreased blood transfusion requirements, less evidence of myocardial ischemia (detected by myocardial enzyme release), diminished acute but not long-term neurocognitive dysfunction, and decreased renal insufficiency. Some studies, however, have shown a lower patency of grafts, potentially necessitating subsequent revascularization with conventional CPB techniques. It is clear that experience and comfort with the OPCAB technique among surgeons, anesthesiologists, and other essential members of the operating team are important for a successful OPCAB program. Nonetheless, due to the absence of large-scale studies that consistently show definitive improvement in perioperative morbidity and mortality associated with OPCAB versus myocardial revascularization with CPB, anesthesiologists must be familiar with managing patients undergoing either procedure.

Suggested readings

Hannan E, Wu C, Smith CR, et al. *Circulation* 2007; 116:1–8.
Jaegere P, Suyker W. *Heart* 2002; 88:313–318.

Kessler P, Aybek T, Neidhart G, et al. *J Cardiothorac Vasc Anesth* 2005; 19(1):32–39.

Mehta Y, Juneja R. *Curr Opin Anesthesiol* 2002; 15:9–18.

Sellke F, DiMaio J, Caplan L, et al. *Circulation* 2005; 111:2858–2864.

Verma S, Fedak P, Weisel R, et al. *Circulation* 2004; 109:1206–1211.

Zangrillo A, Geril C, Landoni G, et al. *Minerva Anestesiol* 2006; 72:827–839.

Chapter 75

Transesophageal echocardiography

Karinne Jervis and Balachundhar Subramaniam

Introduction

Transesophageal echocardiography (TEE) is an important tool for perioperative patient assessment, decision making, and clinical care. The goal of perioperative TEE is to allow assessment of ventricular function and volume status, regional wall motion, structure and function of valvular structures, and evaluation of the great vessels.

American Society of Echocardiography/ Society of Cardiovascular Anesthesiologists standard TEE examination

The American Society of Echocardiography (ASE)/Society of Cardiovascular Anesthesiologists (SCA) published guidelines for performing a comprehensive intraoperative multiplane TEE examination of the heart and great vessels. These guidelines emphasize 20 cross-sectional, two-dimensional views for the recommended comprehensive TEE examination (Fig. 75.1). Each view is based on the transducer location, multiplane angle, and main anatomic structures in the image.

Nomenclature

It is assumed that the imaging plane is directed anteriorly from the esophagus through the heart. Nomenclature exists as follows: A superior indication connotes that the object is in a cephalad position. An inferior position indicates the object is in a caudad direction. Posterior is toward the spine, and anterior is toward the sternum. *Left* and *right* denote the patient's left and right. Advancing the probe refers to moving the tip of the probe distally (Fig. 75.2). Turning to the patient's right refers to the movement of the probe in the clockwise rotation. Turning the probe tip to the patient's left refers to the movement of the probe in the counterclockwise rotation. Anteflexion of the probe allows for the flexing of the probe tip anteriorly with the large control wheel; whereas *retroflexing* is the movement of the tip posteriorly. Axial flexion of the probe tip can be accomplished by means of another control wheel on the probe handle and multiplane rotation from 0° to 180°. Images are displayed in the same manner as radiographic images; in addition, images are shown with transducer angle and near field of the image sector at the top of the display screen and the far field at the base of the screen.

Physics of TEE

The TEE probe is an ultrasound machine mounted to the tip of a gastroscope. The generation of ultrasound is based on the principle of piezoelectricity. Most commonly, materials such as quartz or titanate ceramic are used. Piezoelectric crystals are materials with a distinct property that respond to an applied current with an alignment of polarized particles perpendicular to the face of a crystal, resulting in the expansion of the crystal size. When alternating electric currents are applied, the crystals are compressed and expanded, thereby generating an ultrasound wave. When an ultrasound wave is received by a crystal, an electric current is generated. Crystals in a TEE probe function as a generator and a receiver. In a cycle, transmission duration is 1% of the cycle, whereas reception is 90%. In essence, the ultrasound transducers transmit a burst of ultrasound activity and then switch to receive reflected ultrasound signals. The cycle is repeated temporarily and based on ultrasound transmission and return of the reflected signal.

Guidelines and indications

The American Society of Anesthesiologists (ASA) released practice guidelines for the use of perioperative TEE in 1996. Improved imaging has enabled echocardiographers to use TEE intraoperatively to diagnose myocardial ischemia, confirm the efficacy of valvular reconstruction, determine the etiology of hemodynamic instability, and obtain diagnostic information that could not be obtained preoperatively. Recommendations of the taskforce address indications for the use of TEE, the clinical settings in which TEE should be considered, and the proficiency of the operator performing TEE.

Guidelines delegate the three levels of evidence-based indications for TEE implementation and use. Category I indications are supported by the strongest evidence or expert opinion. TEE frequently is useful for category I indications in improving clinical outcomes, and often is indicated. Category II indications are supported by weaker evidence and expert opinion; TEE may be useful in improving clinical outcomes, but appropriate indications are less certain. Category III indications are based on little current scientific or expert support; TEE is infrequently useful in improving clinical outcomes, and appropriate settings for use are uncertain (Table 75.1).

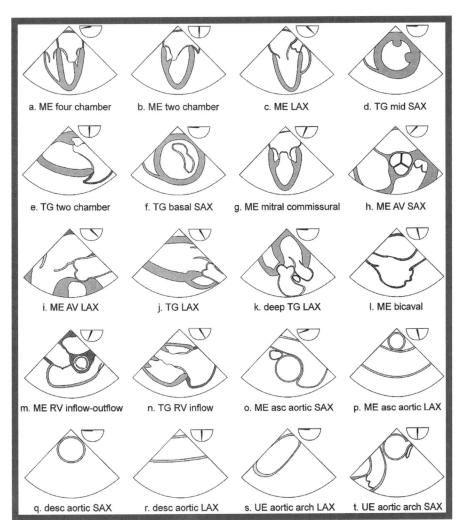

Figure 75.1. ASE/SCA 20 views for comprehensive TEE examination. From Shanewise JS, Cheung AT, Aronson S, et al. ASE/SCA guidelines for performing a comprehensive intraoperative multiplane transesophageal echocardiography examination: recommendations of the American Society of Echocardiography Council for Intraoperative Echocardiography and the Society of Cardiovascular Anesthesiologists Task Force for Certification in Perioperative Transesophageal Echocardiography. *J Am Soc Echocardiogr* 1999; 12:884–900.

a. ME four chamber b. ME two chamber c. ME LAX d. TG mid SAX

e. TG two chamber f. TG basal SAX g. ME mitral commissural h. ME AV SAX

i. ME AV LAX j. TG LAX k. deep TG LAX l. ME bicaval

m. ME RV inflow-outflow n. TG RV inflow o. ME asc aortic SAX p. ME asc aortic LAX

q. desc aortic SAX r. desc aortic LAX s. UE aortic arch LAX t. UE aortic arch SAX

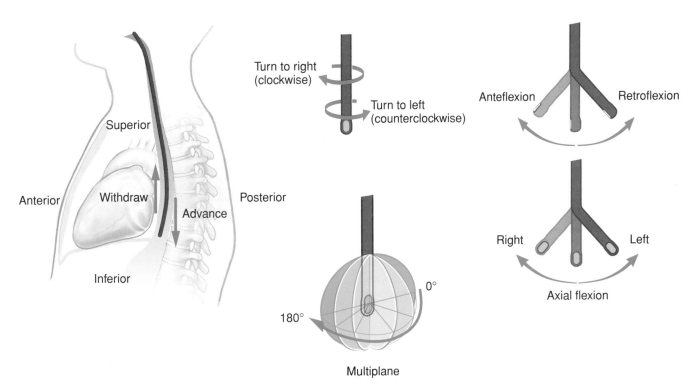

Figure 75.2. Nomenclature of probe positioning.

Table 75.1. Indications for perioperative TEE

Category I	Category II	Category III
Intraoperative evaluation of acute, persistent, and life-threatening hemodynamic disturbances	Perioperative use in patients with increased risk of myocardial ischemia or infarction	Intraoperative evaluation of myocardial perfusion, coronary artery anatomy, or graft patency
Intraoperative use in valve repair	Perioperative use in patients with increased risk of hemodynamic disturbances	Intraoperative use during repair of cardiomyopathies other than HOCM
Intraoperative use in congenital heart surgery requiring CPB	Intraoperative assessment of valve replacements	Intraoperative use for uncomplicated endocarditis during noncardiac surgery
Intraoperative repair of HOCM	Intraoperative assessment of repair of cardiac aneurysms	Intraoperative monitoring for emboli during orthopedic procedures
Intraoperative use for endocarditis when preoperative testing was inadequate or extension of infection is suspected	Intraoperative evaluation of removal of cardiac tumors	Intraoperative assessment of repair of thoracic aortic injuries
Preoperative use in the unstable patient with suspected thoracic aortic aneurysm, dissection, or disruption	Intraoperative detection of foreign bodies	Intraoperative use for uncomplicated pericarditis
Intraoperative assessment of aortic valve function in repair of aortic dissections with possible aortic valve involvement	Intraoperative detection of air emboli during cardiotomy, heart transplants, and upright neurosurgical procedures	Intraoperative evaluation of pleuropulmonary disease
Intraoperative evaluation of pericardial window procedures	Intraoperative use during intracardiac thrombectomy	Monitoring placement of intra-aortic balloon pumps, AICD, or PA catheters
Use in ICU for unstable patients with unexplained hemodynamic disturbances, suspected valvular disease, thromboembolic disease	Intraoperative use during pulmonary embolectomy	Intraoperative monitoring of cardioplegia administration
	Intraoperative use for suspected cardiac trauma	
	Preoperative assessment of patients with suspected acute thoracic aortic dissections, aneurysms, or disruption	
	Intraoperative use during repair of thoracic aortic dissections without suspected aortic valve involvement	
	Intraoperative detection of aortic atheromatous disease or other sources of aortic emboli	
	Intraoperative evaluation of pericardiectomy, pericardial effusions, or evaluation of pericardial surgery	
	Intraoperative evaluation of anastomotic sites during heart and/or lung transplantation	
	Monitoring placement and function of assistive devices	

AICD, automatic implantable cardioverter–defibrillator; CPB, cardiopulmonary bypass; HOCM, hypertrophic obstructive cardiomyopathy; ICU, intensive care unit. American Society of Anesthesiologists and the Society of Cardiovascular Anesthesiologists Task Force on Transesophageal Echocardiography. Practice guidelines for perioperative transesophageal echocardiography. *Anesthesiology* 1996; 84:986–1006.

Common uses of TEE
Evaluation of cardiac function

The midpapillary short-axis view permits the estimation of the global left ventricular function based on the amount of ventricular wall thickening and the difference between end-diastolic volume and end-systolic volume (Fig. 75.3). This view enables the anesthesiologist to assess regional wall abnormalities and determine the presence of myocardial ischemia, and permits the practitioner to postulate the location of coronary artery disease, if present (Fig. 75.3). The ASA guidelines have determined that there is good evidence that the development of regional wall motion abnormalities increases the risk of the development of perioperative myocardial infarction (Fig. 75.4). The ASA

taskforce believes that TEE provides a "more meaningful reference standard for ECG."

As noted in Table 75.1 under category II indications for the use of perioperative TEE, a patient at increased risk for myocardial ischemia is a noted indication for TEE. An increased risk may occur in a patient with an increased risk of myocardial disease, a higher-risk procedure/surgery, or the clinical setting.

The midesophageal four-chamber views give useful information regarding biventricular function, tricuspid and mitral valve visualization, and the major cardiac chambers (Fig. 75.5). In this view, all chamber sizes may be evaluated and may give the practitioner vital information regarding ventricular function.

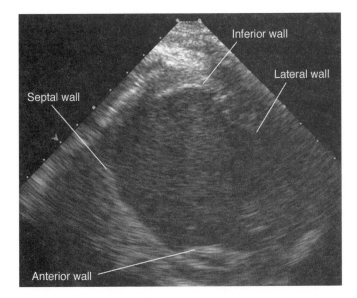

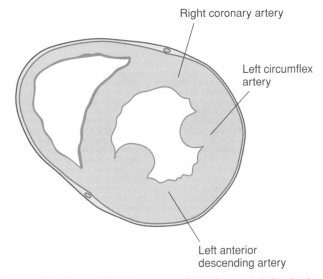

Figure 75.3. Transgastric short-axis view of the left ventricle (LV) and right ventricle (RV).

Assessment of valves

For patients requiring valve surgery, TEE is critical in the evaluation of the diagnosis of valve abnormalities intraoperatively. Surgeons rely on the anesthesiologist to accurately evaluate and confirm preoperative studies, if available, or to initially evaluate valvular anatomy to diagnose abnormal pathology. The ASA taskforce expert opinion confirms that there is indirect evidence that postulates the beneficial use of intraoperative TEE for valve surgery. TEE evaluation appears to have decreased the need for replacement of valves.

Midesophageal aortic valve (AV) short-axis (Fig. 75.6) and AV long-axis (Fig. 75.7) views, along with the transgastric AV long-axis views, are used to evaluate AV lesions such as stenosis and regurgitation.

AV stenosis is commonly seen, and the AV area is calculated using a continuity equation. The flow at the left ventricular outflow tract is a product of its area and the flow at that point. The former is obtained with the midesophageal AV long-axis view (Fig. 75.7). The latter is obtained from the transgastric AV long-axis view (Fig. 75.8).

Left ventricular outflow tract (LVOT) stroke volume

= LVOT area × LVOT velocity time interval (VTI)

Cardiac output = LVOT stroke volume × heart rate.

The pulse wave Doppler cursor is placed at the LVOT, and the velocity time integral is obtained (Fig. 75.9). This product should be equal to that obtained at the AV level. However, the unknown is AV surface area. The flow velocities are higher across a stenotic AV around 4 to 6 m/sec and are obtained with continuous-wave Doppler across the AV (Fig. 75.8).

AV area × AV VTI = LVOT area × LVOT VTI.

The mitral valve is evaluated by the midesophageal four-chamber, commissural, two-chamber, and long-axis views. The transgastric basal short axis view yields plenty of information about the anatomy and location of a lesion such as a regurgitant lesion. A color flow Doppler along with flow Doppler calculations quantifies the mitral valve stenosis and regurgitant lesions. Figure 75.10 shows a transgastric basal short-axis view, and both the anterolateral and inferomedial commissures are seen. The anterior and posterior leaflets are easily recognized. The scallops closer to the anterolateral commissure are A1 and P1 and those closer to the posteromedial commissure are A3 and P3. The mid-scallops are A2 and P2.

Patent foramen ovale is seen in 20% of the population. In normal adults, it may be one of the reasons for right-to-left shunting when the pressure in the right atrium transiently increases more than that in the left atrium. A PFO can be identified by injecting bubbles (i.e. agitated saline) formed in a 10-ml syringe through a central line when Valsalva maneuver (this raises the right atrial pressure transiently more than the left atrial pressure) is released (Fig. 75.11). Presence of several bubbles in the left atrium within three heartbeats signifies the presence of a PFO.

The role of anesthesiologists as primary practitioners and intraoperative echocardiographers

There is continuing debate over the delegation of echocardiographic services intraoperatively: Should the realm of echocardiography be exclusive to cardiologists, or are anesthesiologists equipped to handle the demands of intraoperative treatment and correctly perform and interpret TEEs? In a paper by Mathew et al., the goal was to determine whether diagnostic interpretation of TEE varies widely when the anesthesiologist performing the examination is also providing anesthetic care to the patient. Using continuous quality improvement, an

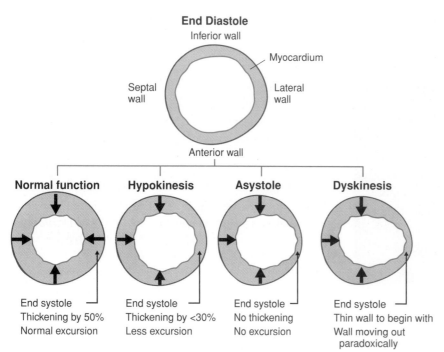

End Diastole

Inferior wall

Myocardium

Septal wall

Lateral wall

Anterior wall

Normal function

End systole
Thickening by 50%
Normal excursion

Hypokinesis

End systole
Thickening by <30%
Less excursion

Asystole

End systole
No thickening
No excursion

Dyskinesis

End systole
Thin wall to begin with
Wall moving out paradoxically

Figure 75.4. Schematic of a transesophageal left ventricle short-axis view showing varying degrees of systolic regional wall motion abnormalities.

educational process to identify problems in health care delivery and to develop solutions to these problems, the authors determined that anesthesiologists responsible for the management of adult cardiac patients and intraoperative TEE were capable of effectively interpreting TEE results. Further results demonstrated that anesthesiologists underestimated the fraction area of change (FAC) compared with radiologist experience in interpretation, but the differences in estimation of the FAC between anesthesiologists and cardiologists and between radiologists and cardiologists were not statistically significant. Finally, as Mathews e. al state "during adult cardiac surgery, the roles of anesthesiologists and the intraoperative echocardiographer need not be mutually exclusive."

Current practice

The literature reports that the use of TEE for cardiac surgery in academic centers averages approximately 91%. ASA practice guidelines consider the use of TEE for coronary artery bypass graft and valve replacement surgery a category II indication, whereas valve repairs, repair of hypertrophic cardiomyopathy, congenital heart surgery, and aortic dissection are category I indications, warranting the use of TEE.

TEE for minimally invasive surgery

The advent of minimally invasive port access during cardiac surgery has enabled patients undergoing cardiac surgery to be placed on cardiopulmonary bypass without the need for median sternotomy for visualization of the heart and great vessels. In the past, placement of catheters was permitted by the use of fluoroscopic guidance, which had limitations. With the increasing proficiency of practitioners using TEE, the use of TEE to aid in the placement of endovascular catheters (coronary sinus

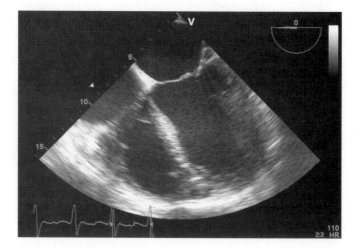

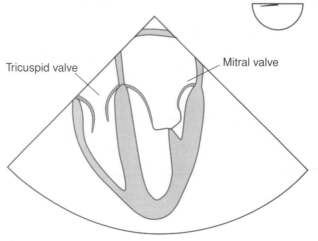

Tricuspid valve

Mitral valve

Figure 75.5. Midesophageal four-chamber view.

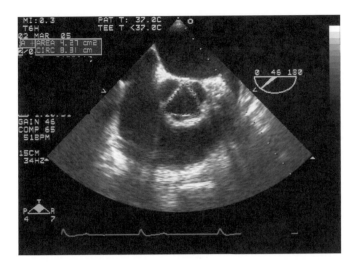

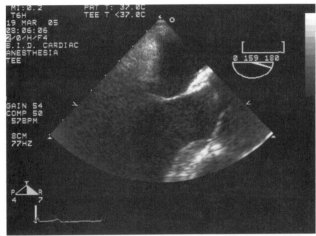

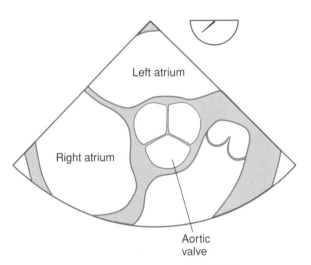

Figure 75.6. Midesophageal AV short-axis (ME AV SAX) view.

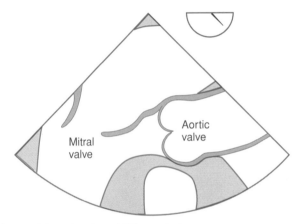

Figure 75.7. Midesophageal AV long-axis view.

catheters, pulmonary artery vent, and venous cannula) has further aided in the progression of minimally invasive surgery. The ability of TEE as an improved, dynamic imaging modality (adequate visualization of cardiac structures) has permitted the placement of catheters without the use of fluoroscopy, with improved success.

TEE in the non–operating room setting

The ASA practice guidelines discuss the use of TEE by anesthesiologists outside the operating room. Common applications include emergent assessment and diagnosis to determine whether surgery is indicated, as well as the postoperative assessment and treatment of patients postoperatively. TEE is useful for recognizing and aiding in the diagnosis of acute hemodynamic instability. Therefore, TEE is critical in nonoperative settings such as the intensive care unit and emergency room. Studies have demonstrated that the impact of TEE on patients with category I indications has been significant, with TEE

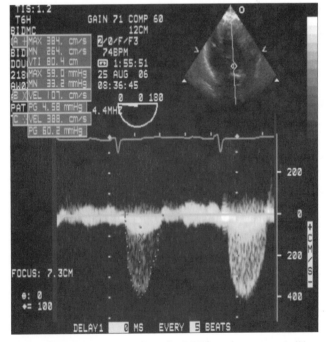

Figure 75.8. Pulse-wave Doppler at the LVOT from the transgastric AV long-axis view.

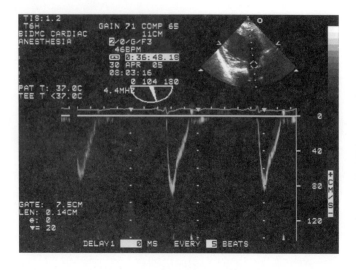

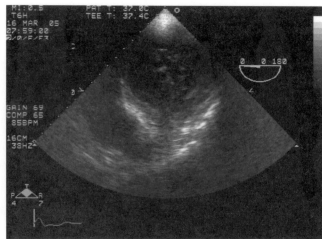

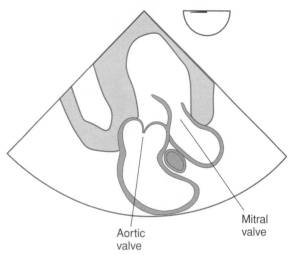

Figure 75.9. Deep transgastric long-axis view of the AV by continuous wave Doppler yields the velocity time integral across the stenotic AV.

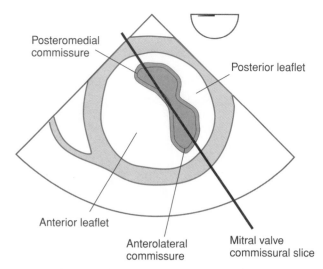

Figure 75.10. Transgastric basal short-axis view of the mitral valve.

altering therapy 60% of the time, compared with the alteration of therapy in category II (31%) and category III (21%).

Pericardial effusion

TEE findings vary depending on the progression of the fluid collection in the pericardial space. Chamber collapse occurs when the pericardial pressure becomes greater than the cardiac chambers' pressures. Thus, it will be noted on TEE that there will be atrial collapse prior to ventricular collapse. Collapse occurs in diastole and in later stages will also occur in systole and is seen on the lower pressure (right) prior to the involvement of the higher (left) sided circulation. The most sensitive diagnostic indicator of pericardial tamponade is right ventricular collapse during diastole in a patient with a pericardial effusion.

Pulmonary embolism

In patients with clinical symptoms suspicious for pulmonary embolism, TEE is a modality that may permit rapid diagnosis of pulmonary embolism (Table 75.2). Although the gold standard

for the diagnosis of pulmonary embolism is pulmonary angiography and/or high-resolution spiral CT, it may be difficult to transport a critically ill and hemodynamically unstable patient to the locations for these emergency diagnostic modalities. TEE has 70% sensitivity and 81% specificity for confirmation of pulmonary embolism. Although visualization of thrombus is infrequent by TEE, the main pulmonary and right pulmonary arteries may be visualized. Because of the location of the trachea and difficulty of ultrasound waves to transmit through air-filled spaces, visualization of the left pulmonary artery remains an obstacle.

Table 75.2. TEE findings of pulmonary embolism

Increased size of pulmonary arteries
Right ventricular dysfunction: flattening of the interventricular septum, basal hypokinesis with apical sparing (i.e., McConnell's sign)
Tricuspid regurgitation: severe – due to right-sided pressure overload
Dilated right atrium
Increased size of inferior vena cava

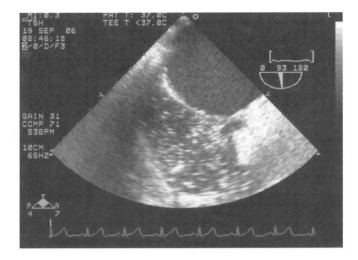

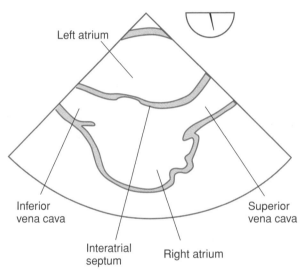

Figure 75.11. A PFO can be indentified by injection of agitated saline.

Table 75.3.	TEE findings of myocardial contusion

Increase in wall thickness of the left ventricle in diastole
Impaired regional wall systolic function
Increased brightness of the ventricular walls

Injuries to the right ventricle typically occur in the right apical wall, whereas injuries to the left ventricle occur along the septal and apical regions.

Massive hypotension

TEE has been used pervasively for the evaluation of hemodynamic instability. Case reports support the usefulness of TEE in diagnosing the etiology of hypotension, with improvements in clinical outcome. The expert opinion of the ASA taskforce is that TEE provides more accurate assessment of preload compared with other monitors, such as central venous and pulmonary artery catheters. TEE determines the etiology of disease in a more rapid manner without the addition of increased adverse effects that occur with other monitors (breach in sterility, damage to the cardiovascular or pulmonary systems). In acute, persistent, and life-threatening hemodynamic disturbances unresponsive to treatment, the emergent use of TEE is considered a category I indication.

Patient risk and complications of TEE

No procedure is without risks and benefits; therefore, it is imperative (unless the use of TEE is emergent) that informed consent be obtained. Although a relatively safe intraoperative monitor, TEE is not without risks or side effects. The rate of complications is <1% (0.2%), with the rate of mortality less than one in 10,000 patients. Prior to TEE examination, it is imperative to ascertain a history of esophageal or gastric disease. There is an increased rate of complications in patients with a history of esophageal pathology and dysphagia. Absolute contraindications to TEE include previous esophagectomy, severe esophageal obstruction, esophageal perforation, esophageal hemorrhage, or cervical trauma (Table 75.4). Relative contraindications include esophageal varices, diverticula, fistulas, previous esophageal surgery, previous gastric surgery, and mediastinal irradiation. In addition to obtaining a history of esophageal or gastric disease, a detailed airway examination must be performed to note the presence of oropharyngeal or dental injuries.

Diagnosis of TEE is often a constellation of findings due to the infrequent visualization of thrombus in the pulmonary arteries. Pulmonary emboli decrease blood flow and result in increased pressures in the right side of the heart. Thus, findings associated with pulmonary emboli would include changes in the vasculature associated with elevated volume or pressure on the right-sided circulation. They include increased size of the pulmonary arteries, right ventricular dysfunction, tricuspid regurgitation, dilated right atrium, and an increase in the size of the inferior vena cava.

Blunt chest trauma

TEE is a safe, reliable, and fast method to diagnosis acute cardiac injury following blunt trauma. Because of its anterior location, the right ventricle is a site of common injury after blunt chest trauma (Table 75.3). Also, because of higher pressures on the left-sided circulation, valve injuries are common. TEE evidence of myocardial injury is an increase in wall thickness of the left ventricle during diastole and impaired systolic function.

Table 75.4.	Contraindication to the use of TEE	

Absolute contraindications	Relative contraindications
Esophagectomy	Esophageal varices
Severe esophageal obstruction	Esophageal diverticula
Esophageal perforation	Esophageal fistula
Esophageal hemorrhage	Previous esophageal surgery
Cervical trauma	Previous gastric surgery
	Mediastinal irradiation

Table 75.5. Complications of TEE

Oral, pharyngeal, laryngeal trauma
Esophageal injury
Hoarseness/sore throat
Dislodgement of endotracheal tube
Thermal injury
Arrhythmias

The placement of the TEE probe is performed by displacing the mandible gently (with or without the use of a laryngoscope), and advancing the probe midline. To prevent trauma, the TEE probe should not be advanced or withdrawn with the probe in the locked position. The TEE probe should not be forced if resistance is met. During insertion or withdrawal, controls should be in the neutral and unlocked position to allow the natural course of the esophagus to be traversed, thus preventing injury.

Complications of TEE are infrequent but do occur (Table 75.5). They include oral and pharyngeal trauma, hoarseness postoperatively, esophageal injury (a serious but rare complication, with high mortality), arrhythmias, and dislodgement of the endotracheal tube. Bioeffects of TEE placement include thermal effects (e.g., heating and thermal injury), cavitation, and torque forces. There have been case reports of splenic injury secondary to TEE placement, and there is a potential risk of endocarditis after TEE placement. In a retrospective study of 7200 cardiac patients, Kallmeyer et al. demonstrated that TEE-associated morbidity occurred in 14 patients (0.2%), with 86% of the complications attributed to oropharyngeal, esophageal, and gastric trauma. One tenth of 1% of patients had clinically significant odynophagia requiring esophagogastroduodenoscopy, which demonstrated linear abrasions. Dental injuries occurred with a frequency of 0.03%, acute upper gastrointestinal hemorrhage occurred in 0.03%, esophageal perforation occurred in 0.01%, and endotracheal tube advancement occurred in 0.03% of patients.

Future direction of TEE

Throughout the years, TEE has been advancing at an enormous pace. Practice guidelines recommended by the American Society of Anesthesiologists and the Society of Cardiovascular Anesthesiologists have recently been updated. (See Suggested Readings.) TEE has fundamentally enabled two-dimensional imaging of the cardiac structures and great vessels. Continued advancement in TEE with three-dimensional imaging, epicardial echocardiography, and epiaortic ultrasound imaging has the potential to enhance the role of the anesthesiologist as a perioperative physician and improve the perioperative outcomes of both cardiac and noncardiac surgical patients.

Suggested readings

American Society of Anesthesiologists and the Society of Cardiovascular Anesthesiologists Task Force on Transesophageal Echocardiography. Practice guidelines for perioperative transesophageal echocardiography. *Anesthesiology* 1996; 84:986–1006.

Applebaum RM, Cutler WM, Bhardwaj N, et al. Utility of transesophageal echocardiography during port-access minimally invasive cardiac surgery. *Am J Cardiol* 1998; 82:183–188.

Denault AY, Couture P, McKenty S, et al. Perioperative use of transesophageal echocardiography by anesthesiologists: impact in noncardiac surgery in the intensive care unit. *Can J Anesth* 2002; 49:287–293.

Kallmeyer IJ, Collard CD, Fox JA, et al. The safety of intraoperative transesophageal echocardiography: a case series of 7200 cardiac surgical patients. *Anesth Analg* 2001; 92:1126–1130.

Mathew JP, Fontes ML, Garwood S, et al. Transesophageal echocardiography interpretation: a comparative analysis between cardiac anesthesiologists and primary echocardiographers. *Anesth Analg* 2002; 94:302–309.

Memtsoudis S, Rosenberger P, Noveva M, et al. Usefulness of transesophageal echocardiography during intraoperative cardiac arrest. *Anesth Analg* 2006; 102:1653–1657.

Shanewise JS, Cheung AT, Aronson S, et al. ASE/SCA guidelines for performing a comprehensive intraoperative multiplane transesophageal echocardiography examination: recommendations of the American Society of Echocardiography Council for Intraoperative Echocardiography and the Society of Cardiovascular Anesthesiologists Task Force for Certification in Perioperative Transesophageal Echocardiography. *J Am Soc Echocardiogr* 1999; 12:884–900.

Thys D, Brooker R, Cahalan M, et al. Practice guidelines for perioperative transesophageal echocardiography. An updated report by the American Society of Anesthesiologists and the Society of Cardiovascular Anesthesiologists Task Force on Transesophageal Echocardiography, *Anesthesiology* 2010; 112:1084–1096.

Chapter 76

Pacemakers and automated implantable cardioverter–defibrillators

Sugantha Sundar and Eswar Sundar

Introduction

Rhythm disturbances can be treated with drugs, devices, or both. Drugs are useful for the management of rhythm disturbances developing in the structurally normal heart. However, in the heart that has undergone considerable remodeling, because of either ischemia or surgery, rhythm management devices such as pacemakers and automatic implantable cardioverter–defibrillators (AICDs) have been proven superior. Treatment of rhythm disturbances may involve the use of pacemakers, internal defibrillators, and ablation therapy or arrhythmia surgery.

Major indications for pacemakers and AICDs are outlined in Table 76.1.

Pacemaker design and codes

Temporary pacing

Temporary pacing has the advantage of immediate, precise control of an arrhythmia without the side effects produced by drugs. It is indicated as prophylaxis in patients at risk of sudden death from high-degree atrioventricular (AV) block, and should be terminated with the resolution of the underlying condition or changed over to an internal pacemaker if the underlying condition is expected to be chronic. Temporary pacing may be endocardial, epicardial, transesophageal, or transcutaneous. Transvenous pacing, the most popular type, may be used in the awake patient. Pacing can also be performed through specialized pulmonary artery catheters. Transcutaneous pacing is easy and noninvasive; however, the pacemaker-stimulated contraction of the chest muscles in a conscious patient may cause considerable discomfort. Sedating patients and minimizing the current strength can help alleviate this problem.

Permanent pacemakers

Modern implantable pacemakers are extremely compact, physiologically shaped, and capable of responding to complex programming. They have lithium ion batteries that usually last at least 10 years. Almost all current implantable pacemakers use transvenous leads that can be individually programmed.

The North American Society for Pacing and Electrophysiology (NASPE) introduced a coding and shorthand system to describe pacing modes. This coding system enables a complete description of the pacemaker to be derived from five letters. Every pacemaker is given a five-letter code based on the following five functions (Table 76.2):

- **Chamber paced:** The chamber that can potentially be paced might be the atrium (A) or the ventricle (V), or both (D); rarely, neither is chamber paced (O).
- **Chamber sensed:** The pacemaker monitors for events in the atrium (A) or ventricle (V), or both chambers (D), or does not perform any sensing function at all (O).
- **Response to the sensed event:** Pacemakers function either by inhibiting themselves (I) when there is a sensed event such as a native depolarization within the sensed chamber, or by triggering (T) a stimulus when they sense the absence of a native depolarization within the sensed chamber. It is important to note that the vast majority of patients with pacemakers have a native rhythm capable of producing an adequate cardiac contraction most of the time. Hence, it is important for pacemakers to be able to sense such native depolarizations within the sensed chambers and inhibit itself if required. However, at the same time, the pacemaker must be able to produce a stimulus (not inhibit itself) in case there is a long pause and a native depolarization is not forthcoming within a programmed time interval.
- **Programmability/rate response:** Modern pacemakers have a feature called adaptive rate pacing (ARP). ARP enables the pacemaker to develop a higher or lower pacing speed depending on activity. Activity sensors sense vibration and acceleration of the body and can increase the pacing speed. Some ARP devices change their pacing rate to the QT interval. Some pacemakers sense minute ventilation changes from changes in thoracic impedance and adapt accordingly. Some of the latest adaptive rate pacemakers can sense variables such as blood pH and oxygen saturation and change the pacing rate accordingly. Some versatile pacemakers fitted on athletes and young patients have more than one mode of adaptive rate sensing in which there is an initial increase in heart rate when an activity is begun based on feedback from movement sensors and then long-term adjustment based on blood pH and other metabolic variables.
- **Antitachycardia function:** Electrophysiologic treatment of tachyarrhythmias involves one or more of the following:

Table 76.1. Major clinical indications for pacemaker and AICD placement[a]

Indications for pacemaker therapy

- 3rd-Degree and advanced 2nd-degree AV block at any anatomic level
- Type 2 2nd-degree AV block; alternating bundle branch blocks
- Persistent 2nd-degree AV block in the His–Purkinje system with bilateral bundle branch block or 3rd-degree AV block within or below the His–Purkinje system after acute myocardial infarction (AMI); transient advanced (2nd- or 3rd-degree) infranodal AV block and associated bundle branch block after AMI; persistent and symptomatic 2nd- or 3rd-degree AV block after AMI
- Sinus node dysfunction with documented symptomatic bradycardia, including frequent sinus pauses that produce symptoms; symptomatic chronotropic incompetence
- Symptomatic recurrent supraventricular tachycardia that is reproducibly terminated by pacing after drugs and catheter ablation fail to control the arrhythmia or produce intolerable side effects; symptomatic recurrent sustained VT as part of an automatic defibrillator system; sustained pause-dependent VT, with or without prolonged QT, in which the efficacy of pacing is thoroughly documented
- Recurrent syncope caused by carotid sinus stimulation; minimal carotid sinus pressure–induced ventricular asystole of more than 3-sec duration in the absence of any medication that depresses the sinus node or AV conduction
- Advanced 2nd- or 3rd-degree AV block associated with symptomatic bradycardia, ventricular dysfunction, or low cardiac output; sinus node dysfunction with correlation of symptoms during age-inappropriate bradycardia; postoperative advanced 2nd- or 3rd-degree AV block that is not expected to resolve or persists at least 7 days after cardiac surgery; congenital 3rd-degree AV block with a wide QRS escape rhythm, complex ventricular ectopy, or ventricular dysfunction; congenital 3rd-degree AV block in an infant with a ventricular rate < 50–55 bpm or with congenital heart disease and a ventricular rate < 70 bpm; sustained pause-dependent VT, with or without prolonged QT, in which the efficacy of pacing is thoroughly documented
- Medically refractory, symptomatic hypertrophic cardiomyopathy with significant resting or provoked left ventricular outflow obstruction
- Symptomatic bradyarrhythmias/chronotropic incompetence after heart transplantation not expected to resolve and other class I indications for permanent pacing

Major indications for AICD therapy

- Cardiac arrest due to ventricular fibrillation (VF) or VT not due to a transient or reversible cause
- Spontaneous sustained VT in association with structural heart disease
- Syncope of undetermined origin with clinically relevant, hemodynamically significant sustained VT or VF induced at EP study when drug therapy is ineffective, not tolerated, or not preferred
- Nonsustained VT in patients with coronary disease, prior myocardial infarction, left ventricular dysfunction, and inducible VF or sustained VT at EP study that is not suppressible by a class I antiarrhythmic drug
- Spontaneous sustained VT in patients who do not have structural heart disease that is not amenable to other treatments

[a] The reader is referred to the American College of Cardiology/American Heart Association guidelines for other indications for pacemaker and AICD therapy.

antitachycardia pacing (P); shock (S): cardioversion or defibrillation; both pacing and shock (D); or no antitachycardia function (O). Overdrive pacing often may be deployed on short runs of ventricular as well supraventricular tachyarrhythmias. Pacing avoids the need for cardioversion or defibrillation, thereby preserving cardiac muscle as well as the AICD battery life. Devices with cardioversion or defibrillation capability (S) fall into the category of AICDs.

Based on NASPE and British Pacing and Electrophysiology Group (NBG) coding there are many varieties of programmable modes. Often, for devices that have only pacing function, the first three letters are used. Thus, a VVI pacemaker will pace the ventricle (V) by not inhibiting itself (I) when it senses a lack of native depolarizations in the ventricle (V). An AAI pacemaker will sense the atrium (A) for depolarizations, and if it does sense a native depolarization, it goes on to pace the atrium (A) by not inhibiting (I) itself. VDD pacemakers pace the ventricle (V) while sensing both the atrium and ventricle (D), and their response could be inhibition or triggering (D) based whether the device senses a native depolarization. The DDD and DDDR (ARP capable) pacemakers are the most widely used mode of pacing, as they are the most versatile and can be used for many indications with only minor programming modifications. The workings of a VVI and DDD pacemaker in various scenarios is illustrated in Figs. 76.1 through 76.4.

Pacemaker programming

Pacemakers are classified as single- or dual-chamber pacemakers depending on whether they pace a single chamber (atrium or ventricle) or both chambers based on programming. The number of leads seen on radiography does not cast any light on whether a pacemaker is single or dual chamber. However, an electrocardiogram (ECG) taken while a dual-chamber pacemaker is functioning usually shows separate atrial and ventricular pacer spikes, unlike a single-chamber pacemaker.

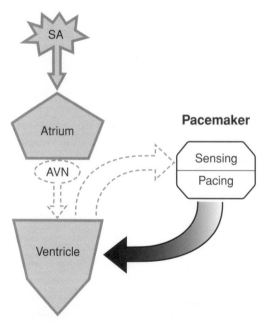

Figure 76.1. This figure shows an atrioventricular node/bundle of His conduction block (AVN unshaded). The sensing unit of the VVI pacer does not sense a depolarization in the ventricle (unshaded arrow). Hence there is no "inhibition" of the pacing unit. This allows the un-inhibited pacing unit to fire and depolarize the ventricle (shaded arrow).

Table 76.2. Pacemaker/AICD codes

I Chamber paced	II Chamber sensed	III Response to sensed event	IV Programmability/rate response	V Antitachycardia function
O = none	**O** = none	**O** = none	**O** = none	**O** = none
A = Atrium	**A** = Atrium	**I** = Inhibit	**R** = Adaptive rate	**P** = ATP
V = Ventricle	**V** = Ventricle	**T** = Triggered		**S** = Shock
D = Dual (A & V)	**D** = Dual (A & V)	**D** = Dual (I & T)		**D** = Dual (P & S)
S = Single	**S** = Single			

ATP = Antitachycardia pacing
From Atlee JL, Bernstein AD. Cardiac rhythm management devices (part II): perioperative management. *Anesthesiology* 2001; 95(5):11265–11280.

Single-chamber pacemakers

Single-chamber pacemakers have a single timing interval between successive depolarizations. This interval is called the escape interval – ventricular escape interval (VEI) or atrial escape interval (AEI) depending on the chamber sensed. This escape interval gets reset if a spontaneous depolarization is sensed within the interval. If no spontaneous depolarizations are sensed within the escape interval, the interval then lapses, triggering a paced depolarization and the initiation of a fresh VEI or AEI.

Dual-chamber pacemakers

Dual-chamber devices have two atrial escape intervals and one ventricular escape interval.

Pacemaker malfunctions

Most modern pacemakers are robust and have excellent shielding properties. Common pacemaker malfunctions and their descriptions are described in Table 76.3. Diagnosis of individual pacemaker malfunction is beyond the scope of this chapter and should be left to electrophysiologists.

AICD design, function, and programming
AICD design and function

An Automatic Internal Cardiac Defibrillator has a microprocessor driven pulse generator that is capable of a biphasic electrical current delivery to minimize the defibrillation energy requirements as well as to conserve battery life. The powering

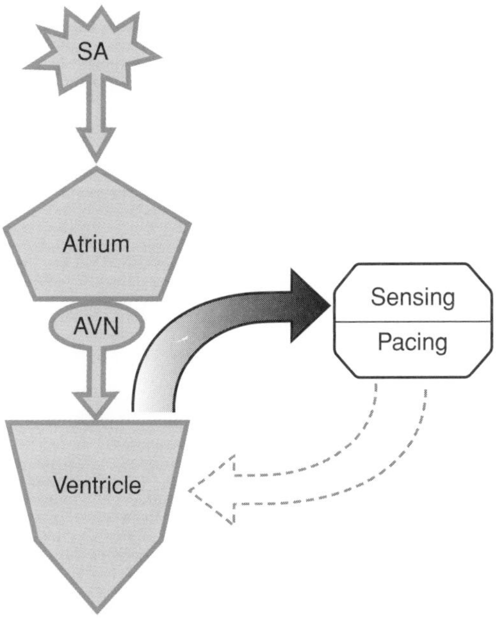

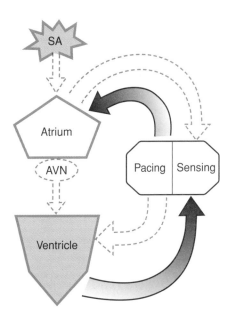

Figure 76.2. In this scenario the patient briefly does not have an atrioventricular nodal (AVN)/bundle of His block. This allows a native depolarization to travel to the ventricle. The sensing unit of the VVI pacer detects this depolarization (shaded arrow) and becomes stimulated. The programmed event of this "stimulation" is the inhibition of the pacer unit (unshaded arrow) allowing native depolarizations to travel through the ventricle and initiate a contraction. SA, sinoatrial node.

Figure 76.3. In this scenario a DDD pacemaker is functioning normally in a patient with sinoatrial node (SA) block: atria and atrioventricular node [AVN] (all unshaded straight arrows); a ventricular escape rhythm (upward facing shaded arrow). Because of the SA block, the sensing unit does not sense an impulse from its atrial lead (unshaded arrow). This results in an atrial pacing beat (downward facing shaded arrow). A few milliseconds later, because of an escape ventricular depolarization (shaded ventricle), the ventricular lead triggers the sensing unit (upward facing shaded arrow) which inhibits further ventricular pacing (left facing unshaded arrow).

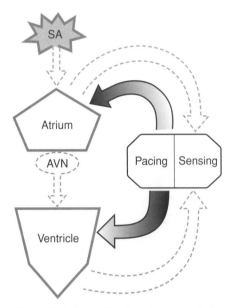

Figure 76.4. Figure 76.4 illustrates a normally functioning DDD pacemaker in a patient with sinoatrial node (SA) and AV node block. However, in this situation, no ventricular escape beat or conduction of the paced atrial beat is forthcoming (unshaded ventricle and unshaded upward and downward facing arrows). Thus, the ventricular lead does not transmit any impulse to the sensing unit (upward facing unshaded arrow). This allows the sensing unit to trigger the pacing unit and the pacing unit induces a paced beat to the ventricle and atria (shaded arrows). In this situation both atria and ventricle are being depolarized by the pacing device. AVN, atrioventricular node.

batteries are often Li-SVO (Lithium Silver vanadium oxide batteries). Batteries are usually changed every 5 to 8 years. The device also has electrolytic storage capacitors to store energy to be used during electrical therapy. The pulse generator attaches to the endocardial surface of the heart by means of transvenous leads that detect and treat arrhythmias.

AICD programming

The first step in the treatment of tachyarrhythmias is the sensing of ventricular depolarizations. The sense amplifier is usually programmed to respond to rates of 50–350 bpm. A band pass filter throws out low and high frequency signals (Electrocautery) and derives an R-R interval. The derived R-R interval is then matched with the set R-R VT/VF detection interval that has been programmed into the device. If the detected R-R interval is less than the programmed R-R detection interval, the device readies itself for electrical therapy. In addition, modern AICDs may take into consideration the morphology of the waveform (chaotic versus regular) and the suddenness of onset (VF is of sudden onset compared to sinus tachycardia) in diagnosing ventricular tachyarrhythmias. Most AICDs have the following electrical treatment capabilities, and the device progresses through the following treatment options:

- Overdrive pacing is the process of increasing the heart rate by means of an artificial cardiac pacemaker in order to suppress certain arrhythmias.
- Cardioversion. The pacemaker synchronizes to the R or S wave of the surface EKG and then shocks are delivered outside these waves to avoid an R-on-T phenomena that can cause the rhythm to degenerate to fibrillation.
- Defibrillation. A process of delivering electrical shocks to a heart in fibrillation or ventricular tachycardia.

The device can be programmed to treat VT with overdrive pacing and if that fails, it progresses on to cardioversion and then defibrillation. The ability to utilize overdrive pacing in the treatment of many tachyarrhythmias helps in the conservation of battery life as well as minimizes the damaging effects of shocks on the myocardium. In tiered therapy, treatment is started with overdrive: atrial tachycardia may be treated with

Table 76.3. Pacemaker malfunctions and descriptions

Malfunction	Description
Failure to sense	Failure to sense is a condition where there may be inadequate cardiac signal strength, and this condition can be diagnosed by the presence of native complexes coexisting with pacing spikes in the same time frame.
Oversensing	In oversensing, the pacemaker becomes exquisitely sensitive to electrical activity outside its zone of surveillance (far-field sensing). Electrocautery, or cross-chamber oversensing can cause the unit to inappropriately trigger or inhibit the pacing unit.
Failure to pace	Failure of a pacemaker to pace maybe the result of battery drain, breakage in the circuit due to lack of contact of the leads at either end, or oversensing.
Failure to capture	In failure to capture, pacing spikes are present appropriately but are not followed by chamber depolarizations. Myocardial ischemia, fibrosis, hyperkalemia, severe acidosis, beta-blockers, hyperglycemia, and some class II and III antiarrhythmics may occasionally cause this type of malfunction.
Pacing at abnormally high rates	Lead disruption, inadequate hysteresis programming, or a dual chamber pacemaker responding to an atrial tachycardia event can lead to pacing at abnormally high rates.
Pacing at abnormally low rates	An abnormally low pacing rate may be caused by excessive hysteresis programming, battery depletion, or an ARP pacemaker responding to deep sleep, or slow respirations.
Pacemaker-mediated tachycardia	Pacemaker-mediated tachycardia is a malfunction unique to dual-chamber pacemakers. Pacemakers can sometimes detect myopotentials from the chest musculature, which may be mistaken for atrial depolarizations and cause the pacemaker to drive ventricular pacing at a high rate.
Crosstalk	Crosstalk occurs when events in the atrial channel are sensed by the ventricular channel, and vice versa, which may lead to inappropriate pacing.

overdrive pacing; ventricular tachycardia (VT) may be preferentially treated initially by cardioversion and ventricular fibrillation (VF) treated by defibrillation.

AICD malfunction

Diagnosing pacemaker malfunction requires a long rhythm strip and a 12-lead ECG, along with a chest radiograph. Information about the pacemaker also can be obtained from the cardiology service that implanted it, or the electrophysiology (EP) service can interrogate the device. If the device appears to be malfunctioning, placement of a magnet over the device usually trips a reed switch; then, if there is a preprogrammed asynchronous pacing mode, the pacer usually reverts to this fixed mode. If a magnet does not seem to fix the problem, then there is a lack of programming of switch behavior, disruption of the leads, or battery failure. In that case, arrangements must be made for urgent transcutaneous or transvenous pacing if there is no time to have the EP interrogate the device.

Failure to deliver effective shocks

Myocardial ischemia and severe acidosis alter the morphology of the rhythm, which may lead to nonrecognition. Recurrent arrhythmias may occur in the context of myocardial ischemia or severe acidosis, leading to repeated shocks; this leads to a degree of "tolerance" by the device, resulting in ineffective therapy. The same conditions may raise the threshold for effective defibrillation, causing the usual current strength to be ineffective. Repeated shocks and depletion of the battery, as well as loss of lead contact, are other causes.

Inappropriate shocks

Electrocautery artifacts, supraventricular tachycardia misdiagnosed as ventricular tachycardia (VT), double counting of R and T waves during pacing, and lead artifacts are some of the reasons for the administration of inappropriate therapy. Sometimes the AICD senses pacer spikes of the pacemaker subunit, leading to miscounting and inappropriate shocks. Conversely, inappropriate AICD shocks may result in the pacemaker failing to sense or capture.

Drug–device interaction

Drugs are often used for rhythm management in patients with an AICD. They may be used for the suppression of nonsustained VT, prophylaxis of atrial fibrillation, or other indications. Such drugs may affect the device function in several ways, including:

- Making the myocardium proarrhythmic
- Increasing defibrillation thresholds (class 1C drugs, phenytoin, amiodarone)
- Altering the ECG morphology, resulting in failure to detect shockable rhythms

Preoperative evaluation of a patient with an AICD or pacemaker

History and physical examination

Patients with rhythm management devices often have coexisting conditions, such as coronary artery disease, cardiomyopathy, valvular heart disease, diabetes, or congenital heart disease. A complete drug history is essential, as some patients may be on antiarrhythmics.

Vitals signs and pulse plethysmography or palpation will confirm that the paced beats do get converted to mechanical contractions of the ventricle. A 12-lead ECG with a rhythm strip may be useful in determining the type of leads and whether the patient is pacemaker dependant. A chest radiograph may be useful in identifying the pacemaker and visualizing any gross malpositioning of the leads. In most cases, a chest radiograph may not shed much light on the status of the pacemakers, and other factors may be taken in account before ordering one. Serum electrolytes may be useful in patients who are extremely ill or on drugs that can alter electrolyte levels, such as diuretics. Electrophysiology or cardiology consults must often be requested before an anesthetic in a patient with a pacemaker or AICD to obtain most of the information listed in Table 76.4.

Evaluating pacemakers

Table 76.4 summarizes the information needed from a pacemaker or AICD before an anesthetic. Some of this information, such as the type of pacemaker and date of the last test, sometimes may be obtained from the patient, EP service consultation and interrogation of the device are necessary to obtain the rest. If needed, the manufacturer may be contacted directly.

Preanesthetic device management

Before the procedure, it is important to answer the following:

- Is the patient pacemaker dependent?
- Is the pacemaker an adaptive rate device?
- How close is the operative site to the device?
- Will monopolar diathermy be used?
- Does the pacemaker need to be reprogrammed?

Patients who are dependent on their pacemakers must have the pacemaker programmed to an asynchronous mode to avoid interference from the electrocautery unit. Adaptive rate pacemakers are known to increase their pacing rate in response to mechanical ventilation; hence, it may be desirable to reprogram the unit to switch off ARP. A patient with an AICD who is pacemaker dependent should have the pacemaker programmed to an asynchronous mode, and the tachycardia sensing mode should be turned off. In such a situation, the anesthesiologist must have the ability to defibrillate externally or internally through an alternate source in case the patient has an episode of unstable tachycardia.

Table 76.4. Preanesthetic pacemaker and AICD evaluation

Determine the indication for and date of placement.

Determine the make and model of the device.

Determine the number of leads and types of leads.

Ascertain the last test date and the status of the battery.

Extract a data log of device events, if any.

Obtain the specifics of the current program residing on the device.

Ensure that pacemaker discharges are converted to peripheral pulses.

Determine the effects of an application of a magnet on the device.

Determine whether the device should be reprogrammed.

Device management during procedures

Place the grounding plate as far as possible from the device. If the cautery is being used less than 6 inches from the device, significant interference may occur. Therefore, consider using bipolar cautery and the lowest-current energy. With simple pacemakers, the use of electric coagulating devices may have serious hemodynamic consequences in pacemaker-dependent patients. Electrocautery may be misinterpreted as native electrical activity and inhibit the pacing function. Placement of the magnet will inhibit device-sensing capabilities and switch the device to automatic pacing at a manufacturer-determined rate. Invariably, this rate is >80 bpm in pacemakers with substantial battery life and cannot be programmed by the electrophysiologist to a lower rate. Limiting the use of monopolar electrocautery to a defined period or use of bipolar electrocautery can minimize periods of elevated heart rates. Also remember that the atrial kick is lost during ventricular pacing and may adversely affect hemodynamic stability.

Modern AICDs are well shielded from electrocautery and have excellent bandpass filters to recognize the high frequencies of the electrocautery unit. However, in some cases failure to use a magnet may result in inappropriate device discharge, because electrocautery may be erroneously interpreted as a malignant rhythm and battery depletion may result from frequent charging. Juxtaposition of a magnet on a combined AICD/pacemaker most likely will disable the defibrillator function but will not affect pacing. The response of the AICD to magnet placement varies and depends on the specific manufacturer. Defibrillation function may be affected by the placement of the magnet, and arrangements for external defibrillation should be at hand.

External electrical therapy

Direct application of defibrillation paddles over a device must be avoided. Paddles should be at least 4 inches from the device, and the lowest possible joule setting with biphasic therapy is recommended. External cardioversion or defibrillation will cause a temporary loss of inhibition of the pacemaker; loss of sensing or failure to capture also may occur, requiring the stimulus strength to be adjusted to a higher setting. All devices must be interrogated after cardioversion or defibrillation.

MRI

Most manufacturers have absolutely contraindicated MRI in patients with an AICD or pacemaker. However, there are published reports of a series of non–pacemaker dependent patients who have safely undergone MRI.

Electroconvulsive therapy

The device (AICD or pacemaker) must be interrogated before the procedure and changed to an asynchronous mode. If a magnet is placed over an AICD during electroconvulsive therapy, then the ability to externally defibrillate must be ensured.

Lithotripsy

Modern lithotripsy units have an ECG input, and the unit fires on the R waves. Lithotripsy units may inhibit the pacemaker or, rarely, damage the circuitry. The following steps minimize the potential for complications:

- Program pacemakers to the VVI or VOO mode.
- Keep the lithotripter focal point at least 15 cm (6 inches) away from the pacemaker, especially in ARP devices.
- If possible, the shockwave delivery should be timed synchronously with the patient's R wave.
- Interrogate the device after the procedure.

Radiofrequency ablation

There have been no reports of electromagnetic interference between a cardiac rhythm management device and radiofrequency ablation. Generally, it is recommended that the cluster electrode be at least 5 cm from the device.

Postprocedure device management

All patients with a pacemaker or AICD who have been exposed to one of the procedures listed previously must have their device interrogated by the EP service in the recovery room. If a magnet was placed over the device, it is reasonable to leave it there until the device has been checked and it is determined that all previously programmed functions are not affected. It is important to have facilities to pace and defibrillate if a situation arises in the recovery room prior to the interrogation of the device.

Suggested readings

Atlee JL, Bernstein AD. Cardiac rhythm management devices (part I): perioperative management. *Anesthesiology* 2001; 95(5):1265–1280.

Atlee JL, Bernstein AD. Cardiac rhythm management devices (part II): indications, device selection, and function. *Anesthesiology* 2001; 95(6):1492–1506.

Practice advisory for the perioperative management of patients with cardiac rhythm management devices: pacemakers and implantable cardioverter-defibrillators: a report by the American Society of Anesthesiologists Task Force on Perioperative Management of Patients with Cardiac Rhythm Management Devices. *Anesthesiology* 2005; 103(1):186–198.

Ventricular assist devices

Amanda A. Fox and John A. Fox

In the United States alone, approximately 5 million people suffer from heart failure, with 300,000 to 800,000 of these patients having advanced heart failure (New York Heart Association class III and IV) despite maximal medical therapy. Although heart transplantation is a very effective treatment for end-stage heart failure, there is an increasing shortage of suitable donor hearts available for patients who need them. In the mid-1970s, the National Institutes of Health established a research initiative to develop mechanical circulatory support devices that could serve as effective alternatives to heart transplantation. Today, there are a variety of mechanical ventricular assist devices (VADs) that can be used to:

1. Provide short-term ventricular support in patients who have suffered acute but potentially reversible myocardial insults
2. Support heart transplant candidates until a donor heart becomes available
3. Provide definitive or "destination" therapy for patients with refractory heart failure who are not heart transplant candidates

What is a VAD?

VADs are mechanical devices that take over all or part of the work of a damaged ventricle to improve patient hemodynamics and end-organ perfusion. VADs have been designed that can provide left, right, or biventricular support. Although there are many types of VADs, they all function according to the same general principles: Blood is removed from a left- or right-sided cardiac chamber via an inflow cannula that then delivers blood to the VAD pumping chamber. Blood is then pumped out of the VAD chamber into an outflow cannula that delivers blood to either the aorta (in the case of a left ventricular assist device [LVAD]) or the pulmonary arteries (in the case of a right ventricular assist device [RVAD]). The VAD therefore decompresses a failing ventricle and simultaneously augments systemic (LVAD) or pulmonary arterial (RVAD) perfusion. Desirable potential outcomes of VAD therapy include improved end-organ function; neurohumoral down-regulation of circulating catecholamines, renin, angiotensin, and other cytokines that are upregulated during end-stage heart failure;

and potential myocyte recovery with related ventricular reverse remodeling. Although improved end-organ function and neurohumoral down-regulation appear to occur relatively consistently with VAD therapy, the propensity for reverse ventricular remodeling has been fairly disappointing. A schematic of a HeartMate vented electric pulsatile LVAD (Thoratec Corp., Pleasanton, CA) is shown in Fig. 77.1.

All VADs currently require some intracorporeal to extracorporeal connection or breach to provide the VAD with power. This need for an extracorporeal power supply makes infection a serious potential complication of VAD therapy. Depending on the type of VAD, external power is supplied by a relatively large electric or pneumatic console. However, some of the newer VAD designs allow for increased patient mobility by allowing power to be supplied from a small battery pack that can be worn in a shoulder holster. VADs may be implanted with the aid of cardiopulmonary bypass (CPB) in a cardiac operative suite, or

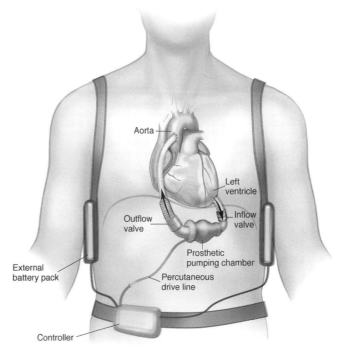

Figure 77.1. Components of the LVAD.

Table 77.1. VAD types

Extracorporeal, nonpulsatile centrifugal flow
- **Short-term support**
  Bio-Medicus[a] – BiVAD potential
  TandemHeart[b] – percutaneous LVAD

Extracorporeal, pulsatile
- **Short-term support or bridge to transplant**
  Abiomed AB5000[c]
  Abiomed BVS 5000[c] – BiVAD potential
  Thoratec[d] – BiVAD potential

Intracorporeal, pulsatile
- **Bridge to transplant**
  Novacor LVAD[e]

HeartMate 1000 implantable pneumatic LVAD[d]
- **Bridge to transplant or destination therapy**
  HeartMate vented electric LVAD[d]

Intracorporeal, nonpulsatile axial flow
- **Short-term support**

Impella percutaneous LVAD[c]
- **Bridge to transplant**
  Jarvik 2000 FlowMaker LVAD[f] (approved in Europe Union;
    investigational in United States)
  DeBakey LVAD[g]
  HeartMate II LVAD[d]

[a] Medtronic, Eden Prairie, MN.
[b] CardiacAssist, Inc., Pittsburgh, PA.
[c] Abiomed, Danvers, MA.
[d] Thoratec Corp., Pleasanton, CA.
[e] World Heart, Salt Lake City, UT.
[f] Jarvik Heart, Inc., New York, NY.
[g] MicroMed Cardiovascular, Inc., Houston, TX.

they may be placed percutaneously in the cardiac catheterization laboratory. Examples of available VADs are listed in Table 77.1. Available VADs may be considered and classified according to whether the VAD:

1. Is intended to be implanted inside or outside the body
2. Generates pulsatile or continuous (axial) flow
3. Is intended for left ventricular support only (LVAD) or is also used for right or biventricular support (BiVAD)
4. Is intended to provide shorter- versus longer-term support

Indications and contraindications for VAD placement

Assuming correction of hypovolemia, acid–base abnormalities, and electrolyte disturbances, VADs are indicated in patients who are in refractory cardiogenic shock despite inotropic or intra-aortic balloon pump support (or both). Although the definition of cardiogenic shock may vary somewhat among institutions, typical criteria include a cardiac index < 2 L/min/m^2, a systolic blood pressure < 80 mm Hg, a pulmonary capillary wedge pressure > 20 mm Hg, and a urine output < 20 to 30 ml/h. When VAD insertion is considered, the goal is to implant the VAD before irreversible multisystem organ failure occurs. Typical contraindications to VAD insertion include patients with renal failure (serum creatinine > 5 mg/dl), severe

hepatic dysfunction (an international normalized ratio that is not correctable to < 1.5), severe lung disease (pulmonary function tests showing forced expiratory volume in the first second of expiration [FEV$_1$], forced vital capacity, or diffusing capacity of lung for carbon monoxide [D$_{LCO}$] $< 50\%$ of predicted), or significant irreversible or progressive neurologic deficits. Because hepatic dysfunction in heart failure patients often reflects right ventricular dysfunction and related hepatic congestion, elevated liver function tests suggest that insertion of a BiVAD might be more successful than an isolated LVAD. Most cancers are also considered contraindications to VAD insertion. Because infection is a significant morbidity after VAD insertion, patient infections should be successfully treated prior to VAD insertion. Some advocate that blood cultures should be negative in such patients for at least a week prior to VAD insertion.

Preoperative assessment of the VAD candidate

When assessing a patient preoperatively before VAD insertion, it is important to recognize that many patients with long-standing heart failure develop concurrent dysfunction of other organs secondary to poor perfusion or vascular congestion. Therefore, it is important to conduct a thorough preanesthetic evaluation of a VAD candidate, paying particular attention to the status of the patient's cardiovascular, renal, hepatic, pulmonary, and neurologic systems. This evaluation will allow the anesthesiologist to identify preoperative organ dysfunction and to discuss with the primary medical team ways in which the patient might be further optimized prior to surgery. Detailed awareness of patient comorbidities also allows anesthesiologists to better anticipate and prepare for related perioperative difficulties.

With regard to the patient's cardiopulmonary and vascular status, it is helpful to know what inotropes and vasopressors the patient is receiving, and at what dosages. It is useful to know whether the patient has been on a stable dosage of a certain inotrope for many months or whether he or she has been requiring rapidly escalating inotrope dosages. This knowledge gives the anesthesiologist a sense of whether VAD surgery is urgent or emergent, thereby dictating how much time (if any) is available for further evaluation or optimization of the patient. Furthermore, if a patient has been reasonably stable on an infusion of a specific inotrope at home and is presenting with gradual deterioration warranting VAD placement, the anesthesiologist would then know that administration of that inotrope may be helpful at preoperatively administered or slightly higher doses during induction of anesthesia as well as during other perioperative phases. In patients undergoing isolated LVAD implantation, knowledge of potentially effective inotropes may be useful for supporting right ventricular function after VAD implantation.

It also is helpful for the anesthesiologist to review the patient's preoperative echocardiogram, as right ventricular dysfunction often occurs in conjunction with left ventricular dysfunction. If the patient has moderate or severe right ventricular dysfunction, it may be useful to discuss with the surgeon the possibility that the patient may require an RVAD as well as an LVAD. Many patients may have significant tricuspid regurgitation that the surgeon may elect to repair as well. This is important for the anesthesiologist to know, as some surgeons may request that the patient's pulmonary artery catheter be withdrawn from the right ventricle before the tricuspid valve is repaired.

Left heart catheterization data are particularly important in LVAD patients who have significant obstructive disease of the right coronary artery, as they indicate that the patient may require a right coronary artery bypass graft as well as LVAD placement. Right heart catheterization data are useful in identifying patients with moderate or severe pulmonary hypertension. Some institutions initiate trials of intravenous inodilators (e.g., milrinone) or vasodilators (e.g., prostaglandins) as well as inhaled pulmonary vasodilators (e.g., nitric oxide) with a pulmonary arterial catheter in place to determine whether a potential VAD candidate has pulmonary hypertension that is "fixed" versus reduced with pharmacotherapy. If such a preoperative evaluation is conducted, it is useful to know which drugs reduce pulmonary hypertension, as those drugs may be useful in the post-CPB period for reducing right ventricular afterload and related right ventricular dysfunction.

It is important to evaluate whether a patient has pulmonary edema, particularly to the degree that it is impairing oxygenation. If a patient has substantial preoperative pulmonary edema, it is worth determining whether he or she might be responsive to further preoperative diuresis. Most VAD candidates are on daily diuretics. It is important to know what diuretics they are on and at what dosages, as, particularly for intraoperative diuresis with loop diuretics, it will be most effective to administer at least, if not more than, the intravenous equivalent of the normal daily dose.

Preoperative renal insufficiency is often associated with diminished renal perfusion secondary to low cardiac output. Many patients experience improved renal function in the weeks and months after VAD insertion. However, patients with preoperative renal insufficiency may develop acute on chronic renal failure in the immediate perioperative period secondary to the insults of surgery and CPB. For patients with moderate to severe preoperative renal insufficiency, it may be useful to consult a renal specialist preoperatively, as such patients may require venovenous hemodialysis during the days after surgery. If this is anticipated, access for such dialysis can be placed sterilely prior to leaving the operating room after VAD placement. It is also important to recognize the potential for uremic platelet dysfunction and to be prepared to transfuse platelets after separating from CPB.

Patients who have elevated liver function tests are more likely to experience significant perioperative coagulopathy. Many VAD candidates have also undergone prior cardiac surgeries. Both of these scenarios increase the patient's risk for substantial bleeding after CPB (one or more patient blood volumes). The anesthesiologist should recognize this and plan for adequate intravenous access for rapid volume resuscitation. It is also useful to communicate with the institution's blood bank preoperatively to ensure rapid access to sufficient packed red blood cells, fresh frozen plasma, cryoprecipitate, and, possibly, recombinant factor VII. Autologous blood scavenging can also be arranged for the intraoperative period. Many VAD candidates have also undergone at least one prior cardiac surgery and therefore also have increased risk for perioperative bleeding secondary to mediastinal scarring and adhesions.

Induction of anesthesia

To maintain hemodynamic stability during induction of anesthesia for VAD surgery, the anesthesiologist must understand the unique physiology of patients with severe left, right, and biventricular failure. A frequent scenario is a patient with severe left ventricular dysfunction (left ventricular ejection fraction of approximately 10%), moderate right ventricular dysfunction, and moderate pulmonary hypertension. Such patients have high levels of circulating endogenous catecholamines as part of the body's attempt to compensate for the failing left ventricle's small, fixed stroke volumes and correspondingly low cardiac output. Increased circulating catecholamines help compensate for this by engendering higher heart rates as well as increased systemic vascular resistance, both of which will improve systemic perfusion. Therefore, it is important for the anesthesiologist to attempt to minimize the sympatholysis that often occurs in response to induction of anesthesia. This can be done in a number of ways. An arterial line should be placed prior to induction to allow blood pressure monitoring with each beat of the heart. If a patient has pulmonary arterial pressures that are approaching systemic pressures, it may be useful to place a pulmonary arterial catheter preoperatively to titrate inodilators and vasodilators during induction. It is also important to minimize hypoxia and hypercarbia by adequately ventilating such patients during induction so as not to exacerbate pulmonary hypertension. Induction drugs such as midazolam and etomidate tend to minimize sympatholysis, but it is important to remember that all drugs administered to VAD candidates prior to VAD insertion will have a slow circulating time before taking effect. Therefore, initial doses of induction agents should be given slowly and patiently before any supplemental doses are given. Higher heart rates are generally desirable for sustaining adequate cardiac outputs in end-stage heart failure patients. Because most end-stage heart failure patients have severe diastolic dysfunction as well as severe systolic dysfunction, these patients generally do not tolerate sudden changes in preload or afterload. Consequently, preoperative inotropes are often continued or increased during induction and maintenance of anesthesia prior to initiating CPB.

Given the potential for hemodynamic collapse with induction of anesthesia, the anesthesiologist inducing the patient should also be ready for urgent initiation of CPB. This means having an adequate heparin dose ready to administer, as well as a primed CPB circuit and an immediately available cardiac surgeon and perfusionist. The Jarvik FlowMaker axial flow VAD (Jarvik Heart, Inc., New York, NY) has been designed so it can be implanted through a left thoracotomy incision with the outflow cannula implantable into the descending thoracic aorta. An advantage of this potential is the ability to avoid scarring and adhesions in patients who have had multiple prior sternotomy incisions. However, the anesthesiologist should be aware of when such a device's implantation and approach are planned, as this situation will require double-lumen endotracheal tube placement or other provisions for lung isolation during VAD implantation.

Anesthetic considerations for the pre-CPB period

The hemodynamic principles discussed earlier with regard to induction of anesthesia also apply to maintenance of anesthesia in the pre-CPB period. Patients are generally continued on inotropes and vasopressors in doses that are equivalent to or higher than those they were receiving preoperatively. Maintenance of anesthesia is usually achieved with low but amnestic doses of volatile agent, as well as slowly administered doses of intravenous narcotics such as fentanyl. If a pulmonary arterial catheter is not placed prior to induction, it should be placed soon thereafter. In patients who have undergone previous heart surgeries, it may be safer to cannulate a femoral artery and vein prior to sternotomy. Some surgeons actually elect to initiate CPB prior to sternotomy, as adhesions and scarring increase the risk of massive bleeding from injury to the right ventricle or other cardiovascular structures that may be adherent to the sternal table. The anesthesiologist should be certain that enough peripheral or central venous access is established to allow for large-volume administration of crystalloids, colloids, and blood products. As discussed in the preoperative assessment section, VAD patients often have hepatic congestion and associated preoperative coagulopathy. Some patients have preoperative uremia and associated platelet dysfunction. When these factors are coupled with the iatrogenic insults to the coagulation system introduced by the overall increased systemic inflammatory response to surgery, as well as by blood exposure to the extracorporeal surfaces of the CPB circuit and the VAD, substantial post-CPB blood loss should be anticipated.

Many institutions also initiate a prophylactic perioperative antibiotic regimen in an attempt to minimize patient risk for serious perioperative infection or sepsis. Intravenous antibiotics such as vancomycin, levofloxacin, rifampin, or fluconazole often are given before skin incision and are regularly redosed throughout the immediate perioperative period. Parts of the VAD are also frequently soaked in antibiotic solution before implantation.

Various aspects of the standard perioperative transesophageal echocardiographic (TEE) examination have particular relevance for identifying cardiac and aortic abnormalities that might contribute to adverse patient outcomes or VAD failure after implantation. When well communicated to the responsible cardiac surgeon, knowledge of such TEE findings can guide additional surgical interventions prior to VAD implantation that might contribute to success. There are several particularly important diagnoses that should be considered by the physician performing the intraoperative TEE prior to VAD implantation:

1. VAD surgeons typically consider correcting greater than mild aortic (in the case of LVAD implantation) or greater than mild pulmonic insufficiency (in the case of RVAD implantation). Such valvular insufficiency is typically addressed surgically by oversewing or replacing the patient's native, incompetent valve. This procedure is necessary with LVAD surgery because the VAD outflow cannula delivers blood to the patient's aorta. Significant aortic insufficiency will result in a substantial percentage of LVAD blood output repeatedly recycling retrograde across the incompetent aortic valve and back through the LVAD pump rather than progressing antegrade to provide systemic perfusion. A parallel concept applies to RVAD placement in the setting of pulmonic insufficiency with regard to retrograde recycling of VAD outflow delivered to the pulmonary artery.

2. Particularly with isolated LVAD surgery, cardiac septal defects such as a patent foramen ovale, atrial septal defects, or ventricular septal defects should be surgically closed to avoid significant right-to-left shunt after VAD support is initiated.

3. Although mitral regurgitation typically improves and becomes insignificant with adequate LVAD function, moderate or severe mitral stenosis may significantly impair VAD filling and should be surgically evaluated and addressed.

4. Because many VAD candidates have severely enlarged cardiac atria and ventricles accompanied by slow or static passage of blood flow through these chambers, TEE examination should assess carefully for intracardiac thrombus to prevent potential embolic events as well as thrombotic complications within the VAD itself. The cardiac surgeon is particularly likely to perform a thrombectomy for left ventricular apical thrombi, as the VAD inflow cannula is often placed directly into the left ventricular apex.

5. As mentioned earlier in this chapter, depending on the type of LVAD inserted, the VAD outflow cannula can be implanted into the ascending or descending thoracic aorta. TEE can be used to assess whether there is significant atheroma in the descending aorta. If descending aortic atheroma is moderate or severe, the surgical approach might be changed to allow for implantation of the VAD outflow cannula in the ascending aorta instead. Because many VAD implantations occur in patients who are undergoing repeat sternotomies that might warrant femoral venous to femoral arterial CPB, knowledge of a

significant descending aortic atheroma might alter the surgical arterial cannulation approach to favor axillary arterial or ascending aortic cannulation. This shift in plan for CPB cannulation might be made out of concern that femoral arterial cannulation might result in significant retrograde embolization of a descending aortic atheroma. With most VAD types, the LVAD outflow cannula is implanted into the ascending aorta, with surgery performed through a midline sternotomy incision. In this case TEE, as well as epiaortic ultrasound, can be used to detect a significant ascending aortic atheroma, which can be addressed surgically by atherectomy or ascending aortic replacement prior to insertion of the LVAD inflow cannula.

6. The VAD candidate should be carefully assessed for severity of right ventricular dysfunction and tricuspid regurgitation. Particularly in the situation of isolated LVAD surgery, cardiac surgeons may conduct tricuspid valve repair for the indication of tricuspid regurgitation. The idea behind such repair is to promote forward flow from the right ventricle to help ensure adequate blood return to the LVAD. Furthermore, knowledge that a patient has moderate or severe right ventricular dysfunction prior to isolated LVAD implantation will allow better planning for right ventricular support with inotropes as well as right ventricular afterload reduction with pulmonary vasodilators. Such knowledge of right ventricular dysfunction also allows preparation for potential additional RVAD implantation.

Anesthetic considerations after VAD insertion

With any open heart surgery, but particularly with VAD placement, complete de-airing of the heart and the VAD takes time. Intraoperative TEE examination is helpful for determining when most of the air has been removed from the left heart and the VAD. TEE is also used to assess proper VAD inflow cannula placement in the left atrium or the more typical apical left ventricular location. If the supported ventricle appears distended rather than decompressed when weaning from CPB to VAD support, inflow cannula malposition should be high on the differential and should be readjusted by the surgeon. If a single VAD is placed, intraoperative TEE may be useful for evaluating function of the non–VAD-supported ventricle. TEE will often guide the care team in deciding when isolated LVAD support has failed and biventricular assistance needs to be implemented through additional implantation of an RVAD.

Before weaning from CPB, a platelet count and fibrinogen level are often sent to help the anesthesiologist anticipate the post-CPB need for fresh frozen plasma, cryoprecipitate, and platelets. This allows such blood products to be readily available in the operating room for early treatment of coagulopathy. When an LVAD has been initiated alone, inotropes are frequently administered to aid right ventricular contractility that is sufficient to tolerate post-CPB blood transfusions and to provide adequate blood return to the left heart and associated VAD. In patients in whom there is particular concern regarding potential volume overload of the right ventricle after LVAD implantation, various modes of ultrafiltration can be implemented while they are on CPB to hemoconcentrate the blood and reduce the overall blood volume to be returned to the patients after being separated from CPB. Also in keeping with the concept of promoting right ventricular output, patients in whom significant pulmonary hypertension is anticipated should be placed on vasodilator therapy such as inhaled nitric oxide. In a patient who receives a large-volume transfusion, has persistent nonsurgical bleeding, or has marginal right ventricular function, the cardiac surgeon may elect to leave the chest open after surgery and allow the patient to recover for several days in the intensive care unit before attempting chest closure again in the operating room. Although many VAD patients hemodynamically tolerate atrial fibrillation and other supraventricular arrhythmias, ventricular tachycardia typically is poorly tolerated, particularly in those receiving an LVAD, and is treated aggressively with cardioversion and pharmacotherapy.

All VADs have an essentially fixed filling capacity. If a pulsatile VAD receives increased blood return, VAD output is increased by increasing the pump ejection rate. If an axial flow or centrifugal VAD receives increased blood return, VAD output is increased by increasing the VAD rotation speed. Unlike with native heart tissue, neither pulsatile nor axial flow–type VADs have the compensatory capacity to increase contractility to improve output. Therefore, VADs are extremely preload dependent. If VAD output decreases, TEE and other hemodynamic monitors should be used to assess whether the patient is hypovolemic, the VAD inflow cannula is malpositioned, or the patient is experiencing significant right ventricular dysfunction that is compromising blood passage to the left heart. The anesthesiologist and surgeon then need to address these causative issues. If the patient has significant right ventricular dysfunction, diuretics can be administered to help mitigate volume overload. Inotropes can be increased or initiated to improve contractility, and pulmonary vasodilators such as nitric oxide can be given to decrease pulmonary hypertension and therefore the afterload against which the right ventricle is contracting. One should not increase the VAD rate or rotation in the setting of low outputs, as this will cause the VAD to exert negative pressure on the supported ventricle as well as the inflow cannula suture line. This scenario may result in air embolization from along the inflow cannula suture line. Increasing the LVAD rate or rotation in the setting of poor filling also may result in a leftward shift of the interventricular septum, which may further perpetuate severe right ventricular dysfunction.

The inflow cannula is inserted into the apex of the left ventricle, and the outflow cannula is anastomosed to the ascending aorta. Blood returns from the lungs to the left side of the heart and exits through the left ventricular apex and across an inflow valve into the prosthetic pumping chamber. Blood is then actively pumped through an outflow valve into the ascending aorta. The pumping chamber is placed within the abdominal wall or peritoneal cavity. A percutaneous drive line carries the electrical cable and air vent to the battery packs (only the pack on the right side is shown in Fig. 77.1) and the electronic controls, which are worn on a shoulder holster and belt, respectively.

Suggested readings

Aaronson KD, Eppinger MJ, Dyke DB, et al. Left ventricular assist device therapy improves utilization of donor hearts. *J Am Coll Cardiol* 2002; 39(8):1247–1254.

Barr ML, Bourge RC, Orens JB, et al. Thoracic organ transplantation in the United States, 1994–2003. *Am J Transplant* 2005; 5(4 Pt 2):934–949.

Chumnanvej S, Wood MJ, MacGillivray TE, Melo MF. Perioperative echocardiographic examination for ventricular assist device implantation. *Anesth Analg* 2007; 105(3):583–601.

Frazier OH, Delgado RM. Mechanical circulatory support for advanced heart failure: where does it stand in 2003? *Circulation* 2003; 108(25):3064–3068.

Frazier OH, Rose EA, McCarthy P, et al. Improved mortality and rehabilitation of transplant candidates treated with a long-term implantable left ventricular assist system. *Ann Surg* 1995; 222(3):327–336; discussion 36–38.

Mets B. Anesthesia for left ventricular assist device placement. *J Cardiothorac Vasc Anesth* 2000; 14(3):316–326.

Mielniczuk L, Mussivand T, Davies R, et al. Patient selection for left ventricular assist devices. *Artif Organs* 2004; 28(2):152–157.

Nicolosi AC, Pagel PS. Perioperative considerations in the patient with a left ventricular assist device. *Anesthesiology* 2003; 98(2):565–570.

Nussmeier NA, Probert CB, Hirsch D, et al. Anesthetic management for implantation of the Jarvik 2000 left ventricular assist system. *Anesth Analg* 2003; 97(4):964–971.

Rose EA, Gelijns AC, Moskowitz AJ, et al. Long-term mechanical left ventricular assistance for end-stage heart failure. *N Engl J Med* 2001; 345(20):1435–1443.

Stevenson LW, Rose EA. Left ventricular assist devices: bridges to transplantation, recovery, and destination for whom? *Circulation* 2003; 108(25):3059–3063.

Chapter 78

Anesthetic considerations for surgical repair of the thoracic aorta

Brian J. Gelfand and Amanda A. Fox

Introduction

Aortic aneurysms and dissections may involve the ascending, arch, or descending segments of the thoracic aorta. Surgical repair of the thoracic aorta involves a variety of perioperative approaches and considerations related to the type, location, and extent of thoracic aortic pathology. Anesthesiologists must understand the full scope of these issues to provide optimal care for patients undergoing thoracic aortic surgeries.

Preparing for urgent or emergent thoracic aortic surgery

In the clinical presentation of thoracic aortic dissection, leaking aneurysm, or contained traumatic transection, a minimum of two large-bore intravenous (IV) catheters must be placed to provide massive volume resuscitation as needed. Placing an arterial line for continuous blood pressure monitoring should be done as soon as possible to allow optimal hemodynamic management. Tight pharmacologic control of a patient's blood pressure and left ventricular ejection velocity should be initiated to help prevent propagation of aortic dissection or aortic rupture. In transporting patients with known or potential acute aortic syndromes to the operating room (OR), it is essential to be prepared for potential acute clinical deterioration and to have appropriate personnel, equipment, drugs, and monitoring available to be able to rapidly intubate the patient (if the patient is not already intubated) and to initiate needed cardiac and volume resuscitation. This is particularly important to remember if the patient is being transported for further diagnostic tests, such as CT imaging, before coming to the OR. Additional venous access or monitoring lines, such as central venous catheters or pulmonary arterial catheters, can be placed in the OR or the intensive care unit when time permits.

In patients with aortic dissections, administering sedatives and pain medication not only will improve patient comfort but should result in better control of high blood pressure and heart rate. However, care must be taken not to oversedate such patients, particularly if they are being monitored for further diagnostic tests prior to going to the OR. The patient needs to be alert enough to respond to serial examinations that would indicate expansion of aortic dissection and the need to go immediately to surgery. Such patients require frequent neurologic assessments for new mental status changes or spinal cord ischemia, as well as abdominal examinations to assess for mesenteric ischemia. A Foley catheter may be placed in the bladder to aid in detecting oliguria related to renal ischemia.

Pharmacologic hemodynamic management

Drugs used for hemodynamic management of patients with suspected or known critical aortic pathology ideally should have few side effects and short half-lives that allow for rapid onset and offset. To prevent extension of aortic dissection or aortic rupture, systolic and diastolic blood pressure should be tightly controlled, with target systolic and mean systemic arterial blood pressures in most patients approximating 100 to 120 mm Hg and 60 to 80 mm Hg, respectively. Vasodilator drugs commonly used to control preoperative hypertension are shown in Table 78.1.

Reducing left ventricular ejection velocity also may be helpful for minimizing expansion of aortic dissections. This can be accomplished by using β-adrenergic receptor antagonists (β-blockers), as this group of drugs will decrease the patient's heart rate (and therefore the number of blood flow pulsations directed toward an intimal tear) and left ventricular contractility (decreasing the force of blood flow pulsations toward an intimal tear). When vasodilators are administered, particularly those that markedly reduce systemic afterload, patients may experience both increased forcefulness of left ventricular ejection and pronounced reflex tachycardia. Therefore, β-blockers are useful alone or as adjuncts to vasodilator therapy in patients with thoracic aortic aneurysms or dissections. Target heart rate for most patients is between 60 and 80 bpm. Commonly used perioperative β-blockers are shown in Table 78.2.

Anticipating bleeding and transfusion requirements

Particularly for patients presenting with acute aortic emergencies, in addition to establishing adequate large-bore intravenous access, the blood bank should be notified regarding the potential for substantial blood loss. Initially, 8 to 10 U of packed red blood cells (PRBCs) should be crossmatched for repair of acute aortic dissections, other potential aortic leak or rupture, or descending thoracic aortic aneurysms. Crossmatching 2 to 4 U of PRBCs may be adequate initially for elective aneurysm

Table 78.1. Common IV vasodilators used to control hypertension

Drug	Common dosages	Comments
Sodium nitroprusside	Start infusion at 0.5–1.0 µg/kg/min and titrate to effect. Cyanide toxicity has occurred with doses of 8–10 µg/kg/min	Rapid onset and offset. Vasodilates both arterial and venous smooth muscle. Central administration is ideal, but can be administered through a large peripheral IV line.
Nitroglycerin	Typical infusion range is 1.0–4.0 µg/kg/min	Rapid onset and offset. Less potent than sodium nitroprusside. May be particularly helpful in settings in which aortic dissection affects coronary arterial flow, as blood flow may be somewhat improved with coronary vasodilation.
Fenoldopam	Start infusion at 0.05–0.1 µg/kg/min and titrate to effect to a maximum dose of 0.8 µg/kg/min	Selective D_1 dopamine receptor agonist with little affinity for D_2 dopamine or other adrenoreceptors. Although fenoldopam results in dilation of many vascular beds, it may have some renal-protective benefits related to increasing renal blood flow.
Nicardipine	Typical infusion range is 5.0–15.0 mg/h and can be titrated to effect; also may be administered as an IV bolus (usually 0.5–2.0 mg)	A dihydropyridine calcium channel blocker that inhibits calcium influx into vascular smooth muscle, thereby causing vasorelaxation. It is marketed as having more selectivity for cerebral and coronary arteries than the other dihydropyridines.

repair of the arch or ascending aorta. Blood warmers and rapid transfusion setups should be ready to use in the OR. Arrangements for intraoperative autologous blood salvaging, such as a Cell Saver (Haemonetics Corp., Braintree, MA), should be coordinated if possible.

Risk of significant bleeding with thoracic aortic surgeries appears to result from multiple factors. In a series of 20 patients with unruptured abdominal aortic aneurysms reported by Balduini et al., platelets were activated in all patients and signs of platelet consumption were present in most patients preoperatively. In another series reported by Fisher et al. in 32 patients scheduled for elective thoracoabdominal aneurysm repair, 9% of the patients had frank disseminated intravascular coagulation, whereas 14% had elevated fibrin degradation products without evidence of consumptive coagulopathy. These findings suggest that patients with thoracic aortic disease may have

subtle preoperative coagulopathy. Coagulopathy is thought to worsen in thoracic aortic surgeries requiring extracorporeal circulation, such as cardiopulmonary bypass (CPB) or left heart bypass. Although these bypass circulation techniques can improve systemic perfusion during aortic repair, they often require anticoagulation (generally with heparin) and also may stimulate inflammatory responses, consumptive coagulopathy, and increased fibrinolysis. Bleeding may also be exacerbated by deep hypothermic circulatory arrest (DHCA), which is conducted in patients requiring aortic arch surgery and may require blood temperatures as low as 16°C to 18°C. Such profound hypothermia may be associated with significant platelet dysfunction. In patients undergoing surgical repair of thoracoabdominal aneurysms, massive blood loss may occur, particularly from back-bleeding through intercostal vessels. Liver ischemia related to aortic cross-clamping above the celiac axis may also

Table 78.2. Commonly used β-adrenergic receptor antagonists (β-blockers)

Drug	Common dosages	Comments
Propranolol	Start with IV bolus of 1 mg, but total doses as high as 8 mg may be required to achieve adequate heart rate control	Nonselective β-adrenergic receptor antagonist (β_1 and β_2) that has been used for many years in the setting of aortic dissection to slow heart rate. However, propranolol use is now often supplanted by β_1-selective adrenergic receptor antagonists (see below). The half-life of the main metabolite of propranolol is 5–7 h, so shorter-acting agents should be considered in patients who are hemodynamically labile.
Labetalol	Loading doses can be administered IV, with initial doses of 5–10 mg. Loading doses should subsequently be doubled approximately every 10 min (up to a maximum total dose of 300 mg) until target heart rate and blood pressure are achieved. Once target heart rate and blood pressure are achieved by IV loading doses, a continuous infusion may be initiated at 0.5–2 mg/min, or the patient may be redosed with small IV boluses approximately every 30 min.	Provides a combination of α_1-, β_1-, and β_2-adrenergic receptor antagonism, and thus can be administered as an alternative to a combination of sodium nitroprusside and β-blocker. The disadvantage of the labetalol approach to blood pressure and heart rate control for aortic dissections is a longer time to onset of desired blood pressure effect and less ease of rapid titration than seen with strict vasodilators.
Esmolol	Bolus IV loading dose of 500 µg/kg over 1 min, then initiate IV infusion at 50 µg/kg/min titrated to effect up to a maximum infusion of 300 µg/kg/min	β_1-Selective adrenergic receptor blocker with rapid onset and short duration of action. Its β_1 selectivity makes it favorable for patients who are prone to bronchospasm. Its short half-life makes it easy to titrate and to terminate if a patient develops bronchospasm or becomes hemodynamically unstable.
Metoprolol	Typical initial IV bolus dose of 2.5–5.0 mg; may be repeated every 5–15 min up to a maximum total dose of 20 mg to achieve target heart rate	β_1-Selective adrenergic receptor blocker with longer duration of action than esmolol, so it can be administered effectively without continuous infusion

worsen bleeding. In addition to red blood cells, the need for potential clotting factor and platelet replacement should be anticipated.

Overview of the surgical objectives for repairing the thoracic aorta

The primary surgical objective for managing acute aortic injury (dissection, ruptured aneurysm, or transection) is to occlude blood flow just proximal and distal to the aortic injury to prevent fatal hemorrhage. The next objective is to restore arterial blood flow to major end organs that are perfused by aortic arterial branches and to repair or replace the region of diseased aorta so that normal antegrade blood flow can resume through the aorta with the ability to provide adequate perfusion to the brain, spinal cord, gut, kidneys, and other tissues.

Aortic aneurysms generally are repaired surgically by replacing the entire length of diseased aorta with synthetic tube graft. Major arterial branches off the replaced aortic segment are individually reimplanted into the synthetic replacement graft, although with aortic arch replacements, an "island" of native aortic tissue containing the ostia for the innominate and the left carotid and subclavian arteries may be reanastomosed to the replacement graft to reduce surgical time. Surgical repairs of thoracic aortic dissections have a somewhat different approach, because often only the region of dissected aorta that actually contains the dissection entry point or intimal tear is replaced with a synthetic interposition graft. The entire length of dissected aorta is generally not replaced; rather, with entry into the false lumen of the dissected aorta now surgically closed, further entry of aortic blood flow into the false lumen should not be possible. The idea is that once continuity of flow is reestablished into only the true aortic lumen, the false lumen will eventually compress and thrombose. In cases of acute aortic transection, the disrupted aortic region is resected, then the aorta is reapproximated to itself. If it is not possible to reanastomose the native aorta to itself, a short interposition graft may be placed.

General anesthetic objectives for repairing the thoracic aorta

In concert with primary surgical objectives to control or prevent aortic hemorrhage and to maintain adequate end-organ perfusion, the anesthesiologist must adequately volume resuscitate patients and monitor and manage the hemodynamics so as to avoid triggering aortic rupture or dissection extension (if they have not already occurred). Anesthesiologists also must take additional measures to monitor and protect the function of organs such as the spinal cord and kidneys that receive blood supply from affected aortic regions. In some emergency situations, massive volume resuscitation may already be underway as the patient enters the OR. To formulate the best overall anesthetic plan for the patient undergoing thoracic aortic surgery, the anesthesiologist should be as aware of significant patient comorbidities as the urgency of surgical presentation will allow. Patients commonly have significant cardiovascular and pulmonary comorbidities, as well as diabetes and renal insufficiency. It is also extremely important for the anesthesiologist to clearly communicate with the surgical team to understand (1) exactly which regions of the aorta are presumed to be involved and (2) how the surgeons plan to approach aortic repair with regard to both the incision site and extracorporeal circulation. As is discussed in detail in the remaining sections of this chapter, these factors have many important implications for anesthetic planning, including where to place arterial lines, what choices to make for other invasive and noninvasive monitoring, the need for lung isolation, and anticipation of blood loss.

Before inducing anesthesia, the anesthesiologist must follow the basic tenets of airway assessment and consideration of a plan to reduce the risk of aspiration. Many patients present as emergencies with a presumed full stomach. In these situations the risk of using rapid-sequence induction, with its associated swings in hemodynamics, must be balanced against the aspiration risk with a "modified" rapid-sequence induction, in which a slower IV induction is conducted in conjunction with gentle manual ventilations done while cricoid pressure is held. Because hemodynamic swings are common with laryngoscopy, drugs such as nitroglycerin and esmolol should be readily available during intubation. Ideally, an arterial line is placed and monitored prior to induction of anesthesia. In conscious patients, administration of a nonparticulate antacid should also be considered before induction.

Prior to placing an arterial line for direct blood pressure monitoring, thought should be given to the location of the aortic pathology. Central venous access is useful in all thoracic aortic surgeries to effectively administer inotropes, vasopressors, and vasodilators as needed. Pulmonary artery catheters, particularly those that can monitor continuous cardiac output and mixed venous oxygen saturation, may provide useful perioperative guidance in the setting of hemodynamic lability and volume shifts, particularly in patients with substantial concurrent cardiopulmonary or renal disease. Transesophageal echocardiography (TEE) also can offer significant direction for intraoperative management. Complementing its preoperative diagnostic capability, TEE is helpful for determining aortic valve involvement, assessing left ventricular function and filling during periods of aortic cross-clamping and unclamping, locating intimal tears and fenestrations within dissection flaps, and discerning whether aortic flow appears to have ceased in the false lumen after dissection repair.

Specific considerations for ascending aortic or aortic arch surgery

Arterial blood pressure monitoring and cannulation for cardiopulmonary bypass

Aneurysms involving the aortic root, proximal aorta, or aortic arch, as well as Stanford type A aortic dissections, are typically repaired through a midline sternotomy incision with use of full CPB. If aortic pathology involves the innominate artery, a left radial or femoral arterial line should be placed. This is also true if right axillary cannulation is anticipated, because in this setting, right radial arterial line blood pressure readings will be inaccurate during CPB. In situations in which the aortic arch needs to be repaired and prolonged DHCA is anticipated, the surgeon may wish to administer antegrade cerebral perfusion through a right axillary arterial cannula and may wish to monitor pressure during administration of antegrade cerebral perfusion through a right radial arterial line. In this situation, a right radial arterial line, as well as a left radial or femoral arterial line, should be placed to allow accurate blood pressure monitoring while on CPB. It is important to make the OR team aware of which arterial line tracing is displaying accurate systemic blood pressure during CPB and which one should be used to monitor antegrade cerebral perfusion during DHCA. Stanford type A dissections may extend into the iliac and femoral arteries, and the possibility of inadvertently monitoring false lumen blood pressures with a femoral arterial line should be considered in this scenario.

Repairs isolated to the aortic root or proximal ascending aorta may permit both cannulation and cross-clamping of an area of nondiseased aorta proximal to the aortic arch. This approach allows the aorta to be repaired on CPB with a bloodless surgical field and concurrent perfusion of the brain and other organs. Arterial cannulation for CPB also may occur in the axillary or femoral arteries, possibly improving surgical exposure for ascending aortic repair.

For surgical repairs involving the aortic arch, a bloodless surgical field cannot be established for portions of the repair with the patient on CPB. Therefore, CPB is initiated by cannulating aneurysmal or normal portions of the ascending aorta, or the axillary or femoral arteries, but patients must undergo periods of cessation of CPB after the heart is arrested for the arch to be repaired. In this scenario, the patient is placed on CPB and is typically aggressively cooled prior to conducting repair of the arch with DHCA. Venous cannulation for CPB is often in the right atrium for both ascending aortic and arch surgeries; however, if the surgeon is concerned that view of the aneurysm will be obstructed or that the aneurysm is too large to allow easy access to the right atrium, a femoral vein can be cannulated.

Cerebral protection strategies

Hypothermia is an important cerebral protection strategy, as it markedly reduces the cerebral metabolic rate of oxygen consumption. Mild to moderate hypothermia on CPB is typically desirable for ascending aortic aneurysm repairs. However, deliberate intraoperative hypothermia is particularly valuable for surgeries involving the aortic arch, as these operations require transient interruption of cerebral blood flow, increasing a patient's risk for postoperative stroke and neurocognitive dysfunction. For aortic arch repairs, profound hypothermia is established on CPB (core temperature of 15°C–20°C) prior to circulatory arrest (DHCA). In this temperature range, a DHCA period of < 40 minutes is generally considered "safe" for the brain. The degree of cooling depends on the anticipated duration of DHCA. During the CPB cooling period prior to DHCA, the heart is arrested and ice is often placed around the patient's head in an effort to more uniformly cool the brain. To avoid thermal injury, care should be taken to avoid direct contact between ice and the ears and nose. Once the target patient temperature for DHCA is reached for the venous return to the CPB circuit, CPB at this temperature should continue until the patient's nasopharyngeal temperature (reflective of brain temperature) is equally cool. Either raw or processed electroencephalogram (EEG) monitoring is often used to verify an isoelectric cerebral state before initiating DHCA. In addition to using hypothermia to establish an isoelectric EEG, a barbiturate such as thiopental is sometimes also administered a few minutes prior to initiating DHCA to further decrease the cerebral metabolic rate. To promote cerebral protection, other pharmacologic measures, including administration of steroids or mannitol (to reduce perioperative cerebral swelling) or magnesium, are sometimes taken prior to initiating DHCA, but there are no strong data to support the efficacy of these measures. Following DHCA, slow rewarming is essential to evenly rewarm the patient's core and periphery; this will better allow the patient to remain warm once separated from CPB, reducing the risk of postoperative bleeding. Slow rewarming also avoids cerebral hyperthermia, which may exacerbate cerebral injury.

To enhance the cerebral protection provided by hypothermia alone during blood flow cessation for aortic arch repair (particularly for complex repairs for which the DHCA period is anticipated to be longer than 40 minutes), selective anterograde or retrograde cerebral perfusion techniques may be employed. Both strategies involve infusion of cold oxygenated blood to the brain. Selective anterograde cerebral perfusion is often administered through a right axillary arterial cannula, with infusion pressure monitored via a right radial arterial line. However, antegrade cerebral perfusate can also be administered directly into the innominate or carotid arteries. Assuming an intact circle of Willis, administering antegrade cerebral perfusate through one arch vessel should provide perfusion to both the ipsilateral and contralateral cerebral hemispheres. Retrograde cerebral perfusion is easily conducted immediately after DHCA is initiated by infusing perfusate through the superior vena cava while the patient is in slight Trendelenburg position.

Specific considerations for descending thoracic or thoracoabdominal aortic surgeries
One-lung ventilation

Repair of descending thoracic or thoracoabdominal aneurysms typically is conducted through a left thoracotomy incision with the patient positioned in full right lateral decubitus position. To optimize surgical exposure, the anesthesiologist usually is asked to ventilate only the right lung during the thoracic portion of the repair. The trachea and left main bronchus may be anatomically distorted in patients with large ascending aortic aneurysms. Placement of a double-lumen endotracheal tube should be done gently to minimize risk of rupturing the aneurysm. Additionally, left-sided double-lumen tubes may be difficult to seat effectively in the left main bronchus. Therefore, some anesthesiologists prefer to place right-sided double-lumen tubes for these operations. For patients potentially difficult to intubate, placing an endobronchial blocker may be preferable to a double-lumen tube, as this avoids the need to change the double-lumen tube to a single-lumen tube at the end of the surgery. This is important, as descending thoracic surgeries may be lengthy and require massive volume resuscitation, factors that both may cause significant airway edema that may make endotracheal tube changes difficult.

Surgical approaches to distal aortic perfusion

One approach to descending thoracic aneurysm repair is to cross-clamp the aorta proximal and sometimes distal to the affected aorta and to conduct subsequent aortic repair as quickly as possible without taking additional measures to provide distal aortic perfusion. This approach has the advantage of not requiring heparin for extracorporeal circulation, which may increase surgical bleeding, but has the disadvantage of increased incidence of hypertension proximal to the aortic cross-clamp, as well as hypotension in the distal aorta and its branches. With this simple cross-clamp technique, the anesthesiologist must prepare to treat proximal hypertension with short-acting vasodilators such as nitroglycerin or sodium nitroprusside to prevent acute congestive heart failure instigated by high left ventricular afterload. Perioperative physicians also should be aware that any prolonged period of distal aortic hypotension presents an increased potential for gastrointestinal, renal, or spinal cord ischemia.

To mitigate the proximal aortic hypertension and distal hypoperfusion that occur with the simple aortic cross-clamp technique, some surgeons use shunts whereas others use extracorporeal circulation to divert aortic blood flow from proximal to the aortic cross-clamp to more distal aortic regions. The Gott shunt is heparin bonded, so generally it does not require additional systemic heparinization. However, these shunts have very small internal diameters (5–6 mm), limiting the degree of decompression and augmentation that can occur for the proximal and distal aorta, respectively. Furthermore, these shunts sometimes can kink. Traditional CPB can be employed with full systemic heparinization and typically is used for descending thoracic aneurysm repairs that will require DHCA because of involvement of the proximal descending aorta or the aortic arch. Full heparinization increases bleeding complications, particularly within the left lung, as this lung is often subjected to surgical manipulation and incidental trauma during repair of the descending thoracic aorta. Traditional full CPB also involves a heat exchanger, which decreases the risk of perioperative hypothermia. Left heart bypass is often used during repairs

of the descending thoracic or thoracoabdominal aorta that are distal to the take-off of the left subclavian artery. Left heart bypass does not require an oxygenator, so required heparinization is typically less than that for full CPB. A heat exchanger may be added to the left heart bypass circuit for cases anticipated to be lengthy and thus at higher risk for hypothermia and related bleeding. Left heart bypass diverts blood from the left atrium, left ventricular apex, or left axillary artery to the distal aorta or femoral artery. The rate of blood flow through the left heart bypass circuit should be titrated according to arterial blood pressure monitoring above and below the aortic cross-clamp, and should be slowed as needed to preferentially provide adequate perfusion of the proximal aorta.

Spinal cord protection

Anterior spinal cord ischemia with resultant paraplegia is a major complication of open repairs of descending thoracic and thoracoabdominal aneurysms. In this scenario, motor function typically is lost but the patient may have some sensation. This complication is caused by compromised blood flow through the anterior spinal artery (the major blood supply to the anterior spinal cord) during aneurysm repair, particularly if this occurs for more than 30 minutes. Significant spinal cord ischemia is more likely to occur if collateral blood flow through vessels such as the intercostal arteries also is compromised during aortic repair. The vertebral arteries fuse to become the anterior spinal artery, and as the anterior spinal artery travels down the spinal cord, it collateralizes with the radicular branches of the intercostal arteries. In many patients, one of these radicular branches, often called the great radicular artery of Adamkiewicz, arises at the T8–L4 spinal cord levels and supplies blood to a major portion of the anterior spinal cord (Fig. 78.1). Unfortunately, this vessel is difficult to locate preoperatively with angiography or during surgical inspection.

Several methods have been tried to prevent hypoperfusion of the spinal cord and resulting paraplegia during repair of the descending thoracic aorta. As mentioned previously, some groups use a passive shunt or extracorporeal bypass to provide some distal aortic blood flow to the mid and lower spinal cord or other end organs. However, although logical, the efficacy of this approach is controversial, as a study conducted by Coselli et al. at a center performing a large volume of descending aortic repairs found that left heart bypass did not reduce that center's incidence of perioperative paraplegia. However, a randomized controlled trial conducted by Coselli et al. at the same center supports the efficacy of perioperative cerebral spinal fluid (CSF) drainage through a lumbar spinal drain in preventing paralysis. At many centers, the lumbar spinal drain is placed preoperatively by anesthesiologists. Commercially available spinal drain catheter kits are available. The technique for placement is similar to lumbar epidural catheter placement at the L3–4 or L4–5 interspaces, but larger-diameter hollow needs are typically used to thread the catheter (12 gauge), and the needle is advanced through the epidural space and into the subarachnoid

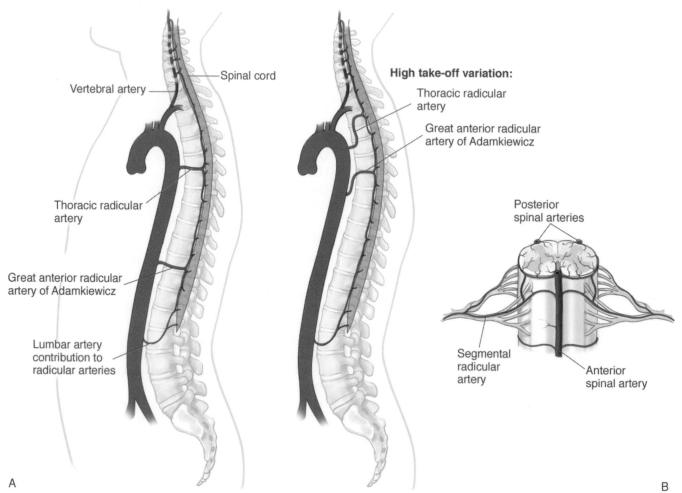

Figure 78.1. Blood supply of the spinal cord. (**A**) Vertical distribution and (**B**) horizontal distribution of the blood supply. Branches of the vertebral, deep cervical, intercostal, and lumbar arteries contribute to three arteries that run the length of the spinal cord: the anterior spinal and the two posterior spinal arteries. The anterior spinal artery arises at the level of the foramen magnum by the junction of two branches, one from each vertebral artery. Each posterior spinal artery arises from the posterior inferior cerebellar artery at the same level. Twenty-one pairs of segmental radicular arteries supply the nerve roots and about half of them contribute to the spinal arteries. Of these larger branches, the largest is the great anterior radicular artery of Adamkiewicz (radicularis magna), which supplies the lower thoracic and upper lumbar parts of the cord. It usually arises from a lower intercostal or a high lumbar artery but may arise as low as L4 or as high as T8. Because it makes a major contribution to the spinal cord blood supply, spinal injury or aortic surgery may compromise the blood supply of the lower part of the spinal cord. Although the other segmental radicular arteries are small, their contributions to the anterior and posterior spinal arteries are important.

space before the lumbar drain catheter is threaded. The lumbar spinal drain is then connected to a manometer and collection bag (Fig. 78.2). The rationale for CSF drainage is that decreasing the external pressure applied to the spinal cord by surrounding CSF will permit increased arterial perfusion of the spinal cord. Spinal cord perfusion pressure (SCPP) can be monitored by using the lumbar spinal drain to transduce CSF pressure around the spinal cord. The equation for SCPP is mean systemic arterial pressure (MAP) minus CSF pressure or central venous pressure (whichever is higher). Some experts suggest maintaining the intraoperative CSF above 10 mm Hg to prevent intracranial hypotension and potential related complications, such as subdural hematoma formation. Additionally, one must monitor for potential lumbar epidural hematoma formation and resultant spinal cord compression at the spinal drain insertion site, particularly in cases that require full systemic

heparinization or otherwise involve extended periods of perioperative coagulopathy. There is no clear evidence-based timing for when spinal drains should be removed postoperatively, but Coselli et al. have reported removing the drains approximately 48 hours after surgery and replacing the drains if delayed paraplegia occurs. Care should be taken to normalize the patient's coagulation profile prior to placing or removing spinal drains.

If paraplegia is noted in the postoperative period, attempts to reverse it by improving SCPP involve increasing MAP pharmacologically or with volume resuscitation in conjunction with increasing CSF drainage. During the surgery itself, such strategies may also be used if spinal cord hypoperfusion is suspected. Some centers try to detect anterior spinal cord function indirectly or directly during periods of potential hypoperfusion by monitoring somatosensory evoked potentials (SEPs) or motor

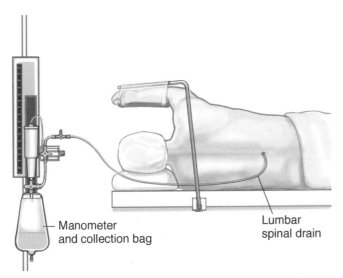

Manometer and collection bag

Lumbar spinal drain

Figure 78.2. Intraoperative CSF drainage during thoracoabdominal aortic repair.

evoked potentials (MEPs), respectively. SEPs monitor the brainstem and cerebral cortex response to peripheral nerve stimulation and therefore directly reflect performance of the posterior sensory columns in the spinal cord. However, the assumption is that if the posterior spinal cord is affected, the anterior spinal cord very likely is underperfused as well. Various anesthetic agents, such as volatile anesthetics, may affect the latency and amplitude of SEPs, so the anesthetic plan must be designed with careful communication with the neuromonitoring team. Several centers have successfully monitored MEPs to gauge anterior spinal cord compromise more directly. Although MEPs can reflect the integrity of the anterior motor horns, transcranial stimulation of the motor cortex is required during thoracic aortic surgery and therefore is an approach that is cumbersome and requires considerable expertise. This approach also may trigger seizure activity.

Conclusions and future directions

Anesthesiologists must have a full appreciation for the wide spectrum of issues associated with urgent or emergent surgical repair of the thoracic aorta to provide optimal perioperative management for these surgeries. The past several decades have seen significant developments in both surgical and anesthetic practice that have improved patient morbidity and mortality from surgical repair of the thoracic aorta. Progression in the arena of less invasive endovascular stent repairs of the thoracic aorta has shown great promise. In addition, continued research efforts directed at understanding the acute physiologic changes encountered with interruption of aortic blood flow should aid in development of measures to reduce end-organ damage from associated ischemia or reperfusion.

Suggested readings

Balduini CL, Salvini M, Montani N, et al. Activation of the hemostatic process in patients with unruptured aortic aneurysm before and in the first week after surgical repair. *Haematologica* 1997; 82:581–583.

Cina CS, Clase CM. Coagulation disorders and blood product use in patients undergoing thoracoabdominal aortic aneurysm repair. *Transfus Med Rev* 2005; 19:143–154.

Coselli JS, LeMaire SA, Conklin LD, Adams GJ. Left heart bypass during descending thoracic aortic aneurysm repair does not reduce the incidence of paraplegia. *Ann Thorac Surg* 2004; 77:1298–1303; discussion 1303.

Coselli JS, Lemaire SA, Koksoy C, et al. Cerebrospinal fluid drainage reduces paraplegia after thoracoabdominal aortic aneurysm repair: results of a randomized clinical trial. *J Vasc Surg* 2002; 35:631–639.

Crawford ES, Saleh SA. Transverse aortic arch aneurysm: improved results of treatment employing new modifications of aortic reconstruction and hypothermic cerebral circulatory arrest. *Ann Surg* 1981; 194:180–188.

Croughwell N, Smith LR, Quill T, et al. The effect of temperature on cerebral metabolism and blood flow in adults during cardiopulmonary bypass. *J Thorac Cardiovasc Surg* 1992; 103:549–554.

Dardik A, Perler BA, Roseborough GS, Williams GM. Subdural hematoma after thoracoabdominal aortic aneurysm repair: an underreported complication of spinal fluid drainage? *J Vasc Surg* 2002; 36:47–50.

de Haan P, Kalkman CJ, Jacobs MJ. Spinal cord monitoring with myogenic motor evoked potentials: early detection of spinal cord ischemia as an integral part of spinal cord protective strategies during thoracoabdominal aneurysm surgery. *Semin Thorac Cardiovasc Surg* 1998; 10:19–24.

Fisher DF Jr, Yawn DH, Crawford ES. Preoperative disseminated intravascular coagulation associated with aortic aneurysms. A prospective study of 76 cases. *Arch Surg* 1983; 118: 1252–1255.

Grigore AM, Grocott HP, Mathew JP, et al. The rewarming rate and increased peak temperature alter neurocognitive outcome after cardiac surgery. *Anesth Analg* 2002; 94:4–10.

Nussmeier NA, Arlund C, Slogoff S. Neuropsychiatric complications after cardiopulmonary bypass: cerebral protection by a barbiturate. *Anesthesiology* 1986; 64:165–170.

Robertazzi RR, Cunningham JN Jr. Monitoring of somatosensory evoked potentials: a primer on the intraoperative detection of spinal cord ischemia during aortic reconstructive surgery. *Semin Thorac Cardiovasc Surg* 1998; 10:11–17.

Shenaq SA, Svensson LG. Paraplegia following aortic surgery. *J Cardiothorac Vasc Anesth* 1993; 7:81–94.

Svensson LG, Crawford ES, Hess KR, et al. Deep hypothermia with circulatory arrest. Determinants of stroke and early mortality in 656 patients. *J Thorac Cardiovasc Surg* 1993; 106: 19–28.

Wan IY, Angelini GD, Bryan AJ, et al. Prevention of spinal cord ischaemia during descending thoracic and thoracoabdominal aortic surgery. *Eur J Cardiothorac Surg* 2001; 19: 203–213.

Chapter 79

Cardiac transplantation in the adult

Martina Nowak, Prem S. Shekar, and Michael N. D'Ambra

Cardiac transplantation is the therapeutic procedure of choice for end-stage heart failure patients. Since South African Christiaan Barnard performed the first allogenic orthotopic (human-to-human) heart transplant in 1967, advances in immunosuppression, early diagnosis, and treatment of rejection and infection have transformed a once experimental intervention into routine treatment.

Nevertheless, heart transplantation in the United States has declined over the past 10 years, leveling at approximately 2200 per year in 2007, mainly because of limited donor organ availability.

The vast majority of patients referred for cardiac transplantation suffer from New York Heart Association class III or IV symptoms and carry a diagnosis of ischemic heart disease or idiopathic dilated cardiomyopathy.

After heart transplantation, 30-day mortality ranges from 5% to 10%, with primary graft failure being the most frequent cause of early death. The 1-year survival rate approximates 80%, with an annual mortality rate of 4% for subsequent years. The most common causes of death in the first 6 months are infection and/or rejection. Accelerated coronary artery disease, allograft vasculopathy, chronic rejection, and posttransplant lymphoproliferative disease are causes of late mortality.

Donor selection and matching

A potential donor is declared brain dead by a medical team that had not been involved in the donor's or recipient's care. Donors are screened and evaluated by the local organ procurement agencies, and donor organs are made available to potential recipients via the United Network of Organ Sharing (UNOS). The accepting transplant center may then evaluate the suitability of the allograft. (See Table 79.1 for complete donor selection criteria.) The donor is matched to the prospective recipient for ABO blood type compatibility and heart size (HLA matching has not shown to improve survival but is still done in some centers). A donor heart size within 20% of the recipient's is preferable. If the recipient has elevated pulmonary vascular resistance (PVR), the increased right ventricular (RV) afterload will require a larger RV muscle mass, which will necessitate a larger donor heart. Care must be taken not to oversize the heart for recipients with acute myocardial infarction or a ventricular assist device (VAD).

Anesthesia management issues for heart transplant donors

Donors normally exhibit major hemodynamic and metabolic disturbances, the main causes of which are hypovolemia (secondary to diuretics or central diabetes insipidus), myocardial impairment (as a result of major catecholamine release during periods of increased intracranial pressure), and insufficient sympathetic tone secondary to absence of brainstem function. Neurogenic ST-T–wave changes, as well as neurogenic arrhythmias, are possible. Volume administration and inotropic support should be guided by invasive monitoring and transesophageal echocardiography if available. Hemodynamic goals are a mean arterial pressure of 80 to 90 mm Hg, central venous pressure (CVP) of 5 to 12 mm Hg, urine output > 100 ml/h,

Table 79.1. Donor selection for cardiac transplantation

Suggested criteria for cardiac donor
  Age < 55 y
  Absence of the following:
    Prolonged cardiac arrest
    Prolonged severe hypotension
    Preexisting cardiac disease
    Preexisting pulmonary hypertension (unresponsive to pharmacologic intervention) with PVR > 5 Wood units and transpulmonary gradient > 15 mm Hg
    Intracardiac drug injection
    Severe chest trauma with evidence of cardiac injury
    Septicemia
    Extracerebal malignancy
    Positive serologies for HIV, hepatitis B or C
    Hemodynamic instability without high-dose inotropic support
Cardiac donor evaluation
  Medical history and physical examination
  Electrocardiogram
  Chest radiograph
  Arterial blood gases
  Laboratory tests (ABO, HIV, hepatitis B and C virus)
  Cardiology consultation (echocardiogram, coronary angiogram)

Source: Data based on information extracted from the following sources:
Cohn LH, Edmunds LH. *Cardiac Surgery in the Adult.* 2nd ed. New York: McGraw-Hill; 2003. Hosenpud JD, Bennett LE, Keck BM, et al. The Registry of the International Society for Heart and Lung Transplantation: Eighteenth Official Report-2001. *J Heart Lung Transplant* 2001; 20:805. Kaplan JA, Reich DL, Konstadt SN. *Cardiac Anesthesia.* 4th ed. Philadelphia: Saunders; 1999.

and normal serum electrolyte levels and arterial blood gas values. Vasopressin administration (0.8–1.0 U/h) might become necessary to limit volume loss from diabetes insipidus. Administration of anesthetic agents to the donor is controversial but recommended to blunt systemic stress responses mediated by functional components of the brainstem, spinal cord, and sympathetic and parasympathetic nervous systems.

Myocardial protection of the donor heart

The donor heart is usually protected with University of Wisconsin (UW) cold crystalloid hyperkalemic cardioplegia during the cardiectomy. The organ is then transported in two sterile plastic bags filled with ice-cold UW solution and carried in an ice chest. The present limit for ex vivo ischemia time is approximately 4 to 6 hours, but new technology to prolong this limit beyond 24 hours is in clinical trials. Prolonged cold ischemia time in conjunction with acute reperfusion injury may lead to tissue necrosis with a fatal outcome, most commonly manifested by RV failure.

Selection and preanesthesia assessment of the recipient

The basic objective of the selection process is to identify patients with end-stage cardiac disease refractory to medical therapies who possess the potential to resume a normal active life and maintain compliance with a rigorous medical regimen after cardiac transplantation.

Each candidate awaiting cardiac transplantation is assigned a *status code* based on UNOS criteria that corresponds to how medically urgent the transplant is:

IA: A patient who has *at least one* of the following in place:

Total artificial heart
Left and/or right ventricular assist device (LVAD/RVAD; Elective 1A time for 30 days)
Intra-aortic balloon pump
Extracorporeal membrane oxygenator
Mechanical circulatory support for more than 30 days with significant device-related complications
Mechanical ventilation
Continuous infusion of two high-dose inotropes in addition to continuous hemodynamic monitoring of left ventricular filling pressures
Life expectancy without transplant of < 7 days

IB: A patient who has *at least one* of the following devices or therapies in place:

LVAD and/or RVAD
Continuous infusion of intravenous (IV) inotropes not meeting the preceding criteria

II: All other waiting patients who do not meet Status Code IA or IB criteria.

Because the preoperative period is often marked by critical time constraints, a focused history including last oral intake, allergies, recent anticoagulant use, recent change in ventricular function, and/or anginal symptoms should be obtained. Physical examination should focus on cardiopulmonary signs of congestive heart failure, airway and access issues, and volume status. A preoperative chest radiograph, as well as a laboratory review, should be examined by the anesthesiologist. Many patients will be admitted on warfarin with therapeutic international normalized ratio levels, and the anesthetic plan will need to address anticoagulation reversal.

Once the organ procurement team has confirmed the acceptability of the donor allograft, the recipient induction may begin. Timing (which is routinely controlled by the harvesting team) is crucial to minimize allograft ischemic time and recipient bypass time. Ideally, the recipient cardiectomy is completed concurrent with the arrival of the cardiac allograft. Catheter placements may be difficult and prolonged because of previous surgery, catheterizations, interventions, and medical care. Be sure to communicate anticipated line placement difficulties.

Anesthesia management of the recipient

The heart transplant recipient is usually very anxious and requires reassurance. If an extended wait is required in the operating room (OR) before induction, consider allowing the patient to use a phone in the OR to speak with close family and significant others. In addition to standard noninvasive monitors, placement of an arterial catheter is required to facilitate a rapid response to hemodynamic events during induction. Symptomatic ventricular tachycardia or fibrillation is the most common cause of sudden cardiac death in patients awaiting heart transplantation and is most common within the first 3 months after referral for transplantation. Therefore, many patients will have an automatic implantable cardioverter–defibrillator (AICD) in place and/or a history of amiodarone use. For that reason, external defibrillation patches are placed before induction. It is important to know what the device setting is for external magnet placement (usually turns off arrhythmic therapy and maintains pacing at a default setting).

Most patients should be considered "full stomach." Therefore, a rapid-sequence induction technique using agents with minimal myocardial depression (etomidate 0.3 mg/kg) and a moderate dose of opioids (fentanyl 10 μg/kg) as well as succinylcholine (1.5 mg/kg) have been used successfully. Inotropic and vasoactive agents should be readily available for the rapid management of induction-induced hypotension and/or arrhythmias. Pre- or postinduction central venous access is obtained (preferably avoiding right internal jugular vein cannulation, which will be used for frequent endomyocardial biopsies postoperatively). A pulmonary artery (PA) catheter can be placed into an introducer, but floating the PA catheter into correct position may be difficult because of cardiac chamber dilation, severe tricuspid regurgitation, VAD cannulae, and AICD hardware. Because the PA catheter will be withdrawn to implant the new heart, it is not a major problem to leave the catheter in the CVP position before cardiopulmonary bypass (CPB). Large-bore IV access is mandatory. Meticulous attention should be paid to sterile technique during all invasive procedures, as these patients are at high risk for postoperative infection, which remains a serious cause of postoperative mortality. A first-generation cephalosporin or vancomycin is administered prior to skin incision.

Anesthesia is maintained with high-dose narcotics and volatile anesthetics. Cross-matched blood (irradiated) should immediately be available once surgery commences. Prior to CPB, the PA catheter should be withdrawn from the right heart and secured in its sterile sheath. It will be refloated after completion of the venacaval anastomoses prior to coming off CPB. Arterial and venous CPB cannulation is performed depending on the surgical technique (see Chapter 73). Aminocaproic acid currently is the antifibrinolytic of choice.

Weaning from CPB may be difficult and prolonged because of acute RV failure, bleeding, and/or hemodynamic instability. The initial bradycardia encountered post bypass should be treated with an infusion of a positive chronotropic agent (isoproterenol or dopamine) or atrial pacing to achieve a heart rate between 90 and 110 bpm. Patients with elevated PVR are at risk for acute RV failure and may benefit from the preemptive use of a low-dose pulmonary vasodilator such as prostaglandin E_1 (0.125–1.0 nanograms/kg/min) during the period of CPB or inhaled nitric oxide. Transesophageal echocardiography (TEE) can provide immediate information about right and left heart function and filling volumes and also assess for restricted anastomotic flow.

Frequently, hemostasis is problematic, and appears related to suppression of clotting factors often exacerbated by preoperative warfarin therapy, Preprotamine warfarin reversal with fresh frozen plasma (FFP) in the CPB circuit may be helpful if the patient is fully anticoagulated upon arrival to the OR. Commonly, FFP, cryoprecipitate, platelets, and, in severe post-CPB hemorrhage, recombinant factor VIIa are administered to normalize coagulation.

Orthotopic heart transplantation

Operative techniques in the recipient are shown in Fig. 79.1.

The surgery begins with a median sternotomy. Frequently, patients will have undergone prior cardiac surgeries. In this case, the groin is prepared and draped to provide rapid access for cannulation to initiate CPB if necessary. The aorta is cannulated as distally as possible, and the superior vena cava and inferior vena cava are cannulated separately. After aortic cross-clamping, the aorta and PA are separated and divided just above the level of their respective valves, and the atria are transected at their grooves.

A complete excision of the right atrium with bicaval anastomoses is the practiced variant of the classic technique described previously and is reported to reduce the incidence of atrial dysrhythmias, better preserve cardiac function by avoiding tricuspid regurgitation, and enhance cardiac output by enhancing right atrial function.

The donor graft is then implanted beginning with the left atrial anastomosis, followed by the aorta. The aortic cross-clamp can be removed while the right-sided anastomoses are carried out. The heart is meticulously de-aired using TEE guidance and then weaned from CPB.

Transesophageal echocardiography

A complete TEE examination may be performed post induction and often reveals useful information not immediately available from other sources, such as the presence of cardiac thrombi, ventricular volume and contractility, and atherosclerosis of the descending aorta. To assess the ascending aorta and the aortic arch for appropriate cross-clamp and cannulation sites, epicardial echocardiography is performed.

Posttransplant management and complications

In the past, a total reverse-isolation environment was maintained in the intensive care unit, but this practice has been replaced by universal precautions. Postoperative monitoring is the same as for all open heart patients. Mechanical ventilation is generally required for up to 24 hours, but extubation is accomplished as soon as possible to minimize infection. Meticulous sterility of all intravascular catheters, suction catheters, and equipment connected to the respirator is maintained. Immunosuppressive therapy is continued. Inhaled nitric oxide can be used to decrease PVR in the face of RV compromise. Severe RV dysfunction refractory to medical therapies may require placement of a mechanical assist device (e.g., RVAD).

The primary etiology for posttransplant RV failure is an increased PVR from preexisting left heart failure. These changes in the pulmonary vasculature are not totally fixed and may normalize with time.

Mediastinal reexploration for bleeding may be required in the immediate postoperative period. Most patients exhibit a mild deterioration in renal and hepatic function, as determined by blood chemistries.

Rejection and antirejection strategies

Hyperacute rejection results from preformed donor-specific antibodies in the recipient. Because of preoperative ABO blood group matching and panel-reactive antibody screening, hyperacute rejection has become a rare but nonetheless catastrophic complication that occurs within minutes to hours.

Immunosuppression following transplantation consists of an early induction phase followed by a long-term maintenance phase. The immunosuppressive regimen at our institution begins with methylprednisolone, 1000 mg IV preoperatively and methylprednisolone/prednisone, cyclosporine, and mycophenolate postoperatively. Because the nephrotoxic effects of cyclosporine place the recipient at increased risk for renal insufficiency, doses should be adjusted in preexisting renal insufficiency.

The gold standard for the diagnosis of acute rejection remains an RV endomyocardial biopsy through the right internal jugular vein. Early signs of impending graft rejection

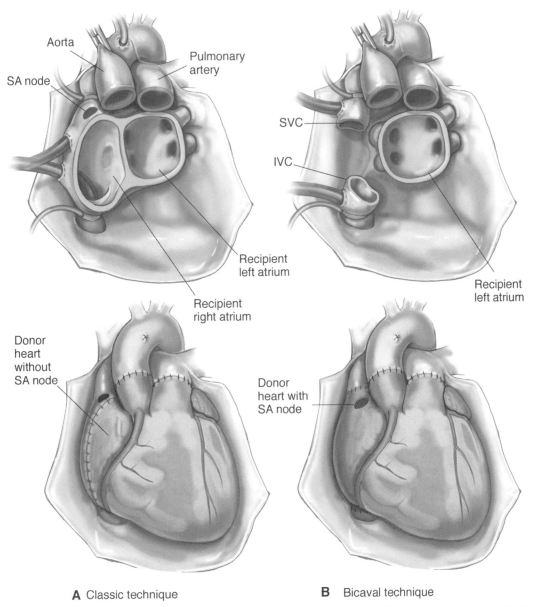

Aorta
Pulmonary artery
SA node
SVC
IVC
Recipient left atrium
Recipient right atrium
Recipient left atrium
Donor heart without SA node
Donor heart with SA node

A Classic technique   **B** Bicaval technique

Figure 79.1. Mediastinum after excision of the heart but prior to allograft placement. (**A**) Classic orthotopic technique. (**B**) Bicaval anastomotic technique.

include a drop in voltage in leads I, II, III, V_1, and V_6 in serial electrocardiograms; abnormal gallop rhythms; urinary output and weight changes; and fever.

Corticosteroids are the cornerstone of acute antirejection therapy. Rescue protocols for recurring or refractory rejection include methylprednisolone plus OKT3 polyclonal antibody therapy, or methotrexate.

Anesthetic management of the patient with a denervated heart

Cardiac denervation is an unavoidable consequence of heart transplantation. A transplanted heart responds atypically to exercise and to certain cardioactive drugs, effects of which are thought to primarily be a result of the lack of direct neuronal control of the allograft.

Denervation substantially alters the response to demands for increased cardiac output. Normally, an increased heart rate can rapidly increase cardiac output. This mechanism is not available in the denervated heart. Heart rate increases only gradually with exercise, an effect mediated mainly by circulating adrenal catecholamines. Increases in cardiac output in response to increased demands are mediated mainly via increased stroke volume. Therefore, maintaining an adequate preload in cardiac transplant recipients is crucial. In certain cases, both donor and recipient sinoatrial nodes are intact and functioning. P waves originating from both sources may be recorded with the recipient's neurally mediated responses intact.

Denervation has important implications for pharmacologic therapy. Drugs that act indirectly through the autonomous nervous system, such as ephedrine, atropine, pancuronium, and edrophonium, generally will be ineffective. Anticholinergic drugs should not be used to treat bradycardia in the setting of hypotension. Hypotensive patients with denervated hearts will respond to anticholinergics, with vasodilation lacking a compensatory tachycardic response and leading to worsening hypotension. Drugs with a mixture of direct and indirect actions will exhibit only their direct heart rate effects (e.g., tachycardia with norepinephrine). The hemodynamic drugs of choice in the transplanted heart are those with direct cardiac effects, such as epinephrine and isoproterenol, dopamine, and dobutamine.

The resting bradycardia in the immediate posttransplant period is probably secondary to sinus node dysfunction and graft-based parasympathetic ganglia and should be treated with a dopamine or isoproterenol infusion or atrial pacing. This bradycardia may persist for up to 7 days postoperatively. Eventually, the resting heart rate of the transplanted heart in the absence of vagal tone is between 90 and 110 bpm. The normal sympathetic responses to laryngoscopy and intubation are absent.

Summary

The anesthetic management of heart transplant patients calls into play all the skill sets of the perioperative physician, ranging from careful attention to managing the psychological stress of the waiting time before induction, to the invasive pharmacology associated with treating life-threatening pulmonary hyperresistance and right heart failure.

Suggested readings

Cohn LH, Edmunds LH. *Cardiac Surgery in the Adult.* 2nd ed. New York: McGraw-Hill; 2003.

Glas KE, Swaminathan M, Reeves ST, et al. Council for Intraoperative Echocardiography of the American Society of Echocardiography; Society of Cardiovascular Anesthesiologists; Society of Thoracic Surgeons. Guidelines for the performance of a comprehensive intraoperative epiaortic ultrasonographic examination: recommendations of the American Society of Echocardiography and the Society of Cardiovascular Anesthesiologists; endorsed by the Society of Thoracic Surgeons. *Anesth Analg* 2008; 106(5):1376–1384.

Hosenpud JD, Bennett LE, Keck BM, et al. The Registry of the International Society for Heart and Lung Transplantation: Eighteenth Official Report – 2001. *J Heart Lung Transplant* 2001; 20:805.

Kaplan JA, Reich DL, Konstadt SN. *Cardiac Anesthesia.* 4th ed. Philadelphia: Saunders; 1999.

Mangano DT, Tudor IC, Dietzel C. Multicenter Study of Perioperative Ischemia Research Group; Ischemia Research and Education Foundation. The risk associated with aprotinin in cardiac surgery. *N Engl J Med* 2006; 354(4):353–365.

Ream AK. *Acute Cardiovascular Management: Anesthesia and Intensive Care.* Philadelphia: Lippincott Williams & Wilkins; 1982.

Steinman TI, Becker BN, Frost AE, et al. Clinical Practice Committee, American Society of Transplantation. Guidelines for the referral and management of patients eligible for solid organ transplantation. *Transplantation* 2001; 71:1189.

UNOS. Allocation of thoracic organs. Available at: http://www.unos .org/PoliciesandBylaws2/policies/pdfs/policy_9.pdf.

Chapter 80

Persistent postoperative bleeding in cardiac surgical patients

Walter Bethune, Michael G. Fitzsimons, and Edwin G. Avery IV

Excessive bleeding after cardiopulmonary bypass (CPB) is associated with cardiac surgical morbidity and mortality. The overall incidence of excessive bleeding after cardiac surgery, commonly defined as the need to transfuse more than 10 U of allogeneic blood in the perioperative period, is commonly reported to be 3% to 5%. Approximately 2% to 4% of patients after CPB require surgical exploration, primarily because of excessive bleeding. Bleeding and surgical reexploration are both established independent predictors of adverse outcomes. Administration of blood products, in the absence of reexploration, may place the patient at risk for transfusion-related complications. Anesthesiologists caring for cardiac surgical patients must understand the risk factors, clinical presentation, diagnosis, and treatment of bleeding after cardiac surgery.

Definition

There is no uniformly accepted definition for excessive bleeding after cardiac surgery. Most patients will demonstrate some bleeding (0.5–1.0 ml/kg/h) within the first 6 hours after surgery. Bleeding in excess of 8 to 10 ml/kg/h generally prompts immediate surgical intervention if there is no response to blood products. Our institutional guideline, based on experience, is that bleeding should not be > 500 ml in the first hour, 400 ml/h for the first 2 hours, 300 ml/h for 3 hours, or 200 ml/h for the first 4 hours. Bleeding in excess of these numbers should prompt strong consideration of surgical reexploration in a normothermic patient, especially if the patient is hemodynamically unstable or if bleeding persists after correction of any coagulopathy.

Risk factors

Risk factors for excessive or persistent bleeding after cardiac surgery may be considered patient specific or surgery specific (Table 80.1). Patient-specific factors include female sex, preoperative cardiogenic shock, renal failure, small body mass, renal insufficiency, and certain preoperative anticoagulants or antiplatelet therapies. Surgery-specific factors include emergency procedures and more complicated heart operations, such as "redo" procedures; combined operations, such as coronary

artery bypass graft (CABG) surgery with valve replacement; and notably, the duration of CPB.

Clinical presentation

Some degree of bleeding after cardiac surgery is expected. Surgeons place chest tubes and mediastinal drains to allow close monitoring of this bleeding and to prevent the complications of concealed blood collection (i.e., cardiac tamponade).

External or free bleeding is evident in the patent, graduated drainage collection system. Blood and fluid that accumulate in the mediastinum from disrupted tissues and suture lines are drained via tubes placed during surgery. Mild bleeding should respond readily to volume replacement. Therefore, it is imperative that the patency of the drainage system be maintained to prevent tamponade and allow an ongoing assessment of blood loss. The color of the drained blood may shed light on the etiology. Blood that is bright red may indicate arterial bleeding from the bed of the internal mammary artery, intercostal arteries or suture lines on the aorta, left atrium, pulmonary veins, or left heart. Darker blood may indicate venous oozing from the chest wall or suture lines on right-sided structures such as the atrial appendage or vena cava. Dilute drainage results from third spacing of fluid in the thoracic cavity.

Concealed bleeding does not appear in the drains. It may result in the accumulation of blood in the pleural or mediastinal space that can simultaneously compromise ventilation or

Table 80.1. Risk factors associated with postoperative bleeding

Patient-specific	Surgery-specific
Female sex	Emergency surgery
Renal insufficiency	"Redo" procedures
Increased age	Combined procedures
Poor nutrition	Long duration of cardiopulmonary bypass
History of excessive bleeding	Excessive operative bleeding
Smaller body mass index	
Preoperative cardiogenic shock	

Source: Data from Ferraris VA, Ferraris S, Saha SP, Hessel EA, et al. Perioperative blood transfusion and blood conservation in cardiac surgery: The Society of Thoracic Surgeons and the Society of Cardiovascular Anesthesiologists Clinical Practice Guideline. *Ann Thorac Surg* 2007;83:S27–86.

hemodynamics, ultimately leading to tamponade. This clinical scenario does not respond as readily to volume replacement and may require surgical reexploration. Chest radiography may demonstrate a widened mediastinum. Transesophageal echocardiography (TEE) may demonstrate classic tamponade or, more commonly, focal compression by hematoma.

A sudden increase in the rate of bleeding, especially in a patient with relatively normal coagulation test parameters who was not bleeding initially, suggests a surgical etiology, as does the presence of clotted blood in the patient's chest tubes. Diffuse, widespread oozing from the skin incision and intravenous catheter sites, however, suggests a platelet abnormality or disseminated intravascular coagulation. Failure of blood within the mediastinal tubes to clot suggests either a platelet or significant coagulation factor abnormality, or both.

Differential diagnosis and pathophysiology

In caring for the patient suffering from excessive bleeding early after cardiac surgery, high priority is given to determining whether the bleeding is attributable to a surgical cause (i.e., tissue injury with inadequate surgical hemostasis or leaking suture lines) or to coagulopathy (i.e., microvascular bleeding). Coagulopathies that may contribute to excessive bleeding may be divided into those related to platelet abnormalities (dilution, depletion, or dysfunction) or clotting factor abnormalities related to inadequate heparin administration during CPB, heparin rebound, or fibrinolysis.

Complicating the diagnosis is the fact that prolonged "surgical" bleeding will inevitably lead to platelet and clotting factor depletion and an associated secondary coagulopathy. Significant causes of postoperative blood loss are listed in Fig. 80.1. Additionally, hypothermia may exacerbate coagulopathy related to either platelet or clotting factor abnormalities.

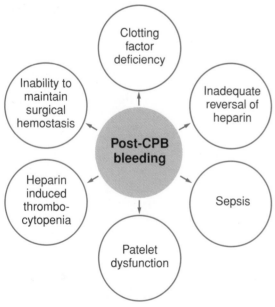

Figure 80.1. Causes of bleeding after CPB.

Preoperative anticoagulation

Platelet abnormalities, either quantitative or qualitative, are the most common causes of postoperative bleeding after surgical procedures using CPB. Patients often receive antiplatelet and antithrombotic agents in the setting of an acute coronary syndrome. These agents may include aspirin, glycoprotein (GP) IIb/IIIa receptor antagonists (tirofiban, abciximab, and eptifibatide), inhibitors of platelet adenosine diphosphate (clopidogrel and ticlopidine), low molecular weight heparins (LMWHs), ultra-pure LMWH (fondaparinux), and warfarin (Table 80.2). Not all have been implicated in increasing the risk of bleeding after cardiac surgery.

Despite numerous retrospective and prospective analyses, it is still controversial as to whether aspirin alone before CABG surgery is associated with an increased risk of postoperative bleeding. The consensus regarding aspirin therapy is that by itself it does not put cardiac surgical patients at increased risk for excessive hemorrhage.

The contribution of newer, more potent antiplatelet agents such as adenosine diphosphate (ADP) receptor antagonists and GP IIb/IIIa inhibitors may increase the risk of postoperative bleeding after cardiac surgery. The consensus is to delay surgery for at least 5 days after cessation of clopidogrel therapy to decrease the risk of excessive hemorrhage after cardiac surgery, if such a delay is clinically feasible.

Abciximab, a GP IIb/IIIa receptor antagonist, is often used to reduce ischemic complications in patients undergoing percutaneous coronary revascularization. Although there is concern regarding increased bleeding risk among the subset of these patients who later require urgent CABG, delaying surgery for at least 24 hours in abciximab-treated patients and for at least 6 hours in tirofiban-treated patients, if clinically feasible, presently is recommended. Enoxaparin used alone is associated with greater overall blood loss and a higher incidence of mediastinal reexploration compared with clopidogrel. The current consensus is to delay cardiac surgery for at least 12 hours in patients who have received LMWH, if clinically feasible.

Patients presenting for cardiac surgery commonly are taking antithrombotic medications in the setting of having in situ artificial valves, atrial fibrillation, or a pulmonary embolism. There is no standard protocol for the cessation of these agents that is guaranteed not to increase the risk of bleeding. The use of warfarin and aspirin has been shown to increase bleeding and the duration of chest drainage. Warfarin generally is stopped 4 to 5 days prior to scheduled surgery.

Bridging agents such as unfractionated heparin (UFH) or LMWH are commonly initiated to prevent thrombosis. Enoxaparin, an LMWH, has been shown to increase mediastinal blood loss and the need for exploration after bypass. Conversion of longer-acting antithrombotic agents (e.g., warfarin or LMWH) to parenteral UFH or direct thrombin inhibitor therapy may provide adequate perioperative anticoagulation if dosing is timed appropriately to the conduct of surgery.

Table 80.2. Drugs that increase perioperative bleeding

Drug	Inhibits	Half-life	Duration of effects	Reversible effects?	Methods to restore function
Aspirin	COX	15–20 min	7 d	No	Platelet transfusion
Abciximab (ReoPro[a])	GP IIb/IIIa receptor	30 min	48 h	Yes	Platelet (partial) transfusion
Eptifibatide (Integrilin[b])	GP IIb/IIIa receptor	2.5 h	4–8 h	Yes	Delay surgery 2 h after stopping drug
Tirofiban (Aggrastat[c])	GP IIb/IIIa receptor	1.5–3 h	4–8 h	Yes	Discontinue drug ASAP before surgery
Clopidogrel (Plavix[d])	ADP receptor	8 h	7 d	No	Blood product transfusion as needed
Ticlopidine (Ticlid[e])	ADP receptor	12 h to 5 d with repeat dosing	7 d	No	Blood product transfusion as needed
Dipyridamole (Persantine[f])	Adenosine uptake; PDE	9–13 h	4–10 h	Yes	Platelet transfusion
Cilostazol (Pletal[g])	PDE III	11–13 h	48 h	Yes	Blood product transfusion as needed
Herbal therapies	Platelet aggregation	Variable	Variable	Variable	Limited data available

[a] Eli Lilly and Co., Indianapolis, IN.
[b] Schering Corp., Kenilworth, NJ.
[c] Merck and Co., Whitehouse Station, NJ.
[d] Sanofi-Aventis, Bridgewater, NJ.
[e] Roche, Nutley, NJ.
[f] Boehringer-Ingelheim, Ridgefield, CT.
[g] Otsuka, Princeton, NJ.
COX, cyclooxygenase; PDE, phosphodiesterase.
From Mashour GA, Avery EG. Anesthesia for cardiac surgery. In: Dunn et al., eds. *Clinical Anesthesia Procedures of the Massachusetts General Hospital.* 7th ed. Philadelphia: Lippincott Williams & Wilkins; 2007:401–440.

Effects of cardiopulmonary bypass on coagulation

CPB affects all elements of the coagulation system, although platelet number and function appear to be the most severely affected. Three factors contribute to a decrease in platelet count while on CPB: dilution, sequestration within the spleen, and destruction. Initiation of bypass results in a dilutional thrombocytopenia related to the volume of pump-priming solution. Hypothermia, commonly utilized for myocardial and vital organ protection, results in a sequestration of platelets within the spleen.

Platelets are also vulnerable to shear stress injury from field suction, roller pumps, balloon bumps, and simple contact with elements of the bypass circuit. Furthermore, regardless of the platelet count, platelet dysfunction in cardiac surgical patients historically has been attributed to CPB-induced platelet activation with subsequent loss of receptors for von Willebrand factor and fibrinogen. Consequently, platelet transfusion has become the primary therapy for nonsurgical (microvascular) bleeding after operations involving CPB.

Prolonged blood contact with the artificial surface of the CPB circuit is known to activate the contact activation and intrinsic coagulation pathways, eventually leading to thrombin formation and consumption of soluble coagulation proteins. CPB requires anticoagulation to prevent blood from clotting within the bypass circuit. UFH is administered to amplify antithrombin III action and prevent thrombin formation. In our center, 350 U/kg of heparin is administered prior to CPB. Additional bolus doses are administered as required to achieve and subsequently maintain the activated clotting time (ACT) values at or above 480 seconds, although this varies among centers. The effects of UFH may persist into the postoperative period, and the activated partial thromboplastin time (aPTT) assay is useful to detect residual heparin effects in cardiac surgical patients.

Protamine sulfate is administered after completion of CPB to reverse heparin-induced anticoagulation. Protamine forms a stable 1:1 complex with heparin, rapidly (<10 minutes) neutralizing its anticoagulant activity. Protamine has a short half-life (~5 minutes), and the effects of UFH may often recur, which is commonly referred to as "heparin rebound." A protamine administration protocol based on plasma heparin concentration measured at the end of CPB has been shown to reduce bleeding into the postoperative period. Commonly, UFH is neutralized empirically with anywhere from 0.5 to 1.3 mg of protamine for every 100 U of UFH administered. Practice patterns vary according to institution, and recently published blood therapy guidelines suggest that lower doses of protamine may help reduce hemorrhage following cardiac surgery.

Blood contact with the foreign CPB surface results in direct extrinsic activation of fibrinolysis. This is caused primarily by the release of tissue plasminogen activator from the vascular endothelium throughout CPB. Thrombin formation, hypothermia, and traumatized endothelial cells also may contribute to fibrinolysis. Unrestricted CPB-mediated thrombin activity and fibrinolysis ultimately lead to consumption of coagulation factors and platelets, further contributing to bleeding.

Finally, CPB induces an intensive activation of the inflammatory system, leading to leukocyte activation. Activated leukocytes release inflammatory mediators that, in turn, activate monocytes, ultimately bringing about tissue factor (TF) expression, thrombin generation, and paradoxic activation and impairment of the coagulation system in many patients.

Surgical factors

The type of surgery and conductance of bypass itself contributes to bleeding after surgery. The combination of a valve repair/replacement with bypass grafting or aortic surgery increases bleeding, as do repeat procedures. Surgeons are vigilant of the common sites of bleeding after cardiac surgery. Cannulation sites such as the right atrial appendage, pulmonary veins, ascending aorta, and vena cava commonly exhibit some minor bleeding after surgery. Other sites, such as the bed of the internal mammary artery, sternum, and anastomosis sites, may exhibit oozing immediately after surgery.

Most surgeons are diligent in examining the mediastinum and thoracic cavity prior to chest closure, but hypertension after surgery may disrupt formed clot. Although the advent of minimally invasive procedures is felt to decrease these risks, this may not be the case, as such patients may exhibit more postoperative blood loss. The duration of CPB has been shown to be strongly associated with transfusion requirements and bleeding after surgery.

Workup
Clinical examination

The evaluation of a bleeding patient in the postoperative setting begins with a detailed clinical history and targeted examination. The rate of bleeding must be determined, and all drains and wound sites should be assessed for the presence of clot. Hemodynamic variables must be considered; hypotension combined with tachycardia, low central venous pressure (CVP), low filling pressures, and a low cardiac index indicates hypovolemia, whereas hypotension combined with an elevated CVP, decreased cardiac index, and equalization of pulmonary artery pressures may indicate concealed bleeding, potentially resulting in cardiac tamponade. The differential diagnosis of tamponade also includes right, left, and biventricular heart failure.

Chest radiography is commonly employed to evaluate for blood collection in the mediastinum; however, its diagnostic value is poor. Only 20% of chest radiographs met the criteria for an enlarged cardiac silhouette, whereas 86% demonstrated an effusion with echocardiography.

TEE is gaining widespread acceptance among physicians in determining the cause of hemodynamic instability in the postoperative setting. In a study of 301 patients requiring TEE in the intensive care unit (ICU), TEE had a direct therapeutic impact in 73% of the cases. Tamponade was diagnosed in 11% and excluded in 12%.

Laboratory and point-of-care testing

Essential elements of the initial laboratory evaluation of the patient bleeding after surgery include the hemoglobin/hematocrit, platelet count, prothrombin time–international normalized ratio (PT-INR), aPTT, and fibrinogen also may be useful. The ACT is widely used to monitor heparin therapy during CPB but is less sensitive than the aPTT to residual heparin concentration post-CPB, limiting its utility in the postoperative setting.

Transient platelet dysfunction is considered the most common and important defect in hemostasis in the early postoperative period. The platelet count from the complete blood count does not necessarily reflect platelet function. Point-of-care (POC) assays are tests performed at the patient's bedside that evaluate coagulation abnormalities without the time delay associated with central laboratory analysis.

Thromboelastography (TEG) is a viscoelastic measure of clot formation and clot dissolution that measures coagulation, platelet function, platelet–fibrinogen interactions, and fibrinolysis. The TEG maximum amplitude parameter has been shown to be more predictive of bleeding after cardiac surgery than other isolated POC tests of platelet function, such as the platelet-activated clotting test or routine coagulation tests such as the platelet , PT, and aPTT. In a randomized, blinded, prospective trial, Shore-Lesserson et al. randomly assigned cardiac surgical patients to either a TEG-guided transfusion algorithm (n = 53) or routine transfusion therapy (n = 52) for intervention after CPB and showed that the algorithm using TEG was effective in reducing transfusion requirements over the first 2 days postoperatively.

Multiple POC assays that evaluate platelet function have been developed. Most preliminary investigations of their potential role in the postoperative management of cardiac surgical patients have shown favorable results, although the full utility of POC testing for patient management in this setting remains to be demonstrated by large randomized controlled trials.

Management

Persistent postoperative bleeding must be managed by providing the appropriate therapy based on the etiology of the blood loss. A bleeding diathesis must be differentiated from a surgical cause requiring urgent reoperation. Instability not responding immediately to volume expansion should prompt immediate reexploration. Management consists of two goals, return of hemodynamic stability and correction of underlying coagulopathy.

Fluids

In the setting of excessive postoperative bleeding, colloids and/or crystalloids should be administered as needed to maintain intravascular volume and hemodynamic stability without worsening coagulopathy. All fluids should be delivered through a warmer to avoid worsening hypothermia. No clear data exist to justify the use of normal saline over Ringer's lactate for volume expansion. Likewise, the benefits of colloid administration for volume expansion are unclear. Hetastarch has been implicated in postoperative bleeding when administered during bypass. A meta-analysis of studies investigating the link between synthetic starch administration and bleeding in cardiac surgery patients has confirmed that use of these solutions significantly increases bleeding.

Blood products

Blood products are the primary means of treatment for postoperative bleeding after cardiac surgery. Red blood cells, platelets, fresh frozen plasma, prothrombin complex concentrates, and/or cryoprecipitate may be necessary, depending on the specific coagulation defect. In practice, the decision regarding when to transfuse must take into account not only numbers but also individual patient characteristics and the anticipated physiologic effects of continued blood loss, including ongoing consumption of coagulation factors and inadequate circulating blood volume.

There is no universally accepted hemoglobin level that demands transfusion. The Society of Thoracic Surgeons and Society of Cardiovascular Anesthesiologists note that red blood cell transfusion for hemoglobin levels < 6 g/dl is reasonable and may be lifesaving. Transfusion for hemoglobin levels < 7 g/dl may also be reasonable, although the data are less clear.

Surgical patients with microvascular bleeding generally do not need platelet transfusion if the platelet count is >100,000/µl but usually do need transfusion for a count <50,000/µl. Current and anticipated bleeding should dictate transfusion when the count is between 50,000 and 100,000/µl. These recommendations are based largely on expert opinion, with little available evidence to guide platelet transfusion in any setting, including the perioperative state.

Fresh frozen plasma should be transfused only as needed to correct specific coagulation factor deficiencies. In cardiac surgical patients, these deficiencies are caused most commonly by dilution secondary to large-volume transfusion. Other causes include warfarin therapy, liver dysfunction, and consumptive coagulopathy. Whenever possible, purified specific factors (instead of plasma) should be administered to patients with single-factor inherited deficiencies who undergo CPB.

Cryoprecipitate, which contains predominantly fibrinogen, factor VIII, von Willebrand factor, factor XIII, and fibronectin, should be used only to treat specific deficiencies of these factors.

Pharmacologic agents to decrease postsurgical bleeding

Several pharmacologic agents are available to treat persistent postoperative bleeding. Tranexamic acid and ε-aminocaproic acid are synthetic lysine analogues that exert their antifibrinolytic effect by displacing plasminogen from fibrin. Desmopressin, an analogue of arginine vasopressin, reduces bleeding by increasing plasma concentrations of factor VIII and von Willebrand factor, thus promoting platelet function.

Recombinant activated factor VII (rVIIa) forms a complex with available tissue factor to activate factor X directly and induce thrombin generation. Recently published guidelines suggest that rVIIa may be considered if administration of blood component therapy fails to reduce bleeding.

Both ε-aminocaproic and tranexamic acids have been shown to reduce bleeding and the need for allogeneic transfusion in heart surgery patients. Although there are potential benefits from the administration of ε-aminocaproic acid and tranexamic acid during surgery, these conclusions cannot be immediately applied when these drugs are started after surgery. No randomized, controlled, blinded studies are available to support the initiation of antifibrinolytic therapy in the postoperative period.

Desmopressin acetate has not been shown to be of benefit if administered in a prophylactic fashion during cardiac surgery, but it is not unreasonable in patients with excessive bleeding after bypass, especially in those with conditions known to respond (uremia, bypass-induced platelet dysfunction, or von Willebrand's disease).

Recombinant activated factor VII (rVIIa) may be effective in the treatment of patients with uncontrolled postoperative hemorrhage after thoracic surgery. Potential drawbacks include a risk of thrombosis and the agent's expense (approximately $4500 for a single dose). Appropriately designed studies to establish the safety of this biologic in cardiac surgical patients do not presently exist.

Resternotomy

Excessive postoperative bleeding or profound hypotension unresponsive to volume and pharmacologic resuscitation – suggesting a significant concealed hemorrhage causing hypovolemia and/or cardiac tamponade – is an indication for immediate surgical reexploration of the chest either in the ICU or in the operating room. In patients undergoing cardiac surgery, rates of reoperation for bleeding vary between 3% and 14%, with approximately 5% of all patients requiring reoperation in the early postoperative period; a surgically correctable source of bleeding is found in 50% to 67% of these patients.

The rates of reexploration, however, are substantially declining. In addition to its association with an adverse effect on patients' morbidity and mortality, bleeding requiring reexploration consumes considerable resources as a result of increased operative time, blood product use, and prolonged ICU and total hospital stays. Reoperation in the ICU, as opposed to the operating room, has been shown to be associated with decreased total hospital charges, quicker time to intervention, and no increase in the wound infection rate compared with no reoperation.

Important points

Important points are as follows:

1. Excessive bleeding is associated with increased morbidity and mortality after heart surgery.

2. Risk factors for excessive bleeding after cardiac surgery include female sex, reoperation, combined procedures, longer duration of CPB, hypothermia, preoperative administration of anticoagulants, renal insufficiency, excessive bleeding during surgery, emergency surgery, and smaller body index.

3. No uniform accepted definition for excessive bleeding after cardiac surgery exists, but bleeding that exceeds 10 ml/kg in the first postoperative hour or an average of >5 ml/kg in the first 3 postoperative hours is abnormal and has been suggested as an indication for reexploration.

4. Bleeding after cardiac surgery can be externally manifested as hypovolemia and continued fluid requirements, or concealed bleeding presenting as tamponade.

5. Preoperative medications such as aspirin, GP IIb/IIIa inhibitors, platelet ADP antagonists, LMWHs, and warfarin may be associated with excessive bleeding after cardiac surgery.

6. CPB may contribute to dysfunction of the hemostatic system through platelet activation, depletion, and hemodilution. CPB may also initiate consumption of coagulation factors, activation of fibrinolysis, and stimulation of the inflammatory system, resulting in a cascade of coagulation and fibrinolysis.

7. Evaluation of bleeding after CPB surgery primarily involves the determination of whether bleeding is surgical or microvascular.

8. Prolonged "surgical" bleeding inevitably leads to platelet and clotting factor depletion and an associated secondary coagulopathy.

9. Chest radiograph analysis is inadequate to evaluate for evidence of concealed bleeding or tamponade. TEE is an increasingly used technique to determine the presence or absence of tamponade after cardiac surgery.

10. Essential elements of initial laboratory analysis of the bleeding patient include PT-INR, aPTT, platelet count, fibrinogen, hemoglobin, and hematocrit.

11. Point of care tests (studies performed at a patient's bedside) avoid the delay associated with central laboratory studies. POC tests are increasingly being used to determine the etiology of bleeding after surgery and employed as part of transfusion algorithms to reduce the administration of allogeneic blood products.

12. The decision regarding when to transfuse must take into account not only numbers and formulaic thresholds but also individual patient characteristics and the anticipated physiologic effects of continued blood loss and inadequate circulating blood volume.

13. No randomized, controlled, blinded studies are available to support the initiation of antifibrinolytic therapy in the postoperative period, but the literature provides support for the pre-CPB administration of antifibrinolytics to reduce blood loss and for the administration of blood products.

Suggested readings

Avorn J, Minalkumar P, Levin R, Winkelmayer W. Hetastarch and bleeding complications after coronary artery surgery. *Chest* 2003; 124:1437–1442.

Bishop CV, Renwick WE, Hogan C, et al. Recombinant activated factor VII: treating postoperative hemorrhage in cardiac surgery. *Ann Thorac Surg* 2006; 81:875–879.

Dacey LJ, et al. Reexploration for hemorrhage following coronary artery bypass grafting: incidence and risk factors. Northern New England Cardiovascular Disease Study Group. *Arch Surg* 1998; 133:442–447.

Despotis GJ, Hogue CW. Pathophysiology, prevention and treatment of bleeding after cardiac surgery: a primer for cardiologists and an update for the cardiothoracic team. *Am J Cardiol* 1999; 83:15B–30B.

Ferraris VA, et al. Aprotinin in cardiac surgery. *N Engl J Med* 2006; 354(18):1953–1957; author reply 1953–1957.

Fiser SM, Tribble CG, Kern JA, et al. Cardiac reoperation in the intensive care unit. *Ann Thorac Surg* 2001; 71(6):1888–1892; discussion 1892–1893.

Levi M, Cromheecke ME, de Jonge E, et al. Pharmacologic strategies to decrease excessive blood less in cardiac surgery: a meta-analysis of clinically relevant endpoints. *Lancet* 1999; 354: 1940.

Mashour GA, Avery EG. Anesthesia for cardiac surgery. In: Dunn et al., eds. *Clinical Anesthesia Procedures of the Massachusetts General Hospital.* 7th ed. Philadelphia: Lippincott Williams & Wilkins; 2007:401–440.

Mehta RH, Roe MT, Mulgund J, et al. Acute clopidogrel use and outcomes in patients with non-ST-segment elevation acute coronary syndromes undergoing coronary artery bypass surgery. *J Am Coll Cardiol* 2006; 48:281.

Paparella D, et al. Coagulation disorders of cardiopulmonary bypass: a review. *Intensive Care Med* 2004; 30(10):1873–1881.

Pleym H, et al. Tranexamic acid reduces postoperative bleeding after coronary surgery in patients treated with aspirin until surgery. *Anesth Analg* 2003; 96:923–928.

Schmidlin D, Schuepbach R, Bernard E, et al. Indications and impact of postoperative transesophageal echocardiography in cardiac surgical patients. *Crit Care Med* 2001; 29(11):2143–2148.

Shore-Lesserson L, et al. Thromboelastography-guided transfusion algorithm reduces transfusions in complex cardiac surgery. *Anesth Analg* 1999; 88:312–319.

Unsworth-White MJ, et al. Resternotomy for bleeding after cardiac operation: a marker for increased morbidity and mortality. *Ann Thorac Surg* 1995; 59:664–667.

Whitlock R, et al. Bleeding in cardiac surgery: its prevention and treatment – an evidence-based review. *Crit Care Clin* 2005; 21(3):589–610.

Woodman RC, Harker LA. Bleeding complications associated with cardiopulmonary bypass. *Blood* 1990; 76(9):1680–1697.

Part 14

Chapter

81

Vascular Anesthesia

Simon Gelman and Stanley Leeson, editors

Carotid endarterectomy

Brian J. Gelfand and Stanley Leeson

Since the introduction of carotid endarterectomy (CEA) for the management of carotid occlusive disease (Fig. 81.1) in the 1950s, the procedure has waxed and waned in popularity, progressively refining its role with the emergence of objective evidence-based support. Operative management of carotid artery stenosis by CEA demands the anesthesiologist's full appreciation of the pathophysiology involved as well as diligent attention to the associated comorbidities of this challenging patient population. CEA can reduce the risk of a fatal or disabling stroke in a selected patient group, but the surgical risk must not outweigh the potential benefits.

Surgical approach

The proper positioning of the patient prior to surgical incision cannot be understated. The patient should be supine with the head comfortably turned toward the nonoperative side, with the patient's neck slightly extended by placement of a roll underneath the shoulders. The anesthesiologist should be aware that hemodynamic instability might result from stimulation of the carotid sinus, presenting as sudden onset of marked bradycardia and severe hypotension. The carotid sinus is located at the carotid artery bifurcation by the initial dilatation of the internal carotid artery. This region contains abundant baroreceptors, which are innervated by the sinus nerve of Hering (Fig. 81.2). This branch of the glossopharyngeal nerve (cranial nerve [CN] IX) synapses in the nucleus tractus solitarius in the brainstem medulla, and its vagal efferents modulate autonomic control of the heart and vasculature.

The surgeon may inject lidocaine 1% into the tissue at the carotid bifurcation to attenuate the afferent limb of this reflex, and the anesthesiologist may administer atropine or glycopyrrolate to diminish the effect of the vagal parasympathetic efferent effects associated with manipulation of this region. The carotid sinus must be differentiated from the carotid body, which also lies within the area of the carotid artery bifurcation. In contrast to the carotid sinus, the carotid body contains a cluster of chemoreceptors, which are sensitive to changes in the composition of arterial blood. Unlike the central brainstem chemoreceptors that are primarily sensitive to changes in CO_2, the type I glomus cells of the carotid body are principally sensitive to changes in the partial pressure of oxygen and increase their output at partial pressures below 100 mm Hg. To a lesser degree, increases in partial pressure of CO_2 and decreases in pH may elicit an increase in glomus activity. These changes are transmitted to the medullary respiratory centers via glossopharyngeal (CN IX) and vagal (CN X) afferents.

Shunting

The decision to use a shunt during CEA still is a focal point of considerable debate. The primary advantage of using a shunt is that during the endarterectomy, ipsilateral cerebral blood flow is continued. Studies have demonstrated that 10% to 15% of patients will have inadequate perfusion crossover to prevent evidence of cerebral ischemia. Without adequate ipsilateral perfusion pressure, cerebral infarction would result. Shunt placement is not without its risks and potential complications; errant placement may result in occlusion or carotid dissection, embolization may occur through the shunt, or thrombus may form because of the shunt, with resultant emboli. In all circumstances, the blood pressure must be sufficient to provide flow through the shunt.

Determination of the need for carotid shunting can be made by several commonly used techniques to assess the adequacy of cerebral perfusion. The first is direct communication with the patient who is awake and anesthetized via regional technique. Communication is usually via a signaling device, such as a "clicker," or by squeezing a ball in the contralateral hand. Voice responses are discouraged to prevent neck movement and disturbing the operative field. The second technique is to determine stump or back pressure by placing a transduced needle or catheter into the carotid artery while the proximal common carotid artery and the external carotid arteries are clamped. In this way, the transduced pressure reflects the internal carotid artery pressure and correspondingly the ipsilateral hemispheric perfusion pressure by means of the contralateral carotid artery pressure across the circle of Willis. This technique has been critically debated in the literature, referencing "safe" stump pressures varying from 25 to 90 mm Hg as indicators of adequate cerebral perfusion. Finally, the gold standard of electroencephalographic (EEG) monitoring by an experienced technician directly compares the ipsilateral and contralateral waveforms and can note any changes at the time of clamping that would indicate inadequate hemispheric perfusion.

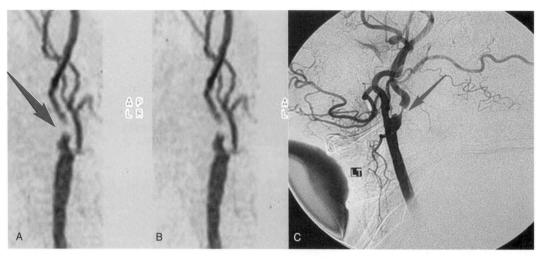

Figure 81.1. (**A and B**) Digital subtraction angiograms with clinically significant internal carotid artery (ICA) stenosis. (**C**) Magnetic resonance angiography demonstrating significant left ICA stenosis. (Images courtesy of Edwin C. Gravereaux, M.D., Brigham and Women's Hospital, Division of Vascular Surgery.)

Anesthetic technique

CEA may be performed under either general or regional anesthesia, with either technique having similar morbidity and mortality rates. The choice of anesthetic must be an appropriate balance among patient selection, the desires of the surgeon, and the expertise of the anesthesiologist. The primary objective in the anesthetic management of the patient undergoing CEA is the prevention of cardiac and cerebral ischemic events. This intention can present as a delicate balance between augmentation of cerebral perfusion pressure and reduction of myocardial oxygen demand. Preparation for and anticipation of hemodynamic fluctuations is essential toward this end. Individual

syringes of low-dose ephedrine (5 mg/ml), phenylephrine (40 μg/ml), and nitroglycerin (40 μg/ml) should be readily available. Additionally, infusions of phenylephrine and nitroglycerin on a preset pump should be in line. Likewise, in treatment, prevention of therapeutic overcorrection by the judicious titration of these short-acting pharmacologic agents is key.

General anesthesia

Proponents of a general anesthetic approach to CEA espouse the ability to control ventilation, maintain a secure airway, and more easily manage the potential intraoperative complications as the major advantages of this technique. Within the

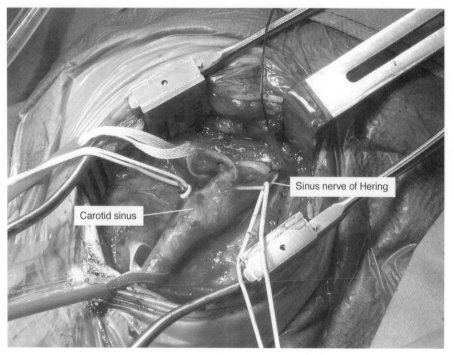

Figure 81.2. Vessel loop denotes the sinus nerve of Hering (branch CN IX) at the carotid artery bifurcation.

Sinus nerve of Hering

Carotid sinus

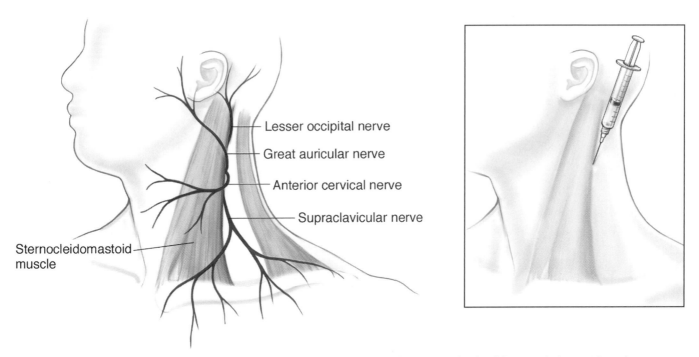

Lesser occipital nerve
Great auricular nerve
Anterior cervical nerve
Supraclavicular nerve
Sternocleidomastoid muscle

Figure 81.3. Superficial cervical block. Local anesthetic is injected along the middle third of the posterior border of the sternocleidomastoid muscle.

broad spectrum of various anesthetic induction and maintenance options, there are no data to absolutely delineate a particular combination of agents.

Ideally, the induction should be designed to maintain hemodynamic stability and avoid the shifts associated with the depressant effects of certain medications or the stimulation of tracheal intubation. It is worth noting that the use of succinylcholine is contraindicated in patients who have had a recent paretic cerebral infarction.

Maintenance anesthesia is usually achieved with the combination of a volatile anesthetic with the addition of an opioid such as fentanyl (2–5 μg/kg), sufentanil (0.5–1.0 μg/kg), or nitrous oxide. The use of nitrous oxide supplementation, although popular, remains controversial because of reports of increases in cerebral metabolic rate and cerebral blood flow (CBF). More recently, there also are reports that the use of nitrous oxide increases serum homocysteine levels during CEA. This association may possibly be correlated with perioperative myocardial ischemic events. Alternatively, a propofol and remifentanil (0.1–1 μg/kg/min) anesthetic may be used. Remifentanil's short half-life permits simple titration during varying levels of stimulation during CEA. The use of easily titratable, short-acting pharmacologic agents also permits a smooth, rapid emergence to facilitate early neurologic assessment.

Regional anesthesia

CEA is commonly performed under regional anesthesia using superficial and deep cervical plexus blocks (Fig. 81.3 and Fig. 81.4). Anesthesiologists may prefer one block to another, although no consensus exists within the literature as to a comparison of efficacy. The necessary region of anesthetic blockade is in the C2–4 dermatomes and may be achieved via either of these blocks, or by subcutaneous infiltration of the peripheral nerves infiltrating the incision site.

Advocates of a regional technique for CEA claim that this approach provides for direct cerebral monitoring, improved hemodynamic stability, and avoidance of endotracheal intubation, as well as its attendant complications in patients with chronic obstructive pulmonary disease or limited cardiac reserves. It should be recognized that this anesthetic approach should be attempted only in a patient likely to remain calm and cooperative throughout the operative procedure with a minimal amount of sedation. These limitations illustrate the disadvantages of a regional anesthetic in this patient group. The onset of seizures, loss of consciousness, or need to control the airway emergently, although uncommon, may present significant difficulty during surgical management.

Monitoring

Intraoperative patient monitoring during CEA should recognize the goals of protection from cerebral and cardiac ischemia. As such, diligent observation of electrocardiographic leads II and V_5, along with ST-segment analysis, provides increased sensitivity in detecting early cardiac ischemic changes. Likewise, direct and continual hemodynamic monitoring by placement of a transduced intra-arterial catheter is recommended. Additional invasive procedures, such as placement of a central venous line to record central venous pressures, or a pulmonary artery catheter, should be dictated by individual patient comorbidities and not used on a routine basis.

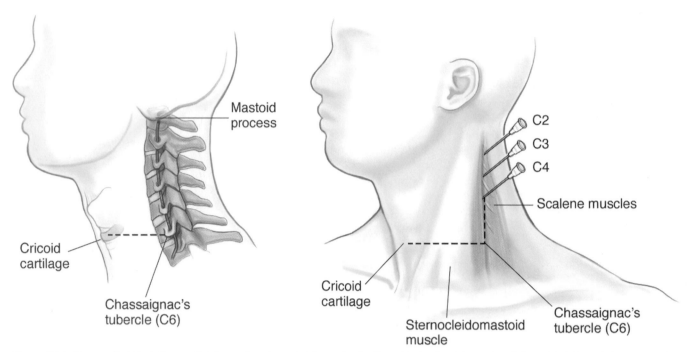

Figure 81.4. Deep cervical block. The needle is inserted on the vertical line at the C2, C3, and C4 level and directed medially and slightly caudad to contact the grove of the transverse processes.

The literature indicates that neurophysiologic monitoring is not associated with a stroke risk reduction or an improvement in outcome. Most perioperative strokes are thromboembolic in origin and not the result of hypoperfusion. The use of various cerebral perfusion monitors, such as the electroencephalogram (EEG), transcranial Doppler (TCD), or cerebral oximetry, may offer guidance in determining the appropriateness of shunt use and more cautious and precise utilization of pharmacologic vasopressors.

The EEG is a graphic representation of the spontaneous electrical activity of the superficial cerebral cortex (Fig. 81.5). Compared with the hemispheres, such as during carotid artery cross-clamping, relative ischemia will demonstrate a decrease in electrical activity and change in regional patterns. This usually will occur below a CBF rate of approximately 15 ml/100 g/min. It should be recognized that EEG monitoring during CEA is not without its limitations. EEG does not monitor deeper structures in the brain, and patients with certain preexisting neurologic deficits may incur a perioperative ischemic event without evidence of EEG changes. In addition, interpretation of the EEG waveforms may be made more difficult by decreases in body temperature, blood pressure, or an increase in anesthetic level, as each of these may mimic an ischemic change in EEG pattern. Therefore, it is absolutely essential to maintain communication between the anesthesiologist and EEG technician when any change is made to the maintenance anesthetic regimen.

TCD presents another modality for assessing the adequacy of CBF. TCD applies the concepts of Doppler ultrasound to determine middle cerebral artery blood flow velocities and embolic events. TCD's utility in the intraoperative evaluation of

the patient undergoing CEA may be somewhat limited in terms of its positive predictive value and may be more useful postoperatively for stroke surveillance or in predicting which individuals may be at risk for cerebral hypoperfusion syndrome following CEA or carotid artery angioplasty and stenting. Likewise, the application of cerebral oximetry during CEA provides a visual measurement of frontal lobe saturation. Limited work has been

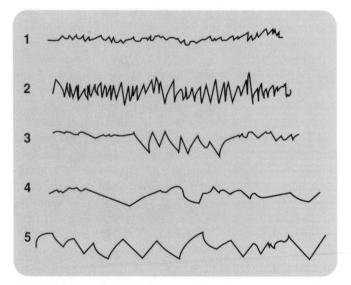

Figure 81.5. Representative EEG patterns. *Line 1*: Beta waves seen in the awake patient. *Line 2*: Alpha waves seen in a relaxed patient. *Line 3*: Theta waves seen in the somnolent patient. *Line 4*: Sleep spindles seen in the sleeping patient. *Line 5*: Delta waves in the relatively deeply anesthetized patient.

done to accurately define a cutoff threshold to indicate when employing a shunt is appropriate.

Postoperative care

The most common postoperative complications following CEA include delayed emergence, hemodynamic instability, respiratory insufficiency, local hematoma, and new evidence of neurologic dysfunction. Although most wound hematomas are relatively small, emergent operative intervention is required for large and rapidly expanding hematomas. The anesthesiologist must be particularly attuned to any evidence of airway compromise that will demand immediate attention. The most common cause of mortality is myocardial infarction, whereas the most common cause of morbidity is stroke. Although seemingly similar to many other procedures and their potentials for postoperative difficulties, the patient undergoing CEA is unique.

In the postoperative setting, approximately 60% of these patients may present with either hypotension or hypertension, with the latter being more common. The etiology of post-CEA hypertension is not exactly clear. It is possible that it could be related to surgical denervation of carotid baroreceptors, and it may be exaggerated in patients with poorly controlled preoperative hypertension. The pattern of postoperative hypertension appears to peak approximately 2 to 3 hours after completion of the procedure, but may persist up to 24 hours. The goal of hemodynamic management in the postoperative period should be directed toward maintaining patients within their usual preoperative range of blood pressures. Postoperative hypertension may be managed with a variety of short-acting agents, such as esmolol, labetalol, and hydralazine, to avoid unnecessary periods of hypotension. In refractory situations, titration of nitroglycerin or nitroprusside may be employed.

In evaluating the postoperative CEA patient for hypotension, it is essential to remember the high correlation with coronary artery disease in this patient population and to exclude myocardial ischemia and infarction as reasons for a decrease in blood pressure in the postanesthesia care unit.

Following CEA, patients may present with varying degrees of neurologic dysfunction, ranging from focal neurologic signs from cranial nerve injury to full-blown cerebral hemispheric insults from carotid artery occlusion, embolic phenomenon, or graft thrombosis. Unilateral recurrent laryngeal nerve injury will appear as transient hoarseness, but preoperative assessment of vocal cord function should be made in any patient who previously underwent contralateral endarterectomy or operative thyroid intervention if the possibility of bilateral recurrent laryngeal nerve injury exists, and as such, an acute airway emergency. Injury to the hypoglossal nerve will result in paresis of the ipsilateral tongue musculature and deviation of the tongue to the side of injury. More commonly, traction injury to the marginal mandibular branch of the facial nerve will manifest as drooping of the corner of the mouth on the ipsilateral side.

Another, less common cause of post-CEA neurologic dysfunction is cerebral hyperperfusion syndrome (CHS) resulting from the rapid restoration of a normal perfusion pressure to areas of brain tissue with impaired autoregulation secondary to chronic ischemic states. The literature reports an incidence of 0.5% to 2.2% and defines CHS as a major increase in ipsilateral CBF, well above the metabolic demands of the brain tissue, following repair of carotid artery stenosis. Occurring between postoperative days 3 and 8, the clinical presentation of CHS may consist of severe unremitting ipsilateral head, facial, or eye pain, with increasing signs of cerebral irritability progressing to seizure activity. Prompt recognition and hemodynamic control are essential for management. The compounding involvement of intracerebral hemorrhage bodes a poor prognosis.

Future trends

The validation studies of the 1990s (North American Symptomatic Carotid Endarterectomy Trial [NASCET], European Carotid Surgery Trial [ECST]) demonstrated absolute risk reduction for the surgical versus medical management of carotid artery stenosis and defined acceptable morbidity and mortality rates. In 2004, the US Food and Drug Administration approved the clinical application of carotid artery angioplasty and stenting systems in the revascularization of symptomatic patients with stenosis ≥ 50% and asymptomatic patients with ≥ 80% stenosis. Early carotid artery stenting literature reported unacceptably high complication rates. The elevated stroke rate in these studies most likely was related to the absence of distal embolic protection filters in the deployment systems. With technologic improvements, further studies such as the SAPPHIRE (Stenting and Angioplasty with Protection in Patients at High Risk for Endarterectomy) and CaRESS (Carotid Revascularization Using Endarterectomy or Stenting Systems) trials demonstrated lower morbidity and mortality rates. Defined complication rates for carotid artery angioplasty and stenting have not been determined yet, pending publication of larger series evaluating longer follow-up and stent durability.

Suggested readings

Badner NH, Beattie WS, Freeman D, Spence JD. Nitrous oxide induced increased homocysteine concentrations are associated with increased postoperative myocardial ischemia in patients undergoing carotid endarterectomy. *Anesth Analg* 2000; 91:1073–1079.

Bove EL, Fry WJ, Gross WS, et al. Hypotension and hypertension as consequences of baroreceptor dysfunction following carotid endarterectomy. *Surgery* 1971; 86:633–641.

CaRESS Steering Committee. Carotid Revascularization Using Endarterectomy or Stenting Systems (CaRESS) phase I clinical trial: 1-year results. *J Vasc Surg* 2005; 42:213–219.

Gelabert HA, Moore WS. Occlusive cerebrovascular disease: medical and surgical considerations. In: Cottrell JE, Smith DS, eds. *Anesthesia and Neurosurgery*. St. Louis: Mosby; 2001.

Herrick IA, Gelb AW. Occlusive cerebrovascular disease: anesthetic considerations. in anesthesia and neurosurgery In: Cottrell JE, Smith DS, eds. *Anesthesia and Neurosurgery*. St. Louis: Mosby; 2001.

Howell SJ. Carotid endarterectomy. *Br J Anaesth* 2007; 99(1): 119–131.

Lam AM, Mayberg TS, Eng CC, et al. Nitrous oxide-isoflurane anesthesia causes more cerebral vasodilation than an equipotent dose of isoflurane in humans. *Anesth Analg* 1994; 78:462–468.

Lineberger CK, Lubarsky DA. Con: general anesthesia and regional anesthesia are equally acceptable choices for carotid endarterectomy. *J Cardiothorac Vasc Anesth* 1998; 12:115–117.

Matta BF, Lam AM. Nitrous oxide increases cerebral blood flow velocity during pharmacologically induced electrical silence in humans. *J Neurosurg Anesthesiol* 1995; 7:89–93.

Moore WS, Yee JM, Hall AD. Collateral cerebral blood pressure: an index to tolerance to temporary carotid occlusion. *Arch Surg* 1973; 106:520–523.

Ogasawara K, Sakai N, Kuroiwa T, et al. Intracranial hemorrhage associated with cerebral hyperperfusion syndrome following carotid endarterectomy and carotid artery stenting: retrospective review of 4494 patients. *J Neurosurg* 2007; 107: 1130–1136.

Pandit JJ, Satya-Krishna R, Gration P. Superficial or deep cervical plexus block for carotid endarterectomy: a systematic review of complications. *Br J Anaesth* 2007; 99(2):159–169.

Piepgras DG, Morgan MK, Sundt TM Jr, et al. Intracerebral hemorrhage after carotid endarterectomy. *J Neurosurg* 1988; 68:532–536.

Rerkasem K, Bond R, Rothwell PM. Local versus general anaesthesia for carotid endarterectomy. *Cochrane Database Syst Rev* 2004; CD000126.

Sundt TM Jr, Sharbrough FN, Piepgras DG, et al. Correlation of cerebral blood flow and electroencephalographic changes during carotid endarterectomy, with results of surgery and hemodynamics of cerebral ischemia. *Mayo Clin Proc* 1981; 56:533–543.

Yadav JS, Wholey MH, Kuntz RE, et al. Protected carotid artery stenting versus endarterectomy in high risk patients. *N Engl J Med* 2004; 351:1493–1501.

Wilke HJ, Ellis JE, McKinsey JF. Carotid endarterectomy: perioperative and anesthetic considerations. *J Cardiothor Vasc Anesth* 1996; 10(7):928–949.

Abdominal aortic aneurysm

Chapter 82

Fred Cobey, Simon Gelman, and Jonathan D. Gates

An arterial aneurysm is a dilation of the artery at least 50% of the expected diameter. The definition of an abdominal aortic aneurysm (AAA) is an aorta with a diameter >3 cm. Approximately 5% of the population older than 50 years has an AAA. These aneurysms are the fifth leading cause of death in men older than 55 years. Prophylactic AAA repair is intended to spare patients the possibility of rupture and death. Ruptured AAAs incur a mortality rate of 70% to 90%, with most deaths occurring before patients arrive at the hospital. Therefore, detection and repair of AAAs prior to catastrophic rupture can prolong the life of many patients. Because atherosclerosis is a systemic disease, severe cardiovascular and other comorbidities frequently accompany these lesions. In the event of an AAA rupture, perioperative homeostasis may be a challenge for anesthesiologists.

Pathophysiology

Although atherosclerosis traditionally was invoked as an etiology for AAAs, this concept has been recently revised. Aneurysms are now believed to result from inflammation that leads to dilation and subsequent plaque formation. Loss of elastin is one of the most common histologic findings, and increased serum activity of elastase has been observed in patients with aneurysms. Alterations in metalloproteinase gene expression and activity also are associated with AAA formation. Smoking also may act synergistically to cause elastin degradation. In addition, the presence of *Chlamydia pneumoniae* in the aortic wall may lead to the degradation of aortic elastin.

Gradual aneurysmal enlargement may be explained on the basis of Laplace's law (Fig. 82.1). The tension (T) on the aneurysm wall is the product of the transmural pressure (P) and the radius (R) of the vessel (T = PR). Therefore, a larger aortic diameter results in increased wall tension at a relatively constant arterial pressure. The tension will increase to a point at which the vessel collagen is incapable of sustaining the transmural pressure. Accordingly, risk of rupture can thus be stratified according to diameter. AAAs enlarge 0.5 cm/y or about 10% per year, so ongoing surveillance is necessary. Lesions <4 cm may be followed with annual imaging, as the risk of rupture at that size is unlikely. Once lesions reach 5 to 6 cm or larger, the risk of rupture increases to 5% to 6% per year, at which point repair is generally indicated. In addition to size, rapid

expansion and female gender also appear to increase the risk of rupture. Patients with lesions 4 to 5.5 cm represent an intermediate group, and the question here may be more of when, rather than whether, to repair them.

Preoperative evaluation

Most AAAs are silent clinically and discovered incidentally. Symptomatic patients may present with back, flank, groin, and abdominal pain. Less commonly, clinicians may discover AAAs during a search for a cause of lower-extremity embolus. On routine physical examination, AAAs that are 4 to 4.9 cm are detected in only 50% of cases. Large lesions often may be more readily palpated; however, large body habitus may render the physical examination unreliable. Ultrasound is a traditional modality for evaluating pulsatile abdominal masses or for following changes in an aneurysm over time. CT provides a better picture of the overall geometry of the lesion and more easily detects iliac artery aneurysms (Fig. 82.2). Formal angiography rarely is used as a preoperative study.

Most patients with AAAs have coexisting cardiopulmonary disease, and their life expectancy generally is shorter than that of age-matched controls. A thorough medical evaluation of patients preoperatively is required to decide whether and what kind of surgery should be done and to ensure that comorbid conditions are addressed. Cardiac complications are the most common complications after vascular surgery, with a myocardial infarction incidence of 12% to 14%. Preoperative cardiac revascularization may not decrease perioperative risk of myocardial infarction or long-term survival. In contrast, use of perioperative β-adrenergic antagonists has been shown to reduce the rate of cardiac complications. There is also evidence

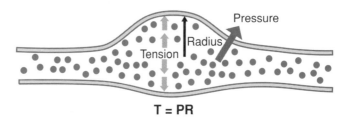

Figure 82.1. Aneurysmal enlargement explained on the basis of Laplace's law. T, tension; P, transmural pressure; R, radius.

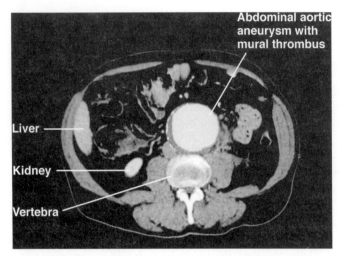

Figure 82.2. CT angiogram of a large AAA with mural thrombus.

that the addition of a statin may further reduce the risk of perioperative cardiac complications beyond β-blockade alone.

Assessment of the patient's tolerance to exercise and notation of any cardiac symptoms are crucial in risk stratification and in determining whether surgery should be delayed for further testing. Cardiac testing can safely be omitted in intermediate-risk patients with acceptable functional status. It is generally recommended that adequate preoperative β-blockade be provided, as evidenced by a patient's heart rate controlled between 60 and 70 bpm.

Since many patients with AAAs have a long history of smoking, pulmonary compromise is common. Patients with productive cough, those with bronchospasm, and those who are CO_2 retainers have higher rates of pulmonary complications. In this group of patients, epidural analgesia is particularly useful. Patients with AAAs also may have coexisting cerebrovascular disease. There is no evidence that correcting asymptomatic carotid disease improves neurologic outcome. Intervention should be entertained in symptomatic patients with transient ischemic attacks or small strokes. However, the timing of the two interventions should be patient specific, based on the relative significance of each lesion. Preoperative renal insufficiency is a strong predictor of increased operative risk, more so than diagnosed cardiopulmonary disease. Diabetes mellitus needs to be addressed and managed preoperatively, as perioperative hyperglycemia has been shown to predispose to cardiac events and may have a role in risk of postoperative infection.

In contemplating AAA repair, one must consider the patient's life expectancy, risk of rupture, and risk of perioperative death. For patients undergoing open operative repair, mortality is inversely related to both surgeon and hospital volume. Operative mortality can actually be predicted using the surgeon's average operative mortality and the patient's comorbidities. Patients who have a high risk of perioperative death and/or a short life expectancy may be managed nonoperatively. β-Adrenergic antagonists should be initiated because of accumulating evidence that they may decrease the rate of aneurysmal expansion.

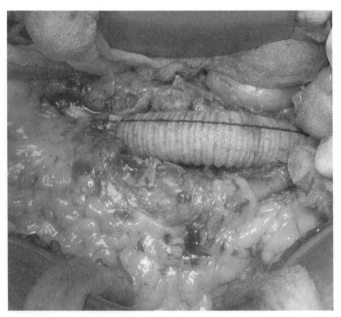

Figure 82.3. Transperitoneal AAA repair with graft in situ.

Surgical approach

There are two basic approaches to open AAA repairs: transperitoneal and retroperitoneal. The transperitoneal approach via a traditional midline laparotomy incision with the patient in the supine position is best for ruptured aneurysms and also provides exposure to the right renal artery (Fig. 82.3). The retroperitoneal approach enables better exposure to suprarenal aneurysms and is the preferred approach in cases of extensive abdominal adhesions or a horseshoe kidney, which would prevent easy access to retroperitoneal structures. The patient requiring this approach is placed in a left-side up, modified decubitus position. This approach avoids violating the peritoneum and may result in faster return of bowel function, although it incurs the risk of an often troublesome postoperative bulge around the incision from denervation of flank muscles.

The development of endovascular repair has changed AAA management, especially for high-risk patients. The anesthetic considerations for patients undergoing the endovascular approach are reviewed in the next chapter. Finally, laparoscopic AAA repair is currently being investigated in Europe. Initial results in the literature are encouraging, with short recovery times similar to those of endovascular techniques. In practice, however, these techniques are not yet viable options.

Intraoperative management
Monitoring

In addition to routine noninvasive monitors, an arterial line is helpful during application and removal of the aortic cross-clamp and in the presence of significant bleeding. A triple-lumen catheter inserted in the subclavian or internal jugular vein may be useful when there is a need to administer multiple medications. Routine placement of pulmonary arterial catheters is unnecessary. The use of such catheters may be restricted to patients with suspected pulmonary hypertension or significant cardiac disease, in whom it may be necessary to know the cardiac filling pressures and output to maintain optimal cardiac function. Intraoperative transesophageal echocardiography (TEE) is often useful in estimating volume status and identifying regional wall motion abnormalities among patients who are hemodynamically unstable.

Anesthetic technique

General anesthesia is required. More important than what drugs are used for induction and maintenance of anesthesia is that they are administered in a manner that ensures hemodynamic stability. It may be wise to avoid ketamine, given the preponderance of coronary artery disease in this group of patients. Epidural analgesia clearly is beneficial in this patient population, given the prevalence of pulmonary disease. Its use decreases postoperative intensive care unit requirements, postoperative pulmonary complications, and hospital stays. The associated decrease in sympathetic tone may complicate hemodynamic management. It seems easier to manage intraoperative hypotension if epidural analgesia is started after the aortic cross-clamp is removed and hemostasis is ensured.

Volume status

Clearly, it is important to assess the volume status of patients undergoing AAA repair throughout the intra- and postoperative course. Aggressive volume resuscitation is required to assist in maintaining optimal hemodynamics and to avoid postoperative renal impairment. Understanding the patient's unique cardiopulmonary status and ability to tolerate fluid shifts is the basis of volume management. Although vasoactive drugs may be needed, their use should be limited. Administration of phenylephrine doubles the incidence of wall motion abnormalities seen on echocardiography compared with patients whose blood pressures are maintained by fluid administration. Urine output cannot be used as an indicator of end-organ perfusion, given the presence of an aortic cross-clamp along with possible administration of diuretics. Even in the infrarenal position, the cross-clamp appears to impair blood flow to the kidneys.

Widespread opinion that central venous pressure (CVP) accurately reflects the volume status of patients is actually incorrect. Values of CVP, as well as those of pulmonary artery occlusion pressure (PAOP), do not correlate with the values of circulating blood volume or with responsiveness to fluid challenge (an increase in cardiac output secondary to the infusion of fluid). Loss of 10% to 12% of blood volume does not change systemic hemodynamic variables, including CVP, to a noticeable degree because such a blood loss is compensated by many mechanisms, including mobilization of blood from the splanchnic vasculature. Adequate CVP is a must for normal cardiovascular function; therefore, the body does everything needed to maintain it at adequate levels. In conditions of normal heart function,

CVP values often remain unchanged despite drastic changes in other variables of systemic hemodynamics. Only extreme values of CVP may have some clinical significance. The PAOP is an even worse indicator of volume status than the CVP, because it is far removed from the action of the mean circulatory filling pressure, which is very close to the pressure in small veins. However, the PAOP is a better indicator of left ventricular function than of volume status.

Dynamic variation in the arterial wave form during positive pressure ventilation may be a better predictor of fluid responsiveness than CVP measurements. Currently, there is discussion that plethysmographic waveform variation obtained from the fingertip, as in the case of systolic blood pressure variations, may predict responsiveness to a fluid challenge. Although such dynamic indices do not provide measurements of intravascular volume or preload, they help answer the clinically relevant question of where patients are on their Starling curves, and whether further volume administration would be helpful. Indeed, using such measures may even improve patient outcomes.

Finally, TEE also may be performed rapidly to evaluate both cardiac function and volume status. As in the dynamic variation seen in arterial waveforms during positive pressure ventilation, fluid responsiveness can also be predicted using respiratory variations in left ventricular stroke area by TEE. Comparing the use of pulmonary artery catheters with echocardiography in high-risk surgery patients, TEE may be the preferred method for rapid intraoperative cardiac evaluation when evaluating hypotension not responsive to volume boluses.

Interestingly, more recently, positive fluid balance after elective AAA repair was retrospectively associated with a higher rate of complications resulting in longer hospital stay. A follow-up prospective randomized trial appears to confirm these findings, arguing for a more restrictive fluid regimen.

Blood loss

The anesthesiologist should resuscitate bleeding patients while being mindful of coagulation parameters. The greatest portion of blood loss during the normal progression of an elective AAA repair usually occurs during the aortotomy, while controlling retrograde bleeding from the lumbar arteries. Although bleeding from graft anastomoses does occur, it generally is not copious. In contrast, inadvertent venous injury to the vena cava, inferior mesenteric vein, iliac veins, or left renal vein, especially at its confluence with its associated lumbar and gonadal veins, may be very difficult to control.

Documented risk factors for blood loss and transfusion in elective AAA repairs include body weight, renal impairment, low hemoglobin and platelet counts, iliac artery involvement, large aneurysm, bifurcated graft, large graft diameter, prolonged aortic clamping time, and long operation time. One can decrease transfusion of allogenic blood by using normovolemic hemodilution and intraoperative cell salvage. There is debate regarding an appropriate target hematocrit and the timing of transfusion. In the absence of acute myocardial ischemia, allowing a hematocrit to fall to the mid-20 range is acceptable. Lower hematocrits leave a narrow margin in case of unexpected blood loss. Frugality with transfusions is important, given the associated immunosuppression and documented increase in nosocomial infections in vascular surgery patients. Massive blood loss and transfusions may result in coagulopathy that can exacerbate bleeding.

In cases of ruptured AAA, the coagulopathy may be severe and portends a poor outcome. There are data suggesting that proactive transfusion of platelets and plasma improves coagulation competence, reduces hemorrhage, and may improve survival in patients with ruptured aneurysms. Patients undergoing elective repair of AAAs demonstrate similar, albeit less dramatic, changes in platelet counts and coagulation parameters. Aortic surgery may lead to thrombocytopenia via platelet sequestration into the graft. Later, patients develop hyperfibrinogenemia and thrombocytosis. These changes may represent a hypercoagulable state that predisposes these patients post-operatively to thrombotic complications.

Cross-clamping

Obtaining proximal control prior to incising the aneurysm requires placing an aortic cross-clamp. This maneuver is the crux of many physiologic alterations specific to aortic surgery (Fig. 82.4). The degree of the changes seen relates to the level and the duration of the cross-clamp. Aortic cross-clamping predictably increases systemic vascular resistance, with an increase in blood pressure above the clamp. This increase not only is the result of a mechanical effect of the cross-clamp increasing resistance, but also is related to activation of the renin/angiotensin axis and release of prostaglandins, catecholamines, and other vasoactive substances. There is a decrease in venous capacity from active venoconstriction distal to the clamp that results in an "autotransfusion" of volume into the circulation proximal to the clamp. A supraceliac position of the clamp produces splanchnic venous constriction and a substantial increase in venous return to the heart. Infraceliac clamping may be associated with a shift in blood volume from veins in the pelvis and lower extremities to the compliant splanchnic veins, which will attenuate preload changes.

The response to the clamp placement also depends on the ability of the heart to handle an increased preload from splanchnic venoconstriction. In healthy hearts, filling pressures appear to remain unchanged. Vasodilators such as nitroglycerin often are not needed to reduce blood pressure, as inhalation anesthetics generally suffice. If the cardiac function is abnormal, then a different hemodynamic profile may ensue. With an acute rise in afterload – and possibly also preload, depending on clamp position – cardiac output may decrease while filling pressures increase. Negative inotropic effects of volatile agents and β-adrenergic antagonists need to be carefully titrated in such patients. Collateral flow maintains some perfusion distal to the clamp, albeit at reduced levels. Any vasodilators given to treat proximal hypertension will exacerbate hypotension and ischemia distal to the aortic clamp. Administering vasodilators may worsen mesenteric and renal perfusion while not necessarily preventing wall motion abnormalities if the aorta is clamped proximal to the renal or celiac arteries. Therefore, the target blood pressure should be carefully selected to perfuse organs distal to the clamp without jeopardizing the myocardium.

Unclamping

Once the aortic graft is sutured in place, the aorta is unclamped, allowing restoration of distal perfusion (Fig. 82.5). This maneuver consistently produces a profound (70%–80%) decrease in vascular resistance and blood pressure. The left ventricular

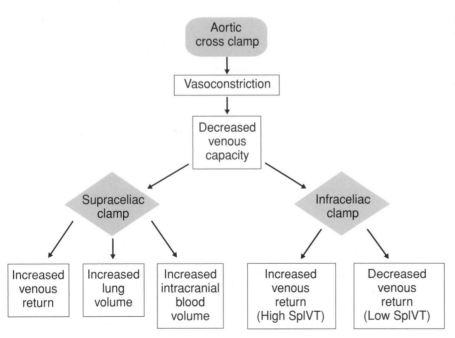

Figure 82.4. Physiologic changes with aortic cross-clamping. SplVT, splanchnic venous tone.

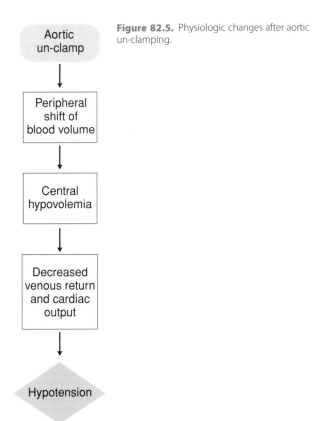

Figure 82.5. Physiologic changes after aortic un-clamping.

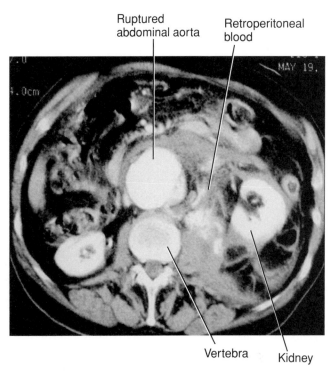

Figure 82.6. CT scan of a ruptured AAA.

filling pressure decreases by 42% compared with baseline values and by 60% compared with values during clamping. Cardiac output may increase, decrease, or remain unchanged. Blood flow through the carotid arteries decreases, whereas blood flow through the femoral arteries increases. Reperfusion of the ischemic distal half of the body liberates products of anaerobic metabolism produced during the cross-clamp period. Prior to removing the cross-clamp, any vasodilators should be minimized or discontinued and the blood pressure should be allowed to rise moderately barring any contraindications. Preemptive loading of the vascular space with intravenous fluids will attenuate the fall in blood pressure with clamp removal.

Some anesthesiologists use nitroglycerin to dilate veins during the cross-clamp period to facilitate fluid loading without causing hypertension. This may decrease the degree of hypotension from aortic unclamping. Perhaps most importantly, the cross-clamp should be removed gradually to allow the body to adjust to the decrease in systemic vascular resistance and reperfusion of the pelvis and lower extremities. The drop in blood pressure with cross-clamp removal is more profound when a tube graft has been used for reconstruction, because both legs are reperfused simultaneously. Sequential clamp removal in a bi-iliac or bifemoral reconstruction is more easily tolerated. In addition to vasoconstrictors for blood pressure, calcium and bicarbonate may be used to offset the effect of potassium and lactate on the heart after reperfusion.

Ruptured aneurysm

Ruptured aortic aneurysms present a more dramatic challenge for the anesthesiologist and surgical team. Rupture of the aneurysm into the peritoneal cavity is often a lethal event, and those patients do not survive to the hospital. Alternatively, a viable blood pressure in a patient with a ruptured aneurysm likely indicates that the rupture is contained in the retroperitoneum (Fig. 82.6). Patients are volume depleted and often hemodynamically unstable. Generally, they are taken immediately to the operating room for exploration and repair, after the suspected diagnosis is confirmed with ultrasound. Induction of anesthesia should be done cautiously, as a rapid induction of general anesthesia with medications that may both decrease vascular tone and have negative ionotropic effects, in addition to positive pressure ventilation, may result in profound hypotension in volume-depleted patients. For this reason, the patient's abdomen is prepped and drapes are placed prior to induction. The surgeon should be poised to enter the abdomen and to gain control of the aorta just below the diaphragm to restore blood pressure. Vasoconstrictors may be needed as a bridge while blood is transfused.

Postoperative care and complications

Postoperatively, patients recover in the intensive care unit. The timing of extubation is decided by the anesthesia and critical care teams. Patients without lung disease or other contraindications may be extubated in the operating room. Epidural analgesia is particularly helpful in patients with poor lung function to minimize pain and achieve adequate ventilation. Preexisting

Table 82.1. Postoperative complications after AAA repair

Prolonged intubation
Hypervolemia
Myocardial ischemia and infarction
Renal insufficiency or failure
Mesenteric ischemia
Spinal cord ischemia
Infection of graft
Pneumonia and atelectasis

poor pulmonary function may be exacerbated by fluid administration and postoperative pain. Although underresuscitation should be avoided, similar care should be taken to avoid fluid overload, as this may result in prolonged ventilatory dependence.

Once patients have demonstrated hemodynamic stability without pharmacologic support and can breathe with only minimal oxygen supplementation, they generally can be cared for on a regular ward. Although some authors advocate advancing patients' diet early, this should be done carefully because postoperative ileus is common. Epidural analgesia can decrease the duration of postoperative ileus. Opioids should be titrated to patient comfort and respiratory rate. Patients generally can be transitioned to patient-controlled analgesia systems and eventually to oral opioid formulations. Nonsteroidal antiinflammatory drugs and acetaminophen should be used, when possible, to reduce opioid requirements. This strategy will decrease the risk of delirium and improve gut motility.

As mentioned, perioperative myocardial ischemia is quite common in patients undergoing AAA repairs, and often occurs during clamp placement (Table 82.1). The anesthesiologist can minimize the risk of cardiac events by administering β-adrenergic antagonists. However, most myocardial infarctions actually occur postoperatively. Relative sympathetic suppression during general anesthesia and lack of such suppression postoperatively might partially explain this phenomenon. Perhaps more attention needs to be given to controlling heart rates in the postoperative period.

Postoperative renal insufficiency is relatively common after aortic surgery. Mortality is four to five times greater in patients with renal failure requiring dialysis than in those without renal impairment. The level of the cross-clamp affects the degree of ischemic insult. There is a 5% rate of renal failure in infrarenal versus 17% in suprarenal clamping. With suprarenal clamping, the renal blood flow decreases by 80%. Renal blood flow is decreased by 45%, with infrarenal occlusion suggesting that endogenous vasoconstrictors play a role in the altered renal perfusion. Altered renal blood flow persists at least an hour after cross-clamp removal. As might be expected, intraoperative urine output is not predictive of postoperative renal function in euvolemic patients. The presence of preoperative renal impairment is the most important factor in predicting postoperative renal failure. Current evidence has not shown the benefit of pharmacologic renal protective strategies. Such approaches have included dopamine, fenoldopam, angiotensin-converting

enzyme inhibition, thoracic epidural analgesia, prostaglandins, furosemide, and mannitol.

The incidence of mesenteric ischemia ranges from 0.6% in elective aortic surgery to 7% in ruptured AAAs. The mortality for postoperative bowel ischemia is about 50% overall, but it rises to 90% with full-thickness gangrene and peritonitis. It is highest in patients with a history of colon resection. In such patients, the collateral blood supply to the rectosigmoid area is compromised. Other factors that contribute to ischemia include the level and duration of aortic occlusion, preoperative renal dysfunction, intraoperative hypotension, the severity of the aortic disease, and lack of attention to bowel retraction during surgical exposure. Given the lethality of mesenteric ischemia, any blood in the stool must be evaluated with endoscopy. Finally, aorto-enteric fistulas are late gastrointestinal complications that may occur months to years after the initial operation. The fistula generally forms between the proximal anastomosis and the overlying duodenum. Patients with a history of AAA repair who present with gastrointestinal bleeding need to be evaluated quickly by endoscopy and possibly arteriography.

There is a paucity of literature on the effect of abdominal aortic cross-clamping on the central nervous system. Spinal cord ischemia occurs 0.2% of the time in elective surgeries involving the distal aorta and is more common in patients presenting with ruptured aneurysms. The spinal cord is supplied by two posterior spinal arteries that supply 25% of the spinal cord's blood flow and one anterior spinal artery that provides 75% of the total perfusion. The anterior spinal artery is supplied by radicular arteries, and collateralization is poor. The artery of Adamkiewicz is a radicular artery that provides blood to thoracolumbar spinal cord and joins the anterior spinal artery between T8 and T12 in 75% of cases and between L1 and L2 in 10% of cases. Thus, high cross-clamping of the aorta may impair spinal cord perfusion. Measures to prevent spinal cord ischemia include a short aortic occlusion time and maintenance of adequate blood pressure while the cross-clamp is in place.

Most postoperative infections involve the skin. Infection of the prosthetic device occurs in about 1% to 6% of patients. This may be a devastating problem requiring prolonged treatment with antibiotics and removal of the prosthesis, with an axillobifemoral reconstruction. Anesthesiologists can reduce the rate of graft infection by adhering to sterile technique during central line placement and ensuring that preoperative antibiotics are administered.

A successful outcome in aortic surgery requires a team approach with attention to detail throughout the entire perioperative period. As the major cause of perioperative mortality is cardiac related, prevention of perioperative myocardial ischemia should be a focus of the anesthesiologist caring for these patients. The use of β-adrenergic blockade, appropriate volume resuscitation, and administration of epidural analgesia affect patient outcome. Finally, the value of clinical experience caring for these patients must be emphasized given the complexity and rapidity with which physiologic changes occur.

Suggested readings

Cannesson M, Slieker J, Desebbe O, et al. Prediction of fluid responsiveness using respiratory variations in left ventricular stroke area by transoesophageal echocardiographic automated border detection in mechanically ventilated patients. *Crit Care* 2006; 10:R171.

Dodds TM, Burns AK, DeRoo DB, et al. Effects of anesthetic technique on myocardial wall motion abnormalities during abdominal aortic surgery. *J Cardiothorac Vasc Anesth* 1997; 11:129–136.

Fleisher LA, Beckman JA, Brown KA, et al. ACC/AHA 2007 guidelines on perioperative cardiovascular evaluation and care for noncardiac surgery: executive summary: a report of the American College of Cardiology/American Heart Association Task Force on Practice Guidelines (Writing Committee to Revise the 2002 Guidelines on Perioperative Cardiovascular Evaluation for Noncardiac Surgery): developed in collaboration with the American Society of Echocardiography, American Society of Nuclear Cardiology, Heart Rhythm Society, Society of Cardiovascular Anesthesiologists, Society for Cardiovascular Angiography and Interventions, Society for Vascular Medicine and Biology, and Society for Vascular Surgery. *Circulation* 2007; 116:1971–1996.

Gelman S. The pathophysiology of aortic cross-clamping and unclamping. *Anesthesiology* 1995; 82:1026–1060.

Gelman S. Venous function and central venous pressure: a physiologic story. *Anesthesiology* 2008; 108:735–748.

Gelman S, Khazaeli MB, Orr R, Henderson T. Blood volume redistribution during cross-clamping of the descending aorta. *Anesth Analg* 1994; 78:219–224.

Gorski Y, Ricotta JJ. Weighing risks in abdominal aortic aneurysm. Best repaired in an elective, not an emergency, procedure. *Postgrad Med* 1999; 106:69–70, 75–80.

Ho P, Ting AC, Cheng SW. Blood loss and transfusion in elective abdominal aortic aneurysm surgery. *ANZ J Surg* 2004; 74: 631–634.

Kalko Y, Ugurlucan M, Basaran M, et al. Epidural anaesthesia and mini-laparotomy for the treatment of abdominal aortic aneurysms in patients with severe chronic obstructive pulmonary disease. *Acta Chir Belg* 2007; 107:307–312.

McArdle GT, McAuley DF, McKinley A, et al. Preliminary results of a prospective randomized trial of restrictive versus standard fluid regime in elective open abdominal aortic aneurysm repair. *Ann Surg* 2009; 250:28–34.

McArdle GT, Price G, Lewis A, et al. Positive fluid balance is associated with complications after elective open infrarenal abdominal aortic aneurysm repair. *Eur J Vasc Endovasc Surg* 2007; 34:522–527.

McFalls EO, Ward HB, Moritz TE, et al. Coronary-artery revascularization before elective major vascular surgery. *N Engl J Med* 2004; 351:2795–2804.

Schermerhorn M, Cronenwett, JL. *Current Surgical Therapy*. 7th ed. 2001:C.V. Mosby; Philadelphia; 807–812.

Schulmeyer MC, Santelices E, Vega R, Schmied S. Impact of intraoperative transesophageal echocardiography during noncardiac surgery. *J Cardiothorac Vasc Anesth* 2006; 20: 768–771.

Steyerberg EW, Kievit J, de Mol Van Otterloo JC, et al. Perioperative mortality of elective abdominal aortic aneurysm surgery. A clinical prediction rule based on literature and individual patient data. *Arch Intern Med* 1995; 155:1998–2004.

Taylor RW, O'Brien J, Trottier SJ, et al. Red blood cell transfusions and nosocomial infections in critically ill patients. *Crit Care Med* 2006; 34:2302–2308; quiz 2309.

Chapter

83 Endovascular abdominal aortic aneurysm repair

K. Annette Mizuguchi

With the introduction of endovascular abdominal aortic aneurysm repair (EVAR) in 1991 by Parodi et al., treatment options for abdominal aortic aneurysms (AAAs) have expanded to conventional open surgical repair or endovascular repair. Clearly, as more vascular surgeons and interventional radiologists overcome the learning curve for the endovascular approach and as endografts with a better long-term record become available, more patients will be offered the endovascular approach.

Surgical considerations

Certain anatomic requirements must be met for a patient to be a candidate for the endovascular approach (Fig. 83.1). The procedure consists of endograft placement in the infrarenal aorta under fluoroscopic guidance and use of digital subtraction angiography (Fig. 83.2). Bilateral iliofemoral arterial access is obtained by either percutaneous or surgical exposure; the vascular sheath is introduced on one side, and arterial access is obtained on the contralateral side for angiography. Systemic anticoagulation is achieved with heparin to an activated coagulation time of 250 seconds (2–2.5 times the baseline value). During the procedure, the breath-hold technique is used to optimize the image quality of digital subtraction angiography.

Anesthetic considerations

All patients scheduled for EVAR have the potential for conversion to an open repair. Therefore, all patients should undergo a thorough preoperative evaluation and optimization of comorbidities similar to patients undergoing open AAA repair.

In addition to standard American Society of Anesthesiologists monitors, an arterial line to monitor the blood pressure and two large-bore intravenous lines are usually placed. The need for central access is dictated by the patient's preoperative status, the need for venous access, and the possibility of converting to an open repair. Blood should be typed, and crossmatched units should be in the room. Inotropic agents, vasopressors, and vasodilators should be readily accessible. Because the procedure is done under fluoroscopic guidance, special attention must be paid to minimizing radiation exposure. After the procedure, most patients are transferred to the recovery room rather than the intensive care unit.

The patient can be managed under local anesthesia with sedation, regional anesthesia (epidural, spinal, or combined spinal/epidural), or under general anesthesia. The surgeon's and anesthesiologist's preferences, as well as patient factors, dictate the choice of anesthetic technique. For local and regional techniques, patient cooperation and motivation are required (especially for the breath-hold technique during digital subtraction angiography). The various anesthesia techniques have not been shown to make a clear difference in intraoperative complication or mortality rates.

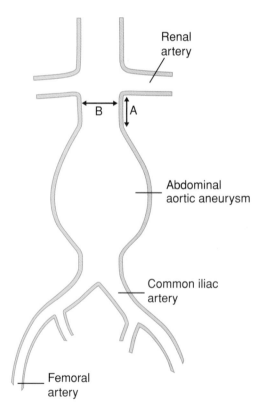

Figure 83.1. Anatomic requirements for infrared EVAR are listed as follows: the aneurysmal aortic neck ("landing zone") should be at least 15 mm (**A**); the infrarenal aortic neck diameter range should be 19 to 36 mm (**B**); one femoral artery must be free from significant occlusive disease and have a diameter > 7.7 mm; if the larger iliac is being used, it must be free from tortuosity or excessive calcification; the distal attachment site must be nonaneurysmal and of sufficient length to accommodate the graft; and there should be at least one straight iliac artery that can be used as a conduit for the delivery system.

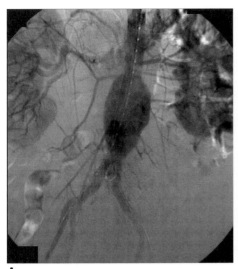
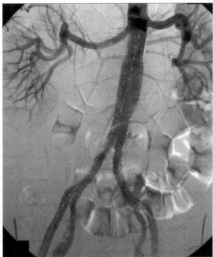

A   B

Figure 83.2. Radiograph showing abdominal aorta pre-repair (**A**) and post-repair (**B**).

Unlike open repair, in which the aorta is cross-clamped and unclamped, EVAR is associated with relative hemodynamic stability. Large fluid requirements are not encountered because of the reduced blood loss and minimal third space fluid losses. Blood loss for EVAR has been reported to be around 100 to 500 ml, compared with 900 to 2300 ml for open repair.

Complications

Although EVAR is minimally invasive, it is associated with several significant complications (Table 83.1). *Endoleak* is defined as the presence of blood flow outside the endograft but within the aneurysmal sac, and it can occur in the acute setting during endograft implantation or anytime during the postoperative surveillance period (Table 83.2). Therefore, patients are subsequently followed up with surveillance CT scans at 1 month, 6 months, 12 months, and annually thereafter. Type I and III endoleaks require fairly urgent interventions because blood flow and sac pressure will continue to increase and lead to rupture. Type IV endoleaks usually resolve with time. The management of type II endoleaks is more controversial, because some will thrombose on their own whereas others will lead to

sac enlargement. Increases in aneurysm diameter and possible device migration are also followed up with surveillance CT scans.

Management of patients coming to the operating room for surgical intervention of a type I or III endoleak may be more complex. In addition to the fact that many of these procedures will be urgent or emergent in nature, and that these patients likely will have more significant comorbidities, which made them endovascular candidates in the first place, they may require a suprarenal or supraceliac cross-clamp for their surgical repair.

EVAR is associated with renal dysfunction, and the etiology is multifactorial. Contrast dye used during the procedure has been implicated, and the prevention of contrast-induced renal dysfunction with the use of hydration, *N*-acetylcysteine, or bicarbonate has been advocated. The position of the graft is another factor. With the use of suprarenal fixation devices, graft material may inadvertently be placed over the renal artery ostium, leading to renal dysfunction. Even with perfect device placement during the procedure, with time, device position may change and alter the relationship of the graft to the renal artery ostium, leading to renal dysfunction that is not seen immediately after the procedure.

Endovascular repair of thoracic aortic aneurysms

Anesthetic considerations for endovascular repair of thoracic aortic aneurysms (TAAs) are similar to those for EVAR. The potential for conversion to an open repair and for major blood loss exists. Transesophageal echocardiography may be used to visualize the undeployed stent–graft in relation to the aortic pathology. Unfortunately, the echo probe interferes with fluoroscopic imaging and can be used only between fluoroscopic examinations. Certain TAAs require a combined approach:

Table 83.1. Complications of endovascular aneurysm repair

- Endoleak
- Migration of stent graft
- Surgical conversion
- Acute rupture: more likely during graft deployment but may occur at any time during EVAR
- Misdeployment, malpositioning, stent graft migration
- Embolic events
- Paralysis
- Local site injury
- Infection
- Groin wound healing problems
- Systemic injury

Table 83.2. Types of endoleaks

Type of endoleak	Causes	Description	Recommended treatments
I	Seal failure	Occurs from the attachment sites at the proximal or distal ends of the graft and is a result of failure to seal attachment sites of the endograft to the native vessels. This type is associated with rupture and is treated aggressively.	Repair in the operating room.
II	Retrograde flow	Occurs from retrograde flow (back-bleeding) from tributaries that have not thrombosed such as lumbars or the inferior mesenteric artery following aneurysm exclusion. Most have a benign course and will resolve spontaneously.	Can be observed for 6 months if there is no sac expansion.
III	Graft defect	Occurs from defect within the graft from module disconnection or fabric tear. This type needs to be repaired immediately with a modular extension or covered stent.	Repair at the time of detection.
IV	Fabric porosity	Occurs through intact but porous fabric.	No specific treatment is necessary.

open surgical repair with cardiopulmonary bypass for the ascending aorta and an endovascular repair for the descending aorta. Similar to the open TAA repair, there is potential for paraplegia. Therefore, many surgeons and radiologists prefer to place a spinal drain prior to the procedure. However, the benefit of perioperative salvage spinal drain placement remains to be determined.

Future

Since its introduction, the field of endovascular repair has greatly advanced. Currently, many centers are treating most of their elective, infrarenal aneurysms endovascularly. Endografts are being developed that will accommodate aneurysms currently excluded because of anatomic restraints. It is foreseeable that with the advancement of the field, endovascular treatment will expand to include patients with ruptured or urgent aneurysms as well, including more complicated patients with various comorbidities and advanced age, who would otherwise have been deemed untreatable.

However, more studies comparing the outcome of long-term morbidity, mortality, and quality of life need to be made before definite conclusions can be made. At present, although randomized controlled studies indicate that short-term mortality is improved by 3% with EVAR, it was associated with a higher number of complications and reinterventions.

Suggested readings

Ghansah JN, Murphy JT. Complications of major aortic and lower extremity vascular surgery. *Semin Cardiothorac Vasc Anesth* 2004; 8:335–361.

Greenhalgh RM. Endovascular aneurysm repair versus open repair in patients with abdominal aortic aneurysms (EVAR trial 1); randomized controlled trial. *Lancet* 2005; 365:2179–2186.

Kahn RA, et al. Anesthetic considerations for endovascular aortic repair. *Mount Sinai J Med* 2002; 69:57–67.

Katzen BT, et al. Endovascular repair of abdominal and thoracic aortic aneurysms. *Circulation* 2005; 112:1163–1675.

Kuchta KF. Endovascular abdominal aortic aneurysm repair. *Semin Cardiothorac Vasc Anesth* 2003; 7:205–211.

Lederle FA, et al. Immediate repair compared with surveillance of small abdominal aortic aneurysms. *N Engl J Med* 2002; 346:1437–1444.

Mehta M et al. Establishing a protocol for endovascular treatment of ruptured abdominal aortic aneurysms: outcomes of a prospective analysis. *J Vasc Surg* 2006; 44:1–8.

Merten GJ, et al. Prevention of contrast-induced nephropathy with sodium bicarbonate: a randomized controlled trial. *JAMA* 2004; 291:2328–2334.

Pannu N, et al. Prophylaxis strategies for contrast-induced nephropathy. *JAMA* 2006; 295:2765–2779.

Parodi JC, Palmaz JC, Barone HD. Transfemoral intraluminal graft implantations for abdominal aortic aneurysms. *Ann Vasc Surg* 1991; 5:491–499.

Prinssen M, et al. A randomized trial comparing conventional and endovascular repair of abdominal aortic aneurysms *N Engl J Med* 2004; 351:1607–1618.

Ruppert V, et al. Influence of anesthesia type on outcome after endovascular aortic aneurysm repair: an analysis based on EUROSTAR data. *J Vasc Surg* 2006; 44:16–21.

Taylor PR, et al. Endovascular abdominal aortic aneurysm repair and renal function. *Nephrol Dial Transplant* 2006; 21:2362–2365.

Tepel M, et al. Prevention of radiographic-contrast-agent-induced reductions in renal function by acetylcysteine. *N Engl J Med* 2000; 343:180–184.

Chapter 84

Peripheral vascular disease

Laura H. Leduc and James L. Helstrom

Atherosclerosis is one of the etiologies of peripheral vascular disease (PVD) and is associated with specific risk factors, including diabetes mellitus, hypertension, hypercholesterolemia, and tobacco use. PVD evolves from lipid deposits at sites of vessel injury that form plaques along the intimal lumen. Further lipid accumulation and hemorrhage into these plaques ultimately result in narrowing of the arterial wall and inadequate blood supply to tissues distal to the lesion. These lesions frequently occur at major arterial bifurcations.

Claudication

Claudication is the clinical description for *functional* ischemia. It is characterized by reproducible lower-extremity muscle pain induced by a defined amount of activity and relieved by rest. The symptoms result from the inability of the vasculature to provide blood flow commensurate with the metabolic demand of the exercising tissue. A subset of patients with claudication will go on to develop pain at rest or *critical* ischemia. In this circumstance, arterial perfusion is inadequate to meet the resting demands of tissue, which is an indication for surgical intervention.

Medical therapy for peripheral arterial disease is essential. Smoking is an independent risk factor for worsening of limb ischemia and continued progression of atherosclerosis.

The overall survival rate for patients with claudication is significantly lower than that for age-matched control subjects. Causes of death are most likely to be coronary and cerebral vascular accidents. In fact, evidence indicates that the incidence of perioperative cardiac events is higher after surgery for peripheral vascular conditions than for open aortic procedures. Therefore, it is imperative that these patients be managed with the same thorough preoperative risk assessment and intraoperative vigilance that would be used for patients undergoing other major vascular procedures.

Preoperative considerations

Patients undergoing peripheral vascular surgery are at high risk for perioperative complications including myocardial ischemia and infarction, respiratory failure, renal failure, graft failure, and death. Infrainguinal arterial bypass surgery is associated with a 30-day mortality rate of nearly 6% and 1-year mortality exceeding 16%. Perioperative myocardial infarction (MI) occurs in 4% to 15% of patients undergoing peripheral vascular surgery and accounts for > 50% of perioperative mortality. Therefore, preoperative evaluation of the patient's cardiac status is of the utmost importance and is based on recommendations by the American College of Cardiology (ACC).

For major vascular procedures, no difference in outcome has been demonstrated between medical management for coronary artery disease (CAD) and interventional management including both percutaneous and surgical coronary artery bypass grafting procedures. Medical treatment typically takes the form of β-blockers, statins, and aspirin, as well as management of hypertension and/or congestive heart failure, if present.

History and examination

The history and physical examination usually focus on the cardiovascular system, as this is a major cause of mortality in this patient population. Specifically, clinicians should elicit a history of nocturnal dyspnea, orthopnea, or anginal symptoms, whereas the examination should elicit evidence of murmurs, heart failure, or bruits. Often, the most useful part of the cardiovascular examination is a conversation with the patient regarding his/her functional status. A patient's ability to achieve a minimum exercise capacity of four metabolic equivalents of task (MET) is consistent with adequate functional status and is a key decision point in the American Heart Association/ACC guidelines.

Preoperatively, blood pressure should be assessed in both arms, as a discrepancy due to subclavian artery stenosis or upper-extremity vaso-occlusive disease may confound intraoperative monitoring and management. A difference of >20% between mean values is considered significant. In these cases, blood pressure monitoring should be undertaken on the side with the higher blood pressure, as this is more likely indicative of aortic root pressure. Beyond the careful cardiac history and examination:

- A baseline electrocardiogram (ECG) should always be obtained as a means of comparison for demand ischemia that may develop intra- or postoperatively.

- A full neurologic examination should be completed, as there may be baseline deficits due to the increased incidence of cerebrovascular disease.
- Diabetic patients should be evaluated for autonomic neuropathies that may be associated with silent myocardial infarction, labile blood pressure, and delayed gastric emptying. In particular, brittle diabetics require intraoperative monitoring of blood sugars with possible insulin administration.
- Renal protection strategies, including hydration, sodium bicarbonate administration, and N-acetylcysteine prophylaxis, should be considered because baseline renal insufficiency may be exacerbated by administration of contrast dye.
- A coagulation profile should be considered given the widespread use of anticoagulation strategies in this population.

In cases of threatened limb loss, a thorough preoperative evaluation may need to be deferred, depending on the urgency of the procedure. In the absence of a thorough history, laboratory, and cardiac evaluation, underlying CAD and other comorbidities should be assumed and managed as carefully as possible without delay of the surgical intervention.

Medications

Patients taking β-blockers for the treatment of previous MI, angina, symptomatic dysrhythmias, or hypertension preoperatively should continue to do so throughout the perioperative period. Additionally, patients undergoing vascular surgery who are at high cardiac risk may also benefit from initiation of β-blocker therapy. Although several case reports have been published suggesting an association between continued statin therapy and postoperative rhabdomyolysis, a cause-and-effect relationship has not been well established. Moreover, given the anti-inflammatory benefits of these agents in the context of atherosclerotic disease and demonstration of clinically worse outcomes following discontinuation prior to major noncardiac surgery and in the presence of ischemia, these agents should be continued through the perioperative period in high-risk patients.

Careful consideration should be given to the decision to discontinue inotropic agents, because such action may precipitate symptomatic worsening of symptoms. Although ACE inhibitor treated patients may be at increased risk for severe postinduction hypotension, abrupt discontinuation may adversely affect blood pressure control. The decision to discontinue these agents perioperatively should be made on a case-by-case basis and weigh the risks of increasing afterload against the benefits of mitigating the potential hypotensive response to induction of anesthesia.

Finally, the decision to continue aspirin therapy perioperatively should be made in conjunction with the surgical team. Although continued aspirin therapy is associated with increased blood loss, this has currently not been linked to increased postoperative morbidity or mortality. Indeed, aspirin discontinuation has been suggested to increase the risk for coronary events, with preliminary data pointing to a maximum risk at 10 to 12 days following cessation. Continued aspirin therapy is not a contraindication to neuraxial anesthesia, although concomitant intraoperative heparinization may increase the risk of epidural hematoma.

Evaluation of PVD

Clinically, PVD is characterized by deteriorating distal blood flow in the lower extremity. This is evaluated by measuring the ankle-brachial index (ABI). The ABI is obtained by comparing the systolic blood pressure in the upper extremity with the corresponding pressure in the ankle.

At this time, fluoroscopic angiography is the gold standard for diagnosis and operative planning for patients with peripheral arterial disease. However, magnetic resonance angiography has the potential to replace invasive angiography because image quality is excellent, yet the procedure is noninvasive, does not require operative time, and reduces the risk of contrast-induced nephropathy.

Surgical approach

Surgical literature suggests that native vein conduits are superior to prosthetic grafts over the long term. Venous mapping may be done preoperatively to identify targets for harvest. Vein harvested from the arms obviates the use of regional techniques for lower-extremity revascularization procedures.

The inflow source is often the common femoral, superficial femoral, or deep femoral artery. The target distal artery is usually at the knee level or below. The distal anastomosis usually is connected first, followed by the proximal anastomosis.

Infrainguinal bypass procedures are indicated for salvage of severely ischemic lower extremities. Patients may present with gangrene, ischemic ulceration, or rest pain. Patients who demonstrate acute symptom onset likely are suffering from thromboembolic disease, whereas those who present with gradual worsening of disease likely are suffering from arterial atherosclerosis causing progressive luminal narrowing. Patients are likely to re-present, as graft patency decreases over the long term.

Arterial embolectomy is likely to be performed under emergent circumstances; bypass revascularization is undertaken after longer periods of ischemia but is less effective. Thromboembolism causes acute arterial insufficiency and is often associated with MI, mitral stenosis, or atrial fibrillation. Thromboembolic disease also may result from thoracic or abdominal aortic aneurysms, severe atherosclerotic disease, or paradoxic emboli via a patent foramen ovale. In the lower extremities, emboli are likely to lodge at the iliac, femoral, or popliteal arteries.

Intraoperative heparinization is used to prevent clot formation associated with vessel cross-clamping. Because of the risk of graft failure, heparinization is often not reversed with protamine. It is essential to consider this in the event of a traumatic needle placement for neuraxial anesthesia, as heparinization with concomitant aspirin use increases the risk of epidural hematoma. As patients return for repeated procedures, it is possible to see an increase in the incidence of heparin-induced thrombocytopenia. Therefore, familiarity with the risks and dosing of thrombin inhibitors will be of increasing importance.

Intraoperative considerations
Anesthetic techniques

Anesthetic options include both general and regional techniques. The decision as to which method is best should take into account patient preference, surgical technique, and operator prowess, as well as each patient's comorbidities. Patients presenting with peripheral artery embolism are likely to be anticoagulated at the time of diagnosis and thus are not candidates for neuraxial anesthesia.

When not contraindicated, administration of neuraxial anesthesia may reduce the incidence of perioperative mortality and cardiac and respiratory morbidity. Epidural anesthesia has been shown to modify the stress response associated with surgery, but there is not enough evidence to indicate whether this is of clinical significance. However, there is limited evidence to suggest an improved graft patency rate with regional anesthesia, which is desirable given an incidence of graft occlusion ranging from 2% to 20%.

Regional anesthesia

Regional anesthesia is an option for patients with a normal coagulation profile. It is worth considering either epidural or spinal catheters, because these allow repeated administration of local anesthetics during these procedures. Fluids must be administered judiciously, as they may lead to congestive heart failure in patients as the vasodilation caused by regional sympathectomy dissipates. Epidural test dosing in this population frequently is based on systolic blood pressure, because heart rate responsiveness is diminished in elderly patients and individuals taking chronic β-antagonists.

General anesthesia

Following adequate preoxygenation, induction of general anesthesia should minimize hemodynamic impact during placement of the endotracheal tube or laryngeal mask airway. This can be done with either propofol, given in incremental doses, or etomidate. The time to peak effect of propofol may approach 2 minutes, and an effective induction often can be achieved with doses of 1 mg/kg. If an arterial line has not been placed, the blood pressure cuff may be cycled every 1 to 2 minutes during periods of hemodynamic instability such as induction and emergence. A phenylephrine infusion may be placed inline prior to the induction of anesthesia, and esmolol and glycopyrrolate are useful adjuncts to traditional emergency medications. In patients with severe CAD or an ejection fraction

< 40%, consideration is given to using norepinephrine instead of phenylephrine because of the transient impairment of left ventricular systolic performance induced by phenylephrine.

Anesthetic maintenance

Anesthetic maintenance can be accomplished in a variety of ways, typically with use of inhaled agents. Recent data suggest that forgoing nitrous oxide is associated with improved wound healing and reduced pulmonary complications. However, these data have not been validated specifically in vascular patients and must be weighed against the hemodynamic stability afforded by nitrous oxide use. Invariably, vascular repair involves arterial cross-clamping, with resultant ischemia in the affected limb. Byproducts of limb ischemia include vasodilatory metabolic products and carbon dioxide. Reperfusion of the affected area causes formation and release of toxic compounds (including oxygen free radicals) that may lead to hemodynamic instability. Clinicians should be aware of these effects and have a plan for the use of vasoactive agents and/or volume infusion to maintain hemodynamics. Patients with obstructive lung disease also may have difficulty eliminating the additional carbon dioxide. This may be a serious issue in patients with underlying pulmonary hypertension and/or right ventricular dysfunction.

Monitoring

Patient comorbidities should determine monitoring requirements. At a minimum, standard American Society of Anesthesiologists monitors should be used. ECG monitoring should include a precordial V_4 or V_5 lead because this lead is particularly sensitive for demonstrating signs of myocardial ischemia. Invasive monitoring of arterial blood pressure often is used, for a variety of reasons; patient comorbidities and the surgical plan should drive decision making. Catastrophic drops in blood pressure may be encountered during anesthetic induction, in the case of loss of proximal arterial control of large vessels, or during reperfusion. Hemodynamic lability also may occur as a result of baseline hypertensive disease, dysrhythmias, or ventricular dysfunction. Central venous and pulmonary artery monitoring is not routine and should be based on individual patient comorbidities.

Postoperative considerations

Postoperative complications may include congestive heart failure, myocardial ischemia, hypothermia, and graft occlusion. Hypothermia should be avoided, as associated vasoconstriction may limit outflow to the graft and compromise graft patency. Patients should continue to be monitored for myocardial ischemia and failure in the postoperative period, because most cardiac complications arise 48 to 72 hours into the postoperative period. If a neuraxial technique has been used, patients should be monitored for formation of epidural hematoma. Moreover, anticoagulation may be important in the postoperative period, and careful communication between anesthetic and surgical teams to allow for the removal of any in situ catheters is critically important. Expeditious workup and intervention are required if epidural hematoma is suspected, because the risk of permanent neurologic damage increases with time.

Suggested readings

Bode RH Jr, Lewis KP, Zarich SW, et al. Cardiac outcome after peripheral vascular surgery. Comparison of general and regional anesthesia. *Anesthesiology* 1996; 84:3–13.

Burger W, Chemnitius J-M, Kneissl GD, Rucker G. Low-dose aspirin for secondary cardiovascular prevention – cardiovascular risks after perioperative withdrawal versus bleeding risks with its continuation – review and meta-analysis. *J Intern Med* 2005; 257: 399–414.

Christopherson R, Beattie C, Frank SM, et al. Perioperative morbidity in patients randomized to epidural or general anesthesia for lower extremity vascular surgery. *Anesthesiology* 1993; 79:422–434.

Coriat P, Richer C, Douraki T, et al. Influence of chronic angiotensin-converting enzyme inhibition on anesthetic induction. *Anesthesiology* 1994; 81:299–307.

Horlocker TT, Wedel DJ, Benzon H, et al. Regional anesthesia in the anticoagulated patient: defining the risks. The Second ASRA Consensus Conference on Neuraxial Anesthesia and Anticoagulation. *Reg Anesth Reg Anesth Pain Med* 2003; 29(9):172–197.

Johnson WC, Lee KK. A comparative evaluation of polytetrafluoroethylene, umbilical vein, and saphenous vein bypass grafts for femoro-popliteal above-knee revascularization: a prospective randomized Department of Veterans Affairs cooperative study. *J Vasc Surg* 2000; 32(2):268–277.

London MJ, Hollenberg M, Wong MG, et al.; the SPI Research Group. Intraoperative myocardial ischemia: localization by continuous 12-lead electrocardiography. *Anesthesiology* 1988; 69:232–241.

McFalls EO, Ward HB, Moritz TE, et al. Coronary artery revascularization before elective major vascular surgery. *N Engl J Med* 2004; 351:2795–2804.

Myles PS, Leslie K, Chan MTV, et al.; the ENIGMA Trial Group. Avoidance of nitrous oxide for patients undergoing major surgery. *Anesthesiology* 2007; 107:221–231.

Poldermans D, Bax J, Kertai M, et al. Statins are associated with a reduced incidence of perioperative mortality in patients undergoing major noncardiac vascular surgery. *Circulation* 2003; 107(14):1848–1851.

Rozner MA. The patient with a cardiac pacemaker or implanted defibrillator and management during anesthesia. *Curr Opin Anaesthesiol* 2007; 20(3):261–268.

Tuman KJ, McCarthy RJ, March RJ, et al. Effects of epidural anesthesia and analgesia on coagulation and outcome after major vascular surgery. *Anesth Analg* 1991; 73:696–704.

Wesner L, Marone LK, Dennegy KC. Anesthesia for lower extremity lower extremity bypass. *Int Anesthesiol Clin* 2005; 43(1): 93–109.

Part 15

Thoracic Anesthesia

Shannon S. McKenna, editor

Chapter

85

Respiratory physiology

Shannon S. McKenna

The primary purpose of the respiratory system is to facilitate uptake of oxygen and removal of carbon dioxide from the blood. This gas exchange is necessary to support the metabolic functions of the cells and organs that comprise the human body.

Functional anatomy of the respiratory system

The thorax

The thorax is a semirigid asymmetric cylinder that increases and decreases in volume during the respiratory cycle. These changes in thoracic volume result in lung inflation and deflation. Bony support comes from the thoracic vertebral column, ribs, and sternum. The superior and inferior borders are the thoracic inlet and the diaphragm, respectively.

Respiratory muscles

The diaphragm is the primary inspiratory muscle. Its descent, with contraction, increases the vertical dimension of the thorax. Contraction of the external intercostal muscles elevates the ribs anteriorly, increasing the diameter of the thorax. The sternocleidomastoid and scalene muscles serve as accessory inspiratory muscles during labored breathing. Normally, expiration is passive and driven by elastic recoil. In some settings, expiration is active and driven by abdominal muscle contraction. The internal intercostals also assist in active expiration by pulling the ribs downward.

Airways and lung parenchyma

The tracheobronchial tree is a complex structure with 23 generations of division. Airways are described by both anatomic location and function. Anatomically, the two lungs are divided into a total of five lobes (three on the right). Each lobe is then divided into segments. There are 42 segments in total: 22 on the right and 20 on the left. Knowledge of the normal segmental anatomy of the lung is essential for proper use of lung isolation techniques during one-lung anesthesia.

From a functional standpoint, the first 17 divisions are progressively smaller conducting airways that carry gas but do not participate in gas exchange. The larger of these airways are supported by cartilaginous rings and have smooth muscle present in their walls. Their mucosa is ciliated columnar or cuboidal.

Around the 17th generation, the mucosa transitions to epithelium and alveoli began to appear, marking the beginning of the respiratory zone. Alveolar walls are thin, allowing close contact between type I alveolar cells and the dense pulmonary capillary network. Oxygen and carbon dioxide are exchanged by diffusion. Type II alveolar cells produce surfactant and can divide to replace damaged type I alveolar cells. The epithelial junctions are tight and water impervious in the absence of lung injury. The interstitial space contains elastin and collagen, providing architectural support and elastic recoil.

Pulmonary circulation

The lungs are supplied by a dual circulation. The bronchial arteries arise from the aorta and provide for the nutritive needs of the conducting airways. The pulmonary arteries carry mixed venous blood from the right ventricle to the pulmonary capillary network, where oxygen uptake and carbon dioxide elimination occur. Relatively large junctions in the pulmonary capillary endothelium permit filtration of large molecules such as albumin, as well as macrophages and neutrophils. Filtered fluid and cells are cleared by the pulmonary lymphatic system. Oxygenated blood is returned to the left atrium via the pulmonary veins. The details of gas transport are discussed in a separate chapter.

Mechanics of breathing

Airflow occurs secondary to the generation of pressure gradients from the upper airway to the alveoli. During spontaneous ventilation, contraction of inspiratory muscles causes an increase in thoracic volume. As a result, pleural pressure decreases. Subsequently, alveolar pressure drops and gas flows along the gradient (Fig. 85.1). During positive pressure ventilation, the ventilator applies positive pressure to the upper airways. Gas flows down the airways until alveolar pressure equilibrates with upper airway pressure. At this point, flow stops. Release, or lowering of the upper airway pressure, allows airflow reversal and expiration to occur.

Determinants of flow and volume

The elastic properties of the pulmonary system determine the lung volume that results from the application of any given static

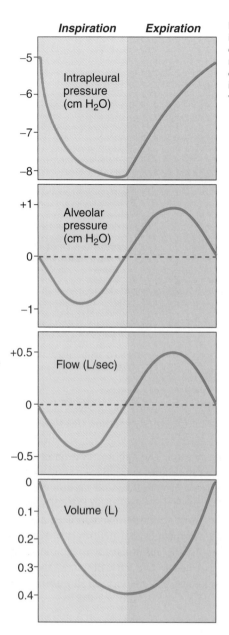

Figure 85.1. Changes in intrapleural and alveolar pressures during normal breathing with corresponding changes in pulmonary flow and volume.

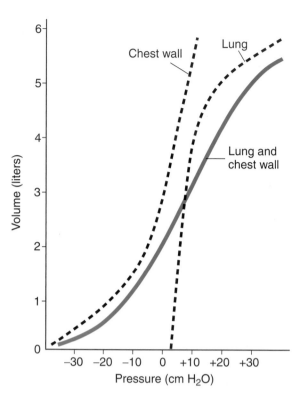

Figure 85.2. Pressure–volume relationships of the lung, chest wall, and lung and chest wall combined.

air, may be used to decrease the resistance to flow in the setting of severe turbulence. Resistance is inversely proportional to the radius to the fourth power, and directly proportional to the length of the airway. Not surprisingly, therefore, bronchospasm, airway stenosis, obstruction, edema, and secretion accumulation all lead to increased resistance.

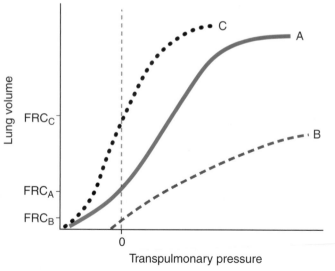

Figure 85.3. Pulmonary pressure–volume relationships in (A) normal lung, (B) severe restrictive disease, and (C) obstructive disease. Note that total lung capacity (indicated by the highest volume achieved), FRC, and compliance (curves) all change with disease.

pressure. The elastic forces of the chest wall and lung move in opposite directions: the chest wall expands outward and the lung collapses inward. *Compliance* is the term that may be used to describe the change in volume that occurs with any given applied pressure. The compliance of both the chest wall and lung can be determined. The combination of the two creates the compliance of the pulmonary system as a whole (Fig. 85.2). Many diseases alter the compliance of the pulmonary system (Fig. 85.3).

Compliance describes the static inflation of the lung. Once flow is present (as is necessary for breathing), resistance to gas flow must be factored in. Gas flow through airways may be either laminar or turbulent. Turbulent flow typically occurs at higher flow rates, branch points, sharp angles, or abrupt changes in diameter. Helium, which has a lower density than oxygen or

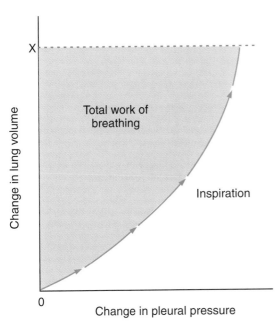

Figure 85.4. Total work of breathing for a single breath to a lung volume of "x" for a pulmonary system with a compliance described by the depicted inspiratory pressure–volume curve.

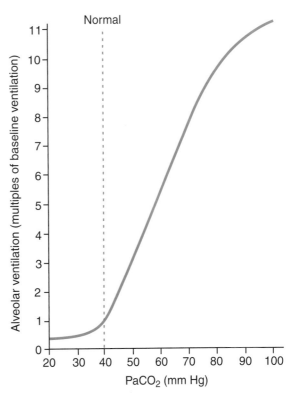

Figure 85.5. Relationship between $PaCO_2$ and minute ventilation.

Work of breathing

Work of breathing represents the total energy used to move the lung and chest wall. In most instances, active work occurs during inspiration only. Expiration is achieved using energy stored in the form of elastic recoil. At high minute ventilation or high resistance, expiration does become an active process. During inspiration, work is needed to overcome the elastic recoil of the lung and chest wall, the resistance to gas flow, and the frictional resistance of the tissue. Work may be calculated as the product of the change in volume and the change in pressure (Fig. 85.4). Normal tidal breathing by a healthy person accounts for only 2% to 3% of total body oxygen consumption. Increased tidal volumes will increase the work needed to overcome elastic recoil, whereas an increased respiratory rate increases the work needed to overcome resistance. As a result, patients with increased airway resistance tend to breathe at slower rates with larger tidal volumes to partially compensate for the increased work of breathing. The converse is true for patients with decreased compliance and stiff lungs or chest walls: they favor a rapid, shallow breathing pattern. Respiratory muscle fatigue, a primary cause of respiratory failure, may occur because of sustained increased loads, muscle atrophy from disease or disuse, or mechanical changes (such as a marked increase in functional residual capacity [FRC]) that foreshorten the muscle fibers and limit excursion with contraction, forcing a sustained increase in the respiratory rate.

Control of breathing

Neuronal control of breathing originates from respiratory centers in the pons and medulla and is influenced by multiple inputs from within the central nervous system. Rhythmic activity of the respiratory muscles maintains normal blood oxygen and carbon dioxide levels. Central chemoreceptors respond to changes in cerebrospinal fluid (CSF) pH. Because CO_2 freely crosses the blood–brain barrier, CSF pH changes with changes in arterial CO_2 concentrations. Minute ventilation increases with increasing arterial CO_2 in a nearly linear fashion (Fig. 85.5). Very high CO_2 levels will depress ventilation, however. Importantly, over time, bicarbonate is transported across the blood–brain barrier and permits the CSF pH to return to normal in the face of sustained hypercarbia. This mechanism is thought to account for the inappropriately low minute ventilation observed in chronic obstructive pulmonary disease (COPD) patients with chronic hypercarbia.

Several peripheral receptors also modulate ventilation. Chemoreceptors in the carotid bodies and aorta detect changes in arterial oxygen and CO_2 tension, as well as pH and perfusion pressure. Minute ventilation is increased in the setting of a falling PaO_2 or pH, or an increasing CO_2 level. The response to oxygen tension is not linear, however, and there is minimal effect until the PaO_2 is < 50 mm Hg (Fig. 85.6). Bilateral carotid body resection can completely ablate the hypoxic ventilatory drive. A variety of receptors located in the lungs themselves also modulate the neuronal control of breathing. Among other functions, these receptors can trigger coughing, bronchoconstriction, and sensations of dyspnea.

Several factors can change the ventilatory response to carbon dioxide and oxygen. The CO_2 response is blunted

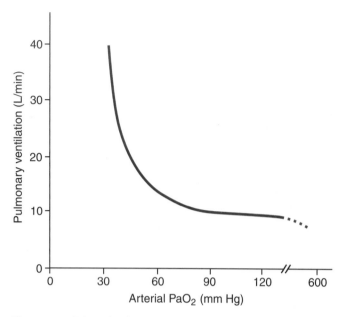

Figure 85.6. Relationship between PaO_2 and minute ventilation.

during sleep, by aging, and by drugs such as opiates, barbiturates, and benzodiazepines. Concomitant hypoxia will increase the response to a given degree of hypercarbia. Interestingly, increased work of breathing, such as seen in the setting of narrowed airways, blunts the hypercarbic ventilatory response.

The matching of ventilation and perfusion

Distribution of ventilation

A portion of the inspired gas never reaches the respiratory zone. This gas occupies the upper airway, trachea, and other conducting airways. It is termed the *anatomic dead space*, and amounts to about 150 ml in an average adult. The remainder of the inspired volume has the potential to participate in gas exchange and is termed the *alveolar ventilation*. Not all gas that reaches the respiratory zone participates in CO_2 elimination, however. For example, gas flow to a set of alveoli that are not perfused contributes additional dead space. The total dead space in the

lung is referred to as *physiologic dead space* and can be calculated using Bohr's equation:

$$\frac{V_D}{V_T} = \frac{Pa_{CO2} - P_{ECO2}}{Pa_{CO2}}.$$

Physiologic dead space represents 20% to 30% of the tidal ventilation during quiet breathing in a healthy person. Certain lung diseases, such as COPD and acute respiratory distress syndrome, markedly increase the physiologic dead space, profoundly decreasing the efficiency of ventilation.

The distribution of ventilation is directly effected by gravity. In an upright individual, the inferior portions of the lung receive the most ventilation and the apical portions the least. When the subject is supine, the highest ventilation occurs in the posterior, most dependent regions.

Distribution of perfusion and the West zones

There is significant asymmetry of distribution of blood flow within the human lung. In the upright position, blood flow is directly influenced by gravitational forces and is lowest at the apex and highest at the base. When body position is changed, the distribution of blood flow tracks the changes in gravitational forces, with the most dependent portions of the lung seeing the greatest perfusion. Additionally, pulmonary capillaries are surrounded by alveoli, which are filled with gas at the alveolar pressure. The West zones describe the relationships among pulmonary alveolar, arterial, and venous pressures (Fig. 85.7). In zone 1, the alveolar pressure is higher than the arterial and venous pressures and the blood vessels are collapsed. This would occur in the setting of low arterial pressure (shock) or high alveolar pressure (positive pressure ventilation) and creates areas that are ventilated but not perfused, thereby increasing the amount of physiologic dead space. In zone 2, arterial pressure exceeds alveolar pressure, but alveolar pressure is still greater than venous pressure. As a result, blood flow is determined by the difference between arterial and alveolar pressures. Once zone 3 is reached, the venous pressure finally is greater than the alveolar pressure and flow is once again determined

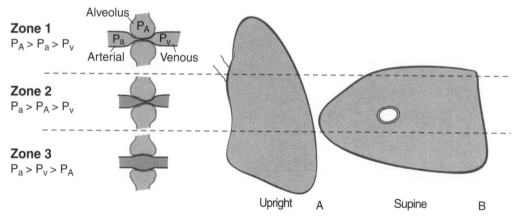

Figure 85.7. West zones of the lung: (A) upright and (B) supine.

by the more customary difference in arterial and venous pressures. Some refer to a zone 4, which occurs in the most dependent areas of the lung where atelectasis and low lung volumes cause compression of the extra-alveolar vessels, resulting in an overall decrease in flow to the region.

Matching ventilation and perfusion

Gravity has an important role in the distribution of both ventilation and perfusion. However, gravity is not sufficient to ensure maximal matching of ventilation and perfusion, which is necessary for efficient gas exchange. This occurs primarily as the result of hypoxic pulmonary vasoconstriction. Through mechanisms not yet fully defined, low alveolar oxygen tension leads to vasoconstriction of the small arterioles supplying that region of the lung. Local blood flow is profoundly reduced. As a result, blood flow is matched to areas of higher ventilation and higher alveolar oxygen content. Inhaled nitric oxide will reverse the vasoconstriction but acts only locally and thus only in the regions where ventilation occurs.

Abnormalities in ventilation/perfusion matching: the primary cause of hypoxemia

Several separate processes may lead to impairment of pulmonary gas exchange. Abnormally low alveolar ventilation, termed *hypoventilation*, results in more oxygen being taken up at the alveolar capillary interface than is supplied to the alveoli, leading to hypoxemia. At the same time, less carbon dioxide is cleared and arterial hypercapnia occurs.

Shunt occurs when blood flows through areas of lung that are not ventilated because of atelectasis or disease of the parenchyma. Additionally, blood may bypass the pulmonary circulation altogether. This occurs via the bronchial circulation, right-to-left shunting in the heart, or coronary venous drainage. This deoxygenated blood mixes with oxygenated blood from the pulmonary veins in the left heart and decreases PaO_2. Hypoxemia due to shunt can be identified by giving a patient 100% oxygen. Because the shunted blood bypasses the respiratory interface, the PaO_2 of the shunted blood does not increase and provision of 100% oxygen will not fully correct the hypoxemia. Shunt is not usually associated with hypercarbia, because even small increases in the PCO_2 result in compensatory hyperventilation, which drives the PCO_2 back to baseline.

Although hypoventilation and shunt both may cause hypoxemia, the most common cause of hypoxemia clinically is regional mismatching of ventilation to perfusion (V/Q). To appreciate the importance of V/Q matching, one must recognize that the concentration of oxygen, or any other gas, in an alveolus is dependent on the rate at which the gas is added (ventilation) and the rate at which the gas is removed (perfusion). End capillary blood exiting an alveolus that is poorly ventilated will have the characteristics of mixed venous blood – a high concentration of carbon dioxide and a low concentration of oxygen. On the other hand, blood exiting an alveolus with high

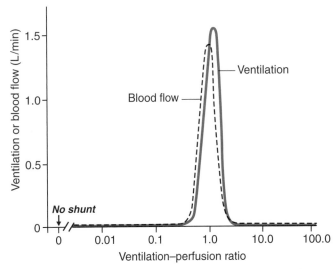

Figure 85.8. Distribution of ventilation and perfusion in a subject with normal lungs.

ventilation but poor perfusion will have a gas content that mirrors the inspired gas – high in oxygen and low in carbon dioxide. In an upright human, the V/Q ratio is highest at the apex and lowest at the base. In a healthy individual, the V/Q ratios in the lung are tightly distributed around the optimum ratio of 1.0, allowing for efficient gas uptake (Fig. 85.8). Pulmonary diseases broaden the distribution of the V/Q ratios, often with increases in the number of alveolar units with both the low and high V/Q ratios (Fig. 85.9). The overall result is worsened gas exchange, with the balance between hypercarbia and hypoxia being determined by the exact nature of the redistribution. A significant increase in the number of low V/Q units will result in hypercarbia, whereas an increase in the number of high V/Q units causes hypoxemia. In vivo, hypercarbia is a potent stimulus for hyperventilation. Most of the time, arterial CO_2 will remain near

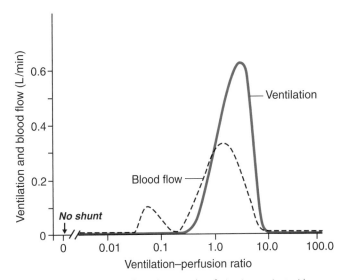

Figure 85.9. Distribution of ventilation and perfusion in a patient with COPD.

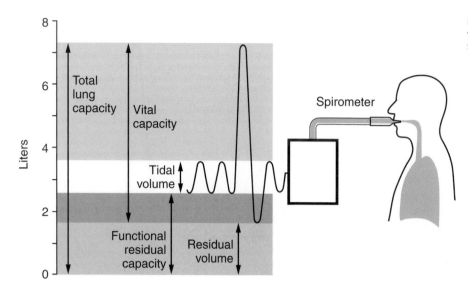

Figure 85.10. Spirometric measurement of lung volumes. RV and FRC cannot be measured by spirometry.

normal at the expense of increased minute ventilation and energy expenditure.

Pulmonary function testing

Pulmonary function tests permit specific, objective evaluation of certain lung functions. They are used to help with diagnosis and also may be used to monitor treatment effects or disease progression. Pulmonary function testing has often been used as part of the preoperative evaluation of patients presenting for major surgery. These tests are most useful when used to evaluate patients with significant underlying pulmonary disease for major lung resection. In most other circumstances, pulmonary function tests do not add significant additional information to that obtained from a careful history and physical examination. They should not be routinely ordered as part of a general perioperative evaluation.

Spirometry measures lung volumes and flows. The tidal volume can be measured during relaxed breathing. A more useful volume is the forced vital capacity (FVC). To make this measurement, the patient is asked to breathe in as deeply as possible and then blow out as hard and fast as he or she can. The exhaled volume is the FVC. There is always some air left in the lung; this is termed the *residual volume* (RV), and it cannot be measured using spirometry. Total lung capacity is the sum of the FVC and RV and also cannot be measured with spirometry (Fig. 85.10).

Several useful measurements of flow can be determined using spirometry. The most commonly used clinically is the forced expiratory volume in the first second of expiration (FEV_1). Normally, 80% of the FVC is expelled in the first second. The combination of the FVC and FEV_1, especially when normalized to the percent predicted based on gender, age, and body size, allows one to distinguish between restrictive and obstructive pulmonary diseases. In the setting of a restrictive disease, such as pulmonary fibrosis, both the FVC and the FEV_1 will be reduced, but the ratio of the two will essentially be unchanged. Obstructive disease, on the other hand, results in a relatively preserved FVC, but the FEV_1 is decreased. Therefore, the ratio of the FEV_1/FVC will be markedly decreased. One problem with the measurement of the FEV_1 is that it is effort dependent. The flow during the middle half of expiration, termed the FEF_{25-75}, also can be measured and is thought to be much more independent of patient effort.

Another way to analyze the flows and volumes obtained via spirometry is to graph the data as flow–volume curves. Both expiratory and inspiratory curves can be displayed. Obstructive disease, restrictive disease, upper airway obstruction, and intrathoracic airway obstruction can be recognized from their classic flow–volume curves (Fig. 85.11 and Fig. 85.12). Of course, many patients have mixed disease and so may have flow–volume curves that are not characteristic of any one disease pattern.

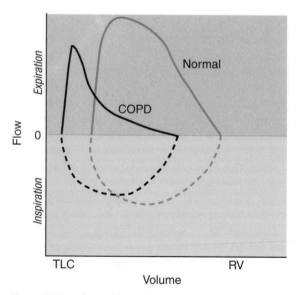

Figure 85.11. Idealized flow–volume loop of a patient with normal lungs and a patient with significant COPD.

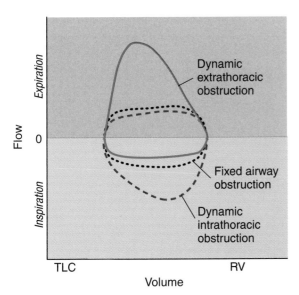

Figure 85.12. Idealized flow–volume loops in three types of upper airway obstruction.

Direct measurement of the RV or FRC can be done using either dilution of an inert gas (usually helium) or body plethysmography. Total lung capacity can also be measured this way. There are subtle differences between the two techniques. In particular, if there is a large portion of pulmonary gas that is trapped and does not communicate with the mouth, the gas dilution technique, which depends on distribution and equilibration of the gas throughout the lung, will yield erroneously low volumes, which would be a particular concern in the setting of significant COPD.

It is important to realize that all the previously described measurements are measurements of ventilation. They do not measure gas exchange at the alveolar–capillary interface. This can be evaluated using the diffusing capacity for carbon monoxide (DLCO). The amount of carbon monoxide taken up in 1 minute will depend on the total area of the alveolar–capillary interface and on the thickness of this membrane. Interstitial lung diseases, such as pulmonary fibrosis and sarcoidosis, which thicken the alveolar interstitium, result in a decrease in DLCO. Likewise, any disease that decreases the total area of the alveolar–capillary interface will result in a decrease in DLCO. Carbon monoxide is taken up by red blood cells, so diseases that reduce the red blood cell flow through the capillaries will affect DLCO, even in the setting of a normal alveolar–capillary interface.

Suggested readings

Morgan GE, Mikhail MS, Murray MJ. Respiratory physiology and anesthesia. In: *Clinical Anesthesiology*. 3rd ed. New York: McGraw-Hill; 2002.

Nunn JF. *Nunn's Applied Respiratory Physiology*. 4th ed. Oxford: Butterworth-Heinemann; 1993.

West JB. *Pulmonary Pathophysiology: The Essentials*. 7th ed. Philadelphia: Lippincott Williams & Wilkins; 2008.

West JB. *Respiratory Physiology: The Essentials*. 5th ed. Baltimore: Williams & Wilkins; 1995.

Oxygen and carbon dioxide transport

Swaminathan Karthik and J. Taylor Reed

This chapter focuses on the transport of oxygen and carbon dioxide at the blood and tissue level.

Oxygen transport
Hemoglobin

Hemoglobin plays a critical role in the transport of oxygen. Ninety-seven percent of oxygen is transported chemically bound to hemoglobin, and 3% is transported dissolved in the plasma.

Each hemoglobin molecule is made up of four chains. Each chain is composed of an iron-containing heme molecule and a polypeptide globin molecule. Variations in the amino acid sequence of the globin yield different hemoglobin chains, such as α, β, γ, and δ. Hemoglobin A (adult) is composed of two α- and two β-chains. Hemoglobin F (fetal) is composed of two α- and two γ-chains. Thus, each hemoglobin molecule has four iron atoms, each of which in their divalent form can bind a single molecule of oxygen. Methemoglobinemia occurs if the iron is oxidized to its trivalent form (Table 86.1). Carbon monoxide poisoning (Table 86.2) occurs when carbon monoxide binds to hemoglobin and displaces oxygen.

Diffusion gradient for oxygen

Oxygen diffuses along its concentration gradient from the alveoli, into plasma, and then into the red cells, where it is bound to hemoglobin (Table 86.3). An alveolar oxygen partial pressure of 104 mm Hg will yield a PaO_2 of about 95 mm Hg secondary to dilution with deoxygenated (shunt) blood from the thebesian and bronchial veins. Oxygen tension in interstitial fluid is around 40 mm Hg, and intracellular PO_2 averages around 23 mm Hg. This concentration gradient causes oxygen to flow into the cells.

Oxygen–hemoglobin dissociation curve

The presence of hemoglobin in blood greatly increases oxygen-carrying capacity. Hemoglobin does not take up oxygen in a linear fashion. With the binding of each successive oxygen molecule, hemoglobin's affinity for oxygen increases. This is referred to as cooperative binding. Plotting the oxygen saturation of hemoglobin against the partial pressure of oxygen yields the classic sigmoid oxygen–hemoglobin dissociation curve (Fig. 86.1). Hemoglobin can be rapidly saturated or desaturated within a narrow range of partial pressures. At a $PaO_2 >$ about 80 mm Hg, hemoglobin saturation is $> 90\%$. At venous PO_2 of about 40 mm Hg, the hemoglobin saturation tends to be around 75%. The P_{50}, or the partial pressure at which hemoglobin is 50% saturated, is 26.5 mm Hg.

Bohr effect

Peripherally, saturated hemoglobin offloads oxygen and binds CO_2 and 2,3-diphosphoglycerate (2,3-DPG). This causes conformational changes at the oxygen binding site, decreasing its affinity for oxygen, further enhancing offloading of oxygen. When desaturated hemoglobin reaches the lung, CO_2 and 2,3-DPG are released and hemoglobin's high affinity for oxygen is restored.

The four common physiologic factors that shift the oxygen–hemoglobin dissociation curve are pH, PCO_2, 2,3-DPG, and temperature. A decrease in pH or an increase in $PaCO_2$ shifts the dissociation curve to the right, facilitating delivery of oxygen to peripheral tissues; this is known as the Bohr effect. An increase in pH, or a decrease in PCO_2, shifts the curve to the left, increasing hemoglobin's affinity for oxygen. Increased temperature shifts the curve rightward, enabling greater oxygen delivery (DO_2) to peripheral tissues in times of greater metabolic need, such as during exercise. Increased 2,3-DPG causes a rightward shift and is produced over hours to days during exposure to

Table 86.1.	Causes and treatment of methemoglobinemia
• Iron in heme moiety is in the ferric (Fe^{3+}) state	
• Results in decreased affinity for oxygen and carbon dioxide	
• Caused by nitrates, nitrites, sulfonamides	
• Treatment: methylene blue (a reducing agent)	

Table 86.2.	Etiology and treatment of carbon monoxide poisoning
• Binds to hemoglobin at same site as oxygen	
• 250 times greater affinity than oxygen	
• A PaCO of 0.6 mm Hg or FiCO of 0.1% may be lethal	
• Treatment includes 100% oxygen and hyperbaric oxygen	

Fico, fraction of inspired carbon monoxide content.

Table 86.3. Partial pressures of gases in different parts of the body[a]

		Partial pressure, *mm Hg*			
	Dry air	Distal airway end inspiration	Alveolar	Arterial	Mixed venous tissue
PO_2	159.7	139.7	100	95	40
PCO_2	0.3	0.3	40	40	46
PN_2	600	573	573	573	573
PH_2O	0	47	47	47	47
Total	760	760	760	760	706[b]

[a] Conditions at sea level. Total atmospheric pressure 760 mm Hg: 21% oxygen, 78% nitrogen, small quantities of CO_2, inert gases (mostly argon, also helium). PO_2 in dry air is 159.7 (760 × 0.21).
[b] $PAO_2 = (760 - 47) × 0.21 - PACO_2/0.8)$. PO_2 decreases more than PCO_2.
$PACO_2$, partial pressure of carbon dioxide, alveolar; PAO_2, partial pressure of oxygen, alveolar; PH_2O, partial pressure of water; PN_2, partial pressure of nitrogen.

hypoxia. This is one of the compensatory mechanisms at high altitudes.

Oxygen delivery and consumption

Each gram of hemoglobin can carry 1.39 ml of oxygen. Thus, a person with a hemoglobin concentration of 15 g/dl carries 20.9 ml (15 × 1.39) of oxygen per 100 ml of blood if the hemoglobin is maximally saturated. Dissolved oxygen accounts for 0.003 ml of oxygen per mm Hg of oxygen per 100 ml of plasma. Venous hemoglobin, with a saturation of 75%, carries 15.7 ml of oxygen per 100 ml of blood. Oxygen consumption (VO_2) therefore is 5.5 ml per 100 ml of blood. Normal oxygen consumption in the resting adult human is approximately 275 ml/min.

$$\text{Content of } O_2 \text{ (CaO}_2) = \text{oxygen bound to hemoglobin}$$
$$+ \text{ oxygen dissolved in plasma}$$
$$CaO_2 = [1.39 × \text{hemoglobin (g/100ml)}$$
$$× O_2 \text{ saturation}] + [0.003 × PO_2].$$

Oxygen extraction ratio

Under normal circumstances, only 25% of oxygen delivered to peripheral tissues is extracted. This is the oxygen extraction ratio (OER); it can be calculated by the equation:

$$OER = VO_2/DO_2$$

or

$$OER = (CaO_2 - \text{mixed venous oxygen content } [CvO_2])/CaO_2.$$

When DO_2 decreases, or oxygen consumption increases, increased oxygen extraction will occur to maintain a constant VO_2 (line *CB* in Fig. 86.2). As DO_2 decreases to a critical threshold, VO_2 starts to fall linearly with falling DO_2 (line *BA* in Fig. 86.2), leading to anaerobic metabolism and an accumulation of lactate. In critically ill patients with impaired cellular respiration, this relationship is altered. Oxygen extraction appears to be impaired even when adequate DO_2 occurs. Thus, increased DO_2 is matched by increased VO_2 (line *EF* in Fig. 86.2). This reflects an oxygen debt that may respond to supranormal DO_2 and has been the basis of goal-oriented therapy.

Exercise physiology

A sixfold increase in cardiac output may occur during exercise. This, combined with a threefold increased oxygen extraction by tissues, results in an almost 20-fold increase in DO_2. Oxygen consumption in muscles is greatly increased, thus this increased DO_2 is needed to prevent lactate buildup.

Fetal oxygen transport

Fetal hemoglobin has greater affinity for oxygen and is thus left shifted compared with adult hemoglobin. This results in a P_{50} of about 19 mm Hg, which is significantly lower than adult hemoglobin. This higher affinity maintains DO_2 to the fetus. Hemoglobin concentration is around 18 mg/dl in the fetus, which allows for a higher content of oxygen to be transported.

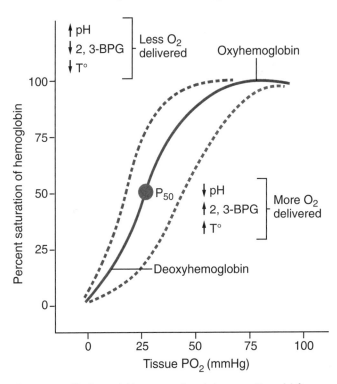

Figure 86.1. The hemoglobin–oxygen dissociation curve. Normal, left-shifted, and right-shifted curves.

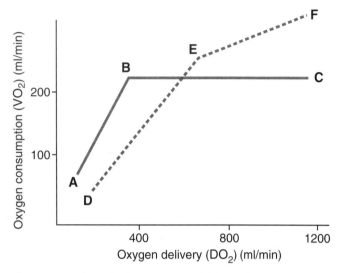

Figure 86.2. Relationship between oxygen delivery and consumption in normal humans (*ABC*) and the critically ill (*DEF*). (From Leach RM, Treacher DF. The pulmonary physician in critical care: 2. Oxygen delivery and consumption in the critically ill. *Thorax* 2002; 57:170–177.)

Mixed venous saturation

Venous PO_2 tends to be around 40 mm Hg with a hemoglobin saturation of around 75%. Venous blood returning to the heart is from three sources: the superior vena cava, the inferior vena cava, and the coronary sinus. The heart and brain have higher extraction ratios. Venous blood from these organs has a lower oxygen saturation. Complete mixing is presumed to occur in the pulmonary artery, hence this saturation is called the *mixed venous saturation*. Mixed venous saturation can be used to calculate cardiac output and shunt fraction.

The Fick principle is a form of indicator dilution that uses oxygen to determine cardiac output. Arteriovenous oxygen content difference multiplied by cardiac output is the amount of oxygen used by tissues. Assuming that a constant amount of oxygen is used by tissue every minute (VO_2), arteriovenous content difference will vary inversely with cardiac output:

Cardiac output = amount of oxygen absorbed/arteriovenous oxygen content difference

or

$$Q = VO_2/(CaO_2 - CvO_2).$$

Solving this for mixed venous oxygen saturation (SvO_2) yields this equation:

$$SvO_2 = \text{arterial oxygen saturation}$$
$$-(VO_2/Q \times 1.39 \times \text{hemoglobin} \times 10).$$

This equation ignores dissolved oxygen, which normally contributes very little to the total content of oxygen. A conversion factor of 10 is used to convert the units of hemoglobin from milligrams per deciliter to milligrams per liter. Oxygen consumption is usually assumed to be 250 ml/min or 4 ml/kg body weight. From this equation, it is clear that the four factors that influence mixed venous saturation are cardiac output, hemoglobin concentration, arterial saturation, and O_2 consumption.

Oxygen toxicity

Complex defense mechanisms have been put in place to control cellular oxygen toxicity. The antioxidant systems are developed meticulously enough that oxygen radicals in fact are being used to defend against invading offenders, such as bacterial endotoxins.

Under normal atmospheric conditions, inspired oxygen fraction can be increased only moderately by hyperventilating or by increasing inspired oxygen fraction up to 100%, as is done routinely when administering anesthesia care (i.e., pre-oxygenation, before extubation, during a single-lung situation). Although this raises the hemoglobin saturation to 100% given normal arterial/mixed venous oxygen content difference, the increase of oxygen in physical solution is almost negligible. Thus, the increase in mixed venous PaO_2 while breathing 100% oxygen is trivial. However, mixed venous PaO_2 closely reflects tissue PaO_2. Target values of oxygen tension on the mitochondrial level are still a matter of debate. Although some argue that men and women are derived from a life without oxygen and are adapted to a rather anaerobic environment in which there is a constant need to defend themselves against oxygen, the bottom line is that mitochondrial oxygen tension is probably very different in different tissues and might range from 3 to 20 mm Hg. Endothelial cells in contact with arterial blood are exposed to much higher oxygen tensions than, for example, bone marrow cells. We can assume that the range of oxygen tensions tolerated on a cellular level is rather wide.

Oxygen radicals

Superoxide radical production occurs in mitochondria through leakage of electrons to molecular oxygen as well as through activated phagocytes and within the hypoxanthine–xanthine oxidase system. Additionally, as a result of ischemia/reperfusion injury, reactive oxygen species (ROS) and reactive nitrogen species (RNS) are produced and widely distributed through the circulation. Biological targets for ROS/RNS are phagocytosed microorganisms, DNA, lipids, and sulfhydryl-containing proteins. Furthermore, ROS play an important role in cell signaling, differentiation, and apoptosis. Inappropriate activation of adherent and migrated neutrophils, however, clearly can produce harm against oneself, as suggested in the pathomechanisms of acute lung injury and other autoimmune diseases. Oxidative stress is increasingly recognized as being involved in several neurodegenerative diseases, such as Alzheimer's dementia, amyotrophic lateral sclerosis, and Parkinson's disease, as well as lipid oxidation and atherosclerosis.

Antioxidant systems

Antioxidant systems such as superoxide dismutase, catalase, the glutathione peroxidase system, and nonenzymatic endogenous antioxidants such as ascorbic acid, vitamin E, and surfactant act as radical scavengers but also protect the integrity of proteins and cell membranes. Their existence allows the sophisticated use of ROS to maintain the organism's integrity. Statins show great promise as regulators of ROS production by reducing NADPH oxidase activity, thus reducing nitric oxide scavenging and causing not only vascular dilation but also inhibition of leukocyte adherence and hence overall immunoregulatory effects. Antioxidants have been trialed as adjuvant therapeutics to adversely affect the impact of oxidative stress such as aging, cardiovascular disease, and cancer. Most nonenzymatic antioxidants can be perceived as a double edged sword because of their potential to act as pro-oxidants in an environment that combines oxygen with metals that may serve as redox-active transition metals (i.e., Fe^{2+}). This antiredox paradox may explain why large doses of supplemental antioxidants so far have failed to significantly alter life expectancy.

Clinical oxygen toxicity

Pulmonary oxygen toxicity has been appreciated for quite some time. Lung tissue is at the forefront of high inspired oxygen fractions. Airway inflammation and reduced vital capacity are known sequelae of breathing high inspired oxygen fractions for 24 hours. Structural changes leading to acute lung injury and pulmonary fibrosis representing irreversible changes of lung function and architecture are predominant in prolonged exposure to normobaric oxygen breathing. Elevated PaO_2 is of more predictive value than fraction of inspired oxygen content (FiO_2). A PaO_2 level of 255 mm Hg has been established as safe.

Reabsorption atelectasis is another pulmonary complication of 100% oxygen breathing, albeit much better established and defined. Lung zones with low ventilation–perfusion ratios collapse only a few minutes after breathing 100% oxygen. This is a frequent occurrence in daily anesthetic practice and remains well established for the induction phase, because preoxygenation and denitrogenization heighten the safety margin when apnea is induced and assisted ventilation commences. Whether the routine increase of FiO_2 to 100% before extubation is necessary or even harmful for reasons stated earlier (why induce atelectasis right before the transition is made from controlled mechanical positive pressure ventilation to spontaneous respiration in a patient at the beginning of recovery from surgery with all the insults to breathing taken together: diaphragmatic dysfunction, decreased functional residual capacity from anesthetic agents, supine position, opioid use, pain, etc.) is being questioned.

Finally, patient factors must be considered as well. The exposure to bleomycin renders a patient susceptible to oxygen-induced pulmonary fibrosis, respiratory failure, and even death when subsequently exposed to high inspired fraction of oxygen. Although the molecular mechanism remains elusive, clinical practice has been not only to limit FiO_2, but also to use intravenous fluids more judiciously, as this is another proposed factor supporting the development of acute lung injury and respiratory failure after bleomycin therapy.

Retrolental fibroplasia

Retrolental fibroplasia still puzzles providers caring for newborns. Initially recognized as a likely result of uncritically generous exposure of newborns to high inspiratory oxygen fractions, it remains the leading cause of blindness and vision impairment in children, even after adjustment of the neonatal resuscitation guidelines and the revelation that in newborns, treating hypoxia is just as critical as avoiding hyperoxia.

Benefits of increased perioperative FiO_2

Increased inspired oxygen tensions at normal atmospheric pressure are usually well tolerated in adults under anesthesia. Recent studies suggest improved outcome with regard to wound infections, partially based on the finding that PaO_2 plays a much more vital role in wound healing than hemoglobin-bound oxygen, because the microvasculature is disrupted and the diffusion-driving force is partial pressure gradient. In conjunction with the avoidance of vasoconstriction and its prerequisites, such as pain, hypothermia, and shock, tissue oxygenation can be optimized without a clinically relevant negative impact of intra- and postoperative delivery of FiO_2 in the range of 80%.

Carbon dioxide transport

Carbon dioxide is produced by the various tissues of the body as a waste product of metabolism. It is a nonpolar molecule that diffuses easily through lipid membranes and, as a result, can travel through the mitochondrial membrane, cytosol, cell membrane, extracellular space, and endothelium until it reaches the plasma. Once in the plasma, it travels in one of three forms: dissolved in plasma, converted to bicarbonate, or as a carbamino compound.

Dissolved in plasma

The solubility of carbon dioxide is 0.075 ml CO_2/dl/mm Hg. When the venous PCO_2 is 45 mm Hg, the amount of dissolved CO_2 is 3.4 ml/dl. This accounts for roughly 9% of all carbon dioxide produced in the body, but can increase to nearly one third of the total amount during strenuous exercise. CO_2 is much too insoluble to be completely eliminated from the body in its unaltered state.

Conversion to bicarbonate by carbonic anhydrase

Once in the bloodstream, carbon dioxide diffuses through the red cell membrane, where it comes in contact with free floating carbonic anhydrase (CA). CA rapidly catalyzes the reaction:

$$\overset{CA}{CO_2 \leftrightarrow H_2CO_3 \leftrightarrow HCO_{3_-} + H^+}.$$

Carbonic acid, the immediate product of this reaction, spontaneously and rapidly dissociates into bicarbonate and a proton. Although CO_2 undergoes this reaction spontaneously, CA greatly accelerates the reaction. CA is well placed in the red blood cell cytosol as hemoglobin buffers the hydrogen ion produced with little change in body pH.

Role of the Bohr effect on CO_2 transport

The affinity of hemoglobin for hydrogen ions is not constant. This is fundamentally important in shuttling carbon dioxide from the periphery to the lung. The Bohr effect (mentioned earlier) refers to the inverse relationship of oxygen and hydrogen ion affinity for hemoglobin. When oxygen dissociates from hemoglobin, the dissociation constant (pK_a) of specific amino acids is increased, causing a greater propensity for hydrogen ions to bind. This favors the transformation of CO_2 to bicarbonate and H^+. This system is driven entirely by the relative concentrations of oxygen and hydrogen ions in the different areas of the body. In the lungs, the concentration of oxygen is high and the concentration of hydrogen ions is low because of the elimination of carbon dioxide. This promotes oxygen binding to hemoglobin and release of hydrogen ions, driving CO_2 formation and elimination. In the tissues, where CO_2 concentration is high because of metabolism, hydrogen ions are created and bound to hemoglobin, and oxygen is released.

Chloride (Hamburger) shift

As bicarbonate is continually being produced in the red cell, bicarbonate levels increase in the cytosol. A transport protein in the red cell membrane rapidly exchanges chloride ions from the plasma for bicarbonate ions. This feature of bicarbonate homeostasis has been termed the *chloride shift*. It prevents progressive intracellular alkalosis while maintaining electrical neutrality.

Carbamino compound formation

Carbon dioxide binds to amino groups on plasma proteins and hemoglobin to form carbamino compounds. The protein concentration in plasma is around 7%. The hemoglobin concentration in the red blood cell is around 30%; therefore, this type of transport is more prevalent inside the red blood cell. Carbamino compound formation accounts for the transport of 5% of the carbon dioxide in arterial blood but 30% of the carbon dioxide taken up in the capillaries.

When a carbamino compound forms, a hydrogen ion is released:

$$R^-NH_2 + CO_2 \leftrightarrow R^-NH^-COO^- + H^+.$$

This hydrogen ion is immediately buffered by the imidazole groups of histidine residues on hemoglobin and on plasma proteins. Once in the lung, O_2 association causes a conformational change that releases H^+ and drives the reaction toward the release of CO_2 from the amino groups.

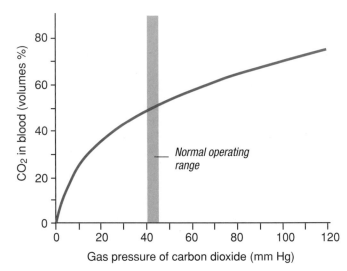

Figure 86.3. Carbon dioxide dissociation curve. The relationship between PCO_2 and total CO_2 content.

Carbon dioxide content versus carbon dioxide tension

Carbon dioxide in the dissolved form varies linearly with its partial pressure in the blood, whereas the total quantity of CO_2 in the blood is graphically illustrated as a flattened hyperbola (Fig. 86.3). In the physiologic range, this relationship is almost linear.

Haldane effect

The Haldane effect describes the relationship between the transport species of carbon dioxide and the binding of oxygen to

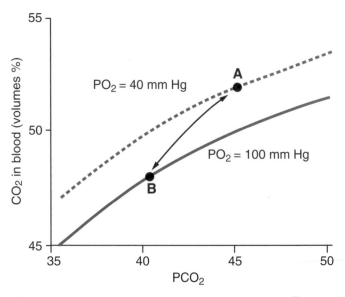

Figure 86.4. Carbon dioxide dissociation curve and the Haldane effect (shift from **A** to **B**). (From Guyton AC, Hall JE. Transport of oxygen and carbon dioxide in the blood and body fluids. In: *Textbook of Medical Physiology*. 10th ed. Philadelphia; 2000:472.)

hemoglobin. Binding of oxygen displaces CO_2 via changes in pK_a of the hemoglobin amino acids. Hydrogen ions bound to hemoglobin are released, favoring release of CO_2 from carbamino compounds. The CO_2 then diffuses down the concentration gradient into the alveoli and is subsequently eliminated via respiration (Fig. 86.4).

Suggested readings

Albert R, Spiro S, Jett J. *Comprehensive Respiratory Medicine.* Philadelphia: Mosby; 2002.

Dempsey JA, Wagner PD. Exercise-induced arterial hypoxemia. *J Appl Physiol* 1999; 87:1997.

Geers C, Gros G: Carbon dioxide transport and carbonic anhydrase in blood and muscle. *Physiol Rev* 2000; 80:681.

Guyton AC, Hall JE. Transport of oxygen and carbon dioxide in the blood and body fluids. In: *Textbook of Medical Physiology.* 10th ed. Philadelphia: Saunders; 2000.

Henry RP, Swenson ER. The distribution and physiological significance of carbonic anhydrase in vertebrate gas exchange organs. *Respir Physiol* 2000; 121:1.

Jones AM, Koppo K, Burnley M. Effects of prior exercise on metabolic and gas exchange responses to exercise. *Sports Med* 2003; 33: 949.

Leach RM, Treacher DF. The pulmonary physician in critical care: 2. Oxygen delivery and consumption in the critically ill. *Thorax* 2002; 57:170–177.

Nikinmaa M. Membrane transport and control of hemoglobin-oxygen affinity in nucleated erythrocytes. *Physiol Rev* 72:301, 1992.

Piiper J. Perfusion, diffusion and their heterogeneities limiting blood-tissue O2 transfer in muscle. *Acta Physiol Scand* 2000; 168:603.

Richardson RS. Oxygen transport and utilization: an integration of the muscle systems. *Adv Physiol Educ* 2003; 27:183.

Roy TK, Popel AS. Theoretical predictions of end-capillary Po2 in muscles of athletic and nonathletic animals at Vo2max. *Am J Physiol* 1996; 271:H721.

Tsai AG, Johnson PC, Intaglietta M. Oxygen gradients in the microcirculation. *Physiol Rev* 2003; 83:933.

Wagner PD. Diffusive resistance to O2 transport in muscle. *Acta Physiol Scand* 2000; 168:609.

West JB. *Pulmonary Physiology and Pathophysiology: An Integrated, Case-Based Approach.* Philadelphia: Lippincott Williams & Wilkins; 2001.

West JB. *Pulmonary Physiology: The Essentials.* Baltimore: Lippincott Williams & Wilkins; 2003.

Wilson WC, Benumof JL. Respiratory physiology and respiratory function during anesthesia. In: *Miller's Anesthesia.* 6th ed. Philadelphia: Churchill Livingstone; 2005.

Lung isolation techniques

Shine Sun and Sarah H. Wiser

The anesthetic management of intrathoracic procedures and the care of critically ill patients who require differential lung ventilation necessitate facility with lung isolation techniques. In its most basic form, the goal of lung isolation is either to selectively interrupt ventilation to a section of the pulmonary tissue or to prevent soilage of the contralateral lung. Isolation may involve a portion of lung, as in lobar isolation, or an entire lung. Familiarity with the tools and techniques of lung isolation is essential. Equally important is the ability to quickly troubleshoot each technique and to know when circumstances favor one technique over another. This chapter focuses on the techniques used for lung isolation and the basic physiology of one-lung ventilation (OLV). Ventilatory settings and management of hypoxemia during OLV are considered in detail in the next chapter.

Indications for lung isolation

The indications for lung isolation are divided into absolute and relative indications (Table 87.1). This designation is somewhat artificial as some surgical procedures, although considered a relative indication, would be difficult if not impossible to perform without lung isolation.

Contraindications

Although no specific contraindications exist, it is important to be mindful of the clinical situation instead of applying a

Table 87.1. Indications for OLV

Absolute
Isolation of lungs to prevent spillage from hemorrhage or infection
Therapeutic need to ventilate only one lung
   Bronchopleural fistula
   Unilateral cysts or bullae
   Unilateral bronchial disruption or trauma
Unilateral lung lavage
Video-assisted thoracoscopic surgery

Relative
Surgical exposure: high priority
   Thoracic aortic aneurysm
   Pneumonectomy
   Upper lobectomy
Surgical exposure: lower priority
   Esophageal surgery
   Middle and lower lobectomies
   Thoracoscopy under general anesthesia

"one size fits all" technique. For example, the use of a left-sided double-lumen tube (DLT) in the setting of an exophytic tumor involving the left mainstem bronchus is not recommended. The decision as to whether lung isolation is necessary and the selection of technique should be intimately tied to the clinical situation.

Anatomy

A basic understanding of the normal tracheobronchial anatomy is essential for successful lung isolation. Often a surgical bronchoscopy is performed at the beginning of a thoracic surgical procedure. This presents an opportunity for the anesthesia practitioner to become familiar with the patient's anatomy. This familiarity is crucial to verify correct placement of the lung isolation device chosen. It has been demonstrated that anesthesiologists with only occasional lung isolation experience malposition the device 40% of the time, despite facility with fiber-optic bronchoscopy and a prior tutorial on lung isolation.

Normal anatomic features in the adult are as follows: The distance from the teeth to the carina averages 20 to 25 cm. From the carina, the left mainstem bronchus continues at a 45° angle before reaching its secondary carina. On average, the left mainstem bronchus is 54 mm long in men and 50 mm in women. The secondary carina of the left mainstem bronchus marks the division of the upper and lower lobar bronchi. Segmental anatomy is depicted in Fig. 87.1. It is important to realize that significant variability exists at the segmental level.

The right mainstem bronchus branches from the carina at a 10° angle and travels, on average, only 19 mm in men and 16 mm in women before dividing into the right upper lobe bronchus and the bronchus intermedius. Classically, the right upper lobe bronchus trifurcates almost immediately, creating what is often referred to as the "Mercedes-Benz" sign. In approximately one in 250 people, a variant known as a tracheal or "pig" bronchus may be present. In this instance, the right upper lobe arises directly from the trachea instead of the right mainstem bronchus. The length of the right mainstem bronchus is an important characteristic and should be noted during bronchoscopy, as a short right mainstem may make lung isolation with a right-sided tube more difficult. Distally, the bronchus intermedius gives rise to the middle and lower lobe bronchi and their respective segmental bronchi.

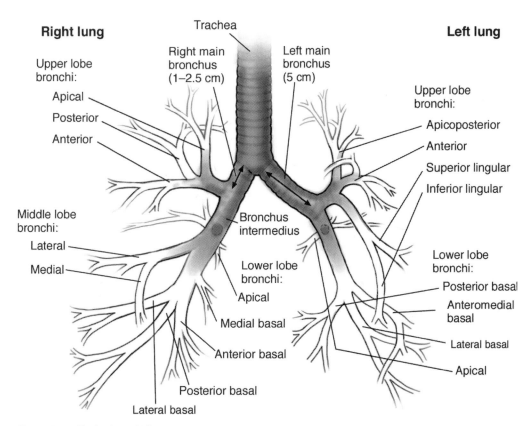

Figure 87.1. Tracheobronchial tree anatomy.

Lung isolation tools
Double-lumen tubes

The most common tool for lung isolation is the DLT. Although it has been through many variations since its initial introduction into clinical use by Carlens 50 years ago, the DLT still retains the basic structure. A DLT consists of two ventilating lumens bound together into one tubular structure. Each lumen, tracheal and bronchial, has a cuff to provide a seal. The bronchial lumen is longer, to allow endobronchial intubation, and its cuff is high pressure/low volume. The tracheal lumen ends above the carina and uses a low-pressure/high-volume cuff (Fig. 87.2).

The proximal take-off from the right mainstem bronchus mandates sidedness in the design of DLTs. The right-sided DLT has a ventilating side port in the endobronchial lumen to allow ventilation of the right upper lobe (Fig. 87.3).

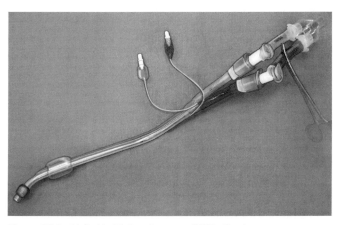

Figure 87.2. A left-sided Robertshaw-type DLT by Rusch.

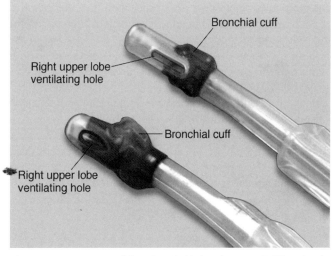

Figure 87.3. Two views of the right-sided Robertshaw-type DLT from Rusch and Mallinkrodt. (Adapted from www.anaesthesiauk.com.)

537

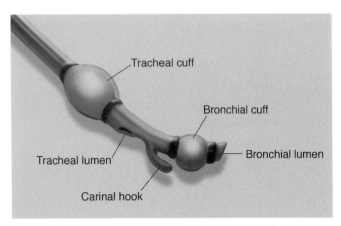

Figure 87.4. Left-sided Carlens double-lumen ETT with carinal hook. (Adapted from Zadrobilek E, Fitzal S. The Robertshaw double-lumen bronchial tubes: fortieth anniversary of the first published description. *Internet J Airway Manag 2* 2002–2003. Available at: http://www.adair.at/ijam/volume02/historicalnote03/default.htm.)

DLT size	35F	37F	39F	41F
Female	≤ 5'1″	5'2″–5'11″	≥ 6'	–
Male	–	≥ 5'5″	5'6″–5"11″	≥ 6'

Table 87.2. Rough DLT sizing guide based on patient height

The presence of a carinal hook, designed to prevent distal migration of the entire tube, is particular to the Carlens type DLT (Fig. 87.4).

Although the carinal hook may help prevent distal migration of the endotracheal tube (ETT), its presence also poses a risk for airway trauma, resulting in tracheobronchial disruption due to "catching" of the hook on tissues other than the carina. Furthermore, the carinal hook can make placement of the DLT through the glottis more difficult.

DLT sizes currently available depend on the manufacturer, but they typically include pediatric (26F, 28F) and adult (35F, 37F, 39F, 41F) sizes. The French catheter gauge size is equal to the external diameter of the DLT in millimeters multiplied by three. For example, a 39F DLT has a total diameter of 13 mm.

Size selection

Proper size selection of the DLT is important to provide good lung isolation while causing minimal trauma to the airway. A correctly sized DLT is one that (a) passes atraumatically through the glottic opening, down the trachea, and into the intended mainstem bronchus; (b) has good alignment of lumens with the appropriate bronchi for ventilation; and (c) provides a good seal at both the tracheal and bronchial cuffs. Despite the obvious importance in proper sizing, there is no consensus as to how to choose the best size. Studies have attempted to correlate DLT size selection with patient criteria including gender and height, left mainstem bronchus size or tracheal diameter on chest radiographs, and left mainstem bronchus measurement on CT scans. There still is no universally accepted method for determining DLT size preoperatively. Many centers choose to use patient height and gender as a guideline for initial DLT size selection. Included here is a rough guide for initial size selection based on patient gender and height (Table 87.2).

Placement

The placement of right- and left-sided DLTs is similar. The tube is packaged with a stylet in the endobronchial lumen to facilitate

placement. The stylet should not be removed, and care should be taken to prevent it from protruding beyond the end of the DLT. Direct laryngoscopy is performed to allow for visualization of the glottis. A Mac blade is preferred, as it provides a greater space in the laryngopharynx for manipulation of the DLT. The DLT is held with the bronchial lumen curved superiorly. The tube is advanced under direct visualization until the bronchial cuff disappears past the vocal cords. At this point, the endobronchial stylet should be removed. Advancement of the DLT with the stylet in place increases the risk of tracheal disruption. The DLT is then rotated toward the desired side of endobronchial intubation and advanced until gentle resistance is felt. The tracheal cuff should now be inflated. The presence of end-tidal CO_2 verifies placement in the airway.

The DLT should not be forced, and stiff resistance should not be "pushed through." Occasionally, it is difficult to advance the DLT once passed through the glottis. This issue can be managed by rotating the DLT 180° toward the desired mainstem bronchus. This directs the tip of the DLT toward the membranous portion of the trachea. If continued resistance occurs, it is advisable to place a fiber-optic bronchoscope through the bronchial lumen and position the DLT under direct visualization. Fiber-optic placement of DLT should be performed for any patient who has an endobronchial mass or extrinsic airway compression. Generally speaking, there should be a low threshold to abandon DLT placement in favor of an alternate plan. The inability to place a DLT may be a result of the patient's inherent anatomy. Tracheal disruption, carinal dislocation, and endobronchial rupture or hemorrhage may occur with DLT placement.

If the initial intubation proved difficult, and a DLT is necessary, a tube exchange catheter may be used to place the DLT. The exchange catheter is placed through the single-lumen tube (SLT) to an average depth of 22 cm. The patient's oropharynx is suctioned, the SLT is removed, and the DLT is threaded over the exchange catheter via the endobronchial lumen and advanced into the airway. Laryngoscopy helps suspend the soft tissues of the oropharynx, promoting passage of the DLT. During placement of the DLT, it is important not to allow the catheter to advance too deeply, as this may cause airway trauma. Bronchoscopy is then used for definitive positioning of the DLT.

Confirmation of placement

Before the widespread availability of fiber-optic bronchoscopes, differential inflation of cuffs and auscultation were the standard for confirmation of correct DLT placement. Although auscultation is rarely used as the primary confirmation technique now, it may be used if fiber-optic equipment is not available. With both

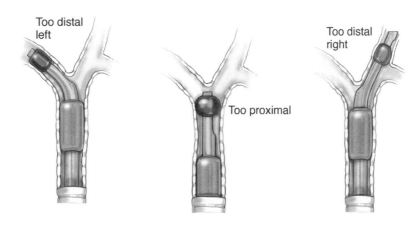

	If DLT is too distal left:	If DLT is too proximal:	If DLT is too distal right:
Action:	**Breath Sounds Heard**	**Breath Sounds Heard**	**Breath Sounds Heard**
Clamp right, both cuffs inflated	Left side only	Left and right	Right side only
Clamp left, both cuffs inflated	None or faint on either side	None or faint on either side	None or faint on either side
Clamp left, deflate distal cuff	Left side only	Left and right	Right side only

Figure 87.5. Types of malposition of the DLT and techniques for identification with auscultation.

cuffs inflated, ventilation of the endobronchial lumen should result in breath sounds only on the endobronchial side. Ventilation of the tracheal lumen should result in breath sounds only in the contralateral lung field. Gross malposition of DLTs can be identified by lung auscultation during differential clamping and balloon inflation, as illustrated in Fig. 87.5.

Multiple studies have demonstrated that auscultation alone is largely insufficient for the confirmation of proper DLT placement. Anywhere from 30% to 80% of DLTs originally confirmed by auscultation are actually malpositioned when evaluated by bronchoscopy. Therefore, fiber-optic bronchoscopy is considered the gold standard for confirmation of DLT placement.

When evaluating DLT positioning by bronchoscopy, one should have a systematic approach. For both left and right DLTs, bronchoscopy through the tracheal lumen should reveal the carina with the bronchial cuff only minimally visible from the orifice of the desired mainstem bronchus (Fig. 87.6a,b). Passing the fiber-optic scope through the endobronchial lumen of a left-sided DLT should reveal the secondary carina (Fig. 87.6c). If these lobar bronchi (which should be roughly equal in size) are not both visible, the endobronchial lumen may be too deep. Bronchoscopy through the endobronchial lumen of a

right-sided DLT should reveal the ventilating side port lined up with the orifice of the right upper lobe and the bronchus intermedius (Fig. 87.6d).

If the location of the DLT is uncertain by initial bronchoscopy, repositioning of the tube under fiber-optic guidance is most expeditious. The bronchoscope is placed down the endobronchial lumen until it emerges from the end of the tube. Both cuffs are deflated, and positive pressure ventilation is suspended. The DLT and bronchoscope are withdrawn as a unit until visualization of the carina is obtained. At this point, the bronchoscope is advanced down the desired mainstem bronchus, and the DLT is advanced over the bronchoscope. This will seat the endobronchial lumen into the desired bronchus. Bronchoscopy via the tracheal lumen will then confirm correct placement and allow for adjustment of the endobronchial portion of the tube.

Fiber-optic confirmation of DLT positioning should be performed after initial placement and following any alteration in patient positioning. Additionally, intraoperative evaluation of DLT positioning may be required, as the tube may become dislodged secondary to external manipulation from the surgical field.

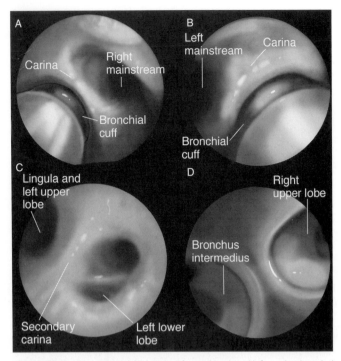

Figure 87.6. Views via bronchoscopy of properly placed left- and right-sided DLTs. (**A**) View through the tracheal lumen of a left DLT in proper position, with the carina visible and the endobronchial cuff barely visible alongside. (**B**) View through the tracheal lumen of a right DLT in proper position, with the carina visible and the endobronchial cuff barely visible alongside. (**C**) View through the endobronchial lumen of a properly seated left DLT with the secondary carina, left upper lobe bronchus, and left lower lobe bronchus visible. (**D**) View through the endobronchial lumen of a properly seated right DLT with the right upper lobe visible through the Murphy eye in the bronchial cuff and the bronchus intermedius visible through the distal hole. (**A** and **C** adapted from Slinger P. http://www.thoracic-anesthesia.com/wp-content/uploads/buffalo-lung-isol-507.pdf; **B** ahd **D** adapted from Campos JH, et al. Devices for lung isolation used by anesthesiologists with limited thoracic experience. *Anesthesiology* 2006; 104:261–266.)

Advantages

DLTs provide excellent lung isolation capabilities. DLTs compare favorably with other lung isolation techniques in a variety of ways. The large internal diameters allow for more laminar airflow patterns and quicker deflation of lung parenchyma. Additionally, the larger lumens facilitate (1) passage of suction catheters for clearance of secretions, (2) application of continuous positive airway pressure (CPAP) to the operative lung in cases in which persistent desaturation occurs during OLV, and (3) passage of a pediatric fiber-optic bronchoscope to directly observe bronchial clamping and suturing, thereby guiding surgical technique.

Disadvantages

Overinflation of the endobronchial cuff may lead to mucosal ischemia. When lung isolation is no longer necessary, it is prudent to deflate the endobronchial cuff to minimize the time of direct pressure on the endobronchial mucosa. If postsurgical pulmonary toilet or evaluation of anastomotic lines is required, bronchoscopy by an adult bronchoscope is best used.

The adult bronchoscope has a larger suctioning lumen and better fiber-optics. The need to use an adult bronchoscope necessitates removal of the DLT for an 8.0 or larger SLT.

Patient comfort for extubation may also be a determining factor for reintubation with an SLT prior to emergence. The large external diameter of the DLT combined with its placement distal to the carina makes the DLT more stimulating for emergence. The smaller lumens also may make breathing more difficult, which may result in coughing, wheezing, and ventilator dyssynchrony.

In cases in which airway edema is a concern, a DLT may be left in place until it is deemed safe to convert to an SLT. The decision to leave a DLT in place postoperatively should be weighed against the risk of mucosal injury, the relative unfamiliarity of intensive care unit personnel with DLTs, and the risk of inadvertent dislodgement of the tube. Typically, in experienced hands, the DLT can be changed safely to an SLT with the use of a tube changer.

Because the DLT is widely used for lung isolation, its large size, relatively rigid construction, and lack of customizability (beyond sidedness and size/length) sometimes preclude its use as the lung isolation technique for a given patient or procedure. In difficult airway situations, extubation from the initially placed SLT may be ill advised. In addition, congenital or surgical anatomic variants may preclude use of a DLT, which relies on relatively conserved anatomic parameters. In these situations, bronchial blockers provide more flexibility for lung isolation.

Bronchial blockers

Bronchial blockers are the other main category of lung isolation tools. There are several variants, including stand-alone devices or those bound to an SLT, but they are conceptually the same. The basic construction of the bronchial blocker consists of a small-diameter catheter with an inflatable occlusive balloon at its distal end. The blocker can be guided via fiber-optic bronchoscopy into the desired location for lung or lobar isolation. Because bronchial blockers must be used in conjunction with an SLT, the blocker can be removed or disabled, allowing for postoperative mechanical ventilation without the necessity for a tube change. The Fogarty catheter, Arndt and Cohen bronchial blockers (Cook Medical, Bloomington, IN), and Univent tube (Fuji Systems Corp., Tokyo, Japan) all fall into this category of lung isolation technology.

Fogarty catheter

The Fogarty embolectomy catheter, although not created for airway use, may be used to provide lung isolation. It has a long track record of use in thoracic procedures, both as a primary lung isolation device and as a rescue device for inadequately functioning DLTs. Commonly employed sizes include 8/14F or 8/22F; both catheters are 80 cm long. The numbers 14 and 22 refer to the inflated balloon diameter in millimeters. The balloons on the Fogarty catheter are low volume/high pressure. Given the ability of the balloon to withstand high pressure without rupture, it is critical to inflate the balloon under direct vision to avoid airway rupture. The catheter itself is made of natural rubber latex and contains a central wire stylet. There is no central communicating lumen from the proximal end to the distal tip.

Placement

Placing a 45° bend in the wire stylet 3 cm from the tip facilitates placement. One of two techniques then may be performed to avoid an air leak around the catheter: (1) During laryngoscopy, the catheter can be placed in the proximal trachea and then an SLT placed alongside the Fogarty catheter, or (2) after intubation with an SLT, a swivel connector with a rubber diaphragm attached to the 15-mm connector of the SLT will allow passage of the embolectomy catheter within the SLT while maintaining ventilation. Proper positioning of the Fogarty catheter requires fiber-optic bronchoscopy. Under direct vision with a bronchoscope, the distal end is directed toward the desired bronchus while the catheter is advanced. Once positioned, the balloon at the distal end should be inflated to create a seal.

Advantages

Fogarty catheters are widely available, and many anesthesiologists have experience with their use for lung isolation. They may be used in a variety of situations, such as with an SLT, through a tracheostomy, nasotracheally, or alongside/inside a DLT. The catheter can be manipulated to provide selective lobar blockade. A Fogarty catheter may be placed within a DLT to rescue a poorly functioning or an ill-fitting DLT.

Disadvantages

Fogarty catheters may be quite difficult to place. Other disadvantages include (1) latex composition, precluding their use in patients with a latex allergy; (2) lack of any guidewire system to help position the balloon tip; (3) lack of a central lumen to allow for delivery of CPAP or suctioning of the distal airway; (4) reliance on absorption atelectasis for lung collapse after placement, and (5) easy dislodgement during positioning and surgical manipulation.

Univent tube

The Univent tube is constructed of medical-grade silicone. It is an SLT with a separate channel fused along the anterior concave surface that houses a sliding bronchial blocker (Fig. 87.7).

The blocker of the Univent tube incorporates a high-pressure/low-volume cuff. The blocker itself slides within the side channel and can be guided into the left, right, or secondary bronchi with the aid of a fiber-optic bronchoscope. It is important to note that even though the insertion of a Univent tube is akin to the placement of a standard SLT, the outer diameter is markedly larger than that of a comparably sized standard ETT. The increased external diameter is the result of the fused channel, which houses the bronchial blocker. The internal diameters of Univent tubes range from 6.0 to 9.0 mm. An 8.0 Univent tube has an external diameter of 13.5 mm.

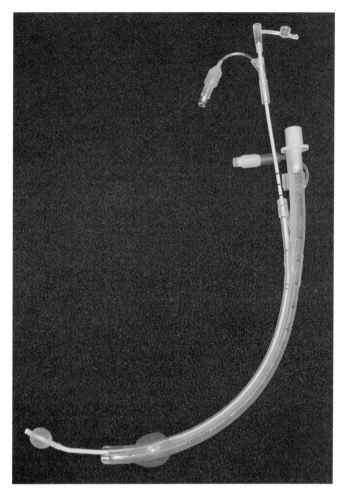

Figure 87.7. A Univent tube.

Placement

Prior to placement, the bronchial blocker should be lubricated to facilitate passage through its channel. The blocker should then be completely retracted into its channel to prevent tracheal trauma. The Univent tube is then placed like a normal SLT into the trachea. The blocker is then guided into place under bronchoscopic visualization. The blocker will preferentially head to the right mainstem bronchus. To facilitate passage into the left mainstem bronchus, the entire Univent tube can be turned 90° to the patient's left so that the inherent curvature in the tube directs the blocker to the left. In lieu of moving the entire Univent tube, the bronchial blocker alone can be twisted to turn the distal tip toward the left. Rotation of the patient's head to the left also helps facilitate this placement. A final option for left-sided blockade is to advance the Univent under fiber-optic guidance so that the tip of the ETT enters the left mainstem bronchus. The bronchial blocker can then be advanced further into the left, and the SLT portion can be withdrawn back into the trachea while the blocker is held in place.

Advantages

Advantages include the ability to convert the Univent tube into a "standard" SLT without replacing the ETT, the ability to provide both CPAP and suction through the small port located within the bronchial blocker, the less bulky nature of the tube relative to a DLT, and the feasibility of its use for fiber-optic intubations in the setting of a difficult airway.

Disadvantages

Unfortunately, even with fiber-optic guidance, placement of the Univent's bronchial blocker may be difficult. Although the small central lumen allows for intermittent application of suction to facilitate lung decompression, deflation still may be a slow process. The high-pressure cuff on the blocker may lead to mucosal ischemia with prolonged use. Last, the larger anterior–posterior outer diameter, created by the separate channel fused to the SLT, has been suggested as a potential source of postoperative vocal cord damage and paresis; therefore, the Univent is not recommended for prolonged postoperative intubation.

Arndt bronchial blocker

The Arndt bronchial blocker is a wire-guided endobronchial blocker, specifically designed as a stand-alone bronchial blocker for bronchial or lobar isolation. It is packaged as a unit including the blocker itself, a multiport connector, a CPAP adapter, and a syringe. The multiport connector is designed to fit onto the 15-mm connector of the ETT. It has a separate port for the fiber-optic bronchoscope, the blocker itself, and connection to the breathing circuit. The blocker port has a Luer-Lok system to allow for ventilation with minimal air leak while the blocker is in place (Fig. 87.8).

The Arndt comes in 5F/50-cm, 7F/65-cm, and 9F/78-cm size configurations, for use with minimum ETT sizes of 4.5, 7.0, and 8.0, respectively. All Arndt blockers are equipped with low-pressure/high-volume cuffs. Integral to the Arndt is a replaceable central flexible nylon wire protruding from the distal end as a loop, which when removed leaves a 1.4-mm lumen.

Placement

Placement of the Arndt bronchial blocker starts with the placement of the bronchoscope and blocker through their respective ports of the multiport adapter. Once the bronchoscope is fed through the wire loop and the loop is cinched tight, the multiport adapter can be connected to the ETT. The bronchoscope is then advanced into the targeted airway for occlusion, and the Arndt is slid off the bronchoscope. If the catheter encounters resistance during advancement, the most likely source is the carina. Repositioning the wire loop at the very tip of the bronchoscope may resolve this problem. Additionally, turning the patient's head contralateral to the desired side also facilitates placement. Once the blocker is in the desired location, the balloon can be inflated under direct vision.

Advantages

The wire is removable, which leaves behind a 1.4-mm central lumen to be used for the provision of CPAP or for suctioning to aid deflation. Akin to the Fogarty catheter, the Arndt shares the

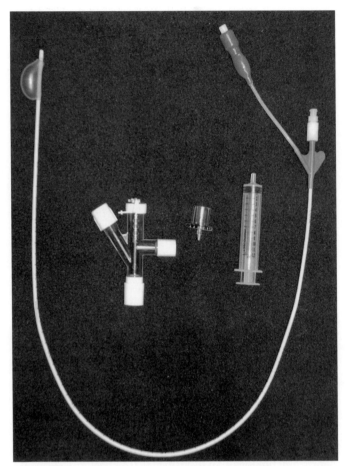

Figure 87.8. An Arndt endobronchial blocker.

characteristics of being deployable in a variety of airway situations, as a DLT rescue device, and also may be used for selective lobar blockade.

Disadvantages

As with all other bronchial blocker devices, the Arndt bronchial blocker suffers from the occasional difficulty of obtaining adequate isolation on the right side (given the proximal origin of the right upper lobe), easy dislodgement during manipulation or patient positioning, slow deflation time, and its difficulty of use in ETTs with an internal diameter smaller than 7.0 mm.

Cohen bronchial blocker

The Cohen bronchial blocker is a relatively new bronchial blocker, approved by the US Food and Drug Administration in 2005 for use in lung isolation and available from Cook Medical, Bloomington, IN. It currently is supplied only in a 9F-circumference/62-cm length size, with a 1.6-mm central lumen and a spherical balloon at the distal end. It performs the same job as the other bronchial blockers but is unique mainly in the method used to control and direct placement.

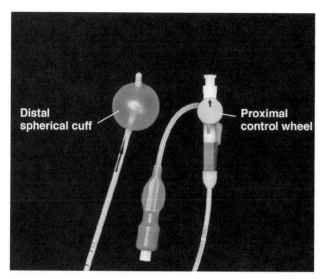

Figure 87.9. A Cohen endobronchial blocker.

Placement

Instead of a wire loop or bend at the distal end of the blocker, the Cohen blocker has a control wheel on the proximal end for bronchial placement (Fig. 87.9).

This control wheel allows a user to turn the distal tip of the catheter toward the desired bronchus. The wheel can be turned counterclockwise only, and the distal tip follows the direction of the wheel. Unfortunately, the movement arc of the distal tip is confined to 90°. The advantages and disadvantages of the Cohen blocker are similar to those of other bronchial blockers. A specific disadvantage may be that the fine motor control needed to manipulate the wheel necessitates two skilled operators for placement: one to operate the bronchoscope and one to steer the blocker.

Fuji bronchial blocker

The manufacturers of the Univent tube have also released the bronchial blocker portion of the Univent as a stand-alone blocker unit, dubbed the Fuji Uniblocker. The Fuji is similar in function, advantages, and disadvantages to the other bronchial blockers discussed. Its unique features include its composition of silicone, the presence of a preformed Coudé tip at the distal end, and the largest central lumen of all the blockers at 2.0 mm. The Fuji blocker currently comes in only one size (9F diameter/51 cm length).

Other options

Centers that routinely perform operations requiring lung isolation will have the tools described earlier readily available. Occasionally, however, lung isolation must be provided in the absence of specialized equipment. It is important to remember that it is possible to advance a single-lumen ETT into the mainstem bronchus, which may provide lung isolation on an emergent basis. Blindly done, the ETT will preferentially favor the

right mainstem bronchus. If it is necessary to continue ventilating the left lung instead, advancement of the ETT can be done by turning the ETT to the left so that the original curvature of the tube angles toward the left. Bronchoscopy can greatly facilitate selective mainstem intubation.

One-lung physiology

Familiarity with the techniques to attain lung isolation is a powerful tool in the anesthesiologist's armamentarium. Equally, if not more important, is an understanding of the physiologic consequences of the lateral decubitus position and OLV.

Lateral decubitus position

The lateral decubitus position is the standard position for pulmonary resection. This position affects both perfusion and ventilation, thereby affecting ventilation–perfusion (V/Q) matching.

Perfusion

Perfusion is directly influenced by gravity. Lateral positioning increases blood flow to the dependent lung by about 10% and decreases flow to the nondependent lung proportionally. Typical redistributions of blood flow with lateral positioning are detailed in Table 87.3. This redistribution of pulmonary blood flow is not altered by the induction of anesthesia or paralysis.

Ventilation

Unlike perfusion, the effect of lateral positioning on ventilation depends on whether the patient is awake, anesthetized, paralyzed, or has an open chest.

Lateral position, awake and spontaneously breathing, closed chest

In a spontaneously breathing, laterally positioned patient with a closed chest, the V/Q ratio is preserved relatively close to 1. On assuming the lateral position, the compliance of the different lung zone changes. The lung is now oriented from superior to inferior (nondependent to dependent) rather than apex to base, but the standard gravitational effect on lung compliance (Fig. 87.10) remains the same. Because the dependent lung is located on the steep portion of the compliance curve, it receives greater ventilation with each breath than the nondependent lung. The combination of greater perfusion of the dependent lung and greater ventilation there as well leads to minimal V/Q mismatch.

Table 87.3. Typical effect of lateral positioning on pulmonary perfusion

Position	Change in perfusion to right lung, %	Change in perfusion to left lung, %
Right lateral decubitus	55 to > 65	45 to > 35
Left lateral decubitus	55 to > 45	45 to > 55

Awake–closed chest

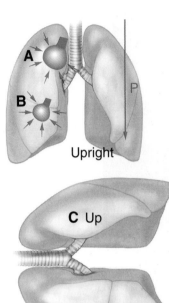

Figure 87.10. Minimal compliance changes in overall lung on assuming the lateral decubitus position. (Adapted from Morgan GE, et al. Anesthesia for thoracic surgery. In: *Clinical Anesthesiology.* New York: Lange Medical Books; 2006:585–613.)

Lateral, anesthetized, spontaneous ventilation, closed chest

Induction of anesthesia leads to a decrease in functional residual capacity. This reduction in lung volume causes a downward shift in the compliance curve for both the dependent and the nondependent lungs. The dependent lung will shift from the steep to the less compliant (horizontal) portion of the curve, and the nondependent lung will shift to the more favorable (steep) portion of the compliance curve (Fig. 87.11). Ventilation will now be greater to the nondependent lung. As a result, V/Q mismatch will increase.

Lateral, anesthetized, paralyzed, mechanical ventilation, closed chest

The introduction of muscle paralysis and mechanical ventilation further increases V/Q mismatch. The weight of the abdominal contents, mediastinum, and chest wall restricts the dependent lung, functionally decreasing its compliance and shifting ventilation to the nondependent lung. Stabilizing devices such as bolsters or bean bags compound this problem. Perfusion remains unchanged.

Lateral, anesthetized, paralyzed, mechanical ventilation, open chest

Opening of the chest wall decreases the confines of the nondependent lung, further increasing ventilation to that lung. The dependent lung remains restricted. Given that the nondependent lung was already receiving proportionately more ventilation than perfusion in the closed chest, opening the operative hemithorax serves only to worsen the V/Q mismatch.

Physiology of OLV

The changes in perfusion and ventilation discussed earlier are independent of lung isolation. Isolation of the operative lung introduces a large right-to-left intrapulmonary shunt. The mixing of deoxygenated with oxygenated blood widens the alveolar–arterial oxygen gradient and manifests as hypoxemia. In addition, shunt and V/Q mismatch exist in the dependent

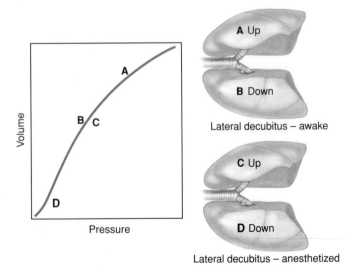

Figure 87.11. Compliance shifts in the lateral decubitus position from awake to anesthetized states. (Adapted from Morgan GE, et al. Anesthesia for thoracic surgery. In: *Clinical Anesthesiology.* New York: Lange Medical Books; 2006:585–613.)

lung secondary to atelectasis and parenchymal disease, further impairing gas exchange.

As mentioned earlier, gravitational forces partially redistribute blood flow away from the operative lung. The remaining shunt is further decreased by hypoxic pulmonary vasoconstriction (HPV). HPV acts as a protective mechanism to diminish blood flow to areas of alveolar hypoxia via pulmonary arteriolar vasoconstriction. HPV can decrease the shunt fraction by 50% and reaches its maximum effect within 15 minutes, reducing a typical 40% shunt fraction to approximately 20%. This shunt is still large enough to cause significant hypoxemia. The fact that many patients tolerate OLV well is likely indicative of chronic redistribution of blood flow away from the diseased lung, which ultimately results in a much lower overall shunt fraction.

Various physiologic and pharmacologic agents may act on the pulmonary vasculature to alter the effects of HPV. Elevated pulmonary artery pressures due to increased airway pressures, hypoxia in the ventilated lung, hypercarbia, heart failure, or preexisting pulmonary hypertension may diminish the effects of HPV. Extremely low pulmonary artery pressures also may hinder HPV if part of the dependent lung exhibits West zone I physiology, in which alveolar pressure exceeds pulmonary artery pressure. Alkalosis globally inhibits HPV, and acidosis globally accentuates it.

Pharmacologic agents may affect the efficiency of HPV. Inhalation agents have been shown to inhibit HPV in in vitro studies; however, in vivo studies have been conflicting at best. Clinically, the overall effect on HPV is felt to be insignificant in the doses used in the operating room. Vasodilating agents such as nitroglycerin, nitroprusside, dobutamine, calcium channel blockers, and hydralazine can hinder HPV. Vasoconstricting agents, if they increase the dependent lung pulmonary artery pressure, may lead to increased perfusion of the operative lung, which will increase the shunt fraction. This, however, may be offset by increased cardiac output, increased mixed venous oxygen saturation, and decreased zone 1 conditions in the dependent lung. Almitrine, a respiratory stimulant, augments HPV at lower doses and improves oxygenation. It is not available clinically in the United States.

Suggested readings

Alliaume B, et al. Reliability of auscultation in positioning of double-lumen endobronchial tubes. *Can J Anesth* 1992; 39: 687–690.

Campos JH. Lung separation techniques. In: Kaplan JA, Slinger PD, eds. *Thoracic Anesthesia*. 3rd ed. Philadelphia: Churchill Livingstone; 2003:159–173.

Campos JH. An update on bronchial blockers during lung separation techniques in adults. *Anesth Analg* 2003; 97:1266–1274.

Campos JH, et al. Devices for lung isolation used by anesthesiologists with limited thoracic experience. *Anesthesiology* 2006; 104:261–266.

Campos JH. Which device should be considered the best for lung isolation: double-lumen endotracheal tube versus bronchial blocker. *Curr Opin Anaesthesiol* 2007; 20:27–31.

Campos JH. Current techniques for perioperative lung isolation in adults. *Anesthesiology* 2002; 97:1295–1301.

Chang PJ, et al. Estimation of the depth of left-sided double-lumen endobronchial tube placement using preoperative chest radiographs. *Acta Anaesthesiol Sin* 2002; 40:25–29.

Chow MY, et al. Predicting the depth of insertion of left-sided double-lumen endobronchial tubes. *J Cardiothorac Vasc Anesth* 2002; 16:456–458.

Cohen E, Neustein SM, Eisenkraft JB. Anesthesia for thoracic surgery. In: Barash PG, ed. *Clinical Anesthesia*. 5th ed. Philadelphia: Lippincott Williams & Wilkins; 2006:813–855.

Farber NE, Pagel PS, Warltier DC. Pulmonary pharmacology. In: Miller RD, ed. *Miller's Anesthesia*. 6th ed. Philadelphia: Elsevier Churchill Livingstone; 2005:155–189.

Ginsberg RJ. New technique for one-lung anesthesia using an endobronchial blocker. *J Thorac Cardiovasc Surg* 1981; 82:542–546.

Gothard J, Kelleher A, Haxby E. Anaesthesia for thoracic surgery. In: *Cardiovascular and Thoracic Anesthesia*. London: Elsevier; 2003:128–143.

Mirzabeigi E, Johnson C, Ternian A. One-lung anesthesia update. *Sem Cardiothorac Vasc Anesth*. 2005; 9:213–226.

Morgan GE, et al. Anesthesia for thoracic surgery. In: *Clinical Anesthesiology*. New York: Lange Medical Books; 2006:585–613.

Neustein SM. Use and limitations of the Cohen endobronchial blocker. *J Clin Anesthes* 2006; 18:400–401.

Slinger P. Lung isolation in thoracic anesthesia, state of the art. *Can J Anesth* 2001; 48:R1–R10.

Wilson WC, Benumof JL. Respiratory physiology and respiratory function during anesthesia. In: Miller RD, ed. *Miller's Anesthesia*. 6th ed. Philadelphia: Elsevier Churchill Livingstone; 2005:679–722.

Wilson WC, Benumof JL. Anesthesia for thoracic surgery. In: Miller RD, ed. *Miller's Anesthesia*. 6th ed. Philadelphia: Elsevier Churchill Livingstone; 2005:1847–1939.

Zadrobilek E, Fitzal S. The Robertshaw double-lumen bronchial tubes: fortieth anniversary of the first published description. *Internet J Airway Manag 2* 2002–2003. Available at: http://www.adair.at/ijam/volume02/historicalnote03/default.htm.

Anesthetic management for pulmonary resection

Sarah H. Wiser and Philip M. Hartigan

Introduction

Pulmonary resection may be performed for a variety of malignant and nonmalignant indications. Broad generalizations can be made based on the specific lesion being resected (Table 88.1), but anesthetic management is largely dictated by the surgical approach, the anticipated extent of resection, and the patient's pathophysiology. Lobectomy is considered here as an archetype for management of pulmonary resection in general. Special considerations for pneumonectomy and for patients with severe lung disease are also discussed. In this broad practical review, emphasis is placed on information germane to anesthetic management.

Lung cancer is now the leading source of cancer-related deaths in North America. In the United States, more than 160,000 deaths from lung cancer occurred in 2008. Without surgery, 5-year survival from lung cancer remains stubbornly fixed at 10% to 15%. Pulmonary resection for lung cancer therefore is considered semi-elective.

Immediate preoperative evaluation

The formal preoperative evaluation generally takes place days to weeks prior to surgery. On the day of surgery, interval changes in health status should be sought, with particular attention paid to pulmonary symptoms (e.g., wheezing, sputum production, dyspnea). Unlike with nonthoracic surgery, the most frequent serious postoperative complications are respiratory in nature (atelectasis, pneumonia, respiratory failure). An experienced pulmonary surgical program should be able to select operable candidates based on published criteria. Risk modification may be accomplished by minor postponements to gain control of acute exacerbations of bronchospasm or significant infections. Malignant pleural effusions may increase in the interval between the preoperative imaging and the day of surgery, and in extreme cases, thoracentesis prior to induction can reduce risk. Cardiac disease is prevalent in this population composed largely of smokers, and interval changes in cardiac status should also be sought. Prior to entering the operating room, the team should have the clearest possible picture of the following:

- The surgical plan, including the best guess at the extent of incision

- The maximum tolerable extent of resection based on respiratory mechanics, cardiopulmonary reserve, and lung parenchymal function
- The plan for lung isolation and postoperative pain control
- The side of surgery, based on radiographic data consistent with written and verbal communications and consents involving surgeon and patient

Assessment of the maximum tolerable extent of resection is an evolving, imprecise science. Most surgeons place the most stock in the predicted postoperative forced expiratory volume in 1 second (ppoFEV$_1$). ppoFEV$_1$ is the preoperative FEV$_1$ proportionally reduced by the amount of proposed lung resection, and can be calculated as follows: ppoFEV$_1$ = preoperative FEV$_1$ [1 − (% functional lung tissue to be removed/100)]. The number of segments removed can be estimated by the location and extent of resection (Fig. 88.1). If ventilation–perfusion scans are available, this can be estimated with greater precision. Lung parenchymal function is assessed by diffusing capacity of lung for carbon monoxide (D$_{LCO}$) or arterial blood gas assessments of gas exchange (PO$_2$, PCO$_2$). Cardiopulmonary reserve is estimated from oxygen consumption (MVO$_2$), exercise tolerance, or extent of desaturation during exertion. Patients are at high risk for postoperative respiratory failure if the extent

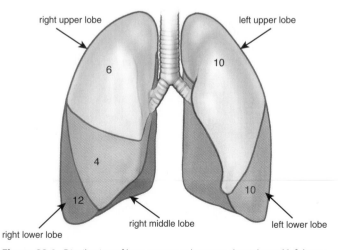

Figure 88.1. Distribution of lung segments between the right and left lungs.

Table 88.1. Anesthetic considerations for pulmonary resection for various lesions

Lesion type	Associated considerations
Squamous cell	Central lesions (predominantly) Mass effects (obstruction, cavitation, compression) Hypercalcemia
Adenocarcinoma	Peripheral lesions Distant metastases Growth hormone, corticotrophin Hypertrophic osteoarthropathy
Small cell	Central lesions (predominantly) Paraneoplastic syndromes Eaton-Lambert (myasthenic) syndrome Proximal limb weakness, improved with activity Increased sensitivity to depolarizing and nondepolarizing relaxants Poor response to anticholinesterases Fast growth rate and early metastases Rarely resectable at diagnosis
Carcinoid	Proximal, intrabronchial lesions Often misdiagnosed as asthma Carcinoid syndrome (rare) (see Table 88.3) "Benign," slow growth rate Prone to bleeding Potentially obstructive, with possible postobstructive pneumonia
Mesothelioma	Pleural based Direct extension to pericardium, diaphragm Often with associated effusion Difficult dissection associated with significant intraoperative hemorrhage Extrapleural pneumonectomy at risk for cardiac arrhythmias, compression effects, cardiac herniation Pleurectomy associated with large postoperative air leak
Thymectomy	Mediastinal location Potential mass effect, but rarely significant Associated with myasthenia gravis Weakness exacerbated by activity Destruction of acetylcholine receptors at neuromuscular junction Clinical behavior depends on state of treatment with anticholinesterases Undertreatment = myasthenic crisis Overtreatment = cholinergic crisis Generally resistant to succinylcholine and highly sensitive to nondepolarizing muscle relaxants Consider preoperative plasmapheresis
Lung volume Reduction surgery/bullectomy	Severe emphysema High risk for air trapping during OLV High risk for dynamic hyperinflation and volutrauma/pneumothorax High risk for hypercapnia High risk for postoperative respiratory failure
Lung abscess	Risk of cross-contamination of contralateral lung
Empyema	Potential septic physiology
Decortication	Potential for hemorrhage
Arteriovenous malformation	Congenital or acquired from trauma, surgery, portal hypertension, schistosomiasis Usually connects pulmonary arteries and veins (right-to-left shunt) Rarely between bronchial arteries and pulmonary veins (left-to-right shunt) Risk of embolic events, stroke, hemorrhage Associated with hereditary hemorrhagic telangiectasias Potential difficulty with one-lung oxygenation (esp. if bilateral arteriovenous malformations)

Lung cysts/bullae	Congenital
	Bronchogenic cysts
	Congenital cystic adenomatoid malformation
	Pulmonary sequestration
	Congenital lobar emphysema
	    Acquired
	    Bullous emphysema
	    Pulmonary hydatid cysts
	    Pneumatocele
	    Potential for mass effects
	    Potential for cross-contamination or septic physiology from infected cysts
	    Potential to trap air during positive pressure ventilation if they communicate with the airway
	    Risk of postoperative air leaks

Adapted from Slinger PD, Johnston MR. Preoperative evaluation of the thoracic surgery patient. In: Kaplan JA, Slinger PD, eds. *Thoracic Anesthesia*. 3rd ed. Philadelphia: Churchill Livingstone; 2003:15.

Table 88.2. Factors associated with desaturation during one-lung ventilation

High proportion of pulmonary perfusion to the operative lung
Low PaO_2 during two-lung ventilation
Significant pathology of the nonoperative lung (pneumonia, prior resection, effusion, edema, restrictive disease, etc.)
Normal or increased ratio of FEV_1/FVC
Right-sided surgery
Supine position

Adapted from Slinger PD, Johnston MR. Preoperative evaluation of the thoracic surgery patient. In: Kaplan JA, Slinger PD, eds. *Thoracic Anesthesia*. 3rd ed. Philadelphia: Churchill Livingstone; 2003:19.

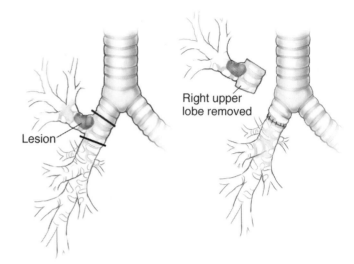

Figure 88.2. Right upper lobe sleeve resection.

of resection would leave them with a ppoFEV$_1$ < 30% of predicted, or if their lung function and cardiopulmonary reserve are significantly limited relative to the proposed amount of resection.

Anesthetic management of pulmonary resection patients needs to consider the anatomic and physiologic effects of the tumor and any associated treatment. Tumors of the chest may effect anesthetic management through mass effects or through metabolic or paraneoplastic effects (Table 88.1). Chemotherapy may leave patients with impaired renal function (cisplatin) or at increased risk of oxygen toxicity (bleomycin). Distorted or anomalous tracheobronchial anatomy may alter the plan for lung isolation. Factors that have been associated with desaturation during one-lung anesthesia are listed in Table 88.2. The most powerful predictor of intolerance of one-lung ventilation (OLV) is a proportionately high perfusion of the operative lung. Prior ipsilateral chest surgery will increase the likelihood of extending a minimally invasive incision because of the presence of adhesions.

Anesthesia for lobectomy and lesser resections

Introduction

Non–small cell lung cancers (NSCLCs; large cell, squamous cell, and adenocarcinomas) are the most common indication for pulmonary resection. Lobectomy is the currently accepted treatment for resectable (stage I–IIIa) NSCLC. Segmentectomy entails the anatomic dissection and excision of sublobar segments of lung, whereas wedge resection implies nonanatomic excision. Segmentectomy or wedge resection may be performed for diagnosis of a nodule, for therapy for very small lesions, or for patients who would not tolerate a lobectomy. Such parenchymal-sparing resections for malignant pulmonary lesions are controversial, although they increasingly are being employed. Sleeve lobectomy entails removal of a portion of the mainstem bronchus along with the lobe, followed by reattachment of the uninvolved lobe(s) (Fig. 88.2). Sleeve lobectomy and right-sided bi-lobectomy are parenchymal-sparing alternatives to pneumonectomy for patients in whom a simple lobectomy would fail to yield clean proximal margins.

Guiding and goals of anesthetic care for lobectomy and lesser resections include obtaining lung isolation, satisfactory one-lung gas exchange, avoidance of lung injury, hemodynamic stability, control of bronchospasm and secretions, rapid emergence and extubation, and excellent pain control. Early extubation with pain control that allows for deep breathing, effective coughing, and early ambulation is considered important to reduce pulmonary complications. High-quality lung isolation is instrumental to the surgeon's ability to visualize and operate through minimally invasive incisions.

Surgical approaches

The traditional posterolateral thoracotomy provides excellent access to the lung and hilum but involves an extensive incision; division of serratus anterior, latissimus dorsi, and intercostal muscles; and possibly resection of portions of the fifth or sixth rib. Increasingly, full posterolateral thoracotomy is reserved for excision of extensive masses or difficult dissections. Video and stapling instrument technology has enabled most resections to be performed via limited muscle-sparing thoracotomy or video-assisted thoracoscopic approaches. Video-assisted thoracoscopic surgery (VATS) generally entails the placement of three ports for the camera and instruments in a triangular pattern (Fig. 88.3). One "utility port" is often extended, as needed, to remove the specimen or to perform operative tasks. Therefore, the extent of the surgical incision varies from porthole to mini-thoracotomy, and may evolve over the course of the surgery as difficulties are encountered. The extent of pain and recovery are only loosely related to the extent of incision, possibly reflecting the influence of other variables, including retraction, intercostal nerve injury, and anesthetic care. Anterior thoracotomy, sternotomy, or clamshell incisions (bilateral anterior thoracotomies with transverse sternotomy) occasionally are used for anterior, mediastinal, or bilateral surgeries, and would entail supine or semi-supine positions.

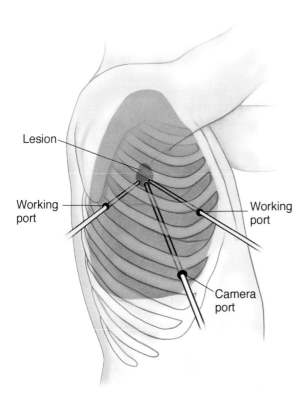

Figure 88.3. Thoracoscopic port placement with triangulation of the lesion of interest.

Preparation for induction

Although most pulmonary resections involve limited blood loss, the potential for major bleeding from hilar vessels must be considered. Invasive arterial blood pressure monitoring is indicated prior to high-risk inductions (see later), for sicker patients, and for more extensive or central surgery. Placement of thoracic epidural catheters and the extent of intravenous (IV) access and invasive hemodynamic monitoring are dictated by the anticipated extent of the surgical trespass and the physiologic fragility of the patient. Radiographic data, history of prior chest surgery (ipsilateral adhesions), and communication with the surgeon help define the risk of significant bleeding or the likelihood that a VATS approach will be extended to a thoracotomy.

Premedication is dictated by the clinical scenario. Sedation, as always, should be tailored to the needs and reserves of the patient. Inhaled bronchodilator treatments given in the immediate preoperative period are advocated for patients with a history of bronchospasm.

Epidural decisions

Thoracic epidural analgesia (TEA) is the most widely used means of controlling postthoracotomy pain. Compared with parenteral opiates, TEA is superior for control of the dynamic pain associated with deep breathing and coughing, and for the preservation of lung function by spirometry. Evidence suggests that many pulmonary and cardiac complications, and possibly chronic postthoracotomy pain, are reduced by effective perioperative epidural pain control. TEA is generally not necessary for lesser resections performed through very limited VATS approaches. The indication for TEA is intermediate for more complicated VATS resections. Generally, any lobectomy (including VATS) requires at least a mini-thoracotomy just to remove the specimen, and the technical challenge of segmentectomy often warrants larger utility ports. Because the extent of the incision may be uncertain upfront, the preoperative decision to place a thoracic epidural catheter may be challenging. One approach is to place epidurals in all patients undergoing pulmonary resection, except those undergoing straightforward wedge resection. TEA should also be considered in the physiologically fragile patient, even when undergoing wedge resection. The usual contraindications for epidural catheters would apply (e.g., coagulopathy, patient refusal, overlying infection).

Not uncommonly, the extent of incision or resection may change intraoperatively in a patient without an epidural. Such patients may be allowed to emerge with reasonable comfort for immediate postoperative awake epidural placement by using intercostal nerve blocks combined with moderate narcotic analgesia. Although not without controversy, a compelling argument has been made that the risk/benefit ratio of TEA placement in the anesthetized patient is unfavorable in adult patients.

Special monitoring considerations for thoracic surgery

Left-sided thoracic procedures preclude formal diagnostic placement of electrocardiographic (ECG) leads. Moreover, the mediastinal shift, which occurs with an open chest and lateral decubitus position, alters the position of the heart relative to the chest wall, potentially further reducing ECG sensitivity to ischemia. Arterial catheters are widely used whenever OLV is prolonged or tenuous, or when hemodynamic management dictates. Central venous pressure (CVP) measurements may be confounded by the open pneumothorax or surgical manipulations and should be followed for trends as opposed to absolute numbers. A central venous line is often primarily indicated for patients with significant cardiac disease, for resuscitation in patients with poor peripheral intravenous access, or for postoperative management. Pulmonary artery (PA) catheters may be problematic during thoracic surgery. If the catheter tip is positioned in the atelectatic lung, both pressure and cardiac output measurements will be unreliable. There also is risk of the catheter getting caught in the surgical staple line. PA catheters are reserved for management of significant pulmonary hypertension or severe cardiac valvular disease. Transesophageal echocardiography may be a superior intraoperative monitor for such situations. The experienced thoracic anesthesiologist will pay close attention to capnogram waveform and lung compliance changes as indicators of the degree of obstruction and early warning signs of tube malposition, accumulating secretions, or developing bronchospasm. Modern anesthesia machines offer continuous spirometry, which also may be very helpful in recognizing changing lung or airway function.

Special induction considerations for thoracic surgery

Aside from the usual considerations for induction (e.g., drug effects, aspiration, a secure airway), four issues deserve special consideration in thoracic patients: (1) bronchospasm, (2) air trapping, (3) mass effects on cardiac output, and (4) mass effects on airway patency. These issues are described as follows:

1. *Bronchospasm.* Smoking and chronic obstructive pulmonary disease (COPD), both of which are highly prevalent in thoracic patients, predispose to airway hyperreactivity. Airway manipulation at induction may be a potent trigger of bronchospasm in predisposed patients. Among the many strategies that have been proposed to circumvent this, adequate depth of anesthesia at the time of airway instrumentation is the most important. Narcotics and inhalational anesthetics have advantages over histamine-releasing agents. Preemptive bronchodilator treatments were mentioned earlier. The theoretic risk of β-adrenergic–blocking drugs is often overstated, and if indicated for cardiac reasons, such drugs should not generally be withheld for fear of bronchospasm. Recent upper respiratory infections or exacerbations of COPD should be under control for 2 weeks prior to surgery, if possible.

2. *Air trapping.* Expiratory flow limitation in patients with obstructive lung disease mandates long expiratory times to prevent air trapping, or auto-positive end-expiratory pressure (auto-PEEP). Failure to remember this during induction may result in sufficient auto-PEEP to cause hemodynamic instability or barotrauma. Patients with bullous emphysema or severe COPD ($FEV_1 < 40\%$ predicted) are particularly prone. Tension pneumothorax and cardiac arrest have been reported with induction of such patients. Bronchospasm, mass-induced dynamic airway obstruction, and the resistance of long, narrow endotracheal tubes (such as double-lumen tubes [DLTs]) also predispose to auto-PEEP.

3. *Mass effect on cardiac output.* Occasionally, thoracic tumors or effusions may affect cardiac output through their mass effect within the thorax. The supine position, induction of general anesthesia, and initiation of positive pressure ventilation may enhance this mechanism. Impaired venous return due to increased intrathoracic pressure, or impaired diastolic filling of the heart due to a tamponade-like effect of a mass or effusion, will be exacerbated by the reduction in functional residual capacity (FRC) associated with anesthesia, as well as the transition from negative to positive pressure ventilation. Preinduction review of the chest CT is important in evaluating the potential effects of a large mass situated anterior to or compressing the heart or great vessels. Preoperative symptoms of positional dyspnea or lightheadedness may be clues. Preemptive vasopressors, careful choice of induction agents, positional adjustments, and fluid loading generally succeed in defending venous return and cardiac output during induction. Superior vena cava (SVC) compression, evident from CT scans or the signs of SVC syndrome, mandates a lower-extremity IV line prior to induction and may require cautious airway manipulation secondary to venous congestion of the head. Patients with large, positionally symptomatic anterior mediastinal masses are at increased risk and are discussed more thoroughly in Chapter 91.

4. *Mass effect on airway patency.* The FRC reduction imposed by the supine position and induction of anesthesia translates to a reduction in the caliber of major airways. Extrinsic compression, or intrinsic obstruction, of airways by masses is thus exacerbated by induction and may result in total obstruction of major airways.

Lung isolation decisions

Many institutions prefer left-sided DLTs (L-DLTs) for most lobectomies or lesser resections of either side. If a left-sided pneumonectomy or sleeve resection is contemplated, the L-DLT may need to be withdrawn somewhat. The potential for disruption of the stump or anastomosis by the L-DLT is not trivial. Therefore, right-sided DLTs are recommended as a preferred option, anatomy permitting. The initial bronchoscopic examination by the surgeon to evaluate or rule out endobronchial pathology is an opportunity for the anesthesiologist to evaluate the anatomy and form a definitive plan for lung isolation. A bronchial blocker placed in the left mainstem will also work well for left pneumonectomies, but must be withdrawn at the time of bronchial cross-clamp to avoid being caught in the staple line. Pros and cons of the different lung isolation options are discussed in the previous chapter.

Positioning

Full lateral decubitus position is used for the vast majority of lung resections (Fig. 88.4). Vulnerable pressure points include the hips, shoulders, ears, and eyes. The neck should be maintained in axial alignment with the spine, using soft padding to support the head, with the ears and eyes protected. An axillary roll is traditionally positioned just below the dependent axilla to offload pressure from the head of the humerus on the neurovascular bundle. The nondependent arm must be supported with attention to avoid stress to the brachial plexus. Tape across the hip theoretically may cause a pressure necrosis of the femoral neck if too tight. The dependent leg is bent, and stabilizers (bolsters or beanbag system) are arranged to prevent anterior or posterior movement. Flexion of the table aids surgical access by widening the spaces between the ribs.

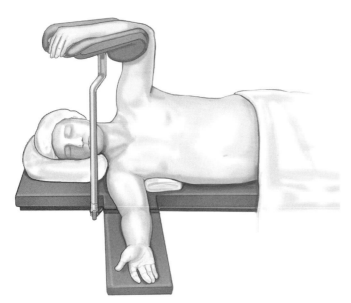

Figure 88.4. Lateral decubitus position.

Choice of anesthetics

No acknowledged "best" anesthetic regimen for thoracic surgery exists. Advocates of inhalation agent–based techniques cite their convenience, ease of titration, and bronchodilating properties. Potential disadvantages are that all current inhalational agents inhibit hypoxic pulmonary vasoconstriction (HPV) and depend on the lungs for their elimination. Despite HPV inhibition in vitro, volatile anesthetics exhibit minimal effects on oxygenation during OLV when used in clinically relevant dosages (<1.5 minimum alveolar concentration). Moreover, excluding enflurane, there is no significant difference among agents with regard to OLV at comparable concentrations. Delayed or unpredictable elimination may occur because of the accumulation of inhalational agents within poorly ventilated lung units. Moreover, end-tidal agent levels may not reflect the presence of such "reservoirs" of agent.

Total IV anesthesia (TIVA) agents (usually propofol plus a short-acting narcotic) do not inhibit HPV and do not rely on the lungs for elimination. Elimination is not confounded by severe obstructive lung disease but may be delayed in prolonged cases if propofol doses accumulate, or if there is liver disease.

Operative events with anesthetic management implications

Incision is an opportunity to assess anesthetic depth, and entry into the chest allows the anesthesiologist to directly view the quality of lung isolation and collapse. If the lung is inflated and ventilating, the tube/blocker position is incorrect or the bronchial cuff is underinflated or ruptured. If the lung is inflated but not ventilating, the delayed collapse may be the result of adhesions, poor elastic recoil (emphysema), secretions, or malposition of the DLT. The inflation of the bronchial cuff should be reassessed, and a bronchoscope should be passed to confirm

tube position, suction secretions, and suction air from the operative lung. Patients with a severely reduced FEV_1 will have very slow collapse, and suctioning will have little beneficial effect because of the principle of flow limitation. If a blocker rather than a DLT was used, the onset of atelectasis may be somewhat delayed. The application of suction to the operative bronchus during apnea with the cuff deflated may encourage air egress in this situation. Insufflation of CO_2 into the chest under pressure to encourage lung collapse generally is not recommended because of the potential for a tension pneumothorax and hemodynamic compromise. Physically compressing the chest with surgical instruments may sometimes improve operative conditions. High-quality atelectasis may be instrumental to the success of a minimally invasive approach.

Often, surgeons must digitally palpate the lung to locate target nodules. When performed through thoracoscopic ports, this may sometimes be a challenge. Occasionally, a Valsalva maneuver to the dependent lung will raise the mediastinum and operative lung to allow the surgeon to reach and locate the nodule, thus avoiding extension of the incision. Evacuation of the stomach with an orogastric tube may also be helpful in allowing the diaphragm to move more caudally, giving the surgeon more room to maneuver. Manipulation of the tumor rarely may result in the release of vasoactive substances, such as with carcinoid tumors (Table 88.3).

The cross-clamping of vessels for lobectomies and lesser resections generally has little impact on hemodynamics, but the field should be observed at this time for bleeding. Stapling instruments have been known to misfire, resulting in incomplete division of vessels. Division of the lobar bronchus during lobectomy is also performed with a stapling instrument. Surgeons may request a bronchoscopic evaluation or a brief reexpansion of the remaining lobe(s) during cross-clamping, but prior to firing the staples, to assure that only the target lobe is within the staple line. Following removal of the specimen, many surgeons request a "leak test." With saline in the chest cavity,

Table 88.3. Carcinoid syndrome

Signs and symptoms	Mediators	Treatment
Cutaneous flushing	Serotonin	Octreotide (somatostatin
Bronchospasm	Histamine	analogue)
Hypotension	Dopamine	Avoid adrenergic stimulation
Hypertension	Substance P	Avoid sympathomimetics
Valvular heart disease	Neurotensin	Avoid tumor manipulation
Diarrhea, nausea, vomiting	Prostaglandins	Less effective agents:
Abdominal pain	Kallikrein	Histamine H_1 and H_2
Hyperglycemia		antagonists
Hypoalbuminemia		Corticosteroids
Pellagra		Glucagon
		5-HT receptor antagonists
		α-Methyldopa

5-HT, selective serotonin 5-hydroxy tryptamine.
Adapted from Hartigan PM. Pulmonary resection. In: Kaplan JA, Slinger PD, eds. *Thoracic Anesthesia.* 3rd ed. Philadelphia: Churchill Livingstone; 2003:238.

such that the staple line is submerged, a brief period of positive pressure (< 30 cm H_2O) is delivered to the operative lung, and the stump is observed for bubbles.

Prior to chest closure, effective recruitment of the remaining lung to maximally obliterate the intrathoracic space is important, but care should be taken not to injure the remaining lung or "blow" open the lobar stump (or parenchymal staple line in the case of a wedge resection). Experience and extrapolation of intensive care unit (ICU) data suggest that exceeding 40 cm H_2O may be imprudent. Less than 30 cm H_2O is widely considered acceptable, but some patients may have tenuous staple lines or more delicate tissue. A bronchoscopic cleanout of secretions may allow more effective recruitment at lower pressures. Following recruitment and chest closure, two-lung ventilation should be resumed at volumes that account for the amount of remaining lung. Chest tubes should be placed on suction for the remainder of the case, unless a pneumonectomy was performed (see later).

Pathophysiology of OLV

Tight matching of pulmonary ventilation (V) and perfusion (Q) is essential for efficient gas exchange. V/Q relationships during typical pulmonary resection surgery are severely disrupted by OLV, the lateral decubitus position, an open pneumothorax, positive pressure ventilation, general anesthesia, paralysis, and underlying lung disease. These factors lead to shunt in the nondependent and dependent lungs, as well as V/Q mismatch in the dependent lung. PaO_2 (at a fraction of inspired oxygen content [FiO_2] = 1.0) in this scenario typically falls from the 400–mm Hg range to approximately 150 mm Hg. On average, nondependent lung blood flow (nondependent lung shunt) is reduced from 45% to 55% to approximately 20% of cardiac output, principally because of gravity and HPV. Shunt occurs in the dependent lung as a result of atelectasis imposed by the weight of the mediastinum, the upward pressure of the dependent hemidiaphragm, and the restrictive forces of the table and anterior/posterior stabilizers. Additional V/Q mismatch occurs in the dependent lung as a result of intrinsic parenchymal disease or disruptions in pulmonary blood flow or ventilation (e.g., DLT malposition, secretions, bronchospasm, inhibitors of HPV).

Hypoxemia during OLV

The reported incidence of hypoxemia during OLV has decreased from $> 20\%$ in the 1970s to $< 1\%$ currently because of improved DLT designs, bronchoscopic positioning of DLTs, and improved understanding of the physiology of OLV. Actions to minimize shunt in the dependent and nondependent lungs are the principal maneuvers to address hypoxemia during OLV, whereas V/Q mismatch due to parenchymal disease is more difficult to manipulate. Treatment of hypoxemia should be individualized based on the most likely cause(s) and the context of the surgery (Table 88.4). An FiO_2 of 1.0 should be assured. If the desaturation is abrupt or severe, reinflation of the

Table 88.4. Treatment of hypoxemia during OLV

Confirm $FiO_2 = 1.0$
Bronchoscopy to rule out obstruction/malposition
Temporary reinflation of operative lung
Recruitment maneuver to nonoperative lung
CPAP to operative lung
PEEP to nonoperative lung
Cross-clamp of pulmonary artery, or branch thereof

nondependent lung should be performed in coordination with the surgeon. If time permits, bronchoscopy should be performed to rule out tube malposition or obstructions from secretions, blood, kinks, and so on. PEEP delivered to the dependent lung may help by combating shunt in that lung, particularly in patients prone to atelectasis (see "Optimal PEEP"). Continuous positive airway pressure (CPAP; 2–5 cm H_2O) delivered to the nondependent lung generally improves oxygenation but may partially reinflate the operative lung. During a thoracotomy, this may be acceptable, but during VATS approaches, it may limit surgical visualization and force extension of the incision. When surgical cross-clamp of the PA branch is imminent, marginal saturations may be tolerated briefly, knowing that cross-clamp likely will improve oxygenation by reducing nondependent lung shunt. The patient with hyperreactive airways may benefit from inline aerosolized bronchodilator treatments.

Hypoxic pulmonary vasoconstriction

During OLV, HPV is critical to reduce nondependent lung blood flow, as well as to fine-tune V/Q matching in the dependent lung. HPV is an exquisitely local phenomenon of the pulmonary microvasculature, responding primarily to low alveolar oxygen tension and secondarily to low mixed venous oxygen levels. Although its precise mechanism remains obscure, HPV is thought to be mediated by voltage-gated potassium channels. HPV is inhibited by most vasodilators and by all currently used inhalational anesthetic agents in a dose-dependent manner (in vitro). Hypercapnia and acidosis enhance HPV, whereas hypocapnia and alkalosis inhibit it. The net effect of any variable on oxygenation during OLV depends on its integrated effects on HPV (direct and indirect), cardiac output, and mixed venous oxygen tension, and cannot be easily predicted. Aside from avoiding obvious offenders (e.g., high-dose nitrodilator infusions), attempts to improve one-lung oxygenation by manipulation of HPV are rarely productive. Because inhalational anesthetic agents inhibit HPV and most intravenous anesthetics do not, TIVA has been proposed to improve oxygenation during OLV. Clinical studies are currently mixed on this matter, which is complicated by secondary effects on cardiac output and mixed venous oxygen saturation. Similarly, inhaled nitric oxide delivered to the dependent lung, which might be expected to improve one-lung oxygenation by reducing nondependent lung shunt, has produced mixed experimental results.

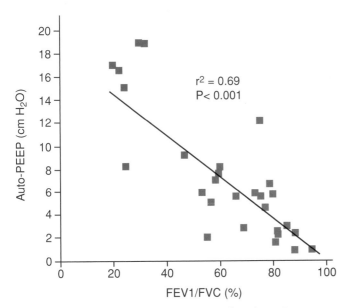

Figure 88.5. Relationship during OLV between airflow obstruction as measured by the FEV_1/FVC percentage and the occurrence of auto-PEEP. (From Ducros O, Moutafis M, Castelian M, et al. Pulmonary air trapping during two-lung and one-lung ventilation. *J Cardiothoracic Vasc Anesth* 1999; 13:35.)

Optimal PEEP

Excessive airway pressures in the dependent lung may redirect blood flow to the nondependent lung, increasing total shunt and reducing oxygenation during OLV. Thus, PEEP to the dependent lung is a double-edged sword. Whether PEEP will result in improvement or deterioration of oxygenation depends on the patient's preexisting physiology. Those with restrictive physiology of the dependent lung (e.g., pulmonary fibrosis, obesity) or young patients with normal lung elastic recoil likely would benefit from some PEEP. Those with severe obstructive disease often have unavoidable levels of auto-PEEP already at or beyond optimal PEEP. The risk of auto-PEEP during OLV is directly proportional to the severity of obstructive lung disease as measured by FEV_1/forced vital capacity (FVC) ratio (Fig. 88.5). The addition of extrinsic PEEP (ventilator delivered) to such patients will neither benefit oxygenation nor increase total PEEP until threshold levels ($\sim$ 75% of preexisting auto-PEEP) are exceeded. Beyond that threshold level, further increases in dependent-lung PEEP will increase airway pressures and nondependent lung shunt to the detriment of oxygenation. The degree of auto-PEEP is not measurable by standard anesthesia ventilators but can be detected by briefly disconnecting the circuit and observing for end-expiratory airflow. A useful strategy is to begin with low levels of extrinsic PEEP ($<$ 5 cm H_2O) and to incrementally increase PEEP using oxygen saturation of hemoglobin (SpO_2) as a guide in patients who are hypoxemic during OLV.

Avoidance of ventilator-induced lung injury

Ventilator-induced lung injury (VILI) results from excessive overdistention (volutrauma) and/or from the shear stresses

Table 88.5. Recommended OLV strategies to avoid VILI

Tidal volume = 6 ml/kg ideal body weight
PEEP in patients without auto-PEEP
Limit plateau pressures to <25 cm H_2O
Limit peak inspiratory pressures to <35 cm H_2O
Intermittent recruitment maneuvers

of repeated collapse and reexpansion of lung units (atelectotrauma). Because the dependent lung during OLV is prone to intermittent atelectasis, and is free to hyperexpand with high airway pressures because of the open pneumothorax, theoretically it is especially vulnerable to VILI. A proportion of patients develop acute lung injury with no apparent cause following pulmonary resection. It has been postulated that VILI may account for some of these cases. Recommendations for single-lung ventilatory settings consequently shifted to lung-protective strategies (Table 88.5). There is no firm prospective evidence at this writing, however, that traditional OLV strategies (tidal volume = 10 ml/kg) are injurious or that protective strategies improve outcome. Isolated perfused rabbit lung preparations displayed reduced stigmata of injury (elevated lung water, PA pressures, and thromboxane A_1) with similar protective ventilatory strategies, compared with conventional OLV. Ultimately, ventilatory settings must be individualized, and a compromise often must be sought between optimal gas exchange and the perceived risk of lung injury. This balance is most tenuous in patients with severe obstructive lung disease, in whom temporary hypoventilation (permissive hypercapnia) is often necessary.

Fluid management and postpneumonectomy pulmonary edema

Barring unusual blood loss, conservative fluid management for pulmonary resection has become a widely entrenched practice. Published recommendations are for a target positive 24-hour fluid balance of $<$ 20 ml/kg. This stems from the recognition that all pulmonary resections are potentially vulnerable to postpneumonectomy pulmonary edema (PPE). PPE occurs in 2% to 4% of pneumonectomies and is a diagnosis of exclusion with a high mortality (50%). Also referred to as acute lung injury (ALI) following pulmonary resection, it manifests in hours to days following pulmonary resection as radiographic pulmonary edema and impaired gas exchange and may progress to acute respiratory distress syndrome. It is more common following right pneumonectomy and less common following lobectomy. Other known causes, including cardiogenic and infectious causes, must be excluded. Low cardiac filling pressures and high protein content in bronchial lavage of such patients speak to an impairment of pulmonary capillary integrity. Postulated etiologies include oxygen toxicity, VILI, and unbalanced chest tube drainage. Impaired lymphatic drainage is undoubtedly contributory and may explain why left pneumonectomies are less vulnerable (lymphatic drainage is better preserved).

Intraoperative fluid administration by anesthesiologists had been postulated to be a cause but is now regarded as only a potentially exacerbating factor. If ALI occurs from any cause, excessive crystalloid would logically exacerbate gas exchange by increasing hydrostatic pressures across leaky pulmonary capillaries. The limited gas exchange reserves and lymphatic drainage of pneumonectomy patients make the process more difficult to reverse. This rationale for conservative fluid management must be individualized and always balanced against the imperative for sufficient intravascular volume to assure adequate end-organ perfusion and to tolerate thoracic epidural sympathetic blockade (if applicable).

Emergence strategies

The conclusion of surgery usually entails resumption of the supine position, exchange of the DLT for a single-lumen tube or laryngeal mask airway, and a cleansing bronchoscopy. The latter also serves to examine the lobar stump and to rule out other issues (e.g., torsion of the middle lobe following right lower lobectomy). The use of a high FiO_2 plus aggressive bronchoscopic suctioning predisposes to atelectasis, and efforts should be made to reexpand the lungs post bronchoscopy. Instrumentation of the airway may provoke bronchospasm. Augmenting anesthetic depth (e.g., with remifentanil) and administering inline inhaled bronchodilators can combat this. Pulmonary mechanics should be optimized by raising the head of the bed prior to extubation. Any splinting from incisional or rib pain should be addressed aggressively with the indwelling epidural catheter, alternative nerve blocks (paravertebral or intercostal), intravenous narcotics, or adjuncts (e.g., nonsteroidal anti-inflammatory drugs, ketamine, dexmedetomidine). Supplemental postoperative oxygen is appropriate for all pulmonary resection patients, with the possible exception of those who received bleomycin therapy. The commonly held fear that oxygen will inhibit the respiratory drive of CO_2-retaining COPD patients is unfounded.

Special considerations for pneumonectomy
Patient selection

Pneumonectomy is most commonly performed for NSCLC that is centrally located, adherent to hilar structures, or crossing a major fissure. Although more frequently the case in developing countries, pneumonectomy may also be performed for intractable hemorrhagic bronchiectasis or to remove a lung destroyed by suppurative disease or trauma. Mortality following pneumonectomy is generally 5% to 7%, compared with 2% to 3% for lobectomy (bi-lobectomy is similar to pneumonectomy). Resectability for pneumonectomy is defined by the stage (no contralateral or distant metastases). Operability is a clinical judgment based largely on perceived cardiopulmonary reserve and ppoFEV$_1$. Criteria considered to indicate high risk are shown in Table 88.6. Violation of any of those criteria necessitates split lung function testing to more accurately assess ppoFEV$_1$, which is the metric most heavily relied upon. In contrast to lesser resections, cardiac complications following pneumonectomy are more frequent than pulmonary complications as causes of perioperative mortality. Complications of pneumonectomy are listed in Table 88.7.

Anesthesia-relevant surgical issues for pneumonectomy

Variants of pneumonectomy include intrapericardial pneumonectomy (in which pulmonary veins are divided proximal to pericardium), carinal pneumonectomy (in which the lung is removed with a sleeve of trachea, carina, and bronchus, and the contralateral bronchus is anastomosed to the trachea), and extrapleural pneumonectomy (EPP). EPP involves

Table 88.6. High-risk criteria for pneumonectomy

$PaCO_2 > 45$ mm Hg (room air)
$PaO_2 < 50$ mm Hg (room air)
$FEV_1 < 2$ L
ppoFEV$_1 < 0.8$ L (or $< 40\%$ predicted)
$FEV_1/FVC < 50\%$ predicted
Max. breathing capacity $< 50\%$ predicted
Max. O_2 consumption < 10 ml/kg/min
Exercise desaturation $> 4\%$
Stair climb < 2 flights with dyspnea
ppoD$_{LCO} < 40\%$ predicted

ppoD$_{LCO}$, predicted postoperative diffusion capacity of the lungs to carbon monoxide.

Table 88.7. Postoperative complications of pneumonectomy

Category	Complication
Cardiovascular	Arrhythmia (esp. atrial fibrillation)
	Myocardial infarction
	Right ventricular failure
	Intracardiac shunt
	Deep vein thrombosis
	Pulmonary embolus
	Postpericardiotomy syndrome
	Cardiac herniation
Pulmonary	Postpneumonectomy pulmonary edema
	Pneumothorax
	Pneumonia
Pneumonectomy space	Bronchopleural fistula
	Empyema
	Postpneumonectomy syndrome
	Hemothorax
	Chylothorax
Oncologic	Recurrence
	Second primary
Neurologic	Recurrent laryngeal nerve injury
	Phrenic nerve injury
	Vagal nerve injury
	Paraplegia
Gastroesophageal	Gastric volvulus
	Esophagopleural fistula

Adapted from Jackson TA, Mehran RJ, Thaker D, et al. Postoperative complications after pneumonectomy. *J Cardiothorac Vasc Anesth* 2007; 21(5):743–751.

en block resection of lung, ipsilateral visceral and parietal pleurae, hemidiaphragm, and pericardium, and is principally performed in selected centers for malignant pleural mesothelioma. All pneumonectomies require at least a muscle-sparing thoracotomy incision.

Catastrophic bleeding from loss of control of hilar vessels is a rare but possible event in any pneumonectomy. Risk increases with tumor proximity to the vessels. Intrapericardial division of vessels is associated with more arrhythmias, and synchronized cardioversion capability should be readily available. Following division of the vessels, the bronchus is divided as proximally as possible. This serves two purposes: it provides the greatest tumor-free margin and results in the shortest stump. Long bronchial stumps are associated with higher rates of breakdown and bronchopleural fistula formation. Bronchoscopic visualization of the carina by the anesthesiologist can help guide the surgeon's positioning of the bronchial cross-clamp. Reinforcement of the bronchial stump with a vascular flap, such as a pedicle of intercostal muscle, frequently is performed. A leak test, described earlier, is performed with the stump submerged in saline. Thereafter, attention to minimize peak inspiratory pressure stress to the staple line is widely considered prudent. Toward this end, immediate postoperative extubation is a priority. Prior to closure, if the pericardium and/or diaphragm have been removed, they are reconstructed with prosthetic patches.

Special monitoring issues for pneumonectomy

Generous IV access and invasive arterial blood pressure monitoring are generally recommended for pneumonectomy. Despite the caveats described earlier, some experts advocate central venous access. At the time of PA cross-clamp, the CVP seldom changes. This is a result partly of the remarkable compliance of the pulmonary vascular tree and partly of the fact that the forces of gravity and HPV largely reduce cardiac output to the operative lung prior to cross-clamp. An abrupt increase in CVP at the time of PA cross-clamp may indicate right ventricular intolerance of the increased afterload, but a failure of the CVP to change is no reassurance that the right ventricle will not subsequently fail. PA catheters are of limited value because of the pitfalls of interpretation discussed earlier.

Cardiac herniation and mediastinal shift

Following pneumonectomy, the chest is closed with a drain in place, but care is taken to prevent the inadvertent attachment of the drain to suction, as this may precipitate cardiovascular collapse from mediastinal shift or cardiac herniation. Cardiac herniation is the abrupt displacement of the heart into the empty hemithorax, resulting in torsion of great vessels and the loss of effective cardiac output. Cardiac herniation is most likely following right pneumonectomy with a pericardial defect that was inadequately reconstructed. Resumption of the supine position is a critical time when cardiac herniation may occur. In its most dramatic form, cardiac herniation results in abrupt cardiovascular collapse. Returning the patient to the lateral position in

Table 88.8. Causes of hypotension at the conclusion of pneumonectomy

Partial cardiac herniation
Tight pericardial patch (if applicable)
Mediastinal shift
Hypovolemia
Recent thoracic epidural bolus
Air trapping, auto-PEEP
Right ventricular failure
Myocardial ischemia
Tension pneumothorax

such a case is the appropriate therapeutic response. This will return the heart to its physiologic position and allow the surgeon to reopen and place or repair an inadequate pericardial patch. Inotropes, vasopressors, and closed chest cardiac massage are of no value to an empty heart herniated into an empty hemithorax.

Rarely, right-to-left intracardiac shunts develop following pneumonectomy as a result of mediastinal shift and rotation of the heart such that the inferior vena caval orifice aligns with the foramen ovale. Such patients may exhibit desaturation in the upright position (platypnea orthodeoxia). Postpneumonectomy syndrome is a rare, late complication from shifting of the mediastinum resulting in the extrinsic compression of the remaining mainstem bronchus.

Emergence

The same emergence strategies described earlier apply to pneumonectomy patients. Because there will always be at least a muscle-sparing thoracotomy incision, aggressive thoracic epidural (or paravertebral) blockade, as tolerated hemodynamically, is advantageous. Mild hypotension at the conclusion of surgery has many potential etiologies (Table 88.8), potentially resulting in diagnostic confusion. Of these causes, mediastinal shift resulting in partial embarrassment of venous return may be especially difficult to rule out. Some surgeons preemptively aspirate up to 200 ml of air from the chest drain. A portable chest radiograph in the operating room is most effective in ruling out mediastinal shift. Following extubation, many patients report a sense of dyspnea despite adequate air movement, which may partly be the result of disruption in their sense of the mechanics of breathing. Even the stable, comfortable, extubated pneumonectomy patient warrants postoperative monitoring in the ICU because of the dire and abrupt potential complications of the operation (Table 88.7).

Suggested readings

Aubier M, Murciano D, Milic-Emili J, et al. Effects of the administration of O2 on ventilation and blood gases in patients with chronic obstructive pulmonary disease during acute respiratory failure. *Am Rev Respir Dis* 1980; 122:747–754.

Ballantyne JC, Carr DC, deFerranti S, et al. The comparative effects of postoperative analgesia therapies on pulmonary outcome: a meta-analysis of randomized, controlled trials. *Anesth Analg* 1998; 86(3):598–612.

Beattie WS, Badner NH, Choi P. Epidural analgesia reduces postoperative myocardial infarction: a meta-analysis. *Anesth Analg* 2001; 93(4):853–858.

Boisseau N, Rabary O, Padovani B, et al. Improvement of 'dynamic analgesia' does not decrease atelectasis after thoracotomy. *Br J Anaesth* 2001; 87(4):564–569.

Drasner K. Thoracic epidural anesthesia: asleep at the wheel? *Anesth Analg* 2004, 99:578–579.

Fernandez-Perez ER, Keegan MT, Brown DR, et al. Intraoperative tidal volume as a risk factor for respiratory failure after pneumonectomy. *Anesthesiology* 2006; 105(1):14–18.

Gamma de Abreu M, Heintz M, Heller A, et al. One-lung ventilation with high tidal volumes and zero positive end-expiratory pressure is injurious in the isolated rabbit lung model. *Anesth Analg* 2003; 96:220–228.

Hanson CW, Marshall BE, Frasch HF, Marshall C. Causes of hypercarbia with oxygen therapy in patients with chronic obstructive pulmonary disease. *Crit Care Med* 1994; 24(1):23–28.

Hurford W, Kolker AC, Strauss HW. The use of ventilation/perfusion lung scans to predict oxygenation during one-lung anesthesia. *Anesthesiology* 1987; 67:841–844.

Jackson TA, Mehran RJ, Thaker D, et al. Postoperative complications after pneumonectomy. *J Cardiothorac Vasc Anesth* 2007; 21(5):743–751.

Karzai W, Haberstroh J, Priebe H-J. Effects of desflurane and propofol on arterial oxygenation during one-lung ventilation in the pig. *Acta Anaesthesiol Scand* 1998; 42:648–652.

Licker M, Perrot M, Spiliopoulos A, et al. Risk factors for acute lung injury after thoracic surgery for lung cancer. *Anesth Analg* 2003; 97:1558–1565.

Nakahara K, Ohno K, Hashimoto J, et al. Prediction of postoperative respiratory failure in patients undergoing lung resection for cancer. *Ann Thorac Surg* 1988; 46:549–552.

Richardson J, Sabanathan S, Shah R. Post-thoracotomy spirometric lung function: the effect of analgesia. A review. *J Cardiovasc Surg (Torino)* 1999; 40(3):445–456.

Saito M, Cho S, Morooka H, et al. Effects of sevoflurane compared with those of isoflurane on arterial oxygenation and hemodynamics during one-lung ventilation. *J Anesth* 2000, 4(1):1–5.

Schwarzkopf K, Schreiber T, Bauer R, et al. The effects of increasing concentrations of isoflurane and desflurane on pulmonary perfusion and systemic oxygenation during one-lung ventilation in pigs. *Anesth Analg* 2001; 93:1434–1438.

Schwarzkopf K, Schreiber T, Preussler N-P, et al. Lung perfusion, shunt fraction, and oxygenation during one-lung ventilation in pigs: the effects of desflurane, isoflurane, and propofol. *J Cardiothorac Vasc Anesth* 2003, 17(1):73–75.

Senturk M, Ozcam PE, Talu GK, et al. The effects of three different analgesia techniques on long-term postthoracotomy pain. *Anesth Analg* 2002; 94(1):11–15.

Slinger P, Scott AC. Arterial oxygenation during one-lung ventilation. A comparison of enflurane and isoflurane. *Anesthesiology* 1995, 82(4):940–946.

Slinger PD. Management of one-lung anesthesia. *Anesth Analg 2005 Review Course Lectures* 2005; 100(3):Suppl 89.

Slinger PD. Perioperative fluid management for thoracic surgery: the puzzle of postpneumonectomy pulmonary edema. *J Cardiothorac Vasc Anesth* 1995; 9(4):442–451.

Slinger PD. Pro: Every postthoracotomy patient deserves thoracic epidural analgesia. *J Cardiothorac Vasc Anesth* 1999; 13(3):350–354.

Slinger PD, Johnston MR. Preoperative assessment: an anesthesiologist's perspective. *Thorac Surg Clin* 2005; 15(1): 11–25.

Sticher J, Scholz S, Boning O, et al. Small-dose nitric oxide improves oxygenation during one-lung ventilation: an experimental study. *Anesth Analg* 2002; 95:1557–1562.

Wilson WC, Kapelanski DP, Benumof J, et al. Inhaled nitric oxide (40ppm) during one-lung ventilation, in the lateral decubitus position, does not decrease pulmonary vascular resistance or improve oxygenation in normal patients. *J Cardiothorac Vasc Anesth* 1997; 11:172–176.

Wittnich C, Trudel J, Zidulka A, Chiu R. Misleading "pulmonary wedge pressure" after pneumonectomy. Its importance in postoperative fluid therapy. *Ann Thorac Surg* 1986; 42:192.

Chapter 89

Lung transplantation

Vladimir Formanek

Lung transplantation is an accepted therapeutic intervention for patients with end-stage lung disease. The anesthesiologist faces many challenges when caring for a patient who presents for transplantation. Individual cases may require the management of hypoxia or hypercapnia, invasive hemodynamic monitoring, treatment of pulmonary hypertension and right ventricular (RV) failure, familiarity with the management of cardiopulmonary bypass, use of inhaled nitric oxide (NO), and transesophageal echocardiography (TEE). Critical incidents are common, and they may challenge even the most experienced anesthesiologist.

Types of lung transplants

Lung transplantation encompasses a group of different operations selected based on recipient factors, donor organ availability, and the transplant center's preferences (Table 89.1).

Single-lung transplantation

The most common indications for single-lung transplantation (SLT) are chronic obstructive pulmonary disease COPD and pulmonary fibrosis. The operation involves a pneumonectomy and transplantation of a single donor lung. The nontransplanted native lung is left in situ. After pneumonectomy, the donor lung is implanted. This requires anastomosis of the bronchus, pulmonary artery (PA), and a cuff of left atrium containing the donor pulmonary veins to the recipient's left atrium. The bronchial circulation, lymphatics, and nerves are not restored. Cardiopulmonary bypass (CPB) is needed in fewer than 10% of cases, but CPB backup should be readily available. CPB may be necessary because of hemodynamic instability, hypoxia, or hypercarbia. SLT allows two recipients to benefit from one donor.

Bilateral lung transplantation

The most common indications for bilateral or double-lung transplantation (DLT) are cystic fibrosis, bronchiectasis, and other infectious processes that would result in soilage of the transplanted lung from the remaining native lung. Pulmonary hypertension is another common indication. Restoration of a normal pulmonary vasculature (via DLT) allows for optimal recovery of the right heart. Evidence shows that long-term

mortality and graft function are better after DLT; therefore, many centers now favor DLT for most patients. The operation is done through a clamshell, subcostal incision (Fig. 89.1) or through a median sternotomy. The anastomoses are the same as for SLT. The procedure may be done with or without CPB.

Heart–lung transplantation

Heart–lung transplantation is usually reserved for patients with pulmonary hypertension and congenital heart disease, Eisenmenger's syndrome, or primary pulmonary hypertension with RV dysfunction. The heart and lungs are transplanted en bloc, from a single donor, with CPB support. At present, heart–lung transplantation is a rare operation. According to the United Network for Organ Sharing (UNOS; http://www.unos.org) data, only 27 heart–lung transplants were performed in the United States in 2008.

Pediatric transplantation

The most common indications for lung transplantation in the pediatric population are cystic fibrosis, primary pulmonary hypertension, bronchopulmonary dysplasia, arteriovenous malformations, and hypoplastic lungs due to congenital diaphragmatic hernia. The procedure invariably is a DLT with the aid of extracorporeal circulation.

Living donor lung transplantation

Living donor lung transplantation involves the transplantation of two lobes from two donors into a single recipient. With the increasing disparity between the number of patients referred for transplant and the availability of suitable cadaveric donor organs, living donor transplantation developed as an alternative to cadaveric lung transplantation. Cystic fibrosis has been

Table 89.1. Types of lung transplantation currently performed in the United States

SLT
DLT (with or without CPB)
Heart–lung transplant
Living donor transplant (2 donors donate one lobe each)
Pediatric lung transplant

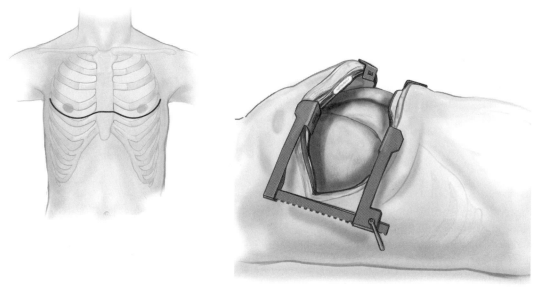

Figure 89.1. Clamshell incision commonly used for DLT transplantation.

the most common indication. These patients are usually smaller in stature, allowing two lobes from average-sized adult donors to provide sufficient pulmonary tissue. The number of living related transplants peaked at 29 in 1999 and declined in subsequent years. According to UNOS data, none was performed in 2008. The operation requires meticulous care of three patients. The perioperative morbidity for donors is not insignificant, nor is the burden on operating room resources.

Donor organs

The Organ Procurement and Transplantation Network (http://optn.transplant.hrsa.gov) and UNOS are government-sponsored organizations that register all patients listed for transplantation. A centralized computer network links all organ procurement organizations and transplant centers. Procurement agencies facilitate matching of organs to recipients throughout the United States. The system is set up to allocate organs to the sickest patients while minimizing ischemic time. Many transplant-related statistics are maintained by UNOS and are available to the public through its Web site.

The lung allocation score system

The lung allocation score system is a relatively new method for allocating lungs. Each candidate is assigned a score of 0 to 100 based on his or her medical urgency and probability of survival after transplant. The system uses several disease-specific parameters and takes into consideration the likelihood of benefit and long-term survival. The information includes laboratory values, use of supplemental O_2, functional status, disease diagnosis, and comorbidities. Each candidate's information must be updated every 6 months. This system appears to better match limited organs to acute need, and may be the reason for the decline in living donor transplants.

Donor lung procurement and preservation

Donor lungs traditionally have come from brain-dead cadaveric donors with preserved lung function. Fewer than 20% of donors of other solid organs are considered suitable for lung donation. Management of the lung donor may involve strict fluid management, bronchoscopy to assess for bronchopulmonary infection, alteration of ventilator settings, arterial blood gas (ABG) monitoring, and chest imaging. Intensive management of marginal donors has been shown to improve the quality and to expand the pool of donor lungs.

Preservation of the lung during harvest requires that the allograft be cooled and flushed with a pulmoplegic solution. Some centers use high-dose steroids and/or pulmonary vasodilators as well. The harvested lungs are kept partially inflated. Ischemic times play a critical role. The time from organ harvest to reperfusion in the recipient should be as short as possible. The number of suitable recipients far exceeds available organ donors; therefore, the expansion of the donor pool is a major concern of all transplant centers. Donation of organs after cardiac death has further expanded the donor pool. Despite about an hour of warm ischemia, early results have been promising.

Recipient selection and indications

Lung transplantation is indicated for patients with end-stage lung disease, those who are failing maximal medical therapy, and those for whom no effective medical therapy exists. Because lung transplantation remains a complex therapy with a significant risk of perioperative morbidity and mortality, potential candidates should be well informed and able to demonstrate adequate behavior and willingness to follow guidelines from health care professionals. Referral for transplant assessment is advisable for patients with <50% predicted 2- to

Table 89.2. Breakdown of SLTs and DLTs according to indication

SLT (%)	DLT (%)
COPD (50)	Cystic fibrosis (28)
Idiopathic pulmonary fibrosis (28)	COPD (24)
α_1-Antitrypsin (7)	Idiopathic pulmonary fibrosis (14)
Cystic fibrosis (2)	α_1-Antitrypsin (8)
Retransplant (2)	Primary pulmonary hypertension (6)
Primary pulmonary hypertension (1)	Retransplant (2)
Other (10)	Other (18)

Data from the International Society for Heart and Lung Transplantation (http://www.ishlt.org) registries for 1995 through 2007.

Table 89.4. Essential studies during pretransplant evaluation

Chest radiography and CT scan of thorax
Pulmonary function test and ventilation–perfusion scan
ABG
Evaluation of renal and hepatic function
Electrocardiogram
Echocardiogram
Cardiac catheterization (as indicated for specific patients)
Complete blood count and coagulation studies
ABO blood typing
Viral serologies (e.g., HIV, hepatitis, cytomegalovirus)

3-year survival. The distribution of lung transplants by indication is reviewed in Table 89.2; contraindications are listed in Table 89.3.

Disease-specific indications

Disease-specific indications are as follows:

Pulmonary fibrosis: Diffusing capacity of lung for carbon monoxide (D_{LCO}) < 39%, a decrease in pulse oximeter saturation to < 88% during the 6-minute walk test, and "honeycombing" on high-resolution CT.

COPD: History of hospitalizations for acute exacerbations with acute hypercapnia, PCO_2 > 50 mm Hg, pulmonary hypertension, cor pulmonale despite O_2 therapy, and forced expiratory volume in the first second of expiration (FEV_1) < 20% predicted.

Connective tissue disorders (eosinophilic granuloma, lymphangioleiomyomatosis, sarcoidosis): Hypoxia at rest and severe impairment of lung function and exercise capacity.

Cystic fibrosis: FEV_1 < 30% or a rapid decline of FEV_1, exacerbations requiring an intensive care unit stay, increasing frequency of exacerbations requiring antibiotic therapy, and recurrent hemoptysis.

Bronchiectasis: Recurrent hemoptysis, pulmonary hypertension, and recurrent infection.

Primary or secondary pulmonary hypertension: Persistent New York Heart Association class III or IV on maximal medical therapy, cardiac index < 2, and failing therapy of intravenous (IV) pulmonary vasodilators.

Workup of the pulmonary transplant recipient

The clinical evaluation and assessment for transplantation should include characterization of the underlying lung disease, evaluation for other organ system dysfunction, and determination of the patient's ability to tolerate long-term immunosuppressive therapy. Essential studies are detailed in Table 89.4. Patients with stable single-vessel coronary disease may still qualify for lung transplantation. Stents or angioplasty may be used in these patients.

Perioperative management
Patient monitoring

Essential and optional monitors are listed in Table 89.5. Most transplant centers routinely use PA catheters for all lung transplants. Continuous monitoring of PA pressures and RV performance is considered essential by most clinicians. Additional evaluation of cardiac performance can be done with TEE. Placement of a central venous line (via a double-stick technique) at the same time the PA line is placed allows flexibility in the timing of removal of the PA line.

Preinduction

Patients usually arrive for the procedure well informed from previous pulmonary clinic visits. Most patients have had a complete workup, allowing the anesthesia care team to do a rapid but complete preanesthetic assessment. It is important to ascertain their NPO status (many have eaten within 8 hours of induction)

Table 89.3. Contraindications to lung transplantation

Contraindications
- Malignancy
- Advanced dysfunction of other organ systems
- Incurable chronic infection (e.g., HIV, hepatitis)
- Psychiatric conditions that preclude the ability to cooperate with posttransplant medical care

Relative contraindications
- Age > 65 y (no hard limit exists)
- Critical unstable condition
- Colonization with highly virulent organism
- Mechanical ventilation or ECMO with small chance for rehabilitation
- Severe chest wall deformity or pleural disease

Table 89.5. Monitors used during lung transplantation

Essential monitors	Additional monitors
Standard ASA monitors (ECG, pulse oximeter, NIBP, ETCO₂)	TEE
Invasive arterial pressure (radial/femoral)	Depth of anesthesia
CVP/PA catheter	Cerebral oximetry
Serial ABGs	

CVP, central venous pressure; ECG, electrocardiogram; ETCO₂, end-tidal carbon dioxide; NIBP, noninvasive blood pressure.

and carefully evaluate the airway, as this component will likely not have been previously evaluated.

Light sedation, antacid prophylaxis, nebulized bronchodilators, and continued supplemental oxygen are likely appropriate. A large-bore IV and an arterial line should be placed. If CPB is unlikely, and time permits, a thoracic epidural catheter also may be placed preoperatively.

Induction and intraoperative management

Before inducing general anesthesia, it is essential to confirm timing with the transplant team. Once a decision is made to proceed, the choice of anesthetic technique and induction or maintenance drugs is less critical than the hemodynamic and pulmonary management.

After initial intubation with a single-lumen endotracheal tube, bronchoscopy is performed to clear secretions and assess anatomy. A double-lumen tube is then placed. Typically, a left-sided tube is used for everything except left SLTs, for which a right-sided tube is indicated if anatomy permits. Central venous and pulmonary artery catheters must now be placed expediently. After induction, prophylactic antibiotics and initial immunosuppression, which typically involves high-dose steroids plus an induction agent such as antithymocyte globulin (if the transplant center uses preimplantation induction), are administered.

Single-lung transplant

For SLT, the patient is positioned for a standard thoracotomy. The lung to be explanted is mobilized. Often, a test clamp of the PA is performed prior to explantation. If the patient does not tolerate one-lung ventilation (OLV) or the test clamp, then CPB will be needed. Once the new lung is implanted, it should be slowly reperfused and ventilated using the lung-protective ventilator setting and low fraction of inspired oxygen content (FiO_2). The bronchial anastomosis can be checked with fiberoptic bronchoscopy. The lymphatics are not anastomosed. Between the capillary leak from reperfusion and the impaired lymphatic drainage, transplanted lungs are very vulnerable to pulmonary edema. For this reason, intraoperative fluids are limited, and diuretics may be given in the operating room.

Double-lung transplant

For DLT, the patient is positioned supine, often with the arms suspended from an ether screen or similar device to allow adequate access for a clamshell incision. Dissection is performed using alternating OLV. If the procedure is done without CPB, one lung is excised and the first donor lung implanted. Then the procedure is repeated on the other side, while the patient is ventilated using the newly implanted lung.

To date, the use of CPB remains inconsistent among transplant centers. Some centers attempt to do most DLTs without CPB and use CPB only if necessary. The usual indications for CPB are high PA pressures, RV dysfunction, severely dilated PAs in primary pulmonary hypertension, severe hypoxia with OLV, and severe hypercarbia and acidosis during OLV. Other centers always use CPB for DLT.

Proponents of CPB cite better vascular control, better hemodynamic stability, better gas exchange, less strain on the right ventricle, easier dissection, and less stress on the first implanted lung. Potential disadvantages are heparin exposure (heparin-induced thrombocytopenia), the potential for greater blood loss, the need for more transfusion, and the inflammatory response to the CPB circuit.

If CPB is used, cannulation may occur through the chest, or the femoral vessels may be used. Unlike during heart surgery, the patient is not cooled and the heart continues to beat. Dysrhythmias must be treated as they occur. Antifibrinolytic agents may be useful to minimize blood loss. The need for slow reperfusion, lung-sparing ventilation, and limited fluid administration are similar to that of SLT.

Treating pulmonary hypertension and RV dysfunction

The basic principles of pulmonary hypertension and RV dysfunction treatment are to avoid hypoxia, hypercarbia, acidosis, light anesthesia, and hypothermia, as all may cause pulmonary vasoconstriction and right heart strain. Systemic pulmonary vasodilator therapy with nitroglycerin, alprostadil, or sodium nitroprusside may be attempted. The major disadvantage is systemic hypotension and, potentially, reversal of hypoxic pulmonary vasoconstriction, resulting in hypoxia. Inotrope therapy to improve RV function and cardiac output may be achieved with dobutamine, milrinone, or epinephrine. Inhaled prostacyclin PGI_2 (iloprost) has been used with success to reduce pulmonary pressures and avoid CPB in select cases. Inhaled NO reduces pulmonary vascular resistance, thereby unloading the right heart. Because NO is rapidly bound to hemoglobin and inactivated, it has no systemic vasodilatory effect. NO also has some attractive anti-inflammatory properties: It interferes with neutrophil adherence to endothelium, inhibits platelet aggregation, and inhibits expression of several inflammatory mediators.

Transesophageal echocardiography in lung transplantation

TEE is used routinely at several transplant centers. It allows assessment of cardiac anatomy and function. Factors commonly assessed include right and left ventricular function, volume status, the interatrial septum for atrial septal defect or patent foramen ovale, pulmonary venous flow, and pulmonary arterial flow. RV dysfunction at the time of PA test clamping may direct the decision to proceed with CPB. TEE can be used to assist in cannulae placement and to confirm that the PA line is in the RV outflow tract or main PA and thus will not end up in the staple line during explant. TEE, of course, provides an excellent assessment of volume status and biventricular function. Finally, pulsed Doppler can be used to assess flow across the pulmonary venous anastomosis. Pulmonary venous obstruction is a rare but potentially fatal cause of postoperative graft failure.

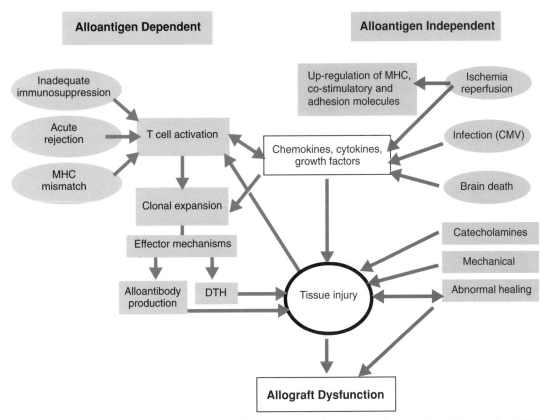

Figure 89.2. Transplant-related lung injury. (Adapted from McRae KM. Pulmonary transplantation. *Curr Opin Anaesthesiol* 2000; 13:53–59.)

Primary graft dysfunction

Primary graft dysfunction (PGD) is a serious complication that causes significant morbidity and mortality. Lung injury caused by ischemia and reperfusion leads to alveolar damage, pulmonary edema, and hypoxemia. Numerous factors, both alloantigen dependent and independent, contribute to the development of PGD (Fig. 89.2). Prevention is the key, but if PGD does occur, treatment is supportive using mechanical ventilation, diuresis, and inhaled NO. If all other measures fail, extracorporeal membrane oxygenation (ECMO) may be lifesaving. Initial ECMO results have improved with advancements in surgical technique, timely institution, and the improvement in membrane oxygenators.

Suggested readings

Bracken CA, Gurkowski MA, Naples JJ. Lung transplantation: historical perspective, current concepts and anesthetic considerations. *J Cardiothorac Vasc Anesth* 1997; 11:220–241.

Janelle GM, Clark TD, Gravenstein N, et al. Cerebral oxygen desaturation during lung transplantation involving CPB. Evidence for a new approach in managing patients with chronic hypercarbia [abstract]. *Anesth Analg* 2003; 96:86.

Marczin N, Royston D, Yacoub M. Lung transplantation should be routinely performed with cardiopulmonary bypass. *J Cardiothorac Vasc Anesth* 2000; 14:739–745.

McIlroy DR, Sesto AC, Buckland MR. Pulmonary vein thrombosis, lung transplantation and intraoperative transesophageal echocardiography. *J Cardiothorac Vasc Anesth* 2006; 20(5)712–715.

McRae K. Con: lung transplantation should not be routinely performed with cardiopulmonary bypass. *J Cardiothorac Vasc Anesth* 2000; 14:746–750.

McRae K, Keshavjee S. The future of lung transplantation. In: Slinger PD, ed. *Progress in Thoracic Anesthesia*. Philadelphia: Lippincott Williams & Wilkins; 2004.

McRae KM. Pulmonary transplantation. *Curr Opin Anaesthesiol* 2000; 13:53–59.

Monk TG, Reno KA, Olsen DC, Koney-Laryea D. Postoperative cognitive dysfunction is associated with cerebral oxygen desaturations [abstract A-167]. Presented at the Annual Meeting of the American Society of Anesthesiologists; 2006.

Myles PS, Snell GI, Westall GP. Lung transplantation. *Curr Opin Anaesthesiol* 2007; 20:21–26.

Myles PS, Weeks AM, Buckland MR. Anesthesia for bilateral sequential lung transplantation; experience of 64 cases. *J Cardiothorac Vasc Anesth* 1997; 11:177.

Orens JB, Estenne M, Arcasoy S, et al. Consensus report. International guidelines for the selection of lung transplant candidates; 2006 update. *J Heart Lung Transplant* 2006; 25:7.

Oto T, Rosenfeldt F, Rowland M, et al. Extracorporeal membrane oxygenation after lung transplantation: evolving technique improves outcomes. *Ann Thorac Surg* 2004; 78:1230–1235.

Starnes VA, Barr ML, Baker CJ, et al. Living donor lung transplantation: selection, technique and outcome. *Transplant Proceed* 2001; 33:3527–3532.

Szeto W, Kreisel D, Karakousis G, et al. Cardiopulmonary bypass for sequential lung transplantation in patients with chronic obstructive pulmonary disease without adverse effect on lung function or clinical outcome. *J Thorac Cardiovasc Surg* 2002; 124:241–249.

Trulock EP, Edwards LB, Taylor DO, et al. Registry of the International Society for Heart and Lung Transplantation: twenty-third official adult lung and heart-lung transplantation report. *J Heart Lung Transplant* 2006; 25:8.

Chapter 90

Bronchoscopy and mediastinoscopy

Sharon L. Wetherall and Philip M. Hartigan

Introduction

Bronchoscopy and mediastinoscopy are surgical procedures commonly performed together under general anesthesia for diagnosis and staging of lung cancer. Bronchoscopy has other applications in and outside the operating room (Table 90.1). The anesthetic management should be tailored to the specific situation. Anesthesia for retrieval of aspirated foreign bodies is considered as an example.

Bronchoscopy involves the use of a lighted instrument to examine the tracheobronchial tree. Flexible fiber-optic bronchoscopes use fiber-optics to deliver the image to the proximal lens of a long, flexible scope. Video-bronchoscopes have a camera at the distal tip of the scope to capture the image, which is delivered by wires to a processor for video display on a monitor. Both use fiber-optics to deliver light to the distal end of the bronchoscope. Most models also have a working channel through which instruments or wires can be passed or suction applied. Rigid bronchoscopy involves the passage of a long, straight, rigid, tubular device through the mouth and glottis into the trachea or a mainstem bronchus (Fig. 90.1). The diameters vary but generally are larger than flexible bronchoscopes, allowing the passage of larger instruments. Indications for rigid bronchoscopy overlap considerably with those for flexible bronchoscopy (Table 90.2).

Anesthesia for flexible bronchoscopy

The anesthetic requirements for bronchoscopy *per se* are limited to blunting or ablating the airway reflexes as well as the powerfully noxious affective response to airway instrumentation. This may be accomplished through general anesthesia or topical anesthesia with sedation. When coupled with mediastinoscopy, general anesthesia with endotracheal intubation is most convenient. Large endotracheal tubes (ETT; >7.5 mm outer diameter) are required to accept adult flexible bronchoscopes without precluding adequate ventilation. Frequent suctioning via the bronchoscope complicates delivery of tidal volumes and anesthetic gases, thus the measurement of return volume and end-tidal CO_2 will be inaccurate. When suctioning is not used, the potential for air trapping due to the reduced functional cross-sectional area of the ETT is a hazard to be aware of. Because

Table 90.1. Indications for flexible bronchoscopy[a]

Staging of lung cancer
   Evaluation of tracheobronchial:
      Stenoses
      Intrinsic obstructions
      Extrinsic obstructions
      Hemoptysis
Persistent, unexplained cough
Persistent, localized wheeze
Bronchoalveolar lavage, brushings, biopsies
Deployment, evaluation, or adjustment of stents
Guide to transbronchial biopsy
Retrieval of foreign bodies
Airway balloon dilatation
Delivery of laser therapy or photodynamic therapy
Placement of brachytherapy cannula
Evaluation of suspected aspiration or burn/chemical injury to airway
Evaluation and potential treatment (e.g., adhesives) of bronchopleural
   fistulae
Evaluation of tracheoesophageal fistulae
Evaluation for rejection of lung transplant recipients
Delivery of agents or devices for bronchoscopic lung volume reduction
   surgery
Anesthetic applications:
   Guide to difficult intubation
   Confirmation of endotracheal tube position (single- or double-lumen)
   Positioning of bronchial blocker or blocker system

[a] Partial list; does not include supraglottic indications.

bronchoscopy is often brief and can be easily interrupted if such problems occur, there is typically limited risk to the procedure. If the bronchoscopy becomes prolonged, use of intravenous anesthetic agents (total intravenous anesthesia [TIVA]) obviates the difficulties of volatile agent delivery.

Issues imposed by the target lesion itself (e.g., mass effect, airway compression, obstruction) or by the patient's coexisting diseases (e.g., severe chronic obstructive pulmonary disease, cardiac disease, pulmonary hypertension) may more profoundly affect anesthetic management decisions. In particular,

Table 90.2. Indications for rigid bronchoscopy

Mechanical core-out of obstructive lesions of the airway
Retrieval of foreign bodies in the airway
Delivery of laser therapy
Deployment, adjustment, removal of airway stents
Evaluation and treatment of hemoptysis
Rescue ventilation of patients with tracheal collapse
Any other surgical indication listed in Table 90.1 in which the flexible
   bronchoscopic approach was inadequate

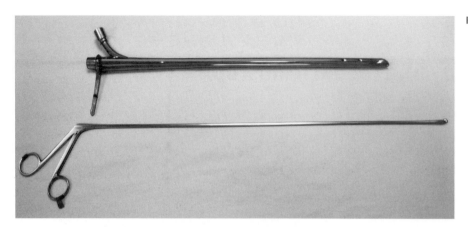

Figure 90.1. Rigid bronchoscope.

induction may convert a subcritical extrinsic tracheal obstruction into a life-threatening one, as the reduction of lung volumes from general anesthesia and the supine position reduce the caliber of airways (see Chapter 91).

Flexible bronchoscopy may be smoothly performed in an awake patient if topical local anesthesia is thorough. The conduit for the bronchoscope may be an oral bite block, an ETT, a laryngeal mask airway (Fig. 90.2), another supraglottic device, or the nasotracheal route. All these techniques allow visualization of the entire trachea. Attention to the recommended maximum tolerable doses of local anesthetics is imperative because of rapid absorption from mucous membranes. It should be assumed that the topically anesthetized airway is unprotected from aspiration for some period following application. Sedation, as always, should be tailored to the reserves, the requirements, and the response of the individual patient. Dexmedetomidine has been used with advantage for bronchoscopy in which preservation of respiratory drive is a premium. An antisialagogue such as glycopyrrolate aids in control of secretions, and preemptive bronchodilator treatments may be of benefit in the patient prone to bronchospasm.

Anesthesia for rigid bronchoscopy

Rigid bronchoscopy is far more stimulating than flexible bronchoscopy, and almost always requires general anesthesia. Positioning with a roll under the patient's back and full neck extension is necessary. Any instability of the cervical spine or any carotid arterial pathology that precludes neck extension is a contraindication. Dental guards should be used to protect the upper teeth. Full muscle relaxation considerably aids insertion of the rigid bronchoscope. As discussed previously, lesion-related or coexisting disease-related issues often dictate specific anesthetic considerations over and above those for rigid bronchoscopy itself. Trauma-related edema of the airway or vocal cords from the rigid scope may be ameliorated by steroids. During insertion of the bronchoscope, ventilation is temporarily interrupted, so hyperventilation and thorough denitrogenation prior to insertion are advised. Complications of rigid bronchoscopy include injury to the neck, teeth, cords, trachea, and bronchus. Pneumomediastinum/pneumothorax or

hemorrhage is possible if biopsy or endobronchial core-out is performed. Loss of airway is the principal risk if there is significant obstruction. Myocardial ischemia and arrhythmias may result from catecholamine surges from the tracheal stimulation. Ischemia is potentially exacerbated by hypoxemia and hypercarbia. Postoperative upper airway obstruction may result from trauma-related edema. If a laser is used, fire hazard issues need to be considered (see Chapter 115 on laser surgery). If stents are being deployed or adjusted, there is a risk of total airway obstruction from a folded or malpositioned stent. Aspiration is also a risk.

Ventilation options during rigid bronchoscopy include (1) spontaneous ventilation, (2) positive pressure ventilation via the side port of a ventilating rigid bronchoscope, (3) jet ventilation or its variants (e.g., high-frequency jet ventilation, oscillatory ventilation), and (4) apneic oxygenation. Spontaneous ventilation may be preferred when variable obstructive lesions threaten loss of airway patency. Anesthetic depth must be sufficient to blunt the sensitive airway reflexes, and may be achieved by inhalational or intravenous agents and/or supplemental topical anesthetics. Most commonly, the anesthetic circuit is attached to the side port of a ventilating rigid bronchoscope. Delivery of oxygen and volatile agents and removal

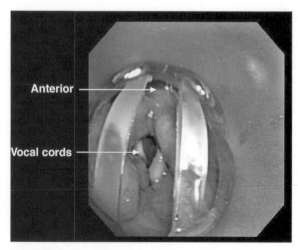

Figure 90.2. View of the glottis through a laryngeal mask airway.

of CO_2 may be disrupted by surgical manipulations and distal airway obstructions, as well as by the intermittent opening of the proximal port by the surgeon. Not infrequently, once the scope is in place to ensure a patent airway, conversion to paralysis and positive pressure ventilation is performed. When side port positive pressure ventilation is employed, the proximal viewing port must be occluded, and moist gauze packing to the posterior pharynx is necessary to minimize the air leak at the glottis. Positive pressure breaths must be timed to coincide with the times the proximal viewing port is closed. With prolonged interruptions in ventilation, the anesthesiologist must estimate the increase in $PaCO_2$ (approximately 6 mm Hg/min during first minute, followed by 3 mm Hg/min thereafter) and communicate with the surgeon when resumption of ventilation is deemed necessary. Use of TIVA avoids interruptions in anesthetic delivery and prevents pollution of the operating room with volatile agent.

Jet ventilation may be performed via an injection needle mounted at the proximal end of a rigid bronchoscope. Oxygen from a high-pressure source exiting the needle entrains room air by the Venturi principle. The resulting fraction of inspired oxygen (FiO_2) and tidal volume is unknown, and exhalation is passive. There is risk of barotrauma as well as unrecognized hypoventilation. Monitoring of ventilation relies on observation of chest rise, arterial blood gas sampling, or transcutaneous CO_2 monitoring. Jet ventilation, in experienced hands, is a viable technique that allows the surgeon uninterrupted access to the working port of the rigid bronchoscope.

Anesthesia for retrieval of foreign bodies in the airway

Management of the patient with a foreign body in the airway requires a flexible approach that is well coordinated with the surgical team. Relevant data are often initially unknown, including the size and shape of the object, the location and extent of obstruction, the duration and degree of reactive mucosal edema, the stability of the object, and whether it impales the mucosa. Children under age 3 are the most common patients presenting with foreign body aspiration (FBA). Therefore, history frequently is limited to parental observation of sudden onset of coughing and dyspnea, or possibly stridor or wheezing. The stable patient should receive a chest radiograph and/or CT scan. Flow–volume loops can define whether the obstruction is intrathoracic (truncated expiratory limb) or extrathoracic (truncated inspiratory limb), but are used rarely because patients are often in respiratory distress and symptomatology often provides the same information. Inspiratory stridor indicates extrathoracic obstruction, whereas expiratory wheezing indicates intrathoracic obstruction. Occasionally, a cooperative, mature patient can be examined under local anesthesia with fiber-optic bronchoscopy. In all cases, general anesthesia, airway management, and rigid bronchoscopy should be immediately available. Coughing or manipulation of the foreign body may convert a partial obstruction to a life-threatening one.

The most common surgical approach to the patient with intrathoracic FBA is a combination of flexible and rigid bronchoscopy. Unlike most other forms of airway obstruction, foreign bodies are at risk of moving to a position that is more obstructive or more difficult to extract. A variety of retrieval tools are available, including baskets, snares, and balloon-tipped catheters that can be passed distal to the foreign body, inflated, and pulled back, as in balloon embolectomy. Aspirated organic matter (e.g., peanuts) may incite reactive mucosal edema that makes extraction more difficult. Friable foreign bodies may break apart with extraction attempts. Rigid bronchoscopy offers greater latitude and is the method of choice for difficult cases. If the object causes life-threatening tracheal occlusion, a solution of last resort is to push the foreign body into a mainstem bronchus and ventilate the contralateral lung. Rarely, it is necessary to surgically open the trachea or bronchus to remove the foreign body.

Anesthetic options range from sedation with local anesthesia for flexible bronchoscopy, to spontaneously breathing inhalation-based general anesthesia, to paralysis with positive pressure ventilation. Pediatric anesthesiologists are often most comfortable and skilled with inhalational inductions. Whether this provides protection against obstruction compared with general anesthesia with positive pressure ventilation is debated. When rigid bronchoscopy is performed, spontaneously breathing volatile agent–based anesthetics may be challenging because of air leak at the glottis and interruptions in gas delivery. Conversion to paralysis and positive pressure ventilation due to desaturation, inadequate depth of anesthesia, or coughing and bucking is frequently required. TIVA is favored by some as a more convenient means of maintaining anesthetic depth during rigid bronchoscopy.

Mediastinoscopy

Mediastinoscopy is a surgical procedure to examine the area between the lungs (mediastinum) using either a rigid or flexible lighted instrument. It is principally used for diagnosis or clinical staging of lung cancer. In some cases, mediastinoscopy has been replaced by other biopsy methods that use CT, ultrasound, or bronchoscopy to guide a biopsy needle to the abnormal tissue. Mediastinoscopy may still be needed when these methods cannot be used or when they do not provide conclusive results.

For cervical mediastinoscopy, the mediastinoscope is passed through an incision just above the manubrium, and advanced along a plane created by blunt dissection between the trachea and the pretracheal fascia (Fig. 90.3).

Anterior mediastinoscopy provides access to lymph nodes of stations 5 and 6 (anterior mediastinal and aortopulmonary window nodes), which typically are not accessible by cervical mediastinoscopy. Blunt dissection to the aortopulmonary window is performed through a 2-cm incision between the second and third ribs. Alternatively, level 5 and 6 nodes can be accessed through the cervical mediastinoscopy incision by creating a more superficial substernal plane beneath the

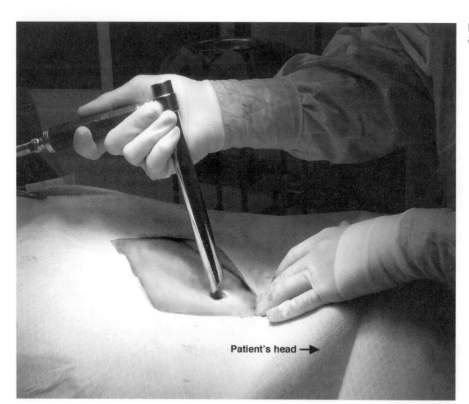

Figure 90.3. Cervical mediastinoscopy; insertion of a cervical mediastinoscope.

Patient's head →

innominate and left carotid arteries, deep to the innominate vein and anterior to the great vessels ("extended mediastinoscopy").

Anatomy of the mediastinum

The mediastinum is the region between the two pleural cavities extending from the thoracic inlet to the diaphragm. This region is further described in Chapter 91.

Anesthesia for mediastinoscopy

Mediastinoscopy patients tend to fall into two groups: those with mediastinal masses (often for biopsy for diagnosis) and those with lymphadenopathy (for cancer staging or diagnosis). Patients with significant masses must be evaluated for compression of the airway, heart, or superior vena cava (see Chapter 91). Mediastinoscopy generally requires general endotracheal anesthesia with muscle relaxation. Subsequent anesthetic considerations are largely intuitive, and are driven by awareness of the potential complications (Table 90.3).

Hemorrhage is the most frequent serious complication. Sources of significant hemorrhage include the azygous vein, the pulmonary artery, and (rarely) the aorta or its major branches. The thin-walled pulmonary artery and azygous vein are vulnerable to avulsion injury as adherent lymph nodes are plucked off their surfaces. The proximity of major vessels emphasizes the importance of a motionless surgical field during biopsy. The response to hemorrhage depends on the magnitude, and ranges from packing and observation to emergent sternotomy or thoracotomy and cardiopulmonary bypass.

Cervical mediastinoscopy often results in compression of the innominate artery with potential compromise of right carotid blood flow. Patients at increased risk are those with coexisting carotid or cerebrovascular disease. A history of cerebrovascular accidents or known left carotid stenosis may warrant electroencephalographic monitoring. Placement of a pulse detector in the right arm (arterial line or pulse oximeter) is widely advocated as an identifier of innominate artery compression, but the actual efficacy of this maneuver is undocumented. Stroke following mediastinoscopy is extremely rare, possibly owing to the generally transient nature of innominate artery compression.

Table 90.3. Complications of mediastinoscopy

Major complications
  Major hemorrhage
  Tracheobronchial laceration
  Esophageal perforation
  Recurrent laryngeal nerve paralysis
  Phrenic nerve paralysis
  Thoracic duct injury
  Cerebrovascular accident
  Air embolus
Minor complications
  Pneumothorax
  Recurrent nerve paresis
  Minor bleeding
  Autonomic reflex bradycardia

Reproduced with permission from Lohser J, Donington J, Mitchell J, et al. Anesthetic management of major hemorrhage during mediastinoscopy. *J Cardiothorac Vasc Anesth* 2005; 19(5):678–683.

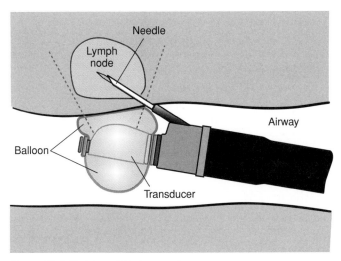

Figure 90.4. Endobronchial ultrasound.

Endobronchial ultrasound-guided transbronchial biopsy

Recent developments have improved the diagnostic resolution of ultrasound while decreasing the diameter of the probe, allowing for a bronchoscope-mounted ultrasound probe. Endobronchial ultrasound (Fig. 90.4) to guide transbronchial biopsy is the most recent development in evaluating mediastinal structures. Anesthetic considerations are similar to those for bronchoscopy, except for two points:

1. There is potential for significant hemoptysis
2. There is potential for tracheal obstruction when the balloon tip is inflated with saline to improve resolution (may require intermittent apnea)

Suggested readings

Kirschner PA. Cervical substernal "extended" mediastinoscopy. In Shields TW, LoCicero J, Ponn RB, eds. *General Thoracic Surgery*. 5th ed. Philadelphia: Lippincott Williams & Wilkins; 2000.

Kumar S, Saxena A, Kumar M, et al. Anesthetic management during bronchoscopic removal of a unique, friable foreign body. *Anesth Analg* 2006; 103(6):1596–1597.

Lohser J, Donington J, Mitchell J, et al. Anesthetic management of major hemorrhage during mediastinoscopy. *J Cardiothorac Vasc Anesth* 2005; 19(5):678–683.

Neuman GG, Weingarten AE, Abramowitz RM, et al. The anesthetic management of the patient with an anterior mediastinal mass. *Anesthesiology* 1984;60:144–147.

Pinzoni F, Baniotti C, Molinaro SM, et al. Inhaled foreign bodies in pediatric patients: review of personal experience. *Int J Pediatr Otorhinolaryngol* 2007; 71(12):1897–1903.

Plummer S, Hartley M, Vaughan R. Anaesthesia for telescopic procedures of the thorax. *Br J Anaesth* 1998; 80:223–234.

Soodan A, Pawar D, Subramaniam R. Anesthesia for removal of foreign bodies in children. *Paediatr Anaesth* 2004; 14(11):947–952.

Chapter

91

Management of mediastinal mass

Ju-Mei Ng

Introduction

The anesthetic considerations for patients with an anterior mediastinal mass vary according to the individual anatomy, pathology, and proposed surgical procedure. Fatal occlusion of the airway and cardiovascular collapse are well-recognized complications. The usefulness of clinical signs and symptoms, radiologic evaluation, and pulmonary function tests to determine perioperative risk are discussed, including some general principles of safe anesthesia for these patients.

Anatomy

The mediastinum extends from the thoracic inlet to the diaphragm and is bounded by the sternum anteriorly, the vertebral column posteriorly, and the parietal pleura laterally. It can be divided into four compartments: superior, anterior, middle, and posterior mediastinum, although the anterosuperior mediastinum may be considered a continuous space (Fig. 91.1).

Pathology

In adults, primary mediastinal masses are generally located in the anterosuperior mediastinum, with a predominance of lymphoma, thymoma, and germ cell tumors. In young children, posterior mediastinal masses of neurogenic origin are most common, whereas in adolescents, lymphomas arising from the anterior mediastinum predominate.

Symptoms and signs

Signs and symptoms are related to mass effect on, or invasion of, surrounding structures (Table 91.1). Most adult mediastinal tumors are asymptomatic or associated with vague complaints such as chest pain, dyspnea, and cough. In contrast, mediastinal masses are symptomatic in 70% of children.

Anesthetic concerns

The three main anesthetic concerns are tracheobronchial tree obstruction; compression of the pulmonary artery and heart, especially the right ventricular outflow tract (RVOT); and superior vena cava (SVC) syndrome. The most common complication during anesthesia for masses involving the vital mediastinal structures is airway obstruction. Each of these

complications is life-threatening and may cause acute deterioration and death during anesthesia if not handled with caution and expertise.

Tracheobronchial tree obstruction

The degree of airway obstruction depends on the location of the mass and extent of compression (Fig. 91.2).

Compression of the pulmonary artery and heart

RVOT obstruction and circulatory collapse may be triggered by altered positioning, induction of anesthesia, institution of positive pressure ventilation, hypovolemia, and reduced cardiac contractility (Fig. 91.3).

Positive pressure ventilation may cause dynamic hyperinflation because of expiratory gas flow obstruction. With

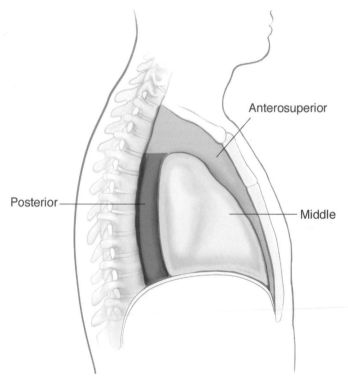

Figure 91.1. Compartments of the mediastinum.

Table 91.1. Signs and symptoms of structural compression by a mediastinal mass

Compression or infiltration of adjacent structures	Symptoms	Signs
Tracheobronchial tree	Cough Stridor Dyspnea Recurrent pulmonary infections Hemoptysis	Wheeze
Esophagus	Dysphagia	
RVOT	Dyspnea Syncope	
Recurrent laryngeal nerve	Hoarseness	Vocal cord paralysis
Sympathetic chain	Horner's syndrome	
Phrenic nerve		Elevated hemidiaphragm
SVC	Dyspnea Cough Syncope Orthopnea Stridor Headache Decreased mentation	Venous engorgement Upper body edema Plethora Cyanosis

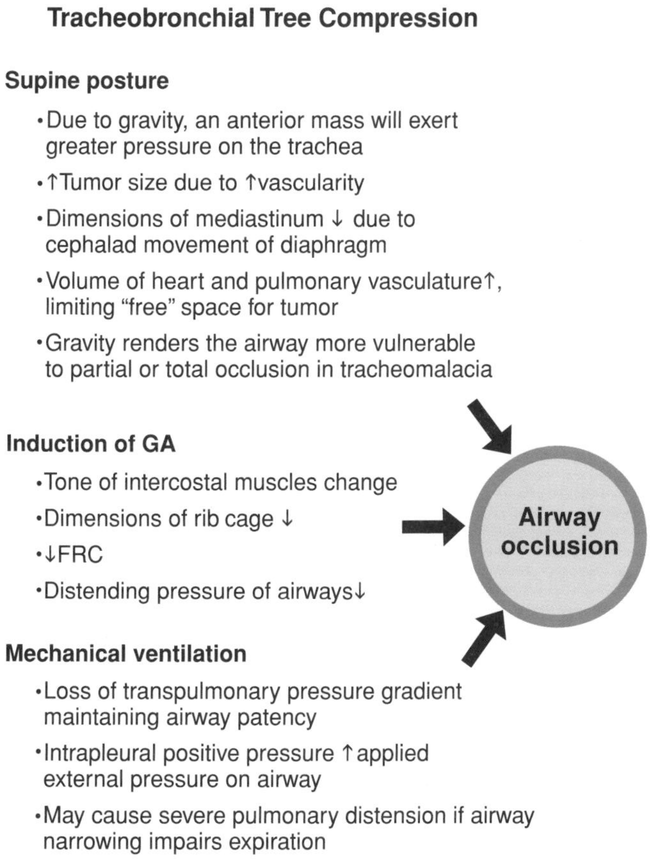

Tracheobronchial Tree Compression
Supine posture
•Due to gravity, an anterior mass will exert greater pressure on the trachea
•↑Tumor size due to ↑vascularity
•Dimensions of mediastinum ↓ due to cephalad movement of diaphragm
•Volume of heart and pulmonary vasculature↑, limiting "free" space for tumor
•Gravity renders the airway more vulnerable to partial or total occlusion in tracheomalacia
Induction of GA
•Tone of intercostal muscles change
•Dimensions of rib cage ↓
•↓FRC
•Distending pressure of airways↓
Mechanical ventilation
•Loss of transpulmonary pressure gradient maintaining airway patency
•Intrapleural positive pressure ↑applied external pressure on airway
•May cause severe pulmonary distension if airway narrowing impairs expiration
Airway occlusion

Figure 91.2. Effects of anesthesia on tracheobronchial tree obstruction.

Compression of the PA and Heart
Increased tumor blood volume and size
Reduced pulmonary blood flow:
Supine
Positive pressure ventilation
Auto-PEEP
Compression of the RVOT/PA
↓Oxygenation
Hypoxemia and hypotension
RV enlargement
↓LV volume → ↓CI
Direct cardiac compression and tamponade
Death

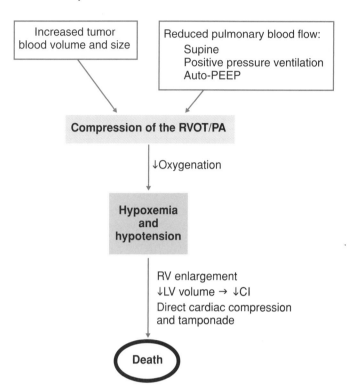

Figure 91.3. Effects of anesthesia on compression of the pulmonary artery and RVOT.

sufficient elevation of intrathoracic pressure, the gradient for venous return is reduced, as are right ventricular pressures, worsening the extent of vascular obstruction.

SVC syndrome

The combination of decreased venous return from the upper part of the body coupled with pharmacologic vasodilatation may result in severe hypotension. Coughing, straining, and supine or Trendelenburg positioning all exacerbate SVC syndrome (Table 91.2).

Preoperative evaluation

The main aims for the anesthesiologist are to delineate the extent of encroachment on other structures and to quantify any functional cardiopulmonary compromise caused by such encroachment. The anesthetic plan is then formulated by taking into account clinical signs and symptoms, radiologic evaluation, and pulmonary function tests (Fig. 91.4).

Table 91.2. Perioperative problems arising from SVC syndrome

	Perioperative concerns
Airway	Edema Airway congestion and hemorrhage
Venous access	Lower extremity Potential for massive hemorrhage

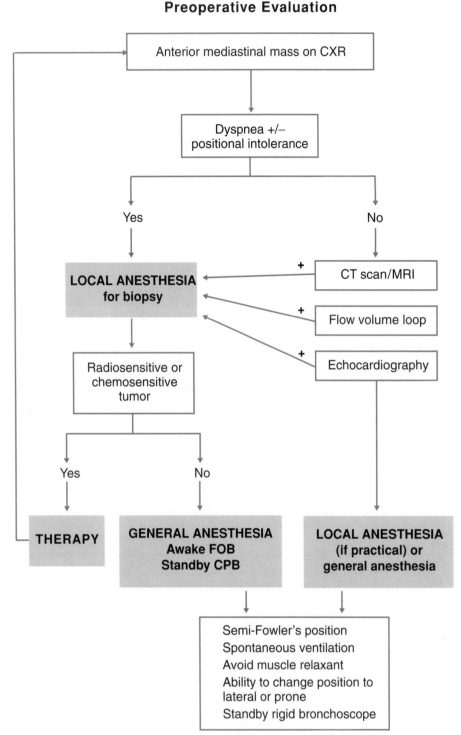

Preoperative Evaluation

Figure 91.4. Preoperative evaluation of a patient with an anterior mediastinal mass.

Radiologic evaluation

A chest CT scan is indicated in all patients and helps identify the location of the mass, delineate margins, define the mass's relationship to adjacent structures, and determine the extent of tracheal or vascular compression. The tracheal cross-sectional area also can be estimated. MRI shows more extensive disease than does CT in 25% of patients, and accurately assesses tumor involvement of cardiac structures.

An increase in the ratio of the transverse diameter of a mediastinal mass to that of the chest has been associated with increased respiratory complications. However, this measurement may be imprecise, and the relation of the mass to the tracheobronchial tree likely is more important. The cross-sectional area of the trachea has been related to the extent of perioperative respiratory complications. There was total airway obstruction in five of eight children under general anesthesia with tracheal area < 50% predicted, but general anesthesia was well tolerated in children with tracheal area > 50% predicted. Postoperative respiratory complications were related to tracheal compression of more than 50% on the preoperative CT scan.

Pulmonary function testing and postural flow–volume loops

Traditionally, part of the preoperative assessment of patients with an anterior mediastinal mass has been to perform postural spirometry. This approach stemmed from the finding that an increased midexpiratory plateau when changing from the upright to the supine position is pathognomonic for a variable intrathoracic airway obstruction and an indicator of patients who are at risk for airway collapse during induction of anesthesia (Fig. 91.5).

Pulmonary function testing gives information about functional impairment but does not accurately predict airway morbidity and does not describe anatomic abnormality. Moreover, studies of flow–volume loops have shown poor correlation with the degree of airway obstruction and may not be any better than symptoms and a CT scan at predicting perioperative complications. In clinical practice, postural spirometry probably does not offer any additive benefit in predicting perioperative complications in a minimally symptomatic population beyond that which is obtained from chest imaging.

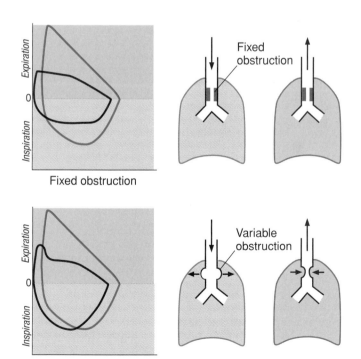

Figure 91.5. Effects of fixed and variable obstructions on flow-volume loops.

Peak expiratory flow rate

The risk of perioperative complications was increased more than 10-fold when the peak expiratory flow rate (PEFR) was 40% or less of predicted. A combination of obstructive and restrictive patterns (mixed pulmonary syndrome) was associated with a high rate of postoperative respiratory complications. In a prospective evaluation of 31 children before 34 procedures, Shamberger et al. found that all patients did well under general anesthesia if their tracheal cross-sectional area and PEFR were > 50%.

Echocardiography

Patients with cardiovascular symptoms, or those unable to give an adequate history, should also undergo transthoracic echocardiography to assess for cardiac, systemic, or pulmonary vascular compression. Echocardiography reliably identifies pericardial thickening and masses adjacent to the pericardium, and can evaluate myocardial dysfunction due to tumor compression or infiltration.

Anesthetic management
Acute management

When a patient presents with acute symptoms, it is important to maintain the sitting posture (or most comfortable position) and provide humidified oxygen. If available, heliox (20% oxygen + 80% helium) may be helpful because it can decrease the density of the inspiratory gas and reduce airway resistance. Steroids have been used successfully to decrease tumor size without affecting the accuracy of histologic diagnosis post administration. The possibility of preoperative chemo- or radiotherapy may be considered. Figure 91.6 shows anesthetic management of anterior mediastinal masses.

Diagnostic procedures

Tissue biopsy is likely the first procedure for most patients, and tissue may be obtained from biopsy of peripheral or metastatic lesions. This avoids an intrathoracic procedure and the need for a general anesthetic. Awake CT-guided needle biopsy (under local anesthesia and sedation as required) and awake anterior mediastinoscopy with local anesthesia in adults are performed relatively frequently.

Induction and intubation

Although there is a need to individualize management on a case-by-case basis, there are some general principles. Depending on the level, extent, and severity of obstruction, awake fiberoptic video-bronchoscopy may be used. This approach allows both the anesthesia and surgical teams to view the lesion and assess the airway dynamics, degree of airway compression, and effect of changes in posture. An appropriately sized endotracheal tube can then be passed beyond the lesion. A routine intravenous induction and intubation may be

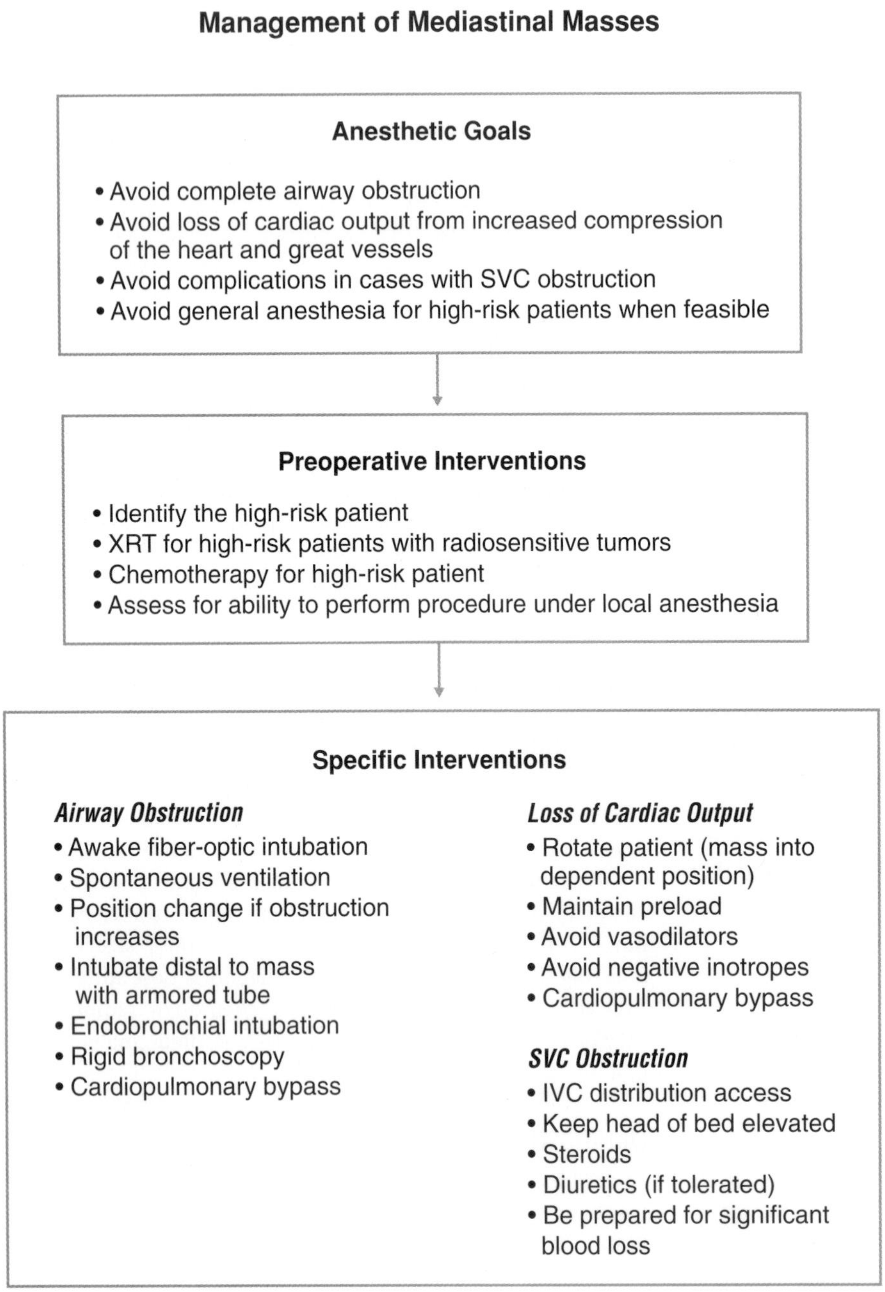

Management of Mediastinal Masses

Figure 91.6. Anesthetic management of an anterior mediastinal mass.

Anesthetic Goals

- Avoid complete airway obstruction
- Avoid loss of cardiac output from increased compression of the heart and great vessels
- Avoid complications in cases with SVC obstruction
- Avoid general anesthesia for high-risk patients when feasible

Preoperative Interventions

- Identify the high-risk patient
- XRT for high-risk patients with radiosensitive tumors
- Chemotherapy for high-risk patient
- Assess for ability to perform procedure under local anesthesia

Specific Interventions

Airway Obstruction
- Awake fiber-optic intubation
- Spontaneous ventilation
- Position change if obstruction increases
- Intubate distal to mass with armored tube
- Endobronchial intubation
- Rigid bronchoscopy
- Cardiopulmonary bypass

Loss of Cardiac Output
- Rotate patient (mass into dependent position)
- Maintain preload
- Avoid vasodilators
- Avoid negative inotropes
- Cardiopulmonary bypass

SVC Obstruction
- IVC distribution access
- Keep head of bed elevated
- Steroids
- Diuretics (if tolerated)
- Be prepared for significant blood loss

performed in patients with no symptomatic, radiologic, or bronchoscopic evidence of airway obstruction. In the pediatric population, an inhalational induction is frequently used. In adults, stage II events may be common during inhalational induction, and it may be difficult to abort midcourse. Other techniques that have been described include the laryngeal mask airway, rigid bronchoscopy, and use of a distal jet ventilation catheter.

Ventilation

It is important to remember that positive pressure ventilation–induced dynamic hyperinflation may worsen obstruction.

Low-frequency or high-frequency jet ventilation has been used successfully. The strategy also depends on the site of compression and whether an appropriately sized single- or double-lumen endotracheal tube or single-lumen endobronchial tube can successfully stent open the airway. Laryngoscopy and rigid bronchoscopy have been used successfully to relieve obstruction. In the postoperative period, corticosteroids, racemic epinephrine, or heliox may be useful.

A stepwise induction of anesthesia is important; it allows the patient to be awakened quickly if airway or vascular compression develops. Repositioning of the patient may be helpful in relieving airway compression.

SVC syndrome

There are no data to support any particular induction and intubation technique. The use of an antisialagogue, a bronchodilator, or racemic epinephrine and maintenance of the sitting position appear to be helpful.

Perils of biopsy under local anesthesia

Anxiety, pain, or high sympathetic tone may increase ventilatory demand and worsen airflow dynamics by inducing turbulent flow across the obstruction. A variety of techniques have been used. Ketamine has been shown to preserve chest wall tone and functional residual capacity.

Suggested readings

Azarow KS, Pearl RH, Zurcher R, et al. Primary mediastinal masses: a comparison of adult and pediatric populations. *J Thorac Cardiovasc Surg* 1993; 106:67–72.

Azizkhan RG, Dudgeon DL, Buck JR, et al. Life-threatening airway obstruction as a complication to the management of mediastinal masses in children. *J Pediatr Surg* 1985; 20(6):816–822.

Bechard P, Letourneau L, Lacasse Y, et al. Perioperative cardiorespiratory complications in adults with mediastinal mass. *Anesthesiology* 2004; 100:826–834.

deSoto H. Direct laryngoscopy as an aid to relieve airway obstruction in a patient with a mediastinal mass. *Anesthesiology* 1987; 67(1):116–117.

Goh MH, Liu XY, Goh YS. Anterior mediastinal masses: an anaesthetic challenge. *Anaesthesia* 1999; 54:670–674.

Keon TP. Death on induction of anesthesia for cervical node biopsy. *Anesthesiology* 1981; 55:471–472.

Levin H, Bursztein S, Heifetz M. Cardiac arrest in a child with an anterior mediastinal mass. *Anesth Analg* 1985; 64:1129–1130.

Lyerly HK, Sabiston DC Jr. Primary neoplasms and cysts of the mediastinum. In Fishman AP, ed. *Pulmonary Diseases and Disorders*. 2nd ed. New York: McGraw-Hill; 1988.

Mancuso L, Pitrolo F, Bondi F, et al. Echocardiographic recognition of mediastinal masses. *Chest* 1988; 93(1):144–148.

Prakash UB, Abel MD, Hubmayr RD. Mediastinal mass and tracheal obstruction during general anesthesia. *Mayo Clin Proc* 1988; 63:1004–1011.

Shamberger RC, Holzman RS, Griscom NT, et al. Prospective evaluation by computed tomography and pulmonary function tests of children with mediastinal masses. *Surgery* 1995; 118:468–471.

Torchio R, Gulotta C, Perboni A, et al. Orthopnea and tidal expiratory flow limitation in patients with euthyroid goiter. *Chest* 2003; 124:133–140.

Turoff RD, Gomez GA, Berjian R, et al. Postoperative respiratory complications in patients with Hodgkin's disease: relationship to the size of the mediastinal tumor. *Eur J Cancer Clin Oncol* 1985; 21:1043–1046.

Principles of neurophysiology

Dennis J. McNicholl and Lee A. Kearse Jr.

Autonomic nervous system: anatomy and receptor pharmacology

The autonomic nervous system (ANS) controls the visceral, involuntary, "auto-pilot" functions of the body – functions that are not under conscious control. Understanding the effects of drugs used in the practice of anesthesia is built on a foundation of the anatomy and physiology of the ANS. Broadly, the ANS is subdivided into the central ANS (hypothalamus, medulla oblongata, and pons) and the peripheral ANS. The peripheral ANS is then further subdivided into the sympathetic nervous system (SNS) and the parasympathetic nervous system (PNS) (see Figs. 92.1 and 92.2).

Sympathetic nervous system ("thoracolumbar" division of the peripheral ANS)

The SNS is a "high-gain" system in the sense that activation of a presynaptic nerve fiber results in mass activation of postganglionic nerve fibers. The ratio of preganglionic to postganglionic fibers in the SNS is approximately 1:200. Sympathetic fibers are distributed throughout the body. Cell bodies in this division of the peripheral ANS originate in the intermediolateral columns of the thoracolumbar spinal cord and travel via spinal nerves T1–L2. Autonomic reflexes function similarly to somatic reflexes with the exception that the efferent limb is unipolar in the somatic arc and bipolar in the autonomic arc (see Fig. 92.3).

Anatomically, synapses in the SNS occur in the paravertebral ganglia (a.k.a. the sympathetic chain or sympathetic trunk ganglia, of which there are 22 pairs) and the prevertebral ganglia (3 unpaired: celiac, superior mesenteric, and inferior mesenteric ganglia). The paravertebral ganglia are connected to the spinal nerves by white rami communicans (myelinated preganglionic fibers which carry signals from the lateral horn cells of the spinal cord into the paravertebral ganglion) and gray rami communicans (unmyelinated postganglionic fibers which continue the signal from the paravertebral ganglion out to the spinal nerves). The paravertebral ganglia are also connected to each other by nerve trunks to form longitudinal chains; this connection allows for nerve fibers to travel up or down several ganglia before synapsing. Preganglionic fibers are short, and

postganglionic fibers are long. One exception is for the adrenal medulla, which has no postganglionic fibers – preganglionic fibers enter the adrenal medulla and synapse on cells that secrete neurotransmitters directly into the bloodstream.

Functionally, all preganglionic fibers in the SNS are cholinergic (i.e., release acetylcholine). Postganglionic fibers in the SNS are adrenergic (i.e., release epinephrine or norepinephrine) or dopaminergic (i.e., release dopamine). Effects of activation of adrenergic receptors are shown in Table 92.1.

Parasympathetic nervous system ("craniosacral" division of the peripheral ANS)

In contrast to the SNS, the PNS is a "low-gain" system; its activation results in a discrete and limited effect. The ratio of preganglionic to postganglionic fibers in the PNS is approximately 1:2. Preganglionic nerves in the PNS are long, and postganglionic nerves are short and are usually located on or in their intended effector organs. Cell bodies in the PNS originate in the midbrain (cranial nerve [CN] III), medulla oblongata (CN VII, IX, and X), and sacral spinal cord (S2–S4). CN X accounts for approximately 75% of parasympathetic activity. The pelvic nerves (S2–S4) supply the distal colon, bladder, and genitalia.

As with the SNS, all preganglionic PNS nerves are cholinergic. All postganglionic nerves of the PNS are also cholinergic. Cholinergic receptors are classified according to their response to nicotine or muscarine. Nicotine is the prototypical ganglionic stimulant, and nicotinic receptors can be further subdivided into N_N (subscript "N" denoting Neuronal-type) receptors found in autonomic ganglia, adrenal medulla, and central nervous system (CNS), and N_M (subscript "M" denoting Muscle-type) receptors located at the neuromuscular junction. Muscarine is a compound isolated from the mushroom *Amanita muscaria* and was the first parasympathomimetic to be studied. The muscarinic receptors have been subdivided into five receptor subtypes (M_1–M_5). Most notably, the M_2 receptor subtype, when activated, leads to a slowing of spontaneous depolarization in the sinoatrial (SA) node and slower conductance through the atrioventricular (AV) node.

A comparison between the SNS and PNS is shown in Table 92.2.

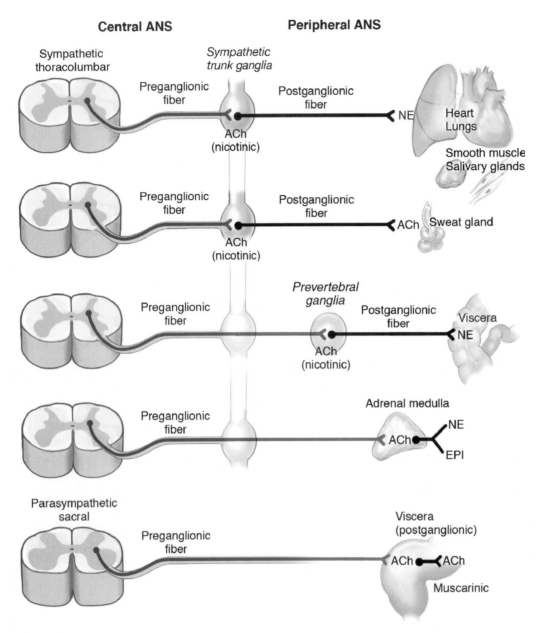

Central ANS   **Peripheral ANS**

Sympathetic   *Sympathetic*
thoracolumbar   *trunk ganglia*

Preganglionic   Postganglionic
fiber   fiber

ACh
(nicotinic)

NE   Heart
            Lungs

            Smooth muscle
            Salivary glands

Preganglionic   Postganglionic
fiber   fiber

ACh
(nicotinic)

ACh   Sweat gland

*Prevertebral
ganglia*

Preganglionic   Postganglionic
fiber   fiber   Viscera

ACh   NE
(nicotinic)

Adrenal medulla

Preganglionic   NE
fiber

ACh

EPI

Parasympathetic   Viscera
sacral   (postganglionic)

Preganglionic
fiber

ACh   ACh

Muscarinic

Figure 92.1. The autonomic nervous system.

Autonomic control of the heart

Cardiac output can increase by more than 100% through sympathetic stimulation of cardiac accelerator fibers (derived from spinal nerves T1–T4); elevation in both the heart rate and contractility contributes to this increase. By comparison, cardiac output can be decreased to almost zero by parasympathetic stimulation. This effect, however, is primarily mediated via heart rate decrease; contractility is less affected by parasympathetic stimulation.

Sympathetic innervation of the heart is diffuse and abundant, resulting in a robust response when activated. Cardiac output can increase two- to threefold with sympathetic stimulation. Parasympathetic input to the heart, via the vagus nerve,

is more discrete (SA and AV nodes). Therefore, parasympathetic/vagal input to the heart affects rate more than pumping capacity – strong vagal stimulation can decrease heart rate to almost zero but the strength of cardiac contraction by only 20% to 30%.

Autonomic control of blood vessels

With the exception of capillaries, all vessels are innervated with sympathetic fibers and can therefore vasoconstrict to cause an increase in blood pressure. This effect is more prominent in the venous system, which contains more blood volume (~64%) at any given time compared with the arterial system. There is no clinically relevant parasympathetic control of blood vessels.

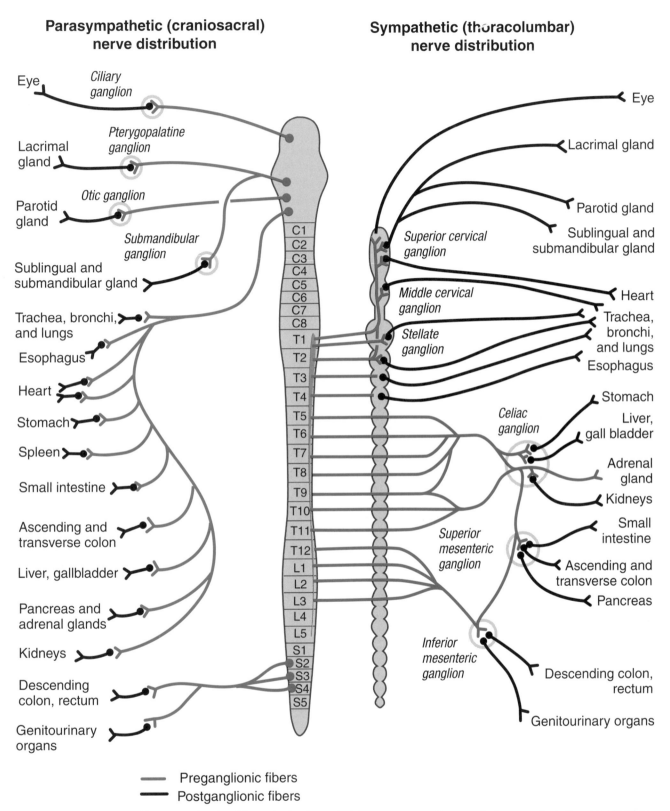

Parasympathetic (craniosacral) nerve distribution

Eye — *Ciliary ganglion*

Lacrimal gland — *Pterygopalatine ganglion*

Parotid gland — *Otic ganglion*

Submandibular ganglion

Sublingual and submandibular gland

Trachea, bronchi, and lungs

Esophagus

Heart

Stomach

Spleen

Small intestine

Ascending and transverse colon

Liver, gallbladder

Pancreas and adrenal glands

Kidneys

Descending colon, rectum

Genitourinary organs

Sympathetic (thoracolumbar) nerve distribution

Eye

Lacrimal gland

Parotid gland

Sublingual and submandibular gland

Superior cervical ganglion

Middle cervical ganglion

Heart

Trachea, bronchi, and lungs

Stellate ganglion

Esophagus

Stomach

Celiac ganglion

Liver, gall bladder

Adrenal gland

Kidneys

Small intestine

Superior mesenteric ganglion

Ascending and transverse colon

Pancreas

Inferior mesenteric ganglion

Descending colon, rectum

Genitourinary organs

C1 C2 C3 C4 C5 C6 C7 C8 T1 T2 T3 T4 T5 T6 T7 T8 T9 T10 T11 T12 L1 L2 L3 L4 L5 S1 S2 S3 S4 S5

— Preganglionic fibers
— Postganglionic fibers

Figure 92.2. The craniosacral (parasympathetic) and thoracolumbar (sympathetic) nervous systems. Parasympathetic preganglionic fibers pass directly to innervate their organ. Postganglionic cell bodies are located near or within the innervated viscera. This limited distribution of parasympathetic postganglionic fibers emphasizes the limited effect of parasympathetic function. In the sympathetic nervous system, the postganglionic neurons begin in either the paired sympathetic ganglia (i.e., the paravertebral ganglia) or one of the unpaired collateral plexuses (i.e., the celiac, superior mesenteric, inferior mesenteric ganglia). One preganglionic fiber influences many postganglionic neurons. Activation of the SNS therefore produces a more diffuse physiologic response.

Table 92.1. Adrenergic receptors

Receptor	Synaptic site	Anatomic site	Action	LV function and stroke volume
α_1	Postsynaptic	Peripheral vascular smooth muscle	Constriction	Decreased
		Renal vascular smooth muscle	Constriction	
		Coronary arteries, epicardial	Constriction	
		Myocardium	Positive inotropism 30%–40% of resting tone	Improved
		Renal tubules	Antidiuresis	
α_2	Presynaptic	Peripheral vascular smooth muscle release	Inhibition of NE	
			Secondary vasodilation	Improved
		Coronaries	?	
		CNS	Inhibition of CNS activity	
			Sedation	
			Decrease in MAC	
	Postsynaptic	Coronaries, endocardial	Constriction	Decreased
		Gastrointestinal system	Inhibition of insulin release	
			Decrease in bowel motility	
		CNS	Inhibition of antidiuretic hormone	
			Analgesia	
		Renal tubule	Promotion of Na^+ and H_2O excretion	
β_1	Postsynaptic (NE sensitive)	Myocardium	Positive inotropism and chronotropism	Improved
		Sinoatrial (SA) node		
		Ventricular conduction		
		Kidney	Renin release	
		Coronaries	Relaxation	
β_2	Presynaptic (NE sensitive)	Myocardium	Acceleration of NE release	Improved
		SA node ventricular conduction vessels	Opposite action to presynaptic α_2 agonism	
			Constriction	
	Postsynaptic (extrasynaptic) (EPI sensitive)	Myocardium	Positive inotropism and chronotropism	
		Vascular smooth muscle	Relaxation	Improved
		Bronchial smooth muscle	Relaxation	Improved
		Renal vessels	Relaxation	Improved
DA_1	Postsynaptic	Blood vessels (renal, mesentery, coronary)	Vasodilation	Improved
		Renal tubules	Natriuresis	
			Diuresis	
		Juxtaglomerular cells	Renin release (modulates diuresis)	
		Sympathetic ganglia	Minor inhibition	
DA_2	Presynaptic	Postganglionic sympathetic nerves	Inhibition of NE release	Improved
			Secondary vasodilation	
	Postsynaptic	Renal and mesenteric vasculature	? Vasoconstriction	

NE, norepinephrine; EPI, epinephrine

Control of circulation is affected by 1) sympathetic chain ganglion (T1–L2), 22 pairs in total, and 2) peripheral nerve fibers originating from T1 to L2 which then travel via the sympathetic chain to the vasculature.

Cerebral physiology
Cerebral metabolic rate

The cerebral metabolic rate (CMR) of oxygen ($CMRO_2$) is defined as the amount of oxygen consumed by the brain in normal, conscious young men (rates are similar for young women). Of all organs, the brain and the heart are at highest risk for ischemia due to their high oxygen utilization and relatively low physiologic reserve. With respect to the brain, this susceptibility stems from its high metabolic demand and its lack of significant anaerobic metabolism to support function in times of decreased oxygen or glucose substrate. The window of time for development of severe irreversible brain damage from hypoxemia is approximately 3 to 8 minutes at normal body temperature. In normal physiology, $CMRO_2$ depends on the functional state (ranging from seizure activity to the comatose or anesthetized state) and body temperature. At normal body temperature, resting $CMRO_2$ is 3.5 ml O_2/100 g/min. Hypothermia decreases $CMRO_2$ significantly. At a body temperature of 18°C to 20°C, complete burst suppression of the electroencephalogram (EEG) can be seen. Conversely, hyperthermia increases $CMRO_2$, however only up to a point (~42°C/103°F). Beyond this range, $CMRO_2$ actually decreases, likely due to neuronal breakdown and enzyme degradation. Therefore, at the extremes of temperature, $CMRO_2$ declines.

Autonomic   **Somatic**

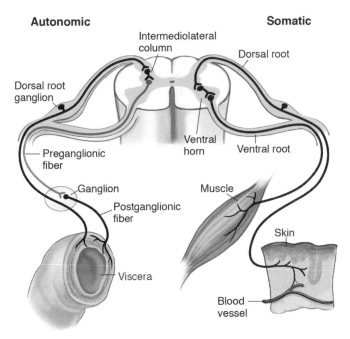

Figure 92.3. Somatic and autonomic reflex arcs. Somatic arcs are unipolar, in contrast to autonomic arcs, which are bipolar.

Cerebral blood flow

Due to the high metabolic demands of the brain (i.e., CMRO$_2$), cerebral blood flow (CBF) is disproportionately high (compared to other organs on a gram-for-gram basis). Distribution of that blood flow will change depending on which regions of the brain are metabolically more active; CBF and metabolism are coupled in normal physiology. Blood flow to the cortex (mostly gray matter) is considerably higher than blood flow to subcortical areas (mostly white matter). The mechanism for this coupling is not completely understood; however, it does allow for manipulation of the CBF by extrinsic influences such as carbon dioxide [CO$_2$] and mean arterial pressure [MAP] regulation (chemoregulation and mechanoregulation, respectively).

CBF is autoregulated in normal patients with MAP between 60 and 150 mmHg. As a starting point, normal homeostasis with a PaCO$_2$ of 40 mm Hg corresponds to a CBF of

$\sim$50 ml/100 g/min. With a PaCO$_2$ increase from 40 to 80 mmHg, CBF would double to $\sim$100 ml/100 g/min. With a CO$_2$ decrease from 40 to 20 mmHg, CBF would be halved (down to $\sim$25 ml/100g/min). In situations in which CBF becomes altered by elevated or depressed CO$_2$ levels, CBF will return to normal after approximately 6 to 8 hours, even if the PaCO$_2$ remains abnormal. In patients who are chronically hypertensive, the CBF autoregulation curve is shifted to the right, and maintenance of higher MAPs is required to avoid relative hypotension and cerebral hypoperfusion. Other circumstances can also disrupt CBF autoregulation: trauma, hypoxia, ischemia, and iatrogenic influences (e.g., anesthetic agents, systemic vasodilators/vasopressors).

Changes in CO$_2$ levels will affect CBF. Hypoventilation leads to elevated levels of CO$_2$, causing a lower pH, cerebral arteriolar vasodilatation, and increased CBF. Under normal conditions, CMRO$_2$ and CBF are inextricably coupled. This arrangement can be negated, however, under circumstances of physiologic disruption. The most common example is that of ischemic stroke. In this setting, early in the course of the stroke, autoregulation of cerebral perfusion is altered in the tissues marked by the damaged ischemic core as well as the "penumbra," the area immediately contiguous with the core. The peri-infarct zone, depending on its size and location, tends not to be uniformly injured, varying between areas demonstrating increases in CMRO$_2$ and those showing distinct reductions in CMRO$_2$ and oxygen extraction fraction (OEF). Postischemic hyperperfusion is a common finding in human stroke imaging studies and animal stroke models, where damaged areas without CMRO$_2$ regulation receive excessive blood flow and volume independent of the metabolic requirements of the area. This luxury perfusion can cause further damage to the area, leading to edema and hemorrhagic extravasation into core ischemic and adjacent areas. Clinical management of CBF by CO$_2$ manipulations may become quite complicated when attempting to provide the optimal blood flow to injured brain in this disorder. Hyperventilation, for example, may vasoconstrict the normal blood vessels and shunt needed nutrients away from the damaged areas that are still viable and have an increased CMRO$_2$ requirement but where blood vessels supplying flow to that area are already maximally dilated. This "inverse steal" or "Robin

Table 92.2. Comparison: sympathetic vs. parasympathetic nervous systems

Anatomic/physiologic parameter	Sympathetic nervous system	Parasympathetic nervous system
Alias	Thoracolumbar (T1–L2)	Craniosacral
Energy mode	Energy expenditure	Energy conservation/restoration
Amplification response	High-gain system	Low-gain system
Target effect density	Diffuse, mass effects	Discrete, limited effects
Preganglionic length	Short	Long
Postganglionic length	Long	Short
Preganglionic neurotransmitter	ACh	ACh
Postganglionic neurotransmitter	ACh, EPI, NE, DA	ACh

ACh, acetylcholine; EPI, epinephrine; NE, norepinephrine; DA, dopamine

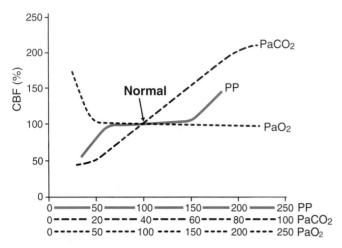

Figure 92.4. Cerebral blood flow is affected by cerebral perfusion pressure (PP), arterial carbon dioxide partial pressure (PaCO$_2$), and arterial oxygen partial pressure (PaO$_2$).

Hood effect" may cause further damage to an already injured but salvageable location.

The effect of hyperventilation on CBF to minimize brain edema and increased intracranial pressure (ICP) has its limits. Cerebral ischemia can result from significant hyperventilation (PaCO$_2$ ~20 mm Hg); therefore, the clinical benefit of hyperventilation to less than 30 mm Hg is lost.

Changes in PaO$_2$ can also affect CBF, but only at the lower end of the PaO$_2$ scale. A PaO$_2$ of less than ~50 mm Hg actually causes a significant increase in CBF, but with one greater than ~60 mm Hg there is no appreciable change in CBF (see Figure 92.4).

Hypothermia decreases neuronal metabolic demand and thereby decreases CBF. Hyperthermia causes the opposite effect.

Hematocrit in the normal range does not have a clinically significant effect on CBF. Some increase in CBF can be seen at lower hematocrit ranges (~30%–34%) due to decreased blood viscosity and decreased cerebrovascular resistance. This relative hemodilution effect can be clinically beneficial in the setting of focal cerebral ischemia, where maximal vasodilatation already exists. By contrast, hemoconcentration is not a particular concern unless at extreme levels (hematocrit ~>55%), in which case it becomes an issue for other organ beds as well.

Cerebral blood volume

Cerebral blood volume (CBV) in the normal brain is approximately 5 ml/100 g of brain tissue, which is approximately 70 ml for a normal adult brain. Changes in CBV and CBF usually parallel each other, especially for ranges of CBF that are autoregulated. At lower MAPs there is an increase in CBV as the cerebral vasculature dilates to maintain constant flow. Similarly, during cerebral ischemia, CBV increases. At higher MAPs, in the range beyond the upper limit of autoregulation, CBV and CBF both increase.

Cerebral perfusion pressure

Normal cerebral perfusion pressure (CPP) is approximately 80 to 100 mm Hg. A somewhat unusual physiologic formula exists for CPP, because the formula itself can change depending on the state of the variables that contribute to it.

For patients with intracranial hypertension, the expression of CPP is:

$$CPP = MAP - ICP \qquad \text{(Eqn. 1)}$$

For patients without intracranial hypertension, the expression for CPP is:

$$CPP = MAP - CVP \qquad \text{(Eqn. 2)}$$

For any case in which the cranium is open, the expression for CPP is:

$$CPP = MAP \qquad \text{(Eqn. 3)}$$

Table 92.3 indicates this difference in how CPP is determined depending on the clinical circumstances. In any case, the factor that contributes most to CPP is MAP.

Table 92.3. Determination of cerebral perfusion pressure

	MAP (mm Hg)	ICP (mm Hg)	CVP (mm Hg)	CPP (mm Hg)
Pt. #1 – normal	80	10	5	70
Pt. #2 – head injury	80	20	5	60
Pt. #3 – heart failure	80	10	20	60
Pt. #4 – open cranium	80	0	5	80

For the supine patient, MAP should be measured at the circle of Willis, which is approximated by zeroing the transducer at the level of the tragus. For a patient undergoing surgery in the seated position, the transducer should be zeroed at the highest point of the skull.

When not maintained in the normal range, CPP can be detrimental due to cerebral ischemia secondary to hypoperfusion at one extreme, and disruption of the blood–brain barrier from vessel rupture with resultant ischemia and cerebral edema at the other extreme.

Intracranial pressure

Normal (ICP) in humans is ≤ 10 mm Hg. Although there is some degree of compliance in the intracranial space, the reserve is limited, and further additions of volume would ultimately result in an exponential increase in pressure. The balance of ICP is dynamically influenced by the three intracranial components – brain, cerebrospinal fluid (CSF), and blood. Swelling of the brain parenchyma or growth of a brain tumor can increase ICP. Blocked drainage of CSF by mass effect on outflow tracts or by decreased absorption through the arachnoid villi can increase ICP. Finally, increased blood volume via vasodilatation, hemorrhage, or hematoma can also increase

ICP. The head-down position in particular will increase ICP solely by allowing gravity to affect cerebral blood volume, an important consideration for placement of central lines into the internal jugular or subclavian veins. Alone or in combination, these effects can rapidly become fatal, either through ischemia from hypoperfusion or by herniation of brain tissue. Although ICP is used to guide clinical management, it does not provide direct information regarding neuronal function or potential for neuronal recovery in the injured brain. Clinically, the fastest method for reducing ICP is CSF drainage via a lumbar or intra-ventricular drain. Other methods include elevation of the head (via gravity-provoked venous drainage), hypocapnia induced by hyperventilation, and medication interventions such as barbi-turates, osmotic diuretics, or corticosteroids selectively used for brain tumors.

Cerebrospinal fluid

Secretion function

Secretion of cerebrospinal fluid (CSF) occurs mainly in the choroid plexus via active transport of sodium ions, which in turn brings chloride and subsequently water (by osmosis) into the subarachnoid space.

Cushion function

The specific gravity of CSF and that of the brain are nearly iden-tical, allowing for flotation of the brain in the CSF medium. The brain and CSF move as a unit when struck, cushioning the insult to the brain parenchyma from its striking the inner surface of the skull.

Excretory function

CSF is reabsorbed by the arachnoid villi, emptying into the sagittal venous sinus and thereby into the bloodstream. There are no true lymphatics in brain tissue, so any protein leakage from parenchymal capillaries in the brain will be absorbed into the subarachnoid space and thus be reabsorbed by the arach-noid villi.

CSF pressure

Normal CSF pressure is 10 mm Hg for a supine patient. This value can range from 5 to 15 mm Hg in normal patients; how-ever, in pathologic states this can increase to 40 mm Hg or higher. Such high pressures can be caused by mass effect from an intracranial tumor compressing the brain, blocking the normal flow of CSF. In other cases the filtering function of the arach-noid villi can become dysfunctional secondary to inflamma-tion or physical blockages of the villi due to increased numbers of cells in the CSF, as is the case with infection or intracranial hemorrhage.

Blood–brain barrier

The first line of defense the brain has against molecules and ionized particles entering the interstitium of the brain is the blood–brain barrier (BBB). Anatomically, this barrier consists of tight junctions between brain capillary endothelial cells, in contrast to fenestrations found in vascular endothelium in other areas of the body. Disruption of this barrier by chronic dis-ease processes (e.g., intracranial tumors, uncontrolled systemic hypertension) or by acute events (e.g., hypertension from direct laryngoscopy, trauma, or inadequately managed acute pain) can have devastating if not fatal consequences. Severe hypertension of even very short duration poses significant risk. Substances that are unimpeded by the BBB include water, lipid-soluble compounds (e.g., volatile anesthetics), and gases (e.g., oxygen [O_2], carbon dioxide [CO_2], nitrous oxide [N_2O]). The BBB is an effective, although not complete, barrier to charged parti-cles (e.g., electrolytes), polar compounds (e.g., glucose, manni-tol, amino acids), and larger molecules (e.g., proteins). Access to the brain interstitium can be obtained by these particles and compounds through facilitated diffusion (as is the case for glu-cose), active transport (as is the case for ions), or pinocyto-sis (as is the case for larger particles such as proteins). Certain areas of the brain are not protected by the BBB, notably the area postrema (with attendant implications for postoperative nausea and vomiting), the pineal gland, and some areas of the hypothalamus.

Anesthetic agents: effects on cerebral physiology

Knowledge of the effects of the various anesthetic agents, alone or in combination with each other, is critical to proper selection of drugs for patients with disturbance of anatomic or physio-logic cerebral function (see Fig. 92.6).

Inhalation agents

Volatile anesthetics

All of the volatile anesthetics cause a dose-dependent decrease in CMR. The effect of volatile anesthetics on CBF is some-what more complicated. CBF is reduced at lower concentrations of volatile anesthetics (~0.5 minimum alveolar concentration [MAC]) due to lower CMR. CBF is increased, however, at higher concentrations of volatile anesthetics (~>1.0 MAC) due to the dilating effects of volatile anesthetics on the cerebral vascu-lature. The balance between these two divergent impacts on CBF is achieved at ~ 1.0 MAC, at which point CBF is neither increased nor decreased; it remains unchanged.

CMR

All of the volatile anesthetics cause a reduction in CMR. The degree of reduction varies somewhat, with isoflurane, sevoflu-rane, desflurane, and enflurane causing similar decrease in CMR of approximately 50%. Maximal reduction occurs at 1.5 to 2.0 MAC, and this corresponds to EEG suppression. Compared to all the other volatile anesthetics, halothane causes the small-est decrease (~25%) in CMR. Another noteworthy exception among the volatile anesthetics is enflurane – while it does cause

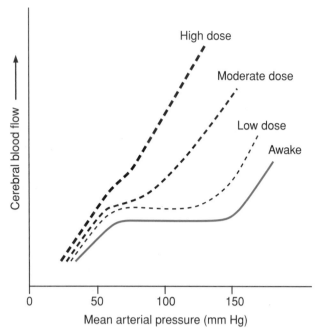

Figure 92.5. Cerebral autoregulation is depressed by the volatile anesthetics in a dose dependent manner.

a reduction in CMR, it also has the capacity to cause seizure-type EEG activity with a concomitant increase in CMR.

CBF

CBF is augmented by volatile anesthetics due to their direct vasodilatory action on the cerebral vasculature. Autoregulation of CBF becomes increasingly blunted with increasing concentrations of volatile anesthetics. The normal autoregulation curve becomes almost linear, with a continuous positive slope, as seen in Fig. 92.5. The approximate order of cerebral vasodilation potency of the volatile anesthetics is halothane (191% increase in CBF at 1.1 MAC) >> desflurane ≈ isoflurane (19% increase in CBF at 1.1 MAC) > sevoflurane. After continued delivery of volatile anesthetic to animals for 2 to 5 hours, CBF returns

to normal levels, but this phenomenon has not been shown in humans. Although all the volatile anesthetics cause an increase in CBF, halothane is notable for causing the largest increase in CBF.

ICP

Isoflurane is unique among the volatile anesthetics in its ability to cause CSF absorption, with resultant decrease in ICP.

N₂O

The effect of N_2O on cerebral physiology depends in large part on the manner in which it is administered; its effects differ if it is administered alone or in combination with an intravenous anesthetic or volatile anesthetic. When administered alone, increases in CBF and ICP do occur and are substantial, owing to the cerebral vasodilation effects of N_2O. These effects, however, are attenuated to negligible levels when N_2O is delivered in conjunction with most intravenous anesthetics (ketamine being the notable exception). When administered with volatile anesthetics, CBF is increased beyond what would be expected if the volatile anesthetic were given alone. This effect can be mitigated by other interventions such as induced hypocapnia (response to CO_2 is preserved with N_2O administration) or barbiturate infusion. In summary, N_2O in the clinical setting of reduced intracranial compliance can be appropriate if used judiciously with other available agents or techniques.

Intravenous agents

Intravenous anesthetics

Parallel reduction in CBF and CMR is the general rule with the effects of intravenous anesthetic agents on cerebral physiology. For this reason, flow and metabolism are said to be "coupled." In contrast, flow and metabolism are not coupled for volatile anesthetics, and this allows for "luxury perfusion" (i.e. increased CBF with decreased CMR) when volatile agents are employed. Intravenous agents also allow for retained response

	Agent											
	Halothane	Isoflurane	Desflurane	Sevoflurane	Nitrous oxide	Barbituate	Etomidate	Propofol	Benzo-diazepines	Ketamine	Opiods	Lidocaine
Cerebral metabolic rate	↓↓	↓↓↓	↓↓↓	↓↓↓	↓	↓↓↓↓	↓↓↓	↓↓↓	↓↓	±	±	↓↓
Cerebral blood flow	↑↑↑	↑	↑	↑	↑	↓↓↓	↓↓	↓↓↓↓	↓	↑↑	±	↓↓
Cerebrospinal fluid production	↓	±	↑	?	±	±	±	?	±	±	±	?
	↓	↑	↓	?	±	↑	↑	?	↑	↓	↑	?
Cerebral blood volume	↑↑	↑↑	↑	↑	±	↓↓	↓↓	↓↓	↓	↑↑	±	↓↓
Intracranial pressure	↑↑	↑	↑↑	↑↑	↑	↓↓↓	↓↓	↓↓	↓	↑↑	±	↓↓

Figure 92.6. Anesthetic agents and their effects on cerebral physiology. *Source:* Morgan & Mikhail, *Clinical Anesthesiology*, Chapter 25, Table 25–1.

Table 92.4 Normal values

Parameter	Normal range/values	Notes
ICP	≤10 mm Hg (≤13.6 cm H_2O)	
CPP	80–100 mm Hg	
CSF volume	150 ml	Approximately half the volume in cranium and the other half in the spinal CSF space
CSF production rate	0.3–0.4 ml/min (18-24 ml/hr)	Daily turnover of approximately 3–4 volumes of CSF. Rate of formation = rate of reabsorption in normal physiology
CSF pressure	5–15 mm Hg (6.8–20 cm H_2O)	Supine position. Average CSF pressure is 10 mm Hg (13.6 cm H_2O)
CNS volume	1600–1700 ml	Space occupied by brain, spinal cord, and CSF
Brain mass – newborn	350 g	
Brain mass – adult	1350 g	
$CMRO_2$ – adult	3.5 ml O_2/100 g/min	
$CMRO_2$ – child	5.2 ml O_2/100 g/min	
Brain – % of body weight	2%	
Brain – % of cardiac output received	15%–20%	
CBF autoregulation	MAP 60–150 mm Hg	
CBF: gray matter	80 ml/100 g/min	
CBF: white matter	20 ml/100 g/min	
CBF: average (adult)	50 ml/100 g/min	~675 ml/min for average adult
CBF: average (child)	95 ml/100 g/min	
CBF: average (infant)	40 ml/100 g/min	
Δ in CBF with Δ in temp.	CBF ↑or↓ 5%–7% per 1°C ↑or↓ in temp.	
Hematocrit range for optimal cerebral O_2 delivery	30%–34%	In the setting of focal cerebral ischemia
CBV	5 ml/100g	~70 ml in a normal brain

to CO_2 as well as retained cerebrovascular autoregulation. One caveat about the barbiturates and propofol is that clinically significant decreases in MAP can result from their use, and consequently CPP can be decreased. Etomidate (0.3 mg/kg) may decrease MAP by up to 15% via decreases in systemic vascular resistance; however, CPP is maintained. Etomidate may be considered the induction agent of choice in high-risk patients with significant cerebrovascular disease in whom preservation of normal blood pressure is critical. Among the intravenous anesthetic agents, ketamine is the notable exception – it causes a parallel increase in CBF and CMR. In fact, ketamine is the only anesthetic agent in clinical practice today that has the ability to increase CMR. In patients with a history of epilepsy, caution is advised with the use of ketamine, etomidate, and methohexital as seizure foci can be activated even with small doses.

Opioids

When added to the anesthetic regimen, opioids have a generally benign effect on cerebral physiology, a finding that is fairly consistent among the various opioids when CO_2 levels are kept constant. CBF is either unchanged or only slightly decreased with opioid administration. Alfentanil (50 mcg/kg) has been reported to activate seizure foci in patients with epilepsy, and meperidine has the known risk of CNS toxicity due to accumulation of its metabolite normeperidine.

Neuromuscular blockers

Efforts should be made to prevent coughing or "bucking" on the endotracheal tube, as this causes significant increases in ICP. Succinylcholine can cause increased ICP, regardless of the state of intracranial compliance. This effect on ICP appears to be mediated by cerebral stimulation caused by increases in muscle afferent activity. Use of succinylcholine in neurosurgical patients is not contraindicated, however. A defasciculating dose of nondepolarizing neuromuscular relaxant may be used in an attempt to mitigate this increase in ICP from succinylcholine. Alternatively, a full paralyzing dose of nondepolarizing muscle relaxant can be used to avoid the ICP increase altogether, as there would be no afferent activity from the muscle spindle. Succinylcholine should be avoided in patients with hemi- or paraplegia due to the risk of hyperkalemia.

Among the nondepolarizing muscle relaxants, histamine release is the prime concern, as this can cause systemic vasodilatation leading to decreased MAP and cerebral vasodilatation leading to increased CBF and ICP – all culminating in lower CPP. Some of the benzylisoquinolinium compounds can cause histamine release. The worst offender in this regard is *d*-tubocurarine. Other benzylisoquinolinium compounds such as mivacurium, metocurine, and atracurium have the potential to release slight amounts of histamine. Cisatracurium, by comparison, has negligible histamine-releasing effect. Atracurium's metabolite laudanosine has been implicated in epileptogenesis in animals but not in humans; thus the impact of this finding is of limited concern in clinical practice.

The steroidal nondepolarizing muscle relaxants lack effect on ICP. Whereas pancuronium can increase heart rate and blood pressure, vecuronium is devoid of such hemodynamic changes and is therefore the muscle relaxant of choice for patients in whom attention to intracranial compliance is warranted.

ICP can be reduced by pharmacologic interventions (e.g., barbiturates, osmotic diuretics, corticosteroids), hyperventilation-induced hypocapnia, or simply by elevation of the head (via gravity-provoked venous drainage). The most expeditious method for reducing ICP, however, is CSF drainage via an intraventricular or lumbar drain (if one is already in place).

Anesthetic agents with inherent seizure risk

Seizure activity can result in dramatic increases in CMR (up to 400%). Anesthetic agents that can pose a potential seizure risk to patients include:

1. Enflurane. Its ability to produce seizures is potentiated by hyperventilation and by inspired concentrations of 2% to 3% (MAC of enflurane is 1.68%). Clinically, this property of enflurane has been used to aid in the surgical resection of silent epileptogenic foci (by activating them) in patients with epilepsy.

2. Sevoflurane (especially in children).

3. Ketamine. It can cause selective activation of the thalamic and limbic areas of the brain.

4. Methohexital. It can activate seizure foci in patients with temporal lobe epilepsy and can be used to accommodate a request by a surgeon performing an awake craniotomy for seizure surgery.

5. Etomidate. In small doses, it can activate seizure foci (without causing convulsant-like motor activity) in patients with a history of epilepsy. Therefore, it can be used for intraoperative mapping of seizure foci. Conversely, etomidate possesses anticonvulsant properties and has been used to terminate status epilepticus.

6. Atracurium. Via its metabolite laudanosine, it has been shown to be epileptogenic in some animal models, although it must be emphasized that epileptogenesis is highly unlikely in humans.

7. Meperidine. Particularly if administered in high doses and/or for extended duration, it has been implicated in CNS toxicity owing to its metabolite normeperidine.

8. Alfentanil. Even in small doses, it can activate seizure foci in patients with a history of epilepsy.

Neurophysiology normal parameters

For a summary of normal parameters for neurophysiologic variables, see Table 92.4.

Suggested readings

Bendo AA, Kass IS, Hartung J, Cottrell JE. Anesthesia for neurosurgery. In Barash PG, ed. *Clinical Anesthesia*. 5th ed. Philadelphia: Lippincott, Williams & Wilkins; 2005.

Cascino GD, So EL, Sharbrough FW, et al. Alfentanil-induced epileptiform activity in patients with partial epilepsy. *J Clin Neurophys* 1993; 10(4):520–525.

Guyton AC, Hall JE. *Textbook of Medical Physiology*. 9th ed. Philadelphia: W.B. Saunders; 1996:116–118.

Lawson, NW, Johnson, JO. Autonomic nervous system: physiology and pharmacology. In Barash PG, ed. *Clinical Anesthesia*. 5th ed. Philadelphia: Lippincott, Williams & Wilkins; 2005.

Michenfelder JD. *Anesthesia and the Brain*. New York: Churchill Livingstone; 1988:94–113.

Modica PA, Templehoff R, White PF. Pro- and anticonvulsant effects of anesthetics (Part I). *Anesth Analg* 1990; 70:303–315.

Modica PA, Templehoff, R, White PF. Pro- and anticonvulsant effects of anesthetics (Part II). *Anesth Analg* 1990; 70:433–444.

Morgan GE, Mikhail MS, Murray MJ. *Clinical Anesthesiology*. 3rd ed. McGraw-Hill; 2002:552–566.

Patel PM, Drummond JC. *Cerebral physiology and the effects of anesthetics and techniques*. In Miller RD, ed. *Miller's Anesthesia*. 6th ed. Philadelphia: Elsevier; 2005:813–857.

Sokoloff L. The metabolism of the central nervous system in vivo. In J. Field, HW Magoun, and VE Hall, eds. *Handbook of Physiology – Neurophysiology*. Washington, D.C.: American Physiological Society; 1960:1843–1864.

Stoelting RK. *Pharmacology & Physiology in Anesthetic Practice*. 3rd ed. Philadelphia: Lippincott, Williams & Wilkins. 1999:146–147.

Chapter 93

Cerebral protection

Grace Y. Kim

Introduction

The brain has a high metabolic demand but is limited in its storage of oxygen, glucose, and adenosine triphosphate (ATP). When cerebral blood flow (CBF) decreases to below the threshold of ischemia, brain ischemia occurs within 3 to 8 minutes. Thus, the window of opportunity for therapeutic intervention is short.

Ion homeostasis

Resting membrane potential is kept negative by the active sodium–potassium pump. Pumping ions against the concentration gradient consumes most of the energy in the brain. Ca^{2+} ions function as second messengers during cell excitation. When the presynaptic terminal is depolarized, voltage-dependent Ca^{2+} channels open and Ca^{2+} ions enter the terminal. Vesicles containing neurotransmitters fuse with the terminal membranes and their content is released into the synaptic cleft. When the postsynaptic neurons are depolarized by excitatory neurotransmitters, action potentials are generated. If the transmitters are inhibitory, however, the neurons are hyperpolarized and action potentials are not generated.

The free Ca^{2+} concentration in the intracellular cytoplasm is much lower because most of the intracellular calcium is stored in mitochondria and endoplasmic reticulum. This gradient is maintained by active transport of calcium out of the cytoplasm and into the mitochondria. During ischemia, the inhibition of this energy-requiring step increases the free Ca^{2+} ions in the cytoplasm and initiates a cascade of reactions.

Cerebral metabolic function

There are two types of metabolic functions in a neuron: electrical activity and basal cellular homeostasis. Fifty-five percent of the total energy is used for electrical activity, and 45% is used for basic cellular homeostasis. The brain has little reserve in high-energy phosphate compounds such as phosphocreatine and is dependent on continuous production of ATP. During ischemia, stored phosphocreatine is preferentially used to preserve ATP levels. Phosphocreatine is depleted within 1 minute, glucose within 4 minutes, and ATP storage within 5 to 7 minutes. Most of the ATP

Table 93.1.	Cerebral ischemia	
Type of ischemia	**Affected area**	**Clinical scenario**
Global ischemia	Whole brain	Cardiac arrest, anoxia
Focal ischemia	Some areas of the brain	Stroke, temporary clipping

is produced from oxidative phosphorylation of glucose in mitochondria.

Cerebral ischemia

Cerebral ischemia is divided into global and focal ischemia. Global ischemia occurs during cardiac arrest when there is complete cessation of blood flow. Focal ischemia occurs when the blood flow is interrupted in a part of the brain (Table 93.1).

Cerebral blood flow during ischemia

When CBF is low, brain cells first increase oxygen extraction to preserve their function. When maximal oxygen extraction occurs, brain cells shut off electrical activity to save energy. This shutoff occurs when CBF is between 15 and 18 ml/100 g/min. Further reduction in CBF to less than 10 ml/100 g/min causes basic cellular functions to cease and ion pumps to fail. The area of the brain with CBF between these two ranges is called the *penumbra*, which has the potential for full recovery if the flow is restored quickly. When CBF decreases below 10 ml/100 g/min, irreversible neuronal death occurs. This catastrophic event occurs during a cardiac arrest if the circulation is not restored in 3 to 8 minutes. Global ischemia progresses so rapidly that neuronal death occurs before a penumbra zone has time to form. The survival of the penumbra depends on the duration and extent of ischemia as well as the efficacy of the collateral circulation. When autoregulation is impaired, CBF becomes pressure dependent and the maintenance of adequate cerebral perfusion pressure (CPP) is critically important. Augmentation of blood flow by induced hypertension or by inverse steal may potentially reduce the extent of focal ischemia (Fig. 93.1).

CBF is regulated by metabolic demand. Cerebral metabolic activity can be measured from jugular bulb blood samples. When CBF is less than the minimal blood flow necessary for survival of neurons, it is called the *ischemic flow threshold*. It

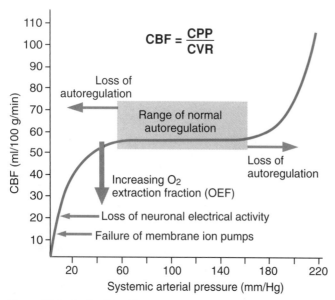

$$CBF = \frac{CPP}{CVR}$$

Figure 93.1. Cerebral blood flow during ischemia. Zabramski JM, Albuquerque FC. Cerebral protection. In: Le Roux PD, Winn HR, Newell DW, eds. *Management of Cerebral Aneurysms.* Philadelphia: Saunders; 2004:548.

occurs at 8 to 10 ml/100 g/min with isoflurane–nitrous oxide anesthesia. In animal studies, reversible paralysis occurs when CBF is less than 23 ml/100 g/min, and permanent paralysis occurs when CBF is less than 8 to 9 ml/100 g/min. Different areas of the brain show selective vulnerability. For example, the limbic system and cerebellum are particularly susceptible to ischemia. This selective vulnerability may be explained by different levels of metabolic activity in different parts of the brain. There is believed to be a 24-to-72-hour window of time between neuronal ischemia and permanent necrosis during which a clinician can intervene.

When ischemia occurs, pyruvate enters an anaerobic pathway and is metabolized to lactate. Cells become acidotic from increased levels of lactic acid and consume more ATPs to maintain the electrochemical gradient in mitochondria. It is not clear whether lactate has direct neurotoxic effects, but the continuous production of lactic acid is postulated as the mechanism of intracellular acidosis, which promotes the cascade reactions of ischemic injury.

Pathophysiology of cerebral ischemia

With the failure of the sodium–potassium pump, the ion concentration gradient is lost, resulting in loss of cellular membrane integrity. When the blood–brain barrier (BBB) is disrupted, cells begin to swell and cerebral edema ensues. Furthermore, Ca^{2+} ions are no longer pumped out of the cell or into the inner membrane of mitochondria. Increasing the intracellular Ca^{2+} level activates phospholipases, proteases, and endonuclease. Phospholipases damage cell membranes, producing free fatty acids (FFA), proteins, and oxygen radicals. Lipid peroxidation is the final outcome of the damage. The release of excitatory neurotransmitters allows further entry of calcium through

excitatory neurotransmitter channels and creates a vicious cycle of neuronal damage.

The level of excitatory neurotransmitters, glutamate and aspartate, is elevated in the ischemic brain. The areas where excitatory neurotransmitter receptors are concentrated are more susceptible to ischemic injury. N-methyl-D-aspartate (NMDA) receptors, one type of glutamate receptor, allow movement of Ca^{2+} and are involved in ischemic neuronal injury. FFA are further metabolized to arachidonic acid, which produces prostacyclin in endothelial cells and thromboxane A_2 in platelets. During ischemia, the activity of prostacyclin synthetase is inhibited, and the amount of thromboxane A_2 is increased. Thromboxane A_2, a potent vasoconstrictor and platelet aggregator, is known to worsen hypoperfusion.

The brain has a limited amount of free radical scavengers. The level of free radicals increases during reperfusion when oxygen becomes available. Free radicals may be formed from iron present in the intracranial blood. Superoxide reacts with hydrogen peroxide to produce highly reactive hydroxyl radicals. This reaction is catalyzed by Fe^{2+}. In addition, when the brain becomes ischemic, the level of nitric oxide (NO) increases dramatically within minutes. The effect of NO is either beneficial or harmful depending on its source of production in that endothelial release of NO is neuroprotective, whereas neuronal release of NO worsens ischemia. NO stimulates the production of excitatory neurotransmitters and, when combined with superoxide radicals, produces the most damaging free radicals called *peroxynitrite.*

For a brief period of time, ischemia is followed initially by reactive hyperemia, which is caused by the release of vasoactive substances during ischemia and the subsequent increased metabolic demand during recovery. During reperfusion, a variety of vasoconstrictive mediators are released contributing to the secondary injury. Ca^{2+} and thromboxane A_2 are particularly implicated in postischemic vasoconstriction. Reperfusion injury includes hypoperfusion secondary to tissue edema, vasospasm, intracellular acidosis, intracellular calcium overload, and production of excitatory neurotransmitters and free radicals. Other vascular changes include platelet activation, prostaglandin synthesis, endothelial swelling, and thrombosis from platelet aggregation. Furthermore, a variety of inflammatory mediators are activated and exacerbate neuronal injury. The role of inflammation can be beneficial or detrimental. It is well-known that the biochemical process during reperfusion perpetuates cellular injury and determines the ultimate outcome.

Neuronal death involves the process of necrosis, apoptosis, or both. Necrotic death starts almost immediately after ischemia and causes significant inflammation that damages the surrounding tissue. In contrast, apoptotic death occurs days after the initial insult and is a more organized form of cell death. In addition, structural reorganization continues for a long period of time through the process called *diaschisis.* Apoptosis and inflammation play important roles in the regeneration of neurons (Fig. 93.2).

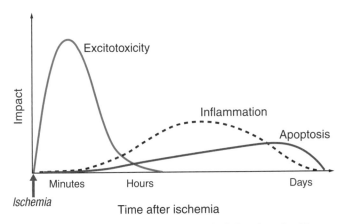

Figure 93.2. The effects of anesthetics on cerebral physiology. Patel P, Drummond JC. Cerebral physiology and the effects of anesthetics and techniques. In: Miller RD, ed. *Miller's Anesthesia*. 6th ed. Philadelphia: Elsevier Churchill Livingstone; 2005:837.

Strategy of cerebral protection

Cerebral protective strategies are focused on two types of injury: ischemic and reperfusion. Each type offers unique opportunities for therapeutic interventions. The main strategies include decreasing cerebral metabolism, inducing hypertension through collaterals, maintaining membrane ion channels, decreasing Ca^{2+} influx, inhibiting excitatory neurotransmission, preventing lipid peroxidation, maintaining BBB integrity, and preventing intracellular acidosis.

Physiologic intervention

Induced hypertension

The theory behind induced hypertension is based on the Hagen–Poiseuille equation:

$$Q = \frac{\Delta P \pi r^4}{8L\eta}, \qquad \text{(Eqn. 1)}$$

where Q = blood flow, ΔP = pressure gradient, r = radius, η = viscosity, and L = length.

During ischemia, cerebral vessels are maximally dilated and become pressure dependent. In contrast, they are constricted during vasospasm. In either case, the diameter of the blood vessel is fixed. The only parameters that can be manipulated are the pressure difference and blood viscosity. Because CBF is linearly proportional to the pressure gradient, induced hypertension improves CBF in the ischemic area.

Induced hypertension is routinely used during burst suppression. The mechanism of action is explained in the following diagrams (Fig. 93.3). When the blood flow is interrupted, CBF is maintained by vasodilation of the collateral circulation (Fig. 93.3b). When the collateral flow becomes insufficient, CBF drops below the ischemic threshold (Fig. 93.3c). If the blood pressure increases, the collateral blood flow increases to above the ischemic threshold (Fig. 93.3d). The major collateral system is the circle of Willis, which is incomplete for most patients.

The blood flow through collateral pathways increases over time during chronic ischemia. In acute ischemia, however, a pressure gradient is necessary, and augmented blood pressure redirects the flow. In global ischemia, blood pressure control has no effect because there is no circulation. In focal ischemia, the vessels in the ischemic area are maximally dilated, and there is no benefit of vasodilators. Further vasodilation may even worsen the ischemia by shunting blood to the normal brain. Induced hypertension is most effective when the cerebral vasculature has impaired autoregulation. There are potential risks of induced hypertension. If the BBB is damaged, it may cause extravasation of fluid and worsen ischemia. Another serious complication is the conversion of cerebral infarct to hemorrhagic stroke.

Hypothermia

Hypothermia has been used as a cerebral protective strategy for many years. Its mechanism of action is a decrease in the energy requirement for electrical and basal metabolic activity. The cerebral metabolic rate (CMR) is temperature-dependent, and the degree of protection is also temperature-dependent. CMR

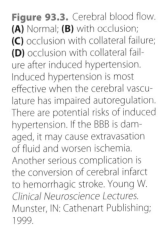

Figure 93.3. Cerebral blood flow. **(A)** Normal; **(B)** with occlusion; **(C)** occlusion with collateral failure; **(D)** occlusion with collateral failure after induced hypertension. Induced hypertension is most effective when the cerebral vasculature has impaired autoregulation. There are potential risks of induced hypertension. If the BBB is damaged, it may cause extravasation of fluid and worsen ischemia. Another serious complication is the conversion of cerebral infarct to hemorrhagic stroke. Young W. *Clinical Neuroscience Lectures.* Munster, IN: Cathenart Publishing; 1999.

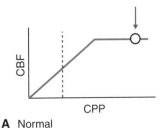

A Normal

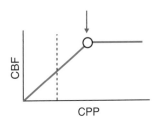

B Occlusion

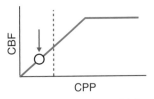

C Occlusion with collateral failure

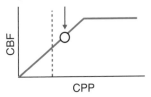

D Occlusion with collateral failure after induced hypertension

decreases 4% for each decreased degree Celsius. The maximum decrease occurs between 27°C and 14°C, the temperature range at which electrical activities cease. With further reduction in the temperature, the basal metabolic rate continues to decrease. At 15°C, the temperature used for circulatory arrest, CMR decreases to 10% of normal. Deep hypothermic circulatory arrest has been used safely for up to 60 minutes. In addition, hypothermia inhibits excitatory neurotransmitters, lipid peroxidation, and free radicals. More recent studies suggest that the role of hypothermia in inhibiting the biochemical steps of ischemic cascade is more significant than its effect on decreasing CMR.

The clinical advantage of mild hyperthermia remains inconclusive. The Intraoperative Hypothermia for Aneurysm Surgery Trial (IHAST) demonstrated no benefit of mild (33°C) intraoperative hypothermia prior to aneurysm clipping in "good-grade patients" with a preoperative World Federation of Neurological Surgeons score of I, II, or III. Furthermore, hypothermia failed to improve neurologic outcome in patients with traumatic brain injury. By contrast, mild hypothermia in comatose survivors of cardiac arrest has demonstrated a better neurologic outcome. The major risk of hypothermia is coagulopathy. Mechanisms include platelet dysfunction, splenic sequestration, and decreased activity of the enzymes involved in the coagulation pathway. Hypothermia also causes sludging of red blood cells and shifts the hemoglobin–oxygen dissociation curve to the left (Table 93.2).

Mild hypothermia in the range of 33°C to 34°C has been used without significant additional morbidity. The temperature is easily controlled with a circulating water blanket underneath and a convection air blanket above the patient's body. A rebound intracranial pressure (ICP) increase should be watched for during rewarming. Brain-injured patients often develop hyperthermia. Even though hypothermia has not conclusively proven to be a cerebral protective strategy, hyperthermia has consistently been shown to produce adverse effects and should be prevented.

Normoglycemia

The brain has limited stores of glucose, which is the only metabolic substrate for the brain in a normal situation. When the blood glucose level is less than 20 mg/dl, an isoelectric line is observed on the electroencephalogram (EEG). With further reduction in the glucose level, neuronal injury ensues. Hyperglycemia has been shown to exacerbate neurologic injury following both focal and global ischemia, although the cause-and-effect relationship has not been clearly established. During ischemia, glucose undergoes anaerobic glycolysis and produces lactate. Pre-ischemic hyperglycemia theoretically provides additional substrates and produces more lactate. Incomplete ischemia continues to provide limited perfusion and produces more lactate compared with complete ischemia, therefore worsening acidosis in the brain. In addition, hyperglycemia during ischemia reduces the level of adenosine in the brain. Adenosine is known to inhibit the release of excitatory neurotransmitters and vasodilate cerebral vessels. The target for glucose levels of between 100 and 180 mg/dl is achieved with insulin infusion. Frequent checks of blood glucose levels are mandatory to avoid hypoglycemia.

Normocapnia

Hypocapnia may increase the risk of cerebral ischemia by reducing CBF, whereas hypercapnia may compromise CPP by increasing ICP. Thus, the goal is to maintain normocapnia. Prophylactic hyperventilation in patients with traumatic brain injury is associated with a worse outcome and is no longer used. When the patient has signs of impending herniation or a tight brain, however, mild hyperventilation may be used temporarily for ICP control and brain relaxation, respectively.

Pharmacologic intervention

Barbiturates

Barbiturates remain the gold standard agent for cerebral protection in focal ischemia. Burst suppression is used to prolong the ischemic time during temporary clipping of a cerebral aneurysm. Barbiturates are also used for refractory intracranial hypertension and cerebral edema. One possible mechanism for cerebral protection is the decreased energy consumption for neuronal transmission. Thiopental decreases CBF and reduces CMR to a maximum of 50%. When all the neuronal activities cease, as demonstrated by isoelectric EEG, there is no further decrease in CMR. There are other protective mechanisms, such as inverse vascular steal, blocking Na^+ channels, reducing Ca^{2+} influx, blocking excitatory neurotransmitter release, and inhibiting free oxygen radical formation. In global ischemia, both neuronal and metabolic activities are shut down by ischemia itself in 30 seconds, and barbiturates have not been shown to be beneficial.

During burst suppression, thiopental is given prior to the placement of temporary clips. Thiopental is titrated with burst-suppression EEG tracing. When burst suppression is achieved, there is no further activity to be suppressed, and an additional dose of barbiturate does not offer more cerebral protection. During this time, blood pressure is maintained at 20% to 30%

Table 93.2. Complications of deep hypothermia (18–22°C)

Cardiovascular	Myocardial depression, arrhythmia, hypotension, ↓tissue perfusion, ↓ADH, ↑viscosity, vasoconstriction
Coagulation	Thrombocytopenia, platelet dysfunction, fibrinolysis, sludging
Metabolism	Slow metabolism of anesthetic agents, prolonged neuromuscular blockade
Shivering	Increased O_2 consumption
Surgical	Increased wound infection

AHD, antidiuretic hormone. Modified from Kass IS, Cottrell JE. Pathophysiology of brain injury. In: Cottrell JE, Smith DS, eds. *Anesthesia and Neurosurgery*, 4th ed. St. Louis, MO: Mosby, 2001: 75.

above the baseline to increase the collateral flow to the potentially ischemic area.

Etomidate and propofol

Etomidate and propofol reduce CMR and CBF, but they lack the protective mechanisms offered by barbiturates. The major advantage of etomidate is its well-known hemodynamic stability. The disadvantages are myoclonic movement that may appear as a seizure activity and potential adrenocortical suppression. Propofol has the advantage of a quick wake-up but has the side effects of seizure-like activity and myoclonus.

Volatile agents

Volatile agents offer some benefits regarding neurologic outcome within the range used clinically. In global ischemia the effect is transient, but in focal ischemia it is persistent. Volatile agents reduce CMR by suppressing neuronal activity and increase CBF. The recent discovery that deep anesthesia may promote apoptosis by blocking synaptic transmission and inhibiting neurogenesis is intriguing, however. Indeed, some studies have suggested that cumulative deep anesthesia time appears to be an independent predictor of increased postoperative mortality. Thus, reducing cumulative deep anesthesia time may offer some cerebral protection.

Calcium channel blockers

Cerebral arteries depend on the extracellular calcium source for their contraction, whereas systemic arteries use the intracellular calcium instead. For this reason, cerebral arteries are sensitive to calcium channel blockers. Two of the most widely studied drugs are nimodipine and nicardipine. Both drugs have a vasodilating effect and improve CBF.

Several randomized studies show that patients treated with nimodipine after subarachnoid hemorrhage (SAH) have a better neurologic outcome than does the placebo group. Nimodipine has been used extensively for the treatment of vasospasm, but cerebral angiography has not demonstrated the improvement of vasospasm. The mechanism of cerebral protection is not clearly understood, but may involve improved regional blood flow and blocking Ca^{2+} into cells and mitochondria. Prophylactic nimodipine is a standard treatment for patients with SAH. In contrast, nicardipine decreased the incidence of clinical vasospasm, but showed no difference in the outcome at 3 months.

Other potential drugs

Neurotransmitter modulators may play an important role in inhibiting the cascade of ischemic reactions. Early clinical studies of glutamate antagonists, especially NMDA receptor antagonists, did not show significant clinical benefit. Ketamine binds phencyclidine-binding sites of NMDA receptors and is found to block the action of glutamate. Magnesium also blocks NMDA receptors and prevents calcium influx and excitatory amino acids. The randomized trial of magnesium loading within 12 hours of acute stroke, however, did not improve the outcome despite the neuroprotective effect shown in several animal models. Free radical scavengers such as vitamins C and E are under investigation. Studies of tirilazad mesylate, a potent free radical scavenger, have not shown a benefit in clinical trials of ischemic stroke. Inhibitors of inducible NO synthase (iNOS) have shown some promise in reducing cerebral ischemia. Lidocaine blocks sodium influx, and in an animal model it has shown benefits in transient focal cerebral ischemia even when administered 45 minutes after the onset of ischemia. It has been found that erythropoietin is produced in the ischemic penumbra. Recombinant human erythropoietin treatment appears to reduce the size of the cerebral infarct.

Conclusion

Many new cerebral protective agents that have shown some promise in laboratories have shown conflicting results or have failed to demonstrate benefits in clinical studies, partly because the window of opportunity for therapeutic intervention is narrow and the injured brain continues to undergo structural reorganization over a long period of time. These observations have led to a new concept of "the neurovascular unit" consisting of neurons, microvessels, and supporting cells as a potential target for cerebral protection instead of neurons alone. Surrounding microvessels, astrocytes, glial cells, and inflammatory mediators in the neurovascular unit are likely to play a critical role in modulating the ultimate outcome of ischemic injury. Other promising concepts include pre-ischemic preconditioning of the brain and enhancing endogenous repair of neurons.

At present, there is no panacea for cerebral protection. The most important strategy is prompt restoration of oxygenation and circulation. Careful surgical planning can also prevent unnecessary ischemic events. It appears that maintaining the physiologic parameters in the optimum range is far more important than any pharmacologic intervention. Further understanding of the pathophysiology of cerebral ischemia will help us to find better cerebral protective strategies in the future (see Table 93.3).

Table 93.3. Cerebral protection strategy

Physiologic	Pharmacologic
Induced hypertension	Barbiturate
Avoid hyperthermia	Nimodipine
Mild hypothermia	Prostaglandin synthesis inhibitor
Normoglycemia	Mg^{2+}
Normocapnea	Vitamins C and E
Normal pH	Lidocaine
Avoidance of seizure	Erythropoietin
ICP control	

Suggested readings

Barker FG, Ogilvy CS. Efficacy of prophylactic nimodipine for delayed ischemic deficit after subarachnoid hemorrhage: a metaanalysis. *J Neurosurg* 1996; 84:405–414.

Bendo AA, Kass IS, Hartung J, Cottrell JE. Anesthesia for neurosurgery. In: Barash PG, Cullen B, Stoelting R, eds. *Clinical Anesthesia*. 5th ed. Philadelphia: Lippincott Williams & Wilkins; 2006:746–789.

Chiari PC, Pagel, PS, Tanaka K, et al. Intravenous emulsified halogenated anesthetics produce acute and delayed preconditioning against myocardial infarction in rabbits. *Anesthesiology* 2004; 101:1160–1166.

Clifton GL, Miller ER, Choi SC, et al. Lack of effect of induction of hypothermia after acute brain injury. *N Engl J Med* 2001; 344(8):556.

Cockroft KM, Meistrell M 3rd, Zimmerman GA, et al. Cerebroprotective effects of aminoguanidine in a rodent model of stroke. *Stroke* 1996; 27:1393–1398.

Collins RC. Selective vulnerability of brain: new insights from the excitatory synapse. *Metab Brain Dis* 1986; 1:231.

Cottrell JE. Techniques and drugs for cerebral protection. *Annual Meeting Refresher Course Lectures*. American Society of Anesthesiologists, Atlanta; 2005:113.

del Zoppo GJ. Stroke and neurovascular protection. *N Engl J Med* 2006; 354(6):553–555.

FAST-MAG Pilot Trial Investigators. Prehospital neuroprotective therapy for acute stroke: results of the Field Administration of Stroke Therapy – Magnesium (FAST-MAG) pilot trial. *Stroke* 2004; 35(5):e106–e108.

Fukuda S, Warner DS. Cerebral protection. *Br J Anaesth* 2007; 99(1):10–17.

Grasso G. Erythropoietin: a new paradigm for neuroprotection. *J Neurosurg Anesthesiol* 2006; 18:91.

Haley EC Jr, Kassell NF, Torner JC, et al. A randomized controlled trial of high-dose intravenous nicardipine in aneurismal subarachnoid hemorrhage. *J Neurosurg* 1993; 78:537–547.

Hossmann KA. Post-ischemic resuscitation of the brain: selective vulnerability versus global resistance. *Prog Brain Res* 1985; 63:3.

Iadecola C. Bright and dark sides of nitric oxide in ischemic brain injury. *Trends Neurosci* 1997; 20:132–139.

Jones TH, Morawetz RB, Crowell RM, et al. Thresholds of focal cerebral ischemia in awake monkeys. *J Neurosurg* 1981; 54:773.

Kass IS, Cottrell JE. Pathophysiology of brain injury. In: Cottrell JE, Smith DS, eds. *Anesthesia and Neurosurgery*, 4th ed. St. Louis, MO: Mosby; 2001:69–82.

Kong DL, Prough DS, Whitley JM, et al. Hemorrhage and intracranial hypertension in combination increase cerebral production of thromboxane A2. *Crit Care Med* 1991; 19:532.

Lam AM. Cerebral aneurysms: anesthetic consideration. In: Cottrell JE, Smith DS, eds. *Anesthesia and Neurosurgery*. 4th ed. St. Louis, MO: Mosby; 2001:367–397.

Lam AM, Winn HR, Cullen BF, et al. Hyperglycemia and neurologic outcome in patients with head injury. *J Neurosurg* 1991; 75: 545.

Lanier W, Stangland K, Scheithauer B, et al. The effects of dextrose infusion and head position on neurologic outcome after complete cerebral ischemia in primates: examination of a model. *Anesthesiology* 1987; 66:39.

Messick JM Jr, Casement B, Sharbrough FW, et al. Correlation of regional cerebral blood flow (rCBF) with EEG changes during isoflurane anesthesia for carotid endarterectomy: critical rCBF. *Anesthesiology* 1987; 66:344.

Milde LN. Cerebral protection. In: Cucchiara RF, Black S, Michenfelder JD, eds. *Clinical Neuroanesthesia*. 2nd ed. New York: Churchill Livingstone; 1998:177–228.

Monk TG, Saini V, Weldon BC, et al. Anesthetic management and one-year mortality after noncardiac surgery. *Anesth Analg* 2005; 100:4–10.

Morales MI, Pittman J, Cottrell JE. Cerebral protection and resuscitation. In: Newfield P, Cottrell JE, eds. *Handbook of Neuroanesthesia*. 4th ed. Philadelphia: Lippincott Williams & Wilkins; 2007:55–72.

Patel P, Drummond JC. Cerebral physiology and the effects of anesthetics and techniques. In: Miller RD, ed. *Miller's Anesthesia*. 6th ed. Philadelphia: Elsevier Churchill Livingstone; 2005:813–857.

Patel, PM. Perioperative neuroprotection: there is no magic bullet. What do I do in my daily practice, and where are we going? Cerebral ischemia–physiologic management. *Annual Meeting Refresher Course Lectures*. American Society of Anesthesiologists, Atlanta; 2005:113.

Sakai H, Sheng H, Yates RB. Isoflurane provides long-term protection against focal cerebral ischemia in the rat. *Anesthesiology* 2007; 106:92–99.

Siesjo BK. Cerebral circulation and metabolism. *J Neurosurg* 1984; 60:883.

The Hypothermia After Cardiac Arrest Study Group. Mild therapeutic hypothermia to improve the neurologic outcome after cardiac arrest. *N Engl J Med* 2002; 346(8):549–556.

Thorens S, Haeusler G. Effects of some vasodilators on calcium translocation in intact and fractionated vascular smooth muscle. *Eur J Pharmacol* 1979; 54:79.

Tirilazad International Steering Committee. Tirilazad mesylate in acute ischemic stroke. A systematic review. *Stroke* 2000; 32:2257–2265.

Todd MM, Hindman BJ, Clark WR, et al. Mild intraoperative hypothermia during surgery for intracranial aneurysm. *N Engl J Med* 2005; 352(2):135.

Warner DS. Perioperative neuroprotection: There is no magic bullet. What do I do in my daily practice, and where are we going? Pathophysiology of cerebral ischemia. *Annual Meeting Refresher Course Lectures*. American Society of Anesthesiologists, Atlanta; 2005:113.

Young W. *Clinical Neuroscience Lectures*. Munster, IN: Cathenart Publishing; 1999.

Zabramski JM, Albuquerque FC. Cerebral protection. In: Le Roux PD, Winn HR, Newell DW, eds. *Management of Cerebral Aneurysms*. Philadelphia: Saunders; 2004:547–562.

Zornow MH, Scheller MS. Intraoperative fluid management during craniotomy. In: Cottrell JE, Smith DS, eds. *Anesthesia and Neurosurgery*. 4th ed. St. Louis, MO: Mosby; 2001:237–249.

Craniotomy

Elizabeth M. Rickerson and Lisa J. Crossley

Preoperative evaluation

A comprehensive evaluation preceding surgery should be conducted for every anticipated craniotomy, as is performed in all major surgeries. Particular attention should be paid to the patient's baseline neurologic examination and functional status, as well as to the location of the lesion(s) and the presence or absence of mass effect. The presence of specific symptoms such as headache, decreased level of consciousness, visual disturbances, papilledema, and seizures should be determined and documented; these symptoms may be indicative of increased intracranial pressure (ICP) or other pathologies. Evaluation of neuroimaging studies to discern the location and size of the lesion as well any subclinical evidence of intracranial hypertension helps with the assessment of operative needs for exposure and the potential for intraoperative hemorrhage. In general, peritumor edema with mass effect great enough to cause a shift in the midline structures will require intraoperative efforts to decrease the ICP. Effacement of the lateral ventricles by tumor burden or expansion of the ventricles by obstructive hydrocephalus indicates that any maneuver resulting in an increased intracranial volume could cause a disproportionate increase in ICP. Small, superficial lesions generally cause minimal difficulty with regard to exposure and hemorrhage, whereas larger lesions or lesions that are deeper in the brain provide a greater challenge for surgical exposure as well as a greater potential for blood loss (Table 94.1).

For non-emergent cases, cardiac optimization prior to surgery is necessary for many reasons. Commonly used techniques used in neuroanesthesia to reduce ICP can stress the heart. Hyperventilation decreases venous return and hypocarbia functionally reduces coronary blood flow. Diuretics ultimately cause further reductions in cardiac output but can transiently increase blood volume and worsen pulmonary function in patients with cardiac failure.

Fluid and electrolyte imbalances are common in craniotomy patients because of poor oral intake, steroids, and diuretics. These imbalances should be optimized prior to surgery. Seizure prophylaxis and treatment may also be required. Patients with seizure disorders are usually on anticonvulsants; blood levels of these drugs should be checked in any patient with signs of toxicity or a history of recent seizures.

Preoperative medications

Sedative medications can blunt the ventilatory drive, leading to hypercarbia and increased ICP, which may not be tolerable in many craniotomy patients. In general, preoperative medications for anxiolysis are given at the discretion of the anesthesiologist when the patent is under direct supervision or upon induction in the operating room. In current clinical practice, the use of preoperative steroids has made it relatively safe to administer sedatives to many patients with brain tumors.

Monitoring and access

Standard American Society of Anesthesiologists monitors should be used for all craniotomy cases. Additional monitors should be used depending on the particular surgery. Intravenous access (preferably on an arm that can be accessed after the patient is prepped and draped) with one or two large bore peripheral intravenous catheters (more depending on anticipated blood loss) is desirable. Arterial catheters are often used in craniotomies and can be placed prior to surgery if tight blood pressure control during induction is a concern; alternatively, the arterial catheter can be placed postinduction. Transduction of the arterial catheter at the level of the external auditory meatus in the supine or prone patient gives a good approximation of the mean arterial pressure (MAP) at the circle of Willis. MAP approximates cerebral perfusion pressure (CPP) until the cranium is open at which time CPP = MAP in the brain (except in the regions of the brain where retractors and packing compress the brain directly). An arterial catheter can also help with the management of blood gases, electrolyte imbalances, and glucose control.

The use of central venous catheters is not routine for craniotomies but is generally helpful in cases when a significant amount of blood loss is anticipated. Central venous pressure (CVP) monitoring can also be useful in the management of intravascular fluid status in patients undergoing resection of large suprasellar tumors who might be at risk for diabetes insipidus. A pulmonary artery catheter may be indicated for patients with severe cardiopulmonary disease. Central venous catheters are often placed in the subclavian veins because access to the neck can be limited and the neck may be rotated substantially, which could obstruct venous outflow.

Table 94.1. Mechanisms of increased intracranial pressure

1. Mass lesions — Hematoma, tumor, abscess
2. CSF accumulations — Hydrocephalus
    a. Impaired absorption – meningitis, subarachnoid hemorrhage, etc.
    b. Obstructive – congenital, due to tumors and other masses
    c. Increased production – choroid plexus Papilloma
3. Cerebral edema — Increased brain water content
    a. Vasogenic – vessel damage (tumor, abscess, confusion)
    b. Cytotoxic – cell membrane pump failure (hypoxia, ischemia, toxins)
    c. Hydrostatic – high transmural pressure (dysautoregulation, postdecompression)
    d. Interstitial – high CSF pressure – e.g., hydrocephalus
4. Congestive (vascular) brain swelling — Increased cerebral blood volume
    a. Arterial vasodilation
    b. Venous obstruction

Albin M. *Textbook of Neuroanesthesia with Neurosurgical and Neuroscience Perspectives.* New York: McGraw-Hill; 1997.

Neuromuscular "twitch" monitors used to guide dosing of muscle relaxants should be used with care for patients with paresis as they can have increased numbers of acetylcholine receptors at the end plates of lower motor neurons. This can make the degree of neuromuscular block with nondepolarizing agents appear less than it actually is. If possible, the twitch monitor should be placed away from the paretic limb(s); if that is not possible, interpreting the twitch monitor results must be done with care to prevent overdoses of neuromuscular blocking agents.

Depending on the location of the lesion, intraoperative monitoring of brainstem evoked potential responses, auditory evoked responses, visual evoked responses, somatosensory evoked responses, motor evoked potentials, and electromyography (EMG) may be useful in guiding surgical resection. Surgery may also be performed under local anesthesia to allow ongoing monitoring of function if areas of the cortex that control speech and/or motor functions are involved.

Induction and maintenance of general anesthesia

There are a variety of approaches to the induction and maintenance of anesthesia for craniotomies. The most commonly accepted methods are designed to accomplish the following goals:

(1) A smooth induction with tight hemodynamic control with minimal coughing and straining;
(2) "Full stomach" precautions in patients undergoing emergency craniotomy;
(3) The ability to achieve hypocapnia quickly and efficiently;
(4) The avoidance of hypoxia and hypercarbia;
(5) Emergence from the anesthetized state with minimal coughing and straining to prevent increased ICP and bleeding in the surgical site; and
(6) A rapid emergence to allow an immediate postoperative neurological examination.

Hypotension during induction usually can be avoided by preinduction volume loading (10 ml/kg normal saline) with adjustments based on the patient's cardiac and volume status. Barbiturates, often used for induction, are potent vasoconstrictors that decrease cerebral blood flow (CBF) and may improve recovery from cerebral ischemia. When consciousness is lost, the patient should be manually hyperventilated until the neuromuscular blocker to facilitate endotracheal intubation has taken effect and it is safe to proceed with intubation. When the dura has been opened, anesthetic requirements are often lower as the brain parenchyma is devoid of sensation. Iso-osmolar fluids such as normal saline are preferable to hypo-osmolar solutions such as lactated Ringer's because of the effect on ICP: Normal plasma osmolarity is 280 to 307 mOsm/L. The osmolarity of lactated Ringer's is 273 mOsm/L, which can cause a transfer of fluid into cells and increased ICP. The osmolarity of normal saline is 308 mOsm/L, and should therefore not increase ICP substantially. Hypothermia may confer some protection from cerebral ischemia (although human trials to date have not shown a benefit of hypothermia). Hyperthermia should be avoided.

Succinylcholine is generally avoided because of the brief increase in ICP during muscle fasciculations; however, in instances of a difficult airway assessment, the use of succinylcholine may be warranted. A defasciculating dose of a nondepolarizing muscle relaxant may decrease or eliminate this transient increase in ICP. Ketamine increases CBF and ICP and is rarely used for craniotomies. Most of the other intravenous anesthetics (opioids, barbiturates, benzodiazepines, etomidate, and propofol) are cerebral vasoconstrictors and thereby reduce CBF. Etomidate has been associated with myoclonic activity and is best avoided in seizure-prone patients. For patients with a history of seizures, atracurium or cisatracurium and meperidine should also be avoided because of their epileptogenic metabolites, laudanosine and normeperidine, respectively. Calcium channel blockers such as nimodipine can improve cerebral vasospasm after subarachnoid hemorrhage.

Nitrous oxide (N_2O) is most likely a cerebral vasodilator; vasodilation can be attenuated by hyperventilation and intravenous agents. There is controversy regarding the use of N_2O and its potential for causing a clinically significant tension pneumocephalus; it should probably not be used in cases where pneumocephalus is known to exist as it diffuses more rapidly into air-filled spaces than nitrogen is able to diffuse out. There is also controversy as to whether N_2O should be used in the sitting position because of the higher risk of venous air embolism (VAE) associated with the sitting position. If a VAE has been detected, it is good practice to discontinue N_2O because of its potential to expand the size of the entrained bubble. Volatile anesthetics produce a dose-dependent reduction in cerebral metabolism. Isoflurane is the most potent of the volatiles in this respect and can produce an isoelectric electroencephalogram (EEG) at lower concentrations.

Elevated ICP tends to force the brain out through craniotomy incisions and can lead to both poor surgical access and neuronal injury. Intracranial hypertension with significant midline displacement might be indicative of increased ICP despite appropriate hyperventilation. Therapy consists of using osmotic diuretics to increase the osmolality of the blood relative to the brain and pull water across the blood–brain barrier (BBB). An intravenous infusion of mannitol at a dose of approximately 0.5 to 1 g/kg before opening the skull is often used when the patient's baseline osmolality is <290 mOsm/kg. Furosemide can be used alone or as an adjunctive therapy with mannitol. Furosemide is usually given prior to mannitol as mannitol can cause an initial increase in ICP by drawing fluid intravascularly. Cerebral spinal fluid (CSF) can also be removed with either a ventriculostomy tube or a spinal catheter placed in the lumbar subarachnoid space to permit drainage.

Available data do not lend support to any one combination of anesthetic maintenance agents as long as the goals stated earlier in this chapter are accomplished. One approach is to infuse a short-acting opioid infusion (sufentanyl, remifentanil, or fentanyl) with 70% N_2O and minimal isoflurane. Remifentanil usage requires that adequate longer acting narcotics be given to prevent postoperative hypertension secondary to inadequate pain control. Before the dura is closed, the blood pressure should be restored to pre-induction levels to verify adequate hemostasis. In instances where the brain is swollen and the dura cannot be closed, the patient should be transported to the intensive care unit (ICU) on controlled ventilation. If new neurological deficits are noted on immediate postoperative examination, immediate surgical re-exploration or a CT scan may be required; this may or may not require re-intubation.

Awake craniotomy

Craniotomies can also be performed under local anesthesia with or without sedation; this is often done for seizure surgery or if the lesion is close to areas of the brain that control speech and motor function. In these cases, an anesthetic should be chosen that both provides anxiolysis and patient comfort and allows for ongoing interaction with the patient. One approach is to use a dexmedetomidine infusion; another option is to use the more traditional conscious sedation combination of midazolam and fentanyl or sufentanil. Access to the airway can be

extremely limited, thus care must be taken to avoid depressing the ventilatory drive entirely.

Fluid management

Fluid management for craniotomies requires an understanding of how fluid shifts across the BBB. In the peripheral vasculature, the endothelial junctions of the capillaries are highly permeable and allow the passage of water, ions, and most low-molecular-weight substances. In these tissues where electrolytes pass freely, water moves in the direction of transcapillary concentration gradient of the larger plasma proteins. In contrast, the brain and spinal cord are isolated from the intravascular compartment, and the endothelial junctions are tight enough to prevent even the passage of ions. Fluid movement is governed by the osmolar gradient, which is determined by the relative concentrations of all osmotically active particles, including the electrolytes. The sodium concentration of the fluid to be infused thus becomes quite important. So-called free-water solutions, i.e., solutions without electrolytes (5% dextrose in water), will lower plasma osmolality, drive water across the BBB into the brain, and increase brain edema and ICP. Dextrose-containing fluids are avoided because of their propensity to worsen neurologic outcome during focal ischemia. Of the isotonic crystalloids, lactated Ringer's solution is mildly hyponatremic, and when large volumes are infused rapidly, ICP can increase. Normal saline is therefore the isotonic crystalloid of choice. When the BBB is intact, mannitol can be used to dehydrate the brain and decrease ICP; doses of 0.25 to 1.5 g/k increase plasma osmolality, and water moves from the brain into the vasculature. Mannitol administration can transiently increase ICP: With the acute increase in plasma osmolality, the cerebral vasculature may initially vasodilate. As stated earlier, furosemide can be given prior to mannitol to attenuate this affect.

Glucose control

The optimal range of serum glucose in traumatic brain injury remains unclear, according to recent studies. In one study, a serum glucose level ≥200 mg/dl was associated with a 3.6-fold increase in mortality. This study recommended maintaining serum glucose levels ≤180 mg/dl, which was associated with only a 4.3% incidence of hypoglycemia compared to an 18.7% incidence of hypoglycemia in patients undergoing intensive insulin therapy.

Transsphenoidal surgery

Pituitary tumors less than 10 mm in diameter are usually approached transsphenoidally. The pituitary gland lies in the sella turcica of the sphenoid bone and is bordered by several important structures including the carotid artery and cranial nerves (CN) III, IV, V_1, and VI. The stalk of the pituitary gland is close to the optic chiasm, and visual evoked potentials may need to be monitored intraoperatively if the tumor involves or lies close to the optic nerve. The surgical approach is through the nasal cavity and nasal septum, then through the roof of the sphenoid sinus to access the sella turcica. There are several problems that can be encountered with the transsphenoidal approach. Prior to surgery, the tumor may actively secrete one or more of the pituitary hormones (anterior pituitary: adrenocorticotropic hormone [ACTH], thyroid-stimulating hormone [TSH], growth hormone [GH], follicle-stimulating hormone [FSH], luteinizing hormone [LH], and prolactin; posterior pituitary: vasopressin and oxytocin). Abnormalities should be investigated prior to any procedure and corrected to the extent possible. Consultation with an endocrinologist may be advisable. As with any surgery in the nasal cavity, the mucosa can bleed heavily and may require topical or injected vasoconstrictive agents. Blood and tissue debris from the nasal cavity can accumulate in the oropharynx, esophagus, and stomach. Risks of the surgery include hemorrhage from damage to the carotid artery or sinus, CSF leak, pituitary hypofunction, and cranial nerve damage. Prophylactic glucocorticoids are usually administered.

Epilepsy surgery

Patients whose seizures are inadequately controlled by medical management undergo extensive noninvasive evaluation including CT, MRI, and PET scanning. A careful evaluation of the patient's concomitant medical problems, as well as an understanding of the ability of anesthetic agents to promote or suppress seizures, is important during management of these patients. Patients may require evaluation of the seizure focus through intraoperative mapping and electrocorticography. For mapping procedures, awake patients are managed using monitored anesthesia care. Low concentrations of propofol or dexmedetomidine can be used for sedation during intraoperative mapping; propofol usage is discontinued before mapping starts. Alternatively, low doses of methohexital or alfentanil can be used to activate seizure foci. Midazolam and high doses of propofol or barbiturates should be avoided during intraoperative mapping procedures as they may impair detection of seizure foci. Surgical procedures used in seizure management consist of craniotomy for placement of grid or strip electrodes, left vagal nerve stimulators (patients with intractable complex partial seizures), resection of specific seizure focus (e.g., anterior temporal lobectomy), and interruption of seizure circuits (e.g., corpus callosotomy). Patients are managed with general anesthetic regimens consisting of either inhaled anesthetics (isoflurane, N_2O/oxygen) and fentanyl, or total intravenous anesthetics using propofol, remifentanil, or fentanyl and muscle relaxants. Complications (hemorrhage, neurologic deficits) seen after surgical resections directly relate to the site of the epileptic focus and are usually independent of the anesthetic technique.

Infratentorial craniotomy

Posterior fossa masses present several challenges not always encountered with surgery for supratentorial masses. First, the posterior fossa is an enclosed space in which the tumor burden/lesion is often in direct contact with highly critical structures, leaving little or no room for error. The posterior fossa contains the cerebellar hemispheres, upper medulla, pons, and the lower midbrain. CN III–XII can be accessed in the posterior fossa. The entire blood supply to neural structures is through the vertebrobasilar system, and the foramina of Magendie and Luschka provide outflow for CSF from the ventricular system. Second, in addition to the risk for neuronal damage, proximity to the brainstem nuclei can trigger significant intraoperative hemodynamic instability usually manifested by bradycardia due to increased vagal tone. Depending on the assessment of the relative risk of cranial nerve damage, intraoperative neurophysiologic monitoring (brainstem auditory evoked potentials [BAEPS], somatosensory evoked potentials [SEP], EMG) may be necessary. Third, the posterior fossa cannot be easily accessed in the conventional supine position, so surgery must be performed in an alternate position which may require different techniques of monitoring and positioning.

Lesions in the posterior fossa can present with a wide variety of symptoms. Elevated ICP may occur because of mass effect or hydrocephalus secondary to obstruction of CSF flow. Nonspecific symptoms include listlessness, headache, fatigue, vomiting, anorexia, personality changes, dysmetria, hemiparesis, and cranial nerve deficits. Bulbar palsies with vocal cord paralysis and swallowing/gag dysfunction can occur. Brainstem involvement can cause respiratory changes including apneustic or ataxic breathing and hyperventilation. Ultimately, herniation will cause loss of consciousness, respiratory changes, bradycardia, hypertension, and death. Tumors of the posterior fossa occur more frequently in children; 50% to 55% of all pediatric brain tumors are infratentorial.

Positioning for craniotomy

A variety of positions are used for craniotomies based on the location and size of the lesion. Each position has its own risks and benefits; close attention must be paid to padding and nerve damage must be avoided in all positions. The eyes should be covered with waterproof protection and be free of external pressure, and the position of the endotracheal tube should be rechecked after final positioning because of limited access to the airway during the procedure. In any head-up position, hypotension during anesthesia may be especially harmful for patients with limited cerebral autoregulation, impaired cerebral perfusion, carotid stenosis, or previous carotid endarterectomy. Zeroing of the transducer for arterial blood pressure requires a different reference point in the sitting position, namely at the highest point of the skull, as opposed to the tragus of the ear for the supine position (see Chapter 93). Intravascular volume depletion is also a consideration, and fluid administration prior to induction as well as lower extremity compression stockings may be useful.

Lateral

This position is good for access to many lateral lesions, the cerebellopontine angle, and the anterior and lateral foramen magnum. Risk for VAE is low in this position, but bleeding from the sinuses can be rapid. Disadvantages of the lateral position also include postoperative brachial plexus and popliteal nerve damage and careful positioning and padding should be performed.

Prone

This position is good for access to midline lesions (especially of the posterior fossa). Disadvantages and complications of the prone position include difficult ventilation, limited access to the endotracheal tube and airway, pressure necrosis, and potential for blindness. The mechanism of blindness after surgeries in the prone position is unclear; it may be due to retinal artery thrombosis. VAE is a potential problem in this position because the head is usually elevated above the heart, but there is a lower incidence as compared with sitting.

Park bench semiprone

This position is useful in emergent cases because positioning can be done rapidly. It allows access to the cerebellar hemispheres but can also be used for midline lesions.

Sitting

This position allows excellent exposure for posterior fossa surgeries, offers improved CSF and venous drainage, and produces less bleeding. The risk of VAE is highest in this position, and monitoring for air embolism is mandatory. Additional risks include quadriplegia, especially in elderly patients with spinal stenosis, and supratentorial hemorrhage in the subcortical white matter (the exact mechanism of this complication is unknown). Relative contraindications to the sitting position – such as intracardiac defects, pulmonary arteriovenous malformations, and carotid stenosis – should not be overlooked. This position has fallen out of favor with most surgeons because of the higher risks associated with it.

Supine

This position allows distribution of the patient's weight over a larger area. The head is often laterally rotated and flexed, which is not always possible with elderly patients or patients with severe joint disease. Risks of this position include impaired jugular venous drainage and brain edema.

Venous air embolism

In the sitting position, the head is elevated above the right atrium, which decreases both dural sinus pressure and venous bleeding. The sinuses are tented open by their attachments to the dura, and. when opened, large volumes of air can be entrained into the venous system. Hypovolemia can contribute to the problem because a lower CVP increases the negative pressure gradient between the head and the right side of the heart.

Morbidity and mortality of VAE are directly related to the amount of air entrained. The lethal dose in humans is estimated to be approximately 300 cc. An air bolus may result in an air lock in the right side of the heart, leading to right ventricular outflow tract obstruction, decreased cardiac output, acute right ventricular dilatation and failure, dysrhythmias, myocardial infarction (MI), cerebral ischemia, and death. There can also be occlusion of the pulmonary vascular bed with resultant increases in pulmonary vascular resistance, pulmonary arterial mean pressure, and right heart afterload. Right ventricular failure causes the cardiac output to decrease, and left ventricular filling is impaired by the displaced interventricular septum. Ventilation–perfusion mismatch is manifested by a falling end-tidal CO_2 and a rising CO_2 concentration. Monitoring for VAE in the sitting position is strongly recommended.

The most sensitive noninvasive monitor for VAE is the precordial Doppler ultrasound. The probe is placed over the right atrium, and its position is tested via injection of air, sodium bicarbonate, or agitated saline. When a VAE occurs, a characteristic "mill wheel" murmur is heard. Transesophageal echo is the most sensitive detector of VAE, but this monitor is invasive, operator dependent, cumbersome and requires continual observation. Because of its sensitivity, noninvasive nature, and ease of interpretation, the precordial Doppler is usually favored over the transesophageal echocardiograph. Capnography is another useful monitor for detecting VAE and is used in conjunction with the precordial Doppler. It is noninvasive and sensitive, but decreases in end-tidal CO_2 are nonspecific. It is of note that a significant decrease in end-tidal CO_2 often occurs with a sudden low cardiac output event. This is caused by decreased pulmonary blood flow and CO_2 elimination during the low cardiac output state, which can be confused with a pulmonary air embolus.

A pulmonary artery catheter can detect the pulmonary hypertension caused by a VAE and is more sensitive than capnography; however, it is quite invasive, and optimal placement for detection may not allow for aspiration in case of air entrainment.

Adequate hydration and the avoidance of drugs that dilate venous capacitance are some of the techniques that the anesthesiologist might use to prevent VAE. In addition, positive end-expiratory pressure (PEEP) may increase the chance of a paradoxic air embolus in a patient with a patent foramen ovale (PFO). If a VAE is detected or suspected, notify the surgical staff to have them irrigate the operative site ("flood the field") and apply material to occlude potential air entry sites. Treatment of VAE also includes placing the patient in the head-down position, discontinuing N_2O, increasing oxygen flow, and attempting to aspirate air via an atrial catheter. Prompt cardiovascular support should be dictated by the clinical picture (increase intravenous fluid administration and start vasopressors as needed). Jugular compression is also recommended to increase cranial venous pressure and cause back bleeding rather than air entrapment, but obstruction of CBF, dislodgement of carotid plaques, venous engorgement leading to cerebral edema and bradycardia are potential consequences. External cardiac massage can disrupt a large air lock if cardiovascular collapse has occurred. The administration of PEEP in this instance might be beneficial in elevating the venous pressure in the head to values greater than zero; however, the entire clinical picture should be taken into account with regard to paradoxical air emboli.

Suggested readings

Albin M. *Textbook of Neuroanesthesia with Neurosurgical and Neuroscience Perspectives*. New York: McGraw-Hill; 1997.

Barash P, Cullen B, Stoelting R. *Clinical Anesthesia*. New York: Lippincott Williams & Wilkins; 2006.

Cottrell J, Smith D. *Anesthesia and Neurosurgery*. Philadelphia: Mosby; 2001.

Morgan GE, Mikhail M, Murray M. *Clinical Anesthesiology*. New York: McGraw-Hill; 2006.

Souter MJ, Rozet I, Ojemann JG, et al. Dexmedetomidine sedation during awake craniotomy for seizure resection: effects on electrocorticography. *J Neurosurg Anesthesiol* 2007; 19:38–44.

Chapter 95

Cerebrovascular diseases

Grace Y. Kim

Subarachnoid hemorrhage (SAH) occurs when a cerebral blood vessel ruptures by trauma or spontaneously. The most common cause of spontaneous SAH is a ruptured cerebral aneurysm. Other causes include bleeding from arteriovenous malformation (AVM) and hypertension.

Cerebral aneurysm

Introduction

Epidemiology

The prevalence of cerebral aneurysms in the United States is estimated at 1% to 5%. Each year 27,000 people sustain ruptured aneurysms in this country. Ruptured aneurysms occur in middle age, between the ages of 40 and 60 years with a slight female predominance. Rebleeding risk is high, and approximately half of all ruptured aneurysms will rebleed in the first 6 months after the initial episode. The overall mortality rate is 25%, and more than 50% of survivors suffer significant neurologic morbidity. The major causes of mortality and morbidity are the direct effects of the initial bleed, rebleeding, vasospasm, and surgical complications. Incidental findings of asymptomatic cerebral aneurysms are not uncommon. Unruptured aneurysms carry a risk of bleeding at 1% to 2% per year. The management of patients with unruptured intracranial aneurysms is controversial. The current recommendation is to clip asymptomatic aneurysms unless the size is less than 3 mm or the risk of surgery exceeds the benefit.

Risk factors

The risk factors of aneurysm ruptures include increasing size, age, hypertension, family history, connective tissue disease (Ehlers–Danlos syndrome and fibromuscular dysplasia), polycystic kidney disease, cocaine use, pregnancy, other intracranial vascular anomalies, coarctation of the aorta, smoking, and strenuous activity.

Presentation

Ruptured aneurysms present as subarachnoid, intracerebral, intraventricular, or subdural hematomas. The common symptoms are sudden onset of severe headache (i.e., "the worst headache I've ever had"), altered mental status, stiff neck, photophobia, neurologic deficits, nausea, and vomiting.

Patients with a giant aneurysm may present with a mass effect of the aneurysm. When a patient with sentinel bleeding develops a mild headache or subtle neurologic changes, early diagnosis and clipping can result in a good outcome. Seizures usually occur shortly after the rupture in up to 13% of cases and pose an increased risk of rebleeding.

The Hunt–Hess classification is used to estimate the prognosis. The World Federation of Neurosurgeons' SAH scale adds the presence of motor deficits and the Glasgow Coma Scale. The important factors determining the final outcome include the Hunt–Hess classification, age, the presence of vasospasm, and the size and location of the aneurysm (Table 95.1).

Diagnosis

A noncontrast CT is the most sensitive imaging method. If the CT is negative, a lumbar puncture is performed to look for xanthochromia. A diagnostic cerebral angiogram is necessary to assess the size, location, and anatomy of the aneurysm and the presence of multiple aneurysms. Negative angiography occurs in 10% to 20% of SAH patients and needs to be repeated. Thrombosed aneurysms may not appear on the angiogram. The amount and distribution of blood in the subarachnoid space are

Table 95.1. Hunt–Hess classification of clinical grade for SAH*

Grade	Description	Mortality, %
0	Unruptured aneurysm	–
I	Minimal headache or slight nuchal rigidity	2
II	Moderate to severe headache, nuchal rigidity, cranial nerve palsy	5
III	Drowsiness, confusion, or mild focal deficit	15–20
IV	Stupor, hemiparesis, early decerebrate rigidity, and vegetative disturbance	30–40
V	Deep coma, decerebrate rigidity, moribund appearance	50–80

*Serious systemic diseases (hypertension, diabetes, coronary artery disease, chronic pulmonary disease) and severe vasospasm seen on arteriography place the patient in the next less favorable category.

Hunt WE, Hess RM. Surgical risk as related to time of intervention in the repair of intracranial aneurysms. *J Neurosurg* 1968; 28(1):14–20.

Newfield P, Bendo AA. Anesthetic management of intracranial aneurysms. In: Newfield P, Cottrell JE, eds. *Handbook of Neuroanesthesia.* 4th ed. Philadelphia: Lippincott Williams & Wilkins; 2007:146.

Table 95.2. Fisher grade

Grade	
1	No blood
2	Diffuse or vertical layers less than 1 mm
3	Localized or vertical layer greater than or equal to 1 mm
4	Intracerebral or intraventricular clot with diffuse or no SAH

Fisher CM, Kistler JP, Davis JM. Relation of cerebral vasospasm to subarachnoid hemorrhage visualized by computerized tomographic scanning. *Neurosurgery* 1980; 6:1–9.

classified by the Fisher grading scale and are the best predictors of vasospasm (Table 95.2).

Types of aneurysm

The blood supply to the brain is divided into anterior circulation from two internal carotid arteries and posterior circulation from two vertebral arteries. Anterior circulation supplies most of the cerebrum, and posterior circulation supplies the visual cortex, cerebellum, and brainstem. The communication between the two systems forms the circle of Willis. Approximately 80% of cerebral aneurysms are located in the anterior (carotid) circulation and 20% in the posterior (vertebrobasilar) circulation. Anterior circulation aneurysms carry a better prognosis compared with posterior circulation aneurysms (Fig. 95.1).

Cerebral aneurysms are divided into three groups: saccular, fusiform, and dissecting. Saccular aneurysms are the most common type. Fusiform aneurysms are often associated with atherosclerosis or degenerative connective tissue disorder. A dissecting aneurysm develops at a tear between the endothelial and medial layers, often due to trauma. Aneurysms caused by trauma or infection are uncommon and are usually located at the distal vessels. An aneurysm is considered large when its size is greater than 12 mm and giant when greater than 25 mm.

Pathophysiology

The etiology of cerebral aneurysms is structural abnormality caused by hemodynamic factors and genetic predisposition. Histologically, cerebral aneurysms are deficient in the middle muscular layer and internal elastic lamina of the vascular wall. According to La Place's law, the tension on the wall of blood vessels is the product of the pressure times the radius of the chamber, and the tension is inversely related to the thickness of the wall. Larger arteries are exposed to higher wall tension than are smaller arteries. When a weak area in a large artery is subjected to high wall tension, it forms an outpouching that gradually forms an aneurysm. As the size of the aneurysm increases, a vicious cycle ensues where the wall compliance decreases further whereas the tension increases, sometimes to the point of rupture. Aneurysms usually occur at the bifurcations of major arteries where the supporting adventitia is thin and the pulsatile pressure is maximal. Increased blood pressure (BP) and turbulent blood flow promote the aneurysm formation and rupture. The location, size, and wall thickness of the aneurysm determine the risk of rupture.

Patients with ruptured cerebral aneurysms present with varying clinical conditions, ranging from a mild headache to a deep coma. Severe headache is due to a sudden increase in intracranial pressure (ICP). Loss of consciousness occurs when cerebral perfusion pressure (CPP) suddenly drops from elevated regional ICP. When the ICP approaches the diastolic BP, the cerebral blood flow (CBF) decreases dramatically and limits further leakage of blood. Some patients regain consciousness as ICP adjusts itself by a compensatory mechanism. When

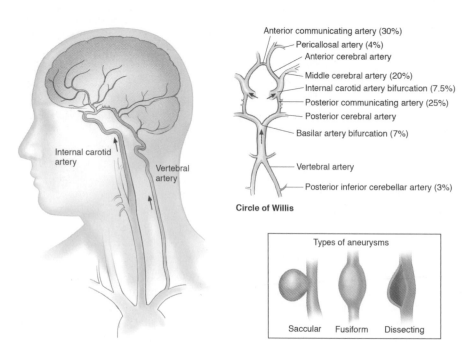

Figure 95.1. The anatomy of cerebral circulation. Adapted from Brisman JL, Song JK, Newell DW. Cerebral aneurysms. *N Engl J Med* 2006; 355(9):929.

the bleeding is extensive, many patients unfortunately continue to have low CBF and progress to a coma.

Patients with poor clinical grades of SAH tend to demonstrate impaired autoregulation, and their cerebral vessels are pressure-dependent. Furthermore, they have impaired cerebrovascular reactivity to carbon dioxide (CO_2) and may not respond to hyperventilation. This group of patients tends to demonstrate higher incidences of vasospasm, intracranial hypertension, and multiorgan dysfunction.

Complications

Rebleeding

The risk of rebleeding is high: 2% to 4% in the first day and 15% to 20% by the second week. The mortality from rebleeding is also high, 60%. There is a high risk of rebleeding during cerebral angiography. The incidence of intraoperative aneurysm bleeding is 6.7% per aneurysm; 5.3% occurring prior to dissection, 39.8% during dissection, 46% during clipping, and 8.8% postclipping.

The risk of rebleeding is proportional to the wall tension of the aneurysm called the *transmural pressure*. It is the pressure difference between the inside and the outside of the aneurysm sac. The transmural pressure has the same numeric value as the CPP, which is the difference between mean arterial pressure (MAP) and ICP.

$$\text{Risk of rebleeding} \propto \text{Transmural pressure}$$
$$= \text{MAP} - \text{ICP} = \text{CPP} \qquad \text{(Eqn. 1)}$$

Transmural pressure increases when there is a sudden change in MAP or ICP. When autoregulation is impaired, CBF becomes pressure-dependent, and an abrupt increase in systolic BP can promote rebleeding. Elevated ICP may protect the aneurysm from rupture to a certain extent. For this reason, ICP should not be decreased too rapidly before the dura is open. The timing of mannitol infusion and cerebrospinal fluid (CSF) drainage is decided carefully to avoid a sudden decrease in ICP.

The International Cooperative Study on the Timing of Aneurysm Surgery showed no differences in the outcome between early (0–3 days) versus late (11–14 days) surgery. The further evaluation of the results from the North American centers, however, indicated that early surgery within 3 days of SAH offered a good recovery in lower grade patients. Most neurosurgeons prefer early surgery to reduce the risk of rebleeding and to treat vasospasm effectively.

Vasospasm

Vasospasm is a leading, but potentially treatable, cause of morbidity after SAH. Vasospasm occurs between days 4 and 12 with a peak at day 6 to 7. With the general trend of early clipping, vasospasm is a postoperative problem in most cases. Patients in vasospasm may present with subtle mental status change or focal neurologic deficits. Whether the neurologic condition is reversible depends on the severity and frequency of vasospasm and the adequacy of the collateral flow.

The diagnosis is made by clinical examinations and confirmed by an angiography. Angiographically detected vasospasm is not always correlated with clinical vasospasm. Angiographic vasospasm occurs in 70% of patients, and symptomatic vasospasm occurs in 30%. A greater than 50% decrease in the diameter of an artery on an angiography is considered severe vasospasm. Vasospasm can occur in the vessels near the ruptured aneurysm as well as in distant vessels. Transcranial Doppler has been used to diagnose vasospasm and to continuously monitor the efficacy of treatment. Flow velocity is expected to decrease as vasospasm improves.

Several vasoactive mediators have been suggested as a cause, particularly the breakdown product of hemoglobin, oxyhemoglobin. Intracranial blood can promote free radicals by using iron in hemoglobin and activate cascade reactions involving vasoactive substances leading to the vasoconstriction of cerebral arteries.

The main strategies for the treatment of vasospasm are early removal of blood clots, triple H therapy (hypertension, hypervolemia, hemodilution), and use of nimodipine. The benefit of triple H therapy is not scientifically proven, yet a good outcome has been reported in some clinical studies. The rationale for triple H therapy is to increase CPP and CBF in the ischemic area through the collateral circulation. Some believe that improving cardiac output is more beneficial than increasing MAP. Triple H therapy has many complications such as pulmonary edema, myocardial ischemia, electrolyte imbalance, cerebral edema, and catheter infection. For patients with neurogenic stunned myocardium, triple H therapy is guided by invasive hemodynamic monitoring to avoid heart failure (Table 95.3).

Hemodynamic management during vasospasm depends on whether the aneurysm has been clipped. If the aneurysm has been clipped, BP is raised to 160 to 200 mm Hg. If the aneurysm has not been clipped, BP is maintained below 120 to 150 mm Hg. Vasopressors such as phenylephrine or dopamine are used to titrate the BP. Intravascular volume expansion is achieved with central venous pressure (CVP) of 10 to 12 mm Hg or pulmonary capillary wedge pressure (PCWP) of 12 to 18 mm Hg. During ischemia, blood viscosity increases secondary to the low flow state. Improved viscosity from hemodilution improves CBF. The hematocrit of 30% to 35% offers the optimum balance between viscosity and oxygen-carrying capacity. If the patient develops vasospasm prior to surgery, maintenance of adequate CPP is critical, and deliberate hypotension is avoided intraoperatively.

Prophylactic use of nimodipine improves the outcome after SAH, even though there is no evidence suggesting that it prevents vasospasm. The mechanism may involve dilation of collateral circulation as well as prevention of calcium influx. Nicardipine decreases cerebral vasospasm, but there was no difference in the neurologic outcome at three months. For

Table 95.3. Treatment of vasospasm

Surgical	Clot removal, early clipping
Hemodynamic	Hypertension, hypervolemia, hemodilution
Pharmacologic	Nimodipine, nicardipine
Endovascular	Intra-arterial verapamil/papaverine, angioplasty

severe vasospasm, intra-arterial injection of verapamil or papaverine relaxes the vessel wall. The effect of papaverine is short-lived, requiring multiple procedures, and is known to be neurotoxic. Refractory vasospasm is treated by transluminal balloon angioplasty, which offers long-lasting effects but carries serious potential complications such as rupture, thrombosis, and dissection of the vessel or displacement of the clip. Stellate ganglion block decreases cerebral vascular tone without affecting chemoreceptor function or autoregulation.. Arterial flow velocities and zero flow pressure decrease, but CO_2 reactivity is maintained. These responses to stellate ganglion block could represent a therapeutic advantage in treating cerebral vasospasms in the future.

Intracranial hypertension

Mild intracranial hypertension is common, and for most patients ICP returns to normal. Acute obstructive hydrocephalus occurs in up to 20% of patients and is commonly due to intraventricular blood clots causing mechanical obstruction of CSF flow. Other causes include the mass effect of intraparenchymal hematoma and ischemic changes from vasospasm. Cerebral vasospasm, when not treated promptly, increases ICP further and exacerbates cerebral edema. Vasospasm can also cause vasodilation in the distal vessels and increase the cerebral blood volume. A comatose patient with dilated ventricles mandates emergency ventriculostomy placement. Because of a risk of herniation, lumbar drain is contraindicated in patients with intracerebral hematoma, however. Hydrocephalus usually presents as a delayed complication from obliteration of arachnoid granulations, the site at which CSF is resorbed (Table 95.4).

In general, the patient with intracranial hypertension arrives in the operating room with an ICP monitor which allows measurement of ICP as well as CSF drainage. Hyperventilation effectively lowers ICP and is used as a temporary measure in an acute setting of intracranial hypertension. Its vasoconstrictive effect dissipates within 12 hours. One important caveat is that an acute decrease in ICP, either by hyperventilation or CSF drainage, increases transmural pressure and risks rebleeding.

Table 95.4. Causes of intracranial hypertension after SAH

CSF obstruction
Mass effect from hematoma
Cerebral edema secondary to ischemia
Loss of autoregulation

Treatment

All ruptured aneurysms require either surgical clipping or endovascular coiling. The decision of clipping versus coiling depends on the anatomy of the aneurysm, neurologic condition, and comorbidity. According to the International Subarachnoid Aneurysm Trial (ISAT), clipping offers a lifetime treatment of aneurysm at a slightly higher risk of neurologic morbidity. Endovascular treatment is a preferable treatment modality for basilar artery aneurysms and for patients with poor Hunt–Hess grades or significant comorbidities. The drawback of an endovascular approach is a higher incidence of incomplete obliteration, recanalization, and rebleeding. New techniques using stent-assisted coils, bioactive coils, and coils of complex shapes are under investigation.

Anesthetic management

Preoperative consideration

Patients with poor clinical grades frequently present with multi-organ dysfunction. Cardiac, pulmonary, and renal systems are commonly affected by the high sympathetic discharge associated with SAH. A thorough assessment of underlying medical conditions (see Table 95.5) and new SAH-related conditions are important in determining the optimum CPP range, the safety of transient hypotension, osmotherapy, and fluid status. The timing of rupture should be noted to assess the perioperative risk of vasospasm.

The CT and cerebral angiogram should be reviewed to assess the size and location of the aneurysm, enlargement of ventricles, and the presence of multiple aneurysms. The overall surgical plan, need for cerebral protection, and positioning are discussed with the surgeon prior to surgery.

Table 95.5. Preoperative evaluation of patients with SAH

History	Onset of bleeding, loss of consciousness, seizure, comorbidity
Medications	Calcium channel blockers, BP medications, seizure medications, osmotherapy
Vital signs	Baseline BP, oxygenation, urine output, central venous pressure, intracranial pressure
PE	Heart and lung, IV access, invasive catheters, ICP monitor
Neurology	Hunt–Hess classification, neurologic deficits
Laboratory tests	Check complete blood count (CBC) and prothrombin time/partial thromboplastin time (PT/PTT), treat coagulopathy, treat electrolyte abnormality, check the baseline renal function, note serum osmolality, treat hyperglycemia, check troponin level
Blood	Type and cross-match four units, plasma or platelets if needed
Chest radiograph	Rule out pulmonary edema or aspiration pneumonia, check the placement of the central line
EKG	Note preoperative EKG changes, arrhythmia
CT	Ventricle size, cerebral edema, Fisher grading
Angiogram	Size and anatomy of aneurysm, presence of multiple aneurysms

Neurologic evaluation

The presence of intracranial hypertension should be noted. Without knowing ICP, the true CPP remains unknown. Even when the patient does not have an ICP monitor, ICP can be estimated by a clinical examination. It is important to document the admission neurologic condition such as mental status, motor deficits, and visual field changes. Seizure medications need to be at a therapeutic level.

Pulmonary evaluation

Neurogenic pulmonary edema (NPE) develops in 1% to 2% of patients with SAH and can be potentially life-threatening. The pathophysiology of NPE is not well known. Pulmonary edema is more common in poor-clinical-grade patients. It is believed that intracranial hypertension stimulates the sympathetic system, and the release of catecholamines from the hypothalamus and medulla appears to be a contributing factor. Elevated pulmonary hydrostatic pressure, leaky membranes, or both have been suggested as an etiology. The patient with NPE presents with dyspnea and hypoxemia. Hypoxemia is due to intrapulmonary shunting and manifests as a wide A-a gradient refractory to oxygen therapy. Hypoxemia dramatically increases CBF and should be corrected immediately. High positive end-expiratory pressure (PEEP), despite a potential detrimental effect on ICP, is recommended to treat hypoxemia whenever necessary. Elevation of ICP from PEEP is more likely due to hypercapnia from an increase in dead space ventilation than to venous outflow obstruction. Unless PEEP is greater than 10 to 12, it is unlikely to increase ICP. As ICP is normalized, NPE resolves in time.

Other differential diagnoses of respiratory failure include aspiration pneumonia. Altered mental status places SAH patients at a high risk of aspiration. The clinical presentation and chest radiograph from aspiration pneumonia may be similar to those of NPE. Pulmonary edema may develop during triple H therapy from overzealous hydration. Patients with SAH are at a moderate risk of developing thromboembolism and may develop pulmonary embolism. Nosocomial pneumonia is another possibility for ventilator-dependent patients.

Cardiac evaluation

Cardiac dysfunction is well-described in patients with a variety of acute intracranial pathology but particularly with aneurysmal SAH. Overactivity of the sympathetic system and an increased level of norepinephrine appear to cause demand ischemia or direct tissue damage. It is postulated that excessive catecholamine release "stuns" the myocardium, causing a reversible wall motion abnormality, usually beyond single coronary vessel territories, which normalizes over time. Severe SAH-induced ejection fraction reduction with large areas of akinetic myocardium coupled with only mild troponin elevations is typical and sets it apart from concomitant acute coronary syndrome. There might be significant overlap with NPE.

More than half of patients show abnormal electrocardiogram (EKG) findings such as ST/T wave changes and prolonged Q-T intervals. EKG changes may be indistinguishable from true myocardial ischemia. EKG abnormalities are correlated with the severity of the neurologic injury, but are not considered an independent predictor of outcome. In contrast, troponin elevation is a good predictor of left ventricular dysfunction and peaks immediately following the SAH. Brain natriuretic peptide (BNP) correlates well with regional wall motion abnormalities as well but also reflects the severity of diastolic dysfunction, reduced ejection fraction, and pulmonary edema. Arrhythmias are present in more than 90% of patients with SAH. Frequent premature ventricular contractions (PVCs) are the most common types of arrhythmia. Atrial flutter, atrial fibrillation, and ventricular arrhythmias are also associated with SAH. Prolonged Q-T increases the incidence of ventricular arrhythmias.

If the patient has an abnormal EKG or elevated troponin, no further workup is necessary unless the patient develops hemodynamic instability or has multiple cardiac risk factors. EKG changes do not affect the surgical outcome and usually normalize within 10 days. For hemodynamically unstable patients, however, cardiac echocardiogram or pulmonary artery catheter placement is considered. The risk of cardiac catheterization and intervention is too high for patients with unclipped aneurysms (Fig. 95.2).

Electrolyte evaluation

A variety of electrolyte abnormalities are common secondary to hypothalamic dysfunction when SAH occurs near the circle of Willis. The most common abnormality is hyponatremia. Other electrolyte abnormalities include hypokalemia, hypocalcemia, and hypomagnesemia and should be corrected promptly.

Hyponatremia is due to either cerebral salt wasting (CSW) or inappropriate secretion of antidiuretic hormone (SIADH). CSW is a more common cause of hyponatremia in SAH patients and is characterized by volume contraction and negative sodium balance. The etiology of CSW is presumed to be due to atrial natriuretic factor (ANF) or brain natriuretic peptide (BNP). In both cases, the urine osmolality is greater than the serum osmolality, and the urine sodium is greater than 20 mEq/L. The major difference between CSW and SIADH is volume status. A central venous catheter is useful in identifying patients with volume depletion. If hyponatremia is present during the vasospasm period, the distinction between these two conditions is critical. The treatment goal is the same, however: euvolemia and correction of hyponatremia with isotonic fluids. The rate of correction should not exceed 0.5 to 1 mEq/L/h to avoid central pontine myelinolysis.

Central diabetes insipidus (DI) is associated with hypothalamic or pituitary dysfunction secondary to hematoma or a mass in the sellar area. The diagnosis is made by hypernatremia, copious urine output, dilute urine, and hypovolemia. Treatment requires replacement of free water loss with hypotonic saline such as half normal saline until euvolemia is maintained. Refractory DI requires treatment with desmopressin.

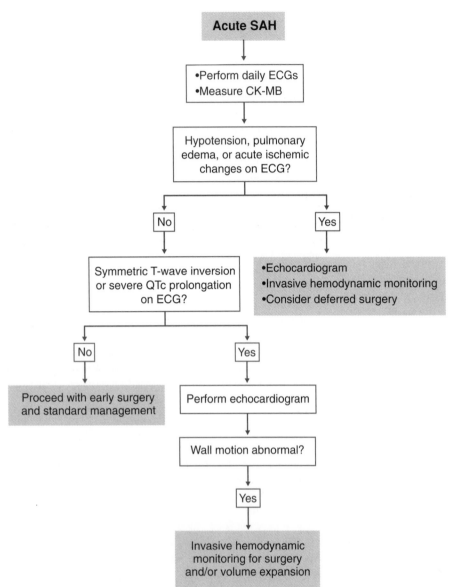

Figure 95.2. Algorithm for the detection of left ventricular dysfunction after SAH. Adapted from McKhann GM II, Mayer SA, Le Roux PD. Perioperative and intensive care of patients with aneurysmal subarachnoid hemorrhage. In Le Roux PD, Winn HR, Newell DW, eds. *Management of Cerebral Aneurysms.* Philadelphia: Saunders; 2004:431–454.

Premedication

Anxious patients with hypertension are sedated in a well-monitored setting. Patients with increased ICP, however, should not be sedated. Hypercapnia caused by respiratory depression is a potent stimulus for cerebral vasodilation and may increase ICP further. For example, a $PaCO_2$ of 60 mm Hg increases CBF by 50%.

Monitoring

In addition to American Society of Anesthesiologists (ASA) standard monitoring, an arterial catheter is indicated prior to induction for a ruptured aneurysm. For an unruptured aneurysm, it can be placed after induction as long as the BP is closely monitored. When an ICP monitor is available, an arterial catheter is zeroed at the level of the foramen magnum, approximately at the level of the circle of Willis. A baseline EKG should be recorded as reference. A CVP catheter is desirable for patients who are at high risk of vasospasm or have underlying cardiovascular conditions. Trendelenburg position during CVP catheter placement should be limited to less than 10% tilt to avoid an increase in ICP.

Neurophysiologic monitors are useful in assessing the adequacy of cerebral perfusion as well as regional ischemia. Commonly used neurophysiologic monitoring devices include electroencephalogram (EEG), somatosensory evoked potential (SSEP), and brainstem auditory evoked potential (BAEP). The choice of neurophysiologic monitoring is based on the vulnerable vascular territory. EEG monitors cortical activity. SSEP assesses sensory conduction to the cortex and is used for anterior and posterior circulation aneurysms. BAEP monitors the auditory pathway through the brainstem and is reserved for posterior circulation aneurysms. Neurophysiologic monitoring

Table 95.6. Cerebral monitoring

Cerebral function	EEG
	SSEP
	BAEP
Cerebral blood flow	Jugular bulb catheter
	Transcranial Doppler

guides the safe duration of temporary clip placement and the adequacy of BP. When cerebral ischemia is suspected, the surgeon may need to reposition the temporary clips, consider temporary reperfusion, or institute the cerebral protective strategy. Despite high false-positive and -negative predictive rates, SSEP and BAEP are the only cortical neurophysiologic monitoring modalities available during burst suppression. The monitoring of CBF with a jugular bulb catheter or transcranial Doppler is less common (Table 95.6).

Induction

The goal of induction is to keep the transmural pressure of the aneurysm at baseline, usually in the range of 60 to 80 mmHg. The risk of rebleeding from hypertension needs to be weighed against the risk of ischemia from hypotension. For patients in vasospasm, the BP is maintained slightly higher than baseline. The attempt to control ICP should not be too vigorous until the dura is open.

Any technique that meets the anesthetic goals is appropriate. A combination of thiopental or propofol, a generous amount of narcotics, and long-acting muscle relaxants is a commonly used technique. Fentanyl at 3 to 5 µg/kg, or sufentanil at 0.4 to 0.6 µg/kg or remifentanil at 0.5 to 1.0 µg/kg are typical doses for induction. Prior to intubation, BP is kept 20% below the baseline to prevent the usual increase in BP with intubation. Esmolol, lidocaine, remifentanil, or an additional dose of thiopental or propofol all effectively blunt the hemodynamic response to laryngoscopy. Propofol does not offer much advantage due to the long duration of the surgery and the additional doses of thiopental that may be used during temporary clipping. Patients who arrive in the operating room with nicardipine infusions tend to develop hypotension upon induction.

Most anesthetics affect cerebral vasculature and change cerebral blood volume. When the compliance of the brain is poor, even a small degree of vasodilation or vasoconstriction has a dramatic impact on ICP. In that situation, the use of intravenous (IV) anesthetics is desirable. The advantage of total IV anesthesia (TIVA) techniques is a reduction in both CBF and cerebral metabolic rate (CMR). If ICP is severely elevated, TIVA with propofol and remifentanil is a good choice as long as CPP is maintained. When volatile anesthetics are used, the cerebral vasodilatory effect is counterbalanced by the simultaneous cerebral vasoconstrictive effect secondary to the decrease in CMR. In fact, CBF remains almost unchanged at 1 minimum alveolar concentration (MAC).

The use of succinylcholine is recommended if the patient has a potentially difficult airway. The transient increase in ICP with succinylcholine is partly due to muscle fasciculation and is blunted by pretreatment with a small dose of nondepolarizing agent. If the patient has signs of impending herniation, rocuronium or mivacurium is an alternative. Laryngoscopy is performed when the patient is fully paralyzed. Coughing and bucking may dramatically increase the ICP. Tapes around the head cannot be used to secure the endotracheal tube for posterior fossa craniotomy. Good venous drainage is checked when the head is positioned. Considering the long duration of the surgery, all pressure points should be carefully padded.

Rebleeding during induction is a disaster. The surgical and nonsurgical stimulation in neurosurgery is highly predictable. Rebleeding occurs most frequently during laryngoscopy, pinning of the head holder, positioning, incision, raising of the bone flap, dural opening, dissection, and clipping. Avoiding an abrupt change in transmural pressure and providing a relaxed brain combined with careful planning of local blood flow may reduce the risk of rebleeding.

If the patient has an ICP monitor in place, it should be observed continuously until the dura is open. Hyperventilation decreases ICP effectively; however, it is not without risk. Hypocarbia increases the risk of ischemia by vasoconstriction, and $PaCO_2$ should never be dropped below 25 mm Hg. Another effective way of controlling ICP is CSF drainage. Accidental drainage of CSF is avoided because it may cause rebleeding or subdural hematoma.

Maintenance

The goal during the maintenance phase is to maintain adequate CPP, provide a "slack brain," offer cerebral protection if necessary, and, most importantly, be prepared for complications. An inhalational agent under 1 MAC with an infusion of fentanyl/sufentanil/remifentanil is commonly used. An opioid infusion provides stable hemodynamics and reduces the use of inhalational agents. The cerebral effects of different volatile agents are similar. The use of nitrous oxide (N_2O) remains controversial. N_2O increases CBF and ICP. Its vasodilatory effect is more pronounced when used with isoflurane in humans. It also increases CMR unlike other volatile agents. If N_2O is used simultaneously with IV anesthetics, however, the increase in CBF and CMR is attenuated. Animal studies have shown that N_2O may increase the risk of cerebral infarction in focal ischemia. For the above reasons, when the patient has a "tight brain" or is at a risk of focal ischemia, N_2O is often omitted.

The brain is unique in that there is little pain perception in the brain parenchyma. This observation is easily made during awake craniotomy. From skin incision to dural opening, however, the surgery is intensely stimulating and adequate amounts of narcotics are needed. Fortunately, the amount of narcotics given during this early period seems to make little difference in the quality of wake-up. After the dura is open, surgical stimulation becomes minimal and the narcotic infusion can be minimized. For closure, β-blockers, lidocaine, and remifentanil effectively blunt the hemodynamic response to stimulation and offer a rapid wake-up. During a posterior fossa craniotomy, sudden changes in BP and heart rate should be watched for when the brainstem or cranial nerves are retracted.

In general, carbon dioxide (CO_2) is maintained in the low end of the normal range. If ICP is elevated, mild hyperventilation is used to maintain $PaCO_2$ between 30 and 35 mm Hg. After the dura is open, ICP is no longer an issue because it becomes 0 mm Hg. At this point, MAP is equal to CPP. The surgeon may still request mild hyperventilation even after the dura is open. The indication for hyperventilation in that setting is for brain relaxation, not for ICP control. Excessive retraction pressure caused by a "tight brain" can cause brain ischemia. A "slack brain" is provided by mild hyperventilation, osmotic diuresis, optimal head positioning, lowering inhalational agent use, and CSF drainage. Hyperventilation should be discontinued as soon as brain relaxation is satisfactory and should not be used during temporary occlusion or vasospasm (Table 95.7).

Hypovolemia is prevalent in 36% to 100% of SAH patients, and the severity of hypovolemia is correlated with the clinical grade. Aneurysm surgery frequently requires diuresis and volume expansion. In a brain with an intact blood–brain barrier (BBB), the plasma osmolality from small ions determines the movement of water. The contribution of oncotic pressure to the total plasma osmolality is negligible, and colloid solution has no additional benefit over crystalloid. The fluid of choice is isotonic crystalloid without glucose. Blood sugar is often elevated from the use of dexamethasone and should be maintained at less than 150 mg/dl with an insulin infusion.

Osmotherapy reduces the bulk of the brain by removing interstitial fluid. Mannitol is usually given after the dura is open because the sudden drop in ICP can potentially cause rebleeding. It is important to keep the patient in a euvolemic state whenever mannitol is used. Mannitol becomes less effective if the patient is dehydrated or if the serum osmolality is greater than 320 mOsm/L. In addition, mannitol causes vasodilation and transiently increases intravascular volume. The usual dose is 0.25 to 1.0 g/kg. For those patients with low ejection fraction or renal failure, a smaller dose should be considered. The onset time is 10 to 15 minutes, and the duration is approximately 2 hours. Mannitol is effective only when the BBB is intact. When the BBB is disrupted, mannitol leaks into the interstitial space and increases the brain water content. Furosemide decreases CSF production and has a synergistic effect with mannitol. The effect of mannitol should be assessed by the improvement of brain relaxation rather than the urine output. Excessive brain relaxation can cause subdural hematoma by tethering bridging veins.

The most serious intraoperative complication during the final stage of dissection by the surgeon is hemorrhage. The incidence of intraoperative rebleeding is 10.7% for ruptured aneurysms and 1.2% for unruptured aneurysms. A transient reduction in MAP to 50 mmHg assists the surgeon in visualizing the field and gaining control over bleeding. If the dissection is near complete, the surgeon may be able to apply temporary clips to the feeding vessel or quickly place a

Table 95.7. Brain relaxation

CSF drainage through lumbar drain or ventriculostomy
Osmotherapy with mannitol and furosemide
Mild hyperventilation
Elevation of head
Metabolic suppression
Adequate venous drainage
Hypothermia
Avoidance of hypertension

permanent clip on the aneurysm. In some situations, the unilateral carotid artery is manually compressed if the aneurysm is located in the anterior circulation. Acute hypotension from hemorrhage or induced hypotension can cause brain ischemia. It is important to restore intravascular volume aggressively whenever hypotensive techniques are used. As soon as the bleeding is under control, BP is increased to the normal range. Communication with the surgeon and vigilant observation of the surgical field through a video monitor is critically important.

If the surgeon decides to use temporary clips, cerebral protection strategies are instituted. The risk of neurologic injury depends on the ischemic time, adequacy of collateral circulation, and cerebral protection strategy. The most commonly used methods are burst suppression, mild hypothermia, and induced hypertension. The frequency and dose of thiopental are titrated based on the EEG monitor. Burst suppression is stopped when the permanent clips are placed. During temporary clipping, the BP is increased to greater than 20% to 30% above the baseline using phenylephrine. Normocapnia is maintained over this period. The efficacy of induced hypertension is improved when the intravascular volume is restored. The transient change in SSEP during temporary clipping is often reversed by induced hypertension. The patient is often allowed to be mildly hypothermic, although a recent study demonstrated that intraoperative mild hypothermia failed to show improved neurologic outcome in "good-grade" patients after SAH.

Blood pressure control

Aneurysm surgery involves meticulous BP control. A history of long-standing hypertension, carotid disease, and renal insufficiency may increase the risk of intraoperative hypotension. In systemic circulation, the activity of the autonomic nervous system plays an important role, but in cerebral circulation, the effect of the autonomic nervous system is less significant. Hypotensive techniques are rarely used with the advances in microsurgical techniques and are used only when the aneurysm is ruptured inadvertently or when bleeding occurs during dissection. When temporary clips are used, BP is increased to improve perfusion in the watershed area through the collateral circulation.

Phenylephrine is the most commonly used drug to increase BP. In the event of hypertensive overshoot after the administration of a vasopressor, vasodilators should be used with

Table 95.8. Common pharmacologic therapy for BP control

Hypotensive agents	Dosage	Action	Advantages/disadvantages
Phenylephrine	0.25–1 µg/kg/min	α-agonist	Rapid onset/offset, reflex bradycardia
Nitroprusside	0.5–10 µg/kg/min	NO-mediated arterial $\gg$ venous, vasodilation	Rapid onset/offset, cyanide toxicity, ICP elevation, rebound hypertension, pulmonary shunting, unsafe in pregnancy, should be protected from light
Nitroglycerin	1–10 µg/kg/min	NO-mediated venous vasodilation	Rapid onset/offset, ICP elevation, rebound hypertension, pulmonary shunting
Esmolol	50–200 µg/kg/min	Selective β_1-blockade	Rapid onset/offset, no effect on cerebral vasculature
Labetalol	0.5–2 mg/min total 300 mg	α_1-, β_1-, and β_2-blockade	Long acting, no effect on cerebral vasculature, bronchospasm, cardiac depression
Nicardipine	5 mg/h, max 15 mg/h	Coronary and peripheral vasodilatation	Slow offset, minimal cardiac depression, reflex tachycardia less common
Volatile agents	Titrate between 0.5 and 1.0 MAC	Vasodilatation, myocardial depression	Increase ICP, cerebral edema

NO, nitric oxide.
Modified from Barash PG, Cullen B, Stoelting R, eds. *Clinical Anesthesia,* 5th ed. Philadelphia: Lippincott Williams & Wilkins, 2006:781.

caution in patients with intracranial hypertension. Nitroprusside and nitroglycerin offer the best BP control. When nitroprusside is abruptly discontinued, rebound hypertension may occur and the anesthesiologist must be prepared to manage it. Nitroglycerin may be used for patients with coronary artery disease or pregnancy, although it does cause an increase in cerebral blood volume and a concomitant increase in CSF pressure. The advantage of β-blockade in the management of acute hypertension is its lack of vasodilation, the ease of use, and the rapid reduction in heart rate and myocardial contractility. This is especially true for short-acting β-blockers such as esmolol, which has a rapid onset and a very brief duration of action. The use of longer acting β-blockers is postponed until blood loss is unlikely. If the patient has left ventricular dysfunction or is treated with triple H therapy, however, β-blockers should be used with caution. Nicardipine is a good alternative when β-blockers are contraindicated (Table 95.8).

Emergence

When the permanent clips are safely placed and the threat of bleeding or rupture is over, a plan for emergence is made. The important factors in considering the need for postoperative intubation are preoperative neurologic condition, intraoperative events such as rupture and hemorrhage, amount of thiopental used during burst suppression, body temperature, total amount of narcotic used, and the possibility of intraoperative ischemic events. For patients with basilar aneurysms, brainstem function needs to be assessed prior to extubation.

The goal for emergence is timely wake-up without BP swings. The patient should be awake enough to allow adequate neurologic evaluation. BP is kept within 20% of the baseline, usually less than 140 mmHg systolic. N_2O is discontinued when the dura is closed to avoid pneumocephalus. Delayed awakening increases the possibility of intraoperative ischemia, hematoma, pneumocephalus, residual hypothermia, and electrolyte abnormality.

The goal for fluid status is euvolemia or slight hypervolemia. Postoperative hypertension is avoided to prevent cerebral edema or bleeding. β-blockers are effective in attenuating the high sympathetic tone. Although mild hypertension is not of great concern when the aneurysm is clipped, the incidence of multiple aneurysms is high, and hypertension needs to be treated promptly. During transport, the patient needs to be fully monitored. Delayed respiratory depression causes hypercapnea leading to high ICP and hypertension.

Surgical considerations

Controlling blood flow into the aneurysm is essential for safe clipping. The common strategies are placement of temporary clips, circulatory arrest, and revascularization.

Temporary clips

When the aneurysm is large, has complex shapes and branches, has a fragile wall, or is present in an area where dissection is difficult, the local blood flow is controlled first. Temporary clip placement avoids the systemic effects of deliberate hypotension and makes the final dissection less risky. It also allows the removal of the thrombus inside and decompression of a giant aneurysm. Temporary clips are placed on the feeding artery or on each side to trap the aneurysm. The disadvantage is the risk of cerebral ischemia, especially when perforators come off the trapped vessel. If the ischemic time is prolonged, intermittent occlusion is an option. The intermittent reperfusion technique is controversial because it may reduce the ischemic injury but increase the reperfusion injury. An ischemic time of 15 to 20 minutes is considered safe (Fig. 95.3).

Circulatory arrest

When the risk of cerebral ischemia is too high, aneurysms are clipped under circulatory arrest. This technique is reserved for giant aneurysms and basilar tip aneurysms. The patient requires cardiopulmonary bypass or complete circulatory arrest with

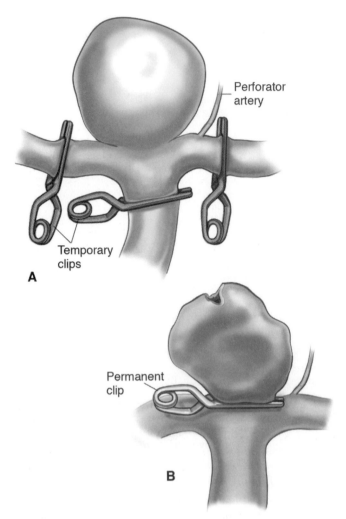

Figure 95.3. Temporary clips. Adapted from Ellegala DB, Day AL. Ruptured cerebral aneurysms. *N Engl J Med* 2005; 352(2):122.

profound hypothermia (<22°C). The patient is prepped for femoral–femoral bypass or open chest bypass. The femoral–femoral bypass with low flow is most commonly used and has lower morbidity. The decision to proceed with circulatory arrest is made after the aneurysm and the nearby perforators are dissected. The circulatory arrest time should be kept to less than 60 minutes.

Revascularization

Revascularization is used when the parent vessel needs to be sacrificed to obliterate the aneurysm. Revascularization anastomosis using an extracranial artery, high flow vein, or adjacent intracranial artery has been used.

Endovascular aneurysm coiling

Interventional neuroradiology has been revolutionized in the past decade and allows treatment of complex neurovascular diseases through peripheral access. Common procedures include diagnostic angiography, coiling of ruptured aneurysm, embolization of AVM, balloon angioplasty, and stenting. The procedure involves placement of a large introducer sheath by a transfemoral artery approach. A guiding catheter is advanced into the carotid or vertebral artery. At that point, a super-selective microcatheter is introduced over a guide wire, with the guidance of road mapping, into the cerebral circulation. Detachable platinum coils of different sizes are advanced through the microcatheter to the aneurysm, and coils are deployed by electrothrombosis. The aneurysm sac is gradually packed with smaller coils until it is completely obliterated (Fig. 95.4).

There is a significant overlap in anesthetic management between clipping and coiling. Diagnostic cerebral angiography is usually done while the patient is awake. Dexmedetomidine is a good choice for sedation because it maintains respiratory drive. General anesthesia with paralysis is used for other procedures. The depth of anesthesia required for endovascular procedures is much less than that for open surgery. The special considerations for endovascular coiling are immobility, anticoagulation, allergy to contrast or protamine, and, most importantly, management of complications. If there is difficulty with an arterial catheter for invasive arterial BP monitoring, the side port of the femoral sheath can be used, but it may underestimate the systolic BP and overestimate the diastolic BP due to the coaxial catheter inside. All IV catheters should have extensions for easy access. N_2O is avoided because of potential enlargement of air bubbles in the microcatheter.

Anticoagulation with heparin is necessary for all neurovascular procedures because a blood clot on a catheter may cause an embolic event. The goal for heparinization is activated coagulation time (ACT) of greater than 250 seconds. The commonly used contrast is nonionic with high osmolality. The incidence of mild reactions with nonionic contrast has decreased, yet life-threatening reactions continue to occur. The risk factors for contrast nephropathy include use of a large amount of contrast, dehydration, concomitant use of other nephrotoxic drugs, and preexisting renal insufficiency. A large amount of fluid from flushing through the catheter needs to be counted as additional fluid intake.

Catastrophic complications may occur during the procedure. The incidence of rupture during coiling is 1.4% to 2.7%, with mortality exceeding 30%. If the aneurysm ruptures, BP should be maintained at the baseline and additional help should be summoned emergently. Rapid correction of anticoagulation is necessary to minimize hemorrhagic complications, whereas mild hypertension with possible thrombolysis is necessary for occlusive complications. Other serious complications are intimal dissection, perforation, and parent vessel thrombosis.

The endovascular approach to treating cerebral aneurysms has become a superior option for selective patient groups and is widely used at present. The technique presents many new challenges to anesthesiologists working in a remote location. Because the microsurgical and endovascular approaches have their advantages and disadvantages, it is likely that both techniques will remain as important treatment options. It is critical

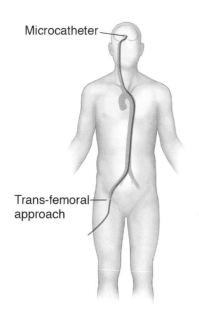
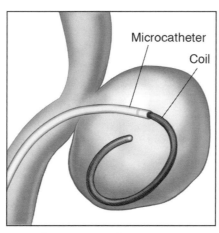
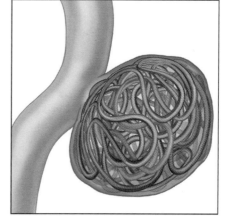

Coil as it enters the aneurysm

Coil completely obliterates the aneurysm

Figure 95.4. Endovascular aneurysm coiling. Adapted from Brisman JL, Song JK, Newell DW. Cerebral aneurysms. *N Engl J Med* 2006; 355(9):928–939.

for anesthesiologists to be familiar with the management of intracranial aneurysms in both settings.

Arteriovenous malformation

Introduction

AVM is a tangle of blood vessels consisting of arteries and veins, but without capillaries (Fig. 95.5). AVM is caused by a congenital vascular anomaly and tends to grow in size over time. Most AVMs become symptomatic and will bleed with age. Patients with AVM usually present with hemorrhage, seizure, and chronic cerebral ischemia. AVM hemorrhages are usually

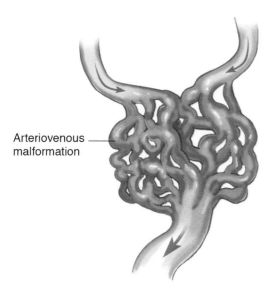

Arteriovenous malformation

Figure 95.5. Arteriovenous malformations of the brain.

intracerebral, but are occasionally subarachnoid and intraventricular. The most common cause of SAH in children is AVM. An infant with the vein of Galen AVM may present as having congestive heart failure and hydrocephalus. AVM occurs in younger patients between ages 20 and 50, and, as a result, the lifetime risk of morbidity and mortality remains high without surgical resection.

The initial workup of choice is a noncontrast CT to detect acute hemorrhage followed by an angiography to evaluate the anatomy of AVM, associated aneurysms, and the pattern of venous outflow.

The risk of rebleeding is slightly higher during the first year. It is reported as 6% to 20% in the first year then 2% to 4% per year thereafter, with overall mortality of 1% per year. Mortality from the initial bleeding is as high as 30%. The risk factors for hemorrhage are previous hemorrhage, deep venous drainage, deep location, intranidal or multiple aneurysms, small size, and high perfusion pressure in the feeding artery or draining vein. In contrast to a ruptured cerebral aneurysm, AVM bleeding rarely causes vasospasm. The recent advances in embolization techniques allow complete obliteration of AVMs even in areas that are surgically difficult to access.

Pathophysiology

AVM is a low-resistance vascular system. Blood is preferentially shunted toward the AVM bed, the pathway of least resistance. The risk of rebleeding is lower than that of cerebral aneurysm because the perfusion pressure in the feeding arteries is only 45% to 70% of the systemic BP. In contrast, the venous system is exposed to higher pressure. As a result, both the feeding and the draining vessels become dilated over time. The feeding arteries gradually develop medial hypertrophy, and aneurysms develop frequently on the feeding arteries in 10% of the patients. When the AVM is large, the low vascular resistance can even lead to high-output cardiac failure. A smaller AVM has higher perfusion pressure and is associated with a higher incidence of hemorrhage compared with a larger AVM.

High blood flow into AVM steals blood from the adjacent brain which compensates for chronic ischemia by maximal vasodilation. The vessels in the surrounding brain lose autoregulation or shift the curve leftward. The hypoperfused brain also promotes angiogenesis, which results in abnormal vessels with impaired autoregulation. When the AVM is resected, blood flow is redirected to other areas where small vessels are unable to vasoconstrict and easily become hyperemic. In contrast, the perfusion pressure in draining veins decreases dramatically after resection and predisposes thrombosis. This phenomenon of cerebral hyperperfusion in the setting of normal CPP is called *normal perfusion pressure breakthrough* (NPPB).

Intracerebral hemorrhage from NPPB carries a high morbidity. The risk of developing NPPB is related to the size and the extent of increased blood flow in the AVM bed. NPPB is more common in large AVMs such as the vein of Galen AVM. Angiographic findings of large, high-flow shunts, multiple large-diameter feeding arteries, and AVMs located in the border zone predict hyperemic complications. Staged embolization allows time for the chronically vasodilated vessels to regain autoregulation.

Treatment options

AVM is treated with microsurgical resection, embolization, stereotactic radiosurgery, or a combination of different modalities. Surgery offers a permanent cure. Embolization is considered for surgically risky AVMs or for patients with major comorbidities. The preoperative embolization for a high-flow AVM can be coordinated with surgery to minimize the risk of intraoperative blood loss. Not all feeding arteries, however, are accessible to an embolization catheter, and the technique is limited by recanalization when used alone. For large AVMs, a staged embolization is considered to avoid sudden restoration of blood flow to the normal brain. A partially embolized AVM carries a higher risk of bleeding than an untreated AVM. Complete resection is important, and an intraoperative angiography is routine for confirmation. Radiosurgery is reserved for small lesions in an eloquent area.

The Spetzler–Martin grading system has been used to assess surgical risk. Spetzler–Martin grade I to II lesions are treated by surgical resection, and grade III lesions are treated by embolization followed by surgical resection (Table 95.9).

Anesthetic management

The risk of rebleeding from AVM is not usually higher immediately after bleeding. Because most of the cases are surgically resected as elective cases, it allows optimization of preexisting medical conditions. On the other hand, when a patient

Table 95.9. Spetzler–Martin grading system of AVMs

Size of AVM	Eloquence of adjacent brain	Pattern of venous drainage
Small (<3 cm) 1*	Non-eloquent 0	Superficial only 0
Medium (3–6 cm) 2	Eloquent 1	Deep component 1
Large (>6 cm) 3		

*The sum of the scores is equal to the grade.
Spetzler RF, Martin NA. A proposed grading system for arteriovenous malformations. *J Neurosurg* 1986; 65:476–483.

presents with severe intracranial hypertension from a large hematoma, the surgery is done on a more urgent basis. The overall anesthetic management of AVM resection is similar to that of aneurysm clipping: careful BP control, slack brain, euvolemia, normoglycemia, and rapid emergence.

Preoperative considerations

The preoperative assessment includes the presence of intracranial hypertension, neurologic deficits, and control of seizures, in addition to the preexisting medical conditions. The size and location of the lesion are noted as well as the presence of other associated aneurysms. Large AVMs with high flow are identified to estimate the risk of NPPB. If the AVM is located in a delicate and risky brain area, the surgery may require two steps: the mapping of the AVM bed under awake craniotomy and the subsequent resection under general anesthesia. Several large-bore IV catheters are needed, and blood products should be available for potential hemorrhage.

Induction

During induction, the risk of rebleeding from systemic hypertension is much lower than that from a cerebral aneurysm because the perfusion pressure within AVM is lower. The frequent presence of an aneurysm in the feeding artery mandates careful BP monitoring, however. In addition, the compliance of the vasculature is abnormal, and avoidance of cerebral vasodilation is recommended. For an elective resection, ICP is usually normalized. The primary goal during induction is to maintain CPP and ICP in the optimum range. An arterial catheter is placed prior to induction. A combination of thiopental/propofol, fentanyl/sufentanil/remifentanil, and long-acting muscle relaxants is commonly used.

Maintenance

A balanced anesthetic technique with an inhalational agent and narcotic infusion has been used most often. Fentanyl/sufentanil/remifentanil infusions provide stable hemodynamics and reduce the requirement for inhalational agents. The concentration of the volatile agent is kept at less than 1 MAC to preserve autoregulation. Judicious use of mild hyperventilation and osmotic therapy provides a relaxed brain and facilitates surgical dissection. Cerebral protective strategies are considered for large AVMs.

Table 95.10. Complications of interventional neuroradiologic embolization/coiling

Complications	Clinical scenario	Treatment
Hemorrhagic	Perforation	Reversal of heparin
	NPPB	Lowering of blood pressure
	Dissection	Rapid delivery of coil, emergency craniotomy
Occlusive	Thromboembolic	Thrombolysis, mechanical lysis, anticoagulation
	Vasospasm	Raising of blood pressure
	Coil fracture	Retrieval/reposition of coil
Miscellaneous	Contrast reaction/nephropathy	Pretreatment, careful fluid management
	Groin hematoma	Compression, evacuation of hematoma

Modified from Varma MK, Price K, Jayakrishnan V, et al. Anaesthetic consideration for interventional neuroradiology. *Br J Anaesth* 2007; 99(1):75–85.

Intraoperative hemorrhage is more common during AVM resection than in aneurysm clipping. Dural arteriovenous fistulas involving major sinuses and the great vein of Galen malformation tend to bleed easily. Vasopressors and vasodilators should be readily available to keep the BP in a tight range. Until the AVM bed is completely resected and adequate homeostasis is obtained, it is prudent to use short-acting drugs such as nitroprusside, nitroglycerin, or esmolol. When massive blood loss occurs, the BP needs to be lowered rapidly to facilitate surgical hemostasis. Preoperative embolization decreases the incidence of major bleeding. The extent of blood-flow increase in the remainder of the brain after AVM resection can be estimated with intraoperative use of transcranial Doppler.

Emergence

Smooth emergence is paramount to avoid hypertension. BP should be maintained at or slightly lower than the baseline during the early postoperative period to avoid NPPB. Postoperative bleeding into the AVM resection bed can cause neurological catastrophe and result in high mortality. Although the vessels surrounding the AVM have impaired autoregulation, they remain responsive to $PaCO_2$. Respiratory depression secondary to excessive narcotics use should be watched for because hypercapnia may worsen cerebral edema. If extensive brain swelling is of concern, the patient should remain intubated and hyperventilated.

Endovascular embolization

Anesthetic management of AVM embolization is similar to that of cerebral aneurysm coiling. Embolization is done under either general anesthesia or monitored anesthetic care. The advantages of general anesthesia are high-quality imaging and the absence of movement. In contrast, monitored anesthetic care allows frequent neurologic examinations and provides the information about the true function of the potentially risky area in the brain. Dexmedetomidine is a reasonable choice because of the lack of respiratory depression. However, its selective α_2-agonist effect tends to cause hypotension and BP monitoring through a radial arterial or femoral coaxial catheter is mandatory. Occasionally, the neurointerventional radiologist may request deliberate hypotension for a brief time to deposit embolic materials in a more controlled manner. If inadvertent embolization into feeding vessels occurs, induced hypertension is necessary to augment perfusion through the collaterals. NPPB may occur when the feeding arteries are obliterated or venous outflow is obstructed due to inadvertent embolization. Hemorrhagic and thrombogenic complications during the procedure are treated as shown in Table 95.10.

Suggested readings

ApSimon HT, Reef H, Phadke RV, et al. A population-based study of brain arteriovenous malformation. *Stroke* 2002; 33:2794–2800.

Barker FG, Ogilvy CS. Efficacy of prophylactic nimodipine for delayed ischemic deficit after subarachnoid hemorrhage: a metaanalysis. *J Neurosurg* 1996; 84:405–414.

Batjer HH, Chander JP, Getch CC, et al. Intracranial aneurysm. In: Rengachary SS, Ellenbogen, RG, eds. *Principles of Neurosurgery.* 2nd ed. Philadelphia: Elsevier Mosby; 2005:215–239.

Bendo AA, Kass IS, Hartung J, Cottrell JE. Anesthesia for neurosurgery. In: Barash PG, Cullen B, Stoelting R, eds. *Clinical Anesthesia.* 5th ed. Philadelphia: Lippincott Williams & Wilkins; 2006:746–789.

Black S, Sulek C, Day AL. Cerebral aneurysm and arteriovenous malformation. In: Cucchiara RF, Black S, Michenfelder JD, eds. *Clinical Neuroanesthesia.* 2nd ed. New York: Churchill Livingstone; 1998:265–318.

Brisman JL, Song JK, Newell DW. Cerebral aneurysms. *N Engl J Med* 2006; 355(9):928–939.

Bulsara KR, McGirt MJ, Liao L, et al. Use of the peak troponin value to differentiate myocardial infarction from reversible neurogenic left ventricular dysfunction associated with aneurismal subarachnoid hemorrhage. *J Neurosurg* 2003; 98:524–528.

Cooper KR, Boswell PA, Choi SC. Safe use of PEEP in patients with severe head injury. *J Neurosurg* 1985; 63:552.

Deibert E, Barzilai B, Braverman AC, et al. Clinical significance of elevated troponin I levels in patients with nontraumatic subarachnoid hemorrhage. *J Neurosurg* 2003; 98:741–746.

Dodson BA. Interventional neuroradiology and the anesthetic management of patients with arteriovenous malformations. In: Cottrell JE, Smith DS, eds. *Anesthesia and Neurosurgery.* 4th ed. St. Louis: Mosby; 2001:399–423.

Ellegala DB, Day AL. Ruptured cerebral aneurysms. *N Engl J Med* 2005; 352(2):121–124.

Fisher CM, Kistler JP, Davis JM. Relation of cerebral vasospasm to subarachnoid hemorrhage visualized by computerized tomographic scanning. *Neurosurgery* 1980; 6:1–9.

Friedlander RM. Arteriovenous malformations of the brain. *N Engl J Med* 2007; 356(26):2704–2712.

Greenberg MS. SAH and aneurysms. In: Greenberg MS, ed. *Handbook of Neurosurgery.* 5th ed. New York: Thieme Medical; 2001:754–803.

Haley EC, Kassell NF, Torner JC. The International Cooperative Study on the Timing of Aneurysm Surgery: the North American experience. *Stroke* 1992; 23(2):205.

Harrod CG, Bendok BR, Batjer HH. Prediction of cerebral vasospasm in patients presenting with aneurismal subarachnoid hemorrhage: a review. *Neurosurgery* 2005; 56(4):633–654.

Hunt WE, Hess RM. Surgical risk as related to time of intervention in the repair of intracranial aneurysms. *J Neurosurg* 1968; 28(1):14–20.

Joshi S, Ornstein E, Young WL. Cerebral and spinal cord blood flow. In: Cottrell JE, Smith DS, eds. *Anesthesia and Neurosurgery.* 4th ed. St. Louis: Mosby; 2001:19–67.

Kassell NF, Torner JC, Haley EC, et al. The International Cooperative Study on the Timing of Aneurysm Surgery. Part I: Overall management results. *J Neurosurg* 1990; 73:18.

Kassell NF, Torner JC, Jane JA, et al. The International Cooperative Study on the Timing of Aneurysm Surgery. Part II: Surgical results. *J Neurosurg* 1990; 73:37.

Kim DH, Joseph M, Ziadi S, et al. Increases in cardiac output can reverse flow deficits from vasospasm independent of blood pressure: a study using xenon computed tomographic measurement of cerebral blood flow. *Neurosurgery* 2003; 53:1044–1051.

Kotapka MJ, Flamm ES. Cerebral aneurysms: surgical considerations. In: Cottrell JE, Smith DS, eds. *Anesthesia and Neurosurgery.* 4th ed. St. Louis: Mosby; 2001:353–365.

Lam AM. Cerebral aneurysms: anesthetic considerations. In: Cottrell JE, Smith DS, eds. *Anesthesia and Neurosurgery.* 4th ed. St. Louis: Mosby; 2001:367–397.

Lam AM, Mayberg TS, Cooper JO, et al. Nitrous oxide-isoflurane anesthesia causes more cerebral vasodilation than an equipotent dose of isoflurane in humans. *Anesth Analg* 1994; 78:462.

Lee L, Lam AM. Anesthesia for patients with intracranial aneurysms. In: Le Roux PD, Winn HR, Newell DW, eds. *Management of Cerebral Aneurysms.* Philadelphia: Saunders; 2004:531–546.

Leipzig TJ, Morgan J, Horner TG, et al. Analysis of intraoperative rupture in the surgical treatment of 1694 saccular aneurysms. *Neurosurgery* 2005; 56:455–468.

Lo EH. A haemodynamic analysis of intracranial arteriovenous malformations. *Neurol Res* 1993; 15:51–55.

McKhann GM II, Mayer SA, Le Roux PD. Perioperative and intensive care of patients with aneurysmal subarachnoid hemorrhage. In: Le Roux PD, Winn HR, Newell DW, eds. *Management of Cerebral Aneurysms.* Philadelphia: Saunders; 2004:431–454.

Molyneux A. International Subarachnoid Aneurysm Trial (ISAT) Collaborative Group. International Subarachnoid Aneurysm Trial (ISAT) of neurosurgical clipping versus endovascular coiling in 2143 patients with ruptured intracranial aneurysms: a randomized trial. *Lancet* 2002; 360:1267–1273.

Murayama Y, Nien YL, Duckwiler G, et al. Guglielmi detachable coil embolization of cerebral aneurysms: 11 years' experience. *J Neurosurg* 2003; 98:959–966.

Nelson RJ, Roberts J, Rubin C, et al. Association of hypovolemia after subarachnoid hemorrhage with computed topographic scans evidence of raised intracranial pressure, *Neurosurgery* 1991; 29:178.

Newfield P, Bendo AA. Anesthetic management of intracranial aneurysms. In: Newfield P, Cottrell JE, eds. *Handbook of Neuroanesthesia.* 4th ed. Philadelphia: Lippincott Williams & Wilkins; 2007:143–172.

Ogilvy CS, Stieg PE, Awad I, et al. Recommendations for the management of intracranial arteriovenous malformations. *Stroke* 2001; 32:1458–1471.

Parsa AT, Solomon RA. Vascular malformations affecting the nervous system. In: Rengachary SS, Ellenbogen, RG, eds. *Principles of Neurosurgery.* 2nd ed. Philadelphia: Elsevier Mosby; 2005:241–258.

Priebe HJ. Aneurysmal subarachnoid haemorrhage and the anaesthetist. *Br J Anaesth* 2007; 99(1):102–118.

Sekhon LH, Morgan MK, Spence I. Normal perfusion pressure breakthrough: the role of capillaries. *J Neurosurg* 1997; 86:519.

Selman WR, Bhatti S, Rosenstein CC, et al. Temporary vessel occlusion in spontaneously hypertensive and normotensive rats. *J Neurosurg* 1994; 80:1085–1090.

Spetzler RF, Hargraves RW, McCormick PW, et al. Relationship of perfusion pressure and size to risk of hemorrhage from arteriovenous malformations. *J Neurosurg* 1992; 76:918–923.

Spetzler RF, Martin NA. A proposed grading system for arteriovenous malformations. *J Neurosurg* 1986; 65:476–483.

The International Study of Unruptured Intracranial Aneurysms Investigators. Unruptured intracranial aneurysms: natural history, clinical outcome, and risks of surgical and endovascular treatment. *Lancet* 2003; 362:103–110.

Todd MM, Hindman BJ, Clarke WR, et al. Mild intraoperative hypothermia during surgery for intracranial aneurysm. *N Engl J Med* 2005; 352(2):135–145.

van Gijn J, Rinkel GJE. Subarachnoid haemorrhage: diagnosis, causes and management. *Brain* 2001; 124:249–278.

Varma MK, Price K, Jayakrishnan V, et al. Anaesthetic consideration for interventional neuroradiology. *Br J Anaesth* 2007; 99(1):75–85.

Young WL, Pile-Spellman J, Isak P, et al. Evidence for adaptive autoregulatory displacement in hypotensive cortical territories adjacent to arteriovenous malformations. *Neurosurgery* 1994; 34(4):601–611.

Zaroff JG, Rordorf GA, Newell JB, et al. Cardiac outcome in patients with subarachnoid hemorrhage and electrocardiographic abnormalities. *Neurosurgery* 1999; 44:34–39.

Chapter 96

Anesthesia for electroconvulsive therapy

Lambertus Drop

Major depressive disorder (MDD) is diagnosed in approximately 14 million adults in the United States each year, and, according to the World Health Organization, depression will be the second most common cause of disability in the world by the year 2020. The consequences of depression are considerable as MDD not only affects quality of life but also increases the severity and mortality of other medical conditions. MDD typically is a relapsing disease, although less frequently with a combination of electroconvulsive therapy (ECT) and antidepressants than with ECT alone. An important clinical problem is intolerance to the side effects of antidepressant drugs. In such cases, ECT may be a suitable and more effective alternative treatment, resulting in a more rapid onset of remission of depressive symptoms, especially in the elderly population.

Although older textbooks advocate that antidepressants be discontinued 14 days prior to the start of ECT, several studies have shown the length of time in that recommendation to be excessive. Generally all antidepressants and benzodiazepines should be discontinued 2 to 4 days prior to the day of the first ECT treatment. Special mention is made of lithium carbonate, which must be discontinued prior to ECT because its combination with ECT is known to produce a state of severe confusion. Also neuroleptics should be discontinued, which are prescribed to many patients with delusional or psychotic depression. Their known side effects include orthostasis and Parkinsonism.

Electroconvulsive therapy

With ECT, an electrical stimulus is applied unilaterally or bilaterally to the scalp with the purpose of eliciting a grand mal motor seizure, which is modified by intravenous (IV) hypnotics and neuromuscular blocking drugs while the lungs are manually ventilated with oxygen.

Physiologic changes with ECT

Seizure activity is associated with profound physiologic changes in the autonomic nervous system and in cerebrovascular and cognitive function.

The hemodynamic response recorded after ECT is biphasic immediate and delayed, and both parts of the response involve both the parasympathetic and sympathetic systems.

Typically, the parasympathetic response comes first, with short-lasting bradycardia because of sinoatrial (SA) node inhibition, and is accompanied by increased salivation. Increased sympathetic tone then follows with self-limited tachycardia and hypertension. To gain insight in their magnitude, a retrospective analysis of 23,000 clinical data points in 227 patients at Massachusetts General Hospital has revealed that post ECT, more than a quarter of patients had systolic blood pressures exceeding 220 mm Hg, heart rate was between 120 and 140 bpm in 20% of patients and between 140 and 160 bpm in 15% of patients. Such a profound hyperdynamic state may be explained by enhanced sympathetic outflow in the brain, augmented by significant increases in circulating norepinephrine and epinephrine. Hypotension after ECT is so rare that, when it occurs, a search for its cause is indicated. This search may reveal inadequate fluid intake (typical for depression), but cardiac pump failure due to cardiac ischemic events must also be considered, especially in the elderly population. The delayed response is manifested as post-ECT bradycardia as a result of sustained enhanced parasympathetic tone. This is most often self-limited, but heart rates occasionally fall below 40 bpm, requiring 0.2 mg of IV glycopyrrolate. The most common arrhythmias during and after ECT are premature ventricular contractions (observed in 30% of patients) and T-wave flattening, which are self-limited. These changes are benign, and cardiac enzyme elevation is notably absent after uncomplicated ECT. In individual patients with previously known coronary artery disease, progressive elevations of the ST segment have been observed, and these changes were key to the diagnosis of myocardial injury.

Pulmonary gas exchange

During both tonic and clonic phases of an unmodified grand mal seizure, there is no effective breathing. With anesthesia and muscle relaxation, controlled ventilation provides adequate oxygenation during the ECT session as shown by pulse oximetry values.

Cerebral blood flow (CBF) is augmented by a factor of up to 5, and cerebral metabolic rate is increased. The degree of cerebral vasodilation is disproportionately greater than the increase in metabolic rate, accompanied by a temporary loss of cerebrovascular autoregulation. There is also increased intracranial pressure, but the magnitude of cerebral hypertension is uncertain, and the CBF adjustment may be inadequate in the presence of cardiac arrhythmias. Besides increased CBF rate there also is increased blood flow velocity as determined by transcranial Doppler ultrasonography, with an increase of 240%. Despite these seemingly ominous events, cellular injury in the brain does not occur with ECT when adequate oxygenation and cerebral perfusion pressure are maintained.

Because of hypothalamic stimulation that occurs with ECT, there is an increased release of several hormones, including adrenocorticotropic hormone (ACTH), vasopressin, prolactin, and cortisol. Effects of ECT on blood glucose levels in diabetic patients are variable, and close monitoring of blood glucose levels is advisable. Diabetic patients maintained on NPH insulin are given half of the daily dose, and an IV infusion with glucose-containing solution is begun. Oral intake is then allowed later in the day. In contrast, some practitioners allow the daily insulin dose to be postponed until shortly after ECT has been administered.

Intragastric pressure

Because ECT is associated with elevation of intragastric pressure, patients with gastric reflux or severe heartburn should receive a proton pump inhibitor alone by mouth or in combination with citric acid/sodium citrate immediately prior to ECT.

Intraocular pressure

Intraocular pressure is reported to more than double during ECT. This can be problematic in patients with glaucoma. Accordingly, an ophthalmologic consult should be obtained when ECT is contemplated in this patient population. Echothiophate, a commonly prescribed drug for glaucoma, is administered in the form of eyedrops. Ecothiophate is a potent inhibitor of plasma pseudocholinesterase and its systemic resorption may cause prolonged apnea from decreased enzymatic breakdown of succinylcholine.

Efficacy and indications

A generalized grand mal motor seizure is essential to the therapeutic efficacy of ECT and clinicians aim for a minimum seizure duration of 20 to 30 seconds. Indications for ECT include the lack of response to antidepressants, intolerance to their side effects, and a good clinical response to ECT previously. Unresponsiveness to antidepressants in the face of severe symptoms of major depressive disorder is an urgent indication for an ECT session, especially when malnutrition and dehydration coexist (secondary to anorexia or in combination with catatonia). Delusional and psychotic depression is a strong indication for ECT before beginning extensive drug treatment. Indications for ECT include the lack of response to antidepressants, intolerance to their side effects, a good response to ECT previously, and an urgent indication is established with unresponsiveness to antidepressants especially when malnutrition and dehydration

Table 96.1. Symptoms of depression

Pessimistic mood
Anorexia
Weight loss
Early awakening
Impaired ability of concentration
Motor restlessness
Speech latency
Constipation
Somatic delusions
Continued fatigue
Feelings of hopelessness
Low self-esteem
Preoccupation with death and suicide

coexist (secondary to anorexia or in combination with catatonia). Delusional and psychotic depression is a strong indication for ECT without extensive drug trials. Although comparative predictors for good responses to a drug regimen versus ECT are not firmly established, a good response to ECT may be expected with symptoms listed in Table 96.1. Central to these symptoms is the loss of interest in activities that used to give pleasure. The efficacy of ECT is dependent on details of the ECT procedure with success rates ranging from 20% to 80%. Such a wide range is possibly related to the total number of treatments that may be arbitrarily limited in some patients to lessen the most important side effect: short-term memory loss. Variables contributing to efficacy also include electrode placement, dosage, and duration – clearly all determined by the treating psychiatrist. Efficacy assessment of ECT may be performed by means of the standard Hamilton rating scale.

Seizure threshold

Seizure threshold for ECT treatment may be defined as the lowest energy level required to elicit an epileptic seizure, and is determined by successive stimulation, starting at a low level of energy with increments until a seizure is produced. Neurotransmitters and their receptors clearly are major determinants of the seizure threshold. The seizure threshold is of major clinical interest for two principal reasons. First, the seizure threshold may be manipulated with drugs or interventions with actions that either elevate or lower it. For example, benzodiazepines, propofol, fosphentoin, and hypoxia elevate the seizure threshold, whereas theophylline, caffeine, hypocapnia, and high partial pressures of oxygen lower it. In young patients, the seizure threshold is lower than in the elderly population and the seizure threshold progressively increases over the course of a series of treatments with ECT. These variables are taken into account when determining the energy level to be delivered. Precise control of the energy level delivered with avoidance of excessive levels, coupled with routine use of unilateral electrode placement are essential to eliminate severe post-ECT mental confusion, agitation, or memory loss. Because reliable predictors of ECT efficacy are not available, lifting of depressive symptoms does not occur in all patients. Improvement of mood after ECT occurs in at least 80% of patients, however.

Patient workup

A proper clinical evaluation includes a detailed history, physical examination, chest radiograph, electrocardiogram (ECG), and routine laboratory tests, including hematocrit and WBC. Tests of hepatic and kidney function may be indicated in elderly and ill patients. The clinical examination of the depressed patient may be limited because detailed information on discomfort or limitation of function often remains hidden or at least is difficult to obtain. Upon indication, specialized consultation and investigations may include cerebral CT and MRI, and study of cardiac function including stress test and echocardiogram. Antihypertensive regimens are optimized if applicable, and, in anticoagulated patients, coumadin is adjusted to yield international normalized ratio (INR) values between 2.5 and 3. The stability of blood sugar levels should be ascertained in diabetic patients. If ECT is offered early in the morning, the insulin dose may be held in diabetic patients until after the treatment. In asthmatic patients, theophylline is discontinued in view of the risk of status epilepticus when a high serum theophylline level is present at the time ECT is to be administered. In most patients there is a favorable response to inhaled corticosteroids or β_2-adrenergic agonists. For pregnant patients, an obstetrical consultation should be obtained. Additional recommendations pertaining to ECT for pregnant patients appear later in this chapter.

Treatment plan

Obtaining informed consent may pose a challenge in a depressed patient, especially when severe motor retardation is present, but the patient, a guardian, or family members must give informed consent for the application of ECT and, separately, for the administration of anesthesia. Brief and ultrabrief pulse stimulation are characterized by a rapid upstroke of the stimulus intensity followed by a rapid offset, with a square waveform. The stimulus is administered by a monitored ECT device (MECTA Corporation, Tualatin, OR) in which individually set variables are stimulus frequency, pulse width, total stimulus duration (depending on age), and number of immediately preceding treatments. The electrical stimulus produces a generalized seizure which spreads throughout the cerebral cortex and is followed by electrical silence of about 1 minute.

Clinically, the ECT patterns of stimulation with brief pulse and ultrabrief pulse predominate, primarily because of a lesser incidence of post-ECT complications, e.g. confusion and amnesia as compared to sine-wave stimulation. Traditionally, an initial series of 6 to 12 treatments on average are given with a sequence every other day (Mon–Wed–Fri), followed by reassessment. If remission is achieved, a regimen with antidepressants is usually required following the ECT treatment. Because ECT is also effective with application spaced at 1- (or more) week time intervals, maintenance ECT is a valuable alternative to maintenance with antidepressants, but comparative

Table 96.2.	Standard anesthesia protocol
Premedication	No atropine
	No benzodiazepines
Monitors	Noninvasive blood pressure
	ECG
	Pulse oximetry
IV access	20–22 gauge IV catheter
Induction	Methohexital 0.75 mg/kg
Muscle relaxation	Succinylcholine 0.75 mg/kg
Mask	Ventilation oxygen
Muscle relaxation confirmed	Foot sole reflex
Bite block	Between molars bilaterally
Terminate seizure (if >2 min)	Propofol, midazolam, lorazepam

data are not available. In the event of incomplete remission, more treatments with the same frequency as the initial series (or on a weekly or biweekly basis) may be indicated.

Augmented seizures

If attempts to induce seizures using standard technique are unsuccessful, several pharmacological interventions are available using agents that can produce or facilitate seizure activity. Some practitioners believe that selecting etomidate (0.2 mg/kg) instead of methohexital is useful. Others have administered caffeine (125–250 mg IV), but it may be remembered that this drug has the potential for an exaggerated response manifested by hypertension, tachycardia, and cardiac arrhythmias.

Anesthesia procedure
Anesthesia protocol

A fasting period of 6 to 8 hours is recommended. Because elderly patients with depression and forgetfulness may not be reliable or cooperative, nursing supervision of the fasting period is important. Hydroxyzine (50–75 mg) or promethazine (25–50 mg) may be administered for pretreatment sedation. Benzodiazepines and barbiturates are not used because of their seizure threshold–elevating effects. A standard anesthesia protocol is shown in Table 96.2. Because the seizure threshold is unknown in the first treatment, it may be necessary to administer more than one stimulus. If the first stimulus fails to elicit a seizure, the power is increased with the subsequent stimulus such that a value at least 50% over threshold is reached. A sequence of more than one stimulus carries the risk of severe bradycardia, however, because the parasympathetic effects of the nonconvulsive first stimulus may not be followed by sympathetic stimulation if a seizure fails to occur on the second attempt. In view of this potentially dangerous possibility, glycopyrrolate is always administered prior to the first ECT. It is preferred over atropine because of a lesser degree of tachycardia and because it is a quaternary compound that does not cause delirium by crossing the blood–brain barrier. IV access is established with a small-bore Teflon catheter configured as a heparin

Table 96.3. Anesthetic agents suitable for ECT

Drug	Dose	Seizure threshold	Seizure duration	Comments
Methohexital	0.5–1 mg/kg IV	Minimal anticonvulsant effects	↔	– Induction agent of choice by APA – Short duration of action – Pain upon injection
Thiopental	2–4 mg/kg IV	↑	↔ ↓	– Longer duration of action
Ketamine	0.5–2 mg/kg IV	↓	↓	– Slower onset – Delayed recovery – Hypersalivation – Ataxia – Increased hemodynamic variability
Propofol	1–2.0 mg/kg IV	↑↑	↓	– Rapid onset – Short duration of action – Use in patients with excessive seizure duration after standard dose of methohexital or with severe PONV
Etomidate	0.15–0.3 mg/kg IV	↓ ↔	↑	– Delayed recovery – Emetogenic – Accentuated hemodynamic response
Opioids	The short-acting opioids remifentanil and alfentanil allow for a reduced dose of barbiturates or propofol and thus prolong seizure duration.			

APA, American Psychiatric Association; PONV, postoperative nausea and vomiting.

lock. A steel needle ("butterfly") is not dependable in the event that IV drugs are needed after ECT. Following IV administration of methohexital (0.75–1.0 mg/kg) and succinylcholine (0.75–1.0 mg/kg), the lungs are manually ventilated by mask with 100% oxygen. (See Table 96.3.) These dosages are remarkably constant throughout the course of treatment in all patients. Suitable alternatives include thiopental (3–5 mg/kg), propofol (1–2 mg/kg), and etomidate (0.15–0.3 mg/kg). Succinylcholine is not given to patients with pseudocholinesterase deficiency, extensive recent burns, patients within 6 months after stroke or with known susceptibility to malignant hyperthermia, or patients with muscular dystrophy. Succinylcholine may have a prolonged action in patients treated with donepezil hydrochloride for Alzheimer's disease or echothiophate for glaucoma. Suitable alternative muscle relaxants are rocuronium (0.6–1 mg/kg), vecuronium (0.1 mg/kg), or mivacurium (0.15–0.25 mg/kg), the effects of which may be reversed with neostigmine. The absence of leg withdrawal in response to stimulation of the foot sole is used to establish adequate muscular relaxation.

Airway management

Dentures should be removed prior to induction of anesthesia. The placement of a face mask for preoxygenation may not be ideal because of heightened anxiety. At the first sign of lowered consciousness, the lungs are manually ventilated with 100% oxygen. A laryngeal mask airway may also be used. Immediately before application of the stimulus, two locally made rolls of cotton gauze are placed bilaterally between the molar teeth to prevent damage to teeth or gums. Placement of a cuffed endotracheal tube may occasionally be necessary in selected patients, including those with a tracheostomy, those who are pregnant, and those with active gastric reflux or a gastric sphincter mechanism that is incompetent because of a gastric feeding tube or a surgical colon interposition procedure relating to a prior suicide attempt with lye ingestion.

Although the motor seizure is essential to the efficacy of ECT, the peripheral manifestations are eliminated with succinylcholine. To monitor the seizure duration and to be certain that the seizure is generalized, a tourniquet or blood pressure cuff is applied around the ipsilateral (in the case of unilateral ECT) arm or leg prior to succinylcholine or a nondepolarizing muscle relaxant administration and inflated to pressures above systolic. This maneuver prevents the neuromuscular blocker from reaching receptors below the tourniquet, thereby allowing observation of the motor seizure activity in this localized peripheral muscle area.

Cardiovascular function

If reduced arterial pressure is present before ECT, sequential blood pressure measurements are taken in supine, sitting, and standing position. If cardiac pump failure relating to ischemic heart disease is the cause of the hypotension, it is prudent to postpone the ECT session and obtain a cardiology consult. The tachycardia and hypertension typically observed after ECT may be effectively attenuated with the β-blocking drugs esmolol and labetalol (mixed α- and β-blocking agent); these drugs also can prevent cardiac arrhythmias. Also remarkable is that their potential side effects, such as exaggerated bradycardia post ECT, unmasking cardiac failure, or asthma, are not seen with these clinical dosages. A clinically useful alternative is sublingual nifedipine (10 mg) approximately 15 minutes before application of the ECT stimulus. Propranolol should not be administered in this setting because of the risk of cardiac arrest immediately after the seizure.

Recovery

After the seizure, patients are taken in the side position to the recovery area, a plastic face mask with an oxygen reservoir is fitted to the face, and ECG, oxygen saturation, and blood pressure are monitored and recorded for 30 minutes.

Side effects and complications of ECT

The most common side effect is a reversible short-term memory loss, which is more often seen with bilateral electrode placement. Post-ECT agitation and confusion, possibly as an expression of a residual seizure, may be successfully treated or prevented with lorazepam (1–2 mg IV), midazolam (1–2 mg IV), or propofol (50–100 mg), alone or in combination.

Complications include congestive heart failure, myocardial ischemia, and augmented hypertension. Cardiac arrhythmias occur in more than 30% of patients.

Pulmonary complications

Because the airway, in almost all patients, is managed with a face mask during ECT, pulmonary aspiration is possible. Endotracheal intubation is therefore performed in patients with known gastrointestinal reflux disease. Patients are turned in lateral decubitus position after ECT. Cognitive complications occur frequently and are primarily those involving memory losses for recent events, which typically are self-limiting. Status epilepticus rarely occurs spontaneously when seizures continue beyond 120 seconds immediately post-ECT stimulus. Headache typically responds well to ketorolac (30 mg IV). Muscle pain is reported by many patients after the first ECT treatment, but not after subsequent treatments.

Special considerations
Recent myocardial ischemic event

Common practice is to observe a 3- to 6-month waiting period before a course of ECT is undertaken in patients with documented myocardial injury, although strong supporting data are not available.

Coronary artery disease

The diagnosis of coronary artery disease is common in many elderly patients presenting for ECT. In such patients, the hemodynamic changes typical for ECT may lead to symptomatic coronary insufficiency with cardiac ischemia as shown by persistent changes in ST segment from baseline on the ECG, followed by cardiac pump failure, even though a given patient may not report any ischemic symptoms before ECT. In these patients, pretreatment with β-blocking drugs may eliminate rate-dependent coronary insufficiency. Clearly, overt chest pain and anginal symptoms require consultation with a cardiologist to advise on additional specific cardiac studies to be performed and on an optimal medical regimen.

A pacemaker may be present in patients with symptomatic bradyarrhythmias, second- or third-degree atrioventricular (AV) block, and sinus node malfunction. An external converter magnet should be readily available, and the serum potassium level should be within the normal range. In addition, the pre-ECT ECG may be examined for a 1:1 capture and a chest radiograph may be examined for intact electrode wires.

Drugs that should be readily available include atropine and isoproterenol. ECT does not ordinarily interfere with pacemaker function because of improved electrical shielding of the pulse generator units; in addition, the ECT stimulus is applied at a distance from the location of the generator unit, and, if interference does occur, the unit changes to a fixed mode. Drugs used in anesthesia for ECT are safe relative to pacemaker function, although, theoretically, the muscle fasciculations after succinylcholine could cause some interference.

Cardiac transplant recipients may receive ECT, but the data are limited. A hypersensitivity of the denervated heart to catecholamines after orthotopic transplantation has been shown not to be of practical concern.

Abdominal aortic and cerebral aneurysms pose an important risk in patients presenting for ECT because of the marked increase in arterial pressure and heart rate typical for ECT. They have been considered contraindications to ECT in the past, but ECT may be successfully administered with special management. Risk factors include marked increased in arterial pressure and blood flow velocity, but a direct correlation between aneurysm rupture and hypertension has not been established. Although the predictors for and mechanism of aneurysm rupture are unknown, the combination of β-blocker pretreatment (atenolol 25–50 by mouth per day, for 2–3 days prior to ECT) to reduce shear stress at the aneurysm site and sodium nitroprusside infusion (to reduce arterial pressure and blood flow velocity) immediately prior to and during treatment has proven useful to successful management and outcome. If sodium nitroprusside is used, it is mandatory that intra-arterial monitoring be employed since the arterial blood pressure may undergo profound changes from moment to moment. Such patients also should be observed for a prolonged period after ECT, possibly staying overnight at the treatment facility or transferred to a hospital setting with appropriate monitoring facilities.

Arteriovenous malformations

Because these lesions are low-pressure lesions (in sharp contrast to aneurysms), they are less likely to have major cerebral consequences in combination with ECT. Close observation with frequent blood pressure measurements is advisable.

Brain tumor

ECT has been successfully administered in the presence of a brain tumor.

In the presence of critical aortic stenosis, ECT poses a challenge because of the catecholamine surge and increased cardiac output. The classic triad of symptoms consists of angina, dyspnea on exertion, and syncope, making ECT quite dangerous in such patients. If ECT must be done, the patient should be extensively monitored and transferred afterward to a hospital or ICU setting for extended observation.

ECT has been successfully administered in the presence of severe pulmonary hypertension.

Pregnancy

ECT produces no complications for pregnancy or delivery and has no adverse effects on growth and development during infancy and beyond.

Case reports suggest that ECT is safe for mother and fetus even in the third trimester of pregnancy, and no premature labor has been reported. With each ECT treatment, fetal well-being may be monitored by means of ultrasonography, and attention is directed to adequate hydration and lateral uterine displacement to prevent hypotension. Antacids and endotracheal intubation are advocated to prevent pulmonary aspiration.

Suggested readings

Abrams R. et al. Electroconvulsive therapy. *Anesthesiology* 1987; 67:367.

Abrams R, Essman WB, eds. Electroconvulsive Therapy: Biological Foundations and Clinical Applications. New York: Spectrum Publications; 1982.

Abrams R. et al. Maintenance ECT. *Convuls Ther* 1994; 10:387.

American Psychiatric Association task force for ECT. The Practice of ECT. Recommendations for Treatment, Training, and Privileging. Washington, DC: American Psychiatric Association.

Beale MD. et al. The effects of electroconvulsive therapy on serial electrocardiograms and serum cardiac enzyme values. *JAMA* 1985; 253:2525.

Castelli et al. Use of electroconvulsive therapy during pregnancy. *Hosp Community Psychiatr* 1994; 45:444.

Crammer J. et al. Ketamine as an anesthetic for ECT. *Br J Psychiatr* 1973; 122:123.

Dec GW. et al. Diagnosis of myocardial injury by real-time recording of ST segments of the electrocardiogram in a patient receiving general anesthesia for electroconvulsive therapy. *Anesthesiology* 1993; 79:383.

Devenand DP. et al. Electroconvulsive therapy in patients taking theophylline. *J Clin Psych* 1993; 54:11.

Drop LJ. et al. Rupture of previously documented small asymptomatic saccular aneurysms. Report of three cases. *J Neurosurg* 1992; 76:1019.

Drop LJ. et al. Anesthesia for electroconvulsive therapy in patients with major cardiovascular risk factors. *Convul Ther* 1989; 5:88.

Drop LJ. et al. Diagnosis of myocardial injury by real-time recording of ST-segments of the electrocardiogram in a patient receiving general anesthesia for electroconvulsive therapy *Anesthesiology* 1993; 79:383.

El-Ganzouri AR. et al. Monoamine oxidase inhibitors: should they be discontinued preoperatively? *Anesth Analg* 1985; 64:592.

El-Ganzouri AR. et al. Stimulus parameters and efficacy of ECT. *Convuls Ther* 1994; 10:124.

Francis A. et al. Supraventricular tachycardia in a patient receiving ECT, clozapine and caffeine. *Convuls Ther* 1994; 10:228.

Green CD. Etomidate anesthesia increases seizure duration during ECT. A retrospective study. *Gen Hosp Psychiatr* 1993; 15:115.

Kellner CH. Status epilepticus following ECT in a patient receiving theophylline. *J Clkin Psychopharm* 1988; 8:153.

Kelly D. et al. ECT-induced asystole from a sub-convulsive shock. *Anaesth Intensive Care* 1988; 16:368.

Khan A. et al. Psychiatric aspects of diabetes mellitus. *Br J Psychiatr* 1981; 139:171.

Know GB. et al. Myocardial stunning after electroconvulsive therapy. *Ann Int Med* 1992; 17:914.

Marks RJ. Intracranial haemodynamics during attenuated responses to electroconvulsive therapy in the presence of an intracranial aneurysm. *J Neurol Neurosurg Psychiatr* 1998; 64:802.

Miller LJ. Hemodynamic responses to electroconvulsive therapy in a patient 5 years after cardiac transplantation. *Anesthesiology* 1995; 83:625.

Pargger H. et al. Headache and electroconvulsive therapy. *Headache* 1994; 34:155.

Rampton AJ. et al. Neuroleptic malignant syndrome and mivacurium: a safe alternative to succinylcholine? *Can J Anaesth* 1993; 41: 845.

Rasmussen KG. et al. Caffeine augmentation of electroconvulsive seizures. *Psychopharmarmacol* 1994; 115:320.

Sackheim HA. et al. *Convuls ther* 1990; 2:85.

Schievink WI. et al. Hemodynamic responses to electroconvulsive therapy in a hypertensive patient with end-stage pulmonary fibrosis. *Anesth Analg* 1998; 87:737.

Selvin BL. Electroconvulsive therapy in depression: a double blind controlled trial. *Brit Med J* 1981; 282:355.

Simpson KH. et al. Comparison of methohexital and propofol for electroconvulsive therapy effects on hemodynamic responses and seizure duration. *Anesthesiology* 1989; 70:412.

Steiner LA. et al. Electroconvulsive therapy induced hemodynamic changes unmask unsuspected coronary artery disease. *J Clin Anesth* 1990; 2:37.

Steiner LA. et al. Hemodynamic responses to ECT in a patient with critical stenosis. *Journal ECT* 2000; 16:52.

Trzepacz PT. et al. Propofol reduces seizure duration in patients having anesthesia for electroconvulsive therapy. *Br J Anaesth* 1988; 61:343.

Viguera A. et al. ECT in patients with intracranial aneurysm. *Journal ECT* 2000; 16:71.

Viguera A. et al. Comparative doses and cost: esmolol versus labetalol during electroconvulsive therapy. *Anesth Analg* 1998; 87:916.

Weiner RD. Electroconvulsive therapy. *Psych Clin North Am* 1993; 16:497.

Weiner SJ. et al. Intracerebral hemorrhage following electroconvulsive therapy. *Neurology* 1991; 41:1849.

Weisberg LA. et al. Electroconvulsive therapy: physiological and anaesthetic considerations. *Can Anaesth Soc J* 1984; 31:541.

Welch CA. Electroconvulsive Therapy in the General Hospital. In: Cassem NH, Stern T, Rosenbaum J, Jellinek M, eds. *Massachusetts General Hospital Handbook of General Hospital Psychiatry*. 4th ed. St Louis, MO: Mosby; 1997.

Welch CA. Electroconvulsive therapy. *New Engl J Med* 2007; 357:1939-45.

Wells DB. et al. Propanolol prior to ECT associated with asystole. *Anesthesiology* 1984; 60:255.

West ED. Seizure threshold in electroconvulsive therapy. Effects of age, sex, electrode placement and number of treatments. *Arch Gen psychiat* 1987; 44:355.

Wulfson HD. et al. Comparative effects of esmolol and labetalol to attenuate hyperdynamic states after electroconvulsive therapy. *Anesth Analg* 1995; 80:557.

Zhy WX. et al. Ect-induced status epilepticus and further ECT. *Am J Psych* 1981; 138:1237.

Renal physiology

Edward R. Garcia

The kidneys are both excretory and secretory organs that tightly regulate the volume and composition of body fluids by precise excretion of excess water and waste products. This chapter describes basic anatomy and physiology of the kidney and ways to measure kidney function.

Anatomy and function

The kidneys are paired organs lying in the retroperitoneal space. Each kidney has an outer cortex and an inner medulla. At the medial border of each kidney is the hilum, which opens into the renal pelvis and continues down as the ureter into the bladder. The renal cortex contains approximately 1 million nephrons, which give it a granular appearance. Each nephron begins in a renal corpuscle, which in turn is composed of a glomerulus, a tuft of capillary loops, enclosed in Bowman's capsule. Plasma is filtered out of the glomerulus (ultrafiltrate = plasma – the proteins), and this filtrate is passed out of the Bowman's space into the proximal tubule ultimately forming urine.

Important homeostatic functions of the kidney include the secretion of erythropoietin (stimulates red cell production in the bone marrow), of renin (regulates extracellular fluid volume), and of vitamin D (active form) and prostaglandins.

The paired kidneys receive blood flow at approximately 1.25 L/min (25% of cardiac output); most of this flow supplies the renal cortex (90%). The majority of this blood flow (1 L/min) goes to the glomeruli and results in the production of 125 ml/min of filtrate (glomerular filtration rate [GFR]). Water, crystalloids, and molecules less than 30,000 daltons are filtered freely through the membranes. GFR is the clinical measure of renal function which gives a gross assessment of the amount of filtration and, therefore, excretion that the kidneys can perform. In normal adults, the GFR averages 90 to 140 ml/min for men and 80 to 125 ml/min for women. GFR normally declines with age, decreasing to approximately 80 ml/min at 60 years of age and to 60 ml/min at 80 years.

Normal age-related decline of GFR is usually of little clinical consequence and does not affect the kidneys' excretory or homeostatic ability under normal conditions. As mentioned earlier in the text, the initial step in the formation of urine is the production of ultrafiltrate at the glomerulus. The efferent arterioles provide the high resistance to blood flow needed to create high glomerular hydrostatic pressure and drive the filtrate into the Bowman's capsule. At 120 ml/min, the total amount of filtrate produced is 173 L/day, whereas normal urine production is approximately 1.5 L/day. Therefore, 99% of the filtrate produced is reabsorbed, and only the remainder is excreted as urine.

Renal blood flow autoregulation

Afferent arterioles likely play a predominant role in renal autoregulation, resulting in near-constant renal blood flow (RBF) and GFR. Autoregulation of RBF in response to blood pressure changes occurs by:

- Native response of smooth muscle cells (myogenic mechanism) that contract in response to increased or decreased stretch. An increase in afferent vascular resistance decreases GFR, whereas a decrease in afferent vascular resistance increases GFR. An increase in efferent vascular resistance increases GFR, whereas a decrease in efferent vascular resistance decreases GFR.
- Tubuloglomerular feedback (TGF) mechanism
- Sympathetic nervous system control (vasoconstriction, T4–L1)
- Renin–angiotensin effect
- Antidiuretic hormone (ADH; vasoconstriction)
- Prostaglandins – prostaglandin E_2 (PGE_2) and prostaglandin I_2 (PGI_2) (vasodilators)

Autoregulation allows RBF and GFR to remain relatively constant as mean arterial pressure (MAP) varies between 80 and 180 mm Hg. The ability to autoregulate blood flow to maintain renal perfusion pressure and GFR becomes impaired when MAP drops below 70 mm Hg.

Reabsorption and secretion

Following the production of ultrafiltrate, a series of reabsorption and concentration steps (Fig. 97.1) occur along the nephron to reclaim water and electrolytes. These steps occur under the control of a number of hormones and factors as discussed in the next section. The renal cortex receives almost 1 L/min of RBF, whereas the medulla receives only 250 to 300 ml/min. The renal medulla, in the region of the tubule, is among the most metabolically active tissues in the body but is relatively poorly perfused. Thus, it is a region of low blood

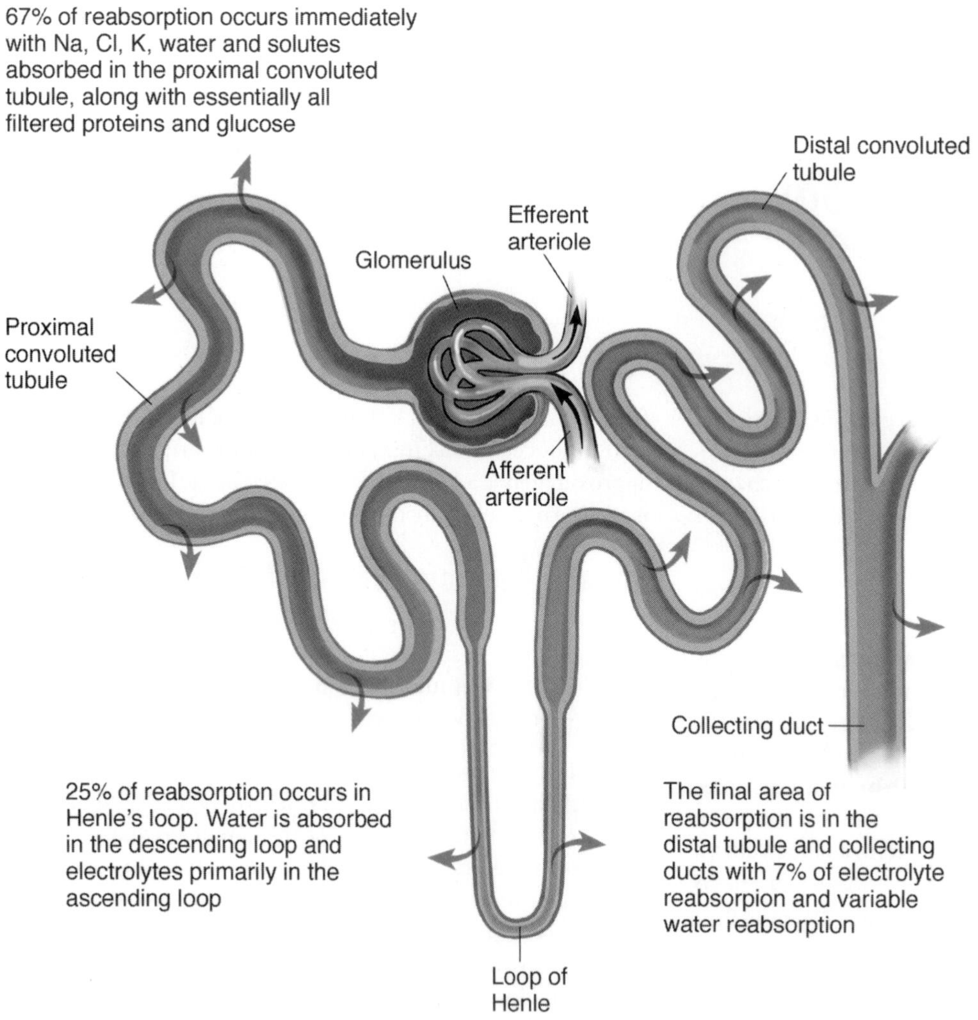

67% of reabsorption occurs immediately with Na, Cl, K, water and solutes absorbed in the proximal convoluted tubule, along with essentially all filtered proteins and glucose

Distal convoluted tubule

Efferent arteriole

Glomerulus

Proximal convoluted tubule

Afferent arteriole

Collecting duct

25% of reabsorption occurs in Henle's loop. Water is absorbed in the descending loop and electrolytes primarily in the ascending loop

The final area of reabsorption is in the distal tubule and collecting ducts with 7% of electrolyte reabsorpion and variable water reabsorption

Loop of Henle

Figure 97.1. Electrolyte and water reabsorption at various locations along the nephron.

flow and relative hypoxia with a high percentage of O_2 extraction ratio, and is vulnerable to ischemic injury from hypoperfusion. The filtration fraction (GFR/RPF) measures the efficacy of reabsorption. Sites of reabsorption and/or secretion of various substances are summarized in Table 97.1.

Table 97.1. Reabsorption/secretion of various substances in the renal tubule

Substance	Proximal tubule	Loop of Henle	Distal tubule	Collecting duct
Glucose	R			
Urea	R (50%)	S		R
Sodium	R (65%)	R (25%)	R	R
Chloride	R	R	R	
Potassium	R (65%)	R (20%)		S
Bicarbonate	R (80%)	R		R
Calcium	R	R		
Magnesium	R	R	R	
Phosphate	R			
Amino acids	R			

R, reabsorption; S, secretion.

Regulation of GFR, tubular reabsorption

Tubuloglomerular feedback (TGF)

The juxtaglomerular apparatus (JGA) is composed of the macula densa of the thick ascending limb (TAL), the extraglomerular mesangial cells, and the granular cells of the afferent and efferent arterioles, which produce renin. As the filtrate flows through the TAL, changes in flow are sensed by the JGA, triggering TGF involving a flow-dependent signal from the macula densa. Increased "distal delivery" results in afferent constriction and decreased GFR, whereas decreased filtrate flow in the TAL increases both RBF and GFR. The $Na^+/K^+/2Cl^-$ cotransporter in the luminal membrane of the macula densa senses changes in luminal electrolyte concentrations (dependent on Na^+ and Cl^- concentration and flow) and initiates TGF. The precise mechanism that then controls this translation of luminal signal into regulation of afferent and efferent arteriolar constriction has yet to be clearly elucidated. Thromboxane, nitric oxide, and angiotensin II have all been identified as possible effectors, though recent studies suggest that adenosine and

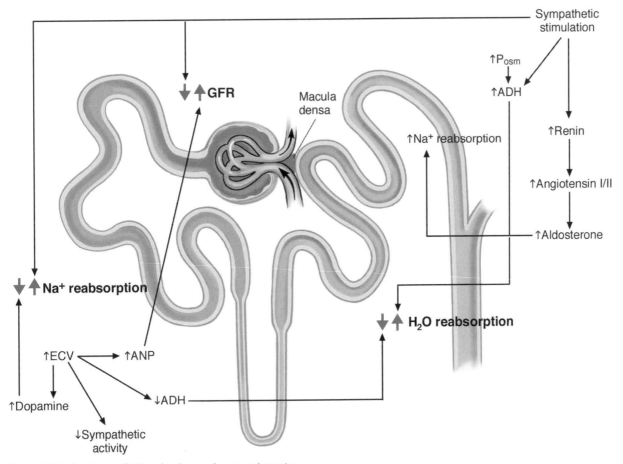

Figure 97.2. Regulation of GRF and sodium and water reabsorption.

possibly ATP may be the primary mediators. Only oscillatory blood pressure signals evoke a regulatory response. Nonpulsatile flow such as that on cardiopulmonary bypass or on ECMO tends to decrease RBF and GFR and increase renin production via TGF.

Renin–angiotensin II

Renin is released from smooth muscle cells in the afferent and efferent arterioles, stimulated by hypotension at afferent arteriolar baroreceptors, increased sympathetic stimulation, and decreased NaCl delivery to the macula densa (Fig. 97.2). Renin catalyzes the conversion of angiotensinogen to angiotensin I for subsequent conversion to angiotensin II. Angiotensin II, a potent arteriolar vasoconstrictor, stimulates (1) aldosterone secretion by the adrenal cortex and (2) ADH secretion and thirst, and enhances NaCl reabsorption by the proximal tubule. Sympathetic stimulation and catecholamine release (e.g., following hemorrhage) stimulates reabsorption of NaCl and water throughout the nephron. The α_1-adrenoreceptors are located primarily on the afferent arteriole, and their activation results in afferent constriction and stimulation of granular cells to release renin.

Measures of renal function

Plasma creatinine is often used as a measure of renal function (Table 97.2). The serum creatinine concentration is dependent on production (dependent on lean body mass and, therefore, relatively constant from day to day) and its elimination by the kidney. Creatinine is also secreted, to a small extent, in the proximal tubule, so this tends to overestimate the GFR. In most clinical situations, however, creatinine clearance and serum creatinine concentration provide a relatively adequate measure of GFR and overall renal function, respectively. A decrease in GFR

Table 97.2. Common parameters to measure renal function

$$\text{Creatinine clearance} = \frac{Cu \times \text{urine flow rate}}{Cp} \quad (\text{Normal} = 110 - 150\text{ml/min})$$

$$\text{RPF} = \text{Clearance of PAH} = \frac{\text{PAHu} \times \text{urine flow rate}}{\text{PAHp}}$$

$$\text{RBF} = \frac{\text{RPF}}{1 - \text{hematocrit}}$$

Cu, urine creatinine concentration; Cp, plasma creatinine concentration; PAHu, para-aminohippurate urine concentration; PAHp, para-aminohippurate plasma concentration.

619

may be the first and only sign of renal dysfunction. Because of renal adaptation, a 50% loss of nephrons will reduce GFR by only approximately 20% to 30%. This decrease in GFR from 125 to 100 ml/min results in an increase in plasma creatinine from 1 to approximately 1.2 mg/dl. This change in creatinine appears to be minor, but reflects a loss of a quarter of GFR and a large percentage loss of nephrons. Contrast this to an increase in plasma creatinine from 1.5 to 2 mg/dl, which correlates to only a 15 ml/min decrease in GFR. If a more precise measure is required, the GFR can be quantified by measuring inulin clearance; inulin is administered by continuous infusion, freely filtered at the glomerulus (neither reabsorbed nor secreted), then its concentration in the urine is measured. This procedure is rarely performed as it is time consuming and expensive, so clinically, nuclear medicine techniques such as iohexol clearance are more practical.

Effective renal plasma flow (RPF) is calculated by measuring para-aminohippurate (PAH) clearance, which is essentially fully cleared (by filtration and secretion) in one passage through the tubules (receiving the plasma flow). RBF is calculated as RPF / 1 – hematocrit. Fractional excretion is the amount of a substance that is excreted from the total that is filtered. A fractional excretion greater than 1.0 indicates net tubular secretion, whereas that less than 1.0 indicates net tubular reabsorption.

Blood urea nitrogen (BUN) is elevated not only in kidney disease but also in dehydration, in gastrointestinal bleeding, and with a high protein diet. Normal BUN levels are 10 to 20 mg/dl, and a normal serum creatinine/BUN ratio is 1:20.

Suggested readings

Epstein M. Aging and the kidney. *J Am Soc Nephrol* 1996; 7: 1106–1122.

Loutzenhiser R, Griffin K, Williamson G, Bidani A. Renal autoregulation: new perspectives regarding the protective and regulatory roles of the underlying mechanisms. *Am J Physiol Regul Integr Comp Physiol* 2006; 290:R1153–R1167.

Navar LG. Renal autoregulation: perspectives from whole kidney and single nephron studies. *Am J Physiol Renal Physiol* 1978; 234:F357–F370.

Sladen RN. Renal physiology. In: Miller RD, ed. *Miller's Anesthesia*. 7th ed. Philadelphia: Elsevier Churchill Livingstone; 2009.

Thalmann M, Schima H, Wieselthaler G, Wolner E. Physiology of continuous blood flow in recipients of rotary cardiac assist devices. *J Heart Lung Transplant* 2005; 24:237–245.

Vallon V. Tubuloglomerular feedback and the control of glomerular filtration rate. *News Physiol Sci* 2003; 18:169–174.

Walker M 3rd, Harrison-Bernard LM, Cook AK, Navar LG. Dynamic interaction between myogenic and TGF mechanisms in afferent arteriolar blood flow autoregulation. *Am J Physiol Renal Physiol* 2000; 279:F858–F865.

Chapter 98

Urology

Naveen Nathan and Tarun Bhalla

Anesthetic care for urologic procedures obligates attention to unique considerations superimposed on basic perioperative patient management. In a broad sense, the anesthesia care provider must have a thorough understanding of (1) the neuroanatomy (Fig. 98.1) subserving pain sensation to the urinary tract; (2) the major vascular structures in association with, or in close proximity to, the renal–urinary axis; (3) renal function and perioperative renal protection; and (4) an appreciation for the medical comorbidities that may be related to or independent of the specific urologic surgical intervention. Because regional anesthesia is often employed during urologic surgery, the anesthesiologist must bear in mind the spinal levels that conduct nociceptive input from the urinary tract (Table 98.1).

Transurethral endoscopic procedures
Diagnostic and therapeutic procedures

Cystoscopy is the most commonly performed urologic procedure. Cystourethroscopy is used to examine and treat lower urinary tract disease involving the urethra, prostate gland, and bladder. Ureteroscopy is used to evaluate the upper urinary tract, including the ureter, renal pelvis, and kidneys. These procedures may be classified as diagnostic when performed for biopsies or radiographic evaluation of the urinary tract and renal collecting system. As such, they are often simple and brief in duration. They involve minimal surgical stimulation, making them amenable to conscious sedation or local anesthetic techniques. More complex endourologic procedures are often therapeutic, involving tumor resection, ureteral dilatation, stenting, or stone extraction. These techniques are used to diagnose and treat many conditions including hematuria, recurrent urinary tract infections, prostatic hyperplasia, nephrolithiasis, trauma, obstruction, and cancer, often necessitating general or regional anesthesia.

Anesthetic technique

The anticipated extent of surgical stimulation, length of procedure, patient comorbidities, and surgeon and patient preference influence the choice of anesthetic management.

General anesthesia

Laryngeal mask airways may be used safely as most healthy patients are able to spontaneously ventilate in the lithotomy and Trendelenburg positions. Alternatively, general endotracheal anesthesia may be indicated for patients at risk for aspiration or for those having procedures of longer duration (>2 h) or procedures requiring muscle relaxation.

Regional anesthesia

If a central neuraxial anesthetic is used, a T6 or a T10 level is necessary for upper tract and lower tract instrumentation, respectively. Both spinal and continuous epidural techniques may be used, although considerable majorities of procedures end well within the finite duration of a single-shot spinal anesthetic.

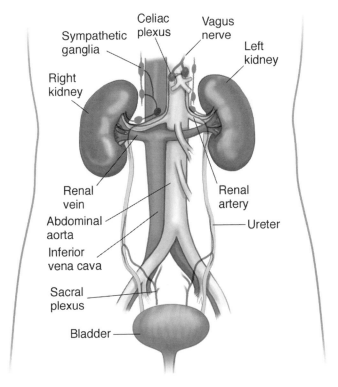

Figure 98.1. Anatomy of the urinary tract.

Table 98.1. Pain conduction in the genitourinary system

Organ	Sympathetic	Parasympathetic	Spinal levels of nociception
Kidney	T4–L1	Vagus nerve	T10–L1
Ureter	T10–L2	S2–S4	T10–L2
Bladder	T11–L2	S2–S4	T11–L2 (dome), S2–S4 (neck)
Prostate	T11–L2	S2–S4	T11–L2, S2–S4
Penis and urethra	L1 & L2	S2–S4	S2–S4
Scrotum (cutaneous)	Not significant for nociception	Not significant for nociception	S2–S4
Testicles	T10–L2	Not significant for nociception	T10–L1

Conscious sedation

This method may be used for certain patients undergoing short procedures, mainly simple cystourethroscopies, depending on surgeon and patient preference.

Local anesthesia

Some minor cystoscopic procedures may be performed using local anesthetic lubricant jelly, which is tolerated particularly well in female patients, owing to the comparatively shorter length of their urethra.

Anesthetic considerations

Lithotomy position

Elevation and abduction of the lower extremities is associated with (1) a decrease in functional residual capacity, (2) an acute increase in venous return, (3) an increase in mean arterial blood pressure without a major change in cardiac output, and (4) the possibility of neuropathies or neuropraxias. The common peroneal nerve is particularly at risk and when injured manifests as foot drop and sensory deficits over the dorsum of the foot. Additionally, both spinal lidocaine (as well as other local anesthetics) and the lithotomy position are observed risk factors for the development of transient neurologic symptoms (TNS). Of note, rapidly lowering the legs at the end of the procedure acutely decreases venous return, resulting in hypotension.

Obturator reflex

Stimulation of the obturator nerve by electrocautery current conducted through the lateral bladder wall may result in abrupt external rotation and adduction of the thigh. An important consideration of using a regional anesthetic technique is that it does not abolish this reflex. The obturator reflex can be reliably blocked by using either nondepolarizing neuromuscular blockers at levels that suppress the twitch response during general anesthesia or an obturator nerve block.

Autonomic hyperreflexia

Individuals who have sustained a prior spinal cord injury characterize a patient population that frequently requires endourologic procedures for the treatment of neurogenic bladder dysfunction, recurrent urinary tract infections, and complications of long-term indwelling urinary catheters. This unique patient demographic is at risk for the development of autonomic hyperreflexia (AH; especially injuries at T6 and above), especially with higher thoracic spinal cord injury. The severe hypertension, bradycardia, and arrhythmias that typify AH are often elicited by mild interventions, such as the mere insertion of a cystoscope. AH can be prevented with general or regional anesthesia and, in the event of its occurrence, treated with intravenous (IV) antihypertensive agents.

Transurethral resection of the prostate

Transurethral prostate resections are primarily indicated for symptomatic benign prostatic hyperplasia (BPH). A resectoscope (a modified cystoscope with a cutting and coagulating metal loop) or a cystoscope with a laser fiber is inserted through the penis into the prostatic urethra. The substance of the prostate gland is then dissected incrementally with the resectoscope or green light laser, and the removal of resected tissue from the surgical field is facilitated through continuous irrigation. As resection proceeds, especially with the resectoscope, prostatic venous sinuses are opened and variable amounts of irrigation fluid can be absorbed into circulation. Several factors influence the degree of systemic absorption of the irrigation fluid (Table 98.2). The procedure ends with irrigation of the bladder to remove residual prostatic debris and placement of an indwelling urinary catheter. The newer surgical techniques employing laser resection and laser vaporization of the prostate have greatly diminished the complications associated with classic resectoscope TURP (transurethral resection of the prostate) procedures.

Anesthetic technique

Regional anesthesia (specifically spinal anesthesia) has been classically advocated as the anesthetic technique of choice for resectoscope TURP. If spinal or epidural anesthesia is used, a T10 dermatome anesthetic level is needed to block the pain from bladder distention by the irrigating fluid. The early mental status changes that result from the progression of TURP syndrome (see next section, Complications of TURP) can be detected promptly with this approach. Despite this advantage,

Table 98.2. Factors influencing the amount of irrigation fluid absorbed during TURP

Duration of resection (20 ml of fluid are absorbed per minute of resection time on average)
Number and size of venous sinuses breached
Prostatic venous pressure
Hydrostatic pressure (height of irrigation fluid relative to patient)

to date no difference in perioperative morbidity and mortality has been shown when comparing regional versus general anesthesia for transurethral prostate resection. Furthermore, the hemostatic proficiency of newer green light laser TURP techniques has increased considerably and has diminished the historic superiority of spinal anesthesia.

Complications of TURP

The breach of prostatic venous sinuses and subsequent intravasation of irrigation solution account for the majority of potential complications of TURP (Table 98.3). In addition, bleeding, mechanical perforation, and bacteremia may also occur. Initial management includes notifying the surgeon and quickly ending the procedure; supporting the patient's airway, breathing, and circulation; measuring serum electrolytes; and obtaining (1) a measurement of arterial blood gas and (2) a 12-lead electrocardiogram (ECG).

Complications that arise from fluid absorption are related to the volume, osmolarity, intrinsic toxicity, and temperature of the irrigation solution used. As such, circulatory overload, hypo-osmolar hyponatremia, glycine and/or ammonia toxicity, hyperglycemia, and/or hypothermia may occur. The term *TURP syndrome* refers to the collective symptoms of volume overload, hyponatremia, and cerebral edema.

All currently available irrigation solutions used to preserve visibility of the surgical field are somewhat hypo-osmolar. Distilled water offers excellent visibility with an osmolality of 0 mOsm/L, but significant absorption can cause severe hemolysis, hemoglobinuria, and hyponatremia. Conversely, crystalloid solutions, such as 0.9 normal saline and balanced salt solutions (lactated Ringer's) are iso-osmolar and cause little (if any) dilutional, hemolytic, or toxic effects when absorbed. The presence of dissociated sodium and chloride ions, however, disperse electric current and render electrocautery ineffective for TURP. Table 98.4 outlines the properties of irrigation solutions currently in use.

Lithotripsy

Urinary calculi in the bladder and lower ureters are usually treated with cystourethroscopy, stone extraction, stenting, and intracorporeal laser lithotripsy (i.e., holmium:yttrium, aluminum, and garnet [Ho:YAG] laser). Stones in the upper two-thirds of ureters or kidneys may be treated with extracorporeal shock wave lithotripsy (ESWL) or percutaneous nephrolithotomy.

Anesthesia technique

1. *Monitored anesthesia care* – Usually is adequate for newer lithotripters, because they cause less discomfort. A variety of techniques are acceptable, including propofol infusion with opioid supplementation.
2. *Regional anesthesia* – Continuous epidural and spinal anesthesia were commonly employed for the first-generation lithotripters using water immersion, as they were associated with high intensities of pain. Regional anesthetic techniques for this procedure require a sensory level of T6.
3. *General anesthesia* – Allows for control of diaphragmatic excursion, as spontaneous ventilation moves the stone in and out of the shock waves focus.

Anesthetic considerations

ESWL relies on high energy, repetitive sound waves focused on renal calculi resulting in stone fragmentation. Tissue destruction can occur if the shock waves are focused at air–tissue interfaces (i.e., lung and gastrointestinal tract). The patient is positioned such that the lung and intestines are out of range from the shock wave focus. If safe positioning proves unfeasible, it is a contraindication to the procedure (Table 98.5). Bruising and ecchymosis of the skin also may occur during ESWL. Rarely, a large perinephric hematoma may develop.

Patients with a history of dysrhythmias and those with pacemakers or internal cardiac defibrillators may be at risk for developing arrhythmias induced by shock waves. Synchronization of the shock waves to approximately 20 ms after the R wave from the ECG, corresponding to the ventricular refractory period, decreases the incidence of arrhythmias during ESWL.

The number of shocks determines the length of the procedure and, in conjunction with the patient's heart rate, predicts the time remaining for the procedure. Adequate IV hydration with occasional diuretic supplementation may aid passage of stone fragments.

Urologic laser surgery

Laser surgery is effective in treating many urologic problems, including condyloma acuminatum, ureteral strictures, interstitial cystitis, BPH, ureteral calculi, and superficial carcinoma of the penis, ureter, bladder, and renal pelvis. A description of the various types of lasers used in urologic procedures is provided in Table 98.6. The application of operative lasers mandates the use of safety goggles and vigilance against the potential for inadvertent thermal injury to the patient and all operating room personnel.

Urologic oncology

Most major, open surgical procedures in urology are performed as a treatment modality for malignancies related to the prostate, bladder, or kidney.

Prostatectomy

Radical prostatectomy has become a common procedure owing to the high prevalence of prostate cancer and improved surgical techniques. The entire prostate gland, bladder neck, ampullae of the vas deferens, and seminal vesicles are removed, after which the bladder is anastomosed to the membranous urethra with an indwelling urinary catheter in place to maintain patency

Table 98.3. Complications of TURP

Complication	Mechanism	Manifestations	Management
Circulatory overload	Excessive intravasation of irrigating solution	Hypertension with compensatory bradycardia. If severe enough to cause LV dysfunction, may manifest as hypotension, dyspnea, pulmonary edema, and elevated PCWP.	Fluid restriction and loop diuretics (furosemide); consider halting the procedure as soon as is feasible. Severe cardiorespiratory compromise may warrant controlled mechanical ventilation and inotropic support.
Hypo-osmolar hyponatremia	Dilution of serum Na^+ concentration and osmolality leading to cerebral edema	CNS effects in order of increasing severity: restlessness, agitation, confusion, seizure, and coma. Cardiovascular effects manifest at Na^+ levels < 120 mEq/L and include hypotension, wide QRS, and dysrhythmias.	Mild cases (Na^+ <120 mEq/L) require fluid restriction and loop diuretics (furosemide). Severe cases (Na^+ <120 mEq/L) may require controlled mechanical ventilation, inotropic support, and 3% hypertonic saline infusion with serial evaluation of Na^+, although rapid correction of Na^+ (>100 ml/h of 3% NS) may cause central pontine myelinolysis.
Glycine toxicity	Glycine may declare its effects as a central inhibitory neurotransmitter when excessive plasma levels are achieved.	Primarily CNS toxicity with transient visual disturbance and blindness	Visual disturbance after TURP mandates immediate attention and an ophthalmology consult. In addition, other causes of perioperative visual loss must be entertained (stroke, acute glaucoma, ischemic optic neuropathy, and corneal abrasion).
Ammonia toxicity	Ammonia is the hepatic metabolite of glycine. Excessive absorption of glycine solution may result in hyperammonemia.	CNS effects causing depressed mental status, delayed awakening, and coma	Depressed mental status requires attention to oxygenation, ventilation, and hemodynamics. Secondarily, blood gas analysis, serum glucose, electrolytes, and ammonia levels should be assessed.
Hyperglycemia	Related to the use of sorbitol irrigation solution. Sorbitol is metabolized to fructose and may cause hyperglycemia, particularly in diabetic patients.	Symptoms are related to hyperglycemia and may include alteration in mental status, DKA, hyperosmolar nonketotic coma, and polyuria.	Insulin therapy guided by serial evaluation of serum glucose concentration. Intravascular volume replacement and supplemental potassium as needed.
Hypothermia	Fluid at room temperature will cause excessive heat loss through continuous irrigation and absorption.	Decreased core body temperature (~1°C/h of surgery), shivering	Prevention is key, and warmed irrigation fluid should be used. Forced-air warming blankets and opiates help treat postoperative shivering.
Bleeding and coagulopathy	Blood loss through prostatic venous sinuses. Systemic fibrinolysis may occur with the release of tissue plasminogen activator and urokinase from the prostate gland. DIC may also occur from absorption of prostate tissue, which is rich in thromboplastin.	Persistent blood loss in surgical field or hematuria postoperatively. Anemia, tachycardia, and hypotension when severe	Serial evaluation of hematocrit, platelets, and coagulation profile. Blood product administration as warranted
Perforation	Inadvertent bladder perforation with resectoscope leading to extraperitoneal leakage of irrigation fluid, blood, and urine. Intraperitoneal leakage may also occur depending on location of bladder and/or prostate perforation.	Extraperitoneal leakage: periumbilical, inguinal, or suprapubic pain; surgeon may note irregular return of irrigation fluid. Intraperitoneal: upper abdominal pain or referred diaphragmatic irritation noted as shoulder pain, pallor, diaphoresis, nausea and/or vomiting, hypotension. Signs are reliable only with spinal anesthetic (<T9 sensory level).	Small perforations may be managed with catheter drainage. Large perforations require prompt open laparotomy for repair.
Bacteremia and sepsis	Bacteria may be introduced directly into circulation through open prostatic venous sinuses.	Fever, chills, rigors, hypotension, and tachycardia	Antibiotic therapy with broad-spectrum agents

LV, left ventricular; PCWP, pulmonary capillary wedge pressure; CNS, central nervous system; NS, normal saline; DKA, diabetic ketoacidosis; DIC, disseminated intravascular coagulation.

Table 98.4. Irrigation fluids used for TURP

Solution	Osmolality, mOsm/L	Precautions
Glycine 1.5%	220	Glycine toxicity, hyperammonemia, transient visual loss
Sorbitol 3.5%	165	Hyperglycemia, infection
Mannitol 5%	275	Acute circulatory volume expansion, osmotic diuresis
Cytal (sorbitol/ mannitol mixture)	178	Same as for sorbitol and mannitol

of the urinary tract. The commonly used retropubic approach involves either a low midline or Pfannenstiel incision with the patient in the supine position. This approach carries the risk of moderate blood loss as the dissection enters the territory of the dorsal venous complex of the penis as well as branches of the hypogastric veins.

Laparoscopic radical prostatectomy offers all the attendant advantages of minimally invasive surgery weighed against the risks of peritoneal insufflation, although no unequivocal difference in mortality has been demonstrated when compared to open prostatectomy. Skilled urologists have gained even greater surgical precision with robot-assisted laparoscopic prostatectomy. This procedure appears to have a lower incidence of ileus and blood transfusion than does the standard retropubic approach.

Anesthetic technique

Open procedures for prostate resection are amenable to both general and regional anesthesia. Although no difference in mortality has been demonstrated between these techniques, employing a central neuraxial block as the primary anesthetic may offer a reduction in blood loss, lower incidence of deep vein thrombosis (DVT), and improved postoperative analgesia, in addition to a potential risk reduction for tumor recurrence. A T8 sensory level should be sought if a spinal or epidural anesthetic is chosen. Lower abdominal operations such as the retropubic approach to prostatectomy may result in as much as a 30% decrement of functional residual capacity (FRC) postoperatively after general anesthesia. Regional techniques may help attenuate this expected degree of pulmonary dysfunction. General anesthesia, however, offers the advantages of predictable

Table 98.5. Contraindications of ESWL

Absolute	Relative
Distal obstruction to the renal calculi	Large calcified aortic or renal artery aneurysm
Bleeding disorder or anticoagulation	Untreated urinary tract infection
Pregnancy	Pacemaker or automated implantable cardioverter-defibrillator (AICD) implant
	Morbid obesity

anesthetic duration and efficient control of oxygenation and ventilation, as well as a lack of visible responses to hypotension associated with rapid blood loss.

Laparoscopic and robotic prostatectomy is best conducted using general anesthesia with endotracheal intubation. The expected physiologic effects of peritoneal insufflation of carbon dioxide (CO_2) mandate airway control and management of ventilation and oxygenation. These effects, in particular decreased pulmonary compliance, are exaggerated in steep Trendelenburg position. Robot-assisted laparoscopic prostatectomy also bears the disadvantage of limited patient access and long surgical duration. Securing all patient monitors, having adequate IV access, and paying strict attention to patient padding and positioning are essential prior to commencing with robot-assisted surgery. Currently, it is believed that laparoscopic approaches to prostatectomy incur less blood loss, provide a faster resumption of bowel function, and expedite hospital discharge.

Orchiectomy

Testicular cancer is the most common malignancy in men between 15 and 34 years of age. Radical orchiectomy is performed for both definitive diagnosis and as the initial step of treatment. Subsequent treatment depends on the histology and stage of the tumor. Radical orchiectomy can be performed with a regional or general anesthetic. It is important to gain at least a T6 level to block sympathetic innervation. Patients with testicular cancer who receive bleomycin chemotherapy are at risk for developing progressive pulmonary fibrosis. These patients may be at increased risk for postoperative respiratory failure with general anesthetic if they are exposed to high concentrations of inspired oxygen or if an excessive amount of IV fluid is administered.

Nephrectomy

Renal cell carcinoma has a peak incidence between the ages of 50 and 60 years with a 2:1 predilection for men. The tumor is frequently associated with paraneoplastic syndromes including hypercalcemia, erythrocytosis, hepatic dysfunction, and hypertension. Surgical removal is the only effective treatment. In approximately 5% of these patients, the tumor invades the inferior vena cava (IVC). Depending on the extent of tumor invasion into the central circulation, cardiopulmonary bypass with deep hypothermic circulatory arrest may be required for complete excision.

The kidney is usually approached via a lumbar flank, transabdominal midline, or thoracoabdominal incision. A radical nephrectomy includes removal of the kidney, surrounding fascia, adrenal gland, and upper ureter. Consequently, the patient should have adequate volume repletion to maintain perfusion to the remaining kidney. Open nephrectomies are usually performed in the "kidney rest position" or lateral flexed position. The patient is placed in lateral decubitus position with the operating table extended for maximal separation between the iliac crest and the costal margin. The kidney rest is then elevated to

Table 98.6. Lasers used in urologic procedures

CO$_2$ laser	Intense heat with vaporization, minimal tissue penetration; unable to penetrate water	Limited to cutaneous lesions of external genitalia
Argon laser	Poorly absorbed by water, but selectively absorbed by Hgb and melanin	Coagulation of bleeding in the bladder
Pulsed dye laser	Generates a pulsed output	Useful for destroying ureteral calculi
Nd-YAG laser	Deep tissue penetration via protein denaturation with minimal vaporization; can be used in water or urine	Excellent for lesions of the penis, urethra, bladder, ureters, and kidneys
KTP-532 laser	Frequency-doubled Nd-YAG laser, does not penetrate tissue as deeply	Better cutting effect for lesions

Hgb, hemoglobin; Nd-YAG, neodymium-doped yttrium aluminum garnet.

raise the nondependent iliac crest for improved surgical exposure. The physiologic effects of patient positioning for radical nephrectomy are outlined in Table 98.7.

A preoperative ventilation–perfusion (V/Q) scan can detect preexisting embolization of the thrombus. A level I thrombus extends into the IVC below the liver. A level II thrombus extends into the IVC, to the liver, but below the diaphragm. Last, a level III thrombus extends into IVC, above the diaphragm, and into the right atrium. A level II or III thrombus suggests the potential for a massive blood transfusion (usually 10–15 units, possibly exceeding 50 units of packed red blood cells [PRBCs]). Therefore, venous access should be obtained accordingly. Central venous cannulation should proceed with caution, however, as the potential to dislodge and embolize tumor thrombus exists. A level III thrombus is a contraindication for flotation of a pulmonary artery catheter. Cardiopulmonary bypass may be employed when the tumor occupies more than 40% of the right atrium.

Anesthetic technique

General endotracheal anesthesia is the customary anesthetic choice for this procedure. A midthoracic epidural (T7–9) may be used adjunctively for postoperative pain control. Extensive fluid shifts and blood loss are to be expected as a result of wide surgical exposure and the manipulation of major vascular structures. Therefore, abundant venous access and direct arterial monitoring are recommended. The patient's baseline hematocrit and renal function should be determined preoperatively. Even in the absence of elevations in blood urea nitrogen (BUN) and creatinine concentration, anesthetic drug doses may need to be adjusted. These dose adjustments address the fact that the

unaffected kidney has yet to initiate compensatory responses to the loss of up to 50% of functional renal tissue.

Cystectomy

Bladder cancer occurs in patients with an average age of 65 years, and it is three times more common in men than in women. Transitional cell carcinoma of the bladder is the second most common cancer of the genitourinary tract. The standard of care for bladder cancer with muscular invasion is radical cystectomy.

Anesthetic considerations

Radical cystectomy is usually performed with a midline incision extending from the symphysis pubis to the xiphoid process. All the anterior pelvic organs, including the bladder, prostate, seminal vesicles, and proximal urethra, are removed in men. In women, the bladder, urethra, uterus, cervix, ovaries, and anterior vaginal wall may also be removed. At the end of the procedure a urinary diversion, which involves implanting the ureters into a segment of bowel, is performed. The bowel is left in situ (ureterosigmoidostomy) or attached to a cutaneous stoma or urethra. The isolated bowel can function as a conduit (ileal conduit), and these channels can be constructed from jejunum, ileum, or colon. The bowel may alternatively be reconstructed to form a reservoir (neobladder). Reservoirs may include ureterosigmoidostomy, small bowel (T-pouch), or large bowel (Indian pouch).

Anesthetic technique

This surgical procedure may be associated with large intraoperative blood loss and fluid shifts, implicating the need for large-bore IV access, and possibly a central venous catheter as well as an arterial line. A minimum time of 4 to 6 hours is usually estimated for this procedure. General endotracheal anesthesia with muscle relaxation is the mainstay of anesthetic management, with optional midthoracic epidural anesthesia for postoperative analgesia. Neuraxial anesthesia may potentially produce hyperactive bowel (from unopposed parasympathetic activity), making the construction of a urinary reservoir technically difficult for the surgeon. This problem may be minimized

Table 98.7. Physiologic changes associated with lateral flexed position

Decreased FRC in the dependent lung
V/Q mismatching as a result of increased blood flow to the dependent lung with greater ventilation to the nondependent lung
Increased dead space ventilation proportional to the duration of procedure
Elevation of kidney rest may decrease venous return by compressing IVC
Inadvertent entry into the pleural space, a potential for a pneumothorax
Venous air embolism may occur through venous structures located above the level of the heart

through the use of glucagon, papaverine, or an anticholinergic (glycopyrrolate). Reduction in urine output from prolonged contact with bowel mucosa may result in hyponatremia, hypochloremia, hyperkalemia, and metabolic acidosis in jejunal conduits. Hyperchloremic metabolic acidosis may occur in colonic and ileal conduits. Ureteral stents, adequate volume replacement, and induced increases in urine output may help alleviate this issue postoperatively.

Suggested readings

Batillo JA, Hendler MA. Effects of patient positioning during anesthesia. *Int Anesthesiol Clin* 1993; 31(1):67–86.

Barash PG, Cullen BF, Stoelting RK. *Clinical Anesthesia.* 5th ed. Philadelphia: Lippincott Williams & Wilkins; 2006.

Gravenstein D. Transurethral resection of the prostate (TURP) syndrome: a review of the pathophysiology and management. *Anesth Analg* 1997; 84:438–446.

Hanson RA, Zornow MH, Conlin MJ, et al. Laser resection of the prostate: implications for anesthesia. *Anesth Analg* 2007; 105(2):475–479.

Jaffe RA, Samuels SI. *Anesthesiologist's Manual of Surgical Procedures.* 3rd ed. Philadelphia: Lippincott Williams & Wilkins; 2004.

Malhotra V. Transurethral resection of the prostate. *Anesthesiol Clin North Am* 2000; 18(4):883–897.

Morgan GE, Mikhail M. *Clinical Anesthesiology.* 4th ed. New York: McGraw-Hill; 2006.

Sprung J, Kapural L, Bourke DL, O'Hara JF Jr. Anesthesia for kidney transplant surgery. *Anesthesiol Clin North Am* 2000; 18:919.

Whalley DG, Berrigan MJ. Anesthesia for radical prostatectomy, cystectomy, nephrectomy, pheochromocytoma and laparascopic procedures. *Anesthesiol Clin North Am* 2000; 18:899.

Kidney and pancreas transplantation

Thomas Edrich and Sayeed Malek

Kidney transplantation

End-stage renal disease (ESRD) requiring hemodialysis (HD) is caused most frequently by diabetes mellitus, glomerulonephritis, polycystic kidney disease, and arterial hypertension. The first attempt at kidney transplantation in humans in 1933 by a Ukrainian surgeon, Voronoy, failed due to organ rejection. Success was achieved in 1954 when the immunologic barrier was circumvented by transplanting between identical twins, at the Peter Bent Brigham Hospital in Boston. It was the introduction of effective immunosuppressants, such as azathioprine, glucocorticoids, antilymphocyte agents, and cyclosporine, however, that improved patient outcome. In comparison to HD, kidney transplantation is now associated with superior quality of life and better patient survival. It is also more cost-effective.

Prospective kidney recipients undergo rigorous preoperative cardiac testing to exclude significant treatable coronary artery disease, because cardiovascular disease is the leading cause of death for adult kidney transplant recipients. Revascularization may be preferable before kidney transplantation because cardiopulmonary bypass would be detrimental to a newly transplanted kidney.

The number of kidney transplants has increased steadily over the past two decades. In 2004, the number of kidney transplants from deceased donors in the United States exceeded 10,000 for the first time. However, both the wait list and wait time have increased as well. According to the United Network for Organ Sharing (UNOS) data, there are more than 72,000 patients on the deceased donor kidney transplant waiting list in the United States.

Preoperative preparations

Patients may arrive for a scheduled transplant (i.e., living related or unrelated donor), or they may be called in on a moment's notice when an organ from a deceased donor becomes available. Close communication with the transplant surgeon is paramount to coordinate the timing as well as preoperative medication.

The current practice at the author's institution includes the preoperative initiation of maintenance immunosuppression using mycophenolate mofetil, which inhibits B and T lymphocytes. One dose is given the night before, and one the morning before surgery. For unanticipated transplants, a single preoperative dose is administered.

Establish which immunosuppressant the surgeon will require intraoperatively: for patients who will receive intraoperative thymoglobulin (rabbit antithymocyte globulin), one dose of acetaminophen should be administered as prophylaxis for commonly occurring fever, chills, headache, and malaise. If an alternative T-lymphocyte antagonist such as basiliximab will be used intraoperatively, then no acetaminophen will be needed.

Intraoperative considerations

Induction of anesthesia should be timed sufficiently early to allow for the possibility of difficult central venous access. This will require tight communication with the surgical team harvesting the organ or with the team transporting the organ from the outside hospital.

Induction of anesthesia should involve medications that do not depend on renal function for their clearance and should take the common comorbidities of renal patients into account, as discussed earlier in Chapter 7. After anxiolysis with midazolam, patients who have not fasted or may have delayed gastric emptying due to diabetic or uremic gastropathy receive gastric acid neutralization with citric acid/sodium citrate followed by rapid-sequence induction (RSI) of anesthesia. Safe medications typically include thiopental, propofol, fentanyl, and hydromorphone. Morphine and meperidine should be avoided, as the active metabolites morphine 3- and 6-glucuronide and normeperidine are dependent on renal excretion and can cause over-narcotization (morphine) and seizures (meperidine). Succinylcholine is administered if the serum potassium level is not elevated and if there are no contraindications, such as concurrent neuromuscular disorders, history of burns, or malignant hyperthermia. Rocuronium can be an alternative to succinylcholine if RSI is required. Otherwise, an awake fiber-optic intubation may be advisable.

Central venous access is used for both intraoperative and postoperative assessment of volume status in an attempt to maximize cardiac output to the new kidney. Patients with ESRD on HD often have had previous central lines, making intravascular thrombi and strictures more likely. Ultrasound may clarify the vascular anatomy and facilitate central venous catheter placement into the internal jugular vein. Occasionally, patients may have an indwelling central line in place already – such lines should be accessed with sterile precautions because their use represents a considerable risk of infection. Also, any heparin-containing locking solution must be withdrawn (withdraw > 5 ml) before use to avoid systemic anticoagulation. An arterial line is not required routinely unless warranted by comorbidities.

Immunosuppressants, such as methylprednisolone sodium succinate and the T-lymphocyte antagonist basiliximab or thymoglobulin, are administered after induction but before the transplanted kidney is reperfused. Diphenhydramine can be given before thymoglobulin to attenuate side effects.

Implantation of the kidney

The kidney is typically placed in a heterotopic position while leaving the native kidneys in place as shown in Fig. 99.1. The right iliac fossa is chosen most frequently because of the more superficial location of the iliac vein on this side. After vascular anastomosis of the renal artery to the external or internal iliac artery and the renal vein to the external iliac vein, the donor ureter is anastomosed to the bladder. A triple-lumen Foley urinary catheter can be used to fill the bladder during the ureteroneocystostomy.

Reperfusion of the new kidney

Before the cross-clamp is released, the intravascular filling and cardiac output should be optimized. Our practice is to administer 4 to 8 liters of crystalloid in the prereperfusion period, attaining a central venous pressure (CVP) of 15 and a systolic blood pressure greater than 140 mm Hg or mean arterial pressure (MAP) greater than 70 mm Hg while avoiding all vasopressor medications. If necessary, a low-dose dopamine infusion (i.e., <5 μg/kg/min) is started. Dopamine is advantageous compared to other inotropes because it improves renal perfusion while minimizing vasoconstriction and graft ischemia.

Postoperative course

Patients are usually extubated and recover in the postanesthesia recovery unit at our institution. Close monitoring of urinary output is recommended. Maintenance of an appropriate intravascular volume optimizes renal function and is facilitated by monitoring the CVP. It is generally wise to avoid the use of medications that may alter the prostaglandin-mediated vasoregulation in the new kidney (these medications include ketorolac, celecoxib, and nonsteroidal anti-inflammatory drugs). Epidural anesthesia is also avoided to minimize risk of hypotension and because the incision is relatively small.

Pancreas and kidney–pancreas transplantation

Type-1 diabetes affects more than 2 million people in the United States with approximately 30,000 new cases diagnosed each year. It is the sixth leading cause of death and the leading cause of kidney failure and blindness (in adults aged 20–74 years). The total estimated cost of diabetes in the United States for 2002 was $132 billion, with $92 billion in direct medical costs.

Simultaneous pancreas–kidney (SPK) transplants from deceased donors are an option for diabetic patients with ESRD, enabling the patient to become insulin- and dialysis-free. Acute rejection rates are lower than those in pancreas transplantation alone (PTA). Other options include pancreas transplantation after living-donor kidney transplantation (PAK), simultaneous deceased-donor pancreas and living-donor kidney transplant (SPLK), and living-donor simultaneous (partial-) pancreas–kidney transplant.

Pancreas transplantation alone is indicated in nonuremic patients in whom complications, such as ketoacidosis or hypoglycemic episodes, continue despite intensive insulin therapy. Here, the risks of transplantation and subsequent chronic immunosuppression may be justified to achieve insulin independence.

Anesthetic management of patients receiving pancreas transplants alone, after, or simultaneously with a kidney transplant is similar to that of patients receiving kidney transplantation, with a few differences as detailed below.

Preoperative initiation of immunosuppression using mycophenolate mofetil is followed by intraoperative immunosuppression with methylprednisolone and thymoglobulin given after induction of anesthesia but before implantation of the

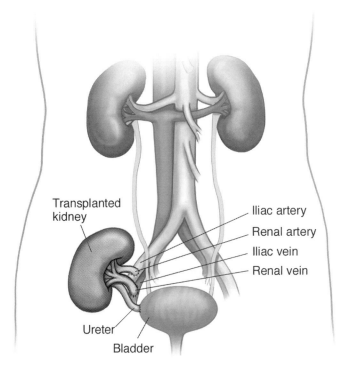

Figure 99.1. Kidney graft in the right iliac fossa.

Transplanted kidney

Iliac artery

Renal artery

Iliac vein

Renal vein

Ureter

Bladder

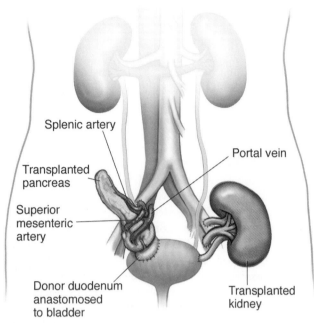

Figure 99.2. Combined kidney and pancreas transplantation. Pancreatic secretions are drained from a short segment of donor duodenum into the jejunum.

Labels on figure: Splenic artery; Transplanted pancreas; Superior mesenteric artery; Donor duodenum anastomosed to bladder; Portal vein; Transplanted kidney.

pancreas and/or kidney (premedicate with acetaminophen and diphenhydramine). In addition, all medications, such as perioperative antibiotics and dopamine, should be available in a dextrose-free form, and any insulin pumps should be discontinued. It is our practice to place both central venous line and arterial line for intraoperative and postoperative management. Baseline lipase and amylase levels should be recorded for reference for later rejection monitoring.

Implantation of the pancreas most frequently occurs into the right iliac fossa with the donor portal vein anastomosed to the recipient iliac vein. Arterial perfusion is supplied via anastomosis from the recipient iliac artery to a brief section of donor iliac artery which is, in turn, anastomosed to the donor splenic artery and donor superior mesenteric artery. As shown in Fig. 99.2 (which shows both pancreas and kidney transplants), the donor pancreas can be maintained in continuity with a section of donor duodenum which is anastomosed to the recipient's small bowel for drainage of the exocrine secretions. Alternatively, the duodenum section can be anastomosed to the recipient's bladder. An advantage of the bladder drainage is the ability to measure the exocrine function of the pancreas in the urine. A drop in urine amylase can indicate rejection and will occur before hyperglycemia occurs. Serum amylase will often increase but is less sensitive than urine amylase. Complications such as acidosis (loss of alkaline pancreas secretions), infection, urethritis, and hematuria are frequent. Drainage into the small bowel (as shown in Fig. 99.2) has fewer long-term complications and is performed more frequently in SPK. In these patients, rejection almost always affects both organs, so serum creatinine is used as an indicator for both kidney and pancreas rejection.

A simultaneously transplanted kidney is typically positioned in the opposite iliac fossa and anastomosed as described earlier in this chapter.

Reperfusion of the new pancreas can cause hypotension from diffuse bleeding from the graft as well as from vasodilation from mediators in the pancreas. It is our practice to maintain a MAP of 70 mm Hg or greater when the cross clamp is removed using crystalloids and blood as needed. In contrast to the kidney transplants, in pancreas transplants overhydration is generally avoided so as to reduce the risk of pancreas edema. Therefore, we use low-dose dopamine (<5 μg/kg/min) if a CVP of 10 to 14 does not suffice to maintain a MAP of 70.

Endocrine function of the pancreas is expected to begin soon after reperfusion, and glucose levels are monitored every 30 minutes. Any glucose or insulin administration should be communicated clearly to the surgical team because it will alter the assessment of the graft. Note that epidural anesthesia is not routinely employed (1) so that risk of hypotension is minimized and (2) because of the possible perioperative use of intravenous heparin.

Anesthesia management for the living-kidney donor

Related or unrelated donors are usually healthy und currently undergo a mortality risk of 0.05%. If possible, the left kidney is explanted due to presence of a longer renal vein. A laparoscopic technique is commonly employed, thus minimizing postoperative pain. Most commonly, general anesthesia is used without a regional technique as these patients can typically be discharged from the hospital on the second postoperative day.

Suggested readings
Cohen DJ, St. Martin L, Christensen LL, et al. Kidney and pancreas transplantation in the United States, 1995–2004. *Am J Transplant* 2006; 6:1153–1169.

The Diabetes Control and Complications Trial Research Group. The effect of intensive treatment of diabetes on the development and progression of long-term complications in insulin-dependent diabetes mellitus. *N Engl J Med* 1993; 329:977–986.

Hamilton DN, Reid WA. Yu Yu Voronoy and the first human kidney allograft. *Surg Gynecol Obstet* 1984; 159:289–294.

Herzog CA, Ma JZ, Collins AJ. Long-term outcome of renal transplant recipients in the United States after coronary revascularization procedures. *Circulation* 2004; 109:2866–2871.

Lentine KL, Brennan DC, Schnitzler MA. Incidence and predictors of myocardial infarction after kidney transplantation. *J Am Soc Nephrol* 2005; 16:496–506.

National Diabetes Fact Sheet, United States 2005. http://www.cdc.gov/diabetes/pubs/pdf/indfs_2005. 2007. Ref Type: Generic

Schaubel D, Desmeules M, Mao Y, et al. Survival experience among elderly end-stage renal disease patients. A controlled comparison of transplantation and dialysis. *Transplantation* 1995; 60:1389–1394.

Wolfe RA, Ashby VB, Milford EL, et al. Comparison of mortality in all patients on dialysis, patients on dialysis awaiting transplantation, and recipients of a first cadaveric transplant. *N Engl J Med* 1999; 341:1725–1730.

Anesthesia for intra-abdominal surgery

Khaldoun Faris and Faraz Syed

Intra-abdominal surgery is a broad term that includes various operations within the abdominal cavity that involve the gastrointestinal (GI) system, genitourinary system, gynecologic system, and endocrine system. This chapter, however, focuses mainly on surgical procedures involving the GI tract and addresses a general approach that may be applicable to many procedures within the abdominal cavity and specific GI disorders.

General principles

Risk of aspiration

Aspiration, with its associated morbidity, is a potential risk in major abdominal surgery, whether elective (bariatric surgery, fundoplication) or emergent (acute abdomen, bowel obstruction) procedures. The incidence of pulmonary aspiration in the perioperative period is rare (<5/10,000 general anesthetic). Measures to prevent pulmonary aspiration of gastric contents are listed in Table 100.1. Perioperative pulmonary aspiration prophylaxis is discussed in Chapter 40. Additional considerations include the following:

- The gastroesophageal sphincter (GES) plays an important role in preventing the aspiration of gastric contents. The GES tone is altered or impaired in clinical conditions such as morbid obesity and hiatal hernia, and during anesthesia. Most anesthetics and analgesics alter the GES tone.
- Impaired gastric emptying due to obesity, bowel obstruction, or other disorders will lead to increased volume and acidity of the gastric contents.

Fluid management

Abdominal surgery may be associated with significant fluid loss as well as significant fluid shifts. These fluid changes may occur preoperatively as well as intraoperatively. Preoperative factors include bowel preparation (elective surgery) and vomiting, gastric decompression and/or drainage, sequestration of fluid, diarrhea, and bleeding (urgent surgery). Intraoperative, factors include insensible losses (traditionally assumed to amount up to 4–8 ml/kg/h for major abdominal surgery, a number that appears grossly overestimated in experimental models, which

show a modest increase from 0.5 ml/kg/h at baseline to approximately 1 ml/kg/h even with extensive surgical exposure of the gut), intraoperative bleeding, gastric drainage, and drainage of ascites. Thus, large-bore peripheral intravenous (IV) access may be necessary. Arterial and central lines may also be chosen to better manage hemodynamic changes associated with fluid shifts even though central venous pressure (CVP) and/or pulmonary capillary wedge pressure (PCWP) measurements do not predict fluid responsiveness and therefore are unable to guide the clinician in optimizing cardiac preload and tissue oxygenation.

Preoperative assessment of fluid status and careful monitoring of volume administration and fluid output during the procedure lead to better assessment of hemodynamic status and prevent complications of under- (as well as over-) resuscitation. The choice of fluid, whether crystalloid or colloid, is left to the judgment of the anesthesiologist and to the clinical condition of the patient. Frequent blood sampling to evaluate hemoglobin concentration, coagulation status, electrolytes, and

Table 100.1. Strategies to prevent pulmonary aspiration

Measure	Comments
NPO for elective surgery	8 h for solid food, 2 h for clear liquids
Decreased gastric acidity	H$_2$ blockers (e.g., ranitidine 50 mg IV or famotidine 20 mg IV), Proton pump inhibitors (e.g., pantoprazole 40 mg IV or esomeprazole 20 mg IV)
Enhancement of gastric emptying	Metoclopramide: 10 mg IV 20–30 min before induction (inject over 1–2 min)
	Contraindicated in patients with obstruction or perforation
Nasogastric decompression	Nasogastric tube itself could impair the GES and would not assure an empty stomach
Rapid sequence induction +/− cricoid pressure	Cricoid pressure should be avoided in cases of active vomiting or if the cervical spine is unstable
Cuffed endotracheal tube	Uncuffed tube or supraglottic airway device such as laryngeal mask airway (LMA) may not prevent aspiration
Awake intubation	Awake intubation should be considered in cases of high risk of aspiration coupled with difficult airway, although topical anesthesia can ablate airway reflexes

arterial blood gases may be needed in prolonged procedures associated with significant blood loss.

Anesthetic technique

General anesthesia continues to be the mainstay of anesthetic management for major abdominal surgery. Although regional anesthesia (continuous epidural or spinal) could be the sole anesthetic in high-risk patients with significant pulmonary disease, this approach is rarely used in modern practice. Low thoracic epidurals are frequently used as adjuncts for intraoperative maintenance of anesthesia and for postoperative pain control. The use of thoracic epidural techniques as adjuncts to general anesthesia for major abdominal surgery has been shown to improve postoperative analgesia, decrease respiratory failure, and enhance ileus resolution, but not to decrease mortality. The risk of epidural hematoma and abscess, with a potential for permanent paralysis, albeit rare, should be kept in mind when deciding to place an epidural for elective abdominal surgery.

A balanced general anesthetic technique with an inhalational agent and an opioid or total IV anesthesia are both suitable anesthetic techniques for abdominal surgery. Muscle relaxation is often needed to improve surgical exposure and to facilitate abdominal closure. The use of nitrous oxide (N_2O) has been debated for years due to its ability to diffuse into gas-containing body cavities, thus theoretically distending the bowel and impairing surgical exposure. Therefore, some anesthesiologists avoid N_2O in major abdominal surgery reasoning that additional bowel distention could be harmful. Data supporting higher inspiratory oxygen concentration combined with mild hypercapnia as a means to improve outcome by reducing anastomotic leaks and wound infections should render obsolete the question as to whether to use N_2O in these cases.

Most patients undergoing abdominal surgery will be extubated successfully in the operating room (OR), but patients who require large amounts of fluid and blood products and who exhibit facial and airway edema and those with hemodynamic or respiratory instability should be kept intubated and ventilated in the intensive care unit (ICU). Extubation should be performed when the edema has resolved and hemodynamic and respiratory stability are achieved.

Intraoperative considerations

Heat loss

Abdominal surgery is associated with significant heat loss; therefore, the patient's temperature should be measured routinely. Items used to prevent hypothermia and associated complications include forced-air warming blankets and humidifiers. The intraoperative use of warming blankets can reduce convective heat loss, has been shown to improve operative outcome, and should be considered in every patient undergoing abdominal surgery. Fluid warmers should be used when large volumes of fluid are to be administered. For certain surgeries with significant heat loss and in children, the ambient temperature of the OR should be raised.

Pulmonary complications

Significant retraction, carbon dioxide (CO_2) insufflation for laparoscopic surgery, and Trendelenburg position will elevate the diaphragm and decrease the functional residual capacity (FRC), potentially leading to hypoxia and hypoventilation. Adding positive end-expiratory pressure (PEEP) increases FRC and may help improve oxygenation and ventilation. The difficulty with ventilation may stem from the causative disorder itself. For example, high peak pressures and difficulty in maintaining adequate tidal volumes may be associated with intra-abdominal processes, such as abdominal compartment syndrome.

Unwanted diaphragmatic movement (hiccup)

Intermittent spasms of the diaphragm due to diaphragmatic irritation and visceral stimulation may be troublesome to the surgeon. They can also interfere with effective mechanical ventilation. If the diaphragmatic movements are significant and immobility is needed, the anesthesia may be deepened or an additional dose of muscle relaxant may be given.

Mesenteric traction syndrome

This syndrome involves sudden onset of tachycardia, hypotension, and flushing associated with excessive traction on the mesentery. Although the exact pathophysiology is unknown, the release of prostacyclin and possibly histamine may play a role in the etiology. Cyclooxygenase (COX) inhibitors such as IV ketorolac may be used to prevent the syndrome, although their use should be discussed with the surgeon, as their platelet-inhibiting effects may be undesirable during surgery. H_1- and H_2- antihistamines also play a role in the prevention of this syndrome.

Postoperative ileus

Ileus is a major complication of abdominal surgery. The etiology involves pain, surgical stress, electrolyte and fluid imbalance, and the use of opioids. Opioids bind to μ-opioid receptors, depressing GI motility and worsening the ileus. Therapeutic options to minimize ileus are mostly supportive and include limiting the use of parenteral opioids, using thoracic epidural analgesia, instituting early feeding and mobility, and using laparoscopic surgery. Epidural analgesia in any location sufficient to provide analgesia for abdominal surgery has a protective role against postoperative ileus by decreasing sympathetic autonomic activity. This decrease in sympathetic autonomic activity leaves parasympathetic autonomic outflow relatively unopposed. Alvimopan and methylnaltrexone, peripherally acting selective μ-opioid receptor antagonists, have been recently shown to accelerate GI tract recovery after bowel resection.

Postoperative infection

Abdominal surgery is an independent risk factor for surgical site infection (SSI). Although many factors contribute to the risk of SSI, several could be manipulated intraoperatively by the anesthesiologist. These factors include hypoxia, hypothermia, hyperglycemia, and blood transfusion. Thus, measures to minimize the likelihood of postoperative infection should be undertaken, including the use of a hyperoxic gas mixture, avoidance of hypothermia, tight glycemic control, and minimizing blood transfusion, and timely administration of appropriate antibiotics.

Specific GI disorders
Bowel surgery

Surgery of the bowel (Table 100.2) is indicated for a variety of disorders including obstruction, perforation, tumor resection, and inflammatory bowel disease. General anesthesia supplemented with a thoracic epidural is often the preferred technique. Postoperative ileus is the most common complication (approximately 7.5%). The mechanism may be multifactorial, but the choice of anesthetic seemingly does not play a role in the development of this complication.

- Bowel obstruction involving the small bowel, the large bowel, or both is associated with volume derangements secondary to severe vomiting and fluid sequestration. Patients with bowel obstruction are treated as having a full stomach, and measures to prevent aspiration should be taken as outlined previously. If time permits, fluid and electrolyte abnormalities should be corrected prior to induction of general anesthesia.
- Patients with bowel perforation may be septic and susceptible to severe hemodynamic changes upon induction. These patients must also be treated as having a full stomach, and fluid and electrolyte abnormalities must be corrected. Invasive monitoring to facilitate tight blood pressure control should be considered.
- Patients with inflammatory bowel disease are often placed on glucocorticoid therapy for flare-ups, and the need for stress dose glucocorticoids must be determined. These patients may also be severely volume depleted secondary to persistent diarrhea. Furthermore, those patients presenting with toxic megacolon may be severely septic and critically ill.

Splenectomy

Patients may undergo elective splenectomy for hematologic disorders (i.e., idiopathic thrombocytopenic purpura) or may require a splenectomy as part of a staging procedure for their malignancy. Patients with hematologic disorders may present with anemia, thrombocytopenia, and/or other coagulopathies. Patients with a prior history of malignancy may be on

Table 100.2. Anesthetic management of GI disorders

GI disorders	Anesthetic management
Bowel obstruction	Correction of fluid imbalance and electrolytes Aspiration precautions Metoclopramide is contraindicated
Bowel perforation	Correction of fluid imbalance and electrolytes if possible, but should not delay surgery Aspiration precautions Metoclopramide is contraindicated Anticipate sepsis and hemodynamic instability
Crohn's/ulcerative colitis	Correction of fluid imbalance and electrolytes Consider glucocorticoids Toxic megacolon may be present
Splenectomy for ITP and malignancies	Anticipate anemia and thrombocytopenia Consider stress dose glucocorticoids Large-bore IV access Transfusing platelets after the splenic vessels are ligated minimizes platelet sequestration
Emergent splenectomy for ruptured spleen	Anticipate multiple injuries with significant blood loss and hemodynamic instability Large-bore IV access Blood products should be available Aspiration precautions
Pancreatitis	Correction of fluid imbalance and electrolytes Anticipate SIRS and organ dysfunction
Whipple procedure for pancreatic tumor	Significant fluid loss, bleeding, hypothermia, and prolonged operative time are all possible Large-bore IV access Consider invasive monitoring Consider thoracic epidural
Carcinoid syndrome	Evaluate for cardiomyopathy Avoid drugs causing histamine release Anticipate need for fluid resuscitation May need central access for potent vasopressors Octreotide blunts much of the carcinoid response
Abdominal compartment syndrome	Large-bore IV access Invasive monitoring Vasopressors Consider an ICU ventilator Anticipate sudden hemodynamic changes following the decompression of the abdomen

ITP, idiopathic thrombocytopenic purpura; SIRS, systemic inflammatory response syndrome.

long-standing glucocorticoid therapy and may have systemic effects from their chemotherapeutic regimens.

Non-elective splenectomy may take place in patients with traumatic ruptured spleen and in those with a spontaneous rupture. These patients may have other considerations, such as difficult airway, multiple severe injuries, hemodynamic instability, and/or full stomach. Large-bore IV access is necessary, as major blood loss is possible. When considering platelet transfusion in thrombocytopenic patients, the patients should be transfused after the splenic vessels are ligated, as the platelets will otherwise be sequestered in the soon-to-be-removed spleen.

Pancreatic surgery

Patients for pancreatic surgery usually have acute pancreatitis, pancreatic cancer, a neuroendocrine pancreatic tumor, or complications of chronic pancreatitis (pseudocyst or abscess).

- Patients with acute pancreatitis are usually managed medically. If surgical intervention is necessary, severe electrolyte abnormalities including hypocalcemia and hyperglycemia may be present and should be corrected preoperatively. Intravascular volume depletion, due to third spacing of fluids and bleeding, systemic inflammatory response syndrome, and organ dysfunction, may be present and should be anticipated.
- The Whipple procedure is usually performed for cystadenocarcinoma of the head of the pancreas, and it consists of partial pancreatectomy, pancreatojejunostomy, gastrojejunostomy, and choledochojejunostomy. The Whipple procedure is historically associated with major intraoperative fluid loss, bleeding, hypothermia, and prolonged operative time, although improved surgical techniques have mitigated these problems. Large-bore IV access and invasive monitoring are usually required for fluid replacement, hemodynamic monitoring, and frequent arterial blood sampling. Epidural analgesia can supplement general anesthesia and provides postoperative analgesia. The epidural infusion of local anesthetic and opioids may be started intraoperatively if the patient is stable hemodynamically. The decision for extubation in the OR should be based on the level of hemodynamic and homeostatic stability. Infusion of large volume loads and the presence of facial edema should temper enthusiasm for immediate extubation.

Carcinoid syndrome

This is a rare syndrome caused by carcinoid tumors that release various hormones, including serotonin. It is characterized by cutaneous flushing, tachycardia, hypotension or hypertension, bronchospasm, and diarrhea. Surgical excision may produce a life-threatening carcinoid crisis but remains the treatment of choice. Patients with untreated carcinoid may develop cardiomyopathy (carcinoid heart disease). Retrospective analyses showed that patients who experienced perioperative mortality had a higher frequency of carcinoid heart disease and had higher urinary 5-hydroxyindoleacetic acid (5-HIAA) levels. Patients who received intraoperative octreotide experienced fewer intraoperative complications than those who did not. There appears to be no role for preoperative octreotide. Intraoperative management involves fluid resuscitation, vasopressors, correction of electrolyte imbalance, octreotide administration, and avoidance of drugs that cause histamine release (morphine, succinylcholine, atracurium, mivacurium). Every patient presenting to the OR with carcinoid tumors should undergo preoperative cardiac imaging (echocardiography) and cardiac function testing to assess cardiac function, particularly function of the right side of the heart. A thorough cardiac assessment is important because 50% of patients with carcinoid tumors develop the typical endocardial plaques of fibrous tissue involving the tricuspid valve, pulmonary valve, the vena cava, and the pulmonary artery and are therefore at risk for right heart failure. Left heart involvement is rare, but if present should raise the suspicion for extensive liver metastasis, bronchial carcinoid, or a patent foramen ovale.

Abdominal compartment syndrome

The abdominal compartment syndrome is defined as intra-abdominal hypertension in association with worsening organ dysfunction. It is caused by a variety of disorders that lead to the elevation of intra-abdominal pressure and consequently hemodynamic instability, decreased lung compliance, and renal impairment. Causes include blunt and penetrating trauma, burns, major abdominal surgery, large fluid resuscitation, and refractory ascites. In addition to the hemodynamic and ventilatory support, prompt surgical decompression is required (see Chapter 172).

The anesthesiologist should be prepared to deal with hemodynamic instability, acute renal failure, and poor ventilation and oxygenation. Large-bore IV access is useful, and a central venous pressure catheter allows measurement of CVP and administration of potent vasoactive agents. In the case of significant ventilatory support requirements, a sophisticated ICU ventilator may be needed in the OR. Fortunately, many modern anesthesia machines feature such capabilities. Blood products should be available if bleeding is anticipated. The hemodynamic status usually improves with restoration of venous return. Sudden hypotension occasionally occurs upon decompression of the abdomen and should be treated promptly with fluid boluses and vasopressors.

Suggested readings

Avgerinos DV, Theoharides TC. Mesenteric traction syndrome or gut in distress. *Int J Immunopathol Pharmacol* 2005; 18:195–199.

Bastidas JA, Angst M. Pancreatic surgery. In: Jaffe RA, Samuels SI, eds. *Anesthesiologist's Manual of Surgical Procedure*. 3rd ed. Philadelphia: Lippincott Williams & Wilkins; 2004:484–494.

Cheadle WG. Risk factors for surgical site infection. *Surg Infect* 2006; 7(Suppl 1):S7–S11.

Delaney CP, Wolff BG, Viscusi ER, et al. Alvimopan for postoperative ileus following bowel resection: a pooled analysis of phase III studies. *Ann Surg* 2007; 245:355–363.

Finfer S, Bellomo R, Boyce N, et al. A comparison of albumin and saline for fluid resuscitation in the intensive care unit. *N Engl J Med* 2004; 350:2247–2256.

Kinney MAO, Warner MR, Nagorney DM, et al. Perianaesthetic risks and outcomes of abdominal surgery for metastatic carcinoid tumours. *Br J Anaesth* 2001; 87:447–452.

Mauermann WJ, Nemergut EC. The anesthesiologist's role in the prevention of surgical site infections. *Anesthesiology* 2006; 105:413–421.

Moore AFK, Hargest R, Martin M, et al. Intra-abdominal hypertension and the abdominal compartment syndrome. *Br J Surg* 2004; 91:1102–1110.

Myles PS, Leslie K, Chan MT, et al. ENIGMA Trial Group. Avoidance of nitrous oxide for patients undergoing major surgery: a randomized controlled trial. *Anesthesiology* 2007; 107:221–231.

Ng A, Smith G. Gastroesophageal reflux and aspiration of gastric contents in anesthetic practice. *Anesth Analg* 2001; 93:494–513.

Ogunnaike BO, Whitten CW. Anesthesia and gastrointestinal disorders. In: Barash PG, Cullen BF, Stoelting RK, eds. *Clinical Anesthesia*. 5th ed. Philadelphia: Lippincott Williams & Wilkins; 2006:1053–1060.

Rigg JR, Jamrozik K, Myles PS, et al. MASTER Anesthesia Trial Study Group. Epidural anesthesia and analgesia and outcome of major surgery: a randomized trial. *Lancet* 2002; 395:1276–1282.

Savas JF, Litwack R, Davis K, et al. Regional anesthesia as an alternative to general anesthesia for abdominal surgery in patients with severe pulmonary impairment. *Am J Surg* 2004; 188:603–605.

Scott AM, Starling JR, Ruscher AE, et al. Thoracic vs lumbar epidural anesthesia's effect on pain control and ileus resolution after restorative proctocolectomy. *Surgery* 1996; 120:695–697.

Shime N, Ono A, Chihara E, et al. Current status of pulmonary aspiration associated with general anesthesia: a nationwide survey in Japan. *Masui* 2005; 54:1177–1185.

Woehlck H, Antapli M, Mann A. Treatment of refractory mesenteric traction syndrome without cyclooxygenase inhibitors. *J Clin Anesth* 2004; 16:542–544.

Chapter 101

Laparoscopic surgery

Kai Matthes and Bhavani S. Kodali

Minimally invasive surgical procedures, when compared to conventional open procedures, are associated with significantly less trauma and the potential advantages of reduced postoperative pain, shorter length of hospitalization, rapid recovery, and decreased health care costs. Laparoscopy produces significant physiologic changes associated with peritoneal carbon dioxide (CO_2) insufflation and alteration in patient position that can have a major impact on cardiopulmonary function, particularly in patients with significant comorbidities.

Physiologic effects of laparoscopic procedures

The physiologic effects of laparoscopy are related to the combined effects of creation of a pneumoperitoneum, alteration of patient position, and effects of systemic absorption of CO_2.

Hemodynamic effects

During laparoscopy, cardiac output decreases to a variable extent depending on intra-abdominal pressure (IAP) and patient position, despite an increase in systemic blood pressure (Fig. 101.1). A characteristic response during the initiation of the pneumoperitoneum is an initial fall of the cardiac index with a subsequent partial recovery. Left ventricular end-diastolic volume is reduced during laparoscopy. Intrathoracic pressure is increased, and that commonly results in increased right atrial and pulmonary artery occlusion pressures.

The heart rate is minimally increased or unchanged. Increased circulating concentrations of catecholamines, renin, angiotensin II, and vasopressin cause an increase in systemic and pulmonary vascular resistance. Compression of arterial vasculature contributes to the increase in afterload. The reduction in splanchnic circulation is an effect of the pneumoperitoneum that may be counterbalanced by the direct splanchnic vasodilating effects of CO_2. Mesenteric ischemia, however, has been reported following laparoscopy.

Effects of CO_2 absorption

CO_2 is used for abdominal insufflation, as it is noncombustible and is more soluble in blood than is O_2, nitrous oxide (N_2O), or air. The absorption of insufflated CO_2, however, may lead to hypercapnia and respiratory acidosis that cause a decrease in myocardial contractility, lowered arrhythmia threshold,

arteriolar dilatation, and decreased systemic vascular resistance. These responses are modulated by mechanical and neurohumoral responses resulting in catecholamine release. The $PaCO_2$ increases progressively to reach a plateau 15 to 30 minutes after insufflation of CO_2 is initiated. This extent of increase in $PaCO_2$ is unpredictable, particularly in patients with severe pulmonary disease. The increase in $PaCO_2$ results in significant decreases in pH and the requirement for an increase in minute ventilation. CO_2 absorption is greater during extraperitoneal (pelvic) insufflation than during intraperitoneal insufflation.

Respiratory effects

During laparoscopy, lung volumes are reduced due to a cephalad shift of the diaphragm caused by abdominal insufflation. The pulmonary compliance is decreased, resulting in increased peak airway pressures and a reduction in functional residual capacity (FRC). There is ventilation-perfusion mismatch that may cause hypoxemia. There is an increase in intrathoracic pressure that adds to the decrease in lung compliance.

Hemodynamic effects of pneumoperitoneum

There is a biphasic cardiovascular response to increases in IAP. At an IAP of less than 10 mm Hg, there is an increase in venous return, probably from reduction in splanchnic sequestration of blood, with a subsequent increase in cardiac output and arterial pressure. This response, however, is blunted by hypovolemia. At an IAP of more than 20 mm Hg, compression of the inferior vena cava leads to a decreased venous return from the lower body and consequent decreased cardiac output. Increased renal vascular resistance at an IAP of more than 20 mm Hg decreases renal blood flow and glomerular filtration rate (GFR).

Urine output during pneumoperitoneum is diminished, but it increases following deflation of the abdomen. An increase in cerebral blood flow velocity and intracranial pressure is observed, which may complicate the anesthetic management of patients with intracranial mass lesions.

Effects of patient positioning

Patient position during laparoscopy varies depending on the procedure performed. For laparoscopic cholecystectomy,

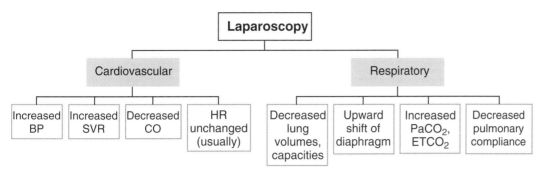

Figure 101.1. Physiologic effects of laparoscopy.

reverse Trendelenburg position with left lateral tilt is chosen to facilitate retraction of the gall bladder fundus and to minimize diaphragmatic dysfunction. This position improves pulmonary dynamics but may result in decreased venous return with a reduction in left ventricular end-diastolic volume. Increased IAP and the head-up position predispose to thromboembolism due to decreased femoral vein blood flow and lower limb venous stasis. The Trendelenburg position (for gynecologic procedures), in contrast, increases central blood volume, decreases diaphragmatic excursion, and causes pulmonary congestion. The ventilation–perfusion mismatch may result in hypoxemia, particularly in obese patients or in patients with pulmonary disease. Care should be taken so that the endotracheal tube does not slip into a mainstem bronchus during position changes.

Capnography during laparoscopic surgery

Capnography has three important applications during laparoscopic surgery. First, it serves as a noninvasive monitor of $PaCO_2$ during CO_2 insufflation and, therefore, can be used to adjust ventilation. Second, it may help in the detection of accidental intravascular CO_2 insufflation. Third, it may also help in the detection of other complications of CO_2 insufflation, such as pneumothorax or pneumomediastinum.

Prolonged intra-abdominal insufflation with CO_2 during upper abdominal laparoscopic surgery does not significantly affect the reliability of partial end-tidal CO_2 ($PETCO_2$) monitoring in predicting $PaCO_2$ in healthy American Society of Anesthesiologists (ASA) I and II subjects and elderly patients. In ASA III and IV patients, however, $PETCO_2$ may not reflect changes in $PaCO_2$ during insufflation due to changes in alveolar dead space consequent to reduced cardiac output or ventilation–perfusion mismatch. Therefore, direct arterial $PaCO_2$ monitoring is recommended in patients with significant cardiorespiratory diseases. An arterial line is reasonable to monitor $PaCO_2$ in ASA III and IV patients for three important reasons:

(1) The end-tidal PCO_2 is not a reliable index of $PaCO_2$;
(2) The normal gradient of 3 to 5 mm Hg between $PaCO_2$ and $PETCO_2$ is increased; and
(3) Even with normal $PETCO_2$, achieved by increasing minute volume, $PaCO_2$ may be as high as 50 mm Hg, resulting in respiratory acidosis.

Occasionally during the course of laparoscopic surgery the arterial-end tidal (a-ET)PCO_2 gradient may be negative in adults, in which case $PETCO_2$ overestimates $PaCO_2$. The incidence of negative gradients is higher in infants and children undergoing laparoscopic surgery. Low frequency, high tidal volume ventilation will open hitherto closed alveoli, the CO_2 from which will now be seen as an increase in the slope of phase III of the capnogram. A low FRC coupled with increased CO_2 delivery to the alveoli can exacerbate this response, thereby increasing the frequency of occurrences of negative (a-ET)PCO_2 values during laparoscopic surgery.

Anesthetic considerations
Choice of anesthetic technique

Although reports about laparoscopic procedures performed under spinal or epidural anesthesia have been documented, the requirement of a pneumoperitoneum and change in patient position commonly limits these procedures to general anesthesia. Endotracheal intubation and controlled mechanical ventilation are required to reduce the increase in $PaCO_2$ and counterbalance the respiratory side effects of the Trendelenburg position. For alternative viewpoints, see Chapter 103.

Recent studies demonstrate the feasibility and safety of using a ProSeal™ laryngeal mask airway (LMA) for laparoscopic procedures with the advantage of a decreased postoperative analgesia requirement and a lower incidence of postoperative nausea and vomiting (PONV). There is supporting evidence that LMAs may be used successfully with positive pressure ventilation, but many anesthesiologists are still reluctant to choose an LMA when positive pressure ventilation is needed. Even though the risk appears to be low, the increased IAP during laparoscopy may predispose to regurgitation and aspiration of gastric contents.

Monitoring

All patients should have ASA standard monitoring. Invasive monitoring may be indicated in ASA III and IV patients to evaluate the cardiovascular response to pneumoperitoneum and during position changes. $ETCO_2$ monitoring as a surrogate for $PaCO_2$ is recommended to adjust minute ventilation. (An increase of approximately 50% in tidal volume and respiratory rate is required to maintain PETCO$_2$ closer to preinsufflation values). Pressure–volume loop monitoring may be helpful in identifying airway complications. PaCO$_2$ monitoring by intermittent blood gas analysis is recommended for patients with severe pulmonary disease.

Maintenance

A balanced anesthetic technique consisting of opioids (fentanyl on induction, and morphine or hydromorphone for long-acting pain control), muscle relaxants, and volatile anesthetic is used. The use of N$_2$O is controversial because it may theoretically diffuse into air-filled spaces and cause distention of the bowel. The diffusion coefficients of N$_2$O and CO$_2$ are similar enough so that there would be no clinically relevant diffusion of N$_2$O into CO$_2$-filled spaces. In addition, the use of N$_2$O may increase the incidence of PONV.

An orogastric tube is inserted to decompress the stomach. A urinary catheter may be inserted to decompress the bladder. The patient is hyperventilated to decrease the ETCO$_2$ to approximately 30 mm Hg prior to abdominal insufflation of CO$_2$. The patient's muscles should be adequately relaxed prior to the initial trocar insertion since it is inserted blindly. Perforation of the inferior vena cava and aorta have been reported to occur during trocar insertion. A vagal response may also occur during trocar insertion.

Intraoperative hypertension should be treated with adequate pain control, deepening of the anesthesia, and administration of an antihypertensive such as labetalol or metoprolol, if indicated. Control of pain may be achieved via a multimodal analgesic regimen combining opioids, COX inhibitors, and local anesthetic infiltration. The nonselective COX inhibitor ketorolac (30 mg) is being increasingly administered near the end of procedures.

Laparoscopic procedures are frequently associated with an increased risk of PONV. Serotonin receptor antagonists (ondansetron, granisetron, dolasetron, and palonosetron), compared with traditional antiemetics, are highly efficacious for PONV. It is likely that combined antiemetics with different sites and mechanisms of action would be more effective than one drug alone for the prophylaxis against PONV, especially in high-risk patients. Adding dexamethasone to ondansetron or granisetron improves antiemetic efficacy in PONV. Dexamethasone should be given early during the surgery, preferably before any emetogens.

Laparoscopy in pregnant patients

The current evidence suggests that laparoscopic surgery is safer than laparotomy during pregnancy and does not have a significant impact on the course of pregnancy or fetus. Contrary to studies in a model using pregnant sheep, maternal PaCO$_2$ can be maintained within reasonable limits during peritoneal insufflations in pregnant patients. Increasing ventilation by about 50% from the baseline during insufflation and maintaining PETCO at approximately 32–34 mm Hg assures that the

maternal PaCO$_2$ is in a similar range. Monitoring arterial blood gases is not necessary unless there are accompanying respiratory and cardiac comorbidities. Cardiac output decreases from baseline values during peritoneal insufflations. Therefore, it is essential to maintain blood pressure within 20% of baseline values with boluses of ephedrine. It is also imperative to place a wedge under the right side of the patient to ensure left uterine displacement to maintain near-normal uterine perfusion during surgery. Our study has demonstrated that the maximum PaCO$_2$ occurs during the immediate postoperative period. Opioids should be administered with caution, since an overdose can depress ventilatory drive, contributing to a further increase in PaCO$_2$.

Laparoscopy in infants and children

Capnography has been proven to be an excellent guide in adjusting ventilation during CO$_2$ insufflation in infants and children. Monitoring PETCO$_2$, however, may overestimate PaCO$_2$ and consequently can result in hyperventilation during laparoscopic surgery in children. PETCO$_2$ often overestimates PaCO$_2$ during laparoscopy in children; thus, arterial blood gas analysis should be performed during long procedures to avoid hyperventilation.

Laparoscopy in obese patients

Laparoscopic procedures usually take longer in obese patients than in patients with a normal body weight and result in a prolonged exposure to the general anesthetic. In overweight patients, the pneumoperitoneum and the Trendelenburg position impair arterial oxygenation, leading to an increased alveolar–arterial oxygen tension difference (AaDO$_2$). Hemodynamic parameters are less affected by body weight.

Cephalad displacement of the diaphragm due to the increased weight of the abdominal wall in obese patients may cause increased airway pressure due to decreased compliance of the lung. Difficulties in ventilation of obese patients undergoing laparoscopic procedures may lead to hypercarbia and hypoxemia due to ventilation–perfusion mismatch. Due to the cephalad shift of the diaphragm, a firmly secured endotracheal tube may be displaced into the bronchial mainstem. Incidence of pulmonary atelectasis in morbidly obese patients is higher than that in nonobese patients.

Complications of laparoscopic procedures

Intraoperative complications during laparoscopic procedures can be a consequence of creation and maintenance of pneumoperitoneum and vascular injuries during surgical instrumentation (Table 101.1).

Postoperative considerations

Laparoscopic procedures have been suggested to reduce the incidence of postoperative pulmonary complications compared to open abdominal procedures. Diaphragmatic dysfunction

Table 101.1. Intraoperative complications during laparoscopy

Traumatic injuries associated with blind trocar or Veress needle insertion	• Injury of vascular structures: aorta, inferior vena cava, iliac vessels, retroperitoneal hematoma • Injury of gastrointestinal structures: small and large bowel, liver, spleen, and mesentery • Minimization of the risk of accidental organ injury by mini-laparotomy insertion of Veress needle
Venous CO_2 embolism	• Inadvertent intravenous placement of the Veress needle • Passage of CO_2 into the abdominal wall or peritoneal vessels during insufflation • Passage of CO_2 into open vessels of the liver surface during laparoscopic cholecystectomy • Symptoms include hypotension with cardiovascular collapse, hypoxemia, mill-wheel murmur, decrease in $ETCO_2$ because of a reduction of pulmonary blood flow • Cerebral CO_2 embolism may result from a patent foramen ovale or atrial septum defect • The incidence of undetected CO_2 embolism may be as high as 79% of patients during laparoscopic cholecystectomy
Pneumothorax, pneumomediastinum, pneumopericardium	• Tracking of insufflated CO_2 around aortic or esophageal hiatus of the diaphragm into the mediastinum with subsequent rupture into the pleural space • Passage of gas through embryogenic defects of the diaphragm • Pleural tears • Rupture of emphysematous bullae • Inadvertent placement of needle in extraperitoneal spaces
Surgical emphysema	• Intentional extraperitoneal insufflation of CO_2 during inguinal hernia repair • Accidental extraperitoneal insufflation of CO_2: subcutaneous emphysema of abdomen, chest, neck, and groin
Vascular injury	• Instrument insertion may cause concealed bleeding, particularly in the retroperitoneal space; may result in delayed diagnosis of vascular injury
Cardiac arrhythmias	• Due to hypercarbia or increased vagal tone; due to peritoneal stretch (bradycardia, asystole)

following laparoscopic cholecystectomy may last for up to 24 hours postoperatively. The increased IAP during the pneumoperitoneum has been reported to cause venous stasis and an increased risk of deep venous thrombosis and pulmonary embolism. Bile duct injuries are more common after laparoscopic cholecystectomy than following an open procedure. Patients with this condition present with pain and jaundice. Same-day laparoscopic cholecystectomy imposes the risk of delayed diagnosis of postoperative complications. Patients who are discharged the same day after their surgery should be selected with care. In addition, it is important to adequately control the pain and any nausea before discharging the patient.

Suggested readings

Amos JD, Schorr SJ, Norman PF, et al. Laparoscopic surgery during pregnancy. *Am J Surg* 1996; 171:435–437.

Bhavani-Shankar K, Philip JH. Defining segments and phases of a time capnogram. *Anesth Analg* 2000; 91:973–977.

Bhavani-Shankar K, Steinbrook RA, Brooks DC, Datta S. Arterial to end-tidal carbon dioxide pressure difference during laparoscopic surgery in pregnancy. *Anesthesiology* 2000; 93:370–373.

Chmielewski C, Snyder-Clickett S. The use of the laryngeal mask airway with mechanical positive pressure ventilation. *AANA J* 2004; 72:347–351.

Darzi A, Mackay S. Recent advances in minimal access surgery. *BMJ* 2002; 324:31–34.

Goodale RL, Beebe DS, McNevin MP, et al. Hemodynamic, respiratory, and metabolic effects of laparoscopic cholecystectomy. *Am J Surg* 1993; 166:533–537.

Hirvonen EA, Nuutinen LS, Kauko M. Ventilatory effects, blood gas changes, and oxygen consumption during laparoscopic hysterectomy. *Anesth Analg* 1995; 80:961–966.

Joris JL, Noirot DP, Legrand MJ, et al. Hemodynamic changes during laparoscopic cholecystectomy. *Anesth Analg* 1993; 76:1067–1071.

Kashtan J, Green JF, Parsons EQ, Holcroft JW. Hemodynamic effect of increased abdominal pressure. *J Surg Res* 1981; 30:249–255.

Michaloliakou C, Chung F, Sharma S. Preoperative multimodal analgesia facilitates recovery after ambulatory laparoscopic cholecystectomy. *Anesth Analg* 1996; 82:44–51.

Nyarwaya JB, Mazoit JX, Samii K. Are pulse oximetry and end-tidal carbon dioxide tension monitoring reliable during laparoscopic surgery? *Anaesthesia* 1994; 49:775–778.

Ogunnaike BO, Jones SB, Jones DB, et al. Anesthetic considerations for bariatric surgery. *Anesth Analg* 2002; 95:1793–1805.

Shankar KB, Moseley H, Vemula V, et al. Arterial to end-tidal carbon dioxide tension difference during anaesthesia in early pregnancy. *Can J Anaesth* 1989; 36:124–127.

Wahba RW, Beique F, Kleiman SJ. Cardiopulmonary function and laparoscopic cholecystectomy. *Can J Anaesth* 1995; 42:51–63.

Anesthesia for esophageal and gastric surgery

Amy L. Kim and Warren S. Sandberg

Introduction

This chapter covers anesthesia for surgery of the upper alimentary tract, namely, the esophagus and the stomach. Anesthesia for esophageal surgery involves many of the specialized techniques of anesthesia for thoracic surgery, and the reader is referred to those chapters for more detailed information (Part 15). Similarly, when considering anesthesia for gastric surgery and many esophageal procedures, the reader will benefit from reviewing the chapter on intra-abdominal surgery (Chapter 100) for more general information. Finally, much gastric reduction surgery is performed laparoscopically, so a review of the chapter on laparoscopy (Chapter 101) as well as the chapter on obesity (Chapter 6) will be useful.

Esophageal surgery

Patients may present for esophageal surgery for numerous reasons. Some of these reasons are reflux disease, esophageal cancer, strictures, motility disorders, and perforation.

Esophagogastrectomy

Multiple surgical techniques are used for the treatment of esophageal carcinoma, depending on the location of the tumor. For tumors of the lower third of the esophagus, a left thoracoabdominal incision is made. An esophagogastrectomy is then performed followed by anastomosis of the jejunum to the proximal esophagus. For lesions of the middle third of the esophagus, an Ivor Lewis approach is generally used. In this approach, the stomach is first mobilized via an abdominal incision with the patient supine. The patient then is repositioned left side down after endobronchial intubation, and a right thoracotomy is performed for esophageal tumor resection. The stomach is then pulled up into the chest and anastomosed to the proximal esophagus. Lesions of the upper third of the esophagus may be managed by combined laparotomy with cervical incision ("blind esophagectomy"). For those lesions in the upper third of the esophagus, when there is insufficient stomach length or the presence of gastric disease, an esophagogastrectomy with colon interposition can be performed in two stages. During the first stage, a midline laparotomy and right thoracotomy are done for the esophagogastrectomy. The patient is then placed supine, and a cervical esophagostomy is performed. In the second stage, at a

second operative sitting, either the right or left colon is used and passed into the retrosternal space where it is anastomosed to the cervical esophagus above and to the stomach remnant below.

Preoperative assessment

The preoperative evaluation of patients with esophageal disease should be a multisystem approach, with focus on the nutritional, hematologic, and cardiopulmonary systems.

Patients with esophageal disease often present with malnourishment, dehydration, and poor synthetic nutritional status (represented by hypoalbuminemia but affecting many synthetic pathways) due to dysphagia. It has been shown that improvement in nutritional status preoperatively has decreased the incidence of wound infections, sepsis, and perioperative morbidity and mortality.

Based on the patient's history and physical examination, additional tests may be necessary to evaluate the cardiopulmonary system Preoperative tests of pulmonary function or arterial blood gases (ABG) may be helpful. They can predict the likelihood of perioperative pulmonary complications and the need for postoperative mechanical ventilation. Patients should also receive a thorough cardiac evaluation due to the possibility of intraoperative hemodynamic instability and ongoing inflammatory and stress responses due to the surgery. The evaluation may include an electrocardiogram (ECG), echocardiogram, or functional cardiac stress testing.

Laboratory tests are indicated based on the patient's history and physical examination; however, a complete blood count (CBC) may be helpful given the ubiquity of anemia with these patients. A blood bank sample should be obtained given the presence of anemia and the possibility of perioperative blood transfusions.

A thorough airway evaluation should be performed preoperatively, with a focus on the presence of mediastinal lymphadenopathy, which may result in airway compression.

The preoperative evaluation should also focus on whether chemotherapy and/or radiation was used in patients with esophageal cancer because they can impact intraoperative patient management. Chemotherapeutic agents such as doxorubicin and bleomycin are commonly used in the management of esophageal cancer. These agents may result in the development of anemia, leukopenia, and thrombocytopenia. Doxorubicin, in addition, may lead to a dose-related cardiomyopathy that can be either acute or slowly progressive and results in heart failure. Thus patients who have been treated with doxorubicin should have a preoperative echocardiogram or nuclear scan to evaluate cardiac function. Bleomycin is another antineoplastic agent that is used to treat esophageal squamous cell carcinoma. It causes minimal myelosuppression but has a high incidence of pulmonary toxicity. With severe toxicity, patients may have resting hypoxemia and interstitial pneumonia and fibrosis. These patients are at increased risk for developing adult respiratory distress syndrome (ARDS) postoperatively possibly due to increased FiO_2 resulting in free radicals.

Radiation is another treatment option that is more effective for squamous cell carcinoma than for adenocarcinoma. Complications of radiation include pneumonitis, pericarditis, bleeding, and tracheoesophageal fistula.

Intraoperative management

Preoperative management focuses on the establishment of adequate intravenous (IV) access, appropriate monitoring, and suitable avenues for effective postoperative analgesia. Sedation and IV analgesia for procedures are also important.

Depending on the patient's anxiety level, premedication with benzodiazepines may be necessary. A large-bore IV (14–16 gauge) catheter should be inserted for volume replacement as needed. Standard monitors including pulse oximeter, temperature, ECG, and blood pressure (BP) cuff are indicated. Additionally, an arterial line may be used for tight BP control and for frequent laboratory sampling. Either central venous or pulmonary artery catheters should be used based on the patient's cardiopulmonary status and the anticipated surgical severity. A Foley catheter is inserted to monitor intraoperative urine output (in this case, as a functional indicator of adequate circulating intravascular volume).

Preoperative placement of a thoracic epidural catheter may be helpful for postoperative pain management and to facilitate early extubation. Chandrashekar and colleagues have shown that patients with good analgesia from a thoracic epidural after a two-stage esophagectomy have been extubated safely postoperatively in the operating room (OR) due to blunting of the stress response from pain. Additionally, postoperative morbidity and mortality secondary to cardiopulmonary complications are reduced when there is adequate analgesia from a thoracic epidural catheter.

Because of the location of surgery, general endotracheal anesthesia (GETA) is the obligatory anesthetic technique, although this may be supplemented by an epidural catheter. Because patients with esophageal disease are often at risk for pulmonary aspiration, patients should be intubated either awake (blind nasal or fiber-optic techniques) with topical anesthesia or after rapid-sequence IV induction with cricoid pressure. A nasogastric tube is typically passed to empty the esophagus and stomach. Maintenance of anesthesia generally uses combinations of volatile anesthetics and local anesthetics

± opioids via the epidural catheter. Nitrous oxide is avoided by some anesthetists, with the goal to minimize bowel distension, thus optimizing surgical exposure. Anesthesia is generally supplemented with nondepolarizing muscle relaxants. The combination of general and epidural anesthesia can dramatically decrease the inhalational anesthetic and muscle relaxant requirements. Pressors and fluids may be needed to treat hypotension.

Depending on the surgical approach, one-lung ventilation with double-lumen endobronchial tubes may be needed to facilitate surgical exposure.

Positioning of the patient is important to prevent pressure injuries, peripheral nerve compression, or stretch injury. If the lateral decubitus position is used, an axillary roll and airplane arm holder should be used. Pressure points, especially of the upper extremities, should be checked to avoid brachial plexus injuries. Radial pulses should be checked to ensure correct placement of the axillary roll. Placement of the oximeter probe on the dependent arm may assist in monitoring the adequacy of perfusion. In addition, eyes and ears should be checked for compression, and the eyes should be taped closed.

Attention to the patient's temperature during long operations is crucial. To prevent hypothermia, consider the use of a forced-air warming blanket, a fluid warmer, and keeping the room temperature warm. Of these options, the forced-air blanket is by far the most effective, and its use obviates the need for any other intervention.

Intraoperative complications of esophageal surgery can include hypotension, bradycardia, dysrhythmias, tracheal damage, hypoxia, and hemorrhage.

The decision to extubate at the end of the surgery is multifactorial, depending on the extent of the surgical procedure and the patient's tolerance of surgery and anesthesia. Patients should be alert, cooperative, hemodynamically stable, and warm, and neuromuscular blockade should be fully antagonized. Those patients who require postoperative ventilation should have the DLT changed to a single-lumen endotracheal tube prior to leaving the OR. Patients can then be weaned from mechanical ventilation and extubated in the intensive care unit (ICU) postoperatively.

Postoperative management

Patients are usually managed postoperatively in an ICU setting, although this depends in part on the degree of surgical insult. In the early postoperative period, patients may have increased fluid requirements. Adequate postoperative pain control is essential to facilitate deep breathing, cough, mobilization of secretions, participation in chest physiotherapy, and early ambulation.

Postoperative complications from esophageal surgery include aspiration, atelectasis, acute lung injury, hemorrhage, pneumothorax, hemothorax, hypoxemia, hypoventilation, recurrent laryngeal nerve injury, deep vein thrombosis (DVT), and esophageal anastomotic leak.

Respiratory problems after esophagectomy are common. ARDS is a major contributor to respiratory morbidity and mortality after esophagectomy. Tandon and colleagues noted that acute lung injury after elective esophagectomy is associated with intraoperative cardiorespiratory instability. They also noted that the longer the one-lung ventilation time and operative time, the greater the incidence of acute lung injury. This may be attributed to the fact that both lungs are subjected to injury during the thoracic phase of the procedure. The dependent lung is exposed to microbarotrauma, whereas the collapsed lung suffers ischemia–reperfusion injury.

Another serious complication is the development of anastomotic leakage. Michelet and colleagues have noted that thoracic epidural analgesia is associated with a decrease in anastomotic leakage. This association may be due to thoracic epidural analgesia allowing intensive chest physiotherapy that helps preserve postoperative pulmonary function and prevent hypoxemia. It has also been shown that thoracic epidural analgesia use during major abdominal surgery increases tissue oxygen, thus improving oxygenation at the wound surfaces.

Nissen fundoplication

Esophageal fundoplication is an operation that increases lower esophageal sphincter pressure to prevent esophageal reflux by wrapping the fundus of the stomach around a 3- to 4-cm segment of the lower esophagus. (See Fig. 102.1.) This operation can be done transabdominally, transthoracically, or laparoscopically. The most commonly used technique is the open or laparoscopic Nissen fundoplication that uses both the anterior and posterior walls of the stomach. Indications for esophageal fundoplication include stricture, respiratory problems, esophageal ulcerations, and Barrett's esophagus, as well as failure of medical management or a patient's unwillingness to submit to a lifetime of medication.

Anesthetic management for open Nissen fundoplication is similar to that for esophageal surgery. Laparoscopic Nissen fundoplication is managed like a typical intra-abdominal laparoscopic case. The potential for carbon dioxide insufflation along the esophagus above the diaphragm is quite high, however, and

it can complicate ventilation management. Surgeons are concerned about the impact of postoperative retching on the viability of the fundoplication. Thus, aggressive postoperative nausea and vomiting prophylaxis is warranted in these patients.

Bariatric surgery

Morbidly obese patients are defined as those who are greater than 100 pounds over ideal body weight or 2 times ideal body weight. Body mass index (BMI) is defined by weight in kilograms divided by height in meters squared. Patients with a BMI greater than 28 are considered obese. Patients with a BMI greater than 35 are considered morbidly obese.

A variety of surgical procedures are used to treat morbid obesity. These procedures can be divided into malabsorptive versus restrictive procedures. Malabsorptive procedures include jejunoileal bypass and biliopancreatic bypass, in which most of the small bowel is bypassed, thus creating a state of chronic malabsorption.

Restrictive procedures include vertical banded gastroplasty and adjustable gastric banding. These procedures work by decreasing the size of the gastric pouch, thus limiting the amount of food that can be consumed at one time. Gastroplasty creates a small upper pouch (15–30 ml) in the stomach, which restricts food intake. The pouch communicates with the remainder of the stomach through a narrow channel, or stoma. Adjustable gastric banding is done by a minimally invasive laparoscopic approach. An adjustable inflatable band is placed around the proximal stomach to limit stomach capacity. The band can be made tighter or less so by adding or removing saline. Roux-en-Y gastric bypass (RYGB) combines gastric restriction with a minimal degree of malabsorption. Restrictive procedures can be performed laparoscopically or via laparotomy.

RYGB is the most commonly performed bariatric procedure in the United States. It is the most effective bariatric procedure to produce safe short- and long-term weight loss in severely obese patients. This procedure involves anastomosis of the proximal gastric pouch to a segment of the proximal jejunum that bypasses most of the stomach and entire

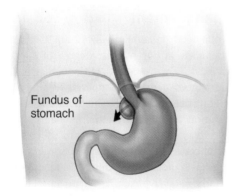
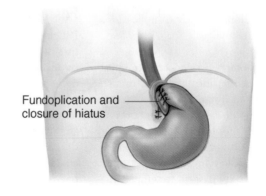

Fundus of stomach

Fundoplication and closure of hiatus

Figure 102.1. Illustration of the key anatomic step in Nissen fundoplication.

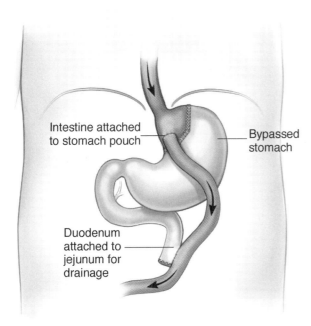

Figure 102.2. Illustration of the RYGB anatomy.

Intestine attached to stomach pouch

Bypassed stomach

Duodenum attached to jejunum for drainage

duodenum (see Fig. 102.2). With RYGB, patients lose an average of 50% to 60% of excess body weight and show a BMI decrease of approximately 10 kg/m^2 during the first 12 to 24 postoperative months. Type 2 diabetes resolves in the majority of patients.

Laparoscopic bariatric surgery is minimally invasive and is associated with less postoperative pain, lower morbidity, and faster recovery. Operative trauma is reduced when compared to open procedures due to smaller surgical incisions and the elimination of mechanical retraction of the abdominal wall. In addition, accumulation of third space fluid is significantly lower after laparoscopic RYGB than after open RYGB. A reduced incidence of wound infection and an early return to daily activities is seen in laparoscopic RYGB patients. Rhabdomyolysis is more common in morbidly obese patients undergoing laparoscopic procedures than open procedures, however. Unexplained elevations in serum creatinine and creatine phosphokinase levels or complaints of buttock, hip, or shoulder pain in the postoperative period should raise suspicion of rhabdomyolysis.

Preoperative assessment

The preoperative evaluation of morbidly obese patients again involves a multisystem approach with focus on the cardiopulmonary status and airway. The incidence of difficult mask ventilation and intubation is high in obese patients. Flexion of the neck in the obese patient could result in difficult intubation due to excessive soft tissue. The presence of submental fat may also limit mouth opening. A large tongue, redundant palate, and pharyngeal tissue may narrow the airway. It has been identified that neck circumference is the single best predictor of problematic intubation in morbidly obese patients. Thus careful airway examination is paramount.

Patients should also be evaluated for systemic hypertension, obstructive sleep apnea with coexisting pulmonary hypertension, signs of right and/or left ventricular failure, and ischemic heart disease. Obesity has serious cardiopulmonary consequences, as outlined in Fig. 102.3. Preoperative tests, such as echocardiogram, ECG, chest radiography, and baseline ABG, may provide useful information for the management of these patients intraoperatively.

This patient population is at risk for pulmonary aspiration of gastric contents due to increased intra-abdominal pressure, gastric volume, and acidity, as well as the increased incidence of hiatal hernia.

Laboratory tests are indicated based on the patient's history and physical examination. A CBC is useful because polycythemia may be present due to chronic hypoxemia. A measurement of fasting blood glucose may be necessary due to the frequent occurrence of glucose intolerance and diabetes mellitus in this patient population. Liver function is often abnormal and drug metabolism may be significantly affected.

Patients' usual medications (with the possible exception of insulin and oral hypoglycemics) should be continued until the time of surgery.

Intraoperative management

Premedication with oral or IV benzodiazepines is reliable for anxiolysis in this patient population, as modest sedative doses cause little or no respiratory depression. However, patients with a history of obstructive sleep apnea may be especially sensitive to sedatives and opioids. H$_2$-receptor antagonists, proton pump inhibitors, and nonparticulate antacids like sodium citrate may be useful preoperatively for reducing gastric volume and acidity, thus reducing the risk and complications of aspiration.

DVT prophylaxis with subcutaneous unfractionated or low-molecular-weight heparin, in addition to pneumatic compression devices, should also be used given the risk for sudden death from acute postoperative pulmonary embolism. Antibiotic prophylaxis is also important because of the increased risk of postoperative wound infection after gastric operations for obesity.

A large-bore (14–16 gauge) IV catheter should be inserted with the anticipation of potential large fluid loss mainly due to fluid shifts. Standard monitors such as pulse oximeter, temperature, ECG, and appropriately sized BP cuff are used for patient monitoring. An arterial catheter may be necessary in those patients with severe cardiopulmonary disease or for those with poor fit of the noninvasive BP cuff. Central venous catheterization may be performed in those in whom peripheral IV access cannot be obtained. Otherwise, central venous cannulation for monitoring and central drug administration is selected on a case-by-case basis, depending on the patient's medical condition and the expected impact of surgery. A urinary catheter is also placed to monitor urine output to guide in fluid management.

Again, the site of surgery necessitates GETA as the anesthetic technique, with or without an epidural catheter for

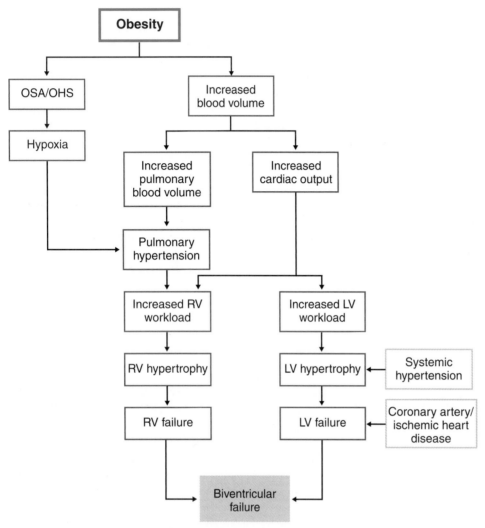

Figure 102.3. Flow diagram of the interrelationships between obesity and cardiopulmonary complications. RV, right ventricle; LV, left ventricle; OSA, obstructive sleep apnea; OHA, obesity hypoventilation syndrome. Redrawn from Figure 36-2, *Clinical Anesthesia*, Barash PG, ed. Philadelphia: Lippincott Williams & Wilkins; 2006.

postoperative analgesia. Preparation should be made for difficult mask ventilation, laryngoscopy, or intubation. Thus, positioning the patient prior to induction by elevating the shoulders and occiput so that the head is in the "sniffing" position greatly facilitates airway access. This can be done by placing towels or folded blankets under the shoulders and head so that the tip of the chin is higher than the chest. Another positioning maneuver known as the head-elevated laryngoscopy position (HELP) can improve laryngoscopic view (see Fig. 102.4). HELP elevates the obese patient's head, upper body, and shoulders above the chest to the extent that an imaginary horizontal line connects the sternal notch to the external auditory meatus. During induction of anesthesia, patients should be positioned in a head-up reverse Trendelenburg position, providing the longest safe apnea period. Adequate preoxygenation is vital in obese patients because of rapid desaturation after loss of consciousness, attributed increased tissue oxygen consumption, and decreased functional residual capacity (FRC).

Because these patients are at risk for aspiration, they should be intubated either awake or after rapid-sequence induction with cricoid pressure. Following successful intubation, a nasogastric (NG) tube should be placed and the stomach contents suctioned. The NG tube may be used later in the surgery to check anastomotic integrity with the injection of saline or methylene blue. The NG tube should also be removed before gastric division to avoid unplanned stapling or transection of the tube.

Anesthesia is generally maintained with inhalational anesthetics. Some providers prefer desflurane due to its rapid recovery profile. Juvin and colleagues have noted that immediate recovery from anesthesia occurred faster with desflurane than with isoflurane or propofol. In addition, postanesthesia care unit (PACU) admission oxygen saturation of hemoglobin (SpO_2) values were significantly higher and patient mobility was significantly better after desflurane. At 30 and 120 minutes postoperatively, sedation was also significantly less pronounced

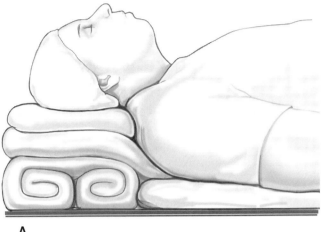

A

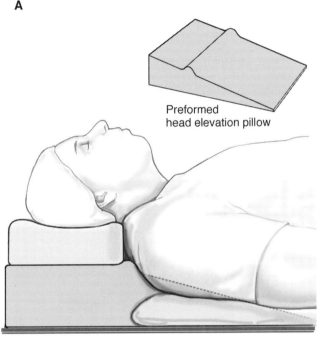

Preformed
head elevation pillow

B

Figure 102.4. Preformed head elevation pillow and its use.

with desflurane. If an epidural catheter is present, it may be used in combination with an inhalational anesthetic. Nitrous oxide is generally avoided to minimize bowel distention as well as due to the high oxygen demand in obese patients. Nondepolarizing muscle relaxants are also used to facilitate adequate ventilation and surgical exposure. Dexmedetomidine infusions can be used to decrease anesthetic and opioid requirements. Infusion of remifentanil, an ultra-short-acting opioid, has been used to supplement a total intravenous anesthesia (TIVA) or an inhalational anesthetic.

Proper positioning is crucial in this patient population. The appropriately sized OR table should be available, and patients should be well secured to the table to prevent falls and injury. Bean bags to help position a patient may also be useful. Protecting pressure areas is important in this patient population given the common occurrence of pressure sores and nerve injuries.

An association exists between ulnar neuropathy and increasing BMI. The supine position, as well as the Trendelenburg position, are generally not well tolerated by the obese patient. The development of ventilation–perfusion abnormalities, left-to-right shunting, and decrease in FRC may result in hypoxemia. Hypotension may also result from supine positioning due to occlusion of the inferior vena cava (IVC), which compromises venous return to the heart.

The decision to extubate at the end of the surgery depends on the patient's underlying cardiopulmonary status and the extent of the surgical procedure. Patients should be hemodynamically stable, warm, alert, cooperative, and fully reversed from any muscle relaxants prior to extubation. The patient should be preferably extubated in the semirecumbent position, which has less adverse effect on respiration. Supplemental oxygen should be administered after extubation.

Postoperative management

These patients – especially those with coexisting diseases – may require ICU admission for postoperative care. There is an increased incidence of atelectasis, which persists into the postoperative period, in morbidly obese patients after general anesthesia. Patients may need continuous positive airway pressure (CPAP) or bilevel positive airway pressure (BiPAP) postoperatively to reduce atelectasis and combat airway obstruction. Postoperative CPAP does not increase the incidence of major anastomotic leakage after gastric bypass surgery despite a theoretical risk.

Pain may cause patients to avoid taking deep breaths and ambulating. Thus adequate pain control is crucial as well as the use of a properly fitted elastic binder for abdominal support in improving pulmonary toilet. Epidural analgesia with local anesthetics, opioids, or both is an effective form of analgesia. Potential advantages of epidural analgesia include DVT prevention, improved analgesia, and earlier recovery of intestinal motility. Patients should be observed, however, for delayed respiratory depression with the use of central neuraxial opioids. Patient-controlled anesthesia (PCA) morphine is equivalent to low thoracic/high lumbar epidural analgesia with continuous infusions of bupivacaine/fentanyl in morbidly obese patients undergoing gastric bypass surgery with regard to the quality of pain control at rest, the frequency of nausea and pruritus, the time to ambulation, time to return of gastrointestinal (GI) function, and the length of hospital stay.

Complications postoperatively include anastomotic leak, gastric pouch outlet obstruction, jejunostomy obstruction, DVT, PE, respiratory failure, GI bleeding, and wound infection. RYGB may also cause a "dumping syndrome" resulting in diarrhea and abdominal cramps secondary to a high-sugar liquid diet.

Suggested readings

Babatunde OO, Jones SB, Jones DB, et al. Anesthetic considerations for bariatric surgery. *Anesth Analg* 2002; 95:1793–1805.

Barash PG, Cullen BF, Stoelting RK. *Clinical Anesthesia.* 5th ed. Philadelphia: Lippincott, Williams & Wilkins; 2006:1045–1051.

Brodsky JB, Lemmons HJM, Brock-Utne JG, et al. Morbid obesity and tracheal intubation. *Anesth Analg* 94: 732, 2002.

Chandrashekar MV, Irving M, Wayman J, et al. Immediate extubation and epidural analgesia allow safe management in a high-dependency unit after two-stage oesophagectomy. Results of eight years of experience in a specialized upper gastrointestinal unit in a district general hospital. *Br J Anaesth* 2003; 90:474–479.

Charghi R, Backman S, Christou N, et al. Patient controlled IV analgesia is an acceptable pain management strategy in morbidly obese patients undergoing gastric bypass surgery. A retrospective comparison with epidural analgesia. *Can J Anesth* 2003; 50:672.

Huerta S, DeShields S, Shpiner R, et al. Safety and efficacy of postoperative continous positive airway pressure to prevent pulmonary complications after Roux-en-Y gastric bypass. *J Gastrointest Surg* 6: 354, 2002.

Juvin P, Vadam C, Malek L, Dupont H, et al. Postoperative recovery after desflurane, propofol, or isoflurane anesthesia among morbidly obese patients: a prospective, randomized study. *Anesth Analg* 2000; 91: 714–719.

Levitan RM, Mechem CC, Ochroch EA, et al. Head-elevated laryngoscopy position: improving laryngeal exposure during laryngoscopy by increasing head elevation. *Ann Emerg Med* 2003; 41:322.

Michelet P, D'Journo X, Roch A, et al. Perioperative risk factors for anastomotic leakage after esophagectomy. *Chest* 2005; 128:3461–3466.

Moghissi K, Hornshaw J, Teasdale PR, et al. Parenteral nutrition in carcinoma of the esophagus treated by surgery: nitrogen balance and clinical studies, *Br J Surg* 64: 125, 1977.

Mognol P, Vignes S, Chosidow D, et al. Rhabdomyolysis after laparoscopic bariatric surgery. *Obes Surg* 2004; 14:19.

Nguyen NT. Open vs. laparoscopic procedures in bariatric surgery. *J Gastrointest Surg* 2004; 8:393.

Rubino F, Gagner M, Gentileschi P, et al. The early effect of the Roux-en-Y gastric bypass on hormones involved in body weight regulation and glucose metabolism. *Ann Surg* 240: 236, 2004.

Tandon S, Batchelor A, Bullock R, et al. Peri-operative risk factors for acute lung injury after elective oesophagectomy. *Br J Anaesth* 2001; 86: 633–638.

Warner MA, Warner ME, Martin JT. Ulnar neuropathy: incidence, outcome and risk factors in sedated or anesthetized patients. *Anesthesiology* 1994; 81:1332.

Anesthesia for gynecologic and breast surgery

Bronwyn Cooper

Introduction

There is a wide range of breast and gynecologic procedures that require anesthesia. This chapter provides an overview of different gynecologic and breast surgeries and their anesthetic requirements that range from local to general anesthesia. In addition, major surgeries often require postoperative hospital admission and regional anesthesia for postoperative pain.

Breast surgery
Breast tumor surgery

The most common breast surgeries are lumpectomy, an enlarged excisional biopsy, and modified radical mastectomy for breast cancer. With axillary dissection, it is often wise to avoid muscle relaxants so that the surgeon may stimulate the long thoracic and thoracodorsal nerves to aid in their identification. Whereas breast biopsy and lumpectomy can be done with local anesthesia (such as bupivacaine or lidocaine) and sedation according to patient preference, major breast cancer surgery is usually done under general anesthesia for patient comfort and surgical ease. Breast surgery, in general, is a low-risk surgery, and perioperative risk is mainly dependent on the presence and severity of comorbidities and the age of the patient.

Nearly 60% of women experience severe pain following breast cancer surgery. One study showed that risk factors associated with pain at 1 month after surgery include non-white race, obesity, and high postanesthesia care unit (PACU) opioid use. It has been suggested by many authors that patients undergoing major surgery for breast cancer experience fewer postoperative side effects if they receive regional rather than general anesthesia for procedures such as mastectomy, lumpectomy, and reconstructive surgery. Lynch and colleagues studied outcomes of thoracic epidural anesthesia after oncologic breast surgery and reconstructive procedures. The conclusion of their retrospective analysis was that lower postoperative nausea and vomiting (PONV) was associated with statistically significant earlier hospital discharge and that thoracic epidural anesthesia is a safe technique not associated with neurologic or respiratory complications that improves patients' recovery while reducing the cost of these procedures. Thoracic epidural anesthesia and analgesia have been described for modified radical mastectomy, breast augmentation, and mastectomy with transverse rectus

abdominus myocutaneous (TRAM) flap reconstruction. It is usually initiated at the T3–T4 interspace (high thoracic), and breast tissue (i.e., augmentation) requires a blockade from T1 through T7. Procedures including the anterior chest wall (i.e., modified radical mastectomy) may require blockade up to C5 to include pectoral nerves. A thoracic paravertebral nerve block can be used to augment, or as an alternative to, general anesthesia in high-risk patients undergoing major breast surgery. Single-injection techniques are limited to the duration of the local anesthetic and are discussed elsewhere in the text. The introduction of disposable infusion pumps has facilitated the use of ambulatory perineural infusions. Preliminary retrospective data suggest a possible advantage of regional techniques in breast cancer surgery beyond decreased postoperative pain and PONV rates. Some retrospective data suggest that the use of regional analgesia and the avoidance of systemic opioids result in lower cancer recurrence rates, possibly due to inhibition of cellular and humoral immune function in humans. Larger prospective studies are under way.

Augmentation mammoplasty

Augmentation mammoplasty is often performed for cosmetic reasons or in patients who have undergone breast cancer surgery. A prosthesis is inserted under or above the pectoralis muscle. The most commonly used anesthetic is general anesthesia, although some patients prefer local with intravenous (IV) sedation. Regional anesthesia choices include epidural, thoracic paravertebral block, or a continuous paravertebral catheter. Local anesthesia includes several techniques, such as subcutaneous injection, intercostal nerve blocks, pump infusions, and "splashing" local anesthetic into the submuscular pocket. Patients who have already undergone breast surgery and chemotherapy may have difficult IV access and a history of exposure to chemotherapeutic agents that can have long-lasting effects on cardiac, pulmonary, and other systems. Commonly used chemotherapeutic agents and their side effects are summarized in Table 103.1.

Gynecological surgery

Since the 1970s there has been a significant increase in gynecologic procedures performed in the ambulatory setting.

Table 103.1. Common chemotherapeutic drugs used in breast cancer

Drug	Significant side effect
Doxorubicin	Cardiomyopathy, nephrotoxicity, hepatotoxicity
Cyclophosphamide	Pseudocholinesterase inhibition, thrombocytopenia, decreased threshold for PONV
Methotrexate	Pulmonary infiltrates, hepatotoxicity, inhibition of folate metabolism
Tamoxifen	Hepatotoxicity
Cisplatin	Peripheral neuropathy, nephrotoxicity
Gemcitabine	Nephrotoxicity, lung toxicity, hepatotoxicity

Table 103.3. Major approaches to gynecologic surgeries

Laparoscopy	Hysteroscopy
Endometriosis	Myomectomy
Ectopic pregnancy	Septum resection
Hysteroscopy	Endometrial ablation
Myomectomy	Polypectomy
Tubal sterilization	Adhesions/Asherman's
Oopherectomy	Proximal tubal cannulation
Ovarian cystectomy	Hysterosalpingogram
Adnexal mass removal	
Salpingostomy/salpingectomy	
Bladder neck suspension	
Infertility	
Sling/Burch procedures	

Vaginal	**Abdominal**
Hysterectomy	Hysterectomy
Myomectomy (rare)	Myomectomy (low transverse incision)
Dilation & curettage	Tumor debulking
Dilation & evacuation	Urinary stress incontinence surgery
Laser therapy	

Table 103.2 shows the different types of anesthesia suitable for common gynecologic procedures. Today, surgeons use improved techniques, such as minimally invasive surgery with small incisions, and new smaller, more flexible scopes and laparoscopic techniques. By the late 1990s, more than 80% of gynecologic surgery for benign pathology was done on an ambulatory basis.

Table 103.3 demonstrates the four major approaches to gynecologic surgery – laparoscopy, hysteroscopy, vaginal, and abdominal – and the different procedures associated with each. Hysteroscopy involves a visual examination of the uterine cavity through a flexible hysteroscope. The uterine cavity is distended with saline, glycine, dextran, or carbon dioxide (CO_2) to inspect the interior of the uterus. IV sedation or paracervical block is adequate for anesthesia as long as prolonged manipulation is not required. Applications include evaluation of abnormal uterine bleeding and polyp or intrauterine device (IUD) removal. Resection of submucosal leiomyomas and endometrial ablation usually require regional or general anesthesia. Often hysteroscopy is done in conjunction with curettage and laparoscopy. The most common complications include uterine perforation, bleeding, and infection. Intravascular extravasation of fluid or gas can become clinically significant only later with onset of hyponatremia, air embolism, cerebral edema, and even death.

The loop electrosurgical excision procedure (LEEP) is therapy for vulvar and cervical lesions, such as vulvar condylomata and cervical dysplasias. Low-voltage, high-frequency alternating current is used to limit thermal damage yet allow good hemostasis. These lesions can also be excised either with a sharp knife or laser, and this procedure can be performed under local anesthesia with IV sedation or general anesthesia.

Tubal ligation is most commonly performed via laparoscopy under general anesthesia. Complications of general anesthesia have been the leading cause of death attributed to sterilization in the United States. The risks of general anesthesia are known to increase during the postpartum period. The use of local anesthesia alone has increased only from 4% to 8 % in the United States. Worldwide, more than 75% of tubal ligation procedures are performed under local anesthesia because a minilaparotomy can be done safely under local anesthesia. The disadvantages, however, can be anxiety and discomfort, both for the patient and the surgeon. It is unknown whether local anesthesia for tubal ligation has a better safety profile than general anesthesia.

Gynecological laparoscopy

Laparoscopy can be either diagnostic or operative. In recent years, the use of laparoscopy in gynecology has expanded dramatically from its use in diagnosis to tubal sterilization, treatment of ectopic pregnancy, and hysterectomy. Compared with laparotomy, laparoscopy offers a shorter hospitalization, less postoperative pain, less morbidity, and a shorter recovery period. The physiologic aspects associated with gynecologic laparoscopy are discussed in detail in the chapter on anesthesia for laparoscopy, Chapter 101.

Anesthetic techniques for laparoscopy

Table 103.4 gives an overview of the different types of anesthetic options for laparoscopic gynecologic procedures. Because more laparoscopic procedures are performed on an outpatient

Table 103.2. Anesthetic options for common gynecologic procedures

Gynecologic procedure	Common anesthetic options
Transabdominal or transvaginal hysterectomy	GA or regional
Diagnostic laparoscopy	GA
LEEP, cervical biopsy	MAC or GA
Dilation & curettage	MAC or GA
Tubal ligation	GA or Regional

GA, general anesthesia; MAC, monitored anesthesia care.
Source: Goulson DT. *Curr Opin Anesthesiol* 2007; 20(3):195–200.

Table 103.4. Possible anesthetic techniques used for laparoscopic gynecologic surgery

GA with ETT
GA/LMA with mechanical ventilation (either classic or ProSeal)
GA with spontaneous ventilation
Regional (spinal, epidural, or CSE)
Local +/− IV sedation
Combined GA/regional

GA, general anesthesia; ETT, endotracheal tube.
Source: Cueto-Garcia J, Jacobs M, Gagner M. *Laparoscopic Surgery.* New York: McGraw-Hill; 2003.

basis, general and regional anesthesia have been successfully and safely used with great emphasis on short-duration drugs, cardiovascular stability, rapid recovery and fast-tracking, mobility, and prevention and treatment of PONV and pain. Most commonly, general anesthesia is used because it allows for controlled ventilation (to counteract the CO_2 absorption), good surgical conditions, and patient comfort. Shorter-acting drugs such as sevoflurane, desflurane, and continuous infusions of propofol are the maintenance agents of choice. An early recovery has been attained with any of these agents. Remifentanil is often used in fast-tracking due to its lack of accumulation with continuous infusion.

Regional anesthesia provides some advantages but can be controversial during laparoscopy. The advantages include decreased PONV, reduced postoperative pain, shorter stay, cost effectiveness, improved satisfaction, fewer hemodynamic changes, and earlier diagnosis of complications. Requirements include a relaxed, cooperative patient, low intra-abdominal pressure, reduced Trendelenburg requirements, and a precise surgical technique. The combined effects of pneumoperitoneum and sedation can lead to hypoventilation and arterial oxygen desaturation. Advances in microlaparoscopy allow these procedures to be performed with local anesthesia alone or supplemented by sedation. Longer laparoscopic procedures may be more suitable for epidural anesthesia, and, if onset time is an issue, a combined spinal–epidural (CSE) anesthetic can be utilized. With the development of gasless laparoscopy and microlaparoscopy, spinal anesthesia will probably take on a greater role in the near future.

Robotic-assisted gynecologic surgery

Robotic-assisted gynecologic surgery is a relatively new technique that is gaining popularity. Fallopian tube anastomosis, hysterectomy, and myomectomy have been successfully performed with this technique. After induction of anesthesia, the abdomen is insufflated with CO_2, and the patient is placed in modified dorsal lithotomy with steep Trendelenburg position. General anesthesia is most commonly used, and continuous muscle paralysis is recommended. It is also advisable to use limited volumes of IV fluids while the patient is in the Trendelenburg position.

Preoperative considerations for gynecologic laparoscopy

Choosing the appropriate patient for laparoscopy and then scheduling an outpatient procedure require careful preoperative assessment to identify increased risk for the individual patient on a case-by-case basis. Most patients will be young and healthy, but, more recently, older, more complex patients have been arriving to the operating room for laparoscopic procedures. In many settings, the surgeon performs such screening, and the anesthesiologist first encounters the patient on the day of surgery.

Induction and maintenance of anesthesia

Induction of general anesthesia is most easily accomplished with an intravenous agent such as propofol, although inhaled agents may also be used. Gynecologic laparoscopy can be performed using a laryngeal mask airway (LMA) in lieu of tracheal intubation, although many anesthesiologists prefer intubation. In gynecologic laparoscopy, devices such as the ProSeal (LMA; San Diego, CA) and its analogs may be useful because they can allow higher airway pressure without leaking. Most studies examining the value of the ProSeal LMA as opposed to tracheal intubation have enrolled healthy American Society of Anesthesiologists (ASA) I-II patients who were not obese and had no airway issues. The choice of an endotracheal tube may also be dictated by the duration of surgery, excess Trendelenburg position, or high intra-abdominal insufflation pressures.

The choice of maintenance technique includes shorter-acting inhalational agents or total IV anesthesia (TIVA). Nitrous oxide (N_2O) is sometimes used to reduce the requirements of inhaled or IV anesthetics, although some studies show an increase in PONV. Muscle relaxants with longer half-lives can still be used, although diagnostic laparoscopy may be brief in duration.

Local anesthesia

In skilled surgical hands, laparoscopic surgery can be accomplished under local anesthesia. Drives toward more office-based procedures may increase the use of local anesthesia for laparoscopy because of its inherent simplicity. The transverse abdominis plane (TAP) block using a "double-pop" technique or ultrasound guidance to advance the needle into the proper neurofascial plane has been reported to provide excellent analgesia after abdominal surgery.

Postoperative analgesia

The multimodal anesthesia model is quickly becoming popular especially in the ambulatory setting, because postoperative pain is one of the most common factors leading to delays in discharge and an increase in hospital admissions. Table 103.5 shows

Table 103.5. Analgesic modalities for laparoscopic surgery

Modality	Clinical
Nonselective COX or selective COX-2 inhibitors	Multimodal approach to pain management, unless contraindicated
Intraperitoneal local anesthesia	More effective for pelvic procedures
Wound infiltration with local anesthesia	Better in combination with above
Removal of gas (and gasless surgery)	Possible decrease in shoulder pain
Intraperitoneal NS irrigation	Need large volumes (25–30 ml/kg) +/− local
Low intra-abdominal pressure	Decrease in analgesic requirements up to a week postoperatively
N_2O pneumoperitoneum	Pain reduction up to 24 h
Heated, humidified CO_2	Less pain and earlier return to activities
Phrenic nerve block	Decrease in the incidence of shoulder pain, but not analgesic requirements
Mesosalpinx/tubal block	Significant decrease in pain post tubal ligation
Rectus sheath block	Earlier discharge and decreased analgesic requirements
Pouch of Douglas block	+/− catheter, especially helpful post bilateral tubal ligation

NSAIDs, nonsteroidal anti-inflammatory drugs; COX-2, cyclooxygenase-2; NS, normal saline.

various analgesic modalities currently being used for laparoscopic procedures.

Prolapse repair

Genital prolapse (i.e., pelvic organ prolapse) includes cystocele, urethrocele, enterocele, and rectocele as well as uterine prolapse. The laparotomy approach has a fairly high risk of operative hemorrhage usually from the laceration of the sacral veins. Bleeding can be difficult to control if the veins retract into the bone. The majority of gynecologists prefer the use of local anesthesia with epinephrine to obtain hydrodissection between the vaginal mucosa and the bladder and rectum that also diminishes bleeding.

Obliterative vaginal operations such as LeFort's procedure and colpocleisis can be performed under local or regional anesthesia. Most patients are elderly or chronically ill and usually present with severe prolapse. There are at least 130 operative procedures described for the treatment of female urinary stress incontinence. The latest modification is the midurethral sling procedure, either retropubic or transobturator with tension-free vaginal tape (TVT). These procedures have been successfully performed under local anesthesia, sedation, or general anesthesia.

Laparoscopic hysterectomy and myomectomy

Ellstrom and colleagues performed a prospective randomized study to evaluate pain with respect to pulmonary function in the first 48 hours after abdominal versus laparoscopic surgery. Pain scores were lower after laparoscopic hysterectomy on both the first and second postoperative days. Although lung function measured as peak expiratory flow, forced vital capacity, and forced expiratory volume in the first second of expiration was impaired in both groups, the patients who had laparoscopic hysterectomy had less impairment in pulmonary function. The influence on pulmonary function is more pronounced in patients having upper abdominal surgery than in those having lower abdominal surgery. For laparoscopic myomectomy, the potential for blood loss due to myometrial vascularity exists

and needs to be monitored. Surgical techniques to minimize blood loss and the need for blood transfusion include applying a tourniquet around the lower uterine segment to compress the uterine arteries, injecting vasopressin intramyometrially, using intraoperative blood-scavenging devices, correcting anemia preoperatively, donating autologous blood, mild overhydration, and requiring (rarely) a simultaneous hysterectomy.

Suggested readings

Brandsborg B, Nikolajsen L, Hansen CT, et al. Risk factors for chronic pain after hysterectomy. *Anesthesiology* 2007; 106(5):1003–1009.

Cueto-Garcia J, Jacobs M, Gagner M. *Laparoscopic Surgery*. New York: McGraw-Hill; 2003.

Cunningham AJ. Anesthetic implications of laparoscopic surgery. *Yale J Biol Med* 1998; 71:551–578.

Ellstrom M, Olsen MF, Nordberg G, et al. Pain and pulmonary function following laparoscopic and abdominal hysterectomy: a randomized study. *Acta Obstet Gynecol Scand* 1998; 77:923–928.

Gerges FJ, Kanazi GE, Jabbour-Khoury SI. Anesthesia for laparoscopy: a review. *J Clin Anesth* 2006; 18:67–78.

Goulson DT. *Curr Opin Anesth* 2007; Jun 20(3):195–200.

Hohlrieder M, Brimacombe J, Eschertzhuber S, et al. A study of airway management using the ProSeal LMA compared with the tracheal tube on postoperative analgesia requirements following gynecological laparoscopic surgery. *Anaesthesia* 2007; 62:913–918.

Hurt WG. Outpatient gynecologic procedures. *Surg Clin North Am* 1991; 71(5):1099–1110.

Karamanlioğlu B, Turan A, Memiş D, et al. Preoperative oral rofecoxib reduces postoperative pain and tramadol consumption in patients after abdominal hysterectomy. *Anesth Analg* 2004; 98:1039–1043.

Kuramochi K, Osuga Y, Yano T, et al. Usefulness of epidural anesthesia in gynecologic laparoscopic surgery for infertility in comparison to general anesthesia. *Surg Endosc* 2004; 18:847–851.

Lynch EP, Welch KJ, Carabuena JM, Eberlein TJ. Thoracic epidural anesthesia improves outcome after breast surgery. *Ann Surg* 1995; 222(5):663–669.

Pay LL, Lim Y. Comparison of the modified airway management device with the ProSeal LMA in patients undergoing gynecologic procedures. *Eur J Anesthesiol* 2006; 23:71–75.

Tong C, Conklin D, Eisanach JC. A pain model after gynecologic surgery: the effect of intrathecal and systemic morphine. *Anesth Analg* 2006; 103(5):1288–1293.

Chapter 104

Anesthesia for liver transplantation

Jason C. Brookman and Warren S. Sandberg

Introduction

The first successful orthotopic liver transplant in a human occurred in 1967. Since then, transplant complexity and survival rates have improved significantly due to enhanced surgical techniques and immunosuppressive drugs. Liver transplant anesthetics are still some of the most complex currently performed because of the surgical and medical criticality of the patients and because of the complexity of the equipment required. Liver transplantation consumes tremendous resources. At least two anesthesiology personnel and at least two additional professional personnel (i.e., perfusionist, monitoring nurse, auto-transfusion nurse) are assigned to each case in most centers. Many of the considerations for liver transplantation anesthesia apply equally to liver resection. Liver resection surgery has tracked with transplantation – trending toward increasing complexity and magnitude of resection, in increasingly sicker patients, while at the same time reducing morbidity and mortality. Accordingly, this chapter is written largely from the transplantation anesthetic perspective, but most of the material is directly applicable to anesthesia for liver resection.

Pretransplant assessments

Indications, contraindications, patient selection

The indications for orthotopic liver transplantation are numerous (Table 104.1). The most common indication is chronic hepatocellular disease due to alcohol and/or hepatitis. Hepatitis B and C both predispose patients to hepatocellular carcinoma. As the prevalence of hepatitis C in the population increases, so does the incidence of hepatocellular carcinoma, which is becoming an increasingly common indication for liver transplantation. Patients with fulminant hepatic failure are relatively rare but require particular attention, as they may develop daily (or even hourly) contraindications to transplantation.

As surgical techniques, risk stratification of potential recipients, and the management of intercurrent diseases all improve, the contraindications to liver transplantation are becoming more nuanced.

Liver transplantation is a grueling process before, during, and after the operation. To be listed as recipients, patients must be screened by a liver transplant listing committee – made up of surgeons, hepatologists, anesthesiologists, psychiatrists,

addiction specialists, social services specialists, family therapists, and financial assistance experts – that will assist in the patients' continued care before, during, and after the transplant has occurred.

Liver transplant candidates must be willing to accept (potentially) massive blood transfusion during and after surgery, although some centers are able to reliably perform liver transplantation with little or no transfusion. Postoperative intubation, mechanical ventilation, and intensive care unit (ICU) admission are likely, and the patient should be aware of these possibilities. Obese patients with a body mass index (BMI) > 30, considered to be a relative contraindication to

---

Table 104.1. Indications for liver transplantation (not exhaustive)

End-stage liver disease (chronic)
  Hepatocellular disease
    Chronic viral hepatitis (mostly hepatitis C)
    Alcoholic liver disease
    "Cryptogenic" cirrhosis
    Chronic drug-induced liver disease
  Cholestatic disease
    Primary sclerosing cholangitis
    Primary biliary cirrhosis
    Biliary atresia (mostly children)
    Other familial cholestatic syndromes
  Vascular disease
    Budd–Chiari syndrome
    Veno-occlusive disease
  Polycystic liver disease
Hepatic malignancies not amenable to other therapy
  Hepatocellular carcinoma (often in setting of hepatitis C)
  Cholangiocarcinoma
  Carcinoid tumor
  Other cancers (e.g., insulinoma)
Fulminant hepatic failure
  Drug induced hepatic failure
  Acute viral hepatitis (A, B, C, delta)
  Metabolic diseases
    Wilson's disease, organic acidurias, others
Metabolic diseases affecting the liver
  Alpha-1 antitrypsin deficiency
  Hemochromatosis
  Other rare diseases (e.g., Alagille syndrome, glycogen storage diseases, urea cycle deficiencies)

Source: Modified from Sandberg WS, Raines DE. Anesthesia for liver surgery and transplantation. In: Longnecker D, Brown D, Newman M, Zapol W. *Anesthesiology.* New York: McGraw-Hill; 2008, with permission.

Table 104.2. Additional preanesthetic history for the patient with liver disease

1. For the patient with known or suspected liver disease, presenting for surgery
   a. Potential inciting agents/events: blood transfusion, infectious diarrhea, travel, jaundice, hepatitis, tattoos, IV drug use, high-risk sexual activities, medication history, alcohol use history, or contact with other jaundiced patients
   b. Signs and symptoms of aggravation of liver disease: worsening fatigue, malaise, or pruritus; hematemesis, abdominal distention
   c. Neurologic manifestations: altered sleep patterns – especially day/night reversal, or behavioral changes – confusion, excitation, lethargy – indicating encephalopathy
2. For the patient presenting for unscheduled surgery, including liver transplantation
   a. Quality and quantity of recent oral intake
   b. Vascular access and history of previous central venous and/or arterial catheter placement
   c. Cardiovascular risk, focusing on recent screening tests of cardiac function and ischemic risk, recent changes in exercise tolerance (although it may be difficult to differentiate between cardiac dysfunction and worsening liver disease), and especially signs or symptoms of angina
   d. Assessment hepatic synthetic function
      i. Changes in abdominal girth or peripheral edema, indicating insufficient albumin and other plasma protein synthesis to maintain plasma oncotic pressure
      ii. History of easy bruising or prolonged bleeding, indicating insufficient hepatic synthetic function of clotting factors
   e. Assessment of neurologic status, including worsening encephalopathy, as well as focal neurologic deficits, as positioning injuries with consequent neurologic deficits are not uncommon

transplantation, are encouraged to lose weight because obesity is associated with increased perioperative mortality.

Preanesthetic evaluation

The prescreening process to place a patient on the liver transplant list is rigorous. Most patients have had an extensive diagnostic and risk stratification assessment in preparation for liver transplant. Patients for hepatic surgery should be evaluated as indicated by their health status and the surgical severity, with the surgery itself being considered "high-risk" or "major" surgery. The immediate preoperative anesthetic evaluation on the day of surgery should be focused on the history and physical examination relevant to the case immediately at hand (Table 104.2).

The physical examination should be tailored for the patient undergoing major intra-abdominal surgery. Special attention should be paid to the assessment of ascites, as it potentiates the possibility of gastric regurgitation and aspiration, and may compromise pulmonary performance, manifesting as dyspnea and atelectasis secondary to ascites, which further reduces the functional residual capacity [FRC]. Attention should also be paid to sites for vascular access. Landmarks for internal and external jugular cannulation, as well as subclavian access, should be examined, as well as peripheral venous and arterial sites on both arms.

Laboratory tests and diagnostic studies should focus on cardiac performance, pulmonary function, hepatic synthetic and excretory function, coagulation status, hemoglobin, and renal function. Table 104.3 summarizes the most pertinent studies.

For liver transplant recipients, cardiac functional testing proximate to the date of surgery is important, as orthotopic liver transplantation is still, physiologically, a highly stressful operation with potential for sudden, massive, and ongoing blood loss complicated by extreme electrolyte derangements. Untreated significant coronary disease is potentially lethal in the setting of liver transplantation. In one study, half of all patients with coronary artery disease who underwent liver transplantation died in the perioperative period, and the morbidity rate was 81%.

Patients should be able to, hypothetically, tolerate variable periods with heart rates greater than 110 bpm, mean arterial pressure (MAP) < 50 mm Hg, hemoglobin of 7 gm/dl, and pH < 7.2. Most transplant programs use a cardiac risk stratification schema similar to that devised by Plevak. The version used by our program, for example, is shown in Fig. 104.1.

Portopulmonary hypertension is an important contributor to morbidity and mortality in liver transplantation. Half of the patients with mean pulmonary pressures between 35 and 50 mm Hg died in the peritransplant period, and mortality was 100% in those with mean pulmonary artery pressure > 50 mm Hg. Because of this result, patients with moderate to severe portopulmonary hypertension are typically refused transplantation.

Perioperative management

Timing of surgery- and anesthesia-related events must be well coordinated, as one donor typically supplies organs to many

Table 104.3. Preoperative laboratory tests and diagnostic studies for liver transplant patients

All patients-
- Serum albumin and bilirubin (hepatic synthetic function)
- Coagulation studies (prothrombin time, partial thromboplastin time, fibrinogen, and platelet count)
- Hemoglobin/hematocrit
- Blood type and antibody screen
- Serum electrolytes (Na^+, K^+, Cl^-, Ca^{2+}, Mg^{2+}, PO_4^-)
- BUN and creatinine
- Electrocardiogram

Liver transplant recipients (and patients for hepatectomy, as indicated)
- ABG measurement (for both pulmonary and renal function)
- Dobutamine stress echocardiogram (or, possibly, exercise stress thallium imaging test)
- Transthoracic echocardiogram (to exclude structural cardiac disease and portopulmonary hypertension)
- Preoperative chest radiograph
- Pulmonary function testing

BUN, blood urea nitrogen; ABG, arterial blood gas.

Diagnostic Approach to Inducible Myocardial Ischemia

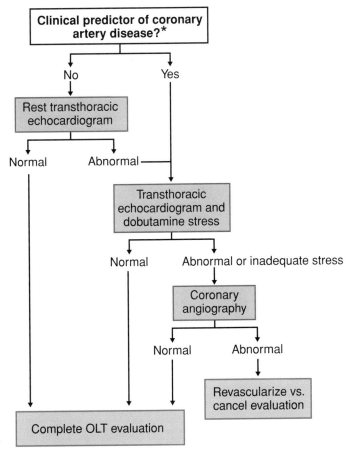

Figure 104.1. Suggested algorithm for assessment of inducible myocardial ischemia. OLT, orthotopic liver transplantation. Modified from Sandberg WS, Raines DE. Anesthesia for liver surgery and transplantation. In: Longnecker D, Brown D, Newman M, Zapol W. *Anesthesiology.* New York: McGraw-Hill; 2008, with permission.

*Clinical predictors
- *History of coronary disease or congestive heart failure*
- *Signs and symptoms of coronary disease or congestive heart failure*
- *Abnormal ECG*
- *Diabetes*
- *Current or prior smoking*
- *Hypertension*
- *Hyperlipidemia*
- *Obesity*
- *Age > 50 for males, > 55 for females
  even in absence of any above*

hospitals, and procedural delays can ripple widely. Liver transplant recipients are usually brought to the operating room (OR) area and undergo several preparatory procedures in advance of knowing whether the donor liver is actually suitable for transplantation. After the harvested organ is deemed suitable, the patient will undergo induction of anesthesia and placement of several invasive monitoring catheters. Concerns and activities during anesthesia for liver transplantation mirror the major phases of the surgery (Table 104.4).

Monitoring and vascular access

Again, many considerations about monitoring apply equally to liver transplant and hepatic resection. Typical monitoring consists of American Society of Anesthesiologists (ASA) standard monitors and selected invasive monitors.

- Blood pressure monitoring is accomplished by an arterial catheter, which is useful for early recognition of hypotension and for obtaining frequent blood samples.
- Central venous pressure (CVP) measurement is useful to guide intravascular volume replacement and to assess right heart pressures when the dissection is expected to be bloody. Central venous access has the added benefit of providing a conduit for potent vasopressor administration.
- A pulmonary artery catheter is sometimes used for measuring pulmonary artery pressures (especially for assessing pulmonary hypertension); assessing left heart

Table 104.4. Liver transplant anesthetic phases

Anesthetic phase	Surgical correlate
• Preinduction	• Beginning of harvest procedure, evaluation of donor organ
• Induction, preparation for surgery, and maintenance	• Donor organ harvest and transport to recipient hospital
• Preanhepatic phase	• Recipient hepatectomy is performed; donor liver is prepared for implantation
• Anhepatic phase	• Vascular anastomoses between the donor liver and recipient's vessels are constructed
• Venous reperfusion of the graft	• Venous clamps removed; surgeon may limit flow of blood through organ to smooth hemodynamic insult
• Neohepatic phase	• Hepatic arterial and biliary anastomoses are constructed; wound is closed
• Emergence/transport to ICU	• Assumption of homeostatic control from the anesthesia team

filling pressures via pulmonary artery occlusion pressure (i.e., wedge pressures); following cardiac output, which is usually elevated to 10 L/min ($\pm$ 2 L/min) in the setting of a hyperdynamic circulation; and guiding pharmacologic therapy in the setting of hypovolemia from dystonic peripheral vasculature.

- Transesophageal echocardiography can also provide information regarding both intravascular volume status and cardiac performance, especially early detection of large embolic events (i.e., air embolus or thrombus).

- Many teams use some form of level-of-consciousness monitoring, often with the goal of minimizing exposure to anesthetic agents and their negative inotropic effects. The interpretation of these data are not straightforward, however, as hepatic encephalopathy itself depresses the bispectral index.

Peripheral vascular access with multiple large intravenous (IV) catheters (i.e., 16 gauge or larger), above the diaphragm, is usually sufficient – this is often the only vascular access placed prior to anesthetic induction. One helpful device is called the rapid infusion catheter (RIC; Arrow International, Reading, PA), an 8.5 French peripherally inserted catheter useful for rapid infusion of large volumes with a high-flow infusion pump. It can be placed in any large peripheral vein. Antecubital or cephalic veins are commonly chosen, but even distal veins on the forearm and hand can be used if they are large enough. The RIC alleviates the need for multiple central lines that might be required to pass a pulmonary artery catheter, run multiple infusions, and accommodate high-flow administration of large volumes.

Another development in the intraoperative management of liver transplant surgery is the use of venovenous bypass (VVB) to decompress the inferior venous systemic and/or portal

circulations. This modality, first described in 1984, maintains venous return to the heart by bypassing the portal circulation after the hepatic vessels have been cross-clamped. VVB is accomplished by actively pumping blood (with flow rates of 1.5–5 L/min) in a circuit usually from the left femoral vein via a percutaneous catheter (inserted by the surgical team), to a large venous vessel that drains into the superior vena cava (SVC) above the liver (i.e., internal jugular vein, subclavian vein, or axillary vein). The anesthesia or surgical team performs the return line cannulation via cutdown to the left axillary vein (by the surgical team) or percutaneously. The portal vein, if accessed, is cannulated intraoperatively via the surgical field. It is important to make sure there is no air in the circuit prior to starting bypass and that all the connections are connected tightly, as any air in the system would be catastrophic.

Induction and maintenance of anesthesia

Liver transplantation produces at least transient hepatic dysfunction, so it may be preferable to choose drugs for which elimination is not completely dependent on hepatic metabolism. In practice, the dose-to-effect mode of administration is almost always sufficient to minimize the interaction between choice of anesthetic and the effect of liver transplantation.

Induction of anesthesia is typically accomplished using standard methods. Careful attention should be directed to adequate denitrogenation, as ascites significantly reduces FRC. Furthermore, patients with ascites should be considered to have a full stomach and receive a rapid-sequence induction with cricoid pressure, if not otherwise contraindicated. Doses of hypnotic drugs, such as propofol or pentothal, should be reduced. Alternately, etomidate may be used to avoid the hemodynamic consequences of propofol. Skeletal muscle paralysis may be achieved either using succinylcholine followed by a nondepolarizing agent (e.g., vecuronium, cisatracurium) or by a rapid-sequence induction dose of rocuronium. Antibiotics directed against skin flora (e.g., cefazolin) should be given no more than 60 minutes before incision and redosed appropriately to account for pharmacologic elimination or loss due to hemorrhage.

Anesthesia is maintained by standard methods. Any commonly used halogenated inhalational agent (e.g., isoflurane, sevoflurane) may be used for maintenance. Many anesthesiologists avoid nitrous oxide, as it can contribute to bowel distension. Intermediate-acting opioids, such as morphine, hydromorphone, or fentanyl, are titrated to meet the patient's needs for analgesia. Paralysis is maintained to facilitate surgical exposure. Like that of antibiotics, readministration of IV drugs must be adjusted to account for losses due to hemorrhage.

Positioning the patient on the operating table is important. The patient is supine, and the right arm is usually tucked to allow for better surgical access. No critical monitors or

Table 104.5. Major foci of intraoperative management during anesthesia for orthotopic liver transplantation

Major focus (problem or organ system)	Subtopics	Related and modifying factors
Cardiac	Ischemic potential Dysrhythmias Right ventricular performance	Hemorrhage (demand and carrying capacity) Acid–base and electrolyte disturbances Emboli, hepatic washout
Portal-to-central venous gradient	Graft perfusion is tenuous	Need to keep CVP adequate to provide cardiac preload during vena cava cross-clamping Need to prevent venous air embolism Sudden hemorrhage
Renal performance	Urine output	Hypovolemia and hypotension Preexisting renal disease Need for intraoperative renal replacement therapy
Anesthesia	Hypnosis Analgesia Muscle relaxation	Patients may not tolerate cardiovascular depression from deep anesthesia
Brain protection	Acute brain herniation can happen, especially in fulminant hepatic failure	Intracranial pressure monitoring risky but helpful Barbiturates and mild hypothermia (34°C) may be helpful
Immunosuppression	Different regimens depending on indication for OLT	
Prophylaxis	Temperature management DVT prophylaxis Preemptive antibiotics	Large incision, large prepped area Dilution due to massive hemorrhage
Glucose management	Coexisting diabetes	Steroid administration Absent gluconeogenesis during anhepatic phase
Coagulation	Hypocoagulable state due to liver failure Platelet sequestration Platelet dysfunction due to uremia	Massive hemorrhage Acute fibrinolysis at graft reperfusion
Electrolytes	Potassium Sodium Calcium	Elevated by K load in blood products Hyponatremic patients at risk for CPM with massive infusions of sodium-rich fluids Citrate in blood products chelates Ca^{2+}
Pulmonary performance	Ventilation Oxygenation Pulmonary vascular resistance	May be impaired by pleural effusions May be impaired by intrapulmonary shunts Acutely elevates in the face of acid load at graft reperfusion
Hemodynamics	Vasodilated hyperdynamic circulation Massive hemorrhage Vena cava compression Possible VVB	

OLT, orthotopic liver transplantation; DVT, deep vein thrombosis; CPM, central pontine myelinolysis.
Modified from Sandberg WS, Raines DE. Anesthesia for liver surgery and transplantation. In: Longnecker D, Brown D, Newman M, Zapol W. *Anesthesiology*. New York: McGraw-Hill; 2008, with permission.

vascular access catheters should be placed in this extremity. The procedure time is long so there is great risk of positioning injuries from many potential pressure points. All pressure points should be supported and padded with viscoelastic gel or soft, compressible foam. The operation is performed through a right-sided subcostal incision extended across the midline to the left subcostal area and sometimes upward along the midline toward the xiphoid.

The surgical preparation for a liver transplant covers the entire abdomen and lower chest, left groin, and, sometimes, the left axilla. This large preparation area makes it initially difficult to maintain satisfactory body temperature. With such a large area exposed, patient warming is important and needed to maintain good clotting performance and to minimize the risk

of surgical site infection. Forced-air warming blankets applied to (1) the lower limbs and (2) the upper chest, left arm, and head and a full under-body unit, all together, are highly effective at maintaining normothermia after the drapes have been applied. IV fluids must be actively warmed during infusion, given the high volume of cooled blood products that are transfused. Warming is usually accomplished by a high-flow warming device which, ideally, has a reservoir for blood products, a debris filter, an air-removal system downstream from the warmer, a pump, and air detectors. Flow capacities are dependent on either the device's pump or the gauge of catheter used.

A summary of the variety of homeostatic goals to which the anesthesia team attends throughout a liver transplant can be found in Table 104.5.

Preanhepatic phase

The preanhepatic phase of the surgery is the point at which a total hepatectomy is being performed.

Surgical approach

After surgical exposure of the hepatic vasculature, the hepatic artery, portal vein, and the common bile duct are clamped and divided in one of two different techniques:

(1) An en bloc technique in which the inferior vena cava (IVC) is clamped above and below the liver, and part of it is resected and replaced with a section of the donor vena cava. This technique causes potentially massive loss of venous return and profound hemodynamic instability. VVB bypass (see Monitoring and Vascular Access above) may be used to minimize these insults.

(2) A "piggyback" technique in which the recipient IVC is preserved and clamped with a side-biting clamp and an end-to-side anastomosis is constructed to the donor liver venous outflow. This method preserves vena cava flow, except for a few minutes during the anastomosis, and may significantly reduce severity of physiologic problems.

While the hepatectomy is being performed, a separate surgical team prepares the graft vessels on the donor liver.

Anesthetic concerns

Clamping the portal triad reduces venous return, although cardiac output and blood pressure do not necessarily decrease. In contrast, cross-clamping the IVC reduces systemic blood pressure and cardiac output secondary to the large reduction in venous return. While moderate decreases in cardiac output and blood pressure can be treated by vasopressor administration, preferably an agent with some inotropic activity (e.g., norepinepherine), and judicious intravascular volume expansion, severe cardiovascular compromise may require institution of VVB. Targeting for CVP between 7 and 10 mm Hg also reduces the incidence of postoperative renal failure and 30-day mortality.

The goals of hemodynamic management (see Table 104.6) are to provide sufficient circulating volume, vascular resistance,

and cardiac output to perfuse the vital organs. This management is guided by urine output, CVP, and minimal vasopressor requirements, except during periods of inadequate venous return.

The goal of volume management and transfusion is to maintain adequate volume to support good circulation. Large-volume hemorrhage requires direct intervention to control the composition of the circulating intravascular volume and coexistent coagulopathy.

Figure 104.2 gives an overview of volume and transfusion management strategies as a function of blood loss during transplantation. Volume replacement therapy should attend to preserving or moving clotting potential toward a normal state as part of the effort to reduce blood loss (see Tables 104.7 and 104.8).

Fluid and blood component replacement strategy

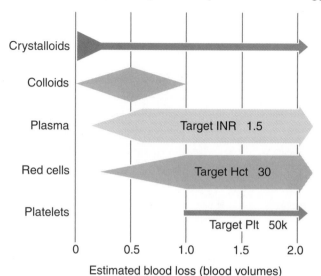

Figure 104.2. High-level overview of one volume and blood component replacement strategy for liver transplantation requiring massive transfusion. All fluids are warmed. The thickness of the bars represents the approximate relative proportions of each fluid in the replacement infusions. Modified from Sandberg WS, Raines DE. Anesthesia for liver surgery and transplantation. In: Longnecker D, Brown D, Newman M, Zapol W. *Anesthesiology*. New York: McGraw-Hill; 2008, with permission.

Table 104.6. Major contributors to hemodynamic changes during liver transplantation

- Episodic alterations in venous return
- Hemorrhage
- Sepsis
- Acidemia
- Hypocalcemia due to citrate toxicity
- Embolism (air or thrombotic)
- Acute right ventricular failure
- Graft reperfusion (due to sudden acid load and temperature decrease)

Table 104.7. Intraoperative transfusion therapies

To maintain intravascular volume	To maintain coagulation capacity
- 5% Albumin - FFP (when coagulopathic) - PRBCs - Good surgical technique	- FFP - Platelets - Epsilon aminocaproic acid (AMICAR; Wyeth-Ayerst, Madison, NJ) – antifibrinolytic - Cryoprecipitate (concentrated source of fibrinogen)

Table 104.8. Serial intraoperative laboratory studies[a]

Parameter	Purpose
Hemoglobin/hematocrit	Gauge volume of blood loss/red cell mass, manage transfusion with RBCs
PT/INR, PTT, platelet count, D-dimer, fibrinogen thromboelastography	Determine coagulation performance (clot initiation, formation, lysis)
ABG	Follow acid–base status, assess/correct acidemia/metabolic acidosis
Electrolytes (Na$^+$, K$^+$, Cl$^-$, Ca^{2+}, Mg^{2+}, PO$_4^-$)	Help assess potentially hemodynamically destabilizing blood levels (i.e., hypocalcemia from chelation by sodium citrate in transfused RBCs and FFP)
Blood glucose	Treat hypoglycemia (or hyperglycemia) during anhepatic phase

[a] Drawn every 30 minutes after the beginning of surgery.
PT, prothrombin time; INR, international normalized ratio; PTT, partial thromboplastin time; ABG, arterial blood gas.

Anhepatic phase

The anhepatic phase of liver transplantation occurs from the point at which the native liver is sufficiently compromised to no longer function (i.e., hepatic artery clamping) until the new liver is reperfused. This is a relatively quiet time, hemodynamically speaking, especially if a piggyback technique or VVB (en bloc resection) is used. Vasopressors may be needed if there is no venous return conduit because of IVC clamping.

The donor liver is brought over from the separate worktable to the surgical field and kept on ice while the vascular anastomoses are completed. It is during the early part of this phase that immunosuppressive drugs are given, usually 100 mg of IV methylprednisolone, to supplement the induction dose of mycophenolate mofetil (CellCept, Roche Pharmaceuticals) given prior to surgery.

Metabolic acidosis may develop in the anhepatic phase due to portal cross-clamping, and partial or complete IVC cross-clamping, in addition to the loss of residual ability to clear organic acids. Ongoing transfusion of low-pH, citrated blood products also contributes to the acidemia, as does a release of an acid load and metabolic waste products during reperfusion. The latter is corrected by hyperventilation and IV sodium bicarbonate.

During the anhepatic phase of liver transplantation, there may be significant changes in potassium balance which favor hyperkalemia. Factors that influence this include infusion of large-volume blood products (e.g., packed red blood cells [PRBCs], fresh frozen plasma [FFP]) with high potassium concentrations, splanchnic ischemia, metabolic acidosis, compromised renal function, and the potassium-rich preservative solution used for the donor liver. Hyperkalemia must be treated to avoid myocardial irritability and cardiac dysrhythmias. Various treatment modalities include potassium-wasting diuretics, bicarbonate, glucose and insulin, and/or continuous venovenous hemofiltration or conventional dialysis in patients with compromised renal function.

Renal failure requiring renal replacement therapy (e.g., dialysis or continuous venovenous hemofiltration) is common after liver transplantation, but is associated with higher mortality rates than in patients who have preserved renal function. Maintaining an adequate circulating volume or a selective medical therapy facilitates preservation of renal function. A commonly used clinical adjunct for assessing renal function is measuring urine output, with a target of 1 ml/kg/h.

Use of large amounts of citrated blood products causes a concomitant reduction in ionized calcium due to chelation. Consequences of hypocalcemia include depressed inotropy and vascular tone and abnormal clotting. Calcium is replaced with calcium gluconate or calcium chloride to achieve the lowest ionized calcium concentration necessary for adequate cardiac performance and coagulation ($\sim$0.9–1.0 mmol/L). After the donor liver is functioning, it readily metabolizes the citrate chelator and may lead to a rebound postoperative hypercalcemia.

Glucose management during liver transplant is usually fairly straightforward. Because the liver is the major site of gluconeogenesis, complete hepatectomy creates the possibility of intraoperative hypoglycemia, although this is rarely a problem in clinical practice.

Neohepatic phase
Graft reperfusion

The neohepatic phase begins with the initial reperfusion of the liver. Volume status and hemodynamic performance must be optimized prior to this event. The perireperfusion period is chaotic, and all potential anesthesia-related distractions (e.g., medication redosing, IV bag/syringe changes, sending laboratory studies) should be addressed prior to this time. Furthermore, abnormalities in pH, K$^+$, and/or Ca^{2+} should be corrected, and sodium bicarbonate, glucose and insulin, and calcium chloride should be prepared and ready for use.

Immediately prior to reperfusion, the donor liver is flushed antegrade from portal vein to hepatic vein with crystalloid, colloid (e.g., 5% albumin) or blood to wash out the potassium- and heparin-rich preservative solution. The venous anastomoses are then sutured closed, and the hepatic vein and portal vein clamps are removed.

Graft reperfusion, with release of residual preservative solution, air, clot, debris, and acidemic blood, is a major insult on cardiovascular performance. Possible consequences include acute pulmonary hypertension causing acute right heart dysfunction with resultant elevation in right heart pressures and CVP, reduced systemic pressure and coronary perfusion pressure due to inadequate left ventricular preload, and, finally, if the multiple insults are significant enough, cardiovascular collapse and cardiac arrest. In preparation for this insult, the patient is often hyperventilated to lower end-tidal carbon dioxide (CO$_2$) and blood pH is increased to induce pulmonary vasodilation. Infusions of vasopressors such as epinephrine, dopamine, and/or norepinephrine should be available and ready for use to support the heart and circulation. Some

Table 104.9. Factors contributing to late blood loss

- Coagulopathy due to synthetic failure
- Thrombocytopenia
- Platelet dysfunction
- Dysfibrinogenemia
- Dilutional coagulopathy
- Hypothermia
- Surgical technical problems with hemostasis
- Acute postreperfusion fibrinolysis syndrome

anesthesiologists also use small prophylactic doses of a vasopressor, such as epinephrine (10-μg boluses), at the time of reperfusion. Selective pulmonary vasodilators, such as inhaled nitric oxide, may be useful at this point. If cardiac arrest occurs, Advanced Cardiac Life Support (ACLS) protocols should be followed, with treatment directed at the presumptive major problem. If necessary, percutaneous venoarterial cardiopulmonary bypass may also be used.

Postgraft reperfusion

After the venous anastomoses are complete and venous reperfusion of the liver has occurred, the hepatic artery anastomosis is constructed to deliver oxygenated blood to the new liver, followed by construction of the bile duct connection, either directly or with a Roux-en-Y anastomosis.

Clotting activity is often deranged during the immediate reperfusion period, as fibrinolysis is increased from reduced clearance of tissue plasminogen activator (t-PA) during the anhepatic phase (see Table 104.9). The anesthesiologist's main goal at this point in the transplant is to stop clot lysis and provide adequate levels of platelets and clotting factors (by way of FFP) to support clotting.

Although controversial in liver transplantation due to concerns of unwanted thrombosis (e.g., clinically significant pulmonary embolism, stroke, myocardial infarction, graft thrombosis), antifibrinolytic agents including aprotinin, tranexamic acid, and epsilon aminocaproic acid have been used to reduce fibrinolysis and transfusion requirements. Use of these agents during liver transplant should be reserved for patients with a high risk of severe hemorrhage. Aprotinin is now of largely historical interest because of an excess morbidity and mortality when used in cardiac surgery.

Postoperative preparations

During the neohepatic phase, the anesthesia team prepares for the postoperative disposition of the patient (see Table 104.10). Most liver transplant recipients are discharged from the OR to an ICU bed. The patient should be transported on an ICU bed, with all necessary infusions running and the patient fully monitored. Although early extubation (i.e., in the OR) is possible and desirable, most patients are left intubated for pulmonary support in the early postoperative period and gradually prepared for extubation within one to two days. Furthermore, although positive end-expiratory pressure (PEEP) may decrease cardiac output, it does not have a major effect on graft function and may be needed to counteract the pulmonary consequences of postoperative intra-abdominal hypertension.

Postoperative pain management is usually relatively straightforward and done with potent opioids (e.g., morphine, hydromorphone). Epidural analgesia is avoided because of the profound perioperative coagulopathy in end-stage liver disease. For some unknown reason, liver transplant patients tend to have less postoperative pain than do hepatectomy patients, although some studies have suggested that immunosuppressive steroids used may have some analgesic effects.

Suggested readings

Biancofiore G, ML Bindi, et al. Fast track in liver transplantation: 5 years' experience. *Eur J Anaesthesiol* 2005; 22(8):584–90.
Bratzler DW, Houck PM. Antimicrobial prophylaxis for surgery: an advisory statement from the National Surgical Infection Prevention Project. *Clin Infect Dis* 2004; 38(12): 1706–15.

Table 104.10. Common complications in liver transplantation and liver surgery

Complication	Consequence	Solution
Massive transfusion	1) Pulmonary edema 2) TRALI 3) Intra-abdominal hypertension 4) Viral infection (e.g., CMV chemoprophylaxis)	Diuresis, controlled phlebotomy Supportive care Leave abdomen open, re-exploration
Anastomotic leaks – Bile ducts – Vascular	Hemorrhage, hematoma, biloma	Re-exploration and anastomotic revision
Vascular anastomotic stenosis/thrombosis	1) Hepatic artery thrombosis (most common) 2) Portal vein thrombosis	1) Diagnosis w/hepatic ultrasound 2) Reoperation for thrombectomy 3) Relisting as Status I for new transplant if defect uncorrectable
Neurologic	1) CPM 2) Peripheral nerve injury	1) Judicious correction of preoperative hyponatremia 2) Proper positioning of retractors, padding

TRALI, transfusion-related acute lung injury; CMV, cytomegalovirus; CPM, central pontine myelinolysis.

Cabezuelo JB, Ramirez P, Acosta F, Torres D, Sansano T, Pons JA, Bru M, Montoya M, Rios A, Sanchez Bueno F, Robles R, Parrilla P. Does the standard vs piggyback surgical technique affect the development of early acute renal failure after orthotopic liver transplantation? *Transplant Proc* 2003; 35:1913–4.

Calne RY, Williams R. Liver transplantation in man. I. Observations on technique and organization in five cases. *Br Med J* 1968; 4(630):535–40.

Figueras J, Llado L, et al. Temporary portocaval shunt during liver transplantation with vena cava preservation. Results of a prospective randomized study. *Liver Transpl* 2001; 7(10):904–11.

Hillingso JG, Wettergren A, et al. Obesity increases mortality in liver transplantation – the Danish experience. *Transpl Int* 2005; 18(11):1231–5.

Krowka MJ, Plevak DJ, et al. Pulmonary hemodynamics and perioperative cardiopulmonary-related mortality in patients with portopulmonary hypertension undergoing liver transplantation. *Liver Transpl* 2000; 6(4):443–50.

Krowka MJ, Mandell MS, et al. Hepatopulmonary syndrome and portopulmonary hypertension: a report of the multicenter liver transplant database. *Liver Transpl* 2004; 10(2):174–82.

Kurz A, Sessler DI, et al. Perioperative normothermia to reduce the incidence of surgical-wound infection and shorten hospitalization. Study of Wound Infection and Temperature Group. *N Engl J Med* 1996; 334(19):1209–15.

Lafayette RA, Pare G, et al. Pretransplant renal dysfunction predicts poorer outcome in liver transplantation. *Clin Nephrol* 1997; 48(3):159–64.

Lentschener C, Roche K, et al. A review of aprotinin in orthotopic liver transplantation: can its harmful effects offset its beneficial effects? *Anesth Analg* 2005; 100(5):1248–55.

Moreno-Gonzalez E, Meneu-Diaz JG, et al. Advantages of the piggy back technique on intraoperative transfusion, fluid compsumption, and vasoactive drugs requirements in liver transplantation: a comparative study. *Transplant Proc* 2003; 35(5):1918–9.

Moretti EW, Robertson KM, et al. Orthotopic liver transplant patients require less postoperative morphine than do patients undergoing hepatic resection. *J Clin Anesth* 2002; 14(6):416–20.

Plevak DJ. Stress echocardiography identifies coronary artery disease in liver transplant candidates. *Liver Transpl Surg* 1998; 4(4):337–9.

Plotkin JS, Scott VL, et al. Morbidity and mortality in patients with coronary artery disease undergoing orthotopic liver transplantation. *Liver Transpl Surg* 1996; 2(6):426–30.

Schumann R. Intraoperative resource utilization in anesthesia for liver transplantation in the United States: a survey. *Anesth Analg* 2003; 97(1):21–8, table of contents.

Schroeder RA, Collins BH, et al. Intraoperative fluid management during orthotopic liver transplantation. *J Cardiothorac Vasc Anesth* 2004; 18(4):438–41.

Shaw BW, Jr, Martin DJ, et al. Venous bypass in clinical liver transplantation. *Ann Surg* 1984; 200(4):524–34.

Spahn DR, Rossaint R. Coagulopathy and blood component transfusion in trauma. *Br J Anaesth* 2005; 95(2):130–9.

Therapondos G, Flapan AD, et al. Cardiac morbidity and mortality related to orthotopic liver transplantation. *Liver Transpl* 2004; 10(12):1441–53.

UNOS website, http://www.UNOS.org, accessed 8/28/07.

Walsh TS, Hopton P, et al. Effect of graft reperfusion on haemodynamics and gas exchange during liver transplantation. *Br J Anaesth* 1998; 81(3):311–6.

Anesthesia for Endocrine Diseases

Balachundhar Subramaniam, editor

Thyroid disorders

Emily A. Singer and Pankaj K. Sikka

Anatomy

The thyroid gland is located in the neck, anterior to the trachea, and between the cricoid cartilage and the suprasternal notch. It consists of a right and left lobe, joined in the middle by the isthmus (see Fig. 105.1). It is a highly vascular organ, fed by the superior and inferior thyroid arteries. It is important to note that the superior thyroid artery is a branch of the external carotid artery and that the inferior thyroid artery is a branch of the thyrocervical trunk, which arises from the subclavian artery. Superior, middle, and inferior thyroid veins are responsible for drainage. It is bordered laterally by the recurrent laryngeal nerves (RLNs), arising from the vagus nerve. In addition, the external branch of the superior laryngeal nerve runs lateral to the upper pole of each lobe. The four parathyroid glands lie posterior to the upper and lower poles of each thyroid lobe.

Physiology

The follicular cells of the thyroid gland produce two circulating hormones, T_3 and T_4. Approximately 80% of circulating thyroid hormone is T_4; however, T_3 is the more active thyroid hormone. The hormones circulate in the blood mainly bound to thyroid binding globulin (TBG) and, to a lesser extent, to albumin. In the periphery, T_4 is converted to T_3 and reverse T_3 (rT_3), which is inactive. T_3 acts on nuclear receptors to influence metabolism. Thyroid hormones increase carbohydrate and fat metabolism, thereby affecting growth and metabolic rate. As a result of their effect on metabolism, they are partially responsible for changes in oxygen consumption, carbon dioxide production, and minute ventilation. They also affect heart rate (HR) and contractility, and therefore, cardiac output.

Thyroid hormone production is dependent on a dietary source of iodine. Lack of iodine produces goiter, and with more severe deficiency, produces hypothyroidism and cretinism. In the gastrointestinal (GI) tract, dietary iodine is reduced to iodide and released into the circulation. Iodide is taken up by the follicular cells of the thyroid gland, where tyrosine is iodinated to form monoiodotyrosine (MIT) and diiodotyrosine (DIT), which are then coupled by an oxidation reaction inside the follicular cells to form T_3 and T_4. This reaction is stimulated by the thyroid-stimulating hormone (TSH) secreted from the anterior pituitary, the production and secretion of which is in turn stimulated by the thyroid-releasing hormone (TRH) secreted from the hypothalamus. Circulating T_3 and T_4 negatively feed back on TSH secretion (Fig. 105.2).

Hyperthyroidism

Hyperthyroidism is a syndrome caused by excessive secretion of thyroid hormones, occurring more commonly in women. The diagnosis is generally made by the presence of a high free T_4 or free T_3 and a low TSH level. Hyperthyroidism is most threatening to the cardiovascular system and can lead to tachycardia, arrhythmias, atrial fibrillation, and congestive heart failure (Table 105.1).

Causes

The most common cause of hyperthyroidism is Graves' disease (multinodular diffuse goiter). The disease is caused by thyroid-stimulating antibody (TSAb), an IgG antibody directed against the TSH receptors of the thyroid follicular cells. Because the TSAb operates outside the normal T_3/T_4–TSH feedback loop, it stimulates the excess production of T_3 and T_4, causing progressive hyperthyroidism that may lead to thyrotoxicosis. Other causes of hyperthyroidism include toxic thyroid adenoma, a functioning thyroid carcinoma, thyroiditis, pregnancy, amiodarone, and radiation therapy.

Treatment

Hyperthyroidism can be treated medically or surgically. Nonemergency surgery, including thyroidectomy, on the hyperthyroid patient should be avoided until the patient is clinically euthyroid. Even after a patient has been rendered euthyroid, antithyroid medications and β-blockers should be given on the morning of surgery.

Medical therapy includes the usage of propylthiouracil (PTU) and methimazole, both of which interfere with thyroid hormone synthesis by inhibiting oxidation and coupling of inorganic iodide. PTU, in addition to its action within the thyroid gland, also inhibits the peripheral conversion of T_4 to T_3. Side effects of antithyroid drugs include agranulocytosis, thrombocytopenia, and hypoprothrombinemia. β-blockers, such as propranolol or atenolol, are effective in controlling the

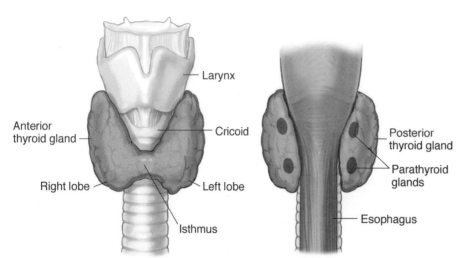

Figure 105.1. Anatomy of the thyroid gland and its relation to the parathyroid glands and the larynx.

adrenergic symptoms of hyperthyroidism. β-blockers decrease tachycardia (goal of HR < 90 bpm), tremor, and anxiety. In addition, they inhibit the peripheral conversion of T_4 to T_3. Nonselective β-blockers should be used cautiously in patients with asthma or congestive heart failure (CHF). Also, glucocorticoids (dexamethasone) may be useful as they inhibit thyroid hormone secretion as well as peripheral conversion of T_4 to T_3.

Medical therapy can be used alone or as a pretreatment to radioiodine thyroid ablation or surgery. Patients should be pretreated with PTU or methimazole prior to radioiodine ablation, in order to diminish the risk of mobilizing the stores of thyroid hormones and therefore worsening the thyrotoxicosis. These medications will need to be stopped approximately 3 days prior to ablation therapy to achieve optimal results. Many patients become hypothyroid after radioiodine ablation and require treatment with levothyroxine (T_4). Subtotal or total thyroidectomy may be used for hyperthyroid patients who have very large goiters, who fail medical or radioiodine therapy, or who are pregnant. Surgery is treatment of choice for thyroid cancer, toxic adenomas, and enlarging thyroid nodules. If a total thyroidectomy is performed, the patient will require levothyroxine therapy postoperatively.

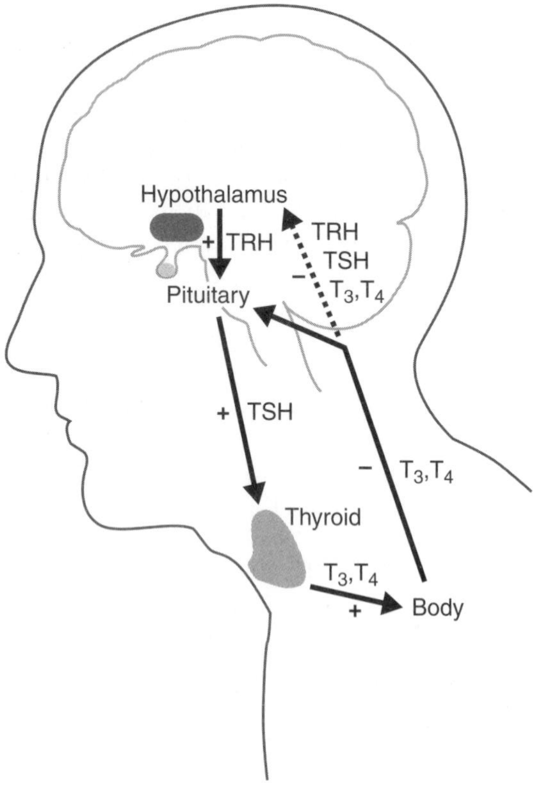

Anesthetic considerations

Patients with goiter should be carefully evaluated for airway difficulties and tracheal deviation. Usually surgery is conducted with endotracheal intubation; however, the use of the laryngeal mask airway (LMA) is becoming increasing popular. The use of LMA allows the visualization of vocal cords in a spontaneously breathing patient. For induction of anesthesia, thiopental, because of its slight antithyroid effect, may be a better choice than other induction agents. Hyperthyroid patients are frequently hypovolemic, and close attention to fluid balance is necessary. In addition, hypovolemia and vasodilation may cause an extreme hypotensive response during induction.

Figure 105.2. Hypothalamus–pituitary–thyroid axis.

Table 105.1. Symptoms and signs of hyperthyroidism

Cardiovascular – Palpitations, tachycardia, elevated systolic blood pressure, CHF, atrial fibrillation, arrhythmias, increased ventricular contractility

Central nervous system – Fine tremor, rapid speech, irritability, restlessness, nervousness, sweating, heat intolerance, hyperactivity, muscle weakness, fatigue

Ophthalmic – Eyelid lag or retraction, proptosis, or exophthalmos

Other – Weight loss, hair loss, diarrhea, oligomenorrhea, leg swelling, pretibial myxedema

If emergency surgery is required for a patient who is currently hyperthyroid, extremely close monitoring of HR, cardiac function, body temperature, and fluid status is critical. Tachycardia, which may induce CHF, can be treated with esmolol (100–300 µg/kg/min IV), titrated to HR, pulmonary artery wedge pressure, and clinical evidence of heart failure. Sympathomimetic drugs (ketamine, pancuronium) should be avoided, as they may cause exaggerated hypertensive and tachycardic responses. Cooling blankets may be necessary for the hyperthermic patient.

Muscle relaxation should be guided by a "twitch monitor" as myopathy and myasthenia gravis are more common in the thyrotoxic patient. Intravenous (IV) steroid administration is recommended to prevent complications from coexisting adrenal suppression. Patients with exophthalmos should have their eyes carefully taped closed to avoid inadvertent corneal abrasion. Although the increased cardiac output may increase the uptake of inhaled volatile anesthetics, MAC (minimum alveolar concentration) is not increased. In addition, the sympathetic blockade provided by regional anesthesia may be beneficial for nonthyroid surgeries in hyperthyroid patients.

Additional anesthetic implications

Because of the intimate physical relationship among the thyroid gland, RLN, and the parathyroid glands, surgical complications can have a direct effect on anesthetic management.

Nerve damage

Damage to only one RLN causes hoarseness, as the paralyzed nerve causes the vocal cord on that side to assume an intermediate position. Damage to both RLNs, a risk associated with total thyroidectomy, causes aphonia and total airway obstruction as the vocal cords fall toward the midline. Damage to the superior laryngeal nerves, which are responsible for sensation above the larynx, causes hoarseness and an increased risk of pulmonary aspiration.

Prevention and early recognition of nerve damage can be pursued through a variety of mechanisms. During surgical dissection, the RLN is identified with the goal of preservation; however, identification can be difficult in a patient with an altered neck anatomy. Endotracheal tubes with external wires to detect electromyographic (EMG) activity from electrical stimulation of the RLN are commercially available. In addition, several studies have shown that the use of a fiber-optic bronchoscope through an LMA can be used by the anesthetist to confirm vocal cord response to electrical stimulation of the RLN by the surgeon. This technique can be used intraoperatively, when working near the RLN territory as well as prior to extubation to confirm patency of the airway. Whether an LMA or endotracheal tube is used, the patient should be asked to phonate (say "e") after extubation. Evidence of bilateral RLN injury should be followed by immediate reintubation, which is often followed by tracheostomy.

Airway issues

Other airway issues may arise from a large goiter, which may cause tracheal compression on induction of anesthesia. These patients should be handled as any other patient with a potential for airway compromise. Sedation should not be excessive, and awake intubation should be considered. A firm endotracheal tube should be used, and should extend past the point of airway compression. Extubation should occur when the patient is fully awake, and the anesthetist should be prepared for reintubation in case the large thyroid gland has caused weakening of the tracheal rings (tracheomalacia) that might lead to airway collapse. Postoperatively, a hematoma at the surgical site can cause airway compromise. Treatment involves opening the wound and evacuating the clot, as well as preparing for intubation or a surgical airway. In addition, extensive neck exploration may lead to an inadvertent pneumothorax, especially in patients with lung disease.

Hypocalcemia

Total thyroidectomy increases the risk of inadvertent parathyroidectomy and resulting hypocalcemia. Hypocalcemia can develop as soon as 1 hour after surgery, but more commonly develops 1 to 3 days postoperatively. Tetany is perhaps the most concerning manifestation of hypocalcemia. The laryngeal muscles are sensitive to hypocalcemia, and inspiratory stridor leading to laryngospasm may be the first sign of hypocalcemia. Treatment includes prompt administration of calcium.

Thyroid storm

Thyroid storm, a life-threatening exacerbation of hyperthyroidism, may occur due to sudden and massive release of thyroid hormones into the circulation. It usually occurs 6 to 24 hours postoperatively, but may occur intraoperatively mimicking malignant hyperthermia. Thyroid storm can also be precipitated by an acute illness or infection, trauma, stroke, surgery, or radioiodine therapy. It is a hypermetabolic state presenting as tachycardia, hyperthermia, and/or arrhythmias and even causes myocardial ischemia or CHF. It is managed (Table 105.2) by administration of PTU (250–500 mg every 6–8 hours) and potassium iodide (250 mg every 6 hours) and by supportive management, including IV fluids, oxygen, and cooling blankets. β-blockers should be used to control the HR, as tachycardia can lead to a high-output heart failure. Steroid administration should be considered: An IV bolus of 10 mg of dexamethasone followed by 2 mg IV every 6 hours decreases peripheral conversion of T_4 to T_3 and treats the relative adrenal insufficiency caused by the hypermetabolic state. The trigger of the thyroid storm should be identified and treated.

Hypothyroidism

Hypothyroidism is a disorder of the thyroid gland associated with a decreased circulation of the thyroid hormones. Diagnosis is made on the basis of an elevated TSH (secreted by the

Table 105.2. Treatment of thyroid storm

Cardiovascular support	• IV hydration with isotonic fluid: D5NS until heart rate (HR) and urine output stable, then D5-1/2NS • Control HR with β-blockers: propranolol in 0.5-mg increments or esmolol drip until HR < 90–100 • Consider corticosteroids: dexamethasone 2 mg q6h or cortisol 100–200 mg q8h

Inhibit thyroid hormone synthesis	• PTU, methimazole
	• Potassium iodide or sodium iodide
	  – 5 drops of potassium iodide (SSKI) q6h starting 1 h after PTU is started
	  – Sodium iodide 1 g over 12 h

Inhibit peripheral conversion	• PTU 600 mg load PO or via NGT, then 200–300 mg q6h • Propranolol
Supportive measures	• Antipyretics, cooling blankets • Oxygen • Nutrition
Enhance clearance	• Cholestyramine (GI clearance) • Plasmapheresis • Hemoperfusion
Treat precipitants	• Treat infection, diabetic ketoacidosis, stroke, etc

D5NS, 5% dextrose in normal saline (0.9% NaCl); D5-1/2NS, 5% dextrose in 0.45% NaCl; PO, by mouth; NTG, nasogastric tube.

pituitary) plus clinical symptoms and signs, which are usually slow to develop (Table 105.3). Thyroid hormone levels may be normal or low. Hypothyroidism often presents in a subacute manner, and its diagnosis is often delayed until symptoms have existed for some time. Often, patients are not aware of their symptoms until after treatment has begun.

Causes

Common causes of hypothyroidism in the United States include autoimmune disease, Hashimoto's (chronic) thyroiditis, and can also be the result of the treatment for hyperthyroidism (drugs, radioiodine, or surgery). Worldwide, iodine deficiency is the most common cause of hypothyroidism. Less common causes include lithium, amyloidosis, sarcoidosis, scleroderma, thyroiditis (postpartum, infectious), pituitary disorders, and hypothalamic disorders.

Table 105.3. Symptoms and signs of hypothyroidism

Slow metabolism – sensitive to drugs

Cardiovascular system – bradycardia, decreased cardiac output and cardiac contractility, pericardial effusion, vasoconstriction, decreased intravascular volume, blunted baroreceptor reflexes, peripheral edema

Central nervous system – lethargy, tiredness, weakness, delayed tendon reflexes, difficulty in concentration, sensitivity to cold, hoarseness of voice, hair loss

Respiratory system – goiter (autoimmune thyroiditis), dyspnea secondary to pleural effusion, sleep apnea, decreased ventilatory drive, weakened diaphragm, decreased production of surfactant

Other – Weight gain but poor appetite, constipation, oligomenorrhea or amenorrhea, carpal tunnel syndrome, decreased cortisol production

Treatment

Hypothyroidism is treated with oral replacement of thyroid hormone (T_4, levothyroxine). An IV preparation is available if oral therapy is not possible or if there is concern that enteral absorption is impaired. The half-life of T_4 is approximately 7 days, and that of T_3 (faster acting than T_4) is approximately 1.5 days. Up to 6 months of replacement therapy may be necessary for full resolution of symptoms. Treatment is guided to a normal TSH value. Angina pectoris may worsen during thyroid hormone replacement, for which the patient may need a cardiac evaluation. Patients with coexisting coronary artery disease are at risk of myocardial ischemia with administration of IV levothyroxine; therefore, emergency coronary revascularization should be considered for those patients with severe hypothyroidism and severe coronary disease.

Anesthetic considerations

As with patients with hyperthyroidism, those with severe hypothyroidism or myxedema coma should not undergo elective surgery until they have achieved a euthyroid state, although mild to moderate hypothyroidism is not an absolute contraindication to surgery. Patients requiring emergency surgery should be treated with IV levothyroxine (100–500 μg IV). Patients with hypothyroidism are sensitive to drug-induced respiratory depression and have decreased response to hypoxia. Therefore, premedication with respiratory depressants, such as benzodiazepines, should be done with caution, and narcotic doses should be minimized in favor of nonopioids, such as ketorolac. Anesthetic requirements (such as minimum alveolar concentration) are not decreased in hypothyroid patients. However, gastric emptying may be delayed in hypothyroid patients; H_2-antagonists and promotility agents, such as metoclopramide, may prove beneficial.

Because hypothyroid patients have decreased cardiac output, decreased intravascular volume, and blunted baroreceptor reflexes, profound hypotension on induction should be prevented. This goal can be achieved by induction with ketamine or by the use of a traditional induction agent (such as thiopental or propofol) with ephedrine (or other vasoactive medications). If hypotension is refractory, steroid administration should be considered, as coexisting adrenal insufficiency is not uncommon. Fluid and electrolyte balance should be monitored carefully and treated with appropriate IV solutions. Because body temperature regulation is altered in hypothyroidism, intraoperatively the patient's temperature should be monitored and maintained in the normal range. As with hyperthyroidism, there is an increased incidence of myasthenia gravis in patients with hypothyroidism. Therefore, neuromuscular blockade should be used with caution. Because recovery from general anesthesia may be prolonged, extubation should be done when the patient is normothermic, awake, and breathing adequately. Regional anesthesia may be a reasonable choice for anesthesia as long as intravascular volume is maintained.

Myxedema coma is a severe form of hypothyroidism and is a medical emergency. It presents with the features of hypothyroidism (Table 105.3) as well as a depressed level of consciousness (stupor, coma), profound hypothermia, hypoventilation, hypotension, hyponatremia, and occasionally seizure activity. The disease is most common in the elderly population and is usually precipitated by sepsis or illness that cause impaired ventilation, such as pneumonia, CHF, stroke, myocardial infarction, or GI bleeding. Sedatives, anesthetics, and antidepressants may also be the precipitating factors. Treatment involves IV levothyroxine and supportive care, which includes ventilatory support, external rewarming, and electrolyte and fluid management. Steroids (hydrocortisone) may be administered, as severe hypothyroidism is associated with impaired adrenal function. Any precipitating illnesses should be aggressively managed.

Suggested readings

Aunac S, Carlier M, Singelyn F, De Kock M. The analgesic efficacy of bilateral combined superficial and deep cervical plexus block administered before thyroid surgery under general anesthesia. *Anesth Analg* 2002; 95:746–750.

Coe NPW, Lytle GH, Mancino AT. Surgical endocrinology: thyroid gland. In: Lawrence PF, ed. *Essentials of General Surgery*. 3rd ed. Philadelphia: Lippincott, Williams, & Wilkins; 2006:386–394.

Eltzschig HK, Posner M, Moore FD. The use of readily available equipment in a simple method for intraoperative monitoring of recurrent laryngeal nerve function during thyroid surgery: initial experience with more than 300 cases. *Arch Surg* 2002; 137:452–457.

Jameson JL, Weetman AP. Disorders of the thyroid gland. In: Braunwald E, Fauci AS, Kasper DL, et al., eds. *Harrison's Principles of Internal Medicine*. 15th ed. New York: McGraw-Hill; 2001:2060–2083.

Mermelstein M, Nonweiler R, Rubinstein EH. Intraoperative identification of laryngeal nerves with laryngeal electromyography. *Laryngoscope* 1996; 106:752–756.

Moore KL, Dalley AF. *Clinically Oriented Anatomy*. 4th ed. Philadelphia: Lippincott, Williams & Wilkins; 2009:1035.

Roizen MF, Fleisher LA. Anesthetic implications of concurrent diseases. In: Miller RD, ed. *Anesthesia*. 6th ed. Philadelphia: Elsevier; 2004:1045–1048.

Scheuller MC, Ellison D. Laryngeal mask anesthesia with intraoperative laryngoscopy for identification of the recurrent laryngeal nerve during thyroidectomy. *Laryngoscope* 2002; 112:1594–1597.

Snyder SK, Roberson CR, Cummings CC, Rajab MH. Local anesthesia with monitored anesthesia care vs general anesthesia in thyroidectomy: a randomized study. *Arch Surg* 2006; 141:167–173.

Stoelting R, Miller R. *Basics of Anesthesia*. 4th ed. Philadelphia: Churchill Livingstone; 2000:310–313.

Anatomy and physiology

The parathyroid glands are responsible for the tight regulation of plasma calcium concentration. They are small (35–50 mg), paired structures located posterior to the thyroid gland, although anatomic variation is not uncommon. The inferior glands, derived from the third pharyngeal pouch, can be found undescended at the carotid bulb, under the thyroid capsule, intrathyroidal, or in the anterior mediastinum within the thymus. The superior glands, derived from the fourth pharyngeal pouch, are more consistent in their location but may migrate down the tracheoesophageal groove into the middle mediastinum or may be retropharyngeal. In addition, some individuals may have fewer or more than four glands.

Parathyroid hormone (PTH) is an 84-amino-acid peptide, the principal effector sites of which are the bone and kidney. Although the interaction of PTH with bone is complex and incompletely understood, PTH has both anabolic and catabolic actions that allow for early rapid mobilization of calcium stores followed by a slow sustained release. In the kidney, PTH acts at multiple sites to increase both calcium reabsorption and phosphate excretion. In addition, it up-regulates the renal enzyme that converts inactive 25-hydroxyvitamin D_3 to the active 1,25 dihydroxyl form, facilitating calcium absorption in the gastrointestinal tract.

The vast majority of the body's calcium stores are found in bone as insoluble hydroxyapatite. Soluble extracellular calcium exists either as a non-ionized albumin-bound form or as a free ion in close to a 1:1 ratio. It is the ionized form that is physiologically active and maintained within a narrow concentration in the plasma (1.0–1.3 mM). Ionized calcium $[Ca^{2+}]$ is sensed by the parathyroids via direct stimulation of a cell-surface, G-protein–coupled receptor. A drop in $[Ca^{2+}]$ is met with a rapid increase in PTH secretion from preformed granules in chief cells. If $[Ca^{2+}]$ is not promptly restored, the hypocalcemic signaling mechanism sequentially works to increase PTH synthesis, PTH mRNA, and ultimately cellular hypertrophy and proliferation. Conversely, when $[Ca^{2+}]$ increases, PTH secretion is suppressed.

Hyperparathyroidism and hypercalcemia
Primary hyperparathyroidism

Primary hyperparathyroidism is the most common cause of hypercalcemia in outpatients. In 80% to 90% of cases a solitary parathyroid adenoma is the culprit. Multiglandular hyperplasia accounts for most of the remaining cases. Parathyroid carcinoma is an uncommon etiology (<1%). Primary hyperparathyroidism is frequently silent or subtle. Early symptoms are nonspecific and may include muscle weakness, fatigue, and vomiting. Early detection and treatment have decreased the incidence of other organ system involvement, which may be widespread and frequently correlates with the degree of hypercalcemia (Table 106.1). Hypercalcemic crisis is a life-threatening condition characterized by profound dehydration, nausea and vomiting, weakness, and mental status changes. If untreated, it will lead to oliguric renal failure, cardiac arrhythmias, and death. Treatment of hypercalcemia is outlined in Table 106.2.

Surgery is the only definitive treatment for primary hyperparathyroidism and has a 95% cure rate. Some controversy remains over which patients should undergo surgery, particularly older asymptomatic individuals. Although treatment options must always be individualized, there is a trend toward recommendation of parathyroidectomy for all patients with a definitive diagnosis of primary hyperparathyroidism.

Table 106.1. Manifestations of hypercalcemia

Cardiac	Hypertension, LVH, arrhythmias, shortened QT interval
Renal	Nephrolithiasis, renal tubular acidosis, polyuria, polydipsia
Gastrointestinal	Nausea and vomiting, anorexia, constipation, peptic ulcer, pancreatitis
Neurologic	Fatigue, confusion, psychosis, decreased pain sensation
Neuromuscular	Muscle weakness, hyporeflexia
Skeletal	Osteopenia, vertebral body fractures, aches and pains

LVH, left ventricular hypertrophy.

Table 106.2. Treatment of hypercalcemia

Rehydration:
  1/2 NS or NS at 250–500 ml/h ± furosemide, 20–100 mg q2h
  Avoid thiazide diuretics
  Vigilant electrolyte monitoring
Bisphosphonates:
  Pamidronate 30–90 mg over 2–4 h
  Zoledronate 2–4 mg over 15 minutes

NS, normal saline.

Secondary hyperparathyroidism

Secondary hyperparathyroidism occurs when chronic hypocalcemia stimulates PTH secretion and parathyroid hyperplasia ensues without intrinsic parathyroid disease. The most common cause is chronic renal failure, owing to deficient vitamin D synthesis and hyperphosphatemia. Deficiency or malabsorption of vitamin D (rickets, osteomalacia) is another possible etiology. Medical treatment is the mainstay of therapy and consists of calcium and vitamin D supplementation as well as phosphate restriction. Surgery is sometimes necessary when conservative measures are inadequate and symptoms are severe (particularly bone manifestations and pruritus). Parathyroidectomy, performed as either a subtotal procedure in which a portion of one gland is left in situ, or rarely as a total parathyroidectomy with autograft placement (typically in the forearm), improves symptoms in 80% of patients.

Tertiary hyperparathyroidism

Tertiary hyperparathyroidism occurs when autonomous oversecretion of PTH persists despite correction of the underlying disease (i.e., after renal transplantation) due to a failure of the hyperactive glands to adapt to a normal renal handling of calcium and phosphate. These glands usually return to normal size and function within 12 months; parathyroidectomy is rarely necessary.

Multiple endocrine neoplasia (MEN) types I or II and non-MEN-related familial hyperparathyroidism may also warrant parathyroidectomy under certain circumstances.

Anesthesia for parathyroidectomy

Conventional parathyroidectomy comprises a bilateral neck exploration, identification of all four parathyroids, and resection of enlarged glands. Adequacy of resection can be assessed using intraoperative PTH monitoring. A decline in PTH by more than 60% 15 minutes after resection of an enlarged gland is highly specific in predicting a cure. Frozen section is useful only to confirm that parathyroid tissue has been resected but is unreliable in distinguishing a normal from a hyperplastic gland.

General anesthesia with endotracheal intubation is most commonly employed, although an LMA could be considered in select patients, acknowledging the potential risk of laryngeal edema with airway compromise. Anesthetic considerations for the hypercalcemic patient include maintaining adequate hydration and urine output and vigilantly monitoring

electrocardiography (ECG). Hypercalcemia can enhance the toxicity of digoxin. Response to nondepolarizing muscle relaxants may be variable as patients with skeletal muscle weakness may have decreased requirements, and hypercalcemia itself may antagonize the drug's effect. Osteoporosis warrants special care in positioning. Given the risk of recurrent laryngeal nerve (RLN) injury, some surgeons advocate evaluating the position of the vocal cords during extubation. Whereas complete paralysis of the nerve leaves the vocal cord in a half abducted position, a partial lesion of the RLN renders the vocal cord in an adducted position, and a bilateral partial RLN injury may be life-threatening. Emergence from anesthesia should be as smooth as possible as hypertension, coughing, and bucking can increase the risk of postoperative hematoma formation.

Given that the majority of cases of primary hyperparathyroidism are due to a solitary adenoma, there has been debate in the surgical literature about the need for a bilateral neck exploration. If a unilateral exploration or minimally invasive parathyroidectomy (MIP) is considered, patients must first undergo preoperative localization with technetium (99mTc) sestamibi scintigraphy. Ultrasound is also frequently used to delineate anatomy. The approach may be open or video-assisted with an endoscope. Randomized controlled trials comparing the techniques have shown that cure rates and complications were no different than the conventional approach, but patients undergoing the unilateral approach had a lower incidence of postoperative hypocalcemia (symptomatic and biochemical) and shorter operating times.

Anesthesia for MIP may be general or regional, using a superficial or deep cervical plexus block, although a block necessitates a considerable degree of patient cooperation. In studies comparing general versus regional anesthesia, patients who underwent MIP with a block had better pain control and less postoperative nausea and vomiting. Length of stay, cure rate, and complications were similar. Furthermore, assessment of the RLN may be performed intraoperatively under regional anesthesia.

Complications of parathyroidectomy

Transient hypocalcemia following parathyroidectomy is common, and symptoms, if present, are usually mild and may include paresthesias of the lips and fingertips. Oral calcium supplementation begun the night of surgery minimizes the incidence and severity of this complication, which is generally self-limiting, resolving in a few weeks. Symptoms of acute hypoparathyroidism and hypocalcemia (tetany, fatigue, seizures) are of particular concern and warrant immediate evaluation and ionized calcium (or albumin-corrected serum calcium) determination. Patients undergoing subtotal parathyroidectomy for secondary or tertiary hyperparathyroidism are at higher risk of developing severe symptoms. Treatment for symptomatic patients consists of an initial bolus followed by a continuous intravenous (IV) infusion of calcium gluconate titrated to resolve symptoms, and possibly oral or IV calcitriol (1,25-OH-vitamin D). Magnesium levels must also be monitored as

Table 106.3. Symptoms and treatment of hypocalcemia

Symptoms of hypocalcemia	Neurologic: Paresthesias (Chvostek, Trousseau signs), tetany, hyperactive reflexes, muscle cramps/weakness, seizures Respiratory: Laryngospasm, bronchospasm Cardiac: Arrhythmias, hypotension, bradycardia, QT prolongation
Treatment of hypocalcemia	$[Ca^{2+}] > 0.8$ mM – Usually asymptomatic $[Ca^{2+}]$ 0.5–0.8 mM – May have mild symptoms; calcium replacement $[Ca^{2+}] < 0.5$ mM – Potentially life-threatening • Ensure an adequate airway is present • IV calcium supplementation required: 100–200 mg of elemental calcium over 10 minutes followed by maintenance 1–2 mg/kg/h until levels normalize (usually 6–12 h), then continue at 0.3–0.5 mg/kg/h • Oral calcium supplementation should be given as soon as possible to supply 1–4 g daily. • Calcitriol, start with 0.25 μg daily, and titrate up to maintain normocalcemia • Vigilant electrolyte monitoring and magnesium repletion
Chemical conversions	1 g of calcium gluconate = 93 mg of elemental calcium 1 g of calcium chloride = 272 mg of elemental calcium

hypomagnesemia aggravates hypocalcemia, rendering the latter refractory to treatment. Treatment of hypocalcemia is outlined in Table 106.3.

Postoperative inspiratory stridor may occur following parathyroidectomy for several reasons that must be considered in the differential diagnosis: laryngeal edema, hematoma, hypocalcemia, and bilateral RLN palsy (Table 106.4). The most common etiology is laryngeal edema. Treatment with inhaled racemic epinephrine is most effective, although corticosteroids may be necessary for refractory cases. Hematoma complicates 0.3% of parathyroid explorations. The diagnosis is made by inspection of the surgical site for neck swelling, pain, pressure, or discoloration. Re-exploration is mandatory and, in the case of severe airway compromise, may need to be performed at the bedside. Acute hypocalcemia after parathyroidectomy must be ruled out, but administration of IV calcium should not be delayed while the ionized calcium level is pending. RLN injury is uncommon (0%–0.8% for unilateral injury), and the use of RLN monitoring is not routinely necessary. Prevention of injury is best accomplished by avoidance of electrocautery, vigorous dissection, or ultrasonic devices near the nerve. Most patients who develop this complication will improve over the course of months, although patients in whom re-exploration was undertaken are at higher risk for permanent paralysis. Bilateral RLN

injury is even rarer but, if present, requires intubation and systemic steroid administration.

Last, operative failure and persistent hyperparathyroidism may complicate up to 5% of initial explorations. Surgical expertise is a significant factor, and surgeons who perform fewer than 10 parathyroidectomies per year had a lower rate of cure than did more experienced surgeons. Failed surgery is nearly always preventable, and patients who require re-exploration have a greater frequency of complications.

Suggested readings

Aguilera IM, Vaughan RS. Calcium and the anaesthetist. *Anaesthesia* 2000; 55:779–790.

Bergenfelz A, Kannigiesser V, Zielke C, et al. Conventional bilateral cervical exploration versus open minimally invasive parathyroidectomy under local anesthesia for primary hyperparathyroidism. *Br J Surg* 2005; 92:190–197.

Black MJ, Ruscher AE, Lederman J, Chen H. Local/cervical block anesthesia versus general anesthesia for minimally invasive parathyroidectomy: what are the advantages? *Ann Surg Oncol* 2007; 14(2):744–749.

Carty SE. Prevention and management of complications in parathyroid surgery. *Otolaryngol Clin N Am* 2004; 37:897–907.

Chen H. Surgery for primary hyperparathyroidism: what is the best approach? *Ann Surg* 2002; 236:552–553.

Fitzgerald PA. Endocrinology. In: Tierney LM, McPhee SJ, Papadakis MA, eds. *Current Medical Diagnosis & Treatment* 2005. New York: McGraw-Hill; 2005:1113–1120.

Guyton AC, Hall JE. Parathyroid hormone, calcitonin and phosphate metabolism, vitamin D, bone, and teeth. In: Guton AC, Hall JE, eds. *Textbook of Medical Physiology*. 9th ed. Philadelphia: W.B. Saunders Company; 1996:985–1002.

Marx SJ. Hyperparathyroid and hypoparathyroid disorders. *N Engl J Med* 2000; 343:1863–1875.

Miccoli P, Barellini L, Monchik JM, et al. Randomized clinical trial comparing regional and general anaesthesia in minimally invasive video-assisted parathyroidectomy. *Br J Surg* 2005; 92:814–818.

Mihai R, Farndon JR. Parathyroid disease and calcium metabolism. *Br J Anaesth* 2000; 85:29–43.

Stoelting RK, Dierdorf SF. Endocrine diseases. In: Stoelting RK, Dierdorf SF, eds. *Anesthesia and Co-Existing Disease*. 4th ed. Philadelphia: Churchill Livingstone; 2002:421–425.

Table 106.4. Postoperative stridor management

Laryngeal edema	• Most common etiology • Treat with inhaled racemic epinephrine, possibly corticosteroids
Hematoma	• Signs: neck swelling, pain, pressure, discoloration • Protect airway; immediate surgical evacuation
Hypocalcemia	• Look for signs and symptoms • Protect airway; IV calcium replacement (do not wait for laboratory result)
RLN injury	• Vocal cord paralysis of varying degree, weak voice, hoarseness • Laryngeal examination to evaluate • Bilateral injury may be life-threatening; protect airway, systemic steroids

Pheochromocytoma

Deborah S. Pederson

Pheochromocytoma is a rare neuroendocrine tumor that can manifest in severe hypertension, cardiac arrhythmias, heart failure, stroke, renal failure, and (rarely) death. Ideally, the diagnosis will be known preoperatively if the patient is scheduled for surgery to remove the tumor, or it may be previously unrecognized. Therefore, it is important that anesthesiologists be familiar with the disease, its presentation, and its management (see Fig. 107.1).

Etiology

Pheochromocytomas are a heterogeneous group of neuroendocrine-secreting tumors that arise from chromaffin cells. Although they are most known for secreting catecholamines, the tumors may secrete a variety of other substances, including neuropeptide Y, dopa, vasoactive intestinal polypeptide (VIP), serotonin, calcitonin, and adrenocorticotropic hormone (ACTH). They are primarily found in the adrenal glands (90%); however, they may occur in extra-adrenal sites along the sympathetic nervous system, where they are referred to as *paragangliomas.*

The annual incidence of pheochromocytoma is two to eight per million per year. The disease may occur at any age, with the peak incidence in the third to sixth decades. Men and women are equally affected. Ten percent of pheochromocytomas are bilateral and 10% are malignant, as defined by distant metastasis. Approximately 25% of pheochromocytomas occur as part of a hereditary disorder, with associated syndromes such as multiple endocrine neoplasia (MEN 2A and MEN 2B), von Hippel–Lindau disease, neurofibromatosis type 1, tuberous sclerosis, and familial paraganglioma (PGL1 and PGL4).

Pathophysiology

The manifestations of pheochromocytoma are the result of elevated levels of plasma catecholamines combined with an up-regulated sympathetic nervous system. These factors lead to increased afterload and decreased capacitance, with subsequent effects on end organs. These effects may include left heart strain with hypertrophy or (rarely) dilated cardiomyopathy, cardiac irritability, pulmonary edema, renal impairment, and stroke. The presentation is variable (see Table 107.1) but can range

from asymptomatic with detection only at autopsy to severe life-threatening disease.

The mechanism of hypertension in pheochromocytoma is not completely understood. Elevated levels of plasma catecholamines are considered the hallmark of pheochromocytoma. This is unlikely the sole mechanism, however. Bravo and Tagle observed a poor correlation between circulating catecholamine levels and the presence of elevated blood pressure. In a series of 34 patients with known pheochromocytoma, they found increased levels of catecholamines in patients with elevated mean arterial pressure; however, the degree of hypertension did not correlate with the plasma catecholamine concentration. Additionally, Bravo published a case report

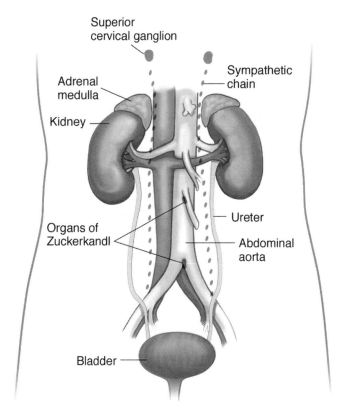

Figure 107.1. Anatomic distribution of pheochromocytomas and paragangliomas.

Table 107.1. Signs and symptoms of pheochromocytoma

Signs	Symptoms
Hypertension – may be paroxysmal	Headache
Weight loss	Palpitations
	Diaphoresis
	Syncope

demonstrating the lack of temporal relationship between catecholamine levels and hypertension. These data suggest that hypertension associated with pheochromocytoma is multifactorial.

Diagnosis

The prevalence of pheochromocytoma is 0.2% to 0.4% among hypertensive patients. Although it must be considered in the differential diagnosis of hypertension, not all patients with pheochromocytoma are hypertensive. In fact, only 50% to 60% of patients with pheochromocytoma have hypertension, and half of these people have paroxysmal episodes. The classic triad of headache, diaphoresis, and palpitations is present in 15% to 25% of patients. Thus, the absence of hypertension or the common clinical symptoms does not exclude the disease.

Traditionally, 24-hour urinalysis with high-performance liquid chromatography (HPLC) for metanephrines and vanillylmandelic acid (VMA) have constituted the laboratory test for pheochromocytoma. More recently, analysis of plasma free metanephrines has proven superior for pheochromocytoma detection with a sensitivity of >95% and a specificity of >80%. Imaging is becoming increasingly useful, particularly in diagnosing metastatic disease. CT, MRI, MIBG (metaiodobenzylguanidine; a functional scan using a guanethidine analogue), and PET scans have all been used to aid in the diagnosis.

The clonidine suppression test can be used to diagnose pheochromocytoma when traditional tests are inconclusive. Studies have suggested that the sympathetic nervous system plays a significant role in producing hypertension. In a study of patients with either essential hypertension or known pheochromocytoma, the administration of clonidine lowered blood pressure in both groups. In the essential hypertensive patients, clonidine lowered catecholamine levels; however, it had no effect on plasma catecholamines in the pheochromocytoma group. This finding suggests that the sympathetic nervous system has a direct role in mediating hypertension in pheochromocytoma. When the sympathetic nervous system is blocked by a centrally acting α_2-agonist agent, the patients are normotensive despite elevated plasma catecholamine levels. This is the basis for the clonidine suppression test to diagnose pheochromocytoma.

Preoperative management

The two issues that must be addressed preoperatively are control of blood pressure and replacement of intravascular volume. The state of chronically increased vascular tone leads to hypovolemia, which is manifest clinically by orthostatic hypotension and elevated hematocrit. Patients with known pheochromocytoma must be evaluated for end organ dysfunction. An elevated serum creatinine level may reveal renal disease and an electrocardiogram arrhythmias, myocardial infarction, or ventricular hypertrophy. Occasionally the presentation can be severe and involve cardiomyopathy. If symptoms of left heart failure, such as dyspnea, orthopnea, or decreased exercise tolerance, are present, an echocardiogram to further assess cardiac function is warranted.

Preoperative antihypertensives (see Table 107.2) combined with volume replacement (either oral or intravenous [IV]) are indicated prior to elective surgery. Traditionally α-blockade was used to decrease peripheral vascular resistance; however, case reports with calcium channel blockers and combined α- and β-blockade have proven to be effective. Given the low incidence of the disease, it is unlikely that randomized controlled trials will ever establish a preferred regimen.

α-Blockers

Historically, nonspecific α-blockade with phenoxybenzamine to achieve preoperative blood pressure control was associated with a decrease in surgical mortality from 40% to 0% to 1%. The drawback of this drug is its long half-life, which may result in hypotension when the tumor is removed. Selective α_1-blockade (prazosin, doxazosin, and terazosin) has the benefit of sparing the presynaptic α_2-receptors; therefore, these drugs do not enhance norepinephrine release and do not lead to reflex

Table 107.2. Medications used preoperatively to control hypertension in pheochromocytoma

Drug	Site of action	Properties
Phenoxybenzamine	Noncompetitive, nonselective α-blocker	Long-acting, risk of hypotension post-tumor excision, reflex tachycardia (due to inhibition of presynaptic α_2-receptors)
Prazosin	Selective α_1-blocker	Decreased incidence of reflex tachycardia due to sparing of α_2-receptors
Labetalol	α- and β-blocker (1:7)	Works predominantly at β-receptors
Propranolol	Nonselective β-blocker	Give only after initiation of α-blockade to avoid unopposed α effects
Atenolol	β_1-blocker	Long-acting selective β_1-antagonist
Nifedipine	Calcium channel blocker	Less likely to produce orthostatic hypotension

Table 107.3. Medications used intraoperatively to control hypertension in pheochromocytoma

Drug	Site of action	Initial dose IV	Properties
Nitroprusside	Direct arteriovenous vasodilator	0.5–2 µg/kg/min; titrate to effect up to 10 µg/kg/min	Short and rapid acting; potent vasodilator
Esmolol	Selective β_1-antagonist	250–500 µg/kg/min IV load followed by infusion (50–300 µg/kg/min)	Short acting; can be used to treat tachydysrhythmias
Phentolamine	Nonselective α-antagonist	Bolus 2–5 mg IV, infusion- 0.5–1 mg/min	Short acting; can result in tachycardia and tachyphylaxis
Magnesium sulfate	Anti-adrenergic and direct vasodilator	Bolus 40 mg/kg, infusion 1–2 g/h, goal 2–4 mmol/L plasma concentration	May prolong nondepolarizing neuromuscular blockade

tachycardia. Additionally, they are shorter acting and therefore less likely to result in postoperative hypotension.

β-Blockers

β-blockade is contraindicated without pre-existing α-blockade to prevent unopposed α_1-mediated vasoconstriction. Nonselective β-blockade is most useful in patients with arrhythmias, but may also be used for blood pressure control. It should be avoided in patients with catecholamine-induced cardiomyopathy as it may lead to heart failure.

Calcium channel blockers

Calcium channel blockers inhibit the norepinephrine-mediated release of intracellular calcium in vascular smooth muscle cells leading to a decrease in peripheral vascular resistance. The primary advantage of using calcium channel blockers is the absence of orthostatic and perioperative hypotension.

When the patient is normovolemic and normotensive for >24 hours and is without significant arrhythmias, it is safe to proceed with elective surgery.

Intraoperative management

The goal of intraoperative management is to maintain normal hemodynamics despite stimulating events such as laryngoscopy, surgical incision, and tumor manipulation. This goal is achieved using a multimodal approach largely based on blockade of the sympathetic nervous system. Regional and general anesthesia techniques have been used, with general anesthesia being most common. Drugs that are known to stimulate the sympathetic system, such as pancuronium or ephedrine, should be avoided.

The surgical approach can be laparoscopic or open. In the case of laparoscopic surgery, the introduction of pneumoperitoneum may stimulate the release of catecholamines and should be anticipated. Studies comparing laparoscopic resection versus open resection of pheochromocytoma have demonstrated equivalent intraoperative hemodynamic control. Laparoscopic resection, however, results in decreased length of stay, decreased intensive care unit (ICU) admission, and decreased postoperative pain. Additionally, laparoscopy allows for superior visualization of the adrenal vein, facilitating ligation. Regardless of

the technique, fluctuations in blood pressure are highly dependent on surgical manipulation. Communication with the surgical team will allow for anticipation of hypertension, as is likely to occur with tumor handling, as well as hypotension, which can be dramatic after ligation of the tumor's venous drainage.

IV access, standard monitors, and invasive blood pressure monitoring are necessary prior to induction. Central venous access may be useful to assess volume status and deliver potent vasoconstrictors. Pulmonary artery catheterization or transesophageal echocardiography is indicated only if it will impact intraoperative management in patients with severely compromised cardiac function.

Preoperative pharmacologic regimens are generally not effective in blunting the hemodynamic response during tumor manipulation and surgical stimulation. Intraoperative blood pressure control is achieved by the use of short-acting modulators of the cardiovascular system as indicated in Table 107.3.

Postoperative management

Postoperatively, the major concern is continued hemodynamic instability; therefore, it is recommended the patient be monitored for hemodynamic lability at least 24 hours postoperatively. Persistent hypertension can result from the release of increased stores of catecholamines. Fluid resuscitation as well as vasopressors are used to treat hypotension. Blood glucose levels should be checked to rule out hyper- or hypoglycemia.

Suggested readings

Barash PG, Cullen BF, Stoelting RK. *Clinical Anesthesia.* 5th ed. Philadelphia: Lippincott, Williams & Wilkins; 2006.

Bravo E, Tagle R. Pheochromocytoma: state-of-the-art and future prospects. *Endocr Rev* 2003; 24(4):539–553.

Bravo EL. Pheochromocytoma: an approach to antihypertensive therapy. *Ann NY Acad Sci* 2002; 970:1–10.

Elder EE, Elder G, Larsson C. Pheochromocytoma and functional paraganglioma syndrome: no longer the 10% tumor. *J Surg Oncol* 2005; 89:193–201.

James MFM. Use of magnesium sulphate in the anaesthetic management of phaeochromocytoma: a review of 17 anaesthetics. *Br J Anaesth* 1989; 62:616–623.

James MF, Cronje L. Pheochromocytoma crisis: the use of magnesium sulfate. *Anesth Analg* 2004; 99:680–686.

Kinney M, Narr B, Warner M. Perioperative management of pheochromocytoma. *J Cardiothorac Vasc Anesth* 2002; 16(3):359–369.

Prokocimer R, Maze M, Hoffman B. Role of the sympathetic nervous system in the maintenance of hypertension in rats harboring pheochromocytoma. *J Pharmacol Exp Ther* 1987; 241:870–874.

Reisch N, Peczkowska M, Januszewicz A, Neumann H. Pheochromocytoma: presentation, diagnosis and treatment. *J Hypertens* 2006; 24(12):2331–2339.

Chapter 108

SIADH, diabetes insipidus, and transsphenoidal pituitary surgery

John Summers and Balachundhar Subramaniam

Antidiuretic hormone (ADH), also known as vasopressin, is a nonapeptide neurohormone synthesized in the hypothalamus and released by the posterior pituitary in response to increases in serum osmolarity and decreased extracellular volume. Osmoreceptors in the hypothalamus can detect changes in serum osmolarity of as little as 1% (normal is 285 mOsm/L), whereas stretch receptors in the left atrium sense changes in blood volume. Many other factors, such as pain, nausea, sympathetic stimulation, positive pressure ventilation, and hyperthermia, also affect ADH release.

One of the most important functions of ADH is to conserve body water. In the absence of ADH, the collecting ducts of the kidney are almost impermeable to water allowing it to flow out as urine. In the presence of ADH, however, aquaporins (water channels) are inserted into the principal cells of the collecting ducts allowing free water to be reabsorbed into the hypertonic renal medulla.

ADH also has other physiologic functions. The term *vasopressin* was coined from the observation that high concentrations of ADH results in widespread constriction of arterioles – primarily in the splanchnic, renal, and coronary vessels. ADH has also been found to play a role in hemostasis by increasing levels of factor VIII and von Willebrand factor. Disruptions in this process from either too much (syndrome of inappropriate ADH secretion [SIADH]), too little (central diabetes insipidus [DI]), or abnormal responses to ADH (nephrogenic DI) will be the subject of this chapter.

SIADH

Too much ADH results in water intoxication. Although there are numerous etiologies of SIADH (Table 108.1), the clinical manifestations remain the same: oliguria, concentrated urine, and signs of hyponatremia. As serum sodium concentrations drop below 125 mEq/L, osmotic fluid shifts lead to cerebral edema and increased intracranial pressure resulting in nausea and anorexia (early signs), followed by confusion, weakness, agitation, muscle cramps, obtundation, seizures, and ultimately coma. As the condition worsens, cardiac and other life-threatening complications may occur when serum sodium concentrations drop below 105 mEq/L. The severity of the symptoms also depends on how quickly hyponatremia develops. Chronic hyponatremic patients with sodium of 120 mEq/L

may show no clinical symptoms. Of note, it has been shown that premenopausal women are more susceptible to the effects of hyponatremia than are men.

Laboratory studies to aid in the diagnosis of SIADH include measuring the osmolarity and sodium levels in both the urine and serum. The presence of hyponatremia and a urine osmolarity higher than maximal dilution (generally >200 mOsm/L) confirm the diagnosis. Other pertinent laboratory test results include a decreased (dilutional) serum uric acid, FeNa >1%, urinary sodium >30 mEq/L, normal potassium (hyperkalemia, hyponatremia, and acidosis may be from adrenal insufficiency rather than SIADH), and normal glucose (serum sodium is decreased by 1.6 mEq/L for every 100 mg/dl increase in glucose). Hyponatremia in the setting of polyuria may indicate cerebral salt-wasting syndrome. Pseudohyponatremia occurs with severe hyperlipidemia and hyperproteinemia (as in multiple myeloma).

Treatment of SIADH is primarily water restriction. Three percent hypertonic saline and furosemide may be needed, however, in symptomatic hyponatremia or when fluid restriction is not possible. Lithium and demeclocycline interfere with the renal tubules' ability to concentrate urine and may be used for chronic hyponatremia. In the event of SIADH from subarachnoid hemorrhage, fluid restriction may worsen the condition as it may promote cerebral vasospasm and infarction secondary to hypotension. The rate of sodium correction should not exceed 12 mEq/L in the first 24 hours so as to minimize the risk of central pontine myelinosis. Calculations for corrections are shown in Table 108.2.

Table 108.1. Causes of SIADH

Paraneoplastic syndromes	Small cell lung cancer
CNS processes	Multiple sclerosis, tumors, head trauma, delirium tremens, Guillain–Barré syndrome, infection
Pulmonary processes	Pneumonia, tuberculosis, positive-pressure ventilation
Drugs	TCAs, chlorpropamide, clofibrate, NSAIDs, nicotine
Endocrine	Hypothyroidism
Sympathetic activation	Postoperative pain

CNS, central nervous system; TCAs, tricyclic antidepressants; NSAIDs, nonsteroidal anti-inflammatory drugs.

Table 108.2. Replacement of sodium

Sodium deficit:
Na deficit = (Desired Na − Measured Na) × 0.6 × (Weight in Kg)
Volume of hypertonic saline needed for correction:
Volume of 3% saline = (Na Deficit)/513 mEq Na/L
Time needed for correction = (Desired Na − Measured Na)/
0.5 mEq/L per hour
Rate of infusion = (Volume of 3% saline)/(Time needed for
correction)

Anesthetic considerations for SIADH include identifying and correcting any underlying disorder as well as optimizing the patient for surgery. In general, elective surgeries should be postponed until the patient's sodium level is corrected to >130 mEq/L, even if he or she is asymptomatic. Lower sodium concentrations may result in cerebral edema, especially in surgeries with large potential fluid shifts, such as in transurethral resection of the prostate.

Diabetes insipidus

Inadequate ADH activity results in water wasting. DI is divided into central and nephrogenic etiologies. Central DI results from decreased production or release of ADH. Nephrogenic DI is caused by the inability of ADH to act normally on the kidneys. Causes of DI are listed in Table 108.3. Clinically, DI is characterized by polydipsia and polyuria, which may be accompanied by hypovolemia and hypernatremia (dehydration) if access to free water is restricted. Laboratory studies include serum sodium and osmolarity along with urine sodium and osmolarity.

Treatment depends on both the cause of DI (central vs. nephrogenic) and the extent of the ADH deficiency. For central DI, serum osmolarity and serum levels should be measured on a regular basis and be treated accordingly. Options for treatment include intravenous (IV) administration of aqueous ADH (100–200 mU/h), intramuscular (IM) vasopressin, and intranasal desmopressin, which has a low incidence of pressor effects. If the patient does not have complete DI, the stress of surgery alone may induce enough ADH secretion to compensate. If plasma osmolarity is less than 290 mOsm/L in a patient with incomplete DI, treatment is usually not necessary during a procedure. On an outpatient basis, clofibrate and

chlorpropamide (an oral hypoglycemic) have been used for incomplete central DI. The best treatment for nephrogenic DI is to treat the underlying disorder (Table 108.3). Thiazide diuretics, however, are known to have a paradoxic antidiuretic action in nephrogenic DI by effecting increased sodium losses.

Anesthetic considerations mainly involve correcting any fluid deficits or existing hypernatremia. Elective cases should be delayed until sodium levels are less than 150 mEq/L.

Anesthetic considerations of transsphenoidal surgery: pituitary tumors

Pituitary tumors are often hypersecretory, and medical therapy is not curative. As a result, surgery for these tumors is commonly performed. These tumors are common in the fifth to seventh decade of life. Tumors more than 10 mm in diameter are called *macroadenomas*. Nonfunctioning tumors tend to present as larger tumors as they are nonsecretory and are detected later. Craniopharyngioma and Rathke cleft cyst are some examples of nonfunctioning tumors. The common functioning tumors are *microadenomas* and can be Cushing disease (hypersecretion of adrenocorticotropic hormone [ACTH]), acromegaly (growth hormone–secreting adenoma), prolactinoma (prolactin hypersecretion), and hyperthyroidism (thyrotrophic hormone oversecretion). These individual diseases have been dealt with elsewhere in this section. The anesthetic considerations of transsphenoidal surgery for pituitary tumor resection will be discussed here.

Anesthetic considerations

The anesthetic considerations include managing the

(a) hypersecretory endocrine systemic effects;
(b) local mass effects, such as increased intracranial pressure, headache, and vision loss;
(c) hypopituitarism due to tumor compression of the anterior pituitary gland; and
(d) understanding of surgical approach, such as endonasal or older sublabial transseptal approach. The endonasal approach has a lower incidence of postoperative DI and a shorter recovery period.

Table 108.3. Causes of diabetes insipidus

Central	Idiopathic (up to 50% of cases)	Autoimmune process with destruction of cells of the hypothalamus
	Surgery	Transsphenoidal resection of an adenoma may result in DI in up to 60% of patients with large tumors
	Trauma	Severe head injury, basal skull fracture, subarachnoid hemorrhage
	Tumors	Craniopharyngioma, pineal tumors
	Other	Hypoxic encephalopathy, anorexia nervosa, sarcoidosis, arteriovenous malformations
Nephrogenic	Drugs	Lithium, demeclocycline, foscarnet, glyburide, methoxyflurane, amphotericin B
	Familial (rare)	Autosomal dominant
	Collecting system insults	Medullary cystic disease, ureteral obstruction

Preoperative evaluation should include:

(a) complete hematological assessment;
(b) airway assessment, especially in patients with acromegaly;
(c) metabolic panel to look for electrolyte and glucose derangements; and
(d) specific endocrine disorders, such as hyperthyroidism, and their systemic effects.

Intraoperative management

The transsphenoidal approach is performed with a mild head-up position to favor venous drainage. Venous air embolism is a possible risk with such a patient positioning. The mucosal surfaces are infiltrated with lidocaine and epinephrine to decrease bleeding and improve surgical dissection. This infiltration has the potential for arrhythmogenicity and hypertension. Hypertensive episodes are common with this type of surgery and should be treated to bring the patient's blood pressure closer to baseline blood pressure. The potential for blood loss is usually limited; however, the proximity of major vessels can lead to massive hemorrhages. There is a potential for cerebrospinal fluid (CSF) leak, and a Valsalva maneuver may be used to check these leaks. The potential for obstructive sleep apnea will mean careful extubation and may be an oral airway left in situ. The nares are packed postoperatively and make the nasal breathing difficult.

Postoperative complications

The postoperative complications are listed below:

- Cranial nerve dysfunction
- CSF leakage
- Nausea and vomiting
- Pain
- DI
- SIADH
- Hypopituitarism

Managing pituitary tumors requires a multidisciplinary approach for successful outcome following surgery.

Suggested readings

Barash PG, Cullen BF, Stoelting RK. *Clinical Anesthesia*. 5th ed. Philadelphia: Lippincott Williams & Wilkins; 2006:1149–1150.

Earley LE, Orloff J. The mechanism of antidiuresis associated with the administration of hydrochlorothiazide to patients with vasopressin-resistant diabetes insipidus. *J Clin Invest*. 1962; 41(11):1988–1997.

Miller RD, Fleisher LA, Johns RA, et al. *Miller's Anesthesia*. 6th ed. Philadelphia: Elsevier Health Sciences; 2005:1766.

Robertson GL. Diabetes insipidus. *Endocrinol Metab Clin North Am* 1995; 24(3):549–572.

Soupart A, Decaux G. Therapeutic recommendations for management of severe hyponatremia: current concepts on pathogenesis and prevention of neurologic complications. *Clin Nephrol* 1996; 46(3):149–169.

Weissman C. The metabolic response to stress: an overview and update. *Anesthesiology* 1990; 73(2):308–327.

Chapter 109

Disorders of the adrenal cortex

John Summers and Balachundhar Subramaniam

The adrenal cortex synthesizes three distinct classes of hormones: glucocorticoid, mineralocorticoids, and androgens. Our main focus will be on disorders of cortisol – the principal glucocorticoid (produced by the zona fasciculata) – and aldosterone – the most important mineralocorticoid (produced in the zona glomerulosa). Androgens, made in the zona reticularis, are less relevant to our anesthetic evaluations and therefore will not be discussed further in this chapter.

Glucocorticoids

Cortisol has many physiologic effects, such as gluconeogenesis, inhibition of glucose uptake in muscle and adipose tissue, mobilization of amino acids from extrahepatic tissues, and stimulation of fat breakdown in adipose tissue. It also has anti-inflammatory and immunosuppressive properties. These effects are mediated by an intracellular glucocorticoid receptor that controls transcription from a number of genes, leading to changes in the cell's phenotype. Therefore, the effects of cortisol last longer than its plasma half-life of 80 to 110 minutes. In the plasma, only approximately 10% of cortisol is free, with the rest bound to plasma proteins – mostly to corticosterone-binding globulin (CBG). CBG is thought to both prolong the life of plasma cortisol and act as a buffer to swings in plasma cortisol levels by serving as a depot. Only free cortisol is available to enter cells and mediate the physiologic effects and therefore is the best marker for cortisol activity. The kidneys excrete unbound cortisol; therefore, a urinary cortisol is the most accurate way to measure its activity.

Regulation of cortisol is mediated via a negative feedback loop (Fig. 109.1). Corticotropin-releasing factor (CRF) from the hypothalamus stimulates the release of adrenocorticotropic hormone (ACTH) from the anterior pituitary, which in turn directly controls cortisol secretion. CRF and ACTH release are stimulated by stress (psychological or physical), inhibited by cortisol, and affected by the sleep–wake cycle. In the absence of stress, ACTH release follows a diurnal pattern with the highest levels just after awakening followed by another lesser peak later in the day. For hospitalized patients, cortisol is dosed twice daily, with a higher dose in the morning so as to follow these natural fluctuations. Glucocorticoids may also exert mild mineralocorticoid effects at high levels.

Cushing syndrome

Cushing syndrome is the result of an excess of glucocorticoid activity. The many causes of Cushing syndrome may be broadly divided between ACTH-dependent and ACTH-independent etiologies. The vast majority of ACTH-independent Cushing syndrome cases are caused by exogenous administration of glucocorticoids. Other causes include adrenocortical adenomas and carcinomas. Cushing disease occurs from an ACTH-secreting pituitary tumor and accounts for 70% of ACTH-dependent Cushing syndrome. The remainder of ACTH-dependent Cushing syndrome cases is due to ectopic secretion of ACTH – usually from tumors of the lung (small-cell), pancreas, or thymus (carcinoid tumors from neuroendocrine cells in those tissues). Only approximately 1% arises from ectopic corticotropin-releasing hormone (CRH) secretion. Signs and symptoms of Cushing syndrome include central obesity, moon facies, muscle wasting and weakness, glucose intolerance, hypertension, and mental status changes. Glucocorticoids may exert some mineralocorticoid effects as well, resulting in hypervolemia and a hypokalemic metabolic alkalosis.

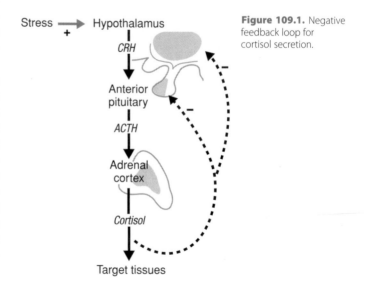

Figure 109.1. Negative feedback loop for cortisol secretion.

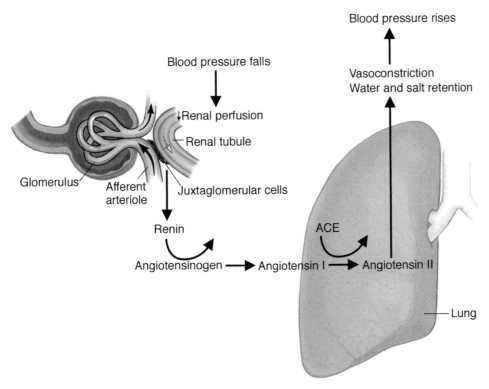

Figure 109.2. Renin–angiotensin system.

Anesthetic considerations

Anesthetic considerations include:

(a) correcting any electrolyte abnormalities, such as hypokalemia;

(b) administering spironolactone (a potassium-sparing diuretic) to deal with volume overload;

(c) potentially difficult airway due to moon facies; mask ventilation may be particularly difficult; and

(d) difficult IV placement due to fragile veins.

Easy bruising may lead to difficulty in positioning these patients. In addition, stress dose steroids should be administered in patients with exogenous steroid use as outlined later in the section "Perioperative steroid use."

Mineralocorticoids

The principal mineralocorticoid is aldosterone, which maintains volume and electrolyte homeostasis by increasing sodium reabsorption and increasing potassium and hydrogen ion excretion. Regulation of aldosterone is primarily influenced by the renin–angiotensin system. Hyperkalemia, prostaglandin E, and ACTH also stimulate aldosterone release. The juxtaglomerular cells surrounding the afferent arterioles release renin in response to decreased renal perfusion pressure and sympathetic stimulation (b_1-adrenoceptors). Renin then cleaves angiotensinogen into the decapeptide angiotensin I, which is then enzymatically cleaved to the octapeptide angiotensin II in the lungs by angiotensin-converting enzyme (ACE).

Angiotensin II is a potent vasoconstrictor and also stimulates the release of aldosterone by the adrenal cortex (see Fig. 109.2). The macula densa adjacent to the juxtaglomerular apparatus inhibits renin release when it senses elevated levels of sodium and chloride in tubular fluid.

Addison disease

Adrenal insufficiency may result from a defect anywhere in the hypothalamic–pituitary–adrenal (HPA) axis. Primary adrenal insufficiency occurs from the destruction of the adrenal cortex and results in depletion of both mineralocorticoids and glucocorticoids. Autoimmune destruction of the adrenal gland is the most common cause of Addison disease in the United States, whereas tuberculosis is the most common cause in developing countries. Other possible etiologies of adrenal gland destruction include infectious (e.g., fungal, HIV, bacterial), neoplastic, traumatic, vascular (e.g., hemorrhage, emboli, thrombus), metabolic (amyloidosis), and iatrogenic (exogenous steroids) events. Patients may remain asymptomatic until 90% of the adrenal gland has been destroyed. Clinical signs of Addison disease include chronic fatigue, muscle weakness, anorexia, weight loss, nausea, vomiting, diarrhea, and hyperpigmentation. Decreased levels of adrenal cortex hormones interrupt the feedback inhibition of the HPA axis and result in elevated levels of corticotropin and melanocyte-stimulating hormone (MSH). MSH is formed when corticotropin is cleaved from its prohormone. Elevated levels of MSH result in the characteristic bronze appearance. Hyperkalemia, hypovolemia, hyponatremia, and metabolic acidosis result from mineralocorticoid deficiency and may lead to associated clinical manifestations, such as cardiac dysrhythmias. Secondary adrenal insufficiency as a result of inadequate ACTH production by the pituitary is not associated with cutaneous hyperpigmentation or mineralocorticoid deficiency. Acute Addisonian crisis presents as refractory hypotension, shock, abdominal pain, severe vomiting, and diarrhea. In critically ill patients, Addisonian crisis may resemble sepsis without a source of infection.

Treatment involves replacement of mineralocorticoids and glucocorticoids. Normal daily endogenous production of cortisol is approximately 20 mg with maximal output at 150 to 400 mg in a day. Usually patients are placed on fludrocortisone and prednisone or hydrocortisone for prolonged therapy.

Anesthetic considerations

Anesthetic concerns involve avoiding acute adrenal insufficiency, which is an emergency and is managed with

(a) an IV bolus of 100 mg of hydrocortisone, followed by an additional 100 mg every 6 hours for 24 hours;
(b) IV isotonic crystalloid fluids; and
(c) correction of any electrolyte abnormalities, such as hyperkalemia and hyponatremia.

The use of stress dose steroids is covered in the section on perioperative steroid use.

Primary hyperaldosteronism

Increased secretion of aldosterone from the adrenal cortex is usually caused by an adrenal adenoma (Conn syndrome) or adrenal hyperplasia. Increased levels of aldosterone result in

(a) hypertension,
(b) hypervolemia (without edema),
(c) suppressed renin activity, and
(d) hypokalemic metabolic alkalosis.

Primary hyperaldosteronism is now thought to be the most common form of secondary hypertension.

Anesthetic considerations

Anesthetic considerations include

(a) correcting any electrolyte abnormalities. This usually involves potassium supplements and spironolactone (an aldosterone antagonist) and
(b) correcting any volume overload.

Patients may also have glucose intolerance from hypokalemia and low ionized calcium secondary to alkalosis.

Hypoaldosteronism

Decreased secretion of aldosterone from the adrenal cortex may be congenital, result from prolonged heparin use, or be caused by certain medical problems, such as renal failure or diabetes. Low levels of aldosterone may result in a hyponatremic, hyperkalemic metabolic acidosis if left untreated. These patients should be treated with 0.05 to 0.1 mg of fludrocortisone preoperatively to correct any electrolyte abnormalities followed by close electrolyte monitoring throughout the surgery.

Perioperative steroid use

In 1952 Fraser and colleagues first described cardiovascular collapse attributed to iatrogenic adrenal insufficiency in the setting of surgical stress. Since that time, many studies have tried to form a consensus on the proper perioperative administration of steroids. Most anesthesiologists have used the recommendations described by Kehlet, Symreng and colleagues, and Salem and colleagues. These state, "New recommendations are proposed which suggest that the amount and duration of glucocorticoid coverage should be determined by: (a) the preoperative dose of glucocorticoid taken by the patient, (b) the preoperative duration of glucocorticoid

Table 109.1. Glucocorticoid treatment regimens

Patients currently taking glucocorticoids	Prednisone 5 mg/d or dexamethasone 1 mg/d or equivalent	Minor surgery (e.g., herniorraphy)	Hydrocortisone 25 mg at induction
		Moderate surgery (e.g., TAH)	Usual daily glucocorticoid dose + hydrocortisone 25 mg at induction + 100 mg/d for 24 h
		Major surgery (e.g., CABG)	Usual daily glucocorticoid dose + hydrocortisone 25 mg at induction + 100 mg/d for 48–72 h
	High-dose immunosuppression	Any surgery	Give usual immunosuppressive doses During perioperative period
Patients who have taken glucocorticoids within the last year	Prednisone 5 mg/d or dexamethasone 1 mg/d or equivalent	Minor surgery (e.g., herniorraphy)	Hydrocortisone 25 mg at induction
		Moderate surgery (e.g., TAH)	Hydrocortisone 25 mg at induction + 100 mg/d for 24 h
	Major surgery (e.g., CABG)	Hydrocortisone 25 mg at induction + 100 mg/d for 48–72 h	

TAH, total abdominal hysterectomy; CABG, coronary artery bypass graft; HPA, Hypothalamic Pituitary Axis.

Table 109.2. Relative potencies of common glucocorticoids

Steroid	Relative glucocorticoid potency	Relative mineralocorticoid potency	Equivalent glucocorticoid dose, *mg*
Short acting			
Cortisol (hydrocortisone)	1.0	1.0	20.0
Cortisone	0.8	0.8	25.0
Prednisone	4.0	0.8	5.0
Prednisolone	4.0	0.8	5.0
Methylprednisolone	5.0	0.5	4.0
Intermediate acting			
Triamcinolone	5.0	0	4.0
Long acting			
Dexamethasone	30.0	0	0.75

Note: Synthetic glucocorticoid varies in both their potencies and mineralocorticoid effects.

administration, and (c) the nature and anticipated duration of surgery." Suggested steroid treatment regimens are outlined in Table 109.1. Current literature states that hypotension in patients previously treated with glucocorticoids is caused by a loss of the permissive effect of glucocorticoids on vascular tone, which may be related in turn to enhanced prostaglandin I_2 (PGI_2) production in the absence of glucocorticoids. It is not caused by mineralocorticoid deficiency. Therefore, if the mineralocorticoid effects are not needed, it seems reasonable to administer the equivalent dose of dexamethasone (Table 109.2) to reap the added benefit of its antiemetic properties.

Physiologic adrenal response to surgery is blunted by anesthesia and will be delayed until the postoperative period. Patients who have taken supplemental steroids greater than 5 mg of prednisone a day for more than a week are theoretically at risk for HPA suppression for up to 1 year. Recovery from short courses of treatment (e.g., 5 days) occurs much more rapidly. Other sources suggest that stress dose steroids are appropriate for a year after a patient takes lower doses (e.g., 5 mg of prednisone) by any route for longer than 2 weeks. Of note, etomidate suppresses adrenal function for at least 24 hours and is affected by both (a) the dose administered and (b) if there is coadministration of an opioid. Long-term use of etomidate may cause severe glucocorticoid deficiency.

Possible side effects of intraoperative steroid use include impaired wound healing, psychiatric disturbances, and glucose intolerance. Topical vitamin A has been shown to decrease the effect of steroids on wound healing by stabilizing lysosomes. All things considered, although the probability of acute adrenal insufficiency is quite small, it is a potentially life-threatening conditioning and therefore skews the risk–benefit curve in favor of providing stress steroids.

Suggested readings

Axelrod L. Perioperative management of patients treated with glucocorticoids. *Endocrinol Metab Clin North Am* 2003; 32(2):367–383.

Barash PG, Cullen BF, Stoelting RK. Endocrine function. In: *Clinical Anesthesia*. 6th ed. Philadelphia: Lippincott Williams & Wilkins; 2009:1279–1304.

Chin R. Adrenal crisis. *Crit Care Clin* 1991; 151(1):185–189.

Ehrlich HP, Hunt TK. Effects of cortisone and vitamin A on wound healing. *Ann Surg* 1968; 167(3): 324–328.

Fraser CG, Preuss FS, Bigford WD. Adrenal atrophy and irreversible shock associated with cortisone therapy. *J Am Med Assoc* 1952; 149(17):1542–1543.

Kehlet H. A rational approach to dosage and preparation of parenteral glucocorticoid substitution therapy during surgical procedures. A short review. *Acta Anaesthesiol Scand* 1975; 19(4): 260–264.

Nicholson G, Burrin JM, Hall GM. *Anaesthesia* 1998; 53(11): 1091–1104.

Oyama T, Taniguchi K, Jin T, et al. Effects of anaesthesia and surgery on plasma aldosterone concentration and rennin activity in man. *Br J Anaesth* 1979; 51:747.

Rivers EP, Gaspari M, Abi Saad G, et al. Adrenal insufficiency in high-risk surgical ICU patients. *Chest* 2001; 119(3):889–896.

Salem M, Tainsh RE Jr, Bromberg J, et al. Perioperative glucocorticoid coverage. A reassessment 42 years after emergence of a problem. *Ann Surg* 1994; 129(4):416–425.

Symreng T, Karlberg BE, Kagedal B, Schildt B. Physiological cortisol substitution of long-term steroid-treated patients undergoing major surgery. *Br J Anaesth* 1981; 53(9):949–954.

Wagner RL, White PF, Kan PB, et al. Inhibition of adrenal steroidogenesis by the anesthetic etomidate. *N Engl J Med* 1984; 310(22):1415–1421.

Malignant hyperthermia

Matthew C. Martinez and John D. Mitchell

Malignant hyperthermia (MH) is a rare, inherited disease involving two or more transmembrane proteins in skeletal muscle that is induced by specific anesthetic agents in almost all cases. The incidence of MH ranges from 1:5000 to 1:50,000–100,000 anesthetics. It affects humans, but can also affect pigs, dogs, cats, horses, and (most likely) other animals. The disease is characterized by hypermetabolism of muscle cells following the administration of a triggering agent, and is thought by some to be associated with heat intolerance.

Etiology

MH was first described by Denborough and Lovell in 1960. They encountered a patient who had 10 of his close relatives die while either under general anesthesia or immediately following a procedure. An investigation into the genetics of this patient's family revealed an inborn error of metabolism that seemed to be inherited as a dominant trait.

Mutations in the skeletal sarcoplasmic reticulum (SR) calcium release channel (ryanodine receptor, RyR1), which is responsible for excitation–contraction (EC) coupling, are the source of the majority of MH cases. EC coupling is the event that translates an action potential into a mechanical event. The action potential depolarizes a muscle cell and allows a conformational change and a small initial influx of calcium via slow voltage-gated calcium channels (dihydropyridine receptors, DHPRs). In skeletal muscle, the conformational change in the DHPR then triggers a large release of calcium stored in the SR through direct signaling to RyR1, and unlike the case in heart and skeletal muscle, this Ca^{2+} release does not require Ca^{2+} entry through the DHPR. The calcium then binds troponin and initiates the interaction of actin and myosin that are translated into a muscle contraction. In cases of MH, one or more of these calcium channels are affected, and large amounts of calcium are released from the SR.

The inheritance pattern in families with MH is thought to be autosomal dominant with variable penetrance. There have been multiple genes linked to MH, with specific mutations found in two of them. The RyR gene, which is found on chromosome 19 and plays a part in EC coupling, is the most studied of these genes. The DHPR gene, which encodes a voltage-gated Ca^{2+} channel, is another gene known to have mutations in MH-susceptible patients. Mutations in these genes can lead to altered function of the calcium release channels, which leads to increased calcium release from the SR. Mutations in the RyR gene were the first to be considered as the cause of MH, but they have been shown to account for just 50% to 80% of the studied cases.

Triggering agents

The two types of drugs known to trigger MH in humans are all depolarizing muscle relaxants (e.g., succinylcholine) and all volatile general anesthetics (Table 110.1). Even in a susceptible patient, however, these drugs will not always cause MH. In at least half of MH cases, the patient has had a previous uneventful exposure to a triggering agent. When MH does occur, there is a rapid release of calcium from the SR in skeletal muscle. This release causes a sudden increase in muscle metabolism, which can cause a contracture when the mechanical threshold is reached. Adenosine triphosphate (ATP) is rapidly consumed, causing an increase in both aerobic and anaerobic metabolism. These hypermetabolic pathways increase oxygen and glucose utilization, leading to an increased carbon dioxide (CO_2) production. This is soon followed by respiratory and metabolic acidosis, hyperkalemia, and dysrhythmias and may result in death.

Presentation
Masseter muscle rigidity

Although a syndrome by itself, one of the first signs of MH can be masseter muscle rigidity (MMR) after the administration of sodium thiopental or halothane (in children) and succinylcholine. MMR is characterized by rigidity of the jaw

Table 110.1. Drugs that can trigger MH

Halogenated general anesthetics
Cyclopropane
Desflurane
Enflurane
Ether
Halothane
Isoflurane
Methoxyflurane
Sevoflurane
Depolarizing muscle relaxants (e.g. succinylcholine)

muscles that prevents the mouth from being opened. Normally, only the jaw is affected, and the remainder of the patient's muscles will be flaccid. The incidence of MH as diagnosed by arterial blood gas abnormalities following MMR is roughly 15%. If the anesthetic is stopped following MMR, there are usually no sequelae. It is uncommon for fulminant MH to occur immediately following MMR, but if the anesthetic is continued with triggering agents, signs of fulminant MH can occur within 20 minutes in susceptible individuals.

Most often the surgery is rescheduled after MMR, but if there are no other signs of MH, some anesthesiologists may elect to continue the case, (particularly if emergent), with non-triggering agents as long as fulminant MH treatment and proper monitoring are immediately available. If MMR is associated with rigid limb muscles, treatment with dantrolene is indicated immediately. Urine should be observed for color change; if cola colored, testing for myoglobin should be undertaken; creatine kinase (CK) studies may also be warranted. Postanesthesia care unit (PACU) observation for at least 12 hours following MMR is also prudent.

Fulminant MH

Unexplained tachycardia and tachypnea may be the first noticeable signs in the operating room that a patient is susceptible to triggering agents. These symptoms are the result of a hyperactive sympathetic nervous system and a sign of the body's increased metabolic state. If the patient has received a muscle relaxant or is mechanically ventilated, tachypnea may not be recognized; however, in its place will be an increase in end-tidal CO_2, even in the face of aggressive hyperventilation. Whole-body muscle rigidity and an increase in body temperature are late signs. At its peak, body temperature can increase as much as $1°C$ to $2°C$ every 5 minutes. Other signs include cyanosis, mottling, sweating, and a warm and quickly discharged CO_2 absorber (Table 110.2).

An arterial blood gas analysis will reveal hypercarbia and a mixed respiratory and metabolic acidosis. Other laboratory findings can include lactic acidemia and, late in the crisis, marked hyperkalemia and hypercalcemia. Serum myoglobin

Table 110.2.	Signs of MH

Tachypnea
Tachycardia
Increased end-tidal CO_2
Cyanosis
Masseter muscle spasm
Mottling
Sweating
Hypertension
Ventricular dysrhythmias
Muscle rigidity
Hyperthermia
Hyperkalemia
Metabolic acidosis
Increased CK

and CK levels increase quickly in the hours following the event. Ventricular fibrillation can occur quickly following the initial presentation of MH, and is the most common cause of death. Later sequelae of a fulminant crisis include renal failure induced by myoglobinuria, congestive heart failure (CHF), acute cerebral edema, and disseminated intravascular coagulopathy (DIC).

Treatment

The mortality rate from a case of MH has dropped from approximately 70% in the 1970s to 5% today. This decrease is a direct result of the availability of dantrolene to treat acute episodes of MH and an increased awareness of the signs and symptoms. Dantrolene is the only available agent that is specifically used for treating MH. It was first synthesized in 1967 and was found to have muscle relaxant properties in animals. Its mechanism of action is unknown, but the end result of its use is a decrease in the resting calcium levels in susceptible muscle to near normal levels, followed by a return to baseline metabolism.

Dantrolene is a hydantoin derivative that is lipophilic and, therefore, has poor water solubility. Dantrolene is available in 20-mg vials that need to be dissolved in 60 ml of water. The dose of dantrolene is 2 to 2.5 mg/kg every 5 minutes up to a total dose of 10 mg/kg, if needed. The half-life of intravenous (IV) dantrolene is approximately 12 hours, but the therapeutic level lasts approximately 4 to 6 hours. Therefore, dantrolene (recommended dose 1 mg/kg) needs to be given at least every 6 hours for the first 24 hours following an event. Recrudescence, or a return of MH symptoms, has been shown to occur in approximately 20% of patients. Dantrolene has few side effects, with muscle weakness (100%), phlebitis (10%), respiratory failure (3%), and gastrointestinal discomfort (3%) being reported.

Treatment for an acute episode of MH is summarized as follows.

- All triggering agents should be discontinued immediately.
- Hyperventilate with 100% oxygen at flows >10 L/min to remove residual anesthetic gases and additional CO_2.
- Call for help, notify surgeons, and obtain dantrolene.
- Administer dantrolene therapy 2.5 mg/kg every 5 minutes up to a total of 10 mg/kg, or until cessation of signs and symptoms of MH.
- Administer sodium bicarbonate (2–4 mEq/kg) for treatment of metabolic acidosis.
- Control fever with surface ice packs, iced gastric and rectal lavage; stop cooling at 38°C to avoid hypothermia.
- Manage hyperkalemia with glucose, insulin, and bicarbonate.
- Follow serial blood gases and laboratory tests and treat as needed.

The patient needs to be followed closely for signs of recrudescence, DIC, and renal failure and should be admitted to an

Table 110.3. Differential diagnosis of MH

Neuroleptic malignant syndrome
Sepsis
Thyroid storm
Pheochromocytoma
Hypoxic encephalopathy
Mitochondrial myopathies
Periodic paralysis disorders
Iatrogenic hyperthermia
Drug-related hyperthermia

intensive care unit. As noted earlier, dantrolene may require redosing every 4 to 6 hours over the first 24 hours. Therapy may need to be initiated to treat rhabdomyolysis and myoglobinuria, including maintenance of high urine output and alkalization of urine.

Differential diagnosis

There are several disorders that cause hyperthermia in the operating room and may therefore be mistaken for MH (Table 110.3). Thyroid storm presents with similar changes in vital signs, but usually occurs postoperatively and is most often associated with hypokalemia instead of hyperkalemia. It is also not associated with respiratory acidosis or muscle rigidity. Sepsis can be confused with MH, but muscle rigidity is rarely seen in sepsis. Unlike with MH, the signs of sepsis can be treated with antibiotics and nonsteroidal anti-inflammatory drugs (NSAIDS). Pheochromocytoma is another disease associated with marked increases in heart rate and blood pressure, but increased end-tidal CO_2 is not a common finding.

Neuroleptic malignant syndrome (NMS) is clinically similar to MH. It presents with tachycardia, hypertension, fever, muscle rigidity, and acidosis. The difference is that it is not triggered by anesthetic agents, but rather after exposure to certain antipsychotic drugs. These drugs cause a decrease in dopaminergic activity in the central nervous system. The onset of symptoms varies from hours to days after the drug is administered. Bromocriptine, a dopamine agonist, may be useful in the treatment of NMS. Dantrolene also seems to be an effective therapy in some cases of NMS but is associated with a higher death rate in some studies.

MH diagnosis

The gold standard test for diagnosis of MH in the United States is the caffeine halothane contracture test (CHCT). The analogous test in Europe is referred to as the in vitro contracture test (IVCT). A muscle biopsy is required to perform this test and is usually taken from the vastus lateralis or the quadriceps. Portions of the biopsy sample are exposed to 0.5 to 10 mM caffeine, 3% halothane, and both in combination. MH susceptible muscle is more sensitive to caffeine and more likely to have a contracture when exposed to halothane than is normal muscle.

The classifications given as a result of the CHCT (US protocol) are either MH susceptible (MHS) or MH normal (MHN). MH susceptibility is diagnosed by an abnormal response to caffeine, halothane, or both in combination. Under the IVCT, three designations are given. MH susceptible (MHS) refers to patients who have abnormal responses to both the caffeine and halothane baths. MH equivocal (MHE) is designated for an abnormal response to either caffeine or halothane, but not to both. MH normal or nonresponders (MHN) have no abnormal response to either caffeine or halothane.

The CHCT (US protocol) has a sensitivity of 97% and a specificity of 78%, whereas the IVCT (European protocol) has been suggested to have a sensitivity of 99% and a specificity of 94%. These rates, however, are highly skewed as the comparison groups are derived only from patients with abnormal responses to anesthesia that resemble MH and not from the general population or a population that includes other muscle disease groups. Despite invasive and expensive testing, patients who have been fully evaluated are often not managed appropriately following a suspected MH crisis. MH normal patients are commonly still given nontriggering anesthetics or subjected to delays in care despite the availability of normal test results, which has made some practitioners question the usefulness of testing, beyond academic interests.

Genetic testing has been proposed as a screening tool, but proves difficult because MH has such a heterogeneous genetic basis. Multiple different mutations have been shown to occur in the RyR gene of some patients. Furthermore, markers may also be present on other chromosomes, making routine screening even more difficult. Finally, discordance has been shown in some patients who have negative genetic screening and a positive IVCT.

Follow-up after presumed MH event

The patient and family should be alerted to the risks and familial nature of MH and referred to the Malignant Hyperthermia Association of the United States (MHAUS). Arrangements should be made for follow-up and, if desired by the patient, a muscle biopsy can be performed for definitive diagnosis. An Adverse Metabolic Reaction to Anesthesia (AMRA; available at www.mhreg.org) report should be completed, and the patient's primary care provider should also be contacted. MHAUS has been operating since 1981 and provides an invaluable resource for physicians and patients. They can be reached at www.mhaus.org, info@mhaus.org, or 1–800–644–9737 (1–315–464–7079 outside the United States).

Suggested readings

Burkman JM, Posner KL, Domino KB. Analysis of the clinical variables associated with recrudescence after malignant hyperthermia reactions. *Anesthesiology* 2007; 106:901–906.
Denborough M. Malignant hyperthermia. *Lancet* 1998; 352:1131–1136.

Deufel T, Golla A, Meindl A, et al. Evidence for genetic heterogeneity of malignant hyperthermia susceptibility. *Am J Hum Genet* 1992; 50:1151–1161.

Jungbluth H. Central core disease. *Orphanet J Rare Dis* 2007; 2:25.

Klinger W, Lehmann-Horn F, Jurkat-Rott K. Complications of anesthesia in neuromuscular disorders. *Neuromuscul Disord* 2005; 15:195–206.

Kozack J, Macintyre D. Malignant hyperthermia. *Phys Ther* 2001; 81(3):945–951.

Krause T, Gerbershagen MU, Fiege M, et al. Dantrolene – a review of its pharmacology, therapeutic use and new developments. *Anesthesia* 2004; 59:364–373.

Malignant Hyperthermia Association of the United States (MHAUS; Web site). Available at: www.mhaus.org

Morgan GE, Mikhail MS, Murray MJ. *Clinical Anesthesiology*. 3rd ed. New York: McGraw-Hill; 2002:869–873.

Robinson R, Carpenter D, Shaw AM, et al. Mutations in RYR1 in malignant hyperthermia and central core disease. *Hum Mutat* 2006; 27(10):977–989.

Rosenberg H, Davis M, James D, et al. Malignant hyperthermia. *Orphanet J Rare Dis* 2007; 2:21.

Rosenberg H, Brandom BW, Sambuughin N, Fletcher JE. Malignant hyperthermia and other pharmacogenetic disorders. In: Barash, PG, Cullen, BF, Stoelting, RK, ed. *Clinical Anesthesia*. 5th ed. Philadelphia: Lippincott, Williams & Wilkins; 2006:529–556.

Scala D, Di Martio A, Cossolino S, et al. Follow-up of patients tested for malignant hyperthermia susceptibility. *Eur J Anaesthesiol* 2006; 3646:1–5.

Steele DS, Duke AM. Defective Mg^2+ regulation of RyR1 as a causal factor in malignant hyperthermia. *Arch Biochem Biophys* 2007; 458:57–64.

Chapter

111

Myasthenia gravis

Tomas Cvrk

Myasthenia gravis (MG) is an autoimmune disease caused by the presence of autoantibodies against the proteins (most often acetylcholine receptor [AChR] of the postsynaptic cell in the neuromuscular junction [NMJ]). It is characterized by the varying degrees of weakness in the muscles of the body. The prevalence of the disease in the general population is 5 to 12.5 per 100,000.

The result of antibody binding to the AChR is a decrease in effective concentration of the receptor in the postsynaptic cell membrane. At least three different mechanisms have been proposed for this to occur: (1) binding and activation of complement at the NMJ; (2) accelerated degradation of AChR molecules by internalization of the antibody-labeled receptor; and (3) functional AChR block that prevents functional binding of ACh.

ACh binding to the AChRs causes an allosteric (conformational) change that increases the AChR channel permeability for Na^+ and K^+, which in turn results in membrane depolarization. This current flowing across the membrane, if sufficient, allows for firing of the action potential and potentially muscular contraction. The reduction in the number of AChRs in MG lowers the generated endplate potential and thus increases the threshold for the number of remaining AChRs that must be activated for triggering an action potential. It is estimated that the presence of the antibody results in an approximately 70% reduction of AChR number, with remaining receptor molecules probably occupied by the antibody. The anti-AChR antibody is present in 85% of tested MG patients. The remaining 15% patients are called *seronegative*. It has been found that the majority of these seronegative patients have antibody against another protein present at the postsynaptic membrane, MuSK, which plays an important role in the process of clustering AChRs during the development of the NMJ.

The cause of MG is still not clear. The majority of patients have an abnormality of the thymus gland, either hyperplasia or thymoma. Several different types of MG have been recognized and are summarized in Fig. 111.1.

Clinical features

MG has a bimodal presentation, affecting women more than men in the third through the fourth decade of life, but there is a higher prevalence in men in the fifth decade onward. The characteristic presentation of MG is fatigability of skeletal muscles with repetitive use. Interestingly, the first muscles that are usually affected by the disease are eyelids and extraocular muscles. As the disease progresses, patients may have difficulty chewing and swallowing. Most of the patients (85%) will develop generalized weakness if not treated. The most serious complication is respiratory failure, either from exacerbation of the stable disease (myasthenia crisis) or from progression of the disease without effective treatment. Patients with anti-MuSK IgG present with bulbar and respiratory weakness rather than limb involvement.

Diagnosis

Initial diagnosis is usually based on a high level of clinical suspicion. The edrophonium (Tensilon) test consists of administration of up to 10 mg of edrophonium with the expectation of a reduction of symptoms in MG patients. The mechanism of action behind this test is that edrophonium is a short-acting acetylcholinesterase (AChE) inhibitor that increases the concentration of ACh at the NMJ, which leads to improvement of the signal transduction and, clinically, increased muscle

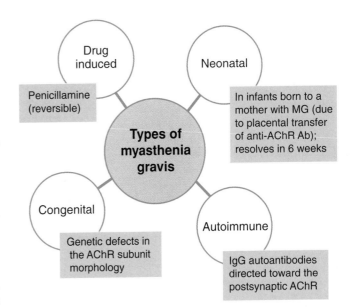

Figure 111.1. Types of MG.

strength within 45 seconds. Although diagnostic, this test has a low sensitivity and specificity.

Another diagnostic modality used for diagnosis is electromyography (EMG). One looks for a >10% decrease in muscle action potential during a 2- to 3-Hz stimulation. Here, single-fiber EMG is more sensitive than compound muscle measurements. The abnormalities that are seen with EMG in MG patients, however, can be caused by other NMJ disorders, such as myopathies or Lambert–Eaton myasthenic syndrome (LEMS). The most specific test is the detection of the circulating autoantibodies.

There is an association between MG and other autoimmune processes like thyroiditis, rheumatoid arthritis, polymyositis, celiac disease, and sarcoidosis. Approximately 75% of MG patients have thymic abnormalities, and 10% of those have thymoma. Thymomas are usually surgically removed because of the risk of invasion.

Treatment

There are two treatment modalities for patients with MG: medical and surgical. AChE inhibitors are usually recommended as the first line of treatment. Pyridostigmine is the most commonly prescribed medication. The dose is slowly titrated up by the effect to avoid overdosing and developing a cholinergic crisis. The disease often can be controlled reasonably well by using drugs, but waxing and waning of symptoms is common with AChE inhibitor treatment.

Steroids are the drugs used most frequently in patients with insufficient control on AChE inhibitors only. Steroid dose is titrated up slowly because a high dose of corticosteroids could cause exacerbation of the disease. After several months of high-dose steroids, dose is reduced for chronic administration. The shortcoming of steroids is a high frequency of side effects associated with their use.

Azathioprine is an immunosuppressant used commonly for MG treatment. As a purine analogue, it interferes with T- and B-cell proliferation. It is as effective as steroids and is often used as a steroid-sparing therapy in patients who do not tolerate high-dose corticosteroids. The disadvantage of its use is that there may be a delay of up to 15 months before the clinical benefit is apparent. Cyclophosphamide is another effective immunosuppressant. It is usually only used in patients who do not respond to other immunosuppressants because it has an undesirable adverse effect profile (hair loss, delayed effect, anorexia, skin discoloration, nausea, vomiting). Less frequently used immunosuppressants are cyclosporine, tacrolimus (FK506), and mycophenolate mofetil, which are usually used as steroid-sparing agents.

Surgical treatment involves thymectomy in patients post puberty. Although the remission of the disease after the surgery has been documented, the clinical efficacy of thymectomy has been questioned because of the lack of solid evidence supporting its use. Moreover, the therapeutic effect can be delayed until months to years after the surgery. One of the reasons why it has been so difficult to establish the benefit of thymectomy is that a lot of patients are treated with corticosteroids and other immunosuppressive medications at the same time, making it impossible to know which treatment is responsible for the remission.

Other treatment modalities that are usually reserved for myasthenia crisis or acute disease exacerbation are plasma exchange and intravenous immunoglobulin (IVIG) therapy. The former directly decreases the titer of the antibodies against AChR by replacing a patient's plasma with albumin, saline, and plasma protein fraction. The mechanism of IVIG is not fully understood, but it involves administration of pooled human IgG for 5 days leading to complex immunomodulatory effects and a decrease in native antibody production. In several randomized clinical trials, neither of these modalities has been shown to have any benefit as a chronic therapy. Thymectomy is a surgical treatment option that involves removal of the thymus gland. This procedure can be quite effective, although it may take time for clinical symptoms to improve.

Anesthetic management of the patient with MG
Preoperative evaluation

Patients with a history of MG present with several preoperative considerations. The history of the disease and its severity should be obtained as well as the current and past therapeutic regimen. Special consideration should be given to assessment of any muscle strength compromise, especially weakness of the respiratory or bulbar muscles. The patient's inability to generate a strong cough to clear secretions is important because it can be a marker for increased risk of aspiration as well as postoperative atelectasis. The baseline preoperative pulmonary function tests should be obtained to identify patients with low forced vital capacity and negative inspiratory pressures that may be at increased risk for postoperative mechanical or noninvasive ventilation.

Most MG patients are managed on AChE inhibitors. The presence of these medications in the body reduces the effect of neuromuscular blockade intraoperatively and diminishes the muscle relaxation effect of inhalational agents in non-muscle-relaxant anesthesia. Therefore, AChE inhibitors are usually discontinued on the day of surgery and resumed postoperatively.

Patients with significant preoperative muscle weakness on AChE inhibitor or other therapy may benefit from a preoperative course of plasmapheresis or IVIG therapy, both of which have been found to result in short-term improvement of functional status.

In patients with MG associated with thymoma, the location, size of the mass, and potential compromise of adjacent structures (airway/vascular) should be evaluated with imaging as well as by pulmonary function flow–volume loops.

Neuromuscular blockade

Succinylcholine

Due to a reduced number of receptors in the postsynaptic membrane, patients with MG usually have an increased requirement for depolarizing agents. A higher concentration of succinylcholine at the NMJ is required to block a sufficient number of receptors that would block the signal transmission. The measured dose response to succinylcholine in MG patients showed that their 95% effective dose (ED_{95}) was 0.8 mg/kg, or 2.6 times higher than that in patients without MG. An administered total dose of 2.0 mg/kg should be sufficient for rapid sequence induction in most MG patients. The duration of action of succinylcholine, however, can be prolonged because of the presence of AChE inhibitors used for treatment. The anesthetist must remember that the high first dose of succinylcholine and/or multiple doses required for intubation put MG patients at increased risk for development of the phase II block.

Nondepolarizing neuromuscular blockers

In general, MG results in increased sensitivity to nondepolarizing neuromuscular blockers (NMBs) because of the lower number of receptors that need to be blocked in the NMJ. It is recommended that the baseline neuromuscular block be tested before inducing anesthesia and again before administration of nondepolarizing NMBs. The train-of-four can be used for that purpose for routine use in the operating room. Other monitoring modalities (electromyography [EMG], mechanomyography) that can be used for neuromuscular monitoring provide more objective data, thus allowing for more precise quantification of the neuromuscular blockade. The set up of these monitoring modalities is more elaborate, however, and therefore often impractical for routine use in the operating room. Patients with a decreased T1/T4 ratio before anesthesia is administered are at increased risk for postoperative weakness and the possibility of prolonged mechanical ventilation.

Because sensitivity to all nondepolarizing NMJ blockers is increased, long-acting NMJ blockers should be avoided. The dose of the agent should be reduced and titrated to effect by giving small increments. A reasonable starting dose of cisatracurium, vecuronium, atracurium, and even rocuronium and mivacurium is approximately 40% of the dose recommended for the normal population given the fact that the ED_{95} for most of these drugs is in the 40% to 60% range of that for normal controls. However, significant variability exists among patients, depending on the natural course of the disease, severity, and treatment.

Choice of anesthesia modality

General anesthesia, regional anesthesia (including peripheral nerve blocks), and the combination of regional with general anesthesia have been used successfully in patients with MG.

Induction

To avoid postoperative complications, some anesthesiologists prefer to avoid use of muscle relaxants all together and use inhalational or IV agents to facilitate muscle relaxation for tracheal intubation as well as surgical relaxation. To avoid using succinylcholine, a rapid sequence technique using propofol and remifentanil for induction has been successfully used in patients with MG who needed emergent surgery. Inhalational induction can be used in patients without indication of rapid sequence induction.

Maintenance

Anesthesia is usually maintained with nitrous oxide and/or volatile gases. The advantage of volatile gases is their ability to provide muscle relaxation in MG patients for many surgical procedures, which may eliminate the need for additional NMBs. The fast elimination of current inhalational agents ensures minimal residual blockade and facilitates prompt extubation. Successful use of total intravenous anesthesia (TIVA) has been reported. Remifentanil has been described as providing great analgesia and hemodynamic stability, especially in older patients, in addition to its rapid and predictable elimination.

Regional anesthesia

Regional anesthesia can provide an excellent level of anesthesia without the need for NMJ blockade. However, it is important to avoid a high level of anesthesia when neuraxial blockade is used, in order to prevent a respiratory muscle compromise. There is a theoretical potentiation of neuromuscular block with the use of local anesthetic; therefore, a reduced dose of local anesthetics for regional anesthesia is recommended. The combination of general anesthesia and epidural anesthesia has been reported for abdominal surgery and thymoma resections. Epidural anesthesia in this case provides analgesia intraoperatively and postoperatively and, in addition, provides muscle relaxation during the surgery.

Postoperative considerations

The majority of patients with MG can be safely extubated at the end of the procedure. Patients with severe, long-standing disease, respiratory compromise (peak inspiratory pressure <-25 cm H_2O; vital capacity <4 ml/kg), and those on high dose pyridostigmine (>750 mg) are predicted to be at higher risk for need of postoperative ventilatory support. All patients with MG need careful monitoring in the postoperative period for signs of muscle weakness and respiratory failure and for the possible need for reintubation. Adequate analgesia should be provided; however, oversedation from narcotic drugs is undesirable.

Any medications that can exacerbate muscle weakness should be avoided intraoperatively and in the postoperative period. These medications include glucocorticoids, lithium,

Table 111.1. Comparison of MG and LEMS

Effect	LEMS	MG
Muscles	Proximal limb weakness (legs > arms)	Extraocular, bulbar, and facial muscle weakness
	Exercise improves strength	Fatigue with exercise
	Muscle pain common	Muscle pain uncommon
	Reflexes absent or decrease	Reflexes normal
Gender	Male > female	Female > male
Coexisting pathology	Small cell carcinoma of the lung	Thymoma
Succinylcholine	Sensitive	Resistant
Nondepolarizing muscle relaxants	Sensitive	Sensitive
AChE agents	Decreased (poor) response	Good response

phenytoin, aminoglycoside antibiotics, clindamycin, ciprofloxacin, propranolol, magnesium, and procainamide. AChE inhibitor therapy should be restarted in the immediate postoperative period. Exacerbation of muscle weakness should be evaluated at once, and any possible residual anesthetic effect should be differentiated from possible myasthenia crisis or cholinergic crisis.

Neonatal myasthenia

Transient neonatal MG occurs in 10% to 20% of infants born to mothers with MG. Maternal AChR antibodies cross the placenta and are responsible for transient MG symptoms in the neonate. The main clinical manifestation of neonatal MG is generalized weakness, and these infants are at increased risk for respiratory insufficiency. AChE therapy is required for 3 to 4 weeks after birth.

Myasthenic crisis versus cholinergic crisis

Both myasthenic crisis and cholinergic crisis can present as respiratory failure. Triggers for myasthenia crisis include disease exacerbations, noncompliance with cholinesterase inhibitor medication, adverse effects of other medications, fever, and emotional stress. Cholinergic crises develop secondarily to an overdose of cholinesterase inhibitor medication. In these cases, excessive ACh stimulation of striated muscles at the NMJ produces a flaccid muscle paralysis that can be clinically indistinguishable from weakness due to myasthenia crisis. Respiratory failure may be present without other cholinergic symptoms (miosis, diarrhea, urinary incontinence, bradycardia, emesis, lacrimation, or salivation).

The edrophonium test can be used to distinguish between cholinergic and myasthenic crises. The initial dose of edrophonium should be 2 mg IV, administered slowly. Atropine is the drug of choice for bradycardia or atrioventricular (AV) block, if encountered. If there is no response or there are no adverse cholinergic effects, another 8 mg IV of edrophonium can be slowly administered, for a total dose of 10 mg. Improved muscle strength after the dose of edrophonium implies myasthenic crisis; increased weakness indicates that it is cholinergic crisis. A myasthenic crisis should be treated with a cautious

administration of appropriate longer acting cholinesterase inhibitors. Treatment for cholinergic crisis is respiratory support, discontinuation of all anticholinesterase drugs, and symptomatic treatment of any associated autonomic dysfunction.

Lambert-Eaton myasthenic syndrome

LEMS is another autoimmune disorder that affects neurotransmitter signaling in the NMJ. In contrast to MG, the autoantibodies are directed toward presynaptic ending, more specifically against voltage-gated Ca^{2+} channels. ACh is released from intracellular vesicles as a result of calcium influx via these channels. The presence of LEMS antibody results in a decrease of ACh release toward the postsynaptic membrane.

In a majority of LEMS patients, the antibody is produced as a part of paraneoplastic syndrome due to underlying malignancy; most commonly it is associated with small cell cancer of the lung (up to 60%). LEMS, however, can exist as a standalone autoimmune disorder. The disease is characterized by lower and upper extremity weakness of variable progressivity, associated with autonomic dysfunction and occasional oculobulbar palsy. The muscle weakness improves with repetitive contraction as more ACh is being released to the endplate.

Diagnosis is usually made based on clinical presentation with increased suspicion in patients with small cell carcinoma and concomitant dysautonomia. A positive calcium voltage-gated channel antibody test confirms the diagnosis. Muscle biopsy most frequently demonstrates a reduction of type 1 muscle fibers. Often the diagnosis of LEMS leads to the diagnosis of previously unrecognized small cell carcinoma.

The only effective medications currently used for treatment of LEMS are guanidine hydrochloride and 3,4-diaminopyridine. The latter increases time of calcium influx into the cells via blockade of potassium. The former inhibits the binding and uptake of calcium into subcellular organelles such as mitochondria, thereby increasing the free intracellular calcium level and facilitating ACh release. Guanidine hydrochloride is hepatotoxic, which limits its use. Plasmapheresis and immunosuppression also have been found to be effective at improving symptoms. A comparison of the clinical symptoms of LEMS and MG is summarized in Table 111.1.

Anesthetic implications

In contrast to MG patients, LEMS patients are characterized by increased sensitivity to both depolarizing and nondepolarizing muscle relaxants. The sensitivity to nondepolarizing agents is more pronounced in LEMS than in MG. An anesthetic strategy that would involve avoidance of muscle relaxants should be strongly considered in patients with known LEMS. When nondepolarizing NMBs are used, the reversal of muscle relaxation in these patients is often incomplete or transient, posing an increased risk for the need for postoperative ventilatory support. As discussed earlier in this chapter regarding MG, volatile anesthetics and/or IV anesthetics are often sufficient in providing muscle relaxation for intubation and maintenance of anesthesia. LEMS should be on the list of differential diagnoses in patients with prolonged paralysis without any evidence of pseudocholinesterase deficiency.

Suggested readings

Eisenkraft JB. Anesthetic implications of myasthenia gravis. *Mount Sinai J Med* 2002; 69(1–2):31–37.

Hirsch NP. Neuromuscular junction in health and disease. *Br J Anaesth* 2007; 99(1):132–138.

Kiran U, Choudhury M, Saxena N, et al. Sevoflurane as a sole anaesthetic agent for thymectomy in myasthenia gravis. *Acta Anaesthesiol Scand* 2000; 44:351–353.

Nilsson E, Muller K. Neuromuscular effects of isoflurane in patients with myasthenia gravis. *Acta Anaesth Scand* 1990; 34:126–131.

O'Neill GN. Acquired disorders of the neuromuscular junction. *Int Anesthesiol Clin* 2006; 44(2):107–121.

Russel SH, Hood JR, Campkin M. Neuromuscular effects of enflurane in myasthenia gravis. *Br J Anaesth* 1993; 71:766P.

Rowbottom SJ. Isoflurane for thymectomy in myasthenia gravis. *Anaesth Intensive Care* 1989; 17:444–447.

Takeda J, Izawa H, Ochiai R, et al. Suppression of neuromuscular transmission by sevoflurane in patients with myasthenia gravis. *Anesthesiology* 1993; 79:A960.

Chapter 112

Muscular dystrophy and myotonic dystrophy

Jason M. Erlich and Sugantha Sundar

Neuromuscular diseases are a group of diseases that include muscular and myotonic dystrophies (Tables 112.1 and 112.2) as well as additional disease states. Many, although not all of the diseases are clinically characterized by the progressive loss of skeletal and cardiac muscle function due to abnormal or insufficient quantities of muscle cell proteins, which affect the integrity of the muscle membrane. As genetic diagnosis of disease becomes more pervasive, new classifications may become the standard. It is possible that neuromuscular disease has been underdiagnosed as clinically mild cases may not arouse suspicion.

The goals of this chapter are to

(1) discuss the different types of muscular dystrophies and their anesthetic implications, and
(2) discuss the anesthetic implications of ion channel myotonias.

Discussion of myasthenia gravis (MG), myasthenic syndromes, multiple sclerosis, motor neuron disease, Guillain–Barré syndrome, mitochondrial disease, and Charcot–Marie–Tooth disease is beyond the scope of this chapter.

Muscular dystrophies

The muscle cell is made up of a variety of proteins, such as dystrophin, merosin, utrophin, syntrophin, dystrobrevin, and sarcoglycans. Errors in production of these proteins lead to abnormalities in the muscle membrane. These are disorders of usually genetic etiology characterized by skeletal muscle necrosis and hence progressive muscle weakness. In some cases, the cardiac muscle is also involved. Muscular dystrophies are often described by their clinical presentation; however the current classification is based on molecular, genetic, and protein biochemistry.

Duchenne muscular dystrophy

Duchenne muscular dystrophy (DMD) is the most common type of childhood muscular dystrophy, occurring at a rate of 1 in 3300 live male births. It primarily affects males via X-linked recessive transmission; however, a milder phenotype can be observed in female carriers. DMD is characterized by a lack of

dystrophin and an imbalance between muscle cell necrosis and regeneration. A mouse model exists and has been scrutinized since the mid-1990s, but a comprehensive mechanism explaining the disease has not been elucidated. There are a number of hypotheses that attempt to explain the mechanism by which absent dystrophin leads to muscle degeneration. The mechanical hypothesis relates the weakened muscle membrane to the fragility of muscle fibers themselves, especially after sustained contraction. This hypothesis has led to the notion that, although physical therapy is still useful in treatment, overexertion may be harmful. The calcium hypothesis states that the poorly controlled calcium influx observed through voltage-independent channels may result in high cytosol calcium levels and destabilization of the cell membrane, which in turn leads to more calcium influx. By age 12, many affected individuals are confined to a wheelchair. Death by age 30 is frequent and is usually secondary to congestive heart failure (CHF) or pneumonia. Cognitive dysfunction is related to the lack of dystrophin in neuronal membranes.

Because there is no curative treatment for DMD, medical management has focused on decreasing the rate of decline of muscle function. Chronic steroid use has an impact on the rate at which DMD progresses and has been shown to slow the progression of disease, improve peripheral muscle function, preserve pulmonary function, and delay wheelchair use by 3 years. Corticosteroids are thought to increase muscle mass via increasing insulin-like growth factor I and promoting skeletal muscle repair and regeneration.

Becker muscular dystrophy

Becker muscular dystrophy (BMD) results from a dystrophin deficiency. The disease course is milder than DMD because the dystrophin protein is present but in insufficient quantity. It is

Table 112.1. Types of muscular dystrophies

Duchenne
Becker
Emery–Dreifuss
Limb-girdle
Congenital muscular dystrophy
Facioscapulohumeral
Myotonic dystrophy: types 1 and 2

Table 112.2. Overview of types of muscular dystrophies

Name	Incidence	Inheritance	Clinical	Treatment	Notes
Duchenne	1:3300 males	X-linked recessive	Progressive proximal muscle weakness beginning in childhood; death possible before 30 y due to cardiac or pulmonary complications	Steroids	Avoid succinylcholine; response to mivacurium is normal
Becker	1:30,000 males	X-linked recessive	Milder form of above; cardiac abnormalities in 75% of 40+ year olds	None	Avoid succinylcholine
Emery–Dreifuss	1:33,000	AD or X-linked recessive	Early contracture of elbows and Achilles tendons, humeropectoral muscle wasting, life-threatening cardiac conduction abnormalities	Implantable defibrillator	Avoid succinylcholine
Limb-girdle	1:20,000	AR > AD	Slowly progressing, relatively benign course; onset 20s–50s; shoulder and pelvic girdle weakness		Avoid succinylcholine; most common in families of North African descent
Oculopharyngeal	Rare		Presents after 30 y; slowly progressive dysphagia; ptosis		Highly sensitive to muscle relaxants; weakness not helped by anticholinesterase agents
Congenital	0.7–1.2:10,000 (Fukuyama form Japan)	AR	Poor prognosis; hypotonia at birth; respiratory difficulty; swallowing abnormalities; CNS involvement; seizures in 50%; death by 10 y; common 10		Avoid succinylcholine; rarely seen outside Japan
Facioscapulohumeral	10–20 per million	AD	Facial, scapulohumeral, anterior tibial, and pelvic girdle muscle weakness beginning in adolescence; cardiac conduction defects, deafness, and retinal disease are also associated		Avoid succinylcholine
Myotonic dystrophy (MD1 and MD2)		AD	Myotonia, insulin resistance, cardiac conduction defects, cataracts, testicular atrophy, frontal balding (males)		Avoid succinylcholine

AD, autosomal dominant; AR, autosomal recessive; CNS, central nervous system.

also caused by an X-linked recessive mutation in the dystrophin gene. Onset is in childhood but may be as late as 16 years.

Emery–Dreifuss muscular dystrophy

Patients with Emery–Dreifuss muscular dystrophy often have implantable defibrillators, as cardiac conduction defects associated with the disease can be fatal. Skeletal muscle manifestations are milder, associated with contractures of the elbows, ankles, and spine. There are two types of Emery–Dreifuss muscular dystrophy associated with defective nuclear proteins: an autosomal dominant type associated with defective lamin and an X-linked recessive type associated with defective emerin.

Limb-girdle muscular dystrophy

Limb-girdle muscular dystrophy is exemplified by shoulder- and pelvic-girdle weakness. It is most common in families of

North African descent. It is associated with a sarcoglycan protein abnormality and is usually inherited as an autosomal dominant or recessive trait.

Facioscapulohumeral muscular dystrophy

Facioscapulohumeral muscular dystrophy is associated with weakness of facial, scapulohumeral, anterior tibial, and pelvic girdle muscles; cardiac conduction defects, deafness, and retinal disease are also associated. It has an autosomal dominant inheritance pattern.

Oculopharyngeal muscular dystrophy

Oculopharyngeal muscular dystrophy is associated with ptosis and dysphagia with onset in late adulthood. The dysphagia is secondary to esophageal smooth muscle dysfunction and pharyngeal skeletal muscle weakness.

Congenital muscular dystrophy

Congenital muscular dystrophy is associated with muscle weakness, mental retardation, feeding difficulties, and respiratory dysfunction with an onset during infancy.

Myotonic dystrophy

This is the most common form of muscular dystrophy in adults. It results from the mutation on either chromosome 19q13 (type 1) or chromosome 3q21 (type 2). Patients present with myotonia, progressive myopathy, testicular atrophy, insulin resistance, defects in cardiac conduction, cataracts, neuropsychiatric illness, as well as frontal balding. Death is usually from cardiac and respiratory complications.

Anesthetic considerations

(1) Patients with DMD frequently require surgical intervention with general anesthesia to correct scoliosis caused by unopposed antagonism of dystrophic muscles. As some diseases such as DMD become multisystemic over time, preoperative testing includes electrocardiography (ECG), echocardiography, chest radiograph, pulmonary function tests and, more recently, cardiac MRI. Postoperatively, patients should be closely monitored for evidence of cardiac and pulmonary dysfunction.

(2) During the administration of general anesthesia, succinylcholine should be avoided in patients with diagnosed or suspected neuromuscular disease, as hyperactive muscle membranes have been associated with rhabdomyolysis, hyperkalemia, and cardiac arrest due to the release of intracellular contents. In addition, there are case reports of both previously unrecognized as well as correctly diagnosed instances of DMD resulting in postoperative rhabdomyolysis, hyperkalemia, and cardiac arrest despite avoiding succinylcholine but using inhalational agents. This has created a debate about the use of inhalational agents previously thought to be acceptable in patients with DMD. Sevoflurane may be the preferred inhalational anesthetic as it may have less of a tendency to release calcium from the sarcoplasmic reticulum. Inhalational anesthetics are better avoided, however, and total intravenous (IV) anesthesia may be indicated in this patient population.

(3) DMD and BMD produce variable cardiac manifestations, such as cardiomyopathy, arrhythmias, and CHF, which generally become clinically significant after skeletal muscle disease develops. Cardiomyopathy can be hypertrophic with potential systolic and diastolic dysfunction. Valvular dysfunction may develop as a result of dilatation. A preoperative echocardiogram is helpful in the intraoperative hemodynamic management of these patients.

(4) Other considerations (not specific to DMD) include intestinal hypomotility and gastroparesis associated with degeneration of alimentary smooth muscle, which increase the risk of aspiration.

(5) Resistance to the effect of nondepolarizing muscle relaxants is due to the reduced sensitivity of the nicotinic acetylcholine receptors. Nondepolarizing muscular relaxants have been noted, however, to have a prolonged effect due to their reduced ability to produce a contractile force from muscle wasting. The response to mivacurium is normal.

(6) Anticholinesterases to reverse nondepolarizing neuromuscular blockers are better avoided because of the variable response noted to these medications.

(7) Notably, blood loss during scoliosis surgery has been shown to be high, possibly due to impaired vasoconstriction from lack of dystrophin as well as reduced neuronal nitric oxide synthase and platelet dysfunction.

(8) Hyperglycemia should be controlled preoperatively as these patients have an insulin resistance syndrome possibly linked to lack of insulin receptors in the muscle fiber membrane.

(9) The patient should be positioned with attention to avoid injury.

(10) When reviewing laboratory test results, it is important to note that persistently elevated serum creatine kinase (CK) is associated with neuromuscular disease states and that it may be the presenting symptom in a mildly symptomatic or asymptomatic patient.

Ion channel myotonias

The ion channel myotonias are a diverse collection of disorders characterized by abnormal sodium, calcium, and chloride channels in muscle. Clinically, myotonia is the result of a prolonged depolarization with a delay in muscle relaxation. Muscle relaxants, general anesthesia, and regional anesthesia do not usually prevent myotonia from occurring.

They are broadly classified as:

(1) Channelopathies: myotonia congenita, paramyotonia, hyperkalemic periodic paralysis, potassium-aggravated myotonia, hypokalemic periodic paralysis, and acquired neuromyotonia

(2) Myotonic dystrophy: type 1 and type 2 (which is classified under muscular dystrophy)

Myotonia congenita

There are two types:

(1) Autosomal dominant: Thomsen

(2) Autosomal recessive: Becker

Both Thomsen and Becker forms of the disease result from mutations in chloride ion channels that decrease Cl^-

Table 112.3. Types of ion channel myotonias

Myotonia congenita (Thomsen and Becker)
Hyperkalemic periodic paralysis
Potassium-aggravated myotonia
Paramyotonia congenita
Hypokalemic periodic paralysis
Acquired neuromyotonia

conductance into the cell. The result is a hyperexcitable muscle membrane that contributes to muscle stiffness. Patients have difficulty initiating muscle movement, which is followed by impaired relaxation of the muscle. When there is sustained activity, the condition improves. Muscle stiffness can be precipitated by the conditions listed in Table 112.4.

Similar to muscular dystrophy considerations, anesthetic considerations in patients with myotonic dystrophy include impaired pulmonary function, cardiomyopathy, delayed gastric emptying, glossal hypertrophy, contractures, and spinal deformity. As the response to nondepolarizing agents is normal to prolonged, using short-acting nondepolarizing neuromuscular blockers such as mivacurium and cisatracurium with close monitoring may be beneficial. Succinylcholine may exaggerate myotonic contracture, and neostigmine may provoke a myotonic episode. Association with MH is uncertain.

Successful anesthetics have included low-dose propofol infusions (high-dose infusions have been associated with prolonged recovery and exaggerated ventilatory depression). Regional techniques have been used with success in both children and adults. Epidural anesthesia has been successful in parturients, although the condition may be exacerbated by pregnancy.

Periodic paralyses

These are of two types:

(1) Hyperkalemic periodic paralysis (paramyotonia congenita) and potassium-aggravated myotonia (mutations of skeletal muscle voltage-gated sodium channel gene)
(2) Hypokalemic periodic paralysis (mutation of skeletal muscle voltage-gated calcium channel gene)

Hyperkalemic periodic paralysis/paramyotonia congenita and potassium-aggravated myotonia

(1) Potassium levels should be reduced before surgery; potassium-free IV solutions are used.
(2) Maintain blood sugar levels with dextrose-rich solutions.

Table 112.4. Conditions that precipitate muscle stiffness with myotonia congenita

1. Cold and shivering
2. Diathermy
3. Succinylcholine
4. Anticholinesterases

(3) Plasma potassium level as well as acid–base status should be monitored.
(4) Short-acting nondepolarizing muscle relaxants are preferred, and succinylcholine is to be avoided.
(5) ECG monitoring for arrhythmia is standard.
(6) Potassium-wasting diuretics may have a role in the preoperative preparation of these patients.
(7) Propofol may be beneficial because it blocks normal and mutant voltage-gated sodium channels.
(8) Spinal anesthesia seems relatively safe in this patient population.
(9) Successful emergency treatment of hyperkalemia includes calcium chloride.

Hypokalemic periodic paralysis

(1) Attacks are triggered by hypothermia, carbohydrate-rich foods, insulin, and vigorous exercise.
(2) Potassium-sparing diuretics may be beneficial in the preoperative setting.
(3) Anxiolytics to avoid preoperative stress should be considered.
(4) Intraoperative K^+ levels should be checked.
(5) Short-acting nondepolarizing muscle relaxants are preferred, and succinylcholine is to be avoided.
(6) Spinal and epidural anesthesia seem relatively safe in this patient population.

Acquired neuromyotonia

(1) Autoantibodies that target the presynaptic voltage-gated potassium channels lead to inhibition of repolarization and hence a hyperexcitable state (i.e., the opposite of MG, although neuromyotonia can coexist with MG).
(2) Symptomatology includes muscle twitching at rest (myokymia); muscle cramps, stiffness, insomnia, mood changes, and hallucinations may be present.
(3) Drugs like phenytoin that increase the sodium pumping action on the nerve may be beneficial.
(4) There is no contraindication to succinylcholine, and no association with MH.
(5) Spinal and epidural anesthesia but not peripheral nerve blocks have been successful in blocking the spontaneous discharges that cause muscle twitching.
(6) Some patients may exhibit resistance to nondepolarizing muscle relaxants, although they are useful in providing muscle relaxation.

Other neuromuscular diseases and malignant hyperthermia

Links between MH and King–Denborough syndrome (KDS) have been made after clinical suspicion was followed up with contracture testing in patients. The inheritance pattern of KDS is not completely understood, and a genetic link has not been made. Contracture testing in some but not all DMD patients has indicated a link to MH as well.

Central core disease (CCD), not usually classified with the myotonic muscular dystrophies, has been shown to be strongly linked to MH with clinical and laboratory evidence. CCD is a distinct disease of the muscle fiber in which "cores" are noted in a significant number of fibers on oxidative enzyme histo-chemical analysis of skeletal muscle. The clinical presentation of CCD varies between being asymptomatic to being severely dis-abled due to skeletal muscle weakness. The association between CCD and MH has been made by analyzing several families with large pedigrees and through genetic analysis. Genetic proof linking CCD to MH comes from the close proximity of the CCD gene to the ryanodine receptor gene (a gene suspected as a cause of MH), both on chromosome 19. Based on this proof, all patients with CCD should be treated as if they are MH sus-ceptible. Hyperkalemic periodic paralysis has also been linked to MH.

Conclusion

Patients with neuromuscular disease are not uncommon, and some of them need repeated surgery for management of compli-cations. Hence adequate knowledge of these clinical situations is vital as there are multiple anesthetic implications. Team collab-oration among the neurologist, surgeon, intensivist, and anes-thesiologist can lead to better patient outcome.

Suggested readings

Barash PG, Cullen BF, Stoelting RK, et al. *Clinical Anesthesia.* Philadelphia: Lippincott Williams & Wilkins; 2006:501–507.

Cho D, Tapscott S. Myotonic dystrophy: emerging mechanisms for DM1 and DM2. *Biochimica et Biophysica Acta* 2007; 1772(2):195–204.

Deconinck N, Dan B. Pathophysiology of Duchenne muscular dystrophy: current hypotheses. *Pediatr Neurol* 2007; 36:1–7.

Elder A, Murray DJ, Forbes RB. Blood loss during posterior spinal fusion surgery in patients with neuromuscular disease: is there an increased risk? *Pediatr Anesth* 2003; 13(9):818–822.

Kerr TP, Durward A, Hodgson SV, et al. Hyperkalaemic cardiac arrest in a manifesting carrier of Duchenne muscular dystrophy following general anaesthesia. *Eur J Pediatr* 2001; 160: 579–580.

McNally E, Towbin J. Cardiomyopathy in Muscular Dystrophy Workshop 28–30 September 2003, Tucson, Arizona. *Neuromuscul Disord* 2004; 14(7):442–448.

Miller RD, ed. *Miller's Anesthesia.* New York: Churchill Livingstone; 2005:534–547.

Rideau Y. Treatment of Duchenne's myopathy with early physiotherapy: critical analysis. *Arch Fr Pediatr* 1985; 42:17–21.

Rifai X, Moxley RT, Lorenson M, et al. Effect of prednisone on growth hormone and insulin-like growth factor I in Duchenne dystrophy. *Neurology* 1993; 43(Suppl.):A202

Warwick A, Hayes J, Crawford M. The role of corticosteroids in Duchenne muscular dystrophy: a review for the anesthetist. *Pediatr Anesth* 2005; 15:3–8.

Wedel D. Malignant hyperthermia and neuromuscular disease. *Neuromuscul Disord* 1992; 2(3):157–164.

Yemen T, Mcclain C. Muscular dystrophy, anesthesia and the safety of inhalational agents revisited; again. *Pediatr Anesth* 2006; 16: 105–108.

Anesthesia for Ocular, Ear, and Throat Diseases

D. John Doyle, editor

Ophthalmic procedures

J. Victor Ryckman and D. John Doyle

Anatomy and physiology

The globe of the eye averages 24 mm in diameter. Its wall has three layers: the inner retina, the middle vascular choroid, and the tough white outer sclera. The iris, ciliary body, and the choroids are referred to collectively as the uveal tract (Fig. 113.1).

Light takes the following path through the eye to the retina:

- Cornea: Moistened by tears, this clear membrane is the outermost surface of the eye. The cornea joins the sclera at the limbus.
- Anterior chamber: Filled with clear aqueous humor, this chamber forms an angle anteriorly where the cornea meets the iris. It is at this location that the trabecular network drains the aqueous humor into Schlemm's canal.
- Pupil: This is the opening in the center of the iris. The muscles of the iris control the papillary size or aperture of the eye by constricting one of two muscle groups. Radial fibers are sympathetically innervated and dilate the pupil when stimulated (mydriasis). Sphincter fibers are circular and parasympathetic innervated; the pupil constricts (miosis) when they are stimulated.
- Posterior chamber: Bathed in the aqueous humor, it is in this chamber that the clear lens is suspended by the zonular fibers to the ciliary body. The ciliary body adjusts the lens shape and acts to focus light on the retina. The ciliary body also secretes aqueous humor.
- Vitreous: This is the transparent, gelatinous material that fills the space between the lens and the retina.
- Retina: It is the retina that converts light to electrical nerve impulses that run via the optic nerve and subsequently radiate to the visual cortex.

Extraocular muscles

The eye is powered by six extraocular muscles. They insert into the anterior sclera 6 mm posterior to the limbus. The inferior oblique's origin is on the nasal side of the maxilla. The superior oblique passes through the trochlea before inserting into the sclera. The superior, inferior, lateral, and medial rectus muscles form a cone that originates at the apex of the orbit where they form the annulus through which the optic nerve leaves the orbit and where the ophthalmic artery, the first branch of the internal carotid artery, enters.

Sympathetic and parasympathetic nerves converge on the ciliary ganglion within this intraconal space prior to innervating the eye. Three cranial nerves innervate these extraocular muscles: III (oculomotor), IV (trochlear), and VI (abducens). Most of the sensory innervations to the eye and orbit are via the ophthalmic branch of the trigeminal nerve, which divides shortly after entering the orbit through the superior orbital fissure into the frontal, lacrimal, and nasociliary nerves.

Intraocular pressure

Because the blood supply to the retina and the optic nerve is related to the intraocular perfusion pressure (defined as the difference between the mean arterial pressure and the intraocular pressure [IOP]), IOP is important in eye surgery. High IOP levels not only impair blood flow but can contribute to loss of eye contents after the globe has been opened. A number of physical factors and drugs will affect IOP. Normal IOP is between 10 and 20 mm Hg; physical factors, such as coughing, vomiting, or even a lid squeeze, can raise IOP to 30 to 40 mm Hg or more.

Similarly, a poorly placed anesthesia mask putting pressure on the eye and even ordinary tracheal intubation can raise IOP. Increases in central venous pressure (CVP) and arterial carbon dioxide tension will also increase IOP and vice versa. To a lesser degree, increases in arterial blood pressure and large decreases in arterial oxygen tension will also increase IOP (and vice versa for arterial blood pressure).

Drugs can also have important effects on IOP. Inhalational agents, barbiturates, and benzodiazepines (and to a lesser extent, opioids) all tend to reduce IOP. Succinylcholine can cause a moderate (6–8 mm Hg) increase in IOP lasting for a few minutes. Consequently, its use in "full stomach" patients with open-globe injuries to facilitate rapid-sequence intubation remains controversial (vide infra). Glaucoma is a condition with increased IOP that is often treated using IOP-lowering drugs, such as timolol (a β-blocker), echothiophate

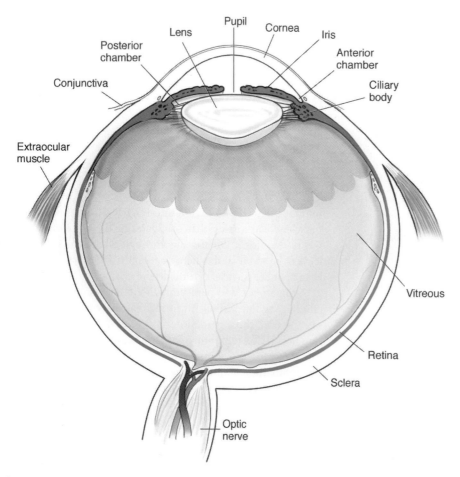

Figure 113.1. Anatomy of the eye.

(an anticholinesterase), acetazolamide (a carbonic anhydrase inhibitor), as well as other drugs (discussed later).

Oculocardiac reflex

A particularly important consideration in eye surgery (and in a number of other procedures) is the oculocardiac reflex. This is a trigeminovagal reflex whose afferent limb extends from the orbital contents to the sensory nucleus of the trigeminal nerve in the brainstem and whose efferent limb is via the vagus nerve to the sinoatrial (SA) node of the heart. The reflex is usually activated by traction on the extraocular muscles (as with strabismus surgery) or with pressure on the eyeball. Although the usual result is bradycardia, more dangerous rhythm disturbances, even asystole, can occur. Should significant bradycardia persist despite the surgeon stopping the eye manipulation, treatment with intravenous atropine or glycopyrrolate can be used. The reflex is accentuated with concomitant hypercarbia and is most predominant in children. Fortunately, the reflex tends to disappear with repeated stimulation.

Clinical issues

Ophthalmic procedures, particularly surgery for cataracts, are commonly carried out. Providing anesthesia for these patients involves a number of special issues. For example, the patients are usually elderly and frequently have comorbidities such as diabetes, hypertension, or coronary disease. In contrast, ophthalmic surgery is low risk, usually involving minimal physiologic trespass, so that mortality after eye procedures is much lower than for the general surgical population. These two conflicting considerations have led to differing philosophies about how ophthalmic patients should be evalutated prior to eye surgery, with one group advocating minimal evaluation beyond a good history and physical examination and another group advocating a more complete evaluation process so that the patient will be fully optimized and be exposed to the lowest risk possible. Regardless, most clinicians would hold that if an untreated reversible condition would be expected to lead to a perioperative complication, then a more complete workup is indicated. A detailed review of the preoperative assessment of the eye surgery patient has been provided by Gordon.

Ophthalmologic drugs

Ophthalmic patients often take eyedrops, some of which have important systemic effects and may interact with anesthetics. Eye drops made with echothiophate, an irreversible inhibitor of cholinesterase used to provide miosis in glaucoma patients, may decrease plasma butyryl- and cholinesterase and consequently may prolong the duration of action of succinylcholine and mivacurium. Phenylephrine, an α-agonist, is often applied topically to dilate the pupil but may also cause severe hypertension with the 10% preparation. Timolol is a topical β-blocker used in glaucoma treatment that may cause systemic β-blockade. Acetazolamide, a carbonic anhydrase inhibitor, is another drug used to lower IOP. It may cause hypokalemia. Mannitol, sometimes given to lower IOP, may distend the urinary bladder from the ensuing osmotic diuresis. Toxicity from atropine drops can result in tachycardia, dry skin, fever, and even agitation. Systemic administration of atropine has fewer mydriatic effects than does that of scopolamine and is not associated with an acute increase in ocular pressure, even in glaucoma patients. Glycopyrrolate, with its quaternary ammonium structure, might be a better choice if anticholinergics are required (i.e., for reversal of neuromuscular blockade).

Nitrous oxide in ophthalmic surgery

In some vitreoretinal procedures the surgeon injects an intravitreal gas bubble (usually sulfur hexafluoride or perfluoropropane) to maintain apposition of the neuroretina to the retinal pigment epithelium. Use of nitrous oxide during or after such cases will cause bubble expansion as nitrous oxide diffuses into the bubble, causing IOP to increase to dangerous levels. Consequently, nitrous oxide should be avoided in future cases until the bubble is resorbed, a period that can be longer than a month for perfluoroethane and 1 to 2 weeks for sulfur hexafluoride (Fig. 113.2). Should you find yourself using nitrous oxide and subsequently end up surprised by a change in surgical plan that now includes the addition of a gas bubble, you must insist

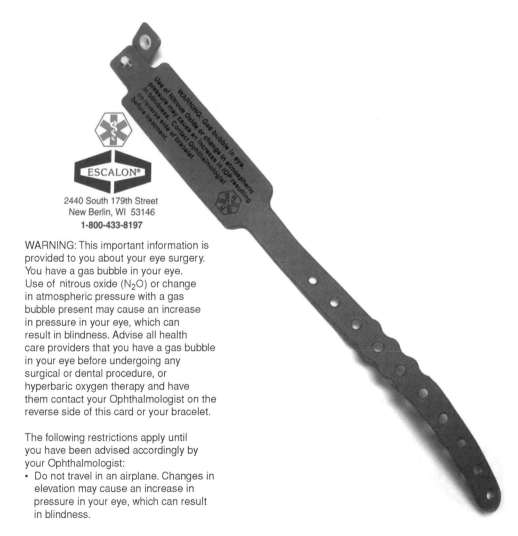

WARNING: This important information is provided to you about your eye surgery. You have a gas bubble in your eye. Use of nitrous oxide (N₂O) or change in atmospheric pressure with a gas bubble present may cause an increase in pressure in your eye, which can result in blindness. Advise all health care providers that you have a gas bubble in your eye before undergoing any surgical or dental procedure, or hyperbaric oxygen therapy and have them contact your Ophthalmologist on the reverse side of this card or your bracelet.

The following restrictions apply until you have been advised accordingly by your Ophthalmologist:
• Do not travel in an airplane. Changes in elevation may cause an increase in pressure in your eye, which can result in blindness.

Figure 113.2. Sample warning information and warning bracelet for patients receiving intraocular gas bubbles.

on having 20 minutes (with a generous fresh gas flow of either 100% O_2 or O_2/air mix) to allow the nitrous oxide to dissipate before a gas bubble is placed.

Topical anesthesia

Cataract surgery and some other eye procedures can often be done using only topical anesthesia, such as tetracaine or lidocaine eye drops. The technique works best when the incision is small and the patients are cooperative, but does not provide akinesis. Consequently, topical anesthesia for cataract surgery has now become more the rule than the exception, as it offers both extreme simplicity as well as the avoidance of the risks associated with retrobulbar and peribulbar injection techniques. Topical eye anesthesia is sometimes supplemented by the surgeon injecting 0.1 ml of 1% preservative-free lidocaine into the anterior chamber (intracameral injection). Topical anesthesia is a poor choice, however, for patients unable or unwilling to follow instructions. Also, there is more eye movement, which may be a disadvantage to the surgeon. Finally, note that the technique is often supplemented with mild to moderate intravenous sedation.

Conduction anesthesia for ophthalmic surgery

A variety of regional anesthetic techniques have been developed for eye surgery. These offer several advantages over general anesthesia: postoperative analgesia, a low frequency of nausea and vomiting, earlier ambulation, and earlier discharge. The primary goals of these blocks are eye anesthesia and eye akinesia (immobility). In addition, patient comfort and anxiolysis must be provided. The former usually involves placing pillows under the knees to keep them flexed, and the latter is usually achieved with judicious intravenous sedation (e.g., midazolam, fentanyl, and/or propofol). In all cases, standard monitors are applied, and oxygen is given via a nasal cannula.

The *retrobulbar* block (Fig. 113.3) provides both eye akinesis and eye anesthesia. As the name implies, it involves injecting local anesthesia behind the globe. The procedure is often done in conjunction with a block of the facial nerve. Retrobulbar hemorrhage is the most common complication of this block. Special care must be taken when performing this block in patients with high myopia because globe perforation is more likely to occur in this situation.

Concerns about retrobulbar hemorrhage with the retrobulbar block have led some ophthalmologists to champion the *posterior peribulbar* block. Disadvantages include a longer onset time and less complete eye akinesia. Another block, the *sub-Tenon* block, avoids sharp needles entirely. The technique uses a blunt cannula that is inserted between Tenon's facia and the sclera under local anesthesia. Local anesthesia (1–2 ml) is then injected into the catheter. Although analgesia with this technique is excellent, and it is less painful than the retrobulbar block, conjunctival edema is a frequent occurrence.

For these blocks, a 1:1 ratio of preservative-free bupivacaine 0.75% and preservative-free lidocaine 2% (without epinephrine) is sometimes used. Hyaluronidase is sometimes added to increase the absorption and dispersion of the local anesthetic. It is not uncommon to "stun" the patient with a small dose of thiopental (50–100 mg) or propofol (30–50 mg) just prior to carrying out a retrobulbar block. Complications of these blocks are usually related to direct needle trauma or local anesthetic toxicity.

- Trauma: retrobulbar hematoma, puncture or perforation of the globe, intraneural injury, intramuscular injury resulting in postoperative strabismus
- Local anesthetic properties: seizures from intravascular (arterial) injection, loss of consciousness and respiratory arrest from local anesthesia entering the central nervous system (epidural, intrathecal) from injection into the sheath of the optic nerve, which is continuous with the dura and arachnoid

General anesthesia for ophthalmic surgery

In patients who are unsuitable for topical or regional anesthesia, general anesthesia is usually used. Unsuitable patients include some anxious patients, patients who are unable to lie still for surgery, mentally challenged patients, patients who are otherwise uncooperative, and much of the pediatric population. Other examples include patients with severe tremors (e.g., from Parkinson's disease), restless leg syndrome, chronic cough, and severe claustrophobia (a patient unable to ride in an elevator due to claustrophobia cannot be expected to tolerate the confinement of surgery while awake).

Strabismus surgery and emergency surgery for an open globe frequently require general anesthesia. It may be wise to use general anesthesia in young, healthy patients undergoing a sclera buckle or in those who may require enunciation of the eye. Other patients who should be considered for general anesthesia include those with high myopia and an intraocular axial length greater than 25 mm (making them at risk for injury to the globe for some eye blocks), monocular patients, patients who have suffered complications from previous regional anesthesia to the eye, anticoagulated patients, and patients with needle phobia.

General anesthesia can be accomplished by using inhalation anesthesia, total intravenous anesthesia, or a "balanced" technique. Muscle relaxants are often used. Use of the laryngeal mask airway (LMA) is popular in Europe for ophthalmologic surgery and is often favored because it is said to provide for a smoother, cough-free emergence. Because the airway is inaccessible during the surgery, however, the technique is shunned by many anesthesiologists in this setting, who are fearful of laryngospasm and other potential airway problems.

Postoperative nausea and vomiting (PONV) is always a concern when general anesthesia is used. Frequently in ophthalmic

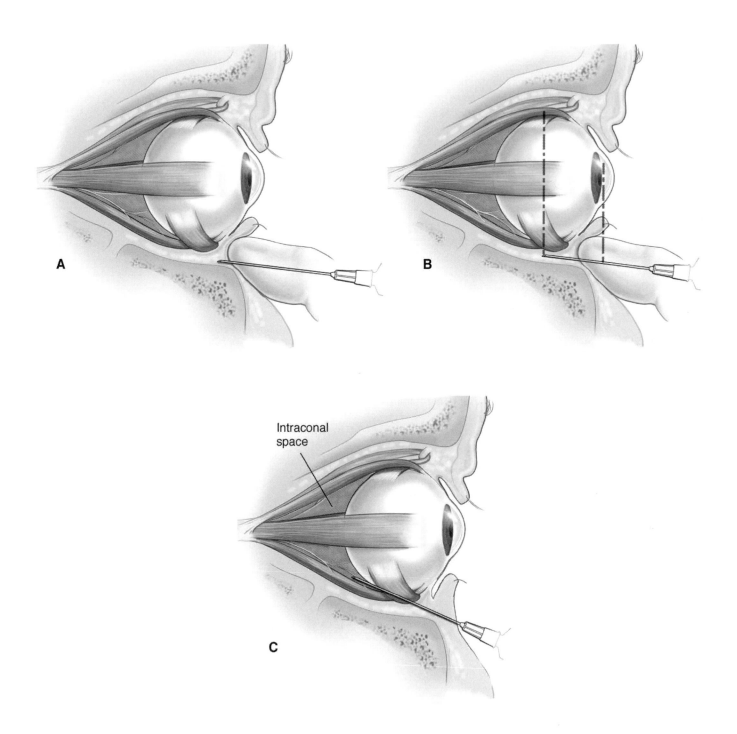

Figure 113.3. Retrobulbar block (inferotemporal intraconal block). (**A**) The needle tip enters at the lower temporal orbital rim slightly up from the orbital floor and passes very close to the bone. (**B**) At 10° elevation parallel to the orbital floor, the needle (e.g., 25 gauge Atkinson needle) passes backward until its mid-shaft is at the iris. The tip is then at the equator of the globe. (**C**) The needle does not pass the midsagittal plane of the globe. It enters the intraconal space after passing through the intermuscular septum. Any movement of the sclera is noted. After test aspiration, 4 ml of anesthetic solution is injected.

surgery prophylactic antiemetic agents, such as ondansetron or droperidol, are used to reduce the likelihood of this happening.

Open globe injury

Globe rupture following blunt injury and globe penetration after a penetrating injury are major emergencies that as a rule require surgery under general anesthesia. (Retrobulbar blocks are contraindicated due to concerns that external pressure might result in extrusion of vitreous.) Unfortunately, these patients usually do not have empty stomachs, necessitating tracheal intubation via rapid-sequence induction if the surgeon is unwilling to delay the surgery until the stomach is empty. Special attention should be paid to the avoidance of applying external pressure to the eye, as with application of a face mask.

Because awake intubation can be associated with considerable coughing and bucking that would be expected to lead to loss of eye content, its use should be reserved to situations in which intubation by direct laryngoscopy would be expected to be difficult. In addition, the use of a supraglottic airway in this setting would usually be inappropriate, as it does not protect the airway against aspiration.

Further complicating matters is the fact that laryngoscopy and intubation are associated with increased IOP, as is the use of succinylcholine as compared to nondepolarizing muscle relaxants. These cases thus present a clinical dilemma that remains unanswered to this day: Is it better to secure the airway more rapidly using succinylcholine, with its typical 6 to 8 mm Hg increase in IOP, or is it better to use a nondepolarizing muscle relaxant that will take longer to work, even in large doses? After years of rigid teaching that the latter is the preferred approach, thinking is now shifting toward the former.

Suggested readings

Ahmad S. Sedation techniques in ophthalmic anesthesia. *Ophthalmol Clin North Am* 2006; 19(2):193–202.

Cass GD. Choices of local anesthetics for ocular surgery. *Ophthalmol Clin North Am* 2006; 19(2):203–207.

Chidiac EJ, Raiskin AO. Succinylcholine and the open eye. *Ophthalmol Clin North Am* 2006; 19(2):279–285.

Cunningham AJ, Barry P. Intraocular pressure–physiology and implications for anaesthetic management. *Can Anaesth Soc J* 1986; 33(2):195–208.

Fraunfelder FW, Fraunfelder FT, Jensvold B. Adverse systemic effects from pledgets of topical ocular phenylephrine 10%. *Am J Ophthalmol* 2002; 134(4):624–625.

Gordon HL. Preoperative assessment in ophthalmic regional anaesthesia. *Contin Educ Anaesth Crit Care Pain* (CEACCP) 2006; 6(5):203–206.

Greenhalgh DL, Kumar CM. Sedation during ophthalmic surgery. *Eur J Anaesthesiol* 2008; 25(9):701–707.

Hoyng PF, van Beek LM. Pharmacological therapy for glaucoma: a review. *Drugs* 2000; 59(3):411–434.

Kumar CM, Williamson S, Manickam B. A review of sub-Tenon's block: current practice and recent development. *Eur J Anaesthesiol* 2005; 22(8):567–577.

Pantuck EJ. Ecothiopate iodide eye drops and prolonged response to suxamethonium. *Br J Anaesth* 1966; 38(5):406–407.

Schimek F, Fahle M. Techniques of facial nerve block. *Br J Ophthalmol* 1995; 79(2):166–173.

Simonson D. Retrobulbar block: a review for the clinician. *AANA J* 1990; 58(6):456–461.

Van Brocklin MD, Hirons RR, Yolton RL. The oculocardiac reflex: a review. *J Am Optom Assoc* 1982; 53(5):407–413.

Venkatesan VG, Smith A. What's new in ophthalmic anaesthesia? *Curr Opin Anaesthesiol* 2002; 15(6):615–620.

Yang YF, Herbert L, Rüschen H, Cooling RJ. Nitrous oxide anaesthesia in the presence of intraocular gas can cause irreversible blindness. *BMJ* 2002; 325(7363):532–533.

Chapter 114

Common otolaryngology procedures

Naila Moghul and D. John Doyle

Otolaryngologic surgery encompasses a wide variety of procedures and an equally wide variety of patients, many with significant comorbidities. It is important to assess the anesthetic risk for the patient and note any history of congenital or acquitted malformations, abscesses or other infections, tumors, a history of head and neck radiation, previous airway trauma, the presence of nasal polyps, proven or suspected obstructive sleep apnea (OSA), and a history of hoarseness, stridor, or hemoptysis.

In all cases, assessment of the airway is particularly vital: Before beginning any case, one must first establish whether problems with ventilation or intubation might be expected. The 11-point airway examination developed by the American Society of Anesthesiology (ASA) is recommended. Additional information may be available from the surgeon in cases in which nasopharyngoscopy has been performed. Many patients will also have recent CT and MRI scans of the head and neck that should be reviewed for possible airway compromise. If there is substantial concern about the airway, an awake intubation (for instance, using a flexible fiberoptic bronchoscope [FOB]) or even a tracheotomy under local anesthesia should be considered.

After induction of anesthesia, it is common that the operating room table be rotated 90° or 180° from the anesthesia setup, necessitating extensions to the patient's breathing circuit. A lower-body or under-body forced-air heating blanket is often placed (e.g., Bair Hugger; Arizant, Eden Prairie, MN), although in long cases body temperature can sometimes become excessive from retained heat from drape use. Inspiratory gases should be humidified. Low-flow anesthesia, over a long period, can help preserve airway heat and humidity. Pressure points must be padded well and frequently checked, and a Foley catheter placed in prolonged cases.

Ear surgery

A number of ear procedures require either general anesthesia or sedation in conjunction with local anesthesia. Myringotomy with tube insertion is an especially common pediatric procedure that is often performed under simple local anesthesia in adults and in older children, although general anesthesia is usually required in younger patients. Ear procedures that usually require anesthesia include acoustic neuroma removal, cochlear implant surgery, otoplasty, tympanoplasty, and stapedectomy.

Use of nitrous oxide

Under normal physiologic conditions, any gas pressure buildup within the middle ear is relieved through an open eustachian tube. This pathway may be partially or completely obstructed in conditions, such as otitis media, upper respiratory tract infection, or sinusitis, preventing the release of gas from the middle ear cavity. This potentiality explains why nitrous oxide can be a problem in ear surgery. Specifically, nitrous oxide diffuses into air-filled cavities more rapidly than the nitrogen present in air is absorbed into the bloodstream. This property results in gas expansion within the middle ear cavity, leading to increased middle ear pressure, possible rupture of the tympanic membrane (eardrum), and even hearing loss. Even in tympanoplasty procedures, during which the middle ear pressure is the same as atmospheric pressure, placement of the tympanic membrane graft converts the middle ear into a closed cavity. If nitrous oxide is either introduced at this point or is discontinued, a change in air pressure in either direction risks dislodgement of the graft. It is therefore recommended that nitrous oxide be avoided entirely during middle ear surgery, or at least discontinued 20 minutes prior to tympanoplasty.

Hemostasis

One of the requirements of microsurgery is that the surgical field be kept clear of blood and secretions to allow good visualization. What may appear to be mere tiny droplets of blood to the naked eye may obscure the operating field when a microscope is in use. Controlled (deliberate) hypotension is one technique occasionally used to counter this problem. The surgical benefits, however, may not always outweigh the inherent risks to the patient.

Nerve injury

In some types of ear operations, nerve stimulators are used to identify nerves. Consequently, intraoperative use of neuromuscular blockade may sometimes predispose to misidentification of anatomic structures and even result in dissection injury to structures such as the facial nerve. In contrast, even the slightest movement under a surgical microscope is magnified. These two aspects must be resolved by a discussion with the surgeon prior to the induction of anesthesia. Not infrequently, an infusion of remifentanil is used as an anesthetic adjunct in such cases.

Postoperative nausea and vomiting

Ear surgery, especially middle ear operations, commonly result in postoperative nausea and vomiting (PONV). PONV prophylaxis is usually employed in such cases, and an anesthetic technique that eliminates or deemphasizes the use of potent inhalational agents and opioids should be considered. Although PONV prophylaxis is detailed elsewhere in this book, commonly used antiemetics include a scopolamine patch, ondansetron, and dexamethasone.

Extubation

Smooth extubation without straining or coughing on the endotracheal tube (ETT) is always desirable, but is particularly important in many ENT cases. Topicalization of the glottic structures with lidocaine at the time of intubation and the intravenous (IV) administration of lidocaine (1–1.5 mg/kg) around the time of extubation may be used to blunt the patient's response to the ETT. Small doses of remifentanil are sometimes also used for this purpose (e.g., 0.2–0.5 μg/kg).

Specific ear operations
Acoustic neuroma surgery

These tend to be long-duration procedures that are often done by a neurosurgical team. A variety of surgical approaches are commonly used (middle cranial fossa approach, retrosigmoid suboccipital approach, translabyrinthine approach), and the function of the facial nerve is often monitored.

Cochlear implant surgery

Cochlear implantation is a common surgical procedure used to treat severe hearing loss, often done in the pediatric population. The procedure usually includes placing an electrode array into the cochlea and inserting the matching signal receiver into the mastoid bone behind the ear.

Mastoidectomy

This surgical procedure is designed to remove pathology, such as a pocket of infection or a cholesteatoma from the mastoid bone. Its purpose is to prevent eventual damage to the hearing apparatus. In a radical mastoidectomy, usually performed to combat extensive spread of a cholesteatoma, the eardrum and middle ear structures may be removed, although the stapes is often spared. The procedure begins with an incision behind the ear. The mastoid bone is then exposed and opened with a drill. The pathology is then removed, followed by closure with

stitches. A drain may be placed. Facial nerve injury is a rare complication.

Myringotomy

Myringotomy is commonly a pediatric procedure and is discussed elsewhere (see Part 24 on pediatric anesthesia).

Tympanoplasty

Tympanic membrane microsurgical repair using homografts is a common otologic procedure. Tissue materials located near the operative field are used to make the graft. Temporalis fascia and perichondrium are two of the more commonly used materials, although artificial materials (e.g., AlloDerm; LifeCell Corporation, Branchburg, NJ) are sometimes used in repeat procedures. Nitrous oxide should be avoided.

Tracheostomy

A tracheostomy creates a surgical airway in the cervical trachea, usually with the intent to place a tracheostomy tube (Fig. 114.1). The procedure is most commonly carried out in patients who could not be weaned off a ventilator, although it is also used for trauma patients, patients who have experienced severe neurologic injury, and patients with head and neck cancers. Although the procedure is often carried out between the second and third tracheal rings, in dire emergencies it is sometimes carried out through the more easily entered but higher positioned cricothyroid membrane (cricothyrotomy).

Some key points to note are as follows:

After the trachea is secured with an ETT, the trachea and the hypopharynx are suctioned, the patient is ventilated with 100% oxygen, and the surgeon dissects down to the trachea. Care must be taken to avoid the use of cautery while 100% oxygen is being administered to prevent an airway fire. The

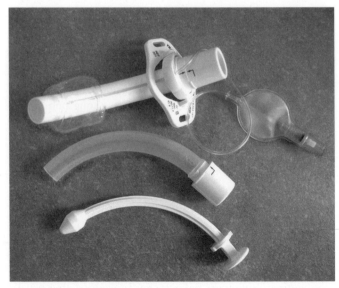

Figure 114.1. Tracheostomy tube assembly. Courtesy Klaus D. Peter, Wiehl, Germany.

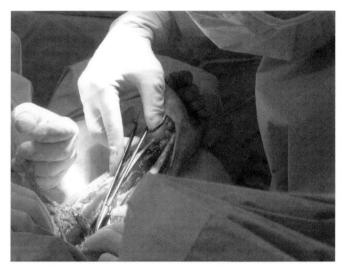

Figure 114.2. Harvesting of a free flap from the upper extremity in a head and neck cancer operation.

ETT cuff is temporarily deflated before the surgeon cuts between the tracheal rings with the scalpel, to avoid cuff perforation. After the tracheal wall is transected and the tracheostomy tube is ready to be placed, the cuff is deflated and the ETT withdrawn until the tip is just cephalad to the incision while the cuff remains distal to the vocal cords.

At this point, the breathing circuit is disconnected from the ETT and handed over to the surgeon, using utmost caution to keep the ETT firmly in place. Only after placement of the tracheostomy tube is confirmed through capnography, chest-rise, and auscultation is the ETT cuff finally deflated and the ETT removed. A reinforced tracheal tube or laryngectomy tube may be temporarily placed when the tracheostomy is part of a cancer operation; otherwise, a regular tracheostomy tube is used (Fig. 114.2).

Possible complications include bleeding (e.g., from a divided thyroid isthmus or other nearby vessels), pneumothorax, subcutaneous emphysema, and tube obstruction from impingement on the posterior tracheal wall, blood clot, or mucus plugging. Inadvertent early decannulation and subsequent difficulty in correctly replacing the tube carry significant mortality. Late complications include tracheal stenosis, tracheoesophageal fistula, and tracheal necrosis. Massive hemorrhage from erosion of the innominate artery can also occur, and is often fatal.

Some individuals favor using a percutaneous tracheostomy technique (e.g., Ciaglia Blue Rhino kit; Cook Medical, Bloomington, IN), especially in some surgical intensive care unit (ICU) wards. In experienced hands this may be a safe and effective alternative to traditional surgical techniques. Regardless of the technique used, it should be emphasized that changing a tracheostomy tube following a fresh tracheostomy is especially perilous as the new tube may enter a false passage. Thus, if a fresh tracheostomy tube is inadvertently removed, a direct laryngoscopy and intubation with an ETT may be necessary to salvage the airway.

For the first 5 to 10 days postoperatively, all tube changes should ideally be carried out in the operating room. After the surgical site has had time to mature, it is no longer necessary to carry out tube changes in an operating room, but a full set of tracheostomy instruments (especially cricoid hooks) should still be available. Changing the tube using a tube exchanger or using an FOB to confirm tracheal placement of a tracheostomy tube prior to attempting positive pressure ventilation may also be useful. Finally, patients should be preoxygenated with 100% oxygen prior to the tube change.

Head and neck cancer surgery, laryngeal surgery, and endoscopy
General considerations

Integrity of the airway is a key concern when evaluating any patient with a neoplastic growth in the head and neck region. Many tumors may enlarge considerably without causing airway compromise, whereas others, due to their location, may lead to problems, such as stridor and aspiration. Highly vascular tumors can hemorrhage with minimal manipulation. Radiation therapy may cause fibrosis of the temporomandibular joint (TMJ) and other structures, adding to difficulty with mouth opening or making it difficult to identify anatomic structures during laryngoscopy.

Surgical treatment of head and neck cancer can include such diverse procedures as laryngectomy, pharyngectomy, hemimandibulectomy, parotidectomy, or radical neck dissection. Because of the extensive nature of these operations and possible complicated postoperative sequelae, most of these patients will have been extensively evaluated prior to presenting for surgery. This patient population tends to be elderly and have various comorbidities, such as hypertension, cardiovascular disease, chronic obstructive pulmonary disease (COPD) from chronic smoking, and heavy alcohol use. Chronic malnutrition, dehydration, and weight loss are also common. The patient's medical history and the anticipated extent and duration of surgery will influence choices of inhalational, opioid, and paralytic agents.

Large-bore IV access is appropriate for most cases. A central venous catheter may also be appropriate if existing IV access is suboptimal. Arterial cannulation for closer monitoring of blood pressure or for frequent blood sampling may be indicated in patients with significant cardiovascular, pulmonary, hepatic, or endocrine disease or in surgeries during which there is a possibility of substantial blood loss or when carotid manipulation may lead to cardiac rhythm disturbances or variations in blood pressure. Manipulation of carotid bodies, sinuses, and the stellate ganglion during radical neck dissection may cause wide swings in blood pressure, arrhythmias, QT abnormalities in the electrocardiogram, and even sinus arrest. In such cases the surgeon must be immediately notified and the procedure must be paused. Infiltration of the carotid sheath with local anesthetic usually produces resolution of these side effects. The denervation of carotid bodies and sinuses, especially in bilateral neck dissection, may result in wide blood pressure variation (hypertension or hypotension) in the postoperative period. Hypoxic drive may be affected as well. The postoperative course may require a stay in the ICU, and the patient is sometimes left intubated due to laryngeal and pharyngeal edema following surgical manipulation.

Radical neck dissection or parotidectomy requires careful surgical dissection of tissues to preserve peripheral nerves, such as the facial and the spinal accessory. Consequently, the anesthesiologist is often asked to withhold neuromuscular blockade after the initial intubating dose. Intubation of trachea may be carried out with succinylcholine or other short-acting agents, after which it is important to document return of neuromuscular function. The planned anesthetic would entail a deeper plane of anesthesia, with the inhalational agents often supplemented by a remifentanil infusion to ensure absence of motor response to surgical stimuli.

In head and neck cases involving free flaps harvested from upper or lower extremities, special attention should be directed at providing adequate flap perfusion. There is substantial uncertainty on how to best achieve this goal. The use of vasopressors, such as phenylephrine, has been questioned because they elicit vasoconstriction. In animal experiments, however, flap blood flow was not altered when phenylephrine was given at low or moderate doses. Maintaining mean arterial pressure solely by means of large amounts of fluid administration can increase tissue edema, jeopardize the integrity of the anastomosis, and ultimately impair tissue oxygenation. Maintaining normothermia and modulating the perioperative inflammation might offer additional means to optimize surgical outcome. Close communication with the surgical team will help to provide appropriate care for every individual case.

Whether a hematocrit at or around 30 provides optimized rheologic properties within the capillaries remains unclear. The negative impact of the transfusion of stored allogenic red blood cells might mitigate this presumed effect.

Airway management

General anesthesia with endotracheal intubation is most commonly used. Distortion of the oropharynx from tumor or tumor-related respiratory compromise may necessitate securing the airway by awake fiber-optic intubation or even awake tracheotomy. Upper airway tissues may be friable following radiation and be prone to bleeding upon manipulation. Alternatively, radiation therapy may lead to tissue fibrosis or spondylosis of the TMJ, resulting in reduced mouth opening.

In cases where there are serious airway concerns, the surgeon should be present in the operating room during induction should emergent cricothyrotomy or tracheostomy become necessary. An inhalation induction with sevoflurane with the goal of maintaining spontaneous ventilation is sometimes a useful alternative to an IV induction or awake intubation.

If an awake fiber-optic intubation is chosen because of significant airway compromise, the oropharynx should be

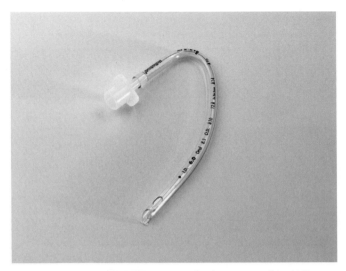

Figure 114.3. An oral RAE ETT. Image used with permission from Nellcor Puritan Bennett LLC, Boulder, Colorado, part of Covidien.

topicalized with lidocaine or benzocaine. In addition, some practitioners will sedate the patient with midazolam, fentanyl, or dexmedetomidine.

As noted earlier, some head and neck procedures, depending on intraoperative requirements and postoperative airway logistics, will require a tracheostomy. If so, the tracheostomy is usually done following the induction of anesthesia, either at the beginning or the end of the main procedure itself. RAE ETTs are popular in ENT surgery as they are designed for secure fixation and easy access. They are available in oral (Fig. 114.3) and nasal (Fig. 114.4) styles.

Airway management issues also arise in laryngoscopy, bronchoscopy, esophagoscopy, and phonosurgery procedures. In head and neck cancer, the first three of these procedures are often carried out in a single session. Intubation is usually accomplished with a small diameter (5.0–6.0 mm) ETT. Another option is to use a microlaryngeal type ETT (MLT).

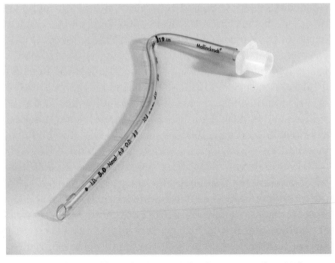

Figure 114.4. A nasal RAE ETT. Image used with permission from Nellcor Puritan Bennett LLC, Boulder, Colorado, part of Covidien.

These ETTs have a narrow shaft (e.g., 4, 5, or 6 mm ID) but are the same length as the adult tube and have a large, high-volume, low-pressure cuff. Naturally, they offer higher resistance to breathing than a regular ETT, and ventilating pressures may need to be higher for a given tidal volume. Phonosurgery involves surgery to the vocal cords and related structures and can be done under sedation to allow the patient to phonate, although it is also commonly done under general anesthesia with an MLT in place.

A mixture of helium and oxygen (heliox) is sometimes used to substantially decrease the pressures needed to ventilate patients with small-diameter endotracheal tubes. Commonly used mixtures include 80%/20% or 70%/30% helium to oxygen. Heliox also offers a potential advantage in patient upper airway obstruction resulting from edema, tumors, or foreign objects. It is the low density of helium that allows it to be useful in such cases.

In some ENT procedures, jet ventilation is used in conjunction with total intravenous anesthesia (TIVA). Typically, the surgeon inserts a special laryngoscope (e.g., Dedo; KARL STORZ Endoscopy-America, Inc., El Segundo, CA) to which a jet ventilation attachment is placed. The patient is ventilated intermittently with bursts of 100% oxygen at 10 to 40 PSI, with special attention to watching the chest rise and fall. (Recall that 1 PSI = 51.71 mm Hg.) Jet ventilation should be done only when the vocal cords are visible through the laryngoscope; consequently, continuous communication with the surgeon is essential. Because barotrauma resulting in pneumothorax is a potential complication, the minimum effective driving pressure should be chosen.

An apneic oxygenation technique can also be used for some short endoscopic procedures, such as tracheal dilatation procedures for tracheal stenosis. The patient is ventilated by mask (or via an ETT) until oxygenation is maximal. The mask is then removed and the surgery performed under apnea until the arterial saturation decreases, and ventilation must again be started.

Nasal and sinus surgery

Common procedures include septoplasty, polypectomy, endoscopic sinus surgery, and maxillary sinusotomy (Caldwell–Luc procedure). Most of these procedures are performed under general anesthesia. These procedures, however, can be tolerated with sedation and local anesthesia in a cooperative patient. Preoperatively, patients should be asked about possible signs of OSA, recent infections, and antibiotic, antihistamine, or aspirin use.

Patients should be assessed for audible or mouth breathing, diminished speech quality, inspiratory stridor, expiratory wheezes, or a prolonged expiration, which may signal partial airway obstruction. Nasal polyps can be associated with allergic disorders and reactive airway disease, such as asthma, or with cystic fibrosis. Aspirin or nonsteroidal anti-inflammatory drug use in association with nasal polyps is of a particular concern.

Premedication may include an antisialogogue, an anxiolytic, and/or antiemetic prophylaxis. Anesthetic induction should always take into account the possibility of existing partial airway obstruction.

Many surgeons like to treat the nose with cotton-tipped pledgets soaked with local anesthetic (e.g., cocaine 4% or 10% to a maximum dose of 3 mg/kg), thereby blocking the sphenopalatine and anterior ethmoidal nerves that provide sensation to the nasal septum and lateral walls. This anesthetic also shrinks the nasal mucosa and reduces blood loss. Intranasal cocaine must be used cautiously in patients with hypertension or with a history of coronary artery disease. Many surgeons also prefer the use of RAE style or reinforced type ETTs. A posterior pharyngeal pack is sometimes used to help prevent blood from trickling down to the trachea. Special care must be taken to tape the patient's eyes because of the proximity of the surgical equipment to the face. These cases are often conducted with the assistance of special surgical navigation equipment.

Coughing, bucking, or straining at the time of extubation can cause increased vascular pressure, thereby risking postoperative bleeding. It is desirable to carry out extubation in as smooth a manner as possible, with the patient having regained consciousness and airway protection reflexes. Smooth extubation is sometimes facilitated using small doses of remifentanil to blunt the patient's reaction to awakening with the ETT in place.

Some anesthesiologists like to employ "deep extubation": The trachea is extubated after establishing spontaneous respiration but before the return of airway reflexes, while the patient is still in a deep plane of anesthesia. This technique is considered to be hazardous by some practitioners because it places the patient at risk for laryngospasm as well as aspiration of gastric contents or bloody secretions. This option may be less attractive for patients who are at high risk for aspiration or who have a history of a difficult intubation. Care must be taken to assist the patient's respiration until all airway reflexes return and full consciousness is regained.

Obstructive sleep apnea

OSA disorder is characterized by the obstruction of the airway during sleep by the oropharyngeal soft tissue. Both anatomic factors (e.g., redundant folds of oropharyngeal tissue, tonsillar hypertrophy, macroglossia, or anomalous positioning of the maxilla and mandible) and neuromuscular factors (e.g., reduced oropharyngeal muscle tone with reduced ventilatory motor output to upper airway muscles during sleep) may be contributing factors. If undetected, OSA can lead to serious health problems and result in important perioperative complications. Patients with OSA may complain of snoring, daytime sleepiness, repeated morning headaches, intellectual impairment, and other symptoms. OSA is also associated with obesity.

The perioperative concerns in patients with OSA are primarily respiratory in nature, and include airway obstruction, the potential for difficult intubation, and an increased sensitivity to opioids. In addition, potential nonrespiratory concerns include a link between OSA and heart failure, ventricular hypertrophy (right-sided first, then left-sided), systemic and pulmonary hypertension, cardiac rhythm disturbances, and vascular disease.

Physiologically, the patency of the upper airway during inspiration requires active muscle tone. When this tone is reduced as a result of sleep, neuromuscular disease, anesthesia, or residual neuromuscular blockade, upper airway obstruction may occur. The velopharynx, a particularly narrow segment of the upper airway, is especially predisposed to obstruction in such settings. Obese patients with large necks often have a more collapsible velopharynx that predisposes to upper airway obstruction. Not surprisingly, OSA apnea events are associated with intermittent hypoxemia, and a potential long-term consequence is pulmonary hypertension and cor pulmonale due to pulmonary vasoconstriction. Heart failure and other complications may follow.

Polysomnography, usually involving an overnight sleep study, is required to formally diagnose OSA. The study is usually performed in a specialized sleep center, where numerous body functions are monitored and scored (e.g., respiratory pattern, pulse oximetry, electroencephalogram [EEG], electrooculogram [EOG], and chin electromyogram [EMG]). In the absence of polysomnography, some specific clinical findings may be helpful in identifying potential OSA patients. In particular, the ASA has recently published guidelines for the perioperative care of OSA patients.

It has been established that the presence of OSA may lead to difficulties in tracheal intubation. Although this does not imply that awake intubation is necessary in OSA patients, clinicians should have immediately available various alternate means to secure the airway should difficulties with intubation be encountered using conventional equipment.

A number of ENT procedures are sometimes used to treat OSA. These may include a uvulopalatopharyngoplasty (UPPP) procedure, tonsillectomy, hyoid myotomy surgery, or other surgical interventions. Postoperative complications such as hypoxemia, hypercapnia, delirium, unplanned ICU days, reintubation, and cardiac events occur disproportionately. It should also be noted that there is a propensity for sedatives to increase the frequency of sleep-related apneic episodes in OSA patients. Although this problem is often highlighted from the perspective of postoperative opioid administration, it should be noted that agents such as benzodiazepines and barbiturates increase the chance of upper airway obstruction by decreasing upper airway muscle tone. In any event, the lowest effective dose of analgesic or sedating drugs should be used, with antagonists such as naloxone and flumazenil being readily available.

Experts surveyed to develop the ASA *Practice Guidelines for the Perioperative Management of Patients with Obstructive Sleep Apnea* suggested that OSA patients be monitored for (a median of) three hours longer than their non-OSA counterparts before discharge from an outpatient facility. In addition, monitoring should continue for (a median of) 7 hours after the last episode of airway obstruction or hypoxemia while the patient is breathing room air in a quiet, unstimulated environment. It is also important that the patient's postdischarge instructions emphasize the continued use of home continuous positive airway pressure (CPAP) in patients who use CPAP preoperatively.

Special situations
Laryngospasm

Laryngospasm is a reflex involving spasm of the glottic musculature. It is triggered to protect the upper airway from exposure to foreign material. Laryngospasm is associated with light anesthesia, is caused by blood or secretions irritating the vocal cords, and may occur after septoplasty and rhinoplasty surgery. This form of airway obstruction is common in children and can occasionally result in profound hypoxia. Although laryngospasm can often be broken using a sustained positive pressure breath or by increasing the depth of anesthesia with propofol or an inhalational agent, muscle relaxation (e.g., succinylcholine 10–20 mg IV) is sometimes needed to break the spasm. Attempts by the patient to breathe in against the glottic obstruction may occasionally produce "negative-pressure" pulmonary edema.

Retropharyngeal abscess

Retropharyngeal abscess formation may occur from a bacterial infection of the retropharyngeal space, which usually results from tonsillar or dental infections. If untreated, the posterior pharyngeal wall may advance anteriorly into the oropharynx, resulting in dyspnea, painful swallowing, trismus, and (eventually) airway obstruction. As abscess rupture can lead to tracheal soiling, contact with the abscess during laryngoscopy and intubation should be minimized. Incision and drainage is the usual treatment, and a temporary tracheostomy is sometimes required.

Ludwig's angina

Ludwig's angina is an infection of the floor of the mouth. The tongue may become elevated and displaced posteriorly, with a resulting concern about loss of the airway. Awake fiber-optic intubation or awake tracheotomy are commonly used to secure the airway in this condition.

Using supraglottic airways

Although the use of an ETT remains customary in most ENT cases, it should be emphasized that there exist a number of reports on the use of supraglottic airways, such as the laryngeal mask airway (LMA), during ENT cases. One advantage of using LMAs and other supraglottic airways is that they can be inserted blindly without the need for paralysis, making them helpful in many cases of difficult intubation. After securing the airway with the LMA, an FOB jacketed with an Aintree intubation catheter (Cook Medical) can be passed through the LMA when there is a need to intubate the trachea. Alternately, one can use supraglottic airways, such as the LMA FastTrac

(The Laryngeal Mask Company, Limited, San Diego, CA), which is specifically designed to aid in tracheal intubation.

Supraglottic airway devices are not only used to facilitate intubation, but can also be used as an alternative to ETTs in some ENT cases. For instance, Webster and colleagues compared use of the flexible reinforced LMA for intranasal surgery to use of an ETT and found that the LMA provided safe conditions with smoother emergence from anesthesia. Use of the flexible reinforced LMA for tonsillectomy procedures has also been reported, and remains popular in some centers.

Suggested readings

ASA practice guidelines for management of the difficult airway. Available at: http://www.asahq.org/publicationsAndServices/Difficult%20Airway.pdf.

ASA standards for basic anesthetic monitoring. Available at: http://www.asahq.org/publicationsAndServices/standards/02.pdf.

ASA practice advisory for intraoperative awareness and brain function monitoring. Available at: http://www.asahq.org/publicationsAndServices/AwareAdvisoryFinalOct05.pdf.

Gan TJ, Meyer T, Apfel CC, et al. Consensus guidelines for managing postoperative nausea and vomiting. *Anesth Analg* 2003; 97(1):62–71.

Gross JB, Bachenberg KL, Benumof JL, et al. American Society of Anesthesiologists Task Force on Perioperative Management. Practice guidelines for the perioperative management of patients with obstructive sleep apnea: a report by the American Society of Anesthesiologists Task Force on Perioperative Management of patients with obstructive sleep apnea. *Anesthesiology* 2006; 104(5):1081–1093; quiz 1117–1118.

Martin JT. *Positioning in Anesthesia and Surgery.* 2nd ed. Philadelphia: W.B. Saunders; 1987.

Webster AC, Morley-Forster PK, Janzen V, et al. Anesthesia for intranasal surgery: a comparison between tracheal intubation and the flexible reinforced laryngeal mask airway. *Anesth Analg* 1999; 88:421–425.

Lasers, airway surgery, and operating room fires

Alvaro A. Macias, Naila Moghul, and D. John Doyle

Laser surgery

It has been several decades since lasers were first introduced into clinical practice (LASER = **L**ight **A**mplification by **S**timulated **E**mission of **R**adiation). Since that time, the laser has become an important tool for surgeons in many specialties, but especially for the ENT surgeon performing laryngeal or tracheobronchial surgery. The use of lasers allows surgeons to concentrate high levels of energy onto a small area, allowing for precise resection of tissue and with the added advantage of providing excellent hemostasis. Different laser types with differing energy properties produce different effects on tissue (Fig. 115.1). With the advent of laser surgery, however, the risk of airway fires as well as fires at other surgical locations has become an important safety issue.

A number of laser technologies are in clinical use. The carbon dioxide (CO_2) laser produces a long-wavelength (10,600 nm) infrared beam that causes instantaneous vaporization of tissue following energy absorption and subsequent internal boiling of the water in cells. Because the beam is not directly visible, a low-energy red targeting laser usually accompanies the beam. In addition, the beam cannot be transmitted via a fiber-optic bundle, a requirement for use in conjunction with a flexible fiber-optic bronchoscope. The CO_2 laser can be used either as a precision cutting instrument or as a tissue vaporizer, depending on the extent to which the beam is focused.

Other popular lasers for clinical use are the Nd-Yag (neodynium-yttrium aluminum garnet) laser, with a beam in the near infrared region at a wavelength of 1064 nm; the KTP-Nd-Yag laser, green colored at a 532-nm wavelength; and the argon laser. All these have beams that can be transmitted fiberoptically. Associated with each laser type is special protective eyewear (goggles) designed to absorb electromagnetic radiation at the wavelength of the laser in use. For example, goggles absorbing radiation at a 532-nm wavelength typically have an orange appearance and would be ineffective in protecting against a laser emitting energy at 1064 nm (Fig. 115.2). CO_2 laser protection eyewear consists of clear glass or plastic lenses that are opaque to far infrared wavelengths. KTP laser protection eyewear distorts color perception significantly in contrast to CO_2 or Nd-Yag laser protection lenses. Glass lenses in general are heavier and more expensive, but provide better protection (higher optical density) and visibility. Note that the

energy of the photons making up a laser beam depend on their wavelength; shorter-wavelength photons (toward the ultraviolet region) have more energy than do longer-wavelength photons (toward the infrared region).

A misdirected laser beam can injure both the patient and the caregiver. Ocular injuries are a special concern, as CO_2 lasers can cause corneal injuries whereas Nd-Yag lasers place the retina at risk. Consequently, the eyes of the patient are protected by taping the eyelids and then applying wet dressings on top, while caregivers wear protective goggles. In addition, laser warning signs should be placed on the outside of any doors leading to the operating room. It should also be emphasized that misdirected laser beams can ignite surgical drapes and other materials. American National Standards Institute (ANSI) standard Z136.3 (Safe Use of Lasers in Health Care Facilities) provides additional information on this and related matters. EN 207 is the European standard for laser safety eyewear.

Anesthesia providers should also be aware that when a laser beam hits tissue, a plume of smoke containing fine particulates is often produced. Because this material has mutagenic and

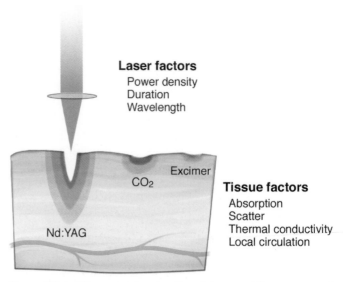

Laser factors
Power density
Duration
Wavelength

Tissue factors
Absorption
Scatter
Thermal conductivity
Local circulation

Figure 115.1. Different wavelengths of laser light cause different patterns of tissue destruction. The destructive effect of laser light on tissue depends on laser parameters and tissue factors.

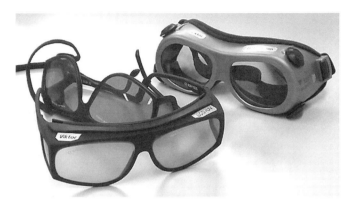

Figure 115.2. Example of three types of laser safety eyewear. *Source:* ttp://en.wikipedia.org/wiki/Image:Laser_goggles.jpg. Reproduced with permission.

teratogenic potential, or may serve as a vector for viral infection, inhalation of the smoke is best avoided by using a smoke evacuator (Fig. 115.3).

Laser-resistant endotracheal tubes

The risk of an airway fire during ENT laser surgery in an oxygen-enriched environment can be reduced by using specially designed laser-resistant ETTs that are less likely to ignite when exposed to intense heat. The traditional polyvinyl chloride tubes, as well as red rubber and silicone tubes, are combustible and potentially toxic. Whereas in earlier years such tubes were often fashioned on the spot using commercially available metallic tape wrapped in a spiral manner to protect standard ETTs, a number of specialized ETTs are now available, such as the Lasertubus tube (Teleflex, Durhan, NC). Another example is the Laser-Flex tube (Cardinal Health, Dublin, OH)

(Fig. 115.4). Only metal ETTs, however, will not ignite when struck by a laser.

Vocal cord polyps and cysts

Vocal cord polyps and cysts can occur in a variety of shapes and sizes but typically occur only on one side. Depending on the characteristics of the lesion, its effects can range from merely causing a voice disturbance to complete airway obstruction. In some cases, awake intubation is the most prudent course. Laser evaporation of these lesions is commonly done, although other techniques are available. A suspension laryngoscope is usually used to expose the glottis.

Frequently a laser-resistant ETT is employed, although some surgeons prefer to avoid using an ETT entirely; in the later case, jet ventilation in conjunction with a total intravenous anesthetic (TIVA) with propofol and remifentanil infusions is useful. The pharmacologic effects of the remifentanil will help to counter the hemodynamic effects (hypertension and tachycardia) from the suspension laryngoscopy. Muscle relaxation is usually achieved using rocuronium and a neuromuscular blockade monitor to guide administration. In addition, IV dexamethasone is sometimes given to help reduce glottic edema.

Airway fires

An airway fire is a potentially deadly complication that may occur during tracheotomy surgery, laser surgery, or a number of other procedures. Several principles apply to reduce the chance of fires in such settings.

- The surgeon should never enter the trachea by using electrocautery.

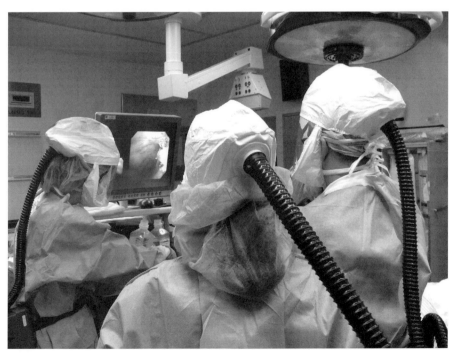

Figure 115.3. Concerns that infectious human papilloma virus (HPV) may be present in the plume of laser-treated recurrent respiratory papillomatosis have led some clinicians to use battery-operated air-purifying hoods, such as those shown here. Such systems typically include a blower, battery, headpiece, and breathing tube, creating a decidedly eerie effect.

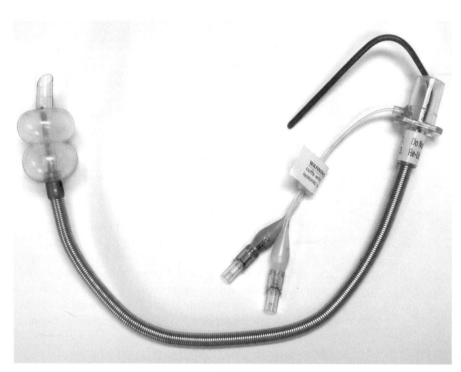

Figure 115.4. Laser-Flex laser-resistant ETT from Cardinal Health. Note the special double cuff arrangement. Some clinicians like to fill the cuffs with dilute methylene blue; in this way, an ETT cuff rupture from a misdirected laser beam can be readily detected.

- The anesthesiologist must maintain special vigilance at the moment of entry into the trachea.
- The anesthesiologist should keep the FiO_2 used to the minimum needed when a significant potential for an airway fire is present.
- Nitrous oxide should not be used during airway surgery, because it supports combustion just like oxygen.

As an example of an airway fire, consider the case described by Chee and Benumof:

A 28-yr-old, 100-kg man was scheduled for elective tracheostomy. The patient's lungs had been ventilated in the intensive care unit for 35 days after emergency craniotomy for a closed head injury. During the course of intensive care unit stay the patient remained comatose and adult respiratory distress syndrome developed, which was now resolving. The airway evaluation revealed an in situ 8.0-mm ID polyvinylchloride ETT, swollen lips, an edematous tongue protruding out of the mouth and an oropharynx filled with secretions.

General anesthesia was induced with 300 mg intravenous propofol and maintained with 0.4% inspired isoflurane and a 35% oxygen/air mixture. The vital signs remained stable within 10% of the baseline values. Electrocautery was used for coagulation by the surgeons. The patient was administered 100% oxygen immediately before insertion of the tracheostomy tube. Suddenly, the surgeons reported a blue flame shooting up vertically from the patient's neck. The breathing circuit was disconnected immediately from the ETT; 20 ml saline, 0.9%, was flushed into the ETT. The fire extinguished promptly.

This case illustrates the kind of situation for which anesthesiologists should always be prepared: a fire in the operating room. Operating room fires are best divided into airway fires and non-airway fires. A recent report by the American Society of Anesthesiologists provides specific guidance for both these scenarios (Fig. 115.5). In addition, Table 115.1 provides specific guidance in the case of airway fires. Note that the prevailing conventional wisdom, at least until recently, holds that cases of airway fire call for immediate removal of the endotracheal tube (ETT). Although this is a reasonable rule of thumb, it should also be noted that there are some patients in whom removal of the ETT would in all likelihood result in irreversible loss of the airway.

Clinicians in such a setting face a particularly difficult choice: leave the ETT in place and risk injury to the patient, or remove the ETT and risk losing the airway entirely. Both

Table 115.1. Airway fire protocol

1. Prevention: Inform the surgical team working on the airway of any situation in which high concentrations of oxygen are being used.
2. Construct an improvised fire extinguisher by filling a 60-ml syringe with saline.
3. In the case of an airway fire:
   a. Inform the surgical team and anesthesia coordinator (control desk).
   b. Stop ventilation.
   c. Discontinue nitrous oxide (which supports combustion) and lower the fraction of delivered oxygen to as little as possible.
   d. Remove ETT.
   e. Put out the fire with your improvised fire extinguisher.
4. When the fire is extinguished:
   a. Ventilate the patient with 100% oxygen via face mask (or supraglottic airway if appropriate).
   b. Assess the extent of any airway damage via laryngoscopy/bronchoscopy.
   c. Reintubate the patient if significant airway damage is found.
   d. Where appropriate, arrange for admission to an intensive care unit.

Note: Removing the ETT may be inappropriate in some cases (see text).

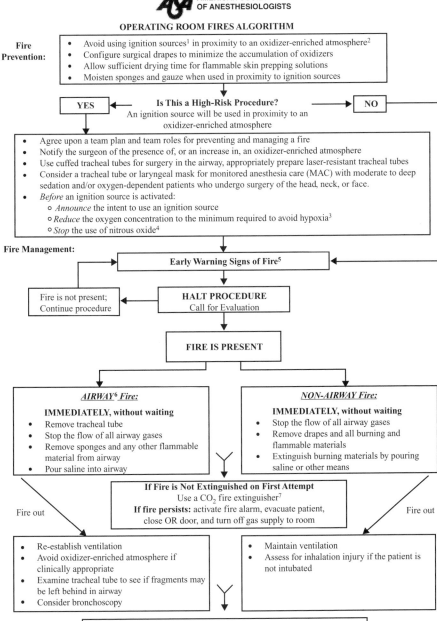

Figure 115.5. American Society of Anesthesiologists operating room fires algorithm.

AMERICAN SOCIETY OF ANESTHESIOLOGISTS

OPERATING ROOM FIRES ALGORITHM

Fire Prevention:
- Avoid using ignition sources[1] in proximity to an oxidizer-enriched atmosphere[2]
- Configure surgical drapes to minimize the accumulation of oxidizers
- Allow sufficient drying time for flammable skin prepping solutions
- Moisten sponges and gauze when used in proximity to ignition sources

Is This a High-Risk Procedure?
An ignition source will be used in proximity to an oxidizer-enriched atmosphere

YES — NO

- Agree upon a team plan and team roles for preventing and managing a fire
- Notify the surgeon of the presence of, or an increase in, an oxidizer-enriched atmosphere
- Use cuffed tracheal tubes for surgery in the airway, appropriately prepare laser-resistant tracheal tubes
- Consider a tracheal tube or laryngeal mask for monitored anesthesia care (MAC) with moderate to deep sedation and/or oxygen-dependent patients who undergo surgery of the head, neck, or face.
- *Before* an ignition source is activated:
  - *Announce* the intent to use an ignition source
  - *Reduce* the oxygen concentration to the minimum required to avoid hypoxia[3]
  - *Stop* the use of nitrous oxide[4]

Fire Management:

Early Warning Signs of Fire[5]

Fire is not present; Continue procedure

HALT PROCEDURE
Call for Evaluation

FIRE IS PRESENT

AIRWAY[6] Fire:

IMMEDIATELY, without waiting
- Remove tracheal tube
- Stop the flow of all airway gases
- Remove sponges and any other flammable material from airway
- Pour saline into airway

NON-AIRWAY Fire:

IMMEDIATELY, without waiting
- Stop the flow of all airway gases
- Remove drapes and all burning and flammable materials
- Extinguish burning materials by pouring saline or other means

If Fire is Not Extinguished on First Attempt
Use a CO_2 fire extinguisher[7]
If fire persists: activate fire alarm, evacuate patient, close OR door, and turn off gas supply to room

Fire out

Fire out

- Re-establish ventilation
- Avoid oxidizer-enriched atmosphere if clinically appropriate
- Examine tracheal tube to see if fragments may be left behind in airway
- Consider bronchoscopy

- Maintain ventilation
- Assess for inhalation injury if the patient is not intubated

Assess patient status and devise plan for management

[1] Ignition sources include but are not limited to electrosurgery or electrocautery units and lasers.

[2] An oxidizer-enriched atmosphere occurs when there is any increase in oxygen concentration above room air level, and/or the presence of any concentration of nitrous oxide.

[3] After minimizing delivered oxygen, wait a period of time (e.g., 1-3 min) before using an ignition source. For oxygen dependent patients, *reduce* supplemental oxygen delivery to the minimum required to avoid hypoxia. Monitor oxygenation with pulse oximetry, and if feasible, inspired, exhaled, and/or delivered oxygen concentration.

[4] After stopping the delivery of nitrous oxide, wait a period of time (e.g., 1-3 min) before using an ignition source,

[5] Unexpected flash, flame, smoke or heat, unusual sounds (e.g., a "pop," snap or "foomp") or odors, unexpected movement of drapes, discoloration of drapes or breathing circuit, unexpected patient movement or complaint,

[6] In this algorithm, airway fire refers to a fire in the airway or breathing circuit.

[7] A CO_2 fire extinguisher may be used on the patient if necessary.

CO_2 = carbon dioxide. OR = operating room.

Chee and Benumoff and Ng and Hartigan provide examples where leaving the ETT in place was probably the best strategy. Chee and Benumoff offer the following commentary: "In certain circumstances, the benefits of leaving the ETT in may outweigh the risks after the airway fire is extinguished. The ETT may still allow acceptable ventilation of the lungs with oxygen, especially when the airway is edematous enough to provide a reasonable seal around the perforated cuff. In addition, the ETT can serve as a conduit for a tube exchanger; this consideration may be extremely important if the airway is difficult to reestablish."

Suggested readings

Caplan RA, Barker SJ, Connis RT, et al. Practice advisory for the prevention and management of operating room fires. *Anesthesiology* 2008; 108(5):786–801; quiz 971–972. Available online at: http://www.asahq.org/publicationsAndServices/orFiresPA.pdf.

Chee WK, Benumof JL. Airway fire during tracheostomy: extubation may be contraindicated. *Anesthesiology* 1998; 89(6):1576–1578.

Ng JM, Hartigan PM. Airway fire during tracheostomy: should we extubate? *Anesthesiology* 2003; 98(5):1303.

Schramm VL Jr, Matoox DE, Stool SE. Acute management of laser-ignited intratracheal explosion. *Laryngoscope* 1981; 91:1417–1426.

Anesthesia for common orthopedic procedures

Patricio Leyton, Gian Paolo Volpato, and Kamen V. Vlassakov

Introduction

Providing optimal anesthesia and perioperative care for orthopedic surgery patients may be quite challenging for the anesthesiologist due to surgical procedure diversity and various coexisting diseases. Most common orthopedic procedures can be performed under regional anesthesia (in the absence of specific contraindications), but because of discomfort in the unanesthetized areas or long surgical duration, a combination of regional and general anesthesia may sometimes be a better choice than regional anesthesia alone. Many orthopedic surgery patients are elderly and present with multiple comorbidities. In addition, the orthopedic procedures themselves predispose to several common complications, such as venous thromboembolism, fat embolism, pneumatic tourniquet- or bone cement-associated hemodynamic instability, and patient positioning injuries. Finally, specific complications could also be related to neuraxial and other regional anesthetic techniques.

General considerations

Anticoagulation

Concomitant thromboprophylaxis presents a unique challenge when planning the optimal anesthetic, especially when neuraxial anesthesia is considered. Careful risk/benefit analysis is warranted when trying to balance possible advantages of the different regional anesthesia techniques against the odds of potentially devastating complications (e.g., epidural or spinal hematoma). The American Society of Regional Anesthesia and Pain Medicine (ASRA) has published a consensus statement addressing patient safety when regional anesthesia is performed in the presence of anticoagulant or antiplatelet drugs. These guidelines are summarized and discussed in Chapter 57.

Management of blood loss

Perioperative blood loss in orthopedic surgery can be high, especially in joint replacements, occasionally exceeding several liters in cases such as complex revision of total hip arthroplasty (THA). Risks and costs associated with blood transfusion are discussed in Chapters 67 and 68.

The term *bloodless surgery* refers to a series of perioperative patient care measures aiming to reduce or avoid the need for allogeneic blood transfusion. Patient assessment and optimization, including accurate history and physical examination, are focused on personal and family history of bleeding disorders and medications that may impair coagulation. Pre-admission testing should be done in advance (e.g., 1 month) to allow time for adequate identification, evaluation, and treatment of any coagulation defect or anemia. Possible corrective measures include the administration of iron, folate, vitamin B_{12}, and recombinant erythropoietin. It is important to plan the intraoperative availability of all equipment necessary to facilitate blood conservation strategies (e.g., cell salvage apparatus).

Surgeons practicing careful hemostasis may help minimize intraoperative blood loss. The use of electrocautery during surgery, a harmonic scalpel, and local hemostatic aids may also help reduce bleeding. Various techniques can also be used to reduce transfusion requirements, including controlled hypotension, acute normovolemic hemodilution, and autologous blood cell salvage. These techniques are discussed in detail in Chapter 69.

Multiple pharmacologic agents are also used to decrease bleeding in high-risk patients. These agents include recombinant activated factor VII, the lysine analogues (ε-aminocaproic acid and tranexamic acid) that inhibit plasmin-mediated fibrinolysis, and desmopressin that stimulates the endothelial release of factor VIII and von Willebrand factor, thereby enhancing platelet aggregation.

Tourniquets

Tourniquets are used frequently in distal extremity procedures to reduce blood loss and provide a bloodless operating field. They may cause systemic effects due to ischemia and reperfusion, as well as local effects from the pressure applied to the tissues. Tourniquet injury has been implicated as a main cause for peroneal and tibial nerve palsies after total knee arthroplasty (TKA), ranging from mild neuropraxia to permanent neurologic deficits. The incidence of tourniquet-induced paralysis is approximately 1 in 8000 operations. Pressurization of the tourniquet above 400 mm Hg is associated with increased risk of transient nerve injury. A retrospective study suggests that patients with mean total tourniquet time of 145 ± 25 minutes have a 7.7% incidence of nerve injury, recovering completely in 89% of the cases. This finding suggests that tourniquet time should not exceed 90 to 120 minutes and tourniquet pressure should not be higher than 150 mm Hg above systolic blood pressure. Controversially, the use of epidural analgesia has been reported to increase the frequency and/or severity of peroneal palsy after tourniquet use. Nevertheless, no explanation other than local anesthetic effects masking sensory and/or motor deficits has been postulated. Similarly, it has been suggested that long-acting sciatic nerve block may also delay the diagnosis of nerve injuries and should be avoided in patients at risk, such as those with preoperative flexion contracture >20° or a valgus deformity, as well as for anticipated complex or prolonged surgeries.

Anesthesia for hip fracture

Hip fracture refers to a femur fracture in the region immediately distal to the articular cartilage of the femoral head to approximately 5 cm below the lower border of the lesser trochanter. An estimated 1.7 million hip fractures occurred worldwide in 1990. In the United States, the incidence is approximately 80 per 100,000 and is increasing each year. Because the majority of these cases are treated surgically, hip fracture surgery has become one of the most commonly performed urgent orthopedic procedures. There is agreement that a delay (more than 24 hours) of surgical management increases the risk of morbidity and mortality.

Preoperative assessment

Most patients presenting with hip fractures are elderly, and many of them have significant coexisting diseases, such as coronary artery disease, arterial hypertension, diabetes, chronic obstructive pulmonary disease, cerebral vascular disease, and/or dementia, all of which may affect the choice of optimal anesthetic and monitoring strategies. Conditions that adversely affect mental status, sensory perception, visual impairment, balance, and locomotion are associated with an increased risk of hip fracture. It is important to evaluate the cause of the fracture because although approximately 90% of hip fractures in both sexes result from a simple "mechanical" fall, sometimes these "falls" can also be the result of syncope due to comorbidities such as dysrhythmias, severe aortic stenosis, cardiovascular collapse, stroke, and so forth. These patients are usually volume-depleted because of low oral intake; in addition, the intravascular volume can be compromised due to occult, but sometimes significant, blood loss.

Another common finding in these patients is the presence of perioperative hypoxia that is usually multifactorial. Possible etiologies include atelectasis due to long periods of bed rest, and pulmonary congestion secondary to heart failure, pneumonia, and rarely fat embolism. Obtaining a thorough medical history, including a review of the tolerated level of preinjury physical activity and medications, as well as a careful physical examination, are also important in assessing the perioperative pulmonary and cardiovascular risk. While patients await surgery, pharmacologic and mechanical

(e.g., pneumatic intermittent compression devices) thromboprophylaxis is strongly indicated for every patient presenting with hip fracture because of the high venous thrombosis risk. Venous thrombosis–associated pulmonary embolism (PE) is the third most common cause of death in hip fracture patients, accounting for 18% of perioperative deaths. As discussed earlier in this chapter, the anesthetic technique choice is influenced significantly by the presence of concomitant pharmacologic thromboprophylactic therapy.

Antimicrobial prophylaxis is usually used for orthopedic surgeries, especially when foreign material is implanted. Prophylactic antibiotics have lowered the incidence of superficial and deep wound infection after hip fracture surgery. Most failures of antibiotic prophylaxis occur because of inappropriate timing (antibiotic blood concentration must be near peak at the time of surgical incision). The Surgical Infection Prevention Guideline Writers Workgroup recommends that infusion of the first antimicrobial dose should begin within 1 hour before the incision. When vancomycin or a fluoroquinolone is used, the infusion may begin 2 hours before incision. If a proximal tourniquet is required, the entire dose should be infused before the inflation of the tourniquet. First-generation cephalosporins have been the agents most commonly used in prophylaxis (e.g., cefazolin 1–2 g). Other methods used to decrease surgical site infection include ultraviolet lights over the field (which require patient and provider skin and cornea protection) or positive pressure laminar flow ventilation systems.

Laboratory testing

Complete blood count, electrolytes, blood urea nitrogen and creatinine values, electrocardiogram, and chest radiography are obtained per standard preoperative protocol. Arterial blood gas analysis may be considered in patients with a history of severe pulmonary disorders or clinical manifestations of fat embolism syndrome. Preoperative cardiac evaluation should be performed in patients with known heart disease, multiple risk factors, and in cases where the mechanism of injury suggests a cardiac event. The American College of Cardiology/American Heart Association (ACC/AHA) guidelines for perioperative cardiovascular evaluation for noncardiac surgery should be followed to stratify the risk in these patients.

Anesthetic management

No consensus exists regarding the best anesthetic technique for hip fracture. Because of insufficient evidence from randomized trials comparing regional versus general anesthesia, clinically important long-term outcomes cannot be confirmed. Differences in protocol and small sample size of many studies limit the validity and power of the conclusions to be drawn. Epidural anesthesia is associated with less acute postoperative confusion, but no definite conclusions can be obtained regarding mortality or other life-threatening postoperative complications, such as PE, myocardial infarction, or pneumonia. Based on existing evidence, epidural analgesia may be superior to systemic opioid analgesia during the first 4 to 6 hours of the postoperative period, but the difference is no longer significant at 18 or 24 hours. To obtain good analgesia and anesthesia of the hip, it is necessary to block the T10 to S2 dermatomes (preferably extending to T8), easily accomplished with spinal or epidural anesthesia. When spinal anesthesia is planned, hypobaric local anesthetic solution might offer some advantages because it permits placing the patient in the lateral decubitus position over the nonfractured side and thus avoids repositioning after the blockade. Isobaric solutions also reliably block the operative side irrespective of patient position. Alternatively, hyperbaric spinal anesthesia is easier to be influenced by position change. The brief repositioning to supine, necessary to obtain adequate anesthesia coverage, is usually used for bladder catheter placement. Some hip fracture operations (transfemoral nail, dynamic hip screw, hip "pinning") are also performed with the patient in the supine position on a traction table.

In addition to standard intraoperative monitoring, arterial pressure monitoring should be considered in patients with a high risk of coronary events or with poorly controlled hypertension. Significant blood loss and potential hemodynamic instability should be anticipated, especially with hip hemiarthroplasty and THA. Large-bore intravenous lines are recommended in preparation for blood transfusion and rapid fluid resuscitation. Patients with hip fracture are at an increased risk for perioperative pulmonary thromboembolism, as well as fat (Table 116.1), air, or methyl methacrylate monomer embolism, resulting in right heart strain, acute ventilation–perfusion mismatch, and decreased oxygen saturation. The presentation may vary, ranging from subclinical to a catastrophe presenting as sudden cardiac arrest, resistant to resuscitation and often necessitating open heart surgical embolectomy. Early transesophageal echocardiography may be useful to confirm or support the diagnosis, and guide the treatment.

Anesthesia for hip arthroplasty

THA is a common orthopedic procedure. In 2002, approximately 343,000 patients underwent 345,000 hip replacement procedures in the United States. Most of these patients suffered from osteoarthritis, rheumatoid arthritis (RA), congenital dislocation, or aseptic/avascular necrosis of the hip.

Preoperative assessment

This group of patients usually presents with limited functional capacity resulting from decreased joint mobility and pain, which potentially masks underlying coronary artery disease and pulmonary dysfunction. These patients should undergo a careful preoperative evaluation to assess their cardiovascular status. RA affects multiple organs, and these patients need to be carefully evaluated prior to surgery (see Chapter 118). Airway management can be difficult and may require awake fiber-optic intubation. If the patient is taking glucocorticoids, a "stress dose" should be given to avoid acute adrenal insufficiency. Moderate to large blood loss, necessitating blood transfusion, is common; therefore, availability of autologous and/or cross-matched homologous blood should be ensured. Thromboprophylaxis and antibiotic prophylaxis recommendations used in hip fracture surgery apply to THA surgery as well.

Laboratory testing

Similar tests as for hip fracture should be obtained. Additionally, dynamic flexion and extension cervical spine radiographs are recommended in patients with RA, as up to 50% have radiographic evidence of cervical spine subluxation. When the atlantoaxial subluxation exceeds 5 mm, neck stabilization and awake fiber-optic intubation reduce the trauma associated with airway management.

Anesthetic management

Patients undergoing THA pose challenges to the anesthesiologist similar to those in patients with hip fracture, such as hemodynamic instability, transfusion requirements, deep vein thrombosis (DVT), or PE (including fat or cement embolism). THA is usually performed with the patient in a lateral decubitus position. The patient's head must be positioned on the side and the cervical spine aligned with the rest of the body. The dependent arm is resting on a padded arm board; an axillary roll should be positioned just caudal to the axilla to relieve pressure on the shoulder and prevent compression of the brachial plexus and vascular structures. The upper arm should be supported on a padded overarm rest. It is important to protect all pressure points in the lower extremities (e.g., inner legs, dependent greater trochanter) to prevent traction or pressure injuries of nerves and skin surfaces. Standard intraoperative monitoring must be used, and invasive arterial blood pressure monitoring should be considered if the patient's comorbidities warrant it, if a hypotensive anesthesia technique is planned, or if the procedure is a revision THA. Large-bore intravenous access for rapid fluid resuscitation and/or blood transfusion is recommended.

Despite the frequency of THA surgery, debates continue regarding which anesthetic technique is best. A recent

Table 116.1. Diagnostic criteria for fat embolism (Two major or one major and four minor criteria are necessary for diagnosis.)

Major criteria	Minor criteria
Petechial rash	Fever
Cerebral involvement	Tachycardia (>120 bpm)
Respiratory distress	Retinal changes (fat or petechiae)
Arterial blood gas abnormalities	Renal changes
$PaO_2 < 60$ mm Hg breathing room air	Jaundice
$PaCO_2 > 55$ or a pH < 7.3	Fat macroglobulinemia
	Hemolytic anemia (a drop of more than 20% of the admission hemoglobin value)

Adapted from Gurd AR, Wilson RI. The fat embolism syndrome. *J Bone Joint Surg Br* 1974; 56B:408–416.

meta-analysis comparing central neuraxial blockade and general anesthesia for elective THA showed statistically significant reductions in the intraoperative blood loss and the number of patients requiring blood transfusions with neuraxial anesthesia. Decreased mean arterial pressure, redistribution of blood flow, and locally reduced venous pressure could all be responsible for this favorable effect. Evidence also suggests that neuraxial blockade might diminish the incidence of DVT when pharmacologic prophylaxis is not used; however, it is not clear if these beneficial effects are still present with the improved pharmacologic DVT prophylaxis today.

Various regional anesthetic techniques have been used for THA. Central neuraxial blockade provides excellent surgical anesthesia. Spinal anesthesia provides rapid and intense anesthesia, with drugs such as bupivacaine and tetracaine providing long surgical block and extended analgesia. When larger doses (particularly of hyperbaric local anesthetic) and higher sensory levels are obtained, deliberate hypotension can be achieved, providing hypotensive anesthesia. Combined spinal–epidural anesthesia offers both the rapid onset and solid block of spinal anesthesia and the extended postoperative analgesia via an epidural catheter.

Lumbar plexus block (single-dose or continuous) is another option. This block can be performed by using different approaches, but the lumbar paravertebral or psoas compartment block is the most reliable in blocking all major lumbar plexus branches (femoral, lateral femoral cutaneous, and obturator nerves). When used for postoperative analgesia after hip replacement surgery, continuous psoas compartment block has shown efficacy similar to epidural analgesia. This technique can be quite challenging, however, and reported complication rates are relatively high; therefore, it is recommended that only anesthesiologists with advanced regional anesthesia training and experience perform it.

Regional anesthetic techniques can be used in combination with general anesthesia. After placement of the epidural catheter or peripheral nerve block, general anesthesia can be induced. This combination of techniques may improve the comfort of the patient in long procedures. When performing a combination of general and neuraxial anesthesia, the amount and concentration of local anesthetics have to be reviewed carefully to lessen hemodynamic derangements.

Complications

Bone cement, polymethyl methacrylate, is frequently used to implant THA prostheses and has been associated with adverse pulmonary and cardiovascular events. Typical clinical signs and symptoms (also described as bone cement implantation syndrome) are similar to those of pulmonary or fat embolism and include tachycardia, hypotension, hypoxemia, tachypnea, dyspnea, bronchoconstriction, pulmonary hypertension (sometimes progressing to heart failure), severe systemic hypotension, and cardiac arrest. In addition, the manipulation, the reaming, and the high pressures reached inside the femoral

canal during the insertion of the cemented (or even uncemented) femoral component, with measured peak pressures as high as 680 mm Hg, cause fat particles and other debris to reach the bloodstream. Eventually, such particles reach the lungs through the medullary venous plexus, resulting in ventilation–perfusion mismatch, pulmonary hypertension, and right ventricular failure, usually manifesting as sudden oxygen desaturation and acute systemic hypotension that may be more dramatic in hypovolemic patients. Strategies to prevent or minimize these complications include increasing the inspired oxygen concentration, optimizing the intravascular volume and proactively treating hypovolemia prior to cementing and using vasoconstrictor drugs to treat hypotension. In addition, drilling a vent hole in the distal femur to relieve intramedullary pressure and removing the debris prior to high-pressure lavage of the femoral canal can help minimize embolism. Treatment of such complications includes timely oxygen administration, ventilation support, and cardiovascular resuscitation, including fluids, inotropic and vasopressor therapy.

Anesthesia for knee surgery

Arthroscopy and partial or total joint replacements are the most frequent knee operations today. Knee arthroscopy is often performed on an ambulatory basis and in mostly younger, active patients. It is used as a diagnostic tool, for removal of loose intra-articular bodies, and to repair ligament and meniscus lesions and/or defects. In contrast, patients who need a total or partial knee replacement are often older and may have significant coexisting disease.

Knee arthroscopy

A routine preoperative visit, history and physical examination, as well as standard testing (as required per protocol) modified by medical conditions and age, are recommended in these usually American Society of Anesthesiologists (ASA) physical status I or II ambulatory patients. In the operating room, the patient is in the supine position, or occasionally with both legs bent at right angles and placed on leg holders. Surgery begins with the intra-articular insertion of two or more ports close to the patellar tendon. An irrigation system is then connected to the portals to improve intra-articular visualization and to wash debris and blood. To provide a bloodless field, surgeons use a pneumatic tourniquet on the thigh and/or arthroscopic pump systems that fluid-distend and pressurize the joint without causing thigh compression. Surgery usually lasts less than 1 hour and is accompanied by little hemodynamic impact and fluid requirements.

Several anesthetic techniques are suitable for knee arthroscopic surgery. Although uncommon, intra-articular injections of local anesthetics have been successfully used for short and purely diagnostic procedures, usually in association with intravenous sedation. Spinal anesthesia is one of the common anesthesia techniques for knee arthroscopy. It provides quick, reliable, and profound anesthesia and short-term postoperative analgesia. With careful choice of local anesthetics and their dose, it does not significantly delay recovery and home discharge. Potential disadvantages of spinal anesthesia include delay in ambulation, urinary retention and pruritus, as well as risk of postdural puncture headache and transient neurologic syndrome (TNS). Faster resolution of the spinal block can be usually achieved by using very low doses of long-acting local anesthetics (bupivacaine or ropivacaine, 4–9 mg) with or without opioids (fentanyl ≤10 µg) or short-acting local anesthetics, such as lidocaine (see Chapter 57). The incidence of TNS is very low with bupivacaine. Peripheral nerve blocks can also be used alone or in combination with spinal anesthesia. Femoral nerve and lumbar plexus blocks are both suitable techniques for knee arthroscopy (for details, see Chapter 61). To achieve functional recovery of the blocked nerves before discharge, short-acting local anesthetics could be used, but this also limits analgesia duration. Finally, general anesthesia with low-solubility inhaled anesthetics (sevoflurane or desflurane) or propofol, often in association with an LMA, is broadly used in ambulatory centers because it is easily accomplished, allows rapid initiation of surgery, and has similar (and often shorter) time-to-home discharge when compared to regional techniques. General anesthesia, however, prolongs emergence time (time from the end of surgery until exit from the operating room), in most cases requires a postanesthesia care unit (PACU) stay, and is associated with higher incidence of nausea and vomiting and lower overall patient satisfaction. With better antiemetic prophylaxis, and especially in combination with preemptive analgesia techniques, general anesthesia is quickly becoming the norm for ambulatory knee arthroscopy.

Pain after knee arthroscopy is usually moderate but can be intense during the first postoperative day. Tourniquet use, type of arthroscopic procedure, and duration of surgery and anesthesia appear to have no significant impact on postoperative pain. Preemptive analgesia confers a better and smoother transition from anesthesia to adequate analgesia, and may permit a faster patient discharge accompanied with better patient satisfaction. A variety of preemptive analgesic techniques have been investigated (including COX inhibitors, intra-articular ketamine, oral or intra-articular opioids, intra-articular local anesthetics, and peripheral nerve blocks). Most of these techniques, to some extent, have been shown to improve postoperative analgesia.

Arthroscopic anterior cruciate ligament repair is a more extensive surgery than knee arthroscopy and causes moderate to severe postoperative pain. Preemptive techniques include oral COX inhibitors, intra-articular local anesthetics, and femoral and sciatic blockade. Postoperative pain is better controlled with peripheral nerve blocks. Postoperative analgesia with continuous peripheral nerve blockades (CPNB) has been used, particularly continuous femoral nerve block (CFNB). A protocol of 2-day home CFNB infusion has shown to maintain pain scores below the moderate range without rebound pain. Careful patient selection and infrastructure, providing support

and potential complication management, are critical for the safety and success of CPNB.

Anesthesia for total knee arthroplasty

Total knee arthroplasty (TKA) is indicated most frequently for patients with osteoarthritis, RA, and hemophilic arthropathy of the knee. Notably, TKA is associated with the highest DVT and PE incidence of all orthopedic procedures (approximately 80% and 20%, respectively). Furthermore, mortality associated with TKA, approximately 0.4% at 1 month and 1.8% at 1 year, is largely attributed to infection and DVT. Therefore, numerous antibiotic and DVT prophylaxis protocols have been used to prevent these complications, presenting the anesthesiologist with specific challenges when choosing the optimal anesthesia and postoperative analgesia approach.

Preoperative assessment

The preoperative evaluation of these patients is similar to what is required for patients undergoing hip arthroplasty. TKA is considered an intermediate risk procedure. Similarly, emphasis should be placed on the cardiovascular and respiratory state, and appropriate tests must be ordered if the clinical condition of the patient warrants it. For RA patients, special focus on airway and cervical spine evaluation is advised.

Anesthetic management

TKA can be performed with general or regional anesthesia. Several studies have suggested lower mortality and morbidity after regional anesthesia; however, recent long-term outcome data for patients undergoing TKA receiving up-to-date medical care do not support this advantage. Nevertheless, regional anesthesia confers superior analgesia and higher patient satisfaction and may improve short-term functional results. In this surgery, associated with significant postoperative pain and need for early and extensive postoperative physical therapy, lumbar epidural anesthesia remains one of the preferred anesthetic choices. Combined spinal–epidural anesthesia is also common, providing fast onset, adequate intraoperative anesthesia including profound motor block, and excellent postoperative analgesia. Aggressive antithrombotic prophylaxis, however, limits the use of postoperative neuraxial techniques in favor of peripheral nerve blocks. General and spinal anesthesia can be used in combination with continuous femoral blockade (with or without sciatic nerve blockade) to provide preemptive analgesia. Peripheral blocks alone (lumbar plexus block combined with sciatic nerve block) are an alternative but a challenging choice, requiring a motivated patient and an expert in regional anesthesia.

TKA takes approximately 1 to 3 hours, and patients are positioned supine. A thigh tourniquet is generally used, and intraoperative blood transfusion is rarely needed. Routine antibiotic prophylaxis is ideally completed 20 to 40 minutes prior to tourniquet inflation and incision. Standard monitoring is complemented in patients with moderate to severe coexisting

Table 116.2. Effects of tourniquet deflation

Hemodynamic	↓ MAP, SVR ↑ Venous capacitance ↑ PVR ↓ CO
Metabolic	Mixed acidosis Hypoxemia/hypoxia ↑ CO_2 production
Embolism	Thrombus Fat Air Cement (methacrylate) Bone marrow debris

MAP, mean arterial pressure; SVR, systemic vascular resistance; PVR, pulmonary vascular resistance; CO, cardiac output; CO_2, carbon dioxide.

cardiovascular and respiratory disease by invasive arterial pressure monitoring. The patients are usually stable during surgery and before deflation of the tourniquet. After cuff deflation, hemodynamic instability, bleeding, and hypoxia may occur (Table 116.2).

Embolism can occur at any time during surgery. It is sometimes observed after inflation of the tourniquet, at the beginning of the surgery, or during cementing of the femur, tibia, or patella. Transesophageal echocardiogram (TEE) detects embolism after release of the tourniquet in most patients. Fortunately, the amount of emboli is usually not clinically significant because PE signs and symptoms are relatively rare. The use of an extramedullary fixed prosthesis is not associated with less visible echogenic embolic material, suggesting that emboli are usually thrombi, not cement or bone marrow. Hemodynamic measurements have demonstrated that mean pulmonary artery pressure (MPAP) and pulmonary vascular resistance (PVR) increase in patients who have large-particle emboli observed by TEE. PVR remains elevated long after mixed venous oxygen saturation (SvO_2) returns to normal values, suggesting that the main cause of the increase in PVR is embolism rather than a drop in SvO_2. Finally, some studies have related the stasis caused by the tourniquet itself to the development of thrombi.

Postoperative analgesia

Most patients experience moderate to severe pain after TKA and may significantly benefit from regional analgesia. Single-injection femoral block has been recognized for more than a decade to provide better analgesia than opioids and COX inhibitors, but it is insufficient in duration (less than 24 hours) and extent (it does not provide analgesia to the posterior part of the knee). Therefore, continuous analgesic techniques have been preferred over single-shot peripheral nerve blockades. Although epidural analgesia provides better coverage of the entire leg, compared to continuous femoral perineural analgesia, it also presents disadvantages, such as urinary retention, pruritus, delayed mobilization, and the inherent risk of

neuraxial hematoma in the aggressively anticoagulated patient. Continuous lumbar plexus or femoral blockades are appealing postoperative analgesia options, offering adequate analgesia with an acceptably low incidence of side effects and complications and allowing for earlier rehabilitation. With these techniques, a supplemental single-injection sciatic nerve blockade can be indicated to complete the analgesia of the knee. It is important to remember, however, that TKA is associated with a significant incidence of surgically induced peroneal nerve palsy that might be masked by a routine use of sciatic nerve blocks. COX inhibitors can be used to supplement postoperative analgesia by reducing opioid consumption and side effects. Selective COX-2 inhibitors such as celecoxib have been shown not to increase blood loss.

Anesthesia for shoulder surgery

Shoulder surgery is frequently performed in patients with osteoarthritis, or in healthy individuals following shoulder trauma. Common shoulder surgeries include diagnostic and therapeutic arthroscopy, acromioplasty, rotator cuff repair, and shoulder arthroplasty.

Preoperative assessment

Routine preoperative evaluation should be performed. Preexisting neurologic deficits must be recognized and documented.

Intraoperative management

Regional anesthesia alone is well suited for most patients undergoing short procedures, as it provides good intraoperative anesthesia, muscle relaxation, and superior postoperative analgesia. Regional anesthesia also allows for faster recovery time and discharge. To block the brachial plexus, one can select among several regional techniques, but to achieve anesthesia of the entire shoulder, it is necessary to perform an interscalene block or a cervical paravertebral block (see Chapter 60). General anesthesia is often considered when prolonged surgery is expected, as well as in patients who refuse regional anesthesia or present other contraindications. Because airway access during shoulder surgery is restricted, one should secure the airway when performing general anesthesia. A laryngeal mask airway can be used easily and safely in individuals breathing spontaneously in association with regional anesthesia. Conversely, endotracheal intubation, which better controls and protects the airway, is recommended in patients undergoing surgery exclusively with general anesthesia, when long procedures are expected, when muscle relaxation is required, and in patients with coexisting respiratory problems.

Patient positioning is an important consideration during shoulder surgery. Almost invariably, surgery is performed with the patient in a modified sitting position, also called the "beach chair position." Typically, the affected shoulder is moved beyond the side of the table and is sometimes elevated with a pad under the scapula. The head and neck are stabilized in a neutral position, avoiding hyperextension of the neck and/or excessive rotation of the head, thus decreasing the risk of injury to the brachial plexus that is already subject to surgical traction. The unaffected arm is secured over a padded arm holder in elbow flexion and slight shoulder abduction to prevent brachial plexus stretch and peripheral nerve injury. The thorax is stabilized with a padded brace or side supports; the legs are slightly flexed at the knees. Elastic compressive stockings and pneumatic compressive devices are used for DVT prophylaxis. Some operating room beds, specially designed for shoulder surgery, have features that improve patient comfort, safety, and surgical accessibility.

Complications

Shoulder surgery is associated with several rare complications. Many complications occur more commonly in the sitting position, including cardiac arrest, stroke, blindness, ophthalmoplegia, and air embolism. Cardiac arrest is rare, but may occur when a hypovolemic patient (especially under general anesthesia) is abruptly moved from the supine to a steep sitting position. Sudden emptying of the ventricles is probably responsible for the extreme bradycardia and hypotension, sometimes progressing to pulseless electrical activity or asystole. Immediate reversal of the sitting position to the Trendelenburg position, rapid fluid resuscitation, and pressor and inotrope support usually quickly reverse the acute circulatory failure spiral.

Stroke in the sitting position can be attributed to postural hypotension, unrecognized decrease in cerebral perfusion pressure, as well as head and neck manipulation that may produce regional changes in cerebral blood flow. Loss of vision and ophthalmoplegia have also been attributed to ischemic events due to low blood pressure. These ischemic events could be related to failure to recognize the perfusion pressure differences, resulting from the sitting position and erroneous choice of blood pressure monitoring reference points. The cerebral blood pressure will differ from the measured pressure by approximately 1 mm Hg for each 1.3-cm difference in height between the brain and the reference point (transducer position for invasive pressure monitor or the blood pressure cuff site for a noninvasive pressure monitor). For example, in an adult patient in the sitting position, the cerebral arterial pressure will be approximately 25 to 30 mm Hg lower than the pressure measured at the arm. Furthermore, the compensatory mechanisms regulating and maintaining cerebral blood flow are affected by general anesthesia. Therefore, blood pressure should be monitored with extreme caution. A noninvasive blood pressure cuff should not be placed routinely at the calf. For invasive blood pressure measurements, the transducer can be positioned at the level of the external auditory meatus for the measured blood pressure to best reflect the cerebral arterial pressure. These considerations are particularly important in patients with a history of cerebrovascular disease and/or chronic hypertension.

Postoperative analgesia

Pain and neurologic complications are important considerations during the postoperative period. Postoperative pain after shoulder surgery ranges from moderate to severe, correlating poorly with the type of surgery performed. In fact, some arthroscopic procedures do not differ from open surgery in postoperative pain scores. Interscalene brachial plexus block provides analgesia superior to all other pain control modalities, reduces opioid use, allows for faster hospital discharge both in the inpatient and outpatient setting, and permits earlier rehabilitation therapy.

Suggested readings

Biboulet P, Morau D, Aubas P, et al. Postoperative analgesia after total-hip arthroplasty: comparison of intravenous patient-controlled analgesia with morphine and single injection of femoral nerve or psoas compartment block – a prospective, randomized, double-blind study. *Reg Anesth Pain Med* 2004; 29(2):102–109.

Bratzler DW, Houck PM. Antimicrobial prophylaxis for surgery: an advisory statement from the National Surgical Infection Prevention Project. *Clin Infect Dis* 2004; 38(12):1706–1715.

Choi PT, Bhandari M, Scott J, Douketis J. Epidural analgesia for pain relief following hip or knee replacement. *Cochrane Database Syst Rev* 2003; (3):3:CD003071.

Eagle KA, Berger PB, Calkins H, et al. ACC/AHA guideline update for perioperative cardiovascular evaluation for noncardiac surgery–executive summary: a report of the American College of Cardiology/American Heart Association Task Force on Practice Guidelines (Committee to update the 1996 guidelines on perioperative cardiovascular evaluation for noncardiac surgery). *Anesth Analg* 2002; 94(5):1052–1064.

Geerts WH, Pineo GF, Heit JA, et al. Prevention of venous thromboembolism: the Seventh ACCP Conference on Antithrombotic and Thrombolytic Therapy. *Chest* 2004; 126 (3 Suppl.):338S–400S.

Gohel MS, Bulbulia RA, Slim FJ, et al. How to approach major surgery where patients refuse blood transfusion (including Jehovah's Witnesses). *Ann R Coll Surg Engl* 2005; 87(1): 3–14.

Hadzic A, Karaca PE, Hobeika P, et al. Peripheral nerve blocks result in superior recovery profile compared with general anesthesia in outpatient knee arthroscopy. *Anesth Analg* 2005; 100(4): 976–981.

Horlocker TT, Hebl JR, Gali B, et al. Anesthetic, patient, and surgical risk factors for neurologic complications after prolonged total tourniquet time during total knee arthroplasty. *Anesth Analg* 2006; 102(3):950–955.

Horlocker TT, Wedel DJ, Benzon H, et al. Regional anesthesia in the anticoagulated patient: defining the risks (the second ASRA Consensus Conference on Neuraxial Anesthesia and Anticoagulation). *Reg Anesth Pain Med* 2003; 28(3):172–197.

Liu SS, Wu CL. The effect of analgesic technique on postoperative patient-reported outcomes including analgesia: a systematic review. *Anesth Analg* 2007; 105(3):789–808.

Mauermann WJ, Shilling AM, Zuo Z. A comparison of neuraxial block versus general anesthesia for elective total hip replacement: a meta-analysis. *Anesth Analg* 2006; 103(4):1018–1025.

Rosencher N, Kerkkamp HE, Macheras G, et al. and OSTHEO Investigation. Orthopedic Surgery Transfusion Hemoglobin European Overview (OSTHEO) study: blood management in elective knee and hip arthroplasty in Europe. *Transfusion* 2003; 43(4):459–469.

Singelyn F, Deyaert M, Joris D, et al. Effects of intravenous patient-controlled analgesia with morphine, continuous epidural analgesia, and continuous three-in-one block on postoperative pain and knee rehabilitation after unilateral total knee arthroplasty. *Anesth Analg* 1998; 87(1): 88–92.

Singelyn FJ, Seguy S, Gouverneur JM. Interscalene brachial plexus analgesia after open shoulder surgery: continuous versus patient-controlled infusion. *Anesth Analg* 1999; 89(5): 1216.

Tziavrangos E, Schug SA. Regional anaesthesia and perioperative outcome. *Curr Opin Anaesthesiol* 2006; 19(5):521–525.

Chapter 117

Rheumatoid arthritis and scoliosis

Kenji Butterfield, Abdel-Kader Mehio, and John D. Mitchell

Rheumatoid arthritis

Introduction

Rheumatoid arthritis is a chronic autoimmune inflammatory disease of unknown etiology, characterized by symmetric poly-arthropathy and significant systemic involvement. It occurs in approximately 1% of the population and has a female pre-dominance. Onset is typically seen in patients between 30 and 50 years of age. Table 117.1 summarizes its effects on organ systems. As discussed below, rheumatoid arthritis causes a variety of systemic disturbances that may present serious perioperative challenges.

Vascular access

Peripheral veins are usually small, brittle and difficult to cannulate – a frequent association with glucocorticoid therapy. The distal arteries are often calcified and placement of a radial arterial catheter could be difficult due to flexion deformities of the wrist joints. Internal jugular venous access may also be challenging due to fusion of cervical vertebrae and/or limited extension.

Airway

Atlantoaxial (C1–C2) subluxation

Cervical spine flexion deformity may limit the degree of neck extension. The majority of subluxations are anterior, but can be in the posterior, lateral, or vertical positions. Anterior subluxation generally presents with flexion of the neck; consequently, great care must be taken with patient positioning to prevent cord compression or vertebral artery compression. Although the "sniffing" position is often recommended for endotracheal intubation, there have been case reports of subluxation associated with this position as well. Lateral neck radiographs or MRI studies revealing a greater than 3 mm gap between the anterior arch of the atlas and the odontoid process can confirm the presence of anterior subluxation (Fig. 117.1).

Temporomandibular joint

Severely limited movement of the temporomandibular joint (TMJ) may make visualization of the glottis by direct laryn-goscopy extremely difficult. Such patients may present with micrognathia and obstructive sleep apnea. When challenges with direct laryngoscopy are predicted, the use of alternative options, such as video-assisted laryngoscopy, fiber-optic laryn-goscopy, or use of the Fastrach LMA (LMA North America, Inc., San Diego, CA), should be considered.

Cricoarytenoiditis

This condition may be present in patients complaining of hoarseness, stridor, odynophagia, or pain when speaking or coughing. Direct laryngoscopy typically reveals bright red swelling over the arytenoids and narrowing of the glottic opening, but normal vocal cords. If the patient presents with mild symptoms, the use of a smaller endotracheal tube (ETT) is recommended. In the presence of severe symptoms, however, oral intubation is relatively contraindicated. Anesthetic alternatives to oral intubation include local anesthesia, regional anesthesia, or presurgical tracheotomy under local anesthesia. These options should be discussed with the patient and the surgeon in the preoperative setting. Due to the possibility of postextubation supraglottic obstruction in these patients, close postoperative observation is of paramount importance.

Neuraxial regional anesthesia

The lumbar spine usually remains unaffected by rheumatoid arthritis. Neuraxial regional anesthesia techniques involving the thoracic spine may be technically challenging. A thorough physical examination should be performed to assess for bony spinal deformities, which if found, may warrant radiographic evaluation. Performing neuraxial anesthesia techniques under fluoroscopic guidance should be strongly considered in such cases.

Scoliosis and spine surgery

Scoliosis is a complex lateral and rotational deformity of the thoracolumbar spine, also resulting in rib-cage deformity. Anterior or posterior deformities, such as kyphosis or lordosis, may also accompany this condition. Approximately 70% of all

Table 117.1. Effects of rheumatoid arthritis on the organ systems

Organ system	Presentation	Evaluation
Cardiac	– Constrictive pericarditis – Pericardial effusion – Aortic root dilatation – Aortic insufficiency – Cardiac conduction abnormalities – Myocarditis – Coronary arteriitis – CAD (chronic steroid use implicated)	– ECG – Consider echocardiography or stress test if cardiac history is significant
Respiratory	– Pleural effusion – Pulmonary fibrosis – Pulmonary vasculitis – Pulmonary nodules – Obliterative bronchiolitis	– Chest radiograph – Consider spirometry or arterial blood gas if history is significant
Neurologic	– Nerve compression (cervical, peripheral) – Muscle weakness due to mononeuritis	– Assess for neuropathies
Renal	– Vasculitis – Amyloidosis – Autoimmune nephropathy	– Baseline BUN and creatinine
Hematologic	– Mild anemia (iron deficiency) – Chronic use of COX inhibitors	– Check pre-op CBC – Anticipate variable platelet dysfunction
Endocrine	– Adrenal insufficiency from chronic steroid use	– Stress-dose steroids may be warranted in case of chronic use

ECG, electrocardiogram; CAD, coronary artery disease; BUN, blood urea nitrogen; COX, cyclooxygenase; CBC, complete blood count.

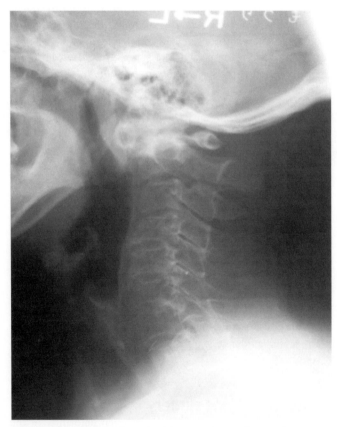

Figure 117.1. Lateral radiograph of the cervical spine, showing the atlantoaxial subluxation and superior migration of the odontoid process into the skull. The atlas has slipped anteriorly on the axis, resulting in the narrowing of the spinal canal.
(Reproduced with permission from Osamu Shirado and *The Journal of Bone and Joint Surgery* / License # 1763730814591)

cases are idiopathic, occurring with a male:female ratio of 1:4. The remaining 30% are secondary to an array of causes, including neuromuscular disease, mesenchymal disorders, infection, trauma, or congenital causes. Surgery is usually considered when the Cobb's angle (lateral curvature) exceeds 50° in the thoracic spine, or 40° in the lumbar spine (Fig.117.2). Surgical intervention aims at halting the disease progression and partially correcting the deformity, thereby improving the quality of life and facilitating care. If left untreated, scoliosis can lead to severe respiratory and cardiovascular compromise, including restrictive lung disease, pulmonary hypertension, and right heart failure.

In general, for patients undergoing cervical spine surgery, gentle neck manipulation is advised while intubating the airway. Direct laryngoscopy with in-line stabilization or awake fiber-optic intubation may be necessary in cases involving cervical spine instability. Thoracolumbar surgery generally involves degenerative disease in older patients who may also present with significant comorbidities.

Preoperative assessment

Scoliosis patients presenting for spinal surgery require a thorough preoperative assessment of their respiratory and cardiovascular systems. The anesthesiologist should be cognizant of the potential for a difficult airway. The possible need for postoperative ventilation and ICU admission should be discussed with the patient, the family, and the surgical team prior to the procedure. As with most spinal surgeries, the need for a wake-up test should be addressed and rehearsed with the patient in advance.

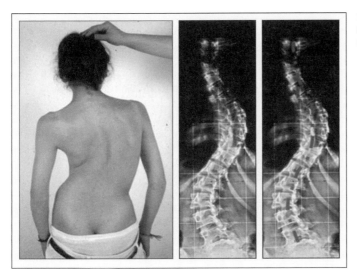

Figure 117.2. Scoliosis is a lateral deviation in the frontal plane associated with rotation. (With *permission from The Spine Society of Europe at eurospine.org*)

Respiratory

The restrictive pulmonary disease caused by scoliosis is related to the following factors:

- Extent of Cobb's angle
- Number of vertebrae involved
- Cephalad location of the curve
- Loss of normal thoracic kyphosis

Both vital capacity and total lung capacity are reduced, but generally the residual volume remains unchanged. In addition, patients often exhibit ventilation/perfusion mismatch due to hypoventilated areas. Physiotherapy and nebulized bronchodilators are the mainstay treatments for these pulmonary conditions.

Cardiovascular

Cardiac disease can occur as a direct result of scoliosis or be indirectly linked to its underlying causes. Distortion of the chest cavity can lead to chronic hypoxemia and pulmonary hypertension, resulting in cor pulmonale. Impaired cardiac contractility can be severely exacerbated by anesthesia and hypovolemia in patients with Duchenne's muscular dystrophy. Table 117.2 summarizes the preoperative planning.

Intraoperative techniques

The most important intraoperative goals include a stable depth of anesthesia, an adequate level of neuromuscular blockade, and a tight control of the patient's hemodynamic parameters. The anesthesiologist can be faced with multiple challenges including (1) significant blood loss, (2) one-lung ventilation during thoracic spine surgery, (3) prone positioning, and (4) the wake-up test.

Hemodynamic management

Several techniques are used to minimize blood loss. The use of antifibrinolytics, such as aminocaproic acid or tranexamic acid, have proven helpful, albeit not risk-free. Intraoperative cell salvage could also be beneficial, yet is often insufficient alone because clotting factors and platelets are lost in the process. Transfusion of fresh-frozen plasma, platelets, and/or cryoprecipitate may be necessary. Controlled hypotension may also be used in some circumstances; although this intervention can play a valuable role, it is not appropriate for all patients. It is therefore important to evaluate each patient for comorbidities that could render controlled hypotenion inappropriate and discuss the limitations with the surgical team.

Table 117.2. Summary of preoperative planning for scoliosis surgery

Airway	– Potentially difficult
	– C-spine movement may be limited
	– Double-lumen ETT may be necessary
Respiratory	– Chest radiograph
	– Arterial blood gas: usually low PaO_2 with normal $PaCO_2$
	– Spirometry
Cardiovascular	– ECG
	– Echocardiogram: LVEF and PA pressures
	– Dobutamine stress echocardiogram considered in patients with limited exercise tolerance
Laboratory Tests	– CBC
	– Electrolytes
	– Coagulation profile
	– Crossmatched blood
IV Access	– Large-bore IVs (possibly central line)
	– Arterial line
Planned Monitors	– Standard
	– Spinal cord monitoring
	– Wake-up test
	– Arterial line
	– TEE (preferable to CVP or PAC)

LVEF, left ventricular ejection fraction; PAC, pulmonary artery catheter.

Intraoperative invasive hemodynamic monitoring can be challenging in the prone position. For example, central venous pressure (CVP) and pulmonary artery (PA) pressure can often yield falsely elevated levels, and only trends can be useful. Transesophageal echocardiography (TEE) allows for better assessment of filling pressures and contractility; however, that modality may also be complicated in the prone position.

Ventilation

Ventilation in such patients can be very challenging due to the difficulties negotiating the specifics of restrictive lung disease management with the surgical positioning constraints. High peak airway pressures are common in these circumstances. Pressure-controlled ventilation may be helpful in managing allowable peak pressures. In some patients, one-lung ventilation with a double-lumen tube or a bronchial blocker is required. Each technique offers its own unique advantages: although a double-lumen tube provides the benefit of optional passive oxygenation to the nonventilated lung, its use often necessitates the eventual exchange to a single-lumen ETT at the end of the procedure. This procedure may be complicated due to postoperative facial and airway swelling from the prone position and major fluid shifts. The use of an endotracheal tube exchanger may be prudent to avoid loss of the airway in this setting. Ultimately, pulmonary function is unlikely to improve immediately after surgery. Indeed, months to years may elapse before improvement can be observed in the patient's respiratory status.

Positioning

Special consideration needs to be made for patients in the prone position, with particular attention to the head, neck, arms and face, especially the eyes. In particular, such patients are at greater risk of developing a postoperative visual deficit. Eye injuries can include corneal abrasion, ischemic optic neuropathy, central retinal artery occlusion, and cortical blindness. Risk factors include prolonged procedures, profound blood loss, anemia, hypotension, hypoxia, in addition to the prone and Trendelenburg positions.

Spinal cord monitoring

Spinal cord monitoring is vital in scoliosis patients undergoing spine surgery. The risk of postoperative neurologic deficits, including paraplegia, is significant. To minimize these risks, three monitoring techniques can be employed: somatosensory evoked potentials (SSEPs), motor evoked potentials (MEPs), and the wake-up test (see Chapter 29).

The monitoring of MEPs can reduce the incidence of neurologic complications, however, it does not completely prevent the risk. When MEPs are monitored, total intravenous anesthesia (e.g., with propofol and opioid infusions) is required with little or no volatile anesthetics. A low-dose infusion of muscle relaxants can also be used, though no muscle relaxation is preferable.

Table 117.3. Summary of intraoperative care for scoliosis surgery

Premedication	– Anxiolytics
	– Bronchodilators may be helpful
Induction	– Guided by patient's condition
	– Avoid succinylcholine in patients with muscular dystrophy
Intubation	– Direct versus fiber-optic laryngoscopy
	– Double-lumen ETT, depending on surgical approach
Maintenance	– Maintain stable depth so that spinal cord monitoring can be interpreted reliably
	– Isoflurane <0.5 MAC with 60% nitrous oxide is compatible with SSEPs
	– Total intravenous anesthesia (preferably with propofol and opioid infusions), especially when MEPs are monitored (avoidance of muscle relaxants preferred)
Positioning	– Often prone; slight reverse Trendelenburg if possible
	– Assess baseline neurologic deficits, including range of motion
Muscle relaxation	– Continuous IV infusion of muscle relaxant
	– Minimal or no muscle relaxants if MEPs monitored
Spinal cord monitoring	– Commonly recommended methods include SSEPs, MEPs, or a wake-up test
	– With wake-up test, use short-acting agents (e.g., remifentanil, propofol, desflurane)
Blood preservation	– Antifibrinolytics
	– Cell salvage
	– Controlled hypotension

The wake-up test is still considered the most reliable evaluation of an intact spinal cord. This test should be planned well in advance. The patient should be warned about the possibility, the concept explained and the scenario rehearsed. Clear communication with the surgical and neurophysiological monitoring teams is vital not only to determine whether a wake-up test will be necessary, but also to allow for appropriate depth of anesthesia. Often, short-acting agents, such as nitrous oxide, propofol, and remifentanil, are used for rapid emergence and resumption of anesthesia. Table 117.3 summarizes the basics of intraoperative care.

Postoperative care

As discussed previously, patients undergoing surgery for scoliosis often have poor preoperative pulmonary function. The need for postoperative ventilation is dependent on a number of patient and surgical factors, including:

- Preoperative forced vital capacity (FVC) <35% of the predicted value
- Preexisting neurologic deficits
- Right heart failure
- Obesity
- Prolonged operative time
- Thoracic surgical involvement
- Blood loss >30 ml/kg

Table 117.4. Postoperative care for scoliosis surgery

| Postoperative ventilation | – Risk factors as above
– Preoperative discussion indicated |
| Postoperative analgesia | – IV PCA opioids, epidural (opioid-based), intrathecal morphine, intrapleural LA/opioids |

PCA, patient-controlled anesthesia.

Patients exhibiting any one or more of these features can be described as the best candidates for postoperative ventilation. In addition, any signs of postoperative visual loss should prompt an urgent ophthalmologic consultation.

Postoperative analgesia is of great importance and is often challenging following scoliosis surgery because of the size of the incision and possible preexisting chronic pain. Moderate to severe pain can be expected for several days postoperatively. Patients who are cognitively impaired or very young may present special challenges in this regard as they are less able to communicate discomfort. If epidural analgesia is used, it should be primarily or entirely opioid-based, because neuraxial local anesthetics can compromise the ability to assess neurologic function. Table 117.4 summarizes the basics of postoperative care.

Suggested readings

Almenrader N, Patel D. Spinal fusion surgery in children with non-idiopathic scoliosis: is there a need for routine postoperative ventilation? *Br J Anaesth* 2006; 97(6):851–857.

Fleisher L. *Anesthesia and Uncommon Diseases.* 5th ed. Philadelphia: Saunders; 2005:144–145.

Kohjitani A, Miyawaki T, Kasuya K, et al. Anesthetic management for advanced rheumatoid arthritis patients with acquired micrognathia undergoing temporomandibular joint replacement. *J Oral Maxillofac Surg* 2002; 60:559–566.

Kolman J, Morris I. Cricoarytenoid arthritis: a cause of acute upper airway obstruction in rheumatoid arthritis. *Can J Anesth* 2002; 49(7):729–732.

MacKenzie CR, Sharrock NE. Perioperative medical considerations in patients with rheumatoid arthritis. *Rheum Dis Clin North Am* 1998; 24(1):1–17.

Miller RD. *Miller's Anesthesia.* 6th ed. Philadelphia: Elsevier/ Churchill Livingstone; 2005:2418–2419.

Raw DA, Beattie JK, Hunter JM. Anaesthesia for spinal surgery in adults. *Br J Anesth* 2003; 91:886–904.

Sloan TB, Heyer EJ. Anesthesia for intraoperative neurophysiologic monitoring of the spinal cord. *J Clin Neurophysiol* 2002; 19:430–443.

Stambough JL, Dolan D, Werner R, Godfrey E. Ophthalmologic complications associated with prone positioning in spine surgery. *J Am Acad Orthop Surg* 2007; 15:156–165.

Stoelting R, Dierdorf S. *Anesthesia and Co-Existing Disease.* 3rd ed. New York: Churchill Livingstone; 1993.

Anesthetic management in spine surgery

Abdel-Kader Mehio and Swapneel K. Shah

Introduction

The spectrum of spine surgery is considerable. There is a significant increase in procedures performed each year, due to both improvements in surgical technique and an increase in patients deemed suitable for surgery.

Spine surgery patients often present with comorbidities, such as serious cardiovascular and respiratory disease. Airway management could be challenging, especially in patients with cervical spine pathology. Spine surgery is frequently associated with significant blood loss, prolonged anesthesia (often in the prone position), and problematic postoperative pain management. The anesthesiologist's role in the perioperative management of these patients is discussed, including techniques to monitor spinal cord function.

Preoperative assessment

When assessing patients before spine surgery, particular care should be given to the respiratory, cardiovascular, and neurologic systems; all may be affected by the pathology for which the spine surgery is proposed.

Airway assessment

The potential for a difficult airway should always be considered, particularly in those patients presenting for surgery of the upper thoracic or cervical spine. Previous intubation history and documentation should be reviewed, and careful assessment of neck flexion and extension should be performed. In addition, the stability of the cervical and thoracic spine should be determined and discussed preoperatively with the spine surgeon.

The cervical spine should be assessed clinically (presence of pain and/or neurologic deficits) and radiographically (lateral or flexion/extension plain films, computer-assisted tomography, or magnetic resonance imaging). The stability of the cervical spine is dependent on ligamental and vertebral elements. Damage to these elements may not be detectable by plain radiographs alone. The adult cervical spine below C2 is unstable or on the brink of instability when one of the following conditions is met:

1. All the anterior or all the posterior elements are destroyed.
2. There is a >3.5-mm horizontal displacement of one vertebra in relation to an adjacent one on lateral radiograph.

3. There is more than 11° rotation of one vertebra relative to an adjacent one.

Above the level of C2, examples of unstable injuries include disruption of the transverse ligament of the atlas and Jefferson burst fracture of the atlas following axial loading that causes atlantoaxial instability. Disruption of the tectorial and alar ligaments and some occipital condylar fractures also cause atlanto-occipital instability.

Some inherited disorders such as Duchenne muscular dystrophy (DMD) may lead to glossal hypertrophy, and previous radiotherapy to tumors of the head and neck can cause difficulty in direct laryngoscopy. A decision must be made whether to intubate the patient awake or asleep.

Respiratory assessment

Patients presenting for spine surgery may have impaired respiratory function. Those who have sustained cervical or high thoracic trauma or who have multiple injuries may be mechanically ventilated preoperatively. Others can suffer from recurrent respiratory infections. Preoperatively, respiratory function should be assessed by a thorough history, focusing on functional impairment, physical examination, and appropriate testing. Scoliosis causes a restrictive pattern on pulmonary function tests (PFTs), with reduced vital capacity and reduced total lung capacity (TLC) (see Chapter 117). The residual volume is unchanged. The severity of functional impairment is related to the angle of the scoliosis, the number of vertebrae involved, cephalad location of the curve, and loss of the normal thoracic kyphosis. The extent of functional impairment cannot, therefore, be directly inferred from the angle of scoliosis alone. The most common blood gas abnormality is a reduced arterial oxygen tension with a normal arterial carbon dioxide tension that is a result of the mismatch between ventilation and perfusion in the hypoventilated lung units (increased shunt). Respiratory function should be optimized by treating any reversible cause of pulmonary dysfunction (including infection) with physiotherapy, nebulized bronchodilators, and antibiotics, as indicated. There is controversy over whether surgery for idiopathic scoliosis improves or worsens pulmonary function.

The type of surgery proposed has also been shown to have a significant effect on PFTs, and may explain some of the contradictory findings in the previously mentioned studies. Spine surgery involving the thorax (anterior approach, combined approach, or rib resection) is associated with an initial decline in forced vital capacity (FVC 19% of baseline values), forced expiratory volume in 1 second (FEV_1 13%), and TLC (11%) at 3 months. These declines are followed by subsequent improvement to preoperative baseline values at 2 years postoperatively. However, surgery involving the posterior approach only, is associated with an improvement in PFTs in 3 months (although not reaching statistical significance) and improvements that are statistically significant at 2-year follow-up: FVC (14% increase from baseline), FEV_1 (14%), and TLC (5%). Older studies have reported that if preoperative vital capacity is less than $30 \pm 35\%$ of predicted, postoperative ventilation is likely to be required.

Cardiovascular assessment

Cardiac compromise may be a direct result of the underlying pathology, such as a muscular dystrophy. Cardiac dysfunction may also occur secondary to scoliosis that causes distortion of the mediastinum, and cor pulmonale secondary to chronic hypoxemia and pulmonary hypertension. Assessment of functional cardiovascular impairment is difficult in patients who are wheelchair-bound. Minimum investigations should include electrocardiography and echocardiography to assess left and right ventricular function and pulmonary arterial pressures. Dobutamine stress echocardiography may be used to assess cardiac function in patients with limited exercise tolerance.

Neurologic assessment

A full neurologic assessment of the patient should be documented preoperatively for the following reasons:

1. In certain patients undergoing cervical spine surgery, the anesthesiologist must minimize neck movement to avoid further neurologic deterioration during airway instrumentation and patient positioning.
2. Muscular dystrophies may involve the bulbar muscles, increasing the risk of perioperative aspiration.
3. In case of spinal cord injury, its anatomical level and the time elapsed from the insult are predictors of possible perioperative cardiovascular and respiratory complications. If surgery is contemplated within the first 3 weeks after the injury, spinal shock may still be present. Later on, autonomic dysreflexia may develop, more likely in injuries above the mid-thoracic level.

Anesthetic techniques

Premedication

In patients with a high spinal cord lesion or those in whom fiber-optic intubation is to be undertaken, administration of anticholinergic agents, such as glycopyrrolate, may be considered to decrease airway secretions. Many patients will present with factors contributing to increased risk of regurgitation and aspiration of gastric contents, such as recent opioid administration, high spinal cord injury, or recent traumatic injury. In these circumstances, it may be prudent to premedicate patients with a histamine H_2 receptor antagonist, or a proton pump inhibitor, and with a nonparticulate antacid, such as sodium citrate. Some patients may have nasogastric tubes in situ that decrease the competence of the lower esophageal sphincter.

Induction

The choice of an intravenous (IV) or inhalation induction is guided primarily by the patient's clinical condition and by the patient's airway assessment. Preoxygenation is advisable in all patients.

The use of succinylcholine in patients with muscular dystrophies may cause cardiac arrest secondary to hyperkalemia. In patients with denervation as a result of spinal cord lesions, the increased number of extrajunctional acetylcholine receptors on skeletal muscle can cause hyperkalemia after administration of succinylcholine. The amount of potassium released may possibly correlate with the extent of the patient's motor deficit. It is usually considered safe to administer succinylcholine within the first 24 hours of injury. The increase in serum potassium is maximal between 4 weeks and 5 months after spinal injury. Serum potassium levels may increase from normal to as high as 14 mEq/L, causing ventricular fibrillation and/or asystole. There are no specific contraindications to the use of nondepolarizing agents, while varying degrees of resistance could be observed.

Intubation

Awake or asleep?

Indications for awake intubation include the need for neurologic assessment following airway management, the risk of aspiration combined with a potentially difficult airway, or the presence of a neck stabilization device (such as halo traction) that prevents adequate access to the airway.

Direct or fiber-optic laryngoscopy?

There is controversy as to whether direct laryngoscopy is a major factor contributing to cord injury in patients with cervical spine instability. Other factors, such as hypotension and patient positioning, may be equally important. Direct laryngoscopy with manual in-line stabilization or a hard collar is an accepted means of intubation for many patients, provided this can be achieved with limited neck movement. Fixed flexion deformities of the upper thoracic and cervical spine may make direct laryngoscopy impossible, requiring a fiber-optic bronchoscope to facilitate intubation.

Anterior approaches to the thoracic spine may necessitate the use of a double-lumen endotracheal tube or a bronchial blocker, optimizing the surgical field by providing single-lung ventilation for portions of the procedure.

Maintenance

To avoid and/or appropriately interpret changes to somatosensory evoked potentials (SSEPs), a stable anesthetic depth is required. Although employing nitrous oxide and volatile anesthetics at combined levels of less than 0.5 minimum alveolar concentration (MAC) is compatible with SSEP monitoring, IV techniques using propofol and an opioid are generally preferred due to their reduced effects on the amplitude and latency of evoked potentials.

Prevention of blood loss

Most of the blood loss in spinal instrumentation and fusion occurs with decortication and disruption of rich vascular networks, and is proportional to the number of vertebral levels involved. During more extensive spine surgery, it can be considerable, varying typically between 10 and 30 ml/kg. Blood loss and transfusion requirements may be reduced through proper positioning and the use of intraoperative blood salvage, induced hypotension, intraoperative hemodilution, and the administration of antifibrinolytic agents, such as tranexamic acid and aminocaproic acid. Induced hypotension is not without risk, and has been reported to cause cord ischemia and neurologic deficits, including blindness.

When patients are placed in the prone or knee–chest position, care must be taken to minimize intra-abdominal pressure. Positioning devices, such as the Relton–Hall frame, which allow the abdominal viscera to hang freely, reduce inferior vena cava (IVC) pressure by one third compared with conventional pads. Elevated IVC pressure is associated with lumbar venous engorgement and increased blood loss. Minor changes to patient positioning on the Wilson frame can reduce blood loss per vertebral level by approximately 50%.

Agents for maintaining deliberate hypotension include volatile anesthetics, calcium channel antagonists, sodium nitroprusside, nitroglycerin, and, in children, the dopamine D_1 receptor agonist, fenoldopam. Mean arterial pressure (MAP) is typically maintained at 60 mm Hg.

Caudal anesthesia has also been shown to reduce surgical bleeding by 50% in patients undergoing lumbar spine surgery. This reduction was thought to be a result of a reduction in sympathetic tone causing a measurable decrease in lumbar vertebral intraosseous pressure. This technique, however, is not as controllable as is continuous IV titration of a short-acting hypotensive agent, nor is it suitable for operations involving the thoracic and cervical spine. It may also hinder early postoperative neurologic assessment.

Thromboembolic prophylaxis

Patients undergoing spine surgery may be at increased risk for thromboembolic complications as a result of prolonged surgery, prone positioning, malignancy, and/or extended periods of postoperative immobilization. The use of compression stockings and/or pneumatic boots is recommended. Many surgeons prefer not to administer anticoagulants because their use may be associated with hemorrhagic complications, including increased blood loss and epidural hematoma.

Muscle relaxation

When the spinal integrity monitoring plan involves motor evoked potentials (MEPs), neuromuscular blocking drugs are best avoided or used sparingly.

Intraoperative monitoring

Cardiovascular monitoring

Prolonged surgery, significant blood loss, the use of controlled hypotension in selected cases, and the hemodynamic and respiratory effects of thoracic spine operations are all indications for invasive arterial pressure monitoring.

In the prone position, central venous pressure (CVP) may be a misleading indicator of right and left ventricular end-diastolic volumes. A study of 12 pediatric patients undergoing surgery for scoliosis in the prone position compared CVP and transesophageal echocardiography (TEE) in the assessment of ventricular filling. Measurements were taken before and after positioning. The results demonstrated that there was no correlation between the measurement of cardiac volume indicators by TEE and CVP or pulmonary artery occlusion pressure (PAOP) in such conditions. High CVP values may be misleading indicators of adequate cardiac filling in the prone position. The changes are probably a result of raised intrathoracic pressure causing reduced ventricular compliance and compression of the inferior vena cava. The dependent position of the lower limbs results in reduced venous return to the heart.

Respiratory monitoring

Patients with severe respiratory dysfunction as a result of scoliosis may have an increased alveolar–arterial oxygen gradient that may be further increased during prolonged surgery because of regional hypoventilation. Serial measurements of arterial oxygen tension are usually recommended.

Temperature monitoring

Thermoregulation may already be impaired in patients with spinal cord lesions secondary to the sympathectomy distal to the lesion. In addition, prolonged surgery is associated with significant heat loss. The use of temperature monitoring, warming of IV fluids, and a warm air mattress device are recommended.

Spinal cord monitoring

When corrective forces are applied to the spinal column, osteotomies are performed, or instrumentation is applied onto the vertebral structures, the spinal cord is at risk of injury. The incidence of motor deficit or paraplegia after surgery to correct scoliosis in the absence of spinal cord monitoring has been quoted to vary between 3.7% and 6.9%. By using intraoperative neurophysiological monitoring (IONM), this percentage can be reduced to 0.5%. The American Academy of Neurology has published guidelines on IONM, concluding that considerable evidence favors the use of neurological monitoring as a safe and efficacious tool in clinical situations in which a significant risk for nervous system injury exists. It is now considered mandatory to monitor spinal cord function during such procedures, while also recognizing the limitations of IONM. The IONM ideally detects perturbations in spinal cord function early, allowing the surgeon to take appropriate corrective steps before irreversible damage occurs. However, the time between a change in the electrophysiologic recordings from the cord after overdistraction and the onset of irreversible ischemic damage is in the order of only 5 to 6 minutes in animal studies. Spinal cord neurophysiological monitoring includes:

- Wake-up test
- SSEPs
- MEPs
- Electromyography

Acute alterations in neurophysiological monitoring (amplitude and/or latency) signify spinal cord compromise and may be the result of direct trauma, ischemia, compression, or hematoma.

Positioning

Patient positioning for spine surgery varies, depending on the level of the spine to be operated on and the type of surgery. Patients may be repositioned intraoperatively. It is important that venous pressure at the surgical site is kept low to reduce bleeding (reverse Trendelenburg tilt and a free abdomen). In addition, peripheral nerves, bony prominences, and the eyes should be protected (see Chapter 51). It is also important to avoid displacement of unstable fractures during patient positioning.

Lumbar surgery

Anterior approaches sometimes require a laparotomy. Minimally invasive surgery with lateral incision has become more popular recently. Posterior surgery requires prone patient position with a decompressed abdomen to keep the epidural venous pressure low (the patient supported on a Wilson frame, for example, or a raised mattress with a hole for the abdomen; see Fig. 118.1). For disc surgery, patients may be placed in the knee–

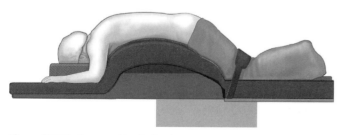

Figure 118.1. Prone position for lumbar surgery.

chest position with a well padded, secure support behind the upper thigh to support the patient's weight. This position results in a horizontal lumbar spine with vertical intervertebral discs.

Thoracic surgery

Anterior approaches to the thoracic spine are via a thoracotomy with the patient supported in a lateral position. One-lung ventilation with a double-lumen endotracheal tube or a bronchial blocker is often used to allow for better surgical retraction of the lung. The optimal tube placement should always be confirmed fiberoptically after the patient is repositioned. Posterior approaches to the thoracic spine require a prone patient with a decompressed abdomen.

Cervical spine surgery

Patients are sometimes positioned with their head away from the anesthesia machine to allow surgical access to the head and neck. Access to the upper extremities is limited and extensions are often needed for the breathing circuit, and arterial and IV lines. Tracheal tubes must be carefully secured without encroaching on the surgical field or the pathway of the C-arm fluoroscopy machine. For anterior surgery, a reinforced tracheal tube may be considered to reduce the risk of airway obstruction as tracheal retraction sometimes occurs during surgery. The head is supported on a padded head ring, or the Mayfield horseshoe headrest. Spine traction may be required by tongs and weights placed into the outer bone plate of the skull for some procedures. Reverse Trendelenburg positioning could minimize venous bleeding and provide counter-traction for the weight attached to the head. Venous pooling in the lower limbs and intraoperative retraction of the carotid artery make an arterial line advisable for some patients, and often practitioners will level the transducer to the level of the head, rather than to the right atrium, to better assess cerebral perfusion. For posterior approaches to the cervical spine, the head of the prone patient can be supported on the gel-padded Mayfield horseshoe headrest or placed in a skull clamp. The orbits, the superior orbital nerve, and the skin over the maxilla are at particular risk of ischemic injury if positioning is incorrect. These problems are avoided by using a skull clamp. The head height and degree of neck flexion may be adjusted intraoperatively, and pressure areas must be rechecked after such maneuvers.

Venous air embolism

Venous air embolism (VAE) is a catastrophic event that may occur during spine surgery. The large amount of exposed bone and the elevated location of the surgical incision relative to the heart predispose to VAE. Incidence of VAE in patients undergoing neurosurgical procedures in the sitting, supine, prone, and lateral positions are 25%, 18%, 10%, and 8%, respectively. The presenting sign in all cases was unexplained hypotension and an increase in the end-tidal nitrogen concentration. If VAE is suspected, the wound should be irrigated with saline, nitrous oxide discontinued, and vasopressors and fluid boluses initiated.

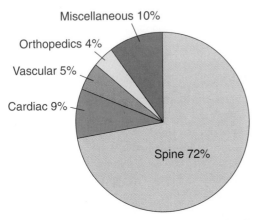

Figure 118.2. Distribution of cases from the ASA POVL Registry. Data were obtained from the study by Lee et al. The American Society of Anesthesiologists Postoperative Visual Loss Registry. *Anesthesiology* 2006; 105:652-9 Figure with permission from Baig M, Lubow M, Immesoete P, et al. Vision loss after spine surgery: review of the literature and recommendations. *Neurosurg Focus* 2007; (5):15.

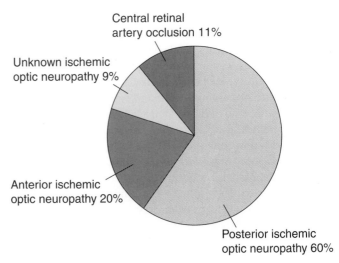

Figure 118.3. Distribution of 93 ophthalmic lesions associated with POVL after spine surgery from the ASA POVL Registry. Data were obtained from the study by Lee et al. The American Society of Anesthesiologists Postoperative Visual Loss Registry. *Anesthesiology* 2006; 105:652-9. Figure with permission from Baig M, Lubow M, Immesoete P, et al. Vision loss after spine surgery: review of the literature and recommendations. *Neurosurg Focus* 2007; (5):15.

Postoperative visual loss

The devastating permanent impairment or loss of sight associated with spine surgery in the prone or lateral position under general anesthesia has led to the creation of a registry by the American Society of Anesthesiologists (ASA) in 1999. In 2006, a review of the first 131 postoperative visual loss cases reported to the registry, of which 93 patients had undergone spine surgery (Fig. 118.2), was completed. A practice advisory was formulated to enhance awareness of postoperative visual loss (POVL) and to reduce its frequency by assisting the clinicians in decision-making when caring for patients undergoing spine surgery under general anesthesia.

The most common causes for POVL associated with spine surgery are ischemic optic neuropathies (IONs), either anterior (AIONs) or (more frequently) posterior (PIONs). AION has been linked to degenerative vaso-occlusive disease involving small arteries, such as the posterior ciliary branches supplying the optic nerve. PION occurs between the optic foramen at the orbital apex and the central retinal artery's point of entry at the midportion of the optic nerve. The perfusion pressure in this section of the optic nerve might be particularly susceptible to increased venous pressure because the supplying arteries consist of small end vessels from the surrounding pia. POVL may also occur from direct trauma to the eye, cortical blindness secondary to hypoperfusion or thromboembolic events, central retinal artery occlusion (CRAO), secondary to direct pressure on the globe or thromboembolic event, or increased intraocular pressure (Fig. 118.3).

The occurrence of ophthalmic complications after spine surgery is reported to be less than 0.2%. There is evidence from one case–control study and several case reports that preoperative anemia and vascular risk factors, such as hypertension and carotid artery disease, as well as smoking, obesity, and diabetes, may be associated with POVL after spine surgery. Patients with these characteristics are referred to as high-risk patients. In addition, careful analysis shows that prolonged surgical procedures >6.5 hours and/or substantial blood loss of an average of 44.7% of estimated blood volume are patient independent risk factors.

The advisory recommends continuous monitoring of blood pressure in high-risk patients and maintaining MAP within 24% of baseline or with a minimum systolic blood pressure of 84 mm Hg. Intravascular volume should be maintained with adequate crystalloid or colloid formulations. Periodic blood sampling to diagnose anemia is advised. There is no recommended threshold for hemoglobin level that may prevent POVL. Therefore, current decision-making strategies for perioperative transfusion therapy apply. CVP monitoring may be considered in high-risk patients. Precautions should be taken when positioning the patient to avoid direct pressure on the eyes and, in high-risk patients, to maintain the head in neutral position above the level of the heart, if possible. Staged procedures could be advised. The advisory committee considers procedures as prolonged when they exceed an average of 6.5 hours (range 2–12 hours).

Postoperative management

Aside from worsened neurologic deficits and continued hemorrhage, airway patency should be a main focus, especially in patients undergoing cervical spine surgery. It is in these patients that a higher incidence of airway obstruction occurs if:

- Surgery involves multiple spinal levels
- Higher spinal levels are involved (C2–C4)
- There is prolonged surgical time
- There is excessive blood loss
- There is significant facial and/or airway edema
- A combined antero-posterior approach is used

Thus, if some of the above criteria are met or if the intubation was difficult, it is usually advised to keep the patient intubated and ventilated in the immediate postoperative period. The use of IV glucocorticoids and head elevation may help to decrease airway edema that could reach a peak on postoperative day 2 or 3. When planning for extubation, a member of the anesthesia team may be present, and the use of a tube-changing stylet may be considered.

Suggested readings

Baig M, Lubow M, Immesoete P, et al. Vision loss after spine surgery: review of the literature and recommendations. *Neurosurg Focus* 2007; 23(5):15.

Kearon C, Viviani GR, Kirkley A, Killian KJ. Factors determining pulmonary function in adolescent idiopathic thoracic scoliosis. *Am Rev Respir Dis* 1993; 148:288–294.

Yadla S, Maltenfort MG, Ratliff JK, Harrop JS. Adult scoliosis surgery outcomes: a systematic review. *Neurosurg Focus* 2010; 28(3):E3.

Chapter 119

Anesthesia for trauma

Bishr Haydar

Introduction

Trauma continues to be a leading cause of morbidity and mortality worldwide. Concerted efforts to prevent secondary injuries and development of algorithmic approaches have improved care and outcomes in patients suffering a wide array of traumatic injuries. The role of the anesthesiologist in the care of trauma patients varies worldwide, from preanesthetic assessment and intraoperative management alone in some regions of the world, to directing the entire continuum from the prehospital resuscitation to the critical care unit in others. This chapter will focus primarily on preanesthetic assessment and intraoperative management, with a brief overview of the overall management of trauma patients.

"Unintentional injuries" continue to be the leading cause of morbidity and mortality in the United States for people aged 1 to 44 years, with the majority of patient deaths due to motor vehicle accidents and other blunt trauma. Homicide, mostly via penetrating trauma, is the next most frequent cause of death in young adults. In adults older than 44 years, trauma continues to contribute significant morbidity and mortality, having been the fourth leading cause of mortality for more than a decade. In the elderly population, hip fractures carry a significant risk of death, and fatal outcomes attributed to other causes (such as pulmonary embolism or sepsis) may have been brought on by the antecedent trauma.

The guiding principles in the care of trauma patients are:

- To treat all potentially life-threatening conditions in order of severity,
- To prevent delay of an indicated treatment, prioritizing it above establishing a definitive diagnosis, and
- To prevent secondary injuries.

Introduction to advanced trauma life support

Advanced trauma life support (ATLS) was developed in the late 1970s to create an algorithmic approach to the resuscitation of the trauma victims. It has become the standard of care in the initial evaluation and treatment of the trauma patient, although it has never been subjected to a randomized trial. The ATLS protocol structures the way the patient is assessed, beginning with the ABCDE mnemonic (see next paragraph); it also gives clear roles and responsibilities to each member of the surgical or emergency medicine team to maximize the efficiency of the initial approach. Life-threatening injuries are treated before the diagnosis is firmly and fully established, with the goal of minimizing any delay. Multiple animal and human studies have shown that, for injuries associated with massive and continuing blood loss, delaying operative treatment in order to further resuscitate or diagnose leads to worsened outcomes. Unstable patients with insufficient vital organ perfusion will suffer from any delay, and the more unstable the patient, the less necessary it is for a definitive diagnosis to be established prior to instituting treatment. Thorough examination, frequent reassessment, and continuous monitoring, however, are critical as these patients often have significant findings missed on initial assessment and can suffer rapid clinical status deterioration.

On arrival to the emergency department, patients may already have an airway device and/or an intravenous (IV) catheter in place and, depending on the perceived initial severity of the injury, may also have a cervical collar and backboard in place. ATLS begins with the primary survey, summarized in the mnemonic ABCDE – Airway, Breathing, Circulation (and hemorrhage control), Disability, and Exposure/Environmental control.

Airway

The need for securing the airway via endotracheal intubation or tracheostomy is determined by assessing both the current status of the patient and the treatment goals. For example, patients may be intubated for obstruction or impending obstruction of the airway due to swelling or hematoma, for mental status changes with failure to protect the airway or respiratory insufficiency, as well as to allow hyperventilation for severe closed-head injuries (see "Airway management" and Table 119.1). If an

Table 119.1. Indications for definitive airway

Airway protection, e.g., GCS < 8 (or vomitus)
Inadequate ventilation, e.g., apnea, hypoxia, hypercarbia, airway bleeding, severe carboxyhemoglobinemia
Severe maxillofacial injury
Impending airway obstruction, e.g., inhalational injury, pulsatile neck mass
Need for hyperventilation

GCS, Glasgow Coma Scale.

airway device is already in place, its correct position must be verified before proceeding further.

Breathing

Establishing, monitoring, and maintaining adequate ventilation are based on the respiratory rate, pulse oximetry, capnography, and physical examination of the thorax and abdomen, including observation, auscultation, palpation, and percussion (ultrasound is also being used increasingly). The goal of the examination is also to rule out tension pneumothorax, open pneumothorax, flail chest, and massive hemothorax. Initial management includes supplemental oxygen, ventilatory assistance with a bag-valve-mask device or endotracheal intubation, placement of a chest tube if necessary, or the decision to perform a thoracotomy emergently.

Circulation

The next goal is to assess for adequate perfusion of vital organs, including identifying sources of potentially exsanguinating hemorrhage. On examination, the level of consciousness, skin color, and pulse quality and rate are immediately assessed; for critically injured patients, mean arterial pressure of 60 to 65 mm Hg is thought to be adequate, although for patients with impaired autoregulation from poorly controlled hypertension or impaired cerebral or coronary vasculature, this value may be insufficient. Rapid circulatory deterioration during the primary survey can be caused by hemorrhage, massive hemothorax, tension pneumothorax, or cardiac tamponade. Until another diagnosis is made, the working assumption for hypotension must be exsanguinating hemorrhage, and resuscitation with lactated Ringer's solution should be immediately instituted. Exsanguinating hemorrhage may occur into five locations – the outside environment, the peritoneum, the retroperitoneal space, the thorax, and fractured long bones and their surrounding tissues. External bleeding is best controlled with direct pressure; internal compartments may require emergent surgical control. Large-bore IV access is established as soon as possible, and resuscitation is initiated with warmed lactated Ringer's solution.

Disability

Disability, or the neurologic status of the patient, is assessed next, by evaluating the patient's best prehospital mental status, Glasgow Coma Scale (GCS) score (see Table 119.2), the ability to move the four extremities, and pupil size and reactivity. Mental status changes may be due to insufficient cerebral oxygenation or perfusion, direct cerebral injury, metabolic derangements, or alcohol or drug intoxication.

Exposure and environmental control

This step is the final one of the primary survey. The patient is undressed and briefly examined from head to toe, and obvious exposures to ingested and environmental toxins are identified.

During the primary survey, monitoring is instituted including electrocardiogram (ECG), blood pressure, and pulse

Table 119.2. GCS

Eye opening	Spontaneous 4
	To speech 3
	To pain 2
	None 1
Verbal response	Oriented 5
	Confused 4
	Inappropriate 3
	Incomprehensible 2
	None 1
Best motor response	Obeys verbal commands 6
	Localizes painful stimulus 5
	Withdraws from painful stimulus 4
	Decorticate posturing (upper extremity flexion) 3
	Decerebrate posturing (upper extremity extension) 2
	No movement 1

Source: Teasdale G, Jennett B. Assessment of coma and impaired consciousness. A practical scale. *Lancet* 1974; 2:81–84.

oximetry. Depending on the patient's status and injuries, a urinary catheter and gastric tube may be placed, and initial blood laboratory samples, often including an arterial blood gas, may be sent. Chest, cervical spine, and pelvic radiographs, along with a diagnostic peritoneal lavage or Focused Assessment with Sonography in Trauma (FAST) examination, are done as soon as possible. The FAST examination is meant to rapidly diagnose hemorrhage by using ultrasonography on four primary views – right upper quadrant, subxiphoid, left upper quadrant, and suprapubic.

The secondary survey begins when the primary survey is complete and resuscitation efforts are well established. This survey includes a head-to-toe evaluation, a complete history and physical examination, and any further laboratory tests and imaging studies. A useful mnemonic for the minimum history required is AMPLE – Allergies, Medications, Past illness/history, Last meal, and the Events and Environment that caused the injury. The patient's vital signs and status are continually reassessed, as yet-undiagnosed injuries may cause rapid deterioration.

During this initial resuscitation, the surgical team seeks to identify immediate threats to the patient's life; these threats define the surgical priorities. Indications for emergent surgery include airway compromise (cricothyroidotomy or emergency tracheostomy), exsanguinating hemorrhage (laparotomy or thoracotomy), or intracranial epidural or subdural hematoma with mass effect. Indications for urgent surgery include limb-threatening injuries, such as a vascular injury or compartment syndrome; sight-threatening globe injuries; or injuries with a high risk of sepsis, such as a bowel perforation.

Blunt trauma

For victims of blunt trauma, the primary ATLS survey should identify obvious severe injuries, such as flail chest or large open wounds. Life-threatening injuries that warrant immediate intervention include exsanguinating hemorrhage into the thorax or peritoneum, tension pneumothorax, and cardiac tamponade. Significant blunt thoracic injuries are common with high-energy motor vehicle collisions but may even occur in falls from standing height in the elderly population. In motor vehicle collisions, blunt thoracic trauma is associated with high-speed, unrestrained collisions with steering wheel deformity or extensive vehicular damage. Fatalities at the scene of a motor vehicle collision, rollover accidents, intrusion into the vehicle, or the victim's ejection from the vehicle are risk factors for more severe injury and mortality. A pronounced initial clinical instability is more predictive of the severity of injury than the mechanism of injury itself. Prehospital death from blunt trauma is usually the result of direct cardiac, aortic, and/or tracheobronchial injury.

Blunt aortic injuries are thought to occur from torsion, deceleration with traction, or "osseous pinch," i.e., compression between bony structures. Predictors of an aortic injury include age greater than 60, high-energy collision with chest wall deformity, multiple rib fractures, pneumothorax, hemothorax, and radiographic chest abnormalities. Such findings should lead to further investigation via chest computed tomography (CT), transesophageal echocardiogram (TEE), or angiography. Suggestive chest radiographic findings include a widened mediastinum, abnormal aortic contour, large hemothorax, or rightward tracheal or esophageal deviation. Initial steps for blunt aortic injury include reducing wall stress by lowering the heart rate, usually below 100 bpm, and systolic blood pressure (SBP) to below 100 mm Hg; common agents for this indication include β-blockade and nitrates until definitive repair can be performed. Contained aortic ruptures are at significant risk of rebleeding within 24 hours.

Cardiac injuries from blunt trauma may include contusion, infarction, or myocardial rupture. Cardiac contusion may present with new bundle branch block, dysrhythmia, or unexplained persistent tachycardia, although hypovolemia must be ruled out first. Myocardial infarction (MI) due to direct trauma may occur due to coronary artery dissection and thrombosis, often in the left anterior descending artery. An MI may also be antecedent to the trauma, whether in a fall or a motor vehicle collision. Myocardial rupture has a significant prehospital mortality; overly aggressive fluid resuscitation may cause further rupture. Myocardial rupture has also been described as occurring several days after admission. Signs of cardiac tamponade physiology, such as hypotension, muffled heart sounds, distended neck veins, and equilibration of central venous and pulmonary artery pressures, may be present. These patients may require emergent thoracotomy, sometimes performed in the emergency department, presenting additional risks for significant injuries and a high mortality rate.

Pulmonary injuries may include pneumothorax, hemothorax, pulmonary contusion, tracheobronchial injuries, diaphragmatic rupture, and lung parenchymal injuries. Pulmonary contusions typically develop over the first 24 hours and may be complicated by pneumonia and acute respiratory distress syndrome. Tracheobronchial injuries in the setting of blunt trauma are highly associated with death in the field; for patients who survive, these injuries are often missed. Persistent pneumothorax despite thoracostomy tube may suggest such an injury. As many as 25% of patients with laryngotracheal injuries have no clinical signs of injury on presentation; signs and symptoms include local contusion, subcutaneous or mediastinal emphysema, voice changes, stridor, and hemoptysis. Cricoid pressure or attempts at endotracheal intubation may dislodge fractured cricoid cartilage causing complete airway obstruction; for these patients, surgical airway backup preparedness is imperative. Although primary repair is most common, there are reports of nonoperative management. Diaphragmatic injuries are associated with hepatic or splenic injuries; herniation of abdominal visceral contents into the thorax is rare, especially after intubation and positive pressure ventilation are instituted. Rib fractures, especially of three or more ribs, and particularly in the elderly population, have been associated with pulmonary contusions and pneumonia. Several studies have demonstrated significant reduction in the incidence of pneumonia and ventilator times in such patients when epidural analgesia is provided. Esophageal rupture is rare in blunt trauma, and is usually associated with high-energy collisions and multiple other injuries; in that context, it could often be overlooked.

Blunt intra-abdominal trauma occurs via direct transmission of energy, such as crush injuries, or through sudden acceleration or deceleration, such as stretch injuries to vascular beds or hollow viscera. Injuries to solid organs are most common, with splenic injuries outnumbering hepatic. Nonoperative management of solid-organ injuries is increasingly favored, so urgent laparotomy for these reasons usually signifies a significant injury or hemorrhage. Urgent laparotomy may also be required when there is persistent hypotension or other signs of continuing internal blood loss, severe gastrointestinal bleeding, evidence of peritoneal irritation, pneumoperitoneum, or diaphragmatic rupture. Massive fluid resuscitation may result in abdominal compartment syndrome, manifesting as hypotension from decreased venous return, increased airway pressures, renal dysfunction, and acidemia.

Crush injuries to the extremities may also precipitate acidemia and renal dysfunction via compartment syndrome, rhabdomyolysis and myoglobinuria. Bone injuries, especially long bone and pelvic injuries, can result in fat embolism syndrome, with the classic triad of petechiae, hypoxia, and neurologic manifestations occurring up to 24 to 72 hours after the fracture. Mental status changes are typical, although focal neurologic findings and seizures have been described. These findings are typically self-limited, although crush injury syndrome is associated with a mortality rate of up to 15%. Treatment is supportive; in one study, prophylactic use of glucocorticids was demonstrated to reduce the incidence of fat embolism syndrome, but no data exist supporting their use after the onset of symptoms.

Penetrating trauma

For patients with penetrating trauma, a brief history may help predict the degree of internal injury. First, there may be associated blunt trauma, including possible cervical spine injury, from falling after the penetrating insult or blast injury. Second, identifying the mechanism of injury is very important. Stab wounds cause less indirect injury than missile injuries. The projectile characteristics, including the type and distance of the firearm from the patient, help to predict the amount of concussive internal injury associated with the missile, separate from the direct lacerating or cutting effect of the missile itself. A military rifle bullet fired at short range, for example, exerts a massive amount of kinetic and concussive energy when compared to a small-caliber pistol bullet or shotgun blast at a greater distance. For penetrating trauma victims with no obvious trauma to the neck, no history consistent with blunt trauma or loss of consciousness, and a normal physical examination of the cervical spine, the incidence of cervical spine injury secondary to this penetrating trauma is exceedingly low. For patients with a direct injury to the trachea, intubation through the airway defect has been described.

Blast injury

Explosions cause four distinct types of injury patterns. Primary blast injury is the direct interaction of the blast wave with the body tissue, whereas secondary blast injury is the interaction of debris energized by the blast with the victim. Tertiary blast injury is the injury sustained by the physical displacement of the body by the blast wind, including tumbling and crush injury, and quaternary injury includes all other types, including burn injuries. Blasts in enclosed spaces are often more severe, as the blast wave may reflect off the walls. Underwater blasts are similarly much more injurious, as water is a better energy transmission medium than is air.

Primary blast injury affects most severely the borders between substances of different densities, for example, at air–tissue junctions in the ear, or air–fluid surfaces in the colon. Blast injury to the thorax typically causes transient apnea, bradycardia lasting up to an hour, and more sustained hypotension. Blast injury to the lung may cause retrosternal chest pain, dyspnea, dry cough, or hemoptysis; hemothorax, pneumothorax, and/or alveolar hemorrhage may ensue. These injuries may, in fact, be more pronounced in victims wearing personal body armor, due to internal reflections of the blast wave. Myocardial ischemia or infarction and arrhythmia may result from coronary emboli, including air. Intestinal injury occurs at the air–tissue junctions and may cause immediate perforation or significant contusion requiring resection to prevent perforation; solid-organ injuries are caused by physical displacement of the body wall. Sensorineural deafness is common, with permanent hearing loss occurring in 55% of patients. Traumatic limb amputations usually occur through a long bone shaft and not through joints.

Secondary blast injuries are similar in character to other high-energy penetrating trauma; any debris in the victim's environment, including radiolucent materials, may be a potential missile. The "blast winds," or the initial wave of energy from the explosion, which may be as fast as 100 mph, can also energize the trauma victim, causing tertiary blast injuries and significant blunt trauma. Quaternary injuries may be immediately identified, such as surface burns and inhalational injury, but may also be significantly delayed, as with acute stress disorder and post-traumatic stress disorder.

Airway management

Victims of severe trauma are often intubated in the field, whereas those with minor trauma may only require intubation with general anesthesia for surgical interventions. For all patients, the first resuscitation step is to confirm that a patent airway is present and that ventilation and oxygenation are adequate. Upper airway obstruction may occur as a direct result of trauma, such as pharyngeal swelling or bleeding, presence of foreign bodies in the airway, laryngeal injury, or hematoma; it may also be due to secondary causes, such as incorrectly applied oropharyngeal airways, unrecognized esophageal intubation, or vomitus in the airway. Inadequate ventilation can result from airway obstruction or other mechanical causes, such as pneumothorax or hemothorax, tracheobronchial injury, aspiration of gastric contents, or bronchospasm. It may also occur as the result of decreased respiratory drive from traumatic brain injury, intoxication, or administered medications (especially opioids and sedatives). Several trauma-specific indications for endotracheal intubation include the need for mechanical hyperventilation to decrease elevated intracranial pressure, to deliver 100% oxygen in patients with carbon monoxide poisoning, or to provide sedation for combative patients unable to comply with urgent diagnostic testing. Importantly, trauma patients should all be considered to be at high aspiration risk ("full stomach"), as the associated catecholamine surge causes significant delay in gastric emptying.

For patients with inadequate ventilation, the initial steps of airway management include application of supplemental oxygen, chin lift, and clearing of the upper airway, with placement of an oropharyngeal airway and/or assisted with bag-valve-mask ventilation. Jaw thrust and cricoid pressure may cause movement of the cervical spine and should be used with caution. Similarly, placement of a nasal airway, NG tube, or nasal intubation should be avoided in patients with suspicion of skull base fracture, as there are reports of intracranial tube placement. For patients who subsequently require a more definitive airway, reproducing operating room (OR) conditions for securing the airway can help minimize complications and number of attempts needed. Basic monitoring such as noninvasive blood pressure (cuff) measurement, 3- or 5-lead ECG and pulse oximetry, along with some form of capnometry, is sufficient. Suction and a functioning IV access are necessary, as well as a laryngoscope with a variety of blades, a backup device for difficult intubation such as laryngeal mask airway, and a bag-mask-valve ventilator with an oxygen source. If emergent intubation is needed, the patient's position should be optimized, with manual in-line stabilization applied if indicated (see Chapters 17 and 18). A succinct airway examination should always

Table 119.3. Causes of hypotension

Hypovolemia (e.g., hemorrhage, "third-space" losses from burns, neurogenic)

Loss of sympathetic tone (high spinal cord injury)

Impaired venous return (tension pneumothorax, pericardial tamponade)

Myocardial dysfunction (myocardial infarction, myocardial contusion, fat or air embolism)

Arrhythmia

Medications, including ingestions or environmental toxins

be performed prior to intubation with the goal of identifying the usual predictors of difficult mask ventilation or difficult intubation, along with trauma-specific considerations, such as facial fractures or markers of inhalational injuries. Surgical airway backup preparedness is vitally important. Please refer to Part 2 for specifics of airway management techniques, including the choice of awake versus anesthetized airway management, induction agents, and use of muscle relaxants.

In patients with facial fractures, the decision to perform an elective tracheostomy is dependent on the individual patient's injury characteristics and surgical plan. In one retrospective review, approximately 12% of patients with facial fractures had a tracheostomy performed concomitantly with the facial fracture repair; tracheostomy was more common in patients with LeFort III fractures or comminuted mandibular fractures and in patients with lower GCS score on admission.

Circulation

In trauma victims, hypotension is most often the sign of significant hemorrhage and empiric treatment is rapidly begun. The list of differential diagnoses, however, must include disease states specific to trauma patients as well as those present in the general perioperative patient population (Table 119.3). Large-bore IV access should be established in the emergency department followed by infusion of 2 L of lactated Ringer's solution, or 20 ml/kg in children; if the hypotension persists, transfusion of uncrossmatched type O blood should be considered.

In young, healthy patients, an acute hemorrhage of up to 40% of the patient's blood volume may have no apparent hemodynamic effects other than tachycardia. In elderly patients or those who take β-blocking agents, a class III (30%–40%) hemorrhage (Table 119.4) may not initially present with any obvious hemodynamic signs either.

Table 119.4. Classes of hemorrhage

	Heart rate	Blood pressure	Pulse pressure	Respiratory rate
Class I: <15% blood volume	—	—/▲	—	—
Class II: 15%–30%	▲	—	▼	▲
Class III: 30%–40%	▲	▼	▼	▲
Class IV: >40%	▲	▼	▼	▲

The goals of resuscitation in the OR setting are to maintain adequate vital organ perfusion and to prevent the cycle of ischemia, capillary leak, acidosis, and immune system activation that leads to further organ dysfunction. To that end, monitoring blood pressure, cardiac output, mixed venous oxygen saturation, urine output, plasma lactate, and other surrogates of perfusion adequacy should permit optimal goal-directed therapy. Delaying definitive control of severe hemorrhage for further resuscitation has been associated with increased mortality. In animal models of uncontrolled hemorrhage, active reduction in blood pressure occurs to decrease the rate of hemorrhage and to allow the formation of a functional clot. In these same studies, resuscitation led to further bleeding and worse outcomes, possibly due to mechanical disruption from higher blood pressures or from dilution of clotting factors. So-called hypotensive resuscitation, or permitting hypotension until definitive hemorrhage control can be obtained, has been demonstrated to reduce mortality in animal models. Bickell demonstrated that, in young men with penetrating thoracic trauma, mortality was reduced by limiting resuscitation prior to the OR. Further studies have demonstrated the safety of hypotensive resuscitation in patients without head trauma. In patients with head trauma, hypotension is clearly associated with significantly increased mortality. Similarly, data on hypotensive resuscitation in patients with impaired autoregulation, such as uncontrolled hypertension, are lacking. After hemorrhage is controlled, prompt resuscitation and establishing adequate perfusion becomes the primary goal. This "under-resuscitation" approach may become more common, even though it is in conflict with the ATLS protocol, which, although never prospectively studied, remains the de facto standard of care.

Significant diffuse hemorrhage, due to trauma-associated coagulopathy, can still occur even after surgical control of bleeding is achieved. Heat loss via conduction, convection and radiation from exposed body areas, evaporation from visceral surfaces, and via cold fluid infusion often causes hypothermia, possibly potentiating platelet and coagulation factor dysfunction. The plasma factor dysfunction may persist after rewarming, due to denaturing of the proteins. Coagulation tests such as prothrombin time and partial thromboplastin time are performed on warmed samples that may overstate the patient's actual ability to form clot. Acidosis can also significantly decrease coagulation factor activity, effects additive to these of hypothermia. Hemodilution and packed red blood cell administration reduce clotting factors, platelets, and fibrinogen. Finally, disseminated intravascular coagulopathy may develop, especially in patients suffering from traumatic brain injury, fat embolism, or multiorgan system failure. Prevention and reversal of worsening coagulopathy is of paramount importance for the survival of trauma victims.

Disability

Trauma to the central nervous system is associated with high morbidity and mortality. Patients with a single episode of

Table 119.5. Traumatic brain injury management goals

Maintain SBP > 90 mm Hg

Maintain O_2 Sat > 90%

Mannitol 0.25–1 gm/kg

No evidence of benefit from hypothermia

ICP monitoring if GCS 3–8 and CT abnormalities

Maintain ICP < 20 mm Hg

Maintain CPP (MAP-ICP) 50–70 mm Hg

Use of barbiturates only for surgically refractory elevated ICP

Use of anticonvulsants to prevent early posttraumatic seizures (<7 d)

Avoidance of hyperventilation – used only as a temporizing measure

No evidence of benefit from glucocorticoids

ICP, intracranial pressure; CPP, cerebral perfusion pressure; MAP, mean arterial pressure.

hypotension, defined as SBP <90 mm Hg, in the setting of cerebral trauma have a 40% higher mortality; long-term neurologic deficits are often the primary concern. When brain or spinal cord trauma is suspected or confirmed, and after airway and exsanguinating hemorrhage are controlled, minimizing further neurologic injury becomes the primary critical care goal. For patients with traumatic brain injuries, guidelines are available from the Brain Trauma Foundation (management goals in Table 119.5).

For patients at risk of having spinal injuries, preventing secondary injury is the mainstay of therapy. Immobilization of patients with possible injury is the first priority; cervical collar placement, manual in-line stabilization during direct laryngoscopy, and logroll movement of the patient are necessary until the injuries can be definitively ruled out, both clinically and radiologically. The use of steroids for acute head trauma is not indicated. The use of steroids for acute spinal cord injury is controversial in the setting of incomplete blunt injury, and is not indicated for penetrating spinal cord injuries. If steroids are used and initiated within 3 hours of injury, administer a methylprednisolone bolus (30mg/kg IV) over 15 min, and after a 45 minute pause initiate an infusion of 5.4 mg/kg/h for 23 hours. If steroid therapy is initiated within 3-8 hours of injury, continue infusion for a total of 47 hours. Although there is some evidence of improved sensory and motor scores in patients who were administered steroids within 8 hours of injury, the use of steroids may significantly increase the risk of infections, and therefore remains controversial.

Suggested readings

American College of Surgeons Committee on Trauma. *ATLS: Advanced Trauma Life Support for Doctors: Student Course Manual.* 7th ed. Chicago: American College of Surgeons; 2004.

The Brain Trauma Foundation. *Guidelines for the Management of Severe Traumatic Brain Injury.* 3rd ed. *Neurotrauma* 2007; 24(Suppl.).

Bickell WH, Wall MJ, Pepe PE, et al. Immediate versus delayed fluid resuscitation for hypotensive patients with penetrating torso injuries. *N Engl J Med* 1994; 331:1105–1109.

Centers for Disease Control and Prevention. Injury prevention & control: data & statistics (WISQARS). Available at: http://www.cdc.gov/injury/wisqars/index.html

Garner J, Brett SJ. Mechanisms of injury by explosive devices. *Anesthesiol Clin* 2007; 25:147–160.

Holmgren EP, Bagheri S, Bell RB, et al. Utilization of tracheostomy in craniomaxillofacial trauma at a level-1 trauma center. *J Oral Maxillofac Surg* 2007; 65:2005–2010.

Shults C, Sailhamer EA, Li Y, et al. Surviving blood loss without fluid resuscitation. *J Trauma* 2008; 64:629–640.

Tieu BH, Holcomb JB, Schrieber MA. Coagulopathy: its pathophysiology and treatment in the injured patient. *World J Surg* 2007; 31:1055–1064.

Teasdale G, Jennett B. Assessment of coma and impaired consciousness. A practical scale. *Lancet* 1974; 2:81–84.

Physiologic changes during pregnancy

Carlo Pancaro and William R. Camann

Pregnancy involves major anatomic and physiologic changes in all the maternal organ systems. The anesthesiologist caring for the pregnant patient must appreciate these physiologic changes, to provide safe analgesia and anesthesia to the mother and enable safe delivery of the fetus.

Cardiovascular system

Hemodynamic changes

Oxygen demand and consumption increase during pregnancy because of the growing fetoplacental unit. To meet these demands, maternal heart rate increases, and peripheral vascular resistance decreases (Table 120.1). The cardiac output increases progressively throughout pregnancy, beginning at 5 weeks and reaching a value 50% greater than that in nonpregnant women by the end of the second trimester. The next significant increase in cardiac output is during the active phase of labor. It reaches its peak increase immediately during the postpartum period, when the uterus contracts and uterine vascular resistance increases. Almost a liter of blood moves through the internal iliac veins and the common iliac vein to the inferior vena cava.

Systemic vascular resistance decreases by 20% primarily because of the development of the placental intervillous space, which is a low-resistance vascular bed. In addition, the vasodilation caused by prostacyclin, estrogen, and progesterone further lowers the systemic vascular resistance. Left ventricular ejection fraction and diastolic function are not significantly changed with pregnancy, nor are central venous or pulmonary arterial and venous pressures. In pregnant patients, the concentrations of markers for the diagnosis of congestive heart failure (e.g., brain natriuretic peptide) or myocardial ischemia (e.g., troponin I) are not different from those concentrations in nonpregnant women.

Aortocaval compression

At approximately the 20th week of gestation, the gravid uterus starts to compress the aorta and the inferior vena cava in the supine position.

Approximately 15% of pregnant patients near term develop the "supine-hypotension syndrome" characterized by a transient tachycardia followed by bradycardia, hypotension, changes in cerebration, nausea, vomiting, sweating, and pallor.

These symptoms are attributed to a lack of venous return to the heart because of the uterus compressing the inferior vena cava. Turning the gravid patient to the left (left uterine displacement) by 15° to 30° generally improves the symptoms (see Fig. 120.1). Left uterine displacement relieves the pressure not only on the inferior vena cava but also on the aorta, which is responsible for uterine perfusion pressure. When the uterus is tilted, uterine perfusion pressure increases and the fetal hemodynamics improve.

Compression of the vena cava diverts blood flow and increases the pressure into the venous azygous system, thereby increasing the pressure and volume of epidural veins. This can increase the likelihood of venous cannulation during epidural placement. Use of the lateral position, during which the epidural veins are less engorged, lessens this risk.

Blood volume

Red-blood-cell volume increases by 30% and plasma volume by 50%, resulting in an increase in the total blood volume of almost 50%. This increase causes a dilutional or physiologic anemia. A greater increase in blood volume occurs with twin pregnancies than with singleton pregnancies, which helps to prepare the parturient for the 500-ml average blood loss during a singleton vaginal delivery or the approximately 1000-ml blood loss during a vaginal delivery of twins or an uncomplicated cesarean delivery.

Table 120.1. Cardiovascular changes in pregnancy

INCREASE
Heart rate
Stroke volume
Cardiac output
Blood, red blood cell, and plasma volume

DECREASE
Systemic vascular resistance
Systolic, diastolic, and mean arterial pressure

UNCHANGED
Central venous pressure
Pulmonary capillary wedge pressure
Left ventricular ejection fraction
Left ventricular diastolic function
Troponin I
Brain natriuretic peptide

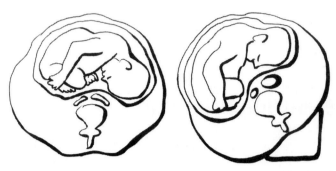

Figure 120.1. Aortic and vena caval decompression demonstrated by lateral tilt. Artwork courtesy of Marlena Bocian.

Auscultation, electrocardiogram, and echocardiogram

An accentuation of the first heart sound occurs with exaggerated splitting of the mitral and tricuspid components. The second heart sound is relatively unchanged. A third heart sound is easily heard during the latter half of pregnancy. Sinus tachycardia is common in pregnancy. Because there is some cardiac enlargement with pregnancy, the tricuspid annulus may enlarge, causing tricuspid regurgitation that can result in a grade I–II early- to midsystolic murmur. The aortic annulus is not dilated. Approximately 94% of term pregnant women exhibit tricuspid and pulmonic regurgitation, and 27% exhibit mitral regurgitation.

Blood pressure

Systolic blood pressure decreases by only 8% during pregnancy due to the increased aortic size and compliance. Diastolic blood pressure decreases by 20% due to the large decrease in systemic vascular resistance.

Hemodynamic changes during labor

Cardiac output increases from prelabor values by 15% in the first stage of labor, 30% in the second stage, and 45% in the third stage (between delivery of baby and placenta). During uterine contractions, cardiac output increases intermittently by an additional 20%, because the contracting uterus forces blood from the intervillous space through the ovarian venous system into the systemic circulation (autotransfusion). A progressive elevation of sympathetic nervous system activity and hence an increase in stroke volume, heart rate, and contractility, combined with the increased blood volume, is responsible for the increased cardiac output throughout labor.

The greatest increase in circulating blood volume occurs immediately after delivery when the uterus is steadily contracted and the obstruction to vena caval and aortic flow is relieved, increasing preload and increasing cardiac output. Patients with cardiac disease are thus most susceptible to worsening of their cardiac function in the postpartum period. In the hour following delivery, cardiac output decreases by 30% because of a decline in both stroke volume and heart rate. Cardiac output declines to prelabor values after 2 days from the delivery and returns to prepregnant levels within 3 to 6 months.

Vasopressors

Ephedrine and phenylephrine are the vasopressors of choice for the treatment of hypotension in pregnant woman, following a regional anesthetic technique. Both drugs will increase maternal blood pressure without significant adverse effects on fetal perfusion or oxygenation. The mechanism of action differs, however, as ephedrine increases cardiac output and phenylephrine increases the peripheral arterial tone to a greater extent. Ephedrine has traditionally been recommended because it may preserve uteroplacental blood flow better in animal models. In clinical practice, however, neonatal condition is identical and umbilical cord blood gases are actually slightly better when phenylephrine is used.

Respiratory system
Upper airway changes

The nasal and oropharyngeal mucosa progressively become engorged early in the first trimester. Nasal endotracheal intubation and direct laryngoscopy should be performed with fine movements and extreme caution because oral, nasal, or pharyngeal bleeding may obscure the laryngoscopic view and make intubation difficult. For the same reason, oral temperature probes and orogastric tubes are preferred over the nasal route after the induction of anesthesia.

The Mallampati score increases during gestation and more so during labor. Because of edema, the pharyngeal volume becomes smaller as labor progresses; this may be responsible for the difficult visualization of the vocal cords under direct laryngoscopy. In addition, the false vocal cords increase in size due to capillary engorgement. Failed endotracheal intubation in obstetric patients is reported to be 1:200 to 1:750, about 10 times more common than the general population. In general, it is prudent to use smaller size endotracheal tubes for general anesthesia during pregnancy.

Changes in respiratory mechanics

The position of the diaphragm rises by as much as 4 cm, which would generally cause a decrease in the vital capacity in pregnancy at term. The chest circumference increases by 5 to 7 cm, which negates the decrease in vital capacity, keeping it unchanged (Table 120.2). Because chest excursions are limited because of the expanded thoracic cage in the resting position, the diaphragm becomes the main inspiratory muscle in term pregnant women. Due to the elevated resting position of the diaphragm and larger diaphragmatic excursions during inspiration, both tidal volume and minute ventilation increase. For these reasons, $PaCO_2$ decreases and PaO_2 increases. These changes and larger tidal volumes decrease physiologic dead space at term.

Table 120.2. Pulmonary changes in pregnancy

INCREASE
Diaphragmatic excursion
Tidal volume
Minute ventilation
Alveolar ventilation
Inspiratory reserve volume
Inspiratory capacity
PaO_2
pH
Oxygen consumption
Mallampati score
False vocal cord size
Rate of induction of inhaled anesthetics

DECREASE
Chest wall excursion
FRC
Expiratory reserve volume
Residual volume
Physiologic dead space
$PaCO_2$
HCO_3
Time to become hypoxemic

UNCHANGED
Respiratory rate
Vital capacity
Small airway resistance
FEV_1
FEV_1/FVC
Closing capacity
Flow–volume loop
Anatomic dead space

The inspiratory reserve volume increases by only 5%, so the inspiratory capacity (inspiratory reserve volume + tidal volume) increases mainly because of the increase in tidal volume. In addition, the diaphragm in the resting position pushes up the bases of the lungs, which causes a reduction in expiratory reserve volume, residual volume, and functional residual capacity (FRC; expiratory reserve volume + residual volume). Because small airway function is unaltered by pregnancy, forced expiratory volume in 1 second (FEV_1), ratio of FEV_1 to forced vital capacity (FVC), closing volume, and flow–volume loops are all unchanged.

The anesthetic implications of these respiratory system changes are profound. FRC is reduced to 80% of the nonpregnant value by term gestation, bringing it closer to closing capacity. For this reason, and due to the increase in oxygen consumption, pregnant women become hypoxemic more rapidly than do nonpregnant women during episodes of apnea. During rapid-sequence induction of general anesthesia, the PaO_2 of parturients decreases at more than twice the rate when compared to nonpregnant women (139 mm Hg/min vs. 58 mm Hg/min). In addition, during induction of anesthesia, the alveolar inhaled anesthetic concentration increases more rapidly in pregnant women, owing to the decreased FRC and the increased minute ventilation. The decrease in $PaCO_2$ and plasma bicarbonate levels lower the plasma-buffering capacity and render the pregnant patient more vulnerable to metabolic acidosis in case of hemorrhage.

Nervous system

During pregnancy, minimum alveolar concentration (MAC) of volatile halogenated anesthetic agents decreases by 30%. In postpartum women, MAC returns to that of the nonpregnant state within 3 days of delivery. Three main factors account for this change during pregnancy:

- Elevated level of progesterone, which acts on γ-aminobutyric acid (GABA) receptors and has sedative effects;
- Increased central serotonergic activity; and
- Activation of the endorphin system.

For the same reasons, the induction dose of thiopental in parturients is reduced by 35% compared to that dose in nonpregnant women. Pregnancy also enhances sensitivity of peripheral nerves to local anesthetics. Despite enhanced neural susceptibility during pregnancy, epidural administration of large doses of local anesthetics (100–150 mg of bupivacaine) results in the same degree of spread in term pregnant and nonpregnant women. With spinal anesthesia, however, pregnant women exhibit a more rapid onset, longer duration of action, and higher spread (25% reduction in the segmental dose requirements) than do nonpregnant women, who receive the same dose of local anesthetic. In addition, women experience an elevation in their threshold to experimental heat pain at term pregnancy, a phenomenon called *pregnancy-induced analgesia*.

Dependence on the sympathetic nervous system for maintenance of blood pressure increases progressively throughout pregnancy. Spinal anesthesia in term pregnant women frequently results in a marked decrease in blood pressure, whereas nonpregnant women experience a lesser decrease.

Endocrine system

Pregnancy is associated with insulin resistance due to the hormone secreted by the placenta – "human placental lactogen." Maternal hyperglycemia may be associated with fetal hyperglycemia, because maternal glucose (but not insulin) crosses the placenta. Near term, oxytocin is secreted by the posterior pituitary (which may initiate labor), and after the birth of the baby, prolactin is secreted by the anterior pituitary, which enhances the production of breast milk.

Approximately 0.1% of pregnancies are associated with a hyperactive thyroid gland. In addition, maternal estrogen and progesterone cause enhanced renin activity, which in turn stimulates the adrenal glands to secrete more aldosterone, resulting in water and sodium retention.

Gastrointestinal system

Pregnancy is associated with an anatomic shift in the position of the stomach caused by the gravid uterus. This shift changes the angle of the gastroesophageal junction, resulting in a decrease of the lower esophageal sphincter tone, which results in heartburn in most pregnant women by term. Many anesthesiologists administer the antacid oral sodium citrate, 30 ml of a 0.3 M solution, prior to anesthesia or labor analgesia, which neutralizes gastric acid and raises its pH. This antacid may ameliorate the consequences of pulmonary aspiration of gastric contents should it occur. In addition, some anesthesiologists administer 10 mg of intravenous metoclopramide, which increases gastrointestinal motility and lower esophageal sphincter tone. It is important to remember that drugs that increase the risk of aspiration, primarily by lowering the esophageal sphincter tone, include glycopyrrolate, succinylcholine, and opioids.

Gastric emptying of liquid and solid materials is not altered at any time during pregnancy, but is slowed markedly during labor. Fentanyl (a 100-µg bolus epidurally or 25 µg intrathecally) and virtually all parenteral opioids also significantly delay gastric emptying during labor. On the other hand, epidural analgesia using local anesthetics and a low dose of fentanyl (e.g., 2 µg/ml) does not delay gastric emptying during labor.

Liver size, morphology, and blood flow do not change during pregnancy, although the liver is displaced upward. Liver enzymes (alanine aminotransferase, aspartate aminotransferase, lactic dehydrogenase) and bilirubin increase to the upper limits of the normal range during pregnancy. The total alkaline phosphatase activity increases two- to fourfold, mostly from production by the placenta. The rate of gallbladder emptying slows, and the bile tends to concentrate, predisposing pregnant women to gallstone formation.

Renal system

The kidneys enlarge and the ureters and renal pelvis and ureters dilate as a result of increased progesterone levels. The dilation of ureters and the pressure on the bladder from the enlarging uterus predispose pregnant women to urinary tract infections. Glomerular filtration rate increases by 50%, resulting in a decrease of blood urea nitrogen (8–9 mg/dl) and serum creatinine (0.5–0.6 mg/dl) concentrations. The resorptive capacity of the proximal tubules for glucose decreases, which leads to mild glucosuria. In addition, increased secretion of erythropoietin by the kidneys leads to an increase in red cell mass.

Coagulation and immune system

Pregnancy is a hypercoagulable state compensated by enhanced fibrinolysis. D-dimer, a specific marker of fibrinolysis, which results from breakdown of cross-linked fibrin polymer by plasmin, increases as pregnancy progresses. The majority of coagulation factor levels are increased. The activated partial thromboplastin time (aPTT) is normal and the prothrombin time (PT) is shortened at term pregnancy. In addition, platelet turnover is increased during pregnancy, although the total count may remain normal or slightly decreased. Pregnancy-induced thrombocytopenia with levels around 100,000 occurs in approximately 8% of all pregnancies and is benign.

Plasma albumin concentration decreases from 4.5 to 3.9 g/dl. Levels of the α_1-acid glycoprotein, the second most important plasma drug binding protein, are not changed during pregnancy. The plasma cholinesterase concentration decreases by 25% in term pregnancy and decreases further postpartum. In individuals with normal cholinesterase enzyme activity, there is no clinically significant change in the duration of action of succinylcholine. The blood leukocyte count increases progressively during pregnancy from 6000/mm³ to 9000 to 11,000/mm³ at term.

Syncytiotrophoblast lacks classic major histocompatibility complex (MHC) antigens, thus creating an immune-privileged surrounding to maintain the fetal allograft. Modulating thymic T-cell selection toward mature T-cell repertoire results in inhibited T-cell activation and tolerance toward paternal HLA as well as interleukin-10 (IL-10) production, which is required for maintenance of pregnancy. Progesterone alters the TH-1/TH-2 ratio toward the immunomodulatory TH-2 subset. These changes set the state for improvement in mainly proinflammatory sustained autoimmune disorders (i.e., multiple sclerosis) but also potential harm by a decrease in immunocompetence and predisposition to infections.

Musculoskeletal system

As the uterus enlarges during pregnancy, lumbar lordosis is enhanced. This change is the primary cause of low back pain that occurs in 50% of pregnant women. A widening of the pubic symphysis and the pelvis results in a head-down tilt when a parturient is in the lateral position. The head-down tilt might increase the rostral subarachnoid spread of hyperbaric local anesthetic solutions when the injection is made with the patient in this position. Pregnancy does not alter cerebrospinal fluid (CSF) pressure, so CSF flow from a spinal needle is unchanged (although uterine contractions during labor do increase CSF pressure).

Suggested readings

Archer GW Jr, Marx GF. Arterial oxygen tension during apnea in parturient women. *Br J Anesth* 1974; 46:358–360.

Carvalho B, Angst MS, Fuller AJ, et al. Experimental heat pain for detecting pregnancy-induced analgesia in humans. *Anesth Analg* 2006; 103:1283–1287.

Christensen JH, Andreasen F, Jansen JA. Pharmacokinetics of thiopental in caesarian section. *Acta Anaesth Scand* 1981; 25:174–179.

Flanagan HL, Datta S, Lambert DH, et al. Effect of pregnancy on bupivacaine-induced conduction blockade in the isolated rabbit vagus nerve. *Anesth Analg* 1987; 66:123–126.

Gaiser R. Physiologic changes of pregnancy. In: Chestnut DH, Polley LS, Tsen LC, Wong CA. *Obstetric Anesthesia: Principles and Practice.* 4th ed. Philadelphia: Mosby; 2009:15–36.

Hellgren M. Hemostasis during normal pregnancy and puerperium. *Semin Thromb Hemost* 2003; 29(2):125–130.

Kodali BS, Chandrasekhar S, Bulich LN, et al. Airway changes during labor and delivery. *Anesthesiology* 2008; 108:1–6.

Porter J, Bonello E, Reynolds F. The influence of epidural fentanyl infusion on gastric emptying in labour. *Int J Obstet Anesth* 1995; 4:261.

Samsoon GLT, Young JRB. Difficult tracheal intubation: a retrospective study. *Anaesthesia* 1987; 42: 487–490.

Stirling Y, Woolf L, North WR, et al. Haemostasis in normal pregnancy. *Thromb Haemost* 1984; 52:176–182.

Chapter

121

Analgesia for labor

Arvind Palanisamy and B. Scott Segal

Labor pain causes extreme discomfort in most parturients, especially nulliparas. Labor pain has been assessed to be among the most severe types of pain. Therefore, to relieve the pain of labor is one of the most important services that an anesthesiologist can provide to parturients.

Pain pathways

Uterine pain, which occurs during the first stage of labor, is transmitted in the sensory fibers accompanying sympathetic nerves that end in the dorsal horns of T10–L1 (Table 121.1). Vaginal and perineal pain, which occurs during the second stage of labor, is transmitted by the afferent fibers of the pudendal nerve (S2–S4). The transmitted signals are relayed to the sensory cortex after processing in the spinal cord.

Anatomic changes in pregnancy

Several pregnancy-related anatomic changes are important for the anesthesiologist to consider. Hormone-induced ligamentous laxity, along with mechanical effects imposed by the enlarging fetus, induces a number of anatomic changes in the lumbar spine, which may lead to the following problems during attempted neuraxial analgesia:

- *Erroneous identification of the intervertebral space* is due to anterior rotation of the pelvis causing Tuffier's line (line connecting the interiliac crests) to cross the lumbar spine at a higher level than the usual L4–L5 interspace.
- *Unintentional head-down tilt* can occur in the lateral position, because the parturient's pelvis is often wider than her shoulders.
- *Increased technical difficulty* is due to a reduction in the physical dimensions of the lumbar intervertebral space as a result of exaggerated lumbar lordosis. Difficulty may be compounded in an actively laboring parturient who is unable to remain still.
- *Enhanced rostral spread of hyperbaric local anesthetics* is due to a cephalad shift of the apex of thoracic kyphosis from T8 to T6 in the supine position.
- *Increased likelihood of vascular cannulation during epidural placement* can occur as a result of the engorgement of the epidural venous plexus, due to inferior vena caval

compression by the gravid uterus and pregnancy-associated increase in plasma volume.

Classification of labor analgesic techniques

Labor analgesia is most commonly provided by regional anesthesia techniques, but there are a number of alternatives available (Table 121.2).

Inhalational analgesia

A mixture of 50% nitrous oxide (N_2O) and 50% O_2 (ENTONOX; The Linde Group, Worsley, Manchester, UK), which is widely used in the United Kingdom, has never become popular in the United States probably due to higher epidural rates along with concerns of bone marrow toxicity from prolonged exposure to N_2O. Halogenated agents, in sub-anesthetic concentrations, have also been shown to possess equianalgesic effects during the first stage of labor. This mode of analgesia requires an anesthetic delivery system in the labor room and the presence of an anesthesiologist. With accumulating laboratory evidence in rodent models implicating N-methyl-D-aspartate (NMDA) antagonists and γ-aminobutyric acid (GABA) agonists in fetal neurodegeneration, the use of such agents will continue to be widely debated.

Systemic opioids

Parenteral opioids are generally safe and reasonably effective analgesics. They are often used in the presence of contraindications to neuraxial techniques or, occasionally, as a means to defer the timing of epidural placement. The commonly used agents include morphine, hydromorphone, meperidine, fentanyl, and, recently, remifentanil. The main disadvantages include sedation, maternal and neonatal dose-dependent respiratory depression, and delayed gastric emptying. The problem

Table 121.1. Stages of labor and dermatomes

Stage I	Uterine contractions to full cervical dilation	T10–L1 (early T11–T12)
Stage II	Full cervical dilation to birth	T10–S4 (addition of S2–S4 – pudendal nerve)
Stage III	Placenta removal	

Table 121.2. Labor analgesic techniques

Non-regional techniques
  Pharmacologic
    Inhalational analgesia
    Systemic opioids, including PCA
  Nonpharmacologic
    Acupuncture
    Transcutaneous electrical nerve stimulation (TENS)
    Hypnotherapy
    Prepared childbirth techniques (Lamaze)
    Hydrotherapy
Regional techniques
  Neuraxial
    Lumbar epidural
    CSE
    Continuous spinal
  Non-neuraxial
    Paracervical nerve block
    Pudendal nerve block

of fluctuating plasma drug levels that are incongruent with analgesic requirements may be attenuated with the use of patient-controlled analgesia (PCA). The favorable properties of fentanyl (quick onset) or remifentanil (unique non-saturable metabolic pathway and easy titratability) make them appealing choices for intravenous (IV) PCA. Unfortunately, most studies comparing neuraxial and IV analgesia find the latter to be far inferior in relieving labor pain. It should be remembered that all opioids (and most sedatives) suppress beat-to-beat variability (indicative of fetal well-being) in fetal heart rate (FHR).

Other methods

A variety of alternative and complementary methods exist for relief of labor pain. The efficacy is variable, risks are low, and, in most circumstances, other than perhaps water immersion, all are compatible with concomitant use of regional analgesic techniques. Because non-neuraxial nerve blocks are experimental (lumbar sympathetic block) or of largely historical interest (paracervical block – abandoned due to high fetal levels of local anesthetic), neuraxial techniques remain the widely used techniques.

Neuraxial analgesia

Indications

Maternal request is a sufficient medical indication for pain relief during labor and is a guideline repeatedly endorsed jointly by the American Society of Anesthesiologists (ASA) and the American College of Obstetrics and Gynecology (ACOG). Recently, the ACOG directly endorsed the provision of neuraxial analgesia without meeting arbitrary milestones of labor progress. More specific indications include:

- Maternal conditions that complicate or contraindicate general anesthesia (e.g., morbid obesity, difficult airway, malignant hyperthermia);

- Obstetric disease, which places the patient at high risk for emergency delivery (e.g., severe pregnancy-induced hypertension);
- Increased likelihood for operative delivery, such as malpresentation and multi-fetal gestation; and
- Maternal coexisting disease (e.g., severe cardiac or respiratory disease), where the sympatho-adrenal consequences of unmitigated labor pain may be detrimental.

Contraindications

Patient refusal, an uncooperative patient, uncorrected coagulopathy, uncontrolled hemorrhage with severe hypovolemia, and epidural site infection qualify as absolute contraindications. All other contraindications (e.g., elevated intracranial pressure, local anesthetic allergy, untreated systemic infection) are relative, and the risks versus benefits need to be carefully considered to make an individualized decision on whether to proceed with a neuraxial technique.

Preparation for neuraxial blockade

The usual preparation for any anesthetic should be undertaken prior to labor analgesia. Because of the unique clinical situation, there are some variations from the routine prior to surgical anesthesia.

- Pre-anesthetic evaluation is obtained, including the patient's medical and anesthetic history, obstetric course, and previous birthing experience, if applicable. A focused physical examination (including the spine) is required, and fetal well-being needs to be documented. The overall plan of care is finalized after discussion with the obstetric care provider.
- Consent is obtained after a detailed explanation of the procedure and a discussion of possible complications and alternatives should regional anesthesia fail. Ideally, consent should be completed prior to the onset of active labor so that the process is unhurried and unencumbered by severe pain.
- Availability of monitoring, resuscitation equipment, and IV access should be verified. It is customary for a majority of labor rooms to be fully equipped for maternal and fetal monitoring and have easy access to resuscitation equipment and drugs. Not all ASA standard monitors may be required for otherwise healthy patients. A large-bore IV catheter, if not already placed, should be secured.
- Aspiration prophylaxis and restriction of oral intake are commonly employed, but controversial. Administration of 30 ml of a nonparticulate antacid, such as sodium citrate, precedes epidural placement. One should generally follow prevailing institutional guidelines regarding restriction of oral intake, as there is no robust evidence to support or refute fasting. ASA guidelines recommend withholding

solid food but allowing moderate amounts of clear liquids in labor. Although it is routine to administer maintenance IV fluids prior to epidural blockade (1–2 liters), fluid preloading is not universally practiced.

- The Joint Commission "safety pause" should be performed prior to beginning the procedure. The name, date of birth of the parturient, and proposed technique should be verbally confirmed by all personnel in the labor room, including the patient.

Monitoring the fetus

FHR is generally monitored either intermittently or continuously during labor, and should be available when performing neuraxial analgesia. The most important features of the tracing are variability and periodic changes in relation to uterine contractions, although one should be aware of the risk of false-positive results. Normal FHR ranges between 120 and 160 bpm. Sympathetic stimulation, prematurity, and maternal fever increase the FHR, whereas parasympathetic (vagus) stimulation, hypoxia, uterine contractions, and fetal head compression decrease FHR. FHR varies constantly from the baseline, which reflects a healthy fetal nervous and cardiac system. FHR variability may be decreased by prematurity, hypoxia, depressant drugs (opioids, magnesium, barbiturates, benzodiazepines), and inadequate uteroplacental blood flow.

FHR decelerations can be classified as *early, late,* or *variable,* according to their characteristics (Fig. 121.1). Early decelerations are normal and are caused by fetal head compression during uterine contractions, resulting in vagal stimulation and slowing of FHR. The onset and offset of the deceleration coincides with the onset and offset of the uterine contraction, producing a mirror image. Late decelerations occur due to any cause compromising uteroplacental blood flow, such as maternal hypotension, acidosis, hypovolemia, and preeclampsia. The FHR usually falls at or after the peak of the uterine contraction and returns to baseline after the contraction has ended. The occurrence of late decelerations calls for urgent evaluation of fetal well-being. Variable FHR decelerations are variable in their duration, timing, and intensity and are often caused by compression of the umbilical cord. Variable decelerations are usually self-limiting and may be mild (<30 sec, FHR > 80 bpm), moderate (30–60 sec, FHR = 70–80 bpm), or severe (>60 sec, FHR < 70 bpm). Persistent or severe variable decelerations may lead to fetal acidosis and call for urgent evaluation and/or intervention.

Description of neuraxial techniques

Neuraxial analgesia for labor can be provided with epidural analgesia, combined spinal–epidural (CSE) analgesia, or continuous spinal anesthesia. Continuous spinal anesthesia is usually done to convert a "wet tap" or unintentional dural puncture into spinal anesthesia.

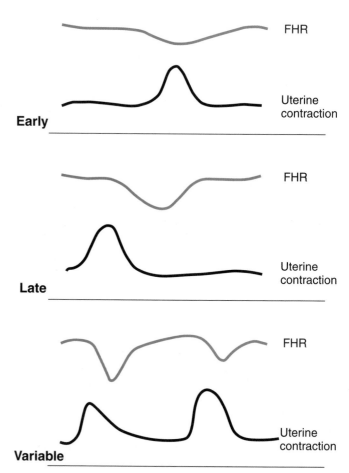

Figure 121.1. Early, late, and variable FHR decelerations.

Epidural analgesia

The anesthesiologist is called at the appropriate time (cervical dilation at 3–4 cm, engagement of fetal head, absence of fetal distress) to administer analgesia for labor. The technique of epidural analgesia is described in Table 121.3.

Table 121.3. Conduct of epidural analgesia for labor

Monitors	On
Position of patient	Supine (usually)/lateral
Back preparation	Povidone-iodine (Betadine; Purdue Pharma L.P., Stamford, CT) × 3 times and draped
Lumbar space	L3–L4/L2–L3
Local infiltration	1–2 ml of 1% lidocaine
Needle	17G or higher gauge Tuohy
Technique	Loss of resistance to air/saline
Wet tap	Remove needle and go one space above
Epidural catheter insertion	2–4 cm into epidural space
Aspiration of catheter	Negative for heme and CSF
Test dose	3 ml of 1.5% lidocaine with 1:200,000 epinephrine
Agent	0.25% bupivacaine 5- to 10-ml bolus
Desirable level of anesthesia	T10

Epidural test dose

Due to the risk of accidental dural puncture or intrathecal migration of catheter and a relatively high incidence of vascular cannulation, it is essential to exclude these in a setting where administration of large volumes of local anesthetics is anticipated, as during the course of labor. A traditional test dose addresses both of these concerns by using a combination of local anesthetic and epinephrine to identify intrathecal migration and intravascular location, respectively. Test dose regimens using air, opioids, or β-adrenergic agonists (e.g., isoproterenol) have also been described.

The commonly used test dose consists of 45 to 60 mg of lidocaine (occasionally bupivacaine, 6–10 mg) with 15 μg of epinephrine. Development of motor block within 5 minutes of injection is considered evidence of intrathecal catheter location; an isolated increase in the baseline heart rate by 25 to 30 bpm 20 to 40 seconds after injection is highly suggestive of intravascular placement. Because of confounding influences associated with uterine contractions, an unpredictable incidence of heart rate elevation with epinephrine, and possible deleterious effects on uteroplacental circulation, employment of a test dose is not ubiquitous. Some authorities suggest that explicit test dosing is unnecessary when dilute concentrations of local anesthetics are used. Given potentially disastrous consequences, however, meticulous fractionation of every bolus dose, along with maintenance of verbal contact with the parturient to identify suspicious symptomatology (perioral tingling, tinnitus), seems prudent.

Local anesthetics

The ideal local anesthetic for labor analgesia should provide excellent sensory analgesia while minimizing motor blockade, have a rapid onset of effect and a long duration of action, and cause no disruption to maternal–fetal physiology. An excellent sensorimotor differential blockade at low concentrations, a reasonably long duration of effect, and an established safety profile in obstetric practice and minimal transplacental transfer make bupivacaine a popular choice. With the use of large-volume, low-concentration mixtures and the addition of opioids to facilitate segmental analgesia, the usual slow onset of action of bupivacaine is not a concern. Due to a reduction in the absolute mass of drug administered, bupivacaine cardiotoxicity is extremely uncommon in labor analgesia.

Ropivacaine, which has a lower potential for cardiotoxicity than does bupivacaine, is a reasonable alternative, albeit a more expensive one. Levobupivacaine (the selective S isomer of bupivacaine) is also less toxic but is currently unavailable in the United States. Lidocaine causes significant motor blockade at analgesic concentrations and has a higher rate of transplacental transfer and the potential to induce tachyphylaxis. For these reasons, lidocaine is not a good choice for maintenance of labor analgesia. Its use as a test for a questionable epidural catheter, or to supplement analgesia (e.g., 5–10 ml of 1.5%–2% lidocaine), is reasonable.

Choice of adjuncts

The addition of neuraxial opioids, which display significant synergism with local anesthetics, enables an overall reduction of local anesthetic dose and minimizes toxicity. Lipophilic opioids (e.g., fentanyl), in particular, also produce segmental analgesia and are shown to reduce the required concentration of local anesthetic. Administration of α_2-adrenergic agonists, such as clonidine, prolongs the duration of analgesia without causing excessive motor blockade. The main side effects are sedation and hemodynamic instability. Vasoconstriction associated with epinephrine use decreases the clearance of epidurally administered local anesthetics and opioids and prolongs the duration of analgesia. It also provides direct analgesic effects through α_2 agonism. Side effects include an increased density of motor block and possible β_2-receptor–mediated tocolysis.

Maintenance of analgesia

Intermittent bolus administrations, either timed or on demand, can provide effective analgesia during labor. High incidence of maternal dissatisfaction, occurrence of dense motor blockade, and an increased anesthetic workload resulted in the use of continuous epidural infusion (CEI) of dilute local anesthetics with or without an opioid. Although CEI provides a more stable level of analgesia and hemodynamic stability, supplemental top-ups are usually required during the course of labor. Patient-controlled epidural analgesia (PCEA), with or without a background infusion, provides better maternal satisfaction as well as decreases the total dose of drug administered. Examples of sample mixtures and parameters are listed in Table 121.4.

Ambulation and progress of labor

Effective analgesia with retention of the ability to ambulate (before placement of an epidural) remains the ideal goal in

Table 121.4. Examples of suggested PCEA regimens

Anesthetic mixture	Infusion rate, ml/h	Bolus dose, ml	Lockout interval, min	Hourly maximum, ml
Bupivacaine 0.125%	6	6	15	30
Bupivacaine 0.125% with 2 μg/ml fentanyl	4–6	6	15	30
Bupivacaine 0.0625% with 2 μg/ml fentanyl	10–15	5	10	45
Bupivacaine 0.08% with 2 μg/ml fentanyl	10	5	15	30
Bupivacaine 0.125% with 1 μg/ml sufentanil	5	5	15	25

most obstetric units. Apart from significantly enhancing maternal autonomy, ambulation is widely believed to reduce the duration of the first stage of labor, but randomized trials support neither this belief nor the common assertion that gravity-mediated increased fetal descent results in a decreased incidence of dystocia. The risk of postural hypotension, subtle motor blockade, and impaired proprioception associated with neuraxial blockade reinforces the need for constant monitoring and nursing supervision during ambulation. Several studies indicate that epidural analgesia does not increase the incidence of cesarean deliveries. Some studies do suggest, however, that it prolongs the first stage of labor, especially in nulliparous women.

Combined spinal–epidural analgesia for labor

Early in labor, especially nulliparous women, may benefit from a CSE analgesia technique (the "walking spinal"). The idea is to inject only opioid (10–25 µg of fentanyl/5–10 µg of sufentanil), or opioid and low-concentration local anesthetic (1 ml of isobaric 0.25% bupivacaine), through the spinal and activate the epidural when needed (when true labor starts). This technique provides a minimal motor block and adequate pain relief in the early stages of labor, allowing the parturient to move about. When active contractions set in, the epidural is activated after a test dose. Alternatively, especially when used in active labor, the CSE technique may be followed by immediate activation of the epidural catheter by beginning a continuous infusion without a bolus. Sufficient local anesthetic usually will be infused by the time the intrathecal analgesia subsides.

The epidural space is reached by using the Tuohy needle. A 4.5-inch to 6-inch, 25G or 27G spinal needle is then introduced through the epidural needle when a give-away sensation is felt (pop) and cerebrospinal fluid (CSF) flow is seen. The two needles are stabilized by one hand, and the spinal agent of choice is administered through the spinal needle. The spinal needle is then withdrawn and an epidural catheter is threaded (2–4 cm) into the epidural space. The patient is then quickly laid supine from the sitting or lateral decubitus position.

Side effects and complications

Serious complications are, fortunately, rare, and only minor side effects are more frequently encountered with labor analgesia. These are listed in Table 121.5.

Table 121.5. Complications of epidural catheter placement for labor analgesia

Hypotension	Pruritus
Inadequate analgesia	Excessive motor block
Urinary retention	FHR abnormalities
Intrapartum fever	Back pain
PDPH	Subdural block
High or total spinal anesthesia	Epidural hematoma or abscess
Accidental IV injection of local anesthetics	

Hypotension

Transient hypotension is one of the commonest side effects occurring with approximately equal frequency during CSE or a standard epidural loading dose. Untreated hypotension causes maternal symptoms, decreases uteroplacental perfusion, and may result in fetal distress requiring prompt treatment. Intravascular volume expansion, left uterine displacement, bolus doses of IV ephedrine (5–10 mg) or phenylephrine (20–40 µg), and supplemental oxygen therapy are required in such cases.

Pruritus

Pruritus following intrathecal and, less commonly, epidural opioids is usually dose-related and transient and requires no pharmacologic intervention. Despite being distressful, reassurance is all that is required in a majority of cases. Although not supported by literature, it may be a good practice to avoid neuraxial opioids in patients with a previous history of severe opioid-induced pruritus and pruritus due to medical conditions in pregnancy, such as symptomatic cholestasis and pruritic urticarial papules and plaques of pregnancy (PUPPP). If treatment is required, administration of either 25 to 50 mg of diphenhydramine, 5 to 10 mg of nalbuphine, or 8 mg of ondansetron may be considered. Severe pruritus may have to be treated with a infusion of dilute naloxone.

Epidural failure

The causes of a failed epidural are numerous and can be arbitrarily classified into early- or late-onset failure. Early-onset failure is usually recognized immediately after epidural placement and can manifest as a unilateral or asymmetric block, a missed segment, or a complete absence of block. Common causes include a malpositioned catheter and altered epidural anatomy (e.g., previous back surgery, severe scoliosis) preventing uniform spread of local anesthetic. Recent evidence suggests that an epidural placed as part of a CSE technique is more likely to result in a successful block.

Late-onset failure manifests as breakthrough pain in a parturient with a previously effective epidural block. A visual inspection to exclude dislodgement of the epidural catheter or disconnection of the maintenance infusion is mandatory before attempting any corrective measures. In the absence of such causes, intravascular migration is the most likely reason, which necessitates replacement of the catheter. Table 121.6 shows approaches to troubleshooting a poorly functioning epidural catheter.

Excessive motor block

With increasing emphasis on the use of dilute local anesthetic solutions for labor analgesia, the incidence of excessive motor block is considerably lower than it has been in the past. Although difficult to predict, it seems to occur more commonly

Table 121.6. Labor epidural troubleshooting

Problem	Presentation	Identification	Remedy
Total failure	No block immediately or at any time following placement	Ambiguous loss of resistance Dislodgement of the catheter Disconnection of the epidural infusion connectors Undetectable block after 10 ml of 0.25% bupivacaine or equivalent	Replace epidural catheter at or above previous site Replace epidural catheter and tape it securely Reconnect after ensuring adequate sterility Replace epidural catheter at or above previous site
Partial failure*	Unilateral block (Patient complains of motor and thermal asymmetry)	Dermatomal pattern with sensory testing	Top-up epidural with painful side in dependent position. If no response in 10 min, withdraw catheter by 1 cm and re-bolus (replace if unsuccessful)
	Missed segment	Usually a subtle unilateral block between T12 and L2 on sensory testing	Same as above, but add an opioid (50–100 µg of fentanyl) for segmental analgesia If in doubt, replace the catheter
	Back pain Perineal pain and rectal pressure	Possible occipito-posterior fetal head position Rapid progress to second stage of labor	Top-up with at least 5–10 ml of 0.25% bupivacaine + opioid in semi-sitting position Check sacral block and then same as above

* Always check PCEA usage, ensure an empty bladder, and verify progress of labor. Exclude possible uterine dehiscence in a parturient undergoing trial of labor after cesarean delivery complaining of disproportionate pain.

in patients who receive multiple boluses during the course of labor. A subjective complaint of excessive lower extremity heaviness is the usual harbinger. Reduction of the infusion rate or temporary discontinuation is the appropriate first step. If PCEA is employed, it may be prudent to discontinue the background infusion while permitting demand boluses so that the possibility of rapid regression of block is minimized.

Urinary retention

Urinary retention commonly accompanies lumbar epidural analgesia, and catheterization is routine in many labor units. Use of neuraxial opioids, in particular, significantly increases its incidence. Urinary retention in the postpartum period, following complete regression of the epidural block, is usually due to obstetric rather than anesthetic factors.

Fetal heart rate abnormalities

Changes in the fetal heart rate (FHR) tracing (decrease in baseline, decelerations) occur with both epidural and CSE techniques. Transient bradycardia, however, is more common with the CSE technique. Although distressing, these FHR changes are usually self-limited and subside with conservative therapy without modifying the obstetric outcome. Nevertheless, its occurrence reinforces the importance of vigilant fetal monitoring during and after the procedure. The mechanisms responsible for FHR changes are not clear, but uterine artery vasospasm due to acute perturbation in maternal catecholamine levels seems to be the most likely explanation. One recommendation is an IV administration of ephedrine.

Intrapartum fever

An observed association between epidurals and intrapartum fever has been confirmed by randomized studies. Maternal pyrexia causes an increase in maternal antibiotic exposure and neonatal sepsis evaluations, and direct toxicity to the fetal brain has been suggested. Although the exact mechanism is still unclear, thermoregulatory imbalances, a suppressive effect of systemic opioids in women without epidurals, and inflammation have all been suggested as possible mechanisms. Recent evidence, however, consistently supports an inflammatory etiology.

Back pain

Forty percent of postpartum women experience lower back pain regardless of the choice of analgesia, neuraxial or otherwise. Multiple studies have consistently shown a poor correlation between epidural analgesia and postpartum backache.

Unintentional dural puncture

The incidence of unintentional dural puncture, the wet tap, is inversely related to the experience of the operator, varying from 1% to 8%. The consequences of a wet tap with the routinely used 17G epidural needle can be quite debilitating. Post-dural puncture headache (PDPH) complicates 50% to 80% of cases. The commonly used management strategies following a wet tap include:

- Placement of an intrathecal catheter: Threading an epidural catheter into the subarachnoid space provides reliable and excellent analgesia. It also obviates the need for replacement of the epidural catheter, which in itself carries a risk of an additional dural puncture. Intrathecal catheters left in situ for more than 24 hours have been suggested to reduce the incidence of PDPH compared to replacement of the catheter, although the data are not consistent. In addition, some anesthetists fear the risk of infection and the potential for iatrogenic disasters on postpartum units where the nursing staff are unfamiliar with such catheters.

Table 121.7. Conduct of an epidural blood patch

Monitors	On
Patient position	Lateral/sitting
Lumbar space	Same or near the first dural puncture site
Skin preparation	Betadine × 3 times, local 1–2 ml of 1% lidocaine
Needle	17G Tuohy
Loss of resistance	Air/saline
Autologous blood collection (15–20 ml)	By assistant with full aseptic precautions (Betadine skin preparation, sterile gloves, and syringe)
Blood injection	Via epidural needle
Patient position	Supine for approximately 1 h

- Replacement of epidural at an alternate interspace: This strategy requires no special precautions compared to an intrathecal catheter, but risks inducing another dural puncture and enhanced drug transfer across the preexisting dural hole during an epidural bolus. Doses, therefore, need to be fractionated and possibly reduced. Prophylactic blood patching has not been shown to give consistent results.

The headache usually occurs after 24 hours and is described as a severe fronto-occipital headache, sometimes with neck pain. Headache improves in the supine position and becomes severe on sitting or standing (traction on the brain). Nausea, vomiting, diplopia, or tinnitus may accompany the headache.

Treatment of PDPH includes conservative measures, such as bed rest, fluids, analgesics, and caffeine (500 mg in a liter of crystalloid) or an epidural blood patch, as described in Table 121.7. Use of saline for a patch (instead of blood) is a less effective means of treating the headache. Recently, fibrin glue has been shown to be an alternative to blood for an epidural patch. Although 85% to 90% of headaches are relieved after one patch, the rest of the patients may need a second blood patch (after 24 hours).

Rare complications

Location of the epidural catheter between the dura and arachnoid membrane results in a subdural block. Although rare, this may also be the cause of patchy epidural blocks. High or total spinal block may occur due to unidentified subarachnoid placement, intrathecal migration of an epidural catheter, or deterioration of a subdural block with rupture of arachnoid induced by a bolus dose. Unappreciated intravascular injection may occur and lead to local anesthetic toxicity.

Suggested readings

ACOG. ACOG Committee Opinion No.295: Pain relief during labor. *Obstet Gynecol* 2004; 104:213.

ACOG. ACOG Committee Opinion No.339: Analgesia and cesarean delivery rates. *Obstet Gynecol* 2006; 107:1487–1488.

Cyna AM, Andrew M, Emmett MS, et al. Techniques for preventing hypotension during spinal anaesthesia for caesarean section. *Cochrane Database Syst Rev* 2006; 4:CD002251.

Guay J. The epidural test dose: a review. *Anesth Analg* 2006; 102(3):921–929.

Leighton BL, Halpern SH. The effects of epidural analgesia on labor, maternal, and neonatal outcomes: a systematic review. *Am J Obstet Gynecol* 2002; 186(5 Suppl Nature):S69–S77.

Ohel G, Gonen R, Vaida S, et al. Early versus late initiation of epidural analgesia in labor: does it increase the risk of cesarean section? A randomized trial. *Am J Obstet Gynecol* 2006; 194(3):600–605.

Palanisamy A, Hepner DL, Segal S, et al. Fever, epidurals, and inflammation: a burning issue. *J Clin Anesth* 2007; 19(3):165–167.

Scavone BM, Wong CA, Sullivan JT, et al. Efficacy of a prophylactic epidural blood patch in preventing post dural puncture headache in parturients after inadvertent dural puncture. *Anesthesiology* 2004; 101(6):1422–1427.

Segal S, Wang SY. The effect of maternal catecholamines on the caliber of gravid uterine microvessels. *Anesth Analg* 2008; 106(3):888–892.

Simkin PP, O'Hara M. Nonpharmacologic relief of pain during labor: systematic reviews of five methods. *Am J Obstet Gynecol* 2002; 186(5 Suppl Nature):S131–S159.

Tsen LC, Thue B, Datta S, Segal S. Is combined spinal-epidural analgesia associated with more rapid cervical dilation in nulliparous patients when compared with conventional epidural analgesia? *Anesthesiology* 1999; 91(4):920–925.

van der Vyver M, Halpern S, Joseph G. Patient-controlled epidural analgesia versus continuous infusion for labour analgesia: a meta-analysis. *Br J Anaesth* 2002; 89(3):459–465.

Chapter 122

Anesthesia for cesarean delivery

Lawrence C. Tsen

The incidence of cesarean delivery (CD), which is defined as the birth of a fetus through incisions in the abdomen (laparotomy) and uterus (hysterotomy), has undergone progressive increases and currently accounts for 15% to 30% of all deliveries in developed countries worldwide.

Indications

The common indications for CD include previous CD, cephalopelvic disproportion, dystocia, fetal malpresentation, placenta previa or abruptio placentae, prematurity, non-reassuring fetal status, and patient request. A prior CD does not require subsequent pregnancies to be delivered in this manner, although a trial of labor after CD (TOLAC; which, if successful, is referred to as a vaginal birth after CD [VBAC]) is an alternative, albeit declining, option.

Conduct and complications of cesarean delivery

CD is usually performed via a low (suprapubic), transverse incision through the skin and uterus (Pfannenstiel incision), which offers improved cosmesis and wound strength as well as a reduction in bowel and omentum adherence, infection rates, and blood loss. Vertical uterine incisions can be used when the lower uterine segment is underdeveloped (prior to 34 weeks of gestation), in the presence of a large-for-gestational-age fetus or multiple fetuses, or in truly emergent cases. Uterine exteriorization following delivery of the fetus and placenta facilitates visualization and repair, particularly when the incision has been extended laterally.

Complications of CD include hemorrhage, infection, thromboembolism, hysterectomy, ureteral tract and vesical injury, abdominal pain, uterine rupture in future pregnancies, and death. Maternal morbidity and mortality still vary widely; however, in most developed nations, maternal death averages 10 to 30 per 100,000 CD, a rate minimally higher than for vaginal delivery. Infant and neonatal mortality follow similar patterns and rates, but are higher following CD, most likely reflecting the conditions prompting non-elective deliveries.

Preparation for anesthesia

A review of the maternal medical, anesthetic, and obstetric history, allergies and medications, an assessment of baseline hemodynamics, and an airway, heart, and lung examination should be performed before providing anesthesia care. Acknowledgment of the risks and benefits of each anesthetic option should be discussed as part of the informed consent. Major hemorrhage can occur at any time in the peripartum period and remains a leading cause of maternal mortality. Risk factors for peripartum hemorrhage should be identified and preparations made. Basic monitors should be applied; invasive hemodynamic monitoring should be considered in women with severe cardiac or renal disease, refractory hypertension, pulmonary edema, or unexplained oliguria. An evaluation of the fetal heart rate by a qualified individual may be useful before and after administration of anesthesia to reduce fetal and neonatal complications.

NPO status and gastric optimization

NPO status should be assessed, although gastric emptying of liquids during pregnancy occurs relatively quickly and similarly in lean or obese, non-laboring, pregnant women. The uncomplicated patient undergoing labor or elective CD can drink modest amounts of clear liquids up to 2 hours prior to induction of anesthesia. Patients with additional risk factors for aspiration (e.g., morbid obesity, diabetes, difficult airway) or patients at increased risk for operative delivery (e.g., nonreassuring fetal heart rate pattern) may have further restrictions of oral intake, determined on a case-by-case basis. Solid foods should be avoided in laboring patients and in those undergoing elective surgery (e.g., scheduled CD or postpartum tubal ligation). A fasting period of 6 to 8 hours for solids has been recommended. A nonparticulate antacid (sodium citrate) is believed to decrease the damage to the respiratory epithelium if aspiration occurs, and is customarily administered. Additionally, metoclopramide may decrease nausea and vomiting and facilitate gastric emptying.

Selection of anesthetic technique

In addition to the urgency and anticipated duration of the case, the most appropriate anesthetic for a CD depends on maternal,

Table 122.1. Advantages/Disadvantages of neuraxial anesthesia

Advantages:
Minimal fetal exposure to drugs
Decreased incidence of maternal pulmonary aspiration
An awake mother with greater bonding with the neonate

Disadvantages:
Greater incidence of hypotension
Exposure to risks of neuraxial anesthesia

fetal, and anesthetic factors. In cases of dire fetal distress, a rapid evaluation of the patient and the situation should be performed as other preparations for the provision of anesthesia are being made. Regardless of the degree of urgency, the anesthesiologist should not compromise maternal safety by failing to obtain critical information, including previous medical and anesthetic histories and allergies, and to quickly assess the airway and basic hemodynamics.

Overall, neuraxial (epidural, spinal, and combined spinal–epidural [CSE]) techniques are the preferred methods for providing anesthesia for CD in both elective and emergent procedures, and specific benefits and risks of each technique dictate the eventual selection. Certain conditions or time constraints, however, may contraindicate their use. Such comorbidities include localized infection or generalized sepsis, severe uncorrected coagulation disorders, severe hypovolemia, or cardiac pathologies where acute onset of hypotension may be detrimental. Severe obstetric hemorrhage in the antepartum period, and severe preeclampsia or hypertension, may also complicate the choice of anesthetic technique. Advantages and disadvantages of neuraxial and general anesthetic techniques are summarized in Tables 122.1 and 122.2.

Spinal anesthesia

This technique is the most common for anesthesia in elective CD. For emergent CD, a general anesthetic is preferred. Spinal anesthesia in emergent situations is administered only if (1) time permits and (2) it is not contraindicated. A simple and reliable technique with rapid onset, spinal anesthesia provides an awake and comfortable patient with minimal risks for aspiration. Despite the lower abdominal cesarean incision, a T4 dermatome level is required to prevent referred pain from traction on the peritoneum and uterus.

Table 122.2. Advantages/Disadvantages of general anesthesia

Advantages:
Rapid onset and reliability
Airway control
Less hypotension than neuraxial
    anesthesia

Disadvantages:
Increased risk of pulmonary aspiration
Drug-induced fetal cardiorespiratory
    depression
Difficult airway management

Table 122.3. Conduct of spinal anesthesia

Monitors	BP measurement every 2 min after spinal administration for 15–20 min, electrocardiogram, pulse oximetry
Patient position	Sitting or lateral recumbent
Back preparation	Betadine or chlorhexidine × 3 times
Lumbar space	L3–4/L4–5
Local infiltration	1–2 ml of 1% lidocaine
Needle	25G or higher (need an introducer)
CSF flow	Free flow; typically no heme or paresthesia
Agent	10–12 mg of hyperbaric (8.25% dextrose) bupivacaine (0.75%)
Additives	Fentanyl 10–25 mcg/morphine 0.2–0.3 mg, epinephrine 1:200,000
Desirable level of anesthesia	T4
Patient position	Supine with left uterine displacement; tilt table toward left and/or put a blanket roll under right hip)
Oxygen supplementation	Nasal cannula/face mask
Hypotension	Phenylephrine 40 μg, ephedrine 5–10 mg, epinephrine if life threatening, fluid supplementation, uterine tilt
Nausea	Check BP (usually due to impending hypotension), metoclopramide, ondansetron

BP, blood pressure; CSF, cerebrospinal fluid.

After a routine preoperative evaluation and obtaining informed consent, the patient is brought into the operating room. Typically, by this time the patient would have already received placement of a large-bore intravenous [IV] catheter, a nonparticulate oral antacid (30 ml of sodium citrate) and frequently a promotility agent (10 mg of metoclopramide IV). Anxiolytics are best avoided until after delivery. Patients are placed on the operating table with a left uterine tilt to prevent aortocaval compression. Supplemental oxygen via a nasal cannula or face mask is routinely provided to the mother, although currently there is some controversy regarding the necessity of this treatment. The conduct of spinal anesthesia is summarized in Table 122.3.

After the baby is born, sedation, if required, can be given to the mother (may interfere with recall). Times for skin and uterine incisions and for the birth of the baby should be recorded in the chart. Antibiotics are administered, per the request of the surgeon. As soon as the placenta is delivered, 20 U of oxytocin are added to each liter of fluid (40 U total) for increasing the uterine tone (may cause hypotension and nausea). Additionally, 0.2 mg of methylergometrine maleate (Methergine; Novartis, East Hanover, NJ) may be given, intramuscularly (IM), if requested by the surgeon. Parturients lose approximately 800 to 1000 ml of blood during the operation.

Epidural anesthesia

The use of epidural anesthesia for CD has increased during the past two decades, primarily due to the growing use of epidural labor analgesia converted to surgical anesthesia for CD (Table 122.4). Although the types of medications used in the spinal and epidural space are similar, epidural doses are 5 to 10 times greater and given in much larger volumes to encourage

Table 122.4. Conduct of epidural anesthesia with an epidural catheter in situ

Monitors	BP measurement every 2 min after spinal administration for 15–20 min, pulse oximetry; electrocardiogram when in the operating room
Patient position	Supine with left uterine displacement; tilt table toward left and/or put blanket roll under right hip)
Level check of existing analgesia	Typically T10
Aspiration of epidural catheter (gentle)	Negative for heme and CSF
Agent	2% lidocaine or 3% chloroprocaine; 5 ml × 4 times = 20 ml, as necessary
Additives	Sodium bicarbonate: 1 ml for each 10 ml of lidocaine or chloroprocaine
Desirable level of anesthesia	T4

adequate spread and subsequent blockade. Advantages of the epidural technique potentially include a lower incidence and range of maternal hypotension, due largely to a gradually developing sympathetic blockade. In addition, catheter-based techniques enable the anesthesiologist to titrate the level, density, and duration of anesthesia. Opioids may be administered via the epidural catheter, including morphine (2–3 mg) and fentanyl (50–100 mcg). Morphine (2–3 mg) or fentanyl (50 mcg) can be used. Sedation, oxytocin, and antibiotic administration are similar to when spinal anesthesia is used.

For CD, the most common epidural agents used are 2% lidocaine, with or without epinephrine (1:200,000), and 3% 2-chloroprocaine, which is the agent of choice for emergent CD due to its rapid onset and rapid maternal and fetal metabolism. Fetal accumulation, especially when acidosis is present, is therefore minimized. By contrast, chloroprocaine is avoided for routine, non-urgent deliveries, as the short duration requires multiple doses, and its use can adversely affect the efficacy of subsequent epidural opioid analgesia. In addition, when used in higher total volumes (>40 ml), chloroprocaine can increase the incidence of back pain. Alkalinization with sodium bicarbonate (1 ml of 8.4% sodium bicarbonate per every 10 ml of 2% lidocaine or 3% chloroprocaine) hastens the onset and increases the intensity of blockade significantly and may be used in urgent or emergent CD. Alkalinization should not be used with certain (particularly longer acting) local anesthetics (e.g., bupivacaine) due to the low threshold for precipitation.

Combined spinal–epidural anesthesia

The principle advantage of the CSE technique is the ability to deliver a quick and reliable spinal anesthetic with the opportunity to augment the density or duration of the anesthesia through the epidural catheter. This technique is particularly useful in obstetrics, where delays in the commencement or increases in the duration of surgery sometimes occur (e.g., possible placenta accreta, history of multiple abdominal surgeries, high index of suspicion for cesarean hysterectomy). The

CSE placement technique is discussed in Chapter 121. Local anesthetic can be given through the epidural catheter if the duration of surgery exceeds that of the initial spinal.

General anesthesia

The mortality and morbidity associated with general anesthesia for CD disfavor its use. It is important to remember that pregnant patients have a 4 to 5 times higher risk of a failed intubation or pulmonary aspiration of gastric contents than does the general population. The speed of the surgeon is important, as skin incision to delivery times greater than 8 minutes or uterine incision to delivery times greater than 3 minutes are associated with greater fetal morbidity and mortality. In a case of failed intubation and in the absence of fetal distress, the patient could be awakened for a fiber-optic intubation or a regional anesthesia technique. If surgery is to be continued, however, the patient could be mask ventilated, a laryngeal mask airway (LMA) could be inserted, or an intubating LMA could be used for airway management. Conduct of general anesthesia is described in Table 122.5.

After the surgical drapes have been applied and the operating personnel are ready at the bedside, the surgeon should be instructed to hold the initial incision until the anesthesia provider secures the correct placement of the endotracheal tube and gives a verbal confirmation to proceed with the operation. A rapid-sequence induction with full cricoid pressure after induction with thiopental at 3 to 5 mg/kg and succinylcholine at 1 to 2 mg/kg is performed. Ketamine at 1 to 1.5 mg/kg or etomidate at 0.2 to 0.3 mg/kg should be substituted for thiopental if hemodynamic instability is present prior to induction. It should be remembered that muscle relaxants do not cross the placenta and, therefore, do not affect the fetus. Oxygen (100% if fetal compromise) or in a 50% mixture with nitrous oxide and a volatile anesthetic as necessary should be provided until delivery. Upon delivery, nitrous oxide can be initiated or its concentration increased to 70%. The concentration of the volatile anesthetic, which causes uterine relaxation, should be reduced after delivery to limit its effect on uterine tone.

Table 122.5. Conduct of general anesthesia

Aspiration prophylaxis	Sodium citrate: 30 ml, within 30 min of induction, if possible
	Metoclopramide: 10 mg IV, preferably 30 min prior to induction; avoid rapid IV push
Position	Supine with left uterine displacement
Preoxygenation	3 min/4–8 deep breaths of 100% oxygen
Induction	Rapid-sequence with cricoid pressure, thiopental 3–5 mg/kg, succinylcholine at 1–2 mg/kg
Incision	If emergent CD as soon as patient is intubated
Intubation	Usually a smaller size endotracheal tube (6- to 6.5-mm diameter), orogastric tube
Maintenance	Oxygen, inhalational agent (low concentration), muscle relaxant
After baby is delivered	Antibiotics, oxytocin, opioids
Reversal of muscle paralysis	Neostigmine and glycopyrrolate
Extubation	Awake

Postoperative recovery

Postoperative recovery includes following the resolution of neuraxial block or recovery from general anesthesia and treating complications or patient concerns.

Pain management

Over the past three decades, the greater efficacy of epidural and spinal opioids for postsurgical analgesia has prompted a shift from a systemic (IV or IM) to a neuraxial route of administration. Morphine has emerged as the leading agent for post–CD analgesia, due to its long duration of action and low cost. Morphine administered intrathecally (0.2–0.3 mg) or epidurally (2–3 mg) appears to provide optimal post–CD pain relief with limited side effects. Due to a low lipid solubility, the peak analgesic effects of morphine are delayed (60–90 minutes), but provide reliable analgesia for up to 24 hours.

The local anesthetic selected for epidural anesthesia may influence the efficacy of epidural morphine. Parturients who received 2-chloroprocaine (a short-acting, rapid-onset local anesthetic used primarily for emergent CD) versus other local anesthetic agents appear to demonstrate significantly shortened duration of epidural morphine analgesia, in some cases to less than 3 hours. Because post-CD pain includes both somatic pain, which can be relieved by local anesthetics and opioids, and visceral pain, which can be more difficult to treat, a multimodal approach to pain relief, include nonsteroidal anti-inflammatory drugs (NSAIDs), such as ketorolac (15–30 mg IV), has been suggested.

Management of anesthetic complications

For a more detailed list of complications of obstetric regional anesthesia, please refer to Chapter 121.

Inadequate neuraxial anesthesia

Approximately 4% to 13% of epidural anesthesia techniques and 0.5% to 4% of spinal anesthesia techniques fail to provide a sufficient anesthetic block for the initiation or completion of the surgical procedure. Epidural techniques are more likely to be associated with failure, given their often earlier placement during labor and the ability of the catheter to migrate out of the epidural space. Factors that may correlate with failed in-situ labor epidural catheter for CD include an increased number of bolus doses for the provision of labor analgesia, patient characteristics (body mass index [BMI], distance from skin to epidural space), initial type of technique used (CSE vs. epidural), and the time elapsed from the initial placement to the CD.

A failed block can be defined as insufficient in height, density, or duration after an appropriate dose of local anesthetic to provide anesthesia for a CD. Steps to reduce a failed block include being meticulous in the technical aspects of the original placement attempt, using solutions consisting of local anesthetics with opioids, and better understanding the characteristics

of an epidural versus spinal blockade. Moreover, the patient should be prepared to expect the sensation of deep pressure and movement, yet be reassured that reports of discomfort or pain will be addressed. Shoulder pain can originate from irritation of the diaphragm or prolonged extension of the arms and is mediated by the phrenic nerve (C3–C5). Additional discomfort can occur from visceral stimulation, such as uterine manipulation, which often involves the greater splanchnic nerve (T5–T10). Also, inadequate anesthesia can result from regression of the block from a cephalad or caudad direction.

If an inadequate, partial block exists in an elective situation prior to incision, either (1) the operative procedure can be postponed to allow resolution of the block, or (2) a repeat neuraxial technique may be performed. After a failed, but partial, epidural or spinal technique, the use (and amount of drug to be used) of a spinal technique is controversial. In this setting, a repeat spinal with more than 10 mg of bupivacaine has been observed to result in a high spinal block. Possible approaches to this problem include reducing the dose of anesthetic, using a semi-sitting (Fowler's) position to limit the cephalad spread of the local anesthetic, employing the CSE technique with a small intrathecal dose and titrating the level with drugs administered through the epidural catheter, or placing an epidural catheter intentionally into the dural sac for use as a continuous spinal catheter.

If the surgery has already commenced and the discomfort is reported, asking the surgeons to temporarily halt surgical manipulation while an assessment is made can be helpful. Low-dose IV opioid (e.g., fentanyl at 1–2 mcg/kg or alfentanil at 5–10 mcg/kg) or nitrous oxide inhalation (50% in oxygen) and anxiolysis (1–3 mg of midazolam) may be helpful. If a neuraxial catheter is in place, additional local anesthetics with opioids should be added. Severe pain may require IV ketamine in 5- to 10-mg increments, with the understanding that significant sedation, loss of consciousness, and psychomimetic and amnestic effects may occur. The obstetrician can use a local anesthetic to infiltrate the wound or instill it intraperitoneally; however, often at this point, the induction of general anesthesia with endotracheal intubation should be considered.

High spinal

It is not uncommon for the parturient to report mild dyspnea or reduced ability to cough, especially if the neuraxial blockade has achieved a T2 level. If impaired swallowing or phonation, unconsciousness, respiratory depression, or significant impairment of ventilation occurs, a conversion to a general anesthetic should be performed. High neuraxial blockade may also result in cardiovascular sequelae, including bradycardia and hypotension. High neuraxial block can be caused by several mechanisms, including an exaggerated spread of spinal drugs or an unintentional dural or subdural puncture with administration of epidural drugs. Although the use of lower doses of local anesthetics has been proposed for patients less than 5 feet tall, patient variability may or may not allow a reduced dose to work with sufficient duration, or be entirely predictable in terms of the cephalad spread.

Hypotension

The incidence of hypotension, defined as a 20% to 30% decrease from the baseline systolic blood pressure or a systolic blood pressure $\leq$ 100 mm Hg, ranges from 30% to 100% following spinal anesthesia in parturients undergoing CD. A lower incidence of hypotension (5%–63%) has been observed following the use of epidural anesthesia for CD, most likely due to the slower onset of sympathetic blockade and the ability to titrate intravenous fluids and vasopressors during this period.

When severe and sustained, maternal hypotension can lead to an impairment of uterine and intervillous blood flow, and can ultimately result in fetal hypoxia, acidosis, and/or neonatal depression. Moreover, hypovolemia can alter maternal well-being (i.e., mental status changes, nausea). The optimization of maternal perfusion should be a primary goal of fluid and vasopressor management throughout the perioperative period.

The frequency of hypotension can be reduced with the use of left uterine displacement and possibly by fluid administration. If hypotension ensues, however, the prompt selection and use of a vasopressor and supplemental oxygen is essential. In the absence of cardiac compromise or conditions that promote capillary leak (i.e., preeclampsia, sepsis), the administration of crystalloid at 10 to 20 ml/kg (approximately 500–1000 ml) within 15 minutes prior to anesthesia is customary. The ability of this maneuver to decrease the incidence of hypotension, however, remains doubtful. The higher cost and possibility of allergic reaction or other side effects of colloids make them less popular. The initiation of anesthesia, in any case, should not be delayed to administer a fixed or arbitrary volume of IV fluid, particularly in urgent or emergent cases. Hypovolemia may also be the result of uterine bleeding, which will continue until surgical correction.

Ephedrine, a mixed α- and β-adrenergic agent, is the most common vasopressor used to treat hypotension, causing less vasoconstriction and uteroplacental blood flow than other agents. Alternatively, phenylephrine (α-adrenergic agent) can also be used for the prevention and treatment of maternal hypotension. Definitive clinical data supporting the use of a single agent, either ephedrine or phenylephrine, are lacking. The restoration of maternal normotension is an important goal, and the best strategy is a proactive response based on the clinical situation. If hypotension is associated with low (<60 bpm) maternal heart rate, ephedrine is indicated; if associated with a relatively high (>80 bpm) heart rate, phenylephrine is indicated. Moreover, if one agent is ineffective, the other should be used. Epinephrine is the agent of choice to treat severe hypotension and bradycardia.

Nausea and vomiting

The incidence associated with CD is variable but as high as 80%, depending on the preexisting symptoms, the anesthetic and obstetric techniques, and the preventative and therapeutic measures taken. Correction of hypotension is an important early step. Nausea may be best prevented by controlling hypotension, optimizing the use of neuraxial and IV opioids, improving the quality of the block, minimizing the surgical stimuli, and judiciously administering the uterotonic agents. Further treatment of nausea and vomiting mirrors that in nonobstetric surgery.

Pruritus and shivering

Although pruritus following neuraxial blockade has a number of postulated mechanisms and treatments, a direct antagonist or partial antagonist, such as IV nalbuphine 5 mg, appears to have a greater effect than some other modalities. Alternately, a dilute infusion of naloxone may be given IV for severe cases. Intra- and postoperative shivering may also have several etiologies and treatments. IV meperidine (12.5–25 mg), clonidine (150 mcg), doxapram (100 mg), ketanserin (10 mg), and alfentanil (250 mcg) have all been demonstrated to be effective, although meperidine appears to be the most consistently effective and popular.

Suggested readings

American Academy of Pediatrics, Committee on Drugs. Transfer of drugs and other chemicals into human milk. *Pediatrics* 2001; 108(3):776–789.

Balki M, Carvalho JC. Intraoperative nausea and vomiting during cesarean section under regional anesthesia. *Int J Obstet Anesth* 2005; 14(3):230–241.

Berghella V, Baxter JK, Chauhan SP. Evidence-based surgery for cesarean delivery. *Am J Obstet Gynecol* 2005; 193(5): 1607–1617.

Bucklin BA, Hawkins JL, Anderson JR, Ullrich FA. Obstetric anesthesia workforce survey: twenty-year update. *Anesthesiology* 2005; 103(3):645–653.

Gadsden J, Hart S, Santos AC. Post-cesarean delivery analgesia. *Anesth Analg* 2005; 101(5 Suppl):S62–S69.

Hepner D, Tsen LC. Fluid management in obstetrics. In: Hahn R, Prough DS, Svensen CH, eds. *Perioperative Fluid Therapy*. New York: Informa Healthcare; 2007:405–422.

Jenkins K, Baker AB. Consent and anaesthetic risk. *Anaesthesia* 2003; 58(10):962–984.

Lee A, Ngan Kee WD, Gin T. A quantitative, systematic review of randomized controlled trials of ephedrine versus phenylephrine for the management of hypotension during spinal anesthesia for cesarean delivery. *Anesth Analg* 2002; 94(4): 920–926.

Lewis G. (Ed.). The Confidential Enquiry into Maternal and Child Health (CEMACH). Saving Mothers' Lives: reviewing maternal deaths to make motherhood safer – 2003–2005. The Seventh Report on Confidential Enquiries into Maternal Deaths in the United Kingdom. London: CEMACH; 2007.

Marx GF, Bassell GM. Hazards of the supine position in pregnancy. *Clin Obstet Gynaecol* 1982; 9(2):255–271.

Mattingly JE, D'Alessio J, Ramanathan J. Effects of obstetric analgesics and anesthetics on the neonate: a review. *Paediatr Drugs* 2003; 5(9):615–627.

Practice guidelines for management of the difficult airway: an updated report by the American Society of Anesthesiologists Task Force on Management of the Difficult Airway. *Anesthesiology* 2003; 98(5):1269–1277.

Practice guidelines for obstetric anesthesia: an updated report by the American Society of Anesthesiologists Task Force on Obstetric Anesthesia. *Anesthesiology* 2007; 106(4):843–863.

Ross BK. ASA closed claims in obstetrics: lessons learned. *Anesthesiol Clin North America* 2003; 21(1):183–197.

Chapter 123

Obstetric hemorrhage

Cosmin Gauran and Lisa R. Leffert

Obstetric hemorrhage is an important cause of maternal and fetal morbidity and mortality. In Western Europe and the United States, it it is the second leading cause of maternal mortality after pulmonary thromboembolism. During pregnancy, uterine blood flow increases from a baseline level of 50 to 100 ml/min to 500 to 800 ml/min at term. Whereas uterine blood flow represents less than 5% of cardiac output before pregnancy, it constitutes roughly 12% of cardiac output at term. As such, obstetric hemorrhage can lead to rapid maternal exsanguination. In addition, the resulting hypotension or disruption of the uteroplacental unit can lead to severe fetal hypoxia with high associated morbidity and mortality.

Antepartum hemorrhage

Placenta previa

Placenta previa is a relatively common condition occurring in 1/200 of pregnancies. It is defined as the implantation of the placenta in advance of the fetal presenting part, often involving partial or complete obstruction of the cervical os. Previa is classified by the degree to which the placenta covers the cervical os (Fig. 123.1): It is "complete" when the os is entirely covered, "partial" when a portion of the os is covered, and "marginal" when the placenta is adjunct to the os. Patients with placenta previa typically present with painless vaginal bleeding in the second or third trimester. Risk factors for placenta previa include multiparity and prior placenta previa and uterine surgery. The diagnosis is usually made by ultrasound examination.

Obstetric management

In general, placenta previa necessitates a cesarean delivery. If the placenta is low lying, with the border more than 2 cm from the cervical rim, then vaginal delivery is often an option. The decision of when to deliver the fetus represents a balance between maximizing fetal gestational age (thus minimizing the fetal morbidity associated with premature delivery) and minimizing maternal bleeding. Patients who are remote from term gestation are typically managed expectantly, with bed rest and occasionally tocolytics, blood transfusion as indicated, and monitoring of fetal well-being. In the event of persistent fetal distress and/or

significant maternal bleeding, prompt cesarean delivery is indicated, regardless of the fetal gestation.

Anesthetic management

As it is not uncommon for patients with placenta previa to present for urgent cesarean delivery, it is crucial that an anesthesia consult, including appropriate airway assessment, is undertaken in a timely fashion. Adequate intravenous (IV) access (usually peripheral, of at least 18G), and an active blood bank sample are indicated. In the case of elective cesarean delivery with a low risk of placenta accreta (see Placenta Accreta section), a regional technique (spinal) is usually preferred. Some practitioners advocate the use of an epidural (or combined spinal–epidural), so that the block can be extended if the surgery is prolonged. Emergent cesarean delivery due to severe fetal distress or maternal instability is best managed by general anesthesia. Etomidate may be indicated for induction if the patient is hypotensive.

Placental abruption

Placental abruption is defined as a premature separation of the placenta prior to delivery. The incidence in the general population is between 3.4 and 7.9 per 1000 pregnancies. This condition is associated with various maternal conditions, such as hypertension, current smoking, cocaine abuse, trauma, premature labor, and prior history of abruption.

The clinical presentation of placental abruption is more variable than that of placenta previa (Table 123.1). Notably, the hemorrhage may be concealed between the uterus and the placenta. In many instances, the accumulated blood serves

Table 123.1. Third-trimester bleeding

Placenta previa	Placental abruption
Painless third-trimester bleeding	Usually painful, third-trimester bleeding
Bleeding usually obvious	Bleeding can be concealed inside the uterus
Risk factors: multiparity, previous uterine surgery, advanced maternal age	Risk factors: smoking, cocaine use, hypertension

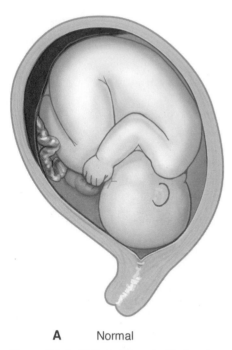 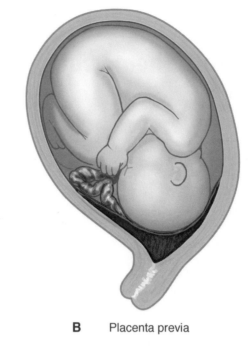

A   Normal   **B**   Placenta previa

Figure 123.1. (**A**) Normal placenta; (**B**) placenta previa.

as a powerful uterine irritant, which in turn leads to uterine contractions and further placental separation. The premature separation of the placenta from the uterine wall can impair placental gas exchange. Depending on the size of the abruption and whether it is acute or chronic, the fetal effects can be minimal or severe, including intrauterine growth restriction (IUGR) or fetal demise.

Obstetric management

The obstetric management of placental abruption depends on the acuity of the presentation and the degree of fetal prematurity. A limited abruption in the premature fetus is usually managed by maternal and fetal monitoring, administration of steroids to the parturient to promote fetal lung maturity, and tocolysis, if needed. Abruption that results in maternal hemodynamic instability or severe fetal distress necessitates expeditious delivery, either cesarean or vaginal (if the patient has been laboring and delivery is imminent).

Anesthetic management

Regional anesthesia is the anesthetic technique of choice if mother and baby are stable. It is important, however, to consider that this patient population has the highest incidence of consumptive coagulopathy among pregnant patients and that routine coagulation tests (prothrombin time [PT], partial thromboplastin time [PTT], platelets) should ideally be checked before regional anesthesia. In the case of a large, acute abruption with fetal distress or maternal hemodynamic instability, general endotracheal anesthesia with a rapid-sequence

induction (RSI) provides for a more expeditious delivery. Invasive monitoring may be needed.

Uterine rupture

Uterine rupture is a relatively rare cause of obstetric hemorrhage, most often occurring during attempted vaginal birth after cesarean delivery (VBAC). Additional risks factors include abdominal trauma, multiparity and multiple gestation, and use of oxytocin for labor induction or augmentation. The typical presentation of catastrophic uterine rupture is sudden and unexplained fetal distress (fetal bradycardia, unexplained tachycardia, or late decelerations). Parturients either (1) may experience abdominal pain that persists between contractions, or (2) be asymptomatic (in some cases). Partial uterine scar dehiscence may occur without significant maternal or fetal consequences. The obstetric management of clinically significant uterine rupture is emergent cesarean delivery.

There is a theoretical concern that a labor epidural will mask the pain of a uterine rupture, thus eliminating an important early warning sign. In clinical practice, however, fetal signs are more reliable, and careful attention to maternal complaint of a sudden increase in character or timing of pain can actually facilitate identification of uterine rupture, even in the presence of labor analgesia. In addition, having an epidural in place that can be quickly dosed for an urgent cesarean delivery may decrease maternal and fetal morbidity associated with an urgent general anesthetic. If there is no epidural in place and/or there is significant fetal or maternal decompensation, then general anesthesia with an RSI is indicated.

Postpartum hemorrhage

Uterine atony

To effect hemostasis after the third stage of labor, the myometrium normally contracts. Uterine atony, the lack of adequate contraction, is the most common cause of postpartum hemorrhage, peripartum blood transfusion, and cesarean hysterectomy. The diagnosis of uterine atony is made clinically in the setting of a soft uterus to palpation and continued hemorrhage after delivery. The degree of blood loss may not be evident as the uterus can conceal a large volume of blood. Risk factors associated with uterine atony include multiparity, multiple gestation, polyhydramnios, prolonged labor requiring oxytocin, and use of tocolytic medications.

Obstetric management

Obstetric management proceeds in a stepwise fashion beginning with medical therapy and uterine massage. If these measures prove unsuccessful, additional options include internal iliac/uterine artery embolization, B-Lynch and other uterine sutures, and hysterectomy in case of hemodynamic instability or refractory bleeding.

The first line of uterotonic therapy is oxytocin, an antidiuretic hormone (ADH)-related polypeptide. It is most commonly administered as a continuous infusion, titrated to effect. Oxytocin produces peripheral vasodilatation resulting in hypotension, especially if given in concentrated boluses. Hypotension can usually be avoided by careful titration of a dilute concentration (e.g., 20 units in 500–1000 cc of lactated Ringer's [LR]) and timely supportive measures (fluid and ephedrine as needed).

The ergot alkaloids ergonovine and methylergometrine maleate (Methergine; Novartis, East Hanover, NJ) are the second line of uterotonic agents. The mechanism of action for these medications is likely α_1-receptor stimulation leading to smooth muscle contraction. Either drug is generally given as 0.2 mg, intramuscularly. Rarely, IV administration, in 0.02-mg increments (1/10 dilution) with careful monitoring of maternal blood pressure, is employed. Systemic and pulmonary hypertension can result, making the two drugs relatively contraindicated for patients with hypertensive disorders, such as preeclampsia, or valvular lesions, such as mitral stenosis. Other side effects include an increased incidence of nausea and vomiting and, rarely, coronary vasoconstriction.

The third line of uterotonic agents are prostaglandins E and F. The 15-methyl prostaglandin $F_{2\alpha}$ ($PGF_{2\alpha}$) derivative, carboprost tromethamine (Hemabate; Pfizer, New York, NY), is available for parenteral administration in the United States. It can be given intramuscularly, sometimes directly into the myometrium, in 250-µg increments every 15 to 30 minutes. The side effects include bronchospasm and pulmonary hypertension, making its use relatively contraindicated in asthmatic patients. Misoprostol (Cytotec; Pfizer) is a prostaglandin E_1 (PGE_1) derivative with uterotonic activity that is typically administered rectally (800–1000 µg) or vaginally in this setting. It is a weak bronchodilator, so its use is relatively safe in asthmatic patients.

Anesthetic management

Administration of uterotonics in the operating room (OR) is typically the responsibility of the anesthesia team in concert with the obstetrician. Other care, such as resuscitation and correction of coagulopathy, is supportive. General anesthesia may be required in cases of severe hemodynamic instability; if volatile anesthetics are used, the concentration should be decreased to ≤ 0.5 minimum alveolar concentration (MAC) after the delivery of the fetus, to minimize interference with uterine contraction.

Retained products of conception

Retained products of conception (POC) can cause insidious or pronounced postpartum hemorrhage, with or without accompanying uterine atony. Diagnosis can be facilitated by careful inspection of the placenta to confirm that it is intact. Obstetric management of retained POC includes either manual or surgical (via dilation and evacuation [D&E]) extraction of retained POC followed by a continuous infusion of oxytocin to minimize uterine atony. These maneuvers can usually be accomplished by extending the block of a labor epidural and adding small IV doses of nitroglycerin (50–200 µg IV or 800 µg sublingually) for uterine relaxation. Alternatively, spinal anesthesia or small boluses of IV ketamine or opioid analgesia can be used in patients who do not have an epidural. In general, extraction of retained POC is best accomplished in the OR where emergency airway and resuscitation equipment are readily available.

Placenta accreta

Placenta accreta is defined by the absence of the decidua basalis layer between the placenta and the myometrium. Depending on the degree of invasion of the myometrium, it is classified as *placenta accreta* with the involvement of the superficial myometrium, *placenta increta* with deep myometrial penetration without violating the serosa, and *placenta percreta* invading the neighboring organs, notably the bladder. The absence of the decidua basalis makes the placenta adherent to the myometrium and impedes the proper separation during the third stage of the labor. Severe bleeding ensues.

The diagnosis can be difficult to make antepartum, as there may be no suggestive signs other than vaginal bleeding. Ultrasound and MRI examination can raise suspicion for the presence of placenta accreta, but usually cannot definitively confirm or exclude the diagnosis unless there is visible invasion of the bladder or associated structures (as in the case of percreta). There is a suggestion that placenta accreta may be associated with increased levels of maternal serum alpha protein (AFP).

Placenta previa and prior cesarean delivery represent the most common risk factors. Isolated placenta previa is associated with a 5% risk of accreta, and the risk increases substantially if the patient has had prior cesarean deliveries; the recent increase increase in the cesarean delivery rate is likely to increase the incidence of placenta accreta.

Obstetric management

Obstetric management of placenta accreta often involves cesarean hysterectomy. To limit intraoperative blood loss, some centers employ uterine or internal iliac arterial balloon catheters with or without preoperative embolization. Whenever feasible, conservative therapy is preferred to preserve fertility. Conservative management, suitable for patients with limited or focal placenta accreta, can involve the use of uterine tonic agents, excision of the involved myometrium, uterine artery ligation or embolization, uterine sutures (e.g., B-Lynch), or medical treatment with methotrexate. Conservatively managed patients are at risk for rebleeding and may require urgent reoperation. Patients with placenta percreta involving other pelvic organs, often the bladder, are typically managed with a cesarean hysterectomy and/or selective arterial embolization.

Anesthetic management

General or regional anesthesia may be employed, even if hysterectomy is required. Irrespective of the anesthetic technique chosen, adequate IV access, typically two large-bore peripheral IVs, should be secured. Contact with the blood bank to ensure ready availability of blood products should be undertaken. Baseline hemoglobin/hematocrit (Hb/Hct) and platelet count should be determined and followed, along with coagulation status, during and after surgery. In more complex cases, an arterial line for blood pressure monitoring and laboratory samples should be considered, as should central venous access for central venous pressure (CVP) monitoring, volume replacement, and vasopressors.

Uterine inversion

Uterine inversion is a rare complication of vaginal delivery, usually in the context of excessive traction on the umbilical cord during the third stage of labor. It can lead to severe hemorrhage and vagally mediated bradycardia and hypotension, if the uterus is not reduced to its anatomic position in a timely fashion. Brief uterine relaxation and pain control are required and can be accomplished with a 50- to 200-μg IV nitroglycerin bolus, IV fentanyl, or use of an existing epidural. Alternatively,

general anesthesia can be induced with rapid-sequence intubation. An oxytocin infusion is typically employed after the uterus is reduced, to prevent persistent uterine atony and to help maintain the uterus in the proper anatomic position.

Genital laceration

Laceration of the genital tract can be encountered after vaginal delivery and may require immediate attention. If an epidural was used for labor, then the block can be augmented for perineal repair. If no regional anesthetic is in place and the lesions are not amenable to repair under local anesthesia, the patient should be taken to the OR and preferentially regional or RSI general anesthesia should be undertaken.

Suggested readings

American College of Obstetrics and Gynecology practice bulletin: clinical management guidelines for obstetrician-gynecologists number 76, October 2006: postpartum hemorrhage. *Obstet Gynecol* 2006; 108:1039–1047.

Clark SL, Koonings PP, Phelan JP. Placenta previa/accreta and prior cesarean section. *Obstet Gynecol* 1985; 66:89–92.

Dyer RA, van Dyk, Dresner DA. The use of uterotonic drugs during caesarean section. *Int J Obstet Anesth* 2010; 19:313–319.

Fong J, Gurewitsch ED, Kang H-J, et al. An analysis of transfusion practice and the role of intraoperative red blood cell salvage during cesarean delivery. *Anesth Analg* 2007; 104:666–672.

Getahun D, Oyelese Y, Salihu HM, Ananth CV. Previous cesarean delivery and risks of placenta previa and placental abruption. *Obstet Gynecol* 2006; 107(4):771–778.

Khan KH, Wojdyla D, Say L, et al. WHO analysis of causes of maternal death: a systematic review. *Lancet* 2006; 367:1066–1074.

Mayer DC, Smith KA. Antepartum and postpartum hemorrhage. In: Chestnut DH, Polley LS, Tsen LC, Wong CA, eds. *Obstetric Anesthesia: Principles and Practice*. 4th ed. Philadelphia: Mosby; 2009: 811–836.

Oylese Y, Scorza WE, Mastrolia R, et al. Postpartum hemorrhage. *Obstet Gynecol Clin North Am* 2007; 34(3):421–441.

Oylese Y, Smulian JC. Placenta previa, placenta accreta, and vasa previa. *Obstet Gynecol* 2006; 107(4):927–941.

Pian-Smith M, Leffert L. *Obstetric Anesthesia*. New York: Cambridge University Press; 2007.

Tikkanen M, Nuutila M, Hiilesmaa V, et al. Clinical presentation and risk factors of placental abruption. *Acta Obstet Gynecol Scand* 2006; 85(6):700–705.

Yao F. *Yao and Artusio's Anesthesiology*. 5th ed. Philadelphia: Lippincott, Williams & Wilkins; 2003:785–806.

In the United States, hypertensive disorders are the second leading cause of maternal mortality, with an estimated rate of 1.5 per 100,000 live births; admissions for hypertensive disorders account for 15% of all antenatal hospitalizations. Hypertensive disorders in pregnancy are a spectrum of diseases that are classified in Table 124.1.

Preeclampsia

Preeclampsia is diagnosed in 3% to 5% of all pregnancies in the United States and is most common in nulliparous women. A patient meets the criteria for a diagnosis of preeclampsia if she has (1) persistently elevated blood pressures after 20 weeks gestation in the setting of previously normal blood pressures, and (2) proteinuria of greater than 300 mg in 24 hours. Preeclampsia can be mild or severe, based on the presence or absence of specific signs, symptoms, and abnormal laboratory values (Table 124.2).

Preeclampsia may be associated with eclampsia and hemolysis, elevated liver enzymes and low platelets (HELLP) syndrome. Eclampsia is defined as the occurrence of seizures in a woman with preeclampsia that cannot be attributed to other causes. Eclamptic seizures may occur antepartum, intrapartum, or postpartum. Eclampsia is a cause of significant maternal and fetal morbidity and is present in approximately 50% of maternal deaths associated with preeclampsia.

HELLP syndrome involves a constellation of laboratory abnormalities and is generally regarded as a subset of severe preeclampsia (Table 124.3). Hypertension, however, may not be present in a substantial portion of patients. The diagnosis of HELLP syndrome is also associated with an increased risk of adverse outcomes including abruption, renal failure, hepatic subcapsular hematoma formation, liver rupture, recurrent preeclampsia, maternal and/or fetal death.

For the fetus, preeclampsia may be associated with growth restriction, preterm delivery, hypoxia, oligohydramnios, neurologic injury, and death.

Etiology and risk factors

Although the precise etiology of preeclampsia remains unknown, it is a disease that occurs only in the presence of placental tissue. The maternal manifestations are consistent with a process of vasospasm, ischemia, and changes in the normal balance of humoral and autocoid mediators.

An imbalance in placental angiogenic and antiangiogenic growth factors is believed to play a central role in the development of preeclampsia. Recent investigations have revealed that increased levels of soluble fms-like tyrosine kinase-1 (sFlt-1) and reduced levels of both phosphatidylinositol glycan anchor biosynthesis, placental growth factor (PGF), and vascular endothelial growth factor (VEGF) shift the balance toward antiangiogenesis and predate the development of the disease. The increased presence of another antiangiogenic protein-soluble endoglin (sEng) has been shown to correlate with the onset of preeclampsia and in vivo causes increased vascular permeability and hypertension. Preeclampsia is also associated with significant alterations in the immune system, and increased levels of circulating inflammatory cytokines in the maternal circulation and placenta have been found.

The earliest clinical manifestation of preeclampsia occurs with placental implantation when there is attenuated trophoblastic invasion into the uteroplacental spiral arteries. The final common feature in preeclampsia is vascular endothelial damage in the maternal circulation. Endothelial dysfunction is manifested in several ways. There is an imbalance between thromboxane, prostaglandins, endothelin, and nitric oxide, resulting in increased vascular reactivity and vasospasm that leads to hypertension and end-organ dysfunction. Endothelial dysfunction also results in increased vascular permeability and subsequent edema, increased sensitivity to endogenous

---

Table 124.1. Hypertensive disorders of pregnancy

Gestational hypertension
Transient hypertension of pregnancy without proteinuria, which resolves after delivery

Preeclampsia: mild or severe
A pregnancy-specific syndrome characterized by elevated blood pressure and proteinuria after 20 weeks gestation

Chronic hypertension
Hypertension present before pregnancy, diagnosed before 20 weeks gestation, or diagnosed after 20 weeks gestation that does not resolve by 12 weeks postpartum

Chronic hypertension with superimposed preeclampsia

Table 124.2. Criteria for diagnosis of preeclampsia

Physical findings	Mild preeclampsia	Severe preeclampsia
Blood pressure	>140/90 but <160/110 mm Hg	>160/110 mm Hg
Proteinuria	0.3–5 g in 24-h urine collection, or 1–2+ on urine dip	>5 g in 24-h urine collection, or 3–4+ on urine dip
Additional signs or symptoms	None	Persistent headache Cerebral or visual disturbances Impaired liver function Epigastric or RUQ pain Thrombocytopenia Pulmonary edema or cyanosis Fetal growth restriction (IUGR) Oliguria < 500 ml in 24 h

RUQ, right upper quadrant.

pressors, and the predisposition to hemolysis and thrombocytopenia. Multiple risk factors have been identified and are listed in Table 124.4.

Physiologic changes in preeclampsia
Cardiovascular system

Physiologic changes in preeclampsia are listed in Table 124.5. Preeclamptic patients have a decreased intravascular volume as a result of decreased oncotic pressure, increased vascular permeability, and elevated peripheral vascular resistance; they also exhibit increased sympathetic nervous system activity and increased sensitivity to endogenous and exogenous pressors.

Preeclamptic patients are usually managed empirically, using measures such as urine output and fetal well-being as signs of adequate organ perfusion. In preeclamptic patients with comorbidities such as anuria, pulmonary edema, massive hemorrhage, or underlying cardiac or pulmonary disease, invasive monitoring with particular focus on trends, rather than absolute values, may be useful.

Pulmonary system

Women with preeclampsia may have a predisposition to upper airway obstruction and difficult intubation from diffuse pharyngolaryngeal edema. Also, they are at risk for development of pulmonary edema, likely due to the combination of increased vascular permeability, decreased oncotic pressure, and a redistribution of intravascular volume into the central compartment.

Table 124.3. Criteria for diagnosis of HELLP syndrome

- Hemolysis: abnormal peripheral blood smear – schistocytes and helmet cells from microangiopathic hemolysis; increased total bilirubin > 1.2 mg/dl
- Elevated liver enzymes: AST > 2 times normal; increased lactic dehydrogenase > 600 U/L
- Low Platelets: Platelet count < 100,000 mm^3

Table 124.4. Risk factors for the development of preeclampsia

Pregnancy-related	Presence of underlying disorders
Multiple gestation Nulliparity Gestational diabetes Hydatidiform mole Structural congenital anomalies	Chronic hypertension and renal disease Obesity Preexisting diabetes Inherited and acquired hypercoagulable states Sickle cell disease
Partner-related	**Other**
Partner who previously fathered a pregnancy complicated by preeclampsia Donor insemination and limited sperm exposure	Age and the interval between pregnancies Family history History of preeclampsia in a prior pregnancy

Renal system

Relative to normotensive non-preeclamptic patients, glomerular filtration rate and renal blood flow decrease by approximately 25% in preeclamptic patients. One proposed mechanism for this finding is glomerular enlargement related to endothelial dysfunction. Fractional urate clearance decreases, and, as a result, serum uric acid levels increase – a frequently measured serum marker for preeclampsia. Nonetheless, because of the significant increase in renal function that occurs with pregnancy, serum creatinine levels may not increase above normal pregnancy levels, and renal insufficiency is uncommon.

Central nervous system

A variety of symptoms may be present in preeclamptic patients, including headache, blurred vision, scotomata, and (rarely) cortical blindness. Focal, lateralizing, neurologic signs are uncommon and warrant prompt evaluation. The precise pathophysiology of eclamptic seizures remains unknown although hemorrhage, edema, and hypoxia are possible mechanisms. If eclamptic seizures occur, they should be promptly treated with magnesium sulfate.

Coagulation

Thrombocytopenia associated with severe preeclampsia is the most common coagulation abnormality. Platelet levels <100,000 mm^3 signal serious disease; if the pregnancy is maintained, platelet levels may continue to fall and increase maternal morbidity. Antithrombin III levels may be decreased,

Table 124.5. Physiologic changes in preeclampsia

Physiologic change	Normal pregnancy	Preeclampsia
Blood pressure	Decreased or normal	Increased
Cardiac output	Increased	Decreased to increased
PVR	Decreased	Increased
Intravascular volume	Increased	Decreased
CVP and PCWP	Normal	Normal

PVR, pulmonary vascular resistance; CVP, central venous pressure; PCWP, pulmonary capillary wedge pressure.

particularly in the setting of significant proteinuria, signaling more severe disease and putting the patient at risk for thrombotic events. Circulating levels of fibrin degradation products may be elevated, but fibrinogen levels are usually normal unless the situation is complicated by placental abruption.

Placental and fetal compartment

In preeclamptic patients the placenta has increased vascular resistance relative to the low-resistance vascular bed typically found in non-preeclamptic pregnancies. This increased vascular resistance is thought to be a result of the attenuated angiogenesis during placental formation and a predisposition to placental infarction. Thus any decrease in uteroplacental blood flow further compromises a fetus that is already predisposed to development of growth restriction, oligohydramnios, abruption, and decreased fetal reserve.

Obstetric management

All patients in whom the diagnosis of preeclampsia is suspected should be evaluated with serial blood pressures, fetal monitoring, and urine and laboratory studies to establish the diagnosis and ensure maternal and fetal well-being.

Delivery

The definitive treatment for preeclampsia is delivery of the fetus and placenta. The decision of when to deliver is made based on the gestational age and the severity of the disease. In preeclamptic patients at or near term, delivery should be initiated after the diagnosis is made. In the setting of prematurity, however, it may be prudent to prolong the pregnancy in an attempt to minimize neonatal morbidity.

In an effort to minimize maternal complications, vaginal delivery is preferred. Cesarean delivery should be reserved for obstetric indications. Because of compromised uteroplacental blood flow, however, the fetus of a preeclamptic patient may tolerate labor poorly, making this patient at increased risk of operative delivery. Additionally, in an unstable patient with an unfavorable cervix, a prompt elective cesarean delivery may be in the patient's best interest. In summary, each patient and clinical situation should be individualized, with a management strategy that seeks to balance and minimize both maternal and fetal morbidity.

Medical management

Eclamptic seizures are a serious complication of preeclampsia and are associated with significant maternal and fetal morbidity and mortality. Although the mechanism of action is unknown, magnesium sulfate is the medication of choice for prophylactic prevention and treatment of eclamptic seizures. Magnesium is administered during labor, delivery, and for up to 24 to 48 hours postdelivery. The treatment is initiated with a 4- to 6-gm intravenous bolus over a 15- to 30-minute period, followed by an infusion of 2 gm/h.

Due to its relaxant effect on vascular and visceral smooth muscle, magnesium therapy may decrease maternal blood pressure and predispose the patient to postpartum atony and hemorrhage. Magnesium also potentiates the effects of nondepolarizing neuromuscular blockers, and caution should be used when administering nondepolarizing neuromuscular blockers in this patient population. Historically, the data have been mixed regarding the interaction between succinylcholine and magnesium; however, more recent studies have shown no potentiation of the depolarizing neuromuscular blockade.

Antihypertensive medications, such as labetalol, hydralazine, and calcium-channel blockers are frequently administered to preeclamptic patients for control of blood pressure. The goal is not to normalize blood pressure, but to keep patients from progressing to a hypertensive crisis, encephalopathy, or stroke. When administering antihypertensive medications, it is important to remember that the placenta lacks the ability to autoregulate flow, and a sudden decrease in maternal blood pressure may decrease placental perfusion and result in significant compromise to the fetus. Dietary supplements of vitamin D, calcium, selenium, and bed rest (with controlled exercise) may be beneficial in the prevention of preeclamptic complications.

Anesthetic management
Labor analgesia

Neuraxial anesthetic techniques have potential benefits in preeclamptic patients, including the reduction of circulating catecholamines and stress hormones and facilitation of blood pressure control. Diminished maternal respiratory response to pain may also improve oxygen delivery to the fetus. In addition, placement of an epidural catheter in labor helps to facilitate expeditious conversion to an operative delivery. The American Society of Anesthesiologists (ASA) Practice Guidelines for Obstetric Anesthesia recommend that practitioners consider early placement of neuraxial anesthesia in high-risk populations (i.e., severe preeclamptic patients), in an effort to reduce the need for general anesthesia. In this situation, the placement of an epidural may precede labor or the patient's request for analgesia.

For placement of neuraxial anesthesia, the same techniques, procedures, and precautions that are practiced in non-preeclamptic patients should be used. More specifically, preeclamptic patients should be routinely monitored with a noninvasive blood pressure (NIBP) monitor and pulse oximetry. Some institutions also advocate the use of maternal electrocardiography (ECG) in this patient population. Because of concern for hypotension and compromised uteroplacental perfusion, continuous fetal monitoring should be performed during placement of neuraxial anesthesia whenever possible. Finally, preeclamptic patients may not be able to tolerate a sitting position for placement because of side effects of magnesium infusion or hemodynamic liability. In this setting the lateral decubitus position may be used.

After initiation of neuraxial analgesia and the onset of sympathetic blockade, preeclamptic patients are at risk for hypotension and impaired uteroplacental perfusion. Epidural labor analgesia in the preeclamptic patient can be initiated with the same medications used for normal labor analgesia, although some experts advocate elimination of epinephrine in the test dose. Although the risk of hypotension may not be significantly affected by pretreatment with intravenous (IV) fluids in normal pregnancy, fluid loading may be prudent in the setting of preeclampsia, as intravascular volume is decreased.

If hypotension occurs after local anesthetic administration, judicious use of IV fluids and pressors is warranted to restore maternal blood pressures. Initial use of reduced doses of pressors (e.g., 2.5 mg of ephedrine or 20 μg of phenylephrine) is recommended by some authorities due to the clinical impression of enhanced sensitivity to vasopressors.

Cesarean delivery

In a small, randomized trial of general, epidural, or spinal anesthesia for cesarean delivery in women with severe preeclampsia, there were no statistically significant differences between the three groups with regard to hypertension, hypotension, and maternal or fetal outcomes attributable to any of the anesthetic techniques.

General anesthesia offers rapid initiation and is an option in patients with a contraindication to a regional technique, but carries the risk of presence of difficult airway and hypertension that may occur with airway management. In contrast, spinal anesthesia affords an almost equally fast onset and blunts the hemodynamic and neuroendocrine responses to pain and stress, but may be associated with significant hypotension. Epidural anesthesia allows the practitioner to titrate the level of neuraxial blockade while carefully monitoring the hemodynamics. Regional anesthesia is contraindicated in the setting of severe thrombocytopenia and is relatively contraindicated in patients with an altered sensorium.

Management of HELLP syndrome

Patients with HELLP syndrome experience progressive thrombocytopenia, and prompt delivery is indicated, perhaps following a course of glucocorticoids to minimize morbidity to the preterm fetus. Administration of glucocorticoids has also been shown to reduce the severity of laboratory abnormalities, resulting in a dose-dependent improvement in platelet count, possibly increasing the use of regional anesthesia.

Although several studies have reported safe neuraxial anesthetic techniques in patients with thrombocytopenia, there is no evidence to support choosing a single value as the appropriate minimum acceptable platelet count. Because no clear correlation exists between the severity of thrombocytopenia and the likelihood of bleeding complications from neuraxial anesthesia, the decision of whether to proceed is typically made on an individual basis. Most anesthesiologists are comfortable at a platelet count of 100,000, and some with counts as low as 70,000 to 80,000. Factors such as the trend in platelet count in addition to other concerns – such as an anticipated difficult airway – should factor into the decision process.

Placement of a prophylactic epidural before the development of worsening thrombocytopenia is an approach that may be of benefit in this patient population. Lastly, some practitioners report that they feel more comfortable in placing a spinal with a 24G to 26G needle in the setting of thrombocytopenia than in placing an epidural that entails a large-bore needle and an indwelling catheter. Although this seems appropriate, there is no good evidence to support this approach.

Obstetric and anesthetic management of eclampsia

Eclamptic seizures are typically self-limited, last 1 to 10 minutes, and are frequently associated with transient fetal distress. The goals of therapy are supportive care and patient safety. The patient should be given supplemental oxygen, protected from injury, and placed in the lateral decubitus position if possible. Magnesium sulfate therapy should be initiated or increased, and blood pressure controlled. Rarely, thiopental or benzodiazepines will be required to control seizures. Although the diagnosis of eclampsia necessitates prompt delivery, immediate cesarean delivery is usually not indicated as fetal well-being will improve with maternal resuscitation and cessation of seizures. Magnesium sulfate should be continued 24 hours postpartum as prophylaxis against additional eclamptic seizures.

Suggested readings

ACOG Practice Bulletin, No 33: Diagnosis and management of preeclampsia and eclampsia. Clinical Management Guidelines for Obstetrician–Gynecologists. January, 2002.

Bosio PM, McKenna PJ, Conroy R, O'Herlihy C. Maternal central hemodynamics in hypertensive disorders of pregnancy. *Obstet Gynecol* 1999; 94:978–984.

Coppage KH, Sibai BM. Hypertensive Emergencies. In: Foley MR, Strong TH, Garite TJ, eds. *Obstetric Intensive Care Manual.* 2nd ed. New York: McGraw-Hill; 2004:51–65.

Hood DD, Curry R. Spinal versus epidural anesthesia for cesarean section in severely preeclamptic patients: a retrospective survey. *Anesthesiology* 1999; 90:1276–1282.

Idama TO, Lindow SW. Magnesium sulphate: a review of clinical pharmacology applied to obstetrics. *Br J Obstet Gynaecol* 1998; 105:260–268.

Levine RJ, Maynard SE, Qian C, et al. Circulating angiogenic factors and the risk of preeclampsia. *N Engl J Med* 2004; 350:672–683.

MacKay AP, Berg CJ, Atrash HI. Pregnancy related mortality from preeclampsia and eclampsia. *Obstet Gynecol* 2001; 97:533–553.

O'Brien JM, Shumate SA, Satchwell SL, et al. Maternal benefit of corticosteroid therapy in patients with HELLP (hemolysis, elevated liver enzymes, and low platelet count) syndrome: impact on the rate of regional anesthesia. *Am J Obstet Gynecol* 2002; 186:475–479.

Polley LS. Hypertensive disorders. In: Chestnut DH, Polley LS, Tsen LC, Wong CA, eds. *Obstetric Anesthesia: Principles and Practice.* 4th ed. Philadelphia: Mosby; 2009:975–1007.

Practice Guidelines for Obstetric Anesthesia: an updated report by the American Society of Anesthesiologists Task Force on Obstetric Anesthesia. *Anesthesiology* 2007; 106(4): 843–863.

Shivalingappa V, Toporsian M, Lam C, et al. Soluble endoglin contributes to the pathogenesis of preeclampsia. *Nat Med* 2006; 12:642–649.

Sibai BM, Akl S, Fairlie F, Moretti M. A protocol for managing severe preeclampsia in the second trimester. *Am J Obstet Gynecol* 1990; 163:733–738.

Wallace DH, Leveno KJ, Cunningham FG, et al. Randomized comparison of general and regional anesthesia for cesarean delivery in pregnancies complicated by severe preeclampsia. *Obstet Gynecol* 1995; 86:193–199.

Pregnant patients with comorbid diseases

Anasuya Vasudevan and Stephen D. Pratt

Anesthetic management of the parturient with comorbid diseases requires a multidisciplinary approach involving the obstetrician, obstetric anesthesiologist, neonatologists, and appropriate medical specialists. Obstetricians should be encouraged to send pregnant patients with major comorbidities to be seen by an obstetric anesthesiologist during pregnancy. The obstetric anesthesia provider must understand the normal pregnancy-related physiologic changes in the affected organ system, how these changes might affect the underlying medical condition, how the conduct of anesthesia for delivery or obstetric procedures might be influenced by the condition, and what medical or surgical interventions might be performed to ensure that the underlying medical condition is well-managed during gestation and parturition.

Cardiovascular disease

Depending on the type and severity of the condition, parturients with cardiovascular disease may tolerate the physiologic changes with little problem (e.g., patients with aortic insufficiency) or may face a 60% risk of maternal death (e.g., patients with pulmonary hypertension). Hypertension and valvular lesions are the most common cardiovascular disease processes seen in pregnancy. Much less commonly, pregnant women may present with complex congenital cardiac lesions, cardiomyopathies, acute or chronic ischemic heart disease, or pulmonary hypertension. Up to 13% of women with heart disease will experience a significant complication during pregnancy. Decreased left ventricular systolic function, significant left-sided valvular obstruction, previous cardiac events (congestive heart failure [CHF], dysrhythmia), and New York Heart Association (NYHA) functional status of II or worse are predictors of adverse cardiac outcomes in parturients with valvular disease.

Unless contraindicated, regional anesthesia is frequently a good choice for the laboring patient with cardiac disease, as it blunts the hormonal response to labor pain and can minimize the cardiac stress. The use of invasive hemodynamic monitoring may be appropriate for some patients, especially during cesarean delivery, when shifts in blood volume may be rapid and significant and the effects of anesthesia (general or regional) are more profound. The use of antibiotics to prevent bacterial endo-

carditis should be considered. Recent guidelines recommend that only patients with significant congenital cardiac lesions, a history of endocarditis, or prosthetic cardiac valves should receive prophylaxis during labor and delivery.

Chronic hypertension

Parturients with chronic hypertension generally tolerate pregnancy well, as blood pressure tends to decrease in early gestation. These patients, however, are at increased risk for developing pregnancy-induced hypertension (PIH). They may present with a relative decrease in their intravascular volume, leading to hemodynamic instability during induction of neuraxial or general anesthesia. Long-standing hypertension can be associated with end-organ damage, including renal or cardiac failure. Finally, many medications used to treat hypertension, including the angiotensin-converting enzyme inhibitors, are contraindicated in pregnancy. No specific changes are necessary in the anesthetic management of the parturient with hypertension without other organ system involvement.

Valvular lesions

In general, left heart stenotic valve lesions are poorly tolerated during pregnancy because the fixed valve lesion prevents the pregnancy-associated increase in cardiac output (CO) and increases the likelihood of pulmonary edema. Invasive monitors are sometimes employed for patients with severe mitral stenosis. Conversely, regurgitant lesions are generally well tolerated through gestation and labor, although acute decompensation can occur after delivery. Many patients with stenotic and some regurgitant lesions may be taking anticoagulants, complicating or contraindicating the use of regional anesthesia. The hemodynamic goals for each valve lesion are outlined in Table 125.1 (also see Chapter 5).

- *Mitral stenosis* is the most common isolated valvular lesion seen in pregnancy, and is the most difficult to manage. The physiologic changes of pregnancy all tend to increase the gradient across the stenotic valve and place the pregnant patient at risk for pulmonary edema. Auto-transfusion following delivery can cause acute decompensation and cardiac failure. Maternal mortality is approximately 1% in

Table 125.1. Optimal cardiovascular physiologic parameters in valvular lesions

	HR	Preload	SVR	Contractility
Mitral stenosis	Avoid tachycardia to allow LV filling; treat atrial fibrillation aggressively (cardioversion)	At risk for pulmonary edema. Keep PCWP ~ 15; avoid hypoxia, hypercarbia, pain ($\uparrow$ PVR)	Keep normal to high	Normal
Aortic stenosis	Avoid extremes of HR; atrial "kick" necessary for LV filling	High pressures are needed to fill noncompliant LV; risk for pulmonary edema	Keep high to maintain LV perfusion pressure (decrease causes hypotension and possibly cardiac ischemia)	Keep normal to high to maintain CO; low if dynamic subvalvular lesion
Mitral regurgitation	$\Uparrow$ HR (decreases regurgitant flow)	Keep normal to low; LV at risk for volume overload	Low SVR augments forward flow	Normal
Aortic insufficiency	$\Uparrow$ HR (decreases regurgitant fraction)	Keep normal to low; LV at risk for volume overload	Low SVR augments forward flow	Normal

LV, left ventricle; PCWP, pulmonary capillary wedge pressure.

the presence of mitral stenosis (although it is much higher if atrial fibrillation occurs).

- *Aortic stenosis* is less common in pregnancy because lesions that predispose to aortic stenosis generally do not become clinically apparent until after childbearing age. The fixed and reduced aortic valve area prevents these patients from increasing their stroke volume or CO.
- Patients with *regurgitant valvular lesions* generally tolerate well the physiologic changes of pregnancy and the effects of regional anesthesia, because increased preload and heart rate (HR), and decreased afterload, help to augment forward flow in these lesions.
- *Pulmonary hypertension,* either primary or secondary, is uncommon during pregnancy, but, if present, maternal mortality may exceed 60%. The anesthetic goals include: (1) prevention of increases in pulmonary vascular resistance (PVR) related to hypercarbia, hypoxia, acidosis, stress, or pain; and (2) prevention of major hemodynamic perturbations, especially decreases in systemic vascular resistance (SVR) or preload.

Rarely, but with increasing frequency, pregnancy may be complicated by congenital cardiac lesions, cardiomyopathy, primary cardiac rhythm disturbances, ischemic heart disease, or cardiac transplantation. Patients with these processes require an individualized, team approach to ensure that the effects of gestation and parturition can be safely navigated.

Pulmonary disease

Chronic respiratory disease, most commonly asthma, and pregnancy-related respiratory distress are often best managed with regional anesthesia, as it limits the increases in ventilation associated with maternal pain avoids the negative consequences of general anesthesia on the lungs. Some caution must be used in patients with severe obstructive lung disease as a dense spinal or epidural anesthesia impairs intercostal muscle function and decreases expiratory volumes. Patients who depend on these accessory muscles of respiration may not tolerate a high regional block.

Asthma

Effect of pregnancy on asthma

Asthma is the most common pulmonary disease in women of child-bearing age and complicates approximately 1% of pregnancies. The course of asthma during pregnancy is highly variable. It has been reported that asthma symptoms are worse during pregnancy in approximately one third of patients, improve in one third, and remain unchanged in one third. A large percentage of those with severe pre-pregnancy asthma, however, will experience an exacerbation during pregnancy. Multiple pregnancy-related factors may influence the course of asthma, including an increase in the production of prostaglandin $F_{2\alpha}$ (a bronchoconstrictor), decreased cellular immunity leading to increased risk of infection, and the bronchodilating effects of progesterone.

Effect of asthma on pregnancy

With appropriate treatment, asthma does not increase risks to the mother or fetus during pregnancy. Severe or poorly controlled asthma, however, has been associated with many adverse obstetric outcomes, including preterm delivery, small-for-gestational-age birth weights, preeclampsia, cesarean delivery, postpartum hemorrhage, and increased neonatal morbidity. It is safer to treat asthma appropriately during pregnancy than to expose the mother and fetus to the negative effects of hypoxia and hypercarbia that may occur with poorly treated disease. Management of asthma during pregnancy should follow the same principles as for the nonpregnant patient, including identification and treatment of triggers (respiratory infections, allergens, etc.) that may precipitate acute exacerbations, appropriate use of inhaled β_2-agonists and steroids, and judicious use of oral steroids or theophylline as indicated. Use of oral corticosteroids in the first trimester may increase the risk for preterm delivery or preeclampsia.

Anesthetic implications

Anesthesia management goals regarding the parturient with asthma in labor should focus on reducing maternal hyperventilation and minimizing physiologic stress. Control of the hyperventilation in response to labor pain is especially important in patients whose asthma is triggered by exercise or stress. Pain relief with neuraxial analgesia is most effective, but systemic opioids or other pain relief techniques, such as pudendal nerve blocks, may also be effective. All asthma medications should be continued throughout labor. Additional concerns during cesarean delivery include the inability to lie flat due to severe disease, respiratory failure due to motor block of accessory muscles of respiration from high regional anesthesia, and life-threatening bronchospasm associated with endotracheal intubation. If general anesthesia is required for cesarean delivery, care must be taken to balance the risk of aspiration against risks associated with bronchospasm from endotracheal intubation. General anesthesia with a laryngeal mask airway (LMA) has been used safely for cesarean delivery in a large series of parturients at low risk for aspiration and might be useful in the parturient with severe reactive airways. Nonsteroidal anti-inflammatory drugs (NSAIDs) should be used with caution for postpartum pain relief in parturients with asthma. Finally, should postpartum hemorrhage occur, 15-methyl prostaglandin $F_{2\alpha}$ and to a lesser extent methylergonovine maleate should be used with caution, as they can precipitate bronchospasm.

Little information exists on other chronic pulmonary diseases and pregnancy. The obstetric anesthesiologist may be asked to help manage parturients with chronic obstructive pulmonary disease, interstitial lung disease, cystic fibrosis, sarcoidosis, and others. A multidisciplinary approach involving obstetricians, anesthesiologists, primary care physicians, and appropriate pulmonary specialists is necessary to adequately care for these patients.

Pregnancy-related pulmonary disease

The parturient is also at risk for acute respiratory failure due to one of many pregnancy-specific disease processes, including pulmonary embolus, amniotic fluid embolus, and pulmonary edema associated with preeclampsia, fluid overload, peripartum cardiomyopathy, sepsis, or massive transfusion after maternal hemorrhage. For each of these disorders, the primary concern is treatment of the underlying disease process. The obstetric anesthesiologist may be required to assist in the management of the pulmonary status until the primary process is stabilized. Management may include aggressive diuresis, bronchodilator therapy, or endotracheal intubation.

Diabetes mellitus

Diabetes mellitus (DM) is a common endocrine disease in pregnancy, complicating approximately 4% of all pregnancies. With optimal glycemic control and multidisciplinary management of the diabetic parturient, the perinatal outcomes are similar to those observed in normal pregnancy.

Effect of pregnancy on DM

Progesterone, human placental lactogen, and cortisol increase during pregnancy and exert an anti-insulin effect. The combination of increased lipolysis, insulin resistance, and ketogenesis renders the diabetic parturient susceptible to metabolic disturbances. Insulin requirements increase during pregnancy and decrease significantly soon after delivery. Diabetic ketoacidosis is more common in pregnancy, particularly in parturients with hyperemesis, infection, steroid therapy (i.e., for fetal lung maturation), or poor medication adherence. Hypoglycemia occurs with increased frequency in the patient with type 1 DM, particularly in the first trimester, probably due to a combination of emesis and reduced calorie intake. The risk of hypoglycemia is higher when tight glycemic control regimes are followed.

Effect of DM on pregnancy

Patients with pregestational DM are at increased risk for gestational hypertensive disorders. Pregestational diabetic nephropathy especially increases the incidence of pregnancy-induced hypertension and intrauterine growth restriction. DM also increases the risk of preterm labor, polyhydramnios, macrosomia, shoulder dystocia, and fetal anomalies. Cesarean delivery is more common in both pregestational and gestational diabetic parturients. Glycosylated hemoglobin has a higher affinity for oxygen, decreasing oxygen transfer to the fetus and increasing the likelihood of fetal asphyxia. Rigorous glycemic control should be instituted from an early gestational age.

Anesthetic implications

Preanesthetic evaluation should include a thorough history, physical examination and laboratory tests focused on identifying end-organ complications related to DM (e.g., neuropathy, nephropathy, retinopathy, gastroparesis, and coronary artery disease). The airway should be carefully assessed, with particular attention paid to the possibility of the stiff joint syndrome involving the cervical spine or temporomandibular joint (TMJ).

The options for pain relief during labor in the diabetic patient are no different from those in the nondiabetic population. Preexisting neuropathy is not a contraindication to neuraxial techniques. In the presence of gastroparesis, it may be prudent to administer a nonparticulate antacid and a prokinetic agent, such as metoclopramide, prior to any anesthetic technique. Severe retinopathy may be a contraindication to maternal pushing during the second stage of labor, and the anesthesiologist may be asked to provide dense epidural anesthesia to prevent maternal expulsive efforts and to facilitate an operative vaginal delivery. Finally, the anesthesiologist must be prepared for an emergent delivery should shoulder dystocia occur.

Regional anesthetic techniques are preferred for cesarean delivery. Preexisting autonomic neuropathy may predispose the diabetic parturient to greater hemodynamic instability after spinal or epidural anesthesia. If general anesthesia is needed, the possibility of a difficult airway should be anticipated. Equipment for advanced airway intubation techniques, including a fiber-optic bronchoscope, various sized laryngoscopes and LMAs, and transtracheal ventilation equipment, should be readily available.

Rheumatoid arthritis

Rheumatoid arthritis (RA) affects 1% of the population and is more common in women.

Effect of pregnancy on RA and of RA on pregnancy

As with most immune disorders, the symptoms from RA improve over the course of pregnancy.

Corticosteroids and NSAIDs are usually continued during pregnancy. Methotrexate, chlorambucil, and cyclophosphamide are teratogenic and are stopped preconception. Women with vasculitis may have intrauterine growth restriction. The combination of pleural effusion and kyphoscoliosis can cause restrictive lung disease, which can further reduce the respiratory reserve in a gravid RA parturient.

Anesthetic implications

The preanesthetic evaluation should focus on the following physical and laboratory findings:

1. Stability of cervical spine: may be asymptomatic; radiograph of cervical spine may be needed.
2. Mobility of the TMJ: more than 45% of RA patients have TMJ ankylosis, causing limited mouth opening.
3. Assessment for cricoarytenoideus: symptoms include dysphonia, dysphagia, wheezing and sore throat; if suspected, obtain an otolaryngologic consult.
4. Evaluation for micrognathia: juvenile RA may be accompanied by mandibular micrognathia.
5. Lumbar or thoracic kyphoscoliosis.
6. Complete blood count to evaluate for thrombocytopenia and anemia.

Patients with mild disease can be managed the same way as a normal parturient. Management of patients with significant disease and joint involvement will need careful planning. The mode of delivery will depend on the severity of skeletal deformity. In a parturient with severe pelvic deformity, a cesarean delivery may be planned.

If a decision is made to proceed with labor in a parturient with a known difficult airway, placement of an epidural catheter early in labor to provide analgesia is ideal. Regional anesthesia, however, may not be possible in patients with severe skeletal deformities. The obstetric team should be made aware of the challenges of the difficult airway, and a plan should be developed to minimize the likelihood of an emergent delivery.

If a cesarean delivery is planned, any regional technique is appropriate but, again, may be difficult. If general anesthesia is required in the parturient with cervical spine involvement or with a difficult airway, an awake intubation may be necessary. The neck should be carefully positioned when the patient is still awake, and excessive flexion and/or extension of the cervical spine should be avoided as it can precipitate spinal cord injury. Extremities should be padded and positioned carefully. Extubation should be carried out only when the parturient is awake, alert, and hemodynamically stable.

Systemic lupus erythematosus

Systemic lupus erythematosus (SLE) is a chronic inflammatory autoimmune disease characterized by the presence of multiple autoantibodies. SLE is more common in women (especially in women of childbearing age).

Effect of pregnancy on SLE

The incidence of SLE flare during pregnancy is low in women who are in remission. Flares in the postpartum period may occur due to an increase of proinflammatory hormones (e.g., prolactin) and reduction of anti-inflammatory steroids. It remains unclear if the flares are more frequent in pregnancy, as flares and remission characterize the natural course of the disease. The drugs used in the treatment of SLE comprise steroids, azathioprine, mycophenolate, cyclophosphamide, and cyclosporines. Steroids can be administered during pregnancy and breastfeeding, but the rest of the cytotoxic drugs should be avoided, even in the preconceptual stage, as they are teratogenic.

Effect of SLE on pregnancy

SLE increases the incidence of gestational hypertension, infection, DM, preterm labor, low platelet count, and thrombotic episodes. Lupus nephritis is likely to worsen during pregnancy in women who experienced nephritis prior to conception. Patients with SLE may have anti-phospholipid antibodies that can cause thromboembolic events (e.g., cerebrovascular accidents, pulmonary embolism). Thrombocytopenia may be a manifestation of SLE and may be difficult to differentiate from the hemolysis, elevated liver enzymes, and low platelets (HELLP) syndrome. Neonatal lupus presents as congenital heart block or lupus rash. It is a rare occurrence in SLE pregnancies. Fetal four-chamber echocardiography is recommended at 16 to 28 weeks gestation to evaluate for neonatal lupus. If heart block is found, treating the mother with steroids may be beneficial.

Anesthetic implications

Management of the parturient with SLE includes a careful history and physical examination focused on identifying evidence of end-organ damage (e.g., cardiac tamponade, pericarditis, endocarditis, nephritis). Activated partial thromboplastin time (aPTT) may be increased in patients with antiphospholipid or lupus anticoagulants. Although the aPTT is prolonged, the antibody has no anticoagulant effect in vivo, and these individuals are at increased risk for thromboembolic events.

The mode of delivery will be determined by the fetal well-being and extent of maternal disease. The incidence of cesarean delivery is higher in the SLE group when compared with normal pregnant women. Regional analgesia can be safely provided for both labor deliveries and cesarean deliveries if the platelet count and the results of coagulation studies are normal. In patients with nephritis, NSAIDs should be avoided as they can precipitate renal failure.

Multiple sclerosis

Multiple sclerosis (MS) generally has a relapsing and remitting course. The common clinical presentations are optic neuritis, diplopia, ataxia, and weakness of the limbs. Physiologic stress, exhaustion, and elevated temperature can all exacerbate the disease.

Effect of pregnancy on MS

Women with MS tend to experience fewer exacerbations during pregnancy (especially in the third trimester), but they are also at an increased risk for exacerbation within the first several months after delivery.

Effect of MS on pregnancy

MS does not have a direct effect on pregnancy or pregnancy-related disease. Patients with bladder involvement may be prone to more urinary tract infections.

Anesthetic implications

Local anesthetics, especially when administered neuraxially, can unmask the symptoms of MS. Even subtherapeutic concentrations of local anesthetics produce a profound conduction block on nerves containing demyelinated plaques, and thus may unmask symptoms. Thus, practitioners may be concerned about performing a regional anesthesia technique for labor or cesarean delivery. Based on the evidence available to date, however, MS by itself is not a contraindication to subarachnoid or epidural anesthesia (and these techniques prevent exposure to the risks of failed intubation associated with general anesthesia). Preexisting neurologic signs and symptoms should be clearly documented.

Hematologic diseases
Idiopathic thrombocytopenic purpura

Idiopathic thrombocytopenic purpura (ITP) is characterized by thrombocytopenia due to increased destruction of the platelets caused by anti-platelet antibodies. ITP can be treated by administering corticosteroids, but splenectomy usually is the more definitive treatment. Some patients require plasmapheresis to

remove the autoantibodies. Platelet transfusion may not be effective in maintaining a normal platelet count as the transfused platelets may be destroyed.

Effect of ITP on pregnancy and of pregnancy on ITP

Maternal ITP can cause neonatal ITP, since the antibodies cross the placenta. The fetal thrombocytopenia can lead to severe fetal or neonatal hemorrhage.

Pregnancy does not appear to influence the course of ITP. This time, however, is common to diagnose subclinical disease. Other causes of thrombocytopenia (HELLP syndrome, thrombocytopenia of pregnancy, etc.) must be excluded.

Anesthetic implications

The platelet count above which it is safe to perform a neuraxial anesthetic has not been established. Current literature frequently cites a cutoff of 100,000/mm^3. It is clear, however, that many practitioners safely administer regional anesthesia when the platelet count is well below this number. In the parturient with thrombocytopenia and no clinical evidence of abnormal bleeding, the obstetric anesthesiologist must balance the risk of epidural hematoma against the risks of general anesthesia. Thromboelastography may prove to be a useful test to determine the adequacy of maternal clotting.

Von Willebrand disease

Von Willebrand disease (vWD) is the most common autosomal inherited coagulation disorder. Von Willebrand factor (vWF) facilitates coagulation by providing multiple bridging sites between platelets and endothelium. There are multiple types of vWD; type 1 accounts for approximately 85% of cases and is simply a low vWF level.

Effect of vWD on pregnancy

There are no specific effects of vWD on pregnancy. As the disease is inherited in an autosomal dominant pattern, however, there is a 50% chance that the fetus will be affected.

Effect of pregnancy on vWD

vWD may be difficult to diagnose during pregnancy as vWF levels tend to normalize. Patients with severe disease, however, may still present in labor with bleeding abnormalities.

Anesthesia implications

Laboratory diagnosis includes vWF level assay, vWF activity (ristocetin-induced platelet aggregation test), factor VIII level, and a prolonged aPTT. Clinical bleeding is often mild with type 1 disease (but may be significant with types 2 and 3). Treatment includes desmopressin acetate (DDAVP; Sanofi-Aventis U.S., Bridgewater, NJ), cryoprecipitate, and pasteurized, fractionated fresh-frozen plasma (Humate-P; CSL Behring, King of Prussia, PA). Patients with untreated vWD may be at an elevated risk for epidural hematoma. Regional anesthesia can be performed in patients with normal aPTT or in desmopressin-sensitive patients 30 minutes after administration of the drug. Even if general anesthesia is used, severe perturbations in clotting should be corrected as laryngoscopy can lead to life-threatening bleeding in the airway.

Suggested readings

ACOG Committee on Practice Bulletins. ACOG Practice Bulletin. Clinical Management Guidelines for Obstetrician-Gynecologists. Number 60, March 2005. Pregestational diabetes mellitus. *Obstet Gynecol* 2005; 105(3):675–685.

Budde U, Drewke E, Mainusch K, Schneppenheim R. Laboratory diagnosis of congenital von Willebrand disease. *Semin Thromb Hemost* 2002; 28(2):173–190.

Dombrowski MP, Schatz M, ACOG Committee on Practice Bulletins-Obstetrics. ACOG Practice Bulletin: Clinical Management Guidelines for Obstetrician-Gynecologists. Number 90, February 2008. Asthma in pregnancy. *Obstet Gynecol* 2008; 111(2 Pt 1):457–464.

Harnett M, Tsen LC. Cardiovascular disease. In: Chestnut DH, Polley LS, Tsen LC, Wong CA. *Obstetric Anesthesia: Principles and Practice.* 4th ed. Philadelphia: Mosby; 2009:881–912.

Hoff JM, Daltveit AK, Gilhus NE. Myasthenia gravis in pregnancy and birth: identifying risk factors, optimising care. *Eur J Neurol* 2007; 14(1):38–43.

James AH, Jamison MG. Bleeding events and other complications during pregnancy and childbirth in women with von Willebrand disease. *J Thromb Haemost* 2007; 5(6):1165–1169.

Kuczkowski KM. Labor analgesia for the parturient with neurological disease: what does an obstetrician need to know? *Arch Gynecol Obstet* 2006; 274(1):41–46.

Lindemann KS. *Respiratory Disease in Pregnancy.* In: Chestnut DH, Polley LS, Tsen LC, Wong CA. *Obstetric Anesthesia: Principles and Practice.* 4th ed. Philadelphia: Mosby; 2009:1109–1124.

Malinow AM, Rickford WJ, Mokriski BL, et al. Lupus anticoagulant. Implications for obstetric anaesthetists. *Anaesthesia* 1987; 42(12):1291–1293.

Ostensen M, Villiger PM. The remission of rheumatoid arthritis during pregnancy. *Semin Immunopathol* 2007; 29(2):185–191.

Petri M. The Hopkins Lupus Pregnancy Center: ten key issues in management. *Rheum Dis Clin North Am* 2007; 33(2):227–335.

Powrie RO, Greene MF, Camann W. (eds). *de Swiet's Medical Disorders in Obstetric Practice.* 5th ed. London: Wiley-Blackwell; 2010.

Reimold SC, Rutherford JD. Clinical practice. Valvular heart disease in pregnancy. *N Engl J Med* 2003; 349(1):52–59.

Rey E, Boulet LP. Asthma in pregnancy. *BMJ* 2007; 334(7593): 582–585.

Stout KK, Otto CM. Pregnancy in women with valvular heart disease. *Heart* 2007; 93(5):552–558.

Chapter 126

Anesthesia for fetal intervention

Roland Brusseau and Linda A. Bulich

Introduction

The development of successful fetal intervention has introduced the possibility of in utero correction or modification of severe developmental defects that, left untreated, would lead to either preterm demise or severe postpartum morbidity or mortality. Powered by advances in fetal imaging and an improved understanding of fetal intervention, the range of diseases, treatments, and intervention types has grown significantly (Table 126.1).

As experience with fetal intervention has grown, so too has knowledge about fetal anesthesia and analgesia. Anesthesia provision for fetal intervention differs from most other anesthetic situations insofar as the anesthesiologist (or anesthesiologists) must care for two, or possibly more, patients – each with potentially conflicting requirements. The first is the mother who can readily indicate discomfort and can be monitored directly, and to whom drugs may be administered directly and easily. For the fetus (or fetuses), nociception must be assumed or inferred indirectly, monitoring is limited at best, and drug administration is complicated and often indirect. Both fetal and maternal hemodynamic stability must be assured, and a plan to resuscitate the fetus, should problems occur during the procedure, must be developed.

Types of fetal intervention

Fetal interventions may be roughly divided into three categories. Open midgestational (or hysterotomy-based) procedures are generally performed between 18 and 26 weeks and typically involve exteriorization of the fetus (or affected body part) with subsequent replacement in the uterus, allowing further maturation. Such procedures are generally performed on fetuses with well-defined lesions and for whom there is the expectation of preterm demise or significant postpartum morbidity or mortality without intervention.

Ex utero intrapartum therapy (EXIT) procedures, also known as operations on placental support (OOPS), are generally performed on term or near-term fetuses with significant airway obstruction or pulmonary insufficiency. In such cases, surgical intervention is performed with intact uteroplacental function prior to cord clamping. EXIT-to-ECMO (extracorporeal membrane oxygenation) cases similarly depend on intact placental function prior to ECMO cannulation and

initiation. Congenital diaphragmatic hernia (CDH) patients with poor predicted lung volumes are often managed by an EXIT-to-ECMO strategy to avoid unnecessary hypoxemia and pulmonary barotrauma.

Finally, there is an ever-increasing variety of techniques for minimally invasive fetal procedures. Fetoscopic, ultrasound guided, and fetal transesophageal echocardiographically assisted procedures may be undertaken at nearly any gestational age for the ligation or ablation of aberrant fetoplacental vessels, the placement of shunts or plugs, or modification of cardiac anatomy. Such techniques are typically employed in situations in which severe morbidity will result and other therapeutic options (typically medical) have failed.

Maternal anesthetic considerations

For procedures requiring hysterotomy and the maintenance (even if only briefly) of uteroplacental function, general anesthesia is the technique of choice. High concentrations of inhaled anesthetics, typically in the range of 2 times minimum alveolar concentration (MAC), are required to maintain appropriate uterine relaxation for maintenance of fetal perfusion, to optimize fetal exposure, and to provide continuous tocolysis. Such anesthetic depth also assures appropriate fetal anesthesia prior to hysterotomy and intervention. This anesthetic depth, however, may compromise maternal blood pressure, requiring pressor support to maintain maternal blood pressure within 10% of baseline and thus provide appropriate myometrial and placental perfusion for fetal oxygenation. In addition, consideration must be given to the multiple maternal physiologic changes associated with pregnancy that are discussed elsewhere in this volume.

Uteroplacental anesthetic considerations

Uterine and umbilical blood flow, as well as placental barriers to diffusion, govern fetal oxygen delivery. As noted, volatile anesthetics beneficially decrease myometrial tone but also decrease maternal blood pressure, leading to decreased maternal placental blood flow. This diminution of flow has been shown to result in decreased fetal oxygenation and underlies the recommendation to maintain maternal blood pressure within 10% of baseline.

Table 126.1. Diseases eligible for fetal intervention

Disease	Intervention type(s)
CCAM (cystic adenomatoid malformation)	EXIT, EXIT-to-ECMO (if significant airway obstruction)
CDH	EXIT, EXIT-to-ECMO, or minimally invasive (ultrasound or fetoscopically guided tracheal plug placement and removal)
Cervical teratoma	EXIT, EXIT-to-ECMO (if significant airway obstruction)
CHAOS (congenital high airway obstruction syndrome)	EXIT, EXIT-to-ECMO (if significant airway obstruction)
Congenital goiter	EXIT, EXIT-to-ECMO (if significant airway obstruction)
Cystic hygroma	EXIT, EXIT-to-ECMO (if significant airway obstruction or high-output cardiac failure)
HLHS (hypoplastic left heart syndrome)	Minimally invasive (ultrasound-guided percutaneous aortic valve dilatation)
Hydronephrosis and bladder outlet obstruction	Minimally invasive (ultrasound or fetoscopically guided shunt placement)
MMC (myelomeningocele)	EXIT, minimally invasive (fetoscopic patch application)
Pulmonary sequestration, bronchogenic cysts, and mixed or hybrid pulmonary lesions	EXIT
SCT (sacrococcygeal teratoma)	EXIT, EXIT-to-ECMO (for high-output cardiac failure)
TRAP (twin reversed arterial perfusion sequence)	Minimally invasive (fetoscopic laser/photoablation of aberrant vasculature)
TTTS (twin–twin transfusion syndrome)	Minimally invasive (fetoscopic laser/photoablation of aberrant vasculature)

Studies in both animals and humans have demonstrated that maternal hypocapnia may also influence fetal oxygenation via umbilical venous flow. Maternal hypocapnia significantly reduces umbilical venous blood flow and has been shown to produce fetal hypoxia and metabolic acidosis. Conversely, maternal hypercapnia and acidosis have been demonstrated to increase umbilical venous flow and increase fetal arterial PO_2.

Although umbilical venous flow is clearly dependent on intrinsic factors, as above, it is also influenced by extrinsic factors, such as umbilical cord compression or kinking. During open procedures, the loss of amniotic fluid and its impact on fetal and umbilical buoyancy may lead to inadvertent cord compression or kinking and profound fetal hypoxemia. To avoid this complication, amniotic fluid or warmed saline should be continuously infused into the uterine cavity and appropriate volumes should be assured at myometrial closure.

Fetal anesthetic considerations

Fetal dependence on the placenta for oxygenation, gas, drugs, and waste exchange makes maintenance of uteroplacental circulation the highest priority for fetal anesthetic management. As the fetal pulmonary system is essentially offline in utero, enhanced umbilical blood flow is the chief determinant of increased fetal oxygenation. Fetal cardiac output is almost entirely rate-related, making the maintenance of fetal heart rate a similar priority to ensure adequate umbilical blood flow. The disproportionately vagal tone of the fetal nervous system, as well as the immaturity of baroreflex mechanisms, adds a further challenge, as fetal distress, including hypoxemia, will often present as a decreased fetal heart rate. Volatile anesthetics, which function as myocardial depressants and vasodilators, further complicate fetal hemodynamics and oxygen delivery. Indeed, fetal pH is routinely depressed by volatile anesthetics, furthering myocardial depression.

Surgical conditions also threaten the fetus during open repairs. Fetal blood volume is approximately 100 to 110 ml/kg, but given the small size of most intervention patients, even a small amount of blood loss can lead to severe hemodynamic compromise. Immature fetal hepatic and hematologic function may lead to impaired hemostasis and enhanced surgical losses. Such coagulopathy may be worsened by fetal cooling during open interventions. Great care must be taken to limit fetal heat loss.

Rationale for fetal anesthesia and analgesia

The proliferation of minimally invasive fetal interventions and the apparent lack of a requirement for maternal general anesthetics in such cases has called into question the need for fetal anesthesia and analgesia. In such cases, anesthetized mothers could be considered an anesthetic conduit for the fetus, placing them at unacceptable levels of risk for a questionable fetal benefit. A significant body of evidence, however, has grown to suggest the importance of mitigating the fetal stress response to enhance fetal outcome and possibly limit preterm labor.

It is clear that the fetus is capable of mounting a physiochemical stress response to noxious stimuli as early as 18 weeks gestation. Given the state of current knowledge, it is impossible to know exactly when the fetus first becomes capable of experiencing pain, although most agree that the gestational age range in which this occurs is between 20 and 30 weeks. It so happens that this range coincides with the gestational ages during which most fetal interventions occur. Indeed, the fetal experience of pain may be even greater than that of the term neonate or young child, due to the immaturity of systems of descending inhibition. Descending inhibition is the process whereby ascending nociceptive signals in the ascending spinal neurons are dampened via inhibitory descending neurons of the dorsal horn of the spinal cord. These inhibitory tracts develop late in gestation and are still immature at birth.

For this reason, most practitioners provide fetal anesthesia or analgesia of some sort during both open and minimally invasive procedures. Because access to the fetus is limited in the latter cases, alternative routes of administration are frequently required (Table 126.2).

Table 126.2. Routes for fetal drug delivery

Route	Disadvantages	Notes
Transplacental	Delayed delivery; significantly higher maternal levels required to achieve therapeutic fetal concentrations	Fetal isoflurane levels reach 70% of maternal isoflurane levels in 60 min; most commonly used induction agents rapidly cross the placenta
IM	Variable absorption, bleeding, tissue damage	Fentanyl (20–50 µg/kg) and pancuronium (200 µg/kg) may be given for open procedures and with ultrasound guidance during minimally invasive procedures
IV	Difficult to obtain access, bleeding, vessel thrombosis	Standard neonatal doses may be delivered; blood may be given via this route
Intracardiac	Difficult to establish, may produce arrhythmias, may lead to pericardial effusion and tamponade	Best reserved for emergent resuscitation; dose volumes should be as small as possible, generally between 0.2 and 0.5 ml
Intraamniotic	Experimental; correct dosing currently unknown	Allows for minimally invasive drug delivery; may be useful for sustained delivery of medications

Challenges of fetal monitoring

Fetal monitoring provides another significant challenge for the anesthesiologist. Access to the patient and the presence of amniotic fluid greatly limit available monitoring modalities. In open cases, during which a fetal limb may be exposed, fetal pulse oximetry can serve as a marker of general oxygenation and cardiovascular state (via heart rate). Fetal arterial oxygen saturation (SaO_2), even with a maternal fraction of inspired oxygen content (FiO_2) of 1.0, rarely exceeds 70%, and an intraoperative SaO_2 greater than 40% is generally considered acceptable. Whereas fetal electrocardiography has proven notoriously difficult to reliably obtain and assess, fetal transesophageal echocardiography in both open and minimally invasive procedures may provide information about heart rate, stroke volume, and cardiac function. Surface or transmyometrial echocardiography may also be of use. In situations in which fetal blood may be aspirated, fetal blood gas sampling and analysis may help in the assessment of fetal well-being.

Doppler ultrasonographic measurement of fetal cerebral blood flow, as well as experimental use of near infrared spectroscopy (NIRS), may help to reveal the adequacy of cerebral blood flow and cerebral oxygenation during fetal interventions. Fetuses will preferentially redistribute circulation to the brain and other vital tissues during hypoxemic and generalized fetal distress. These technologies may reveal signs of fetal distress and provide early indications of fetal compensatory failure.

Intrauterine fetal resuscitation

Given the immaturity of fetal organ function, the fetal disposition to cardiovascular instability and collapse, and the multiple stresses of surgery and its associated anesthetics on fetal compensatory mechanisms, a plan for fetal resuscitation must always be prepared in advance (Table 126.3).

Both maternal and fetal factors may contribute to fetal decompensation, and both maternal and fetal interventions may contribute to effective fetal resuscitation. Whether or not uteroplacental insufficiency is implicated, measures should be undertaken to maximize oxygen delivery to the fetus. These maternal measures include left lateral positioning to relieve aortocaval compression, FiO_2 of 1.0 if intubated, or high-flow oxygen administration with a face mask to increase fetal oxygen saturation. A rapid intravenous (IV) fluid infusion, possibly including vasopressor administration, may be employed to improve uterine blood flow. If there is evidence of uterine contraction, efforts must be undertaken to enhance uterine relaxation, including tocolysis if necessary.

Limited access to the fetus with hemodynamic decompensation may complicate resuscitation measures. Hemodynamic compromise may result from hypoxemia, acute fetal hemorrhage or routine surgical bleeding, preexisting fetal cardiac disease and/or anemia, electrolyte abnormalities, hypothermia, and/or other forms of generalized fetal distress. Open procedures lend direct access to the fetus and allow direct cardiac compressions (100–150 compressions per minute),

Table 126.3. Fetal resuscitation interventions

Intervention	Dose	Notes
Atropine	20 µg/kg (minimum dose 0.1 mg)	Useful to counteract significant fetal vagal responses to stress and hypoxemia; useful as prophylaxis prior to intervention
Epinephrine	10–20 µg/kg	May be repeated every 3 min; increasing doses may be of limited benefit
Calcium gluconate	100 mg/kg	Calcium chloride (20 mg/kg) may be substituted
Sodium bicarbonate	1–2 mEq/kg	Of unclear benefit; given acidemia inherent to anesthesia with volatile anesthetics, may be reasonable to enhance efficacy of epinephrine
PRBCs	10–15 ml/kg to achieve an Hb increment of 2–3 g/dl	Generally reserved for acute loss of > 25% estimated blood volume

Hb, hemoglobin.

intravascular (IV) or intramuscular (IM) delivery of routine resuscitation medications (epinephrine, atropine, sodium bicarbonate), and packed red blood cells (PRBCs). When giving PRBCs, consideration should be given to their pH correction to limit excess potassium delivery. Calcium gluconate may be needed to limit citrate-induced hypocalcemia. To assure normothermia and prevent umbilical kinking, the fetus should be continuously bathed in warm fluids.

During minimally invasive procedures, similar medications may be given, but delivery is generally limited to IM or intracardiac administration under ultrasound guidance. Even PRBCs may be delivered via an intracardiac route, but special care must be taken to adjust blood pH and temperature as well as to deliver volume slowly so as not to distend the fetal heart or produce excessively hypoxemic cardiac output. Large pericardial effusions should be drained. If resuscitation fails, maternal transabdominal or transmyometrial compressions may also be considered, although utility may be limited. Consideration should also be given to emergent delivery in viable fetuses, although preparation for such should be a part of preprocedure planning.

Postoperative considerations

Preterm labor poses the greatest risk to the postoperative fetus. Maternal and fetal stress, and hysterotomy in particular, greatly increase the risk of preterm delivery, compromising fetal well-being directly via preterm delivery and limiting the maturational efficacy of the intervention. Maternal prophylaxis with tocolytic agents and aggressive pain control are standard therapy following open interventions. There is some suggestion in an animal model that IV opioid analgesia provided to the mother may inhibit postoperative myometrial contractions. Epidural anesthesia using a low concentration of local anesthetics and a high concentration of opioids may provide effective maternal and fetal analgesia, but the effect on preterm labor is not yet known.

Fetal assessment is more difficult. Fetal heart rate analysis in the immediate postoperative period may be useful for determining fetal distress; echocardiography may also reveal the fetus's general cardiovascular state, and cerebral artery pulsatility indices may further help to assess fetal well-being. The fetal ductus arteriosus should also be monitored for patency and diameter change following indomethacin exposure.

A look to the future

Clearly, with advances in surgical and anesthetic techniques and technologies, significant progress may be made in midgestation fetal intervention. Already there is movement toward expanding treatment to include not only life-threatening fetal pathologies but also preemptive management of fetal disorders that are not necessarily life-threatening but have significant, disabling postpartum morbidities.

The particular challenges for anesthesiologists are to develop methods to provide selective fetal anesthesia and analgesia as well as techniques of targeted uterine relaxation so that safer, specifically tailored anesthetics may be provided to all patients involved in the fetal intervention. Enhanced fetal monitoring will help the anesthesiologist provide better care for the fetus during both the procedure and the postoperative period. With such advances, the provision of fetal anesthesia may become a more routine part of pediatric surgical and anesthetic practice, bringing with it new opportunities for practice and research and new problems to be solved.

Suggested readings

Boris P, Cox PBW, Gogarten W, et al. Fetal surgery, anaesthesiological considerations. *Curr Opin Anaesthesiol* 2004; 17:235–340.

East CE, Colditz PB. Intrapartum oximetry of the fetus. *Anesth Analg* 2007; 105(6 Suppl):S59–S65.

Fisk NM, Gitau R, Teixeira JM, et al. Effect of direct fetal opioid analgesia on fetal hormonal and hemodynamic stress response to intrauterine needling. *Anesthesiology* 2001; 95:828–835.

Golombek K, Ball RH, Lee H, et al. Maternal morbidity after maternal-fetal surgery. *Am J Obstet Gynecol* 2006; 194:834–839.

Kohl T, Muller A, Tchatcheva K, et al. Fetal transesophageal echocardiography: clinical introduction as a tool during cardiac intervention in a human fetus. *Ultrasound Obstet Gynecol* 2005; 26:780–785.

Lakhoo K. Introduction: surgical conditions of the fetus and newborn. *Early Hum Dev* 2006; 82:281.

Myers LB, Cohen D, Galinkin J, et al. Anesthesia for fetal surgery. *Paediatric Anaesth* 2002; 12:569–578.

Okutomi T, Saito M, Kuczkowski KM. The use of potent inhalational agents for the intrapartum treatment (exit) procedures: what concentrations? *Acta Anaesthesiol Belg* 2007; 58:97–99.

Robinson MB. Frontiers in fetal surgery anesthesia. *Int Anesthesiol Clin* 2006; 44:1–15.

Tame JD, Abrams LM, Ding X, et al. Level of postoperative analgesia is a critical factor in regulation of myometrial contractility after laparotomy in the pregnant baboon: implications for human fetal surgery. *Am J Obstet Gynecol* 1999; 180:1196–1201.

Basic considerations for pediatric anesthesia

Alina Lazar and Patricia R. Bachiller

Anesthetic care of infants and children requires an understanding of the differences that exist between the adult and pediatric population with respect to anatomy, physiology, and pharmacology. It also requires attention to the unique psychology of the child and family, which has an effect on the conduct of anesthesia.

Anatomy and physiology relevant to pediatric anesthesia

Respiratory

By approximately 24 weeks gestation, the lung has developed primitive gas exchange. Over 26 to 35 weeks of gestation, respiratory epithelial cells begin to form terminal sacs (which will later become mature alveoli), and the cells begin to differentiate and to produce surfactant. Mature alveoli develop beginning at 35 weeks gestation. At birth, children have approximately one sixth of their adult number of alveoli; this helps to explain the sensitivity of premature and newborn lungs to mechanical ventilation and other insults. The majority of alveoli are formed by the age of 2 years, and the adult number is reached by ~8 years. Relative to body size, infant tidal volumes approximate adult values (7–10 ml/kg). Respiratory rate is higher to match the infant's greater oxygen consumption (6 ml/kg/min vs. 3 ml/kg/min in adults) and metabolic rate. (See Table 127.1 for normal pediatric vital signs by age.) The infant chest wall lacks rigidity, and the lung has poorly developed elastic fibers, which leads to less negative intrapleural pressure and predisposes to early airway closure and decreased functional residual capacity (FRC). Compensatory mechanisms are abolished by anesthesia, causing FRC to fall markedly. High compliance of the infant chest wall means that less positive airway pressure is required during mechanical ventilation. The infant's increased alveolar ventilation to FRC ratio and greater oxygen consumption results in faster oxygen desaturation during ventilatory depression. Lung mechanics approach the adult state by 1 year of age.

Rhythmic breathing begins at approximately 30 weeks gestation, and control of breathing matures over the first month of life. *Periodic breathing* (5- to 10-second episodes of apnea without hemoglobin [Hb] desaturation) is common in full-term and especially in premature neonates, up to 12 months of age.

Apnea of prematurity is defined as apnea $\geq$ 20 seconds or a shorter apnea episode ($\geq$10 seconds) associated with bradycardia (heart rate $<$ 100) or oxygen desaturation to $<$ 80% to 85%. Apnea is more common in premature infants and in infants with upper respiratory tract infection (URI). See further discussion in Chapter 128.

Cardiovascular

At birth, the fetal circulation changes to the neonatal as pulmonary vascular resistance (PVR) decreases and systemic vascular resistance (SVR) increases. As a series circulation is established through the lungs and body, there is normally functional closure of the foramen ovale and the ductus arteriosus, which will close anatomically over the next few months. The foramen ovale closes anatomically over months to years but remains patent in up to 25% of adults. Hypoxemia, acidosis, or elevated pulmonary pressures can return a neonate's circulation to a fetal-like circulation with shunting. Changes in myocardial function, conduction, and autonomic innervation also occur during the first days and months of life. The cardiac output of neonates is especially dependent on heart rate because the less compliant myocardium limits increases in stroke volume. Neonates have less cardiac reserve than older infants and children because of higher baseline preload, afterload, and decreased contractility. Hypoxemia, acidosis, and large anesthetic doses can profoundly depress the neonatal myocardium. The development of the cardiac conduction

Table 127.1. Normal vital signs in children, by age

Age	Respiratory rate	Heart rate	Systolic blood pressure	Diastolic blood pressure
Preterm	60	140 (90–180)	50	35
Neonate	45–50	140 (90–180)	60	45
6 mo	35–40	120 (80–150)	70	55
1 y	25–30	110 (80–150)	80	65
6 y	20–25	100 (60–110)	90	60
10 y	20	90 (50–90)	100	65
16 y	12–16	80 (50–90)	120	70

Modified from Chapters 2 and 3 of Motoyama EK, Davis PJ (eds.). *Smith's Anesthesia for Infants and Children.* 7th ed. Philadelphia: Mosby Elsevier; 2006.

Table 127.2. Estimated circulating blood volume

Patient age	Estimated blood volume, ml/kg
Premature neonate	90–100
Full-term neonate	80–90
3–12 mo	75–80
1–6 y	70–75
>6 y	65–70

Modified from Chapter 11, p. 367, of Motoyama EK, Davis PJ (eds.). *Smith's Anesthesia for Infants and Children.* 7th ed. Philadelphia: Mosby Elsevier; 2006.

system is less well studied, but it is worth noting that the premature infant and neonate have shorter refractory periods. Arterial baroreceptors and chemoreceptors are mature at birth, and autonomic–cardiovascular interactions are well developed although they continue to mature over the first 6 months of life.

Hematologic

At birth, the Hb concentration averages 17 g/dl with approximately 80% HbF, which has a higher oxygen affinity than does adult HbA. At birth, levels of *2,3-diphosphoglycerate* (2,3-DPG) increase, compensating for this high oxygen affinity to allow oxygen unloading in the tissues. The high PaO_2 after birth reduces erythropoiesis, and Hb decreases to a nadir of approximately 10 to 11 g/dl at 2 to 3 months (7–10 g/dl at age 6 weeks in premature infants). Over the first 6 months of life, the switch to HbA occurs. Coupled with the higher 2,3-DPG levels in infants, the switch to HbA leads to Hb oxygen affinity lower than that of adults (arterial PO_2 at which hemoglobin is 50% saturated with oxygen [P_{50}] of ~30 mm Hg vs. 27 mm Hg in an adult). These factors slowly approach adult levels over the first decade of life, and, because they allow more tissue unloading of oxygen, they may be the reason that children normally have lower Hb levels than adults (11.5–12 g/dl from age 3 months to 2 years, increasing to adult levels by puberty). Estimated blood volumes by age are shown in Table 127.2. The coagulation system matures slowly over the first decade of life. Platelet function improves over the first few days of life. Vitamin K–dependent coagulation factors at birth are ~50% of adult values; a single prophylactic dose of vitamin K is generally given to newborns. Preterm neonates are especially at risk for bleeding.

Neurologic

Neuronal growth and development continue throughout childhood. The sympathetic nervous system matures more slowly than the parasympathetic, leading to exaggerated vagal responses to stimuli, such as airway manipulation or hypoxia, in infants. In animal studies, it has been found that young neurons are more sensitive to therapeutic and toxic effects of local anesthetics. Studies in rodents also show apoptosis of neonatal brain cells after exposure to several types of anesthetics, including ketamine, isoflurane, and midazolam. Other studies in humans show, however, that pain and surgical stress in neonates lead to long-term effects on pain sensitivity,

behavior, and cognition. Current recommendations are to provide appropriate anesthesia in neonates for necessary procedures with care to avoid excessively high doses.

The neonatal brain is less tolerant of extremes. In neonates, the blood–brain barrier is more easily injured by hypoxemia. Premature infants are at risk for intracerebral and intraventricular hemorrhage, which can be triggered by high blood pressure, hypoxia, hypercarbia, anemia, overtransfusion, and rapid administration of hypertonic fluids (e.g., bicarbonate, glucose). Similarly, the premature and neonatal retina is sensitive to high oxygen, and retinopathy can result from oxygen supplementation in infants up to 44 weeks post-conceptual age (PCA).

Renal and hepatic

Nephrogenesis is complete in the term neonate. Renal blood flow and glomerular filtration rate are low at birth and increase to adult levels by 2 years of age. Concentrating and diluting capacity are also low at birth and mature during early childhood. Neonates, especially preterm, are sensitive to fluctuations in fluid and solute loads and are prone to dehydration, hyponatremia (which can lead to cerebral edema), hyperkalemia, hypocalcemia, and hypo- and hyperglycemia.

The fetal and neonatal liver stores glycogen, makes and metabolizes proteins, metabolizes drugs and toxins, and is the site of hematopoiesis (up to 6 weeks of age). Protein synthesis and protein and drug metabolism are decreased in neonates, reaching adult levels by approximately 1 year of age.

Temperature regulation

Infants and young children are more easily cooled or warmed because of increased surface area-to-volume ratio, a thinner subcutaneous fat layer, less keratinized skin, and high minute ventilation. They are thus more susceptible to hypothermia under anesthesia. Nonshivering thermogenesis is the major mechanism of heat production in neonates and is gradually replaced by the more effective shivering thermogenesis by approximately 2 years of age.

Pharmacology

Pharmacokinetic and pharmacodynamic differences between children and adults are most pronounced and clinically significant in infants up to the age of 3 to 6 months. In this population, the volume of distribution is larger, protein binding is reduced, and hepatic metabolism and renal excretion are diminished, whereas the sensitivity to various drugs may be enhanced.

Inhaled anesthetics

The minimum alveolar concentration (MAC) of most volatile anesthetics is greater in infants than in older children and adults, but is lower in term neonates and especially preterm neonates (see Table 127.3). The MACs of sevoflurane for neonate and infant are similar. The MAC of sevoflurane for endotracheal intubation (the inhaled anesthetic concentration

Table 127.3. MAC value (%) and age

	Sevoflurane	Isoflurane	Desflurane	Halothane
Neonate	3.3	1.3–1.7	9.2	0.87
Infant	3.3	1.7	9.4	1.1
Child	2.5	1.6	8.0	0.9
Adult	2.0	1.2	6.0	0.75

Modified from Chapter 11, p. 368, Motoyama EK, Davis PJ (eds.). *Smith's Anesthesia for Infants and Children.* 7th ed. Philadelphia: Mosby Elsevier; 2006.

Table 127.4. Intubating doses of neuromuscular blockers in children[a]

Drug	Dose, mg/kg	Minutes to intubation	Minutes to recovery, T_{25}[b]
Succinylcholine	IV: 2.0	<1.0	3–5
	IM: 4.0	3.0	20
Vecuronium	IV: 0.1	2.0	73 (infants) / 35 (children) / 53 (adults)
Rocuronium	IV: 0.6	1.0	10–30
	IV: 1.2	0.5	40–75
Cisatracurium	IV: 0.2	1.5	43 (infants) / 36 (children)
Pancuronium	IV: 0.1	2.5	45–60

[a] Maintenance doses (one-fourth of the intubating dose) may be given when one twitch is present.
[b] T_{25} is the time from injection to recovery of 25% of baseline neuromuscular transmission or three to four twitches to a train-of-four stimulus.

that would allow intubation with no coughing or movement in 50% of pediatric patients) is 2.8%, and the MAC for extubation is 2.3%. Similarly, the MAC of sevoflurane for laryngeal mask airway (LMA) placement and removal are 2.0% and 1.5%, respectively. In children, nitrous oxide has a blunted effect on the MAC of sevoflurane and desflurane (60% inspired nitrous oxide reduces the MAC by only 25%).

Inhaled anesthetic drugs increase in concentration in the alveoli more rapidly in children than in adults due to a higher minute ventilation-to-FRC ratio and higher blood flow to vessel-rich organs. High concentrations of potent inhalational agents can cause bradycardia, hypotension, or cardiac arrest in infants and young children, particularly when ventilation is controlled. Halothane causes more pronounced bradycardia and is more of a myocardial depressant than is sevoflurane; halothane also sensitizes the myocardium to catecholamines. In addition, the halothane vaporizer allows more MAC-equivalents than does the sevoflurane vaporizer, which may have contributed to the reported cases of halothane overdose.

The lack of pungency of sevoflurane and halothane makes these agents useful for inhalational induction. Induction of anesthesia is slightly shorter with sevoflurane than with halothane due to sevoflurane's lower solubility in blood. The incidence of coughing, breath holding, laryngospasm, and bronchospasm may be slightly lower with sevoflurane. Isoflurane and desflurane are not used for induction due to airway irritation. Emergence agitation, primarily in preschool-age children, may be more common after administration of insoluble anesthetic gases such as sevoflurane and desflurane, although the literature is not conclusive.

Muscle relaxants

The use of succinylcholine in pediatric anesthesia has declined primarily because of life-threatening complications, such as malignant hyperthermia, and hyperkalemic cardiac arrest in children with undiagnosed muscular dystrophy. The administration of succinylcholine is accompanied by varying degrees of masseter muscle rigidity and/or spasm in 1% of children. Mild rigidity may represent a normal response to succinylcholine, especially if underdosed. Fifty percent of patients with severe masseter rigidity test positive for malignant hyperthermia. If definitive masseter spasm occurs, triggering agents should be discontinued and the surgical procedure postponed, unless urgent.

Bradycardia, junctional rhythm, and sinus arrest may be seen after succinylcholine in pediatric patients, but pretreat-

ment with atropine (0.02 mg/kg) reduces this complication. Fasciculations are often not seen because of the small muscle mass. Succinylcholine may increase intraocular pressure. Despite its drawbacks, succinylcholine remains valuable when immediate securing of the airway is necessary or for treatment of laryngospasm. It may be used for rapid-sequence induction (RSI) in patients with a full stomach; RSI with rocuronium (1.2 mg/kg intravenously [IV]) is also acceptable if succinylcholine is contraindicated. Infants and young children require a larger dose of succinylcholine because of a larger volume of distribution (see Table 127.4), and the duration of action is shorter partly because the drug is more rapidly distributed away from the effector site by a greater cardiac output.

Neonates are more sensitive to nondepolarizing muscle relaxants: Vecuronium, rocuronium, and pancuronium have a lower 95% effective dose (ED_{95}) and a longer time to recovery in infants; cisatracurium has a longer recovery time in infants, but the ED_{95} is the same as in children or adults. The vagolytic effect of pancuronium prevents bradycardia associated with fentanyl administration for cardiac and other high-risk procedures in infants when a longer duration is appropriate. Nondepolarizing blockade may be reversed with neostigmine (0.07 mg/kg) administered with atropine (0.02 mg/kg) or glycopyrrolate (0.01 mg/kg).

Opioids

Fentanyl is the most commonly used opioid in pediatric anesthesia. Because of its lipid solubility, its brain concentration is not affected by the immaturity of the blood–brain barrier, but neonates metabolize fentanyl more slowly than infants do. The initial dose is typically 1 to 5 μg/kg IV, depending on the duration and magnitude of surgery. High-dose fentanyl (10–50 μg/kg) is sometimes used as the major component of anesthesia for cardiac surgery or in sick neonates to provide cardiovascular stability and to blunt the stress response. Intranasal fentanyl (1–2 μg/kg) may be given for analgesia when an IV is not used, such as in myringotomy. Oral transmucosal fentanyl is formulated for premedication, but its utility is limited by respiratory depression, nausea and/or vomiting, dysphoria, and oversedation. The initial IV dose of morphine is 0.05 to 0.1 mg/kg. Due to decreased clearance and immaturity of the blood–brain barrier, morphine should be administered with caution in infants less than 1 month of age (0.025–0.05 mg/kg IV). Significant histamine release may follow an IV bolus of morphine. Infants and young children require higher bolus and infusion doses of remifentanil than do adults, reflecting the larger volume of distribution and increased elimination clearance, respectively. Bolus doses of 1 to 2 µg/kg administered over several minutes are followed by an infusion dose of 0.1 to 0.5 µg/kg/min titrated to effect. If remifentanil is chosen as the major intraoperative opioid, adequate longer-acting opioid must be administered for postoperative analgesia.

Sedatives and hypnotics

Thiopental may be used for IV induction in pediatric anesthesia as its injection into small veins is painless. Due to a higher volume of distribution, the induction dose is higher in infants and young children than in adults (5–7 mg/kg). Neonates require a lower dose (3–4 mg/kg), reflecting a higher free fraction of the drug. The elimination half-time (6 ± 3 hours) is significantly shorter than in adults (12 ± 6 hours). Propofol is used for induction in doses of 3 to 5 mg/kg for infants and 1.5 to 2.5 mg/kg for older children. Maintenance doses are also larger in children because of greater elimination clearance. Infusion doses of 150 to 250 µg/kg/min preserve spontaneous ventilation and can be used for nonpainful procedures that require immobility (CT, MRI). When used for general anesthesia in conjunction with opioids or other agents, ventilatory assistance may be required. Long-term infusions (>12 hours) in the intensive care unit (ICU) setting have been associated with metabolic acidosis, myocardial failure, and death. Propofol produces more suppression of pharyngeal and laryngeal reflexes than an equipotent dose of thiopental. Etomidate (0.2–0.4 mg/kg) may be used for induction in cases of severe hypovolemia or decreased cardiovascular function. The potential for adrenal suppression should be noted.

Ketamine is used in pediatric anesthesia as intramuscular (IM) premedication for extremely uncooperative patients, as oral premedication, for brief sedation for painful procedures, or as an adjunctive intraoperative analgesic. It may also be used for induction in patients with a difficult airway, severe bronchospasm, or marginal cardiovascular status as respiration and blood pressure are usually preserved. Anesthesia after a single IV dose lasts 5 to 10 minutes and can be maintained with repeated doses of 0.5 to 1.0 mg/kg; 0.25 to 0.5 mg/kg IV may be adequate to provide analgesia. Infants <6 months old may require up to fourfold higher doses than older children. For premedication, ketamine is administered in doses of 2 to 3 mg/kg IM, or 4 to 10 mg/kg orally (PO). A small dose of midazolam may prevent distressing nightmares and hallucinations associated with ketamine use. Ketamine increases intracranial pressure for approximately 15 minutes and intraocular pressure

for approximately 30 minutes. Ketamine stimulates salivation and may predispose to laryngospasm; an antisialogogue is often given.

Midazolam is administered for preoperative sedation in doses of 0.5 to 0.7 mg/kg PO, not exceeding a 20-mg total dose, with minimal incidence of respiratory depression. The clinical effect begins at ~10 minutes, peaks at 15 to 30 minutes, and dissipates by ~45 minutes. It can also be administered intranasally (0.2 mg/kg) with faster onset, or IV (0.05–0.1 mg/kg).

Initial studies suggest that the α_2-receptor agonists clonidine and dexmedetomidine may have utility in pediatric anesthesia. As premedication, oral clonidine (4 µg/kg) requires approximately 40 minutes until peak effect. IV clonidine (1 to 2 µg/kg) or IV dexmedetomidine (0.1–0.3 µg/kg, slowly over 10 minutes) may augment analgesia and reduce the incidence of emergence agitation. Dexmedetomidine is given by infusion in some centers as a sole agent for pediatric procedural sedation. Clonidine and dexmedetomidine are alternatives to meperidine for treatment of postoperative shivering at doses of 1 and 0.5 µg/kg, respectively, given as a single bolus slowly IV.

Anticholinergic agents are used infrequently with modern anesthetics but may be used to reduce oral secretions or to prevent vagally mediated bradycardia during induction. The doses are (1) atropine IV or IM at 0.02 mg/kg, or (2) glycopyrrolate IV or IM at 0.01 mg/kg. Potential side effects include temperature elevation, central nervous system (CNS) irritation, and flushing.

Nonopioid analgesics and other adjuvant medications

Acetaminophen is a useful nonopioid analgesic. The oral loading dose is 20–30 mg/kg followed by 10–15 mg/kg every 4 to 8 hours; an initial oral dose may be given in combination with sedative premedication. The rectal loading dose is 30 to 40 mg/kg (20 mg/kg in neonates) followed by 20 mg/kg every 6 to 8 hours. Absorption following rectal administration is variable, with peak concentration reached 1 to 3 hours after administration. Maximum daily doses, which should be followed scrupulously due to the risk of hepatotoxicity, are 100 mg/kg for children > 1 year old, 75 mg/kg for infants (age 1 month to 1 year), 60 mg/kg for neonates > 32 weeks PCA, and 40 mg/kg for preterm neonates ≤ 32 weeks PCA; the dosage interval is longer in neonates due to decreased metabolism. An IV form of acetaminophen was recently approved by the Food and Drug Administration and is given in a dose of 15 mg/kg.

Ketorolac doses of 0.5 mg/kg IV every 6 hours for less than 5 days have been used successfully for postoperative pain control in neonates, infants, and children. Bleeding potential and renal dysfunction are relative contraindications to nonsteroidal anti-inflammatory agents.

Ondansetron (0.05–0.15 mg/kg) and dexamethasone (0.15–0.5 mg/kg, up to a maximum of 10 mg) are often used for prophylaxis during procedures with a high risk of postoperative nausea and vomiting (PONV; ophthalmic surgery, inner ear surgery, tonsillectomy, or adenoidectomy) or in patients with a history of PONV or motion sickness.

Patient preparation

Preoperative preparation of pediatric patients must take into account their psychological development as well as the family dynamics. The goals of preoperative preparation are to reduce anxiety and stress before induction and minimize behavioral problems that may occur days and weeks after surgery, such as temper tantrums, separation anxiety, enuresis, and sleep and appetite disturbances. Parental anxiety reduction and satisfaction with the perioperative experience are also important.

Many preoperative preparation techniques have been evaluated in the literature. Individualized preoperative interventions, such as seeing a child-life specialist at age-appropriate times before surgery (approximately 1 week for children >6 years old, a shorter time for ages 3–6, and probably no preparation for those <3 years old), are most likely to successfully diminish patient anxiety in the holding area. Listening to music may reduce anxiety in the holding area and possibly during anesthesia induction, especially if live-interaction music is provided by a music therapist. Limiting sensory stimulation (using dim lighting and soft music and interacting with only one person, usually the anesthesiologist) may also alleviate anxiety during induction. Sedative premedication reduces preoperative anxiety and improves cooperation with mask induction in the majority of children.

Reducing parental anxiety can be helpful in calming pediatric patients as anxious parents are less able to respond to their children and may increase the child's anxiety. Informational videotapes and acupuncture for parents have been shown to allay anxiety about anesthesia preoperatively. Being invited to be present for their child's anesthesia induction also increases parental satisfaction with the perioperative experience but has not been shown to reduce parental or patient anxiety (preoperatively or postoperatively) or to change the incidence of postoperative behavioral disturbances in pediatric patients, although it may be beneficial in a subset of child–parent pairs.

Induction

Inhalation induction of anesthesia is the most common choice for pediatric patients in the United States because most children dread needles, and it is practical due to the rapid onset in children. Maintaining spontaneous ventilation during induction allows the patient to self-regulate anesthetic depth and may protect against overdose. When an inhalational induction is inappropriate (full stomach or intestinal obstruction, risk of malignant hyperthermia, acutely elevated intracranial pressure) IV induction is performed. The pain of venipuncture can be reduced by EMLA cream (eutectic mixture of local anesthetics) applied 45 minutes ahead of time or lidocaine delivered via a needleless injection system immediately before IV placement. Sedative premedication or nitrous oxide (70% in oxygen) may also help to facilitate IV placement.

The anesthesiologist should adapt the induction to fit the child's age, temperament, and personality; the family dynamic; and any relevant medical issues. Common methods to calm a child include allowing parental presence during induction, applying a scent to the inside of the mask, and distracting the patient with songs, storytelling, games, jokes, and so forth. Options for inhalation induction range from starting with a pre-filled breathing circuit of 70% nitrous oxide and 8% sevoflurane in oxygen (pungent smelling but rapid-acting) to starting with just 70% nitrous oxide in oxygen for a few minutes, slowly introducing sevoflurane, and increasing the concentration every few breaths (often better tolerated initially but slower).

A larger tongue, smaller oral cavity, and smaller nasal passages predispose children to obstruction after anesthesia is induced. Airway obstruction is managed by applying gentle chin lift and jaw thrust, opening the mouth (ensuring that the tongue is not against the roof of the mouth), obtaining a tight mask fit, and slightly closing the pop-off valve to generate 5 to 10 cm of continuous positive airway pressure (CPAP). One hand should remain on the breathing bag as much of the time as possible to confirm adequate, easy gas exchange. When the patient is sufficiently anesthetized, an oral airway can be inserted if necessary. IM doses of succinylcholine (4 mg/kg) and atropine (0.02 mg/kg) should be readily available in case laryngospasm or bradycardia develops prior to securing IV access. After the patient has passed through the excitatory stage and is more deeply anesthetized, an IV cannula is inserted, the concentration of the agent is decreased, and nitrous oxide is discontinued in preparation for securing the airway.

Securing the airway

Intubation can be facilitated with muscle relaxant, deep inhalational anesthesia, a bolus of propofol, or a short-acting opioid. For all but the shortest cases, endotracheal intubation is usually chosen for infants less than 6 months of age because of potential difficulty in maintaining upper airway patency, decreased FRC with faster oxygen desaturation, and higher likelihood of inflating the stomach during mask ventilation. For some procedures, in children 6 to 12 months or older, maintenance of anesthesia with a mask or LMA is acceptable. Due to the relative cephalad location of the pediatric larynx, adequate positioning of the LMA is more difficult in pediatric patients, and delayed airway obstruction may occur in up to 25% of the patients. Indications for endotracheal intubation are otherwise similar to those in adults.

There are major anatomic differences in the airway anatomy of infants and children that should be taken into consideration for pediatric intubation. Infants have a larger occiput, obviating the need for neck flexion to attain the "sniffing position"; a shoulder roll may allow better ability to extend the head and open the mouth.

The more cephalad larynx (C3–4 in infants vs. C4–5 in adults) and the proximity of the tongue lead to a more acute angle between the plane of the tongue and the plane of the larynx (see Fig. 127.1). The epiglottis is short and omega-shaped

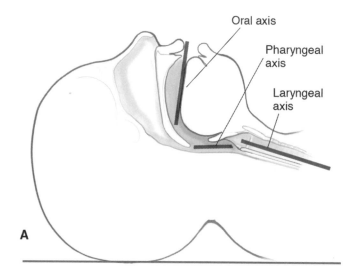

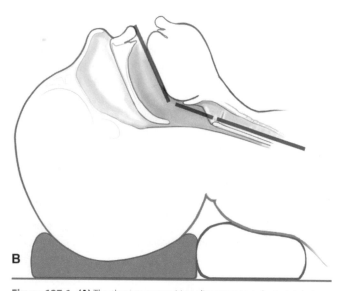

Figure 127.1. (A) The three axes requiring alignment in order to intubate the trachea via direct laryngoscopy. **(B)** Alignment of the axes with proper positioning.

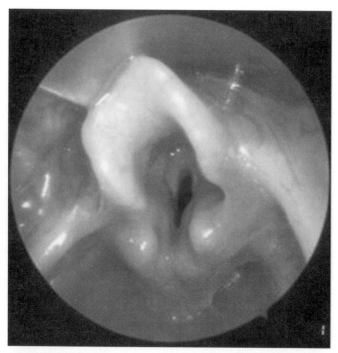

Figure 127.2. Appearance of the infant glottis. Courtesy A. Inglis, MD.

in the infant and small child, and longer and U-shaped in the older child. It is stiffer, and angled into the lumen of the airway, making it more difficult to displace during laryngoscopy. A straight laryngoscope blade displaces the tongue anteriorly, lifts the epiglottis out of the way, and improves the angle between the tongue and larynx. It may be difficult to lift the epiglottis without its slipping off the laryngoscope blade. If this happens, the blade should be advanced further into the hypopharynx and slowly withdrawn until only the glottis slips off the blade. The infant glottis is shown in Fig. 127.2. The vocal cords have a lower insertion anteriorly than posteriorly, and occasionally the endotracheal tube (ETT) is held up at the anterior commissure. Pushing the tube posteriorly or flexing the head will facilitate advancement. Excessive laryngoscopic lifting can angle the trachea forward and impede advancement of the tube.

The narrowest part of the infant larynx is the cricoid ring. As the child grows (at approximately 10–12 years of age), the triangle-shaped glottis becomes the narrowest part of the larynx. A small degree of mucosal edema can significantly increase the airway resistance in smaller children. The appropriate ETT size (see Table 127.5) is approximately the diameter of the child's fifth finger or nostril. The modified Cole's formula may also be used for patients > 2 years old:

$$\text{Internal tube diameter (mm)} = \left[\frac{age(years) + 16}{4}\right].$$

Because there is great variability in tracheal size, ETTs 0.5 mm larger and smaller than predicted should be readily available. A tight ETT may cause trauma, whereas a loose tube may not protect against aspiration or permit adequate ventilation. The pressure at which a leak is audible (auscultating over the neck or mouth) approximates the pressure against the tracheal wall. Because tracheal damage occurs with pressures exceeding capillary pressure (20–25 mm Hg), it is recommended to avoid leak pressures exceeding 30 cm H_2O. The use

Table 127.5. ETT size guidelines for patients less than 2 years old

Age	Weight, kg	ETT ID, mm
Premature	<2	2.5–3.0
Term	3–4	3.0–3.5
0–6 mo	3–5	3.5
6–12 mo	5–10	4.0
1–2 y	10–14	4.5

Table 127.6. Simplified pediatric transfusion guidelines

Component	Indication	Volume to transfuse	Change in parameter expected from transfusion
Packed RBCs	Hb <7–8 g/dl with symptoms Acute blood loss ≥15% of total blood volume Hb <12 g/dl with severe cardiopulmonary disease (<15 g/dl for neonates and premature infants)	10–15 ml/kg	Hb increase of 2–3 g/dl
Platelets	<10,000 per μl <50,000 per μl if active bleeding or major surgery planned <100,000 per μl with CNS bleeding or planned CNS surgery or in sick, premature infant with active bleeding	5–10 ml/kg	Platelet increase of 50,000–100,000 per μl
FFP	Emergency reversal of warfarin PT >1.5 × midrange of normal value or PTT > 1.5 × top range of normal value; Replacement for specific factors when their concentrates are unavailable	10–15 ml/kg	Factor activity increase of 15%–20%
Cryoprecipitate	Hypofibrinogenemia or dysfibrinogenemia with active bleeding or invasive procedure; If DDAVP or factor VIII is unavailable; in a patient with von Willebrand disease with active bleeding or invasive procedure	1–2 U per 10 kg of patient weight	Fibrinogen increase of 60–100 mg/dl

PT, prothrombin time; PTT, partial thromboplastin time; FFP, fresh frozen plasma.
Modified from Roseff SD (ed.). *Pediatric Transfusion: A Physician's Handbook.* 1st ed. Bethesda, MD: American Association of Blood Banks; 2003.

of oversized tubes is associated with postintubation croup, especially in young children with a URI or a prior history of croup. If, however, the passage of the ETT was without resistance and the procedure is expected to be short, a tight tube may be kept in place, considering the additional tracheal trauma associated with reintubation. Mucosal swelling may be reduced by dexamethasone (0.5 mg/kg).

Traditionally, uncuffed tubes have been used in patients less than 8 years of age, based on the fact that, in this age group, the cricoid ring provides a natural seal around the ETT. The slightly larger lumen obtained by creating a seal with an uncuffed tube was also considered an advantage. The use of cuffed ETTs (internal diameter [ID] 0.5–1.0 mm smaller than that of uncuffed tubes) has been shown to be safe in all ages, and their use has become more popular in recent years to avoid multiple intubation attempts, allow lower fresh gas flows, and decrease operating room pollution. The ability to adjust cuff pressure may decrease the incidence of mucosal trauma compared to sealing with an uncuffed tube, particularly with prolonged intubation. Care must be taken not to inflate the cuff with pressures higher than 20 to 25 mm Hg and to position the cuff in the midtrachea, not straddling the larynx. The pressure of the cuff should be checked periodically, especially when using nitrous oxide.

The ETT insertion distance (measured at the teeth or gums) is roughly equal to the size of the ETT multiplied by 3, but the insertion distance should be confirmed by visually noting, during direct laryngoscopy, the point at which the ETT is 2 to 3 cm past the vocal cords. Some ETTs have black line markings designed to rest at the level of the vocal cords. An easy estimate of the appropriate length of the tube at the gums is 10 cm for a newborn, 11 cm for a 1-year-old, and 12 cm for a 2-year-old. The ETT may be positioned by advancing it until no breath sounds are heard in the left axilla (right mainstem intubation) and then withdrawing the ETT to 2 cm above the point where bilateral breath sounds are again noted (the carina). In neonates, the distance from carina to vocal cords is only 4 to 5 cm, increasing the risk of accidental extubation and mainstem intubation with neck extension and flexion, respectively.

Fluid management and transfusion

Healthy term neonates and infants can often be managed for routine anesthetics using an hourly maintenance fluid guideline of 4 ml/kg for the first 10 kg, 2 ml/kg for the next 10 kg, and 1 ml/kg for the remainder of the body weight. Glucose supplementation is important in premature or debilitated infants and in term neonates within the first few days of life, and should be considered separately from fluid boluses. Although healthy term neonates and infants have higher glucose requirements than do older children, the stress response to surgery usually increases the serum glucose under anesthesia, and hypoglycemia (glucose < 45 mg/dl) is rare in older children.

Guidelines for intraoperative transfusion are listed in Table 127.6. In general, signs of hemodynamic instability (hypotension, tachycardia), coupled with significant observed blood loss, strongly suggest the need for red-blood-cell transfusion. In procedures during which it is more difficult to measure blood loss accurately, the anesthesiologist must have increased suspicion, especially in neurosurgical, craniofacial, and major orthopedic (e.g., scoliosis) operations.

Maintenance and emergence

Anesthesia is maintained with the same agents used in adult patients. (See Pharmacology section earlier in this chapter). Meticulous care should be taken to maintain fluid and temperature homeostasis and to monitor for accidental extubation or mainstem intubation, ETT kinking or occlusion by secretions, infiltration of the IV line, and excessive pressure by equipment or the surgical team.

At the end of the procedure, all anesthetics are discontinued, muscle relaxants are reversed, and the stomach is emptied if indicated. Tracheal extubation may take place after the patient is fully awake or during deep anesthesia, depending on the patient and care setting. Before awake tracheal extubation, the child should be able to maintain regular nonparadoxical breathing, demonstrate adequate muscular tone (sustained hip flexion, forceful cough, grimace using the eyebrows) and spontaneously open the eyes or perform purposeful movements. During emergence through the second stage of anesthesia, infants and young children may exhibit breath holding, bronchospasm, and chest wall rigidity or desaturation. Bucking on the tube may lead to postintubation croup if extubation is unnecessarily delayed; however, full return of reflexes and a regular respiratory rate must be sustained prior to extubation. After careful oropharyngeal suctioning, the ETT is removed, the facemask is applied, and oxygen is administered. If the patient is not moving air, laryngospasm should be suspected and treated with positive pressure and a small dose of succinylcholine if needed (see section below on laryngospasm).

Some anesthesiologists favor deep extubation for patients with severe reactive airways disease and for those in whom severe coughing could jeopardize surgical outcome (e.g., ophthalmic surgery). Adequate depth must be confirmed prior to extubation (e.g., no reaction to movement of the ETT). After removal of the breathing tube, an oral airway is placed to prevent upper airway obstruction and the mask is held for a few minutes to verify ventilation. The patient is placed in the lateral decubitus position to keep the airway clear; it is important to understand that these patients remain at risk for laryngospasm and aspiration until full consciousness is regained.

Compared with adults, children develop more coughing, laryngospasm, and breath-holding during emergence. Therefore, in children, LMAs are often removed during deep anesthesia, followed by insertion of an oral airway as described earlier in this chapter. A small bolus of propofol (1 mg/kg) may also facilitate smooth removal of the LMA while preserving spontaneous respirations.

Pediatric anesthesia risk and complications

Respiratory complications, such as laryngospasm, bronchospasm, or oxygen desaturation, represent the most common intraoperative adverse events (Fig. 127.3). Factors identified as being predictors of respiratory complications are asthma, URIs, passive smoking, younger age, anesthetic care by a nonpediatric anesthesiologist, ENT surgery, and tracheal intubation not facilitated by the use of a muscle relaxant.

Cardiovascular causes, followed by respiratory causes, account for the highest proportion of anesthesia-related cardiac arrests. The most frequent cardiovascular cause seen in cases submitted to the POCA (Pediatric Perioperative Cardiac Arrest) registry between 1998 and 2004 was hypo-

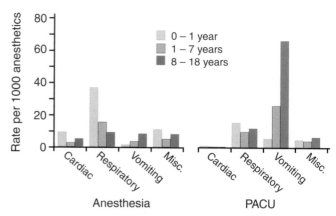

Figure 127.3. Rate of adverse events during anesthesia and in postanesthesia care unit (PACU) in different age groups. Adapted from Murat I, Constant I, Maud'huy H. Perioperative anaesthetic morbidity in children: a database of 24,165 anaesthetics over a 30-month period. *Pediatr Anesth* 2004; 14:158–166 (Fig. 1, p. 161).

volemia related to blood loss (e.g., scoliosis surgery, craniofacial surgery), usually as a result of underestimation of bleeding, insufficient peripheral venous access, and/or inadequate monitoring of hemodynamic parameters. The two second-most-common causes of cardiac arrest were (1) laryngospasm and (2) hyperkalemia resulting from rapid transfusion of old or irradiated blood. Use of fresh red blood cells (RBCs) as well as washing old blood (stored > 2 weeks) and RBCs irradiated more than 48 hours prior to administration reduces the incidence of transfusion-related hyperkalemia. The decline of halothane use in favor of sevoflurane over the past decade has led to a significant reduction in the proportion of medication-related arrests although medications remain the most common cause of anesthesia-related cardiac arrests in ASA 1–2 children.

Laryngospasm

Children are at higher risk than adults are for laryngospasm, and this risk is increased by an ongoing or recent respiratory infection. Laryngospasm represents reflex closure of the glottis triggered during light anesthesia by stimuli such as blood, secretions, or a foreign body in the airway or by other stimuli, such as manipulation of the neck, venipuncture, removal of adhesive tape, and surgical incision. The obstruction can be partial (manifested by inspiratory stridor) or complete (manifested by loss of ventilation and paradoxical movement of the chest). Partial laryngospasm is treated by applying chin lift and jaw thrust, which stretch and widen the partially obstructed airway, ventilating with 100% oxygen, and maintaining moderate CPAP while squeezing the bag synchronously with inspiratory efforts of the patient. Small amounts of propofol (1–2 mg/kg), succinylcholine (0.25–0.3 mg/kg), or a nondepolarizing muscle relaxant may be administered if these maneuvers fail to break laryngospasm. Complete laryngospasm may also resolve with a short trial of CPAP but otherwise requires rapid administration of propofol (IV only) or succinylcholine (IV or IM, if no intravascular access has been obtained). Negative-pressure pulmonary edema may develop after upper airway obstruction.

Pulmonary aspiration

The risk of aspiration in children is low (1–10:10,000) but slightly higher than that in adults, according to several studies. Factors that may make infants and young children more susceptible to regurgitation are a shorter esophagus, lower gastroesophageal sphincter tone, excessive swallowing of air during crying, and a tendency for upper airway obstruction complicated by insufflation of air into the stomach during positive pressure ventilation. There is a higher incidence of aspiration in patients with intestinal obstruction or ileus, higher American Society of Anesthesiologists (ASA) status (3 and 4), emergency surgery, and severe obesity. Pulmonary aspiration may cause bronchospasm, laryngospasm, atelectasis, and chemical pneumonitis; however, clinical effects in healthy patients may be minimal or short-lived. If the patient remains asymptomatic with normal oxygen saturation for at least 4 hours after emerging from anesthesia, it is unlikely that symptoms will appear later. Chest radiography is indicated in the presence of respiratory distress or persistent hypoxemia.

Emergence agitation/delirium

Children ages 2 to 5 years are at the highest risk for emergence agitation/delirium, a state of hyperexcitation that includes disorientation, inconsolable crying and/or screaming, and violent movements (flailing, kicking, rolling). Patients may demonstrate increased sensitivity and reactivity to their environment. The causes are unknown but appear to be related to untreated pain, preoperative anxiety, volatile anesthetics, and patient temperament. This agitation usually appears immediately after emergence but can occur up to 30 minutes afterward. It is self-limited, lasting 5 to 20 minutes (rarely longer).

Certain medications given preoperatively or intraoperatively may help to reduce the incidence of emergence delirium. Ensuring that patients awaken pain-free by using regional anesthesia, opioids, α_2-receptor agonists, or ketorolac has been associated with less emergence agitation. In several studies, premedication with oral midazolam also reduced emergence delirium without increasing length of stay. Other approaches include premedication with ketamine or melatonin.

The primary goal of treating emergence agitation/delirium is to keep the patient safe from self-injury. Often treatment is best limited to holding the child in a comforting and gentle manner while avoiding stimuli such as noise or bright light. If pain is suspected as a potential cause, a small dose of IV fentanyl (1 µg/kg) can be effective. Bringing a parent to the bedside may help to resolve the agitation. If the agitation/delirium is especially severe or prolonged, it may be treated with sedatives such as midazolam (0.02–0.1 mg/kg), propofol (0.5–1 mg/kg), or dexmedetomidine (0.5 µg/kg), along with careful monitoring.

Pediatric facility requirements and credentialing of providers

Patient care facilities that wish to provide anesthesia for pediatric patients must have a full selection of pediatric equipment

Table 127.7. Pediatric anesthesia equipment and drugs

- Airway equipment for all ages of pediatric patients: ventilation masks, tracheal tubes, oral and nasopharyngeal airways, laryngoscopes with pediatric blades, fiber-optic airway equipment
- A separate, fully stocked "difficult airway cart" containing specialized equipment for management of the difficult pediatric airway
- Positive-pressure ventilation systems appropriate for infants and children
- Devices for the maintenance of normothermia (e.g., warming lamps, circulating warm-air devices, airway humidifiers, and fluid-warming devices)
- IV fluid administration equipment including pediatric volumetric fluid administration devices, intravascular catheters in all pediatric sizes, and devices for intraosseous fluid administration
- Noninvasive monitoring equipment for electrocardiography, measurement of blood pressure, pulse oximetry, and capnography
- Equipment for the measurement of arterial and central venous pressures in infants and small children
- Pediatric resuscitation cart, including pediatric defibrillator paddles
- Resuscitation cardiac drugs in appropriate pediatric concentrations

and drugs (see Table 127.7), laboratory and radiology capabilities, as well as nursing and physician staff with documented competence in the care of these patients. The only exception is an operative procedure required in a life-or-death emergency. Pediatric patients designated as being at increased anesthesia risk (e.g., neonates, patients requiring postoperative intensive care, patients with other coexisting medical conditions) should be under the care of an anesthesiologist with special training in pediatric anesthesia or a provider with documented, demonstrated competence in the care of this population. The general anesthesiologist should be able to provide safe anesthesia for routine pediatric surgery; recognize when the clinical condition of the patient requires skills, facilities, or support beyond the capabilities of the anesthesiologist or institution; and be able to resuscitate neonates, infants, and children. All other health care providers involved in the perioperative care of an infant or child, such as nurses and respiratory therapists, should be trained and experienced in routine and emergent pediatric care.

Suggested readings

American Academy of Pediatrics. Guidelines for the pediatric perioperative anesthesia environment. *Pediatrics* 1999; 103:512–514.

Berde CB, Sethna NF. Analgesics for the treatment of pain in children. *N Engl J Med* 2002; 347(14):1094-103.

Bhananker SM, Ramamoorthy C, Geiduschek JM, et al. Anesthesia-related cardiac arrest in children: update from the pediatric perioperative cardiac arrest registry. *Anesth Analg* 2007; 105:344–350.

Borland LM, Sereika SM, Woelfel SK, et al. Pulmonary aspiration in pediatric patients during general anesthesia: incidence and outcome. *J Clin Anesth* 1998; 10:95–102.

Brandom BW. Neuromuscular blocking drugs in pediatric patients. *Anesth Analg* 2000; 90(5 Suppl):S14–S18.

Cote CJ, Lerman J, Todres ID. *A Practice of Anesthesia for Infants and Children*, 4th ed. Philadelphia: Saunders Elsevier; 2009.

Finer NN, Higgins R, Kattwinkel J, Martin RJ. Summary proceedings from the apnea of prematurity group. *Pediatrics* 2006; 117(3):S47–S51.

Flick RP, Schears GJ, Warner MA. Aspiration in pediatric anesthesia: is there a higher incidence compared with adults? *Curr Opin Anesthiol* 2002; 15:323–327.

Gregory GA. (ed). *Pediatric Anesthesia*. 4th ed. New York: Churchill Livingstone; 2001.

Holzman RS, Van Der Velde ME, Kaus SJ, et al. Sevoflurane depresses myocardial contractility less than halothane during induction of anesthesia in children. *Anesthesiology* 1996; 85:1260–1267.

Keenan RL, Shapiro JH, Kane FR, Simpson PM. Bradycardia during anesthesia in infants: an epidemiologic study. *Anesthesiology* 1994; 80:976–982.

Khine HH, Corddry DH, Kettrick RG, et al. Comparison of cuffed and uncuffed endotracheal tubes in young children during general anesthesia. *Anesthesiology* 1997; 86:627–631.

Leelanukrom R, Cunliffe M. Intraoperative fluid and glucose management in children. *Pediatric Anaesthesia* 2000; 10:353–359.

Litman RS. *Pediatric Anesthesia: The Requisites in Anesthesiology*. Philadelphia: Mosby Elsevier; 2004.

Mamie C, Habre W, Delhumeau C, et al. Incidence and risk factors of perioperative respiratory adverse events in children undergoing elective surgery. *Pediatr Anesth* 2004; 14:218–224.

Motoyama EK, Davis PJ (eds.). *Smith's Anesthesia for Infants and Children*. 7th ed. Philadelphia: Mosby Elsevier; 2006.

Murat I, Constant I, Maud'huy H. Perioperative anaesthetic morbidity in children: a database of 24,165 anaesthetics over a 30-month period. *Pediatr Anesth* 2004; 14:158–166.

Roseff SD (ed.). *Pediatric Transfusion: A Physician's Handbook*. 1st ed. Bethesda, MD: American Association of Blood Banks; 2003.

Sadler TW. Respiratory system. In: Sadler TW. *Langman's Medical Embryology*. 10th ed. Philadelphia: Lippincott, Williams & Wilkins; 2006:195–202.

Snyder LS, Martinez FD. Developmental anomalies of the respiratory tract manifesting in the adult. In: Crapo JD, Glassroth J, Karlinsky JB, King TE, eds. *Baum's Textbook of Pulmonary Disease*. 7th ed. Philadelphia: Lippincott, Williams & Wilkins; 2004:1343–1355.

Soriano SG, Anand KJ. Anesthetics and brain toxicity. *Curr Opin Anaesthesiol* 2005; 18:293–297.

Tait AR, Malviya S. Anesthesia for the child with an upper respiratory tract infection: still a dilemma? *Anesth Analg* 2005; 100:59–65.

Tait AR, Pandit UA, Voepel-Lewis T, et al. Use of the laryngeal mask airway in children with upper respiratory tract infections: a comparison with endotracheal intubation. *Anesth Analg* 1998; 86:706–711.

Vlajkovic GP, Sindjelic RP. Emergence delirium in children: many questions, few answers. *Anesth Analg* 2007; 104:84–91.

Voepel-Lewis T, Malviya S, Tait AR. A prospective cohort study of emergence agitation in the pediatric postanesthesia care unit. *Anesth Analg* 2003; 96:1625–1630.

Preoperative evaluation of the pediatric patient and coexisting diseases

Scott A. LeGrand and Thomas M. Romanelli

The practice of pediatric anesthesia may be particularly challenging because the formulation of an appropriate perioperative technique requires not only a physiologic assessment of the patient and the disease processes that have prompted surgical intervention, but a reasonable understanding of the child's and family's emotional state as well. The increasing frequency of pediatric outpatient procedures may limit the time that an anesthesiologist has to conduct a thorough review of all the issues pertinent to the pediatric patient. This chapter will focus on the psychological and physiologic assessment of the pediatric patient with an emphasis on commonly encountered issues affecting their management. Evaluation of the child with congenital heart disease is detailed in a separate chapter.

Psychological assessment

Many factors will influence how a patient and his or her family respond to the prospect of having anesthesia. These factors include the child's age and medical history, cultural issues, experience with previous anesthetics, and the reasons for which surgery is needed. Anticipating and recognizing these factors may aid in forming a trusting bond with the patient and family and relieving anxiety. It is helpful if information regarding the anesthetic is available in advance through books, pamphlets, videos, and so forth that can provide education without disrupting perioperative flow. It is important to reassure patients and their families, and time should be spent to explain the process from induction to postprocedure care. Children tend to interpret words literally, and it is best to use simple language to explain procedures. Prior to administering any preoperative sedation, discuss with parents its risks and benefits and what they can expect after the medication is given. Encourage the child to hold a comfort object such as a toy, doll, or blanket. Consider allowing the parents to be present for induction of anesthesia (in accordance with hospital policy); calm, well-prepared parents can provide emotional support for the child. The inclusion of child-life specialists, if available, may also smooth the induction period.

Physiologic assessment

Physiologic assessment of a child about to undergo anesthesia begins with a thorough history of present illness, a review of the indication for surgery and presenting symptoms, and pertinent organ system involvement. Current medications and hyperalimentation (if any) must be recorded, and the patient's NPO status confirmed.

Features of the past medical history that are of particular importance to pediatric patients include gestational age and birth weight, any complications of labor and delivery, the presence of congenital disorders, prior hospitalizations, a history of apneic or bradycardic spells, and previous anesthesia and any side effects. Drug, food, or latex allergies should be documented. Additionally, inquire about sick contacts and an up-to-date immunization schedule. Seek out symptoms of upper respiratory tract infection (URI) and environmental smoke exposure, because both may result in increased airway sensitivity. Ask the parents if the child's physical activity is normal or decreased. Difficulties with feeding in young infants may indicate cardiorespiratory embarrassment. Previously diagnosed cardiopulmonary dysfunction (e.g., known patent foramen ovale, pulmonary hypertension, congenital heart disease, sleep apnea, tracheal stenosis) should be assessed for current severity. Family history is of particular importance in pediatric patients and should include history of malignant hyperthermia (MH), sickle cell, von Willebrand disease, hemophilia, plasma cholinesterase deficiency, muscular dystrophies, and cystic fibrosis.

General assessment of the patient's mental status, level of alertness, and ease of interaction can be made during the preoperative interview. Physical examination in most healthy children may be limited to a cardiopulmonary focus. Airway assessment includes the presence of micrognathia, loose teeth, or obvious caries. Dysmorphic facial features may indicate a congenital syndrome associated with a difficult airway. Signs of respiratory compromise include nasal flaring, nasal discharge, wheezing, stridor, and retractions. Heart murmurs or cyanosis should be noted as these may indicate congenital heart disease. Abdominal distention or emesis may influence management of the airway in addition to indicating possible gastrointestinal disease. Bruising, oozing, or pallor from anemia may be signs of hematologic disease.

Laboratory studies should be ordered based on the presenting illness, anticipated surgery, and postoperative course. Baseline hemoglobin values are useful for surgery with potential for large blood loss. Coagulation studies are indicated for hemophiliacs or for long surgeries with significant blood volume replacement. Glucose levels should be monitored in newborns due to their higher metabolic rates and limited stores. Pulmonary function tests are useful to quantify the severity of chronic lung disease (e.g., cystic fibrosis). Echocardiogram results should be reviewed in patients with congenital heart disease. Other imaging studies and relevant anatomy should be reviewed based on the presenting complaint.

Coexisting disease in the pediatric patient
Respiratory
Apnea of prematurity

Apnea of prematurity is common among newborns born at less than 34 weeks gestation with its incidence being inversely related to both gestational and postconceptual age. Central apnea is related to central nervous system (CNS) immaturity as well as abnormal responses to hypercapnia and hypoxia. Obstructive apnea may also occur in which uncoordinated upper airway musculature causes cessation of airflow. Apnea of prematurity is often mixed apnea (i.e., a combination of both central and obstructive apnea).

Therapy for apnea of prematurity includes patient positioning to prevent airway obstruction, gentle tactile stimulation to elicit arousal responses in the setting of brief apnea, and respiratory stimulants such as aminophylline, theophylline, or caffeine for chronic therapy or in the perioperative period.

Volatile agents, opioids, and hypnotic drugs used in anesthesia have the potential to worsen apnea as many decrease the ventilatory response to hypercarbia and hypoxia. Central apnea may be exacerbated by hypothermia, hypoglycemia, and anemia. Although they are thought to be associated with a lower risk of apnea than is general anesthesia, regional techniques have also been associated with postoperative apneic spells. Therefore, for newborns less than 60 weeks post-conceptual age who are at risk for apnea of prematurity, outpatient surgery is generally not recommended, and appropriate cardiorespiratory monitoring should be available, regardless of anesthetic technique.

Bronchopulmonary dysplasia

Bronchopulmonary dysplasia (BPD), sometimes referred to as chronic lung disease of the newborn, has changed in its presentation since it was first described in 1967. The diagnosis of BPD is based on the need for oxygen therapy and/or ventilatory support in relation to the infant's developmental age and birth weight. This consensus definition has not yet been universally accepted, however, and the strength of its correlation to long-term pulmonary and neurodevelopmental outcomes remains unclear.

The older form of BPD resulted from aggressive mechanical ventilation and the delivery of high concentrations of oxygen in the premature newborn. The constellation of edema and

Table 128.1. Causes of chronic lung disease and definition of BPD

Causes of chronic lung disease:
Premature newborns
  BPD (old or new)
  Prematurity
  Status after respiratory distress syndrome
Term and near-term newborns
  BPD (old)
  Pneumonia or sepsis
  Aspiration syndromes
  Persistent pulmonary hypertension of the newborn
  Pulmonary hypoplasia
  Diaphragmatic hernia
  Congenital heart disease
Current definitions of BPD:
Diagnosis
  Oxygen dependence for at least 28 postnatal days
Grading at 36 postmenstrual wk for infants born at <32 wk or at 56 d of
    life for infants born at ≥32 wk
  Mild: $FiO_2 < 0.21$
  Moderate: FiO_2 0.22–0.29
  Severe: $FiO_2 \geq 0.30$ or continuous positive airway pressure or mechanical
    ventilation required

FiO_2, fraction of inspired oxygen. The definition of BPD was adapted from Jobe and Bancalari.; also adapted from Bimkrant DJ, Panitch HB, Benditt JO, et al.

inflammatory processes in the conducting airways resulted in pulmonary fibrosis and emphysematous changes in many of the survivors. These patients developed smooth muscle hypertrophy and pulmonary hypertension with associated right-sided cardiac dysfunction.

The introduction of corticosteroid therapy as well as exogenous surfactant replacement and gentler modes of ventilatory support have advanced the survival of premature, low-birth-weight infants. Surprisingly, the overall incidence of BPD has not changed, but rather a new pattern of lung injury has emerged. This change in pathophysiology has led to the present form of BPD. (See Table 128.1.)

Premature infants younger than 30 weeks gestational age may display evidence of pulmonary developmental arrest. The disruption of parenchymal organization leads to fewer alveoli and a reduced surface area for effective gas exchange. There is also evidence that microvascular angiogenesis is adversely affected. Some recent studies suggest that BPD may be influenced by genetic and environmental factors. The preterm survivors who grow into adulthood may develop chronic respiratory symptoms and pulmonary volumetric abnormalities, but, unlike the prior cohort, tend not to suffer from pulmonary hypertension or fibrosis.

It is important to consider the persistence of pulmonary dysfunction when conducting anesthesia for these patients, especially because BPD represents a spectrum of disease and physiologic embarrassment. A focused history and physical, documenting baseline symptoms and limitations of physical activity, is critical for planning. It is also important to note that airway hyperreactivity is common, and patients are prone to respiratory infections. Preoperative consultation with pulmonary and intensive care specialists may be useful for those patients with severe BPD.

Supportive care in these patients has focused on limiting barotrauma (e.g., modes that closely regulate mean airway pressures and I:E ratios), techniques and medications that enhance secretion clearance, inhaled corticosteroids, β_2-agonists, and diuretics. Invasive monitoring for serial blood-gas measurements should be considered, especially for those patients with severe disease. Appropriate postprocedure care, including admission to an intensive care setting, should be considered on an individual basis. Regional anesthesia, whether used as the primary anesthetic or for supplemental postoperative pain control, may be appropriate for selected patients.

Asthma

Asthma results in reversible airway obstruction, inflammation, and increased reactivity to a variety of stimuli. Common symptoms include wheezing, coughing, breathlessness, and chest tightness. With severe cases, however, air movement may be so minimal that wheezing is no longer audible. Airway obstruction causes air trapping and hyperinflation of the lung, and impairs ventilation–perfusion matching. Initially, hyperventilation causes a decreased $PaCO_2$. With worsening obstruction and fatigue of respiratory muscles, however, $PaCO_2$ begins to increase. Therefore, a normal $PaCO_2$ level in a child with a severe asthma attack is an ominous sign. Management of asthma includes supplemental oxygen, inhaled agents (including albuterol and ipratropium bromide), epinephrine, and intravenous steroids.

The history of a child with asthma should include the documentation of asthma triggers; frequency of inhaler use; history of hospitalization, intubation, or pneumothorax; and need for systemic steroids. Asthma medications should be continued until the time of surgery. As endotracheal intubation may cause bronchospasm, adequate depth of anesthesia should be ensured, and bronchodilators should be available for administration intraoperatively. Additionally, if full stomach precautions are not necessary, deep extubation may help to limit bronchospasm.

Upper respiratory tract infection

URIs are extremely common in pediatric patients, with most children having at least six to eight infections per year. The majority of URIs are viral, with rhinovirus being the most common cause. Other infections, such as croup, influenza, and streptococcal pharyngitis, may mimic URI. Additionally, non-infectious etiologies, such as allergic rhinitis, may cause URI-like symptoms. Although URI is typically self-limited, airway hyperreactivity may persist for weeks following infection. Thus, controversy exists as to the timing of surgery for children with current or recent URI. Tait and colleagues examined 1078 children (1 month to 18 years old) who presented for elective surgery, and found that children with a URI within 4 weeks prior to surgery had significantly more episodes of breath holding, oxygen desaturation, and overall adverse respiratory events

than did children without URI, although incidence of laryngospasm and bronchospasm were no different between groups. Risk factors for adverse respiratory events in children with URI included use of an endotracheal tube, history of prematurity, history of reactive airway disease, paternal smoking, surgery involving the airway, presence of copious secretions, and nasal congestion. There were no long-term adverse sequelae for the children with adverse respiratory events. A suggested algorithm for the management of children with URI is presented in Fig. 128.1.

Anesthetic management for children with current or recent URI is aimed at reducing the risk of airway complications. To that end, avoidance of endotracheal intubation in favor of a mask airway or even a laryngeal mask airway (LMA) may be beneficial. If the nature of the surgical procedure necessitates use of an endotracheal tube, sufficient depth of anesthesia should be ensured prior to intubation. If a volatile anesthetic is used for maintenance, it is preferable to use a non-irritating agent, such as sevoflurane or halothane. Deep versus awake extubation may be appropriate depending on the specific patient situation and the experience or preference of the anesthesiologist.

Secondhand smoke exposure

Exposure to secondhand smoke is known to have negative health consequences. Recent studies have shown anesthetic complications to be among these deleterious effects. Jones and colleagues performed a prospective study of a cohort of 405 children who had outpatient procedures performed under mask anesthesia. The children with secondhand smoke exposure were at increased risk for nearly all airway complications examined, including laryngospasm, bronchospasm, hypersecretion, and airway obstruction, both during anesthesia and in the recovery room. For this reason, it is prudent to screen for secondhand smoke exposure in the preoperative evaluation for all children scheduled to undergo general anesthesia.

Sleep apnea

Sleep apnea is discussed in detail in the section on pediatric otolaryngologic procedures. Although this is an obvious component of the preoperative evaluation of the child presenting for tonsillectomy, it is important to remember that children with enlarged tonsils or sleep apnea of other etiologies may present for other types of procedures. History of snoring, disordered sleep, and daytime somnolence are important historic features. Children with sleep apnea may require overnight admission for monitoring and may also exhibit an exaggerated response to opioids.

Cystic fibrosis

Cystic fibrosis is an autosomal recessive disorder seen in the Caucasian population. Typical manifestations of the disease include meconium ileus, inadequate weight gain, protein malabsorption, recurrent pulmonary infections, nasal polyps, and pancreatic insufficiency. Early in the course of cystic fibrosis,

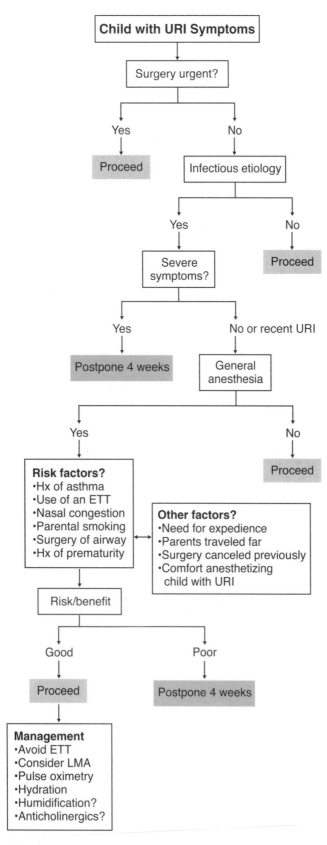

Figure 128.1. Suggested algorithm for the assessment and anesthetic management of the child with a URI. Hx, history; ETT, endotracheal tube. Reproduced with permission from Tait, AR, et al, *Anesth Analg* 2005; 100: 59–65.

Staphylococcus aureus is typically isolated from the respiratory tract; with disease progression, however, *Pseudomonas aeruginosa* becomes more common. Treatment of the disease includes pancreatic enzyme replacement, chest physiotherapy, and treatment of respiratory infections.

Anesthetic management of patients with cystic fibrosis begins preoperatively with an evaluation of the manifestations of disease for the particular patient. Preoperative pulmonary function studies may help to quantify the degree of pulmonary disease and difference from baseline; these results often show an obstructive pattern. Additionally, any pulmonary fibrosis or intraluminal secretions can cause increased alveolar–arterial oxygen tension differences on arterial blood gas analysis. Increased arterial carbon dioxide concentrations may be seen in advanced disease. Liver involvement may lead to impaired synthesis of clotting factors. Other preoperative tests that are useful include a complete blood count, electrolyte analysis, liver function tests, chest radiograph, and sputum culture results.

Intraoperative management is dependent on the severity of the patient's cystic fibrosis and the nature of the surgical procedure. Local anesthetic techniques offer the advantage of maintaining spontaneous respiration but may not be appropriate, depending on the operation and the child's ability to cooperate. If general anesthesia is required, induction may be by inhalational or intravenous routes. Sevoflurane, due to its bronchodilating properties, is probably the best choice for maintenance of anesthesia. Given the risk of pneumothorax in patients with cystic fibrosis, nitrous oxide may be avoided. Intraoperative monitoring should be guided by the severity of disease and the extent of the surgical procedure, but may include an arterial catheter and a central venous line. In the case of pulmonary hypertension and right heart failure, use of a pulmonary artery catheter or transesophageal echocardiography may be considered.

Postoperatively, patients with cystic fibrosis need close monitoring for respiratory compromise. Clearance of secretions is essential, and the use of humidified oxygen or nebulized hypertonic saline is often of benefit.

Neurologic

Seizure disorder

Seizures may result from a variety of pathologies in the pediatric population, including fever, trauma, infection, toxic ingestion, electrolyte disturbance, and hypoglycemia, in addition to idiopathic seizure disorder. They may be partial (limited to a focal region of one cerebral hemisphere) or generalized (involving both hemispheres). Partial seizures are further classified as simple or complex based on impairment of consciousness. Generalized seizures may be convulsive or nonconvulsive.

Anesthetic care of patients with seizure disorder should focus on the patient's presenting symptoms and pattern, the pharmacologic treatment regimen, and information regarding the degree of control that drug therapy provides. Blood levels, if available, should be reviewed as well as any side effects or end-organ effects from the seizure medications. Antiseizure medications should typically be continued during the perioperative period. Several anesthetic drugs or metabolites may lower the seizure threshold, including the meperidine metabolite normeperidine, and laudanosine, a metabolite of atracurium and cisatracurium. Ketamine and methohexital may also precipitate seizures. Increased doses and shortened dosing intervals of nondepolarizing neuromuscular blockers may be necessary due to enzyme induction from antiseizure medications. In addition, children with refractory seizures may be on a ketogenic diet, in which case dextrose administration is relatively contraindicated.

Muscular dystrophy

Muscular dystrophy refers to a group of progressive muscle disorders that result in differing patterns of muscle weakness. Of the muscular dystrophies, Duchenne muscular dystrophy is the most common, with an incidence of approximately 1 in 3500 male births. This X-linked disorder results in a lack of dystrophin, a muscle cell membrane protein, and causes weakness starting in the proximal muscle groups of the pelvic and shoulder girdles. Symptoms generally occur before the age of five and may include frequent falls, difficulty standing, and gait abnormalities. Progression of the disease leads to these patients becoming wheelchair bound prior to their teenage years. Cardiac involvement is common and may include arrhythmias and dilated, hypertrophic cardiomyopathy. Additionally, musculature of the pulmonary system, including the diaphragm and accessory muscles, may be involved, leading to decreased lung capacity, weakened cough, and hypoventilation.

A recent consensus statement has been published to help guide care for patients with Duchenne muscular dystrophy who are undergoing anesthesia or sedation. Suggestions for preoperative care include evaluations by anesthesiologists, pulmonologists, cardiologists, and nutritionists for the optimization of patient status prior to the procedure. Preoperative pulmonary function testing is also recommended. Discussion with the patient and family should include risks and benefits of anesthesia as well as advance directive planning. Intraoperative suggestions include avoidance of both volatile anesthetics and succinylcholine given the possibility of acute rhabdomyolysis with exposure to these agents. Use of an endotracheal tube, LMA, or noninvasive positive pressure ventilation are all acceptable and should be guided based on the clinical status of the patient and the surgical procedure. Postoperatively, patients with compromised respiratory function, defined as a forced vital capacity (FVC) less than 50%, may be extubated directly to noninvasive positive pressure ventilation. Adequate pain control should be ensured. If analgesics lead to hypoventilation or sedation, extubation may be delayed. Assisted cough, as well as an aggressive bowel regimen, may be necessary postoperatively.

Table 128.2. Representative mitochondrial disorders

Mitochondrial syndromes caused by known mutations
  MELAS: mitochondrial encephalopathy with lactic acidosis and stroke-like episodes
  MERRF: myoclonic epilepsy with ragged red fibers
  LHON: Leber hereditary optic neuropathy
  NAPR: Neuropathy, ataxia, and retinitis pigmentosa
  Chronic progressive ophthalmoplegia
  MNGIE: Mitochondrial neurogastrointestinal encephalomyopathy
Syndromes based on clinical features
  Lethal infantile mitochondrial disease
  Leigh syndrome
  Cardiomyopathy and myopathy
  Sengers syndrome (congenital cataracts, hypertrophic cardiomyopathy, mitochondrial myopathy, and lactic acidosis)
  Barth syndrome (left ventricular noncompaction, skeletal myopathy, 3-methylglutaconic aciduria, and diminished statural growth)
  Nonspecific encephalomyopathy

Summarized from Scaglia F, Towbin J, Craigen W, et al. Clinical spectrum, morbidity, and mortality in 113 pediatric patients with mitochondrial disease. *Pediatrics* 2004; 114:925–931.

Metabolic and genetic disorders

Malignant hyperthermia

MH is a genetic, hypermetabolic disorder of calcium reuptake triggered by volatile anesthetic agents and succinylcholine. The pathogenesis, clinical features, and treatment are described elsewhere in this text.

Mitochondrial disease

Mitochondrial disease encompasses a genetically diverse group of enzyme-complex defects that result in altered energy metabolism. The energy-intensive organ systems (brain, heart, and muscle) are most commonly affected. There is an estimated incidence of 1 in 5000 patients with a variable age of onset and presentation. Specific clinical syndromes are listed in Table 128.2.

Symptoms reflect the organ systems that are affected by the impairment of adenosine triphosphate (ATP) production. Neurologic sequelae include seizures, spasticity, ataxia, and developmental delay. Muscle weakness and hypotonia are common. Cardiomyopathies, conduction defects, failure to thrive, and gastrointestinal dysmotility may present in various combinations.

Many anesthetic techniques have been successfully applied in children with mitochondrial diseases with no adverse effects. Previous concerns about an association between MH and mitochondrial disease have not been firmly established, and the current literature does not support the avoidance of volatile agents. It is possible that children with mitochondrial disorders may have an increased sensitivity to volatile agents, presenting with cardiovascular depression in the usual clinical dose ranges. There is also some concern that the use of propofol may be associated with metabolic acidosis in some of these patients because of further impairment of mitochondrial function in the setting of impaired fatty acid oxidation.

Patients with mitochondrial disorders do not metabolize lactate well; administration of normal saline may be preferable to lactated ringers. In addition, these patients require availability of sugar or carbohydrate substrates and so do not tolerate prolonged fasting; dextrose supplementation is recommended.

Trisomy 21

Trisomy 21, also known as Down syndrome, is a common chromosomal disorder with an estimated incidence of 1 in 600 to 800 live births. Manifestations of the disease vary from patient to patient but typically include some degree of developmental delay and a characteristic facial appearance. Children with Down syndrome frequently have a large tongue and small pharynx, predisposing them to both sleep apnea and difficult mask ventilation. The trachea may also be somewhat smaller than expected based on age. Cardiac defects, particularly those of the atrioventricular canal, are present in approximately 40% of children with Down syndrome. Therefore, an echocardiogram, particularly in a newborn with a heart murmur, may be indicated prior to surgery. Intestinal obstruction (e.g., duodenal atresia) may also be present.

Atlantoaxial instability, wherein laxity of the transverse ligament allows C1 to sublux anteriorly on C2 causing spinal cord compression, is another relatively common finding in children with Down syndrome (estimated incidence 10% to 20%). A preanesthetic examination focusing on signs and symptoms of cord compression is important. Positive findings warrant postponing elective surgery for further cervical spine evaluation. If the child has never had radiographic imaging of the cervical spine, particularly if there is an anticipated or known difficult airway or if the surgery requires patient positioning in a nonneutral position, flexion and extension views of the cervical spine may be useful. Even in the presence of normal radiographs, however, cervical spine movement should be minimized during the course of the anesthetic.

Diabetes

Type 1 (juvenile) diabetes is marked by a failure of appropriate insulin secretion resulting in hyperglycemia. The mechanism is believed to be an autoimmune reaction that destroys the islet cells of the pancreas. Diabetes in this setting may accelerate macrovascular disease, leading to early-onset coronary atherosclerosis as well as microvascular disease and end-organ damage (retinopathy, neuropathies, etc.).

The ability to achieve normoglycemic control in young children is confounded by sensitivity to insulin, variability in physical activity, and unpredictable eating patterns. The recognized increase in childhood obesity is yet another complicating factor, with significant implications in long-term outcomes.

The preanesthetic interview should focus on the current insulin regimen(s) and a review of the patient's daily glucose measurements. The time of last meal and most recent dose of hypoglycemic agent should be documented. The threshold for additional glucose measurement (bedside glucometer testing) should remain low.

Some pediatric patients with diabetes may have an implanted subcutaneous pump as part of their therapy. Most anesthesia providers will not discontinue its use in the intraoperative period, but will perform frequent (every hour) glucose measurements to avoid potential complications.

Hematologic

Sickle cell disease

Sickle cell disease is an autosomal recessive disorder common among African Americans, which results from abnormal hemoglobin production. A valine for glutamate substitution at position 6 on the β-globin chain of hemoglobin produces a molecule, hemoglobin S, that is prone to polymerization (i.e., sickling) during periods of deoxygenation, acidosis, hypothermia, or dehydration. The aggregation of hemoglobin molecules leads to capillary occlusion and hemolysis. The disease frequently becomes apparent at approximately 6 months of age, when hemoglobin F levels decline and production of hemoglobin S begins. At this point, a hemolytic anemia may be noted. Vaso-occlusive crises may be frequent during childhood and are caused by ischemia from capillary occlusion. This ischemia precipitates further polymerization and can result in pain and tissue infarction. Strokes may be caused by vaso-occlusion of the cerebral vasculature. Sickled red blood cells may be sequestered in the spleen, resulting in splenomegaly. Repeated splenic infarction may cause splenic dysfunction and susceptibility to infection from encapsulated organisms. Thus, vaccination against organisms such as *Streptococcus pneumoniae* and *Haemophilus influenzae* is of particular importance in these patients. Acute chest syndrome, a medical emergency, is the leading cause of death in patients with sickle cell disease. Precipitating causes are not fully understood but may include fat embolism and community-acquired pneumonia. Patients may present with chest pain, fever, hypoxia, wheezing, or pain in the arms and legs. Neurologic complications or respiratory failure may develop. Treatment is supportive and includes blood transfusion (and possibly exchange transfusion), bronchodilator therapy, analgesics, broad-spectrum antibiotics, and supplemental oxygen therapy.

Anesthetic considerations for patients with sickle cell disease include ensuring adequate oxygenation, maintaining sufficient intravascular fluid volume, and avoiding acidosis. For procedures with large anticipated blood losses, preoperative transfusion to a hematocrit of 30% has been advocated. Intraoperatively, hypotension should be promptly treated to prevent prolonged periods of inadequate tissue perfusion. Normothermia is also important to prevent hemoglobin aggregation. Adequate analgesia is important to prevent splinting, but careful monitoring and supplemental oxygen are required in the postoperative period.

Sickle cell disease is distinguished from sickle cell trait in which a child is heterozygous for the sickle cell gene. Patients with sickle cell trait are typically phenotypically normal, although some of them may have painless hematuria and be unable to concentrate their urine. They do not, however, experience anemia, vaso-occlusive crises, acute chest syndrome, or any of the other features of sickle cell disease.

Hemophilia

Hemophilia refers to a group of X-linked disorders resulting in insufficient production of a coagulation factor. Hemophilia A is the more common type and causes low to absent levels of factor VIII, whereas hemophilia B results in deficient or absent levels of factor IX. These clotting factors are necessary for the conversion of fibrinogen to fibrin; therefore, these patients are unable to stabilize platelet plugs. Signs and symptoms of the disease are variable and depend on the degree of factor insufficiency. Patients may present with joint or muscle hemorrhages which, in children, frequently start after they begin to ambulate. Laboratory tests will show a prolonged partial thromboplastin time and low to absent concentrations of the deficient factor. Treatment involves replacement of the appropriate factor. For patients with mild hemophilia A, desmopressin (which causes release of factor VIII from endothelial cells) may also be used. Anesthetic considerations include avoidance of intramuscular injection of medications and of regional anesthesia. For patients undergoing major operations, perioperative factor replacement is required.

Von Willebrand disease

Von Willebrand disease is the most common inherited bleeding disorder and results in qualitative and/or quantitative abnormalities of von Willebrand factor, a glycoprotein necessary for platelets to adhere to damaged endothelium. Type 1 von Willebrand disease, the most common form, is caused by insufficient production of normal von Willebrand factor. Its severity depends on the degree of factor insufficiency, and patients range from being asymptomatic to having frequent mucosal bleeding. Frequently, these patients may be undiagnosed until they have excessive bleeding following mucosal surgery. Patients with type 1 disease typically respond to desmopressin, which causes release of factor VIII and von Willebrand factor from endothelial cells. Type 2 von Willebrand disease is further divided into five subtypes but is generally caused by both qualitative and quantitative defects in von Willebrand factor. Desmopressin is generally not effective for patients with type 2 disease, and treatment with cryoprecipitate is often necessary. Type 3 is the most severe form of the disease and results in little, if any, functional von Willebrand factor. As with type 2 disease, type 3 von Willebrand disease does not respond to desmopressin, necessitating use of cryoprecipitate.

Anesthetic concerns for patients with von Willebrand disease vary depending on which type of disease is present and the nature of the surgical procedure. For patients with asymptomatic disease undergoing minor surgical procedures, no intervention may be necessary. For more complex procedures, however, pretreatment with desmopressin or cryoprecipitate, depending on disease type, may be necessary during the perioperative period.

Aspiration risk

Full stomach

Pediatric patients, like adults, may present for emergent surgery without a sufficient period of preoperative fasting, or they may have pathologies that predispose them to aspiration. In these patients, as in adults, full stomach precautions must be used, with placement of an intravenous catheter prior to induction of anesthesia. Induction may be performed with propofol or thiopental, without mask ventilation, followed by either succinylcholine or rocuronium. Given the potential for bradycardia with succinylcholine, atropine may also be administered. Cricoid pressure is traditionally performed, although its efficacy has been questioned; it is maintained until confirmation that the airway is secure. Extubation should not be performed until the full return of airway reflexes. Depending on the nature of the surgical procedure and the age and cooperation of the child, regional techniques with minimal sedation may also be used when full stomach precautions are necessary.

NPO guidelines

In 1999, the American Society of Anesthesiologists published guidelines for preoperative fasting for healthy patients undergoing elective procedures. For pediatric patients, the recommendations are as follows: 2 hours for clear liquids, 4 hours for breast milk, 6 hours for infant formula or nonhuman milk, 6 hours for a light meal (e.g., toast and clear liquids), and 8 hours for solid foods. These recommendations, however, may be modified, depending on each patient's individual pathology.

Suggested readings

American Society of Anesthesiologists Taskforce of Preoperative Fasting. Practice guidelines for preoperative fasting and the use of pharmacologic agents to reduce the risk of pulmonary aspiration: application to healthy patients undergoing elective procedures. *Anesthesiology* 1999: 90:896–905.

Baraldi E, Filippone M. Chronic lung disease after premature birth. *N Engl J Med* 2007; 357:1946–1955.

Berhe T, Postellon D, Wilson B, Stone R. Feasibility and safety of insulin pump therapy in children aged 2 to 7 years with type 1 diabetes: a retrospective study. *Pediatrics* 2006; 117:2132–2137.

Bimkrant DJ, Panitch HB, Benditt JO, et al. American College of Chest Physicians consensus statement on the respiratory and related management of patients with Duchenne muscular dystrophy undergoing anesthesia or sedation. *Chest* 2007; 132:1977–1986.

Cote CJ, Todres ID, Ryan JF, Goudsouzian NG. *A Practice of Anesthesia for Infants and Children.* 3rd ed. Philadelphia: W.B. Saunders, 2001.

Della Rocca G. Anaesthesia in patients with cystic fibrosis. *Curr Opin Anaesthesiol* 2002; 15:95–101.

Driessen J, Willems S, Dercksen S, et al. Anesthesia-related morbidity and mortality after surgery for muscle biopsy in children with mitochondrial defects. *Pediatr Anesth* 2007; 17:16–21.

Hata T, Todd MM. Cervical spine considerations when anesthetizing patients with Down syndrome. *Anesthesiology* 2005; 102:680–685.

Hayes J, Veyckemans F, Bissonnette B. Duchenne muscular dystrophy: an old anesthesia problem revisited. *Pediatr Anesth* 2008; 18:100–106.

Jobe AH, Bancalari E. Bronchopulmonary dysplasia. *Am J Respir Crit Care Med* 2001; 163:1723–1729.

Jones DT, Bhattacharyya N. Passive smoke exposure as a risk factor for airway complications during outpatient pediatric procedures. *Otolaryngol Head Neck Surg* 2006; 135:12–16.

Scaglia F, Towbin J, Craigen W, et al. Clinical spectrum, morbidity, and mortality in 113 pediatric patients with mitochondrial disease. *Pediatrics* 2004; 114:925–931.

Section on Ophthalmology, American Academy of Pediatrics, American Academy of Ophthalmology and American Association for Pediatric Ophthalmology and Strabismus. Screening examination of premature infants for retinopathy of prematurity. *Pediatrics* 2006; 117:572–576.

Stoelting RK, Dierdorf SF. *Anesthesia and Co-Existing Disease*. 4th ed. Philadelphia: Churchill Livingstone.

Tait AR, Malviya S. Anesthesia for the child with an upper respiratory tract infection: still a dilemma? *Anesth Analg* 2005; 100:59–65.

Tait AR, Malviya S, Voepel-Lewis T, et al. Risk factors for perioperative adverse respiratory events in children with upper respiratory tract infections. *Anesthesiology* 2001; 95: 299–306.

Vichinsky EP, Neumayr LD, Earles AN, et al. Causes and outcomes of the acute chest syndrome in sickle cell disease (erratum appears in *N Engl J Med* 2000; 343(11):824). *N Engl J Med* 2000; 342: 1855–1865.

Wilson W. Prevention of infective endocarditis: guidelines from the American Heart Association. *Circulation* 2007; 116: 1736–1754.

Chapter 129

Anesthetic considerations for common procedures in children

Tonya L. K. Miller, Noah E. Gordon, and Mary Ellen McCann

A number of procedures occur frequently in pediatric anesthesia. Building on the basics discussed in prior chapters, anesthetic considerations for some common surgical procedures are presented in this chapter. Anesthesia for other diagnostic and therapeutic procedures is also discussed. This chapter concludes with a summary of considerations in pediatric recovery, including postoperative nausea and vomiting (PONV).

General pediatric surgery
Anesthesia for hernia and hydrocele in young infants

Inguinal hernias in infants are indirect hernias in which abdominal contents protrude through the internal inguinal canal. Hydrocele includes the presence of fluid in the potential space of the processus vaginalis. Hernias are 20 times more common in infants weighing less than 1500 grams than in the general population, and are often repaired in infants to prevent incarceration of the hernia contents. Clinically, most hernias or hydroceles present as a unilateral, nonpainful bulge in the inguinal area, which may be intermittent in nature. Surgery is indicated if there is a bulge noted during consultation or if there is a history of a bulge and the surgeon notes a thickening of the cord structures. An incarcerated hernia, occurring when abdominal contents become trapped in the hernia sac, can lead to a cycle of swelling and pain, impaired venous return, and impaired arterial inflow. Eventually, strangulation can occur, which can lead to bowel perforation, sepsis, and death. Thus, an incarcerated hernia that can not be manually reduced is a surgical emergency.

The most common surgical repair of inguinal hernias is a through a small inguinal incision and involves reducing abdominal contents and ligating the processus vaginalis at or above the internal ring. Many surgeons explore or laparoscopically examine the contralateral inguinal area because inguinal hernias are found bilaterally in 10% of infants. Recently, a technique of completely repairing inguinal hernias laparoscopically (the hernia sac is closed at the neck with a suture) has been pioneered in Europe.

Inguinal herniorrhaphy can be performed under regional (spinal block, spinal with single shot caudal block, continuous caudal block) or general anesthesia with an ilioinguinal or single shot caudal block for postoperative analgesia. Regional anesthesia as an adjunct may allow for a lighter plane of general anesthesia and eliminate the need for opioids. Spinal anesthesia may be the preferred anesthetic for infants with a history of apnea or bradycardia. The success rate of spinal anesthesia depends on the anesthesiologist placing the spinal and on the surgeon doing the surgery. Spinal anesthesia has a low risk of postoperative apnea and bradycardia; however, addition of any sedative or hypnotic agents confers the same risk as general anesthesia. Spinal anesthesia is generally performed with hyperbaric bupivacaine (0.75%) or tetracaine (1.0%) dosed at 0.8 to 1.0 mg/kg, mixed with an equal volume of 10% dextrose in patients who weigh up to 5 kg.

General anesthesia may be preferred for emergency cases (strangulated or nonreducible incarcerated hernias), when the patient is uncomfortable and unable to easily be positioned for a spinal, and also for cases done completely laparoscopically. Preterm or former preterm infants less than 60 weeks post conception have an increased risk of apnea and bradycardia, and a small percentage of them may need postoperative ventilatory support. Caffeine given prophylactically in a dose of 10 mg/kg intravenously (IV) has been shown to decrease the incidence of apnea and bradycardia, although some neonatologists have concerns about the long-term safety of caffeine on the neurodevelopment of preterm infants. Overnight apnea monitoring is advised after anesthesia in all former preterm infants under the age of 60 weeks postconceptual age; the need for monitoring in term infants is controversial. The advantages and disadvantages of regional and general anesthesia are summarized in Table 129.1.

Table 129.1. Advantages and disadvantages of regional and general anesthesia for infant hernia

Regional anesthesia	General anesthesia
Advantages:	*Advantages:*
Minimal infant exposure to general anesthetics	Rapid onset and reliability
Minimal disruption in feeding schedule	Airway control
Disadvantages:	*Disadvantages:*
Limited duration (spinal)	Postoperative apnea and bradycardia in preterm or former preterm infants
Failure rate in infants ranges from 5% to 30% (spinal)	Risk of pulmonary complications (e.g., atelectasis)

Pediatric neurosurgical procedures

Hydrocephalus

Hydrocephalus is dilatation of the cerebral ventricles with an excessive amount of cerebrospinal fluid (CSF). It usually occurs when there is a blockage to the absorption of CSF. This blockage can lead to increased CSF pressure, which can cause neurologic symptoms. Communicating hydrocephalus refers to hydrocephalus in which the blockage to flow occurs outside the ventricular system, and noncommunicating hydrocephalus occurs when the blockage occurs within the ventricular system.

Congenital causes of hydrocephalus include intrauterine infections, such as syphilis, toxoplasmosis, cytomegalovirus, and rubella; isolated aqueductal stenosis; Dandy–Walker malformation; and Chiari type 2 malformation. Acquired causes of hydrocephalus in childhood include infections of the nervous system, such as bacterial meningitis, tumors that obstruct CSF flow, and intracranial hemorrhage, including intraventricular hemorrhage of premature and newborn infants.

Chronic obstruction of CSF flow in infants with open cranial sutures will lead to head enlargement, bulging fontanelles, frontal bossing, ventricular dilatation, and a gradual loss of cerebral white matter. Rapid obstruction to CSF flow results in nonspecific findings, such as headaches, often accompanied by nausea and vomiting. Patients may be irritable at first, and eventually they will become lethargic and drowsy. Papilledema and diplopia from compression of the third and sixth cranial nerves may occur. Cushing's triad (bradycardia, hypertension, and disordered breathing) indicates impending herniation.

Surgical therapy consists of mechanically shunting CSF to bypass the normal pathways. Usually, a catheter is placed in a lateral ventricle and connected to a one-way valve that opens when the pressure reaches a preset value. The distal end of the shunt is usually placed within the peritoneal space but occasionally is placed within the atrium. Third ventriculostomy, which may be performed endoscopically, can be used to treat some forms of hydrocephalus. Shunts can become disconnected, obstructed, infected, or outgrown by the patient; revision may need to be done emergently if there is rapid obstruction to CSF flow.

Shunt placement is done under general anesthesia. Intravenous induction with full stomach precautions should be performed in patients who are exhibiting signs and symptoms of increased intracranial pressure. These cases are true emergencies, and the patients need to be thoroughly evaluated by the neurosurgical and anesthesia teams. Emergence after any neurosurgical case should be as smooth as possible with careful assessment that the patient has a regular and adequate respiratory pattern.

Pediatric brain tumors

Fifteen percent of all pediatric solid tumors consist of brain tumors. The most common tumor is astrocytoma, accounting for almost 50% of the brain tumors in children. Other common types include ependymoma, medulloblastoma, and craniopharyngioma. Many children with brain tumors will eventually be treated with a shunting procedure as well as resection. Brain edema may be treated acutely with dexamethasone, but patients should be considered to be at risk for increased intracranial pressure. Large tumors may require urgent resection if the clinical condition deteriorates.

Craniopharyngioma is a benign tumor arising from the anterior portion of the sella turcica which causes neurologic complications, such as headache, hydrocephalus, visual loss, and pituitary and hypothalamic failure. A full endocrine workup is required prior to surgery, and patients who are found to be hypothyroid or hypoadrenal need to have replacement therapy prior to surgery because these conditions have been linked to increased intraoperative mortality. In infants and young children, a frontal craniotomy approach between the frontal lobes provides the best access to the pituitary gland. Transsphenoidal surgery is generally performed only in adolescents and older children with pituitary adenomas. In many patients, a subtotal resection followed by radiation is done to avoid damaging crucial neurologic structures. Nonetheless, postoperatively, it is common for patients to exhibit transient or permanent pituitary failure and for some patients to exhibit diabetes insipidus. Up to a third of children will demonstrate recurrence of this tumor and will need to have another resection.

Any pediatric craniotomy requires general endotracheal anesthesia with adequate venous access as well as arterial monitoring. If the patient is not exhibiting signs of hydrocephalus and increased intracranial pressure, then a mask induction with a parent present is permitted. Central access and precordial Doppler monitoring may be considered, depending on the risk of air embolus in the individual patient. Normal saline for replacement of intraoperative fluid loss is generally preferable to Ringer's lactate solution. Depending on the location of the tumor, and particularly with pituitary tumors, diabetes insipidus or secretion of antidiuretic hormone (SIADH) may develop intraoperatively.

Anesthesia for pediatric otorhinolaryngology surgery

Otorhinolaryngology (ORL) procedures are some of the most common procedures in pediatrics. These are typically short in duration, requiring a deep level of anesthesia and immobility, followed by prompt awakening with modest postoperative pain requirements. Pediatric patients presenting for routine ORL procedures are often American Society of Anesthesiologists (ASA) physical status 1 or 2 and appropriate for an ambulatory setting. Any hospital can also see pediatric airway emergencies, including foreign body (FB), croup, or acute epiglottis. (See Table 129.2.) Airway bleeding after tonsillectomy can present emergently and require capable airway management skills provided by an experienced anesthesiologist. When planning the anesthetic management of any airway procedure, whether emergent or elective, one should consider the perioperative

Table 129.2. Common conditions causing airway obstruction in children

Diagnosis	Onset	Breathing on examination	Miscellaneous	Typical presenting age
Croup (laryngotracheobronchitis)	Insidious with prodrome of URI; also seen postoperatively after traumatic intubation	Inspiratory stridor, barky cough, slow inspiratory phase	Stridor and respiratory compromise worsened with increased respiratory rate	Infants, children younger than 3 years
Epiglottitis, acute supraglottitis	Rapid, fulminant onset with sore throat and dysphagia	Sitting up, drooling, dysphonia or aphonia, dysphagia with inspiratory obstruction	Limited air flow from the obstruction can muffle or obviate the inspiratory stridor	Children 2–7 years
Subglottic stenosis	Congenital, posttrauma, or prolonged intubation	Respiratory distress, notable retractions, biphasic stridor	Most common cause is prolonged intubation	Neonates, infants, or children of any age after prolonged intubation
Foreign body	Insidious or rapid	Decreased air exchange and/or wheezing	Organic foreign bodies cause more inflammation; small, inert foreign bodies may cause chronic wheeze or cough	Toddler

expertise and resources that are needed. In some cases, transport of a stabilized patient to a more specialized facility may be required.

Although pediatric patients presenting for ORL procedures are usually healthy, they frequently have recurrent upper respiratory infections (URIs) or other respiratory issues. Elective ORL cases may be performed despite the patient having a current or recent URI because the enlarged tonsils and adenoids predispose these children to upper airway congestion which is only relieved by the surgery. Special focus on the history of breathing symptoms, including sleep apnea, and careful attention to the respiratory examination are important to planning the intraoperative and postoperative care of these patients.

Tonsillectomy and adenoidectomy

The vast majority of tonsillectomy and adenoidectomy (T&A) procedures are performed for treatment of obstructive sleep apnea (OSA), with a significant minority performed for the treatment of recurrent streptococcal throat infections. OSA is defined as "a disorder of breathing during sleep characterized by prolonged partial upper airway obstruction and/or intermittent complete obstruction (obstructive apnea) that disrupts normal ventilation during sleep and normal sleep patterns." The incidence of OSA is approximately 2% to 3% of the pediatric population, with the peak incidence occurring between the ages of 2 and 6 years. There is a continuum between snoring and OSA, but there also exist variations on thresholds for arousal, as well as degrees of obstruction that lead to hypopnea or apnea. The incidence of habitual snoring is up to 10% of the pediatric population, but the majority of these patients do not show symptoms of OSA, such as sleep disturbance, excessive daytime somnolence, attention disturbances, emotional instability, and headaches. Children with disordered breathing by clinical symptoms and history or by diagnostic polysomnog-

raphy (sleep study) may present for T&A to improve airway patency by removal of the enlarged lymphoid tissue. It is important to recognize that these patients may also have some degree of altered ventilatory response to hypercarbia and hypoxia and increased sensitivity to opioids and sedatives. Because of edema, the airway obstruction may not be completely resolved in the initial postoperative period. Children with significant sleep apnea, especially those younger than 3 years or those with concurrent diseases, should be observed overnight after tonsillectomy.

With anesthesia induction, these patients are at risk for partial or complete obstruction as the pharyngeal muscle tone decreases. During inhalation induction, holding continuous positive airway pressure (CPAP) by mask until the patient reaches a deeper plane of anesthesia may minimize the obstruction, or an oral airway may be required. Airway management is with either a midline endotracheal tube (ETT) or a flexible laryngeal mask airway [LMA]). Attention must be paid to not kinking or dislodging the ETT on placement and removal of the surgical instrument such as a Boyle–Davis mouth gag (Fig. 129.1). Maintenance of anesthesia can be achieved with inhaled or IV agents along with narcotic or by use of muscle relaxant to lessen the amount of anesthetic agent needed. In patients with a history of significant OSA, it is prudent to avoid sedative premedication and use morphine at 0.05 mg/kg or fentanyl at 1 µg/kg as intraoperative analgesia, and then titrate in more narcotic if needed after the patient is awake. Acetaminophen is routinely administered; there is also some interest in other analgesic adjuncts, such as small doses of ketamine or dexmedetomidine. Upon completion of the procedure, the surgeon may pass an orogastric tube to eliminate any blood that may have accumulated in the stomach; the oropharynx should be suctioned carefully to avoid initiating bleeding. Many anesthesiologists prefer awake extubation of tonsillectomy patients with OSA.

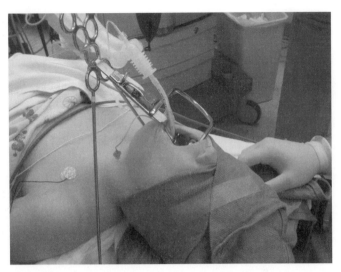

Figure 129.1. Patient positioning for tonsillectomy, with mouth gag in place.

Bronchoscopy

Bronchoscopy is performed to evaluate structural or functional airway abnormalities (subglottic stenosis, laryngomalacia) or for emergency situations, such as to remove a FB or to secure the airway in epiglottitis. Paramount to a safe anesthetic and successful operation involving a shared airway is close communication between the anesthesiologist and surgeon to discuss surgical objectives and patient comorbidities and to decide on an airway management plan prior to the procedure. Preparation includes having any equipment that could potentially be needed present and ready to use. Spontaneous ventilation may be preferable in some situations, relaxation and controlled ventilation in others. If cautery or laser is to be used, oxygen concentration should be decreased to minimize the potential for airway fire. If postoperative airway swelling is likely, dexamethasone at 0.25 to 0.5 mg/kg (maximum of 12 mg) should be considered.

Sevoflurane is frequently used for mask induction because it is the least pungent to the airways and is less arrhythmogenic in the presence of frequently used hemostatic sympathomimetics. It may be used by insufflation for airway procedures with spontaneous ventilation; however, patients will not remain in a deep plane of anesthesia for long if the agent is turned off, and operating room (OR) pollution may be an issue. Propofol's ability to blunt laryngeal reflexes and its antiemetic qualities make it useful in airway surgery, often in conjunction with remifentanil infusion or a small dose of fentanyl.

Understanding of the specific bronchoscopic system to be used is crucial, and the anesthesiologist must know how to use it to deliver oxygen and agents or to ventilate. Jet ventilation can be used with a suspension laryngoscope from a supraglottic position, where the risk of barotrauma is minimized. In this position, the adequacy of the ventilation is assessed by watching the chest rise and recoil; an inspiratory:expiratory (I:E) ratio of 1:3 (at a minimum) is suggested. Topical anesthesia by the

anesthesiologist or surgeon prior to starting the procedure may be accomplished by application of 1% to 4% lidocaine to the larynx, cords, and trachea (maximum of lidocaine at 4 mg/kg without epinephrine). Whether or not neuromuscular blocking agents are used, immobility of the patient is critical during both suspension of the larynx and, especially, when the trachea is instrumented to avoid tracheal injury and rupture. A laser may be used for treatment of laryngeal clefts, papillomas, or other airway lesions. Goggles should be worn by OR personnel to avoid retinal injury from direct or indirect laser beams, and the patient's eyes should be covered with a flame-retardant, light-impenetrable barrier. The airway device should be nonflammable, such as metal tubes or reinforced and/or wrapped tubes, and the cuff should be filled with water.

Some specific concerns exist for location and removal of a FB in the airway. FBs may not be radio-opaque and so may not be seen on chest radiograph; air trapping may also be indicative of a FB. A FB lodged in an airway can cause complete or partial fixed obstruction of all airways distal to its location or a dynamic obstruction creating a ball–valve obstruction leading to distal air trapping. The anesthesiologist must be prepared for bronchospasm, difficult ventilation, and possible hypoxemia during the time it takes for FB retrieval. The anesthetic technique of paralysis and controlled ventilation, or keeping the patient breathing spontaneously, is best chosen by preference consensus between the anesthesiologist and surgeon to optimize patient safety and surgical outcome. After the surgeon has grasped the FB with the surgical instrument, it is important to minimize patient movement or cough, which could cause the FB to be dislodged during removal. Nuts, like any organic FB, can cause a severe inflammatory reaction, and can also be very friable and difficult to extract. Postoperative care for these children can involve prolonged respiratory support in an intensive care unit (ICU) setting and treatment of acute respiratory distress syndrome (ARDS). A sharp FB can cause airway injury and bronchopleural fistulas. If the FB cannot be retrieved, open thoracotomy may be required.

Ear procedures

The most common procedure on the ear is bilateral myringotomy (BMT) with placement of ventilation tubes (tympanostomy tubes or grommets). Ear tubes are generally placed while the patient is under a brief mask anesthetic; the anesthesiologist must ensure a patent airway with the head turned and be able to maintain a still working field at critical points. Analgesia is usually provided with oral (PO) or rectal (PR) acetaminophen, or nasal fentanyl, because intravenous (IV) catheters are not usually inserted unless the patient has underlying medical issues such as cardiac disease.

Cochlear implant or cosmetic ear reconstruction may involve having the patient's head a significant distance away from the anesthesiologist and turned to the side; for this reason, and because of procedure duration, the patient is usually intubated. Patients having cosmetic ear reconstruction may have hemifacial microsomia or other syndromal abnormalities and should be evaluated carefully for possible difficult airway. Middle ear surgery requires a still and bloodless field for microscopic dissection, ability to monitor facial nerve function (avoidance of muscle relaxants), and avoidance of nitrous oxide during closure. Smooth emergence is desirable to minimize bleeding and disruption of the tympanic membrane.

Nasal surgery

Patients presenting for nasal surgery typically have some degree of nasal obstruction and often come for revision of a congenital anomaly (e.g., cleft lip or palate) or correction of a traumatic injury. Nasal surgery or manipulation of nasal bones may cause bleeding, so protecting the airway from nasal secretions with an LMA or oral ETT (OETT) is recommended. If significant bleeding is expected, a throat pack may be placed after the patient is intubated. The operative team must have a group approach to ensure that the pack is removed at the end of surgery. Careful vigilance to eye care is important as the eyes are often in the surgical field. Likewise, care should be taken to avoid placing too much pressure on a repaired nose with a face mask during airway management.

Choanal atresia (present in 1:7000 births) can occur incidentally or associated with other syndromes, such as CHARGE syndrome or association (coloboma of the eye, heart anomaly, choanal atresia, retardation, and genital and ear anomalies, and often including facial palsy, cleft palate, and dysphagia). Bilateral choanal atresia produces respiratory distress immediately after birth and requires respiratory support because infants are obligate nose breathers. Partial or unilateral atresia can sometimes be picked up from a history of cyanosis or respiratory distress when feeding.

Patients with nasal polyps or with chronic sinusitis will present for functional endoscopic sinus surgeries (FESS) to debride and clear soft tissue and bone and to open up the sinus cavities. Patients with cystic fibrosis are a large percentage of FESS patients, and, hence, associated perioperative concerns with this disease entity must be considered. To ensure adequate visualization for the surgeon, careful management of blood pressure with the use of controlled hypotension may be beneficial.

Topical vasoconstrictors (oxymetazoline, epinephrine, phenylephrine, and cocaine) are frequently used during nasal procedures, and the anesthesiologist must be aware of the potential for systemic absorption with cardiovascular side effects. The total dose should be appropriate for weight; phenylephrine should not exceed 20 μg/kg for 25 kg or less or 0.5 mg total for 25 kg and over. The use of pure β-blockade to treat elevated blood pressure from phenylephrine has caused cardiovascular collapse.

Neck surgery

Excision of thyroglossal duct or brachial cleft cysts, neck mass biopsy or excision, or removal of hemangiomas or other vascular malformations typically require general anesthesia with an OETT. Preoperative imaging is often available to view to ascertain if there is any airway compromise from the lesion. An array of ETT sizes is useful to have at hand in the event that the airway anatomy is not as anticipated. Also, if external hemangiomas exist, one should have a high suspicion that they may also exist within the airway. Airway hemangiomas or other vascular malformations can create blood in the airway on instrumentation. Induction and maintenance of anesthesia can be with IV or inhalational agents. Intra- and postoperative analgesia requirements are usually mild to minimal but may depend on the extent of the lesion excised. In the absence of patient comorbidities, these procedures can typically be day surgery in the absence of unusual findings or intraoperative airway events.

Pediatric anesthesia in remote locations

There is an increasing demand for anesthesiologists to provide anesthesia and sedation to children for therapeutic and diagnostic procedures that adults might tolerate with minimal or no sedation. Typically these locations are far removed from the OR in both physical location as well as type of environment. Provision of anesthesia or sedation in remote locations requires careful planning and coordination, as well as appropriately trained staff. The ASA has standards that should be met for non-OR anesthesia locations.

Institutions vary on specifics of who may provide pediatric sedation, but all should comply with guidelines from the American Academy of Pediatrics and the ASA as well as with individual institutional guidelines. In general, these guidelines speak to the need for an individual not involved in the procedure to monitor the patient, appropriate training and credentialing, appropriately sized equipment, and appropriate patient evaluation, monitoring, and discharge criteria. Clear consensual definitions of different levels of sedation within the institution are imperative for the safe care of patients. Understanding of the pharmacology and ability to "rescue" from a deeper-than-intended level of sedation are also hallmarks of the safety guidelines. Goals of sedation include minimizing physical discomfort and pain; controlling anxiety, minimizing psychological trauma, and providing amnesia; controlling behavior and/or movement to allow safe completion of the procedure; guarding the patient's safety and welfare throughout the procedure; and returning the patient to a state allowing safe discharge as determined by recognized criteria. Potential "red flags" for sedation by non-anesthesia providers include apnea, unstable cardiac disease, respiratory compromise (including recent URI), active gastroesophageal reflux or vomiting, hypotonia, tremor, allergy to barbiturates, and prior failed sedation. Medications used in pediatric sedation are listed in Table 129.3.

The choice of anesthetic technique for maintenance of general anesthesia during procedures in remote locations depends on patient, equipment, and procedural factors. Frequently, anesthesia can safely consist of spontaneous ventilation using a propofol infusion with nasal cannula oxygen and carbon

Table 129.3. Commonly used sedative medications

Drug	Usual dosing
Chloral hydrate	PO/PR: 25–50 mg/kg
Fentanyl	IV: 0.5 μg/kg
Midazolam	PO: 0.25–0.5 mg/kg
	IV: 0.025–0.05 mg/kg
Pentobarbital	IM/PO: 2–6 mg/kg
	IV: 2 mg/kg
Ketamine	IM: 3–7 mg/kg IV: 0.5–2 mg/kg

IM, intramuscular.

dioxide (CO_2) detection. For procedures that are long, involve pain, or affect the airway, or for patients with airway concerns, increased risk of aspiration, or cardiopulmonary or neuromuscular comorbidities, alternative strategies must be employed. Other considerations during the procedures include airway access, patient positioning, ability of the anesthesiologist to be in the room during the procedure, drugs or contrast agents used during the procedure, risks for life-threatening blood loss, and possible postoperative implications from the procedure. Adequate IV access, appropriately secured airways, availability of resuscitation medications and blood products, and possibly invasive pressure monitoring, urinary catheters, and temperature maintenance equipment should be used when appropriate. Anaphylactic reactions are rare for PO or IV agents but should be watched for and appropriately treated when contrast or other exogenous agents are used.

Postoperative management requires recovery staff experienced in the care of children and also familiar with issues that may arise after particular procedures. Small recovery locations within the radiology suite may be useful, but using the OR postanesthesia care unit (PACU) may be appropriate after hours or for complicated patients.

Anesthesia related to specific off-site locations

Computerized tomography

For these short, painless procedures it is not uncommon for PO as well as IV contrast to be given. The oral contrast is typically a clear iodine-containing solution that is diluted to an iso-osmolar liquid and given in a relatively large volume. Most anesthesiologists prefer waiting 2 hours before sedating or anesthetizing patients who have received oral contrast; in general, the quality of the scans is not adversely affected by this wait. CT scans that require only the briefest of immobility and no contrast may be done with mask sevoflurane and spontaneous ventilation.

Magnetic resonance imaging

MRI scans typically last 30 to 90 minutes and frequently involve IV contrast, such as gadolinium. Side effects of MRI contrast are relatively rare and mild but include nausea, vomiting, hives, or irritation at the injection site. Recent literature suggests that renal complications may occur with preexisting renal insufficiency, so patients should be screened clinically (and by laboratory evaluation if indicated) prior to gadolinium administration. Airway access is more limited than in other procedures especially in patients getting brain or spine imaging. Care should be taken to ensure that the airway device of choice is not kinked or dislodged after the coils are positioned.

Also of note are routine magnet safety issues and contraindications. Equipment incompatibilities can lead to patient burns or injury, magnet interference, and malfunction of implantable devices, such as pacemakers. Induction of general anesthesia and resuscitation of patients in the MRI suite can pose unique equipment-limiting problems. All equipment must be checked for compatibility. If at any time a patient needs to be resuscitated, he or she should be removed from the MRI room and the resuscitation should ensue in an area without magnet safety concerns.

Interventional radiology

Typical cases in the interventional radiology (IR) suite include angiography, image-guided biopsies and drain placements, placement of peripherally inserted central catheter (PICC) lines or indwelling central lines, and sclerotherapy or embolization of vascular or lymphatic malformations. Anesthetic management is tailored for variable lengths of procedures that often require controlled ventilation to facilitate breath holding for cineangiography or manipulation of CO_2 levels to control the amount of cerebral vasodilation. Maintaining temperature for a pediatric patient in the IR suite can be challenging because the IR suite must be maintained at a low ambient temperature to ensure proper function of the imaging equipment. Forced air warmers, fluid warmers, and warm blankets should be available.

Gastrointestinal endoscopy

Gastroenterology suites are designed to do esophagogastroduodenoscopies (EGDs) and colonoscopies in an efficient manner. As with any remote location, careful patient selection is paramount. Routine EGDs can be done with the patient in a lateral position, O_2 via nasal cannula, and routine monitoring including CO_2 detection. In straightforward patients, maintenance anesthesia may be by an IV technique using propofol with or without an opioid (fentanyl or remifentanil). Airway vigilance is crucial as complications of apnea, respiratory distress, and airway obstruction can occur during or after the EGD. Patients at high risk for aspiration, small patients, or those needing a larger endoscope may need intubation for upper endoscopy.

Radiation therapy

Daily treatments for several days at a time can create much patient anxiety and family stress. Planning should be done with the family to ensure that the NPO times are not excessive to ensure that patients maintain their nutrition during treatments. These treatments, although usually short, require complete immobility of the patient. To avoid staff exposure to radiation, the patient is monitored from a separate room via video cameras and remote monitors. The airway is typically not instrumented to minimize tracheal damage, and frequently a body mold or head mask, even for prone patients, is used to ensure consistent patient positioning for treatments. Oxygen delivery and CO_2 detection are accomplished by nasal cannula or by taping the mask and sampling line to the outside of the head mask.

Postanesthetic considerations for the pediatric patient

Skilled PACU nurses appropriately treating pain and nausea, and orienting patients with a parent, can ensure an uncomplicated recovery. PONV is frequent in middle ear surgeries or in cases in which blood collects in the stomach. Emergence delirium can complicate the recovery phase in young children. The etiology of this phenomenon is not clearly understood, but it occurs most frequently in patients from 2 to 5 years old and, more frequently, with volatile anesthetics. Comfort measures and adequate analgesia may be adequate in some patients, but in others resedation may at times be required. An anesthesiologist available to the PACU is important for appropriate respiratory vigilance and potential airway management. For more involved procedures or for patients with comorbidities, facilities should have the appropriate resources to care for the postoperative needs of these children (e.g., intensive care unit capability for patients with difficult airways or OSA).

Pediatric postoperative nausea and vomiting

PONV is seen commonly in pediatric patients. Despite the fact that PONV may be associated with significant complications, including wound dehiscence, pulmonary aspiration of gastric contents, bleeding, dehydration, and electrolyte disturbances, many reports and reviews in the literature suggest that PONV may be undertreated. Even mild PONV may lead to delayed hospital discharge, decreased parental satisfaction, and increased use of resources (physician and nursing care, administration of IV fluids and medications). PONV remains a major cause of unanticipated admission to the hospital after day surgery; consequently, prevention and management are seen as increasingly important (see Table 129.4).

Pediatric patients have a higher incidence of PONV than adults do, with a peak incidence of 30% to 50% in school-age children. The lowest incidence occurs in infants (5%), whereas preschool-age children have an intermediate incidence (20%). For prepubertal children, female sex is not consistently associated with an increased risk for PONV, although, in teenage patients, studies show that girls vomit significantly more often than boys do after general anesthesia. Children undergoing adenotonsillectomy, strabismus repair, orchidopexy, herniorrhaphy, middle ear surgery, dental procedures, or laparotomy are at

Table 129.4. Strategies to reduce baseline PONV risk

Perioperative period	Strategy	Evidence
Preoperative	Premedication (clonidine or midazolam)	Weak
Intraoperative	Avoidance of general anesthesia through use of regional anesthesia	Strong
	Use of propofol for induction and maintenance of anesthesia	Strong
	Avoidance of nitrous oxide	Strong
	Avoidance of volatile anesthetics	Strong
	Minimization of opioids	Weak
	Minimization of neostigmine	Weak
	Adequate hydration	Strong
Postoperative	Minimization of opioids	Strong
	Minimization of movement	Weak
	Timing of oral intake	Weak
	Adequate hydration	Strong

increased risk of PONV. The risk of PONV increases with duration of surgery and anesthesia. Pain has been shown to increase PONV, but opioid therapy is also a risk factor. Practitioners have long maintained that gastric distention, early movement, early drinking, and dehydration all contribute to a higher incidence of PONV.

Recently, Eberhart and colleagues published a study of a large series of pediatric patients in which a multivariable analysis was applied to identify PONV risk factors in children. This study identified four independent predictors of PONV: duration of surgery of at least 30 minutes, age of at least 3 years, strabismus surgery, and a positive history for PONV in the patient, sibling, or parent. Depending on the presence or absence of these factors, Eberhart and colleagues demonstrated that the risk for PONV was 9%, 10%, 30%, 55%, and 70% for 0, 1, 2, 3, or 4 of the independent predictors, respectively. Kranke and colleagues later validated this score, demonstrating comparable predictive value to the results in adult patients.

Benzodiazepines, particularly midazolam, have been shown to reduce PONV in children after strabismus repair and adenotonsillectomy. Clonidine has also been noted to have an antiemetic effect when given as a premedication during strabismus surgery. Not surprisingly, opioid analgesics used for preoperative and preprocedural sedation lead to increased PONV. Etomidate and ketamine are both associated with increased PONV, and several barbiturates, including methohexital and thiopental, have been shown to be more emetogenic than propofol. A large systematic review of propofol, involving several thousand pediatric patients, suggested that the best results may be achieved by using propofol for both induction and maintenance of anesthesia. Omission of nitrous oxide seems to lower the incidence of vomiting for some types of surgery, with less effect for other types of surgery. This practice has little effect, however, on the incidence of late PONV. Possible explanations for the greater emetogenic effect of nitrous oxide include diffusion of the gas into the middle ear or bowel, which through distention of these confined structures (vestibular apparatus

Table 129.5. Properties of antiemetic drugs

Class	Drug	Receptor antagonism	Dose, mg/kg	Antiemetic efficacy	Relative cost	Timing of administration
Corticosteroids	Dexamethasone	?	0.1–0.25	✓✓✓✓	$$	At induction
Anti-serotonins	Dolasetron	5-HT$_3$	0.035	✓✓✓✓	$$$$	Timing not important
	Granisetron	5-HT$_3$	0.04	✓✓✓✓	$$$$$	End of surgery
	Ondansetron	5-HT$_3$	0.05–0.1	✓✓✓✓	$$$$	End of surgery
	Tropisetron	5-HT$_3$	0.1	✓✓✓✓	$$$$	End of surgery
Antihistamines	Dimenhydrinate	Histamine	0.5	✓✓✓✓	$	End of surgery
	Diphenhydramine	Histamine	1.0–1.25	✓✓	$	End of surgery
	Hydroxyzine	Histamine	1.0	✓✓✓	$	End of surgery
Butyrophenones	Droperidol	Dopamine	0.025–0.075	✓✓✓✓	$$	End of surgery
Phenothiazines	Prochlorperazine	Dopamine	0.125	✓✓✓	$	End of surgery
	Promethazine	Dopamine	0.25–0.5	✓✓✓	$	At induction
	Perphenazine	Dopamine	0.025–0.07	✓✓✓	$	End of surgery
Anticholinergics	Scopolamine	Muscarinic acetylcholine	0.006	✓✓	$$$	Prior evening or 4 h before
Benzamides	Metoclopramide	Dopamine	0.1–0.25	✓	$$	End of surgery

and loops of bowel) might lead to activation of the medullary dopaminergic system and increased endogenous cerebrospinal opioid receptor agonists. Potent volatile anesthetic agents are all associated with a higher risk of nausea with few differences among the modern agents.

The cost effectiveness of therapy is one of the primary considerations governing whether or not to use PONV prophylaxis (see Table 129.5). In general, pharmacologic prophylaxis against PONV with older, less expensive antiemetics is cost-effective when the risk of emesis is as low as 10%, whereas prophylaxis with the more expensive agents may not be cost-effective until the risk of emesis is as high as 30% to 60%. A suggested hierarchical approach to managing PONV based on a child's calculated risk is to give no prophylaxis for low-risk patients, a selective serotonin 5-hydroxytryptamine type 3 (5-HT$_3$) antagonist for medium risk, and combination therapy (a serotonin antagonist and dexamethasone or a serotonin antagonist and a butyrophenone) or multimodal therapy (antiemetics from additional classes, use of strategies to minimize baseline risk for PONV, and nonpharmacologic prophylaxis) for high-risk patients.

The 5-HT$_3$ receptor antagonists (ondansetron, dolasetron, granisetron, and tropisetron) are most effective in the prophylaxis of PONV when given at the end of surgery. The 5-HT$_3$ antagonists for the most part have a favorable side-effect profile, although this class of drugs can prolong the QT interval. By a mechanism yet to be elucidated, the glucocorticoid dexamethasone effectively prevents nausea and vomiting. Droperidol, a neuroleptic antagonist of central dopamine receptors and a butyrophenone, is an effective drug for the prevention of PONV. One meta-analysis evaluating prophylaxis for children undergoing strabismus repair revealed that droperidol had the greatest antiemetic benefit with a number needed to treat (NNT)

of 4. Although sedation, lethargy, agitation, and extrapyramidal effects have been reported with the commonly used pediatric doses, the most serious adverse effects are estimated to occur in less than 1% of all children. The 2001 US Food and Drug Administration (FDA) black box warning regarding possible QT prolongation leading to torsades de pointes has limited the use of droperidol. Some initial adult studies have shown the efficacy of haloperidol, another butyrophenone, but without large enough numbers to suggest that it is safer from a cardiovascular standpoint. Antihistamines, such as dimenhydrinate, have shown moderate efficacy in some studies but not in others; they can also have profound sedative effects, but are inexpensive and therefore have a relatively favorable cost/efficacy ratio. Central nervous system antimuscarinics effectively prevent emesis related to vestibular stimulation, one of the proposed mechanisms for morphine-induced PONV. Transdermal scopolamine has been found useful for the control of nausea in the setting of morphine PCA in older children but is not recommended in children < 40 kilograms in weight. Drugs with a lack of evidence of effect include metoclopramide in standard clinical doses, ginger root, and cannabinoids. Examples of agents with possible efficacy but too little evidence include the phenothiazines (promethazine and prochlorperazine) and ephedrine. A new class of antiemetic drugs, the neurokinin-1 (NK$_1$) receptor antagonists, has been shown to provide protection against multiple different emetogenic stimuli (motion, chemotherapy, radiation therapy, narcotics, other emetogenic drugs and treatments), whereas other conventional antiemetic drugs are typically effective against only a few of these stimuli. In addition, preliminary evidence shows promising results with opioid antagonists (naloxone, nalmefene) for reduction of nausea, vomiting, and a need for rescue antiemetic medication in children and adolescents.

In adults, a meta-analysis of nonpharmacologic PONV prophylaxis demonstrated antiemetic efficacy with acupuncture, transcutaneous electrical nerve stimulation, acupoint stimulation, and acupressure. Pressure, puncture, or stimulation of the P6 or Neiguan point located on the anterior surface of the wrist approximately three finger breadths above the distal skin crease of the wrist and between the tendons of the flexor carpi radialis and palmaris longus muscles reduced the incidence of nausea and vomiting and need for rescue medication in adults. In children, acupuncture after induction of anesthesia was ineffective in reducing PONV after strabismus repair, although the antiemetic efficacy of this technique may in fact depend on the timing and duration of therapy. Further studies in children are needed to confirm the beneficial antiemetic effect that these nonpharmacologic techniques are reported to have in randomized controlled trials for adults.

Suggested readings

American Society of Anesthesiologists. Guidelines for nonoperating room anesthetizing locations, 2003. Available at: http://www. asahq.org/publicationsAndServices/standards/14.pdf. Accessed June 1, 2008.

American Society of Anesthesiologists Task Force on Management of the Difficult Airway. Practice guidelines for management of the difficult airway: an updated report. *Anesthesiology* 2003; 98:1269–1277.

American Society of Anesthesiologists Task Force on Sedation and Analgesia by Non-Anesthesiologists. Practice guidelines for sedation and analgesia by non-anesthesiologists. *Anesthesiology* 2002; 96:1004–1017.

American Thoracic Society. Standards and indications for cardiopulmonary sleep studies in children. *Am J Respir Crit Care Med* 1996; 153:866–878.

Bisonnette B, Dalens BJ. (eds.). *Pediatric Anesthesia.* New York: McGraw-Hill; 2002.

Bolton CM, Myles PS, Carlin JB, et al. Randomized, double-blind study comparing efficacy of moderate-dose metoclopramide and ondansetron for the prophylactic control of postoperative nausea and vomiting in children after tonsillectomy. *Br J Anaesth* 2007; 99:699–703.

Bolton CM, Myles PS, Nolan T, et al. Prophylaxis of postoperative vomiting in children undergoing tonsillectomy: a systematic review and meta-analysis. *Br J Anaesth* 2006; 97:593–604.

Brown KA, Moss IR. Opiate usage in children with obstructive sleep apnea syndrome. *Anesth Analg* 2007; 105:547–548.

Chin T, Liu C, Wei C. The morphology of the contralateral internal inguinal rings is age-dependent in children with unilateral inguinal hernia. *J Pediatr Surg* 1995; 30:1663–1665.

Cote CJ, Wilson S, American Academy of Pediatrics Work Group on Sedation. Guidelines for monitoring and management of pediatric patients during and after sedation for diagnostic and therapeutic procedures: an update. *Pediatrics* 2006; 118:2587–2602.

Diaz JH. Croup and epiglottitis in children: the anesthesiologist as diagnostician. *Anesth Analg* 1985; 64: 621–633.

Diez L. Assessing the willingness of parents to pay for reducing emesis in children. *Pharmacoeconomics* 1998; 13:589–595.

Eberhart LH, Geldner G, Kranke P, et al. The development and validation of a risk score to predict the probability of postoperative vomiting in pediatric patients. *Anesth Analg* 2004; 99:1630–1637.

Edler AA, Mariano ER, Golianu B, et al. An analysis of factors influencing postanesthesia recovery after pediatric ambulatory tonsillectomy and adenoidectomy. *Anesth Analg* 2007; 104:784–789.

Gan TJ. Risk factors for postoperative nausea and vomiting. *Anesth Analg* 2006; 102:1884–1898.

Gan TJ, Meyer TA, Apfel CC, et al. Society for Ambulatory Anesthesia guidelines for the management of postoperative nausea and vomiting. *Anesth Analg* 2007; 105:1615–1628.

Groudine SB, Holliner I, Jones J, DeBouno BA, the Phenylephrine Advisory Committee. New York State guidelines on the topical use of phenylephrine in the operating room. *Anesthesiology* 2000; 92:859–864.

Hackel A, Badgwell JM, Binding RR, et al. Guidelines for the pediatric perioperative anesthesia environment. *Pediatrics* 1999; 103:512–515.

Henderson K, Sethna NF, Berde CB. Continuous caudal anesthesia for inguinal hernia repair in former preterm infants. *J Clin Anesth* 1993; 5:129–133.

Hopper N, Albanese A, Ghirardello S, Maghnie M. The pre-operative endocrine assessment of craniopharyngiomas. *J Pediatr Endocrinol Metab* 2006; 19(Suppl 1):325–327.

Kaatsch P, Rickert CH, Kuhl J, et al. Population-based epidemiologic data on brain tumors in German children. *Cancer* 2001; 92:3155–3164.

Katz ES, D'Ambrosio CM. Pathophysiology of pediatric obstructive sleep apnea. *Proc Am Thorac Soc* 2008; 5:253–262.

Kemmotsu H, Oshima Y, Joe K, Mouri T. The features of contralateral manifestations after the repair of unilateral inguinal hernia. *J Pediatr Surg* 1998; 33:1099–1102.

Kovac AL. Management of postoperative nausea and vomiting in children. *Paediatr Drugs* 2007; 9:47–69.

Kumar VH, Clive J, Rosenkrantz TS, et al. Inguinal hernia in preterm infants (< or = 32-week gestation). *Pediatr Surg Int* 2002; 18:147–152.

Lumeng JC, Chervin RD. Epidemiology of pediatric obstructive sleep apnea. *Proc Am Thorac Soc* 2008; 5:242–252.

Schier F. Laparoscopic inguinal hernia repair–a prospective personal series of 542 children. *J Pediatr Surg* 2006; 41:1081–1084.

Thomas M, Woodhead G, Masood N, et al. Motion sickness as a predictor of postoperative vomiting in children aged 1–16 years. *Paediatr Anaesth* 2007; 17:61–63.

Watcha MF, Smith I. Cost-effectiveness analysis of antiemetic therapy for ambulatory surgery. *J Clin Anesth* 1994; 6:370–377.

Watcha MF, White PF. Postoperative nausea and vomiting: its etiology, treatment, and prevention. *Anesthesiology* 1992; 77:162–184.

Welborn LG, Rice LJ, Hannallah RS, et al. Postoperative apnea in former preterm infants: prospective comparison of spinal and general anesthesia. *Anesthesiology* 1990; 72:838–842.

Welborn LG, Hannallah RS, Fink R, et al. High-dose caffeine suppresses postoperative apnea in former preterm infants. *Anesthesiology* 1989; 71:347–349.

Wisselo TL, Stuart C, Muris P. Providing parents with information before anaesthesia: what do they really want to know? *Paediatr Anaesth* 2004; 14:299–307.

Neonatal surgical emergencies

Noah E. Gordon and Mary Ellen McCann

Introduction

The impact of congenital malformations in pediatrics is significant. Three percent of newborns are born with congenital malformations, and 20% of neonatal mortality is secondary to congenital malformations. The care of a neonate with a major congenital malformation is resource-intensive. In one study, newborns with congenital malformations accounted for one-fourth of all neonatal intensive care unit (NICU) referrals, one-third of total NICU days, and nearly half of NICU costs. Surgical interventions and their accompanying sequelae are major contributors to the costs, morbidity, and mortality of these neonates. The disease processes, anesthesia, and surgery all can interfere with developmental changes and threaten survival.

General approach to the neonate

Preanesthetic considerations

Neonates requiring urgent or emergent surgical intervention are approached in the standard fashion, with steps taken to gain an understanding of the patient's physiology, the disease process, and implications of the surgical plan. A detailed history and physical examination are essential. Of particular interest in the history are the mother's pregnancy, the course of labor and delivery, and events over the first hours to days of life. Depending on the results of the history and physical, it may be important to do laboratory and radiologic assessments as well. (See Table 130.1.)

Transitional circulation

Many newborns requiring urgent or emergent surgical procedures arrive in the operating room (OR) with a transitional circulation – so-called because it has aspects of both the adult series circulation and fetal parallel circulation owing to the presence of a patent ductus arteriosus (PDA), as well as possible interatrial and/or interventricular communications. There is the potential for these nonrestrictive shunts to lead to large right-to-left or left-to-right shunts, depending on the balance between the pulmonary and systemic vascular resistances (PVR and SVR, respectively). With left-to-right shunting, overcirculation of the pulmonary vascular bed can lead to pulmonary edema, a low-cardiac-output state (with impaired flow to the cerebral, coronary, renal, and splanchnic beds), and, eventually, pulmonary vascular occlusive disease. With right-to-left shunting, bypassing the pulmonary bed leads to impaired oxygenation and ventilation with ensuing cyanosis.

Apnea

Unlike older infants, premature and term neonates paradoxically decrease their respiratory rates in response to hypoxia (a response that is further exacerbated by hypothermia) and exhibit little, if any, increased minute ventilation in response to increasing arterial carbon dioxide levels. Risk factors for true apnea in the postoperative period include a postconceptual age of 60 weeks or less and anemia in ex-premature neonates. Caffeine is a centrally acting respiratory stimulant that, in doses of 10 mg/kg (20 mg/kg caffeine citrate), can prevent or reduce apnea in this population.

Hypoglycemia

Glycogen stores are small in premature infants and neonates; therefore, newborns are at a high risk for hypoglycemia when

Table 130.1. Perinatal conditions and their associated potential perioperative problems

Condition	Perioperative problems
Asphyxia	Hypoglycemia, hypocalcemia, hyperkalemia, impaired cerebral autoregulation, depressed myocardial function, decreased gut perfusion, shock, coagulopathy
Infants of diabetic mothers	Hypoglycemia, hypocalcemia
Maternal IV drug use	Opioid withdrawal, infectious agents (hepatitis B/C, human immunodeficiency virus), seizures
Prematurity	Hypoglycemia, respiratory distress syndrome, postoperative apnea, ROP, temperature instability
Small for gestational age	Hypoglycemia, hypocalcemia, polycythemia/hyperbilirubinemia, temperature instability, congenital anomalies, increased incidence of pulmonary aspiration/pneumonia
Large for gestational age	Birth injury (brachial/phrenic nerve, fractured clavicle), hypoglycemia, hypocalcemia, polycythemia/hyperbilirubinemia, meconium aspiration

Table 130.2. Glucose and electrolyte requirements in the premature and term newborn

Nutrient/ Electrolyte	Requirement	Comment
Glucose	2–4 mg/kg/min	Most newborns
	8–10 mg/kg/min	SGA/LGA infants
	>15 mg/kg/min	Infants of diabetic mothers
Sodium	None	For first 24h for most newborns
	2–4 mEq/d	Day 2 and beyond
	>4 mEq/d	GI, renal, skin losses
	Variable	Drug and metabolic effects
Potassium	None	First 24–48 h for most newborns
	1–3 mEq/d	Day 2–3 and beyond, ensure normal urine output
	<1 mEq/d	Requirements lower in VLBW and ELBW infants
	>3 mEq/d	GI, renal, iatrogenic losses – replace cautiously
Calcium	200–400 mg/kg/d	Calcium gluconate dosing (calcium chloride contains three times as much elemental calcium)
	Variable	Premature, SGA/LGA infants

LGA, large for gestational age; SGA, small for gestational age; VLBW, very low birth weight; ELBW, extremely low birth weight.

exogenous glucose is not administered. The threshold for defining hypoglycemia in the neonate is controversial but the American Academy of Pediatrics suggests an operational definition of <36 mg/dl in an asymptomatic neonate with the goal of maintaining the plasma glucose level of 45 mg/dl or greater. There are no recent data to support a lower threshold for premature infants.

In the newborn, hypoglycemia has profound consequences, including apnea, hypotension, bradycardia, seizures, and neurologic injury. If a bolus of glucose is needed, dextrose 10% in water ($D_{10}W$) at 1 to 2 ml/kg should be administered, followed by careful monitoring of serum glucose. Whereas term neonates need glucose at 5 to 8 mg/kg/min to prevent hypoglycemia, premature and small-for-gestational-age newborns generally require an infusion rate of 8 to 10 mg/kg/min. Intraoperative infusion of D_{10} at maintenance rates will deliver glucose at approximately 7 mg/kg/min and should be adequate to avoid hypoglycemia. Fluids for replacement of insensible, deficit, and blood losses should not contain glucose, to avoid hyperglycemia. (See Table 130.2.)

Retinopathy of prematurity

Retinopathy of prematurity (ROP) is a progressive vascular overgrowth of the retinal vessels eventually leading to intraocular hemorrhage, retinal detachment, and blindness. Seen primarily in premature newborns exposed to a high fraction of inspired oxygen content (FiO_2), ROP has also been described in term babies on room air or in infants with cyanotic congenital heart disease. Despite the fact that prematurity and oxygen exposure are just two of many (mostly unknown) risk factors for ROP, it is recommended that the inspired oxygen concentration

be minimized for babies less than 44 weeks postconceptual age to achieve a target oxygen saturation in the low to mid-90s.

Temperature management

Neonates lose heat rapidly because of a reduced amount of subcutaneous fat and a large surface area. With limited ability to maintain their body temperatures through shivering or even nonshivering thermogenesis, the newborn is at risk for significant temperature fluctuations in the perioperative period – with transport, exposure during placement of intravascular lines and invasive monitoring, and heat losses during surgery. Measures must be taken to protect against heat loss. During transport to the OR, the neonate should remain covered with care taken to continue adequate monitoring and access in a heated isolette. The OR should be warmed to greater than 27°C. A radiant heat warmer is useful during line placement and preparation. Forced-air warming blankets are now available that go under the entire infant and include plastic drapes to cover noninvolved areas. Other intraoperative strategies include heating and humidifying inspired gases, warming intravenous (IV) fluids and blood products, and warming the surgical prep and irrigation solutions.

Monitoring

Two pulse oximeter probes should be available – one preductal (right hand) and one postductal (either foot) – to measure and compare the magnitude and direction of possible shunting across a PDA. Capnography may be unreliable owing to a large dead space in the breathing system, which can be reduced with specialized endotracheal tubes and low-volume connections. A precordial or esophageal stethoscope will permit detection of changes in heart rate or intensity of heart sounds, which may serve as useful indicators of cardiac function, intravascular volume status, and depth of anesthesia. A urinary catheter is of assistance for fluid balance in long cases. Neuromuscular monitoring is often challenging in small, premature newborns.

Invasive monitoring, principally an intra-arterial catheter, should be placed for cases with anticipated sudden or dramatic changes in hemodynamics, acid–base status, or oxygenation and ventilation to allow beat-to-beat monitoring of blood pressure and repeated sampling of hemoglobin and platelet counts, coagulation status, electrolytes, and arterial blood gases. Central venous catheters are infrequently used, and pulmonary artery catheters are rarely used in neonates for hemodynamic monitoring; however, the anesthesiologist can gain valuable information from the arterial line tracing. In hypovolemia, the arterial waveform is narrow, suggesting low stroke volume from inadequate preload, and there is marked respiratory variation in the tracing, suggesting collapse of great veins and changes in preload during the respiratory cycle. The dicrotic notch is present in the middle third of the downstroke in euvolemia, but in the outer third (or absent) in hypovolemia. A sluggish increase and decreased slope of ascent of the arterial waveform suggests diminished left ventricular function or the presence of aortic valve disease. Low amplitude and a rapid rate of increase of ascent suggests low SVR.

Fluid requirements

Intraoperative fluid therapy has four main components: maintenance fluid, replacement of fluid deficit, replacement of blood loss, and replacement of insensible and other losses. Maintenance fluid covers the normal insensible water loss from the respiratory epithelium and evaporative losses from the skin. Based on estimations of the interaction between metabolic rate and fluid requirements, this maintenance fluid can be calculated as: 4 ml/kg for the first 10 kg, 2 ml/kg for the next 10 kg, and 1 ml/kg for each additional kg over 20 kg. Fluid deficits are simply calculated by multiplying the hourly maintenance deficit by the number of hours since the last fluid intake, and can be replaced in most cases over 3 hours: 50% of the fluid deficit is given in the first hour, 25% in the second hour, and the final 25% in the third hour in the OR. Greater insensible losses above maintenance can take place from surgical trauma resulting in translocation of extracellular fluid from the intravascular space into the interstitial space, producing edema in the bowel wall and mesentery or in the subcutaneous tissues and muscle. Initial guidelines for replacement of these "third-space" losses are as follows: 2 to 5 ml/kg/h for peripheral or superficial surgeries, 5 to 10 ml/kg/h for open abdominal or thoracic surgery, and greater than 10 ml/kg/h for extensive abdominal surgery, titrated to heart rate and perfusion. As in older children and adults, hemorrhage can be acutely replaced with 3 ml of crystalloid per 1 ml of estimated blood loss to re-expand the intravascular blood volume. If colloids, such as albumin, are preferred, this can be accomplished using a 1:1 volume ratio.

Management of surgical urgencies and emergencies

Gastroschisis and omphalocele

Gastroschisis and omphalocele are defects of the abdominal wall at or near the umbilicus. Gastroschisis is a defect of the abdominal wall that occurs to the right of the umbilicus and lacks a peritoneal covering (see Fig. 130.1). It is hypothesized that this defect results from a weakening of the abdominal wall as the right umbilical vein regresses during development. Gastroschisis is typically not associated with major congenital anomalies or syndromes, although as many as 10% of affected infants will suffer intestinal atresia secondary to vascular compromise of the affected segment arising from a constricting fascial defect. In contrast, omphalocele (Fig. 130.2) is considered to be a more serious abdominal wall defect, given that associated anomalies are common (trisomies 18 and 21, other midline defects including bladder exstrophy, and congenital heart disease). Pathophysiologically, omphalocele is a herniation of abdominal viscera through the base of the umbilical cord and possesses a covering of peritoneum. Like gastroschi-

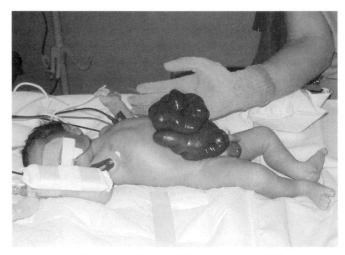

Figure 130.1. Gastroschisis Courtesy of Roberta E. Sonnino, M.D.

sis, the intestines fail to rotate normally prior to returning to the abdominal cavity during development.

Newborns presenting for repair of abdominal wall defects require urgent surgery, as the large exposed surface area allows for substantial evaporative fluid and heat losses and presents a significant infection risk. For patients with omphalocele, there is a 20% incidence of cardiac anomalies, and there should be a low threshold for an echocardiogram, particularly if a murmur is noted. In addition, omphalocele may be seen in Beckwith–Wiedemann syndrome, with associated hypoglycemia, which requires frequent glucose monitoring during the perioperative period and macroglossia, which can make intubation challenging.

If not already intubated, these babies should be treated as having full stomachs, and gastric decompression should be undertaken prior to induction and intubation. Given the possible depleted intravascular volume status, care should be exercised by using an induction agent that would further reduce preload (propofol, thiopental) or contractility in patients with

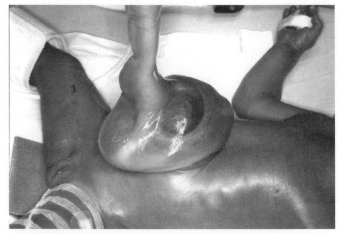

Figure 130.2. Omphalocele Courtesy of Roberta E. Sonnino, M.D.

congenital heart disease (where etomidate would be the better choice). If blood cultures are negative, an epidural catheter can be inserted and used intraoperatively in conjunction with a light general anesthetic or for postoperative analgesia, threaded via either the lumbar or caudal route. If an epidural is not placed, an opioid-based technique with some vapor may be most hemodynamically stable (these patients will remain intubated). Good IV access should be established for the large anticipated third-space fluid losses (use crystalloid and/or colloids such as 5% albumin) and possible bleeding.

In general, surgical planning will involve either reducing the defect through staged procedures or undertaking primary closure if possible. If there is insufficient space in the abdomen, reduction may cause bowel ischemia and deleterious respiratory mechanics from increased intra-abdominal pressure leading to difficulties with oxygenation and ventilation. The anesthesia team will need to effectively communicate any observed decreases in pulmonary compliance (increased peak inspiratory pressures [PIPs], decreased tidal volumes, decreased minute ventilation) or increases in central venous pressure (if a central line is present) with surgical manipulation, placement of packing and retractors, or attempted abdominal closure. A primary repair is typically aborted if bladder pressures are transduced at greater than 20 mm Hg or if PIPs are noted at 35 mm Hg. Clinical changes suggestive of decreased peripheral perfusion or impaired venous return may also indicate inability to successfully reduce these defects during the initial procedure. In the case of staged closure, a prosthetic material is applied to the edges of the defect, creating a tubular silo. After gradually being reduced in the NICU over a period of several days, the abdomen is finally closed primarily. Intestinal function typically returns within a week for omphalocele and within a couple of weeks to a month for gastroschisis. Given the obvious nutritional concerns with this delayed bowel function in a catabolic newborn, a central line is often placed during the initial operation for parenteral nutrition.

Congenital diaphragmatic hernia

Congenital diaphragmatic hernia (CDH) is a posterolateral defect of the diaphragm that occurs in 1:4000 live births. A Bochdalek hernia results from a failure of the normal closure of the pleuroperitoneal canal during the eighth week of gestation, leading to a communication between the abdominal and thoracic cavities. Consequently, the intestine migrates into the chest as it returns from the umbilical cord. (See Fig. 130.3.) Resultant compression of the developing lung leads to a small and abnormally developed lung or lungs. Because the bowel is in an abnormal location, malrotation may occur (as mentioned earlier in the case of abdominal wall defects). Whereas more than 90% of hernias are on the left side, only 5% are on the right, which typically contain only a portion of the liver and a small amount of intestine. The earlier in gestation the hernia occurs, the greater the degree of ensuing pulmonary hypopla-

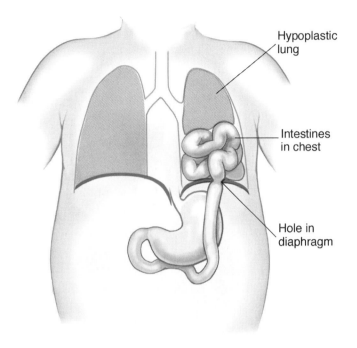

Figure 130.3. Congenital diaphragmatic hernia.

sia on both sides – with mediastinal shift, the development of the contralateral lung is restricted as well. As the hypoplastic lung contains fewer alveolar and capillary units; the pulmonary vasculature is also abnormal. Both undeveloped and composed of abnormally increased smooth muscle, the pulmonary circulation may be highly reactive to factors affecting PVR (see Table 130.3). One-quarter of afflicted babies have associated congenital diseases.

Now that immediate surgical repair is no longer routine, these patients are stabilized in the NICU (sometimes requiring extracorporeal membrane oxygenation [ECMO] if oxygenation and ventilation are significantly impaired), where additional cardiac and pulmonary evaluation and optimization can be performed preoperatively. For initial intubation, the stomach

Table 130.3. Factors affecting PVR and SVR in the premature and term newborn

PVR		SVR	
Increase	**Decrease**	**Increase**	**Decrease**
↑ Hematocrit	↓ Hematocrit	↑ Hematocrit	↓ Hematocrit
↑ $PaCO_2$	↓ $PaCO_2$	Vasopressin	Nitrates
α-agonists	Vasopressin	α-agonists	PDE-inhibitors
↓ FiO_2/PaO_2	↑ FiO_2/PaO_2	↓ Temperature	↑ Temperature
High PIPs, PEEP	Nitrates	Ca^{2+}	β-agonists
↓ pH	PDE-inhibitors		
↓ Temperature	Ventilation at FRC		
Ca^{2+}	↑ pH		
	β-agonists		

PDE, phosphodiesterase; FRC, functional residual capacity; PEEP, positive end-expiratory pressure.

should be decompressed and mask ventilation avoided. The approach to ventilatory management of the infant with CDH has changed over the last decade, with the recognition that barotrauma probably caused the most significant morbidity and mortality. Thus management has evolved from maintaining adequate oxygenation and normocarbia at all costs to permissive hypercapnia and early use of therapies to minimize mean airway pressure. Whereas small defects may be closed primarily, larger defects may require use of a thin patch of synthetic material. During transport and in the OR, inotropes and pressors (dopamine and epinephrine) should be available for boluses and infusions, while avoiding overaggressive volume administration. Good IV access and an arterial line should be available for surgery and are frequently in place from ICU care. Assuming normal coagulation (check coagulation if the liver is up in a right-sided CDH), an epidural catheter can be threaded via the caudal or lumbar region and used for both intraoperative and postoperative analgesia. If no epidural is planned, an opioid-based technique can be used for sympathetic suppression to control potentially deleterious surges in PVR.

In the OR, it should be remembered that overaggressive ventilation can lead to pneumothorax (usually of the overdistended "good lung" opposite the herniation), manifesting as sudden respiratory embarrassment or cardiovascular collapse. This diagnosis should always be at the top of the differential.

Ventilation should be managed by mimicking the ventilator settings that were successful preoperatively (if applicable), and it should be realized that pressures and tidal volumes will change as the compliance changes when the intestines are returned to the abdominal cavity. Muscle relaxation should be continued to optimize chest wall compliance and pulmonary mechanics. After the abdominal contents are reduced, the lungs should be expanded with manual ventilation (limiting PIPs to 35 mm Hg to avoid the potential for barotrauma, volutrauma, and/or possible pneumothorax). As always, good communication in the OR is essential: Alert the surgeons if abdominal closure leads to worsening PIPs, oxygenation, or ventilation. All but the most minimal of these defects will require postoperative ventilation and ongoing management of PVR.

Tracheoesophageal fistula and esophageal atresia

Esophageal atresia (EA) encompasses a spectrum of anomalies that occur early in gestation (22–36 days), as the trachea buds from the primitive foregut. Failure of the normal development of the esophagus and separation of the trachea from the esophagus result in one of five possible outcomes: EA with distal tracheoesophageal fistula (TEF; 85%), isolated EA (8%), TEF without EA (5%, also referred to as "H-type"), EA with proximal TEF (1%), or EA with proximal and distal TEF (1%). (See Fig. 130.4.) Because other developing organs are vulnerable to the

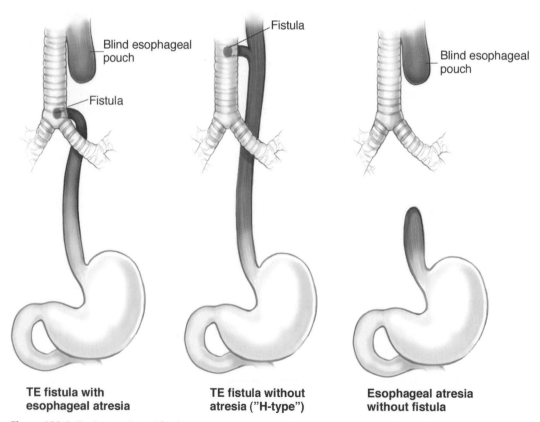

TE fistula with esophageal atresia **TE fistula without atresia ("H-type")** **Esophageal atresia without fistula**

Figure 130.4. Tracheoesophageal fistula types.

same insult, associated anomalies are common (50% or more), particularly vertebral, anal atresia and other GI abnormalities, cardiac (ventricular septal defect [VSD], PDA, tetralogy of Fallot, atrial septal defect [ASD], coarctation of the aorta), renal abnormalities, and limb malformations otherwise known as the VACTERL associations. There is also a high incidence of TEF among children born with trisomy 21. The diagnosis is made presumptively when a nasogastric tube cannot be advanced past 10 cm and gas is present in the stomach on radiograph. These babies get into trouble because they aspirate from pooling oropharyngeal secretions and because increasing amounts of stomach gas can worsen pulmonary compliance and lead to atelectasis, hypoxemia, and impaired ventilation. The risk of aspiration can be minimized if repair is undertaken within a few days of birth. Repairs are performed all at once or in a staged manner (for babies weighing less than 1000 g, with pure EA, or critical anomalies, often a gastrostomy tube is placed first, followed by patient stabilization, and deferred repair). The operation is typically performed in the left lateral decubitus position for a right thoracotomy (90% of cases), via a retropleural or transpleural approach. Some isolated TEF (H-type) can be approached through a neck incision.

General anesthesia is used, but can be augmented with a caudal or lumbar epidural catheter after the airway is secured. To minimize gastric distention, spontaneous ventilation is maintained or minimal pressures are used if mask ventilation is required prior to intubation. It is important to position the endotracheal tube to avoid ventilating into the fistula. Classically, the endotracheal tube is advanced to the right mainstem bronchus and slowly withdrawn until breath sounds are heard bilaterally, at which point the tip will be just above the carina (hopefully distal to the fistula), and the tube is rotated so that the bevel opens anteriorly – away from the posteriorly positioned fistula. If a large fistula exists, bronchoscopy with placement of a Fogarty catheter prior to intubation may improve ventilation. A gastrostomy tube, if placed, may help by serving as a pop-off valve for the gastric air, but can also encourage ventilation into the stomach as gases follow the path of least resistance (in which case the gastrostomy tube may have to be clamped or placed to water seal).

Blood loss is typically minimal, and an arterial line is typically placed for monitoring blood gases as well as perfusion with potential compression of great vessels. If no epidural is placed, muscle relaxation and moderate-to-high dose opioid is used (unless spontaneous ventilation is still being used until ligation of the fistula). At the point where the surgeon is approaching the fistula, it may be necessary to pass an orogastric tube to identify the proximal pouch. At the end of the repair, a nasogastric tube is passed under direct visual inspection by the surgeon and carefully taped in place. At the end of the case, extubation may be considered with competing pros and cons: immediate extubation in the OR would limit the time the endotracheal tube spends lying against the suture line, but the need for urgent reintubation might compromise a new esophageal anastomosis. If not extubated in the OR, the baby is typically sedated and ventilated for a few days in the NICU to allow healing.

Necrotizing enterocolitis

Necrotizing enterocolitis (NEC) results from ischemia and/or inflammation of the GI tract. It most commonly affects the terminal ileum and occurs in stressed, premature infants, with a severity of symptoms, complications, and a mortality rate that is inversely proportional to gestational age. Although its specific etiology is not completely understood, NEC is linked to mucosal injury from decreased mesenteric blood flow, which may be caused by reduced cardiac output from fetal asphyxia, a PDA, postnatal apnea, heart failure, arrhythmia, or severe bradycardia and hypoxemia. Other factors include enteral feeding of small preterm infants, use of hyperosmolar formula, bacterial infection, intestinal dysfunction, gram-negative endotoxemia, polycythemia, congenital heart disease, and a history of umbilical artery catheterization or exchange transfusion. The combination of bacteria and ischemia seems to be critical, with a wide range of organisms associated with NEC, including *Escherichia coli, Enterobacter, Klebsiella,* and *Pseudomonas.*

Although NEC may resolve with conservative management (antibiotics, gastric decompression, no enteral feeds), it may progress to necrosis and perforation requiring either laparotomy with bowel resection and stoma formation or a drainage procedure, according to surgeon preference (evidence supports drains for weight < 1500 g). Absolute indications for operation include pneumoperitoneum and intestinal gangrene (positive paracentesis). Relative indications for surgical intervention include signs of clinical deterioration (e.g., worsening metabolic acidosis, respiratory failure, oliguria or hypovolemia, thrombocytopenia, leucopenia or leukocytosis), portal vein gas or dilated loops of bowel on abdominal imaging, erythema of the abdominal wall, or discoloration of the abdominal wall (suggestive of intraperitoneal meconium).

Most infants will be intubated for stabilization in the NICU, but, if not, full-stomach precautions should be employed after effective preoxygenation. Atropine may be considered prior to laryngoscopy. With concern for ROP, avoid excessive inspired oxygen concentration with an oxygen–air mixture during the maintenance. Consider use of a NICU ventilator if high ventilator support settings are needed. Because extubation will not usually be planned, a hemodynamically stable opioid-based anesthetic is appropriate. An arterial line, preferably preductal, is needed for hemodynamic monitoring, to follow oxygenation and ventilation, and for sampling laboratory tests. Good IV access is needed for volume resuscitation (a central line may be necessary if access is difficult). Five percent albumin boluses, at 10 to 20 ml/kg at a time, are typically needed to maintain intravascular volume, although dopamine and even epinephrine may be needed for additional hemodynamic support. Fluid therapy is geared to attempt to maintain intravascular volume but minimize bowel wall edema, which may make ventilation difficult with closure. Transfusion of packed cells

Table 130.4. Anesthetic considerations for various surgical urgencies and emergencies

Surgical diagnosis	Preoperative considerations	Intraoperative considerations	Postoperative considerations
Gastroschisis and omphalocele	RDS if premature Cardiac anomalies (omphalocele) Sepsis Intestinal atresia Hypovolemia Hypoglycemia	Hypovolemia Hypothermia Hypercarbia Hypoxemia Respiratory acidosis Metabolic acidosis Atelectasis Volume overload/pulmonary edema	Oxygenation/ventilation problems Bowel ischemia Renal failure Peritonitis Sepsis Metabolic acidosis Hypothermia Analgesia (epidural or opioid)
CDH	Overexpanded contralateral lung Hypoplastic ipsilateral lung Pneumothorax and barotrauma Pulmonary HTN May be on ECMO Respiratory acidosis Metabolic acidosis IVH Hypoglycemia Hypokalemia if on diuretics	Epidural or opioid-based technique Pneumothorax Hypovolemia Pulmonary HTN Suprasystemic RVBPs Hypoventilation Hypothermia Metabolic acidosis Right-to-left shunting Volume overload	Analgesia (epidural or opioid) Pneumothorax and barotrauma Hypovolemia Pulmonary HTN Suprasystemic RVBPs Hypoventilation Hypothermia Metabolic acidosis Right-to-left shunting Volume overload May require HFOV or ECMO after "honeymoon period" within 24–48 h of repair
TEF	Aspiration Gastric distention RDS if premature Cardiac anomalies GI anomalies Renal anomalies	Epidural or opioid-based technique Aspiration Hypothermia Metabolic acidosis Respiratory acidosis Pneumothorax Atelectasis/hypoxemia Mucus plugging Gastric distention Extubate in OR if possible	Analgesia (epidural or opioid) Pneumothorax Apnea Hypoventilation Tracheal leak Weakness RLN injury Pneumonia
NEC	Respiratory compromise from abdominal distention Respiratory and metabolic acidosis Sepsis Volume depletion Hypoglycemia Hypocalcemia DIC	No epidural if septic Minimize FiO$_2$ (retinopathy) Vasopressors/ionotropes Hypovolemia Metabolic acidosis Hypoglycemia Hypocalcemia Bowel wall edema Respiratory compromise with abdominal closure	ROP Hypovolemia Metabolic acidosis Sepsis Pulmonary edema with fluid remobilization Opioids for postoperative analgesia

RDS, respiratory distress syndrome; HTN, hypertension; ECMO, extracorporeal membrane oxygenation; IVH, intraventricular hemorrhage; RVBP, right ventricular blood pressure; HFOV, high frequency oscillatory ventilation; RLN, recurrent laryngeal nerve; DIC, disseminated intravascular coagulation.

and possibly fresh frozen plasma (FFP) and platelets may be required. Epidurals are generally not used because of the concern for sepsis and are not needed if the patient is intubated for several days. Potential complications in the OR include hypothermia, metabolic acidosis, hypovolemia, hypocalcemia, hypoglycemia; postoperatively, pulmonary edema may be seen as fluid mobilizes. (See Table 130.4.)

Pyloric stenosis

Pyloric stenosis is caused by idiopathic hypertrophy of the muscular layers of the antrum and pylorus, and usually manifests in the 2nd to 8th week of life. Occurring more frequently in boys (and perhaps first-born boys), this lesion has an incidence of approximately 1:500 live births. Neonates present with nonbilious projectile vomiting, and the hypertrophied muscular layers can often be palpated as an olive-sized mass

located between the midline and right upper quadrant. Radiologic diagnosis was historically accomplished with barium swallow, and is now increasingly performed with the widespread availability of ultrasound. Clinical awareness has also led to earlier diagnosis, leading to less severe physiologic derangements of these babies when they present for preoperative evaluation before the definitive surgical treatment, pyloromyotomy – division of the hypertrophied fibers.

Pyloric stenosis is not a surgical emergency, but fluid resuscitation may be urgent depending on the severity of dehydration. Chloride and hydrogen ions are lost from the GI tract through severe vomiting, and this loss is accompanied by a renal response that begins with excretion of bicarbonate, sodium, and potassium. With ongoing depletion of sodium and potassium, conservation of these electrolytes in the distal tubules leads to excretion of hydrogen ions and a resultant worsening of the metabolic alkalosis. With protracted vomiting, these infants can have a mixed metabolic alkalosis (from GI and renal proton losses) and metabolic acidosis (lactic acidosis from pronounced intravascular depletion from the dehydration accompanying ongoing vomiting and decreased effective enteral intake), with hypokalemia and hypochloremia. Prior to a patient's arrival in the OR, his or her electrolytes should be checked to ensure that they have been normalized, and volume status should be assessed to ensure adequate preoperative fluid resuscitation (sometime requiring as much as 50–100 ml/kg in fluid boluses if severely dehydrated).

Pyloromyotomy is performed through either an open approach or laparoscopically. If open, the operation involves either a right upper quadrant or periumbilical incision. If laparoscopic, three trocar incisions are typically made for cameras, tools, and intraperitoneal carbon dioxide insufflation. After being identified, the serosa and hypertrophic muscle of the pylorus are divided with a scalpel or electrocautery, with care not to advance the division so deep as to cause a tear of the fragile gastric mucosa. Adequate myotomy is usually indicated by visible herniation or bulging of the submucosa into the myotomy site.

Anesthetic preparation is as for most neonatal cases, including warming the room. To minimize the risk of aspiration, the stomach is emptied by passing a large-bore orogastric tube prior to induction and suctioning with the baby in the right lateral, left lateral, and supine positions. Atropine at 20 µg/kg, with a minimum dose of 100 µg may be given before induction to minimize bradycardia if succinylcholine is used and as an antisialogogue. The two usual approaches to intubation include (1) an awake technique or (2) a rapid sequence or modified rapid-sequence induction after careful preoxygenation. Maintenance is achieved with a balanced technique of volatile agent delivered in either an air–oxygen mixture or a nitrous oxide–oxygen mixture (the latter probably best avoided in laparoscopic procedures). Even term infants with pyloric stenosis may be more sensitive to postoperative apnea with opioids, probably related to residual central nervous system (CNS) acid–base changes; adequate postoperative analgesia can be achieved by local anesthetic infiltration of the incision site in conjunction with acetaminophen and possibly ketorolac. Emergence is accompanied by adequate reversal of muscle relaxation (hip flexion is a good indicator for return of strength in an infant) and extubation when fully awake. Postoperatively, the neonate should be monitored for apnea for 12 to 24 hours given the risk of apnea after general anesthesia (and perhaps greater risk if opioids are also administered).

Meningomyelocele

Neural tube defects occur with an incidence of 0.5/1000 to 1/1000 live births and are more common in female infants than males; they are generally diagnosed prenatally by ultrasound and are associated with elevated maternal serum alphafetoprotein levels. Low levels of maternal folate and maternal ingestion of valproic acid have been associated with these

defects. Spina bifida occurs when the posterior neural tube fails to close properly starting in the 4th week of fetal life. The least severe form of spina bifida is spina bifida occulta, which is a failure of the vertebral arches to form, usually with a normal spinal column; this defect may be detected by skin dimpling or a lipoma in the area. Another form of spina bifida is a meningocele, in which a fluid-filled sac composed of skin and meninges protrudes from the back. The spinal cord function may remain normal in a patient with a meningocele. A third type is a meningomyelocele, in which the fluid-filled sac also contains neural elements. Spinal cord function is never normal in patients with meningomyelocele, although patients with low lumbar or sacral meningomyeloceles can learn to walk with braces. Finally, in raschisis, much of the spinal cord is abnormal and covered with skin and meninges. This birth defect is usually incompatible with life.

These defects may be associated with lower extremity weakness, bowel and bladder dysfunction, orthopedic abnormalities such as hip dysplasia and club feet, and congenital heart disease. Some lumbar meningomyeloceles are associated with an Arnold–Chiari type 2 malformation, which consists of displacement and elongation of the brainstem and protrusion of the cerebral tonsils through the foramen magnum. The fourth ventricle is also displaced below the level of the foramen magnum, which may be small. This malformation is almost always accompanied by hydrocephalus and usually requires surgical shunting. Cranial nerve difficulties are also common and include vocal cord paresis, stridor, apnea, facial weakness, and strabismus.

Although clinical trials of intrauterine repair of meningomyelocele are being done, the majority are repaired within 48 hours of birth. A cesarean delivery is advised because it is associated with less perinatal infection. At delivery, the sac should be covered with a moist, occlusive, antibiotic dressing, and great care should be taken to maintain the sac's integrity. Surgical repair is done with the patient in the prone position, and the goal of surgical treatment is create a repair with secure dural coverage, free of cerebrospinal leaks and tension. Primary closure is often done, but, for large defects, musculocutaneous or cutaneous flaps or grafts may be required and involve the services of plastic surgeons in addition to neurosurgeons. Patients with symptomatic hydrocephalus may have a ventriculoperitoneal shunt placed during their initial meningomyelocele repair.

Meningomyelocele repair is usually done with a general anesthetic, although there are case reports of spinal anesthesia being used for repair. It is critical to preserve the integrity of the sac prior to repair, and thus the patient should not be positioned in the supine position if possible. For induction and intubation, the patient can be either positioned lateral or placed on a foam "donut" (or on rolls under the shoulders and hips) to allow the sac to hang free from all pressure. Most infants will have an IV catheter in place for fluid replacement and antibiotics, but there is no contraindication to inhalation induction. Because of both multiple surgical procedures and some atopic predisposition, this patient population is at increased risk for development of latex allergy, so latex precautions are generally taken from birth.

Because infants have the potential for cranial nerve dysfunction, it is critical to extubate these patients at the conclusion of the surgery only if they demonstrate alertness, a normal breathing pattern, and the ability to protect their airway. These patients are initially cared for in an intensive care setting. Opioids are used with caution in this patient population. Positioning for extubation is as for induction; the patient is generally positioned prone again after extubation after it is clear that there are no airway issues.

Suggested readings

Andropoulos DB, Heard MB, Johnson KL, et al. Postanesthetic apnea in full-term infants after pyloromyotomy. *Anesthesiology* 1994; 80:216–9.

Andropoulos DB, Rowe RW, Betts JM. Anaesthetic and surgical airway management during tracheo-oesophageal fistula repair. *Paediatr Anaesth* 1998; 8:313–9.

Azarow KS, Ein SH, Shandling B, Wesson D, et al. Laparotomy or drain for perforated necrotizing enterocolitis: who gets what and why? *Pediatr Surg Int* 1997; 12:137–9.

Brett CM, Davis PJ, Bikhazi G. Anesthesia for neonates and premature infants. In *Smith's Anesthesia for Infants and Children*, 7th edition. St. Louis: Mosby-Year Book; 2006:521–70.

Cook-Sather SD, Tulloch HV, Cnaan A, Nicolson SC, et al. A comparison of awake versus paralyzed tracheal intubation for infants with pyloric stenosis. *Anesth Analg* 1998; 86:945–51.

Cook-Sather SD, Tulloch HV, Liacouras CA, Schreiner MS. Gastric fluid volume in infants for pyloromyotomy. *Can J Anaesth* 1997; 44:278–83.

Goh DW, Brereton RJ. Success and failure with neonatal tracheoesophageal anomalies. *Br J Surg* 1991; 78:834–7.

Grosfeld JL, Molinari F, Chaet M, Engum SA, et al. Gastrointestinal perforation and peritonitis in infants and children: experience with 179 cases over ten years. *Surgery* 1996; 120:650–5.

Holzki J. Bronchoscopic findings and treatment in congenital tracheoesophageal fistula. *Paediatr Anaesth* 1992; 2:297–303.

Lindower J, Atherton H, Kotagal U. Outcomes and resource utilization for newborns with major congenital malformations: the initial NICU admission. *J Perinat* 1999; 19: 212–9.

Liu LM, Pang LM. Neonatal surgical emergencies. *Anesth Clin North Am* 2001; 19:272–6.

Moss RL, Dimmitt RA, Barnhart DC, Sylvester KG, et al. Laparotomy versus peritoneal drainage for necrotizing enterocolitis and perforation. *N Engl J Med* 2006; 354:2225–34.

Shaer CM, Chescheir N, Schulkin J. Myelomeningocele: a review of the epidemiology, genetics, risk factors for conception, prenatal diagnosis, and prognosis for affected individuals. *Obstet Gynecol Surv* 2007; 62:471–9.

Wilson JM, Lund DP, Lillehei CW, Vacanti JP. Congenital diaphragmatic hernia: a tale of two cities: the Boston experience. *J Pediatr Surg* 1997; 32:401–5.

Wilson JM, Lund DP, Lillehei CW, Vacanti JP. Congenital diaphragmatic hernia: predictors of severity in the ECMO era. *J Pediatr Surg* 1991; 26:1028–33.

Yaster M, Buck JR, Dudgeon DL, Manolio TA, et al. Hemodynamic effects of primary closure of omphalocele/gastroschisis in human newborns. *Anesthesiology* 1988; 69:84–8.

Yaster M, Scherer TL, Stone MM, Maxwell LG, et al. Prediction of successful primary closure of congenital abdominal wall defects using intraoperative measurements. *J Pediatr Surg* 1989; 24:1217–20.

Chapter 131

Congenital heart disease

Denise M. Chan and Annette Y. Schure

Introduction

Congenital heart disease (CHD) is the most common congenital defect. It affects 4 to 9 per 1000 live-born, full-term infants and is two to three times more common in premature babies. There are currently more than 1.2 million patients with CHD living in the United States, and 300,000 of them are younger than 21 years. Over the last few decades, mortality rates have declined dramatically, and more and more of these patients will require both cardiac and noncardiac surgical procedures. Thus it is imperative for all anesthesiologists, not only cardiac specialists, to understand the basic principles of managing patients with CHD.

Classification

Congenital heart defects can be broadly categorized as cyanotic ("blue babies") or acyanotic ("pink babies") and then can be further classified according to the underlying pathophysiology into shunts, obstructions, and complex lesions with mixing of pulmonary and systemic blood flow (Table 131.1).

The most common congenital cardiac lesions are ventricular septal defect (VSD), transposition of the great arteries (TGA), tetralogy of Fallot (TOF), and coarctation of the aorta. Together these comprise approximately half of all CHDs.

Pathophysiology
Left-to-right shunts

Children with significant left-to-right shunts will demonstrate increased pulmonary blood flow as soon as the initially high pulmonary vascular resistance (PVR) of the perinatal period starts to decline, usually around 6 to 8 weeks of age. The pulmonary overcirculation leads to increased pulmonary artery (PA) pressures and progressive left ventricle (LV) volume overload, which will eventually result in congestive heart failure (CHF), low cardiac output, and pulmonary congestion or edema. Clinically this will manifest as poor peripheral circulation with cold extremities and mottled skin, as well as tachypnea, rales, increased work of breathing, and hepatomegaly. Persistent increases in pulmonary blood flow and pressure provoke changes in the pulmonary microvasculature that cause vasoconstriction and, ultimately, the development of

pulmonary vascular obstructive disease (PVOD). Initially, these changes are reversible, but they can be fixed as early as 6 months, depending on the type and size of the defect. If left untreated, increasing PA pressures will eventually compromise right ventricle (RV) function. With further increases in PVR, either sudden or gradual, PA pressure may exceed LV pressure and can lead to reversal of the shunt, resulting in right-to-left flow and cyanosis (Eisenmenger syndrome).

Right-to-left shunts

In cardiac defects with a right-sided flow obstruction and a connection between the right and left sides of the heart, venous blood will be shunted away from the pulmonary circulation and directly mixed with arterial blood, leading to hypoxemia and cyanosis. To maintain adequate tissue oxygenation, these patients develop polycythemia. Unfortunately, this compensatory mechanism causes significant hyperviscosity and increases the risk for spontaneous thrombus formation and ischemic strokes. These negative effects on blood rheology can be further exacerbated by dehydration and prolonged fasting periods. Depending on the location and extent of the right-sided flow obstruction, the pressure load on the RV can result in marked hypertrophy and progressive RV dysfunction and arrhythmias.

Table 131.1. Classification of CHD (incidence of lesion as percentage of all CHD)

Cyanotic	Acyanotic
Right-to-left shunts	**Left-to-right shunts**
Tetralogy of Fallot (10%)	VSD (20%–25%)
Pulmonary atresia (1%)	ASD (5%–10%)
Tricuspid atresia (<1%)	Endocardial cushion defect (AV canal) (4%–5%)
	PDA (5%–10%)
Complex "mixing" lesions	
Transposition of the great vessels (5%)	
Total anomalous pulmonary venous return (1%)	
Truncus arteriosus (1%)	
HLHS (1%)	
Double-outlet RV (<1%)	
Obstructive lesions (right-sided)	**Obstructive lesions (left-sided)**
Pulmonary stenosis (5%–8%)	Coarctation of the aorta (8%–10%)
	Aortic stenosis (5%)

Table 131.2. Manipulation of PVR

Factors increasing PVR	Factors decreasing PVR
• PEEP	• No PEEP
• High airway pressure	• Low airway pressure
• Atelectasis	• Normal FRC
• Low FiO$_2$	• High FiO$_2$
• Acidosis and hypercapnia	• Alkalosis and hypocapnia
• Increased hematocrit	• Low hematocrit
• Sympathetic stimulation	• Blunted stress response
• Pain and agitation	• Nitric oxide
• Epinephrine, dopamine	• Vasodilators (milrinone)
• Direct surgical manipulation	

PEEP, positive end-expiratory pressure.

Obstructive lesions

Left- or right-sided outflow obstructions impose primarily pressure loads on the respective ventricles, resulting in significant hypertrophy and increased oxygen consumption. With critical stenosis or obstruction, cardiac output and tissue perfusion are markedly decreased, leading to hypoxemia and metabolic acidosis. Decreased coronary perfusion can manifest as ventricular failure and arrhythmias. During the neonatal period, adequate systemic or pulmonary blood flow is often maintained through a patent ductus arteriosus (PDA). Closure of the PDA can lead to sudden decompensation.

Complex "mixing" lesions

Defects in which venous and arterial blood are mixed at various levels before reaching the systemic circulation are known as complex mixing lesions. Often additional intra- or extracardiac flow obstructions are present. Arterial oxygen saturation and adequate tissue perfusion are highly dependent on a well-balanced ratio of pulmonary and systemic blood flow. Pulmonary overcirculation will initially lead to high saturations (>90%), but it will also result in inadequate systemic cardiac output and metabolic acidosis. Predominance of the systemic circulation and poor pulmonary perfusion will result in hypoxemia and cyanosis. This form of circulation is described as "parallel circulation" in contrast to the "series circulation" of a normal heart. PVR and systemic vascular resistance (SVR) are important determinants for a heart with parallel circulation (Tables 131.2 and 131.3).

Table 131.3. Manipulation of SVR

Factors increasing SVR	Factors decreasing SVR
• Sympathetic stimulation	• Adequate sedation and analgesia
– Pain and agitation	• Vasodilators
– Epinephrine, dopamine	
– Norepinephrine	– Milrinone, dobutamine
– Ketamine	– Nitroprusside
• Negative intrathoracic pressure	– ACE inhibitors
• Hypothermia	• Positive pressure ventilation
	• Fever, sepsis

Preoperative evaluation of patients with congenital heart disease

A thorough understanding of the anatomy and pathophysiology of the cardiac defect is important for the safe perioperative management of patients with CHD. For complex lesions it can be useful to contact the pediatric cardiologist. Table 131.4 highlights the important aspects of the preoperative assessment. However, all evaluations must be adjusted for the specific lesion and planned procedure; not all patients need cardiac catheterization or MRI.

For patients with repaired congenital heart defects who present for cardiac or noncardiac procedures, specific information about the type and outcome of previous surgeries is important. Palliative repairs (e.g., PA banding, Blalock–Taussig shunts) with significant residual pathophysiology must be differentiated from definitive repairs. The anesthesiologist should be aware of any residual defects, such as patch leaks or outflow obstructions, surgical complications, or altered anatomy and physiology. A history of frequent interventional procedures can be a strong indicator of residual problems. All patients should be specifically asked about signs and symptoms of exercise-induced ventricular dysfunction or arrhythmias. In addition, sites of previous vascular shunts and cut-downs for access need to be documented.

The indication for perioperative endocarditis prophylaxis has to be assessed on an individual basis, according to the latest guidelines published by the American Heart Association (http://www.americanheart.org). The current version recommends prophylaxis only for CHD with the highest risk of adverse outcome from endocarditis and for specific surgical procedures.

General considerations for anesthetic management

Premedication in children with complex CHD is desirable, as it improves oxygen saturation, decreases myocardial oxygen consumption, and facilitates a smooth induction. Opioids and benzodiazepines, alone or in combination with ketamine, may be used, but care must be taken to avoid oversedation, because hypoventilation and bradycardia are often poorly tolerated.

Induction of anesthesia may be accomplished using a variety of techniques, depending on the type of cardiac defect and extent of ventricular dysfunction. For patients with well-preserved ventricular function, a careful inhalation induction is an option. Of note, a significant right-to-left shunt can slow down an induction with inhaled anesthetics. When a substantial portion of the cardiac output is shunted away from the lungs, the uptake of inhaled anesthetics is decreased, and the time to reach adequate partial pressures in the brain is prolonged. This effect is more pronounced for insoluble gases.

Patients with significant ventricular dysfunction and poor cardiac reserve may be unable to tolerate the cardiodepression

Table 131.4. Important aspects for the preoperative evaluation

History	• Signs and symptoms of CHF:
	  – Failure to thrive (FTT), poor feeding, tachypnea, sweating
	  – Recurrent pulmonary infections (secondary to congestion)
	  – Decreased activity level and fatigue in older patients
	• Palpitations or syncope
	• Additional congenital anomalies (e.g., airway, genitourinary)
	• Recent and current medications (e.g., diuretics, digoxin, ACE inhibitors)
	• Review of previous surgeries and interventional procedures
	• Last follow-up with the patient's pediatric cardiologist

Physical examination	• Characteristic heart murmur, precordial thrill, arrhythmias • Tachypnea, increased work of breathing, rales • Poor peripheral perfusion, delayed capillary refill • Bounding or diminished pulses • Cool extremities, mottled skin, sweating • Hepatomegaly • Peripheral edema
Laboratory studies	• CBC: polycythemia (secondary to cyanosis), anemia (secondary to malnutrition) • Electrolytes: hypokalemia, hyponatremia (secondary to diuretic therapy) • Coagulation profile
Additional tests	• Echocardiography: cardiac function and intracardiac anatomy • EKG: rhythm, signs of atrial or ventricular hypertrophy • CXR: cardiomegaly, pulmonary edema, or infiltrates
Specific studies	• Cardiac catheterization: anatomy, pressure gradients, saturations, shunts • Cardiac MRI: anatomy, pulmonary blood flow, RV and LV function

CBC, complete blood count; EKG, electrocardiography; CXR, chest radiograph.

and hypotension that are often associated with inhalation induction. For intravenous (IV) induction, a combination of benzodiazepine, opioid, and a small dose of an induction agent is frequently used. Maintaining a good airway for effective oxygenation and ventilation as well as an optimal ratio of PVR to SVR are also extremely important.

The plan for maintenance of anesthesia will depend on many factors, including the type of CHD; the age, condition, and comorbidities of the patient; the surgical procedure; the expected duration; the use of cardiopulmonary bypass (CPB); and the need for postoperative ventilatory support. In general, more complex or fragile patients should be maintained with an opioid-based anesthetic, whereas patients with simple or straightforward defects and preserved cardiac function can be anesthetized with a balanced technique with inhalation agent and opioid.

The risk and benefits of invasive monitoring are determined by the complexity of the cardiac defect, the patient's condition, and the surgical procedure. For patients with complex lesions having extensive procedures with possible hemodynamic instability, major fluid shifts, or poor vascular access, central venous cannulation and invasive blood pressure (BP) monitoring should be established prior to the procedure. Additional monitoring modalities include intraoperative transesophageal echocardiography and cerebral oximetry.

Depending on the patient's history and condition, the need for inotropic support, nitric oxide, or antiarrhythmic therapy (e.g., defibrillation, adenosine, or amiodarone) must be anticipated.

Common congenital heart defects
Ventricular septal defect
Incidence and pathophysiology

VSDs are the most common form of CHD, affecting 20% to 25% of CHD patients; 30% to 40% of VSDs will close spontaneously within the first year of life.

VSDs are differentiated according to location: perimembranous (80%), outlet (just beneath the pulmonary valve; 5%–7%), inlet (posterior and inferior; 5%–8%), or muscular (within the trabecular area; 5%–20%). Muscular VSDs are often multiple and have a "Swiss-cheese" appearance (Fig. 131.1).

The resulting left-to-right shunt is dependent on the size of the defect and the pressure gradient across the septum, which is determined by LV and RV pressures, PVR, and SVR. Large left-to-right shunts lead to pulmonary overcirculation, CHF, and poor cardiac output.

Signs and symptoms

Small VSDs can be completely asymptomatic and found incidentally on physical examination. Infants with a large VSD will usually develop CHF at 6 to 8 weeks of age when PVR declines. Cardiac examination may reveal a holosystolic murmur and possibly a systolic thrill at the left sternal border. Poor cardiac output results in tachypnea, mottled skin, and cool extremities. Additional signs and symptoms include failure to thrive (FTT), poor feeding, and delayed growth and development, as well as recurrent pulmonary infections due to pulmonary overcirculation and congestion.

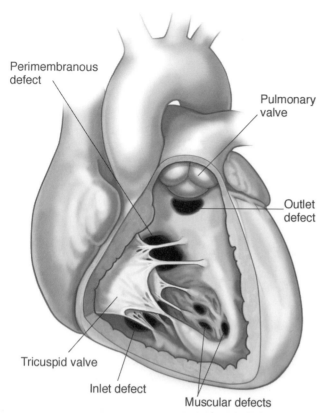

Perimembranous
defect

Pulmonary
valve

Outlet
defect

Tricuspid valve

Inlet defect

Muscular defects

Figure 131.1. Location of various types of ventricular septal defects.

Associated anomalies

Fewer than 5% of VSDs are associated with chromosomal abnormalities, such as trisomy 13, 18, and 21.

Treatment

Medical treatment of CHF may include digitalis, angiotensin-converting enzyme (ACE) inhibitors, and/or diuretics. VSD closure may be performed either with a device placed by an interventional cardiologist or surgically. Surgical management is considered in infants with CHF and FTT who are unresponsive to medical treatment or in patients with large left-to-right shunts with a ratio of pulmonary to systemic flow > 2:1. Asymptomatic children may undergo elective repair at approximately 2 years of age to prevent long-term complications. Direct patch closure is performed via an atrial approach or a ventriculotomy. Infants who are unable to tolerate CPB may alternatively undergo PA banding to reduce pulmonary blood flow.

Anesthetic considerations

Patients with a small VSD and no obvious CHF will usually tolerate a careful inhalation induction; however, one must still be aware of reduced cardiac reserve. Conversely, patients with a large VSD and significant CHF should have a careful IV induction aiming for a stable PVR/SVR ratio and normoventilation. Hyperventilation and high fraction of inspired oxygen content

(FiO$_2$) will increase left-to-right shunting and therefore should be avoided. Severe hypotension or an increase in PVR places the patient at risk for shunt reversal (i.e., right-to-left).

Considerations for patients with repaired VSDs

Endocarditis prophylaxis should be given for the first 6 months after patch repair. Dysrhythmias and conduction defects, such as right bundle branch block (RBBB), ventricular arrhythmias, and heart block, may persist, as well as ventricular dysfunction after ventriculotomy.

Patent ductus arteriosus

Incidence and pathophysiology

The ductus arteriosus is a normal fetal structure that connects the main pulmonary artery and the upper descending aorta. In utero, approximately 60% of RV output bypasses the lungs via the ductus arteriosus. In full-term infants, functional closure (i.e., smooth muscle contraction) usually occurs 10 to 15 hours after birth as a result of lung expansion, decreases in PVR, exposure to increased PaO$_2$, decreased prostaglandin levels, and the release of vasoactive substances. Permanent closure is completed by the first 2 to 3 weeks of life, leaving a fibrosed band (the ligamentum arteriosum), which is the only remnant of this intrauterine connection. In approximately 1:2500 live births, however, the ductus fails to close.

The degree of left-to-right shunting via the PDA depends on the size of the PDA and the ratio of PVR to SVR. Small PDAs are often hemodynamically insignificant and asymptomatic. Left-to-right shunting through medium PDAs increases as PVR decreases over the first few months of life. With large PDAs, a significant left-to-right shunt leads to LV overload and progressive CHF, usually within the first few weeks of life, and, eventually, pulmonary hypertension. Additionally, sudden increases in PVR can lead to shunt reversal with right-to-left shunting and cyanosis.

Signs and symptoms

The classic finding on physical examination is a continuous machine-like murmur best heard at the left sternal border. Signs of CHF include tachypnea, hepatomegaly, poor peripheral perfusion, and FTT. A widened pulse pressure with low diastolic pressures may be seen, due to a "steal effect" from left-to-right shunting. Patients also commonly have pulmonary congestion or edema and recurrent respiratory infections.

Associated anomalies

A PDA is often essential for pulmonary or systemic blood flow in patients with complex cardiac lesions (see sections on TGA and hypoplastic left heart syndrome [HLHS]).

In preterm infants, the cardiovascular changes associated with a PDA can exacerbate conditions such as necrotizing enterocolitis, intracranial hemorrhage, or respiratory distress syndrome.

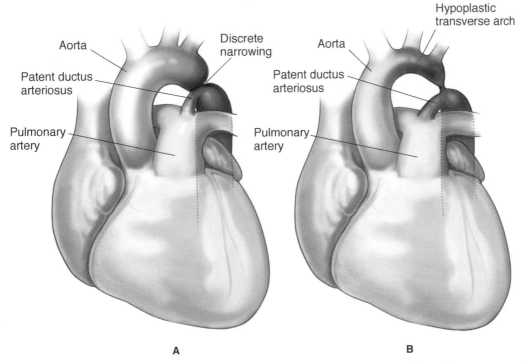

Figure 131.2. Coarctation of the aorta. Anatomic spectrum of coarctation of the aorta, ranging from a discrete narrowing **(A)** to a diffuse hypoplasia of the transverse arch **(B)**.

Treatment

Medical treatment in preterm infants includes a trial of indomethacin, as well as treatment of CHF and pulmonary edema. Device closure may be performed by the interventional cardiologist but has a high incidence of residual shunts (∼5%–10%). Surgery is indicated for neonates who fail medical therapy and for older asymptomatic children, usually at 2 to 4 years of age. Current surgical options include PDA ligation or division via posterolateral thoracotomy or hemoclip occlusion via video-assisted thoracoscopic surgery (VATS).

Anesthetic considerations

Pre- and postductal pulse oximetry are important tools to detect ligation of wrong vessels, and upper and lower extremity BP monitoring are used to determine pressure gradients. Upon PDA closure, the diastolic pressure should increase and the murmur should disappear. In older children, lung isolation with an endobronchial blocker or a double lumen tube may be requested.

In preterm infants, PDA ligation is often performed at the bedside to avoid transport and the risks associated with it (e.g., hypothermia, respiratory changes, or accidental extubation). Surgical exposure and retraction cause "functional" single-lung ventilation. Short periods of desaturation may have to be accepted to complete the procedure.

Considerations for patients with repaired PDAs

Recurrent laryngeal nerve injury is a potential complication of surgical repair. In cases of late repair, pulmonary hypertension and ventricular failure may develop.

Endocarditis prophylaxis should continue for the first 6 months after device closure or for residual shunts.

Coarctation of the aorta

Incidence and pathophysiology

Coarctation of the aorta is present in 5% to 10% of patients with CHD. Most patients have a discrete stenosis of the upper thoracic aorta, but the anatomic spectrum can range from a long tubular hypoplasia of the transverse arch to bandlike strictures in the descending aorta (Fig. 131.2). The hemodynamic picture is highly dependent on the severity of the stenosis and the presence of associated cardiac defects and collateral circulation. For instance, a newborn with critical stenosis may decompensate acutely when the ductus arteriosus closes. In contrast, older patients with mild and slowly progressive pressure gradients will develop systemic hypertension and compensatory LV hypertrophy. Later in childhood, some form of collateral arterial circulation often supports the perfusion in the distal descending aorta.

Signs and symptoms

There are two major clinical presentations of patients with coarctation of the aorta. An infant with severe coarctation has CHF and low cardiac output. A child or adolescent with mild to moderate coarctation presents with hypertension and a murmur; these patients, although often asymptomatic, may occasionally have exercise-induced claudication or headaches. A systolic pressure gradient exists between upper and lower extremities.

Associated anomalies

Coarctation of the aorta is often associated with other congenital anomalies: Fifty percent of patients have an additional intracardiac lesion; 85% have a bicommissural aortic valve. In addition, variations of the brachiocephalic vessels with an abnormal origin of the subclavian arteries may occur, and 3% to 5% of patients have berry aneurysms of the circle of Willis. Patients with Turner syndrome have a high incidence of coarctation; other congenital malformations are present in 25% of patients.

Treatment

Prostaglandin E is used to establish or maintain ductal patency in infants. Older children are placed on β-blockers for treatment of hypertension prior to repair. Symptomatic neonates will undergo surgery as soon as possible, usually after a 12- to 24-hour period of stabilization. Otherwise, asymptomatic patients should have their defect corrected after 3 months of age to reduce the risk of long-term sequelae (e.g., persistent hypertension, increased cardiovascular morbidity). Balloon angioplasty and stenting, although the procedure of choice for recoarctation, is controversial for primary treatment of coarctation because of the higher incidence of restenosis and complications.

Anesthetic considerations

Newborns and infants with CHF usually need a careful IV induction and an opioid-based maintenance technique. Older infants and children will generally tolerate an IV or inhalation induction and maintenance. Invasive BP monitoring should be placed in the right radial artery (the left subclavian artery may be clamped during repair), unless there is an anomalous right subclavian artery. Additional BP monitoring and pulse oximetry are placed in lower extremities. During cross-clamping, isoflurane and short-acting vasoactive agents (e.g., esmolol, nitroprusside, or nitroglycerin) decrease wall tension and oxygen consumption. Upon unclamping, goals include correction of metabolic acidosis and volume replacement. In the postoperative phase, it is important to watch for hypertension and postcoarctectomy syndrome (e.g., abdominal pain, vomiting).

Considerations for patients with repaired coarctation

Endocarditis prophylaxis should continue for the first 6 months following patch repair. Patients are at risk of recoarctation and exercise-induced pressure gradient, as well as persistent hypertension and myocardial hypertrophy with diastolic dysfunction. Patients with coarctation repaired late in life are at higher risk of premature coronary artery disease.

Atrial septal defect

Incidence and pathophysiology

In its isolated form, atrial septal defects (ASDs) comprise 5% to 10% of congenital heart defects, but they are part of more

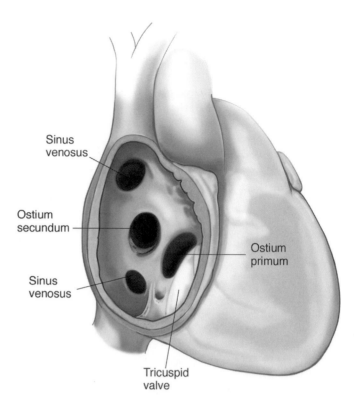

Figure 131.3. Location of the different types of atrial septal defects.

complex cardiac defects in 30% to 50% of CHD patients. There are three basic categories of ASDs: an ostium secundum defect (50%–70%) is located in the fossa ovalis; an ostium primum ASD (15%–30%) is an endocardial cushion defect and is commonly associated with a cleft mitral valve and mitral regurgitation; and a sinus venosus ASD (10%–30%) is most commonly located at the junction of the superior vena cava (SVC) and right atrium (RA), and is often found in combination with partial anomalous pulmonary venous return (Fig. 131.3). Occasionally, an unroofed coronary sinus may be considered as a form of ASD.

The underlying pathophysiology is a left-to-right shunt with slowly progressive RA and RV dilation and eventually development of pulmonary hypertension. More than 80% of ASDs, especially those < 8 mm in size, will close spontaneously within the first 2 years of life.

Signs and symptoms

Most patients are asymptomatic; large, untreated ASDs may cause CHF and significant pulmonary hypertension in the third or fourth decade of life. ASDs are often incidental findings on physical examinations or later in life during the evaluation of supraventricular tachyarrhythmias or paradoxic embolization. Cardiac examination classically reveals a widely split and fixed S2 and a II-III/VI systolic murmur along the left sternal border. Patients may have a slender body build and exhibit decreased exercise tolerance and dyspnea on exertion. Later in life, they may have palpitations, atrial flutter, or atrial fibrillation.

Associated anomalies

ASDs may be associated with virtually any congenital anomaly. The most commonly associated cardiovascular defects include pulmonary stenosis, partial anomalous venous return, and VSD. There is a higher incidence of secundum ASDs in patients with Holt–Oram, Noonan, Marfan, and Turner syndromes.

Treatment

Device closure may be performed by the interventional cardiologist for patients with suitable anatomy. Surgery is usually indicated for infants with CHF and FTT who are too small for device closure. Surgery may also be performed electively in asymptomatic children around 2 to 5 years of age to prevent long-term complications (e.g., arrhythmias, Eisenmenger syndrome). Via a mini or full median sternotomy and an atrial approach, the defect is directly closed with a suture or a pericardial patch.

Anesthetic considerations

Careful removal of all air bubbles from lines is essential to prevent paradoxic air embolus. Inhalation induction is usually well tolerated, except in sick infants with CHF. Most patients can be extubated at the end of the surgical repair.

Consideration for patients with repaired ASDs

Endocarditis prophylaxis should be given during the first 6 months after device or patch closure. These patients frequently have perioperative dysrhythmias, and they may have persistent RV dilation or pulmonary hypertension if the repair has been delayed.

Tetralogy of Fallot

Incidence and pathophysiology

Approximately 5% to 10% of all CHDs are classified as TOF. It is by far the most common cyanotic lesion.

Embryologically, TOF is caused by an underdevelopment of the RV infundibulum and malalignment of the infundibular septum, leading to the classic tetrad: RV outflow tract (RVOT) obstruction; a large, nonrestrictive VSD; an overriding aorta; and RV hypertrophy (Fig. 131.4). The most important pathophysiologic aspect of TOF is the obstruction to pulmonary blood flow, which leads to a right-to-left shunt via the VSD and subsequent hypoxemia and cyanosis.

The obstruction to pulmonary blood flow can be located at any level of the pulmonary outlflow tract: in the area of the RV infundibulum, the pulmonary valve or annulus, the main PA, or even the branch PAs. The vast majority of cases will have a combination of infundibular and valvular stenosis, where the degree of obstruction can be highly dependent on RV contractility and preload. Dehydration, tachycardia, and positive inotropes are usually not well tolerated.

Signs and symptoms

Depending on the morphology, the clinical presentation can vary significantly, from a severely cyanotic newborn to a "pink

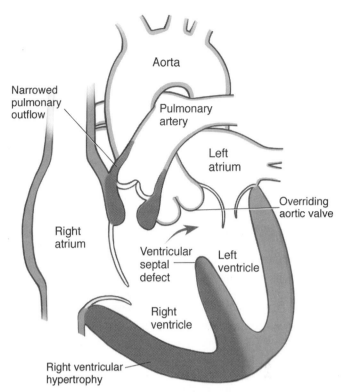

Figure 131.4. Typical features of tetralogy of Fallot: RV hypertrophy, RV outflow tract obstruction, large VSD and overriding aorta.

Tet" with CHF. Physical examination reveals a pansystolic murmur at the left upper sternal border, representing flow through the VSD. Patients often have cyanosis and hypoxemia, with oxygen saturations between 70% and 90%, as well as decreased exercise tolerance, dyspnea on exertion, and easy fatigability. Squatting increases SVR and arterial oxygenation. Chronic hypoxemia leads to polycythemia and an increased risk of spontaneous thrombosis and ischemic strokes. Hypercyanotic spells or "tet spells" (episodes of severe cyanosis, abnormal respirations, and altered level of consciousness) occur in 20% to 30% of patients, with a peak incidence at 2 to 3 months of age.

Associated anomalies

Only 68% of TOFs are isolated cardiac lesions. Associated chromosomal abnormalities include trisomy 13, 18, and 21; genetic syndromes such as DiGeorge, CHARGE (Coloboma of the eye, Heart defects, Atresia of the choanae, Growth retardation and/or developmental delay, Genital and/or urinary abnormalities, Ear abnormalities and deafness), and VACTERL association (Vertebral, Anal, Cardiac, Tracheal, Esophageal, Renal, Limb anomalies) are also associated with TOF. TOF is often seen with other cardiac anomalies, such as a right-sided aortic arch and coronary anomalies, which may affect the surgical approach to repair.

Treatment

Asymptomatic infants with minimal cyanosis are initially managed conservatively. Some patients may be given prophylactic propranolol to prevent hypercyanotic spells while waiting for surgery. Treatment of hypercyanotic spells includes "knee-chest position" or abdominal compression to increase venous return; supplemental oxygen; volume expansion with crystalloid or colloids; vasoconstrictors (e.g., phenylephrine); β-blockade with esmolol or propranolol; and sedation with morphine or ketamine.

Surgical management

Historically, surgical treatment involved a multistage approach: palliation in infancy via an arterio-pulmonary shunt to provide adequate flow to the lungs and definitive repair later in life. More recently, with improved bypass and surgical techniques, the one-stage repair has been the procedure of choice. For stable patients with a favorable anatomy, most centers will plan surgery for 3 to 4 months of age.

Depending on the specific morphology, definitive surgical repair consists of the following components: patch closure of the VSD; excision of RVOT muscle bundles; ventriculotomy versus an atrial and transpulmonary approach; transannular or infundibular patch; or complex repair with an extracardiac RV to PA conduit for TOF with pulmonary atresia.

Anesthetic considerations

Polycythemia predisposes these patients to strokes, especially during periods of dehydration and prolonged fasting. Optimal timing of procedures and adequate rehydration are important. Care should be taken to remove all air bubbles from lines to avoid systemic air embolism. The potential for "hypercyanotic spells" must also be considered. Generally, a gentle IV induction is used to maintain SVR and preload; in patients with mild forms of TOF, a careful inhalation induction is possible.

Considerations for patients with repaired tetralogy of Fallot

These patients may need continued endocarditis prophylaxis, depending on the presence of residual VSDs, RVOT obstructions, or pulmonary valve regurgitation and RV dilation (after transannular patch repair). There is also a potential for arrhythmias and significant RV dysfunction after ventriculotomy due to scarring and fibrosis. LV dysfunction can result from ischemic injury in patients with anomalous coronaries. In addition, aortopulmonary collaterals may persist, especially in patients with TOF and pulmonary atresia.

Transposition of the great arteries

Incidence and pathophysiology

TGA is a complex mixing lesion that comprises 5% to 7% of all CHDs. It is the most common cyanotic CHD diagnosed in the newborn period. Abnormal rotation and septation of the arterial truncus results in transposition of the aorta and pulmonary artery. The aorta arises anteriorly from the RV and transports deoxygenated blood to the body, whereas the PA originates posteriorly from the LV and carries oxygenated blood back to the lungs. Thus, pulmonary and systemic circulations are in parallel

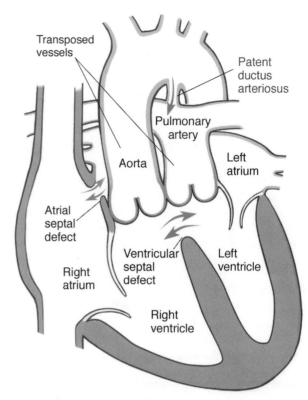

Figure 131.5. Transposition of the great arteries. Aorta arises from the RV and the PA originates from the LV: Deoxygenated blood from the SVC and IVC is transported back to the body via the aorta; and oxygenated blood from the pulmonary veins goes back to the lungs via the PA. Complete separate and parallel circulations, compatible with life only if some mixing of blood occurs via an ASD, VSD, or PDA.

(Fig. 131.5). This situation can be fatal if it is not coupled with another defect to provide a connection between the two circulations; an associated ASD, VSD, or PDA will allow for some mixing of oxygenated and deoxygenated blood. The RV has to support the relatively high-pressure systemic circulation, whereas the LV is exposed only to the slowly declining PVR. Over time this situation will lead to RV failure and LV underdevelopment.

Signs and symptoms

Clinical manifestations are determined by the extent of mixing and the presence of associated cardiac defects. Cyanosis is present within hours of birth, and arterial hypoxemia and acidosis may be unresponsive to oxygen inhalation. Signs of CHF develop over the first few weeks, especially in TGA patients with a large VSD.

Associated anomalies

Associated cardiac defects that provide mixing between the two circulations are necessary for survival; in more than 50% of patients, it is a PDA or patent foramen ovale (PFO), whereas in 40% a VSD is present. Coronary anatomy variances and ventricular outflow tract obstructions can complicate the picture (e.g., subpulmonary stenosis is seen in 30% of patients). TGA is rarely associated with extracardiac anomalies or syndromes.

Treatment

Prostaglandin E_1 infusion is used to maintain ductal patency if necessary. CHF and metabolic acidosis are treated accordingly. Balloon atrial septostomy can be performed to increase mixing at the atrial level as the patient awaits surgical correction.

TGA can be repaired with the so-called "switch" procedures, which redirect blood flow to the appropriate circulation. Switch procedures can be done at all levels within the heart but with different physiologic consequences. With a Senning or Mustard procedure, an intra-atrial baffle redirects flow from the SVC and inferior vena cava (IVC) to the left atrium (LA) and from the pulmonary veins to the RA. The RV remains the systemic ventricle, however, and complications can include baffle obstructions, arrhythmias and RV failure later in life.

In a Rastelli or Damus–Kaye–Stansel procedure, an intraventricular baffle and an RV-to-PA conduit are used to redirect the blood flow. These patients are at risk for conduit stenosis, ventricular scars, and arrhythmias.

Last, an arterial switch or Jatene procedure involves the switching of the great vessels just above the ventricles – transection of the aorta and PA, transfer of coronary arteries, and reanastomosis over the appropriate ventricle. Kinking or obstruction of the coronary arteries may occur.

Historically, TGA was repaired using the Senning or Mustard technique, which was often associated with poor longterm results. Currently the procedure of choice is the arterial switch operation. When performed within the first week of life, before the LV is "deconditioned," it has by far the best long-term results.

Anesthetic considerations

Goals for induction and maintenance include careful preservation of cardiac output and intercirculatory mixing. Decreases in contractility, heart rate, or preload can lead to further impairment of tissue oxygenation, increased oxygen extraction, and venous desaturation, and thereby cyanosis. Additionally, increases in PVR relative to SVR should be avoided. Elevated PVR will reduce pulmonary blood flow, whereas decreases in SVR will promote systemic recirculation. Both can result in inadequate mixing and lower arterial oxygen saturation.

Considerations for patients with repaired TGA

Patients who have undergone an atrial switch are susceptible to progressive RV dysfunction, tricuspid regurgitation, and right heart failure. They are at increased risk of arrhythmias, sick sinus syndrome, and sudden death, as well as baffle obstruction, which leads to pulmonary edema and/or SVC syndrome. Conversely, long-term problems are rare in arterial switch patients. Supravalvular pulmonary stenosis or regurgitation into the neoaorta is possible. Occasionally patients may have asymptomatic occlusion of coronary arteries.

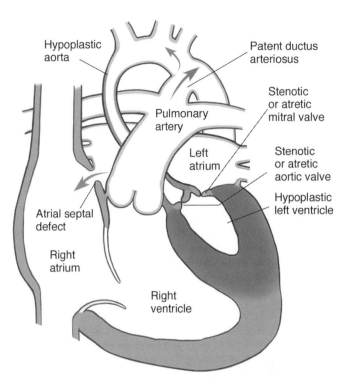

Figure 131.6. Hypoplastic left heart syndrome. Severe underdevelopment of all left-sided structures: mitral valve stenosis or atresia, aortic valve stenosis or atresia, hypoplastic left ventricle, ascending aorta and aortic arch. Systemic perfusion via PDA including retrograde perfusion of coronary arteries.

Hypoplastic left heart syndrome

Incidence and pathophysiology

HLHS accounts for ~1% of all CHDs. It is the most common cause of death from CHD within the first month of life. This syndrome involves a wide spectrum of cardiac anomalies characterized by a combination of severe mitral and aortic valve stenosis/atresia and marked hypoplasia of the LV, ascending aorta, and aortic arch (Fig. 131.6). In utero, impaired blood flow through the stenotic left-sided valves prevents adequate growth of the LV and aortic arch. Typically, left-to-right shunting via a PFO or ASD decompresses the left atrium, and a large PDA provides flow to the descending aorta as well as retrograde flow to the ascending aorta and coronary arteries. This anatomy results in a classic univentricular physiology with parallel systemic and pulmonary circulations. Oxygenated and deoxygenated blood mixes in the single ventricle and may enter, depending on the PVR/SVR ratio, either the pulmonary or systemic circulation. Pulmonary overcirculation will lead to decreased systemic output and acidosis, whereas systemic overcirculation will result in significant cyanosis and hypoxemia. Therefore, a careful balance between PVR and SVR must be maintained.

Signs and symptoms

Signs and symptoms of cardiogenic shock manifest within the first few hours of life as the PDA closes.

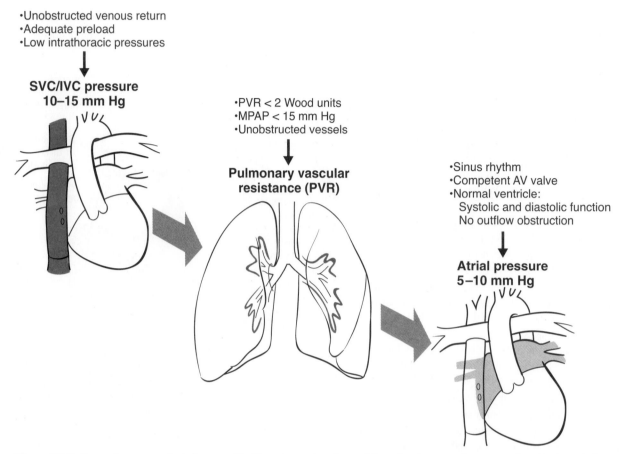

- Unobstructed venous return
- Adequate preload
- Low intrathoracic pressures

**SVC/IVC pressure
10–15 mm Hg**

- PVR < 2 Wood units
- MPAP < 15 mm Hg
- Unobstructed vessels

**Pulmonary vascular
resistance (PVR)**

- Sinus rhythm
- Competent AV valve
- Normal ventricle:
  Systolic and diastolic function
  No outflow obstruction

**Atrial pressure
5–10 mm Hg**

Figure 131.7. Transpulmonary gradient after a modified Fontan procedure. Factors influencing the transpulmonary gradient: Unobstructed venous return, adequate preload, and low intrathoracic pressure on the "venous side," unobstructed PAs with low pressures and PVR in the pulmonary circulation and low atrial pressure on the "ventricular side," requiring normal sinus rhythm, a competent atrio-ventricular valve and normal ventricular function without residual outflow obstruction.

Associated anomalies

In addition to the associated cardiac defects (PDA, ASD, and coarctation), 12% of patients with HLHS have extracardiac anomalies (e.g., trisomy 12 or 18, Noonan or Turner syndrome, and agenesis of the corpus callosum).

Treatment

Ductal patency is maintained with prostaglandin E_1. Stabilization of the patient may require intubation, inotropic support, and correction of metabolic acidosis. It is important to balance pulmonary and systemic blood flow distribution, maintaining arterial oxygen saturation at approximately 80% to 85%. Atrial balloon septostomy is occasionally needed to enlarge a PFO and decompress the LA.

Early surgical intervention within the first few days of life is necessary for survival. Surgical options are basically cardiac transplantation or palliative surgery (the "Fontan pathway"). Neonatal cardiac transplantation is usually limited by the lack of adequate donors, so most patients are initially treated with several staged surgeries. Palliative procedures in the neonatal period aim for balanced systemic and pulmonary blood flows, allowing the baby to grow for several months despite cyanosis and volume load on the ventricle.

The first stage (Norwood procedure), is performed within the first week of life. This procedure includes the creation of a neo-aorta originating from the RV using the main PA and patch augmentation of the hypoplastic aorta, an atrial septectomy, ligation of the PDA, and a modified Blalock–Taussig (mBTS, subclavian artery-to-PA) or Sano (RV-to-PA) shunt to provide pulmonary blood flow. The goal is to secure systemic perfusion independent of the PDA and allow for adequate maturation of the pulmonary vascular bed while preserving the function of the single ventricle.

The second stage (bidirectional Glenn procedure), is performed at 3 to 6 months. The mBT or Sano shunt is replaced by a direct anastomosis between the SVC and right pulmonary artery, providing passive pulmonary blood flow. The IVC remains connected to the heart. As a result, the volume load on the ventricle is significantly reduced, but oxygenated and deoxygenated blood still mix, and oxygen saturation remains in the low 80s.

The third and final stage (modified Fontan procedure), is performed at 18 to 24 months. With adequate growth and maturation of the pulmonary vascular bed, the resistance should be low enough to allow for complete separation of systemic and pulmonary flow. The IVC is now also connected to the pulmonary artery, via either a lateral tunnel in the atrium or an extracardiac conduit, with or without a small fenestration. Pulmonary blood flow is completely passive, driven only by the pressure gradient across the pulmonary vascular bed. A fenestration can act as a pop-off valve and provide a residual right-to-left shunt in case of sudden increases in PVR.

Anesthetic considerations

Induction and maintenance are aimed at preserving a careful balance of pulmonary and systemic circulations. The goal is a normotensive, well-perfused, nonacidotic patient with an arterial oxygen saturation ~80% to 85%. Pulmonary overcirculation with poor cardiac output should be treated by increasing the PVR with controlled hypoventilation and low FiO_2 and providing inotropic support. Systemic overcirculation with profound cyanosis can be addressed by decreasing PVR and optimizing afterload. Systemic hypotension can lead to poor coronary perfusion, cardiac ischemia, and sudden ventricular fibrillation. Patients are mechanically ventilated for at least 3 to 5 days postoperatively. During CPB for the first stage of repair, significant total body edema develops; the chest is usually left open for a few days until the edema resolves.

Considerations for patients after the modified Fontan procedure

Pulmonary blood flow and cardiac output are dependent on the transpulmonary pressure gradient, which is determined by several factors: adequate preload and venous return, low PVR, and good ventricular function (Fig. 131.7). All factors that increase PVR (e.g., acidosis, atelectasis, hypoxia, hypercapnia, hypothermia) need to be corrected immediately.

In addition, prolonged dehydration and fasting periods should be avoided. These patients have a high incidence of arrhythmias, thrombosis, strokes, and clot formation. They are also susceptible to sudden right-to-left shunting if a fenestration is present.

Suggested readings

Adult Congenital Heart Association Web site. Available at www.achaheart.org.

American Society of Anesthesiologists (ASA) 2005 Annual Meeting Refresher Course Lectures, *Perioperative Issues in Patients with Congenital Heart Disease.*

Emmanouilides GC, Allen HD, Riemenschneider TA, Gutgesell HP (eds.). *Clinical Synopsis of Moss and Adam's Heart Disease in Infants, Children and Adolescents Including the Fetus and the Young Adult.* 1st ed. Baltimore: Williams & Wilkins; 1998.

Hoffman JIE, Kaplan S. The incidence of congenital heart disease. *J Am Coll Cardiol* 2002; 39:1890–1900.

Huntington JH, Malviya S, Voepel-Lewis T, et al. The effect of a right-to-left intracardiac shunt on the rate of rise of arterial and end-tidal halothane in children. *Anesth Analg* 1999; 88:759–762.

Lake CL, Booker PD (eds.). *Pediatric Cardiac Anesthesia.* 4th ed. Baltimore: Lippincott, Williams & Wilkins; 2005.

Lovell AT. Anaesthetic implications of grown-up congenital heart disease. *Br J Anaesth* 2004; 93(1):129–139.

Mavroudis C (ed.). *Pediatric Cardiac Surgery.* 3rd ed. St. Louis: Mosby; 2003.

Miller RD (ed.). *Miller's Anesthesia.* 6th ed. Burlington, MA: Elsevier; 2005.

Motoyama EK, Davis P (eds.). *Smith's Anesthesia for Infants and Children.* 7th ed. St. Louis: Mosby; 2006.

Murphy JG et al. Long-term outcome after surgical repair of isolated atrial septal defect. Follow-up at 27 to 32 years. *N Engl J Med* 1990; 323(24):1645–1650.

Nichols DG, Cameron DE. *Critical Heart Disease in Infants and Children.* 2nd ed. Philadelphia: Mosby-Elsevier; 2006.

Park MK. *Pediatric Cardiology for Practitioners,* 4th ed. St. Louis: Mosby; 2002.

Prevention of Infectious Endocarditis: Guidelines from the American Heart Association: A Guideline from the American Heart Association Rheumatic Fever, Endocarditis, and Kawasaki Disease Committee, Council on Cardiovascular Disease in the Young, and the Council on Clinical Cardiology, Council on Cardiovascular Surgery and Anesthesia, and the Quality of Care and Outcomes Research Interdisciplinary Working Group. *Circulation* 2007; 116:1736–1754.

Rivenes SM, Lewin MB, Stayer SA, et al. Cardiovascular effects of sevoflurane, isoflurane, halothane, and fentanyl-midazolam in children with congenital heart disease: an echocardiographic study of myocardial contractility and hemodynamics. *Anesthesiology* 2001; 94:223–229.

Russell IA, Hance WCM, Gregory G, et al. The safety and efficacy of sevoflurane anesthesia in infants and children with congenital heart disease. *Anesth Analg* 2001; 92:1152–1158.

Sarner J, Levine M, Davis PJ, et al. Clinical characteristics of sevoflurane in children: a comparison with halothane. *Anesthesiology* 1995; 82:38–46.

Strafford MA. Management of the patient with repaired or palliated congenital heart disease. In: Coté CJ, Todres ID, Goudsouzian NG, Ryan JF, eds. *A Practice of Anesthesia for Infants and Children.* 3rd ed. Philadelphia: Saunders-Elsevier; 2001.

Williams GD, Jones TK, Hanson KA, Morray JP. The hemodynamic effects of propofol in children with congenital heart disease. *Anesth Analg* 1999; 89:1411–1416.

Chapter 132

Management of postoperative pain in children

Rahul Koka and Navil F. Sethna

Introduction

Acute postoperative pain in adults and children is a well-recognized inherent consequence of tissue damage no matter how minor the procedure or trauma might be. Considerable efforts have been made in recent years to standardize and improve acute pain management through the establishment of guidelines. Historically, management of acute pain has been undervalued for a variety of reasons, including a lack of adequate training. A recent nationwide survey from Sweden demonstrated that a large proportion of children had poor pain relief after surgical procedures (23%) and from nonsurgical conditions (31%) due mainly to organizational deficiencies rather than knowledge deficiency or lack of time or other burdens on health care providers.

The Joint Commission and other organizations have mandated systematic pain assessment, informing patients of their right to pain relief, prompt and effective treatment of unrelieved pain, access to specialists in pain management, and hospital-wide efforts at continuous quality improvement in pain treatment. These initiatives develop a set of pain protocols specifically for pediatric care, foster combined use of nonpharmacologic and pharmacologic approaches, and promote collaboration of multiple disciplines to manage a child's anxiety and fear as well as pain. These goals are best achieved through implementation of an acute pain management consult service to provide 24-hour consultation and supervise and administer analgesics requiring specialized interventions, such as epidural analgesia, continuous peripheral nerve blocks (PNBs), or complex pharmacologic management. Such a service is usually staffed by anesthesiologists, anesthesia trainees, and trained nurses.

Practitioners should strive to alleviate pain whenever possible to minimize the complex sequence of events that sets up an intense nociceptive afferent input, sensitizes peripheral and central nociceptive neurons, releases inflammatory mediators, and activates adrenocortical responses. Pain has psychological as well as physiologic effects and causes anxiety, fear, and insomnia in children. It is not always possible to eliminate all forms of pain, fear, anxiety, or distress, and no ideal analgesic strategies exist for controlling acute postoperative pain. Optimal pain management requires striking a balance between analgesia and adverse effects and risks. Considering these challenges, a multi-modal analgesia approach is embraced to improve recovery and resume normal activities of daily living.

Assessment of pain

As with adults, considering the subjective nature of pain experience, direct measurement of pain is not feasible, and so children should be permitted to self-report pain by using developmentally appropriate pain assessment scales. Family members should report their observations regarding the child's pain, and special approaches of surrogate measures should be used for the assessment of pain in children with special needs (those who are neurologically impaired and/or noncommunicating). For newborns and infants, validated composite measures that combine physiologic (heart rate, respiratory rate) and behavioral (facial expression, position) parameters are available for use at the bedside to assess pain during procedures and in the postoperative period. Pain assessment remains a challenge in premature and critically ill infants. Consideration should always be given to provide analgesia as these infants have adequately mature nociceptive pathways and the neural substrates to process pain stimuli at the level of spinal cord and supraspinal nociceptive centers.

Analgesic strategies

A combination of cognitive–behavioral and various pharmacologic strategies is useful for successful control of postoperative pain. It is well-recognized that the extent of tissue damage does not necessarily correlate with the patient's report of pain intensity after surgery as many other factors contribute to the pain experience, including interindividual variability in analgesic pharmacokinetics, pharmacogenetics, pharmacodynamics, mood state, and trait reaction.

Nonpharmacologic strategies

Cognitive behavioral therapy (CBT) is an effective strategy for supporting children with developmental maturity (usually 7 years or older) to deal with an acute painful event such as procedural pain by addressing factors, such as cognition, affect, and behavior, that may affect the individual child's pain experience. The more a person is aware of his or her illness and what to expect during a painful procedure, the more control

Table 132.1. Recommended doses of IV opioids for moderate to severe pain[a]

Opioid	Age	IV bolus and PRN frequency dose/kg	Continuous infusion, microgram/kg/h
Morphine	Preterm neonates	4 µg q2h or 8 µg q4h	2–10
	Term neonate	15 µg q2h or 30 µg q4h	5–20
	>6 mo	50 µg q2h or 100 µg q4h	15–30
Hydromorphone	>6 mo[b]	0.015 mg q4–6h	No data available
Fentanyl	Preterm neonates	0.25–0.5 µg q1–2h	0.5–1
	Term neonate	0.5–1 q1–2h	0.5–2
	>6 mo	1 µg q1–2h	1–2
Meperidine	<6 mo	See text	Not recommended[c]
	>6 mo	0.5 mg q2h or 1mg q4h	No data available
	Adults	0.5–1 mg q2–3h	2.5 mg/h
Methadone	Children >1 y	0.5–1.0 mg q4h for 24 h, followed by 0.5 mg q4–6h prn[c]	

[a] All IV doses should be administered slowly over 10 to 15 minutes, at lower starting doses in infants from 0 to 3 months old. There should be close monitoring for respiratory depression in infants younger than 6 months.
[b] Morphine clearance approaches that of adult values between the ages of 6 and 12 months.
[c] Prolonged elimination half-life; suggests the need for longer observation periods.
PRN, as needed.

that person has; with appropriate knowledge and techniques, episodes of emotional distress occur less often and are usually less severe in intensity and duration. Other strategies, such as acupuncture, acupressure, transcutaneous electrical nerve stimulation (TENS), distraction, play therapy, and so forth, are also useful but of limited value in early postoperative pain control.

Pharmacologic strategies

There is a wide variability in drug response among infants and children based on age and genetic, environmental, and disease processes that may influence absorption, distribution, metabolism, and excretion. The larger extracellular and total body water and a higher water to adipose ratio lead to a larger volume of distribution and therefore lower initial plasma concentration of drugs. The lower concentration of total plasma proteins (including albumin and α-1 glycoprotein) increases the biologically free active fraction of protein-bound drugs. In neonates, the circulating fetal albumin, which has an affinity to strong acids, binds to bilirubin and free fatty acids and can displace drugs from albumin-binding sites, leading to a higher free fraction of biologically active drug (e.g., diazepam).

The bioavailability of extensively metabolized drugs (e.g., acetaminophen) administered by the rectal route may be increased in neonates and infants due to the immaturity of their hepatic metabolism.

Delayed maturation of phase II drug-metabolizing enzyme (e.g., glucuronidation of morphine) decreases clearance. The total body clearance reaches 80% that of adults by 6 months and 96% of that predicted in adults by 1 year. Similarly, delayed maturation of phase I drug-metabolizing enzymes, hepatic cytochrome P-450 isoforms, decreases the clearance of drugs metabolized by these systems. Both glomerular filtration and tubular secretion are immature at birth and reach adult capacity at 8 to 12 months.

Opioids

Opioids are commonly used postoperative analgesics in patients of all ages. If dosed correctly, opioids produce excellent analgesia with a reasonable margin of safety. Morphine is the most commonly used opioid in children and has been extensively studied in all ages, including premature infants. Infants younger than 6 months clear total body morphine at rates up to 80% of the adult value. Morphine-3-glucuronide is the predominant metabolite. Suggested dosing guidelines are presented in Tables 132.1 and 132.2. Opioids are administered by a variety of routes: orally, intravenously (IV), rectally, transdermally, or transmucosally. Several opioids are available in elixir form for children who are not able or willing to swallow pills. Recently, the fentanyl patch and oral transmucosal fentanyl citrate (the fentanyl "lollipop") have garnered support among physicians for their usefulness in the treatment of cancer pain; these formulations may also be used for preoperative sedation and postoperative analgesia.

Table 132.2. Recommended oral opioids for acute pain management

Opioid	Age	Dose, mg/kg	Daily frequency	Maximum daily dose, mg/kg
Tramadol	≥7 y	1–2	q4–6h	8 (maximum 400 mg/d)
Oxycodone	>6 mo	0.05–0.15	q4–6h	NA*
Codeine	>1 y	0.5–1	q4–6h	NA
Morphine	<6 mo	0.1	q4h	NA
	>6 mo	0.2–0.5	q4–6h	NA
Morphine ER	>6 mo	0.3–0.6	q12h	For chronic use
Hydromorphone	>6 mo	0.03–0.08	q4–6h	NA

* Data on dosing schedule is lacking for infants younger than 6 months, and half-life of elimination varies widely (2.4–14 hours). The dose must be titrated to a lowest effective dose individually.
NA, not available; ER, extended release.

Table 132.3. Close clinical and cardiorespiratory monitoring is mandatory for children at risk for opioid-induced respiratory depression in conditions including (but not limited to) the following:

Term infants <6 months old or infants <1 years old with history of apnea and/or bradycardia
Compromised airways
Muscle weakness (e.g., neuromuscular disorders)
Somnolence
Opioid naïve and concurrent use of sedative agents
Significant lung disease (e.g., obstructive, restrictive)
Neurologic impairment
All children receiving epidural morphine and hydromorphone

Table 132.4. Minimum assessments for patients who receive patient- or nurse-controlled IV opioids[a]

Assessment items	Assessment frequency
Pain assessment	4 h
Level of consciousness score	4 h
Respiratory rate and depth	1 h
Heart rate, blood pressure, temperature	4 h
Side effects of analgesia	4 h

[a] Continuous electronic monitors (electrocardiogram [EKG]–apnea monitor system and pulse oximetry) are used in children at risk for respiratory compromise, infants younger than 6 months, and children receiving epidural hydrophilic drugs, such as morphine and hydromorphone.

Patient-controlled analgesia in children

Maintaining steady-state serum concentrations of opioids has been at the core of postoperative pain relief. In years past, pain relief consisted mainly of opioids given via ineffective routes such as by intramuscular injections, with needle sticks causing anxiety and pain. This mode of opioid administration caused periods of inadequate pain control between the peaks of plasma concentrations, leading to the distressing cycle of sedation, analgesia, and discomfort. Many young patients were reluctant to report pain because of fear of receiving injections. Continuous infusions of low-dose opioids have been used and offer some advantages, particularly in neonates, as these opioids maintain a nearly constant plasma drug concentration. This method, unfortunately, does not consider dynamic changes in analgesic need or variation in drug clearance or effective plasma concentration. In addition, routine use of opioid infusions in ventilated premature newborns has become controversial. Opioid-induced respiratory depression is the most concerning side effect and should be monitored, particularly in those children who have conditions that may predispose to airway and ventilatory compromise (Table 132.3).

Patient-controlled analgesia (PCA) has been used effectively in the pediatric population. The theory of PCA is that only patients know when they are in pain, so they can titrate their own analgesic requirements (within a window of safety) based on their fluctuating needs. It has been demonstrated that children older than 7 years (as well as some mature children ages 5 and 6) can understand the concept, purpose, and instructions of PCA use and use it appropriately to derive adequate pain relief. Patients appear to learn quickly to administer medication before painful procedures or activities and tend to accept some degree of incomplete analgesia with minimal adverse effects rather than achieving no pain.

Controversy exists in the adult and pediatric literature regarding the use of PCA with a continuous background infusion as it does increase the incidence of brief episodes of hypoventilation and hypoxia, particularly during night sleep. Although PCA therapy is used safely in children, respiratory depression remains a major concern with any IV administration of opioid. Therefore, all children receiving PCA therapy should be assessed periodically as outlined in our institutional monitoring policy (Table 132.4). The prescription of the vari-ous doses of opioids and parameter settings depends on institutional policies and type of PCA equipment used. Our regimen for routine initial postoperative and acute pain management is outlined in Fig. 132.1.

Nurse-/parent-controlled analgesia

Some pediatric institutions allow nurse-controlled analgesia (NCA), which can provide a reasonable, effective alternative to PCA in children younger than 6 years and in those with developmental or physical disability. This form of drug delivery does sidestep one of the inherent safety features, that sedated patients will not trigger the device. Fear of overmedicating patients by the analgesic provider remains stronger and the repercussions remain greater than the fear of undermedicating patients in pain, however. Fear of respiratory depression, addiction, and lack of confidence in titration to relieve a patient's pain may result in persistent reports of inadequate pain management.

Parent-assisted PCA is a useful mode of effective pain control in children who are incapable of self-administration of PCA because of age or severity of illness (e.g., cancer patients). For safety reasons, parents are allowed to administer opioids via a parent-activated delivery system after demonstrating that the child is not opioid-naïve and that the parents are well-informed in assessing the child's pain and monitoring adverse effects.

Nonopioid adjuvant agents

Adjuvants such as N-methyl-D-aspartate (NMDA) receptor antagonists (low-dose IV or subcutaneous ketamine), α-2 agonists (clonidine via oral, IV, transdermal, epidural, intrathecal, or PNB), anticonvulsants (oral gabapentin, pregabalin), tricyclic antidepressants (e.g., oral amitriptyline), and sodium channel blockers (e.g., IV lidocaine) are proposed as a component of multimodal postoperative pain management to minimize sensitization and reduce hyperalgesia and allodynia in postoperative pain. Adjuvant use is also proposed to diminish the development of acute neuropathic pain after surgery and trauma as well as for its opioid-sparing effect. Limited data are available on improved outcomes with the use of these agents in children. Several studies in children reported that the addition of clonidine (1–5 µg/kg) to caudal local anesthetic increased the duration of analgesia by 2 to 3 hours, whereas others showed

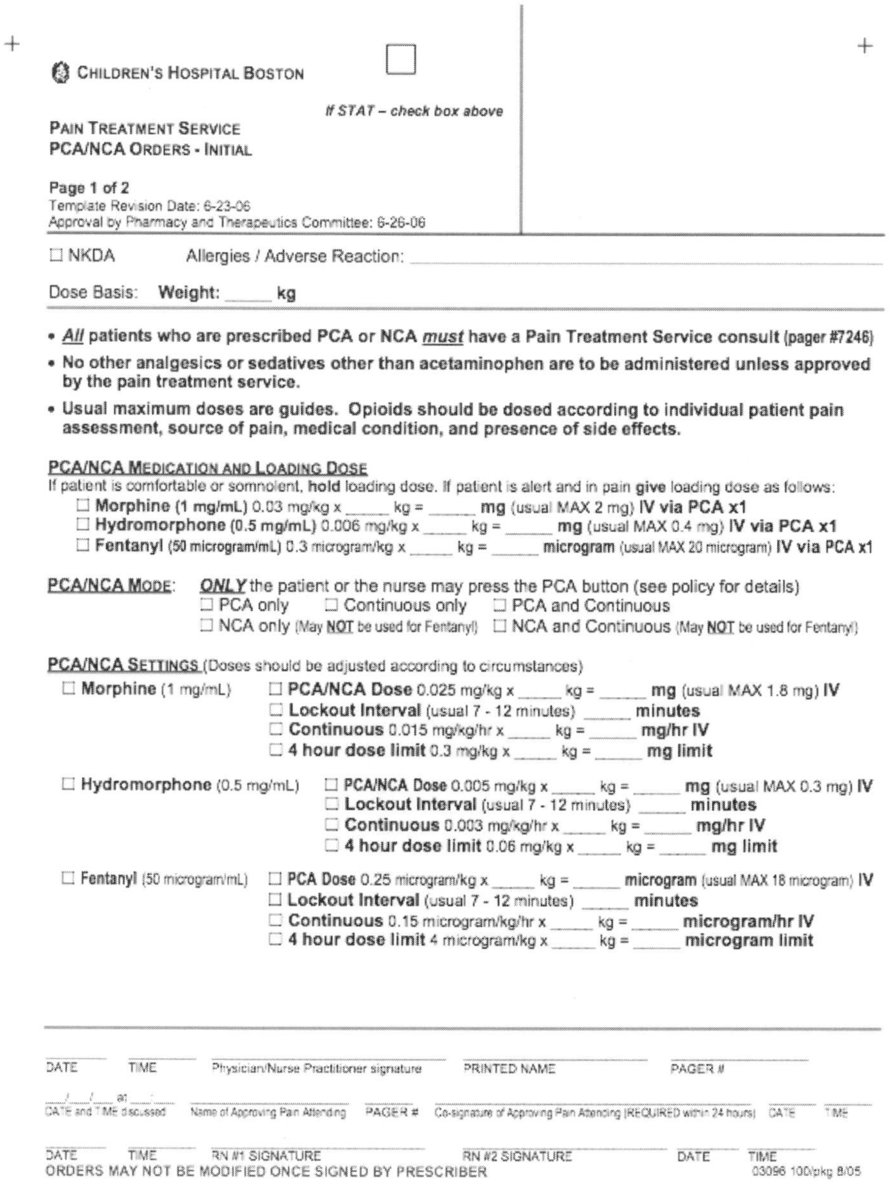

Figure 132.1. Patient-/nurse-controlled IV opioid orders.

+

☺ CHILDREN'S HOSPITAL BOSTON   ☐   *If STAT – check box above*

PAIN TREATMENT SERVICE
PCA/NCA ORDERS - INITIAL

Page 1 of 2
Template Revision Date: 6-23-06
Approval by Pharmacy and Therapeutics Committee: 6-26-06

☐ NKDA   Allergies / Adverse Reaction: _____

Dose Basis: Weight: _____ kg

- *All* patients who are prescribed PCA or NCA *must* have a Pain Treatment Service consult (pager #7246)
- No other analgesics or sedatives other than acetaminophen are to be administered unless approved by the pain treatment service.
- Usual maximum doses are guides. Opioids should be dosed according to individual patient pain assessment, source of pain, medical condition, and presence of side effects.

PCA/NCA MEDICATION AND LOADING DOSE
If patient is comfortable or somnolent, **hold** loading dose. If patient is alert and in pain **give** loading dose as follows:
    ☐ **Morphine** (1 mg/mL) 0.03 mg/kg x _____ kg = _____ **mg** (usual MAX 2 mg) **IV via PCA x1**
    ☐ **Hydromorphone** (0.5 mg/mL) 0.006 mg/kg x _____ kg = _____ **mg** (usual MAX 0.4 mg) **IV via PCA x1**
    ☐ **Fentanyl** (50 microgram/mL) 0.3 microgram/kg x _____ kg = _____ **microgram** (usual MAX 20 microgram) **IV via PCA x1**

PCA/NCA MODE: *ONLY* the patient or the nurse may press the PCA button (see policy for details)
        ☐ PCA only   ☐ Continuous only   ☐ PCA and Continuous
        ☐ NCA only (May **NOT** be used for Fentanyl)   ☐ NCA and Continuous (May **NOT** be used for Fentanyl)

PCA/NCA SETTINGS (Doses should be adjusted according to circumstances)
    ☐ **Morphine** (1 mg/mL)   ☐ **PCA/NCA Dose** 0.025 mg/kg x _____ kg = _____ **mg** (usual MAX 1.8 mg) **IV**
                    ☐ **Lockout Interval** (usual 7 - 12 minutes) _____ **minutes**
                    ☐ **Continuous** 0.015 mg/kg/hr x _____ kg = _____ **mg/hr IV**
                    ☐ **4 hour dose limit** 0.3 mg/kg x _____ kg = _____ **mg limit**

    ☐ **Hydromorphone** (0.5 mg/mL)   ☐ **PCA/NCA Dose** 0.005 mg/kg x _____ kg = _____ **mg** (usual MAX 0.3 mg) **IV**
                    ☐ **Lockout Interval** (usual 7 - 12 minutes) _____ **minutes**
                    ☐ **Continuous** 0.003 mg/kg/hr x _____ kg = _____ **mg/hr IV**
                    ☐ **4 hour dose limit** 0.06 mg/kg x _____ kg = _____ **mg limit**

    ☐ **Fentanyl** (50 microgram/mL)   ☐ **PCA Dose** 0.25 microgram/kg x _____ kg = _____ **microgram** (usual MAX 18 microgram) **IV**
                    ☐ **Lockout Interval** (usual 7 - 12 minutes) _____ **minutes**
                    ☐ **Continuous** 0.15 microgram/kg/hr x _____ kg = _____ **microgram/hr IV**
                    ☐ **4 hour dose limit** 4 microgram/kg x _____ kg = _____ **microgram limit**

DATE _____ TIME _____ Physician/Nurse Practitioner signature _____ PRINTED NAME _____ PAGER # _____

__/__/__ at ____
DATE and TIME discussed   Name of Approving Pain Attending   PAGER #   Co-signature of Approving Pain Attending (REQUIRED within 24 hours)   DATE   TIME

DATE _____ TIME _____ RN #1 SIGNATURE _____ RN #2 SIGNATURE _____ DATE _____ TIME _____
ORDERS MAY NOT BE MODIFIED ONCE SIGNED BY PRESCRIBER   03096 100/pkg 8/05

no significant benefit. A recent controlled trial suggests that caudally administered clonidine is likely absorbed systemically and acts centrally rather than at the dorsal horn level. Potential benefits are an opioid-sparing effect and reduction of postoperative agitation, shivering, and vomiting. Doses ≥ 2 µg/kg may produce dose-dependent sedation, hypotension, bradycardia, and respiratory depression, particularly in infants younger than 1 year. Administration of epidural ketamine and midazolam cannot be recommended because of lack of safety data on neurotoxicity.

There is conflicting evidence on the analgesic effect of IV ketamine in children. The use of low dose ketamine (most commonly 0.25 or 0.5 mg/kg) in pediatric trials of tonsillectomy is shown to be effective in some and equivocal in others. The risk of psychomimetic adverse effects of hallucinations

remains a major deterrent to its use. Addition of benzodiazepines may minimize this risk but also prolong recovery time.

Nonsteroidal anti-inflammatory drugs

Nonsteroidal anti-inflammatory drugs (NSAIDs) are effective analgesics and appealing substitutes for opioids in the management of moderate to severe pain because they lack the common opioid-related side effects of nausea, emesis, pruritus, sedation, and respiratory depression. Their use is limited, however, by adverse effects, including inhibition of platelet function in patients who are at risk for postoperative bleeding, renal impairment, gastric irritation, and inhibition of osteoblast function that may impede growth of new bone and healing. The lowest effective dose should be chosen, then used for the shortest

Table 132.5. Recommended doses of acetaminophen for oral and rectal routes[a]

Age	Oral maintenance dose, mg/kg	Rectal loading dose, mg/kg	Rectal maintenance dose, mg/kg	Maximum daily dose, mg/kg	Duration, days[b]
28–32 wk postconceptual age	15 mg q12h	20	15 mg q12h	35	2
33–37 wk postconceptual age	20 mg q8h	30	20 mg q12h	60	2
Term to 3 mo	20 mg q8h	30	20 mg q12h	60	2
>3 mo	15 mg q4h	40	20 mg q6h	90	3

[a] The relative bioavailability of the rectal route is formulation-dependent and decreases with age.
[b] The proposed doses may cause hepatotoxicity in some infants if used for longer than 2 to 3 days or in the event of drug interactions.

possible duration while monitoring effects on gastrointestinal, renal, and hepatic functions. Reports of severe bronchospasm have been observed in adults and in adolescents with severe asthma. Although bleeding after tonsillectomy has been reported, a Cochrane review showed that NSAIDs were not associated with an increase in bleeding requiring return to the operating room for hemostasis.

Ketorolac is an NSAID available in IV form; it reversibly inhibits cyclooxygenase (COX)1 and 2, limiting prostaglandin synthesis and thereby decreasing inflammation and the pain response centrally and peripherally. It can provide excellent analgesia, is used routinely to manage acute pain, and is available in IV form. A pharmacokinetic study in children ages 1 to 16 years found that ketorolac disposition is similar to that reported in adults, and a recent study of pharmacokinetics of ketorolac in infants and toddlers ages 6 to 18 months showed no accumulation, rapid elimination of ketorolac isomers, and no clinical or laboratory adverse effects. The recommended dose in children is 0.5 mg/kg IV every 6 hours with a possible need for a shorter dosing interval in infants.

The NSAID of first choice is ibuprofen because of its safety profile. It is available over the counter in a variety of forms (pills, suspension) as an antipyretic and analgesic.

Acetaminophen

Acetaminophen (paracetamol) is an effective antipyretic and analgesic that has been used for many decades. It is often used alone for mild to moderate pain or in combination with opioids for patients with moderate to severe pain, and is the most commonly used analgesic and antipyretic in the pediatric population, including premature infants. Its popularity burgeoned after the withdrawal of pediatric aspirin formulations because of their association with Reye syndrome in the 1980s. It is thought to have an analgesic effect on NMDA receptors in the spinal cord. The therapeutic plasma concentration for analgesia with acetaminophen is unknown, but it is assumed to be similar to that of the concentration range required for antipyresis (10–20 µg/ml). Recent research has shown the existence of an isoenzyme of COX3 found only in the brain and spinal cord, which is selectively inhibited by acetaminophen.

Acetaminophen is administered via oral and rectal routes (Table 132.5); an IV preparation was recently approved in the United States. Acetaminophen has few contraindications or side effects in therapeutic doses, but should be used with caution in children with hepatic disease or in critically ill children, particularly in the larger loading doses in current use. Neonates are capable of producing the reactive intermediary by conjugating acetaminophen to the sulfate metabolite rather than the glucuronide metabolite, which causes hepatic damage in overdose.

Regional anesthesia

The majority of regional anesthesia techniques used in adults are applied in children and infants. With a refinement in technique and use of suitably sized equipment, these techniques can be adapted to the pediatric population. Regional anesthesia techniques are used as an analgesic adjunct to general anesthesia or primarily to manage postoperative pain (Table 132.6). Unlike in adults, in the pediatric population regional techniques are often performed after the induction of general anesthesia for safety reasons. Lack of cooperation of most children during needle insertion and use of nerve stimulation requires that they be anesthetized or heavily sedated. There are no reports or studies

Table 132.6. Indications and types of central blocks and PNBs in children

Type of block	Type of surgical indication
Caudal epidural single injection block	Inguinal herniorrhaphy, penile surgery, perineal and anorectal surgery, muscle biopsy, lower extremity orthopedic surgery
Lumbar-to-thoracic epidural catheter block	Lower and mid-abdominal surgery, urologic surgery, renal and bladder surgery, pelvic and lower extremity surgery
Thoracic epidural catheter block	Upper abdominal surgery, thoracotomy, pectus repair, sternotomy, renal surgery
Femoral nerve block (with/without catheter)	Femur fractures and surgery, quadriceps muscle biopsy, anterior knee surgery (arthroscopic surgery)
Sciatic nerve block (subgluteal, distal, popliteal nerves) supplemented with sensory femoral nerve block	Foot surgery

Table 132.7. Caudal epidural anesthesia/analgesia in infants

Prerequisites	Skills and experience in performing adult epidural techniques
Indications	Surgical procedures below T10
Benefits when combined with general anesthesia	Reduces neuroendocrine responses, amount of inhaled anesthetics requirement, perioperative opioids, and postoperative vomiting
Position	Lateral decubitus and hips and knees flexed
Entry site	Sacral hiatus is identified as a slit cephalad to coccyx tip and flanked by sacral cornua. In newborn, the dural sac ends at S4 and spinal cord at L3, and both recede to S2 and L1, respectively, by age 1 y
Needle	22- or 20-gauge blunt stylet needle inserted at 60° and directed cephalad to sacral surface
End point	"Give" as the needle pierces the sacrococcygeal ligament and enters the epidural space; further advancement of the needle at 60° results in contact with anterior table of sacral bone; cephalad advancement of the needle is unnecessary once the sacral epidural space is entered; to avoid complications such as dural puncture and intravascular and marrow entry can be avoided
Test dose: lidocaine 1% or 1.5% with epinephrine 1:200,000	0.1 ml/kg maximum 3 ml; positive test dose in anesthetized child = HR increase of 10 bpm or change of 25% in T-wave amplitude
Local anesthetics: bupivacaine 0.25% or ropivacaine 0.2%	Administer fractionated dose with repeated aspiration for blood and CSF detection; duration of analgesia 4–6 h; significant postoperative motor block if administered at the end of surgery
Bupivacaine 0.125%	Minimal motor block particularly when administered at end of the surgery; may be inadequate for longer procedures
Dose	0.7 ml/kg (0.06 ml/spinal segment/kg) for children younger than 8 y and < 20 kg
Complications (many of these may occur with use of sharp or overly long needles, or cephalad advancement after the epidural space is entered)	Subcutaneous injection; bloody tap; inadvertent intravascular injection; intraosseous injection; hematoma (the sacral canal is wide and neurologic consequence from hematoma is less of an issue than other epidural sites); dural puncture; total spinal; local and epidural infection (with lack of adequate sterile precautions); some believe that use of hollow needles can result in implanting devascularized skin with microorganisms into the epidural space; rectal perforation and pelvic entry with forceful advancement through the soft anterior table of the sacrum which could be mistaken for sacral ligament "give"

HR, heart rate; CSF, cerebrospinal fluid.

to suggest that heavy sedation or general anesthesia increases the risk of neurologic complications or local anesthetic toxicity in children. Therefore, practice of regional anesthesia in anesthetized patients is universally accepted in this population with appropriate attention to technique.

Both peripheral and neuraxial (central) regional anesthetic (RA) techniques have an important and evolving place in the practice of pain management in infants and children. RA may afford many of the same advantages for pediatric patients as it does for adult patients, but there are few controlled clinical trials evaluating the its advantages and adverse effects in children

compared to conventional analgesic strategies. The safe and successful performance of central and peripheral neural blockade techniques in infants and toddlers demands specific knowledge of anatomic, pharmacologic, and psychological domains of development (Tables 132.7 and 132.8). A thorough knowledge of the developmental differences and sufficient prior skills in practice of regional neural blockade in adults greatly enhance the safe and successful application of these techniques in the pediatric population. Hepatic degradation of amide-type local anesthetics involves aromatic hydroxylation, *N*-dealkylation, and amide hydrolysis. Hepatic clearance is slower in newborn

Table 132.8. Pediatric lumbar and thoracic epidural anesthesia technique

Epidural access most easily achieved	Midline via intervertebral space to avoid injury to venous plexus and nerve roots
Needles: Tuohy (lumbar) and Crawford (thoracic)	18- or 20-gauge
Needle angle	15°–20° to median plan to avoid dural puncture and to freely thread the catheter cephalad through the widest part of the epidural space
LOR to saline	LOR to air can produce air embolism and potential for serious hemodynamic and neurologic changes if inadvertently injected into a vein
Catheter (20- or 22-gauge) advancement	2–3 cm if epidural space is accessed at the target spinal segments; threading the catheter at a greater length is unpredictable; it may coil, exit intervertebral foramina, and enter a blood vessel, subarachnoid, paravertebral, or pleural space
Aspiration test	May not be reliable in infants and young children due to low IV pressure; expect slow reflux of blood or CSF by gravity and aspiration may collapse the vein
Test dose: lidocaine 1% or 1.5% with epinephrine 1:200,000	0.1 ml/kg, maximum 3 ml; positive test dose in anesthetized child = HR increase of 10 bpm or change of 25% in T-wave amplitude
Epidural infusion rates; volume per spinal segment of anesthesia/analgesia for children ≤ 8 y[a]	Lumbar and lower thoracic (T10–S1): 0.06 ml/kg; mid-thoracic (T6–T9): 0.03 ml/kg; upper thoracic (T1–T5): 0.02 ml/kg

LOR, loss of resistance; CSF, cerebrospinal fluid; HR, heart rate.
[a] The proposed dosing should be calculated for ideal body weight. The infusion rates are average starting doses that may require adjustment based on an individual child's response and proper placement of the epidural catheter within the spinal segments innervating the surgical zone.

Table 132.9. Representative epidural amide and ester local anesthetic doses in children

Local anesthetics	Age in reference studies	Maximum single injection, mg/kg	Maximum continuous infusion rate, mg/kg/h
Bupivacaine	Premature–term neonate[a]	1.5	0.15–0.2
Levobupivacaine	1–3 mo	2	0.25
Ropivacaine	3–6 mo	2.5	0.3
	Children	2.5	0.4
2-Chloroprocaine 1.5%	Preterm and term neonates (via lumbar route)	15	7.5–12
	Preterm and term neonates (via thoracic route)	7.5	3–6

[a] Limited data are available on use of local anesthetics for premature infants, thus smaller dose regimen is advised in preterm infants and in those with impaired hepatic metabolism.

infants and approaches adult functional capacity by 3 to 6 months of life. Bupivacaine and lidocaine, the most commonly used amide local anesthetics, have prolonged elimination half-lives in infants younger than 6 months; repeated doses or continuous infusions of local anesthetics should be administered at lower dose ranges (Table 132.9).

RA (skin infiltration, epidural, PNBs) is commonly used in daily clinical practice as an adjunct to general anesthesia and for management of postoperative pain. Potential benefits include a reduction in the requirements for both volatile anesthetics and opioids both intra- and postoperatively, thereby minimizing adverse effects such as nausea, vomiting, pruritus, ileus, and urinary retention.

Peripheral nerve block

In the past decade, the application of PNB has increased in pediatric anesthesia practice. The advent of ultrasound-guided PNB has improved the success rate, quality of block, and ease of placement of continuous perineural catheters. In addition, it has facilitated the performance of PNB, which was until recently performed only in adults and only as infraclavicular, brachial plexus, popliteal, and rectus sheath nerve blocks. PNB may be associated with a lower incidence of neurologic and systemic toxicity compared to neuraxial blocks when performed under general anesthesia. Preliminary safety studies of continuous PNB via an indwelling catheter in both the inpatient and outpatient settings show encouraging results.

Local infiltration

Local anesthetic infiltration of the skin and subcutaneous tissue, or field blocks, are technically easy, minimally time-consuming, highly effective, and safe. Local infiltration or field blocks can be used to prevent incisional pain and for suturing lacerations. These techniques produce a low plasma blood concentration of local anesthetics and minimal motor block, demand no special equipment, require minimal postoperative care, and yet are quite underused in daily practice. Both ester and amide local anesthetics are used for local infiltration with longer duration of action with bupivacaine and ropivacaine. Addition of

epinephrine improves hemostasis and prolongs duration of analgesia but should be avoided at end artery sites, such as the nose, fingers, and penile shaft.

Neuraxial analgesia

Caudal blocks may be used in pediatric anesthesia as an adjunct to general anesthesia and to provide postoperative analgesia for common pediatric surgical cases below the umbilicus. Anatomy and landmarks are shown in Figs. 132.2 and 132.3, and the technique is summarized in Table 132.7.

Continuous lumbar or thoracic epidural infusion may be used as an adjunct to general anesthesia (balanced anesthesia) to effectively control severe pain with medical diseases and extensive surgery and trauma, avoid the need for systemic opioids, allow early tracheal extubation, and for continuation of the infusion for management of postoperative pain. Such a combination technique is appealing where postoperative intensive care support is scarce. Epidural analgesia is particularly useful in children undergoing upper abdominal and thoracic procedures and in those children with chronic restrictive and obstructive chest wall and lung disease, such as neuromuscular disorders, cerebral palsy, and encephalomyopathies. It can prevent a serious decline in pulmonary function after upper

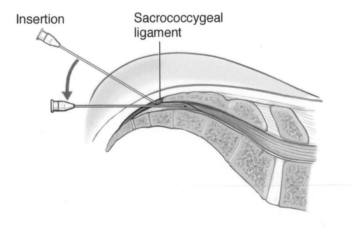

Figure 132.2. Anatomy of the caudal space.

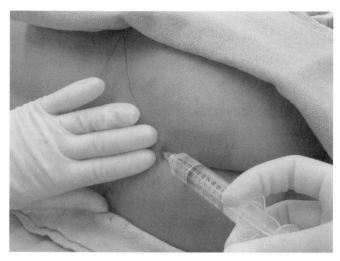

Figure 132.3. Caudal block.

abdominal and thoracic surgery by rapid restoration of functional residual capacity (FRC) to normal values, and it decreases the duration of ileus after upper abdominal surgery. The incidence of common side effects of opioids, such as nausea, vomiting, and pruritus, can be significantly diminished by using local anesthetic with an adjuvant such as clonidine, reducing or eliminating the dose of opioid. Common postoperative epidural infusions use dilute bupivacaine (0.1%–0.0625%) with opioid (fentanyl or hydromorphone) or clonidine. Target hourly opioid doses by the epidural route are fentanyl at 0.5 µg/kg/h or hydromorphone at 1 to 2 µg/kg/h. Hemodynamic side effects (hypotension and bradycardia) are rare in younger children.

Considering the higher failure rate with both the advancement of caudal-to-thoracic and lumbar-to-thoracic catheters (7%–83%), several approaches are proposed to improve the reliability and safety of epidural catheter placement in infants and children. Radiographic guidance (fluoroscopy and/or epidurography), electrical motor nerve stimulation guidance, or ultrasound techniques have been recommended. In infants undergoing thoracotomy, an epidural catheter may be placed directly into the thoracic epidural space or the extrapleural paravertebral space prior to closure.

Complications

As with adults, complications associated with RA in children and infants are rare. A large prospective trial involving 24,409 infants, children, and adolescents reported an overall complication rate of 9 per 10,000. These complications were generally minor and temporary, with no residual morbidity and no mortality, but did include a few cases of inadvertent intravascular injection and of total spinal blockade. More than half of these complications were avoidable by the use of proper equipment and techniques (e.g., oversized needle, avoidance of excessive threading of epidural catheters) and appropriate doses of local anesthetics and epidural opioids.

Conclusion

In summary, proactive prevention and control of pain before it is established by surgical and medical procedures can offer both short- and long-term benefits. Pain that is established and severe is difficult to control. Although it may not be realistic to entirely abolish procedural and disease-related nociception and pain, various safe and effective analgesic strategies are available to reduce pain to a magnitude that is tolerable and least disruptive to the resumption of normal functioning.

Suggested readings

Anand KJ. Consensus statement for the prevention and management of pain in the newborn. *Arch Pediatr Adolesc Med* 2001; 155:173–180.

Anderson BJ, van Lingen RA, Hansen TG, et al. Acetaminophen developmental pharmacokinetics in premature neonates and infants: a pooled population analysis. *Anesthesiology* 2002; 96:1336–1345.

Ansermino M, Basu R, Vandebeek C, Montgomery C. Nonopioid additives to local anaesthetics for caudal blockade in children: a systematic review. *Paediatr Anaesth* 2003; 13:561–573.

Bartocci M, Bergqvist LL, Lagercrantz H, Anand KJ. Pain activates cortical areas in the preterm newborn brain. *Pain* 2006; 122:109–117.

Berde CB, Lehn BM, Yee JD, et al. Patient-controlled analgesia in children and adolescents: a randomized, prospective comparison with intramuscular administration of morphine for postoperative analgesia. *J Pediatr* 1991; 118:460–466.

Bouwmeester NJ, Anderson BJ, Tibboel D, Holford NH. Developmental pharmacokinetics of morphine and its metabolites in neonates, infants and young children. *Br J Anaesth* 2004; 92:208–217.

Chambers CT, Reid GJ, McGrath PJ, Finley GA. Development and preliminary validation of a postoperative pain measure for parents. *Pain* 1996; 68:307–313.

Chen E, Joseph MH, Zeltzer LK. Behavioral and cognitive interventions in the treatment of pain in children. *Pediatr Clin North Am* 2000; 47:513–525.

Cucchiaro G, Adzick SN, Rose JB, et al. A comparison of epidural bupivacaine-fentanyl and bupivacaine-clonidine in children undergoing the Nuss procedure. *Anesth Analg* 2006; 103: 322–327.

Dsida RM, Wheeler M, Birmingham PK, et al. Age-stratified pharmacokinetics of ketorolac tromethamine in pediatric surgical patients. *Anesth Analg* 2002; 94:266–270.

Elia N, Tramer MR. Ketamine and postoperative pain – a quantitative systematic review of randomised trials. *Pain* 2005; 113:61–70.

Epstein RH, Mendel HG, Witkowski TA, et al. The safety and efficacy of oral transmucosal fentanyl citrate for preoperative sedation in young children. *Anesth Analg* 1996; 83:1200–1205.

Ganesh A, Rose JB, Wells L, et al. Continuous peripheral nerve blockade for inpatient and outpatient postoperative analgesia in children. *Anesth Analg* 2007; 105:1234–1242.

Giaufre E, Dalens B, Gombert A. Epidemiology and morbidity of regional anesthesia in children: a one-year prospective survey of the French-Language Society of Pediatric Anesthesiologists. *Anesth Analg* 1996; 83:904–912.

Goobie SM, Montgomery CJ, Basu R, et al. Confirmation of direct epidural catheter placement using nerve stimulation in pediatric anesthesia. *Anesth Analg* 2003; 97:984–948.

Hansen TG, Henneberg SW, Walther-Larsen S, et al. Caudal bupivacaine supplemented with caudal or intravenous clonidine in children undergoing hypospadias repair: a double-blind study. *Br J Anaesth* 2004; 92:223–227.

Hewitt M, Goldman A, Collins GS, et al. Opioid use in palliative care of children and young people with cancer. *J Pediatr* 2008; 152:39–44.

Chapter 133

Neonatal resuscitation: clinical and practical considerations

Denise M. Chan, Thomas J. Mancuso, and McCallum R. Hoyt

Introduction

There are more than 4 million babies born in the United States each year. Approximately 10% of them will need some assistance with ventilation at birth, and approximately 1% will need extensive resuscitation. Birth asphyxia accounts for nearly 1 million deaths each year worldwide. As a vital member of the labor and delivery team, the anesthesiologist should be skilled in the techniques of neonatal resuscitation. Although our primary focus is the care of the mother, we may be called on to care for the newborn as well.

Initial assessment

Evaluation of the newborn should begin as soon as the baby is handed over, and what to do next is determined by the condition of the child as well as knowledge of predisposing conditions. The fundamental ABCs (Airway, Breathing, and Circulation) underlie the initial steps and are the core of determining ongoing efforts.

Assessment begins with answering the following questions:

- Is the oropharynx clear of meconium?
- Is the baby breathing or crying?
- Is there good muscle tone?
- Does the baby have good color?
- Is the baby full term?

If the answer is yes to all of these questions, routine care can proceed with warming and drying the baby and clearing the airway as needed. If the answer is no, give additional stimulation while warming and drying, and position and clear the airway while providing supplemental oxygen. See Table 133.1 for a list of recommended supplies and equipment for neonatal resuscitation. Prevention of heat loss is important, as cold stress can increase oxygen consumption. Hyperthermia, however, is associated with perinatal respiratory depression.

Although evaluation begins prior to assigning the 1-minute Apgar score (Table 133.2), this score can be helpful in determining whether interventional steps need to be initiated or maintained. The Apgar score is conventionally performed at 1 and 5 minutes after birth. If the 5-minute score is less than 7, ongoing evaluation and the assignment of scores continue every 5 minutes, up to 20 minutes. There are no consistent data on the significance of the Apgar score in preterm infants.

The need for resuscitation can often be predicted prior to delivery, as certain risk factors increase the likelihood of difficulties at birth (Table 133.3).

Airway, breathing, circulation

Although the current recommendation is to use 100% oxygen in the resuscitation of the newborn, recent studies have suggested that this may be of no benefit, and perhaps even harmful, when compared to resuscitation with room air. In a Cochrane Database meta-analysis of five studies comparing resuscitation with room air versus 100% oxygen, four of the studies showed a significant reduction in the rate of death in the room air group, whereas one study showed no significant differences in rates of adverse neurodevelopmental outcomes at 18- to 24-month follow-up. If resuscitation is performed with room air, supplemental oxygen should be readily available, especially if central cyanosis is present. Additionally, the fraction of inspired oxygen content (FiO_2) that is delivered should be determined by the neonatal saturation of peripheral oxygen (SpO_2), which should read in the low 90s. The FiO_2 should be increased only as necessary to reach this goal, noting that 100% saturation is *not* the goal.

If meconium is present (as is seen in approximately 12% of deliveries), but the infant is vigorous (i.e., strong respiratory effort and good muscle tone), suctioning may not be necessary beyond the usual need to clear the oropharynx and nose. If meconium is present at delivery and the baby is not vigorous, the trachea should be intubated and suctioned via the endotracheal tube (ETT) as the ETT is withdrawn. Ideally this process is performed only once, as trauma to the trachea from repeated suctioning and hypoxemia may occur. In addition, care must be taken not to suction too vigorously as pharyngeal stimulation may cause a vagal reflex resulting in severe bradycardia and/or apnea.

Evaluate the newborn for respiration, heart rate, and color within 30 seconds of birth. If the baby is apneic or has a heart rate of < 100 bpm, give positive-pressure ventilation (PPV) at 40 to 60 breaths per minute for 30 seconds. Peak inspiratory pressures of 30 to 40 cm H_2O are often needed for initial expansion because of fluid-filled lungs, but subsequent breaths for healthy lungs require only 15 to 20 cm H_2O. Endotracheal intubation may be considered at any point; for example,

Table 133.1. Neonatal resuscitation supplies and equipment

Suction equipment
  Bulb syringe
  Wall suction and tubing
  Suction catheters, 5F or 6F, 8F, and 10F or 12F
  8F feeding tube and 20-ml syringe
  Meconium aspiration device
Bag-and-mask equipment
  Neonatal resuscitation bag with a pressure-release valve or pressure
    manometer (the bag must be capable of delivering 90%–100%
    oxygen)
  Face masks, newborn and premature sizes (masks with cushioned rim
    preferred)
  Oxygen with flowmeter (flow rate up to 10 L/min) and tubing (including
    portable oxygen cylinders)
Intubation equipment
  Laryngoscope with straight blades, No. 0 (preterm) and No. 1 (term)
  Extra bulbs and batteries for laryngoscope
  Tracheal tubes 2.5, 3.0, 3.5, and 4.0 mm ID
  Stylet
  Scissors
  Tape or securing device for tracheal tube
  Alcohol sponges
  CO_2 detector
  Laryngeal mask airway (optional)
Medications
  Epinephrine 1:10,000 (0.1 mg/ml) – 3-ml or 10-ml ampules
  Isotonic crystalloid (normal saline or Ringer's lactate) for volume
    expansion – 100 or 250 ml
  Sodium bicarbonate 4.2% (5 mEq/10 ml) – 10-ml ampules
  Naloxone hydrochloride 0.4 mg/ml – 1-ml ampules; or 1.0 mg/ml – 2-ml
    ampules
  Normal saline, 30 ml
  Dextrose 10%, 250 ml
  Normal saline "fish" or "bullet" (optional)
  Feeding tube, 5F (optional)
  Umbilical vessel catheterization kit or supplies
  Sterile gloves
  Scalpel or scissors
  Povidone–iodine solution
  Umbilical tape
  Umbilical catheters, 3.5F, 5F
  Three-way stopcock
  Syringes, 1, 3, 5, 10, 20, and 50 ml
  Needles, 25-, 21-, and 18-gauge or puncture device for needleless system
Miscellaneous
  Gloves and appropriate personal protection
  Radiant warmer or other heat source
  Firm, padded resuscitation surface
  Clock (timer optional)
  Warmed linens
  Stethoscope
  Tape, 1/2 or 3/4 inch
  Cardiac monitor and electrodes and/or pulse oximeter with probe
    (optional for delivery room)
  Oropharyngeal airways

ID, internal diameter.

Table 133.2. Apgar score

Physical examination	0	1	2
Heart rate	None	<100/minute	100/minute
Respiratory effort	Apnea	Irregular, slow	Crying, good effort
Muscle tone	Limp	Flexed extremities	Actively moving
Irritability	No response	Facial grimace	Cough, cry
Color	Blue or pale	Peripheral cyanosis	All pink

other reasons despite endotracheal intubation, such as mechanical blockage of the airway (e.g., choanal atresia, meconium, or mucus plug) or impaired lung function (pneumothorax, pleural effusion, pneumonia, congenital diaphragmatic hernia, pulmonary hypoplasia, or extreme prematurity).

If the heart rate is < 60 bpm, chest compressions should be started at 90 compressions per minute. Ventilation and chest compressions (see Fig. 133.1) should be synchronized at a 3:1 ratio (i.e., 30 breaths and 90 compressions per minute, performed simultaneously).

Medications and fluids

If, after 30 seconds of chest compressions, the heart rate is still less than 60 bpm, epinephrine may be given via either the ETT or the umbilical vein while compressions and ventilations continue (Table 133.5). Fewer than 0.2% of newborns will need epinephrine during resuscitation, and care must be taken when giving it, as the subsequent hypertension and increased cerebral

Table 133.3. Risk factors associated with birth of a depressed newborn

Antepartum factors	
Maternal diabetes	Significant maternal cardiac, renal, pulmonary disease
Maternal hypertension (chronic or pregnancy-induced)	Polyhydramnios
Maternal infection	Oligohydramnios
Fetal anemia	Multiple gestation
Fetal hydrops	Post-term gestation
Fetal anomalies	Premature or preterm rupture of membranes
Decreased fetal activity	Maternal substance abuse
Second- or third-trimester bleeding	No prenatal care
	Maternal age < 16 or > 35 years
Intrapartum factors	
Chorioamnionitis	Placenta previa
Nonreassuring fetal heart rate tracing	Placental abruption
Emergent caesarian delivery	Uterine hyperstimulation
Use of general anesthesia	Prolapsed cord
Forceps or vacuum-assisted delivery	Breech or other abnormal presentation
Premature labor	Meconium-stained amniotic fluid
Precipitous labor	Significant intrapartum bleeding
Prolonged rupture of membranes	Opioids administered to mother within 4 h of delivery
Macrosomia	
Prolonged labor	
Prolonged second stage of labor	

low-birth-weight infants may be difficult to mask ventilate and may need to be intubated early. A colorimetric carbon dioxide (CO_2) detector should be used to ensure proper ETT placement: Remember that there may be no color change in the detector if the baby's cardiac output is low.

Although still controversial, a laryngeal mask airway may be considered if bag-mask ventilation or endotracheal intubation is unsuccessful. In addition, ventilation may be inadequate for

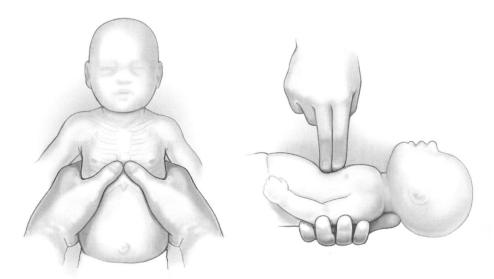

Figure 133.1. Chest compressions in the neonate. The preferred manner for chest compressions is the thumb-over-thumb technique with the fingers wrapped about the thorax for further support. This is preferred because it is considered to be more stable. The other acceptable technique is the two-finger technique with the other hand beneath the chest for further support. It is more useful for smaller hands and when an umbilical catheter is being placed.

blood flow may be associated with intracranial bleeding, especially in the fragile region of the germinal matrix.

Chest compressions should continue until the heart rate is >60 bpm; PPV should continue until the heart rate is >100 bpm and the baby is breathing. After 3 to 5 minutes, the dose of epinephrine may be repeated.

If the baby is not responding to resuscitation, consider that the neonate may be hypovolemic. Isotonic crystalloid or O-negative blood cross-matched with the mother's blood (10 ml/kg) should be given intravenously (IV) over 5 to 10 minutes. Albumin is no longer the fluid of choice for initial volume expansion and should not be considered. If hypovolemic shock is indeed the diagnosis, the neonate should respond quickly.

Sodium bicarbonate (2 mEq/kg) is sometimes given IV to correct metabolic acidosis, although no clear reduction of morbidity or mortality has been shown. This medication must be given slowly to reduce the risk of developing an intraventricular hemorrhage. It is also recommended that it not be given without an ETT in place. Refer to Table 133.4 for normal umbilical venous and arterial blood values.

Naloxone (0.1 mg/kg IV) may be given for severe respiratory depression if there is documented administration of an opioid to the mother within the past 4 hours. If the baby's mother is a chronic opioid user, however, naloxone should not be given because it may cause the baby to go into opioid withdrawal.

If ongoing resuscitative efforts have not resulted in clinical improvement, there are several unusual clinical problems that should be considered. Pneumothorax may have occurred at some point during delivery and resuscitation. Hypoglycemia can be ruled out by checking the glucose level. Congenital diaphragmatic hernia can present with unequal breath sounds in the setting of unsuccessful resuscitation. If the infant has severe undiagnosed central nervous system (CNS) anomalies, resuscitation may not succeed.

After resuscitation

After a baby has been successfully resuscitated, ongoing care and monitoring should be provided to assess for complications as noted in Table 133.6. For instance, if meconium was present in the amniotic fluid, the newborn is at risk for development of meconium aspiration syndrome with respiratory distress, hypoxemia, hypercarbia, and pulmonary artery hypertension. In addition, complications may occur as a direct result of resuscitation efforts, such as a pneumothorax from broken ribs or a ruptured liver or spleen from improperly performed chest compressions.

Discontinuing resuscitation efforts is a difficult decision that involves all members of the team, including parents, physicians,

Table 133.4. Umbilical venous and arterial blood gas values

	pH	PO$_2$	PCO$_2$	Saturation (%)
Umbilical vein	7.30–7.35	30	40	70
Umbilical artery	7.24–7.29	20	50	28

Table 133.5. Medications for newborn resuscitation

Medication	Dose	Notes
Epinephrine IV	0.01–0.03 mg/kg	Can repeat q5min
Epinephrine ETT	Up to 0.1 mg/kg	Give with PPV
IV fluid	10–20 ml/kg	NS, LR, or blood
Naloxone	0.1 mg/kg IV or IM	Give in the setting of acute maternal opioid use after other considerations are eliminated
NaHCO$_3$	2 mEq/kg IV	Give slowly

NS, normal saline; LR, lactated Ringer's; IM, intramuscularly.

Table 133.6. Potential complications in newborns

Pulmonary hypertension
Respiratory distress syndrome
Pneumonia
Hypotension
Acute tubular necrosis
Electrolyte imbalances
Syndrome of inappropriate antidiuretic hormone secretion
Feeding problems
Seizures
Necrotizing enterocolitis
Intracranial hemorrhage
Hypothermia
Hypoglycemia

and social workers. Some infants will not be able to be resuscitated. After 10 minutes of asystole, the chance of survival is slim, and, in those who survive, the incidence of severe disability is almost universal.

An intimate knowledge of the techniques of neonatal resuscitation is essential for the practicing anesthesiologist. Preparation, organization, and communication among team members will facilitate the best outcome for the baby.

Suggested readings

American Academy of Pediatrics, Committee on Fetus and Newborn, American College of Obstetricians and Gynecologists and Committee on Obstetric Practice. The Apgar score. *Pediatrics* 2006; 117:1444–1447.

Arkoosh, Valerie A., 2005 ASA Annual Meeting Refresher Course Lectures, *Neonatal Resuscitation: What the Anesthesiologist Needs to Know,* American Society of Anesthesiologists, Park Ridge, IL.

Beveridge CJE, Wilkinson AR. Sodium bicarbonate infusion during resuscitation of infants at birth. *Cochrane Database Syst Rev* 2006;1. CD004864. DOI: 10.1002/14651858.CD004864. pub2.

Camann W. Obstetrics – never a dull moment! *American Society of Anesthesiologists Newsletter* 2003; 67:13–14.

Datta S. *Obstetric Anesthesia Handbook.* 4th ed. New York: Springer; 2006.

Goldsmith JP, Zaichkin J, eds. *Textbook of Neonatal Resuscitation.* 5th ed. Elk Grove Village, IL: American Academy of Pediatrics and American Heart Association; 2006.

Grein AJ, Weiner GM. Laryngeal mask airway versus bag-mask ventilation or endotracheal intubation for neonatal resuscitation. *Cochrane Database Syst Rev* 2005;2:CD003314.

Harrington D, Redman C, Moulden M, Greenwood C. The long-term outcome in surviving infants with Apgar zero at 10 minutes: a systematic review of the literature and hospital-based cohort. *Am J Obstet Gynecol* 2007; 196(5):463.e1–463.e5.

International Guidelines for Neonatal Resuscitation: An Excerpt from the Guidelines 2000 for Cardiopulmonary Resuscitation and Emergency Cardiovascular Care: International Consensus on Science. *Pediatrics* 2000; 106(3):e29.

Keenan WJ. Neonatal resuscitation: what role for volume expansion? *Pediatrics* 2005; 115:1072–1073.

Perondi MB, Reis AG, Pavia EF, et al. A comparison of high-dose and standard-dose epinephrine in children with cardiac arrest. *N Engl J Med* 2004; 350:1722–1730.

Tan A, Schulze A, O'Donnell CPF, Davis PG. Air versus oxygen for resuscitation of infants at birth. *Cochrane Database Syst Rev* 2005;2. CD002273.

Toker-Maimon O, Joseph LJ, Bromiker R, Schimmel MS. Neonatal cardiopulmonary arrest in the delivery room. *Pediatrics* 2006; 118:847–848.

Saugstad OD, Ramji S, Vento M. Oxygen for newborn resuscitation: how much is enough? *Pediatrics* 2006; 118:789–792.

Wyckoff MH, Perlman JM, Laptook AR. Use of volume expansion during delivery room resuscitation in near-term and term infants. *Pediatrics* 2005; 115:950–955.

Ambulatory and Remote Location Anesthesia

Beverly K. Philip, editor

Introduction to ambulatory anesthesia

McCallum R. Hoyt and Naila Moghul

Over the past three decades, anesthesia techniques and strategies for ambulatory surgery have grown considerably. Freestanding surgery centers have become common, and in some hospitals as many as 80% of all surgeries performed are on an ambulatory basis.

From a cost-based perspective, ambulatory centers are designed to offer improved case efficiency, better use of limited resources, and less expensive care. Choice of anesthetic technique and perioperative management play an important role in how the center functions, as do procedures and personnel appropriate to the center's marketplace strategy, available equipment, and facility design. Rapid induction and emergence as well as a thorough knowledge of anesthetic techniques to minimize common postoperative complications, such as postoperative nausea and vomiting (PONV), require a thorough understanding of the pharmacology and principles behind the choices made.

As the specialty has refined itself, cases of increasing complexity as well as patients with more significant medical issues are being considered for ambulatory settings. Precisely which cases are appropriate as well as what disqualifies a patient for procedures in an ambulatory setting remain to be fully defined, but the expectation is that the trend toward greater complexity will continue.

Patient selection

An ambulatory procedure can occur in either a free-standing center or as part of a hospital-based service. To categorize the procedures that match the facility resources and personnel expertise, some free-standing centers develop guidelines on appropriate procedures but also describe the suitable patient population that will match the abilities of the center's personnel. Guidelines may only propose which patients may be appropriate to the center, and, as the range and complexity of ambulatory surgical cases have increased over the years, so has the complexity of the patients being managed in such settings. As a result, appropriate patient selection remains an evolving concept.

The basic principles for preoperative patient evaluation are the same for ambulatory patients as they are for inpatients. Healthy patients or those with minor medical issues do not necessarily need to go through an on-site preoperative evaluation. They can fill out a form, partake in a phone screen, or fill out an online form that is reviewed by someone from the preoperative clinic. For patients with more significant health issues that require active medical management, an evaluation at a preoperative clinic is usually recommended. This evaluation should be done several days in advance of the planned surgery as it often takes time to obtain records, review tests, or perform more assessment. It is also practical to discuss the probable anesthetic choices and initiate the informed consent process during this initial meeting so that patients have time to consider any questions they may have for the anesthesia provider on the day of surgery. Additionally, patients should be informed of the requirement that they will not be allowed to drive themselves home after surgery but will need to arrange for a responsible adult to take them home. Patients should understand that not having adequate arrangements before their surgery will likely disqualify them for ambulatory status, resulting in their surgery being rescheduled or plans made for an overnight stay.

Special considerations

There are some medical conditions or patient populations that raise questions as to their appropriate selection or require forethought unique to the ambulatory setting. These conditions and populations will be mentioned here. Although ambulatory centers may choose to include or exclude pediatric or pregnant patients, there is nothing about these populations that contraindicate their inclusion as ambulatory cases. Their basic management principles are discussed elsewhere.

Patients with significant comorbidities

No single factor determines whether a patient with significant health comorbidities requiring active medical management can be appropriately chosen for an ambulatory procedure in a free-standing center. Hospital-based centers may be better equipped both with personnel and facility resources to deal with the potential complications such a patient brings, making an unplanned inpatient admission far easier to address and manage. Regardless, cases should be decided within the context of facility and personnel capabilities. For instance, a stable American Society of Anesthesiologists (ASA) IV patient may have a cataract operation carried out safely in a free-standing ambulatory setting, yet a morbidly obese asthmatic for liposuction may not be appropriate for the same facility.

Elderly patients

There are no published guidelines on age limits for elderly patients, but rather each patient should be selected based on his or her medical status and the proposed procedure. Studies have not confirmed that advanced age alone is a risk factor, and elderly patients are scheduled for a broad range of procedures at most ambulatory centers. Although one study identified an age greater than 85 years as a predictor for hospital admission in the immediate postoperative period, pre-existing comorbidities and surgical length may have contributed to their results. Other studies have not confirmed this finding.

Morbid obesity

The percentage of patients who meet the body mass index (BMI) definition of morbid obesity is increasing at a rapid pace. Many of these patients have a comorbid history of cardiovascular, endocrine, pulmonary, or gastrointestinal disease. Difficulty with intravenous and airway access should be anticipated, and, when combined with the logistical considerations of proper equipment for higher BMIs, such patients may not be suitable for that facility. Although there is no evidence that adverse perioperative events leading to unplanned admissions are more frequent for patients with BMI greater than a particular number, centers may choose to set a limit above which patients are considered unsuitable candidates.

Obstructive sleep apnea syndrome

Obstructive sleep apnea (OSA) is estimated to be present in 2% of women and 4% of men, and is expected to increase severalfold over the next decade. Although OSA is almost always a consideration in the morbidly obese population, it can be present in persons with a normal body habitus, regardless of gender. Intraoperative airway management as well as postoperative somnolence, desaturation, hypertension, and dysrhythmias are more common complications encountered in this population. Although the literature acknowledges these complications, it does not exclude this population from the ambulatory setting. Current management strategies recommend matching the patient to the procedure, and suggest the use of neuraxial techniques, judicious use of opioids, both neuraxial and systemic, to avoid the potential respiratory depressant effects, and use of local field blocks and nonopioid analgesics for postoperative pain management. These patients should be placed in a nonsupine position while in recovery and discharge delayed until advancement into a nonmonitored environment is safe.

Respiratory disease

Patients with preexisting but well-controlled reactive airway disease are at low risk for postoperative respiratory complications and can routinely be managed at most ambulatory surgery centers. The risk for adverse postoperative events is higher if there are active symptoms and signs of bronchospasm preop-eratively. If bronchospasm is present, any elective procedure should be rescheduled until it is adequately managed.

Cardiovascular disease

Patients with stable, preexisting cardiovascular disease routinely have procedures done at ambulatory centers. The literature does not suggest that well-managed patients are at increased risk. The patient's cardiac medication should be continued throughout the perioperative period, and there is no evidence that prolonged cardiac monitoring is required or beneficial. For laparoscopic procedures, there should be a clear understanding of the effects on the cardiovascular system, but these changes are resolved within an hour of the recovery period. Obviously, patients with unstable cardiovascular status or a history of a recent myocardial infarct are not considered suitable candidates.

Anesthetic options

Any anesthetic technique may be considered for the ambulatory patient as long as it is appropriate for the procedure and adheres to the goals of a rapid recovery.

General anesthesia

In selecting whether to use inhalational agents or avoid them by using a total intravenous anesthetic (TIVA), several concerns that apply to the ambulatory patient should be considered. As the pharmacologic properties of the medications discussed are covered elsewhere, only clinical considerations will be covered here.

Inhalation agents

The newer volatile agents of desflurane and sevoflurane work well for the ambulatory patient as the drug profiles show a fast onset and recovery with few side effects. Indeed, recovery indices are achieved more quickly when compared with popular TIVA agents, such as propofol. Randomized, controlled trials (RCTs), however, show that the use of volatile agents provides a risk factor for PONV, which may delay discharge of patients at risk despite the use of appropriate antiemetics. Nitrous oxide is also a popular adjunct to the inhalational technique, but systematic reviews also suggest that it may predispose the patient to PONV, if used.

A common practice is to try to achieve the benefits of one drug or method by combining techniques or switching volatiles; for example, using an isoflurane-based technique and then switching to desflurane to achieve the faster recovery profile it provides. This only serves to expose the patient to two agents unnecessarily as the observed recovery profile is that of an isoflurane-only technique. The same misconception is at play when propofol is used at the beginning and end of an anesthetic that uses a volatile in between – the so-called "propofol sandwich." The goal is to achieve the antiemetic effects of the propofol; however, the recovery profile more closely resembles that of the volatile agent.

Total intravenous anesthetics

Propofol provides the cornerstone for this technique, and opioids such as sufentanil or remifentanil are often added (see Chapter 49). By itself, propofol can provide antiemetic effects, but its recovery profile can be more prolonged when compared with profiles of the newer volatiles. Should an opioid be added, the risk of PONV increases and may delay discharge. Initial profiles suggest that opioid use in this manner may not be well-suited to the ambulatory patient; further research will be necessary to make that determination.

Neuraxial and regional anesthesia, field blocks, and pain management

One of the most common reasons for an unplanned hospital admission after ambulatory surgery is intractable pain. The use of neuraxial anesthesia (i.e., spinal, epidural, or a combined spinal epidural) in the ambulatory setting is somewhat controversial as it may delay discharge as the block recedes, but that does not mean that its use is not an appropriate choice if the patient and/or procedure are correctly selected. Regional blocks, as are used for surgery on the peripheral limbs, can correlate with a timely discharge and good pain management well into the postoperative period. Increasingly, continuous nerve blocks are being used to provide analgesia beyond the first 24 hours. Ambulatory patients receiving these techniques are often alert, comfortable, and discharged in a timely manner. A field block, which is the infiltration of local anesthetics along the incision by the surgeon, can also be an effective way to manage pain. Whether it is best to have the surgeon employ a field block before the incision, at the time of the closure, or both is unclear.

Whether some form of block is used or not, successful pain management is generally of a multimodal nature. Although the use of intraoperative opioids may be necessary, continuation of those same medications should not be the sole source of pain management. Intraoperative, but particularly postoperative, opioid use has been associated with PONV and is a specific risk factor. Attempts to reduce the use of opioids or avoid them altogether in the postoperative period can be achieved through the use of a multimodal analgesic approach. Medications, such as nonsteroidal anti-inflammatory drugs (NSAIDs) and cyclooxygenase (COX)-2 inhibitors (a subset of NSAIDs), are reasonable choices, as is acetaminophen. An N-methyl-D-aspartate (NMDA) antagonist such as ketamine may also be a reasonable choice when used judiciously. The goal is to provide effective analgesic management that is comprehensive, of adequate duration, and with minimal side effects. Additionally, preemptive pain management with opioids has not been shown to reduce postoperative pain requirements. The preemptive use of nonopioid medications, such as the NSAIDs, has been shown, however, to significantly reduce postoperative analgesic needs.

Discharge criteria

Established algorithms and predetermined protocols are frequently used during the recovery of patients in the postoperative unit. The nursing staff use these criteria to ensure that the patients are stable and ready for discharge. It is also their responsibility to make sure that the patients understand the discharge orders and have adequate transport and coverage for the required period. As outlined below, there are three distinct phases of recovery from anesthesia and surgery that apply to ambulatory patients.

Phase I

This phase immediately follows the removal of the patient from the operating area. Initial monitoring is intensive with one-to-one or two-to-one nursing coverage, and the patient is watched for maintenance of his or her own airway, stabilization of vital signs, and a return to baseline alertness. Blood pressure and oxygenation saturation are monitored as is the electrocardiogram (ECG). After the patient is considered to be stable and has met the defined criteria, he or she is moved to the second phase of recovery.

Phase II

When the patient is considered hemodynamically stable and alert and does not require the previous monitors, he or she advances to the second phase of recovery. Family members can now be present and often are in the ambulatory setting. Ambulation is monitored, voiding is encouraged, and, although liquids and solids may be offered, for ambulatory patients it is often prudent to not encourage intake because of the issues of PONV and travel. Analgesia should be achieved with nonopioid medications and ideally with over-the-counter analgesics. It is from this phase that the patient is discharged home, and patients must be discharged into the care of a responsible adult.

Fast-tracking

Fast-tracking is the term used for patients who are awake enough to bypass phase I recovery. Any variety of procedures may qualify a patient for this if he or she has had minimal anesthesia or any of a range of anesthetic techniques. Although the layout of the ambulatory recovery facility as well as nursing resources may impact the availability of such a program, the criteria used to fast-track a patient into phase II recovery directly from the operating room (OR) are the same criteria used to advance the patient from phase I into phase II recovery by the nursing staff. The exact criteria may vary slightly by facility, but generally the patient should be awake; with stable vital signs and minimal dizziness, pain, or nausea; and able to maintain a saturation of 92% or greater on room air. Patient satisfaction surveys have shown that patients, families, and surgeons respond favorably to an early discharge as it contextualizes a well-conducted, well-tolerated, and well-planned anesthetic experience.

Postoperative issues

A true complication from anesthetics for ambulatory patients is rare, but side effects are common. Two issues, pain management and PONV, are the leading causes of an unplanned hospital admission when they occur to the extreme. Pain management principles have already been discussed. Emetic management involves patient hydration, limiting intake of solids postoperatively, recognizing the risk factors and minimizing them as much as possible, and giving appropriate antiemetics as indicated. Risk factors for PONV can be broken down into surgical, anesthetic, and patient-specific. Anesthetic factors have already been addressed. These involve the use of multimodal analgesics to reduce or avoid opioids in the intraoperative and especially the postoperative phase, the avoidance of volatiles and nitrous oxide, and the use of a regional technique or field blocks by the surgeon as appropriate. The surgical factors are less controllable and involve the type and duration of the surgery. The Apfel score, which is a simplified PONV risk score, applies one point for each of the following factors: female, nonsmoker, history of PONV, and use of postoperative opioids. With zero risk factors, the incidence for PONV is 10%. With each additional factor, the incidence increases to 20%, 40%, 60%, and 80%, respectively. Prophylactic treatment of PONV is also a multimodal approach, and some of the recommended antiemetics are selective serotonin 5-hydroxytryptamine type 3 (5-HT$_3$) receptor antagonists, steroids, anticholinergics, and butyrophenones. Dosing algorithms are beyond the scope of this chapter, but two rules to follow are (1) if the medication has not worked, do not give more but move to another class of antiemetic; and (2) if PONV returns ≥ 6 hours after treatment, the dose that was successful may be repeated.

Other side effects that may delay the discharge of the ambulatory patient or his or her return to normal activity are drowsiness, dizziness, headache, sore throat, and general aches. Although many of these side effects are difficult to avoid, the incidence of sore throat can be reduce by using a smaller endotracheal tube than is normally used for inpatients.

Suggested readings

Benumof JL. Obstructive sleep apnea in the adult obese patient: implications for airway management. *J Clin Anesth* 2001; 13:144–156.

Bryson GL, Chung F, Cox R, et al. (CAARE Group). Patient selection in ambulatory anesthesia – an evidence-based review: Part 1. *Can J Anesth.* 2004; 51(8):768–781.

Bryson GL, Chung F, Cox R, et al. (CAARE Group). Patient selection in ambulatory anesthesia – an evidence-based review: Part 2. *Can J Anesth* 2004; 51(8):782–794.

Chikungwa M, Smith I. Controversial issues in ambulatory anesthesia. *Anesthesiol Clin N Am* 2003; 21:313–327.

Chung F, Mezei G, Tong D. Pre-existing medical conditions as predictors of adverse events in day-case surgery. *Br J Anaesth* 1999; 83:262–270.

Crews J. Multimodal pain management strategies for office-based and ambulatory procedures. *JAMA* 2002; 288:629–632.

Gan TJ, Meyer TA, Apfel CC, et al. Society for Ambulatory Anesthesia guidelines for the management of postoperative nausea and vomiting. *Anesth Analg* 2007; 105:1615–1628.

Marshall SI, Chung F. Discharge criteria and complications after ambulatory surgery. *Anesth Analg* 1999; 88:508–517.

Practice Guidelines for Management of Patients with Obstructive Sleep Apnea. A report by the American Society of Anesthesiologists Task Force on Perioperative Management of Patients with Obstructive Sleep Apnea. *Anesthesiology* 2006; 104:1081–1093. Available at: http://www.asahq.org/publicationsandservices/sleepapnea103105.pdf.

Springman SR, Hines R (eds.). *Ambulatory Anesthesia: The Requisites in Anesthesiology.* 1st ed. St. Louis: Mosby Press; 2006.

Twersky RS, Philip BK (eds.). *Handbook of Ambulatory Anesthesia.* 2nd ed. New York: Springer; 2008.

White PF, Song D. New criteria for fast-tracking after out-patient anesthesia: a comparison with the modified Aldrete's scoring system. *Anesth Analg* 1999; 88:1069–1072.

Chapter 135

Anesthesia outside the operating room

Wendy L. Gross and Ramon Martin

Nonsurgical approaches to treatment outside the operating room (OR) often require the participation of anesthesiologists. Cases performed outside of the OR occur in areas that lack the infrastructure of the OR and are often unfamiliar to anesthesiologists. Medical practitioners and anesthesiologists practicing outside the OR are frequently faced with chronically or acutely ill patients whose medical conditions have not been or cannot be optimized. Existing comorbidities may go unnoticed and untreated unless an anesthesiologist points them out. Medical proceduralists are focused on getting the cases done and are likely to be unfamiliar with the risks of anesthesia in this environment. It is the task of the anesthesiologist to step back and evaluate the "big picture."

Comorbidities such as obesity, (coronary artery disease [CAD], chronic obstructive pulmonary disease [COPD], hypertension [HTN], diabetes mellitus [DM], arthritis, etc.), significant opioid intake, solid tumors that compress and/or invade major organs, and psychosocial issues are some common complicating patient characteristics that are as important as airway evaluation in the anesthetic care of these patients. Consideration of these issues should be a component of ongoing discussions with participating medical interventionalists and constitute the key features of deciding how to take the best care of a patient during the procedure at hand.

A complete medical history is essential. Good communication skills and a thorough understanding of pathophysiology are required of any anesthesiologist practicing in a remote location because the OR support network may not be readily available and the procedure may be unfamiliar or new. Many interventionalists rely upon imaging modalities that anesthesiologists are unfamiliar with. Therefore, it is incumbent on the anesthesiologists outside the OR to establish an environment in which there is succinct, frequent, and clear communication between anesthesiologist and interventionalist regarding both the procedural plan and the progress of the intervention.

The change in venue creates technical, communication, and operational difficulties for anesthesiologists. This chapter addresses practice standards, problems encountered, and recommended approaches for procedures frequently performed in some common non-OR anesthetizing locations.

Non-OR standards of care

The OR model of care should be extended to all cases performed in non-OR locations and includes the following fundamental features:

1. Thorough preprocedure assessment and informed consent;
2. Standardized monitoring and anesthetic equipment consistent with maximal patient safety and comfort;
3. Clearly marked and readily available emergency equipment (code cart, defibrillator, and difficult airway cart);
4. Adequate backup (equipment and personnel) in case of emergencies and/or difficulties;
5. Available postoperative care in a postanesthesia care unit (PACU) setting with the oversight of an anesthesiologist and a dedicated nursing staff; and
6. A clear and understood procedure and anesthetic plan.

Any procedure performed in a non-OR area can degenerate into a complex or unmanageable situation for logistical or medical reasons. Adherence to the standards just mentioned is even more critical when an anesthetic is administered away from the support structure of the OR. The American Society of Anesthesiologists (ASA) guidelines for non-OR anesthesia care are summarized in Fig. 135.1.

Non-OR anesthetizing locations

In this section, we highlight seven commonly encountered non-OR locations where anesthetic care is provided regularly. Each of these will be discussed in terms of typical procedures performed and commonly encountered problems.

Angiography/interventional radiology

The angiography/interventional radiology (angio/IR) suite encompasses a wide range of procedures. Up to 70% of the procedures are urgent or emergent and are booked less than 48 hours ahead of time. Even though most of these cases are performed with a nurse providing sedation to the patient, there is a continual discussion between the anesthesiologists and angio/IR staff about how best to keep patients comfortable. Patient assessment before the procedure is critical to determine

GUIDELINES FOR NONOPERATING ROOM ANESTHETIZING LOCATIONS

(Approved by House of Delegates on October 19, 1994,
and last amended on October 15, 2003)

These guidelines apply to all anesthesia care involving anesthesiology personnel for procedures intended to be performed in locations outside an operating room. These are minimal guidelines which may be exceeded at any time based on the judgment of the involved anesthesia personnel. These guidelines encourage quality patient care but observing them cannot guarantee any specific patient outcome. These guidelines are subject to revision from time to time, as warranted by the evolution of technology and practice. ASA Standards, Guidelines and Policies should be adhered to in all nonoperating room settings except where they are not applicable to the individual patient or care setting.

1. There should be in each location a reliable source of oxygen adequate for the length of the procedure. There should also be a backup supply. Prior to administering any anesthetic, the anesthesiologist should consider the capabilities, limitations and accessibility of both the primary and backup oxygen sources. Oxygen piped from a central source, meeting applicable codes, is strongly encouraged. The backup system should include the equivalent of at least a full E cylinder.

2. There should be in each location an adequate and reliable source of suction. Suction apparatus that meets operating room standards is strongly encouraged.

3. In any location in which inhalation anesthetics are administered, there should be an adequate and reliable system for scavenging waste anesthetic gases.

4. There should be in each location: (a) a self-inflating hand resuscitator bag capable of administering at least 90 percent oxygen as a means to deliver positive pressure ventilation; (b) adequate anesthesia drugs, supplies and equipment for the intended anesthesia care; and (c) adequate monitoring equipment to allow adherence to the "Standards for Basic Anesthetic Monitoring." In any location in which inhalation anesthesia is to be administered, there should be an anesthesia machine equivalent in function to that employed in operating rooms and maintained to current operating room standards.

5. There should be in each location, sufficient electrical outlets to satisfy anesthesia machine and monitoring equipment requirements, including clearly labeled outlets connected to an emergency power supply. In any anesthetizing location determined by the health care facility to be a "wet location" (e.g., for cystoscopy or arthroscopy or a birthing room in labor and delivery), either isolated electric power or electric circuits with ground fault circuit interrupters should be provided.*

6. There should be in each location, provision for adequate illumination of the patient, anesthesia machine (when present) and monitoring equipment. In addition, a form of battery-powered illumination other than a laryngoscope should be immediately available.

7. There should be in each location, sufficient space to accommodate necessary equipment and personnel and to allow expeditious access to the patient, anesthesia machine (when present) and monitoring equipment.

8. There should be immediately available in each location, an emergency cart with a defibrillator, emergency drugs and other equipment adequate to provide cardiopulmonary resuscitation.

9. There should be in each location adequate staff trained to support the anesthesiologist. There should be immediately available in each location, a reliable means of two-way communication to request assistance.

10. For each location, all applicable building and safety codes and facility standards, where they exist, should be observed.

11. Appropriate postanesthesia management should be provided (see Standards for Postanesthesia Care). In addition to the anesthesiologist, adequate numbers of trained staff and appropriate equipment should be available to safely transport the patient to a postanesthesia care unit.

Figure 135.1. Guidelines for non-OR anesthetizing locations. With permission from ASA.

what is needed for the patient to comfortably tolerate (i.e., hold still, breathe, and have no pain) a procedure. As a result, a member of the anesthetic team is often involved in evaluating even those patients who are not anticipated to require anesthesia. Such evaluation should begin with morning rounds in the angio/IR suite, when all the patients for the day are presented to the entire group of radiologists, nurses, and anesthesiologists. Discussion should continue during the day among providers.

Most of the procedures require that the patient lie supine. Pain from arthritis and surgical incisions; respiratory compromise from COPD, pneumonia, pleural effusions, or obstructive sleep apnea; and inability to cooperate because of dementia, language differences, or psychiatric disturbances can make a seemingly simple procedure extremely difficult or impossible. Some procedures (portal sclerotherapy, placement of a lumbar dialysis catheter, angiography and/or embolization for gastrointestinal (GI) bleeding in a hypotensive patient) clearly require the involvement of an anesthesiologist. Other procedures, such

as percutaneous nephrostomy tubes, biliary drainage catheters, hemodialysis catheters, arteriovenous (AV) graft declotting, and major vessel stenting, cause little pain after the placement of the intravascular catheter. The patient, however, does have to lie still and be able to cooperate when asked. Patient comorbidities and the scope of the procedure determine the choice of analgesia/anesthesia.

Increasing caseloads may make it cost-effective to have a nurse practitioner involved as a member of the anesthesia team to assist with patient assessments (from airway evaluations in patients with obstructive sleep apnea to comprehensive evaluations in complicated patients). The nurse practitioner interfaces with both the anesthesiologist assigned to angio/IR and the nurses and radiologists in the suite. This nurse practitioner assessment allows for timely and comprehensive patient-information gathering that might otherwise not occur and expedites implementation of treatment by both the radiologist and the anesthesiologist.

Particular issues of concern in the angio/IR area include temperature and radiation exposure. Elderly or chronically ill patients tolerate cold temperatures poorly. Hypothermia is a particularly serious complication of long procedures. Procedure rooms, traditionally kept at 60°F, are now maintained at 68°F. Longer procedures and a high acuity patient population make cold temperatures unacceptable. In addition, forced warm-air heaters are available in all rooms and are used for all patients. Several models that surround the patient but do not interfere with instrumentation are available. Fig. 135.2 shows a typical interventional radiology procedure in the CT scanner.

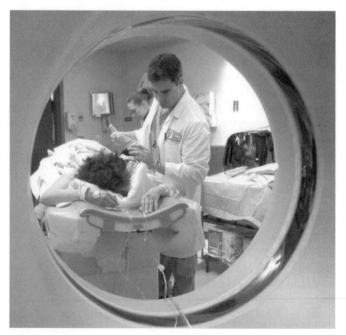

Figure 135.2. Typical interventional radiology procedure in the CT scanner (Source: Brigham and Women's Hospital Web site).

The anesthesiologist should be educated about radiation exposure and the need to wear lead. In some cases, anesthesiologists who staff this area on a regular basis have been provided with their own lead because chronic use of lead that is too heavy or ill-fitting can lead to injury or exposure. There are often challenges related to maintaining a safe distance from the fluoroscopy equipment cone while still adequately monitoring the patient.

Endoscopy

Despite efforts by some insurers to curtail payment for anesthesia services provided in the endoscopy suite, there has been growing use of anesthesia care for those patients. This is due not only to patient requests, but more so to the increasing number of patients with multiple comorbidities, including obesity and chronic narcotic use. Esophagogastroduodenoscopy (EGD), retrograde endoscopy of the bile and pancreatic ducts (ERCP), and colonoscopies normally require only nurse-administered intravenous conscious sedation (IVCS), but medical comorbidities can make a patient an anesthetic candidate. The challenge has been to determine the need for anesthesia services well ahead of time. Because most of the procedures are scheduled electively, patients who are known to require anesthesia care are sent to the preadmitting test center for evaluation and then present on the day of their procedure with a preanesthetic evaluation and plan. The GI staff and the anesthesiologists assigned to the endoscopy suite should discuss individual outpatients and the plan for keeping them comfortable during their procedure. Sometimes outpatients who are scheduled to be cared for by an anesthesiologist have already unsuccessfully attempted the procedure with conscious sedation alone. Inpatients often present as add-on or emergent cases. A thorough preanesthetic assessment will determine what is needed. A patient with ischemic cardiomyopathy who is on the transplant list, a patient with complex congenital heart disease, or a patient with a left ventricular assist device may need to be cared for in the OR with a cardiac anesthesiologist either present for the case or available nearby for consultation. Anesthesiologists may be needed for unstable patients in either the medical intensive care unit (MICU) or the cardiac care unit (CCU) who cannot be moved but require endoscopy.

Most upper and lower endoscopies can be performed with mild to moderate sedation by anesthesiologists or properly trained nonanesthesiologists. Commonly used medications include benzodiazepines, short-acting opioids (such as fentanyl), and propofol. Intubation is rarely necessary and should be dictated by the patient's comorbidities. More complicated, lengthy, and painful procedures such as ERCP are more likely to require deep sedation or general anesthesia (GA).

Increasingly innovative procedures that are lengthy and require deep sedation also contribute to the increasing numbers of endoscopy cases requiring the involvement of anesthesiologists. Gastric bypass repair and double balloon enteroscopy are performed with GA. The anesthetic choice for other procedures, such as laser treatment of Barrett's esophagus, percutaneous endoscopic gastrostomy (PEG) placement, or secretin test to assess bile and pancreatic duct function, are determined by the patient's overall condition.

Radiation oncology

The treatment of surgically unresectable cervical and uterine carcinoma has evolved from a 3-day tandem and ovoid application with continuous radiation therapy and the patient confined to bed, to short outpatient treatments over several days. GA is used for most of these cases. After induction of GA, the patient is placed in the lithotomy position for placement of tandem and ovoids. CT imaging confirms placement and provides the basis for the dosimetry calculations that take place next. Treatment is then carried out, the instrumentation is removed, and the patient is awakened and taken to the PACU. She is discharged later in the day. Some patients have undergone MRI for dosimetry planning. The magnetic resonance scanner being in a different location requires transporting the patient for the 20-minute scan. Occasionally, the authors have used epidural anesthesia with intravenous sedation for such cases, to minimize transport of intubated patients through the hallway.

Epidurals with either intravenous sedation or GA are used for interstitial implants. Because the radiation is given continuously for 48 to 72 hours after placement of the implants, epidurals are left in place and a continuous infusion of dilute local anesthetic and opioid (hydromorphone) is maintained until the course of radiation is completed and the instrumentation removed.

Prostate brachytherapy is a procedure chosen by men who wish to avoid surgical resection. After induction of GA, the patient is placed in lithotomy position and an ultrasound probe is used to guide the placement of needles that hold irradiated seeds. The CT scanner is used for dosimetry. After the seeds are placed and instrumentation removed, the patient is awakened and taken to the PACU. Discharge is usually the next morning.

GA is needed for patients who cannot hold still for conventional external beam radiation therapy. Severe tremors caused by Parkinson's disease or myotonic dystrophy can make external beam radiation impossible unless the patient can be immobilized. Each patient is handled individually with a meeting of all members of the care team as well as by a discussion with the patient and family to review all available options. Every attempt is made to find an alternative technique, distraction, or medication change before embarking on a lengthy course of a short anesthetic (5 days a week for 5–7 weeks).

Computed tomography

Diagnostic CT scans are quite quick and do not require sedation, analgesia, or anesthesia, with the exception of intubated patients from the OR or an ICU. CT-guided cryoablations of solid tumors require anesthetic support. Lesions of the liver and kidney can be accomplished with intravenous analgesia. Comorbidities that render the patient unable to lie flat or keep relatively still for prolonged periods will occasionally necessitate the use of GA. Lung lesions require more careful consideration, and GA is used more frequently. If the lesion is close to a bronchus, a double-lumen tube is placed after induction of GA, and its position is confirmed with a fiber-optic bronchoscope prior to the start of a case. A pneumothorax is expected to some degree in most patients undergoing lung cryoablation, so close attention is paid to respiratory mechanics and the extent of the pneumothorax prior to extubation. If the pneumothorax is large enough to compromise pulmonary function, a chest tube is promptly inserted.

With rising patient acuity, the number of patients who cannot lie flat or hold still is increasing. As a result, the number of cases requiring anesthesia support is growing as well, even for simple procedures such as biopsies or placement of drainage catheters under CT guidance. As in other non-OR locations, the main goal is to screen patients to identify those who are not sedation candidates. We prefer, whenever possible, to schedule these patients for interview at our preoperative evaluation center prior to their procedure. In this way, patients undergo complete assessment and are booked electively with anesthesia care, which avoids the potential of a failed attempt to perform a procedure carried out with nurse-administered sedation only.

Magnetic resonance imaging

Magnetic resonance scanners are unique among non-OR locations because they are used solely for diagnostic testing. Patients who require anesthetic support to get through this imaging comprise a wide variety of patients who simply cannot lie still in the bore of the scanner for 25 minutes to 2 or 3 hours (depending on how much of the body is scanned). As with other non-OR areas, patient evaluation is of primary importance to determine the underlying causes of the MRI intolerance so that the intolerance can be effectively treated. Mental retardation, severe claustrophobia, anxiety disorders, pain from arthritis or physical injuries, and dementia or confusion from an intracerebral bleed are some of the underlying problems routinely seen. When paired with organ system dysfunction, these patients require thought and discussion before proceeding with intravenous analgesia or GA. It is sometimes necessary to discuss the risks and benefits of GA with the patient, family, and primary care team about when the possible information gained from the scan might not change the patient's outcome. This discussion must also include the MRI technicians who have a full schedule and are used to moving patients quickly through their scans.

MRI scanners present specific and unique challenges to anesthesiologists. First, all anesthesia equipment – including the anesthesia machine, laryngoscopes, pumps, and anesthesia cart – must be MRI compatible. In addition, the noise level in the 3-Tesla (3T) units is considerably higher than in 1.5T machines. It is so high that one cannot hear monitor signals and alarms. Remote monitoring from just outside the machine using a slave unit for vital signs and video images of the patient from ceiling-mounted cameras is therefore needed. It remains

to be seen whether this increased noise level will result in more patients being uncomfortable while lying in the scanner. With the advent of the 3T units, there are plans to begin performing procedures just as in CT: biopsies and cryoablation of solid tumors. This will generate more anesthetic cases in the MRI suite.

Unstable cardiovascular disease cannot be monitored with any precision in an MRI scanner and can possibly exclude some patients from having an anesthetic in that location. Although there have been improvements in the consistency of displaying the electrocardiogram (ECG) tracing, it is still not reliable when looking for changes in the ECG, particularly when the patient has been moved all the way into the bore of the magnet.

The magnet's impact on ferrous material precludes any patient with such material implanted from undergoing a magnetic resonance scan. Danger arises from dislodgement or malfunction of vascular clips, pacemakers, automatic implantable cardioverter–defibrillators (AICDs), mechanical heart valves, and implanted biological pumps. Shrapnel is another contraindication. The use of nonferrous materials such as titanium for vascular clips is considered MRI-safe. Some tattoo inks contain high amounts of ferrous oxide and have been reported to cause burn injury.

Interventional neuroradiology

The interventional neuroradiology suite is essentially an offshoot of the neurosurgical OR. Diagnostic cerebral angiograms are performed electively prior to aneurysm clippings. Vascular tumors or large meningiomas are imaged and embolized prior to surgical resection. The neuroradiology suite is also the main source of unplanned urgent cases. Patients often arrive with a subarachnoid hemorrhage for diagnostic angiography to look for a ruptured or leaking aneurysm or arteriovenous malformation (AVM) to determine whether it can be coiled or to map the vascular supply for clipping in the OR. After a craniotomy, if mental status changes ensue, patients are sent to the interventional neuroradiology suite for imaging to look for vasospasm and for possible treatment with intra-arterial verapamil.

Aside from the diagnostic cerebral angiograms (which are done with sedation only), all other procedures require GA, usually with arterial blood pressure monitoring. Because of the need to maintain cerebral perfusion pressure, blood pressure management is an important part of the anesthetic technique and requires communication with the IR staff about target blood pressure and whether anything is given by the proceduralist that might decrease blood pressure (i.e., intra-arterial verapamil). Communication must be maintained with the main OR anesthesia staff about any patients who might end up in the OR for open surgery.

Orphan non-OR cases

Not infrequently, anesthesiologists receive requests to provide "a little bit of propofol" to help get patients through procedures in the MICU, the CCU, the emergency department (ED), or diagnostic areas (PET/CT and ultrasound). These requests are usually urgent or emergent, without prior warning. The patients are generally quite ill with multiple medical problems and no preprocedure assessment. The physicians making the requests are usually internists or radiologists who are not aware of the constraints that the patient's comorbidities place on the performance of the procedure or the administration of sedation or anesthesia. It is important for the anesthesiologist to ascertain that the procedure room has proper equipment, gas supply, and monitors for the safe provision of anesthesia.

The requests from the MICU, CCU, and ED present a dilemma because often these are truly emergencies. An anesthesiologist is sent to evaluate the patient and talk to the care team about what needs to be done. If the patient cannot be moved to the OR, then a limited amount of analgesia, with appropriate monitoring in place, is given to help get the patient through the procedure.

Cardioversions are sometimes necessary in intensive care units and in the electrophysiology (EP) or catheterization laboratories. Cardioversions require the presence of an anesthesiologist because the patient receives intravenous GA for the procedure, which can be short in duration but quite painful while the electrical shock is being delivered. Standard ASA monitoring should be used, including ECG, blood pressure cuff, pulse oximetry, and capnography. Equipment for emergency airway support must be immediately available at the bedside. Usually propofol or etomidate is administered for hypnosis while the patient is maintaining spontaneous ventilation. If the patient becomes apneic and requires ventilatory support, bagmask ventilation is initiated. If the patient's airway is potentially difficult and minimal sedation is desirable, it is reasonable to give midazolam initially, so that the patient has amnesia for the event, and fentanyl for analgesia. The patient should be monitored postcardioversion for at least 30 minutes by a nurse until the vital signs return to baseline and the patient is fully awake.

Summary

Non-OR anesthetizing locations are a diverse, growing area that presents both challenges and opportunities for anesthesiologists. Non-OR procedures are becoming a significant aspect of hospital practice and patient care. As the perimeter of anesthesiology moves from the OR to encompass these new arenas, anesthesiologists must be involved in the planning of procedure rooms so that they are safe and are in compliance with basic ASA standards. We will need to expand the scope of preanesthetic evaluation to non-OR locations.

Transport of patients from ICUs to procedure areas and back is often more challenging than the procedure itself and may well become the routine responsibility of the anesthesiologist. In addition, transport requires good communication with nursing staff both in the procedure area and in the patient care unit. Transport monitoring should ensure that the anesthesiologist has all the information necessary to treat the patient should problems develop en route to the procedure area or back to the unit.

Each health care facility needs to create guidelines for the definition and administration of safe moderate and deep sedation and be able to clarify and discuss the risks and benefits of GA with nonsurgical medical practitioners. Anesthesiology has successfully spearheaded patient safety initiatives and advanced surgical practice in the OR, and it is critical to import those principles to the non-OR arenas.

Suggested readings

Aisenberg J, Brill JV, Ladabaum U, et al. Sedation for gastrointestinal endoscopy: new practices, new economics. *Am J Gastroenterol* 2005; 100:996–1000.

Bhananker SM, Posner KL, Cheney FW, et al. Injury and liability associated with monitored anesthesia care: a closed claims analysis. *Anesthesiology* 2006; 104(2):228–234.

Campo R, Brullet E, Montserrat A, et al. Identification of factors that influence tolerance of upper gastrointestinal endoscopy. *Eur J Gastroenterol Hepatol* 1999; 11:201–204.

Cohen LB, Delegge MH, Aisenberg J, et al. AGA Institute review of endoscopic sedation. *Gastroenterology* 2007; 133:675–701.

Cohen LB, Wechsler JS, Gaetano JN, et al. Endoscopic sedation in the United States: results from a nationwide survey. *Am J Gastroenterol* 2006; 101:967–974.

Frakes JT. Outpatient endoscopy. The case for the ambulatory surgery center. *Gastrointest Endosc Clin N Am* 2002; 12:215–227.

Holzman RS, Cullen DJ, Eichorn JH, Philip JH. Guidelines for sedation and analgesia by nonanesthesiologists during diagnostic and therapeutic procedures. *J Clin Anesth* 1994; 6:255–274.

Holzman RS, Cullen DJ, Eichorn JH, Philip JH. Guidelines for sedation by nonanesthesiologists during diagnostic and therapeutic procedures. The Risk Management Committee of the Department of Anaesthesia of Harvard Medical School. *J Clin Anesth* 1994; 6(4):265–276.

Hussain N, Alsulaiman R, Burtin P, et al. The safety of endoscopic sphincterotomy in patients receiving antiplatelet agents – a case-control study. *Aliment Pharmacol Ther* 2007; 25:579–584.

Kelly JS. Sedation by non-anesthesia personnel provokes safety concerns; anesthesiologists must balance JCAHO standards, politics, & safety. Available at: http://www.apsf.org/resource_center/newsletter/2001/fall/07personnel.htm. Accessed May 25, 2008.

Mathew A, Riley TR 3rd, Young M, et al. Cost-saving approach to patients on long-term anticoagulation who need endoscopy: a decision analysis. *Am J Gastroenterol* 2003; 98:1766–1776.

Payen JF, Chanques G, Mantz J, et al. Current practices in sedation and analgesia for mechanically ventilated critically ill patients. *Anesthesiology* 2007; 106:687–695.

Pike IM. Open-access endoscopy. *Gastrointest Endosc Clin N Am* 2006; 16:709–717.

Pino, RM. The nature of anesthesia and procedural sedation outside of the operating room. *Curr Opin Anaesthesiol* 2007; 20:347–351.

Practice guidelines for sedation and analgesia by non-anesthesiologists. *Anesthesiology* 2002; 96(4):1004–1017.

Soto RG, Fu ES, Vila H Jr, Miguel RV. Capnography accurately detects apnea during monitored anesthesia care. *Anesth Analg* 2004; 99(2):379–382.

Chapter 136

Office-based anesthesia

Fred E. Shapiro

Office-based anesthesia (OBA) refers to the practice of ambulatory anesthesia in the office setting. OBA is a relatively new and growing field as the number of requests to provide anesthesia services by practitioners who have their own outpatient office-based operating facilities have grown at an exponential rate.

OBA marries convenience with financial incentive. It has attraction for both surgeon and patient; the former benefiting from greater control over schedule, operating costs, and revenue generation, and the latter gaining in comfort, convenience, and privacy. One need look no further than recent national statistics for evidence of the popularity of this emerging subspecialty. In 2005, The American Society of Anesthesiologists estimated that more than 10 million surgical procedures were performed in doctors' offices. This number has doubled since 1995 and continues to steadily grow. Today nearly 80% of all surgeries are currently performed in an outpatient facility, either connected to a hospital or in a separate surgical center, and approximately 1 in 10 surgeries are office-based. However, despite the large numbers of procedures, such facilities generally have little regulation at the local, state, or federal level – only 22 of 50 states have any regulations regarding OBA.

The most common procedures performed in the office include gastrointestinal (GI) endoscopy, ophthalmology, and cosmetic surgery. Other specialties (e.g., gynecology, urology, orthopedics, interventional pain, neurosurgery, pulmonary and cardiac procedures) are increasingly represented.

There has also been an increase in the complexity of the cases being performed in the office as well as an increase in the number of patients with major medical problems and risk factors undergoing these procedures. Therefore, the tremendous growth of OBA has been accompanied by concerns for patient safety. These concerns have been escalated by media reports of tragedies that may have been precipitated because the physician's office lacked the same resources (i.e., personnel, equipment, drugs, administrative policies, and facilities) that are present in an ambulatory surgical center or hospital. There must be one standard of care, no matter where the surgery is performed.

Advances in both surgical and anesthesia technology enable the office to be a very desirable place to perform numerous surgical procedures. In a properly accredited site with qualified, licensed, and trained personnel, the office-based setting can provide a safe, pleasant, comfortable, and cost-effective experience for all.

The office-based anesthesia practice: creating a safe, pleasant, and comfortable experience

At this point one can easily see how anesthesia in the nonhospital setting is a unique subspecialty with its own particular challenges and concerns. This chapter is intended to familiarize the reader with the most crucial issues and to impart a knowledge basis for anyone delving into an OBA practice. We begin by discussing three key principles underlying OBA – to facilitate an experience that is safe, pleasant, and comfortable for both the patients and the personnel involved in the process.

How to keep it safe

Accreditation of office-based surgical facilities is currently performed by the following three organizations:

- The American Association for Accreditation of Ambulatory Surgery Facilities (AAAASF);
- The Accreditation Association for Ambulatory Health Care (AAAHC); and
- The Joint Commission (TJC).

The commonly used classification of surgical facilities focuses on the level of anesthesia provided. The source of these classifications is the American College of Surgeons (ACS), as found in its booklet *Guidelines for Optimal Ambulatory Surgical Care and Office-based Surgery*. The ACS definitions are:

Class A (also known as Level I): Provides for minor surgical procedures performed under topical and local infiltration blocks with or without oral or intramuscular preoperative sedation. Excluded are spinal, epidural, stellate ganglion interscalene, supraclavicular, infraclavicular blocks, and intravenous regional anesthesia.

Class B (also known as Level II): Provides for minor or major surgical procedures performed in conjunction with oral, parenteral, or intravenous sedation or under analgesic or dissociative drugs.

Class C (also known as Level III): Provides for major surgical procedures that require general or regional block anesthesia and support of vital bodily functions.

Safety features that are taken for granted or even unnoticed in an acute care hospital must be carefully built into a new office operating suite or retrofitted into an existing one.

To promote safety and encourage states to develop guidelines, the American Medical Association (AMA), with input from the ACS and the ASA, published a consensus list of principles. Entitled the "AMA Core Principles for Office-Based Surgery," this list is summarized as follows (for full text, see http://www.asahq.org/Washington/AMACorePrinciples.pdf):

1. Guidelines or regulations for office-based surgery should be developed by states according to levels of anesthesia defined by the ASA.
2. Physicians should select patients for OBA by specified criteria including the ASA Physical Status Classification System.
3. Where available, offices that perform surgery should be accredited by a state-recognized entity.
4. Physicians involved in office-based surgery should have admitting privileges at a nearby hospital or maintain an emergency transfer agreement with a nearby hospital.
5. Informed consent guidelines should be followed.
6. Continuous quality improvement and adverse incident–reporting programs should be kept.
7. All physicians in an office-based setting should be board certified and fully trained.
8. Physicians performing office-based surgery may show competency by maintaining privileges at an accredited hospital or ambulatory surgical center for the procedures they perform in an office setting.
9. At least one physician who is credentialed in advanced resuscitative techniques (advanced trauma life support [ATLS], advanced cardiac life support [ACLS], or pediatric advanced life support [PALS]) must be present or immediately available with appropriate resuscitative equipment until the patient has met discharge criteria.
10. Physicians administering or supervising the anesthetic should have appropriate education and training.

How to make it pleasant

The next dictum for establishing a good OBA practice is to make the entire office-based perioperative experience pleasant. The ability to reinvent the traditional surgical experience is one of the most important reasons behind the emergence of anesthesia in the office setting. Office-based surgery can offer the convenience of having procedures performed in a more comfortable setting with an expedient return home.

Advances in analgesic drugs and a growing awareness of complementary techniques, when carried out in the hands of skilled personnel, can help ease a patient smoothly into post-surgical recovery. The aim should be a pleasing experience for patient, family, and friends.

How to make it comfortable

The anesthesiologist plays an integral role in helping to make the perioperative experience pleasant for the patient. A well-conceived, well-structured office environment is essential. One would not want to walk into an office if the equipment and infrastructure are antiquated, cumbersome, or ill-functioning. Building an effectively functioning office-based practice can be a challenging business, but, when properly executed, the office-based environment can be the ideal place of work for an anesthesiologist.

Patient and procedure selection

There are two major issues that the anesthesiologist needs to address prior to initiating an anesthetic in the office: first, whether the patient would be an appropriate candidate for the proposed procedure, and second, whether the proposed surgical procedure would be appropriate for an office-based setting. The ASA *Guidelines for Office-Based Anesthesia* specifically address these issues.

In 2007, the ASA published the *Manual for Anesthesia Department Organization and Management* (MADOM; available from the www.ASAhq.org). Chapter 5 (Ambulatory Anesthesia) contains relevant TJC, AAAHC, and AAAASF accreditation standards, as well as the following additional ASA statements:

1. Guidelines for Ambulatory Anesthesia and Surgery
2. Statement on Qualifications of Anesthesia Providers in the Office-Based Setting
3. Guidelines for Nonoperating Room Anesthetizing Locations
4. Position on Monitored Anesthesia Care
5. Continuum of Depth of Sedation: Definitions of General Anesthesia and Levels of Sedation/Analgesia
6. Statement on Safe Use of Propofol
7. Statement on Granting Privileges for Administration of Moderate Sedation to Practitioners Who Are Not Anesthesia Professionals
8. Statement on Granting Privileges to Non-Anesthesiologist Practitioners for Personally Administering Deep Sedation or Supervising Deep Sedation by Individuals Who Are Not Anesthesia Professionals
9. Outcome Indicators for Office Based and Ambulatory Surgery

Sedation by non-anesthesiologists is addressed in *Practice Guidelines for Sedation and Analgesia by Non-Anesthesiologists*.

The administration of sedatives, hypnotics, analgesics, as well as anesthetic drugs commonly used for the induction and maintenance of general anesthesia is often, but not always, a part of monitored anesthesia care (MAC). In some patients who may require only minimal sedation, MAC is often indicated because even small doses of these medications could precipitate adverse physiologic responses that would necessitate acute clinical interventions and resuscitation. If a patient's condition and/or a procedural requirement is likely to require sedation to a deep level or even to a transient period of general anesthesia, only a practitioner privileged to provide anesthesia services should be allowed to manage the sedation. Due to the strong likelihood that deep sedation may, with or without intention, transition to general anesthesia, the skills of an anesthesia provider are necessary to manage the effects of general anesthesia on the patient as well as to return the patient quickly to a state of deep or lesser sedation.

In summary, MAC is a physician service that is clearly distinct from moderate sedation due to the expectations and qualifications of the provider who must be able to use all anesthesia resources to support life and to provide patient comfort and safety during a diagnostic or therapeutic procedure.

What types of drugs are used in the office?

Anesthesia for office-based surgery can be accomplished using a variety of approaches. Induction and maintenance of sedation or anesthesia can include intravenous and inhalational techniques. Short-acting agents are most appropriate. Central and peripheral regional anesthetic techniques can also be valuable.

More important than the choice of specific agents or techniques, the anesthesiologist must focus on providing an anesthetic that will provide for a rapid recovery to normal function, with minimal postoperative pain, nausea, or other side effects.

We might suggest a word of caution about using various drug combinations to accomplish adequate levels of sedation. It is reasonable to use drug combinations to provide synergy of effects, decrease the dose of each drug, and decrease the side effects. In the current environment, however, both the case complexity and patient comorbidities are increasing as well as the number of non-anesthesia personnel administering sedation in the office-based setting. We have to ask ourselves, "Are there any limits to this type of practice?"

In a recent article, Bhananker and colleagues performed a closed claims analysis of the injuries associated with MAC. These data refer to procedures performed in all kinds of health care settings, such as offices, ambulatory surgical centers, and acute care hospitals. The authors examined closed malpractice claims in the ASA Closed Claims Database since 1990 and found that more than 40% of claims associated with MAC

involved death or permanent brain damage similar to general anesthesia claims, and that respiratory depression was the most common (21%) mechanism of injury. They concluded that almost half (46%) of the claims could have been prevented by better monitoring, including capnography, improved vigilance, and audible alarms.

Which is the safest choice of anesthesia recommended for the office-based setting? Because the main focus of office-based anesthesia practice is to provide safety and comfort while facilitating a fast-track recovery, it is important to highlight the discharge criteria from the ASA–Society for Ambulatory Anesthesia (SAMBA) manual, *Office-Based Anesthesia: Considerations for Anesthesiologists in Setting Up and Maintaining a Safe Office Anesthesia Environment*. Here are a few excerpts:

> The attention to patient safety issues provided by these standards and guidelines should apply to all postanesthesia care regardless of facility location.
>
> Wherever the recovery of the patient is to occur, the area designated must provide an environment that ensures that space, equipment and staffing adequately meet the intent of current postanesthesia care guidelines and standards.
>
> Policies and procedures specific to the postanesthesia care of the patient should be developed and routinely reviewed by all office staff members. Regardless of facility site, all patients shall be observed and monitored by methods appropriate to the patient's medical condition by appropriately trained staff. The qualifications of these staff are clearly delineated in the following documents: ASA Statement on the Anesthesia Care Team, Statement on Qualifications of Anesthesia Providers in the Office-Based Setting, Practice Guidelines for Sedation and Analgesia by Non-Anesthesiologists, Statement on granting Privileges for Administration of Moderate sedation to practitioners who are not Anesthesia Professionals.
>
> Patient discharge is a physician responsibility. Appropriate written criteria for discharge should be applied and should conform to any specific state regulations that govern the provision of office anesthesia. Ambulatory Discharge Criteria require that the patient's vital signs be stable, the patient is fully oriented, is able to ambulate without dizziness, has minimal pain, nausea, vomiting, bleeding; and the patient must have a responsible "vested" adult escort. Personnel with training in advanced resuscitation techniques should be immediately available until all patients are discharged home. A standardized scoring system such as the Modified Aldrete Score may be used. Fast-Tracking Criteria may use the same scoring criteria with two additional assessments: postoperative pain and postoperative emetic symptoms.

Suggested readings

American Society of Anesthesiologists. Practice guidelines for sedation and analgesia by non-anesthesiologists. *Anesthesiology* 2002; 96:1004–1017. Available at: http://www.asahq.org/publicationsAndServices/practiceparam.htm#sedation

ASA Guidelines For Office-Based Anesthesia (2009). Available at: http://www.ASAhq.org/publicationsAndServices/standards/12.pdf

Bhananker SM, Posner KL, Cheney FW, et al. Injury and liability associated with monitored anesthesia care: a closed claims analysis. *Anesthesiology* 2006; 104:228–234.

Clayman MA, Seagle BM. Office surgery safety: the myths and truths behind the Florida moratoria – six years of Florida data. *Plast Reconstr Surg* 2006; 118:777–785.

Shapiro FE (ed.). *Manual of Office-Based Anesthesia Procedures.* Philadelphia: Lippincott Williams & Wilkins; 2007.

Twersky RS, Philip BK, Shapiro FE (eds.). *Office-Based Anesthesia: Considerations for Anesthesiologists in Setting Up and Maintaining a Safe Office Anesthesia Environment.* Washington, DC: American Society of Anesthesiologists; 2008.

Vila H, Desai MS, Miguel RV. Office based anesthesia. In: Twersky RS, Philip BK, eds. *Handbook of Ambulatory Anesthesia.* New York: Springer Science + Business Media, LLC; 2008:283–324.

Management Aspects of Anesthesia Practice

Ross J. Musumeci, editor

Patient safety, quality assurance, and risk management

Miriam Harnett and Jeffrey B. Cooper

Quality and safety – the concepts

Patient safety, quality assurance, and risk management are related concepts, but they differ in important ways. Patient safety is primarily concerned with the prevention of injury. Quality assurance includes safety, but it is a broader term that also includes measures of the failure and success of medical treatments at levels beyond safety. Modern risk management focuses on proactive prevention of adverse outcomes and managing potential liability in their aftermath. Prevention of injuries via error reduction and system improvements is a primary means to reduce the adverse events that would otherwise lead to malpractice or compensatory claims.

It is important to remember that anesthesia is not primarily therapeutic. Thus, it must be the goal of every anesthetic that *no patient should sustain an injury or complication from the anesthetic encounter.*

Dimensions of quality

Quality is an abstract concept. Numerous definitions of quality exist, but perhaps the most widely accepted definition is that of the Institute of Medicine (IOM) – quality is the "extent to which health services for individuals and populations increase the likelihood of desired health outcomes and are consistent with current professional knowledge."

Donabedian proposed that the quality of health care could be measured by observing its major components: structure, process, and outcomes. *Structure* involves the facilities and environment in which the care is delivered; *process* involves how care is actually delivered, including the interactions between clinicians and patients; and *outcomes* involves measuring the results of medical care. When making these observations, it is important to remember that it is the patient's perspective on the quality of care that is most important.

Causes of preventable adverse events

The cause of accidents is almost always multifactorial and can include failures of the organization, the care team, the individual, technology, or process design. Poor communication is one of the most common root causes of major adverse events, and it can have many underlying causes. Factors that contribute to failures by the individual practitioner are:

1. Production pressure
2. Fatigue or sleep deprivation
3. Failure to check equipment
4. Lack of supervision
5. Unfamiliarity with equipment or with drug
6. Failure to follow routine
7. Unawareness of a protocol
8. Failure to follow protocol
9. Distraction

Improving safety: from individual events to systems

Safety requires continual vigilance and a culture that makes safe practice the highest priority. It is not enough to consider individual actions. The organization must also consider working conditions, facilities, procedures, and work flow so that all aspects of anesthesia care are addressed.

The review of closed malpractice claims, peer review, clinical conferences, and incident reports can be helpful in identifying areas for improvement. These methods do not quantify the incidence of a particular event, but they may identify problems that can be corrected.

Historically, adverse events in medicine have been dealt with in a punitive fashion. There is now an increasing realization that these events are most frequently the result of bad systems and that blaming individuals is counterproductive. Attention is now being turned toward understanding the deeper causes of adverse events and correcting problems with the system of care in an attempt to reduce the likelihood of errors.

Practical elements for producing safe, high-quality patient care

Teamwork – Effective teamwork improves safety, so each individual must learn to work as a team member rather than as an individual.

Preparation of equipment and medication – Failure to adequately prepare for the administration of anesthesia often contributes to critical incidents. Preparation includes ensuring availability of emergency drugs and equipment, ensuring that equipment is functional, and having a plan in the event of an emergency.

A pneumonic (SOAP M) is an example of a checklist for setting up the operating room (OR).

- **Suction** – Make sure it is working.
- **Oxygen** – Do you have it? Can you measure it? Can you deliver it?
- **Airway** – Check laryngoscope and have an endotracheal tube ready even if you do not plan to use it.
- **Pharmacy** – Check vial before and after drawing up drugs, have emergency drugs ready, and make sure that vaporizers are full.
- **Machines/Monitors** – Perform negative and positive pressure checks and check ventilator function.

Preoperative assessment and planning

Preoperative assessment and planning include a thorough medical evaluation of the patient and development of the anesthesia care plan with attention to addressing any comorbidities or other issues that might contribute to an adverse event. The plan should include the anesthetic technique and requirements for monitoring and for postoperative care, all of which must be consistent with the wishes of the patient, the needs of the surgeon, and the resources of the facility.

Monitoring

The safe practitioner should follow the standards promulgated by the American Society of Anesthesiologists (ASA; see "Suggested readings"). Critical alarms must never be disabled.

Safety in care transitions

Transitions in care present special risks for adverse events because key information can easily be lost and practitioners may become distracted during this process. Transitions include handoffs for breaks during cases or transfers between the OR and the postanesthesia care unit (PACU) or intensive care unit (ICU). It is important to develop specific protocols for conducting handoffs and to be especially mindful at such times.

Control for human factors

It is imperative to be organized and consistent in the layout of your emergency airway equipment and emergency drugs so that they are easily accessible. Ritualizing simple safety routines is a good idea because it makes them instinctive and harder to forget. When drawing up a drug from a vial, the vial must be checked both before and after the drug is drawn, and syringes should always be labeled immediately. One of the most important routines that must be followed without exception is to read the drug label three times before a drug is administered. Keeping lines well organized and drug infusions clearly and obviously labeled, maintaining an uncluttered workspace, and minimizing distractions are all important safety measures.

Applying systematic crisis management techniques

Anesthesia Crisis Resource Management (ACRM) is an organized set of principles for managing crisis situations in anesthesia. Adapted from CRM in aviation by Gaba and colleagues, it consists of the following principles:

- Seek assistance as soon as unusual circumstances are recognized, inform others on the surgical team, and call for extra assistance.
- Establish clear roles for each person involved in management of the event, and identify who will manage the event (the leader).
- Use effective communication processes, including reading back instructions before they are carried out, and clearly identifying who should carry out the instructions.
- Use resources effectively and identify what additional resources (people, supplies, equipment, transportation, etc.) are available to manage the situation.
- Maintain situational awareness and avoid fixations. One person should act as the event manager who observes the big picture rather than becoming immersed in details.

Following standards and practice guidelines

Standardizing practices is now widely accepted as a critical component for safety and reliability, and the ASA has established a large set of standards and guidelines. A list of common practice standards can be found on the ASA Web site listed in the "Suggested readings" section at the end of this chapter. Practitioners should be familiar with such guidelines and should know how and where to access them and apply them when necessary.

Periodic training

Because critical events are relatively rare, it is important to practice skills periodically. Schwid demonstrated that advanced cardiac life support (ACLS) skills are generally maintained for only approximately 6 months. Simulation is being used increasingly for such training in anesthesia, and in some specialties simulation has already become part of the evaluation processes of accrediting agencies.

Involving the patient in safety and quality

Anesthesia providers can involve patients in their own care, thus improving patient satisfaction and safety by

- Giving the patient information about the process of anesthesia care that he or she will experience;

- Encouraging the patient to speak up if he or she sees things that he or she does not understand or that may not seem appropriate (e.g., drugs that are being given, absence of hand washing or wearing gloves);
- Involving the patient's family members in care whenever practical;
- Giving the patient your contact information so he or she can notify you if he or she has any concerns or side effects after the anesthetic; and
- Encouraging a policy of disclosing errors and adverse events (a strategy that enhances trust and decreases skepticism in concerned patients).

Risk management
Background

In its 1999 report – "To Err Is Human" – the IOM declared that medical injury is a major cause of preventable deaths and called on the health care industry to make the reduction of medical errors a priority. The IOM emphasized evidence from other industries showing that faulty systems are the major cause of errors and accidents, and it strongly recommended that health care organizations focus their safety efforts in this area. In response, a major national movement has been launched to redesign health care systems.

In a subsequent report – "Crossing the Quality Chasm" – the IOM called on health care organizations to provide care that is safe, effective, patient-centered, timely, efficient, and equitable. There are two principles underlying the IOM recommendations for responding to incidents:

1. We must commit ourselves to relentless self-examination and continuous improvement.
2. Medical care must be patient-centered. After an incident, the primary objective should be to support the patient and maintain open communication by providing patients and families with the details of incidents and their implications.

How should an institution respond?

A serious incident should trigger a cascade of responses. The first concern should be the prevention of further harm and relief of suffering. Members of the health care team and appropriate administrative and clinical leadership should be promptly notified of the event. The patient and family should be told about the event as soon as possible and provided with only the facts that are known. They will probably need emotional and psychological support, so this should be readily available. Finally, the medical record should clearly document not only the event, but also the disclosure and all supportive measures that are provided to the patient and the family. It is important to note that caregivers may also require psychological support, depending on the type of event.

As soon as practical, all involved parties should participate in an analysis of the event, in which they search for the underlying systems failures. The goals of the analysis should be to gain a full understanding of the circumstances involved in the event, identify contributing factors, and develop practical recommendations for systems changes designed to prevent a recurrence.

There are four essential steps in the full communication of adverse events:

1. Tell the patient and family *what* happened, but leave details of how and why for later. Determining the causes of an adverse event requires careful analysis and is time-consuming. Patients and their families are likely to want immediate answers when you disclose the event to them, but it is important to limit your discussion to known facts and avoid speculation.
2. Take responsibility. Taking responsibility for an adverse event is an essential step in the full communication of that event.
3. Apologize. When there has been an error, one of the most powerful things a caregiver can do to heal the patient and him-/herself is to apologize. Even when the caregiver is not at fault and system failures are responsible for the error, an expression of sorrow for the undesirable outcome can be helpful. Explaining the event, communicating remorse, and making a gesture of reconciliation can do much to defuse the hurt and anger that follows an injury.
4. Explain what will be done to prevent future events. After the investigation is completed and corrective changes are planned, it is important to inform the patient and family of these plans. Injured patients have a strong interest in seeing to it that what happened to them does not happen to someone else.

Reporting

Incidents should be reported promptly to supervisors, risk management, and other concerned parties to ensure appropriate treatment and communication with the patient and family and to facilitate institutional learning. Reporting is also necessary to comply with specific mandates established by various external regulatory agencies, such as the local department of public health, state board of registration in medicine, the US Food and Drug Administration, or the Joint Commission. Practitioners should be aware of such requirements in their area. Providers and hospitals also have an obligation to notify their liability insurance carriers of certain types of incidents, especially if there is a potential for future malpractice claims or compensation.

Summary and conclusions

The delivery of care should be recognized as a complex matrix of multiple providers, including both clinicians and facilities, all interacting with one another. There are many opportunities to improve patient care, and the pressure to improve the quality of perioperative care will continue to increase. The specialty of anesthesia is recognized as a leader in patient safety, and anesthesia providers can continue to provide leadership by implementing the IOM recommendations and adopting a patient-centered approach to dealing with adverse events.

Suggested readings

American Society of Anesthesiologists. Standards, guidelines and procedures. Available at: http://asahq.org/publicationsAnd Services/sgstoc.htm. Accessed August 9, 2010.

Cooper JB, Longnecker D. Safety and quality. In: Longnecker D, ed. *The Guiding Principles of Patient-Centered Care.* New York: McGraw Hill Medical Publishing; 2007:20–37.

Cooper JB, Newbower RS, Kitz RJ. An analysis of major errors and equipment failures in anesthesia management: considerations for prevention and detection. *Anesthesiology* 1984; 60:34–42.

Donabedian A. Evaluating quality of medical care. *Millbank Q* 1996; 44:166–206.

Gaba D, Fish K, Howard S. *Crisis Management in Anesthesiology.* Philadelphia: Churchill Livingstone; 1994.

Institute of Medicine. Crossing the quality chasm. Washington, DC: National Academies Press; 2001.

Joint Commission. Crafting an effective apology: what clinicians need to know. *Joint Commission Perspectives on Patient Safety* 2005; 4:7–8.

Kohn KT, Corrigan JM, Donaldson MS. To err is human: building a safer health system. Washington, DC: National Academies Press; 1999.

Morell RC, Eichhorn JH. *Patient Safety in Anesthetic Practice.* New York: Churchill Livingstone; 1997:270.

Chapter 138

Operating room management: core principles

Richard D. Urman and Sunil Eappen

The operating room (OR) is an important part of the hospital because it is typically one of the biggest sources of revenue and one of the largest areas of expense. Until the 1980s, OR suites generated large profits and hospital administrators were able to allow them a great deal of autonomy despite their inefficiency. This situation has changed dramatically due to increasing requirements for cost containment in health care and a demand for accountability to the federal and state government, insurance companies, hospital administrators, surgeons, and patients. Whereas there was little centralized leadership in ORs of the past, OR management is now a critical feature of successful hospitals. A good management team must bring together many diverse components of the hospital to function together efficiently and effectively. Figure 138.1 shows a typical hospital organizational structure and the parties involved in day-to-day OR management.

OR manager

There are at least four distinct stakeholders in the OR: hospital administration, nursing, anesthesiology, and surgery. Each of these stakeholders has its own interests, and the OR manager must be able to balance the needs of these different groups to maximize productivity and minimize conflict. The key characteristics of an effective OR manager are listed in Table 138.1.

A more detailed job description of the OR manager can be found on the Web site of the American Association of Clinical Directors (AACD; www.aacdhq.org).

Anesthesiologists who have the characteristics listed in Table 138.1 are particularly well-qualified to fill the OR manager position because they typically have a constant presence in the OR without the need for office hours, and they usually have a clear understanding of OR processes. Hospital administrators may prefer anesthesiologists or nurses for the OR manager position because their economic interests are often aligned with those of the hospital.

A successful OR manager must have the support of the hospital CEO and the chairpersons of the departments of surgery, nursing, and anesthesiology. It is necessary for all departments to give up some of their own authority and control so that the OR manager can run the OR in a manner that benefits everyone. The OR manager must also have the support of his or her own group, because the position will require time that could otherwise be spent on group activities. For this reason, and also to emphasize the neutrality of the OR manager position among all departments, the OR manager and/or the manager's practice should be compensated by the hospital.

Scheduling and efficiency measures

The amount of revenue that an OR generates is dependent on the number of surgical cases that are performed, so a significant amount of time in OR management is spent on scheduling. Surgical scheduling rules must be established, and a daily schedule for both cases and OR staff must be generated. Both of these schedules are frequently modified to account for emergency cases and differences between booked and actual case times. The American Society of Anesthesiologists (ASA), The American College of Surgeons, and the American Organization of Registered Nurses have accepted the terminology presented by the AACD in their glossary of operating room measures. The complete glossary and standardized abbreviations are published on their Web site, and individuals interested in accurately measuring OR times should consult this comprehensive glossary. Many of the terms that are seen in the anesthesia literature are either AACD terms or are derived from AACD glossary terms. We have included an abbreviated list of commonly used terms in Table 138.2.

OR utilization is a popular concept that can be used differently depending on the desired analysis. *Adjusted OR utilization* is defined as the amount of time an OR is used (in-OR

Table 138.1. Characteristics of an effective OR director

Has strong problem solving and organizational skills
Is even-tempered
Is able to commit a significant amount of nonclinical time
Is a strong clinician garnering respect of other clinicians
Has strong interpersonal and negotiation skills
Is able to understand business/financial concerns of institution and
   physicians
Understands perioperative processes
Understands scheduling systems and information technology
Understands organizational dynamics and is able to understand divergent
   needs and concerns of different stakeholders and bring them together
Is committed to overall performance of OR suite rather than individual
   department

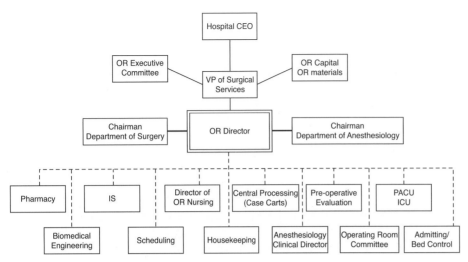

Figure 138.1. Typical organizational chart for management of OR.

time + turnover time) divided by the total amount of time the OR is staffed and available for the day (resource hours). The AACD term for adjusted OR utilization is "adjusted-percent utilized resource hours" (AURH). This measure tells you how much of the day has been filled with scheduled OR time. *Raw OR utilization* excludes turnover time in the calculation (in-OR time/resource hours). Raw OR utilization gives a ratio of billable to total OR hours, and either unbooked time or excessive turnover time will drive this value down. Decisions about the allocation of OR time for a surgeon or a service are often based on OR block utilization. *Block utilization* is defined as the amount of time that an OR is scheduled by a particular surgeon or service, divided by the total amount of block time

that this surgeon or service has been granted. This value may exceed 100% because it typically includes hours that services operate outside of their block time. A service that is consistently at greater than 80% block utilization will typically have trouble scheduling cases, so this number is frequently used as a guide as to when the service should be granted more OR time.

It is important to remember that factors other than block utilization may need to be considered for decisions regarding more or less OR time. For example, trauma services that are important to the community may require an unscheduled OR that is always ready for an emergency. The resulting low utilization rates will be acceptable if trauma is part of the hospital's mission.

Table 138.2. Sample of OR efficiency terms

Resource hours *or* Allocated OR time	Time scheduled for OR to be staffed and available for performance of procedures
In-OR time	Total time that ORs have patients in them per day during resource hours
Raw OR utilization	(In-OR time/resource hours) × 100
Adjusted OR utilization *or* Adjusted-percent utilized resource hours	(In-OR time + turnover time) × 100/resource hours
Block utilization *or* Adjusted-percent service utilization	(In-OR time + turnover time) for day's cases × 100/block time
Induction complete *or* Anesthesia ready	Time when patient handed over to surgeon for positioning, surgical prepping, and draping
Induction time	Time from when patient enters OR to Induction complete
Surgical controlled time	Time from induction complete to when last dressing is placed
Emergence time	Time from last dressing is placed to when patient is ready to transfer
Anesthesia controlled time	Induction time + emergence time
Turnover time	Time from when one patient leaves the OR to when the next patient arrives into the OR
First case starts	Routinely measured as percentage of ORs in which the first scheduled patient arrives into the OR prior to or at scheduled start time

Open scheduling versus block scheduling

Traditionally, OR schedules were filled on a "first-come, first-served" basis that assumed that any case could be performed in any room and that all anesthesiologists and nurses could handle the different surgeries equally well. Increasingly complex cases with specialized equipment and teams have led to a more organized system of assigning rooms to specific surgeons or services and guaranteeing them specific time slots. This method of scheduling allows specialized equipment to remain in designated ORs (e.g., cardiopulmonary bypass circuits, laparoscopic equipment/displays) and for specific teams to work in these areas consistently. Block scheduling smoothes the variability in OR case volume by giving greater predictability to surgeons when booking their cases. It also creates more accountability when evaluating case volume expectations and targets for hospitals, surgeons, nurses, and anesthesiologists. In general, blocks appear to work more efficiently when they are assigned to specific services rather than to surgeons. Additionally, full day blocks are preferable to partial day blocks because they eliminate the possibility of delayed starts for a second service due to preceding cases running longer than expected. Block booking may not work well in ORs with high numbers of emergent cases that disrupt the schedule; in such situations, open scheduling for one or more rooms may lead to higher OR utilization and patient satisfaction.

A key part of block scheduling is having specific rules in place that govern how OR time is allocated. *Release time* is defined as the number of hours before the scheduled time of surgery when a block of time must be either booked or released for use by others. Release times for specific services should reflect the nature of their cases. For example, cardiac surgery typically has short release times due to the urgent nature of many of their cases, whereas plastic surgery has longer release times because their cases are almost exclusively elective.

Turnover time

Much energy and money has been expended on decreasing *turnover time,* which is defined as the time between when one patient has left the OR and the next one arrives. From a business perspective, it makes sense to reduce turnover time, because no revenue is generated while there is no patient in the OR. Unfortunately, a number of studies have revealed that even maximal improvements in turnover time will usually not open enough time in the schedule to allow additional case bookings later in the day. Efficient turnover during the course of the day, however, may lessen overtime in a busy OR leading to lower expenses and improved morale of the staff.

A number of functions need to be completed during turnover time:

- Room cleaning;
- OR table setup with sterile equipment;
- Anesthesia equipment cleaned and restocked;

Table 138.3. OR efficiency metrics to be measured

Overtime hours of OR staff
Scheduled start times to actual start time difference for all scheduled cases
Case cancellation rate
Contribution margin per hour or per OR per day
Turnover times
Prolonged turnover times (turnover times > 60 min)
PACU or ICU admission delays (cumulative number of minutes)
Scheduled case time to actual case time difference for all scheduled cases

- Patient taken to PACU/ICU, vital signs checked, patient signed off to PACU nurse;
- Medications reconciled and new ones checked out;
- Next patient greeted (anesthesiologist and OR nurse);
- Preoperative assessment including surgical and anesthesiology consent, surgical reassessment, review of plans, and site verification;
- Intravenous lines/block placed; and
- Anesthesia equipment checkout performed.

From the list above, it should be apparent that turnover time is dependent on many different factors.

OR efficiency

OR efficiency is a difficult concept to contain in any one single measurement. Macario and colleagues recently described a set of criteria and a scoring system that hospitals and OR managers may consider in determining the overall efficiency of their ORs. Table 138.3 lists the suggested metrics. All of these factors may not apply to every OR suite, but this is the first set of metrics that has met with some acceptance and uses measures that are readily available in most ORs. Hospital administrations are now beginning to benchmark their metrics against comparable institutions to identify opportunities and techniques that may improve efficiencies.

Additional cost-control measures

In 1994, the ASA formed an ad hoc committee on value-based anesthesia care to promote the best patient outcomes at the most reasonable costs. The committee wrote that the optimal choice of anesthesia management depends on maximizing the positive aspects of health, function, and satisfaction while minimizing the negative aspects of mortality, morbidity, and expense. Indeed, health care realities mandate that the costs of drugs, equipment, and time be incorporated into every anesthesiologist's decision-making process. Anesthesiologists control large amounts of expensive resources, and their decisions affect the finances of patients, hospitals, and insurers. It is important to practice evidence-based anesthesia, promote departmental discussions of costs and goals, define permissible activities for sales representatives, minimize waste, and develop practice guidelines for expensive drugs and technologies. Practitioners should also be provided with personalized anesthetic usage costs and patient outcomes feedback, including peer comparisons.

Physician credentialing

Diligence in physician credentialing and privileging is critical to high-quality care in the OR. The purpose of credentialing is to assure patients and third-party payers that the highest quality of health care is being provided by a professional staff selected according to a rigorous evaluation process based on qualifications and other objective criteria. Critical elements in the credentialing process include professional degrees conferred by accredited educational institutions, current and unrestricted professional licensure, postgraduate residency training, fellowship training, specialty board certification, professional standing as judged by peer review processes, physical health, and psychological well-being. Specific OR privileges for surgeons and anesthesiologists are determined by specialty training, certification, experience, and demonstrated competence. Recredentialing and repriviliging are required regularly and should be based on a critical appraisal of professional performance through peer review and continuous quality improvement (CQI) monitoring. The ASA Guidelines for Delineation of Clinical Privileges in Anesthesiology are referenced for the reader's convenience.

Suggested readings

Dexter F, Macario A, Quian F, et al. Forecasting surgical groups' total hours of elective cases for allocation of block time. Application of time series analysis to operating room management. *Anesthesiology* 1999; 91:1501.

Eappen S, Flanagan H, Lithman R, Bhattacharyya N. The addition of a regional block team to the orthopedic operating room does not improve anesthesia-controlled times and turnover time in the setting of long turnover times. *J Clin Anesth* 2007; 19:85–91.

Glenn DM, Macario A. Management of the operating room: a new practice opportunity for anesthesiologists. *Anesthesiol Clin North Am* 1999; 17:365.

Guidelines for Delineation of Clinical Privileges in Anesthesiology, American Society of Anesthesiology (approved by House of Delegates on October 15, 1975, and last amended on October 15, 2003). Available at: http://www.asahq.org/publicationsAnd Services/standards/08.pdf. Accessed June 4, 2008.

Harris AP, Zinzman WG (eds.). *Operating Room Management: Structure Strategies and Economics*. St. Louis: Mosby; 1998.

Kulli JC, Lee SB, Spratt DG, et al. *Operating Room Management*. Boston: Butterworth-Heinemann; 1999.

Malangoni M (ed.). *Critical Issues in Operating Room Management*. Philadelphia: Lippincott-Raven; 1997.

Orkin FK. Moving toward value-based anesthesia care. *J Clin Anesth* 1993; 5:91.

Overdyk FJ, Harvey SC, Fishman RI, et al. Successful strategies for improving operating room efficiency at academic institutions. *Anesth Analg* 1998; 86:896.

Valenzuela RC, Johnstone RE. Cost containment in anesthesiology: a survey of department activities. *J Clin Anesth* 1997; 9:93–96.

Willock M. Management of the operating room. *Int Anesthesiol Clin.* 1998; Winter; 36(1):1–115.

Chapter 139

Practice management

Ross J. Musumeci

Introduction

Practice management includes the functions that are necessary to support the business and clinical operations of an anesthesia practice. The complexity of business operations that are required for each practice and the mix of physicians and non-physicians that fill those roles will vary depending on the size and objectives of the practice. This chapter describes the different components within practice management and acquaints the reader with important aspects of each one.

Contracting

Contracting is the process of negotiating a formal agreement with outside entities that defines the nature of your business relationship. Anesthesia practices typically negotiate professional service contracts with health care facilities, insurers, and employees. It is the role of the practice management team to negotiate these contracts with the aid of legal counsel.

Professional service agreements negotiated with a health care facility define the relationship between the anesthesia group and the facility. Among other things, these contracts usually describe the expectations that the hospital has of the anesthesia group, the methods that the anesthesia group will use to fulfill those expectations, the resources that the hospital will provide in support of the group's efforts, and the options that each side has if the other does not fulfill its side of the agreement. When structuring hospital contracts it is a good idea to carefully define which services the practice is obligated to provide and to clarify those services that are not included. Hospital contracts may also include an agreement about the level of financial support that the hospital will provide to the anesthesia group. The more time you spend up front creating a contract that is specific, the less likely it is that you will encounter a misunderstanding later.

Agreements must be secured with insurers to determine the level of reimbursement to which the practice will be entitled and the nature of the interaction among the insurer, its clients, and the practice. Collectively, these contracts define the level of income to which the practice is entitled, so a great deal of emphasis should be placed on securing the most favorable contracts possible.

Employment agreements form the basis for the relationship between the practice and its employees, and they typically specify compensation and the responsibilities of the employer and employee. It is worth spending some time to create good employment agreements to avoid misunderstandings after employment begins.

Billing and collections

Whereas contracting determines the level of revenue to which the practice is entitled, the billing and collections department performs the activities necessary to actually collect the money associated with the physician's services. The medical industry is unlike many others in that the actual amount received for a service is indeterminate at the time the service is rendered, making aggressive and thorough follow-up on claims important.

The typical activities within a billing and collections department are outlined in Table 139.1. It is important to make sure that providers are credentialed with each insurer. If credentialing is not completed prior to providing services, the insurer may deny reimbursement.

Anesthesia records generated when services are rendered typically provide the basis for charges that are submitted to third-party payers. These records, along with any necessary supplemental documentation, are forwarded to the billing office for processing. There should be a mechanism to reconcile records that the billing office receives against cases that were actually performed on any given day to ensure that no charts are lost during transport. After charts are received by the billing office, patient demographic information is entered and the charts are then scanned for the relevant diagnoses and procedures.

Table 139.1. Billing and collections

Insurer credentialing
Demographics entry
Coding
Chart auditing
Claims processing
Cash posting
Collections and follow-up
Reporting

The diagnoses and procedures must be "coded" by converting diagnoses and procedures to Current Procedural Terminology (CPT) codes, *International Classification of Diseases, 9th Revision, Clinical Modification* (ICD-9-CM) codes, and American Society of Anesthesiology (ASA) codes. CPT codes describe the medical, surgical, and diagnostic services that are performed by physicians and other health care providers. ICD-9-CM codes are used to code signs, symptoms, injuries, diseases, and conditions. The diagnosis indicated by the ICD-9-CM code must support the medical necessity of the procedure defined by the CPT code. CPT codes may be used when a flat fee is charged for services, such as arterial line placement, but all time-based billing requires that the CPT code be converted or "cross-walked" to a corresponding ASA code. The ASA updates and publishes ASA codes each year and structures them so that almost every CPT code has at least one corresponding ASA code, but in most cases ASA codes are further broken down to allow for greater anatomic specificity. It is extremely important to code accurately so that the practice can avoid rejections, which cause a delay in reimbursement. Prior to submission, charts should also be audited to ensure that they are in full compliance with documentation and billing guidelines as required by the American Medical Association and the Centers for Medicare and Medicaid.

After coding has been performed, claims processing can begin. This processing consists of charge capture, where information and coding are transferred from the chart to the actual billing instrument, and submission of the billing instrument to third-party insurers. Claims personnel should (1) have a mechanism for tracking the status of outstanding claims, and (2) follow up quickly on those that have either been rejected or have not received a timely response. Cash-posting personnel process all payments and match them to outstanding claims. They should ensure that payment amounts match the fee schedule agreed to by the insurer and should appeal any low or inaccurate payments. Given the varied ways in which claims are processed by different insurance companies, and the fact that many claims still require human intervention for processing, it is imperative that the practice have an effective way to monitor payer contract performance. Specifically, an allowable monitoring system is a required function of the billing department (with oversight from the finance department) in which all reimbursements are matched against contracted rates to ensure that there are not underpayments or overpayments made by payers. After a correct payment has been received, the claim is closed. In the event that payment is not received within a reasonable time frame despite appropriate follow-up, the claim is submitted to the collections department. Many groups outsource this function for older claims so that they can free resources to pursue more current claims that they are more likely to collect.

Billing and collections departments should also be able to provide the practice with reports of their activities. Some of the common reports that a billing department can provide are shown in Table 139.2. Basic performance of the billing and collections department can be readily ascertained by examining

Table 139.2. Reports and descriptions

Report	Description
Gross revenue	Gross charges prior to contractual allowances
Contractual allowances	Discounts given to insurers off of full rates
Net revenue	Charges net of contractual allowances
Net income	Excess of all revenues and gains over all expenses and losses for a period
Net collection ratio	Total collections divided by net charges
Bad debt	Uncollectible accounts
AR	Claims against payers (or other debtors) that are not yet collected
Average collection period	Average number of days from time of service to collection; also referred to as Days Outstanding in AR or Days Sales Outstanding (DSO)
Aging report	Breaks AR into buckets based on time since service provided
Payer mix ratio	Ratio of each payer's gross charges to total gross charges; can also be calculated with net charges

the size of accounts receivable (AR), average collection period, the percentage of bad debt, and the age of AR. Upward trends in any of these metrics are undesirable and should prompt an investigation into the causes.

In general, an average collection period of less than 60 days is desirable, but it is not uncommon to see practices with average collection periods of more than 100 days. It is advisable to keep this value as low as possible. A typical aging report shows the amount of AR in the categories of up to 30 days, 60 days, 90 days, and older than 120 days. In general, the older the claim the harder it is to collect, so an increase in older claims is a significant finding that should be examined immediately.

It is advisable to evaluate the payer mix ratio of a hospital and to follow it over time. The significant disparity between governmental and nongovernmental payers that currently exists in reimbursement for anesthesia services makes it essential that the practice administrator knows exactly what this ratio is and understands its implications for profitability and the possible need for financial support from the hospital.

Scheduling

The scheduling department controls clinical personnel – the primary asset a practice uses to generate revenue and also its largest expense. It follows that this department has a major impact on expenses, revenues, and net income. In small practices, the scheduling function will be easier, but, as practice size increases, the complexity of scheduling can increase rapidly and can require significant resources.

There are several types of schedules that must be completed for the routine operation of an anesthesia practice. A daily schedule must be created to determine the personnel who are allocated to a given hospital each day and the locations to which they are assigned within that hospital.

Methods for creating on-call and vacation schedules must incorporate safeguards to ensure fairness. Aside from the

Table 139.3. HRM functions

Recruiting and hiring
Hospital credentialing
Maintaining a positive workplace environment
Personnel development and training
Ensuring that personnel and management practices conform to various regulations
Managing company's approach to compensation and benefits
Maintaining employee records and personnel policies
Performing employee evaluations
Dealing with employee relations, performance issues, and termination

obvious need to schedule these two items in a way that is consistent with safe and efficient practice operations, the most important aspect of the scheduling system is that it is perceived to be fair by the individuals that it affects. Anything that can be done to make the process and the results transparent to the involved individuals usually helps. A lack of transparency and perceived unfairness in these areas can cause a decrease in morale.

Human resources

The primary product of an anesthesia practice is the service that its personnel provide. Without good personnel, the product suffers. Good human resource management (HRM) is essential to a successful practice, especially in the competitive personnel market of today. An effective HRM department can improve employee retention leading to better customer service and a competitive advantage for the company. The essential functions of an HRM department are broad and include the items shown in Table 139.3.

Shortages of both anesthesiologists and nurse anesthetists have made recruiting and hiring qualified personnel an increasingly difficult and important task, and a good HRM department will devote a significant amount of time to this task. It is important to remember that the cost of hiring a new employee and orienting and training him or her is usually greater than retaining existing employees. For this reason, the HRM department should also spend a significant amount of time on employee retention.

Development, training, and continuing education are a means to keep employees stimulated and interested and can lead to improved productivity and better morale. Retention is also dependent on maintaining a workplace that is pleasant and free of hostility. Issues of discrimination and harassment have implications for both employee retention and company liability, and it is the job of the HRM department to manage any issues that arise in this area.

Competing for personnel on the basis of salary alone is difficult and costly, but a flexible and creative benefits package may attract employees despite a lower salary offer. It is important that employees understand their total compensation, so the HRM department must both structure the benefits program well *and* communicate its contents and value effectively. Without good communication, the practice may be wasting its money on the program. Employee evaluations

provide an opportunity for the practice to improve the quality of the service its employees provide, but only if the process is managed in a professional and fair manner. Evaluations must be done as objectively as possible and with a means for appeal in the event that an unfavorable evaluation is delivered. Results should be delivered in a sensitive and confidential manner and with constructive intent. In the event that evaluations are not successful in altering poor performance and termination is considered, it is the job of the HRM department to ensure that (1) the employee is treated fairly and in accordance with all applicable laws, and (2) appropriate documentation is obtained prior to termination. For employees who self-terminate, HRM departments will frequently try to obtain competitive information by conducting exit interviews with departing employees. Issues related to termination, discrimination, or any type of harassment in the workplace should cause a practice's manager to consider early consultation with a labor attorney. The applicable law is complex, court decisions can result in treble damages, and the losses are not insurable. Furthermore, conflicts related to employment disagreements are usually fraught with emotion. For all of these reasons, issues related to termination, discrimination, and harassment in the workplace are dangerous to address without professional advice.

Human resource information systems are frequently used and can be helpful. When choosing a system, make sure that it is multifunctional and reduces redundant processing of information such as payroll and accounting. A good system should also track compliance items, such as the continuation of health insurance under Consolidated Budget Reconciliation Act (COBRA) or Family and Medical Leave Act (FMLA) issues, because noncompliance can be costly.

Finance

The finance department is responsible for managing all financial aspects of the practice, including accounts payable, payroll, expense reimbursement, revenue and expense tracking, creation of financial reports, and preparation of tax documents. This department is also responsible for helping to create and enforce financial controls, which are policies and procedures meant to safeguard assets within the company.

To understand financial reports, the practice manager must understand the difference between cash-based and accrual-based accounting. Cash-based accounting requires that revenue be recognized when money is received and expenses be recognized when payment is made. This idea is in contrast to that of accrual-based accounting, in which revenue is recognized when it is earned by providing a service, and expenses are recognized when they are incurred regardless of when money actually changes hands. Smaller practices may use cash-based accounting, but larger practices will almost exclusively use accrual-based accounting because it is considered to be more accurate and better able to give a clear picture of practice performance at any given time. Analysis of financial reports should be undertaken with the intent of understanding past performance and finding ways to improve future performance. Reports should be analyzed on a regular basis, and attention should be paid to trends as well as to overall amounts in both expense and revenue line items. Good reports should be timely, accurate, and simple (but with enough detail to provide necessary information). The financial reports that are most commonly reviewed are the balance sheet, the income statement, and the statement of cash flows. The balance sheet is prepared on a single date, and it gives the reader a snapshot of the financial condition of the practice at that single moment in time. In contrast, the income statement reports revenues, expenses, and net income over a defined time period, so it provides a moving picture of the company's performance. Finally, the statement of cash flows reports on sources and uses of cash over a defined time period and tells the reader what the change in cash balances was during the time period. This statement is useful in accrual accounting because the other statements do not directly report on the cash status of the company.

The finance department is also responsible for assisting management in forecasting revenue and budgeting expenses. The process of budgeting and forecasting can be time-consuming, but it is time well spent. It requires thoughtful consideration of the current business environment, the resources that the practice will need, as well as existing opportunities and the likelihood that the practice will be able to capitalize on them. Considering all of these elements and their financial implications at a time when the information is actionable is far better than waiting to analyze financial data after the fact.

The creation of pro forma cash flow and income statements can also be useful if the practice is considering new hospital contracts or new investments of any kind. Pro forma statements are projected financial statements that are targeted to a specific initiative and are meant to show the expected cash flows, revenues, expenses, and net income from the project under consideration. Creation and analysis of these reports, along with a critical review of the assumptions that go into creating them, lessen the chance of the practice making an unprofitable decision on a new project or contract.

Risk management

Risk management is covered in another chapter, so comments here will be limited to those that apply directly to the business operations of the anesthesia practice. The risk management department is responsible for dealing with the possibility that future events may cause harm to the practice. Every anesthesia practice engages in some form of risk management, but the complexity of risk management activities varies widely based on the size of the practice and its organizational goals. Smaller practices tend to have simple structures with minimal personnel. They may have physicians perform many of the routine risk management activities and depend on their hospital's professional risk manager or the risk manager for their professional liability carrier in the event of an adverse outcome. Larger practices are likely to have a more complex arrangement, up to and including employment of their own risk manager and the creation of a captive insurance company.

At its most basic level, risk management involves examining an organization to determine what can go wrong, what should be done to prevent adverse events, what should be done to manage adverse events after they occur, and how the practice will pay for adverse events that are compensable. This examination usually involves establishing and managing formal quality assurance–quality improvement programs, conducting analyses of adverse events, managing litigation, performing risk analysis of policy and procedure, and engaging in communication and education for the purposes of risk reduction. The key components of a properly structured risk management program include a user-friendly reporting system, a method for collection and review of data with the ability to identify trends and implement strategies to decrease risk, access to a risk manager and counsel, and strict attention to evidentiary protections when structuring the program. Some states provide limited protection for work products related to peer review or quality improvement, but this protection differs from state to state and is subject to judicial interpretation and balancing the plaintiff's interest in discovery against the public policy interest in peer review and quality improvement. The risk manager who is structuring your program should make sure that he or she is familiar with the particular evidentiary protections available in your state and must alter the program to keep up with any changes in these laws so that documents created as part of your risk management program will not be discoverable in a malpractice case.

Although not all risk managers work directly with brokers for the purpose of securing the organization's insurance, it is essential for the risk manager to play a role in this process. A broker will usually secure bids from multiple vendors to obtain cost-effective malpractice insurance and will present the bids to the risk manager and other designated individuals within the organization. When examining bids from malpractice insurers it is important to consider all aspects of the potential insurer including size, financial strength, reputation, length of time writing malpractice policies, and ratings by independent insurance rating organizations. It is also important to consider the level and quality of service they provide when claims are made. The best way to determine level and quality of service is to contact colleagues who have been sued while covered by the company. Additional weight should be given to bids from companies whose main product is professional liability insurance, particularly those that have provided at least 10 years of professional liability service in the same geographic area as the practice because experience with the local court system and defense attorneys is valuable when mounting a malpractice defense.

Some larger practices have attempted to gain more control over their malpractice costs and administration by self-insuring using on- or offshore captive insurance companies. Commercial malpractice insurance rates are partially dependent on the history of claims throughout the entire malpractice market.

Self-insuring can result in malpractice insurance rates being more dependent on the claims history of the practice being insured, so a practice with a good claims history may be able to lower malpractice insurance rates. It is important to note that setup and ongoing administrative costs are considerable and that a practice that is not already paying at least 1 million dollars in malpractice insurance premiums will probably not find it cost-effective to self-insure. The practice must also be large enough and have a long enough history for the actuarial analysis that determines its premiums to be reliable.

The Health Insurance Portability and Accountability Act of 1996

The Health Insurance Portability and Accountability Act of 1996 (HIPAA) deserves special mention because it has a significant impact on many aspects of practice management. Title II of the act addresses the security and privacy of health data stating that "reasonable and appropriate" safeguards must be taken to protect the integrity and confidentiality of health information. Following from the requirements of Title II, the Department of Health and Human Services (DHHS) has created five rules: the Privacy Rule, the Transactions and Code Sets Rule, the Security Rule, the Unique Identifiers Rule, and the Enforcement Rule. These five rules apply to all covered entities, which include health plans, billing services or health care clearinghouses of other types, and health care providers.

The Privacy Rule requires covered entities to protect the privacy of certain individually identifiable health data called Protected Health Information (PHI). It also establishes regulations for the use and disclosure of PHI, which includes any part of a patient's medical record or payment history. PHI must be disclosed to the patient on request, when required by law, or to facilitate treatment or payment or to third parties when consent has been given by the individual, but disclosure must be limited to the minimum amount necessary to achieve the required purpose. When PHI is disclosed, the disclosing entity is required to notify the individual and to keep track of any such disclosures.

The Security Rule deals specifically with electronic PHI and it requires the practice to institute administrative, physical, and technical safeguards. Administrative safeguards include policies and procedures that show how the practice will comply with the act. Physical safeguards protect against unauthorized access to hardware and software, and technical safeguards should protect against interception of PHI that is transmitted electronically.

The Enforcement Rule sets monetary penalties for noncompliance with any of the above rules. It is important that the prac-

tice manager be aware of all rules pertaining to the protection of PHI and to enact policies and procedures that will ensure compliance so that enforcement actions are avoided.

A full discussion of HIPAA is beyond the scope of this text, but practice managers should be fully versed in all aspects of Title II. All five of the above rules are relevant to practice management, and this chapter has only highlighted some of the major requirements of these rules. The reader is referred to the Centers for Disease Control and Prevention (CDC) and DHHS Web sites for further information.

Suggested readings

Adessa J. Endangered species, hospital based anesthesia groups. *ASA Conference on Practice Management* 2008; Tampa, FL, pp. 65–83.

Bierstein K. Anesthesia and Pain Medicine Coding Changes for 2003. *ASA Newsletter*, Nov 2002, Vol. 66(11). Available at: http://www.asahq.org/Newsletters/2002/11_02/pracMgmt.html.

Centers for Disease Control and Prevention (CDC). HIPAA Privacy Rule and Public Health Guidance from CDC and the U.S. Department of Health and Human Services. Available at: http://www.cdc.gov/MMWR/preview/mmwrhtml/su5201a1.htm.

Centers for Medicare & Medicaid Services (CMS). HIPAA General Information. Available at: http://www.cms.hhs.gov/HIPAAGenInfo/.

Davis KS, McConnell JC. Data management. In: Carroll R (ed.). *Risk Management Handbook for Health Care Organizations*. 2nd ed. Chicago: American Hospital Publishing; 1997:353.

Hagg-Rickert S. Elements of a risk management program. In: Carroll R (ed.). *Risk Management Handbook for Health Care Organizations*. 2nd ed. Chicago: American Hospital Publishing; 1997:35–37.

Hawawini G, Viallet C. *Finance for Executives-Managing for Value Creation*. 2nd ed. Cincinnati: South-Western; 2001.

Manuel BM. How to select professional liability insurance. *Bull Am Coll Surg* 2000; 85(2):17–19. Available at: http://www.facs.org/ahp/proliab/manuel0200.pdf.

McNamara C. Human Resources Management. Free Management Library. Available at: http://www.managementhelp.org/hr_mgmnt/hr_mgmnt.htm#anchor722373.

Riebolt JM. *Financial Management of the Medical Practice*. 2nd ed. Chicago: AMA Press; 2002.

CRICO/RMF. *Risk Management Essentials*. RMFInteractive, October 2004; Issue 5. Available at: http://www.rmf.harvard.edu/research-resources/articles/risk-management-essentials.aspx.

Schlotter W. Role of the practice administrator. *ASA Conference on Practice Management* 2008; Tampa, FL, 190–198.

Stickney CP, Weil RL. *Financial Accounting: An Introduction to Concepts, Methods, and Uses*. 9th ed. Orlando, FL: The Dryden Press; 1997:912.

ASHRM. Strategies and tips for maximizing failure mode and effect analysis in your organization. White Paper, July, 2002. Available at: http://www.ashrm.org/ashrm/resources/files/FMEAwhitepaper.pdf.

Chapter 140

Principles of medical ethics

Robert J. Klickovich and Rae M. Allain

Anesthesiologists are obligated to adhere to basic ethical principles in their practice. These principles primarily serve to protect the patient's interest, but are also applicable to other areas of professional conduct, including interactions with colleagues. This chapter will discuss basic medical ethics and describe common situations for the anesthesiologist in which ethical issues are paramount. Knowledge of ethical behavior is important given the anesthesiologist's role when patients are rendered unconscious and thus vulnerable due to either illness or intentionally administered medications.

Principles of consent

Autonomy, derived from the Greek roots *autos* (self) and *nomos* (rule), is widely accepted in our society, and it follows that patients have a right to self-determination. Patients may accept or refuse treatments after being presented with the necessary information, including the expected risks, benefits, and possible alternatives to a procedure. This dialogue between patient and physician is part of the informed consent process, which precedes the induction of anesthesia in elective circumstances. An inherent assumption of informed consent is that the patient understands the information and has the capacity for decision making. If the anesthesiologist questions whether a patient has this capacity (such as in the demented or delirious patient), then a formal assessment by a psychiatrist may be warranted. In such circumstances, a surrogate decision maker can be called on. This surrogate may be the patient's health care proxy (sometimes termed "durable power of attorney for health care") if the patient had designated such an individual previously. Alternatively, the patient's next of kin or close friend may be designated as the surrogate decision maker. It is incumbent on this individual to make decisions congruent with the patient's prior expressed wishes or values and not to choose based on what he or she would wish for him- or herself. If the patient has prepared advance directives (written documents describing what treatments or goals of care the patient would wish if incapacitated), these wishes should be respected by surrogates in the decision-making process. Advance directives may include a health care proxy designation and/or a "living will." The special circumstance of the pediatric patient mandates a surrogate decision maker for consent, usually a parent or legal guardian. Depending on the child's age, he or she may participate in the informed consent discussion and render preferences. For example, a child may choose between an inhalation and an intravenous induction. Similarly, this dictum of involving patients in the explanation of the procedure and inviting their input where appropriate may be applied to patients lacking full capacity, such as the adult patient with developmental delay whose guardian provides consent for the procedure.

The informed consent process requires the anesthesiologist to disclose information regarding the anesthetic procedure. The consent process should meet the "reasonable person standard." This means that any reasonable person would be satisfied that the patient was fully informed of all material information prior to signing the consent form. The specifics of the level of disclosure and the amount of detail cannot be precisely defined and will vary with the individual patient and procedure. The anesthesiologist should be aware that informed consent is a process of communication between provider and patient and that no rote or standardized form can guarantee protection against legal recourse by the patient. A prudent approach seeks to offer the patient as much information as he or she wishes, with ample opportunity to answer the patient's questions at the conversation's conclusion.

Emergency circumstances may preclude the informed consent process. In such situations, both surgeon and anesthesiologist should agree that the procedure requires emergent intervention to prevent permanent harm to the patient, and this should be documented in the medical record. In the absence of known advance directives, full treatment options should be pursued until such time as the patient's directives become clear.

Religious and cultural beliefs

Modern medicine dictates respect for varying cultural and religious beliefs. For the anesthesiologist, a common situation is the refusal of blood transfusions by patients who are Jehovah's Witnesses. Members of this religion may interpret biblical scripture as prohibitive of transfusion, including the strict penalty of loss of eternal salvation. Interpretation of this prohibition of blood transfusion varies among Jehovah's Witnesses and, therefore, a careful and private discussion should take place between the anesthesiologist and the Jehovah's Witness presenting for surgery. The purpose of this discussion is to delineate the patient's wishes regarding transfusion. The discussion should include preoperative preparation for blood conservation, consideration of deliberate hypotension or hypothermia, hemodilution, autologous donation, erythropoietin, and transfusion of synthetic colloid preparations (e.g., albumin). Many Jehovah's Witnesses will allow the use of red blood cell salvage, especially if the circuit is kept in continuity with the patient's circulation in a "closed" fashion. Finally, a frank discussion of the possible consequences of blood refusal, including death, is necessary. Legal precedent exists that allows the physician to administer a blood transfusion despite patient objections in some situations. Examples include the patient who is the sole parent of dependent children or the pediatric patient whose parents object to transfusion. It is prudent to involve legal counsel preoperatively in these circumstances whenever possible.

Cultural respect may require the anesthesiologist to make inquiries before interviewing the patient. For example, women of the Muslim faith may request a same-sex translator to discuss health-related issues. These patients may also require that the male head of household render health care decisions for them. To engender trust, enhance communication, and ensure understanding, it is beneficial to approach patients of different cultural backgrounds in an open-minded, nonjudgmental fashion.

Occasionally, the provision of care may provoke conflict with the anesthesiologist's personal ethics. For example, some practitioners object to providing anesthesia for procedures to terminate a pregnancy. There is controversy about the proper professional approach in this type of situation, but most ethical experts suggest that patients should be provided information about all legal and medically acceptable treatment options and that the practitioner has an obligation to help the patient find an alternate provider (e.g., anesthesiologist) if he or she cannot continue the physician–patient relationship due to ethical objections. A similar strategy may be invoked for the provider who is unwilling to respect a Jehovah's Witness patient's right to refuse blood transfusion. Open communication with the patient and with colleagues is usually the best approach in these situations, with the goal being adherence to the ethical principles of all involved parties. Emergency procedures that involve ethical conflict may be more difficult to resolve, but providing necessary care to the patient until an alternate provider is available is advisable.

Do not resuscitate (DNR) orders

The administration of anesthesia for a procedure frequently involves provision of measures that would be considered to be "resuscitation" in another setting. For example, hypnotic agents administered during the induction of general anesthesia commonly render a patient apneic, necessitating airway support to prevent imminent death. Similarly, muscle relaxants are commonly administered as part of an anesthetic to achieve optimal operating conditions for the surgeon, but the effects of these agents may require endotracheal intubation. In the past, these "resuscitative" measures were considered necessary for anesthesia care, and DNR orders were rescinded while a patient underwent anesthesia. In today's increasingly complex medical environment, this approach no longer holds. The American Society of Anesthesiologists (ASA) recognizes that respect for patient autonomy requires an open discussion with the patient or patient's surrogate regarding do not resuscitate (DNR) orders prior to anesthetic care and suggests three possible approaches. First, the DNR orders may be revoked for the anesthetic and perioperative period, allowing full resuscitation. Second, limited resuscitation may be performed to include certain measures (e.g., endotracheal intubation) but not others, based on the patient's preferences. With this approach, the anesthesiologist may play a role in educating the patient, helping him or her to weigh the relative risks (or burdens) versus benefits of each intervention. Third, a goal-directed approach to resuscitation may be adopted for the anesthetic course. This approach seeks to define the goals of care and allows the anesthesiologist to use his or her judgment to determine if resuscitation is likely to achieve those goals. For example, a patient with end-stage cardiomyopathy may not wish to undergo treatment of dysrhythmias. If this patient were to develop a bradycardia judged easily reversible and directly attributable to the anesthetic, it might be treated with a drug, whereas development of ventricular tachycardia attributable to myocardial ischemia might not be treated at all. Regardless of the approach to resuscitation status under anesthesia, the anesthesiologist must participate in a discussion in advance with the patient or patient's surrogate to understand the patient's preferences, goals, and values. Involvement of the surgeon or proceduralist and/or the patient's primary physician in the discussion is ideal, and a detailed documentation of the discussion should be provided in the patient's medical record.

Death under anesthesia care

Advances in anesthesia care have made death related to anesthesia an uncommon event, with estimates ranging from 5 to 7 per 100,000 anesthetics. Mortality rates are higher for patients of ASA physical status III or greater. Although death in the operating room or procedure suite is rare, anesthesiologists who specialize in critical care medicine are more accustomed to caring for the dying patient. Approximately 10% to 25% of patients admitted to an intensive care unit (ICU) will not survive, so it is incumbent on the intensivist to be familiar with care of the dying patient. When the chance of a cure or meaningful recovery is poor, the patient or patient's surrogate may choose *comfort care* rather than further life-sustaining measures. The role of the physician at this time is to provide relief from pain, anxiety, or distress and to allow the patient to die in a dignified fashion. Optimal care under these circumstances involves the collaborative efforts of the patient, family, and an interdisciplinary health care team. Care should focus not only on the medical and psychological aspects of dying, but also on the emotional and spiritual needs of surviving family members.

Medications (e.g., opiates, hypnotics, benzodiazepines) commonly employed for anesthesia may be useful to treat symptoms in the dying patient. These medications should not be withheld for fear of hastening death in such circumstances. To justify such treatment, some experts cite the ethical principle of *double effect,* where the intended good of the action (relief from pain) permits the potential harm (hastened death). Literature from the study of critically ill patients suggests that, despite clinicians' fears, medications administered to treat symptoms do not cause an earlier death.

Futility

Futility is a controversial topic that may arise in end-of-life discussions. Medical futility is perhaps best defined in the context of a particular treatment or intervention that scientific evidence shows will not achieve the goals of therapy. By this strict definition, physicians are not obligated to provide futile care. Sometimes futility is invoked as the reason to withdraw or limit life-sustaining treatments. This invocation may prove problematic because the wide variety of patient expectations, goals, values, and religious beliefs makes it difficult to define futility. In addition, society has provided no consensus definition of *futile care.* A more pragmatic approach to these situations is for the anesthesiologist to assist patients and their families in weighing the relative benefits and burdens of a given therapy within the context of the patient's beliefs and values. Using this approach, therapies that are likely to increase pain, suffering, or morbidity and those that diminish quality of life as appreciated by the patient are more likely to be refused.

Organ donation

The concept of organ donation is a medically and ethically acceptable option in our society but is one that may provoke ethical conflict. Most organ procurements derive from brain-dead donors (i.e., patients who are legally dead due to failure of whole brain function, but whose hearts are still beating). The exact criteria for determining brain death are locally determined and publicized in most hospital policy and procedure manuals; commonly, involvement of a physician specialized in neurologic illness is required. Although the legal concept of brain death is no different than death, this concept may be difficult for some families of religions or cultures that only recognize death as the cessation of the heartbeat. In such situations, efforts should be made to facilitate understanding in families who have a conflict with the withdrawal of care. A thoughtful, compassionate approach to the family may promote the consideration of organ donation in situations in which it would otherwise be refused.

Another option for organ donation is donation after cardiac death (DCD). This route may be considered by the patient or patient's surrogate if devastating injury or disease precludes an acceptable recovery and involves a controlled removal of the patient from life-sustaining treatments with the intention of organ procurement at some time interval (usually 2–5 minutes) following asystolic death. The withdrawal of life support (usually mechanical ventilation) may occur in the ICU or in the operating room and requires careful orchestration of a multidisciplinary team to assure proper adherence to ethical principles. Specifically, there should be a clear distinction between the physician caring for the patient (often the intensivist) and the procuring transplant surgeons. Care for the dying patient should be paramount with the same attentiveness to treating pain and distress as would be provided to the non–organ donor patient. Because these patients die due to cessation of cardiopulmonary function, an anesthesiologist may not be required for the procurement. If the procurement of intrathoracic organs (heart, lungs) is planned, then reintubation and ventilation of the patient following pronouncement of death may be desirable and the attendance of an anesthesiologist may be requested. Finally, plans must be in place to treat the patient who does not die within the time frame (usually 2 hours) necessary for organ donation. Usually, the patient is then transported back to the ICU to continue treatment until death does occur.

Ethics consultation

Many hospitals offer clinicians and patients the assistance of a hospital ethics committee when confronting difficult ethical problems or a nonnegotiable conflict around ethical issues. An ethics consultation should provide a reasoned opinion and often recommends a specific course of alternative actions. The opinion offered by the consult is a recommendation and not a mandate, and acceptance is always voluntary. If a given dispute cannot be resolved, the anesthesiologist may inquire if the hospital has a resolution of conflict policy and follow the prescribed path. Finally, if a given dispute cannot be resolved, judicial involvement may be requested but often requires a great deal of time and expense. In general, US courts support the settlement of ethical conflicts within the medical environment.

The impaired anesthesiologist

Chemical dependence is a chronic, relapsing disease affecting individuals at all social levels. The impression that the disease is more common among anesthesiologists as compared to other health care providers has been disproved, but anesthesiologists are unique in administering drugs to patients themselves rather than entering an order for a medication to be administered by another professional. As a result, controlled substances are immediately available to the practicing anesthesiologist. If a colleague demonstrates the signs of addiction, including a loss of interest in activities, problems at home, problems at work, obvious changes in work habits (including the overadministration of opiates, frequent unexplained absences, inappropriate volunteering for extra work, or witnessed self-administration), then intervention is necessary.

Intervention should take place in a formal setting and should be conducted by an expert. It must include irrefutable documentation of the behavior, willingness of colleagues to describe events demonstrating the behavior, and a specific treatment plan. If the individual should deny the behaviors despite irrefutable evidence, he or she should be informed that the state medical board will be advised of the suspected chemical dependence.

Anesthesiologists who have a history of addiction to opioids are statistically more likely to lapse than are those who have addictions to other substances. Legally, addiction is a disability. Recovering addicts who have been drug-free may not be refused employment solely on the basis of their disability, but state medical boards carefully weigh the risk to patients before allowing a recovered physician to return to practice and usually require that strict criteria for reentry be met. The anesthesiologist must have received treatment at a skilled facility with recommendations from treating providers stating that there is a low likelihood of relapse. A recovering provider must adhere to a detailed program of recovery, which may include the use of naltrexone, and he or she must abide by a written aftercare contract. The health care provider must be committed to a lifelong recovery. Family, partners, hospital staff, and administrators must accept the physician's return to work, and current recommendations suggest that a returning anesthesiologist should have 5 years of continuous monitoring.

While chemical dependence is an incurable disease, it may remain in long-term remission. Relapse is not a given, but may occur. Colleagues should provide the assistance and advocacy necessary to reinstitute treatment, aftercare, and recovery in the event of relapse.

Suggested readings

American Medical Association, Council on Ethical and Judicial Affairs. Medical futility in end-of-life care. *JAMA* 1999; 281:937–941.

Arnold W III. Chemically impaired anesthesiologist: reentry? In: Bready LL, ed. *Decision Making in Anesthesiology: An Algorithmic Approach.* 3rd ed. St Louis: Mosby; 2000:70–71.

Lagasse RS. Anesthesia safety: model or myth? A review of the published literature and analysis of current original data. *Anesthesiology* 2002; 97:1609–1617.

Truog RD, Campbell ML, Curtis JR, et al. Recommendations for end-of-life care in the intensive care unit: a consensus statement by the American Academy of Critical Care Medicine. *Crit Care Med* 2008; 36:953–963.

Truog RD, Waisel DB, Burns JP. DNR in the OR: a goal-directed approach. *Anesthesiology* 1999; 90:289–295.

Van Norman GA. Another matter of life and death: what every anesthesiologist should know about the ethical, legal, and policy implications of the non-heart-beating cadaver organ donor. *Anesthesiology* 2003; 98:763–773.

Waisel DB, Truog RD. Informed consent. *Anesthesiology* 1997; 87:968–978.

Chapter

141

Risks in the operating room

Jie Zhou

The operating room (OR) contains safety risks for both patients and staff. This chapter discusses safety risks that are relevant to anesthesia providers.

Needle safety

The Centers for Disease Control and Prevention (CDC) estimates that there are approximately 1000 *sharps-related injuries* per day sustained by hospital-based health care personnel in the United States. Sharps-related injuries include those that are due to needles, scalpels, or invasive medical devices. Hollow-bore devices create more of a concern, because they are more likely to transmit pathogens. According to the CDC, hepatitis B virus (HBV), hepatitis C virus (HCV), and HIV are the most commonly transmitted pathogens during patient care. Other pathogens include herpes, malaria, and tuberculosis.

The decrease in HBV infections, from approximately 12,000 in 1985 to 500 in 1997, is largely attributed to widespread immunization. Susceptible health care workers still have a 6% to 30% likelihood of HBV infection without postexposure prophylaxis, especially if the source patient is hepatitis B e antigen (HBeAg) positive. The number of transmissions of HCV to health care workers is unknown, but studies suggest that the transmission rate from an HCV-positive source to a healthy individual through a hollow needle ranges from 0% to 7%. HCV and HIV can also be transmitted through splash contamination of the conjunctiva or nonintact skin. The risk of HIV transmission following needlestick or mucous-membrane exposure is estimated to be 0.3% and 0.09%, respectively.

Data from the National Surveillance System for Health Care Workers (NaSH) suggest that 25% of hospital exposures to bloodborne diseases occur in the OR.

Several injury prevention strategies have been deployed over the past two decades, including the use of barrier-focused universal precautions for all OR personnel, the Bloodborne Pathogens Standard published by the Occupational Safety and Health Administration (OSHA), and the Needlestick Safety and Prevention Act of 2000. In addition, many engineering controls, such as retractable needles or blunt needles, have been developed, but work-practice controls are the most effective means of preventing blood exposure. The CDC recommends the following procedures in the OR:

- Using instruments, rather than fingers, to grasp needles, retract tissue, and load/unload needles and scalpels;
- Giving verbal announcements when passing sharps;
- Avoiding hand-to-hand passage of sharp instruments by using a basin or *neutral zone*;
- Using alternative cutting methods, such as blunt electrocautery and laser devices, when appropriate;
- Substituting endoscopic surgery for open surgery when possible; and
- Using round-tipped scalpel blades instead of sharp-tipped blades.

Anesthesia gases

There are two current classes of inhaled anesthetic agents: nitrous oxide and halogenated gases, including sevoflurane, desflurane, halothane, and enflurane. A US Food and Drug Administration (FDA) review in 2005 associated methoxyflurane with serious, irreversible, and even fatal nephrotoxicity and hepatotoxicity in humans, so it has been withdrawn from the market.

The National Institute for Occupational Safety and Health (NIOSH) issued "Criteria for a Recommended Standard. Occupational Exposure to Waste Anesthetic Gases (WAGs) and Vapors." The NIOSH criteria are highlighted in Table 141.1.

The 2007 update of the NIOSH criteria that is listed at the end of this chapter encourages raising awareness of WAG hazards among health care workers and suggests strategies to minimize exposure. OSHA published the "Guideline for Workplace Exposures" (GWE) in 2000. This guideline lists operational procedures, engineering controls, and work practices for WAGs in the OR. Its Web address is also listed at the end of this chapter.

More recently, the Task Force on Trace Anesthetic Gases (TFTAG) of the American Society of Anesthesiologists (ASA) issued "Information for Management in Anesthetizing Areas and the Postanesthesia Care Unit." TFTAG analyzed the literature on WAGs regarding their mutagenicity, carcinogenicity, organ toxicity, and reproductive effects. TFTAG concluded that there is not adequate evidence to prove adverse health effects caused by exposure to trace levels of WAGs in the OR. However, TFTAG does support the use of scavenging systems for WAGs,

Table 141.1. The NIOSH criteria

No worker is exposed to halogenated anesthetic agents at concentrations > 2 ppm when used alone or > 0.5 ppm when used in combination with nitrous oxide over a sampling period not to exceed 1 h.

No worker is exposed to nitrous oxide when used as the sole anesthetic agent exceeding a time-weighted average concentration of 25 ppm during anesthetic administration.

Anesthetic gas machines, non-rebreathing systems, and T-tube devices shall have an effective scavenging device that collects all WAGs.

WAG disposal systems are in place prior to starting an anesthetic.

Low-pressure leaks shall be < 100 ml/min at 30-cm water pressure.

High-pressure leaks from the gas supply (cylinder or pipeline) to the flow control valve should be a maximum of 10 ml/min.

Anesthetic gas flows shall not be started prior to induction of anesthesia.

Anesthetic flow meters shall be turned off or the Y-piece sealed when the breathing circuit is disconnected from the patient after administration of the anesthetic agent has started.

Before the reservoir bag is disconnected from the anesthetic delivery system, it shall be emptied into the scavenging system.

Comprehensive medical and occupational histories shall be obtained on each employee prior to employment and maintained in the employee's medical record.

Employees shall be provided with information and training on hazardous chemicals.

Any abnormal outcome of pregnancies of employees or of the spouses of employees exposed to WAGs shall be documented as part of the employee's medical records, and these records shall be maintained for the period of employment plus 20 years.

Upon employment and at least yearly thereafter, each worker shall be informed of possible health effects of exposure to WAGs.

Air monitoring shall be performed in all locations with the potential of worker exposure to WAGs.

Results of air sampling methods, locations, dates, and concentrations measured and results of leak tests shall be maintained for at least 20 years.

not only in the OR, but also in other locations where inhaled anesthetic gas is administered.

Chemical hazards

Latex

Latex has become a common source of allergic reactions in OR personnel, and it is estimated that 8% to 12% of health care workers are latex-sensitive. Latex can trigger an IgE-mediated cutaneous, respiratory, and systemic reaction, ranging from irritant contact dermatitis (Type IV) to immediate, life-threatening sensitivity (Type I). The prevalence among anesthesiologists is reported to be approximately 12.5% to 15.8%. Latex allergy is associated with allergies to avocado, potato, banana, tomato, chestnut, kiwi fruit, and papaya. People with spina bifida are also at increased risk for latex allergy.

Latex allergy should be suspected in anyone who develops allergic symptoms after latex exposure. Irritant or contact dermatitis is the most common reaction from a latex encounter. Certain medications may reduce the allergy symptoms, but complete latex avoidance is the most effective approach.

Halothane

There are two distinct forms of liver damage from halothane. Type I hepatitis occurs commonly and presents with minor elevations of liver enzymes. Type II hepatitis, which is thought to be immune-mediated, is rare and unpredictable and can result in severe, fulminant hepatitis with a high mortality.

Hepatitis induced from occupational exposure to halothane has been reported in pediatric anesthesiologists. There is also a reported case of isoflurane hepatotoxicity in a patient with a previous history of halothane-induced hepatitis. This case suggests that personnel with a history of liver injury from one haloalkane should not be exposed to another. Occupational safety and health guidelines for halothane are available at the OSHA Web site.

Methyl methacrylate

Methyl methacrylate (MMA) is an organic compound used to cement prostheses in orthopedic surgery. The most common effect of overexposure to MMA is irritation of the skin, eyes, nose, throat, or lungs, but it can also affect the nervous system. OSHA has established a permissible exposure limit of 100 ppm, 410 mg/m^3 time-weighted average (TWA).

Severe cardiopulmonary complications, such as hypotension, bradycardia, and cardiac arrest, have been reported in patients with the use of MMA. The direct myocardial depressant effect of MMA seems to be caused in part by depression of Ca^{2+} influx across the cardiac membrane. MMA may also cause direct relaxation of venous and arterial smooth muscle.

Fire safety

OR fires are rare but potentially disastrous. Current literature estimates that there are approximately 100 surgical fires in the United States each year, but the real incidence may be higher.

Most surgical fires involve the airway. For a fire to occur, three components, known as the "fire triad," must be present: an oxidizer, an ignition source, and a fuel. In the OR, oxidizers include oxygen and nitrous oxide; ignition sources include lasers, drills, electrocautery sets, and fiber-optic light sources; and fuels include endotracheal tubes, flammable solutions, sponges, and drapes.

In May 2008, ASA issued a Practice Advisory for the Prevention and Management of Operating Room Fires. The advisory recommends providing fire safety education and training to anesthesiologists, and it lists the methodology for preparation, prevention, and management of OR fires. The ASA Operating Room Fires Algorithm contained within the full advisory summarizes important aspects of fire prevention and fire management. Recommendations for prevention include keeping ignition sources away from oxidizer-enriched atmospheres, configuring surgical drapes to minimize the accumulation of oxidizers, and allowing sufficient drying time for flammable skin-prepping solutions. They also recommend that the surgical team determine preoperatively whether the procedure is high risk and that appropriate precautions be identified and put in place prior to the start of surgery. The fire management section calls for immediate evaluation if an "early warning sign of fire" is identified, and discusses the management of both airway and nonairway fires. The full ASA advisory is listed at the end of the

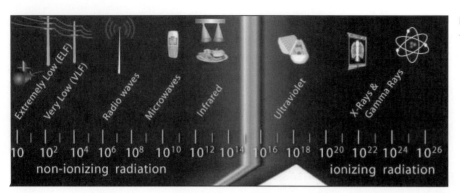

Figure 141.1. Radiation scale. From http://www.osha.gov/SLTC/radiation.

chapter; all anesthesia practitioners should be familiar with its contents.

Radiation safety

Radiation is used in a variety of areas in the OR. In general, there are two types of radiations: non-ionizing radiation and ionizing radiation. Non-ionizing radiation comprises electromagnetic radiation ranging from extremely low frequency (ELF) to ultraviolet (UV). Ionizing radiation consists of particulate (alpha, beta, neutrons) and electromagnetic (x-rays, gamma rays) radiation. Anesthesiologists may be exposed to any of them (see Fig. 141.1).

Non-ionizing radiation

Laser safety

Laser is the acronym for "light amplification by stimulated emission of radiation." The four major properties of laser light are monochromaticity, spatial coherence, high energy, and focusability (directionality).

Clinical usefulness of each laser is determined by the degree of thermal effect when it strikes the tissue, which in turn is determined by three variables: the absorptive and reflective properties of the tissue at the laser wavelength, the power density, and the duration of exposure. The absorption of laser energy is determined by the wavelength of the light and the physical characteristics (pigmentation, hemoglobin, and water content) of the tissue. There are four types of lasers that are used clinically: the carbon dioxide (CO_2) laser, the argon laser, the neodymium:yttrium–aluminum–garnet (Nd:YAG) laser, and the potassium titanyl phosphate (KTP) laser (green laser).

The CO_2 laser has a wavelength of 10,600 nm, which is in the invisible infrared region. A low energy helium–neon (HeNe) 633-nm laser was added to provide visibility during clinical use. CO_2 laser emissions are completely absorbed by cellular water and produce tissue destruction to a depth of 100 to 200 microns, which is approximately half the thickness of the epidermis.

The argon laser emits at a wavelength of 488 nm and 514 nm, which carries a visible blue-green color. It is absorbed by hemoglobin and pigmented tissue and is poorly absorbed by water. It can be used to effectively coagulate vessels.

The Nd:YAG laser is in the near-infrared range with a wavelength of 1064 nm. It is commonly used for eye, bladder, and synovial capsule surgery.

The KTP laser is generated by passing the Nd:YAG laser through a potassium titanyl phosphate crystal. The beam is at a wavelength of 532 nm and has a green color. It is commonly used in prostate surgery.

Risks of laser use include thermal burns, eye injuries, electrical hazards, fires, and explosions. Ophthalmic safety is one of most common concerns with laser use because a reflected laser beam could create significant ocular trauma. Protective eyewear should be worn by all OR personnel any time that the laser is in use. Effective protection from laser injury requires a unique lens that absorbs the particular wavelength of the laser in question, so there is no universal eyewear that provides protection against all lasers. Eyewear is rated for optical density (OD), which is the base-10 logarithm of attenuation. For example, eyewear with OD 3 will reduce the beam power in the specified wavelength range by a factor of 1000.

Smoke plumes resulting from the thermal destruction of tissue by laser and electrocautery devices have received increased attention as a safety concern in recent years. Research studies have confirmed that this smoke plume can contain toxic gases and vapors such as benzene, hydrogen cyanide, and formaldehyde; bio-aerosols; dead and live cellular material (including blood fragments); and viruses. At high concentrations, the smoke causes ocular and upper respiratory tract irritation in health care personnel and creates visual problems for the surgeon. NIOSH released a Health Hazard Alert on the danger of smoke plumes in 1996.

UV safety

Studies of indoor UV-emitting fluorescent lamps have demonstrated a 3.9% increase in the risk of skin malignancies over solar UV exposure. The level of risk is associated with the specific frequency within the UV range. UVB (290–320 nm) radiation directly damages DNA and is highly mutagenic and carcinogenic in animal experiments compared to UVA (320–400 nm) radiation, which indirectly damages DNA through the formation of reactive oxygen radicals.

No OSHA standard exists for UV radiation (UVR), but both NIOSH and the International Commission on Non-Ionizing

Radiation Protection (ICNIRP) have made varying recommendations for UV light within the spectral region of 200 to 400 nm with the most restrictive limits on the UVB region between 200 and 315 nm. Exposure limits are dependent on both the frequency and intensity of the radiation and must be determined using tables that can be found in the NIOSH or ICNIRP information at the end of this chapter.

Ionizing radiation

Anesthesiologists may encounter various types of ionizing radiation, including particulate radiation with alpha, beta, or neutrons in a radiology oncology treatment suite, gamma rays at a Gamma Knife center, or x-rays in a fluoroscopy or neuroradiology suite.

Ionizing radiation is carcinogenic at high doses. Its effects include direct chromosomal changes, indirect free radical formation, and cataract formation. Total radiation exposure is determined by three factors: (1) intensity and time of exposure, (2) distance between the anesthesiologist and the source of radiation, and (3) the use of shielding. The latter two factors can be modified by the anesthesiologist. Radiation exposure is inversely proportional to the square of the distance from the source, so increasing distance is an effective way of decreasing exposure.

Common lead aprons leave several vulnerable spots of the human body, including both the thyroid and the eyes. Thyroid shields and eye protection should be worn along with lead aprons to minimize the risk of thyroid cancer or cataract formation.

The U.S. Nuclear Regulatory Commission (NRC) has established the current occupational exposure limits for both shallow and deep doses in adults:

(1) An annual limit, which is the more limiting of

  (i) the total effective dose equivalent being equal to 5 rems (0.05 Sv) or
  (ii) the sum of the deep-dose equivalent and the committed dose equivalent to any individual organ or tissue other than the lens of the eye being equal to 50 rems (0.5 Sv).

(2) The annual limits to the lens of the eye, to the skin of the whole body, and to the skin of the extremities, which are

  (i) a lens dose equivalent of 15 rems (0.15 Sv) and
  (ii) a shallow-dose equivalent of 50 rem (0.5 Sv) to the skin of the whole body or to the skin of any extremity.

The limits for fetal radiation exposure vary between agencies from 100 mrem/y (1 mSv/y) to 500 mrem/y (5 mSv/y) or less during the gestational period.

Suggested readings

Alleva R, Tomasetti M, Solenghi MD, et al. Lymphocyte DNA damage precedes DNA repair or cell death after orthopaedic surgery under general anaesthesia. *Mutagenesis* 2003; 18(5):423–428.

American Optometric Association. Occupational Vision Manual. Available at http://www.aoa.org/x5358.xml (accessed August 15, 2010).

ASA Task Force on Operating Room Fires. Practice Advisory for the Prevention and Management of Operating Room Fires. *Anesthesiology* 2008; 108(5):786–801. Available at: http://www.asahq.org/publicationsAndServices/orFiresPA.pdf. Last accessed August 2010.

ASA Task Force on Trace Anesthetic Gases. Waste Anesthetic Gases: Information for Management in Anesthetizing Areas and the Postanesthesia Care Unit. Available at http://www.asahq.org/publicationsAndServices/wasteanes.pdf (accessed August 15, 2010).

Baden JM, Simmon VF. Mutagenic effects of inhalational anesthetics. *Mutat Res* 1980; 75(2):169–189.

Behrman AJ. Latex Allergy eMedicine. Available at http://www.emedicine.com/emerg/topic814.htm (accessed August 15, 2010). Last updated August 7, 2008.

Bell DM. Occupational risk of human immunodeficiency virus infection in healthcare workers: an overview. *Am J Med* 1997; 102(5B):9–15.

Beltrami EM, Kozak A, Williams IT, et al. Transmission of HIV and hepatitis C virus from a nursing home patient to a health care worker. *Am J Infect Control* 2003; 31(3):168–175.

Berry A, Katz J. Occupational health. In: Barash P, Cullen B, Stoelting R, eds. and trans. *Clinical Anesthesia*. Philadelphia: Lippincott Williams & Wilkins; 2006:76–98.

Bolus NE. Review of common occupational hazards and safety concerns for nuclear medicine technologists. *J Nucl Med Technol* 2008; 36(1):11–17.

Bozkurt G, Memis D, Karabogaz G, et al. Genotoxicity of waste anaesthetic gases. *Anaesth Intensive Care* 2002; 30(5):597–602.

Brown RH, Schauble JF, Hamilton RG. Prevalence of latex allergy among anesthesiologists: identification of sensitized but asymptomatic individuals. *Anesthesiology* 1998; 89(2):292–299.

Caplan RA, Barker SJ, Connis RT, et al. Practice advisory for the prevention and management of operating room fires. *Anesthesiology* 2008; 108(5):786–801; quiz 971–972.

Centers for Disease Control and Prevention. Overview: Risks and Prevention of Sharps Injuries in Healthcare Personnel. Available at http://www.cdc.gov/sharpssafety/ (accessed August 15, 2010). Last updated July 27, 2010.

De Vane GG. AANA journal course: new technologies in anesthesia: update for nurse anesthetists–lasers. *AANA J* 1990; 58(4):313–319.

Fishman SM, Smith H, Meleger A, et al. Radiation safety in pain medicine. *Reg Anesth Pain Med* 2002; 27(3):296–305.

Garvin M. Making the Operating Room a Safer Place. Virgo Publishing, LLC. Available at http://www.infectioncontroltoday.com/articles/2002/10/making-the-operating-room-a-safer-place.aspx (accessed August 15, 2010). Last updated October 1, 2002.

Government agency issues surgical smoke hazard control. *AORN J* 1996; 64(6):1045.

Gruber F, Peharda V, Kastelan M, et al. Occupational skin diseases caused by UV radiation. *Acta Dermatovenerol Croat* 2007; 15(3):191–198.

Hasan F. Isoflurane hepatotoxicity in a patient with a previous history of halothane-induced hepatitis. *Hepatogastroenterology* 1998; 45(20):518–522.

Herd RM, Dover JS, Arndt KA. Basic laser principles. *Dermatol Clin* 1997; 15(3):355–372.

Hernandez ME, Bruguera M, Puyuelo T, et al. Risk of needle-stick injuries in the transmission of hepatitis C virus in hospital personnel. *J Hepatol* 1992; 16(1–2):56–58.

Ichihashi M, Ueda M, Budiyanto A, et al. UV-induced skin damage. *Toxicology* 2003; 189(1–2):21–39.

International Commission on Non-Ionizing Radiation Protection (ICNIRP). Guidelines on Limits of Exposure to Ultraviolet Radiation of Wavelengths Between 180 NM and 400 NM (Incoherent Optical Radiation). *Health Physics* 2004; 87(2):171–86. Available at: http://www.icnirp.de/documents/UV2004.pdf. Accessed August 15, 2010.

Ippolito G, Puro V, De Carli G. The risk of occupational human immunodeficiency virus infection in health care workers. Italian Multicenter Study. The Italian Study Group on Occupational Risk of HIV infection. *Arch Intern Med* 1993; 153(12): 1451–1458.

Ippolito G, Puro V, Petrosillo N, et al. Simultaneous infection with HIV and hepatitis C virus following occupational conjunctival blood exposure. *JAMA* 1998; 280(1):28.

Karlsson J, Wendling W, Chen D, et al. Methylmethacrylate monomer produces direct relaxation of vascular smooth muscle in vitro. *Acta Anaesthesiol Scand* 1995; 39(5):685–689.

Kashimoto S, Nakamura T, Furuya A, et al. Cardiac effects of methylmethacrylate in the rat heart-lung preparation with or without volatile anesthetics. *Resuscitation* 1995; 30(3):269–273.

Kelley P, O'Hara M, Bishop J, et al. Flammability of common ocular lubricants in an oxygen-rich environment. *Eye Contact Lens* 2005; 31(6):291–293.

Kim KJ, Chen DG, Chung N, et al. Direct myocardial depressant effect of methylmethacrylate monomer: mechanical and electrophysiologic actions in vitro. *Anesthesiology* 2003; 98(5):1186–1194.

Kiyosawa K, Sodeyama T, Tanaka E, et al. Hepatitis C in hospital employees with needlestick injuries. *Ann Intern Med* 1991; 115(5):367–369.

Konrad C, Fieber T, Gerber H, et al. The prevalence of latex sensitivity among anesthesiology staff. *Anesth Analg* 1997; 84(3):629–633.

Korniewicz DM, Chookaew N, Brown J, et al. Impact of converting to powder-free gloves. Decreasing the symptoms of latex exposure in operating room personnel. *AAOHN J* 2005; 53(3):111–116.

Kuczkowski KM. Anesthesia machine as a cause of intraoperative "code red" in the labor and delivery suite. *Arch Gynecol Obstet* 2008; 278(5):477–478.

Lanphear BP, Linnemann CC Jr, Cannon CG, et al. Hepatitis C virus infection in healthcare workers: risk of exposure and infection. *Infect Control Hosp Epidemiol* 1994; 15(12):745–750.

Laser Safety. Wikipedia. Available at http://en.wikipedia.org/wiki/Laser_safety (Accessed August 15, 2010). Last updated August 12, 2010.

Luleci N, Sakarya M, Topcu I, et al. [Effects of sevofluran on cell division and levels of sister chromatid exchange]. *Anasthesiol Intensivmed Notfallmed Schmerzther* 2005; 40(4):213–216.

Lytle CD, Cyr WH, Beer JZ, et al. An estimation of squamous cell carcinoma risk from ultraviolet radiation emitted by fluorescent lamps. *Photodermatol Photoimmunol Photomed* 1992; 9(6):268–274.

National Institute for Occupational Safety and Health (NIOSH). Control of Smoke From Laser/Electric Surgical Procedures. Available at http://www.cdc.gov/niosh/hc11.html (accessed August 15, 2010). Last updated March 2, 1998.

National Institute for Occupational Safety and Health (NIOSH). Criteria for a recommended standard occupational exposure to waste anesthetic gases and vapors. Available at http://www.cdc.gov/niosh/pdfs/77-140a.pdf (accessed August 15, 2010).

National Institute for Occupational Safety and Health (NIOSH). Guidelines for protecting the safety and health of health care workers. Available at http://www.cdc.gov/niosh/docs/88-119/health.html (Accessed August 15, 2010).

National Institute for Occupational Safety and Health (NIOSH). Waste Anesthetic Gases – Occupational Hazards in Hospitals. Available at http://www.cdc.gov/niosh/docs/2007-151/pdfs/2007-151.pdf (accessed August 15, 2010). Last updated September 2007.

Njoku DB, Greenberg RS, Bourdi M, et al. Autoantibodies associated with volatile anesthetic hepatitis found in the sera of a large cohort of pediatric anesthesiologists. *Anesth Analg* 2002; 94(2): 243–249.

Njoku DB, Mellerson JL, Talor MV, et al. Role of CYP2E1 immunoglobulin G4 subclass antibodies and complement in pathogenesis of idiosyncratic drug-induced hepatitis. *Clin Vaccine Immunol* 2006; 13(2):258–265.

Occupational exposure to bloodborne pathogens; correction–OSHA. Final rule, correction. *Fed Regist* 1992; 57(127):29206.

Otedo AE. Halothane induced hepatitis: case report. *East Afr Med J* 2004; 81(10):538–539.

Puro V, Petrosillo N, Ippolito G, et al. Occupational hepatitis C virus infection in Italian health care workers. Italian Study Group on Occupational Risk of Bloodborne Infections. *Am J Public Health* 1995; 85(9):1272–1275.

Rathmell JP. Imaging in regional anesthesia and pain medicine: we have much to learn. *Reg Anesth Pain Med* 2002; 27(3):240–241.

Romig CL, Smalley PJ. Regulation of surgical smoke plume. *AORN J* 1997; 65(4):824–828.

Sadoh DR, Sharief MK, Howard RS. Occupational exposure to methyl methacrylate monomer induces generalised neuropathy in a dental technician. *Br Dent J* 1999; 186(8):380–381.

Sartori M, La Terra G, Aglietta M, et al. Transmission of hepatitis C via blood splash into conjunctiva. *Scand J Infect Dis* 1993; 25(2):270–271.

Situm M, Buljan M, Bulic SO, et al. The mechanisms of UV radiation in the development of malignant melanoma. *Coll Antropol* 2007; 31(Suppl 1):13–16.

Spence AA, Cohen EN, Brown BW Jr, et al. Occupational hazards for operating room-based physicians. Analysis of data from the United States and the United Kingdom. *JAMA* 1977; 238(9): 955–959.

U.S. Food and Drug Administration. FDA Notice: Determination that penthrane (methoxyflurane) inhalation liquid, 99.9 percent, was withdrawn from sale for reasons of safety or effectiveness. Available at http://www.asahq.org/news/alert090605.htm (accessed August 15, 2010). Last updated Sept. 6, 2005.

U.S. Nuclear Regulatory Commission. Standards for protection against radiation. Available at http://www.nrc.gov/reading-rm/doc-collections/cfr/part020/ (accessed August 15, 2010).

U.S. Occupational Safety & Health Administration (OSHA). Laser Hazards. Available at http://www.osha.gov/SLTC/laserhazards/index.html (accessed August 15, 2010). Last updated October 6, 2008.

U.S. Occupational Safety and Health Administration (OSHA). Latex Allergy. Available at http://www.osha.gov/SLTC/etools/hospital/hazards/latex/latex.html (accessed August 15, 2010).

U.S. Occupational Safety and Health Administration (OSHA). Occupational Safety and Health Guideline for Halothane. Available at http://www.osha.gov/SLTC/healthguidelines/halothane/recognition.html (accessed August 15, 2010).

U.S. Occupational Safety and Health Administration (OSHA). Radiation. Available at http://www.osha.gov/SLTC/radiation/ (Accessed August 15, 2010).

U.S. Occupational Safety and Health Administration (OSHA). Anesthetic Gases: Guidelines for Workplace Exposures. Available at http://www.osha.gov/dts/osta/anestheticgases/index.html (Accessed August 15, 2010). Last updated May 18, 2000.

Weber SM, Hargunani CA, Wax MK. DuraPrep and the risk of fire during tracheostomy. *Head Neck* 2006; 28(7): 649–652.

Statistics for anesthesiologists and researchers

Samuel M. Galvagno Jr. and Kamal K. Sikka

An elementary understanding of statistics is essential to help the evidence-based practitioner address common problems encountered throughout the vicissitudes of daily anesthetic practice.

The medical literature has an abundance of studies that use statistics, but there are few available books devoted to the use of statistics in anesthesiology. Because statistical techniques are complicated, researchers and practitioners of anesthesia should be aware of the misuse of statistics to promulgate flawed conclusions. The data in the numerical examples described in this chapter are adapted from Jensen, Wernberg, and Andersen.

This chapter is not a comprehensive dissertation on statistics. For more comprehensive studies, the reader is referred to two excellent texts: one by Freedman, Pisani, and Purves and the other by Dawson and Trapp.

Basic math review

Logarithms

Logarithms are used to describe the power to which a number must be raised to get another number. For example, the Henderson–Hasselbalch equation describes how plasma partial pressure of carbon dioxide (PCO_2), plasma bicarbonate concentration ($[HCO_3^-]$), the negative logarithm of the apparent dissociation constant (pK) for plasma carbonic acid (H_2CO_3), and the solubility (S) of CO_2 in plasma interact to determine plasma pH.

$$pH = pK_1 + \log[\text{bicarbonate}]/0.03 \times PCO_2$$

A logarithmic scale is a scale of measurement that uses the logarithm of a physical quantity instead of the quantity itself. Presentation of data on a logarithmic scale can be helpful when the data cover a large range of values. The logarithm reduces this range to a more manageable range. On most logarithmic scales, *small* values, or ratios of the underlying quantity, correspond to *small* values of the logarithmic measure. Well-known examples of such scales are:

- Richter scale for earthquake magnitude,
- Decibel for acoustic power, and
- Logit for odds in statistics.

One example of the use of logarithms is Lagasse's depiction of the trend of anesthesia-related deaths from 1954 through 2001. The death rate was extrapolated from either a power or logarithmic fit of these figures (1/5000–1/10,000). By using logarithmic methods, the death rate from anesthesia for plastic surgery can be more accurately estimated because previous nonlogarithmic methods cited the risk to be falsely low – 1/300,000.

Graphs of simple equations

It is a frequent practice in anesthesiology and critical care medicine to estimate the human body surface area (BSA). BSA is one example of a linear regression equation that can be applied clinically. Linear regression is a statistical method that involves determining an equation to predict a value based on other known values. The determination of BSA is useful in several areas related to the body's metabolism, such as ventilation, fluid requirements, extracorporeal circulation, and drug dosages. The following formula estimates BSA and is demonstrated in Fig. 142.1.

Basic exponential functions are depicted as hyperbolic or parabolic curves. These mathematical functions are used to determine the value of y when x is known, or vice versa. Fig. 142.2 demonstrates a basic exponential function ($y = b^x$).

Linear Regression of Body Surface Area vs. Weight

BSA = 1321 + 0.3433 × Wt
$r^2 = 0.9715$

Figure 142.1. An example of linear regression.

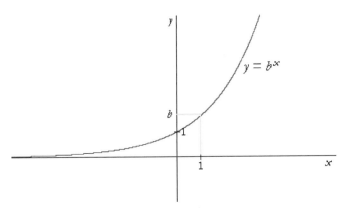

Figure 142.2. An example of an exponential function.

Table 142.1. Blood glucose levels of 25 preoperative children undergoing anesthesia

Patient	mg/dl	Patient	mg/dl	Patient	mg/dl
1	36	11	70	21	86
2	47	12	72	22	88
3	52	13	74	23	93
4	56	14	75	24	97
5	61	15	76	25	106
6	63	16	77		
7	66	17	79		
8	67	18	83		
9	68	19	83		
10	69	20	83		

Two common graphical representations of data, the histogram and the percentage cumulative frequency distribution, are shown in Fig. 142.3 for the data from Table 142.1.

The histogram graphically represents the type of distribution exhibited by the data, whether they is balanced around the mean or skewed to one side. The percentage cumulative frequency represents the percentage of data occurrences below a given percentage value. The percentage cumulative distribution in Fig. 142.3 shows that only 4% of the children undergoing preoperative starvation had a blood glucose level less than 40 mg/dl, which can be classified as hypoglycemic.

Table 142.2. Examples of interval and categorical data

Type of data	Description	Example
Interval	Discrete: Integer-only scale	Number of toes, number of nostrils
Interval	Continuous: Constant scale interval	Temperature, weight, blood pressure
Categorical	Dichotomous: Binary data	Male/Female, Alive/Dead
Categorical	Nominal: Qualitative; cannot be ranked	Eye color, type of surgery
Categorical	Ordinal: Data that are ranked but do not have a consistent scale interval	ASA class, Mallampati class, VAS pain score

Basic statistics

Data classification

Samples of populations are described with different terms. Interval data are composed of discrete and continuous variables. Categorical variables refer to observations the values of which are categories. Examples are provided in Table 142.2. Classification of data becomes important when choosing the correct statistical test.

Probability

The probability (Pr) of an event (A) is the proportion of times it occurs in a long sequence of trials. Probabilities always lie between 0 and 1.

$$Pr(A) = N_A/N$$

N = mutually exclusive outcomes

N_A = equally likely outcomes

p value

The *p* value is the probability of obtaining a test statistic that is as extreme or more extreme as the one actually observed, assuming that the null hypothesis is true. The *p* value is a measure of the probability that a difference between groups during an experiment happened by chance. For example, a *p* value of

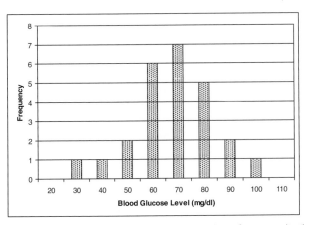
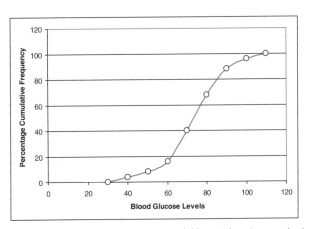

Figure 142.3. Histogram and percentage cumulative frequency distribution of blood glucose levels of preoperative children undergoing anesthesia.

Table 142.3. Ways to prevent Type I and Type II errors

Raise the level of alpha (not commonly done)
Reduce population variability
Make the difference between the conditions greater
Increase the sample size (most common method used)

.01 ($p = .01$) means that there is a 1 in 100 chance that the result occurred by luck. The lower the p value, the more likely it is that the difference between groups was caused by the experimental intervention.

Type I (α) and Type II (β) error

Type I (α) error is the probability that the data will indicate that the null hypothesis is wrong. Stated another way, Type I error is the probability that a difference will be found between two groups when none actually exists. Type I error (α) is usually set at .05, which means that there is a 5 in 100 chance that a given result occurred purely by chance.

Type II (β) error is the probability that a difference actually does exist between two conditions but the data erroneously indicate that no difference exists. By convention, Type II (β) is usually set at .2. (See Table 142.3.)

Statistical power

The power of a test is $1 - \beta$, which usually equals 80%. Statistical power is the probability that one will detect a meaningful difference, or effect, if one were to occur. Ideally, studies should have power levels of .80 or higher, which means that there will be an 80% chance or greater of finding an effect if one is really there.

Measures of central tendency and dispersion

Given a population of data, there are several numeric measures for characterizing the information represented by the data. The population of data can be represented by measures representing the central tendency or dispersion of the data.

Mean (or average) represents the central tendency of the data, defined as

$$\overline{x} = \sum_{j=1}^{N} x_j,$$

where x_j is the jth sample in a total population of N samples. For the sample size of $N = 25$ in Table 142.1, the mean is 73.1 mg/dl.

The median is the central sample when the data are ordered in an ascending or descending order. For $N = 25$, the 13th sample of the data from Table 142.1, when arranged in an ascending or descending order, is the median and is equal to 74 mg/dl. For distributions that are composed of an even number of samples, the median is the arithmetic average of the two central samples. For example, when $N = 20$, the median is the arithmetic average of the 10th and 11th sample.

The mode is the most frequently occurring sample in the population. The mode of the data in Table 142.1 is 83 mg/dl.

The standard deviation is a measure of dispersion and is the root mean square (RMS) deviation of values from their arithmetic mean. It is expressed as

$$\sigma = \sqrt{\frac{1}{N} - 1 \sum_{j=1}^{N} \left(x_j - \overline{x} \right)^2}.$$

The standard deviation of the population in Table 142.1 is 15.78 mg/dl.

The range is another measure of dispersion and is the difference between the maximum and minimum values in a distribution. The range in Table 142.1 is 70 mg/dl.

The variance is the square of the standard deviation.

Standard deviation and standard error of the mean

The standard deviation is a measure of spread, scatter, or dispersion of a sample. When data are distributed normally, 1, 2, and 3 standard deviations from the mean encompass 68%, 95%, and 99% of the population, respectively (Fig. 142.4).

The standard error of the mean is a measure of the precision with which the population center (mean) is known. If the data from a sample are distributed in the standard bell-curve fashion (normal distribution), a formula can describe the spread of the data around the mean. The standard error of the mean is calculated by dividing the standard deviation by the square root of the sample size. It is always smaller than the standard deviation. The choice between using the standard deviation or the standard error of the mean is controversial.

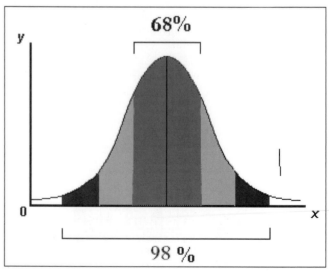

Figure 142.4. Standard deviations.

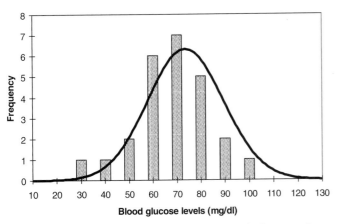

Figure 142.5. Normal distribution of blood glucose levels of preoperative children undergoing anesthesia superimposed over the histogram from Fig. 142.3.

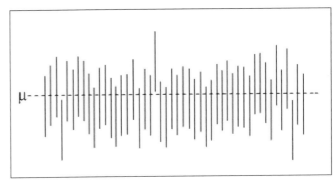

Figure 142.6. Fifty realizations of a CI for μ. See text for explanation.

Normal statistical distribution

Also known as the Gaussian distribution, or the bell curve, the normal distribution is commonly used in statistical analyses. It is characterized by the mean and variance of the data. When the distribution is normalized to a mean of 0 and a variance of 1, it is termed as the standard normal distribution. The probability distribution for the normal distribution is represented as

$$f(x) = \frac{1}{\sigma\sqrt{2\pi}} \exp\left(-\frac{(x - \overline{x})^2}{2\sigma^2}\right).$$

In Fig. 142.5, the normal distribution is superposed on the histogram from Fig. 142.3. It can be observed that the normal distribution accurately represents the data in Table 142.1.

Confidence intervals

Confidence intervals (CIs) define a range of values within which the population mean is likely to lie. A CI is the probability that a number will be between an upper and lower limit. CIs are usually reported as a 95% CI, which is the range of values within which one can be 95% sure that the true value for the whole population lies. The 95% (p value $= .05$) and 99% (p value $= .01$) CIs are the most commonly used.

Figure 142.6 demonstrates 50 realizations of a CI for μ. A CI can be considered as the range, or interval, of results in which the researcher has confidence. As seen from the figure, there is a fair chance that an interval that actually contains μ will be picked; however, there is still a chance that the wrong interval may be picked.

Statistical techniques

Student's t test

The Student's t test can be used to examine the effect of a controlled experiment on a population distribution by a comparison of the means. If each subject in a study has one measurement (blood pressure, heart rate, temperature), as in before and after some event, than a *one sample* or *paired t test* should

be used. This pairing of measurements reduces variability and increases the power of the test. When two separate groups are compared to each other (one group gets one drug, another group gets a placebo or standard treatment), *a two sample* or *unpaired* t *test* should be used. Unpaired t tests have less power than do paired t tests due to increased variability.

Nonparametric tests

When data are *not* normally distributed or when they are on an *ordinal* level of measurement (i.e., American Society of Anesthesiologists [ASA] class, visual analog scale [VAS] pain score), nonparametric tests should be used. A common mistake in medical research is using the wrong class of statistical test, such as a parametric test in place of a nonparametric test. The basic rule is to use a parametric test (t test) for data normally distributed and a nonparametric test for skewed data. The Mann–Whitney U test is the nonparametric equivalent of the unpaired t test. It is used to compare two groups, but unless the data are skewed or ordinal, it is best to use a t test. The Wilcoxon rank-sum test is almost identical to the Mann–Whitney U test (see Table 142.4).

Analysis of variance

An analysis of variance (ANOVA) is a parametric statistical test that is used when there is more than one group that requires analysis. The t test tells one if the variation between two groups is significant. When multiple groups require analysis, multiple t tests are not the answer because, as the number of groups grows, the number of needed paired comparisons grows quickly. For seven groups there are 21 pairs. If 21 pairs were compared, one would not be surprised to observe that events happen only 5% of the time. Thus, in 21 pairings, a p value of .05 for one pair

Table 142.4. Commonly used parametric and nonparametric tests

Parametric	Nonparametric
Student's t test	Mann–Whitney U test
One-way ANOVA	Kruskal–Wallis H test
Paired t test	Wilcoxon signed-rank test
Correlated F ratio	Friedman ANOVA by ranks

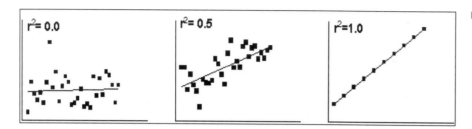

Figure 142.7. Examples of correlation coefficients.

cannot be considered significant. An ANOVA puts all the data into one number (F) and provides one probability for the null hypothesis.

Chi-square

The chi-square test (χ^2) is a statistic used to compare the frequencies of two or more groups. Researchers often use chi-squares to test *nominal* data (e.g., eye color, type of surgery). This nonparametric test provides a rough estimate of confidence; it accepts as input data that are weaker and less accurate than are the data accepted by parametric tests (e.g., *t* tests and ANOVAs). Therefore, it has less status in the hierarchy of statistical tests.

Regression analysis

It is often important to relate the effect of an input parameter to the output parameter of an experiment. The correlation between input and output parameters is achieved through regression analysis. The correlation can be used for prediction of the output parameter through interpolation for input parameters within the range of the experiment or by extrapolation outside the range of the experiment. Regression can be single variable or multivariable, linear or nonlinear.

Linear regression

Linear regression analyzes the relationship between two variables, X and Y. In general, the goal of linear regression is to find the line that best predicts Y from X. The term *regression*, like many statistical terms, is used in statistics quite differently than it is used in other contexts.

The value r^2 is a fraction between 0 and 1.0, and has no units (see Fig. 142.7). An r^2 value of 0.0 means that knowing X does not help predict Y. There is no linear relationship between X and Y, and the best-fit line is a horizontal line going through the mean of all Y values. When r^2 equals 1.0, all points lie exactly on a straight line with no scatter, and knowing X allows one to predict Y perfectly.

A simple linear regression between the blood glucose levels (B) and the ages (A) in Fig. 142.3 can be represented as

$$B = mA + c,$$

where *m* is the slope and *c* is the intercept of the solid line in Fig. 142.3. The slope *m* and intercept *c* are obtained from the formulae

$$m = \frac{\sum \left(B_j - \overline{B} \right) \left(A_j - \overline{A} \right)}{\sum \left(B_j - \overline{B} \right)^2} \quad \text{and}$$

$$c = \overline{B} - m\overline{A},$$

where the subscript *j* represents a patient, $\overline{B}$ is the mean blood glucose level, and $\overline{A}$ is the mean age of all patients in Table 142.2. If a limit of 40 mg/dl is used, it can be observed that children younger than 4 years would be susceptible to hypoglycemia and an intervention would be required. (See Fig. 142.8.)

Multiple regression

In multiple regression, there is more than one variable. For example, in predicting a difficult airway, a study might look at Mallampati classification, thyromental distance, and mouth opening. Some board questions may ask one to choose between an ANOVA or multiple regression given the scenario presented. All ANOVA models can be solved using multiple regression, but the reverse is not true. ANOVA is used for independent variables that are *categorical* (e.g., male/female, alive/dead, blue/brown eyes), whereas multiple regression models can be used with categorical, continuous, or a mix of both types of variables.

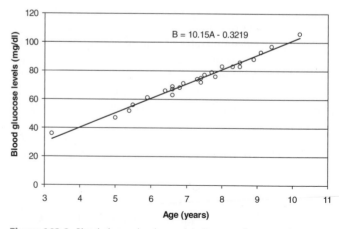

Figure 142.8. Blood glucose levels correlated to age of preoperative children undergoing anesthesia.

Regression draws a line that relates changes in one variable to changes in another. On the left-hand side, multiple regression also has one variable, but the right-hand side can have more than one. For two independent variables, multiple regression draws a plane, and for more than two a *surface* or *hyperplane*.

The data showed a correlation among the systemic vascular resistance index (SVRI), hematocrit, and MFV in the MCA. As SVRI increased and hematocrit decreased, MFV appeared to increase. Multiple regression analysis showed that SVRI and hematocrit explained 46% of the variance of MFV in patients without vasospasm. These results suggest that, in addition to already accepted variables (a hematocrit of 33%–38%, a central venous pressure of 10–12 mm Hg, a pulmonary wedge pressure of 15–18 mm Hg, and a systolic arterial pressure of 160–200 mm Hg), SVR/SVRI might be of value to more appropriately adjust triple-H-therapy.

Odds ratios

Odds are a ratio of events to non-events. For example, if the event rate for a disease is 0.2 (20%), the non-event rate is 0.8 (80%), and its odds are 0.2/0.8 = 0.25. The odds ratio is the odds of an experimental patient suffering an event relative to the odds of a control patient.

The odds ratio can be defined as the ratio of the odds of an event occurring in one group to the odds of it occurring in another group. These groups might be men and women, an experimental group and a control group, or any other dichotomous classification. An odds ratio of 1 indicates that the condition or event under study is equally likely in both groups. An odds ratio greater than 1 indicates that the condition or event is more likely in the first group; an odds ratio less than 1 indicates that the condition or event is less likely in the first group. The odds ratio must be greater than or equal to zero. As the odds of the first group approaches zero, the odds ratio approaches zero. As the odds of the second group approaches zero, the odds ratio approaches positive infinity.

For example, in a study of 185 adult patients who had retromastoid craniectomy with microvascular decompression of cranial nerves, use of desflurane was an independent predictor for postoperative nausea and vomiting (PONV). The odds ratio was 2.8; therefore, patients who received desflurane were 2.8 times more likely to have PONV than were patients who did not receive desflurane.

Risk ratios

The risk ratio is the ratio of the risk in the experimental group (EER: experimental event rate) to the risk in the control group (CER: control event rate). The risk ratio is equal to the EER divided by the CER. Risk ratios are used in randomized trials and cohort studies.

Miscellaneous statistical definitions

Sensitivity: True positives / (true positives + false negatives). The probability of the test finding disease among people who have the disease or the proportion of people with disease who have a positive test result.

Specificity: True negatives / (true negatives + false positives). The probability of the test finding NO disease among those who do NOT have the disease or the proportion of people free of a disease who have a negative test.

Positive predictive value (PPV): True positives / (true positives + false positives). The percentage of people with a positive test result who actually have the disease.

Negative predictive value (NPV): True negatives / (true negatives + false negatives). The percentage of people with a negative test who do *not* have the disease.

Suggested readings

American Board of Anesthesiologists. ABA Content Outline: Joint Council on In-Training Examinations, American Board of Anesthesiology Examination Part 1. September 2006 Revision. Retrieved on August 10, 2009, from: http://www2.asahq.org/publications/p-175-in-training-examinations.aspx.

Cruickshank S. *Mathematics and Statistics in Anesthesia*. Cambridge: Oxford University Press; 1998.

Dawson B, Trapp RG. *Basic and Clinical Biostatistics*. 4th ed. New York: Lange Medical Books/McGraw-Hill; 2004.

Freedman D, Pisani R, Purves R. *Statistics*. 4th ed. New York: W.W. Norton; 2007.

Goodman NW, Powell CG. Could do better: statistics in anaesthesia research. *Br J Anaesth* 1998; 80:712–714.

Jensen BH, Wernberg M, Andersen M. Preoperative starvation and blood-glucose concentrations in children undergoing inpatient and outpatient anesthesia. *Br J Anaesth* 1982; 54(10):1071–1074.

Lagasse RS. Anesthesia safety: model or myth? A review of the published literature and analysis of current original data. *Anesthesiology* 2002; 97(6):1609–1617.

Meng L, Quinlan JJ. Assessing risk factors for postoperative nausea and vomiting: a retrospective study in patients undergoing retromastoid craniectomy with microvascular decompression of cranial nerves. *J Neuro Anesth* 2006; 18(4):235–239.

Nates JL. Monitoring hypervolemic-hemodilution and hypertensive therapy in subarachnoid hemorrhage. *Internet J Anesth* 2001; 1–5.

Sokal RR, Rohlf FJ. *Biometry: The Principles and Practice of Statistics in Biological Research*. 2nd ed. New York: W.H. Freeman; 1995.

Part 27

Chapter

143

Pain Management

Pradeep Dinakar and Edgar L. Ross, editors

Neurophysiology of pain

Edgar L. Ross

The ability to sense, interpret, and modulate pain is vital to survival. René Descartes proposed one of the first descriptions of the sensory system more than 300 years ago. Descartes' theory envisioned a direct, single-channel system that coursed via nerves to the spinal cord with a direct synapse in the brain. This theory implied that our central nervous system is hard-wired and unchanging. This approach adversely impacted our approach to pain management for centuries. Descartes' approach to pain was unquestioned and not critically examined until the second half of the 20th century. This theory did not take into account our understanding of various other influences in pain, such as the psychological, environmental, biological, social, and genetic factors in an individual, and suggested treatment approaches, such as neurolytic procedures, which were believed to be universally curative and were widely practiced without an understanding of the possible consequences. Improvement in our understanding of chronic pain now provides evidence that this approach was to the detriment of the patients. With the publication of the gate theory of pain by Melzack and Wall in 1965, research was rekindled, leading to a complete reexamination of perception and modulation of pain. This research has significantly improved our understanding of treatment approaches and opened entire new vistas of potential treatment options.

Definition

What has become apparent from our new insights and understanding is that pain as a sensation is a complex phenomenon. The two basic terminologies that are needed to explain this clinical phenomenon include nociception and pain. The International Association for the Study of Pain (IASP) defines these two different terms as follows:

- *Nociception* is a noxious stimulus or a stimulus that would become noxious if prolonged. Activity induced in a nociceptive pathway by a noxious stimulus triggers pain.
- *Pain* is an unpleasant sensory and emotional experience, which we primarily associate with tissue damage or describe in terms of such damage, or both.

These two terms speak to both the complexity of our nervous system and its perception of pain. Most important, what is implied by this definition is that nociception is not equivalent to pain. Nociception can take place without the patient experiencing pain, and perception of pain is understood as a protective response from our body required for survival. In fact, under certain circumstances, we all have a profound ability to suppress nociception to the point that we would not even sense pain, even in the presence of significant injuries. There are times, however, when pain would be distracting and even detrimental to survival. Patients can have severe, unremitting pain without significant pathology that explains their pain. Centrally originating inhibitory systems are thought to have evolved for these situations. With the increased understanding of these inhibitory systems, treatment approaches have been developed that take advantage of and enhance this inhibition to manage pathologically painful states.

Neuronal plasticity

Normal sensation, which is the absence of pain, requires a balance between both the inhibitory and excitatory pathways of the central and peripheral nervous systems. This balance is changed in a process called *sensitization*. Sensitization leads to increased sensitivity of all stimuli. Two clinical phenomena that can be noted clinically are considered the hallmarks of this process (Fig. 143.1).

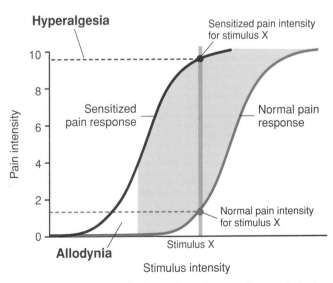

Figure 143.1. Sensitization leading to change in responsiveness of stimulus.

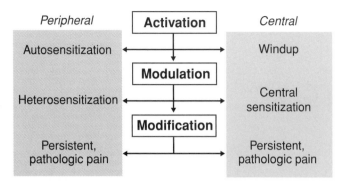

Figure 143.2. Steps leading to central sensitization.

- Hyperalgesia – an increased response to what is usually a painful stimulus
- Allodynia – a painful response to what is ordinarily a non-painful stimulus, such as light touch

Various specialized sensory receptors including free nerve endings are located at the end of the peripheral nervous system. Injuries to tissue can release numerous substances that sensitize these receptors leading to a decreased threshold and increased responsiveness to all stimuli, such as light touch instead of just pain (Fig. 143.2).

The peripheral sensory nervous system is composed of two distinct classes: larger rapid conducting myelinated A delta and beta fibers and slower smaller unmyelinated C fibers. Under normal circumstances, the larger rapid conducting fibers responding to cold sensations are able to localize pain sensation quickly and precisely. The C fibers, which are normally stimulated by heat or mechanical stimuli, poorly localize the site of pain. They are connected to both the sympathetic nervous system and the spinal cord. These two nerve classes are responsible for pain transmission and stimulation of a protective reflex arc.

Pain-processing mechanisms

Sensory nerve fibers course into the dorsal horn where multiple different mechanisms have been found to modulate noxious stimuli. Three important types of modulating influences are

1. Nonpainful sensory inputs,
2. Descending inhibitory inputs, and
3. Central processing.

The ascending sensory information is transmitted up the spinal cord to the supraspinal processing areas. The spinothalamic tracts are the primary but not the only tracts responsible for this. Wall and Melzack's gate theory proposes that this ascending, nonpainful sensory input helps to gate the painful stimulus and forms the basis for the spinal cord stimulator's mechanism of action.

Inhibiting descending pathways are primarily based on noradrenergic, opioid, and serotonergic neurotransmitters and exert their inhibitory action on the lamina II of the dorsal horn. This inhibitory influence acts either directly through neural connections from higher centers, such as rostral ventral

medulla or nucleus raphe magnus, or by the release of endorphins and other inhibitory neurotransmitters. There also appear to be descending facilitatory pathways that serve to enhance transmission of nociceptive impulses in the spinal cord. The origins of these pathways are found in the rostral ventral medulla. This pathway is active during peripheral tissue injury and produces hyperalgesia. This effect is achieved through maintenance of central sensitization and enhancement of active neurons. Glutamatergic neurotransmitters appear to be important in this process. With persistent injury, repeated C fiber stimulation leads to increased sensitivity of the dorsal horn to further stimulation. This phenomenon is known as the *windup*. This process contributes to initiation and perpetuation of central sensitization. Glutamate plays a major role in this process as well. Activation of these pain inhibitory processes, either from higher centers or through the use of medications such as opioids, tricyclic antidepressants, N-methyl-D-aspartate (NMDA) receptor antagonists, α-adrenergic antagonists, or electrical stimulation using a transcutaneous electrical nerve stimulation (TENS) unit or a spinal cord stimulator, helps in shutting down the nociceptive gate.

From the dorsal horn, the ascending pathways consist of the spinothalamic, spinoreticular, and spinomesencephalic tracts. These tracts synapse in supraspinal modulatory centers. Neurons found in selected centers of the cerebral cortex respond to and process the nociceptor input. These centers include the somatosensory cortex, thalamus, cingulate gyrus, and the insular cortex. These multiple areas are involved in the central processing of the pain experience, including affective responses, responsiveness to stress reduction (such as hypnosis), and stress management approaches.

Other factors that affect pain processing include central nervous system immune responses initiated by endothelial and glial cells. This immune response serves to enhance production of a variety of inflammatory mediators and sustain pain and hypersensitivity found in acute injuries as well as to perpetuate chronic pain states. Gender differences in pain have been well documented. Multiple studies have suggested that women have greater pain sensitivity compared to men. In addition, cyclical changes found in women change pain perceptions as well. Responsiveness to analgesics, including receptor differences and responsiveness, has also been documented. Continued research into gender differences, including genetic factors, will likely lead to differences in treatment approaches.

Types of pain

There are three different etiologies of pain that can be described. These include:

1. Nociceptive pain without tissue damage or sensitization. In this model, a noxious stimulus is detected, but no physiologic change occurs to change the nervous system (Fig. 143.3a).
2. Inflammatory pain from tissue damage leading to sensitization. In this situation, tissue damage releases

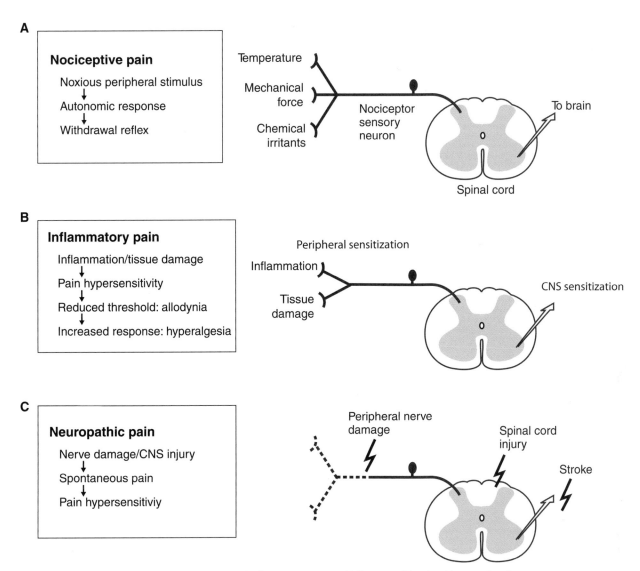

Figure 143.3. Types of pain: **(A)** nociceptive pain; **(B)** inflammatory pain; and **(C)** neuropathic pain without nociception.

factors that lead to sensitization in both the peripheral and central nervous systems. This sensitization leads to a physiologic change, which decreases the discriminatory ability of peripheral nociceptors as well as heightens sensitivity to all stimuli, including spontaneous pain. These changes are usually temporary and part of the healing process. In small numbers of patients, these changes are permanent and lead to chronic pain (Fig. 143.3b).

3. Neuropathic pain results from damage to either the peripheral or central nervous system. This damage could come about from unchecked sensitization or physical damage. Many chronic pain syndromes are neuropathic in nature. In addition, this neuropathic process points to the fact that pain can be reported without any nociception or tissue damage. Neuropathic pain is commonly not reversible and is often considered to be much more severe and resistant to treatment (Fig.143.3c).

Summary

Pain physiology is much more complex than the original René Descartes idea. With the growing understanding of how pain is modulated and perpetuated, new therapeutic targets are now understood with the promise of improvement in treatment.

Suggested readings

DeLeo JA. Basic science of pain. *J Bone Joint Surg Am* 2006; 88(Suppl 2):58–62.

Gottschalk A, Smith DS. New concepts in acute pain therapy: preemptive analgesia. *Am Fam Physician* 2001; 63(10): 1979–1984.

Sivilotti LG, Thompson SW, Woolf CJ. Rate of rise of the cumulative depolarization evoked by repetitive stimulation of small-caliber afferents is a predictor of action potential windup in rat spinal neurons in vitro. *J Neurophysiol* 1993; 69(5):1621–1631.

Thompson SW, Woolf CJ, Sivilotti LG. Small-caliber afferent inputs produce a heterosynaptic facilitation of the synaptic responses evoked by primary afferent A-fibers in the neonatal rat spinal cord in vitro. *J Neurophysiol* 1993; 69(6):2116–2128.

Wiesenfeld-Hallin Z. Sex differences in pain perception. *Gend Med* 2005; 2(3):137–145.

Woolf CJ. Pain: moving from symptom control toward mechanism-specific pharmacologic management. *Ann Intern Med* 2004; 140(6):441–451.

Woolf CJ, Salter MW. Neuronal plasticity: increasing the gain in pain. *Science* 2000; 288(5472):1765–1769.

Zhuo M. Neuronal mechanism for neuropathic pain. *Mol Pain* 2007; 3:14.

Postoperative acute pain management

Darin J. Correll

The Joint Commission mandates that all patients have the right to adequate assessment and management of pain. Better pain control, depending on the agent(s) and modalities used, leads to benefits not only in terms of cardiovascular and respiratory complications but also in endocrine, immunologic, gastrointestinal, and hematologic outcomes. Other reasons to control pain in the postoperative setting are that patients are often more concerned about being in pain than they are about the primary reason for being in the hospital, quality of recovery is improved, and acute pain may become persistent if not treated properly.

Basic pain management guidelines

Listen to and believe the patient: Pain is always subjective, and the provider must accept the patient's report of pain. Assess the patient's level of pain and degree of pain relief using appropriate tools on a regular basis. A multimodal approach for managing pain is always better than using a single modality to its limit. This approach may include both pharmacologic and non-pharmacologic measures and allows for the best possible analgesia with the lowest incidence of side effects. Always discuss the analgesic plan with the patient and family, understand the patient's expectations of pain management, and offer reasonable goals for the therapy. If pain is present most of the time or expected to last for an extended period of time (e.g., longer than a few weeks), dose around-the-clock or with long-acting agents. As-needed (PRN) dosing of immediate-release agents is also needed for breakthrough pain. If pain is intermittent or expected to last a short time (e.g., less than a couple of weeks) then PRN dosing of immediate-release agents can be used. Communication with the patient's primary care provider regarding the discharge analgesic plan is helpful, especially if there has been an alteration to a chronic analgesic regimen. Ensure that the patient has adequate follow-up for the effectiveness of the analgesic regimen and the development of possible side effects on discharge from the hospital, as well as a plan for a taper off of analgesics; if the patient was not on chronic analgesics before.

Pain assessment and mechanism of pain

It is important to ask the patient about his or her prior analgesic history, what therapies have either worked or not worked in the past, as well as if he or she was taking any analgesic agents prior to admission, and, if so, the exact doses. Ask about all the locations where the patient is experiencing pain and any radiation from the primary location(s). Have the patient rate the intensity of the pain using scales appropriate to the patient and situation.

The most commonly used measurement tools for intensity of pain in the postoperative setting are the single-dimension scales. A frequently used variation of this scale is the verbal numeric scale. Patients are asked to verbally state a number between 0 and 10, where 0 is "no pain at all" and 10 is "the worst pain imaginable," to correspond to their present pain intensity. Variations of the single-dimension scales that may be of benefit in elderly or cognitively impaired populations are scales that use drawn faces ranging from a content-looking smiling face to a distressed-looking face (e.g., Faces Pain Scale or Wong–Baker Faces Scale) instead of relying on the patient choosing a number for his or her pain.

The benefits of single-dimension scales are that they are quick and easy to use – this is important in the acute setting, where repeated measures are needed over a brief period of time. One disadvantage of single-dimension scales is that they attempt to assign a single value to a complex, multidimensional experience. Another disadvantage is that patients can never know if the present experience is the "worst." A final disadvantage is that these scales have a ceiling at the uppermost end, so if a value of "10" is chosen and the pain worsens, the patient officially has no way to express this change.

To choose the correct therapy for treating pain, the underlying mechanism or generator of the pain needs to be determined (Table 144.1). One of the best ways to make this determination is to have the patient use adjectives to describe the character of the pain (e.g., aching, burning, dull, electric-like, sharp, shooting, stabbing, tender, throbbing). In the postoperative period it is still important to determine the impact of the pain on the patient's functional ability. Specifically, does the pain affect the patient's ability to cough, get out of bed, and ambulate while in the hospital?

Analgesic modalities

It is important to remember that pain can be helped with non-pharmacologic measures. In general, the scientific data on the

Table 144.1. Mechanisms of pain

Pain mechanism	Character	Examples	Treatment options
Somatic	• Usually well localized • Constant • Aching, sharp, stabbing	• Laceration • Fracture • Burn • Abrasion • Localized infection or inflammation	• Heat/cold • Acetaminophen • NSAIDs • Opioids • Local anesthetics (topical or infiltrate)
Visceral	• Not well localized • Constant or intermittent • Ache, pressure, cramping, sharp	• Muscle spasm • Colic or obstruction (GI or renal) • Sickle cell crisis • Internal organ infection or inflammation	• NSAIDs • Opioids • Muscle relaxants • Local anesthetics (nerve-blocks)
Neuropathic	• Localized (i.e., dermatomal) or radiating, can also be diffuse • Burning, tingling, electric shock, lancinating	• Trigeminal • Postherpetic • Postamputation • Peripheral neuropathy • Nerve infiltration	• Anticonvulsants • Antidepressants • NMDA antagonists • Neural/neuraxial blockade

NSAIDs, nonsteroidal anti-inflammatory drugs; GI, gastrointestinal. (From Correll, DJ, *Pain Management in Hospital Medicine: Just the Facts*, McKean, Bennett, Halasyamani.)

use of these measures are limited; however, most of the measures have little risk, and, if the patient believes that the therapy is going to help, then it is likely to be of at least some benefit, due to the cognitive and affective nature of pain. In terms of pharmacologic measures, many different agents are available in three basic categories: non-opioid analgesics, opioids, and adjuvant analgesics. There is no one correct way to treat a patient in pain. It is best to individualize therapy for each patient, developing a regimen that uses a multimodal approach with the addition or alteration of agents when pain control is inadequate and an adjustment or diminishing of agents as the pain resolves.

Nonpharmacologic measures

Application of cold (to reduce inflammation) or heat (to reduce spasms) to muscles or joints is a commonly employed technique, but the evidence for an actual analgesic benefit is mixed. Hypnosis has been shown to reduce pain associated with medical procedures; however, it requires specific training and

time to administer. Transcutaneous electrical nerve stimulation (TENS) has shown conflicting results in terms of an analgesic benefit in the acute setting, but it has been shown to reduce the need for pharmacologic analgesics. There is limited evidence of a benefit in the acute setting for relaxation and guided imagery. Acupuncture and electro-acupuncture have been shown to be of benefit in the acute setting both to improve pain and to reduce common side effects of opioid analgesics; however, they require specific training and time to administer.

Pharmacologic measures

The various pharmacologic options have been discussed in other chapters. Table 144.2 lists some of the available non-opioid analgesics. Ketorolac is available in the intravenous (IV) form for patients who are unable to take anything by mouth.

A detailed discussion on opioids for management of pain can be found in other chapters. Other than asking the patient if a particular agent has worked or not worked in the past, it is not possible to determine which opioid may work best

Table 144.2. Select nonopioid analgesics

Agent	Adult dosing	Maximum dose	Comments
Acetaminophen	650–1000 mg q 6 h PO/PR	4000 mg	Single doses > 1000 mg do not improve analgesia
Choline magnesium trisalicylate	1000–1500 mg BID PO	3000 mg	Caution in liver disease, avoid in severe liver disease
Diclofenac	50 mg BID–QID PO	200 mg	Low GI effect incidence, but possible increased renal effects; recent data suggest increased negative CV effects
Etodolac	200–400 mg q 6–8 h PO	1000 mg	Low GI and renal effect incidence; safest NSAID in liver disease
Ibuprofen	400–600 mg q 4–6 h PO	3000 mg	< 1,500 mg QD has low risk of GI effects, possible increased renal effects, inhibits CV benefits of aspirin when given concomitantly
Ketorolac	30 mg q 6 h IV	120 mg	High risk of renal and GI complications; use for no more than 5 days; 15 mg q 6 h in renal impairment, age > 65 y, weight < 50 kg
Nabumetone	750–1500 mg QD or BID PO	1500 mg	Low GI effect incidence
Naproxen	250–500 mg q 6–12 h PO	1500 mg	Possible increased liver and renal effects, probably least negative CV effects
Celecoxib	100–200 mg QD PO	200 mg	Use 100-mg dose if possible; long-term use has increased negative CV effects

CV, cardiovascular; PO, oral; PR, rectal. (From Correll, DJ, *Pain management in Hospital Medicine: Just the Facts*, McKean, Bennett, Halasyamani.)

Table 144.3. Recommended starting doses of opioids for adults over 50 kg

Agonist	Oral	IV
Codeine	15–60 mg q 3–4 h	n/a
Hydrocodone	5–10 mg q 3–6 h[a]	n/a
Tramadol	50–100 mg q 4–6 h[b]	n/a
Oxycodone	5–10 mg q 3–4 h	n/a
Morphine	10–30 mg q 3–4 h	5–10 mg q 2–4 h
Hydromorphone	2–6 mg q 3–4 h	1–1.5 mg q 3–4 h
Oxymorphone	10–20 mg q 4–6 h[c]	1 mg q 3–4 h

n/a, Not applicable

[a] Daily dose limited by acetaminophen component in available preparations.

[b] Maximum recommended 24-hour dose: 400 mg in adults ≤ 75 years; 300 mg in adults > 75 years old.

[c] Recent US Food and Drug Administration (FDA) approval of oral form; therefore, limited clinical experience. (From Correll, DJ, *Pain management in Hospital Medicine: Just the Facts*, McKean, Bennett, Halasyamani).

for a given patient. Whenever possible, the enteral route of administration is best as it is the easiest route and offers the most stable pharmacokinetics. If the enteral route is not available or if adequate analgesia is not able to be obtained in a timely manner, then IV administration should be used. Intramuscular administration is not recommended because it is painful and has variable pharmacokinetics. With a competent patient, the use of an IV patient-controlled analgesia (PCA) has been demonstrated to offer the best overall pain management option (see sections on PCA later in this chapter).

The pronounced individual variability in opioid response, combined with changes in responsiveness over time, mandates individualization of opioid doses based on a continuing process of assessment (analgesia and adverse effects) and dose titration. Table 144.3 lists the recommended starting doses for moderate to severe pain in the opioid-naïve patient.

There are, however, some agents that should not be used, at least first-line, in the postoperative setting. Codeine is not a good first choice because it is possible that approximately 10% to 20% of the population does not have an active form of the enzyme (i.e., cytochrome P450 2D6) necessary to convert codeine into the active drug, morphine. Morphine is relatively contraindicated in patients with severe renal insufficiency due to the accumulation of the metabolite morphine-6-glucuronide, which can lead to sedation and respiratory depression. Meperidine is not recommended as its active metabolite, normeperidine, can accumulate in a day or two to levels that cause nervous system excitation (tremors, muscle twitching, convulsions). In addition, it causes a strong euphoric feeling, especially when given as an IV push, and it usually causes more nausea than do other agents. Hydrocodone use needs to be monitored closely because of the acetaminophen component in the available preparations that can lead to acetaminophen toxicity. Also, non-medical uses of hydrocodone combination preparations lead to emergency department visits more frequently than any other pharmaceutical agent.

If a patient is not receiving enough pain relief at a given dose, increase the dose by 25% to 50%. If a patient is having pain before the next dose is due, reduce the interval and/or increase the dose.

Rotation from one opioid to another may be necessary in several circumstances. The first situation is when a few attempts have been made at increasing the dose of an opioid and the patient is still not receiving any pain relief, in this case, rotation to a different opioid may provide better analgesia. A second situation is one in which a patient is having intolerable side effects; again, rotation to a different opioid may provide a better side effect profile. A third situation occurs when a particular opioid is not available by the route of administration required in a given patient. A fourth situation would occur if a patient has been on an opioid for an extended period of time and is demonstrating signs of tolerance to the analgesic effects, again, rotation to a different opioid may provide better analgesia, usually at less than the expected equianalgesic dose due to incomplete cross-tolerance, which means that the patient will not be "as tolerant" to the new opioid agonist as he or she was to the one previously taken. Thus, when converting between opioids, for any of the reasons mentioned above, the calculated equianalgesic dose of the new agent must be reduced by 25% to 75% to prevent oversedation and/or respiratory depression.

Sustained-release formulations should generally only be initiated in the acute setting if pain is present most of the time and it is assumed that the pain generator will last for an extended period of time (e.g., >2 weeks). If the pain is more incident-related or expected to be of a brief duration, then immediate-release agents should be employed. When using a sustained-release opioid, also provide doses of an immediate-release opioid equivalent to 10% to 15% of the 24-hour total, to be used every few hours for breakthrough pain. While on a sustained-release opioid, if the need for breakthrough pain medications is high (e.g., if more than four rescue doses are needed in 24 hours) then increase the dosage of the sustained-release agent by 50% to 100% of the total 24-hour breakthrough dose used.

Transdermal fentanyl is not appropriate for acute pain, especially in opioid-naïve patients. There is a black box warning against its use in the acute setting due to the risk of severe respiratory depression from the delayed peak effect of the drug as the pain level decreases. It is intended for use in patients who are already tolerant to opioids of comparable potency.

Methadone is not appropriate as the first-line agent in the acute setting, especially in opioid-naïve patients. Its use requires an understanding of the unique pharmacology of the drug, especially its extended duration of action and its dose-dependent potency. Also, as it takes a few days to reach a stable plasma concentration, patients will need to be followed closely to monitor for effectiveness and side effects. It must also be realized that methadone is a racemic mixture of a μ-agonist and an *N*-methyl-D-aspartate (NMDA) antagonist, which makes patients have a lesser degree of analgesic tolerance development.

A detailed discussion of the various adjuvant medication in pain management will be discussed in additional chapters.

Acute pain in the opioid-tolerant patient

In patients with chronic pain on opioids, post-surgical pain adds to the pain burden, thus opioid use can be expected to be higher than just replacement of what the patient was on before coming in to the hospital, and can be significantly higher than in opioid-naïve patients. More pain complaints and higher pain scores should be expected. Discussion of reasonable goals and expectations of analgesic therapy with the patient is crucial. These patients often know what agents have either worked or not worked for them in the past. The use of multimodal therapy in this patient population is especially important.

IV patient-controlled analgesia

IV PCA is an excellent therapy for the maintenance of already established analgesia. Therefore, if a patient is in moderate to severe pain, health care provider-delivered doses of an opioid must be used to reach an acceptable level of analgesia first because the incremental dosing of a PCA will not allow patients to achieve comfort in a reasonable period of time.

PCA may be used in any patient requiring IV opioids provided that he or she is alert, oriented, and able to understand how to use the equipment appropriately.

PCA parameters

All PCA machines allow for the setting of the following parameters: demand (bolus) dose, lockout interval, hourly limit, continuous (basal) infusion, and rescue (loading) dose.

Demand (bolus) dose

The demand dose is the amount of opioid that the patient receives each time he or she activates the machine. The appropriate choice for the amount of the demand dose should be small enough so that side effects are minimized yet large enough to provide effective analgesia.

Lockout interval

The lockout interval is the amount of time following a successfully delivered demand dose during which the patient can administer no further opioid even if the system is activated. Lockout intervals between 5 and 10 minutes are commonly used. Even though the time to peak effect for certain opioids may be longer, there do not appear to be any data suggesting that any specific time is more or less effective or safe, regardless of the opioid chosen.

Hourly limit

An hourly limit sets the maximum amount of opioid that can be administered in the given time period. The proposed purpose for this setting is to add a level of safety to the system; however, no data support this claim. An hourly limit is automatically determined by the setting of a demand dose and lockout interval. The use of an hourly limit less than the predetermined limit based on bolus dose and lockout interval does not make logical sense, as the patient would be able to get a dose of opioid on schedule for only a part of every given time period and then not be able to receive anything for the remainder of the time period.

Continuous (basal) infusion

A continuous infusion delivers a set amount of opioid every hour without the need for the patient to activate the system. Continuous infusions are not commonly used, as no documented benefits have been shown for most patients. Continuous infusions are not recommended in high-risk populations such as elderly patients, opioid-naïve patients, patients concomitantly using other sedatives, and patients with obstructive sleep apnea or morbid obesity. The use of continuous infusions increases the overall opioid consumption and has been identified as an independent risk factor for respiratory depression. Continuous infusions have not been shown to improve patient satisfaction or pain rating scores, and they do not decrease the frequency of demand dose use.

It may appear to make sense to use a continuous infusion at night when the patient is sleeping and therefore unable to activate the PCA; however, studies have shown that nighttime basal infusions do not improve sleep or analgesia.

Continuous infusions may be needed in opioid-tolerant patients, especially those who are chronically taking continuous-release agents. If the patient cannot take his or her usual doses of opioid enterally, then a continuous infusion should be used. Determine an IV equivalent for the amount of opioid that the patient takes in a day (taking into account incomplete cross-tolerance if switching to a different agent), divide this amount by 24 hours, and administer as the hourly continuous infusion rate.

Rescue (loading) dose

Rescue doses are specific amounts of opioid delivered by a health care provider that are generally in excess of the patient's demand dose given when the level of analgesia from the PCA is inadequate. These doses can also be administered at the initiation of PCA therapy to initially achieve an adequate level of analgesia at which point they are more commonly referred to as *loading doses*.

Patients may require a rescue dose for a variety of reasons while they are on a PCA. There may be brief periods of increased nociceptive input beyond the ability of the demand dose to be effective (e.g., dressing changes). If patients forget to or cannot use the PCA for a period of time (e.g., long period of sleep) they may get behind on their analgesia and require a larger amount of opioid to catch up.

PCA opioid choices

There does not appear to be a clearly superior opioid for use in PCA devices. Because morphine has an active metabolite

Table 144.4. Initial PCA demand doses in opioid-naïve patients

Opioid agonist	Demand dose
Morphine	1–2 mg
Fentanyl	20–30 µg
Hydromorphone	0.2–0.3 mg
Methadone	1–2 mg
Sufentanil	2–5 µg
Meperidine	10–20 mg

there can be an accumulation of effects, especially in elderly patients and/or patients with renal failure, so it is generally best to avoid in these patients. Fentanyl has a shorter duration of action than morphine, which is good if one is concerned about accumulating effects, but bad in that patients must frequently activate the PCA. Meperidine should be used only in rare cases in which a patient has documented intolerance to all other opioid choices, and then it is recommended to limit the total dose to 600 mg in a 24-hour period for no more than 3 days. Methadone is especially useful in patients who take methadone chronically, whereas it is not appropriate as a first-line agent in others because the conversion from methadone to another agent when the patient is taking oral analgesics is difficult given the dose-dependent potency of methadone.

Table 144.4 lists the recommended starting demand doses to be used in opioid-naïve patients. In the opioid-tolerant patient, these doses will need to be individualized based on the amount of opioid the patient takes per day leading to higher initial demand doses and possibly the initial use of continuous infusions (see the Continuous (basal) infusion section.) High-risk patients – identified as elderly (age 70 or older), morbidly obese, or with a history of obstructive sleep apnea – should have lower initial demand doses (e.g., one half the usual demand dose).

PCA management

If the patient does not receive adequate pain relief with a given demand dose, increase the dose of opioid per activation using the parameters suggested in Table 144.5.

A small subset of opioid-naïve patients may prove that they need and can be safe with a continuous infusion. For example, if, following several demand dose increases over several hours, a patient continues to need to use the PCA frequently to maintain analgesia without evidence of side effects (i.e., sedation or respiratory depression) and repeatedly gets behind, because he or she falls asleep, and then awakens in severe pain not adequately treated with the demand doses or easily treated with

Table 144.5. Usual PCA demand dose changes for inadequate analgesia

Opioid agonist	Demand dose increase
Morphine	0.5–1 mg
Fentanyl	5–10 µg
Hydromorphone	0.1 mg
Methadone	0.5–1 mg
Sufentanil	2 µg
Meperidine	5–10 mg

rescue doses, then a low-dose continuous infusion may be appropriate. The starting continuous infusion for the opioid-naïve patient should generally not be more than a single demand dose per hour (e.g., 1–2 mg/h for morphine).

If a continuous infusion is being used in any patient, one must be cautious if the amount of pain is assumed to be decreasing with time (e.g., continued healing following surgery). If a patient has a continuous infusion and does not need to activate the PCA, or if side effects (i.e., pruritus, nausea, sedation) begin to increase, then the basal rate should be decreased or discontinued. This downward adjustment or discontinuation of the basal rate allows for the maintenance of the inherent safety of the PCA device in that the patient controls the amount of opioid received as opposed to it being on an opioid infusion, to help reduce the chance of respiratory depression.

PCA safety and efficacy

One of the major benefits of PCA is that it helps overcome the wide interpatient variation in opioid requirements by allowing each individual patient to titrate the amount of opioid that he or she receives based on the response experienced. In addition, there is some degree of a placebo effect imparted by the use of a PCA enhancing the overall pain control. The patient-controlled aspect is also one of the major safety features of the PCA in that it is assumed that if a patient is getting sedated, he or she will not activate the PCA, thereby limiting the possibility of respiratory depression.

Based on the results of several meta-analyses, when PCA is compared to conventional nurse-administered opioids on a PRN basis it has been shown to provide slightly better pain control and improved patient satisfaction and is preferred by patients. Patients with PCA use slightly more opioid and experience a higher incidence of pruritus but have similar rates of other opioid-related side effects (e.g., nausea, vomiting, sedation, and respiratory depression). There is also a slight (nonsignificant) reduction in the length of hospital stay in patients using PCA. Finally, there appears to be a lower incidence of pulmonary complications in patients using PCA.

The reason that PCA is proposed to be more effective than nurse-delivered opioid administration is termed the *PCA paradigm* (Fig. 144.1). Analgesia is obtained when the plasma concentration of an opioid is within a certain range, which is specific to each individual. The lowest value of this range is known as the minimum effective analgesic concentration (MEAC). When the concentration of opioid goes above this range no further analgesia is obtained and side effects (i.e., sedation and respiratory depression) occur. When the opioid plasma concentration falls below the MEAC, the patient experiences pain. The assumed course of events is that patients will be able to maintain their own plasma opioid concentration around the MEAC by administering a demand dose every time they experience pain, which is in contrast to conventional nurse-administered boluses that result in much larger fluctuations in opioid plasma concentration with time spent above

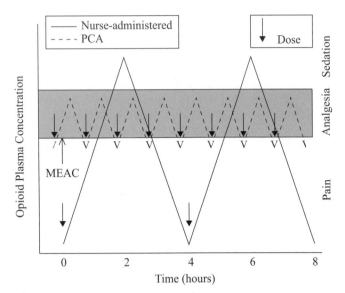

Figure 144.1. Intermittent nurse-administered opioids versus PCA-administered opioids. *Shaded area:* analgesic plasma concentration range. Adapted from: Ferrante FM, Orav EJ, Rocco AG, Gallo J. A statistical model for pain in patient-controlled analgesia and conventional intramuscular opioid regimens. *Anesth Analg* 1988; 67:457–461.

the analgesic range as well as significant time spent below the MEAC.

PCA monitoring

Although there are no actual guidelines for how to monitor patients on PCA, a recent statement by the Anesthesia Patient Safety Foundation (APSF) offered recommendations. The APSF advocates the use of continuous monitoring of oxygenation (i.e., pulse oximetry) and ventilation in patients receiving PCA. The reason for monitoring both oxygenation and ventilation is that pulse oximetry has reduced sensitivity as a monitor of hypoventilation when supplemental oxygen is administered. Therefore, when supplemental oxygen is used, monitoring of ventilation should be undertaken with a technology designed to assess breathing or estimate arterial carbon dioxide concentrations. Continuous monitoring is most important for high-risk patients (e.g., patients with obstructive sleep apnea, morbidly obese patients) but likely should be applied to all patients.

Patient-controlled epidural analgesia

Although this section focuses on the use of patient-controlled epidural analgesia (PCEA) for the postoperative patient, the concepts can be used in other settings as well (e.g., women in labor, cancer patients). A PCEA may be used in any patient requiring epidural analgesia provided that he or she is alert, oriented, and able to understand how to use the equipment appropriately.

PCEA parameters

All PCEA machines allow for the setting of the same parameters as described for a PCA.

Demand (bolus) dose

The optimal demand dose for PCEA is not known but is usually set at 2 to 4 ml. There is no information that a particular demand dose works best with a certain analgesic regimen.

Lockout interval

Lockout intervals between 10 and 20 minutes are commonly used. These times are more in line with the peak effect of the analgesics than are the lockout intervals used for PCA.

Hourly limit

If an hourly limit is used it should be the amount mathematically determined by the choice of demand dose, lockout interval, and continuous infusion rate. This determination will ensure that the patient receives analgesics continuously.

Continuous (basal) infusion

Continuous infusions are commonly used for PCEA management. Continuous infusions are usually started at 4 to 6 ml per hour with the usual upper limit of 14 ml per hour. Height of the patient does not appear to be a determinant of the correct infusion rate. There are some data to suggest that weight is positively correlated and age is negatively correlated with PCEA requirements. It is the location of the surgery, however, that appears to have the strongest correlation with PCEA requirements in that thoracoabdominal operations need higher rates than do lower extremity surgeries. This increased anesthetic requirement is likely a function of the number of dermatomes that need to be covered.

Rescue (loading) dose

The amount of a rescue dose to be used will be determined by a number of factors including the specific analgesics being used, the number of dermatomes that need to be covered, and potentially the hemodynamic status of the patient (see "PCEA management" section later in text).

PCEA analgesic agents

There does not appear to be a clearly superior regimen for use in PCEA devices. Local anesthetics are the most commonly used analgesic agents. Classically, bupivacaine is the most commonly used local anesthetic due to its relative resistance to tachyphylaxis. The cardiotoxicity of bupivacaine has led some practitioners to the use of levobupivacaine or ropivacaine instead. The usual ranges of concentration for the various local anesthetics are listed in Table 144.6. Often the higher range of concentrations is used for lower extremity orthopedic procedures and the less concentrated solutions used for thoracic surgery; however, there are no conclusive data to support this practice.

The next most common agents used for PCEA therapy are the opioids. They are commonly used in combination with a local anesthetic. There seems to be no benefit of administering

Table 144.6. Local anesthetic choices for PCEA

Local anesthetic	Concentration range
Bupivacaine	0.0625%–0.2%
Levobupivacaine	0.0625%–0.2%
Ropivacaine	0.1%–0.2%

Table 144.8. Other agents for PCEA

Analgesic	Concentration range
Clonidine	1–3 µg/ml
Epinephrine	2–5 µg/ml
Neostigmine	1–7 µg/ml

lipophilic opioids (i.e., fentanyl or sufentanil) solely via the epidural route. The site of action of lipophilic opioids when given epidurally is not clear. Studies looking at the efficacy of fentanyl and sufentanil given epidurally versus IV are contradictory. Most studies measuring the plasma concentrations of these opioids when given via an epidural or IV have shown no difference in levels, thus suggesting that the major site of action is not at the spinal cord but rather due to systemic absorption.

Hydrophilic opioids (i.e., morphine or hydromorphone), in contrast, maintain high cerebrospinal fluid levels for an extended period of time and therefore can act at the opioid receptors in the spinal cord. Table 144.7 lists concentrations documented in the literature for the various opioids when administered via the epidural route; the "correct" dose is not known. The total 24-hour dose of opioid must be kept in mind if high, continuous-infusion rates or large, frequent-demand doses are used, especially for high-risk patients. When used in combination with local anesthetics, the lower end of the concentration ranges are suggested.

Other agents have been studied as adjuvant medications added in combination with local anesthetics and/or opioids for epidural use; however, they are not used extensively in most clinical practices. This is likely because the studies are limited and show equivocal results. The major proposed benefits are improved analgesia and an analgesic sparing effect (i.e., the ability to use lower concentration of the other agents, specifically local anesthetics and opioids). Table 144.8 lists the adjuvant agents and offers suggested concentrations from the literature as the "correct" doses have not been determined.

A major concern with the addition of clonidine has been an increased incidence of hypotension and sedation. Use of epinephrine has shown improved analgesia with activity, although it may lead to an increased incidence of motor block. Epinephrine use also has been shown to reduce plasma concentrations of lipophilic opioids by allowing them to remain in the neuraxis for long enough to actually bind to the opioid receptors in the spinal cord. The concern with neostigmine is that, when used for intrathecal administration, a dose-dependent incidence of nausea and vomiting occurs as well as sedation,

Table 144.7. Opioid choices for PCEA

Opioid	Concentration range
Fentanyl	1–4 µg/ml
Hydromorphone	10–50 µg/ml
Morphine	20–100 µg/ml
Sufentanil	0.5–1 µg/ml

but epidural use does not seem to have the same increased incidence of nausea and vomiting, and only minimal sedation occurs, if at all. Also, when neostigmine is started preoperatively it may provide some degree of a preemptive analgesic effect.

PCEA complications/side effects

Epidural infusions are associated with complications related to the placement of epidural catheters and medications used. The incidence of serious, permanent neurologic complications is exceedingly rare, and data comprise mostly a handful of case reports. The incidence of spinal hematoma has classically been thought to be 1:150,000 in the presence of normal coagulation, although recent studies have suggested that it may be more common. The incidence of epidural hematoma formation in a patient who is anticoagulated is not known, but it is estimated at 1:3000 in patients receiving therapeutic low-molecular-weight heparin. A full discussion of epidurals and anticoagulation is beyond the scope of this chapter; the most recent guidelines can be found on the American Society of Regional Anesthesia and Pain Medicine Web site (www.asra.com). Epidural abscess incidence is not known but is considered rare (at most 0.05%). Risk factors for abscess formation may be longer times of having the epidural in place (possibly > 6 days) as well as use in immunocompromised patients. Intrathecal or intravascular migration of an epidural catheter is estimated at approximately 0.2%, although it is likely much less frequent. The incidence of premature catheter dislodgement is estimated at approximately 6%.

The major side effects due to local anesthetics in epidurals are hypotension, central nervous system (CNS) toxicity, and motor block. The probability of hypotension from an epidural does not rise above 1% to 2% until the spread of the epidural is beyond 14 sympathetic dermatomes. In most instances, the band of analgesia, plus another 6 dermatomes for the spread of the sympathetic blockade beyond the analgesic level, is less than 14 dermatomes. The major mechanism by which an epidural might cause hypotension is through decreased venous return (preload) from reduced venous capacitance; therefore, the most appropriate treatment is increasing cardiac preload by increasing intravascular volume. Hence, hypotension is rarely seen in the supine normovolemic patient. Thus it is often the fluid status of the patient that is more of a causative factor than the epidural itself. This is evidenced by the fact that stopping the epidural infusion in a patient often does not improve blood pressure unless the pain becomes so great that a large sympathetic response occurs.

CNS toxicity (seizures) from systemic accumulation of local anesthetics is obviously based on the total amount of the drug used over time and has an estimated incidence of 0.01% to 0.1%. Motor block of the lower extremities is estimated at less than 3% when lower concentrations of local anesthetic are used and greater than approximately 25% with higher concentrations. In addition, the level of epidural insertion has much to do with the actual incidence in that lumbar epidurals are more likely than thoracic epidurals to cause motor block.

The incidence of nausea and/or vomiting with opioid-containing PCEA therapy is estimated at between 4% and 15%, although higher incidences have also been reported. The incidence of severe pruritus is between 2% and 17%, with the incidence of any degree of pruritus likely being well over 50%. Sedation is reported to occur in approximately 15% of patients. Respiratory depression is estimated to occur in 0.1% to 0.4% of patients. A higher incidence (approaching 1.5%) of respiratory depression is seen in some studies using morphine.

The respiratory depression seen with epidural opioids is biphasic. Early respiratory depression (within an hour of epidural initiation) is thought to be due to systemic absorption of the opioids via epidural veins and is thus more likely with the lipophilic opioids. Delayed respiratory depression (occurring 4–8 hours after epidural initiation) is seen especially when using the hydrophilic opioids and is thought to be due to the cephalad spread of the opioids in the cerebrospinal fluid.

PCEA management

Inadequate pain relief with an epidural can be due to a number of reasons, and an evaluation of the patient needs to be done to determine the best course of action. When a local anesthetic is part of the epidural solution, this evaluation should entail a determination of where the band of analgesia is located, either by testing for pinprick sensation or temperature differentiation. If the level of analgesia is more, or completely, one-sided the epidural catheter can be pulled out of the epidural space in 0.5- to 1-cm increments in an attempt to make the block bilateral. The optimal depth of multiorifice catheters is 3–5 cm in the epidural space. If the level of analgesia is not adequate to cover the entire extent of the surgical incision, then the rate of the continuous infusion can be increased, usually in increments of 2 ml/h, or the concentration of the local anesthetic can be increased. Either change will increase the number of dermatomes covered as the total quantity of local anesthetic, in milligrams, is the major factor in the amount of spread. If the patient has an adequate number of dermatomes covered but is still having pain, then the block is not dense enough. In this case, change the epidural solution to a more concentrated local anesthetic and/or add other agents (i.e., opioid and/or adjunct). If at any point the patient is in severe pain, a rescue dose of either the epidural infusion (4–8 ml) or a more concentrated local anesthetic bolus (e.g., 3–6 ml of 0.25% bupivacaine) can be used to achieve comfort faster.

Lower-extremity motor block can be of any degree from mild to complete. If the level of analgesia does not need to cover the lumbar nerves and it more than adequately covers the surgical incision, then the rate of the continuous infusion can be decreased (usually in increments of 2 ml/h). If the level of analgesia needs to cover the lumbar nerves or if the level of analgesia is just covering the extent of the surgical incision, then the local anesthetic concentration should be decreased to attempt to make the motor block less pronounced. If the patient is not going to be getting out of bed, for reasons other than the motor block from the epidural, then no change in therapy is really necessary, especially if the motor block is not bilateral and complete.

The concern with a complete motor block, especially one that occurs after the epidural has been running for some time with normal motor function previously, is that it may be a sign of the development of an epidural hematoma. Motor block, the most common presenting symptom of epidural hematomas, is seen in 46% of cases, followed by back pain in 38% of cases. If an epidural hematoma is suspected, the epidural should be stopped and motor function evaluated over the next 2 hours. If no resolution of the motor block occurs in this time, the patient should be sent for an MRI to rule out hematoma formation. The best chance for recovery of neurologic function from an epidural hematoma is to undergo a decompression laminectomy within 8 hours of the onset of symptoms.

As stated in the PCEA complications /side effects section, if hypotension is seen it is usually best to treat with intravascular volume expansion. If this is not possible, then the analgesic level should be established to ensure that the spread is not too excessive for the surgical incision; if it is, then a reduction in the continuous infusion rate can be made. If the hypotension is so severe that the epidural infusion needs to be turned off, one should ensure that the patient has another means of analgesia (e.g., IV PCA). In addition, if the blood pressure does not increase significantly after approximately 2 hours, then it is not likely that the epidural was contributory to the hypotension and the infusion can be restarted.

If the patient is having the opioid-related side effects of nausea and/or vomiting or pruritus, the options are to treat the particular side effect with a specific therapy or remove the opioid from the epidural solution. To treat nausea and/or vomiting, any of the available antiemetics can be tried as none has been proven to be the most effective. The pruritus caused by epidural opioids is generally not due to histamine release, instead being a central μ-receptor–related phenomenon. Thus it is best treated with a medication that has μ-receptor antagonist properties (e.g., 5 mg of IV nalbuphine every 4 hours PRN) – not an antihistamine.

Sedation or respiratory depression from epidural opioids definitely requires at least the removal of the opioid from the solution. If either is severe, especially respiratory depression, then naloxone administration may be necessary. Careful titration of naloxone (40-μg increments every couple of minutes) is necessary to minimize the chance of complete reversal of analgesia and the development of hypertension, tachycardia, and pulmonary edema. Naloxone has a relatively short duration of action (about 1 hour); therefore, patients should be monitored for return of respiratory depression as the opioid effects can last as long as 12 hours after discontinuation. Therefore, repeat doses of naloxone may need to be given. Another option is to begin a naloxone infusion.

PCEA efficacy versus parenteral opioids

Based on the results of several studies and meta-analyses, epidural analgesia is better than PCA with opioids in a number of ways. Pain control is improved for general surgery, orthopedic, and gynecologic patients. All epidural regimens (except hydrophilic opioids alone) when compared to PCA provide improved analgesia. There is statistically better analgesia at rest and during activity for all types of surgery (through postoperative day 4), as well as clinically appreciable differences in pain with activity through postoperative day 1. Greater improvements in analgesia are seen when epidurals contain a local anesthetic and when the insertion level is matched to the surgery (i.e., epidural insertion site around the mid-dermatome of the incision).

There is a reduction in pulmonary and cardiac complications (including postoperative myocardial infarction) in major vascular surgery and in high-risk patient populations with the use of thoracic epidurals. In addition, there is a reduction in the time of postoperative ileus (by 1–1.5 days) following abdominal surgery with the use of epidural regimens that contain local anesthetics. There has also been the suggestion that epidurals decrease the time to mobilization, duration of intensive care unit stay, and time to discharge. In lower-extremity revascularization, epidurals have been shown to improve the incidence of graft survival. Historically, epidurals have reduced the incidence of deep vein thrombosis (DVT) and pulmonary embolism (PE); however, no studies have been done recently comparing epidural infusions to newer pharmacologic thromboprophylaxis. Epidural therapy is more expensive than PCA therapy. In terms of side effects, PCA therapy has a higher incidence of nausea and sedation, whereas epidurals have a higher incidence of pruritus, urinary retention, and motor block (although this will vary with the agents and concentrations chosen).

PCEA efficacy versus continuous epidural infusions

It has been suggested that PCEA compared with continuous epidural infusion (CEI) optimizes pain control by allowing the patient to top-up him- or herself when there is an increase in pain or in anticipation of a painful event (e.g., prior to getting out of bed or having physical therapy) as opposed to having to wait for a health care provider. Some studies have shown that PCEA compared to CEI provides improved analgesia, whereas others have only shown a decreased requirement for provider-administered boluses. Some data are contradictory in terms of whether PCEA or CEI provides improved analgesia, but PCEA has been suggested to improve patient satisfaction, and PCEA does reduce the total amount of analgesics required. Additionally, PCEA has a decreased risk of motor block and nausea but an increased incidence of pruritus when compared to CEI.

PCEA safety and monitoring

Tubing that is clearly marked and differentiated from IV tubing (e.g., different color) is essential to prevent medications other than the intended epidural solution from being injected into the epidural space. Although there are no actual guidelines for how to monitor patients on a PCEA, the APSF does offer some recommendations if the infusion contains an opioid as described in the section PCA monitoring.

Suggested readings

American Pain Society. *Principles of Analgesic Use in the Treatment of Acute Pain and Cancer Pain.* 5th ed. Glenview, IL: American Pain Society; 2003.

Block BM, Liu SS, Rowlinson AJ, et al. Efficacy of postoperative epidural analgesia. A meta-analysis. *JAMA* 2003; 290:2455–2463.

Carr DB, Goudas LC. Acute pain. *Lancet* 1999; 353:2051.

Chang KY, Dai CY, Ger LP, et al. Determinants of patient-controlled epidural analgesia requirements. *Clin J Pain* 2006; 22:751–756.

Gordon DB, Dahl JL, Miaskowski C, et al. American Pain Society recommendations for improving the quality of acute and cancer pain management. *Arch Intern Med* 2005; 165:1574.

Grass JA. Patient-controlled analgesia. *Anesth Analg* 2005; 101:S44–S61.

Hudcova J, McNicol E, Quah C, Carr DB. Patient controlled opioid analgesia versus conventional opioid analgesia for postoperative pain. *The Cochrane Database of Systemic Reviews* 2006; (4):CD003346.

Liu SS, Wu CL. Effect of postoperative analgesia on major postoperative complications: a systemic update of the evidence. *Anesth Analg* 2007; 104:689–702.

Macintyre PE. Safety and efficacy of patient-controlled analgesia. *Br J Anaesth* 2001; 87:36–46.

Morrison RS, Meier DE, Fischberg D, et al. Improving the management of pain in hospitalized adults. *Arch Intern Med* 2006; 166:1033.

Weinger MB. Dangers of postoperative opioids. *Anesthesia Patient Safety Foundation Newsletter* 2007; 21:61–63.

Wheatley RG, Schug SA, Watson D. Safety and efficacy of postoperative epidural analgesia. *Br J Anaesth* 2001; 87: 4–61.

Chapter 145

Multidisciplinary approach to chronic pain management

Pradeep Dinakar and Edgar L. Ross

Pain is the most common presenting symptom and accounts for the majority of visits to the physician's office. Acute pain can usually be treated with oral, intravenous, or epidural administration of analgesics, both opioid and non-opioid. Unlike the treatment of acute pain, that of chronic pain is usually more complex given the bio-psycho-socio-genetic influences on the development of chronic pain. A common mistake and reason for treatment failure is the tendency to simplify the treatment of chronic pain by trying these approaches individually and sequentially rather than simultaneously. A multimodality approach addressing these complex interrelated factors leads to the best possible outcome. Several other treatment barriers have been identified that lead to these poor outcomes (Table 145.1).

The evaluation process should identify the various problems, and the treatment plans formulated must address these problems concurrently. Individual treatment plans addressing all of the problems maximize the potential for improved outcomes. Treatment plans for chronic pain should consist of the following components tried concurrently:

- Pharmacologic management;
- Interventional pain management;
- Pain-related psychological symptom management along with behavioral therapy; and
- Rehabilitation directed toward improving the patient's function and endurance.

Table 145.2 enumerates the various treatments available for chronic pain.

Pharmacologic management

Many different classes of medications have been used in the treatment of pain. Given the varying pain physiologies, rarely can one single medication be completely effective in all types of pain. The most common approach is to try various different classes of medications, both individually and in combination, until optimal pain relief is obtained. Polypharmacy can lead to both synergistic analgesic effects as well as a reduction in individual medication side effects due to dose reduction. Good knowledge of the pharmacodynamics, pharmacokinetics, and adverse effects of these medications is essential in the treatment of these conditions.

Analgesics can be classified as either primary or adjuvant medications based on the pain etiology. In most of the nociceptive pain conditions the primary medications are usually opioid or nonopioid drugs, and adjuvants are anticonvulsants, antidepressants, N-methyl-D-aspartate (NMDA) antagonists, muscle relaxants, or topical medications. In neuropathic pain syndromes, these adjuvants serve as the primary medications and the opioid and nonopioid medications work as adjuvants given their lack of efficacy in neuropathic pain. Table 145.3 lists some of the more common classes of medications used in pain management.

Opioid analgesics

Opioid analgesics are μ-receptor agonists, which are the oldest class of medication used in the management of both cancer and noncancer pain. Multiple routes of administration include oral,

Table 145.1.   Chronic pain management treatment barriers

Treatment barrier	Solution
Inadequate or wrong type of analgesics	Defining the types of pain and using appropriate agents are important for successful treatment.
Allowing patients to overuse analgesics	Use treatment contracts for controlled substances, and monitor effects of medication and improvement in the patient's function with the use of these analgesics.
Failure to use polypharmaceutical approaches	Often no single analgesic can be effective by itself. The use of multiple pharmaceutical agents enhances analgesia and can decrease individual side effects.
Failure to recognize patient's psychological symptoms, such as depression and anxiety	Psychological symptoms are common and enhance pain perception.
Failure to recognize a patient's loss or lack of a social support system	Social isolation and loss of a job is common. Distraction is an easy and effective approach for chronic pain.
Failure to recognize deconditioning and other rehabilitative needs	Deconditioning and muscle weakness lead to further pain if activity is inappropriate for ability. Energy conservation principles are important for successful treatment.

From Ross EL. *Pain Management. Hot Topics.* 1st ed. Philadelphia: Hanley & Belfus; 2003.

Table 145.2. Multidisciplinary modalities for pain treatment

Treatment modality	Description
Medications	Medication management for different types of pain and associated symptoms; see Table 146.3 for more specific management discussion.
Nerve blocks	Interventional treatments that can be helpful even when patients have not responded to noninvasive therapies.
Surgery and implantable devices	In certain well-selected patients, implantable devices, such as spinal cord stimulators and intrathecal pumps, can be helpful as part of a comprehensive treatment plan.
Relaxation training	Anxiety and unmanageable stress enhance a patient's pain perception.
Biofeedback	These approaches can provide patient-initiated nonpharmacological treatment and help to give patient a sense of control.
Support and education, groups and individual	Using groups and individual approaches, learning about what chronic pain is and how a patient can restore self-control can be helpful.
Psychotherapy	Depression and other comorbid psychological conditions can stand in the way of meaningful progress in chronic pain management.
Vocational counseling	Helpful for treatment plans that call for return to work; should be obtained early in the treatment course to facilitate goal-directed treatment.
Occupational and physical therapies	A must for almost all chronic pain patients to restore function.
Transcutaneous electrical nerve stimulation (TENS)	Noninvasive device that can be helpful for select patients where electrical energy is applied to the skin through electrodes.
Acupuncture and other alternative medicine approaches	Alternative medicine therapies have been helpful for relaxation and analgesia in well-selected patients as part of the treatment plan.
Nutrition counseling	Many chronic patients are obese and require weight loss as part of a treatment plan.

Modified from Ross EL. *Pain Management. Hot Topics.* 1st ed. Philadelphia: Hanley & Belfus; 2003.

intravenous, epidural, intrathecal, topical patch, buccal, rectal, and inhalational. Given the inherent risk of abuse and dependence, these drugs are classified as Schedule II and III drugs. Tolerance and dependence are common among all opioid medications. Reducing analgesia due to tolerance can be countered by opioid rotation. The initial management of nociceptive pain is with noncombination or combination short-acting opioids. Long-acting opioids are useful when the short-acting opioids fail to effectively control pain. These long acting opioids provide a baseline pain control, and short-acting opioids are used for breakthrough pain. These short-acting opioids are dosed at 10% to 15% of the total opioid dose. Breakthrough doses should ideally not exceed four doses per day. Opioid side effects are common with increasing doses and in more sensitive patients. The first strategy is opioid rotation, which can often improve

a patient's tolerance to this therapy. The more common side effects and their treatments are listed in Table 145.4.

Nonopioid analgesics

Nonopioid medications include the nonsteroidal anti-inflammatory drugs (NSAIDs), corticosteroids, and acetaminophen. NSAIDs are the most commonly prescribed medications for pain. They work by inhibiting cyclooxygenase (COX) 1 and 2. This COX1 inhibition also forms the basis for their gastrointestinal (GI) side effects. COX2 inhibitors are selective in controlling inflammation and have minimal GI side effects. Acetaminophen is now thought to work on a recently identified COX3 receptor. Both classes of NSAIDs should be used with caution in patients with a history of hypertension,

Table 145.3. Medication classes useful in management of chronic pain

Drug class	Pain treated
Opiates (oxycodone, OxyContin, Percocet, hydrocodone, morphine, methadone)	Used for nociceptive pain; helpful with appropriate adjuvants for neuropathic pain.
NSAIDs (aspirin, naproxen, ibuprofen, celecoxib)	Mainly useful for nociceptive pain; the COX2 inhibitors have increased the variety of clinical settings where they can be used with reduced GI discomfort.
TCAs (amitriptyline, nortriptyline, doxepin, imipramine)	Neuropathic pain, can improve sleep and mood.
SSRIs (citalopram, fluoxetine, fluvoxamine, paroxetine, sertraline)	Some studies have suggested that these might be helpful in neuropathic pain syndromes. They are helpful for depression, which is common in chronic pain.
Anticonvulsants (gabapentin, pregabalin, tegretol, valproic acid, valium, topiramate, levetiracetam, zonisamide, lamotrigine)	Primarily used for neuropathic pain syndromes; can be useful as adjuvant for opiates and improvement in quality of sleep.
NMDA receptor antagonists (ketamine, memantine dextromethorphan)	Useful as opiate adjuvants, might help to improve responsiveness of neuropathic pain to opiates; might be helpful to manage opiate tolerance
Muscle relaxants (baclofen, valium, cyclobenzaprine)	Myofascial pain from muscle spasms and headaches.
μ-2 agonists (tizanidine, clonidine)	Useful for opiate withdrawal, can be helpful for neuropathic pain.
Topical medications (lidocaine patch, desipramine cream, capsaicin)	Localized neuropathic pain or dysesthesias.

Modified from Ross EL. *Pain Management. Hot Topics.* 1st ed. Philadelphia: Hanley & Belfus; 2003.

Table 145.4. Opioid-induced complications and their treatments

Side effect	Treatment approach	Comments
Nausea	Antiemetics or pro-peristaltic agents	Ensure that the patient is not constipated.
Sedation	Psychostimulants such as methylphenidate or modafinil	Use low doses and administer in AM to avoid sleep difficulties. Consider depression with this side effect.
Euphoria	Trial of methadone	This can be a troubling side effect for many patients.
Constipation	Laxatives, stool softeners, oral naloxone	Use prophylactic measures to avoid this routine side effect.
Loss of libido	Hormone replacement therapy	High-dose opiates cause suppression of the hypothalamic pituitary axis.
Loss of appetite	Anabolic steroids or dronabinol (Marinol; Abbott Laboratories)	Also a symptom of depression
Dizziness	Consider scopolamine patch.	Opioids can have an effect on the inner ear balance mechanism.
Urinary retention	Trial of bladder muscle stimulant such as bethanechol (Urecholine; Duramed Pharmaceuticals)	If using a tricyclic or other anticholinergic, consider stopping or changing medication.
Respiratory depression	Usually not needed, tolerance builds rapidly	If respiratory depression is noted, look for new developing pathology.
Myoclonus	GABA agonists, such as baclofen, benzodiazepines	Rare with oral routes; consider reducing opioid doses if able, opioid rotation or alternate routes such as epidural or intrathecal route

From Ross EL. *Pain Management. Hot Topics.* 1st ed. Philadelphia: Hanley & Belfus; 2003.

concurrent use of prednisone, coronary artery disease, pre-existing renal disease, peptic ulcer disease, or concurrent use of other highly protein-bound drugs, such as coumadin. The routes of administration include oral, intravenous, rectal, and topical.

Antidepressants

Antidepressants are used in the management of pain and depression in chronic pain. Their use is limited by debilitating side effects as seen in Table 145.5. When using these medications, the effective approach is to pick the drug with the side-effect profile that may be a secondary benefit to the patient. Tricyclic antidepressants (TCAs) exert their analgesic effect by restoring inhibitory controls through blockade of noradrenaline and serotonin reuptake. Unfortunately, the tricyclics are limited by significant anticholinergic side effects that many patients find intolerable. Newer antidepressants, such as the selective serotonin reuptake inhibitors (SSRIs) and selective norepinephrine reuptake inhibitors (SNRIs), lack anticholinergic side effects.

Anticonvulsants

The various generations of anticonvulsants have neuropathic pain action (Table 145.6). They are commonly used as adjuvants in nociceptive pain and as primary agents in neuropathic pain unless limited by side effects or lack of efficacy. Carbamazepine

Table 145.5. Side effects of TCAs

Side effect	Drug class and examples	Comments
Cardiovascular effects	TCAs cause postural hypotension, nortriptyline and doxepin less than imipramine, amitriptyline, desipramine, clomipramine	Most serious in elderly patients with increased risk of falling and hip fractures
	TCAs have also been shown to increase the incidence of cardiac arrhythmias in patients with existing cardiac disease.	There might even be a risk of this side effect in patients without evidence of cardiovascular disease.
Sedation	Common with all TCAs; nortriptyline less common and the SSRIs and desipramine can produce insomnia	The sedating TCAs are often used at night to take advantage of their sedation. To avoid falling, care should be taken with patients who frequently get up at night.
Anticholinergic effects	Imipramine, amitriptyline, and doxepin show strong effects, less so with nortriptyline, desipramine; SSRIs lack this effect	Manifested by dry mouth, constipation, and urinary retention
Weight change	TCAs cause increased appetite, SSRIs can lead to anorexia and some weight loss.	Consider drug class based on weight goals for patient
Sexual dysfunction	TCAs and SSRIs have all been reported to have sexual side effects.	Consider dose reduction or plan sexual activity with trough levels of drug.
Psychiatric complications	Use TCAs with caution in suicidal patients; can trigger mania in bipolar patients.	Seek psychiatric help for patients with complicated psychological history.
Withdrawal symptoms	Both SSRIs and TCAs	Wean all antidepressants; avoid abrupt discontinuation.
Central serotonin syndrome	Can be caused by combinations of SSRIs and TCAs	Use these combinations with caution.
Analgesic effects	Strong analgesics include imipramine, amitriptyline, nortriptyline, and desipramine. Less analgesic are the SSRIs. Venlafaxine and bupropion might have some analgesic activity.	Balance dose, side effects, and analgesic activity; consider adding anticonvulsant to lower antidepressant doses when partial response to antidepressant alone

From Ross EL. *Pain Management. Hot Topics.* 1st ed. Philadelphia: Hanley & Belfus; 2003.

Table 145.6. Types of anticonvulsants used in pain management

Drug	Dose	Frequency	How supplied, *mg*	Comments
First-Generation Anticonvulsants				
Carbamazepine (Tegretol, Novartis Pharmaceuticals)	100–1000	BID to QID	100, 200, 20 mg/ml suspension, also 200 and 300 CR tablets	Requires monitoring for liver toxicity and anemia
Phenytoin (Dilantin, Pfizer Pharmaceuticals)	100–300	QD	50, 100, also 100 CR capsule, 25 mg/ml suspension	Not helpful for neuropathic pain; significant side effects
Valproic acid (Depakote, Abbot Laboratories)	150–1000	TID	125, 250, 500 coated tablets	Not helpful for neuropathic pain; indicated for third-line migraine prophylaxis
Clonazepam (Klonopin, Roche Laboratories)	.25–2 mg/d	TID	0.5, 1.0, and 2.0 tablets	Limited evidence for efficacy as an analgesic; must be weaned off slowly because of potential of seizures
Second-Generation Anticonvulsants				
Gabapentin (Neurontin, Pfizer Pharmaceuticals)	900–3600	TID	100, 300, 400 capsules, 600 and 800 tablets	Indicated for PHN; doses should titrated upward to 3600 mg at least before determining to be ineffective
Lamotrigine (Lamictal, Glaxo SmithKline)	150–500	BID	25, 100, 150, 200 tablets and 5, 25 mg dispersion tablet	Slow titration at 25 mg/wk to avoid Stevens–Johnson syndrome; also associated with nausea, vomiting, and visual disturbances
Topiramate (Topamax, Ortho-McNeil Pharmaceuticals)	25–200	BID	15, 25 capsules, 25, 100, 200 tablets	No consistent evidence for neuropathic pain; good support for headache management; associated with weight loss
Oxcarbazepine (Trileptal, Novartis Pharmaceuticals)	150–300	BID–QID	150, 300, 600 tablets	Monitor sodium levels
Levetiracetam (Keppra, UCB Pharma)	1000–4000	BID–QID	250, 500 tablets	Well tolerated, little evidence for efficacy
Zonisamide (Zonagran, Elan Biopharmaceuticals)	100–400	QD	100, 200, 300, 400 tablets	Titrate slowly, to avoid sedation; little evidence for efficacy
Tiagabine (Gabitril, Cephalon)	2–32 mg	BID–QID	2, 4, 12, 16 tablets	Small trials show some efficacy

CR, Controlled release; PHN, Post-herpetic neuralgia.
From Ross EL. *Pain Management. Hot Topics.* 1st ed. Philadelphia: Hanley & Belfus; 2003.

may produce bone marrow depression, phenytoin causes undesirable cosmetic effects (gum hyperplasia, hirsutism) and ataxia at high doses, valproate can produce hepatotoxicity, and neurontin causes weight gain and sedation.

NMDA antagonists

The various medications in this class are ketamine, memantine, dextromethorphan, and methadone. Ketamine has shown considerable efficacy in treating neuropathic pain. Methadone is effective in weaning heroin and other narcotic abusers in detoxification.

Muscle relaxants

Muscle relaxants are a varied group of medications that involve depression of the central nervous system (CNS). The various classes of muscle relaxants are shown in Table 145.7. The γ-aminobutyric acid (GABA) agonists and other CNS depressants have been shown to have analgesic effects in both chronic and acute pain. The mechanism of action is thought to be through the depression of the descending reticular activation system and not peripheral inhibition. Benzodiazepines and carisoprodol have long-term dependency liability. Sedation is a common side effect with most of the muscle relaxants. Clonidine acts by potentiating the effects of opioids. It is most commonly used intrathecally along with opioids. Cyclobenzaprine is related to

TCAs. Its mechanism of action is through a reduction in activity of both the gamma and alpha motor systems.

Topical medications

Topical medications have the potential advantage of providing effective therapy without the side effects of systemic absorption. Topical medications would have the promise of being effective adjuvants against peripheral sensitization, which is a significant

Table 145.7. Types of muscle relaxants

Drug class	Trade name	Generic name
GABA agonists	Lioresal (Novartis Pharmaceuticals)	Baclofen
	Valium (Roche Laboratories)	Diazepam and other benzodiazepines
CNS depressants	Soma	Carisoprodol
	Parafon Forte	Chlorzoxazone
	Skelaxin (King Pharmaceuticals)	Metaxalone
	Robaxin (Schwarz Pharmaceuticals)	Methocarbamol
Antihistamines	Norflex (3M Pharma)	Orphenadrine
Central μ2-adrenergic agonists	Catapres	Clonidine
	Zanaflex	Tizanidine
TCA-like drug	Flexeril	Cyclobenzaprine

From Ross EL. *Pain Management. Hot Topics.* 1st ed. Philadelphia: Hanley & Belfus; 2003.

Table 145.8. Behavioral therapy for chronic pain

Therapy	Description
Hypnosis and visualization	The patient is taught to visualize relaxing mental images, such as a secluded beach or a peaceful meadow. This helps to decrease anxiety, and facilitates deep relaxation.
Guided imagery	Directed visualization focuses on specific psychological issues using pain-decreasing images.
Biofeedback	Relaxation technique measures a physiologic phenomenon, such as muscle tension, and provides audible or visual feedback indicating a state of relaxation.
Cognitive-behavioral therapy	This teaches various techniques, such as distraction training, cognitive restructuring, role-playing, or mental imagery.
Group therapies	When well planned and with appropriate patient dynamics, group therapy is helpful. The interaction is planned to share important breakthroughs in insight, discuss progress with treatment, and different strategies for overcoming everyday obstacles to improvement.
Family therapy	Patients and their families often feel angry at each other. The family can be a significant stressor but is an important source of support that is needed for progress. This approach attempts to bring insight into how to provide support without enabling continued disability.

From Ross EL. *Pain Management. Hot Topics.* 1st ed. Philadelphia: Hanley & Belfus; 2003.

mechanism for the maintenance of a chronic pain condition. Limitations of topical agents include (1) the ability to treat only relatively small areas and (2) systemic absorption. Examples of topical medications include NSAIDs, local anesthetics (EMLA cream: eutectic mixture of lidocaine and prilocaine), and capsaicin, a vanilloid agonist that causes conduction analgesia not associated with suppression of motor or sensory function unrelated to pain.

Interventional pain management

Interventional approaches to pain management and their complications are described in detail later. They are almost always used in conjunction with other conservative modalities of treatment.

Psychological approach

Coexisting psychological problems including depression, anxiety, mood disorders, personality disorders, anger, and history of abuse are commonly associated with chronic pain. Table 145.8 lists some of the psychotherapy approaches to deal with these problems.

Rehabilitation

Rehabilitation is as important as medical management and psychological therapy in the successful management of chronic pain. It helps in restoring better daily function and quality of life, reducing psychological comorbidities, and even discontinuing pain medications. Without rehabilitative therapies, the likelihood of improvement is low and the chance of reoccurrence for disability is high. Patients are taught that pain should not dictate the level of activity and the same level of activity should be maintained irrespective of the level of pain. The basics of the rehabilitative strategies described in Table 145.9 include general aerobic conditioning and focused therapy directed at the injured part of the body. Given that therapy is difficult in this patient population, maintaining motivation is key to a better outcome. Group activities, keeping logs of progress, and involvement in miscellaneous recreational activity can be of help to improve compliance. The initial part of acute rehabilitation involves 3 to 5 days of intense therapy. Aggressive therapy can result in noncompliance due to worsening of pain. After patients start meeting the initial goals, visits can be gradually decreased in frequency and intensity. An overview of the treatment of chronic pain is presented in Fig. 145.1.

Table 145.9. Rehabilitative therapies for chronic pain

Rehabilitative therapy	Description of treatment and goals
Modalities such as heat, ice, ultrasound	These are temporary, short-lasting therapies and therefore should only be used as adjuvant to an active rehabilitation.
Stretching	Mild and controlled stretching prepares the patient for further activity. Care should be taken to avoid injuring tight muscles that have not been active for a long period of time.
Cardiovascular exercise	Chronic pain patients are often deconditioned. A general aerobic program can increase endurance and activity tolerance. Aerobic exercise has antidepressant effects.
Work conditioning	This is a specific program that is used to prepare for a return to work. A job description is obtained, and the goals of therapy should lead to the physical demands of that type of work.
Strength training	This is usually focused on the portion of a chronic pain patient that is significantly weakened by the original insult. This approach is also used to train alternate muscle to supplement the site of original injury. Care should be taken to keep the goals realistic and avoid further injury.
Orthotics and prosthetics	Adaptive aids are often useful for return to function. The benefits of truly understanding a patient's impairments and creatively designing adaptive aids can be extremely helpful in enhancing function.

From Ross EL. *Pain Management. Hot Topics.* 1st ed. Philadelphia: Hanley & Belfus; 2003.

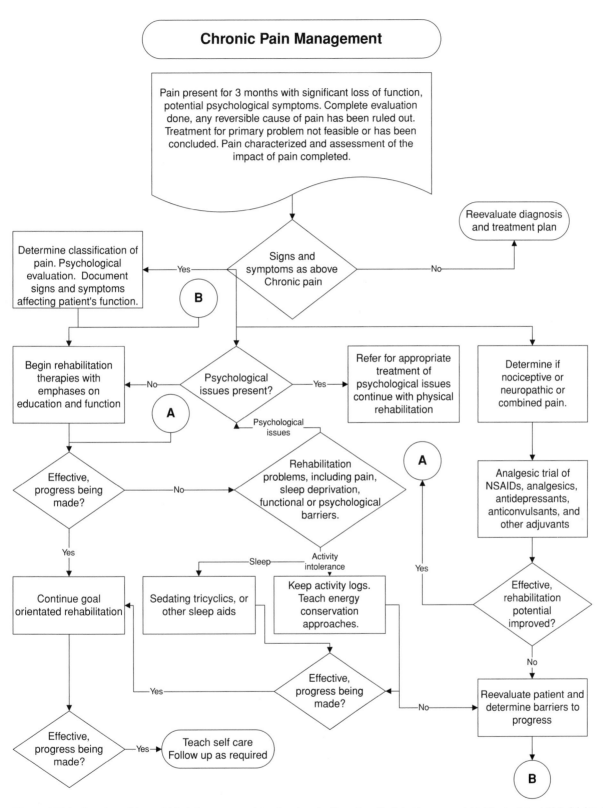

Figure 145.1. Overview of the multidisciplinary approach to chronic pain. (From Ross EL. *Pain Management. Hot Topics.* 1st ed. Philadelphia: Hanley & Belfus; 2003.)

Suggested readings

Grzesiak RC. Strategies for multidisciplinary pain management. *Compendium* 1989; 10(8):444, 446–448, 450.

Guay DRP. Adjunctive agents in the management of chronic pain. *Pharmacotherapy* 2001; 21(9):1070–1081.

Kottke, TE, Caspersen CJ, Hill CS. Exercise in the management and rehabilitation of selected chronic diseases. *Prev Med* 1984; 13(1): 47–65.

Loeser JD, Cousins MJ. Contemporary pain management. *Med J Aust* 1990; 153(4):208–212, 216.

McQuay H. Opioids in pain management. *Lancet* 1999; 353(9171):2229–2232.

McQuay HJ, Moore RA, Eccleston C, et al. Systematic review of outpatient services for chronic pain control. *Health Technol Assess* 1997; 1(6):1–135.

Portenoy RK. Current pharmacotherapy of chronic pain. *J Pain Symptom Manage* 2000; 19(1 Suppl):S16–S20.

Ross EL. *Pain Management. Hot Topics.* 1st ed. Philadelphia: Hanley & Belfus; 2003.

Sullivan MD, Turner JA, Romano J. Chronic pain in primary care. Identification and management of psychosocial factors. *J Fam Pract* 1991; 32(2):193–199.

Chapter 146

Psychological evaluation and treatment of chronic pain

Robert N. Jamison

Introduction

The International Association for the Study of Pain defines *pain* as "an unpleasant sensory and emotional experience associated with actual or potential tissue damage or described in terms of such damage." This definition recognizes that pain is an emotional as well as a sensory phenomenon. Pain is the most common reason to see a physician, and epidemiologic studies have independently documented that chronic noncancer pain is seen as an international problem of immense proportions.

Chronic pain influences every aspect of a person's functioning. Profound changes in quality of life are associated with intractable chronic pain. Significant interference with sleep, employment, social function, and daily activities is common. Chronic pain patients frequently report depression, anxiety, irritability, sexual dysfunction, and decreased energy. Family roles are altered, and worries about financial limitations and future consequences of a restricted lifestyle abound. Patients with chronic back pain generally present with a history of multiple medical procedures yielding minimal physical findings.

Psychological assessment of chronic pain

Important components of chronic pain that must be evaluated as part of a psychological assessment include pain intensity, functional capacity, mood and personality, coping and pain beliefs, and medication usage. In addition, a behavioral analysis should be conducted, and information on psychosocial history, adverse effects of treatment, and health care utilization should be obtained.

Semistructured interview

The most popular means of evaluating the psychological state of the patient is a semistructured interview. Pertinent information acquired during an interview is frequently given significant weight when a decision regarding treatment is made. Before meeting with the patient, the interviewer should review all referral information, including discharge summaries, psychological testing results, previous physicians' notes, and medical history reports. Each of the following categories should be assessed during the interview: (1) pain description; (2) aggravating factors; (3) daily activity level; (4) relevant medical history; (5) past and current treatments; (6) education and employment history; (7) compensation status; (8) history of drug or alcohol abuse; (9) history of psychiatric disturbance; (10) current emotional status and social support; and (11) perceived directions for treatment. These areas have been identified as important in assessing candidacy for medical interventions for pain. Whenever possible, the spouse, the significant other, or a close family member of each patient should be interviewed.

Pain intensity measures

One of the primary goals of treatment for chronic pain is to decrease the intensity of the pain. As a result, it is important to monitor pain intensity both for a period before treatment and throughout the course of treatment. There are a number of ways to measure pain intensity, including numeric pain ratings, the visual analogue scale (VAS), and verbal rating scales (Table 146.1).

Numeric pain ratings often involve the patient's rating of his or her pain on a scale of 0 to 10 or 0 to 100. Descriptive anchors that help the patient understand the meaning of each numeric value improve the measure. Another popular means of measuring pain intensity is the VAS, which uses a straight line (often 10 cm long) with extreme limits of pain at either end (e.g., "no pain" to "worst pain possible"). The pain patient is instructed to place a mark at the point on the line that best indicates present pain severity. Scores are obtained by measuring the distance from the end labeled "no pain" to the mark provided by the patient. The disadvantages of this method are that it is time-consuming to score and that its validity for older patients is questionable. Handheld computers enable VAS entry by screen touch with a stylus, and electronic diaries can aid in more complete and timely collection of patient diary data.

There are a number of verbal rating scales, which consist of words (as few as four or as many as 15, often ranked in order of severity from "no pain" to "excruciating pain") that are chosen by the patients to describe their pain. Verbal scales not only measure pain intensity but also assess sensory and reactive dimensions of the pain experience. Verbal scales can be used to measure the descriptive nature of pain; the patient chooses words from a list that best describe the pain experience (e.g., piercing, stabbing, shooting, burning, throbbing).

Of all of the self-report measures, numeric rating scales are most popular among professionals. There is no evidence to

Table 146.1. Pain rating scales*

Example of numeric pain rating scale

0		1	2	3	4	5	6	7	8	9	10
No pain											Worst pain possible

Example of VAS

No pain   Worst pain possible

Examples of verbal rating scales of pain intensity.

1. No pain	1. None	1. No pain	1. Not noticeable	1. None	
2. Mild	2. Mild	2. Mild	2. Just noticeable	2. Extremely weak	
3. Moderate	3. Moderate	3. Discomforting	3. Very weak	3. Just noticeable	
4. Severe	4. Severe	4. Distressing	4. Weak	4. Very weak	
	5. Very Severe	5. Horrible	5. Mild	5. Weak	
		6. Excruciating	6. Moderate	6. Mild	
			7. Strong	7. Moderate	
			8. Intense	8. Uncomfortable	
			9. Very strong	9. Strong	
			10. Severe	10. Intense	
			11. Very intense	11. Very strong	
			12. Excruciating	12. Very intense	
				13. Extremely intense	
				14. Intolerable	
				15. Excruciating	

* Karoly P, Jensen MP. *Multimethod Assessment of Chronic Pain.* New York: Pergamon Press; 1987.

suggest that the VAS or verbal rating scales are any less sensitive to treatment effects, however. All of these measures have been shown to be acceptable in the quantification of clinical pain. The McGill Pain Questionnaire (MPQ) is a frequently used comprehensive questionnaire that includes 20 subclasses of descriptors as well as a numeric pain intensity scale and a dermatomal pain drawing. A short form of the MPQ is also popular. The MPQ measures various aspects of the pain experience and is sensitive to treatment effects and differential diagnosis.

Mood and personality assessment

Pain patients often show signs of depression and anxiety. Psychopathology and/or extreme emotionality have been seen as a contraindication for certain therapies. There is ongoing debate among mental health professionals about the best way to measure psychopathology and/or emotional distress in chronic pain patients. Most measures are helpful in ruling out severe psychiatric disturbance. Unfortunately, no measure can boast validity in predicting treatment outcome. The measures most commonly used to evaluate personality and emotional distress include the Minnesota Multiphasic Personality Inventory (MMPI-2), the Symptom Checklist-90-Revised (SCL-90-R), the Millon Behavioral Health Inventory (MBHI), the Illness Behavior Questionnaire (IBQ), and the Beck Depression Inventory (BDI).

Functional capacity and activity interference measures

Some clinicians consider pain reduction meaningless if there is no noticeable change in function. Thus, some reliable measurement of functional capacity should be used before the onset of therapy. A noticeable increase in level of activity helps to justify continued therapy and supports treatment efficacy. A

number of self-report measures can be used to assess activity level and function: the Sickness Impact Profile (SIP), the Short-Form Health Survey (SF-36), the Multidimensional Pain Inventory (MPI), and the Pain Disability Index (PDI). Automated measurement devices, such as the portable up-time calculator and the pedometer, are useful in obtaining accurate measures of activity. These devices should be used in conjunction with self-monitoring assessment techniques.

Performance measures of function include the Modified Symptom Limited Treadmill Test and the Fingertip to Floor Distance Test. The first test has much in common with the 6-minute treadmill walking test, where distance is measured by how fast a patient is able to walk on a treadmill in 6 minutes. In the latter test, patients are asked to bend forward as far as possible without bending the knees and the distance from the tip of the middle finger to the floor is measured. These tests assess aerobic capacity and range of motion in the lumbar spine but are not always highly correlated with pain or disability.

Pain beliefs and coping measures

Pain perception, beliefs about pain, and coping mechanisms are important in predicting the outcome of treatment. Unrealistic or negative thoughts about an ongoing pain problem may contribute to increased pain and emotional distress, decreased functioning, and greater reliance on medication. Certain chronic pain patients are prone to maladaptive beliefs about their condition that may not be compatible with the physical nature of their pain. Patients with adequate psychological functioning exhibit a greater tendency to ignore their pain, use coping self-statements, and remain active to divert their attention from their pain.

Because efficacy expectations have been shown to influence the efforts that patients will make to manage their pain, measures of self-efficacy or perceived control are useful in assessing a patient's attitude. A number of self-report measures assess coping and pain attitudes. The most popular tests used to measure maladaptive beliefs include the Coping Strategies Questionnaire (CSQ), the Pain Management Inventory (PMI), the Pain Self-Efficacy Questionnaire (PSEQ), the Survey of Pain Attitudes (SOPA), and the Inventory of Negative Thoughts in Response to Pain (INTRP). Newer instruments currently being tested include the Pain Beliefs and Perceptions Inventory (PBPI), and the Chronic Pain Self-efficacy Scale (CPSS). Patients who catastrophize, who are passive in coping with pain, who demonstrate low self-efficacy regarding their ability to manage their pain, who describe themselves as disabled by their pain, and who report frequent negative thoughts about their pain are at greatest risk for poor treatment outcome. It is suspected that patients who have unrealistic beliefs and expectations about their condition are also poor candidates for pain treatment.

Monitoring of medication and adverse effects

Compliance is an important component in decisions about whether to continue, discontinue, or modify treatment for chronic pain. Clinicians ask patients to comply with their treatment protocol but rarely come up with a way to monitor compliance, particularly medication usage. A patient's retrospective report of use of medication, although of value, is subject to inaccuracies. Recall can be enhanced if the patient continuously monitors usage. In addition, both compliance and accuracy in reporting are improved if a family member assists with the monitoring. Medication records kept by patients should include the name of the medication, the date and time when it is taken, and the dosage.

Adverse effects should be monitored regularly during treatment for chronic pain. The monitoring of side effects related to medication use is often neglected in clinical practice, yet can be as important as the monitoring of pain intensity. Periodic monitoring of adverse effects by means of a checklist can provide relatively objective criteria useful in the assessment of treatment. Such a checklist may include drowsiness, dizziness, coordination impairment, irritability, depression, headache, memory lapse, dry mouth, visual distortions, nausea or vomiting, sweating, constipation, heart palpitations, itching, breathing problems, nightmares, and difficulty urinating. Although patients frequently report adverse reactions to medication during the initial stage of treatment, many of these reactions diminish over time.

Portable monitors using customized software have made the collection and storage of serial data about health behaviors both convenient and affordable. Electronic diaries allow two-way communication between patients and providers and may be an efficient means of evaluating and tracking medication use and associated symptoms. With the advent of palm-top computers (PTCs) and the ability to capture time-stamped data and store them for uploading to a larger computer, more investigators are exploring options of capturing data throughout the day. Ecologic momentary assessment (EMA) refers to frequent data captured from subjects in their natural environment. Studies have shown that natural data are less prone to fabrication and may be a truer indicator of patient responses in the environment. Patients are shown to demonstrate remarkably high compliance with electronic diary monitoring.

Neuropsychological testing

As part of a comprehensive psychological assessment, a patient's neuropsychological status must first be determined. In cases of physical trauma (such as head injury) or in cases of decreased cognitive functioning, neuropsychological assessment may be indicated. Such an assessment is important in the evaluation of potential organic pathology that may limit the usefulness of cognitive interventions. A number of neuropsychological assessment tools exist for such evaluations.

Substance abuse assessment

Structured interview measures have been published for the assessment of alcoholism and drug abuse. Whenever possible, the patient's family members and/or significant other should also be interviewed. The Structured Clinical Interview for the *Diagnostic and Statistical Manual of Mental Disorders, 4th Edition* (DSM-IV), SCID, is a semistructured diagnostic interview that assigns current and lifetime diagnoses based on DSM-IV criteria. For each positive identification of a symptom, the SCID follows a question sequence to determine whether the symptom meets severity criteria for diagnosis. Other substance abuse measures include the CAGE Questionnaire, the Michigan Alcoholism Screening Test (MAST), and the Self-Administered Alcoholism Screening Test (SAAST).

Psychological approaches to pain management
Goals of psychological interventions

Patients with chronic pain who consult their primary care physicians, pain specialists, pain services, or pain management programs are usually experiencing a significant degree of psychological distress that requires intervention. Regardless of the setting, a number of treatment goals are relevant to the care of the chronic pain patient: reduction of pain intensity; increased physical functioning; control of medication use; improvement in sleep, mood, and interaction with others; and eventual return to work or to normal daily activities.

Reduction of pain intensity

A persistent pain problem is the reason most patients enter a pain management program. In such a program, however, patients are taught not to set pain reduction as their primary treatment goal. Instead, they are encouraged to focus on other, more attainable goals. Although the elimination of pain is rarely reported, patients often describe a reduction in the intensity of their pain by the conclusion of a structured pain program.

Increased physical functioning

Most interventions support regular exercise, including stretching, cardiovascular reconditioning, and weight training. Patients are encouraged to exercise regularly and to increase their activity at a progressive rate while under supervision. The goal is to gradually increase function without exceeding predetermined limits of pain and discomfort.

Control of medication use

Through education and daily monitoring, most patients are able to use prescription pain medication responsibly. Patients are frequently requested to monitor and record their daily medication use as a way to become aware of patterns and any associated side effects.

Improvement in sleep, mood, and interaction with others

Most patients report depression, problems relating to other people, and difficulties with memory and attention. Techniques aimed at decreasing emotional distress and increasing self-esteem should be considered in these instances.

Return to work or to normal daily activities

Patients who set as their goal an eventual return to work often are successful. Follow-up helpfulness ratings indicate that patients who have a positive experience in a pain management program tend to return to work and/or maintain an active, productive lifestyle.

Psychological interventions and program components

Education

Most people with chronic pain have an inadequate understanding of the nature of their painful condition. It is important for them to be knowledgeable about their pain and the treatments designed for them. Information can be conveyed through patient manuals on chronic pain, video presentations, handouts, or individual sessions. An optimal way to educate patients is through didactic groups; however, individual psychoeducational training may be useful as well. Topics for these educational sessions may include the physiology of pain, medication for chronic pain, exercise and pain, stress management, sleep disturbance, assertiveness training, posture and body mechanics, problem solving, weight management and nutrition, vocational rehabilitation, sexual issues, positive thinking, and relapse prevention. In general, patients who understand their condition and who have been exposed to relevant management techniques maintain a perception of control over their pain and show higher rates of success in meeting their goals. Active learning techniques, including the completion of homework such as periodic surveys, checklists, diaries, or questionnaires and brainstorming, should be emphasized.

The ultimate goal of any intervention is to increase the patient's perceived control over pain. Several themes critical to a pain management approach should be highlighted throughout a structured program:

1. You will most likely not be "cured."
2. You need to expect ups and downs.
3. Rarely does pain intensity remain exactly the same over time.
4. You need to have a fall-back plan for those times when you have a flare-up of pain.
5. What you do about your pain may be as beneficial as anything that is done to you.
6. You need to work toward gaining control over your condition with the help of medical treatments and psychological pain management strategies.

Repetition will ensure that patients leave with an understanding of these important principles.

Relaxation training

Chronic pain patients tend to experience substantial residual muscle tension as a function of the bracing, posturing, and emotional arousal often associated with pain. Such responses, maintained over a long period, can exacerbate pain in injured areas of the body and can increase muscular discomfort. For example, it is common for patients with low back pain or limb injuries to develop neck stiffness and tension-type headaches. Relaxation training has been recommended as a way to reduce pain through the relaxation of tense muscle groups, the reduction of symptoms of anxiety, the use of distraction, and the enhancement of self-efficacy. In addition, this training can increase the patient's sense of control over physiologic responses. In a pain management intervention, patients are taught and encouraged to practice a variety of relaxation strategies, including diaphragmatic breathing, progressive muscle relaxation, autogenic relaxation, self-hypnosis, and cue-controlled relaxation. Biofeedback training may also be employed. Live demonstrations of these techniques are preferable to verbal explanations. All patients should be encouraged to practice each technique at home. Compact discs can be made or purchased for practice purposes.

Cognitive/behavioral therapy

Pain patients frequently show signs of emotional distress, with evidence of depression, anxiety, and irritability. Therapy with a cognitive/behavioral orientation is designed to help patients gain control of the emotional reactions associated with chronic pain. Specific problem-solving strategies can be offered during therapy sessions, including (1) identifying maladaptive and negative thoughts, (2) disputing irrational thinking, (3) constructing and repeating positive self-statements, (4) learning distraction techniques, (5) working to prevent future catastrophizing, and (6) examining ways to increase social support. Personal relationship issues can also be explored. The patient's strengths and positive coping mechanisms should be emphasized.

Cognitive/behavioral therapy has a number of objectives. The first is to help patients change their view of their problem from overwhelming to manageable. Patients who are prone to catastrophize benefit from examining the way they view their situation. What might otherwise be perceived as a hopeless condition can be reframed as a difficult yet manageable condition over which the patient can exercise some control.

The second objective is to help convince patients that treatment is relevant to their problem and that they need to be actively involved in their own treatment and rehabilitation. Patients need to understand how relaxation training, cognitive restructuring, adaptive coping skills, and pacing behaviors can help decrease their pain. They also need to reorient their view away from that of passive victim and toward that of proactive, competent problem solver. When individuals are successful in managing difficult painful episodes, their views change. They eventually begin to believe themselves capable of overcoming any acute flare-up of pain.

The third objective is to teach patients to monitor maladaptive thoughts and substitute positive thoughts. Persons with chronic pain are plagued, either consciously or unconsciously, by negative thoughts related to their condition. These negative thoughts have a way of perpetuating pain behaviors and feelings of hopelessness. Demonstrating how and when to attack these negative thoughts and when to substitute positive thoughts and adaptive management techniques for chronic pain is an important component of cognitive restructuring. Patients are encouraged to attribute success to their own efforts; they need to know that they are responsible for the gains they make. Finally, future problems and lapses need to be discussed so that the patient will have a "game plan" to manage short-term setbacks.

Group therapy

Group therapy presents an opportunity to discuss concerns or problems that patients have in common. The specific problem-solving strategies used may be the same as in individual supportive therapy and cognitive behavioral therapy. Unlike psychotherapists in traditional group sessions, group therapists in a pain management program are encouraged to be active facilitators. They may need to redirect the discussion so that every member has an opportunity to speak and no one individual monopolizes the session. Participants should be offered individual therapy sessions in which to deal with personal issues.

Certain group members may initially be reluctant to discuss personal problems related to their pain. The group therapist must prevent other group members from being overly judgmental and negative. Group members should be told that they are there to learn from one another and to support one another in gaining control over their pain.

Family therapy

Chronic pain significantly impacts all members of a family. Family members need to be educated about the goals of therapy and should have an opportunity to share their concerns. Moreover, active involvement of family members helps to ensure the patient's long-term success. Therefore, both patients and members of their families should be invited to attend family therapy sessions during which the facilitator encourages them to ask questions about the pain management program, to discuss their concerns and expectations, and to express their feelings. Besides enhanced communication, important outcomes of these sessions are that family members learn how to help the person in pain to achieve and maintain goals and that they come to understand that they are not alone in dealing with the person in pain.

Physical activity and exercise

Most patients are deconditioned because of their reluctance to exercise and because of a perceived need to protect themselves. Some patients have been medically advised to restrict activity when pain increases. Patients with chronic pain need to know that exercise is important. Some stretching, cardiovascular activity, and weight training should be encouraged. Each patient should be asked to keep track of his or her activity in an exercise record. It is important to set an exercise quota so that the patient will work to meet a weekly goal. The exercise plan should initially be determined by the patient and reviewed and supervised by a physical therapist or exercise physiologist. Patients should be instructed to stretch before and after each exercise session.

Any attempt by chronic pain patients to exercise is bound to entail some disappointment and perceived failure. Patients may make excellent gains, only to experience a flare-up of their condition. These setbacks should be anticipated so that the patient does not become excessively disappointed. Behavioral research suggests that compliance with exercise is best in a structured setting where each person is monitored and given encouragement for his or her accomplishments. Unfortunately, many persons with chronic pain tend to discontinue a regular exercise regimen within 6 months after a treatment program is concluded. Ways to encourage perseverance, such as organizing an exercise period with others, joining a health club, or combining exercise with another everyday activity, should be explored.

Vocational counseling

The goal of vocational rehabilitation is a return to work. After an extended period out of work, patients become both physically and psychologically deconditioned to the demands and stresses of the workplace. Together, a vocational rehabilitation counselor and the patient can develop a plan that incorporates both long-range employment goals and short-term objectives based on medical, psychological, social, and vocational information. Vocational rehabilitation counselors are specialists in the assessment of aptitudes and interests, transferable skills, physical capacity, modifications in the workplace, skills training, and job readiness.

Many chronic pain patients receive workers' compensation benefits or social security disability income. Patients may fear that their benefits will be jeopardized if they return to work. A vocational rehabilitation counselor can help a patient negotiate with an employer a return-to-work trial that will not jeopardize the patient's income. Through counseling strategies and assessment tools, a patient's suitability for returning to work or retraining can be determined. Patients should be familiar with the Americans with Disabilities Act to know their rights regarding discrimination due to a pain-related disability.

Relapse prevention

Most chronic pain patients need continued support if they are to maintain their gains. Patients should be encouraged to identify and anticipate situations that place them at risk for returning to previous maladaptive behavioral patterns. They should also be encouraged to rehearse problem-solving techniques and behavioral responses that will enable them to avoid a relapse. The goals of relapse prevention are to help the patient (1) maintain a steady level of activity, emotional stability, and appropriate medication use; (2) anticipate and deal with situations that cause setbacks; and (3) acquire skills that will decrease reliance on the health care system.

Follow-up has been shown to be a vital factor in the prevention of relapse. A specific written follow-up plan should be made for each patient before the end of treatment. The participant should be offered structured follow-up services, such as participation in a monthly support group session and/or in individual sessions.

Multidisciplinary team

Chronic pain involves a complex interaction of physiologic and psychosocial factors, and successful intervention requires the coordinated effort of a treatment team with expertise in a variety of therapeutic disciplines. Although some clinics offer a single treatment approach, most pain programs use a blend of medical, psychological, vocational, and educational techniques. Treatment modalities for chronic pain generally include medical assessment, medication management, pain-reduction treatments, didactic instruction, relaxation training, biofeedback, physical therapy, psychotherapy, and vocational counseling.

An interdisciplinary staff coordinates efforts to rehabilitate the pain patient and provides a comprehensive discharge and follow-up plan designed to meet the patient's short- and long-term needs. The patient's active participation in the treatment plan is strongly encouraged. Among the predictors of success in a multidisciplinary pain program are the patient's motivation to cope with pain and his or her external support systems.

Benefits of a pain management program

Pain programs are cost-effective. Patients who complete a multidisciplinary pain program return to work or undergo voca-

tional rehabilitation more often than do patients who do not enter a pain program. Multidisciplinary pain programs also produce marked subjective and functional improvements in chronic pain patients: Pain ratings decrease from admission to discharge, reliance on medication decreases, and physical functioning increases. These positive treatment outcomes are often maintained 2 to 3 years after discharge.

Future studies

There has been a rapid change in the way health care services are offered in the United States. More and more decisions about treatment are made by employees of insurance carriers on the basis of financial resources rather than need. An increasing need for accountability and efficacy has encouraged the implementation of cost-saving measures and program evaluation. Preference is given to programs that are tailored to the individual rather than to programs in which all group participants receive every treatment.

In light of the attention given to these changes, the economic efficiency of treatment for chronic, nonmalignant pain is worthy of discussion. Although evidence exists for the cost-effectiveness of therapy for chronic pain, such treatment may not meet the criterion of increased benefit with little cost. Prior classification of patients may help in identifying those individuals who will most benefit from pain therapy. No reported studies have satisfactorily addressed this issue, and outcome data are needed. Documentation of increased function and decreased health care utilization among certain patients as a result of pain therapy would support the continuation of pain management programs. The field of remote data entry through personalized technology holds much promise for clinicians in the future. Currently available technologic methods of tracking can address the need for improved evaluation and treatment of persons with chronic pain.

Suggested readings

Fishman SM, Ballantyne JC, Rathmell JP. *Bonica's Management of Pain* (4th ed.). New York: Lippincott Williams & Wilkins; 2010.

Jamison RN. *Learning to Master Your Chronic Pain*. Sarasota, FL: Professional Resource Press; 1996.

Jamison RN. *Mastering Chronic Pain: A Professional's Guide to Behavioral Treatment*. Sarasota, FL: Professional Resource Press; 1996.

Turk DC, Gatchel RJ (eds.). *Psychological Approaches to Pain Management: A Practitioner's Handbook* (2nd ed). New York: Guilford Press; 2002.

Turk DC, Melzack R (eds.). *Handbook of Pain Assessment* (2nd ed.). New York: Guilford Press; 2001.

Chapter 147

Interventional pain management I: epidural, ganglion, and nerve blocks

John C. Keel and Alina V. Bodas

General patient care considerations

Patients who undergo interventional procedures for pain, such as single-shot epidural steroid injections (ESIs), or ganglion or nerve blocks, should be instructed in advance to prepare for the procedure. They should not have the procedure in the event of recent febrile illness or if there is risk of bacteremia because of the risk of bacterial seeding of the epidural space and other structures. They should take only clear liquids for 4 hours prior to the procedure, to avoid aspiration in the event of loss of airway protection. For neuraxial procedures, any anticoagulant use must be stopped according to established guidelines, under the supervision of the prescribing physician, to reduce risk of bleeding and epidural hematoma. Standard guidelines regarding anticoagulants include the consensus statement of the American Society of Regional Anesthesia and Pain Medicine. An escort must be available on the day of injection. Written, informed consent must be carefully documented. During neuraxial procedures, the patient will generally be monitored with a blood pressure cuff and pulse oximeter. Certain patients will require a peripheral intravenous (IV) line. Sedation is generally not recommended for elective pain procedures, as it is important for the patient to be able to provide feedback and cooperation.

Pharmacology

Injectates typically include local anesthetic and adrenocortical steroids (glucocorticoids). Local anesthetics are reversible sodium channel binders, and they produce varying degrees of neural blockade. Most often used are the amino amides lidocaine 1% to 2% and bupivacaine 0.25 % to 0.5%. Higher concentrations of lidocaine can be associated with neurotoxicity. Lidocaine for anesthetizing skin can be mixed in a 9:1 ratio with 0.9% bicarbonate to enhance onset speed and reduce discomfort. Bupivacaine should not be mixed with bicarbonate because of resulting precipitate formation. Epinephrine is generally not included in chronic pain procedures, as it could exacerbate sympathetically mediated pain (SMP).

Glucocorticoids reduce inflammation by stabilizing leukocytes, inhibiting macrophages, decreasing edema, and reducing scar formation. Steroids also decrease the activity of irritated nerves. In interventional pain medicine, long-acting depot steroid is used, such as triamcinolone or methylprednisolone. Interestingly, such agents are US Food and Drug Administration (FDA) approved for intramuscular use, so they are usually used "off-label" for chronic pain procedures. The typical dose is 40 mg (1 ml) for transforaminal epidural injections, and 80 mg (2 ml) for interlaminar and caudal injections. At these doses, four to six ESIs per year can be administered, if appropriate. ESIs performed in series, however, are not routinely indicated (e.g., "series of three"). As little as 40 to 80 mg of intramuscular triamcinolone acetonide can suppress the hypothalamic–pituitary–adrenal axis for 2 to 4 weeks. All glucocorticoids have systemic effects, such as fluid retention and increased insulin requirement in diabetes, but the degree of systemic effect in neuraxial pain procedures is not well understood. Although rare, even *single doses* of injected steroid have been reported to cause Cushing's syndrome its devastating sequelae such as avascular necrosis, e.g., in patients who take ritonavir for HIV.

Neurolytics are most often used in patients with cancer pain. Alcohol 50% to 95% and phenol 6% to 10% produce long-lasting neurolysis by protein denaturation, coagulation, and precipitation. Phenol acts as an anesthetic at lower concentrations, is more viscous, and is less painful on injection than is alcohol. Alcohol is hypobaric in cerebrospinal fluid (floats on top), whereas phenol is hyperbaric (sinks) in cerebrospinal fluid. Neurolysis of peripheral nerves with a cutaneous sensory distribution should be avoided, as this can result in neuropathic pain.

Fluoroscopy

In blind techniques, using only surface landmarks, 30% of lumbar and 50% of cervical ESIs may miss the intended target. Controversy exists regarding outcomes of ESI, in part because earlier studies did not include fluoroscopic guidance. Fluoroscopy greatly enhances accuracy of needle placement, and is now the standard of care in the performance of ESI. Contrast agents are often used with fluoroscopic imaging. Contrast can be injected under live fluoroscopy to visualize potential unintended intra-arterial injection. The method of aspirating and looking for blood return should not be used alone, as it has up to a 50% false-negative rate. Contrast can detect intrathecal or subdural placement. Contrast can demonstrate location and extent of intended injectate distribution. Non-ionic monomeric contrast agents are used for interventional pain procedures, as these are stable in solution and are less toxic. Gadolinium can be used in patients at risk of allergic reaction.

Epidural steroid injections

Interventional pain practitioners use fluoroscopically guided ESIs to place steroid in this space near the nerve roots to suppress local inflammation that is thought to be the cause of radicular pain. Radicular pain is neuropathic pain in the distribution of spinal nerve roots, whereas radiculopathy involves conduction block in the spinal nerve, with resulting neurologic deficit, with or without pain. Radiculitis is inflammation of the nerve root. Radicular pain can arise from mechanical or chemical irritation due to a herniated nucleus pulposus or spondylosis with stenosis of nerve pathways. Varieties of ESI include interlaminar, transforaminal, selective spinal nerve block, and caudal.

Evidence-based indications for ESI include treatment of pain radiating in the distribution of spinal nerves. Spinal stenosis and neurogenic claudication may also be treated with ESI. Axial back pain is usually not an indication for ESI, except in discogenic back pain, which may be mediated by the sinuvertebral nerves. Interlaminar and transforaminal ESI are indicated to treat cervical and lumbar radicular pain. Selective nerve root blocks (SNRBs) are used as diagnostic procedures to determine if a specific nerve root is the source of pain, in the setting of inconclusive or inadequate imaging, often in anticipation of surgery. Caudal ESIs can treat lumbosacral radicular pain and back pain attributed to failed back surgery syndrome. The various complications of ESIs are described in subsequent chapters.

Interlaminar epidural steroid injections

Interlaminar ESIs are performed in the cervical and lumbar spine using the loss of resistance (LOR) technique. The patient is placed prone on the fluoroscopy table. In anteroposterior (AP) view, the 22-gauge Touhy needle tip is directed just lateral to the spinous process, toward the interlaminar space. As the tip nears the ligamentum flavum, lateral views are used to check depth, as the LOR indicates the exact place of the epidural space

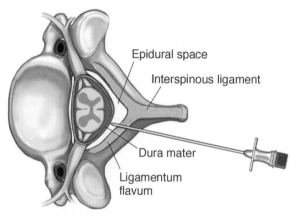

Figure 147.1. Interlaminar epidural steroid injection. (Adapted from Waldman SD. *Atlas ofInterventional Pain Management.* 2nd ed. Philadelphia: Elsevier; 2004.)

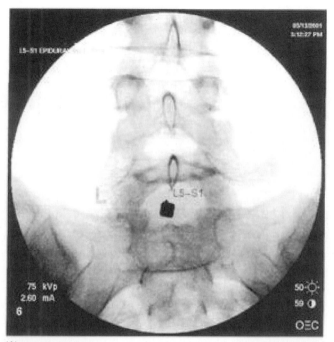

(A)

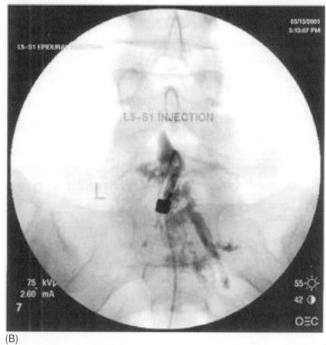

(B)

Figure 147.2. Fluoroscopy views. (**A**) AP view of coaxial needle placement in lumbar epidural steroid injection. (**B**) Epidural spread of contrast. (From Waldman SD. *Atlas of Interventional Pain Management.* 2nd ed. Philadelphia: Elsevier; 2004.)

(Fig. 147.1). Non-ionic contrast is used to confirm epidural flow before injecting steroid (Fig. 147.2). Typical injectate is 80 mg (2 ml) of triamcinolone. Injectate in the lumbar region may include a small amount of local anesthetic, but local anesthetic is usually not used in the cervical spine (Fig. 147.3). This interlaminar ESI technique cannot be performed if there has been a laminectomy at that level, as there are no reliable landmarks for

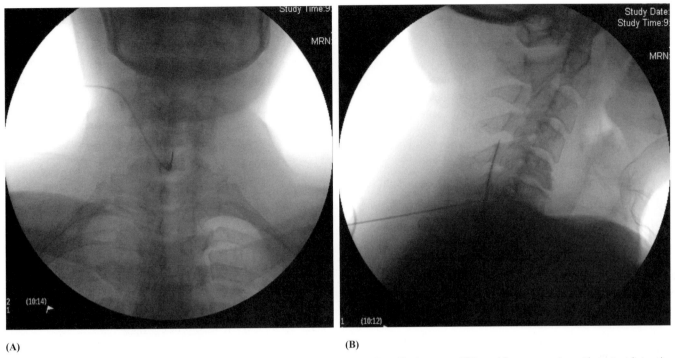

Figure 147.3. Cervical interlaminar epidural steroid injection. (**A**) AP fluoroscopy view of needle placement. (**B**) Lateral fluoroscopy view with contrast lining the epidural space. Courtesy of Pradeep Dinakar, M.D.

the interlaminar epidural space. In such cases, transforaminal or caudal approaches should be used.

Transforaminal epidural steroid injections

Transforaminal ESIs are most commonly performed in the lumbar spine. For lumbar transforaminal ESIs, the patient is placed prone on the fluoroscopy table. Oblique views are used to identify the pedicle over the target nerve root and the superior articular process of the vertebra below the nerve. The tip of a 25- to 22-gauge spinal needle is directed at the "six o'clock" position of the pedicle, within the "safe triangle," outlined by the inferior border of the pedicle, the spinal nerve itself, and the lateral border of the vertebral body (Fig. 147.4). AP views are used to check the medial extent of the needle, then lateral views are used to guide the needle transforaminally (Fig. 147.5). Nonionic contrast under live fluoroscopy is used to confirm epidural flow and to rule out intravascular uptake before injecting steroid. Typical injectate is 40 mg (1 ml) of triamcinolone, with or without a small amount of local anesthetic. The transforaminal approach has a much greater chance of delivering injectate to the anterior epidural space, the site of presumed pathology in disc herniations. Cervical, thoracic, and sacral transforaminal ESIs are sometimes performed. Cervical and thoracic transforaminal injections have high complication rates and are not as commonly used. Sacral transforaminal ESIs, most often accomplished at S1, are similar to lumbar ESIs. During the sacral transforaminal ESI, the spinal needle is advanced through the posterior sacral foramen until it is in proximity to the exiting S1 nerve root. Contrast is used to confirm the position and

the steroid is injected around the nerve root with an epidural spread.

Selective spinal nerve blocks

A selective spinal nerve block – an SNRB – is similar to a transforaminal ESI. An SNRB is used as a diagnostic procedure to

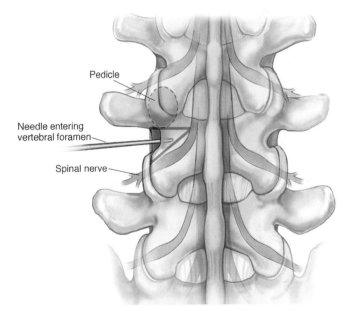

Figure 147.4. Lumbar transforaminal epidural steroid injection. (Adapted from Waldman SD. *Atlas of Interventional Pain Management.* 2nd ed. Philadelphia: Elsevier; 2004.)

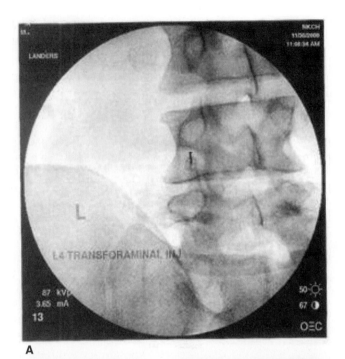

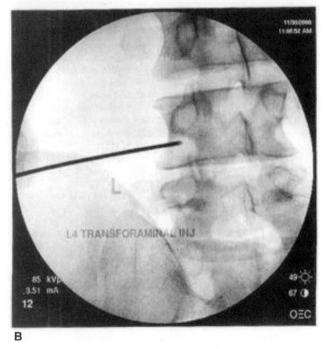

Figure 147.5. Fluoroscopy views (**A** and **B**) of needle placement in a lumbar transforaminal epidural steroid injection. (From Waldman SD. *Atlas of Interventional Pain Management.* 2nd ed. Philadelphia: Elsevier; 2004.)

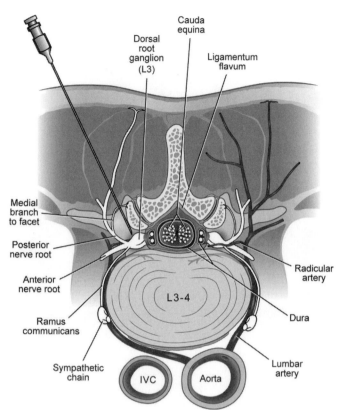

Figure 147.6. SNRB. (From Waldman SD. *Atlas of Interventional Pain Management.* 2nd ed. Philadelphia: Elsevier; 2004.)

Caudal epidural steroid injections

Caudal ESIs are performed by introducing a needle through the sacral hiatus, past the sacrococcygeal ligament. The patient is placed prone on the fluoroscopy table. Using lateral views, the needle is advanced, not past the lower aspect of S3 (avoiding dural puncture). Non-ionic contrast under live fluoroscopy is used to confirm epidural flow and to rule out intravascular uptake before injecting steroid (Fig. 147.7).

Ganglion blocks

Sympathetic blocks have utility in the diagnosis and treatment of pain that is mediated by the sympathetic nervous system. Positive response to sympathetic block may be diagnostic of SMP. The therapeutic effect of blocks may be due to interruption of central sensitization. The effect of sympathetic blocks may even predict outcomes with implanted spinal cord stimulators.

Sympathetic nervous system anatomy

The cell bodies of the preganglionic nerve fibers of the sympathetic nervous system arise in the intermediolateral cell column from T1 through L2. After exiting the spinal cord, these fibers either synapse or pass through the sympathetic chain. The sympathetic chain is composed of ganglia containing the cell

determine if a specific root level is the source of pain. The needle tip is placed just outside of the neural foramen, lateral to the position for transforaminal ESIs. There should not be epidural spread of injectate. This procedure is often performed to locate a target for surgery (Fig. 147.6).

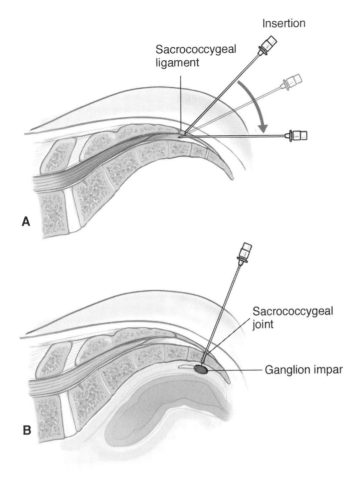

Figure 147.7. Caudal epidural steroid injection.

bodies of sympathetic postganglionic fibers, and is located on both sides of the vertebral column. Anatomic variation exists in the preganglionic pathways. For example, preganglionic sympathetic axons may travel up to 12 segments intraspinally before exiting the spinal cord. Axons of the thoracic ganglia remain ipsilateral, but axons in the lumbar ganglia take both ipsilateral and contralateral pathways. The cervical sympathetic ganglia include the superior, middle, and inferior cervical ganglia. The inferior cervical ganglion is often fused with the first thoracic ganglion (82% of cases) to form the stellate ganglion. Sympathetic afferent and efferent innervation of the head, neck, and upper limbs travels through this stellate ganglion. Eleven sympathetic ganglia lie in the thoracic region juxtaposed to the necks of the ribs. In both of these regions, the sympathetic chain lies in close proximity to the somatic nerves. Sympathetic innervation of the abdominal viscera is supplied by the celiac plexus. The preganglionic sympathetic nerves pass through the paravertebral sympathetic chain without synapsing. They then synapse at the celiac plexus, anterolateral to the abdominal aorta at T12–L1. Postganglionic fibers follow branches of the aorta to respective visceral structures.

Efficacy of sympathetic blocks

A number of methods have been devised to determine the effectiveness of a sympathetic block. One example is surface temperature monitoring. For upper limb blocks, temperature change can be monitored on the shoulder, forearm, and dorsum of hand or digit (preferably the thumb). For lower limb blocks, temperature can be monitored along the anterior thigh, dorsum of the foot, or the great toe. After a sympathetic block, the skin temperature should increase by at least 1°C to 2°C. Other methods involve psychogalvanic response, or sweat testing, wherein various chemicals that detect the presence of sweat are used to test a limb postblock. If a sympathetic block is successful, no sweat should be detected.

Stellate ganglion block

The stellates ganglion lies in front of the neck of the first rib with the vertebral artery passing over it. The sympathetic innervation to the head and neck arise from T1 and T2 and passes through the stellate ganglion on its way to more cephalad ganglia. The sympathetic innervation to the upper extremity arises from T2 through T8. Some of these fibers may synapse at the second thoracic ganglion and therefore may not be fully affected by a stellate ganglion block. Stellate ganglion blocks are indicated for pain, vascular spasm, and other various conditions of the head, neck, and upper extremities (Table 147.1).

To perform a stellate ganglion block, first position the patient supine with a roll under the shoulder for extension of the head and neck. This position draws the cervical spine more superficially, making it easier to reach while drawing the esophagus behind the trachea. Next, palpate the space between the carotid pulsation and the lateral trachea as low as possible in the neck. Another method is to retract the sternocleidomastoid muscle laterally and palpate the transverse process of the sixth cervical vertebra, called Chassaignac's tubercle. Generally, the sixth cervical vertebra is located at the level of the cricoid cartilage. Then make a skin wheal with local anesthetic over the medial border of the carotid pulsation. Direct a 22- to 25-gauge, 1.5-inch needle caudally and medially toward the junction of the lateral portion of C7 through T1 (Fig. 147.8). When bone is encountered, withdraw the needle 1 mm and inject 1 ml of contrast medium. Confirm contrast spread with fluoroscopy. Inject

Table 147.1. Stellate block indications

Pain	Vascular	Other
Complex regional pain syndrome type I or II	Vasospasm	Hyperhidrosis
Postherpetic neuralgia	Occlusive and embolic vascular disease	Ménière disease
Phantom limb pain	Scleroderma	Vascular headaches
Paget's disease		
Neoplasm of upper extremity		
Postradiation neuritis		
Intractable angina pectoris		

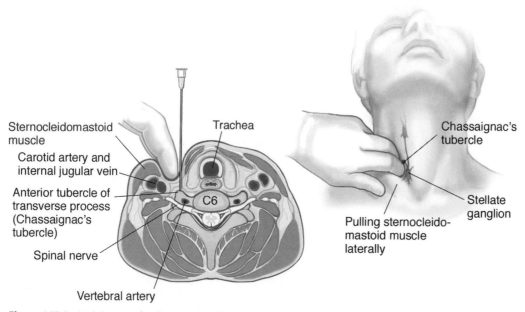

Figure 147.8. Axial diagram of stellate ganglion block. The great vessels of the neck are gently retracted laterally, and the needle is placed on the anterior tubercle of the transverse process of C6 (Chassaignac's tubercle). Note the position of the vertebral artery within the foramen transversarium, the spinal nerve root and dural cuff, and the carotid artery and jugular vein.

5 to 10 ml of local anesthetic. Use of fluoroscopy in the performance of stellate ganglion blocks is the standard of care. Prior to the use of fluoroscopy, larger volumes of local anesthetic were injected because the exact location of injection could not be assessed. Larger volume insured wider spread but increased risk of adverse events. Signs of a successful block include ipsilateral Horner syndrome along with nasal congestion, venodilation of the limb, and increase in temperature of the limb by at least 1°C to 2°C (Table 147.2).

Celiac plexus blocks

Sympathetic innervation to the abdominal viscera is composed of preganglionic axons from the T5 through T12 level that leave the spinal cord, pass through the sympathetic chain, and synapse at distal sites. A network of ganglia, including the celiac ganglia, superior mesenteric ganglia, and the aorticorenal ganglia compose the celiac plexus. This plexus is located at the T12 through L1 level, anterior to the aorta, epigastrium, and crus of the diaphragm.

Celiac plexus block is indicated for treatment and diagnosis of pain from visceral structures innervated by the celiac plexus. These structures include the pancreas, liver, gallbladder, omentum, and mesentery and alimentary tract from the stomach

Table 147.2. Signs of successful stellate ganglion block

Horner syndrome (ipsilateral)
Nasal congestion
Venodilation of the ipsilateral limb
Increase in temperature of the limb by at least 1°C–2°C

to the transverse colon. Use of celiac plexus block for chronic relapsing pancreatitis is controversial, but there may be some role, including the use of celiac plexus steroid injection. Neurolytic celiac plexus block is indicated as a palliative measure in upper abdominal malignancies, such as pancreatic carcinoma, where there is intractable pain. Celiac plexus neurolysis may lead to some diarrhea due to unopposed parasympathetic activity. It may, however, also decrease nausea and vomiting in these patients.

Current practice involves the use of fluoroscopy or CT for guidance of celiac plexus block. The block can also be performed using ultrasound, gastroscopy, or direct visualization intraoperatively. All approaches have the goal of depositing injectate anterior to the aorta, at the location of the plexus. For example, a fluoroscopically guided diagnostic block can be accomplished with a transcrural approach (crosses the diaphragmatic crura) or a retrocrural approaches (Fig. 147.9). In the transcrural approach, the patient is positioned prone with a pillow under the epigastrium. For the left side, an 18-gauge introducer needle is inserted 2 to 3 cm lateral to the L1 spinous process and aimed at the upper lateral margin of the L1 body. A 22- to 25-gauge needle with a curved tip is inserted through introducer and advanced medially to the celiac plexus. In the lateral view, the needle is then passed 2 to 3 cm beyond the edge of the L1 vertebral body. Continuous aspiration is maintained. Blood aspirate indicates penetration of the aorta, in which case a transaortic approach should be used. In this approach, needle advancement is simply continued through the anterior wall of the aorta. Contrast should indicate a pulsatile pattern anterior to the aorta. If bilateral spread is not seen, for the right

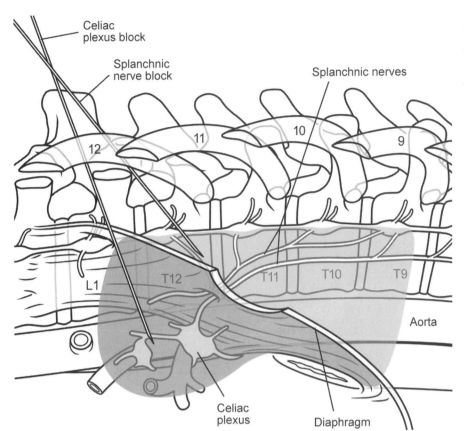

Figure 147.9. Anatomy of the celiac plexus and splanchnic nerves. *Shading* indicates the pattern of solution spread for each technique. (Reproduced with permission from Rathmell JP. *Atlas of Image-Guided Intervention in Regional Anesthesia and Pain Medicine*. 1st ed. Philadelphia: Lippincott Williams & Wilkins; 2006. Figure 11-1, p. 124.)

side, a 20-gauge, 15-cm needle tip is directed to the upper lateral border of L1, then directed 2.5 cm anterolaterally and caudad. Contrast is injected again to assess spread. If spread is adequate, the 10 to 15 ml of local anesthetic is injected intermittently (e.g., 0.5% lidocaine or 0.25% bupivacaine). If a neurolytic block is being considered, a diagnostic celiac plexus block must be performed well in advance, using local anesthetic, to determine if a neurolytic block would be effective. The splanchnic nerve block is essentially the retrocrural approach to a celiac plexus block. The needles are directed toward mid-T12 (versus cephalad L1). This technique avoids the aorta, and has similar effects as the celiac plexus block.

Lumbar sympathetic blocks

The lumbar sympathetic chain is located along the anterolateral border of the lumbar vertebral bodies. There are a variable number of ganglia, with blockade of the second and third ganglia resulting in close to complete sympathectomy of the lower limb.

Lumbar sympathetic block is indicated for several SMP and neuropathic pain conditions (Table 147.3). The patient is positioned prone with a pillow beneath the epigastrium. Fluoroscopy is used to identify L2 transverse process and vertebral body. A 20-gauge, 5-inch needle is placed roughly 4 to 8 cm lateral to the L2 spinous process and advanced until it is 1 to 2 mm posterior to the vertebral body. Contrast medium is

injected to confirm spread prior to injection of local anesthetic. A large volume (15–20 ml) is injected incrementally. Successful block is indicated by venodilation and temperature increase in the involved lower limb. This procedure can be performed bilaterally (Fig. 147.10).

Hypogastric plexus block

The superior hypogastric plexus, just below the aortic bifurcation, anterior to the L5 vertebral body, innervates organs in the pelvis and pelvic floor. The hypogastric plexus carries sympathetic and parasympathetic fibers. Hypogastric plexus block is performed for diagnosis of pain from pelvic viscera and for treatment of pain from pelvic malignancies. With the patient prone, a 22-gauge long needle is directed to the inferior anterolateral aspect of L5. Contrast should spread just anterior to

Table 147.3. Lumbar sympathetic block indications

Complex regional pain syndrome type I and II of the lower limb
Pain due to peripheral vascular insufficiency for diffuse distal disease not amenable to surgical intervention
Herpes zoster/postherpetic neuralgia
Phantom limb pain
Cancer pain from lower extremity or gastrointestinal tract distal to the transverse colon
Outcome predictor for spinal cord stimulator

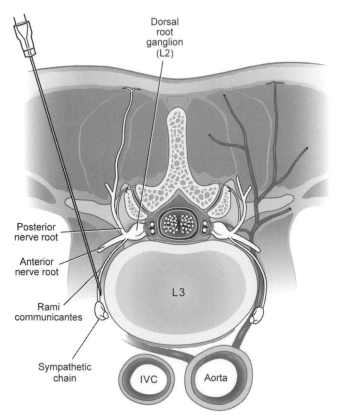

Figure 147.10. Axial diagram of lumbar sympathetic block. A single needle passes over the transverse process, and the tip is in position adjacent to the lumbar sympathetic ganglia over the anteromedial surface of the L3 vertebral body. (Reproduced with permission from Rathmell JP. *Atlas of Image-Guided Intervention in Regional Anesthesia and Pain Medicine.* 1st ed. Philadelphia: Lippincott Williams & Wilkins; 2006. Figure 12-2, p. 137.)

L5 through S1 (Fig. 147.11). Bilateral, unilateral, diagnostic, or neurolytic blocks can be performed. For a diagnostic block, 5 to 10 ml of local anesthetic is injected incrementally, per side.

Ganglion impar block

The ganglion impar represents the termination of the sympathetic chain. It rests anterior to the sacrococcygeal junction. Various techniques are described to block this ganglion, including a bent needle technique during which the needle enters at the level of the anococcygeal ligament. Given the close proximity of the rectal canal to this entry site, however, the easiest and safest approach is to traverse the sacrococcygeal ligament itself. Injection of contrast agent under fluoroscopy confirms proper needle placement. The technique can be performed with local anesthetic and steroid for nonmalignant pain conditions, such as coccygodynia, or perirectal pain from tumor involvement. Neurolytic blockade should probably be performed only for malignant pain conditions, and only after a diagnostic block is performed. The advantage of the ganglion impar block over other neurolytic procedures for rectal pain is that bowel and bladder function is generally unaffected. A local anesthetic

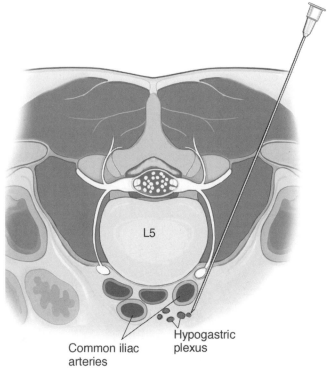

Figure 147.11. Sagittal view of the superior hypogastric block.

block should be done prior to a more permanent neurolytic blockade.

Peripheral nerve blocks

Single injections to block peripheral nerves can be used for diagnosis and treatment in chronic pain conditions. Local anesthetic can provide several hours of relief and can aid in diagnosis or the ability to participate in physical therapy. Steroids can provide lasting relief in entrapment syndromes where pathology includes inflammation. Some of the common peripheral nerve blocks for chronic pain are described in this section.

Trigeminal nerve block

Trigeminal nerve blocks help reduce pain in trigeminal neuralgia. The trigeminal nerve and Gasserian ganglion are accessed via a similar approach for diagnostic and neurolytic blocks, as well as via radiofrequency ablation. With the patient supine, a long 20-gauge needle is inserted 2.5 cm lateral to the corner of the mouth. The needle is directed to the pupil of the eye, into the foramen ovale. Fluoroscopy and contrast are used to confirm position (Fig. 147.12).

Greater and lesser occipital nerve blocks

These blocks are usually performed using surface landmarks. The posterior occipital protuberance and the mastoid process are identified, and the injection sites aresites are at the one-third and two-thirds points on the line between these landmarks. The greater occipital nerve (mostly C2) is medial,

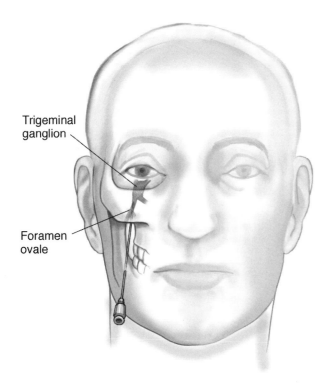

Figure 147.12. Trigeminal nerve block. Sagittal view of the Gasserian ganglion block.

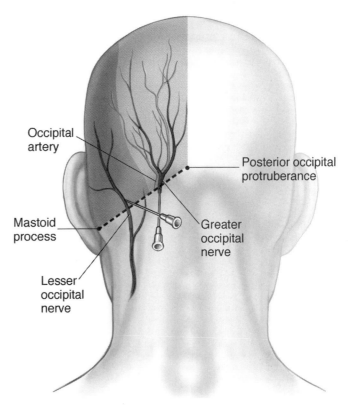

Figure 147.13. Occipital nerve blocks.

and the lesser occipital nerve (C2 or C3) is lateral. Care is taken to avoid the occipital artery by entering medial to the artery. Steroid and local anesthetic are typically injected. This procedure is performed to treat occipital headaches or occipital neuralgia. Tension-type headache may not respond to occipital nerve blocks (Fig. 147.13).

Cervical plexus block

Cervical plexus block provides analgesia to the head and neck region. Both superficial and deep cervical plexus can be blocked. The deep cervical blocks help with surgeries such as carotid endarterectomy and thyroid surgeries. These blocks also have a role in pain management of the upper extremity, including postoperative pain, pain from trauma, complex regional pain syndrome (CRPS), and neuropathic pain (Fig. 147.14).

Suprascapular nerve block

This block can be performed with landmarks or with fluoroscopy. A short, 22-gauge needle is directed to the suprascapular notch, at the location of the nerve. Steroid and local anesthetic are typically injected. This injection can be used for any painful condition of the shoulder, such as arthritis or adhesive capsulitis (Fig. 147.15).

Intercostal nerve block

An intercostal nerve block is an injection of a steroid or local anesthetic around the intercostal nerves that are located under each rib (Fig. 147.16). It is used to treat neuropathic chest pain

secondary to postthoracotomy syndrome, postherpetic neuralgia, and other neuropathic chest pain syndromes. This procedure can be performed blindly, under ultrasonography and fluoroscopy. Pneumothorax is a possible complication of which the physician should be cognizant during and after the procedure.

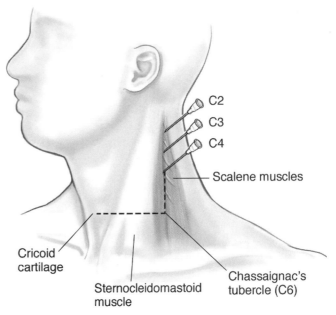

Figure 147.14. Cervical plexus block.

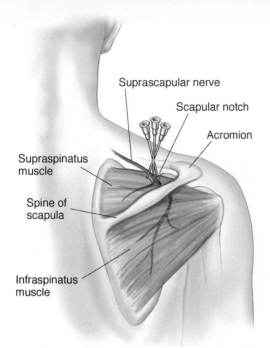

Figure 147.15. Suprascapular nerve block. Posterior view of blocking the suprascapular nerve.

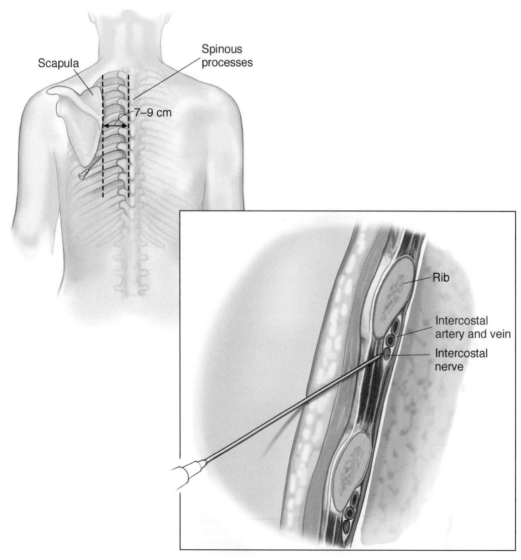

Figure 147.16. Intercostal nerve block.

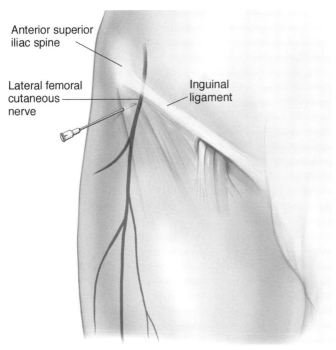

Figure 147.17. Lateral femoral cutaneous nerve block. Anterior view of the nerve block 2 cm below and medial to the anterior superior iliac spine.

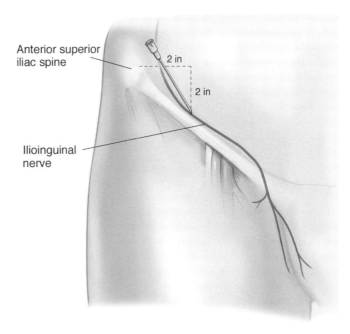

Figure 147.18. Ilioinguinal nerve block. Anterior view of the nerve block 2 inches below and medial to the anterior superior iliac spine over the inguinal ligament.

Paravertebral nerve block

Paravertebral block is an injection of local anesthetic adjacent to the vertebral body close to the exit of the spinal nerves from the intervertebral foramina. This injection causes both an ipsilateral somatic and sympathetic nerve blockade in multiple contiguous thoracic dermatomes above and below the site of injection. Indications include postoperative and surgical analgesia in breast, thoracic, renal, and abdominal surgeries. Other indications include fractured ribs and postherpetic neuralgia. The advantages include avoidance of thoracic epidural injection, low risk of pneumothorax, and multiple levels of analgesia with a single injection.

Lateral femoral cutaneous nerve block

With the patient supine, a 25-gauge short needle is directed 2 cm medial and 2 cm inferior to the anterior superior iliac spine, deep to fascia. A 10-ml volume of steroid and local anesthetic is injected in a field block pattern. This block is used to treat meralgia paraesthetica (Fig. 147.17).

Ilioinguinal and iliohypogastric nerve blocks

With the patient supine, a 25-gauge, 1.5-inch needle is inserted 2 inches medial and inferior to the anterior superior iliac spine, directed toward the symphysis pubis. When the needle enters the external oblique fascia a mixture of steroid and local anesthetic is injected in a field block pattern without violating the peritoneal cavity (Fig. 147.18). This block may be used in posthernia pain secondary to ilioinguinal neuropathy. Iliohypo-

gastric block is done in a similar fashion, but the needle entry point is 1 inch medial and below the anterior superior iliac spine (Fig. 147.19). The iliohypogastric and ilioinguinal nerves have overlapping cutaneous distributions (Fig. 147.20).

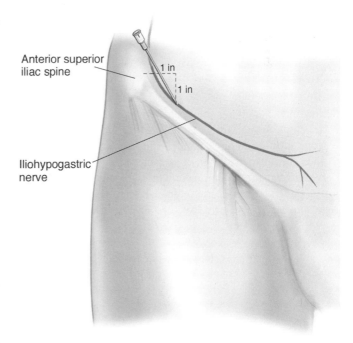

Figure 147.19. Iliohypogastric nerve block. Anterior view of the nerve block 1 inch below and medial to the anterior superior iliac spine over the inguinal ligament.

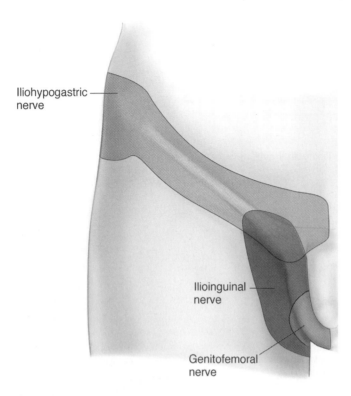

Figure 147.20. Overlapping dermatomes of the ilioinguinal, iliohypogastric, and genitofemoral nerves.

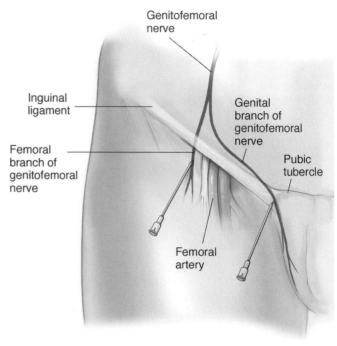

Figure 147.21. Genitofemoral nerve block. Anterior views of the nerve block at both the femoral and genital branches are shown.

Genitofemoral nerve block

With the patient supine, the genital branch is injected at the junction of the inguinal ligament and pubic tubercle. The femoral branch is injected below the midpoint of the inguinal ligament after avoiding the femoral artery. A mixture of local anesthetic and steroid is injected. This is typically done in post-hernia or scrotal pain (Fig. 147.21).

Pudendal nerve block

Pudendal nerve block provides analgesia to the S2 through S4 dermatomes supplying the anal, perineal, and genital areas. It can be performed transvaginally or transperineally by fluoroscopy, ultrasound or CT-guided approaches. The indications include chronic pelvic or perineal pain secondary to pudendal nerve entrapment or compression by sacrospinous ligament or in the pudendal canal. The pudendal nerve terminates in the right and left dorsal nerve of the penis. Penile nerve blocks provide analgesia in release of paraphimosis, dorsal slit of the foreskin, penile lacerations, and circumcisions.

Suggested readings

Ballantyne JC. *The Massachusetts General Handbook of Pain Management*. 3rd ed. Philadelphia: Lippincott Williams & Wilkins; 2006.

Brown DL. *Atlas of Regional Anesthesia*. Philadelphia: Elsevier; 2006.

Fenton DS, Czervionke LF. *Image-Guided Spine Intervention*. Philadelphia: Elsevier; 2003.

Lennard TA. *Pain Procedures in Clinical Practice*. 2nd ed. Philadelphia: Hanley & Belfus Inc.; 2000.

Rathmell JP. *Atlas of Image-Guided Intervention in Regional Anesthesia and Pain Medicine*. Philadelphia: Lippincott Williams & Wilkins; 2006.

Slipman CW, Derby R, Simeone FA, Mayer TG. *Interventional Spine: An Algorithmic Approach*. Philadelphia: Elsevier; 2008.

Waldman SD. *Atlas of Interventional Pain Management*. 2nd ed. Philadelphia: Elsevier; 2004.

Chapter 148

Interventional pain management II: implantable and other invasive therapies

Christian D. Gonzalez, Pradeep Dinakar, and Edgar L. Ross

Interventional techniques were developed to interrupt the transmission of pain. It makes the healing process more tolerable. The fundamentals of interventional pain medicine can be traced as far back as the American Civil War. During that time, Silas Weir Mitchell performed amputations of limbs that were extremely painful after nerve injury, a phenomenon he termed *causalgia*. In Europe it would be René Leriche who would follow Mitchell's steps during World War I. He based his hypothesis on sympathetic dysfunction as an etiology for causalgia.

Scientific advancements have allowed for the development of newer techniques to treat pain. The use of fluoroscopy and its advancements have created a more effective and safer practice. This chapter is dedicated to the discussion of more invasive and implantable techniques in the management of pain.

Medial branch nerve blocks

Medial branch nerve blocks (MBBs) are a diagnostic tool for the pain physician (Refer to figure in Chapter 147). With age, we develop arthritic changes of the spine. These changes are accelerated by trauma, obesity, weight lifting, and work-related stress on the facet joints. We start seeing degenerative changes in the spine by the third and fourth decade of life. The loss of cushion from the disc causes the facets to bear more weight. The end result is hypertrophied facets that can be painful. MBB is performed using just a local anesthetic or in combination with steroids to determine if the patient obtains pain relief. If the block is positive (there is pain relief), the patient is scheduled for radiofrequency lesioning (RFL) of the medial branch nerves. RFL gives a longer lasting pain relief than the block. The need to perform diagnostic blocks and the number of diagnostic blocks, if any, prior to the RFL are controversial. There are no adequate data to support either practice.

Intra-articular facet blocks

Intra-articular facet block involves the deposition of medications inside the facet joint (Refer to figure in Chapter 147). The drawback of performing these injections is the repetitive use of corticosteroids. Some practitioners argue, however, that it is a therapeutic injection and only requires one step. Others consider a positive finding enough of a criterion to performing RFL when the pain returns.

Sacroiliac joint injection

The sacroiliac joint is a major culprit of axial back pain, especially in the elderly population. These joints become degenerative and cause pain as the degeneration progresses. Imaging of the joint is not accurate in determining if the changes observed correlate with pain. Also, physical examination has been under debate to determine the most accurate test to diagnose sacroiliac joint pain. Most practitioners will agree that combinations of examinations, with or without imaging, are the best tool for the diagnosis. New studies show that tenderness to palpation over the sacroiliac joint may be the single most accurate examination. Others argue that, if it is suspected, a diagnostic/ therapeutic block can be performed (Fig. 148.1). If the pain worsens, then it can be repeated as necessary versus consideration of an RFL of the joint.

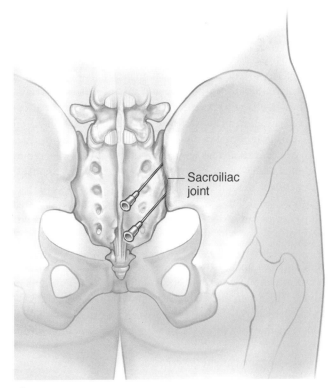

Figure 148.1. Sacroiliac joint injection.

Radiofrequency lesioning

Conventional RFL is used for many different therapies in the management of pain. Today it is mostly used for the treatment of axial back pain produced by facet arthropathy and sacroiliac joint arthropathy. After obtaining a positive diagnostic block, which is a reported pain relief of greater than 50% to 75%, the decision is made as to whether to proceed to RFL. This procedure is therapeutic and (at least in theory) gives pain relief for greater than 6 months, which is the nerve regeneration time. RFL causes the lesion by the passage of current from an active electrode in the tissue (insulated cannula with a bare tip) to the dispersive electrode (grounding pad/cannula). Voltage on the cannula generates an electric field around its tip. Heat is then generated in the tissue. The lesion size is dependent on the time, temperature, and tip diameter. The radius of the lesion increases until thermal equilibrium is reached. Monitoring the tip temperature enables control of the lesion size. The nervous tissue withstands temperatures up to 42.5flC, whereas temporary cessation of neural functions occurs at 42.5flC to 44flC. In conventional RFL, we cause permanent damage to the nerve by increasing the temperature to 80°C, thus causing thermal injury.

Pulsed RFL, in contrast, is used to treat facet joints, sacroiliac joints, dorsal root ganglion, stellate ganglion, Gasserian ganglion, and intervertebral discs. Pulsed RFL causes voltage fluctuations, but there is no heating of the tissue or tissue damage. Even though the exact mechanism of action of pulsed RFL is unknown, a presumed theory states that persistent increase of c-Fos expression in the dorsal horn neurons causes possible inhibition of the synaptic activation of the C fibers.

Vertebral body augmentation therapy

Indications are recent vertebral body compression fractures secondary to osteoporosis or malignancies that have failed conservative therapy. In both conditions there is skeletal disease that is characterized by low bone mass and architectural deterioration of bone tissue. These changes lead to an increase in bone fragility and increased susceptibility to fractures. It is estimated that approximately 44 million people in the United States are at high risk for vertebral body compression fractures. Ten million are related to osteoporosis, whereas the other 34 million are related to low bone mass. The vast majority of osteoporotic cases are in women, with a predominance of a 4:1 ratio. Fifty-five percent of this population at risk is older than 55 years. In 2002, the National Osteoporosis Foundation estimated that osteoporosis-related expenditures in the United States account for more than 20 billion dollars per year. Silverman and colleagues showed that approximately 20% of osteoporotic patients who have suffered a vertebral fracture in the past will present with another fracture within 1 year.

Evaluating the patient for vertebral body compression fracture involves a thorough history and physical examination.

Most patients can tolerate the acute period of the fracture and require no therapy. The first step in patient care is to allow 6 weeks of conservative therapy. The patient is given analgesics, usually opioids, and placed on minimal exercise recommendations. However, if after 2 weeks the patient is bedridden, in severe pain, or not tolerating the analgesics, then the therapy is recommended to prevent adverse outcomes. It is important to rule out any contraindications for treatment, including allergies, severe spinal stenosis, retropulsion of fracture fragments, or nerve root compromise. It is also important to obtain appropriate imaging. MRI with a STIR sequence is the imaging modality of choice. Acute inflammatory processes will be bright, whereas normal tissue and fat will be dark. This allows us to best determine the approximate time of injury (old vs. new fracture) and also the extent of inflammation in the area. If MRI is contraindicated, then a bone scan study would be the next option.

There is a debate between the use of a balloon to create a cavity for the injection of cement (kyphoplasty; Fig. 148.2) versus injection of the cement without a cavity (vertebroplasty; Fig. 148.3). The major difference between the two is the extravasation of cement, which is less common with the creation of a cavity. Also, a major advantage of using the balloon and creating the cavity is the thickness of the cement that can be injected. If no cavity is created, thin, liquefied cement is injected. Extravasation of cement intravascularly can cause unwanted major complications, including pulmonary embolism and death. Studies have shown that both procedures are effective in treating the fracture and pain. Recent randomized, controlled trials (RCTs) have not shown a significant long-term improvement between patients undergoing vertebroplasty and those undergoing sham procedures.

Discography

Discography is a study performed for the diagnosis of a suspected painful disc. It also serves as an anatomical study of the disc by using contrast and imaging the disc afterward. The main reason to use this study is to help determine which disc is causing the pain before the patient undergoes further therapy. Most practitioners use this technique prior to the patient having fusion surgery of the spine. Outcome studies show a better outcome from fusion surgery if the affected disc was first identified with the use of discography.

Some institutions inject a determined volume, some follow a pressure-guided study, and others inject until a painful response is obtained and compared this at other levels. With the development of newer technology, we can assess the opening disc pressure, volume injected, and changes in pressure during the study at different levels. If no concordant pain is achieved, it is a negative study. If there is concordant pain, it is a positive study and the level(s) affected is identified (Fig. 148.4). The outcomes from fusion surgery or other therapies improve if one single level is affected (vs. multiple level involvement).

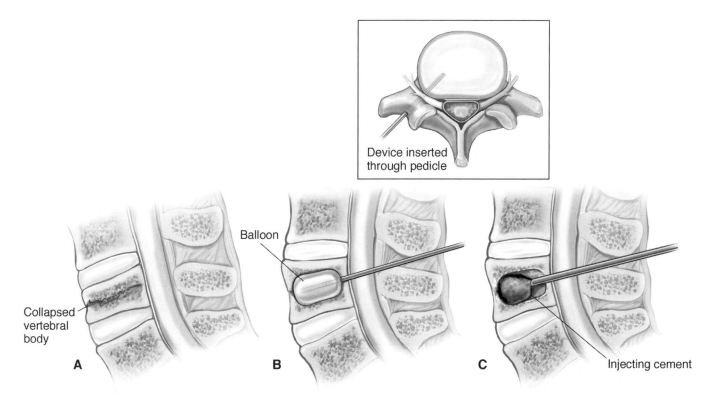

Device inserted through pedicle

Balloon

Collapsed vertebral body

Injecting cement

A   **B**   **C**

Figure 148.2. Kyphoplasty.

Intradiscal electrothermal therapy

Approved by the U.S. Food and Drug Administration (FDA) in 1998, more than 50,000 intradiscal electrothermal therapy (IDET) procedures have been performed to date. Periprocedural costs are less than one-fifth of those for fusion surgery. IDET works by causing thermal modification of the annular collagen fibers (Fig. 148.5). It is used for chronic discogenic back pain. Discogenic pathology must be established prior to performing the therapy. Candidates should (1) have failed at least 6 months of comprehensive conservative therapy and (2) be facing surgery as the sole therapeutic option. Two major RCT studies have shown that IDET is beneficial for patients who are younger than 50 years, have a lesser than 30% disc height loss, have no major disc herniation (>4 mm), do not have central canal stenosis, and have only one disc affected with a positive-concordant discogram.

Implantable therapies for pain

Implantable therapies have long held a role in the treatment of the most refractory pain patients. These therapies hold the promise of relief in well-selected patients, even when all other approaches have not been helpful. There are several different approaches that are selected based on clinical circumstances.

Figure 148.3. Vertebroplasty.

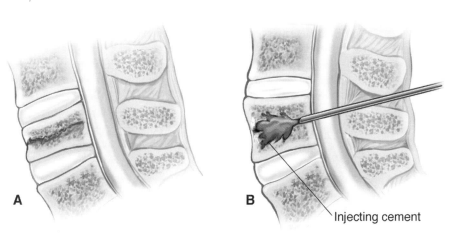

A   **B**   Injecting cement

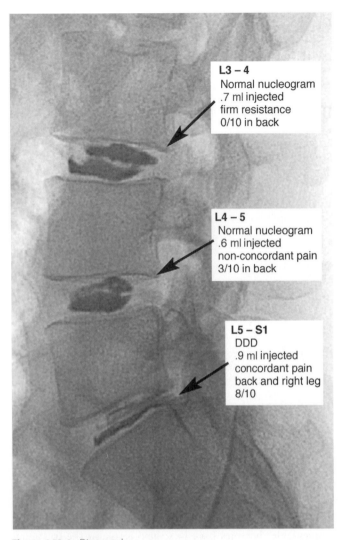

L3 – 4
Normal nucleogram
.7 ml injected
firm resistance
0/10 in back

L4 – 5
Normal nucleogram
.6 ml injected
non-concordant pain
3/10 in back

L5 – S1
DDD
.9 ml injected
concordant pain
back and right leg
8/10

Figure 148.4. Discography.

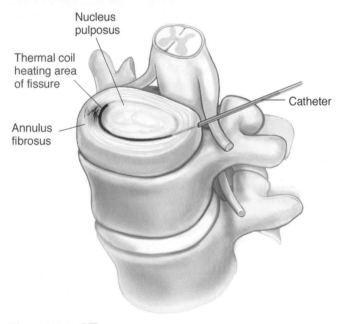

Nucleus
pulposus

Thermal coil
heating area
of fissure

Catheter

Annulus
fibrosus

Figure 148.5. IDET.

Epidural catheters

There are two types of epidural catheters and multiple techniques for implantation and anchoring. This is usually used in conditions requiring short-term analgesia. These catheters are tunneled subcutaneously a distance from the insertion site. Some epidural catheters have Dacron sleeves that reduce the incidence of infection migrating to the epidural space.

Subcutaneous reservoir or port-a-cath

This device consists of two parts: (1) a subcutaneous port attached to (2) a catheter, which is placed into either the epidural or intrathecal space. This procedure is indicated for either malignant or nonmalignant pain states after oral medications have proven ineffective. This procedure is generally reserved for intermediate-length therapy, particularly for patients with malignancies and less than 3 months of life expectancy. This procedure can also be used in the treatment of complex regional pain syndrome (CRPS), and can facilitate aggressive rehabilitation. The device can subsequently be removed after treatment has concluded. The procedure for catheter placement is identical to the one used for epidural or intrathecal catheter placement. The catheter is tunneled subcutaneously to a silicone access port, which is placed in a pocket over the anterior of the rib cage. This reservoir can be accessed percutaneously to provide either intermittent injections or continuous infusions of analgesics.

Intrathecal infusion pump implantation

There are two types of pumps: fixed flow and programmable. Fixed flow pumps are usually less costly and can hold more medication; however, dosing changes require pump refills. Programmable pumps can provide various programming options, including complex infusion programs. Dosing changes are easily done, with programmed increases in the pump's infusion rate. The indications for these pumps are refractory pain secondary to either malignant or nonmalignant pain in a patient who is not a candidate for surgical approach or has not responded to oral medications. Psychological screening is recommended. The placement of these infusion pumps is similar to catheter placements as described earlier in text. An additional step is required to surgically create a pocket, usually on the anterior abdominal wall. The spinal catheter is tunneled subcutaneously from the posterior site to the pump pocket and attached to the pump. Radiographs of pump and catheter are shown in Fig. 148.6.

Neurostimulation

Electrical stimulation of the central nervous system (CNS) has long been used for analgesia in neuropathic pain states. Electrodes can be used for both peripheral and central stimulation. Epidural placement of multielectrode arrays can be effective for a variety of conditions, including neuropathic pain syndromes and pain from vascular insufficiency. Electrodes have also been

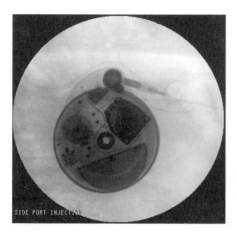 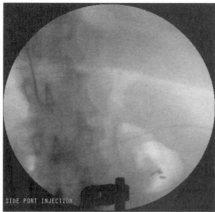

Figure 148.6. Programmable intrathecal pump and intrathecal catheter radiographs.

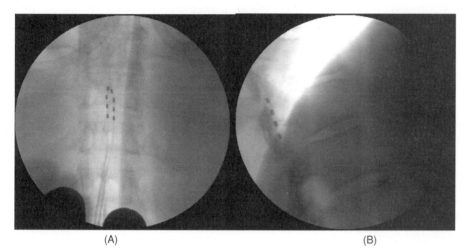

(A)   (B)

Figure 148.7. (**A**) Radiograph of thoracolumbar SCS leads. (**B**) Radiograph of lumbosacral leads.

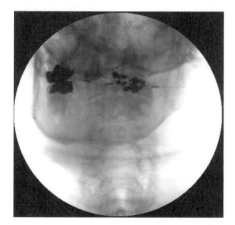

Figure 148.8. Occipital electrodes: anteroposterior view.

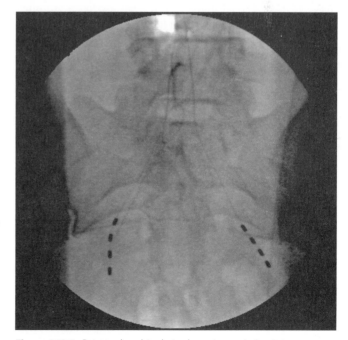

Figure 148.9. Retrograde pelvic electrodes: anteroposterior view.

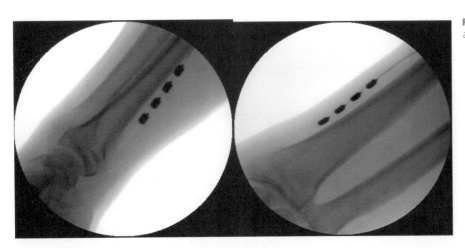

Figure 148.10. Peripheral nerve stimulator anteroposterior and lateral radiographs.

implanted along peripheral nerves, such as the median, radial, sciatic, tibial, and peroneal nerves. More recent approaches have used a suboccipital approach for occipital neuralgia and transsacral approaches for pelvic pain and bladder dysfunction. Deep brain stimulation has been used to a limited extent for various central pain syndromes and Parkinson's disease. To be effective, spinal cord electrodes must be placed in the epidural space. Intrathecal placement is painful and causes unwanted motor stimulation. The location of peripheral nerves determines placement of stimulating electrodes. Suboccipital electrodes are placed transversely in the subcutaneous tissue at the C1 or C2 level. Transsacral placement of electrodes relies on the visualization of sacral foramen.

Peripheral nerve stimulator placement requires visualization of the affected nerve. Either a percutaneous approach using a needle or a direct approach using a cut down to the nerve to allow the placement of a flat or paddle lead alongside the desired nerve is used. Fascial grafts in the open approach are often used to protect the nerve. For epidural stimulation, the placement of the electrode is similar to the placement of epidural catheters. Trial stimulation determines efficacy prior to implantation of the system. Fixation of the electrode is important to avoid movement. Two types of pulse generators exist: an external system that relies on radiofrequency current for power or a battery-operated implantable pulse generator (IPG). Recently, rechargeable systems have been introduced that have largely replaced radiofrequency units. The IPG is usually implanted in the buttock, over the greater trochanter, or in the abdominal wall (see Figs. 148.7–148.10).

Suggested readings

Aldrete JA. Extended epidural catheter infusions with analgesics for patients with noncancer pain at their homes. *Reg Anesth* 1997; 22(1):35–42.

Birkenmaier C, Veihelmann A, Trouillier HH, et al. Medial branch blocks versus pericapsular blocks in selecting patients for percutaneous cryodenervation of lumbar facet joints. *Reg Anesth Pain Med* 2007; 32(1):27–33.

Boswell MV, Colson JD, Sehgal N, et al. A systematic review of therapeutic facet joint interventions in chronic spinal pain. *Pain Physician* 2007; 10(1):229–253.

Eck JC, Nachtigall D, Humphreys SC, Hodges SD. Comparison of vertebroplasty and balloon kyphoplasty for treatment of vertebral compression fractures: a meta-analysis of the literature. *Spine J* 2008; 8(3):488–497.

Kumar K, Nath R, Wyant GM. Treatment of chronic pain by epidural spinal cord stimulation: a 10-year experience. *J Neurosurg* 1991; 75(3):402–407.

Martin DC, Willis ML, Mullinax LA, et al. Pulsed radiofrequency application in the treatment of chronic pain. *Pain Pract* 2007; 7(1):31–35.

Rainov NG, Heidecke V, Burkert W. Long-term intrathecal infusion of drug combinations for chronic back and leg pain. *J Pain Symptom Manage* 2001; 22(4):862–871.

Chapter 149

Complications associated with interventions in pain medicine

Christopher J. Gilligan and James P. Rathmell

Overview

As with virtually all medical treatments, interventions used to treat acute and chronic pain may result in complications. To prevent adverse outcomes during these treatments, it is essential to have detailed knowledge of the anatomy of the structures that lie near the target site for each intended treatment and a clear understanding of technical aspects of the procedure that are devised to minimize the risk of harm to these structures. The widespread use of fluoroscopy has increased both the precision and the safety of many techniques. When complications do arise, prompt recognition and treatment can often prevent serious sequelae. This chapter will review complications that may arise from common treatments used in pain medicine.

Complications associated with epidural, transforaminal, facet joint, and sacroiliac joint injections

Direct injection of local anesthetic, with or without long-acting corticosteroid suspensions, is widely used in the diagnosis and treatment of pain arising from spinal structures. Among the most common procedures are epidural steroid injections and transforaminal injections for radicular pain associated with acute lumbar disc herniation and spinal stenosis, zygapophyseal (facet) injections aimed at treating axial back pain associated with facet arthropathy, and sacroiliac (SI) joint injections for treatment of SI-related low back pain. The American Society of Anesthesiologists (ASA) maintains an ongoing surveillance of malpractice claims that have been settled through the ASA Closed Claims Project. A recent report stemming from this project detailed 114 complications associated with chronic pain treatment (Table 149.1). Neurotoxicity, direct neurologic injury, and the pharmacologic effects of corticosteroids have all been reported.

Neurotoxicity

The intrathecal injection of radiographic contrast, anesthetics, or steroids for meningeal inflammation from the breach of the spinal canal during surgery with or without direct neural injury can result in arachnoiditis or cauda equina syndrome. The typical signs and symptoms of arachnoiditis are shown in

Table 149.2. There is little evidence that any of the components of the available long-acting corticosteroid preparations are neurotoxic. Following the appearance of arachnoiditis during the intrathecal injection of methylprednisolone acetate, polyethylene glycol was suggested as the offending agent, which was subsequently disproved. It is important for practitioners to realize, however, that, despite their widespread use for epidural injection, these steroid preparations are not labeled for epidural use by the US Food and Drug Administration or any other regulatory agency. The concern regarding arachnoiditis appears to be limited to intrathecal administration (e.g., following inadvertent dural puncture in the course of attempted epidural placement). Thus, it is advisable to use all available means to avoid intrathecal injection of corticosteroid.

Neurologic injury

Direct mechanical injury to the spinal nerves or the spinal cord itself can occur during needle placement for epidural injection. The most common presentation of such nerve injuries is persistent paresthesia. Surprisingly, needle penetration into the cord is not always catastrophic and may even occur without the patient reporting symptoms. More significant injury occurs if there is subsequent bleeding into the spinal cord or if anything is injected through the needle into the parenchyma of the spinal cord. The risk of direct injury to the spinal cord is greatest when epidural injection is carried out at the high lumbar, thoracic, or cervical level with deep sedation; these patients are unable to report symptoms on needle contact with the cord. Large disc herniations at the level of the injection, which narrow or obliterate the epidural space anteriorly, displace the spinal cord

Table 149.1. Primary outcome for claims related to epidural steroid injections

Nerve injury	28
Infection	24
Death/Brain damage	9
Headache	20
Increased pain/No relief	10

Fitzgibbon DR, Posner KL, Caplan RA, et al. Chronic pain management: American Society of Anesthesiologists Closed Claims Project. *Anesthesiology* 2004; 100:98–105.

Table 149.2. Symptoms of adhesive arachnoiditis

Constant, burning pain in low back and legs
Urinary frequency and incontinence
Muscle spasm in the back and legs
Variable sensory loss
Variable motor dysfunction

posteriorly, predisposing the cord and dorsal root ganglion to injury (Fig. 149.1). Immediate neurosurgical consultation and diagnostic imaging are warranted in cases where injury to the spinal cord is suspected; consideration should be given to administration of a course of high-dose intravenous corticosteroids, as this approach has proven somewhat beneficial in reducing neuronal injury following blunt traumatic spinal cord injury.

Vascular injury

The most concerning risk of transforaminal injection is unintentional vascular injection of the steroid suspension.

Intravenous injection is an innocuous event during transforaminal injection; particulate steroid injected intravenously will simply be carried away from the site of inflammation, thus reducing any local anti-inflammatory effect. In contrast, intra-arterial injection is far less common, but may cause catastrophic neurologic injury. In the cervical spine, the vertebral artery, the ascending cervical artery, and the deep cervical artery all furnish spinal branches that enter the intervertebral foramina. These spinal branches supply the vertebral column but also give rise to radicular arteries that accompany the dorsal and ventral roots of the spinal nerves (Fig. 149.2). Frequently, anterior radicular arteries are of significant caliber and reinforce the anterior spinal artery. Such reinforcing arteries can occur at any cervical level, but appear to be more common at lower cervical levels. If particulate steroid is injected into a reinforcing radicular artery during transforaminal injection, infarction of the cervical spinal cord could ensue. Radicular arterial branches arising from the vertebral artery can also join the arterial supply that reaches the anterior spinal artery; it is possible that injectate placed within a radicular artery during

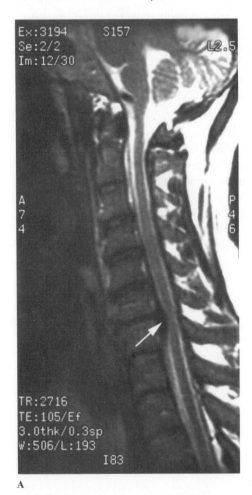

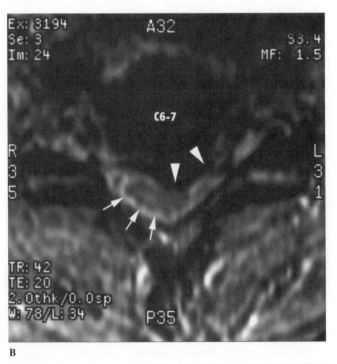

A   B

Figure 149.1. Cervical MRI of large disc herniation causing effacement of the epidural fat and CSF surrounding the spinal cord. (**A**) Midline sagittal, T2-weighted MRI showing large disc herniation at the C6/7 level (*arrow*) that effaces the epidural fat and CSF signal both anterior and posterior to the spinal cord. (**B**) Axial, T1-weighted MRI, showing a large central and left-sided disc herniation (*arrowheads*) displacing the spinal cord (*arrows*) to the right posterolateral limits of the spinal canal. (Reproduced with permission from Field J, Rathmell JP, Stephenson JH, Katz NP. Neuropathic pain following cervical epidural steroid injection. *Anesthesiology* 2000; 93:885–888.)

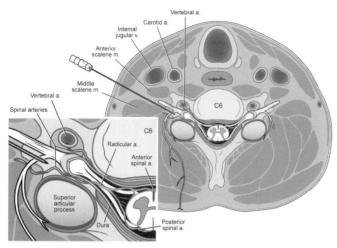

Figure 149.2. Axial view of cervical transforaminal injection at the level of C6. The needle has been inserted along the axis of the foramen and is in final position against the posterior aspect of the intervertebral foramen. Insertion along this axis places the needle behind the spinal nerve and behind the vertebral artery, which lies anterior to the foramen. *Inset:* A spinal artery arises from the vertebral column. It supplies the vertebral column. Another spinal artery enters the intervertebral foramen from the ascending cervical artery or deep cervical artery. It furnishes radicular branches that accompany the nerve roots and ultimately reach the anterior and posterior spinal arteries of the spinal cord. (Modified with permission from: Rathmell JP. *Atlas of Image-Guided Intervention in Regional Anesthesia and Pain Medicine.* 1st ed. Philadelphia: Lippincott Williams & Wilkins; 2006, Figure 6–1, p. 54.)

transforaminal injection could reach the vertebral artery via retrograde flow through an arterial anastomosis. If particulate steroid reaches the vertebral artery during transforaminal injection, infarction of the posterior circulation of the brain, including the cerebellum, could result. Published guidelines for performing cervical transforaminal injections are designed to prevent these complications (Table 149.3).

Epidural catheters are usually used in conditions requiring short-term analgesia The major vascular complication with lumbar transforaminal injections involves the reinforcing radicular artery, known as the artery of Adamkiewicz, which typically arises at thoracic levels but in 1% of individuals it arises as low as L2, and more rarely as low as the sacral levels. In patients with a low-lying radicular artery, the artery can be entered during lumbar transforaminal injections. The more frequently reported minor complications include transient headaches, increased back pain, facial flushing, increased leg pain, and vasovagal reaction.

Pharmacologic effects of corticosteroids

The administration of exogenous corticosteroids can lead to both hypercortisolism and suppression of the adrenal cortex's normal production of endogenous glucocorticoids. The long-acting corticosteroid preparations used for epidural steroid injection slowly release the active steroid over 1 to 3 weeks. Fluid retention, weight gain, increased blood pressure, congestive heart failure, and Cushingoid side effects have been reported after epidural steroid injections. Glucocorticoid administration reduces the effect of insulin and results in increased blood glucose levels and insulin requirements in diabetics for 48 to 72 hours. Although rare, allergic reaction to systemic administration of corticosteroid has also been documented.

Bleeding complications

Epidural injection for pain treatment carries the risk of epidural or subdural bleeding in patients without any apparent coagulopathy. Significant bleeding within the epidural space can cause compression of neural structures, potentially resulting in paraplegia or quadriplegia. The risks of neuraxial injections for pain treatment in patients taking anticoagulants are similar to those in such patients receiving perioperative epidural analgesia. Epidural injection of steroids should be avoided in patients receiving systemic anticoagulants (e.g., coumadin or heparin) or potent antiplatelet agents (e.g., clopidogrel or ticlopidine). Nonsteroidal anti-inflammatory drugs (NSAIDs), including aspirin, do not appear to increase the risk of epidural hematoma formation due to epidural injection.

Infectious complications

Injection therapy for pain treatment carries a small risk of both superficial and deep infection, including neuraxial infection, such as epidural abscess, which has potentially devastating complications, including permanent sensory and motor deficits and bladder and bowel dysfunction. Table 149.4 shows a recent review of epidural abscess following various types of epidural steroid injections. Other complications include meningitis, osteomyelitis, and septic arthritis of the facet joints. Considerations regarding sterile technique and use of disinfectant solutions are similar to those recommended for single-shot regional anesthetic techniques performed in the perioperative period. Most experts recommend the use of an iodine-based skin

---

Table 149.3. Preventing complications during cervical transforaminal injection

- Advance the needle using fluoroscopic guidance from an anterior oblique approach.
- Ensure that the needle remains over the superior articular process along the posterior aspect of the intervertebral foramen. The vertebral artery lies anterior to the foramen. Keeping the needle posterior avoids risk of penetrating the vertebral artery.
- Use anteroposterior radiography to adjust final needle depth. Do not advance the needle more than 50% across the medial-lateral dimension of the foramen to avoid penetrating the dural sleeve.
- Once the needle is in final position, inject a small volume of radiographic contrast under "live" or "real-time" fluoroscopy to ensure that injection into an artery does not occur. Digital subtraction angiography is a fluoroscopic technique that offers advantages over conventional fluoroscopy by subtracting out the overlying radiodense structures and improving visualization of contrast spread.

Rathmell JP, Aprill C, Bogduk N. Cervical transforaminal injection of steroids. *Anesthesiology* 2004; 100(6):1595–1600.

Table 149.4. Data regarding cases of epidural abscess following epidural steroid injections

Total number of cases	15
Onset ≤1 wk	9
Onset >1 wk	6
Patients with diabetes	5
Caudal epidural injection	1
Lumbar epidural injection	10
Thoracic epidural injection	1
Cervical epidural injection	3
Required laminectomy	11
Deaths	2
Residual motor dysfunction	5

Huang RC, Shapiro GS, Lim M, Sandhu HS, Lutz GE, Herzog RJ. Cervical epidural abscess after epidural steroid injection. *Spine (Phila Pa 1976)* 2004; 29(1):E7–9; Hooten WM, Kinney MO, Huntoon MA. Epidural abscess and meningitis after epidural corticosteroid injection. *Mayo Clin Proc* 2004; 79(5):682–686.

preparation solution, routine use of sterile drapes and gloves, and strong consideration of use of face masks and hats. Routine use of preprocedure antibiotics does not appear to be warranted in the majority of single-shot spinal and perispinal injections. Pain practitioners should establish written postprocedural instructions for their patients that provide a clear description of the signs and symptoms of evolving infection and a clear process for contacting pain clinic personnel in the event of any worrisome signs or symptoms. Whereas some isolated paraspinous infections have been treated with needle aspiration, most will require open surgical incision and drainage along with the administration of systemic antibiotics.

Complications associated with sympathetic blocks

Sympathetic blocks, including stellate ganglion, celiac plexus, and lumbar sympathetic blocks, have been used for more than half a century. The various complications described earlier in this chapter, including neurotoxicity, neurologic injury, vascular injury, bleeding, and infectious complications, also apply to sympathetic blocks. The specific complications that are associated with these blocks are described in the following sections.

Stellate ganglion block

Complications from stellate ganglion block can arise from vascular complications, unintended nerve blocks, epidural or intrathecal injection, or inadvertent injury to the surrounding structures.

Several arteries and veins lie in close proximity to the intended injection site, the anterior tubercle of C6 or C7. Intravenous injections into the neck veins do not commonly result in sequelae because the low volume and concentration of local anesthetic do not produce a toxic effect. In contrast, intraarterial injections can give rise to catastrophic complications. Vertebral artery injections can occur when the needle is inserted too medially and posteriorly. The practitioner typically contacts

bone, but mistakes the posterior tubercle for the anterior tubercle. Slight withdrawal of the needle from the posterior tubercle, particularly if in a medial position, can lead to vertebral artery injection. The carotid artery and the spinal radicular artery also lie near the needle path during a stellate ganglion block. Intraarterial injections can cause seizures or embolic stroke of the brain. Complications of aspiration during a seizure can be minimized by maintaining an NPO status prior to the procedure. The embolic stroke complication can be minimized by not using particulate steroids during a stellate block, given the lack of evidence suggesting added benefit with steroids.

Unintended block of the cervical spinal nerves, recurrent laryngeal nerve, phrenic nerve, and brachial plexus are more commonly seen complications associated with the stellate block. Cervical spinal nerves traversing the intervertebral foramen near the location for a stellate ganglion block results in a selective cervical motor and sensory nerve root block. Recurrent laryngeal and phrenic nerve blocks are frequent side effects of stellate ganglion block. They occur from local anesthetic injection that spreads from the area of the ganglion. Because diffusion of drug is required to obtain a satisfactory block, it can be expected that these nerves will often be temporarily blocked. Symptoms of a recurrent laryngeal nerve block include hoarseness and, occasionally, stridor. Patients often complain of difficulty in catching their breath and the sensation of a lump in their throats. Symptomatic treatment is sufficient along with reassurance that these sensations will resolve when the local anesthetic effect ends. Patients should be cautioned to drink clear liquids initially after a stellate ganglion block to make sure that their upper airway reflexes are not compromised. When they feel comfortable swallowing liquids, they can progress to regular food. Unilateral phrenic nerve block rarely presents as a problem for patients unless they have preexisting severe respiratory compromise. The potential for producing phrenic nerve block is one reason why bilateral stellate ganglion blocks are rarely performed simultaneously. Most practitioners wait several days or a week between injections. Horner's syndrome is often observed following a stellate ganglion block. Horner's syndrome is, theoretically, a side effect, because a stellate ganglion block is most commonly performed for patients with upper extremity pain (to establish the diagnosis of sympathetically mediated pain [SMP] or therapeutically for complex regional pain syndrome [CRPS] type I or II). Horner's syndrome consists of miosis, ptosis, and enophthalmos. In fact, many practitioners look for Horner's syndrome as evidence of sympathetic denervation following stellate ganglion injection of local anesthetic. Brachial plexus block can occur following a stellate ganglion injection and occurs most commonly when the needle has been inserted too deep, bypasses the anterior tubercle, and rests on the posterior tubercle. After retraction from the posterior tubercle, the injection of local anesthetic will commonly block one or more of the roots of the brachial plexus.

Intrathecal injection of local anesthetic at this site typically produces a total spinal block accompanied by loss of airway reflexes and phrenic nerve function. Intubation and assisted ventilation will be required until the block abates. The duration of the block depends on the drug and the total dose injected. Verbal reassurance of the patient can further calm fears and assure him or her that the effects experienced are temporary.

The pleural dome of the lung extends variably above the first rib. Most commonly, this dome passes laterally to the intended C6 injection site for the stellate ganglion block. Pneumothorax can result despite careful attention to anatomy and technique, and patients should be warned of this potential complication prior to a posterior approach to the sympathetic chain or stellate ganglion. Paratracheal hematoma causing airway obstruction and death has been reported as a complication of stellate ganglion block. Infections are uncommon following stellate ganglion injections, but there are case reports of cervical vertebral osteomyelitis. Other rare complications include transient locked-in syndrome following the stellate ganglion block.

Celiac plexus block and lumbar sympathetic block

Complications that have been reported include intravascular injection, intraspinal injection, infection (including discitis), postdural puncture headache, and hematoma formation.

On the left side of the spine, the aorta lies close to the needle-placement site. The inferior vena cava lies near the placement site for needles on the right side. Large volumes of local anesthetic, particularly bupivacaine, can cause seizures and/or cardiovascular collapse if injected into either vessel. Resuscitation can be prolonged and difficult, especially in cases where bupivacaine is injected. Careful, frequent aspiration and intermittent injection are recommended. If the solution contains epinephrine, changes in heart rate may serve as a warning sign of intravascular injection.

Accidental lumbar nerve root block, epidural, intrathecal, or intraspinal injections occur rarely now that fluoroscopy is more commonly used. The intervertebral disc lies near the path of a lumbar sympathetic block needle. Unintentional injury to the disc usually does not cause any complications. Occasionally it can cause discitis. Postdural puncture headache after a lumbar sympathetic block has been reported, most likely occurring as a result of the needle passing near a nerve root sleeve that contained spinal fluid. Severe bleeding, including both subcutaneous and retroperitoneal hematomas, have been reported. Considerations for performing these blocks in patients taking antiplatelet or anticoagulant medications are similar to those proposed for performing neuraxial blockade.

Complications associated with neurolytic blockades

Chemical neurolytic blockade

Neurolytic blocks are performed in patients with severe pain secondary to advanced cancer or occlusive vascular disease. Their use in nonmalignant chronic pain (e.g., chronic relapsing pancreatitis) remains controversial. The potential complications of neurolytic blockade can be devastating to the patient and must be carefully weighed against the anticipated benefits.

The different types of neurolytic blocks include local injections, peripheral nerve blocks, lumbar sympathetic blocks, celiac plexus blocks, and epidural and intrathecal blocks. Neurolytic blocks can be done using ethyl alcohol, phenol, or hypertonic saline.

Local complications of neurolytic blocks include skin and subcutaneous tissue necrosis and sloughing secondary to vascular damage and ischemia. Peripheral neurolytic blocks are rarely performed because they can cause motor deficit when mixed nerves are blocked. Neuritis and deafferentation pain are potential consequences, and the block is not predictably permanent. Anesthesia dolorosa is also seen as a complication in neurolytic blocks. Neuraxial blocks can result in prolonged motor and sensory blocks, bladder and bowel dysfunction, and saddle-shaped anesthesia. Systemic complications can result from any of the blocks and include hypotension, central nervous system (CNS) excitation, and cardiovascular collapse.

Neurolytic celiac plexus block (NCPB) has been shown to be an effective analgesic technique for management of pain in patients with intra-abdominal malignancies, particularly pancreatic cancer. Celiac plexus block using a transcrural approach places the local anesthetic or neurolytic solution in direct contact with the celiac ganglion anterolateral to the aorta. In contrast, splanchnic nerve block or retrocrural technique avoids the risk of penetrating the aorta, uses smaller volumes of solution, and is unlikely to be affected by anatomic distortion caused by extensive tumor of the pancreas or metastatic lymphadenopathy. Many of the minor complications of NCPB are the result of effective sympathetic block due to neurolysis of the celiac ganglia. Neurolytic blockade of these sympathetic structures results in the relative increase in parasympathetic tone to the splanchnic region. Subsequent vasodilation of the splanchnic vasculature can result in orthostatic hypotension. Bowel hypermotility causes diarrhea. Major complications – significant neurologic deficits, such as loss of sensation or motor function of the lower extremities, or vascular events, including uncontrolled bleeding, arterial dissection, or injury to the artery of Adamkiewicz – are extremely uncommon. Hematuria and pneumothorax are complications from incorrect needle trajectory or placement. Acetaldehyde dehydrogenase deficiency resulting in sensitivity to ethanol has been reported. Following ethanol injection, individuals with aldehyde dehydrogenase deficiency have increased systemic levels of acetaldehyde causing skin flushing, nausea, headache, tachycardia, hypotension, and drowsiness.

In the event of a major vascular complication, such as significant arterial bleeding or aortic dissection, immediate radiographic imaging coupled with emergent surgical evaluation is recommended. If neurologic deficits occur during the NCPB, emergent consultation with a neurologist is indicated. There are no known remedies for relieving arterial spasm after it has occurred, but at least one case of transient paraplegia following NCPB has been reported and attributed to arterial spasm.

Cryoneurolytic blockade

Cryoneurolysis uses a low temperature to create nerve injury resulting in long-lasting analgesia. The mechanism of nerve injury is unclear. Given the intact nerve sheaths, the nerves tend to slowly regenerate and pain returns to baseline. The complications associated with cryolesioning are secondary to improper insertion of the cryoprobe and thermal injury. Frostbite and ulcerations are the more common complications. When mixed nerves are cryolesioned, reversible paresthesias and motor deficits are not uncommon.

Radiofrequency neurolytic blockade

Radiofrequency (RF) generators use high-frequency waves in the range of 300 to 500 kHz to produce tissue lesions via ionic means. Because high frequencies in this range are also used in radio transmitters, the current was named RF current. Conventional RF treatment uses a constant output of high-frequency electric current, produces controllable tissue destruction surrounding the tip of the treatment cannula, and, when placed at precise anatomic locations, has demonstrated success in reducing a number of different chronic pain states, including facet arthropathy, whiplash injury, and trigeminal neuralgia. Pulsed RF, in contrast, uses brief pulses of high-voltage, RF range (~300 kHz) electrical current that produce the same voltage fluctuations in the region of treatment that occur during conventional RF treatment, but without heating to a temperature at which tissue coagulates. Conventional wisdom holds that the usefulness of RF stems from the ability to produce a small lesion of precise dimensions in a specific anatomic location.

Despite the widespread use of RF thermoablation for facet-related pain, there are limited data regarding the safety of this technique and its associated complications. As may occur with any technique that requires needle placement, complications may result from direct injury to neural or vascular structures in the vicinity of treatment or from thermal destruction during the RF treatment.

The anatomic configuration of the sensory nerves to the facet joints allows safe destruction without damage to the sensory or motor nerves to the extremities. Precise radiographic guidance allows placement of the RF cannula, and lesions can be produced without affecting the anterior primary ramus, which supplies the sensory and motor innervation to the trunk and extremities (Fig. 149.3). Thermal injury caused by incorrect positioning of the RF cannula has also been reported. Even with proper technique, conventional RF lesions are associated with sensory loss and onset of neuropathic pain in a subset of patients secondary to either direct tissue, periosteal, or spinal nerve injury. The frequency and severity of these neural changes vary with the specific site of treatment, and are common after intracranial RF lesioning of the trigeminal ganglion. Injury to adjacent nerves can also occur; the frequency of these complications is minimized by the proper use of sensory and motor stimulation before lesioning.

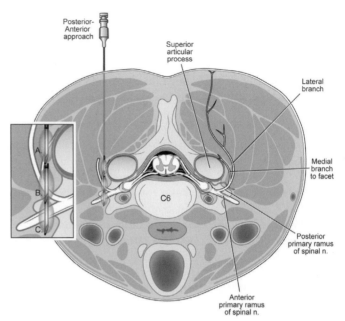

Figure 149.3. Mechanism of complications that arise during lumbar RF medial branch neurotomy. Axial diagram of lumbar RF medial branch neurotomy. A 22-gauge, 10-cm RF cannula with a 5-mm active tip is advanced just anterior to the base of the transverse process where it joins with the superior articular process. (**A**) An RF cannula in correct position for lumbar RF medial branch neurotomy. The point of bifurcation of the posterior primary ramus of the spinal nerve into medial and lateral branches is variable, and conventional RF treatment commonly destroys both nerves. The medial branch supplies sensation to the facet joint, and the lateral branch provides motor innervation to the paraspinous musculature and a small and variable patch of sensory innervation to the skin overlying the spinous processes. (**B**) Neurolysis of the lateral branch does not have any demonstrable effect on strength of the paraspinous muscles; however, cutaneous hyperesthesia and/or hypoesthesia do occur infrequently. (**C**) Placement of the RF lesion directly on the anterior primary ramus of the spinal nerve can cause severe and persistent radicular pain. (Reproduced with permission from: Neal JM, Rathmell JP. *Complications in Regional Anesthesia and Pain Medicine*. Philadelphia: Saunders Elsevier; 2007, Figure 29–3, p. 295.)

The most common complications associated with cervical medial branch neurotomy include postoperative pain (97%); ataxia, unsteadiness, and spatial disorientation (23%); and vasovagal syncope (2%) (Table 149.5). Lord found that brief postoperative pain was the only side effect of lower cervical procedures, but ataxia occurred when the third occipital nerve was treated. Because the third occipital nerve carries a large proportion of fibers involved in cutaneous innervation, numbness routinely accompanies lesioning of this nerve. In patients whose treatment was successful, this numb patch regressed over 1 to 3 weeks and was replaced by dysesthesia and pruritus, followed by the return of normal cutaneous sensation and pain. The incidence of expected treatment-related adverse effects and complications associated with lumbar RF medial branch neurotomy is markedly lower than that observed following treatment at cervical levels.

Major complications have been described mainly in the form of case reports. Serious complications appear to be rare, and the available data prevent meaningful systematic analysis.

Table 149.5. Observed complications of cervical medial branch neurotomy

Complication	Observed frequency, %	95% CI, %
Vasovagal syncope	2	0–6
Postoperative pain	97	94–100
Ataxia, unsteadiness, spatial disorientation	23	14–32
Cutaneous numbness		
TON procedures	88	75–100
C3/4 procedures	80	55–100
Lower levels	19	8–30
Dysesthesias		
TON procedures	56	37–75
C3/4 procedures	30	2–58
Lower levels	17	6–27
Dermoid cyst	1	0–4
Transient neuritis	2	0–6

CI, confidence interval; TON, third occipital nerve.
Lord SM, Bogduk N. Radiofrequency procedures in chronic pain. *Best Pract Res Clin Anaesthesiol* 2002; 16:597–617.

Minor burns due to insulation breaks in electrodes and improper function of grounding pads have been reported. There is no evidence of any significant risk of infection, hemorrhage, or neurologic deficit.

Separate consideration should be given to the emerging use of pulsed RF techniques that do not cause neurodestruction. Complications with this type of neurolysis are limited to direct needle injury and not thermal injury, because the temperature is not high enough to cause nerve damage. Despite the enthusiasm for pulsed RF because it does not appear to be neurodestructive, the nature and extent of lesions made by these methods have not been described, and little evidence has been published to demonstrate their efficacy.

Most sequelae following RF medial branch neurotomy are self-limited and require nothing more than reassurance and time to resolve. Patients should be warned to expect a transient increase in pain for several days to weeks following treatment. Providing a brief course of oral analgesics can obviate unnecessary return visits. If new-onset radicular pain with or without allodynia appears, spinal nerve injury should be suspected, and oral neuropathic pain treatment with a tricyclic antidepressant or anticonvulsant should be started. Localized allodynia described as a sunburn sensation is common, particularly following RF treatment of the high cervical medial branch nerves. Topical 5% lidocaine patches can prove invaluable for symptomatic management in these cases, which also tend to resolve within days to weeks of treatment. Persistent numbness is also common and rarely requires specific treatment.

Complications associated with implantable therapies for pain

Subcutaneous reservoirs or port-a-cath

Complications are similar to those described for tunneled intrathecal or epidural catheters. There is a 1% to 5% reported risk of infection. As in any external infusion system, late-onset neuraxial infection is a constant risk and appropriate care is required. The presentation of an epidural abscess with the potential of spinal cord compression requires appropriate clinical vigilance. Minor complications can include pocket seromas, hygromas, and spinal headaches from cerebrospinal fluid (CSF) leaks. Inadvertent intrathecal placement may lead to inappropriately high doses of medication. Spinal cord injury and unrecognized catheterization of epidural veins can lead to inadvertent intravascular injection of local anesthetic into the epidural veins. Because of the delayed onset of epidural hydromorphone hydrochloride and morphine, respiratory depression many hours after injection has been reported. Spinal opiates can cause nausea and vomiting, urinary retention, pruritus, sedation, and respiratory depression. These side effects are usually transient and can be symptomatically treated.

Intrathecal infusion pump implantation

Complications are similar to the complications seen with the epidural port-a-cath. Additional complications associated with high-dose opioids are intrathecal granulomas. The incidence of these is not well established, but vigilance is needed to avoid potential devastating spinal cord compression and permanent neurologic changes. Complications involving refilling these pumps include inadvertent side port injections, especially in older pumps that lack safety screens. This mistake may deliver a fatal intrathecal dose of medication initially starting with respiratory and cardiovascular collapse and finally death if left unrecognized and untreated.

Neurostimulation

Specific complications from stimulators depend on the location of the device. Spinal cord injuries from misplaced epidural leads can occur during the procedure or later if dural erosion occurs. Risks from surgical infections are present and are similar in incidence to those from the other implantable devices. Fractured electrodes are the most common complications requiring replacement. Programming errors resulting in painful stimulation are temporary and rarely have long-term consequences. Caution with a turned on stimulator while driving should be discussed with the patient. This problem occurs particularly early after surgery while the stimulation still varies with body position. Lead displacement is also possible and can lead to the need for surgical revision to establish effective stimulation.

Summary

There is a low incidence of serious complications associated with the majority of interventional techniques currently in use for the treatment of chronic pain. Careful history and physical examination will help to identify risk factors such as diabetes, immunosuppression, coagulopathy, and occult infection. Knowledge of the anatomy relevant to each treatment technique and coupling this knowledge with meticulous use of radiographic guidance can minimize complications. The use of intravenous sedation during these procedures remains controversial. While modest levels of sedation that allow the patient to communicate verbally with the operator throughout the procedure seem reasonable, the use of heavy sedation or general anesthesia that compromises verbal communication with the patient is imprudent. Patients should be informed of the most serious complications as well as common minor complications, such as accidental dural puncture and postdural puncture headache. They should be instructed to report promptly any neurologic changes, new or increasing pain, headache, and fever. There are several complications that arise in the course of pain treatment that, when recognized and treated early in their course, may well result in less catastrophic outcomes; foremost among these are evolving epidural abscess and hematoma. A system of night and weekend coverage should be available, and patients should be instructed how to contact the on-call physician, such that any adverse sequelae of these treatment techniques can be promptly recognized and treated.

Suggested readings

Abram SE. The use of epidural steroid injections for the treatment of lumbar radiculopathy. *Anesthesiology* 1999; 91:1937–1941.

Delport EG, Cucuzella AR, Marley JK, et al. Treatment of lumbar spinal stenosis with epidural steroid injections: a retrospective outcome study. *Arch Phys Med Rehabil* 2004; 85:479–484.

Fitzgibbon DR, Posner KL, Caplan RA, et al. Chronic pain management: American Society of Anesthesiologists Closed Claims Project. *Anesthesiology* 2004; 100:98–105.

Lord SM, Bogduk N. Radiofrequency procedures in chronic pain. *Best Pract Res Clin Anaesthesiol* 2002; 16:597–617.

Neal JM, Rathmell JP. *Complications in Regional Anesthesia and Pain Medicine*. Philadelphia: Saunders Elsevier; 2006.

Rathmell JP. *Atlas of Image-Guided Intervention in Regional Anesthesia and Pain Medicine*. 1st ed. Philadelphia: Lippincott Williams & Wilkins; 2006.

Standards Committee of the International Spine Intervention Society. Cervical transforaminal injection of corticosteroids. In: Bogduk N (ed.). *Practice Guidelines for Spinal Diagnostic and Treatment Procedures*. San Francisco: International Spine Intervention Society; 2004:237–248.

Chapter 150

Back pain

John C. Keel

Introduction

Painful disorders of the spine are some of the most frequently encountered conditions in the pain clinic. Back pain is also a leading cause of any type of medical visit. In particular, low back pain is one of the most common medical complaints, thereby accounting for millions of primary care physician visits annually, and is a leading factor in disability and lost productivity. This chapter focuses on basic concepts of low back pain, including specific definitions, functional anatomy, epidemiology, and natural history. An overview of diagnosis and treatment is included and will be discussed in more detail in other chapters.

Definitions

The technical term for low back pain is *lumbosacral spinal pain*. The International Association for the Study of Pain (IASP) has defined spinal pain based on the perceived location of pain. Lumbosacral spinal pain can arise from the lumbar or sacral spine (Fig. 150.1). *Lumbar spinal pain* originates in an area of the low back below the T12 spinous process, above the S1 spinous process, and medial to the lateral borders of the erector spinae muscles. *Sacral spinal pain* originates in the sacrum below the S1 spinous process, above the sacrococcygeal joints, and medial to a line between the posterior superior and inferior iliac spines.

Radicular pain is closely associated with lumbosacral spinal pain. Lumbosacral radicular pain is perceived as arising from the lower limbs due to ectopic activation of sensory fibers at a spinal root level. Radicular pain is typically distributed in a bandlike dermatomal pattern corresponding to the affected spinal nerve (Fig. 150.1) and is distinguished from *radiculopathy*, which requires a focal neurologic deficit in the distribution of a spinal nerve. *Neurogenic claudication* is intermittent pain in the buttock, thigh, or leg, exacerbated by prolonged walking or standing. Neurogenic claudication is due to stenosis of the central spinal canal.

Epidemiology and risk factors

Epidemiologic studies of back pain report varying numbers of incidence and prevalence, but studies confirm that lumbosacral spinal pain is a widespread medical condition. As many as 50% to 80% of adults experience at least one significant episode of low back pain in their lifetime. In a single year, 15% to 20% will have back pain, and 2% to 5% of the entire population will seek medical attention for back pain. One fifth of all physician visits may be prompted by low back pain. Back pain affects children, adolescents, and adults. Among older adults, back pain is more prevalent in women than in men. Back pain has less prevalence with advanced age, decreasing in women older than 85 years and men older than 90 years. Low back pain is the most common cause of disability in persons younger than 45 years and is the third leading cause in other age groups. Up to 1% of the population is disabled at any time due to low back pain. Approximately 25% of workers' compensation costs are due to low back pain. As a leading cause of absenteeism, temporary disability, lost productivity, and workers' compensation claims, back pain has a great cost to society.

Numerous risk factors for low back pain have been described (Table 150.1). Recurrent episodes of back pain and a history of back pain strongly predict recurrence. New-onset back pain is most common in the third decade of life, and incidence rates are highest in the third through sixth decades.

Table 150.1. Risk factors for back pain

Demographic factors
Age
Gender
Socioeconomic status and education level

Health factors
Body mass index (BMI)
Tobacco use
Perceived general health status

Occupational factors
Physical activity, such as bending, lifting, or twisting
Monotonous tasks
Job dissatisfaction

Psychologic factors
Depression

Spinal anatomy factors
Anatomic variations
Imaging abnormalities

Rubin DI. Epidemiology and risk factors for spine pain. *Neurol Clin* 2007; 25(2):353–371.

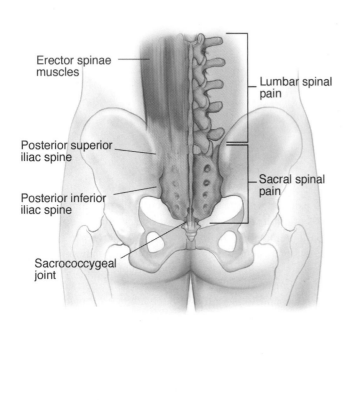
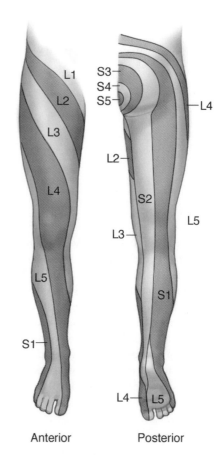

Anterior   Posterior

Figure 150.1. Lumbosacral spinal and radicular pain.

Women may be more likely to seek medical care for back pain and develop chronic back pain. Lower socioeconomic status and level of education are associated with markedly increased rates of disability due to back pain. Body mass index greater than 30 is a risk factor for back pain, especially in women. Smoking may be a risk factor for back pain, but studies have not clearly identified it as being independent of other associated factors. Patients with chronic back pain are approximately six times more likely to have depression, and patients with depression are twice as likely to develop back pain. Anatomic risk factors for back pain may include congenital and acquired abnormalities of the spine, but evidence is conflicting, as many subjects have such abnormalities but do not have pain. For example, several studies have demonstrated a high incidence of lumbar disc abnormalities in asymptomatic individuals.

A third or more episodes of low back pain are related to occupational risk factors. Conditions involving heavy lifting; bending or twisting of the back; long-term static positions, such as sitting, prolonged standing, or walking; or low-frequency, whole-body vibration may be risk factors for back pain. Perception of high physical demand may be more of a risk factor than actual demand. Workplace dissatisfaction may be a significant risk factor. A study of a large population of aircraft employees revealed that subjects who had low work satisfaction were 2.5 times more likely to report a back injury than were those who had high job satisfaction.

Natural history

Acute low back pain is usually a self-limited episode that will resolve without intervention. Approximately half of disabling episodes recover in 2 weeks, 70% are recovered by 4 to 6 weeks, and 90% are recovered by 12 weeks. The definition of *chronic* low back pain is typically pain that has persisted for 3 months. Fewer that half of patients who have disabling back pain for 6 months will return to work. Almost none who experience disabling back pain for 2 years ever return to work.

Several age-related and mechanical changes in the spine are important in understanding the development of low back pain. The intervertebral discs lose water content with age, which is associated with loss of disc height. Repeated loading may lead to circumferential tears in the annulus fibrosus, also known as *internal disc disruption*. Such tears may be painful in themselves, as they occur most often in the posterior outer third of the disc, known to have sensory innervation. Internal disc disruption weakens the annulus and may allow herniation of the nucleus pulposus. The lumbar facet joints may develop synovitis, then articular surface degradation, capsular abnormalities, and joint hypertrophy.

Table 150.2. Bogduk's postulates

An anatomic structural cause of back pain must meet these criteria:
1. The structure must have a nerve supply.
2. The structure should be capable of causing pain similar to what is clinically observed (e.g., when provoked in normal volunteers).
3. The structure should be susceptible to painful disease or injury; such disorders should be detectable by clinical, imaging, biomechanical, or postmortem tests.
4. The structure should be shown to be a source of pain in actual patients, using reliable and valid diagnostic tests.

Anatomy

Anatomic structures of the lumbosacral spine that are responsible for pain are often referred to as *pain generators*. Several conditions are required for a structure to be considered a pain generator, as described in-depth by Nikolai Bogduk (Table 150.2): There must be a nerve supply, because insensate structures are not typically sources of pain. Provocation or irritation of the structure in normal volunteers should produce a distribution of pain that is similar to what is observed in patients. The structure must be naturally susceptible to injury or disease, which may activate or sensitize local nociceptors mechanically or chemically (e.g., via inflammation). Finally, the structure must be demonstrated, using diagnostic techniques of known reliability and validity, as a source of pain in patients.

Specific anatomic causes have been described for lumbosacral spinal pain (Table 150.3). A precise anatomic cause, however, may not be discovered in as many as 90% of individual cases of chronic lumbosacral pain. Well-established pain generators include zygapophyseal (facet) joints, sacroiliac joints, and discs. Incidence of internal disc disruption is estimated to be 39% in chronic lumbosacral pain. Incidences of facet and sacroiliac joint pain are 15% each.

Pain due to facet joints is typically deep aching of gradual onset located near the midline of the lumbar spine, over the location of the actual joints. Lumbosacral facet joint pain may be referred to the buttocks and thighs, but usually not past the knee. Pain may be exacerbated by compression of the joint surfaces or stretching of the joint capsule.

Sacroiliac joint pain is usually deep aching of gradual onset, located in the lower back and upper buttock, over the posterior margin of the joint. Pain may be referred to the thigh, but again,

Table 150.3. Generators of lumbosacral spinal pain

Structure	Example
Vertebral body	Osteoporotic fracture
Muscle, fascia, ligaments	Trigger points
Meninges	Epidural hematoma
Sacroiliac joint	Sacroiliitis
Zygapophyseal joints	Osteoarthritis
Intervertebral disc	Internal disc disruption

usually not past the knee. Numerous physical examination techniques have been described to assess the sacroiliac joint, but the diagnostic block with local anesthetic is the best test.

Pain due to the discs themselves, known as *discogenic pain*, is characterized by deep aching in the lumbosacral midline. As with facet and sacroiliac joint pain, referral can be to the buttock and thigh, but not past the knee. The most distinguishing historic feature of discogenic pain is intolerance to prolonged sitting. Prolonged standing and forward flexion of the lumbosacral spine also exacerbate discogenic pain.

The anatomic cause of radicular pain is most often attributed to herniation of nucleus pulposus of the intervertebral disc. Such ectopic disc material can mechanically irritate the nerve root and can also cause an inflammatory reaction. Radicular pain can also arise from epidural, meningeal, or neurologic disorders, as well as from any cause of foraminal stenosis. Causes of foraminal stenosis other than disc herniations include osteophytes, degenerative changes of ligamentum flavum, cysts, tumors, and infections (Fig. 150.2). *Failed back surgery syndrome* is a nonspecific description of persistent or recurrent pain after lumbar spinal surgery.

Diagnosis and treatment

Initial evaluation of back pain requires screening for potentially dangerous conditions, often referred to as the "red flags" of back pain (Table 150.4). For example, bowel or bladder dysfunction or saddle anesthesia can be associated with *cauda equina*

Table 150.4. The red flags of back pain

History

Gradual onset of back pain
Age < 20 y or > 50 y
Thoracic back pain
Pain lasting longer than 6 wk
History of trauma
Fever/chills/night sweats
Unintentional weight loss
Pain worse with recumbency
Pain worse at night
Unrelenting pain despite supratherapeutic doses of analgesics
History of malignancy
History of immunosuppression
Recent procedure known to cause bacteremia
History of intravenous drug use
Physical examination
Fever
Hypotension
Extreme hypertension
Pale, ashen appearance
Pulsatile abdominal mass
Pulse amplitude differentials
Spinous process tenderness
Focal neurologic signs
Acute urinary retention

Winters ME, Kluetz P, Zilberstein J. Back pain emergencies. *Med Clin North Am* 2006; 90(3):505–523.

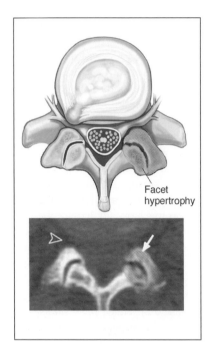

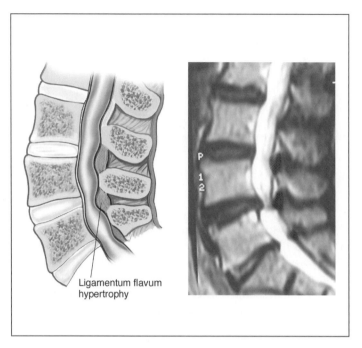

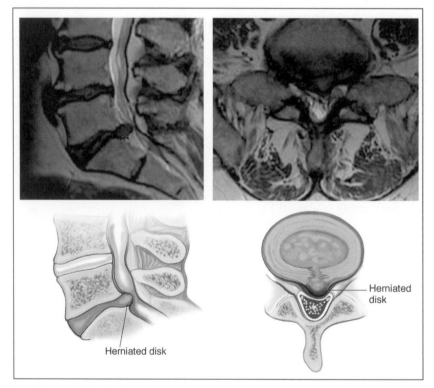

Figure 150.2. Anatomic sources of back pain.

syndrome, which may require emergency surgical decompression to prevent permanent neurologic injury. Urinary retention and overflow incontinence are pathognomonic of cauda equina syndrome (90% sensitivity, 95% specificity), and absence of a postvoid residual urine has a 99.99% negative predictive value. History or examination suggesting compression of the spinal cord is critical, as 20% of patients with spinal metastases will present with these features as the first evidence of their malignancy. MRI is the gold standard diagnostic test in such cases. Unexplained weight loss or fever can also be suggestive of infection or malignancy. Pain that is unrelenting when recumbent has also been associated with spinal tumors. Red flags can indicate serious conditions that need immediate imaging or surgical consultation.

After exclusion of red flags, the general algorithmic approach to back pain begins with determining if the predominant pattern of pain is lumbosacral or radicular, then deciding if the episode is acute or chronic. Physical examination is beyond the intended scope of this chapter (the reader is referred to several existing sources in the "Suggested readings" section), but a few common tests should be mentioned here. The straight leg raise, also known as Lasègue's test, consists of passive hip flexion with knee extended, with passive ankle dorsiflexion. This sensitive maneuver causes traction of L4, L5, and S1 nerve roots, and provokes radicular pain extending past the knee in the elevated leg. The crossed straight leg is a more specific test that provokes radicular pain in the symptomatic leg when lifting the asymptomatic leg. Facet loading tests are usually positive in facet arthropathy. The flexion, abduction and external rotation (FABER) test and Gaenslen's test are characteristic signs in diagnosis of sacroiliitis.

Acute lumbosacral or radicular pain may initially respond to a brief course of nonsteroidal anti-inflammatory drugs (NSAIDs) or acetaminophen, with a centrally acting muscle relaxant. Acute lumbosacral pain that persists may respond to physical therapy and patient education. Lumbar epidural steroid injections may speed resolution of acute radicular pain in the 2- to 6-week timeframe (level 2 evidence). Bed rest is no longer advised for back pain.

Diagnostic imaging is not generally used in the first 6 weeks of an episode of lumbosacral spinal pain. If there is evidence of acute nerve root compression, it is reasonable to obtain a lumbosacral MRI in preparation for performing an epidural steroid injection. In cases of prior back surgery or failed back surgery syndrome, the MRI should be ordered with gadolinium. Flexion and extension radiographs can identify mobile segments due to pseudoarthrosis in patients who have had spinal fusion. CT and CT myelogram can be used when MRI is not possible, but CT cannot distinguish causes of compression as is possible with MRI.

Patients with chronic radicular pain may benefit from neuropathic pain medications, such as tricyclic antidepressants, selective norepinephrine reuptake inhibitors, or antiepileptic medications as described in Chapter 145. Interventional options including epidural injections, transforaminal injections, selective nerve root blocks, and pulsed radiofrequency lesioning of the dorsal root ganglion, will be considered as a part of multidisciplinary care for worsening pain. In cases of chronic radicular pain refractory to more conservative treatments, implantable spinal cord stimulation may be an option.

Facet joint treatment can be considered for chronic lumbar spinal pain. Diagnostic blocks of the medial branch nerves (or posterior primary ramus at L5) that innervate the facet joints can determine if these joints are pain generators. If a series of blocks significantly relieves pain for the duration of injected local anesthetic, it suggests that facet joints mediate the pain. Following this, radiofrequency lesioning of the same nerves can be performed, potentially providing 3 to 6 months of relief.

A similar approach can be used for the chronic sacral spinal pain. For facet and sacroiliac joints, diagnostic injections are the gold standard for determination of the pain source. If such blocks do not determine the source of chronic lumbosacral spinal pain, provocative discography can be used to determine if a disc is the source of pain, in cases where treatment options would include intradiscal electrothermal therapy (IDET) or surgical fusion. Multidisciplinary pain programs that incorporate physical therapy and cognitive behavioral therapy are also indicated for chronic lumbosacral spinal pain.

Use of long-term opiate therapy for back pain remains controversial. Evidence does exist for efficacy and improved function in chronic noncancer pain; however, there is also evidence of difficulties with chronic opiate therapy, including addiction, hyperalgesia, and hormonal imbalance.

Surgery is sometimes indicated for painful disorders of the lumbosacral spine. The patient must be healthy enough otherwise to undergo surgery. Surgical indications include cauda equina syndrome, progressive or severe motor deficit, or persistent motor deficit that does not improve after 6 weeks of conservative treatment. Reflex or sensory abnormalities are not indications for surgery. Severe, intractable radicular pain may also be an indication for surgery.

Conclusion

Lumbosacral spinal pain is one of the most common and costly medical problems in the world. Most episodes, however, will resolve without treatment within 6 weeks. A specific anatomic source of pain is often not found in individual cases. For chronic painful disorders of the lumbar spine, good evidence exists for multidisciplinary comprehensive treatment, including activity and physical therapy, psychological treatments, medications, and interventional techniques.

Suggested readings

Ballantyne JC. *The Massachusetts General Handbook of Pain Management*. 3rd ed. Philadelphia: Lippincott Williams & Wilkins; 2006:366–390.

Benzon HT, Rathmell JP, Wu CL, et al. *Raj's Practical Management of Pain*. Philadelphia: Mosby; 2008:368–387.

Bogduk N. *Clinical Anatomy of the Lumbar Spine and Sacrum*. 4th ed. Philadelphia: Elsevier; 2005.

Hoppenfeld S. *Physical Examination of the Spine and Extremities*. East Norwalk, CT: Appleton-Century-Crofts; 1976.

Magee DJ. *Orthopedic Physical Assessment*. Elsevier Canada; 2002.

Merskey H, Bogduk N (eds.). *Classification of Chronic Pain: Descriptions of Chronic Pain Syndromes and Definitions of Pain Terms*. 3rd ed. Seattle, WA: IASP Press; 1994.

Rathmell JP. A 50-year-old man with chronic low back pain. *JAMA* 2008; 299(17):2066–2077.

Rubin DI. Epidemiology and risk factors for spine pain. *Neurol Clin* 2007; 25(2):353–371.

Slipman CW, Derby R, Simeone FA, Mayer TG. *Interventional Spine: An Algorithmic Approach*. Philadelphia: Elsevier; 2008.

Winters ME, Kluetz P, Zilberstein J. Back pain emergencies. *Med Clin North Am* 2006; 90(3):505–523.

Chapter

151

Complex regional pain syndrome

Omid Ghalambor

Complex regional pain syndrome (CRPS) refers to a group of pain conditions that are characterized by continuous, intense neuropathic pain out of proportion to the severity of the injury. Typical features include burning pain and dramatic changes in the color and temperature of the skin over the affected limb or body part, accompanied by hyperesthesia, hyperhydrosis, edema, and, rarely, ulceration (see Fig. 151.1). Early in the course of the syndrome, the skin may be warm and erythematous. As the process becomes chronic, the involved extremity is usually cool and pale or cyanotic. Dystrophic changes manifest as bone demineralization, and skin in the affected area becomes smooth and glossy. Joints in the affected extremity become stiff and painful. The exact etiology of CRPS is yet to be determined. In some cases, the sympathetic nervous system seems to play an important role in sustaining the pain. Several pathophysiologic concepts have been proposed to explain the complex symptoms of CRPS: (1) facilitated neurogenic inflammation; (2) pathologic sympatho-afferent coupling; and (3) neuroplastic changes within the central nervous system (CNS). Furthermore, there is accumulating evidence that genetic factors may predispose for CRPS. Another theory postulates that CRPS is caused by a triggering of the immune response, which leads to the characteristic inflammatory symptoms of redness, warmth, and swelling in the affected area.

CRPS is classified into two types: CRPS type I (formerly referred to as reflex sympathetic dystrophy [RSD]) includes cases in which the nerve injury cannot be immediately identified, and CRPS type II (formerly referred to as causalgia) in which a distinct major nerve injury has occurred. Generally, CRPS type II provides more objective evidence of disease due to neurologic changes (numbness and weakness). Because there is no single laboratory test to diagnose CRPS, an arbitrary set of criteria has been suggested to establish the diagnosis.

Criteria for diagnosing CRPS

1. The presence of an initiating noxious event, or a cause of immobilization in CRPS type I or signs of major nerve damage in CRPS type II
2. Continuing pain, allodynia, or hyperalgesia with which the pain is disproportionate to any inciting event
3. Evidence at some time of edema, changes in skin blood flow (skin color changes, skin temperature changes more

than 1.1°C different from the homologous body part), or abnormal sudomotor activity in the region of the pain
4. Change in tissue growth; atrophy or dystrophy

The diagnosis is excluded by the existence of conditions that would otherwise account for the degree of pain and dysfunction.

Patients do not need to meet all of these criteria for the diagnosis. Also, one should remember that many of these symptoms, especially the temperature differences, are not static. The involved body region may be hotter or colder than the contralateral region. Moreover, in any one patient, the same region may fluctuate from hot to cold. The skin temperature can undergo dynamic changes in a relatively short period of time (within minutes), depending critically on room temperature, local temperature of the skin, and emotional stress. In some cases, the

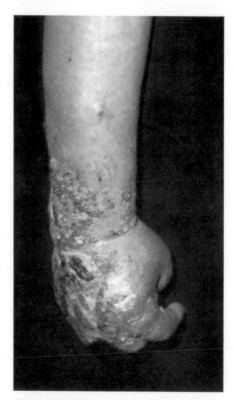

Figure 151.1. Hand exhibiting features of CPRS, including significant focal skin changes and contractures from disuse.

differences in temperatures may fluctuate spontaneously even without any apparent provocation.

Historically, CRPS type I had been described to have three phases. The staging system is now abandoned because many patients do not follow the described phases. In fact, only a minority of patients have symptoms and signs of trophic changes corresponding to the described stage III of the disease.

There is a natural tendency to rush to the diagnosis of CRPS with minimal objective findings, although early diagnosis is critical. If undiagnosed and untreated, CRPS can spread to all extremities, making the rehabilitation process a much more difficult one. It seems that the speed with which therapy is commenced after the precipitating event or onset of symptoms determines the outcome of the disease. If untreated, CRPS can lead to permanent deformities and chronic pain.

Treatment

As with all pain conditions, an interdisciplinary approach has the most chance for success. The key disciplines needed for the management of CRPS include pharmacotherapy, psychotherapy, interventions, and physiotherapy. The cornerstone in the treatment of CRPS is normal use of the affected part as much as possible. Therefore, all other modalities of therapy are employed to facilitate movement of the affected region of the body.

Medications

Pulse doses of corticosteroids for 2 weeks have been reported to be beneficial in CRPS type I patients. For constant pain associated with inflammation, nonsteroidal anti-inflammatory drugs (NSAIDs), such as ibuprofen, may prove beneficial. For constant pain not caused by inflammation, centrally acting medications by an atypical mechanism, such as tramadol, could be used. Tricyclic antidepressants, such as amitriptyline and nortriptyline, have been tried with some success. Anticonvulsants (in particular, gabapentin) have been shown to provide good results for controlling the pain symptoms of CRPS patients and are becoming more and more popular given excellent safety and side-effect profile. Intranasal or intramuscular calcitonin, intravenous (IV) bisphosphonates, as well as free-radical scavengers (dimethyl sulfoxide or acetylcysteine) have been reported to successfully reduce symptoms. In patients determined to have sympathetically maintained pain (SMP), clonidine patches have shown some benefit. Oral lidocaine (mexiletine) has proven to be beneficial in patients in whom IV lidocaine infusions have helped. For muscle cramps (spasms and dystonia) in the involved extremity, muscle relaxants, such as clonazepam and baclofen, are useful. Recently, promising results have been described using ketamine and midazolam in anesthetic doses in severe spreading and refractory CRPS cases.

Psychotherapy

The psychiatrist's role is to identify comorbid psychiatric conditions, such as depression, posttraumatic stress disorder, and anxiety disorder, and to treat them if needed. Moreover, psychological treatment approaches include cognitive behavioral techniques and supportive psychotherapy, with the goal of teaching the patient chronic pain coping skills, biofeedback, and relaxation techniques.

Interventions

For patients who are significantly impaired in their ability to mobilize their extremity, it is important to offer the patient the opportunity to determine the contribution of their sympathetic nervous system to their pain. This determination can be made by a sympathetic nerve block to the affected extremity. Future therapeutic options for the patient will depend on whether the pain is determined to be SMP or sympathetically independent pain (SIP). A patient with CRPS who reports pain relief after a sympathetic block is defined to have SMP. Published reports suggest that the best response to sympathetic blocks will occur if the blocks are given as soon as possible during the course of the disease. Blockade of the sympathetic nervous system is performed at the level of the stellate ganglion for upper extremity involvement or at the level of lumbar sympathetic chain for lower extremity involvement. The pain relief following sympathetic nerve block (SNB) generally outlasts the effects of the local anesthetics and, in the case of the SMP group, may be long lasting.

IV regional anesthetic (IVRA) blocks in the affected extremity have been performed using guanethidine, lidocaine, clonidine, droperidol, bretylium, and reserpine, with the first two being more extensively studied.

Neurostimulation

Spinal cord stimulation (SCS) has been shown to be effective in reducing pain and improving the function and quality of life in patients with CRPS in the upper extremities. This option should be considered when alternative therapies have failed.

Physiotherapy

The primary goal of physiotherapy is the restoration of function through activity. Interventions include passive and active assisted range-of-motion work and strengthening exercises aiming to improve motor control as well as to build functional tolerance to activities such as standing, sitting, walking (in cases of lower extremity involvement), and weight-bearing (for upper extremities).

Suggested readings

Burton AW, Hassenbusch SJ 3rd, Warneke C, et al. Complex regional pain syndrome (CRPS): survey of current practices. *Pain Pract* 2004; 4(2):74–83.

Janig W, Stanton-Hicks M (eds.). Reflex sympathetic dystrophy: a reappraisal. In: *Progress in Pain Research and Management*. Volume 6. Seattle: IASP Press; 1996.

Kiefer RT, Rohr P, Ploppa A, et al. Complete recovery from intractable complex regional pain syndrome, CRPS-type I, following anesthetic ketamine and midazolam. *Pain Pract* 2007; 7(2):147–150.

Loeser JD, Bonica JJ. *Bonica's Management of Pain.* 3rd ed. Philadelphia: Lippincott Williams & Wilkins; 2001: 388–411.

Raja SN, Grabow TS. Complex regional pain syndrome I (reflex sympathetic dystrophy). *Anesthesiology* 2002; 96:1254–1260.

Reflex Sympathetic Dystrophy Syndrome Association (RSDSA). Complex regional pain syndrome: treatment guidelines. Milford (CT): RSDSA; 2006.

Chapter

152

Cancer pain

Assia Valovska and Robert J. Klickovich

Introduction

According to the American Society of Anesthesiologists (ASA) Task Force, cancer pain is defined as "pain that is attributable to cancer or its therapy." Cancer is the cause of approximately 10% of deaths globally and 20% of deaths nationally. Each year several thousands of patients suffer from cancer pain, including 25% of patients in active treatment and 90% of those with advanced disease. Although cancer pain can be relieved, surveys have shown that pain is often undertreated in as many as 50% of patients. Barriers to adequate treatment of cancer pain include underreporting by patients and family members, lack of provider knowledge regarding current treatment standards, inadequate assessment of the patient by health care providers, fear of prosecution by federal and state agencies for the prescription of opioids, lack of accountability regarding failure to control pain, and inadequate reimbursement or excessive paperwork required by payers for the treatment of pain by health care providers. The World Health Organization (WHO) and other governmental agencies have recognized the importance of pain management as part of routine cancer care.

Etiology and pathophysiology

Cancer pain may occur in different parts of the body. There are three types of pain, depending on where in the body the pain is felt:

1. *Somatic pain* is caused by the activation of pain receptors in either the cutaneous (body surface) or deep tissues (musculoskeletal tissues) and could be caused by metastasis in the bone (an example of deep somatic pain) or involve postsurgical pain from a surgical incision (an example of surface pain). It is usually sharp and well localized.
2. *Visceral pain* is caused by activation of pain receptors from infiltration, compression, extension, or stretching of the thoracic (chest), abdominal, or pelvic viscera. Visceral pain is not well localized and is usually described as pressure-like, deep, squeezing.
3. *Neuropathic pain* is caused by injury to the nervous system as a result of either a tumor compressing nerves or the spinal cord or cancer actually infiltrating the nerves or spinal cord. It also results from chemical damage to the nervous system that may be caused by cancer treatment

(chemotherapy, radiation, surgery). This type of pain is severe and usually described as burning or tingling. Tumors that lie close to neural structures are believed to cause the most severe pain that cancer patients feel.

Somatic, visceral, and neuropathic pain can occur separately or together and can be felt at the same time or at different times. Somatic and visceral pains are easier to manage than neuropathic pain.

Cancer pain can be acute or chronic. Acute cancer pain is caused by nociceptor stimulation from actual damage to tissues. It is arbitrarily defined as lasting from the time of insult to the tissues to about 3 months. It can occur intermittently (episodic or intermittent pain) or constantly. Chronic cancer pain is defined as pain lasting for more than 3 months. It is much more subjective and not as easily described as acute pain. According to the American Cancer Society, chronic cancer pain may involve persistent (constant and sustained) pain or breakthrough pain. Breakthrough pain is a brief superimposed episode of severe pain that occurs while the patient is regularly taking pain medication. It usually comes on quickly and lasts from a few minutes to an hour. Many patients experience a number of episodes of breakthrough pain each day.

Cancer pain can be also categorized into three basic subtypes:

1. Pain associated with the tumor: bone lesions, metastases, local infiltration, hollow viscera obstruction, organ capsule distension, mono- and polyneuropathies, leptomeningeal metastases, cauda equina syndrome, and paraneoplastic syndrome;
2. Pain associated with the therapy: postradiation enteritis, radiation fibrosis, osteoradionecrosis, cystitis; chemotherapy and posthormonal related arthralgia, myalgia, avascular necrosis, chronic abdominal pain, mucositis, neuropathy; postsurgical phantom limb pain, posthoracotomy pain; and
3. Pain not specifically related to the malignancy: preexisting chronic pain problem; headaches, muscles strains, other aches and pains associated with arthritis, kidney stones (these conditions can normally be treated along with cancer pain).

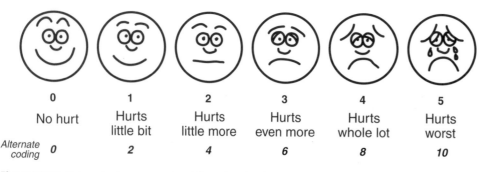

Figure 152.1. Universal pain assessment tool. Reproduced with permission, Mosby press.

Assessment and evaluation

The following items are essential to the initial assessment: detailed history of the pain, physical examination, including a complete neurologic examination, diagnostic testing, and development of a management plan.

The patient history should include information about the premorbid chronic pain, drug or alcohol use, medications, cancer diagnosis, staging of the tumor, progression of malignancy, and specific characteristics of treatments. Evaluation of cancer pain involves many features: duration of the pain (acute vs. chronic), intensity of the pain (mild, moderate, or severe), quality of the pain (neuropathic, nociceptive, or mixed), and temporal pattern (continuous, breakthrough, or both); initiating factors (pain related to posture, position, or activity); radiation; previous therapy; and associated psychological and emotional components. If there is more than one pain complaint, each source of pain should be considered independently. The intensity of the pain should be determined. Common forms of measurement include facial expression scale (Fig. 152.1) or linear analog scale from 0 to 10 in which 0 is no pain and 10 is the worst pain level imaginable. Scales may be verbal or written (which can be colors, numbers, or lines).

Patients who identify themselves as having pain should thereafter be evaluated with a more thorough assessment, such as the Brief Pain Inventory. A psychosocial evaluation is necessary, including the patient's as well as the family's objectives in treatment of pain as well as cancer.

Comprehensive physical examination should include weight, vital signs, determination of nutritional status, thorough examination of the site of pain and referring sites, complete musculoskeletal and neurologic examination, and auscultation of heart and lungs. Provocative bedside maneuvers reproducing pain help to better identify the pain-sensitive structure and should be a routine part of the comprehensive assessment of cancer pain patients. Patients should also be evaluated for associated physical symptoms, such as fatigue, constipation, and changes in mood.

The data obtained from the history and physical examination may prompt further diagnostic workup to exclude the presence of medical emergencies requiring rapid specialist consultation and intervention. Diagnostic testing should be used only when it will contribute to the treatment of the patient or confirm a suspected diagnosis. Plain films and CT should be used to determine fracture or visceral pathology. Radionucleotide studies will reveal changes in bone growth or destruction of bone. MRI should be used for the evaluation of soft tissue changes. The amount of the diagnostic testing should be decreased or eliminated with progression of disease, especially in terminally ill patients.

Formulating a plan of care is essential, including a substitute plan in case of resistant pain. Discussion with the patient is essential, and the patient may need assurance that the first plan is not the only option available.

Management

Treatment goals for cancer pain patients should be geared toward cure or prolonging life, maintaining function, and providing comfort. They should include inhibition of the transmission of pain as well as modulation of the patient's perception of pain. Although it has been suggested that more than 85% to 95% of cancer patients can be treated by the use of appropriate pharmacologic and anticancer therapy, some patients require invasive interventions to relieve their pain or to assist in the management of their pain when the secondary effects of the opioids are so significant as to compromise the cancer patient's quality of life. Frequent reevaluation of the patient is required.

Pharmacologic management

There are a number of suggested algorithms for pharmacologic treatment of cancer pain. The best known of these is the WHO's three-step analgesic ladder and the four-step modified analgesic ladder. The WHO's analgesic ladder provides adequate analgesia in the majority of cases.

1. Step one – mild pain: nonopioid analgesics including nonsteroidal anti-inflammatory drugs (NSAIDS) +/− adjuvant therapy, such as anticonvulsants and acetaminophen

Freedom from Cancer Pain

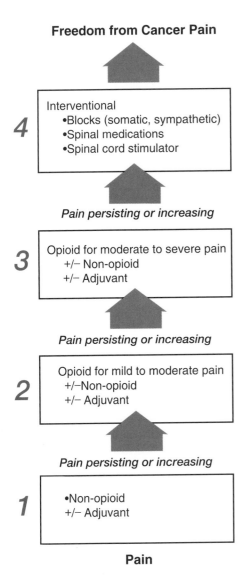

4 Interventional
   •Blocks (somatic, sympathetic)
   •Spinal medications
   •Spinal cord stimulator

Pain persisting or increasing

3 Opioid for moderate to severe pain
   +/– Non-opioid
   +/– Adjuvant

Pain persisting or increasing

2 Opioid for mild to moderate pain
   +/–Non-opioid
   +/– Adjuvant

Pain persisting or increasing

1 •Non-opioid
   +/– Adjuvant

Pain

Figure 152.2. Modified analgesic ladder for cancer pain, including interventional management. Adapted from World Health Organization. *World Health Organ Tech Rep Ser* 1990; 804:1–73; Miguel R. *Cancer Control* 2000; 7:149–156; and Krames E. *Med Clin North Am* 1999; 83:787–808.

2. Step two – mild to moderate pain: opioids +/– nonopioid analgesics and adjuvant therapy
3. Step three – moderate to severe pain: strong opioids, such as long acting opioids, in addition to short-acting opioids +/– adjuvant therapy
4. Severe to intractable pain/failure-to-treat persistent pain with increasing doses of opioids warrants interventional therapies as mentioned in the modified analgesic ladder (Fig. 152.2).

Medication management in cancer pain uses all the drug classes including nonopioid, opioid, and adjuvant medications. The doses required are much higher, and the side-effects profile seen is more severe. Breakthrough medications should be fast acting.

Adverse effects management

Side-effect management is an integral part of any cancer pain treatment regimen and requires a proactive approach. Patient education should be implemented to decrease apprehension about the use of opioids and clear concerns regarding issues of addiction, dependence, tolerance, and pseudoaddiction. Reassurance should be used to decrease underreporting of pain. Goals should include reduction of pain to tolerable levels, titration of dose to effect, and use of the minimum amount of medication required to achieve analgesic goals without significant side effects.

Nausea is the most common side effect, affecting approximately one third of patients. In most cases, nausea is mild or resolves spontaneously, but in a small number of patients it may become unremitting, and failure to manage it may limit the patient's use of the most effective form of treatment. Evaluation of nausea in the cancer patient on opioids should begin with review of the bowel function. Many factors can be considered as a cause of nausea including opioid therapy, bowel obstruction from disease progression or increase in the intracranial pressure from tumor growth. Chemotherapy and radiotherapy frequently lead to nausea. Treatment of nausea should be based on the associated symptom reported by the patient. Alternatives include phenothiazines, serotonin antagonists, or atypical antipsychotics. Other options include intestinal motility agents, antivertiginous agents, and oral dexamethasone. In patients who develop anorexia secondary to opioids, one should consider hormonal therapy, such as dronabinol, megestrol acetate, corticosteroids, or anabolic steroids. Patients should also be evaluated for mood disorders.

Opioid-induced constipation is the second most common side effect of opioid therapy. Treatment of constipation should be started prophylactically with the initiation of opioid therapy. Stool softeners, strong laxatives, and dietary adjustments should be implemented to ensure regular bowel habits. Orally administered naloxone, a pure opioid antagonist, improves idiopathic constipation. Opioid agonist–antagonists exhibit a lower frequency of constipation than do the pure agonists.

Opioid therapy can cause a wide range of effects on the central nervous system (CNS). Patients may exhibit drowsiness, confusion, dysphoria, or euphoria. Sedation could be minimized by decreasing the dosage, changing the medication, slow dose titration, and using psychostimulants such as methylphenidate and methylphenidate modafinil.

The excitatory effects on the CNS may present with hyperalgesia, myoclonus, or seizures. Opioid-induced hyperalgesia was recognized as an emerging side effect of opioid therapy. Patients experiencing hyperalgesia complain of pain out of proportion to physical findings, which is a common cause for loss of efficacy of these medications over time. As it can be difficult to distinguish from tolerance, opioid-induced hyperalgesia is often compensated for by escalating the dose of opioid, potentially worsening the problem by further increasing sensitivity to pain.

It may develop in response to both chronic and acute exposure to opioids. This side effect can be severe enough to warrant discontinuation of opioid treatment.

Chronic opioid use may lead to the development of tolerance to the analgesic effect. The patient becomes less susceptible to the effect of the opioid as a consequence of its prior administration. Tolerance to one opioid, however, does not lead to tolerance to an equianalgesic dose of another opioid. Due to this concept of "incomplete cross tolerance," it is necessary to decrease the equianalgesic dose of a drug in a naïve patient by 30% to 50%.

Physical dependence is the term used to describe the phenomenon of withdrawal when an opioid is abruptly discontinued or an opioid antagonist is administered. Both tolerance and physical dependence are predictable pharmacologic effects seen in response to repeated administration of an opioid and can be easily managed after being identified. These effects are distinct from psychological dependence or addiction. Psychological dependence describes a pattern of drug use characterized by a continued craving for an opioid, manifested as compulsive, drug-seeking behavior and overwhelming involvement in drug procurement and use.

Pseudoaddiction is a term describing behavior that appears to be drug-seeking in a patient who has been undertreated or in whom the disease has progressed. Such behavior should prompt review of the therapeutic plan or further investigation of the disease.

Less common side effects of opioid therapy include urinary retention, respiratory depression, pruritus, and miosis. Whereas tolerance to nausea, vomiting, sedation, euphoria, and respiratory depression occur rapidly, there is minimal development of tolerance to constipation and miosis.

Palliative therapy

The use of external beam radiation therapy in the treatment of painful metastasis is particularly important. Radiation for bone pain, pain secondary to apical lung mass, and so forth, can lead to a quick and lasting pain relief. Therapeutic radionuclides, such as strontium-89 chloride and samarium-153-ethylenediaminetetramethylene phosphonic acid (EDTMP), are useful in patients with multiple bony metastases, such as those in breast cancer. The agents are picked and concentrated within the bone. They exhibit little toxicity except mild sedation. The expected effects occur within a week and can be used to supplement external beam radiation. They also might prevent formation of new metastases.

Chemotherapy reduces the size of the targeted tumors and can be helpful with pain due to compression, stretching, or ischemia. Bisphosphonates are helpful as analgesics. These drugs bind to the hydroxyapatite crystals within bone and inhibit osteoclastic activity. Prospective randomized studies in patients with myeloma and metastatic breast cancer show that bisphosphonates improve pain and reduce morbidity secondary to bony pathology.

Interventional therapies

If pharmacotherapy for pain associated with malignancy is inadequate or is found to cause intolerable secondary effects, interventional techniques should be considered. These modalities include antitumor therapy, neural blockade with or without neurolytic drugs, CNS opioid therapy, electrical stimulation, or surgery.

Local anesthetic blocks can be used for diagnostic, prognostic, or therapeutic purposes. A diagnostic nerve block can help to determine which anatomic structure is responsible for generation and transmission of the pain and to distinguish between somatic, visceral, sympathetic, and central pain. The effects from the block should be carefully analyzed, and the results used to determine the potential for more permanent ablative procedure. A diagnostic block should always precede an ablative block. Such a trial block will enable the patient to be aware of the effect and possible side effects of the block and also will identify any neurologic deficits that may be intolerable to the patient.

Therapeutic blocks are often administered to treat pain caused by tumor compression of nerve structures; neuropathies and neuralgias from direct nerve damage such as postthoracotomy pain or post-herpetic neuralgias; and trigger points from muscle spasm.

Neurolytic blocks involve injection of a destructive substance close to a spinal or peripheral somatic nerve and the sympathetic nervous system. It may be beneficial for targeted areas of pain, such as head and neck cancer, pancreatic cancer, pelvic malignancies, and pain related to the perineum.

The most common neurolytic agents used are alcohol and phenol. They both produce equal effects. Alcohol causes severe pain on injection that may be alleviated by pretreatment with local anesthetic. A phenol injection is better tolerated and causes almost immediate sensation of numbness and pain relief.

Specific applications

Neurolytic sympathetic blocks can be helpful in controlling pain that is either visceral or dysesthetic (causalgic) in origin. Visceral pain occurs when sympathetic nerves or visceral structures are stretched, traumatized, or invaded by the cancer. The patient complains of dull, burning pain that is poorly localized. Referred pain can occur (e.g., shoulder pain from tumor invasion of the diaphragm). In some cases, the causalgia can respond to a blockade alone, but in others ablation of involved ganglia or surgical rhizotomy may be necessary.

The various other ganglion blocks include the stellate ganglion block, celiac plexus block, hypogastric plexus block, and ganglion impar block. These blocks are described in detail in other chapters.

Chest and abdominal wall pain can be treated with neurolytic intercostal nerve block. The intercostal nerves provide sensory innervation to the skin of the chest and abdomen anterolaterally. They travel in the inferior part of the ribs posterior to the intercostal artery. Subcostal nerve comes from the ventral ramus of T12 and is equivalent to the intercostal nerve at the above levels. For diagnostic block, 1 to 2 ml of bupivacaine 0.25% to 0.5% is injected. For neurolytic block, 4 to 5 ml of phenol 10% can be injected. Alcohol should be avoided because of the risk of intercostal neuritis after the block. Most clinicians now favor the use of radiofrequency lesion of the intercostal nerves instead of injecting neurolytic medications. Common complications include pneumothorax and potential local anesthetic toxicity. Postprocedural intercostal neuropathy may occur, which can be treated with a transcutaneous electrical nerve stimulation (TENS) unit, transdermal lidocaine patch, or neuropathic medication.

Subarachnoid neurolytic block is suitable for patients who have significant cancer pain that is not controlled by any other modalities. The pain should be localized into few sensory segments of the spinal cord. The main goal of the block is selective destruction of the corresponding dorsal root ganglia. This destruction is accomplished by positioning the patient in a way that permits the neurolytic material (either hypo- or hyperbaric) to remain localized in the dorsal surface of the spinal cord. Extremely important for the lower thoracic and lumbar neurolysis is the fact that thoracic and lumbar nerves leave the spinal cord at a higher level than the exiting neural foramina. For example, pain at the level of T9 nerve distribution requires neurolysis at T6, T7, and T8 levels. The usual dose of either agent is 0.6 ml and is injected within 80 to 90 seconds for each level. Complete neurologic examination before and after the block is mandatory to evaluate any neurologic deficits. Common side effects include temporary or permanent weakness of the urinary or rectal sphincters. Postdural puncture headache may occur and is most common in younger patients. Radiofrequency lesioning is the application of electrical current to achieve coagulation of proteins and nerve destruction. It is used to ablate pain pathways in the trigeminal ganglion, spinal cord, dorsal root entry zone, dorsal root ganglion, sympathetic chain, facet joints, and peripheral nerves. Because it causes nerve destruction, this technique is used only as an end-of-the-line therapeutic modality when other measures have failed. Fluoroscopic guidance is a requirement for proper needle placement. Common complications include pneumothorax, postlesioning neuritis, motor paralysis, numbness, and incomplete pain relief.

Neuraxial opioid therapy is often effective for treating cancer pain that has not been adequately controlled by systemic treatment. The close proximity of the opioid receptors in the spinal cord to the injected neuraxial opioids ensures maximum effect with small doses of medication. The preservative-free drug can be delivered via epidural, intrathecal, or intraventricular approach. Opioids can be used alone or in combination with local anesthetics, α-adrenergic agents, or baclofen to achieve synergistic effect and optimal pain relief. The intraventricular approach is used infrequently for neck and head cancer pain.

A tunneled epidural catheter can be placed at any level in the lumbar, thoracic, or cervical level. The indications include cancer pain anywhere from the neck to the lower extremities and a life expectancy of 3 to 6 months or less. This technique is more advantageous than the nontunneled epidural catheter because of the low incidence of infections. A tunneled epidural catheter can be either a simple, one-piece catheter or consist of two pieces with a Dacron cuff and antibiotic cuff. Administration of epidural medications can be accomplished by continuous infusion via a standard portable infusion pump connected to a port. Patient-controlled epidural analgesia (PCEA) allows delivery of intermittent boluses by the patient or the family and thus some degree of control over the pain management.

Intrathecal delivery of opioids into the CNS has certain advantages over epidural catheters. The doses of medications needed are significantly lower; opioid requirements are approximately 10% of those for epidural administration. The intrathecal drugs act quicker and last longer. Patients experience fewer side effects due to decreased systemic absorption. Implantable intrathecal pumps are considered for patients whose pain becomes increasingly more difficult to manage, who experience significant side effects with increasing doses of enteral and parenteral medications, who cannot tolerate large doses of epidural infusions, and whose life expectancy is longer than 6 months. Morphine is the only opioid approved for intrathecal use by the US Food and Drug Administration (FDA) for treatment of chronic and cancer pain. Other opioids have been used, such as hydromorphone, fentanyl, and sufentanil. The most common nonopioid medications used are clonidine, ziconotide, bupivacaine, and baclofen. Usually one or more of these drugs are added to opioids in the intrathecal delivery system. The infusion regimen is individualized, based on the results from the patient's pain assessment and oral or intravenous opioid requirements. Several companies produce intrathecal pumps. Codman's model 400 (Raynham, MA) is a nonprogrammable, constant-flow infusion pump. Medtronic's Isomed and Synchromed II (Minneapolis, MN) allow the physician to change the daily rate (mg/d), including options of single bolus, timed-specific boluses, or a complex continuous delivery of drug. Changing the rate is easily performed with a programmer. The implanted pumps require infrequent drug refills.

Surgery

Finally, in some cases, it may be appropriate to perform neurosurgical destructive procedures. Examples include anterolateral cordotomy, stereotactic mesencephalotomy, and midline myelotomy.

Conclusion

Despite the multiple options available for the management of cancer pain, many patients are undertreated or suffer limiting secondary effects. Pain may result from the primary disease process, secondary to treatment, or from sources unrelated to malignancy.

Secondary effects of opioids should be anticipated in all patients and screened for in each encounter as they may affect a patient's ability to use opioids. Opioids are the mainstay of treatment for cancer pain and should be used at any stage of the disease without concern for life expectancy.

Suggested readings

Abrahms JL. *A Physician's Guide to Pain and Symptom Management in Cancer Patients*. 2nd ed. Baltimore: The Johns Hopkins University Press; 2005.

Christrupp LL. Morphine metabolites. *Acta Anesthesiol Scand* 1997; 41(1 Pt 2):116–122.

Foley K. Changing concepts of tolerance to opioids: what the cancer patient has taught us. In: Chapman CR, Foley KM, eds. *Current and Emerging Issues in Cancer Pain: Research and Practice.* New York: Raven Press; 1993:331–350.

Gabriel SE. *Cancer Pain Relief: With a Guide to Opioid Availability.* 2nd ed. Geneva: World Health Organization; 1996.

Hagen N. Reproducing a cancer patient's pain on physical examination: bedside provocative maneuvers. *J Pain Symptom Manage* 1999, 18:406–411.

Kanner RM. The scope of the problem. In: Portenoy RK, Kanner RM, eds. *Pain Management, Theory and Practice*. Philadelphia: FA Davis; 1996:40.

Raj PP. *Pain Medicine: A Comprehensive Review*. Boca Raton, FL: CRC Press; 1996.

Ross EL. *Hot Topics. Pain Management.* Philadelphia: Hanley & Belfus; 2004.

Rowe DS. Neurolytic Techniques For Pain Management. Available at: http://www.dcmsonline.org/jax-medicine/1998journals/october98/neurolytic.htm.

Vainio A, Auvinen A. Prevalence of symptoms among patients with advanced cancer: an international collaborative study. Symptom prevalence group. *J Pain Symptom Manage* 1996; 12: 3–10.

Intensive Care Unit

Gyorgy Frendl, editor

Cardiopulmonary resuscitation

Samuel M. Galvagno Jr.

Introduction

In 2010, the American Heart Association (AHA) revised guidelines for cardiopulmonary resuscitation (CPR) and emergency cardiovascular care (ECC). Employing an evidence-based approach, these guidelines are based on the best available scientific evidence and were the result of an international collaboration amongst resuscitation experts. Several changes were made to simplify CPR instructions and ECC algorithms and to emphasize critical, evidence-based assessments and interventions recommended for cardiac arrest or other life threatening conditions. A thorough discussion of topics covered in courses such as advanced cardiac life support (ACLS), pediatric advanced life support (PALS), or the Neonatal Resuscitation Program (NRP) is beyond the scope of this chapter. An introduction to the essential guidelines for CPR and ECC is presented with an emphasis on critical actions that are most likely to be used within the operating room or intensive care unit.

Basic life support (CPR)

The 2010 guidelines recommend a "Circulation-Airway-Breathing" approach ("C-A-B") as opposed to the classically taught "Airway-Breathing-Circulation" sequence. Fig. 153.1 depicts the sequence of steps to be followed for an unresponsive adult patient.

For all single rescuers of infant, child, and adult victims (excluding newborns), a universal compressing-ventilation ratio of 30:2 is recommended. This ratio may be altered to 15 compressions to 2 breaths for infant and child 2-rescuer CPR. Rescuers should "push hard and fast," compressing the chest at least 100 times a minute, while allowing complete chest recoil between compressions and minimizing interruptions. Incomplete recoil during compressions is associated with high intrathoracic pressures and impaired hemodynamics, including decreased coronary perfusion, decreased cardiac index, and decreased myocardial blood flow. Layperson bystanders not trained in CPR should provide "hands only" CPR. A summary of basic life support maneuvers for infants, children, and adults is presented in Table 153.1.

It should be noted that, after an advanced airway is secured, rescue breaths for adults, children, and infants should be delivered at a rate of approximately 8 to 10 breaths per minute. Hyperventilation during CPR for victims with advanced airways has been shown to decrease cardiac output, decrease coronary perfusion pressure, increase gastric inflation, and worsen outcomes. When an advanced airway is placed, chest compressions should not be interrupted to deliver ventilations. During CPR, cardiac output may be reduced to 25% of normal; hence, lower minute ventilation can maintain effective oxygenation and ventilation. Tidal volumes of 500 to 600 ml (6–7ml/kg) are recommended, and an effective way to ensure adequate tidal volume is to produce a visible chest rise. Vigilance is required during bag-mask ventilation as adult ventilating bags typically contain volumes of 1 to 2 liters. There is inadequate evidence to define the optimal timing of advanced airway placement in relation to other interventions for cardiac arrest. Some studies have shown that patients had better neurologic outcomes after cardiac arrest when intubation was delayed and combined with minimally interrupted chest compressions.

Sudden cardiac death is a leading cause of death in North America, and most victims demonstrate ventricular fibrillation (VF) at some point during their arrest. Early defibrillation is most likely to be effective if delivered during the first 5 minutes of collapse; however, many patients will not be defibrillated within this narrow therapeutic window. CPR performed immediately before and after shock delivery after VF-induced collapse has been shown to confer a nearly threefold improved chance of survival. Consequently, the 2010 guidelines continue to strongly emphasize the proper performance of CPR for victims of cardiac arrest.

Electrical therapies

Survival rates for VF are highest when CPR is initiated promptly with defibrillation within 3 to 5 minutes. For every minute that passes between witnessed VF cardiac arrest and defibrillation, survival rates decrease by approximately 10%; when CPR is provided, the decrease is less rapid and averages approximately 4% per minute from collapse to defibrillation. Whereas CPR may maintain minimal oxygen and substrate delivery to the heart and brain, basic CPR, by itself, is not likely to eliminate VF.

Defibrillation is defined as termination of VF for at least 5 seconds following a monophasic or biphasic electrical shock.

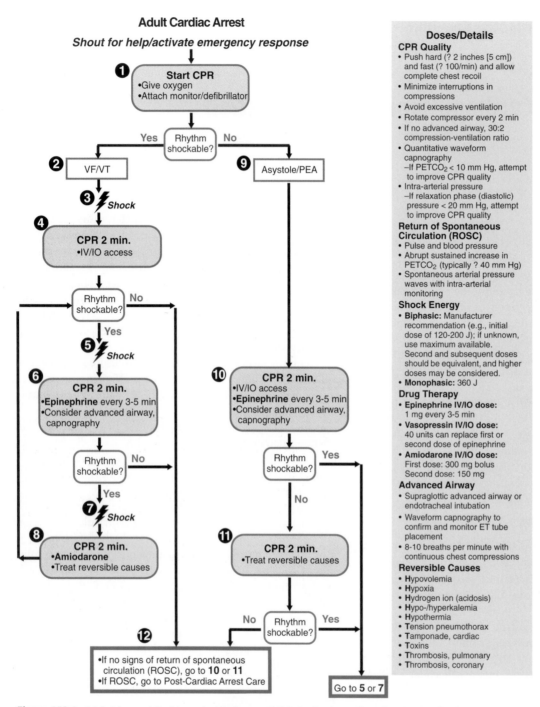

Adult Cardiac Arrest

Shout for help/activate emergency response

❶ Start CPR
•Give oxygen
•Attach monitor/defibrillator

Rhythm shockable?
Yes — **❷ VF/VT**
No — **❾ Asystole/PEA**

❸ ⚡ Shock

❹ CPR 2 min.
•IV/IO access

Rhythm shockable? — No

❺ ⚡ Shock

❻ CPR 2 min.
•**Epinephrine** every 3-5 min
•Consider advanced airway, capnography

Rhythm shockable? — No

❼ ⚡ Shock

❽ CPR 2 min.
•**Amiodarone**
•Treat reversible causes

❿ CPR 2 min.
•IV/IO access
•**Epinephrine** every 3-5 min
•Consider advanced airway, capnography

Rhythm shockable? — Yes / No

⓫ CPR 2 min.
•Treat reversible causes

Rhythm shockable? — No / Yes

⓬
•If no signs of return of spontaneous circulation (ROSC), go to **10** or **11**
•If ROSC, go to Post-Cardiac Arrest Care

Go to **5** or **7**

Doses/Details
CPR Quality
• Push hard (? 2 inches [5 cm]) and fast (? 100/min) and allow complete chest recoil
• Minimize interruptions in compressions
• Avoid excessive ventilation
• Rotate compressor every 2 min
• If no advanced airway, 30:2 compression-ventilation ratio
• Quantitative waveform capnography
  –If PETCO$_2$ < 10 mm Hg, attempt to improve CPR quality
• Intra-arterial pressure
  –If relaxation phase (diastolic) pressure < 20 mm Hg, attempt to improve CPR quality

Return of Spontaneous Circulation (ROSC)
• Pulse and blood pressure
• Abrupt sustained increase in PETCO$_2$ (typically ? 40 mm Hg)
• Spontaneous arterial pressure waves with intra-arterial monitoring

Shock Energy
• **Biphasic:** Manufacturer recommendation (e.g., initial dose of 120-200 J); if unknown, use maximum available. Second and subsequent doses should be equivalent, and higher doses may be considered.
• **Monophasic:** 360 J

Drug Therapy
• **Epinephrine IV/IO dose:** 1 mg every 3-5 min
• **Vasopressin IV/IO dose:** 40 units can replace first or second dose of epinephrine
• **Amiodarone IV/IO dose:** First dose: 300 mg bolus Second dose: 150 mg

Advanced Airway
• Supraglottic advanced airway or endotracheal intubation
• Waveform capnography to confirm and monitor ET tube placement
• 8-10 breaths per minute with continuous chest compressions

Reversible Causes
• Hypovolemia
• Hypoxia
• Hydrogen ion (acidosis)
• Hypo-/hyperkalemia
• Hypothermia
• Tension pneumothorax
• Tamponade, cardiac
• Toxins
• Thrombosis, pulmonary
• Thrombosis, coronary

Figure 153.1. Adult Advanced Cardiovascular Life Support (ACLS) Cardiac Arrest Algorithm. Reprinted with permission. 2010 American Heart Association Guidelines for Cardiopulmonary Resuscitation and Emergency Cardiovascular Care, Part 8: Adult Advanced Cardiovascular Life Support. *Circulation* 2010; 122[suppl 3]: S736, Figure 1. ©2010 American Heart Association, Inc.

Investigators have proposed different hypotheses regarding the mechanism of action; however, the exact mechanism of effective defibrillation is unknown. Defibrillating shocks may cause transient depolarization of myocardial tissue or prolong the refractory period of the cardiac action potential. The ability of an electrical shock to defibrillate the heart depends on its waveform and energy. Cardioversion, as opposed to defibrillation, involves delivery of a shock synchronized with the QRS complex.

Regardless of the timing, a defibrillation waveform describes the energy, or current, mathematically as a factor of time. A monophasic waveform has a single positive phase that

Table 153.1. Summary of key basic life support components for adults

Component	Recommendation
Pulse check	No more than 10 seconds, healthcare providers only (laypersons should not check for a pulse)
CPR sequence	C-A-B (Circulation/Chest Compressions-Airway-Breathing)
Compression rate	100 compressions/minute
Chest wall recoil	Full chest wall recoil should be allowed between compressions
Compressor rotation interval	Healthcare providers should rotate compressors every 2 minutes to avoid fatigue
Compression-to-ventilation ratio	30:2 (1 or 2 rescuers)
Ventilations (rescue breathing)	1 breath every 6-8 seconds (8-10 breaths/min)
	1 second per breath
	Visible chest rise should be observed
	Asynchronous with chest compressions

either rapidly or gradually returns to zero voltage with current flowing in the direction between defibrillation electrodes (Fig. 153.2).

Biphasic waveforms have a positive and negative phase reflecting a reversal of current flow between the defibrillation electrodes. Recent clinical trials have compared the use of monophasic and biphasic shocks for external defibrillation, but neither has been consistently associated with a higher rate of return of spontaneous circulation or survival. Biphasic shocks have shown a trend toward equivalent or higher success for termination of VF and are now the standard waveform used in most commercial defibrillators. Multiple prospective studies have failed to demonstrate the ideal biphasic energy level. Current recommendations are to deliver the initial shock at 150 J for biphasic truncated waveforms. If the defibrillator is designed to deliver a rectilinear biphasic waveform, 120 J can be used. For subsequent shocks, the same or a higher energy level can be used. Directions for selection of the appropriate energy level are provided with each specific model of defibrillator. If the type of defibrillator is unknown, current guidelines recommend delivering the first shock at 200 J. Previous guidelines recommended three-shock initial sequences for VF, but because the first shock is most likely to be the most effective, especially when biphasic waveforms are used, the current recommendation is to deliver single shocks in between sequences of high-quality CPR.

Defibrillator electrodes, including automated external defibrillators (AEDs), should be placed in an anterolateral (sternal–apical) position. If an implantable medical device is present, the electrode pads should be positioned at least 1 inch (2.5 cm) away from the device. Pads should never be placed over transdermal medication patches. Several case reports of fires, ignited by defibrillator current arcing, have been described in the presence of oxygen-rich environments, such as the operating room or intensive care unit. Rescuers should take precautions to minimize arcing by using self-adhering defibrillation pads and by minimizing the flow of oxygen across a patient's chest during defibrillation attempts.

Pulseless cardiac arrest

The four most common lethal rhythms encountered during cardiac arrest include VF, rapid ventricular tachycardia (VT), pulseless electrical activity (PEA), and asystole.

The most critical intervention during the first minutes of pulseless arrest is immediate CPR. Chest compression interruptions should be minimized, and defibrillation should be accomplished as soon as possible. Central venous access for drug administration is not required for most resuscitation attempts, and, if access is identified as a problem, endotracheal administration of drugs or intraosseous (IO) cannulation are reasonable alternatives. IO cannulation is safe and effective for initial fluid resuscitation, drug delivery, and blood sampling. IO access is attainable in all age groups and is likely to be a better route for emergency drug administration than the endotracheal route because multiple studies have shown that lidocaine, epinephrine, atropine, naloxone, and vasopressin are absorbed poorly with lower blood concentrations than would be expected with intravenous (IV) administration.

The survival rate for cardiac arrest from asystole and PEA is poor. A successful resuscitation in such cases is most likely when a reversible cause can be identified and treated. As opposed to treatment for VF and VT, defibrillation is not effective. CPR, with early establishment of an advanced airway, remains the mainstay of treatment.

Despite the prolific use of vasopressor and antiarrhythmics for ECC over the past several decades, to date, there is no evidence that any of these agents increase the rate of neurologically intact survival to hospital discharge. For all lethal arrhythmias encountered during pulseless arrest, high-quality CPR and defibrillation should be initiated before

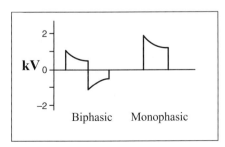

Figure 153.2. Biphasic and monophasic defibrillation waveforms.

Table 153.2. Pharmacologic agents for use in pulseless arrest

Drug	Initial dose	Frequency	Mechanism	Comment
Epinephrine	1 mg IV/IO for adults (0.01 mg/kg of 1:1000 for children or 0.1 mg/kg of 1:10,000)	Every 3–5 min	α- and β-adrenergic; increases cerebral and myocardial perfusion	High-dose epinephrine is no longer recommended
Vasopressin	40 Units IV/IO	One-time dose only	Nonadrenergic peripheral vasoconstrictor	One dose may replace either first or second dose of epinephrine
Atropine	1 mg IV/IO (0.02 mg/kg IV/IO for children, minimum dose 0.1 mg)	Every 3–5 minutes; maximum dose 3.0 mg for adults, 1.0 mg for children	Reversal of cholinergic-mediated decreases in heart rate, systemic vascular resistance, and blood pressure	Only indicated in children with bradycardia due to increased vagal tone or primary AV block
Amiodarone	300 mg IV/IO for arrest (5 mg/kg for children)	First dose can be followed by 150 mg	Sodium, potassium, calcium channel blocker; α- and β-adrenergic blocker	If successful, should be followed with a continuous infusion
Lidocaine	1.5 mg/kg first dose IV/IO (1 mg/kg for children)	1.0 mg/kg at 5- to 10-min intervals to maximum dose of 3 mg/kg	Sodium channel blocker	No proven short-term or long-term efficacy in cardiac arrest
Magnesium	1–2 g IV/IO (50 mg/kg IV/IO, maximum dose 2 g for torsades in children)	Give in 10 ml of D_5W over 5–10 min	Calcium channel blocker	Effective for termination of polymorphic VT (torsades de pointes)

AV, atrioventricular; D_5W, 5% dextrose in water.

pharmacotherapeutic therapy. CPR should not be interrupted to give medications. Drugs can be administered before or after defibrillation in a *CPR-RHYTHM CHECK-CPR-SHOCK* sequence, repeated as needed. Epinephrine is the first drug of choice in all instances of pulseless arrest. A summary of medications for cardiac arrest is provided in Table 153.2.

Interventions that are not supported by available evidence include pacing in asystole, norepinephrine, and the precordial thump. Procainamide was shown to be effective in a small study of 20 patients, but its use is limited by the need for slow infusion and limited evidence for effectiveness in emergent situations.

Management of symptomatic bradycardia and tachycardia

The management of symptomatic tachycardia and bradycardia is discussed in Chapter 155. Figures 153.3 and 153.4 are the current algorithms for symptomatic tachycardia and bradycardia taught in ACLS.

Pediatric advanced life support

In children, sudden cardiac arrest is uncommon and usually results from a respiratory rather than cardiac event. Impending respiratory failure is indicated by increased respiratory rate, nasal flaring, retractions, gasping, diminished breath sounds, or grunting. Shock is another cause of cardiac arrest in the pediatric population with the most common cause being hypovolemia. The signs of compensated and decompensated shock in pediatric patients are summarized in Table 153.3. Knowledge of the signs of shock and imminent respiratory failure is imperative because early recognition may lead to interventions that can prevent cardiac arrest in pediatric patients. Many of the signs of

shock may be confused with other etiologies, such as pain, fever, or anxiety.

Management of the pulseless arrest in the pediatric patient is similar to management of adults insofar as prompt advanced airway management and CPR remain the cornerstones of care (Fig. 153.5).

Initial electrical shocks, when indicated, should be delivered with 2 J/kg. AEDs are preferred for patients 1 to 8 years of age. Vasopressin is not indicated for pediatric patients. Possible causes should be considered and treated (Table 153.4).

If an intubated pediatric patient's condition deteriorates precipitously, the mnemonic "DOPE" should be considered to identify the most common culprits:

D – Displacement of the endotracheal tube
O – Obstruction of the tube
P – Pneumothorax
E – Equipment failure

During CPR, interruptions in chest compressions should be minimized and hyperventilation should be avoided because pediatric patients, like adults, tend to be overventilated during resuscitation. For a complete review of PALS, it is recommended that anesthesiologists who provide care for pediatric patients take the course offered in conjunction with the American Academy of Pediatrics and the AHA.

Neonatal resuscitation

Approximately 10% of newborns require some assistance with breathing at birth, and 1% require formal resuscitation. Guidelines for neonatal resuscitation are provided in the NRP course offered by the American Academy of Pediatrics. Initial management of a neonatal resuscitation, as taught in the NRP, is outlined in Fig. 153.6.

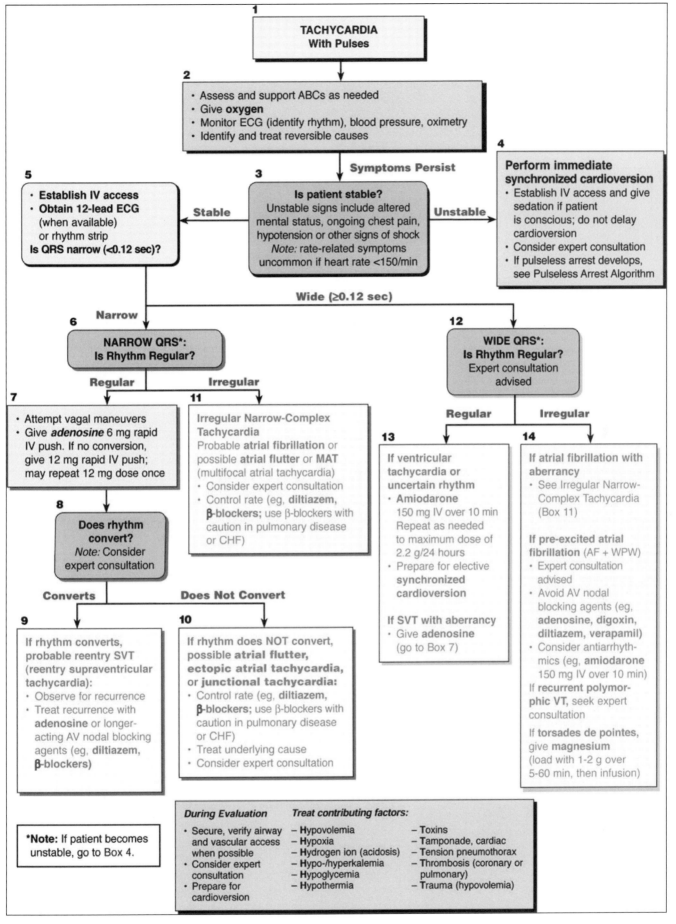

Figure 153.3. Adult Tachycardia (with pulse). Reprinted with permission. 2010 American Heart Association Guidelines for Cardiopulmonary Resuscitation and Emergency Cardiovascular Care, Part 8: Adult Advanced Cardiovascular Life Support. *Circulation* 2010; 122[suppl 3]: S751, Figure 4. ©2010 American Heart Association, Inc.

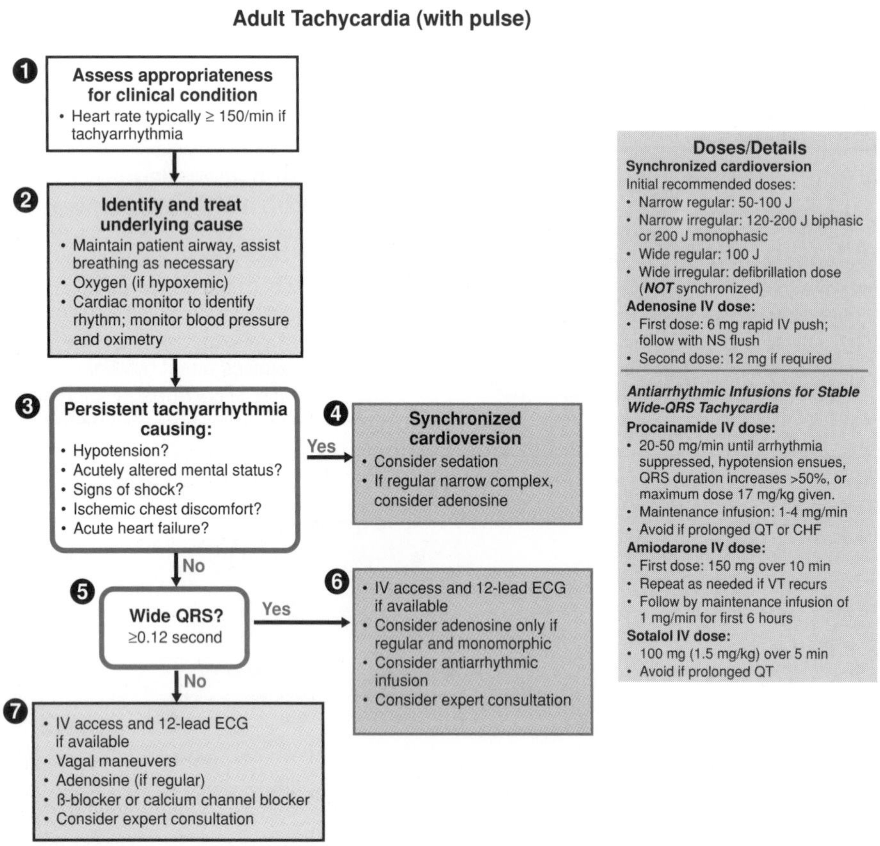

Adult Tachycardia (with pulse)

❶ Assess appropriateness for clinical condition
- Heart rate typically ≥ 150/min if tachyarrhythmia

❷ Identify and treat underlying cause
- Maintain patient airway, assist breathing as necessary
- Oxygen (if hypoxemic)
- Cardiac monitor to identify rhythm; monitor blood pressure and oximetry

❸ Persistent tachyarrhythmia causing:
- Hypotension?
- Acutely altered mental status?
- Signs of shock?
- Ischemic chest discomfort?
- Acute heart failure?

→ **Yes** → **❹ Synchronized cardioversion**
- Consider sedation
- If regular narrow complex, consider adenosine

↓ **No**

❺ Wide QRS? ≥0.12 second

→ **Yes** → **❻**
- IV access and 12-lead ECG if available
- Consider adenosine only if regular and monomorphic
- Consider antiarrhythmic infusion
- Consider expert consultation

↓ **No**

❼
- IV access and 12-lead ECG if available
- Vagal maneuvers
- Adenosine (if regular)
- ß-blocker or calcium channel blocker
- Consider expert consultation

Doses/Details

Synchronized cardioversion
Initial recommended doses:
- Narrow regular: 50-100 J
- Narrow irregular: 120-200 J biphasic or 200 J monophasic
- Wide regular: 100 J
- Wide irregular: defibrillation dose (**NOT** synchronized)

Adenosine IV dose:
- First dose: 6 mg rapid IV push; follow with NS flush
- Second dose: 12 mg if required

Antiarrhythmic Infusions for Stable Wide-QRS Tachycardia

Procainamide IV dose:
- 20-50 mg/min until arrhythmia suppressed, hypotension ensues, QRS duration increases >50%, or maximum dose 17 mg/kg given.
- Maintenance infusion: 1-4 mg/min
- Avoid if prolonged QT or CHF

Amiodarone IV dose:
- First dose: 150 mg over 10 min
- Repeat as needed if VT recurs
- Follow by maintenance infusion of 1 mg/min for first 6 hours

Sotalol IV dose:
- 100 mg (1.5 mg/kg) over 5 min
- Avoid if prolonged QT

Figure 153.4. Adult Bradycardia (with pulse). Reprinted with permission. 2010 American Heart Association Guidelines for Cardiopulmonary Resuscitation and Emergency Cardiovascular Care, Part 8: Adult Advanced Cardiovascular Life Support. *Circulation* 2010; 122[suppl 3]: S749, Figure 3. ©2010 American Heart Association, Inc.

Table 153.3. Compensated and decompensated shock

Compensated shock	Decompensated shock
Tachycardia	Depressed mental status
Cool extremities	Decreased urine output
Prolonged capillary refill	Metabolic acidosis
Weak peripheral pulses	Tachypnea
Normal blood pressure	Weak central pulses
	Systolic pressure:
	<60 (0–28 d)
	<70 in infants (1–12 mo)
	<70+ (2 × age in years) in children 1–10 y
	<90 in children over age 10

Table 153.4. Possible etiologies for pulseless arrest in both adult and pediatric patients

6 "H's"	5 "T's"
Hypovolemia	Toxins
Hypoxia	Thrombosis (coronary or pulmonary)
Hydrogen ion (acidosis)	Tension pneumothorax
Hypoglycemia	Trauma
Hyper- or hypokalemia	Tamponade, cardiac
Hypothermia	

Source: International Liaison Committee on Resuscitation. 2005 International Consensus on Cardiopulmonary Resuscitation and Emergency Cardiovascular Care Science with Treatment Recommendations. Part 4: Advanced life support. *Resuscitation* 2005. 67:213–247.

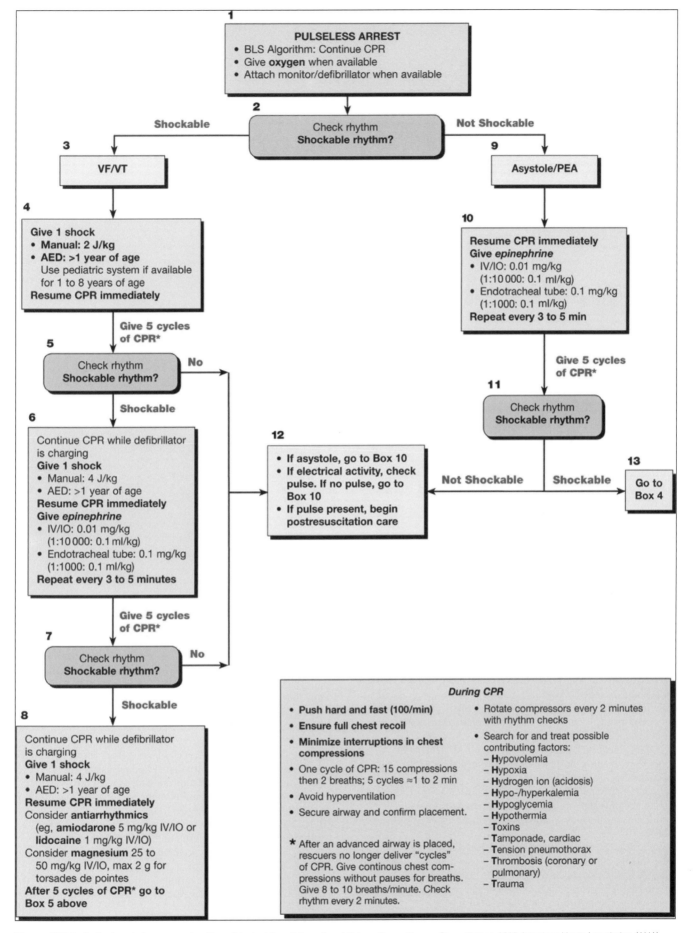

Figure 153.5. Pediatric pulseless arrest algorithm. Adapted from International Liaison Committee on Resuscitation. 2005 American Heart Association (AHA) guidelines for cardiopulmonary resuscitation and emergency cardiovascular care of pediatric and neonatal patients: pediatric advanced life support. *Pediatrics* 2006; 117(5):1005–1028.

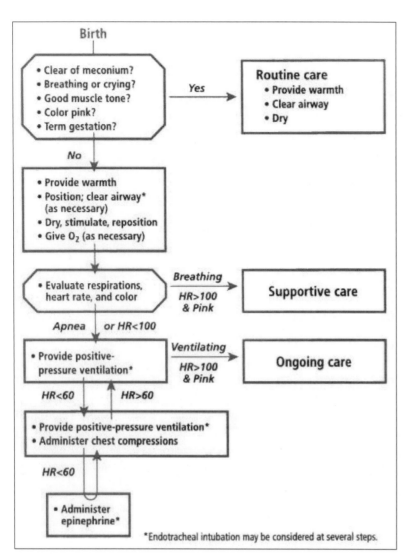

Figure 153.6. Resuscitation algorithm for neonates. Adapted from Katwinkel J. *Neonatal Resuscitation Textbook*, T1, American Heart Assocation, 2006.

Suggested readings

2010 American Heart Association guidelines for cardiopulmonary resuscitation and emergency cardivascular care. *Circulation* 2010; 122[suppl 3]:S729–S676.

Aufderheide TP, Sigurdsson G, Pirrallo RG, et al. Hyperventilation-induced hypotension during cardiopulmonary resuscitation. *Circulation* 2004; 109:1960–1965.

Cobb LA, Fahrenbruch CE, Olsufka M, Copass MK. Changing incidence of out-of-hospital ventricular fibrillation, 1980–2000. *JAMA* 2002; 288:3008–3013.

Gabrielli A, O'Connor MF, Maccioli GA. Anesthesia advanced circulatory life support. Available at: http://www.asahq.org/clinical/Anesthesiology-CentricACLS.pdf. Accessed April 14, 2008.

Galvagno SM. *Emergency Pathophysiology*. Jackson, WY: Teton NewMedia; 2004.

Hickey RW, Billi JE, Nadkarni VM, et al. 2005 American Heart Association guidelines for cardiopulmonary resuscitation and emergency cardiovascular care. *Circulation* 2005; 112(24):IV-1–IV-84.

Johnston C. Endotracheal drug delivery. *Pediatr Emerg Care* 1992; 8:94–97.

Larsen MP, Eisenberg MS, Cummins RO, Hallstrom AP. Predicting survival from out-of-hospital cardiac arrest: a graphic model. *Ann Emerg Med* 1993; 22:1652–1658.

Niemann JT, Stratton SJ, Cruz B, Lewis RJ. Endotracheal drug administration during out-of-hospital resuscitation: where are the survivors? *Resuscitation* 2002; 53:153–157.

Sayre MR, Berg RA, Cave DM, et al. International Liaison Committee on Resuscitation. 2005 International Consensus on Cardiopulmonary Resuscitation and Emergency Cardiovascular Care Science with Treatment Recommendations. *Circulation* 2005; 1112:III-1–III-136. 3.

Stiell IG, Wells GA, Hebert PC, et al. Association of drug therapy with survival in cardiac arrest: limited role of advanced cardiac life support drugs. *Acad Emerg Med* 1995; 2:264–273.

Young KD, Seidel JS. Pediatric cardiopulmonary resuscitation: a collective review. *Ann Emerg Med* 1999; 33:195–205.

Multiorgan failure and its prevention

K. Annette Mizuguchi and Gyorgy Frendl

Introduction

As anesthesiologists, we are routinely asked to care for patients with multiple and complex comorbidities. Few situations, however, can be more challenging than caring for patients with multiorgan dysfunction. These patients are challenging because they have acute functional changes and the potential to deteriorate dramatically. They also present with various combinations of organ involvement and with varying degrees of severity adding another layer of complexity to their management.

Definition of multiorgan dysfunction syndrome and failure

Multiorgan dysfunction syndrome (MODS) and multiorgan failure (MOF) are most commonly seen in the context of critical illness or injury that is often due to sepsis or trauma. Most commonly affected organs are the lungs, kidneys, liver, heart, brain, and the hematopoietic system, but involvement of any organ is possible, and the severity of dysfunction is variable. Unlike other disease processes, organ dysfunction is not caused by a direct disease process involving a particular organ (like infection or trauma); rather the patient's diseased state is thought to indirectly affect the organ.

Incidence, morbidity, and mortality

MOF develops in 15% of all hospital admissions and contributes to up to 80% of all deaths. Patient survival is inversely related to the number of failing organs involved (Table 154.1). When three or more organs are involved, mortality reaches 50%. After five organ systems are affected, mortality is >80%. Therefore, preventing the development of MOD and MOF is desirable and can significantly impact patient survival. Unfortunately, early detection of organ dysfunction by clinical signs and symptoms or by reliable biomarkers is not possible for all organs involved. Early detection of cardiac injury, however, is now possible with the use of troponin as a biomarker.

A MOD score of 5 through 8 is associated with 5% mortality, which increases to 30% with scores of 9 through 12 (Table 154.3). Mortality is further increased to 70% with scores of 13 through 16 and 91% for scores of 17 through 20. Certain combinations of organ dysfunction (i.e., pulmonary and hepatic dysfunction or cardiac and hepatic dysfunction) carry a high risk of early mortality (Table 154.3).

Dysfunction of key organs

Isolated organ dysfunction is rare. In general, patients with MODS or MOF have combinations of involved organs. Key organs and systems involved are noted in this section.

Lungs

Acute lung injury (ALI), with moderate impairment of lung function, is defined as a PaO_2/FiO_2 ratio of < 300 ($[SpO_2/FiO_2] \leq 315$ if $SpO_2 \leq 97\%$, where SpO_2 is the oxygen saturation). Severe lung injury is defined as a ratio of $PaO_2/FiO_2 < 200$ (or $SpO_2/FiO_2 \leq 235$ if $SpO_2 \leq 97\%$), and it is also known as acute respiratory distress syndrome (ARDS). A detailed discussion of this disease state can be found in Chapter 159.

Cardiovascular

Cardiovascular dysfunction is associated with significantly increased mortality. In mild cardiac dysfunction, elevation of serum troponin is often seen without significant decrease in pump function. In advanced cardiac dysfunction, however, an often severe decrease in left ventricular (LV) pump function (measured as decreased LV ejection fraction [LVEF]) is seen.

Vascular dysfunction manifests as hypotension, due to a profound vasodilatory state that accompanies most forms of MODS or MOF. The combined dysfunction of the cardiac and vascular systems is often apparent as these patients frequently require inotropic agents (i.e., dobutamine) to support their LV pump function as well as vasoconstricting agents to counteract peripheral vasodilation (i.e., norepinephrine or dopamine).

Table 154.1. ICU survival is related to the number of failing organ systems involved

Failing organ systems, *n*	Mortality, %
0	0.8%
1	6.8
2	26.2
3	48.5
4	68.8
5	83.3

Table 154.2. Risk, injury, failure, loss, and end-stage (RIFLE) kidney criteria

Class	Glomerular filtration rate criteria	Urine output criteria
Risk	Increase in serum creatinine × 1.5 from baseline	<0.5 ml/kg/h × 6 h
Injury	Increase in serum creatinine × 2 from baseline	<0.5 ml/kg/h × 12 h
Failure	Increase in serum creatinine × 3 from baseline, or serum creatinine ≥ 4 mg/dl with an acute rise > 0.5 mg/dl	<0.3 ml/kg/h × 24 h, or anuria × 1
Loss	Persistent acute renal failure = complete loss of kidney function > 4 wk	
End-stage kidney disease	End-stage kidney disease > 3 mo	

Adapted from Bellomo R, Kellum JA, Ronco C. Defining and classifying acute renal failure: from advocacy to consensus and validation of the RIFLE criteria. *Intensive Care Med* 2007; 33:409–413.

Kidneys

Acute kidney injury (AKI) is a major cause of morbidity and mortality in hospitalized patients, and it is consistently associated with increased mortality. AKI can be defined as elevation of serum creatinine greater than 0.3 mg/dl from baseline (pre-diseased state) or the doubling of baseline creatinine. Although there are various definitions for AKI, the two widely accepted criteria are the RIFLE (Table 154.2) and the AKIN classification. The RIFLE criteria provides a graded definition of AKI severity that correlates with outcomes.

Liver

The primary function of the liver is detoxification of internal toxins as well as the production of proteins. It is hypothesized that in MODS or MOF a sepsis-related increased gut permeability and bacterial translocation lead to the development of liver dysfunction. Signs of liver dysfunction consist of persistent elevation of aspartate aminotransferase (AST) and alanine aminotransferase (ALT), elevation of bilirubin to greater than 1.2 mg/dl (mostly due to cholestasis), and persistent unexplained elevation of prothrombin time (PT) indicating a synthetic dysfunction of the liver. Liver failure is noted by hypoglycemia, persistent coagulopathy, ongoing elevation of bilirubin, and elevation of liver enzymes (AST and/or ALT).

Gastrointestinal tract

Gastroparesis (impaired gastric emptying) and postoperative ileus are commonly seen in MODS and/or MOF. Stress ulcers (Curling ulcers) used to occur commonly, but they have been almost completely eliminated with the routine use of acid-suppressing agents (H_2 blockers or proton pump inhibitors).

Brain

Mental status is altered in mild forms of brain dysfunction, and delirium is the most frequent presentation. Delirium is a disoriented state of mind characterized by fluctuation of mental status, inattention, and disorganized thinking. It can be diagnosed with the CAM-ICU (confusion assessment measurement in the intensive care unit) method developed by Ely and colleagues. The benefit of this method is that it can be applied in ventilator-dependent patients. In more severe forms, mental status can deteriorate to somnolence, stupor, or even coma, even in the absence of organic brain damage.

Hematopoietic system

The most common form of hematologic dysfunction is thrombocytopenia and elevation of prothrombin time (PT) and international normalized ratio (INR). In disseminated intravascular coagulation (DIC), thrombocytopenia and increased PT are seen. Leukocytosis is common, but leukopenia frequently accompanies severe sepsis and septic shock.

Musculoskeletal system

Seen less frequently than other forms of organ dysfunctions, variable degrees of skeletal muscle weakness can develop in the context of critical illness, and it is often referred to as *critical illness myopathy*. Although the cause is often unclear, in certain cases, longer-term use of neuromuscular blocking agents has been suspected.

Assessing the severity of MODS and/or MOF

Two scoring systems have been developed to assess the degree of combined organ dysfunction in MODS and MOF: the MOD score (Table 154.3) and the sequential organ failure assessment

Table 154.3. MOD scores

Organ system	Score				
	0	1	2	3	4
Respiratory: PaO₂/FiO₂	>300	226–300	151–225	76–150	≤75
Renal: creatinine (μmol/L)	≤100	101–200	201–350	251–500	>500
Hepatic: bilirubin (μmol/L)	≤20	21–60	61–120	121–240	>240
Cardiovascular: PAR[a]	<10.0	10.1–15	15.1–20.0	20.1–30.0	>30.0
Hematologic: platelet count	>120	81–120	51–80	21–50	≤20
Neurologic: Glasgow Coma Scale score	15	13–14	10–12	7–9	≤6

[a] PAR (pressure-adjusted heart rate) is the product of the heart rate and the ratio of the right atrial pressure to the mean arterial pressure.
Adapted from: Marshall JC, Cook DJ, Christou NV, et al. Multiple organ dysfunction score: a reliable descriptor of a complex clinical outcome. *Crit Care Med* 1995; 23:1638–1652.

Table 154.4. SOFA scores

Organ system	Score				
	0	1	2	3	4
Respiratory: PaO$_2$/FiO$_2$	400	≤400	≤300	≤200	≤100
Renal: creatinine (μmol/L)	≤110	101–170	171–299	300–440; urine output ≤500 ml/d	>440; urine output <200
Hepatic: bilirubin (μmol/L)	≤20	20–32	33–101	102–204	>204
Cardiovascular: hypotension	No hypotension	MAP < 70 mm Hg	Dopamine ≤ 5[a] dobutamine (any dose)	Dopamine > 5[a] or epinephrine ≤0.1[a] or norepinephrine ≤ 0.1[a]	Dopamine >15[a] or epinephrine >0.1[a] or norepinephrine > 01[a]
Hematologic: platelet count	150	≤150	≤100	≤50	≤20
Neurologic: Glasgow Coma Scale score	15	13–14	10–12	6-9	<6

[a] Adrenergic agents administered for at least 1 h (doses given are in μg/kg/min). MAP, mean arterial pressure.

(SOFA) score (Table 154.4). Both of these score the same six organ systems, using physiologic data, but in a slightly different manner. The SOFA score is calculated based on the most abnormal value during a 24-hour period, whereas the MOD score is calculated using physiologic values measured at the same point in time every day (i.e., first morning values). Importantly, both of these scores, when indicating more severe injury, were found to correlate with poorer outcome and survival.

Clinical conditions commonly leading to MODS and MOF

The most common cause of organ failure is sepsis, and sepsis triggered by a localized inflammatory process can lead to systemic inflammatory response syndrome (SIRS). In 1992, the American College of Chest Physicians and Society of Critical Care Medicine (ACCP/SCCM) consensus conference established the diagnostic criteria for SIRS.

SIRS is present when two or more of the following conditions are met: temperature >38°C or <36°C; heart rate >90 beats/min; respiratory rate >20 breaths/min or PaCO$_2$ <32 mm Hg; and white blood cell count >12,000/mm^3, <4000 cells/mm^3, or >10% immature (band) forms. This definition of sepsis (Table 154.5) recognizes the progression of disease status from early inflammation to sepsis, and through severe sepsis and septic shock, ultimately, to MOF (Table 154.3).

Certain critical events seem to be associated with SIRS and MOF: cardiac arrest, congestive heart failure, infection, pneumonia, upper gastrointestinal bleed, surgery, trauma, and thermal injury. Common surgical procedures associated with SIRS and MOF include surgery for head trauma, elective abdominal aortic aneurysm repair, aortic dissections or ruptures, cardiac valvular surgery, and gastrointestinal surgery for perforation, inflammatory disease, or carcinoma. Other factors associated with the development of SIRS and MOF include delayed or inadequate resuscitation, persistent infection or inflammation, surgical "misadventure," presence of hematoma, age > 64 years, prior organ dysfunction, steroid use, chronic health problems (i.e., alcoholism, malnutrition, and diabetes), and serious physiologic abnormality on ICU admission.

Other forms of significant (noninfectious) tissue injury (i.e., poly-trauma) can also lead to the development of MODS or MOF in which organ dysfunction develops as a result of tissue hypoperfusion without overwhelming inflammation. Cytokines released from damaged tissues are suspected to play a role in this form of MODS and MOF.

Pathogenesis and suspected mechanism of MODS and/or MOF

Although there is evidence that sepsis- and injury-related hypoperfusion (hypoxemia) of the tissues, in combination with release of mediators, play a role in MODS and MOF, it is yet unclear which of these factors are most important. In fact, it is likely that each of these factors plays a role in the different forms of complex, critically ill states that lead to MODS and MOF. It is hypothesized that both capillary leakiness and the cytokine-induced impaired oxygen extraction further aggravate organ dysfunction and facilitate organ failure.

Sepsis is a disease of the microvascular endothelium that leads to tissue hypoxia and dysoxia even when sufficient oxygen is delivered through the blood. In sepsis, patients are unable to adequately extract oxygen from the blood. Thus, this impaired ability to extract oxygen leads to worsening organ dysfunction. Most likely the combination of tissue hypoxia and inflammatory mediator release triggers the development of organ dysfunction as the clinical signs of sepsis develop.

Table 154.5. Definitions

Sepsis = SIRS as a result of infection
Severe sepsis = sepsis + 2 or more organ dysfunction
Septic shock = severe sepsis + hypotension refractory to volume infusion
MODS = abnormal function in more than one vital organ
MOF = failure in more than one vital organ

Prevention and management

The prevention of MOF requires effective and early management of SIRS. For the management of MODS or MOF related to sepsis, evidence-based guidelines have been developed and are detailed in Chapter 161. These guidelines include early administration of broad-spectrum antibiotic following the submission of appropriate microbial cultures, elimination of known infections focus (i.e., source control), and early, appropriate fluid resuscitation. The success of early volume resuscitation in sepsis is likely due to improved microcirculation and interruption of the vicious cycle of tissue dysoxia, hypoperfusion, and cytokine release. The primary resuscitative fluids should be crystalloids, with judicious supplementation with colloids. Studies have shown that volume resuscitation with albumin can be harmful, particularly for head injured trauma patients, and therefore should be avoided for this patient population. The use of albumin in other populations seems to carry an equipoise and can be used at the discretion of the physicians.

For the management of ALI or ARDS, evidence-based guidelines recommend that a tidal volumes of 6 to 8 ml/kg of ideal body weight be delivered, while keeping the mean airway plateau pressures < 30 mm Hg, combined with the judicious increases of positive end-expiratory pressure (PEEP) to support adequate oxygenation.

For trauma patients, early stabilization of fractures and adequate cardiopulmonary resuscitation play a key role. In burn patients, aggressive fluid resuscitation can significantly reduce secondary organ damage and MODS or MOF.

Early and accurate detection of AKI could lead to improved survival. However, currently available diagnostic tests, which include serum creatinine and blood urea nitrogen, are suboptimal markers for AKI because they are neither sensitive nor specific for detecting early changes in kidney function. New biomarkers are being evaluated, but none have been approved yet.

The most common cause of AKI is decreased renal perfusion followed by administration of nephrotoxin, contrast administration, and major surgery. Therefore, early institution of prevention strategies in these patients may be helpful. Such strategies include maintenance of adequate blood volume and renal blood flow by providing adequate hydration and avoidance of nephrotoxic drugs. Routine use of diuretics has not been shown to be helpful. Certain forms of AKI (i.e., contrast-induced nephropathy) may benefit from the administration of antioxidants, such as N-acetylcysteine.

When AKI progresses to renal failure, renal replacement therapy can be instituted. Continuous renal replacement therapy is commonly used to manage critically ill patients because it seems to be associated with less hemodynamic changes compared to conventional, intermittent hemodialysis. No prospective, randomized studies to date, however, have documented that continuous renal replacement therapy improves clinical outcome when compared with intermittent hemodialysis.

The precise and timely assessment of cardiac dysfunction is difficult even if one uses the combination of hemodynamic and echocardiographic data in combination with vasopressor requirement. The testing of several biomarkers that will provide early detection of cardiac dysfunction is under way. Troponin I and T levels seem to be associated with increased catecholamine requirement, decreased stroke work index, decreased LVEF, and increased mortality. Thus, some institutions follow troponin levels for the assessment of cardiac dysfunction in the ICU. B-type natriuretic peptide has been investigated as another potential biomarker but, as with the troponins, further studies are needed to prove its utility.

At present, the prevention and treatment of cardiovascular dysfunction rest on adequate and early fluid resuscitation with a combined approach of judicious fluid replacement and inotropic support. Maintaining normoglycemia may be beneficial as studies suggest that normoglycemia protects the endothelium, possibly by inhibiting nitric oxide release, and may contribute to the prevention of organ failure and death. Preventative use of statins and β-blockers seem to show promise, but further studies are required.

The future

Prevention and treatment of MOF will improve with availability of acute biomarkers that provide early diagnosis of SIRS and specific organ dysfunction. Such biomarkers could potentially be used to follow disease progression and treatment as well. Development of real-time polymerase chain reaction assays that identify the presence of bacterial or viral infection may replace our current reliance on blood cultures and permit earlier and appropriate antibiotic therapy.

Suggested readings

Barie PS, Hydo LJ. Epidemiology of multiple organ dysfunction syndrome in critical surgical illness. *Surg Infect (Larchmt)* 2000; 1:173–185; discussion 185–186.

Bellomo R, Kellum JA, Ronco C. Defining and classifying acute renal failure: from advocacy to consensus and validation of the RIFLE criteria. *Intensive Care Med* 2007; 33:409–413.

Bone RC, Balk RA, Cerra FEB, et al. Definitions for sepsis and organ failure and guidelines for the use for innovative therapies in sepsis. The ACCP/SCCM Consensus Conference Committee. American College of Chest Physicians/Society of Critical Care Medicine. *Chest* 1992; 101:1644–1655.

Dellinger RP, Levy MM, Carlet JM, et al. Surviving sepsis campaign: international guidelines for management of severe sepsis and septic shock. *Crit Care Med* 2008; 36:296–327.

Ely EW, Inouye SK, Bernard GR, et al. Delirium in mechanically ventilated patients. Validity and reliability of the confusion assessment method for the intensive care unit (CAM-ICU). *JAMA* 2001; 286(21):2703–2710.

Finfer S, Bellomo R, Boyce N, et al. A comparison of albumin and saline for fluid resuscitation in the intensive care unit. *N Engl J Med* 2004; 350:2247–2256.

Marshall JC, Cook DJ, Christou NV, et al. Multiple organ dysfunction score: a reliable descriptor of a complex clinical outcome. *Crit Care Med* 1995; 23:1638–1652.

Mehta RL, Kellum JA, Shah SV, et al. Acute Kidney Injury Network: report of an initiative to improve outcomes in acute kidney injury. *Crit Care* 2007; 11:R31.

Nash K, Hafeez A, Hou S. Hospital-acquired renal insufficiency. *Am J Kidney Dis* 2002; 39:930–936.

Rivers E, Nguyen B, Havstad S, et al. Early goal-directed therapy in the treatment of severe sepsis and septic shock. *N Engl J Med* 2001; 345:1368–1377.

Russell JA, Walley KR, Singer J, et al. Vasopressin versus norepinephrine infusion in patients with septic shock. *N Engl J Med* 2008; 358:877–887.

van den Berghe G, Wouters P, Weekers F, et al. Intensive insulin therapy in the critically ill patients. *N Engl J Med* 2001; 345:1359–1367.

Chapter

155

Supraventricular arrhythmias

James P. Hardy and Thomas Edrich

Supraventricular arrhythmias are frequently encountered in the operating room, recovery room, and intensive care unit (ICU). The anesthesiologist and intensivist must recognize the type of arrhythmia and decide on appropriate management, which will depend on the hemodynamic stability of the patient and should be guided by the advanced cardiac life support (ACLS) principles as outlined in Chapter 153. This chapter describes the rationale behind the treatment options and helps prioritize treatment goals.

Classification

A supraventricular tachyarrhythmia is one in which the focus of the dysrhythmias starts above the His bundle. In most cases it provides the ventricles with excitation along the usual pathways (His–Purkinje conduction system), leading to a narrow complex QRS. There may be aberrant conduction of excitation into the ventricles in the case of accessory bundles and rate-responsive bundle blocks leading to wide complex QRS. Fig. 155.1 displays possible mechanisms of the most common supraventricular arrhythmias, and Table 155.1 lists common treatment options.

Sinus tachycardia

Sinus tachycardia is the most common tachycardia seen in the ICU and may have causes listed in Table 155.2.

Identifying characteristics of sinus tachycardia are heart rate (HR) > 100 bpm in an adult and presence of P waves that may be difficult to visualize at a high HR. Uncertainty regarding the P waves may cause difficulty differentiating from paroxysmal supraventricular tachycardia (PSVT) and atrial flutter with 2:1 block. Slowing the HR by vagal maneuvers (carotid sinus massage, Valsalva maneuver) or by medications (β-blocker, adenosine, diltiazem) may help to identify the rhythm via the following mechanisms:

1. Slowing true sinus tachycardia enough to reveal the P waves;
2. Slowing AV-nodal conduction enough to reveal underlying atrial flutter; and
3. Interrupting and possibly terminating PSVT.

Sinus tachycardia is often well tolerated. Tachycardia, however, can lead to poor ventricular filling and compromise cardiac output. Also, the percentage of time that the heart spends in diastole is reduced, thereby reducing perfusion especially to the left ventricle. This reduction can lead to coronary ischemia especially in the setting of left ventricular hypertrophy.

Treatment should focus on reversing underlying mechanisms. Patients perceived as moderate or high risk for rate-related coronary ischemia should receive β-blockade. Frequently used medications are esmolol (short-lasting and easily titratable) or metoprolol.

Atrial fibrillation

Atrial fibrillation (AF) represents chaotic activation of the atria due to the presence of multiple foci of excitation as shown in Fig. 155.1a. The electrocardiogram (ECG) shows irregularly spaced QRS complexes and lacks regular P waves. The ventricular rate depends on the conduction of the irregular atrial depolarizations across the AV-node and into the His bundle. Most often, the QRS will be narrow because the ventricular activation occurs in an orderly fashion along the His–Purkinje conduction system. If the ventricular rate is high enough, a rate-dependent bundle branch block may cause the QRS to widen. AF is the most common dysrhythmia encountered in the surgical ICU. The estimated prevalence is 0.4% to 1% in the general population, and 8% in patients older than 80 years. It occurs in up to 40% after coronary artery bypass graft (CABG) and with a similarly high incidence (8%–60%) after major thoracic surgical procedures. Often, AF will terminate spontaneously when the underlying cause is treated and therefore does not require aggressive attempts at rhythm conversion back to sinus rhythm. Table 155.3 lists common conditions associated with AF.

Symptoms depend on the stiffness or diastolic function of the ventricle. A ventricle with hypertrophy will depend more heavily on the diastolic filling contribution of atrial contraction (the "atrial kick") and the onset of AF may reduce the stroke volume by 20%.

Postoperative AF has several significant clinical implications:

• Perfusion pressure to vital organs may be lowered critically, requiring more aggressive fluid resuscitation to correct.

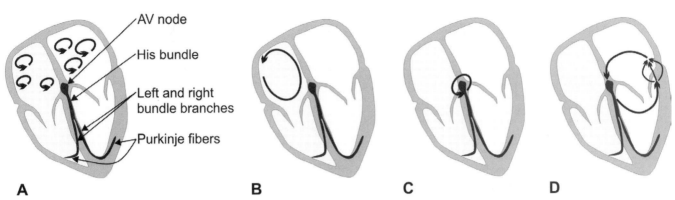

Figure 155.1. Simplified mechanisms of common supraventricular tachycardias. (**A**) AF is caused by multiple reentry wavelets that provide high-frequency impulses to the atrioventricular (AV) node that are conducted in an erratic fashion. (**B**) Atrial flutter is caused by a larger reentry circuit within the atrium that provides impulses to the AV node at a rate of approximately 300 beats per minute. Conduction is often regular and limited by a 2:1 or 3:1 blockade due to the refractory period of the AV node. (**C**) AV nodal reciprocating tachycardia (AVNRT) is entertained by two pathways within the AV node that have different refractory periods and conduction velocities. One premature atrial contraction can suddenly initiate this circular pattern of activation (paroxysmal tachycardia), thus activating the ventricles in a rapid regular fashion. (**D**) AV-reentry tachycardia (AVRT) requires an accessory pathway through which excitation can be conducted back to the AV node. Anterograde conduction through the AV node and then circling back through the accessory pathway causes a regular tachycardia with a narrow QRS. Alternatively, conduction may proceed down the accessory pathway first and return retrogradely through the AV node causing a wide-complex tachycardia.

Table 155.1. Treatment options for supraventricular tachycardias (SVTs)

Principle	Intervention	Comments
Mechanical vagal stimulation leading to AV conduction slowing	Carotid sinus massage (CSM)	*Method:* Steady or pulsatile pressure applied to the carotid sinus for 5–10 s. The carotid sinus is located below the angle of the mandible at the level of the thyroid cartilage. *Contraindications:* CSM should be avoided in patients with a carotid bruit, a known carotid stenosis > 50%, a history of myocardial infarction or stroke within the preceding 3 months, or a history of ventricular arrhythmias or symptomatic bradyarrhythmias. The risk of neurologic complications attributed to arterio-arterial embolization is low following CSM ranging from 0.28% to 0.9% in patients older than 50 yrs, with most deficits resolving within 24 h (persistent deficits 0.1%).
	Valsalva maneuver	A randomized study of 148 patients with SVT showed termination of the SVT in 18% with Valsalva maneuver compared to 11.8% with CSM. A smaller study of 35 patients also showed that the Valsalva maneuver was more effective than CSM or facial immersion.
Medications blocking fast AV conduction[a]	Esmolol Metoprolol	Short lasting (10 min) – use 20–40 mg IV push or infuse and titrate to effect. Initial dose 1–5 mg IV Onset of action: oral, 20–40 min; IV, within minutes Duration of action: oral, 3–6 h; IV, 2–4 h Conversion IV to PO is 1:2.5 although commonly converted more aggressively (1:5)
	Diltiazem	Initial dose 10–20 mg IV, or infuse 5–15 mg/h Onset: 3 min; duration: 1–3 h Caution: risk of complete AV-block is high when combining both IV metoprolol and IV diltiazem
	Adenosine	Initial dose 6 mg IV rapid push, may repeat with 12 mg Onset: 20 s; duration: <1 min. Note: heart transplant patients are very sensitive.
	Ibutilide	Caveat: Torsades de pointes risk = 1.7%. Pretreatment with magnesium may reduce this risk.
	Amiodarone and procainamide	Useful for tachycardia with wide QRS of uncertain etiology that could be supraventricular with conduction aberrancy, WPW or ventricular. Choose amiodarone if low EF (<45%). Caveat: lung toxicity (2%–7%) and hepatic toxicity (<3%) with amiodarone
	Electrical cardioversion	Recommended energy levels are not yet uniform for biphasic defibrillators. Biphasic 50–100–200 J for AF, atrial flutter, and wide complex tachycardia Biphasic 100–200 J for SVT Monophasic energy levels are approximately 2x higher (ceiling at 360 J). Caveats: Sedation before cardioversion if possible. Remember to SYNCHRONIZE before shocking to avoid shocking in the vulnerable phase of the T wave, which could induce ventricular fibrillation. It is important to recheck for synchronization before each new shock as the defibrillator may default to a nonsynchronized mode.

IV, intravenous; PO, oral; WPW, Wolff–Parkinson–White syndrome
[a] β-blockers, diltiazem, verapamil, adenosine, and digoxin may enhance conduction through accessory pathways in WPW and other pre-excitation syndromes and are therefore contraindicated.

Table 155.2. Causes of sinus tachycardia

Pain, anxiety
Absolute or relative intravascular volume depletion (e.g., hemorrhagic, neurogenic, or septic shock)
Exposure to positive chronotropic medications, such as dopamine
Fever
Heart failure, acute coronary ischemia
Uncommon: hyperthyroidism, pheochromocytoma

Certain patients, such as those who have had lung resections, may not tolerate the increased intravascular volume and develop edema leading to non-compliant lungs, increased work of breathing, and respiratory failure. Alternatively, vasopressors may become necessary but may compromise perfusion of vital organs with complications such as acidosis.

- Prolonged AF raises the risk of clot formation in the atria, leading to embolic complications such as strokes. The annual risk of stroke is 3% to 8%. Anticoagulation may become necessary, but increases the risk of bleeding complications in the postoperative patient.

Prevention of postoperative AF

Studies of patients undergoing cardiac surgery have shown an overall reduction in the rate of postoperative AF following the use of prophylactic β-blockade and, to a lesser extent, calcium channel blockers. Dosing schedules and type of β-blocker vary in these studies. Ideally, preoperative β-blockade should be initiated in collaboration with the patient's primary care physician, if indicated.

In general, perioperative β-blockade has been shown to reduce postoperative cardiac complications for *high-risk* patients undergoing *high-risk* surgery. However, titration is critical to avoid morbidity due to hypotension. Patients who already take β-blockers should continue them in the perioperative period, as withdrawal of these medications doubles the risk of postoperative AF. Contraindications to perioperative β-blockade include patients who are hemodynamically unstable and possibly requiring inotropic support and patients with second- or third-degree AV block. Cardioselective β-blockers that predominantly antagonize β-1 receptors (e.g., esmolol, metoprolol, atenolol) have been found to be safe even in patients

Table 155.3. Risk factors for atrial fibrillation

Electrolyte disturbances (hypokalemia, hypomagnesemia)
Hyperadrenergic state
β-adrenergic drugs, such as dopamine
Absence of β-blocker therapy or withdrawal of previous β-blockade
Atrial manipulation (cardiac or thoracic surgery)
COPD
Obesity
Atrial enlargement (e.g., mitral stenosis)
Age
Valve surgery

with chronic obstructive pulmonary disease (COPD) and reactive airway disease, with no changes in forced expiratory volume in the first second of expiration (FEV_1) or symptoms in a large meta-analysis.

Treatment of AF
Patients with hemodynamic instability

Rapid AF may compromise perfusion severely, with hypotension leading to mental status deterioration, oliguria, chest pain, or signs of coronary ischemia in the ECG. These patients should be treated emergently with electric cardioversion as described in Table 155.1. Vasopressors, such as phenylephrine, that do not increase HR may be useful to restore adequate perfusion pressure while awaiting cardioversion. If possible, a heparin bolus and infusion to attain a 1.5- to 2-fold prolongation of PTT should be performed concurrently with cardioversion, unless contraindicated due to risk of post-surgical bleeding. Anticoagulation is recommended for 4 weeks even after successful cardioversion, as will be discussed below.

Patients who are hemodynamically stable – rate control versus rhythm control

A decision must be made whether to lower the HR to a tolerable range without converting to sinus rhythm (rate control), or to attempt electrical or chemical cardioversion back to sinus rhythm (rhythm control). Even when pursuing rate control only, a large proportion of postoperative patients will spontaneously convert back to sinus rhythm once the insult of surgery has passed without requiring anti-arrhythmic medications. A review of the largest prospective randomized trials found that pharmacologic rhythm control was not superior to rate control, but did result in a higher rate of hospitalization and a trend towards more strokes although the increased stroke rate did not become apparent until following patients for 3.5 years. Certain malignant dysrhythmias were significantly more likely to occur in the rhythm control group. A subsequent review of electrical cardioversion compared to rate control did not show a mortality difference but found a non-significant increase in strokes in the cardioversion group. Several indices of quality of life, however, improved significantly after cardioversion. These studies may be less applicable to the surgical patient population where the insult of surgery, and presumed cause of AF, is expected to resolve over time.

Rate control

Most frequently, rate control is initiated with a β-blocker (e.g., metoprolol) or calcium antagonist (e.g., diltiazem). These agents lower the HR but have no intrinsic ability to cardiovert. Nevertheless, spontaneous cardioversion to sinus rhythm often occurs after hours or days as the conditions underlying the arrhythmia resolve (see Table 155.3). Once in sinus rhythm, β-blockers or calcium antagonists are known to reduce the likelihood of recurrent AF (secondary prevention).

Rhythm control

Unsatisfactory rate control in patients with an elevated risk posed by tachycardia (e.g., coexisting coronary artery disease) may necessitate cardioversion. Both electrical and chemical cardioversion carry the risk of dislodging blood clots from the heart and causing a stroke. The risk of stroke increases after AF has persisted for more than 48 hours. Thus, after the 48-hour limit, patients require either 3 weeks of full anticoagulation before the cardioversion attempt or, alternatively, transesophageal echocardiography (TEE) to rule out a clot before immediate cardioversion. Even when using TEE, initiation of heparin therapy with an IV bolus and infusion to attain an elevated PTT (1.5–2 times normal) is recommended immediately before cardioversion (unless contraindicated). Thrombi can be found in the left atrial appendage where inadequate atrial contraction has allowed stasis of blood. Thus, TEE is the best method to rule out clots because the esophageal positioning of the probe brings it closest to the left atrium for optimal imaging quality.

Special considerations for patients with AF and Wolff–Parkinson–White Syndrome (WPW)

As described below, patients with WPW syndrome have an accessory conduction pathway between the atria and the ventricles. They may exhibit a delta wave on a resting ECG. Agents that slow conduction across the AV node are contraindicated in patients with WPW and AF. These include β-blockers, adenosine, calcium channel blockers, and digitalis. Slowing AV conduction in these patients can enhance anterograde conduction along the accessory pathway during AF, leading to acceleration of the ventricular rate with subsequent hypotension and possible degeneration into ventricular fibrillation. Hemodynamically unstable patients should be cardioverted. Stable patients may be treated with amiodarone, procainamide, or ibutilide.

Anticoagulation after AF

AF carries the risk of clot formation and subsequent thromboembolism due to loss of mechanical function of the atrium and stasis of blood. Return to sinus rhythm enhances the risk of dislodging a clot, particularly from the left atrial appendage. This risk exists after both electrical and chemical cardioversion. In both cases, the complete recovery of atrial mechanical function may be delayed by several weeks. In addition, there is an elevated risk of recurrent AF, which may be asymptomatic and therefore go unnoticed. Thus, these patients require full anticoagulation for 4 weeks after cardioversion. If AF recurs, the need for continued anticoagulation will depend on the patient's risk factors for stroke, and either full anticoagulation (e.g., coumadin) or aspirin will be needed.

Atrial flutter

Atrial flutter most commonly results from a macro-reentry phenomenon with an excitatory wave-front circling through the right atrium in a regular pattern as illustrated in Fig. 155.1b. The ventricular rate can appear regular because atrioventricular conduction may be blocked for every second or third atrial beat leading to 1:2 or 1:3 conduction. Symptoms, management, and prevention of perioperative atrial flutter are similar to AF. Treatment typically begins with a β-blocker. Rate control can be challenging because a lower atrial rate may match the AV-refractory period better and actually cause a 3:1 block to "improve" to a 2:1 block with an undesirable *increase* in ventricular rate. This is more likely when using class I antiarrhythmic drugs, such as procainamide, flecainide, or propafenone, because these agents do not prolong the AV-node refractory period and thus do not protect against the switch to a lower conduction ratio. Therefore, simultaneous rate control with AV-nodal blocking agents, such as esmolol, metoprolol, or diltiazem, is advisable. Although the risk of stroke may be lower with atrial flutter than with AF, the same anticoagulation strategies are recommended. Atrial flutter can be treated with catheter ablation.

Atrioventricular nodal reciprocating tachycardia

Atrioventricular nodal reciprocating tachycardia (AVNRT) is the most common cause of narrow-QRS tachycardia with a regular rate, accounting for up to 60% of cases (see Fig. 155.1c). In AVNRT there are two functionally different pathways within the AV node: one with a short refractory period and slow conduction, and the other with a longer refractory period but faster conduction. In sinus rhythm, only the faster pathway is used. An irregular atrial contraction (e.g., a premature atrial beat), however, can be transmitted to the ventricle via the slow pathway if the fast pathway is still refractory and then circle back through the fast pathway when it has recovered from its refractory period. This triggers a sudden onset of tachycardia, typically at a rate of 140 to 250 beats per minute. The QRS remains narrow because the ventricular activation is triggered from the AV node, unless a rate-dependent bundle branch block also occurs. Because the atria and ventricles are activated almost simultaneously, the P wave is obscured by the QRS and cannot be seen on the surface ECG. Acute management is the same as for AVRT and will be discussed in the next paragraph.

Atrioventricular reentry tachycardia

Atrioventricular reentry tachycardia (AVRT) requires the presence of both the normal AV node, as well as an anatomically distinct conduction pathway between the atria and the ventricles called an accessory pathway (see Fig. 155.1d). The most common such accessory pathway is the Kent bundle. Both the AV node and the accessory pathway can conduct in both directions so that paroxysmal onset of circular excitation is possible. When excitation progresses down the regular AV node to the ventricles and then returns to the atria via the accessory pathway, it is termed *orthodromic* AVRT. The QRS complex is typically narrow because the ventricles are depolarized in an orderly fashion starting with the AV node and progressing through the His–Purkinje conduction system. In *antidromic* AVRT, anterograde conduction occurs via the accessory pathway and returns via retrograde conduction through the AV node. Because depolarization of the ventricles is initiated outside the His–Purkinje system, the QRS is wide. When an accessory pathway allows anterograde conduction *at rest* while the HR is normal, the QRS can be slightly widened with a slurred upstroke of the QRS complex called a *delta wave*. This occurs because there is fusion of ventricular depolarization emanating from both the His–Purkinje system (narrow QRS) as well as via the accessory pathway (pre-excitation of the ventricle causing widening of the QRS via the delta wave). If the accessory pathway allows only retrograde conduction at rest, then there is no manifestation on the surface ECG. This is called a *concealed accessory pathway*. The combination of delta waves and a short PR interval in the ECG at rest, and a history of palpitations is referred to as the Wolff–Parkinson–White (WPW) syndrome.

Treatment of AVNRT and AVRT

If initial assessment indicates an unstable hemodynamic state or if tachycardia poses a significant risk of exacerbation of underlying disease such as coronary artery disease, then immediate cardioversion may be indicated. Otherwise, therapy hinges on the assessment of the ECG and the patient's previous medical history.

Narrow QRS complex

Regular tachycardia with a narrow QRS complex poses a diagnostic dilemma because it could represent orthodromic AVRT, AVNRT, or atrial flutter with a fixed conduction ratio. Adenosine can be considered the first choice for all regular narrow complex tachycardias. The other nodal blocking agents listed in Table 155.1 (esmolol, metoprolol, diltiazem) are also appropriate. In patients with pacemakers, overdrive atrial pacing may also terminate narrow complex tachycardias, but with the risk of inducing AF.

Wide QRS complex

Differential diagnosis of regular tachycardia with a wide QRS is more problematic, and management depends on the etiology. Possibilities include:

- Ventricular tachycardia
- Antidromic AVRT
- Orthodromic AVRT, AVNRT, atrial flutter, or atrial tachycardia, all with coexisting bundle branch block (preexisting block or a rate-dependent block)

If in doubt regarding the etiology of regular-rate wide-complex tachycardia, ventricular tachycardia (VT) should be assumed and treated with amiodarone (150 mg IV over 10 minutes, repeated as needed to a total of 2.2 g over 24 hours) or elective synchronized cardioversion. Treatment with nodal-blocking agents, particularly verapamil or diltiazem, may be deleterious because they may precipitate hemodynamic collapse in a patient with VT.

With antidromic AVRT, nodal blocking agents (e.g., adenosine, esmolol, metoprolol, diltiazem) do not slow conduction via the accessory pathway but may actually enhance conduction over the accessory pathway. This can lead to ventricular arrhythmia, even ventricular fibrillation, in AVRT as well as in the setting of AF/flutter or atrial tachycardias. Procainamide is the drug of choice because it slows conduction over the accessory pathway more than over the AV node, although amiodarone is preferred in patients with a low ejection fraction (EF). Cardioversion is an alternative.

Treatment for known orthodromic AVRT, AVNRT, atrial flutter, or atrial tachycardia remains as described in the previous sections regardless of the presence of a bundle branch block.

Multifocal atrial tachycardia

Multifocal atrial tachycardia (MAT) is an uncommon arrhythmia usually seen in critically ill patients with electrolyte abnormalities or COPD. It is an irregular narrow complex tachycardia, with a variable P-wave appearance and is considered to be a transitional rhythm between atrial tachycardia and AF. Treatment should be focused on correction of precipitating causes. β-blockers or channel blockers may be used for rate control.

Suggested readings

Andrews TC, Reimold SC, Berlin JA, Antman EM. Prevention of supraventricular arrhythmias after coronary artery bypass surgery. a meta-analysis of randomized control trials. *Circulation* 1991; 84:III236–III244.

Blomstrom-Lundqvist C, Scheinman MM, Aliot EM, et al. ACC/AHA/ESC guidelines for the management of patients with supraventricular arrhythmias–executive summary. A report of the American College of Cardiology/American Heart Association Task Force on Practice Guidelines and the European Society of Cardiology Committee for Practice Guidelines (writing committee to develop guidelines for the management of patients with supraventricular arrhythmias) developed in collaboration with NASPE-Heart Rhythm Society. *J Am Coll Cardiol* 2003; 42:1493–1531.

Davies AJ, Kenny RA. Frequency of neurologic complications following carotid sinus massage. *Am J Cardiol* 1998; 81:1256–1257.

Echahidi N, Pibarot P, O'Hara G, Mathieu P. Mechanisms, prevention, and treatment of atrial fibrillation after cardiac surgery. *J Am Coll Cardiol* 2008; 51:793–801.

Fuster V, Ryden L, Cannom D, et al. 2006 ACC/AHA/ESC guidelines for management of patients with atrial fibrillation: A Report of the American College of Cardiology/American Heart Association

Task Force on Practice Guidelines and the European Society of Cardiology Committee for Practice Guidelines (Writing Committee to Revise the 2001 Guidelines for the Management of Patients With Atrial Fibrillation): Developed in Collaboration With the European Heart Rhythm Association and the Heart Rhythm Society. *Circulation* 2006; 114:e257–e354.

Go AS, Hylek EM, Phillips KA, et al. Prevalence of diagnosed atrial fibrillation in adults: national implications for rhythm management and stroke prevention: the AnTicoagulation and Risk Factors in Atrial Fibrillation (ATRIA) Study. *JAMA* 2001; 285:2370–2375.

Hart RG. Atrial fibrillation and stroke prevention. *N Engl J Med* 2003; 349:1015–1016.

Mead GE, Elder AT, Flapan AD, Kelman A. Electrical cardioversion for atrial fibrillation and flutter. *Cochrane Database Syst Rev* 2005:CD002903.

Salpeter S, Ormiston T, Salpeter E. Cardioselective beta-blockers for chronic obstructive pulmonary disease. *Cochrane Database Syst Rev* 2005:CD003566.

Singer DE, Albers GW, Dalen JE, et al. Antithrombotic therapy in atrial fibrillation: the Seventh ACCP Conference on Antithrombotic and Thrombolytic Therapy. *Chest* 2004; 126:429S–456S.

Wolf PA, Abbott RD, Kannel WB. Atrial fibrillation as an independent risk factor for stroke: the Framingham Study. *Stroke* 1991; 22:983–988.

Wyse DG, Waldo AL, DiMarco JP, et al. A comparison of rate control and rhythm control in patients with atrial fibrillation. *N Engl J Med* 2002; 347:1825–1833.

Chapter 156

Cardiac failure in the intensive care unit

Maxwell Weinmann

Introduction

There are more than 1 million hospital admissions per year in the United States of patients suffering from acute decompensated congestive heart failure (CHF); the most common etiology is ischemic heart disease. As pump failure develops, the physician is often confronted with competing therapeutic demands to optimize oxygenation and perfusion in an attempt to prevent organ failure and reduce mortality, This is of particular importance when the anesthesiologist is faced with stabilizing the uncompensated cardiac failure patient requiring emergent surgery.

Epidemiology

CHF affects approximately 2% of the population. Almost half a million new cases are diagnosed nationally per annum – 10 times that of newly diagnosed HIV infection and twice that of breast carcinoma. Despite advances in the field, admission rates have actually grown over time and are responsible for in excess of more than $20 billion in health care expenditures annually in the United States alone.

Etiology

The most common etiology of CHF is underlying ischemic heart disease. While these patients frequently have a history of angina, myocardial infarction, and an array of associated risk factors (e.g., diabetes, hypertension, smoking), coronary vascular disease often progresses silently, and CHF can be the first clinical manifestation of the disease. Other less common conditions include idiopathic dilated cardiomyopathy, valvular heart disease, myocarditis, drugs (e.g., doxorubicin, cocaine), HIV infection, and so forth.

Pathophysiology
Neurohumoral dysregulation

A neurohumoral cardio–cerebro–renal axis exists that regulates cardiovascular homeostasis through cardiac filling/output and systemic perfusion. In CHF, this homeostatic mechanism breaks down. As the heart begins to fail, its output declines, as does systemic organ perfusion. The body interprets this low cardiac output as hypovolemia, and compensatory mechanisms are initiated which produce vasoconstriction and fluid retention. Consequently, sympathetic activity is increased to maintain cardiac output, via elevated catecholamine levels, while the renin–angiotensin–aldosterone system (RAAS) acts to retain fluid and Na^+. In the setting of progressive cardiac disease, a chronic hyperstimulatory state results which is self-perpetuating, leading to progressive myocardial wall stress, fibrosis, and ventricular remodeling. These changes culminate in a shift to anaerobic myocardial metabolism, electrolyte abnormalities and diminished myocardial reserve, leading to a propensity for arrhythmias, worsening cardiac failure, and increased mortality.

Diastolic dysfunction

Diastolic dysfunction refers to an abnormality of ventricular relaxation that impairs filling, and can occur in the presence or absence of an abnormal left ventricular ejection fraction. Ventricular relaxation is an active process and thus energy dependent. Myocardial ischemia will therefore lead to nonhomogeneity of diastolic filling.

It is estimated that up to one-third of patients presenting in decompensated heart failure (HF) demonstrate diastolic dysfunction. This estimate rises with increasing age such that approximately 70% of patients older than 70 years of age have findings consistent with this condition.

Systolic dysfunction

Classically, systolic dysfunction and failure refer to the progressive decline in left ventricular ejection fraction due to ventricular remodeling in the face of injury or increased afterload. The most common etiologies contributing to ventricular remodeling are coronary vascular disease and hypertension.

Myocardial injury is characterized by an imbalance of collagen degradation and production, perivascular fibrosis, and myocardial scarring, which may occur despite recanalization of the infarct-related vessel. Myocardial scarring is, in part, due to changes in the neurohumoral environment with activation of the renin–angiotensin system, which has been shown to be profibrotic and proinflammatory. In the absence of intervention, a chronic inflammatory state and ongoing myocardial remodeling ensue. Ultimately, the left ventricle begins to fail both mechanically and in terms of its electrophysiologic integrity and homogeneity.

Systolic and diastolic dysfunction have emerged as two distinct clinical entities such that diastolic failure demonstrates initial preservation of ejection fraction in the absence of ventricular dilatation, whereas systolic failure is characterized by profound remodeling and progressive decline in output.

Right ventricular failure

Unlike the left ventricle, the right ventricle functions in a relatively low-pressure milieu. Functioning as a crescentic "bellows" adjacent to the more muscular left ventricle, its pressure–volume relationship is much flatter, demonstrating that it can accommodate large variations in venous return in the absence of large pressure swings. This relationship also has implications for contractility, which is preload-dependent. In the presence of acute increases in afterload, but in the absence of changes in preload, the ventricle responds with increased inotropy. As afterload continues to increase, however, right ventricular dilatation will occur, and its declining mechanical reserves will lead to right heart failure. At this point, the elevated right ventricular pressure will impair coronary perfusion, and worsen mechanical failure. Although ischemia does affect the right ventricle, it is extremely rare in isolation (the anterior wall of the right ventricle has dual blood supply from both the right coronary and the left anterior descending arteries), and it occurs more commonly in association with inferior wall ischemic events (up to 50% of cases).

Cardiogenic shock

Cardiogenic shock is life-threatening ventricular failure and a sign of a profound acute myocardial decompensation. Cardiogenic shock is typically due to acute ischemia or infarction. This can occur with or without preexisting ventricular dysfunction. Measuring systemic vascular resistance and cardiac contractility may help discern where in the clinical spectrum ranging from ventricular dysfunction to failure a particular patient lies. For these patients the therapeutic goal in the intensive care unit (ICU) will be myocardial preservation, optimization of function, and organ salvage.

Diagnosis

Electrocardiogram

While an electrocardiogram (ECG) is not diagnostic of CHF, it does allude to the underlying etiology, associated complications, and need for intervention. The left ventricular hypertrophy of chronic hypertension, the S-T changes of acute ischemia, and the evolution of conduction abnormalities which would benefit from pacing are some examples. Additionally, evolutionary changes are particularly helpful if an acute ischemic event is suspected, such that serial ECGs may be clinically relevant on admission to the ICU, in addition to biochemical markers, such as troponins, to confirm one's clinical suspicions. Furthermore, as therapy is initiated and progresses, continuous ECG monitoring is important due to the inherent risk of arrhythmias, which may be exacerbated by the electrolyte shifts accompanying therapy.

Chest radiograph

The radiologic findings accompanying CHF are well known. The heart may appear enlarged and globular, which may suggest the presence of pericardial fluid which, if suspected, should prompt echocardiographic investigation. Interstitial pulmonary edema may range from blunting of the costophrenic angles through to gross CHF with pleural effusions and fluid in the fissures.

Hemodynamic monitoring

The pulmonary artery catheter is less frequently used in the ICU due to its associated morbidity, the lack of outcome benefits, and the availability of less invasive measures of heart function, such as echocardiography. While the pulmonary artery catheter does provide an assessment of the left ventricular end diastolic *pressure*, its correlation with left ventricular end diastolic *volume* is skewed by acute changes in ventricular compliance, especially in the setting of an acute ischemic syndrome. The intensivist should take this into account when titrating volume status to a particular wedge pressure.

Echocardiography

Both transthoracic and transesophageal echocardiography are useful, noninvasive tools to measure contractility and wall motion, wall thickness, valvular and intraluminal pathology, as well as any pericardial disease. Both may be performed within the ICU rapidly, easily, and without the need for transport of a critically ill patient. It is, nevertheless only a snapshot of an evolving clinical syndrome and does not exclude the absence of transient ischemia should wall motion be seen to be normal.

Biochemical markers

Troponin

The I and T subunits of troponin are considered specific for myocardial injury and should be evaluated whenever failure is considered secondary to acute ischemia. However, the intensivist should be wary of other clinical situations that may complicate the interpretation of elevated levels, such as severe sepsis, renal failure, pulmonary embolism, pulmonary hypertension, and acute liver failure, to name a few. The exact mechanisms of troponin elevation in these noncardiac diseases remain unclear but include myocardial injury and inflammation due to elevated free fatty acid levels in sepsis, reduced filtration of troponin fragments in renal failure, and endothelial injury or dysfunction in critical illness and systemic inflammatory response syndrome (SIRS). Of importance, however, is recent evidence supporting that critical illness–related troponin elevation is of prognostic value, implicating incipient organ failure and increased mortality.

Brain natriuretic peptide

Progressive understanding of the mechanisms of action of natriuretic peptides has demonstrated their key role in a cardio–cerebro–renal axis of fluid and electrolyte homeostasis within the body. Natriuretic peptides gained particular relevance in the diagnosis, management, and prognostication of patients with CHF. Levels > 100 pg/ml are considered to have good sensitivity and specificity in diagnosing CHF in acutely dyspneic patients who present to the emergency room.

Additionally, natriuretic peptides have been implicated in the regulation of myocardial perfusion by promoting coronary vasodilation in the presence of ischemia. This theory has been supported by elevations of brain natriuretic peptide (BNP) proportional to underlying coronary vascular disease even in the absence of ventricular dysfunction. Presumably, by stimulating both coronary vasodilatation and systemic afterload reduction, myocardial work is reduced and the effects of ischemia blunted. Similarly, successful revascularization has been associated with a reduction in BNP levels postoperatively.

Therapy
Airway management and oxygenation

The application of positive airway pressure (via both noninvasive or invasive modes delivering continuous positive airway pressure [CPAP] or bilevel positive airway pressure [BiPAP]) has been shown to be effective in the acute management of decompensated CHF. By reducing work of breathing, increasing afterload reduction, and improving oxygenation, there is a marked reduction in intubation rates, mortality and improved cardiac performance compared to oxygen by mask alone. Adequacy of oxygenation should be determined not only by pulse oximetry, but also by arterial blood gas studies, which can provide information on the adequacy of circulation (through pH, lactate, the presence of associated carbon dioxide retention, and so forth). If work of breathing and hypoxia do not respond to noninvasive ventilatory support, the patient should be intubated to optimize systemic oxygenation.

Pharmacotherapy

Reperfusion strategies

Treatment of CHF in the ICU is governed by optimizing myocardial function, perfusion, preservation, and salvage. If acute ischemia or infarction is identified as the underlying etiology, then the patient should be assessed as a potential candidate for reperfusion via percutaneous coronary intervention (PCI), thrombolysis, or even surgery. Previous studies have demonstrated that in patients with ST elevation myocardial infarction PCI is superior to thrombolysis in terms of mortality and morbidity, leading to the conclusion by some investigators that reperfusion by stenting should be the standard approach.

Although primary intervention with thrombolysis is relatively easy compared to PCI, it nevertheless presents challenges in terms of the risk of hemorrhagic complications (particularly in elderly patients), the relatively short window of optimal opportunity (4 hours), re-occlusion rates, inadequate restoration of flow in the infarct-related segment, and the lack of efficacy in those patients who present with cardiogenic shock. PCI or coronary artery bypass grafting is recommended in the latter. In those patients not considered candidates for thrombolysis, emergent PCI offers a significant opportunity for myocardial salvage.

Diuretic therapy

Although diuretics have not been shown to affect mortality, they are typically used to alleviate the symptoms of volume overload. Outpatient oral dose may be changed to the intravenous dose by dividing the oral dose by 2 to 2.5 and observing the response. Diuretics reduce left ventricular filling pressures, and commencement of diuretic therapy will also enhance the action of angiotensin-converting enzyme (ACE) inhibitors through volume contraction. Although bolus dosing diuretics is commonly implemented, an infusion is also an alternative if one wishes to titrate a response or achieve a gentler, consistent diuresis in a fragile patient. Electrolyte imbalances must be watched for, as arrhythmias may be easily precipitated in these patients. By evaluating urinary K^+, for example, K^+ replacements may be preempted. Additionally, K^+ losses may be ameliorated by aldosterone antagonists.

Digoxin

Although well known, digoxin is certainly not outmoded in the approach to CHF. It has been shown to provide symptomatic relief even in the presence of a conventional therapeutic regimen including ACE inhibitors, diuretics, and low dose β-blockers. It was not, however, found to improve survival. Anuric renal failure is not a contraindication to fully loading digoxin, and serum levels should be used to assess and follow the potential for toxicity, particularly in the presence of renal dysfunction.

Vasodilators
Nitroglycerin

Nitrates are typically part of the first line of therapy in acute decompensated HF. They serve to produce venodilatation predominantly, although they are active, but weaker, arteriodilators. This is particularly relevant to the coronary arteries. The combined result is a reduction in preload, reduced ventricular wall tension, enhanced myocardial perfusion, and, ultimately, reduced myocardial oxygen consumption. In acute syndromes, perfusion is also enhanced by their antiplatelet activity, which is mediated via nitric oxide (NO) mechanisms, a property of all nitrovasodilators. Unfortunately, tolerance develops rapidly, particularly to high doses of nitrates, such that these medications cannot be relied on to provide a sustained clinicopharmacologic impact.

ACE inhibitors

ACE inhibitors are potent vasodilators. Through their action on aldosterone and antidiuretic hormone (ADH), salt and water reabsorption are inhibited in CHF patients. The consequent increase in angiotensin-I levels acts to reduce norepinephrine release by binding to sympathetic nerve terminals. Acute administration also helps to correct myocardial β-sympathetic insensitivity associated with CHF, reduces myocardial inflammation and remodeling, and helps to restore endothelial NO responsivity and synthesis.

Abundant evidence exists confirming the decreased mortality benefits of these agents in the chronic patient and recently in the asymptomatic high-risk patient as well. These agents should be administered cautiously, however, in patients with renal dysfunction and in those who may already be volume-depleted by concomitant diuretic administration. Additional concerns have been raised perioperatively where ACE inhibitors may potentiate the renal toxicity of aprotinin (note that aprotinin is no longer in clinical use). Cessation is not associated with rebound phenomena.

Nitroprusside

A potent "balanced" vasodilator, nitroprusside is administered as an infusion. A half-life measured in minutes translates to rapid titratability clinically. Its metabolites, although pharmacologically inactive, are potentially toxic. Nitroprusside is metabolized by combining with hemoglobin to form cyanmethemoglobin and cyanide ions. The intensivist must, therefore, monitor for the development of metabolic acidosis and methemoglobinemia in these patients. Although uncommon in the acute phase (<48 hours), it is more common in patients with renal insufficiency. Methemoglobinemia responds rapidly to vitamin B12 and/or thiosulfate administration.

β-blockers

CHF is characterized, in part, by a chronic sympathetic hyperautonomic state. This has been shown to lead to a down-regulation of myocardial β-receptor number and sensitivity with a reduction in myocardial performance, altered myocardial energetics, and reduced myocardial efficiency. This biochemical and metabolic disarray can be modulated by the introduction of low-dose β-blockade. By affecting substrate utilization, energetics are improved, allowing enhanced myocardial performance. The intramyocardial inflammatory state is also antagonized, with a reversal of myocardial remodeling. As a result, morbidity and mortality are reduced. Importantly, impact on morbidity and mortality appears to be drug specific, rather than an inherent feature of all β-blockers (Table 156.1).

Nesiritide

Characterization of the physiologic actions of natriuretic peptides has demonstrated that they appear to be extremely important to cardiovascular homeostasis. Properties include potent vasodilator activity, with preferential arterial activity via modulation of Ca^{2+} through cyclic guanosine monophospate (cGMP) and NO synthesis. They also produce renal afferent vasodilatation and efferent vessel vasoconstriction that culminates in an enhanced glomerular filtration rate (GFR). Suppression of renin and aldosterone and modulation of sympathetic activity is also evident. Most recently, modulation of coronary artery vasculature, through NO, implicates them as part of the myocardial paracrine response to ischemia. Studies of nesiritide have remained controversial, in part due to the lack of any clear dose–response relationship for the agent. These findings hindered therapeutic predictability and limited the use of nesiritide. New evidence using more circumspect dosing is emerging, suggesting that the peptide possesses a dose–response relationship that warrants reinvestigation of its utility.

Inotropes

Inotropes are usually considered when end-organ damage has evolved due to persistent hypoperfusion. Unfortunately, there is no method to determine the inherent physiologic cost to the myocardium (induction of ischemia) by pharmacologically induced increased performance. Therefore, the intensivist risks stressing oxygen dynamics in an already compromised myocardium and may exacerbate underlying ischemia and arrhythmogenesis. Such detrimental effects were borne out by previous trials in which morbidity was found to increase with the administration of milrinone thus raising questions regarding the safety of this agent in CHF. Indeed, in a recent comparison of therapy in acutely decompensated HF patients, nesiritide was found to be more innocuous, being associated with less morbidity and mortality, reduced length of stay, and a lower likelihood of readmission with recurrent symptoms when compared to treatment with milrinone or dobutamine.

Mechanical support

Intra-aortic balloon counterpulsation

Should medical therapy be unsuccessful in providing adequate circulatory support, mechanical means may be considered. The utility of intra-aortic balloon counterpulsation (IABP) depends on the overall salvageability of the myocardium. In other words, can the etiology of the refractory HF or cardiogenic shock ultimately be reversed by revascularization, valve repair, or even transplant in an appropriate candidate? IABP therapy produces a reduction in ventricular wall tension with an associated reduction in myocardial oxygen demands. In fact, in those patients undergoing emergent revascularization or acute myocardial infarction complicated by shock, the implementation of an IABP has been shown to be associated with a lower mortality. Efficacy of the balloon is dependent on correct placement and timing of insufflation and deflation. The balloon is placed just distal to the origin of the left subclavian artery to avoid ischemic complications. Contraindications to placement include severe aortic regurgitation, where augmentation cannot be achieved and the regurgitant fraction is increased. The presence of severe atheromatous disease, aortic dissection, aortic aneurysm, and mild aortic regurgitation are relative contraindications. The physician must be vigilant for potential complications related to placement of the IABP, including ischemia, vascular injury, and bleeding. The overall complication rate is $< 8\%$.

Table 156.1. Large-scale, placebo-controlled mortality trials of β-blockade in HF

Trial	Drug	HF severity	Patients, *n*	Target dose, mg	Effect on all-cause	
					Mortality	Hospitalization
US Carvedilol (94)	Carvedilol	NYHA II-III	1094	6.25–50 BID	↓ 65%	↓ 27%
CIBIS-II (18)	Bisoprolol	EF ≤ 35; NYHA III-IV	2647	10 QD	↓ 34%	↓ 20%
MERIT-HF[a]	Metoprolol CR/XL	EF ≤ 40; NYHA II-IV	3991	200 QD	↓ 34%	↓ 18%
BEST (95)	Bucindolol	EF ≤ 35; NYHA III-IV	2708	50–100 BID	NS	↓ 8%
COPERNICUS[b]	Carvedilol	EF ≤ 25; NYHA IV	2289	25 BID	↓ 35%	↓ 20%

NYHA, New York Heart Association; EF, ejection fraction.
From Groban L, Butterworth J. Perioperative management of chronic heart failure. *Anesth Analg* 2006; 103:557–575.
[a] Effects of controlled-release metoprolol on total mortality, hospitalization, and well-being in patients with heart failure: the Metoprolol CR/XL Randomized Intervention Trial in congestive heart failure (MERIT-HF). MERIT-HF Study Group. *JAMA* 2000; 283:1295–1302.
[b] Effect of carvedilol on the morbidity of patients with severe chronic heart failure; results of the canvedilol prospective randomized cumulative survival (COPERNICUS) study. *Circulation* 2002; 106:2194–2199.

Table 156.2 Current and emerging devices[a]

	General description	Types on market	Advantages	Disadvantages
Extracorporeal pulsatile	• Pump located outside body • Provides pulsatile flow (compression pusher plate surounds a reservoir of blood and compressed by pneumatic or compressed air technology)	• Abiorned BVS 5000[b] and AB 5000[b] (Abiorned, Inc.: Danvers, MA) • Thoratec PVAD[b,c] (Thoratec Corp.: Pleasanton, CA)	• Wide range body types • May provide biventricular support • Less expensive • Insensitive to electromagnetic interference	• Usually not discharged to home
Extracorporeal nonpulsatile	• Centrifugal (heart-lung machine/ECMO) • Continuous flow • Often used emergently with resuscitation	• Levitronix CentriMag[b,d] (Levitronix LLC; Waltham, MA) • TandemHeart System[b] (CardiacAssist, Inc.: Pittsburg, PA) • Heart-Lung Machines[b]/ECMO[b]	• Rapid, percutaneous access (TandernHeart) • Utilizes cardiopulmonary bypass cannulae (Levitronix)[d] • Operates without mechanical bearings or seals	• Often requires patient to be ventilated and sedated • Requires anticoagulation • Use limited to days/week
Implantable pulsatile	Fully or partially implanted within the body (energy supply and control system extracorporeal)	• HeartMate IP[c] and XVE[c,d] (Thoratec Corp.: Pleasanton, CA) • Thoratec IVAD[b,c] (Thoratec Corp.: Pleasanton, CA) • Novacor IVAS[c,d] and Novacor II[c,d] (WorldHeart Corp.: Oakland, CA)	• May be discharged to home • Increased mobility • May not require anticoagulation • Magnetically driven; completely implantable with transcutaneous energy system (Novacor II)[d]	• Susceptible to electromagnetic interference • Must have a sufficient BSA (approximately ≥ 1.5 m²)
Implantable nonpulsatile	Centrifugal or axial-flow pump powered by an impellar rotating at high revolutions per minute	• Jarvik 2000[c,d] (Jarvik Heart Inc.: New York) • DeBakey VAD[c,d,e] (Micromed Inc.: Woodlands, TX) • HeartMate II IVAS[b,c,d,e] (Thoratec Corp.: Pleasanton, CA) • CorAide[b,c,d,e] (Arrow International, Inc.: Reading, PA)	• Reduced size and noise • High flows that can provide all or part of heart's cardiac output • Only one moving part (ompellar) • May be less expensive • Energy efficient • Easier to replace • May be fully implantable	• Requires anticoagulation

[a] Refer to device manufactures for device-specific information such as flow rates, RPMs, device weight etc. ECMO indicates extracorporeal membrane oxygenation; BSA, body surface area.
[b] Bridge to recovery short-term use.
[c] Bridge to transplant.
[d] Investigational, in clinical trials.
[e] Destination therapy.
From Richards NM, Stahl MA. Ventricular Assist Devices in The Adult. *Crit Care Nurs Q* 2007; 30;104–18.

Ventricular assist devices

The application of ventricular assist devices (VADs) in patients with refractory CHF has increased with time, particularly as recent evidence has indicated that survival and quality of life are enhanced. Indeed, at 1 year, survival has been shown to be 52% versus 25% with conventional medical therapy ($P = 0.002$). As a result, the devices are used not only as bridges to transplantation or to facilitate heart recovery, but also as "destination" therapy.

Presently, devices are defined by position (extracorporeal [external] pumps or implantable pumps) and by the nature of flow (pulsatile or nonpulsatile) (Table 156.2).

VAD insertion is associated with improved myocardial metabolic profiles. Additionally, local neurohumoral activity and adrenergic receptor density and responsivity return, facilitating myocardial function. Complications include hemorrhage, hemolysis, sepsis, malfunction, embolic phenomena, and infection. The latter may predispose to HLA sensitization. Overall, outcome is determined by the indication for VAD support and the associated comorbidities.

Future therapies

Novel therapies are on the horizon for the treatment of CHF. These therapies range from the delivery of stem cells used to enhance myocardial recovery and healing postacute infarction to neurohormonal manipulation. Even myocyte reprogramming of energy metabolism through gene transfer therapy is currently being investigated in the laboratory as a novel and unique therapeutic option. All present both controversy and promise but reflect the aggressive and imaginative pursuits required to address a medical epidemic that challenges the intensivist.

Summary

- CHF is a medical epidemic.
- Etiology is typically due to the advancement of coronary artery disease.
- The pathophysiology can be considered in terms of intrinsic myocardial and extrinsic factors. Intrinsically, there is no longer an ability to contract and relax normally due to inflammation, ischemia, and loss of actual myocytes. Extrinsically, disordered neurohumoral homeostatic mechanisms contribute to fluid accumulation and loss of cardio–renal balance.
- There are a host of investigational tests that can confirm CHF. None can replace clinical history and examination.
- Primary critical care therapy is always aimed at organ preservation and salvage through oxygenation and restoration or preservation of perfusion
- No therapy is without potential side effects. One example is arrhythmogenesis due to inotropes.

- Try to avoid polypharmacy, which often leads to drug combinations that are conflicting. Rationalize the use of medications, realizing that dose response is often altered by disease and, as the intensivist, you may have to titrate to effect.
- Be clear with therapeutic goals and communicate closely with the family and patient.

Suggested readings

Arnold LM, Crouch MA, Carroll NV, Oinonen MJ. Outcomes associated with vasoactive therapy in patients with acute decompensated heart failure. *Pharmacotherapy* 2006; 26(8):1078–1085.

Arnold JM, Yusuf S, Young J, et al. Prevention of heart failure in patients in the Heart Outcomes Prevention Evaluation (HOPE) study. *Circulation* 2003; 107(9):1284–1290.

Bersten AD, Holt AW, Vedig AL, et al. Treatment of severe cardiogenic pulmonary edema with continuous positive airway pressure delivered by facemask. *N Engl J Med* 1991; 325:1825–1830.

Dyub AM, Whitlock RP, Abouzahr LL, Cinà CS. Preoperative intra-aortic balloon pump in patients undergoing coronary bypass surgery: a systematic review and meta-analysis. *J Card Surg* 2008; 23(1):79–86.

Kastrati A, Mehilli J, Nekolla S, et al. A randomized trial comparing myocardial salvage achieved by coronary stenting versus balloon angioplasty in patients with acute myocardial infarction considered ineligible for reperfusion therapy. *J Am Coll Cardiol* 2004; 43:734–741.

NAPA Trial. Effects of perioperative nesiritide in patients with left ventricular dysfunction undergoing cardiac surgery. *J Am Coll Cardiol* 2007; 49(6):716–726.

Opie LH. The neuroendocrinology of congestive heart failure. *Cardiovasc J S Afr* 2002; 13(4):171–178.

Palazzuoli A, Gennari L, Calabria P, et al. Relation of plasma brain natriuretic peptide levels in non-ST-elevation coronary disease and preserved systolic function to number of narrowed coronary arteries. *Am J Cardiol* 2005; 96(12):1705–1710.

Palazzuoli A, Poldermans D, Capobianco S, et al. Rise and fall of B-type natriuretic peptide levels in patients with coronary artery disease and normal left ventricular function after cardiac revascularization. *Coron Artery Dis* 2006; 17(5):419–423.

Rose EA, Gelijns AC, Moskowitz AJ, et al. Long-term use of a left ventricular assist device for end-stage heart failure. *N Engl J Med* 2001; 345(20):1435–1443.

Sabbah HN. Biologic rationale for the use of beta-blockers in the treatment of heart failure. *Heart Fail Rev* 2004; 9(2):91–97.

Silver MA, Maisel A, Yancy CW, et al. BNP Consensus Panel 2004: a clinical approach for the diagnostic, prognostic, screening, treatment, monitoring and therapeutic roles of natriuretic peptides in cardiovascular diseases. *Congest Heart Fail* 2004; 10:1–30.

Wu TT, Yuan A, Chen CY, et al. Cardiac troponin I levels are a risk factor for mortality and multiple organ failure in noncardiac critically ill patients and have an additive effect to the APACHE II score in outcome prediction. *Shock* 2004; 22(2):95–101.

157

Sedation in the surgical intensive care unit

David A. Silver

Introduction

Most patients admitted to the surgical intensive care unit (SICU) require analgesia as part of their treatment; many also require sedation and anxiolysis. The medications used to provide analgesia and sedation are not without significant side effects, however, and the intensivist must at all times be mindful of the overall goals of care both in choosing which medications to use and in dosing these medications.

The following recommendations are intended to apply primarily to intubated patients. Although most of the medications discussed may be safely administered to spontaneously breathing patients in need of analgesia and anxiolysis, the focus of this chapter is the effective maintenance and weaning of sedation in the mechanically ventilated patient.

Goals of sedation

Patient safety and comfort are the two primary concerns in the titration of sedation in the ICU. A patient is ideally sedated if he or she lies quietly, without attempting to remove lines or tubes; does not pose a threat to his or her own safety; and has a fairly normal sleep–wake cycle. Several objective instruments have been designed as tools to help guide ICU sedation, including the Ramsay Sedation Scale and sedation–agitation scales. In our SICUs, we use the Richmond Agitation–Sedation Scale (RASS) (Table 157.1), which is easy to perform, has excellent inter-rater reliability, and has been clinically well-validated. Our goal for most patients is a RASS score of 0 to −2.

Commonly used pharmacologic agents

Analogous to the concept of a balanced anesthetic, the appropriate sedation regimen usually comprises a combination of medications. Opioids and other analgesics minimize pain and relieve a sense of dyspnea or the need to cough, both common in patients undergoing mechanical ventilation. Central neuraxial and regional anesthesia techniques, in particular epidural analgesia, can be vital in ensuring patient comfort while minimizing exposure to systemic opioids, which can contribute to delirium. Propofol, benzodiazepines (BZDs; lorazepam and midazolam), and dexmedetomidine add sedation and anxiolysis, important in critical illness, which is inherently fraught with

emotional stress. Traditional antipsychotic medications, such as haloperidol, and atypicals, such as olanzapine, risperidone, and quetiapine fumarate, may be added to treat delirium and agitation. In addition, ketamine hydrochloride, a phencyclidine derivative, is a potent analgesic and sedative at low doses and is a useful adjunctive agent in certain situations.

Analgesia

SICU patients have obvious needs for analgesia related to surgical procedures as well as to pain related to care (e.g., mechanical ventilation, dressing changes, suctioning) and rehabilitation (physical therapy, limited mobility). Many surgical patients, especially those with malignancy, have chronic pain issues as well. The approach to the agitated patient in the SICU must begin with an assessment of analgesic requirement; undertreated pain is common in the critically ill, especially those who are hemodynamically unstable, and administration of adequate analgesia can significantly reduce sedation requirements.

We begin our approach to analgesia with regional anesthetic options. Where appropriate and not contraindicated, our patients have epidural catheters (especially after major thoracic, abdominal, or orthopedic surgery and in trauma patients with rib fractures or pulmonary contusions). In elderly patients, most epidural infusions contain only local anesthetic, typically dilute bupivacaine. In younger patients, we add a small amount of hydromorphone, but systemic levels are still far lower than those seen with parenterally administered opioids. Nerve block catheters may be appropriate for patients whose anticoagulation status precludes central neuraxial blockade; this approach includes the use of paravertebral catheters as well as peripheral nerve blocks in thoracic surgery and trauma patients. Many of our cardiac surgery patients have pumps that continuously infuse bupivacaine through surgically placed catheters at the site of sternotomy. Finally, where appropriate, we often apply transdermal lidocaine patches to identifiable sites of patients' pain.

For enteral and parenteral analgesia, we begin with non-opioid medications, such as acetaminophen, ketorolac tromethamine, and ibuprofen. We supplement these medications with opioids as needed, whether via a nurse-titrated continuous infusion, intermittent dosing, or a patient-controlled

Table 157.1. The Richmond Agitation-Sedation Scale (RASS)

Term	Description	Score
Aggressive	Overly combative, violent, immediate danger to staff	**+4**
Very agitated	Pulls or removes tube(s) or catheter(s); aggressive	**+3**
Agitated	Frequent nonpurposeful movement, fights ventilator	**+2**
Restless	Anxious but movements not aggressive or vigorous	**+1**
Alert + calm		**0**
Drowsy	Not fully alert, but has sustained awakening (eye opening/eye contact) to voice (10+ seconds)	**−1**
Light sedation	Briefly awakens with eye contact to voice (under 10 seconds)	**−2**
Moderate sedation	Movement or eye opening to voice (but no eye contact)	**−3**
Deep sedation	No response to voice, but movement or eye opening to physical stimulation	**−4**
Unarousable	No response to voice or physical stimulation	**−5**

Procedure for RASS assessment

1. Observe patient
   Patient is alert, restless, or agitated. — Score 0 to +4

2. If not alert, state patient's name and instruct the patient to open eyes and look at speaker
   Patient awakens with sustained eye opening and eye contact — Score −1
   Patient awakens with eye opening and eye contact, but not sustained — Score −2
   Patient has any movement in response to voice but no eye contact — Score −3

3. If there is no response to verbal stimulation, physically stimulate patient by shaking or rubbing shoulder
   Patient has any movement to physical stimulation — Score −4
   Patient has no response to any stimulation — Score −5

Adapted from Ely EW, Shintani A, Truman B, et al. Delirium as a predictor of mortality in mechanically ventilated patients in the intensive care unit. *JAMA* 2004; 291(14):1753–1762.

analgesia (PCA) device for the awake patient. Due to its attractive pharmacokinetics, a fentanyl infusion is our preferred method of providing analgesia to intubated patients with ongoing opioid requirements. Similarly, fentanyl's rapid onset and short duration make it the opioid of choice for brief procedures, such as bronchoscopy, dressing changes, and burn debridement. It is important to remember, however, that intermittent boluses of fentanyl are generally *not* appropriate for analgesia in the patient being weaned off an infusion: A longer-lasting opioid, such as morphine or hydromorphone, should be used to ensure consistent analgesia.

For patients with chronic opioid requirements, we continue their home regimens as much as possible and add additional medication for acute pain. For those who use morphine or hydromorphone at home, we generally respond to acute pain issues by increased doses of the medications they are already taking. Oral-to-parenteral conversion instruments are useful tools and are easily located on the Internet and elsewhere.

Finally, we find that a low-dose continuous infusion of ketamine (0.1–0.3 mg/kg/h) can be an excellent supplemental agent for patients who may complain of significant pain despite maximal opioid therapy limited by respiratory depression or other side effects or who require escalating doses of sedatives. Ketamine provides potent analgesia without respiratory depression, can significantly reduce both opioid and BZD requirements, and can be continued through extubation in patients weaning from mechanical ventilation. Careful monitoring for hallucinations and other psychiatric side effects is important, especially at the upper end of the infusion range; if these develop, we decrease or stop the infusion.

Anxiolysis and sedation

Once adequate analgesia has been established, the addition of sedatives helps the intensivist achieve the desired level of sedation to ensure the patient's comfort and safety.

The most commonly employed sedatives in the ICU are propofol, midazolam, and lorazepam – all of which are relatively inexpensive and effective. None of these drugs has any analgesic properties, and they should not be used as sole agents in patients who have significant pain.

Propofol (and a prodrug form currently undergoing testing, fospropofol) is an intravenous anesthetic agent that is particularly attractive as a sedative because its short redistribution half-life (on the order of minutes) allows for rapid lightening of sedation to allow frequent assessment of patients' mental status, which is particularly useful in patients with neurologic injuries. In addition, daily lightening of sedation (a sedation "holiday") has been demonstrated to reduce duration of mechanical ventilation and ICU stay and is easily achieved with propofol sedation.

In contrast to the other sedative agents discussed later in this chapter, propofol is primarily a general anesthetic agent that has sedative effects at low doses. For its safe use and titration, it should be administered only by persons experienced in its use.

Disadvantages of the use of propofol include pain on peripheral injection, hypotension (at least in part due to dose-dependent vasodilatation), elevated serum triglycerides with long-term infusion, and risk of infection and bacterial contamination of the emulsion. A rare but serious complication, *propofol infusion syndrome*, has been described in patients undergoing long-term propofol infusion at high doses. Prominent features of the syndrome include cardiac and renal failure, rhabdomyolysis, and severe metabolic acidosis, and it has been reported most frequently in patients (especially children) receiving corticosteroids and catecholamines in addition to propofol. Clinicians should be cautious in administering high doses of propofol (in the range of 5 mg/kg/h) for >48 hours, especially in patients receiving these concomitant medications.

Propofol is initially redistributed to peripheral tissues, then metabolized in the liver via the cytochrome P450 system (CYP450) to inactive conjugates that are renally excreted. Significant hepatic dysfunction may lead to prolonged effects, but if infusions are titrated via the RASS, hepatic and renal dysfunction often do not mandate significant dosing adjustments.

BZDs, in particular lorazepam and midazolam, have long been mainstays of ICU sedation as they are potent anxiolytic and sedative agents. These drugs exert their effects primarily through binding to inhibitory γ-aminobutyric acid (GABA)-A receptors (as does propofol), have anticonvulsant properties, and can be used to treat the withdrawal syndrome associated with ethanol dependence.

Midazolam traditionally has been used in short-term sedation, whereas lorazepam, historically less expensive and with a longer half-life, has been used for long-term sedation. Each has advantages and disadvantages: Midazolam is a more potent amnestic agent, a "hypnotic" BZD, whereas lorazepam is primarily an "anxiolytic" BZD. Although the amnestic effect of midazolam may be initially desirable in critically ill patients, it may contribute to disorientation and the development of delirium over time. The long half-life of lorazepam can be a disadvantage in attempts to lighten sedation, and its preparation in a base of propylene glycol can lead to toxicity and acidosis when administered over time at high doses. Midazolam can also demonstrate prolonged sedative effects, however, particularly in elderly patients and in patients with hepatic dysfunction, and the variability of the effects of midazolam is greater than that seen with lorazepam.

Midazolam has useful properties as a long-term infusion or when bolused for procedures (rapid onset, rapid offset), but like fentanyl, it is inappropriate to use bolus administration for sedation in the patient being weaned from mechanical ventilation; however, abrupt withdrawal after long-term infusion of BZD is well-described and should be avoided. A smooth transition may be accomplished by switching from midazolam to propofol approximately 24 hours before the anticipated discontinuation of sedation or by initiating a tapered regimen of intermittent doses of lorazepam after the discontinuation of the midazolam infusion (because the goal is to prevent withdrawal symptoms, not to provide ongoing sedation).

Midazolam and lorazepam are both metabolized via CYP450 and excreted in the urine. Significantly impaired hepatic or renal function should lead the clinician to reduce the doses used or to select another sedative agent.

Dexmedetomidine, a highly specific α_2-agonist with both anxiolytic and analgesic properties, is quickly gaining acceptance in ICU care and in many ways has begun to revolutionize the approach to ICU sedation. The use of dexmedetomidine requires an initial paradigm shift regarding the perception of adequate sedation: Whereas patients receiving opioids plus propofol or BZDs are often asleep or unresponsive (RASS < −2), patients receiving dexmedetomidine are commonly awake and respond to questions and commands. Appropriate dosing means that the patient is not uncomfortable, trying to remove lines or tubes, or expressing pain. Many critical care nurses at first find dexmedetomidine anxiolysis to be disquieting, perceiving it as inadequate sedation, but with experience they come to prefer it as facilitating patient assessment and avoiding overmedication.

Although dexmedetomidine is significantly more expensive per dose than propofol, midazolam, or lorazepam, it has recently been shown in mechanically ventilated patients to result in more days alive without delirium or coma than lorazepam, with no overall increase in cost, adding to literature showing the agent to be cost-effective when overall costs of hospitalization are considered. Dexmedetomidine is US Food and Drug Administration (FDA)-approved for 24 hours of use at doses up to 0.7 µg/kg/h, although longer infusions and higher doses have both been documented to be well-tolerated. Common side effects include initial hypertension and bradycardia with rapid bolus dosing (avoided by administering the initial loading dose [1 µg/kg] over 30–45 minutes), followed by bradycardia and hypotension during the maintenance phase.

In contrast to propofol and opioid–BZD combinations, dexmedetomidine is not a respiratory depressant. This makes its use in nonintubated patients safer than use of the other agents and allows for weaning and discontinuation of mechanical ventilation without adjusting or stopping the sedative/analgesic agent, which may enhance patient comfort and smooth the transition to spontaneous, unassisted ventilation.

Like propofol and the BZDs, dexmedetomidine undergoes hepatic CYP450 metabolism and renal excretion, and dosing should be carefully adjusted to clinical targets in patients with significant dysfunction of these organs.

Ketamine is a useful adjunct to sedative as well as analgesic medications. We add it to the regimen when the standard approach is not providing adequate analgesia and sedation, and wean it in parallel with other medications or with the development of undesirable side effects, especially delirium. Ketamine has sympathomimetic effects, which can be especially problematic in patients with significant cardiovascular disease, and, like the sedatives listed earlier in text, dosing should be reduced in patients with significant hepatic and renal dysfunction.

Processed electroencephalograph monitoring

For patients whose condition requires the administration of neuromuscular blockers (NMBs), which preclude traditional

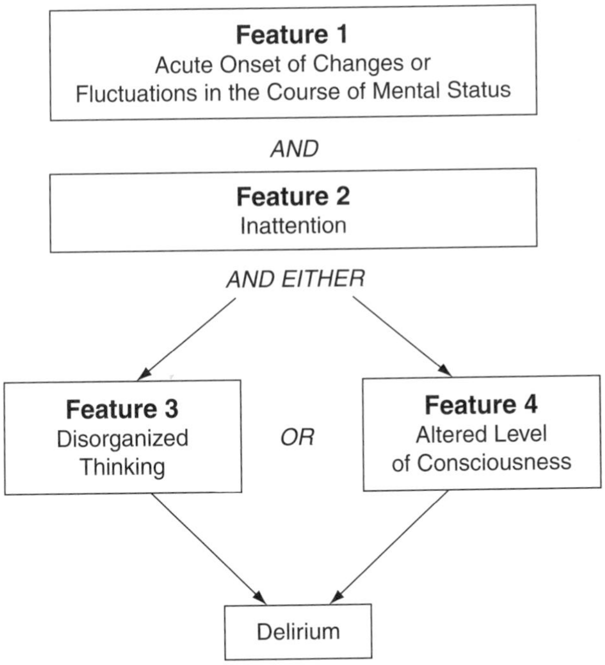

Feature 1
Acute Onset of Changes or
Fluctuations in the Course of Mental Status

AND

Feature 2
Inattention

AND EITHER

Feature 3
Disorganized
Thinking

OR

Feature 4
Altered Level
of Consciousness

Delirium

The diagnosis of delirium requires the presence of acute onset of changes or fluctuations in the course of mental status, and inattention, and either disorganized thinking or an altered level of consciousness.

Figure 157.1. Flow diagram of CAM-ICU. From Ely EW, Inouye SK, Bernard GR, et al. Delirium in mechanically ventilated patients: validity and reliability of the confusion assessment method for the intensive care unit (CAM-ICU). *JAMA* 2001; 286(21):2703–2710.

assessment of adequacy of sedation through patient movement and interaction, the processed electroencephalograph (EEG) score provided by the BIS monitor (Aspect Medical Systems, Newton, MA) or similar devices can be helpful in reassuring clinicians that the patient's level of sedation is adequate and that recall is unlikely to occur.

Delirium in the ICU

ICU delirium (also referred to as *acute brain dysfunction*) is an increasingly appreciated contributor to morbidity and mortality in critically ill patients, with a prevalence of up to 85% and long-term implications for patient outcomes. Hyperactive delirium, formerly known as "ICU psychosis," is more dramatic but less common than hypoactive delirium (characterized by negative symptoms [inattention, flat affect]), which is associated with a worse prognosis. Delirium is more common in the elderly population and among patients with underlying neurologic disease, and its causes are multifactorial. Frequent assessment for the presence of delirium as well as efforts to minimize patients' exposure to medications known to cause delirium should be part of daily rounds.

To screen for delirium, we combine the RASS with the Confusion Assessment Method for the Intensive Care Unit (CAM-ICU) tool (Fig. 157.1 and Table 157.2), administered at least once per shift by our critical care nurses.

Restoring a normal sleep–wake cycle is important in preventing or treating delirium, and this restoration may be approached in various ways. Nocturnal ambient lighting in the ICU should be reduced to a minimum, as should noise and other stimuli. The administration of a sedating psychoactive medication at bedtime (trazodone, olanzapine, quetiapine) can help patients fall asleep without the disruption of delta-wave sleep and risk of delirium associated with the use of BZDs. Propofol anesthesia has been shown to be restful and to share EEG traits with normal sleep, and we sometimes use nocturnal propofol infusions to help our critically ill patients "sleep" at night.

Finally, the conventional antipsychotic medication haloperidol remains a mainstay in the treatment of ICU delirium, particularly in agitated patients, and has been joined in recent years by the atypical antipsychotic medications mentioned earlier in this text. Haloperidol has the advantage of easy intravenous or intramuscular administration, which is

Table 157.2. The Confusion Assessment Method for the Intensive Care Unit (CAM-ICU) part i

1. **Acute onset or flucuating course**
   Is there evidence of an *acute change in mental status* from the baseline?
   Or, did the (abnormal) behavior fluctuate during the past 24 hours, that is, tend to come and go or increase and decrease in severity as evidenced by fluctuations on the Richmond Agitation Sedation Scale (RASS) or the Glasgow Corna Scale?

2. **Inattention**
   Did the patient have *difficulty focusing attention* as evidenced by a score of less than 8 correct answers on either the visual or auditory components of the Attention Screening Examination (ASE)?

3. **Disorganized thinking**
   Is there evidence of *disorganized or incoherent thinking* as evidenced by incorrect answers to 3 or more of the 4 questions and inability to follow the commands?
   Questions:
     1. Will a stone float on water?
     2. Are there fish in the sea?
     3. Does 1 pound weigh more than 2 pounds?
     4. Can you use a hammer to pound a nail?
   Commands:
     1. Are you having unclear thinking?
     2. Hold up this many fingers. (Examiner holds 2 fingers in front of the patient.)
     3. Now do the same thing with the other hand (without holding the 2 fingers in front of the patient)
   (If the patient is already extubated from the ventilator, determine whether the patient's thinking is disorganized or incoherent, such as rambling or irrelevant conversation, unclear or illogical flow of ideas, or unpredictable switching from subject to subject.)

Adapted from Ely EW, Inouye SK, Bernard GR, et al. Delirium in mechanically ventilated patients: validity and reliability of the confusion assessment method for the intensive care unit (CAM-ICU). *JAMA* 2001; 286(21):2703–2710.

Table 157.3. Summary points on management of delirium in the ICU

Monitor delirium regularly in ICU patients using a valid, reliable tool (e.g., the Delirium Screening Checklist or the CAM-ICU). Remember that the most is hypoactive and will be missed if not actively "looked for."

Discuss results of delirium assessments on all petients daily on interdisciplinary rounds.

Identify patients with a high number of risk factors for the development or persistence of delirium (e.g., electrolyte imbalance, fever, addition of new medications; especially those with anticholinergic properties, uncontrolled pain, new onset of congestive heart failure or nosocomial infection, prolonged immobility and restrain use, sleep/wake cycle disturbance).

Review sedation and analgesia therapy, and ensure that the patient is receiving the minium doses needed to achieve comfort, reading that narcotics are often used for the double effect of analgesia and sedation. Implement strategies for tight titration (e.g., nurse-driven, patient-targeted sedation delivery with daily sedation vacations).

Consider the benefit and risk profile of adding medications that might spare the use of sedatives and avoid respiratory suppression (e.g., haloperidol or atypical antipsychotics).

Adapted from Pun BT, Ely EW. The importance of diagnosing and managing ICU delirium. *Chest* 2007; 132:624–636.

useful in the agitated patient, although the risk of QT prolongation and precipitation of torsades de pointes, a potentially lethal arrhythmia, must be recognized and the electrocardiogram (ECG) monitored. Our preference is to avoid the use of antipsychotic medications, but when their administration is deemed necessary, we use haloperidol in patients who require parenteral administration, and switch to enterally administered atypical medications as soon as possible, basing our choice on desired attributes, such as degree of sedation, and so forth. For a summary of management of delirium in the ICU, see Table 157.3.

The ICU patient in the operating room

Critically ill patients may require various surgical procedures, from the relatively minor (tracheostomy and percutaneous enteral access) to more significant (exploratory laparotomy, wound debridements, completion of staged procedures). The anesthesiologist will often find it easiest to continue the patient's existing regimen through the operating room course, integrating it into the general anesthetic plan, as long as the patient's clinical stability allows it. Often the anesthesiologist will simply add a small amount of volatile anesthetic and an NMB to the ICU sedation regimen to achieve an adequate balanced anes-

thetic. For longer procedures, it may be more appropriate to suspend the ICU sedation during the general anesthetic and restart it for the return to the ICU.

Weaning sedation

As mentioned previously, a daily wake-up test has been shown to improve outcomes in sedated, critically ill patients. A ventilator bundle, which includes frequent reassessment of the patient's readiness to separate from mechanical ventilation, should also drive a regular assessment of the ability to lighten or discontinue sedation. Critically ill patients metabolize and recover from the effects of sedating medications differently over time, and frequent reassessment of mental status and depth of sedation are critical to avoiding overmedication and its attendant ill effects, including prolonged ventilation and ICU stay, increased risk of ventilator-associated pneumonia and acute brain dysfunction, and poor long-term outcome. The increasing use of validated sedation scales, delirium screening tools, and algorithm-driven sedation and ventilator weaning protocols have all helped to improve outcomes in critically ill patients.

Suggested readings

Ely EW, Inouye SK, Bernard GR, et al. Delirium in mechanically ventilated patients: validity and reliability of the confusion assessment method for the intensive care unit (CAM-ICU). *JAMA* 2001; 286(21):2703–2710.

Ely EW, Shintani A, Truman B, et al. Delirium as a predictor of mortality in mechanically ventilated patients in the intensive care unit. *JAMA* 2004; 291(14):1753–1762.

Ely EW, Truman B, Shintani A, et al. Monitoring sedation status over time in ICU patients: reliability and validity of the Richmond Agitation-Sedation Scale (RASS). *JAMA* 2003; 289(22):2983–2991.

Kahn DM, Cook TE, Carlisle CC, et al. Identification and modification of environmental noise in an ICU setting. *Chest* 1998; 114:535–540.

Kress JP, Pohlman AS, Hall JB. Sedation and analgesia in the intensive care unit. *Am J Respir Crit Care Med* 2002; 166:1024–1028.

Kress JP, Pohlman AS, O'Connor MF, Hall JB. Daily interruption of sedative infusions in critically ill patients undergoing mechanical ventilation. *N Engl J Med* 2000; 342:1471–1477.

Pandharipande PP, Pun BT, Herr DL, et al. Effect of sedation with dexmedetomidine vs lorazepam on acute brain dysfunction in mechanically ventilated patients: the MENDS randomized controlled trial. *JAMA* 2007; 298(22):2644–2653.

Pun BT, Ely EW. The importance of diagnosing and managing ICU delirium. *Chest* 2007; 132:624–636.

Weaning from mechanical ventilation

Maxwell Weinmann

There is little agreement regarding the optimal method for weaning patients from mechanical ventilator support. No single mode has been identified as ideal for this purpose other than that which achieves optimal patient comfort while not sacrificing gains in oxygenation and ventilation made during the acute illness. Indeed, it has been estimated that some patients spend approximately 40% of their ventilator time committed to the weaning process. Additionally, the literature is replete with the search for indices which can predict patient weaning capability from mechanical ventilation; however, a gold standard has yet to emerge. It is not surprising therefore that no single test has supplanted clinical evaluation, possibly because such tests represent physiologic "snapshots" rather than an evaluation of pulmonary reserve. The capacity to wean is not merely a function of pulmonary status but is a codependent dynamic process affected by fluid balance, cardiac function, neurologic status, coexistent abdominal pathology, and associated therapy (such as sedatives), to name a few. This has led some clinicians to challenge the practicality of such indices which are considered to be only modest predictors of the need for reintubation, tracheostomy and mortality, and in some cases thought only to prolong the weaning process.

In light of the ongoing confusion, a collaboration among the American College of Chest Physicians, the Society of Critical Care Medicine, and the American Association of Respiratory Physicians produced evidenced-based guidelines for weaning from mechanical ventilation.

Pathology of ventilator dependence

All aspects of the underlying disease which necessitated intubation, potential reversibility, and associated complications must be identified and treated. Prolonged mechanical ventilation may be associated with ventilator-induced lung injury, respiratory muscle deconditioning, pneumonia, tracheal injury, prolonged sedation, and so forth. Removal from ventilatory support, must be balanced against the patient's ability to protect his/her airway, clear secretions, demonstrate a consistently clear sensorium, maintain hemodynamic stability, and cope with the often increased work of breathing. For example, regarding the latter, many patients with underlying chronic obstructive pulmonary disease (COPD) develop a compensated hypercapnic acidosis during their acute illness that persists in the recovery phase despite ventilatory support. Acetazolamide has been used in these cases to produce a metabolic acidosis to stimulate respiratory drive. The potential for success of such a strategy, however, is a function of the underlying physiologic reserve of the patient. The physiologic cost of "normalizing" gas values often translates to increased work of breathing, which may not be sustainable due to diminished pulmonary reserve. This may be secondary to incomplete resolution of the patient's illness, respiratory muscle deconditioning, and/or complicating pathology. This approach has had limited success and demonstrates the potential dangers of "treating the numbers."

Assessing patient potential to wean

With resolution of the acute phase of the illness and stabilization of the patient, the clinician must determine if those factors necessitating implementation of mechanical ventilation have resolved sufficiently for the commencement of weaning. This determination is fraught with clinical subjectivity and the absence of any clear predictor.

Today, central to the success of liberating patients from ventilator support is regular and meticulous clinical assessment. The following indices have been developed and tested, with varying successes, for the ventilator weaning process (Table 158.1).

Frequency-to-tidal volume ratio: rapid shallow breathing index (RSBI)

Application of this parameter is based on the observation that those patients who failed weaning demonstrated increasing respiratory rates with declining tidal volumes. Although the sensitivity and specificity of this parameter have varied within the literature, it remains among the most common evaluations and is considered quite reliable. A threshold of approximately 100 breaths/min/L is becoming generally accepted as predictive of successful weaning. Clinical reliability, however, will depend on additional factors, such as the presence or absence of ongoing support, the level of support, the size of the endotracheal tube, and so forth.

Minute ventilation

Normal minute ventilation is approximately 6 L/min. Its use as a predictor of weanability has a sensitivity and specificity of

Table 158.1. Selected recommendations from the ACCP–SCCM–AARC Evidence-Based Weaning Guidelines Task Force

Recommendation 1: Patients receiving mechanical ventilation for respiratory failure should undergo a formal assessment of discontinuation potential if the following criteria are satisfied:

1. Evidence of some reversal of the underlying cause of respiratory failure
2. Adequate oxygenation: PaO_2/FiO_2 150–200 mm Hg, required PEEP $\leq$ 5–8 cm H_2O, $FiO_2 \leq$ 0.4–0.5, and pH $\geq$ 7.25
3. Hemodynamic stability as defined by the absence of clinically important hypotension and requiring no vasopressors or only low-dose vasopressors (e.g., dopamine or dobutamine < 5 μg/kg/min)
4. Patient is able to initiate an inspiratory effort

The decision to use these criteria must be individualized. Some patients who do not satisfy all the criteria may, nevertheless, be ready for an attempt to discontinue mechanical ventilation.

Recommendation 2: Formal discontinuation assessments should be done during spontaneous breathing rather than while the patient is still receiving substantial ventilatory support. An initial brief period of spontaneous breathing can be used to assess the patient's ability to do a formal SBT.

Criteria to assess patient tolerance during SBT are the respiratory pattern, adequacy of gas exchange, hemodynamic stability, and subjective comfort. Patients who tolerate a 30- to 120-min SBT should promptly be considered for ventilator discontinuation.

Recommendation 3: With patients whose ventilatory support has been successfully discontinued, the decision of whether to remove the artificial airway should be based on assessment of airway patency and the patient's ability to protect the airway.

Recommendation 4: If the patient fails an SBT, determine the reasons the patient continues to require ventilatory support. When the reversible causes of failure are corrected, an SBT should be performed every 24 h.

Recommendation 5: Patients who fail SBT should receive a stable, nonfatiguing, comfortable form of ventilatory support.

Recommendation 6: Weaning/discontinuation protocols designed for nonphysician clinicians should be developed and implemented by ICUs. Protocols should aim to optimize sedation.

Recommendation 7: Critical care practitioners should be familiar with facilities in their communities or units in their hospital that specialize in managing patients who suffer prolonged ventilator dependence, and practitioners should stay abreast of peer-reviewed reports from such units. When medically stable enough for transfer, patients who have failed discontinuation attempts in the ICU should be transferred to facilities that have demonstrated success and safety in accomplishing ventilator discontinuation.

Recommendation 8: Unless there is evidence of clearly irreversible disease (e.g., high spinal cord injury, advanced amyotrophic lateral sclerosis), a patient who requires prolonged ventilatory support for respiratory failure should not be considered permanently ventilator-dependent until 3 months of weaning attempts have failed.

Recommendation 9: With a patient who requires prolonged ventilation, the weaning should be slow paced and should include gradually lengthening SBTs.

ACCP, American College of Chest Physicians; SCCM, Society for Critical Care Medicine; AARC, American Association for Respiratory Care; PaO_2/FiO_2, ratio of arterial partial pressure of oxygen to fraction of inspired oxygen; SBT, spontaneous breathing trial.
Adapted from Meade M, Guyatt G, Cook D, et al. Predicting success in weaning from mechanical ventilation. *Chest* 2001; 120(6 Suppl):400S.

approximately 0.96 and 0.47, respectively, and while considered to be a reflection of the potential of the patient to deal with a respiratory burden, it nevertheless has to be placed in the perspective of how the patient achieves it. In other words, if the minute ventilation is >6 L/min but predominantly due to a high respiratory rate, then sustainability and potential for successful weaning must be questioned.

Vital capacity

Vital capacity is not considered particularly reliable as it depends, in part, on patient cooperation and does not correlate with sustainability.

Maximum inspiratory pressure

Measurements of this parameter demonstrate substantial variability, and it has not become clearly established as a reliable guide for weaning. The ratio of the inspiratory pressure to the airway occlusion pressure has been proposed as more reliable (the latter reflecting ventilatory drive and muscle strength), but requires further assessment.

Work of breathing

Typically, indirect markers have been used as surrogates of work of breathing, such as respiratory rate, use of accessory

muscles, and tachycardia. Direct measures have proven to be rather cumbersome and clinically impractical. A definitive predictive value has remained elusive. Consequently, the interactions between Compliance, Respiratory rate, Oxygenation and inspiratory Pressure have been proposed as an alternative, the the so-called CROP index. Its clinical utility remains to be determined.

Arterial blood gases

Contrary to what might be expected, arterial blood gas values have not been shown to correlate with weanability, despite their reflection of underlying gas exchange capacity. One would not attempt, however, to reduce the level of support and consider weaning if hypoxia and/or hypercapnia were ongoing issues.

Overall

No single parameter has been shown to be the gold standard by which successful weaning and liberation from mechanical ventilation can be predicted. Nor has any been shown to impact on or predict in-hospital mortality, extubation failure, or need for tracheostomy. The key to effective weaning is regular assessment of the patient's comfort, in close collaboration with intensive care unit (ICU) nursing staff and respiratory therapists, and individualized care tempered by clinical perspective (Fig. 158.1).

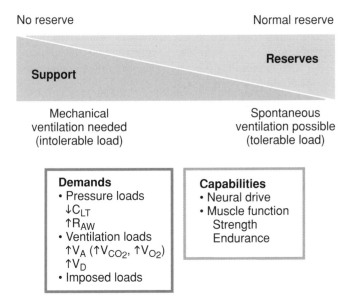

Figure 158.1. Determinants of need for mechanical ventilatory support.

Weaning strategies

A key to determining the appropriateness and success of a particular mode of support during weaning is patient comfort. A balance must be achieved between patient demand and the level of support. This should be achieved in the absence of distress and deterioration in physiologic function and therapeutic gains that accompany change in ventilator settings. Patient synchrony, indirect markers of work of breathing, cardiovascular status, oxygenation and ventilation status must be regularly evaluated to avoid the onset of fatigue and derecruitment. Potential traps include "treating the numbers" (e.g., when patients demonstrate abnormal blood gases but are nonetheless well compensated despite diminished pulmonary reserve). Many algorithms have been proposed to achieve weaning. These algorithms vary from regularly exercising the respiratory muscles, to rapidly reducing support to avoid respiratory muscle deconditioning, to T-tube trials and extubation. No single approach has been shown to be superior to another. The physician must, therefore, tailor a therapeutic strategy based on patient capabilities. Clearly, the respiratory reserve of a patient with an uncomplicated drug overdose may allow rapid weaning to extubation, whereas a patient with Guillain–Barré syndrome provides an ongoing challenge of progressive slow reduction in support during neurologic recovery and rehabilitation. Similarly, basing weaning to an acceptable respiratory rate of 18 to 24 may be impossible in a patient who has developed restrictive lung physiology following severe acute respiratory distress syndrome (ARDS).

Traditional weaning methods

Pressure support

Pressure support ventilation (PSV) is a pressure targeted, or limited, mode supporting each patient breath in a synchronized fashion. Detection of the onset of inspiration is either by the generation of a negative pressure or a rapid increase in flow, whereas the onset of expiration is indirectly heralded by a reduction in inspiratory flow. It is the patient who regulates rate and has partial control over tidal volume. PSV has been shown to efficiently reduce work of breathing as evidenced by increased tidal volumes, reduced respiratory rates, and parallel reductions in transdiaphragmatic pressure swings. Support is not necessarily linear, such that above a certain pressure, volume increments are not as great, and work of breathing is not decreased. To wean, therefore, the physician must establish sustainable patterns of respiratory rate and tidal volume confirming that patient comfort may be achieved. If successful, a strategy of progressive scheduled reductions in support can be instituted until extubation is accomplished while the patient is closely monitored. It is important to recall that this includes regular blood gas analysis, as pulse oximetry is not a measure of ventilatory status.

Synchronized intermittent mandatory ventilation

In this mode, an underlying mandatory rate is set, at a fixed volume. The rationale is that the patient's respiratory muscles are progressively exercised and reconditioned during spontaneous effort, while resting during mandatory breaths. Typically, the mandatory rate is gradually reduced as the patient's work progressively increases to the point of extubation. Pressure support has recently been added to the spontaneous cycle to further assist in patient work of breathing. Evaluation of this mode has shown, however, that the theoretical impact on work of breathing is not borne out in practice and that effort is similar in both assisted and unassisted breaths. This has been attributed to the inability of the respiratory center to adapt to breath-to-breath changes in work load, culminating in ventilator dyssynchrony and respiratory muscle fatigue.

Spontaneous breathing trials

T-piece weaning is the oldest weaning technique. It consists of the initiation of progressively increasing intervals of spontaneous breathing while the patient is connected to a T-piece circuit consisting of a high flow, humidified gas source. During the evaluation, the patient is not connected to the ventilator, hence the term *spontaneous breathing trial*. Typically, evaluation was based on repeated efforts over hours; however, the current understanding that respiratory muscle recovery requires approximately 24 hours has limited such trials to once a day for periods of less than 2 hours.

Currently, spontaneous breathing trials are the recommended final step in the weaning process and for evaluating patient readiness for extubation. These are most commonly performed while the patients are on the ventilator. This provides the advantage that all parameters of respiration can be continuously monitored and evaluated during the weaning process. Such trials are performed once daily and only for eligible patients who meet standard criteria (RSBI<105, adequate oxygenation [PaO_2>60 mm Hg on FiO_2 of 40%, presence of spontaneous effort for breathing, PEEP<5-10, PaO$_2$/FiO$_2$ >300], stable cardiovascular status, T<38°C, no significant respiratory acidosis, adequate mentation, no other contraindications [such as intracranial hypertension, etc.]). When performed via the ventilator, the patient is placed on continuous positive airway pressure (CPAP) mode with activation of alarms providing additional monitoring benefits. On occasion, positive end-expiratory pressure (PEEP) has been added to compensate for the perceived loss of any physiologic PEEP, but in reality is of no benefit and counterintuitive to our current understanding of respiratory physiology.

Role of PEEP

Conventionally, PEEP is used as a tool to optimize oxygenation by alveolar recruitment. It is therefore considered more physiologic than merely increasing FiO$_2$ by achieving greater homogeneity within the lung. It does so at some cost, however, and may potentially impact on cardiovascular function by impeding venous return and therefore cardiac output. This impact is in part dependent on lung compliance and may be estimated by esophageal pressure measurements and fluctuations in the central venous pressure (CVP). The more compliant the lung, the more likely it is that pressure changes will be transmitted to the central veins. PEEP has also been purported to potentially increase intracranial pressure (ICP); however, this increase can only occur when venous pressure exceeds intracerebral tissue pressure.

In terms of its relationship to weaning, PEEP can also impact on work of breathing. This is particularly true in patients with obstructive lung disease who demonstrate gas trapping due to delayed expiration, with a failure to exhale down to functional residual capacity (FRC) of the lung. As volume accumulates, expiratory pressure increases and effectively splints open the airways until a new equilibrium is reached at both a higher overall pressure and FRC. The resultant pressure is termed *auto PEEP*, or *intrinsic PEEP*, as it acts much in the same way as extrinsic or ventilator-derived PEEP. At end expiration, total PEEP is therefore the sum of both these values: one set by the operator, the other, an inadvertent consequence of impaired exhalation, due to intrinsic lung and/or airway disease or an inappropriate adjustment of inspiratory and/or expiratory times. In weaning such a patient, airflow will not commence until the intrinsic pressure is exceeded. This becomes an added respiratory muscle load and increases the work of breathing, thereby hampering weaning unless the physician is vigilant for its presence. This may be clinically apparent as ventilator asynchrony or dyspnea, as there is a delay between overcoming auto-PEEP and triggering the ventilator.

Overall assessment of traditional methods

Studies have failed to demonstrate the superiority of any particular mode over another in terms of successful extubation, in-hospital mortality, ventilator-associated complications, or the requirement for reintubation. The key is patient comfort and titrating weaning parameters in a physiologically sensitive manner. This translates to the clinician's assessment of the patient's underlying respiratory reserve and the patient's response to reduced support, in collaboration with respiratory therapists and ICU nursing staff.

New modes of ventilation

Some new modes of ventilation may ease the process of weaning due to their enhanced responsiveness to the patient's needs. However, it is yet unclear if these new modes can help shorten the time patients spend on the ventilator.

Tube compensation

Tube compensation was designed to overcome the problem of breathing against the resistance of an artificial airway and its accompanying work load. The flow resistance qualities of the endotracheal tube size are known and are associated with a pressure drop across the length of the tube during inspiration. The ventilator, in turn, compensates for this pressure drop, making tracheal pressure constant, depending on the degree of assist required by the patient (100% and lower). Potentially, this mode enhances patient ventilator synchrony, increases patient comfort, reduces risk of gas trapping (through expiratory resistance by the tube), and reduces respiratory muscle fatigue.

Proportional assist

The level of assistance in this new mode of ventilation is proportional to patient effort and is therefore a positive feedback loop. The patient determines pressure, flow, and volume, which are then amplified according to clinical assessment. This mode is considered by some investigators to be more physiologic but its superiority as a support and a weaning mode has yet to be demonstrated.

Mandatory minute ventilation

Mandatory minute ventilation was one of the earliest forms of closed loop ventilation support. The clinician presets minimum minute ventilation; should the patient be unable to achieve or maintain it, the ventilator augments support by increasing either respiratory rate or tidal volume (depending on the machine). Alternately, if the patient begins to exceed the minimum preset level, support diminishes. Unfortunately, the ventilator is indifferent to how minute ventilation is achieved, so that 10 breaths per minute of 450 ml each would be viewed as identical to 30 breaths per minute of 150 ml each.

Airway pressure release ventilation

Two levels of positive pressure are applied for preset times; the high pressure dictates lung volumes during inhalation, which is longer in duration than exhalation (and is therefore a form of inverse ratio ventilation), whereas the lower pressure is the exhalation baseline. Due to the very short duration of the expiratory phase, the lung does not completely deflate such that auto PEEP maintains alveolar recruitment. The patient may breathe spontaneously during the inspiratory phase, but no additional support is provided, unlike bilevel ventilation (see below). This mode, despite being an inverse ratio, is well tolerated by patients.

Bilevel ventilation

Unlike airway pressure release ventilation, bilevel ventilation is not necessarily an inverse mode, although it is an option depending on the inspiratory time, which the clinician may determine. It may be easier to consider bilevel ventilation as a pressure-regulated synchronized intermittent mandatory ventilation (SIMV) mode that runs in the background, while any additional spontaneous breaths may be supported by the addition of pressure support. Weaning is achieved by a reduction in the mandatory rate and high pressure level (which determines tidal volume) with a transition to pure pressure support.

Pressure-regulated volume control and/or volume support

Here a set tidal volume is predetermined by the clinician while the ventilator delivers the volume to a maximum pressure level; in other words, it is volume targeted and pressure regulated. The ventilator delivers a pressure-controlled breath to calculate the patient's lung compliance. Based on this calculation, the ventilator delivers the appropriate pressure to generate the desired volume. The ventilator will continue to titrate pressure to volume within its set pressure range. If the rate is set, the mode is identified as "volume control," while if the rate is determined solely by the patient, it is termed "volume support." Although this method is attractive, if the patient increases tidal volume in response to worsening of the underlying pathology, the ventilator will interpret this increase as an improvement in lung status and consequently reduce support.

Assessment of new weaning modes

Many new modes incorporate a closed loop system in which the ventilator reacts to changes in a target variable by the initiation of a rapid compensatory response (as in volume support, mentioned earlier in text). These techniques are therefore considered to be more physiologic than traditional methods, and hold promise. Their overall superiority in terms of weaning, or reducing the time spent on the ventilator, remains to be determined.

Extubation

After the patient has demonstrated that he or she meets weaning criteria, extubation follows. The clinician must be wary of the facts that such criteria (as outlined earlier in the text) do not necessarily correlate with sustainability of liberation from the ventilator and that close monitoring must continue if reintubation is to be avoided. Additionally, problems may surface that were not readily apparent during weaning, such as subglottic edema, postextubation laryngospasm, and aspiration, to name a few. Edema and laryngospasm often respond to nebulized racemic epinephrine, and the risk of aspiration may be diminished by discontinuing feeds prior to extubation. Some clinicians also perform a cuff leak test to evaluate postextubation airway patency. This test has not been shown to be reliable because leak volume is also a function of system compliance, inspiratory flow, and expiratory resistance.

For those patients who still struggle postextubation, noninvasive positive pressure ventilation may be a temporizing measure rather than resorting to immediate reintubation. To be effective, however, the patient must be cooperative, anxiety should be minimal, the patient must have an effective cough, secretions should be minimal, and the condition that necessitates the ventilator support has to be reversible in the short term (hours to days). Finally, nonrespiratory factors should always be evaluated and treated in the patient who either struggles to meet extubation criteria or develops respiratory distress on extubation as outlined in Table 158.2.

Tracheostomy

Tracheostomy should be considered when it is evident that the patient requires either long-term ventilator support or airway protection, despite the capacity to wean, and is at risk of ongoing aspiration. Tracheostomies may be performed either surgically or at the bedside using the percutaneous technique. The patient may be reassured that comfort and tolerance of an artificial airway is greater with a tracheostomy and that it is not necessarily permanent and can be easily removed when normal respiratory function returns.

Summary

- As yet, no particular method has emerged as the gold standard for successful patient weaning.
- Similarly, there is no ideal index of weanability.
- Indices reflect moments in time rather than a true assessment of respiratory reserve and the capacity to remain extubated for a protracted period.
- Liberating the patient from mechanical ventilator support requires regular and meticulous assessment of the patient's readiness to separate from the ventilator, and observation postextubation.
- Weaning presupposes that the acute precipitating event has resolved.
- Weaning is a collaborative effort involving the physician, respiratory therapist, ICU nursing staff, and the patient.
- Patient comfort is the key that dictates the methodology and rate of declining support.
- Clinical acumen determines timing, avoidance of complications, and reversibility of confounding factors.

Table 158.2. Nonrespiratory factors in weaning patients from mechanical ventilation

Category	Factor	Mechanism	Clinical presentation
Cardiac status	Acute left-ventricular failure	Inreased preload because of increased venous return and decreased pulmonary capillary compression as intrathoracic pressure is reduced	Patient fails weaning, often after initially doing well for 30-60 minutes; may develop acute respiratory and/or metabolic acidosis, hypoxemia, hypotension, chest pain, and cardiac dysrhythmias
Acid-base status	Acute alkalosis in patient with underlying carbon dioxide (CO_2) retention	Loss of preexisting metabolic compensation for hypercapnia; inability to sustain required V_E and WOB	Patient with COPD or other cause of chronic respiratory acidosis before acute insult fails weaning after several days of ventilation to a PCO_2 lower than the patient's pH-compensated level
	Respiratory alkalosis	Depression of ventilatory drives by hypocapnia and alkalemia	PCO_2 rises and pH falls during weaning attempt; patient is said to fail weaing if some arbitrary change in these values (e.g. 10 mm Hg increase in PCO_2) is used as a criterion for failure.
	Metabolic acidosis	Increase in ventilatory demand to compensate for respiratory alkalosis	Patient may be unable to sustain required increase in V_E and WOB to maintain a lower PCO_2 to compensate for a lower HCO_3
Metabolic status	Hypophosphatemia and hypomagnesemia	Ventilatory muscle weakness	Patient fails weaning because of rapid shallow breathing, respiratory distress, and acute respiratory acidosis; maximal inspiratory pressure is decreased.
	Hypothyroidism	Decreased ventilatory drive with possible ventilatory muscle weakness	Rare cause of weaning failure that occurs because of acute respiratory distress.
Drugs	Narcotics, sedatives, tranquilizers, and hypnotics	Depression of ventilatory drive	Patient fails weaning because of acute respiratory acidosis in the absence of tachypnea and respiratory distress
	Neuromuscular blocking agents	Ventilatory muscle weakness; delayed clearance in patient with rental insufficiciency	Patient fails weaning because of rapid shallow breathing, respiratory distress, and acute respiratory acidosis; maximal inspiratory pressure is reduced.
		Ventilatory muscle weakness caused by acute myopathy, especially in patients who have received high-dose systemic corticosteroids	Same as above; may have elevated muscle enzymes; can last for weeks or months.
	Aminoglycosides	Neuromuscular blockade	Very rare cause of weaning failure that occurs because of rapid shallow breathing, respiratory distress, and acute respiratory acidosis; maximal inspiratory force is reduced.
Nutrition	Overfeeding	Increased CO_2 production, especially with excessive carbohydrate calories	Patient fails weaning because of excessive ventilatory demand (high V_E requirement to keep PCO_2 normal); unusual cause of weaning failure unless very large caloric loads are administered.
	Malnutrition	Effects of acute illness; preexisting nutritional deficiencies	May contribute to ventilatory muscle weakness, decreased ventilatory drive, impaired immunologic function, fluid retention, depression, distinguishing this from other factors is difficult
Psychological status	Agitation: "psychological ventilator dependence"	Anxiety, fear, delirium, ICU psychosis, or influence of preexisting personality factors	Patient becomes agitated and panicky during attempt to reduce or discontinue ventilatory support; can be said to cause weaning failure when other factors are absent
	Lack of motivation	Depression, effects of drugs, organic brain dysfunction, or influence of preexisting personality factors	Patient refuses to participate in care (e.g., mobilization, bronchial hygiene, physiologic measurements); flat affect and immobility in bed; considered when other factors are absent

V_E, minute ventilation; WOB, work of breathing; PCO_2, partial pressure of carbon dioxide; pH, hydrogen ion concentration; HCO_3^-, bicarbonate.
Adapted from Pilbeam SP, Cairo JM *Mechanical Ventilation: Physiological and Clinical Applications*. 4th ed. Philadelphia: Mosby Publications; 2006: 461–2.

Suggested readings

ACCP/AARC/SCCM Task Force. Evidenced based guidelines for weaning and discontinuing mechanical ventilatory support. A collective task force facilitated by the American College of Chest Physicians; the American Association of Respiratory Care; and the American College of Critical Care Medicine. *Chest* 2001; 120(Suppl 6):375S–484S.

Fabry B, Haberthur C, Zappe D, et al. Breathing pattern and additional work of breathing in spontaneously breathing patients with different ventilatory demands during inspiratory pressure support and automatic tube compensation. *Intensive Care Med* 1997; 23:545.

Grasso S, Ranieri VM. Proportional assist ventilation. *Respir Care Clin N Am* 2001; 7(3):465–473.

Hess DR. Mechanical ventilation strategies; what's new and what's worth keeping? *Respir Care* 2002; 47:1007–1017.

Hörmann C, Baum M, Putensen C, et al. Biphasic positive airway pressure (BIPAP)–a new mode of ventilatory support. *Eur J Anaesthesiol* 1994; 11(1):37–42.

Kenney BD. Airway pressure-release ventilation. *Respir Care* 2008; 53(7):922–923.

Jones PW, Greenstone M. Carbonic anhydrase inhibitors for hypercapnic ventilatory failure in chronic obstructive pulmonary disease. *Cochrane Database Syst Rev* 2001;1:CD002881.

MacIntyre NR. Respiratory mechanics in the patient who is weaning from the ventilator. *Respir Care* 2005; 50(2):275–286.

Meade M, Guyatt G, Cook D, et al. Predicting success in weaning from mechanical ventilation. *Chest* 2001; 120(6 Suppl):400S.

Vitacca M, Bianchi L, Zanotti E, et al. Assessment of physiologic variables and subjective comfort under different levels of pressure support ventilation. *Chest* 2004; 126(3):851–859.

Chapter 159

Acute lung injury and acute respiratory distress syndrome

David A. Silver

Diagnostic criteria

The clinical syndromes of acute lung injury (ALI) and acute respiratory distress syndrome (ARDS) represent degrees of severity along the continuum of noncardiogenic respiratory failure, and present significant management challenges to the anesthesiologist and intensivist.

ALI is a clinical syndrome defined by the rapid onset of severe hypoxemia (PaO_2/FiO_2 [P/F ratio] ≤ 300) regardless of positive end-expiratory pressure (PEEP), bilateral infiltrates on frontal chest radiograph, and lack of cardiogenic etiology for these findings. In the presence of a pulmonary artery catheter (PAC), this "noncardiogenic" is generally defined by a pulmonary artery occlusion pressure (PAOP) ≤ 18 mm Hg; otherwise, the diagnosis is based on absence of stigmata of elevated left atrial pressure. ARDS is defined by the same criteria, but with more severe hypoxemia, a P/F ratio ≤ 200 (Table 159.1).

A recent study from the National Institutes of Heath, National Heart, Lung, and Blood Institute ARDS Network (ARDSnet) has validated the use of pulse oximetric saturation in a ratio of SpO_2/FiO_2 (S/F ratio) in patients with $SpO_2 \leq 97\%$, with an S/F ratio of 315 correlating with a P/F ratio of 300, and an SpO_2/FiO_2 (S/F) ratio of 235 correlating with a P/F ratio of 200. This new convention appears to have excellent sensitivity and fair specificity and may allow less invasive screening for and rapid diagnosis of ALI/ARDS, facilitating the initiation of appropriate therapy and entry into clinical trials of patients at the onset of the disease syndrome. It is also consistent with the concerns in modern critical care to minimize blood draws (and resultant iatrogenic anemia) as well as the costs associated with processing arterial blood gas (ABG) samples.

Many patients will meet some criteria for both clinical heart failure (e.g., due to volume overload after resuscitation for severe sepsis) and for ALI. Thus there may be uncertainty as to how to categorize respiratory failure in patients with multiorgan system failure. The diagnosis of ALI is not based on purely objective tests, and lacks a pathognomonic clinical finding. As a result, for instance, since different clinicians interpret patients' chest radiographs differently, they may or may not make the diagnosis of ALI. In clinical practice, it is important to have a high index of suspicion for the development of ALI and to treat patients appropriately as soon as the diagnosis is made. It is also crucial, however, to ensure that another disease process with a specific treatment is not missed (Table 159.2).

Markers of inflammation

Although levels of various biomarkers of inflammation, including tumor necrosis factor-alpha (TNF-α), transforming growth factor-beta-1 (TGF-β1), angiostatin, and interleukins 1 and 8 (IL-1 and -8), are elevated in bronchoalveolar lavage (BAL) specimens from ALI patients, their roles in the pathophysiology of the disease process are still under investigation, and routine BAL is not required for the diagnosis of ALI. It is clear that pulmonary neutrophils are important in the development of ALI, as their increased activation of the transcriptional regulatory factor nuclear factor-kappa B (NF-κB) leads to the increased production of many of the factors listed above, as well as the kinases p38 and phosphoinositide 3-kinase (PI3-K).

Epidemiology

Risk for the development of ALI/ARDS is particularly high in older patients, in patients with significant medical comorbidities (such as chronic hepatic and pulmonary disease), and possibly in patients with a genetic predisposition to severe inflammation. Once labeled "adult respiratory distress syndrome" to distinguish it from the infant respiratory distress syndrome, it is now called "acute" and is well-described in patients 15 years of age or older.

Recent studies of the epidemiology of ALI have demonstrated that it is much more common than previously thought,

Table 159.1. Defining ALI and ARDS

Timing: Acute onset
Hypoxemia (regardless of PEEP)
ALI: $PaO_2/FiO_2 \leq 300$ (or $SpO_2/FiO_2 \leq 315$ if $SpO_2 \leq 97\%$)
ARDS: $PaO_2/FiO_2 \leq 200$ (or $SpO_2/FiO_2 \leq 235$ if $SpO_2 \leq 97\%$)
Frontal chest radiograph: Bilateral infiltrates present
Noncardiogenic: PAOP (when measured) ≤ 18 mm Hg; otherwise, no clinical evidence of elevated left atrial pressure

From Bernard GR, Artigas A, Brigham KL, et al. The American-European consensus conference on ARDS: definitions, mechanisms, relevant outcomes and clinical trial coordination. *Am J Respir Crit Care Med* 1994; 149:818–824.

Table 159.2. Differential diagnosis of ALI

Left ventricular failure
Intravascular volume overload
Mitral stenosis
Veno-occlusive disease
Lymphangitic carcinoma
Interstitial and airway diseases
● Hypersensitivity pneumonitis
● Acute pneumonia
● Bronchiolitis obliterans with organising pneumonia

From Wheeler AP, Bernard GR. Acute lung injury and the acute respiratory distress syndrome: a clinical review. *Lancet* 2007; 369:1553–1565.

Table 159.3. Risk factors in the development of mortality from ALI

Obesity	Decreased mortality
Diabetes	Decreased risk of developing ARDS
Chronic alcoholism	Increased risk of developing ARDS
Increasing age up to 69 y	Increased incidence and mortality
Worse physiologic severity of illness	Increased mortality
Shock on hospital admission	Increased mortality
African-American race	Increased mortality
Low body mass index (below-average weight)	Increased mortality
Male gender	Increased mortality
Longer hospitalization before ALI	Increased mortality
Shorter ICU stay with ALI	Increased mortality
Increased radiographic opacity	Increased mortality
Immunosuppression	Increased mortality
Various genetic factors	Variable effects

From Rubenfeld GD, Herridge MS. Epidemiology and outcomes of acute lung injury. *Chest* 2007; 131:554–562.

and represents a significant public health issue. The reported incidence of and mortality associated with ALI and ARDS vary significantly among trials.

In 2002, the Australian and New Zealand Intensive Care Society Clinical Trials Group reported an overall incidence of ALI and ARDS of 34 and 28 cases per 100,000 per annum, respectively. The overall 28-day intensive care unit (ICU) mortality rate was 28% for patients with ALI/ARDS; mortality was 30% with the subgroup that met ARDS criteria, and mortality was only 10% (a significant difference) in the ALI without ARDS group.

The King County Lung Injury Project (KCLIP) reported in 2005 a higher incidence of ALI/ARDS (combined) of 78.9 cases per 100,000 person-years, with an age-adjusted incidence of 86.2 per 100,000 person-years, and an overall in-hospital mortality of 38.5%. This study confirmed a dramatic increase in incidence with age, from 16 per 100,000 person-years for patients 15 to 19 years old to 306 per 100,000 person-years for those 75 to 84 years old. Mortality similarly ranged from 24% for teenagers to 60% for patients 85 years or older. The authors extrapolated their findings to estimate 190,600 cases of ALI in the United States each year, associated with 74,500 deaths and 3.6 million hospital days. Although the incidence the authors describe is higher than that reported from the Australia/New Zealand group, their standardized methods of review may have uncovered a much higher incidence of these syndromes than had previously been appreciated, and they reinforce an appreciation for the persistently high mortality of ALI/ARDS even after the advent of low-tidal-volume ventilation.

As the diagnosis of ALI may not be made in up to 48% of patients who meet criteria, the KCLIP study results are credible in revealing a significant incidence of ALI. Various risk factors have been examined in epidemiologic studies, and investigation continues into the genetic and other factors involved in a complex and heterogenous disease process. Table 159.3 lists some factors that have been implicated as risk factors for the development of, or mortality from ALI/ARDS. Some are not surprising – for instance, patients admitted to the hospital with greater severity of illness (as measured by the Acute Physiology And Chronic Health Evaluation II [APACHE-II] or similar scores) have a higher mortality. Others, such as a seemingly protective effect of diabetes, are less clear. It may be that diabetic patients

are more likely to have nonpulmonary (and more easily treated) sources of sepsis (e.g., genitourinary, soft tissue infections), but there may be another yet-unelucidated protective effect. Obese patients diagnosed with ALI may have better reserves to deal with critical illness, or they may not have lung injury at all, just significant atelectasis, the rapid resolution of which may lead to the appearance of lower mortality in this patient population.

Pathophysiology

ALI is not a primary disease process, but is rather a reaction to a direct or indirect insult to the lungs (Table 159.4).

Direct injury (e.g., pneumonia, aspiration) or indirect injury due to systemic inflammation (especially with severe sepsis) leads to a common pathway of generalized inflammation and subsequent increased pulmonary vascular permeability. In early ALI, a protein-rich pulmonary edema characterizes what has been called the *exudative phase*, during which inflammation

Table 159.4. Causes of ALI

Direct injury
Pneumonia
Gastric aspiration
Drowning
Fat and amniotic-fluid embolism
Pulmonary contusion
Alveolar haemorrhage
Smoke and toxic gas inhalation
Reperfusion (pleural effusion drainage, embolectomy)
Unilateral lung re-implantation

Indirect injury
Severe sepsis
Transfusions
Shock
Salicylate or narcotic overdose
Pancreatitis

From Wheeler AP, Bernard GR. Acute lung injury and the acute respiratory distress syndrome: a clinical review. *Lancet* 2007; 369:1553–1565.

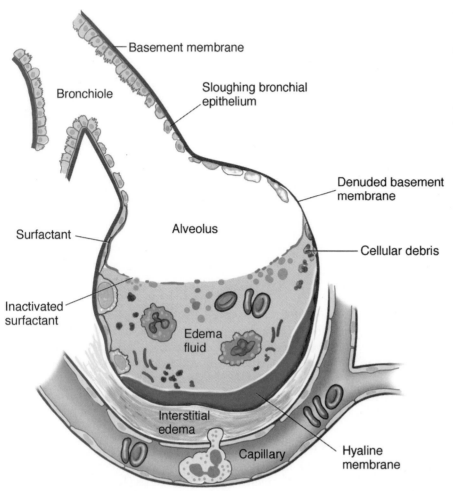

Figure 159.1. The Alveolus in Acute Lung Injury. In the acute phase of the syndrome, there is sloughing of both the bronchial and alveolar epithelial cells, with the formation of protein-rich hyaline membranes on the denuded basement membrane and filling of the air space with protein-rich edema fluid which inactivates surfactant. Macrophages in the air space secrete cytokines, which (among other effects) stimulate chemotaxis and activation of neutrophils and a subsequent inflammatory cascade.

predominates, surfactant production decreases, existing surfactant is inactivated, and widespread atelectasis results (Fig. 159.1). Elastases damage the structural framework of the lung (both alveolar–capillary and epithelial cell injury are seen), and a procoagulant environment likely leads to capillary thrombosis.

In some patients, the histopathologic changes of ALI resolve completely after the acute phase. In others, the disease progresses to a prolonged *fibroproliferative phase*, characterized by chronic fibrosing alveolitis, increased alveolar dead space, persistent hypoxemia, and, in some patients, pulmonary hypertension and right ventricular failure.

In the *recovery phase*, improvements in lung compliance and oxygenation are seen. Pulmonary function may return to normal, as may the appearance of the chest radiograph. Long-term recovery and prognosis after ALI vary.

Treatment

The ARDSnet trial, published in May 2000 in the *New England Journal of Medicine*, showed great benefits of low-tidal-volume ventilation to patients with ALI/ARDS. The trial was stopped early, after the enrollment of 861 patients, when an interim analysis showed significantly decreased mortality (31.0% vs.

39.8%, $P = 0.007$) in the low-tidal-volume group. This group also had significantly more ventilator-free days (days 1–28), a significantly better chance of being off the ventilator by day 28, and a significant reduction in nonpulmonary organ failure. The ARDSnet protocol assigned to patients in the intervention group a target tidal volume of 6 cc/kg of predicted body weight, to be reduced to as little as 4 cc/kg if inspiratory plateau pressures exceeded 30 cm H_2O. PEEP and FiO_2 were adjusted per the protocol (and Table 159.5), as was pressure support weaning.

Whereas the ARDSnet publication demonstrated the efficacy of low-tidal-volume ventilation in the management of patients with ALI/ARDS, many investigations have attempted to find the best levels of PEEP, acceptable hypercapnia, and so forth, in these critically ill patients.

Although high PEEP levels have been associated with deleterious effects, such as circulatory compromise and overdistension, PEEP may help with recruitment of some areas of atelectasis and improve oxygenation. Following the observation that the ARDSnet low-tidal-volume strategy resulted in intrinsic PEEP and higher PEEP$_{total}$ in patients in the study, the ARDSnet investigators pursued a comparison of a high- versus low-PEEP strategy in patients with ARDS. They found no

Table 159.5. ARDSnet protocol[a]

Variable	Group receiving traditional total volumes	Group receiving lower total volumes
Ventilator mode	Volume assist–control	Volume assist–control
Initial tidal volume (ml/kg of predicted body weight)[b]	12	6
Plateau pressure (cm of water)	< 50	< 30
Ventilator rate setting needed to achieve a pH goal of 7.3 to 7.45 (breaths/min)	6–35	6–35
Ratio of the duration of inspiration to the duration of expiration	1:1–1:3	1:1–1:3
Oxygenation goal	PaO_2, 55–80 mm Hg, or SpO_2, 88–95%	PaO_2 55–80 mm Hg, or SpO_2, 88–95%
Allowable combinations of FiO_2 and PEEP (cm of water)[c]	0.3 and 5	0.3 and 5
	0.4 and 5	0.4 and 5
	0.4 and 8	0.4 and 8
	0.5 and 8	0.5 and 8
	0.5 and 10	0.5 and 10
	0.6 and 10	0.6 and 10
	0.7 and 10	0.7 and 10
	0.7 and 12	0.7 and 12
	0.7 and 14	0.7 and 14
	0.8 and 14	0.8 and 14
	0.9 and 14	0.9 and 14
	0.9 and 16	0.9 and 16
	0.9 and 18	0.9 and 18
	1.0 and 18	1.0 and 18
	1.0 and 20	1.0 and 20
	1.0 and 22	1.0 and 22
	1.0 and 24	1.0 and 24
Weaning	By pressure support; required by protocol when FiO_2 < 0.4	By pressure support; required by protocol when FiO_2 < 0.4

[a] PaO_2 denotes partial pressure of arterial oxygen, SpO_2 oxyhemoglobin saturation measured by pulse oximetry, FiO_2 fraction of inspired oxygen, and PEEP positive end-expiratory pressure.
[b] Subsequent adjustments in tidal volume were made to maintain a plateau pressure of < 50 cm of water in the group receiving traditional tidal volumes and < 30 cm of water in the group receiving lower tidal volumes.
[c] Further increases in PEEP, to 34 cm of water, were allowed but were not required.
From The Acute Respiratory Distress Syndrome Network. Ventilation with lower tidal volumes as compared with traditional tidal volumes for acute lung injury and the acute respiratory distress syndrome. *N Engl J Med* 2000; 342:1301–1308.

difference in clinical outcome (breathing unassisted, death before hospital discharge) in patients assigned to a high- versus low-PEEP strategy, as long as plateau pressures remained ≤ 30 cm H_2O. The study was stopped early for futility, although some feel that this was a premature termination based on careful post-unblinding assessment of the patient groups in the study. Perhaps the most important information from this study was the reinforcement of a mortality benchmark of 25% to 30% in patients treated with low-tidal-volume ventilation, much lower than the expected mortality of approximately 40% in the pre-ARDSnet ICU.

Rouby and colleagues have urged that "a pragmatic, rather than a dogmatic approach" be used to select the "right" level of PEEP for each individual patient, balancing the clinician's assessment of the need for recruitment against the risk of over-inflation. They recommend considering three clinical elements: the lung morphology pattern (much better demonstrated by CT of the chest than by plain-film chest radiograph), the shape of the pressure–volume (P–V) curve, and the changes in gas exchange resulting from different PEEP levels. We find that this practical approach of "building a PEEP curve" for each individ-

ual patient helps to fine tune ventilator settings and guides the continual process of reassessment as the patient's disease progresses.

The use of esophageal balloon manometry to calculate transpulmonary pressure (as [airway pressure – pleural pressure]) also can be useful in guiding ventilator adjustment, as many of the most critically ill patients have markedly increased intra-abdominal pressures, diminished chest wall elastance, and so forth. Balloon measurements of pleural pressure can reassure the intensivist that, although total airway pressures may be high, the transpleural (and thus the transalveolar) pressure is not dangerously elevated. Esophageal balloon manometry thus may help to guide recruitment maneuvers and PEEP adjustment in patients with ALI/ARDS.

Further attempts at recruitment through the use of cyclic "sighs," prone positioning of patients, the use of chest weights or sandbags, high-frequency oscillatory ventilation (HFOV), airway pressure release ventilation (APRV), and biologically variable or "fractal" ventilation using low tidal volumes have variously been shown to improve oxygenation, and continue to attract research attention as potentially beneficial. None of these small studies, however, has shown improvement in mortality as has the ARDSnet protocol, which must still be considered the gold standard treatment in this patient population.

It is interesting that, while volume- and pressure-limited ventilation has been convincingly shown to reduce morbidity and mortality in patients with ALI/ARDS, the preemptive use of this ventilatory strategy in patients at high risk for lung injury has not been shown to be beneficial, and may actually increase morbidity.

Permissive hypercapnia (PHY) is the concept of allowing the partial pressure of carbon dioxide to exceed normal levels to maintain low-tidal-volume ventilation, even when patients develop moderate associated acidemia. Hypercapnia is not a therapeutic goal in itself – indeed, many patients will tolerate a high enough respiratory rate that they will not become hypercapneic, with tidal volumes limited to 6 ml/kg. With the large amount of dead-space ventilation and limited gas exchange common in ARDS, allowing the $PaCO_2$ to increase and the pH to decrease may be necessary to enable a lung-protective ventilatory strategy. As long as right heart failure does not develop, even sudden PHY and its associated transitory hyperdynamic cardiovascular state and pulmonary hypertension are well-tolerated, especially by younger patients.

Pharmacologic interventions
Steroids and ARDS

The use of steroids in ARDS remains controversial. In 2006, the ARDSnet investigators reported no mortality benefit from administration of methylprednisolone (2 mg/kg × 1, followed by 0.5 mg/kg every 6 hours for 14 days), although patients who received steroids had more ventilator-free and shock-free days during the first 28 days, improved oxygenation and respiratory system compliance, and more days free of vasopressor therapy. Patients who were started on steroids after 14 days of ARDS had higher mortality than those randomized to placebo. The authors concluded that the routine use of methylprednisolone for persistent ARDS was not supported by the results of the study.

In 2007, however, Meduri and colleagues reported the results of a multicenter, randomized, double-blind, placebo-controlled study of methylprednisolone infusion (1 mg/kg/d) in early severe ARDS which showed reductions in ventilation time, ICU stay, and ICU mortality. In an accompanying editorial, Djillali Annane argued that, despite the attributable risks of gastrointestinal (GI) bleeding, ICU myopathy, hyperglycemia, and so forth, the results of this and several other studies justify the routine use a of low-dose steroid infusion in patients with severe ARDS of < 2 weeks duration.

The use of exogenous surfactant in ARDS has not been shown to improve ventilator-free days or mortality, although, in a 2004 report in the *New England Journal of Medicine*, patients randomized to surfactant had greater improvements in gas exchange than did those receiving standard therapy. Similarly, exogenous nitric oxide therapy has not been shown to provide survival or other significant benefit in the management of ventilated patients with ARDS.

Fluid management and transfusion

A conservative fluid-management strategy is increasingly supported by evidence in ARDS as improving oxygenation and ventilator-free days, although no mortality benefit has yet been shown. Fluid resuscitation may of course be needed for the appropriate treatment of an underlying disease process, such as pancreatitis, sepsis, and so forth, but as soon as is practical, a conservative approach to fluid administration to minimize pulmonary edema and optimize oxygenation seems prudent. Guidance of resuscitation with a central venous line (CVL) alone is adequate; a trial of PAC use in ARDS has added to the overwhelming weight of evidence against PAC use, showing approximately twice as many catheter-related complications and no outcome benefit in the PAC group.

Transfusion of red blood cells and other blood products is well-recognized as a risk factor for the development of ALI/ARDS in critically ill patients, and the body of evidence demonstrating poor outcomes with aggressive transfusion practices continues to grow. Evidence-based conservative transfusion practices are certainly warranted, and blood products should never be used to "spare" crystalloid infusion in fluid-requiring patients with ALI/ARDS.

Outcomes

Several investigators are now looking at quality of life and outcomes in survivors of ARDS and have found significant physiologic, neurocognitive, and emotional deficits that persist for years after ICU discharge and result in decreased quality of life. Many patients show a significant loss of body mass (average 18% loss of baseline body weight), complain of persistent muscle weakness and fatigue, and, although they have normal lung volume and spirometric measurements by 6-month follow-up, DLco (diffusing capacity of lung for carbon monoxide) generally remains low a year after discharge, reflecting abnormal gas exchange capacity at the alveolar level. Patients usually do not require supplemental oxygen at follow-up, but may have significant desaturation with exercise to below 88%. Patients who did not receive corticosteroids, did not acquire additional illnesses during their hospital stay, and had rapid resolution of their multiorgan and pulmonary dysfunction have better functional status at 1-year follow-up.

A Canadian study has reported that 85% of patients who are discharged from the ICU survive to 2-year follow-up, and the initial hospital stay accounts for the majority of the costs associated with the disease. Although 65% of these patients had returned to work at 2-year follow-up, most continued to have exercise limitation, and although emotional and mental health improved in the 1- to 2-year postdischarge interval, all other quality-of-life measures remained below those of the general population and did not show statistically significant improvement from 1 to 2 years.

Future study

Although significant improvements in the management of ALI/ARDS and its underlying causes have been made in the past decade, mortality remains high at 30% to 50%. The National Heart, Lung, and Blood Institute Working Group, among others, is working to develop new approaches to the management of this heterogeneous disease process through a multimodal approach combining the use of biologic, genomic, and genetic approaches in animal and clinical studies, with the goal of improving detection and treatment of the disease syndrome.

Suggested readings

Acute Respiratory Distress Syndrome Network. Ventilation with lower tidal volumes as compared with traditional tidal volumes for acute lung injury and the acute respiratory distress syndrome. *N Engl J Med* 2000; 342:1301–1308.

Annane D. Glucocorticoids for ARDS: just do it! *Chest* 2007; 131:945–946.

Anzueto A, Baughman RP, Guntupalli KK, et al. Aerosolized surfactant in adults with sepsis-induced acute respiratory distress syndrome. *N Engl J Med* 1996; 334:1417–1421.

Bernard GR. Acute respiratory distress syndrome: a historical perspective. *Am J Respir Crit Care Med* 2005; 172:798–806.

Bernard GR, Artigas A, Brigham KL, et al. The American-European consensus conference on ARDS: definitions, mechanisms, relevant outcomes and clinical trial coordination. *Am J Respir Crit Care Med* 1994; 149:818–824.

Bersten AD, Edibam C, Hunt T, et al. Acute respiratory distress syndrome in three Australian states. *Am J Respir Crit Care Med* 2002; 165:443–448.

Boker A, Graham MR, Walley KR, et al. Improved arterial oxygenation with biologically variable or fractal ventilation using low tidal volumes in a porcine model of acute respiratory distress syndrome. *Am J Respir Crit Care Med* 2002; 165:456–462.

Carvalho CRR, Barbas CSV, Medeiros DM, et al. Temporal hemodynamic effects of permissive hypercapnia associated with ideal PEEP in ARDS. *Am J Respir Crit Care Med* 1997; 156:1458–1466.

Chan KPW, Stewart TE, Mehta S. High-frequency oscillatory ventilation for adult patients with ARDS. *Chest* 2007; 131:1907–1916.

Cheung AM, Tansey CM, Tomlinson G, et al. Two-year outcomes, health care use, and costs of survivors of acute respiratory distress syndrome. *Am J Respir Crit Care Med* 2006; 174:538–544.

de Durante G, del Turco M, Rustichini L, et al. *ARDSNet* lower tidal volume ventilatory strategy may generate intrinsic positive end-expiratory pressure in patients with acute respiratory distress syndrome. *Am J Respir Crit Care Med* 2002; 165:1271–1274.

Eisner MD, Thompson BT, Schoenfeld D, et al. Airway pressures and early barotrauma in patients with acute lung injury and acute respiratory distress syndrome. *Am J Respir Crit Care Med* 2002; 165:978–982.

Fan E, Needham DM, Stewart TE. Ventilatory management of acute lung injury and acute respiratory distress syndrome. *JAMA* 2005; 294:2889–2896.

Ferguson ND, Frutos-Vivar F, Esteban A, et al. Acute respiratory distress syndrome: underrecognition by clinicians and diagnostic accuracy of three clinical definitions. *Crit Care Med* 2005; 33:2228–2234.

Ferguson ND, Meade MO, Hallett DC, Stewart TE. High values of the pulmonary artery wedge pressure in patients with acute lung injury and acute respiratory distress syndrome. *Intensive Care Med* 2002; 28:1073–1077.

Gattinoni L, Chiumello D, Carlesso E, et al. Bench-to-bedside review: Chest wall elastance in acute lung injury/acute respiratory distress syndrome patients. *Crit Care* 2005; 8:350–355.

Gerlach H, Keh D, Semmerow A, et al. Dose-response characteristics during long-term inhalation of nitric oxide in patients with severe acute respiratory distress syndrome: a prospective, randomized, controlled study. *Am J Respir Crit Care Med* 2003; 167:1008–1015.

Girard TD, Bernard GR. Mechanical ventilation in ARDS: a state-of-the-art review. *Chest* 2007; 131:921–929.

Guerin C, Gaillard S, Lemasson S, et al. Effects of systematic prone positioning in hypoxemic acute respiratory failure – a randomized controlled trial. *JAMA* 2004; 292:2379–2387.

Hamacher J, Lucas R, Lijnen R, et al. Tumor necrosis factor-α and angiostatin are mediators of endothelial cytotoxicity in bronchoalveolar lavages of patients with acute respiratory distress syndrome. *Am J Respir Crit Care Med* 2002; 166:651–656.

Hebert PC, Wells G, Blajchman MA, et al. A multicenter, randomized, controlled clinical trial of transfusion requirements in critical care. *N Engl J Med* 1999; 340:409–417.

Herridge MS, Angus DC. Acute lung injury – affecting many lives. *N Engl J Med* 2005; 353:1736–1738.

Herridge MS, Cheung AM, Tansey CM, et al. One-year outcomes in survivors of the acute respiratory distress syndrome. *N Engl J Med* 2003; 348:683–693.

Hildebrand F, Pape HC, van Griensven M, et al. Genetic predisposition for a compromised immune system after multiple trauma. *Shock* 2005; 24(6):518–522.

Hopkins RO, Weaver LK, Collingridge D, et al. Two-year cognitive, emotional, and quality-of-life outcomes in acute respiratory distress syndrome. *Am J Respir Crit Care Med* 2005; 171:340–347.

Khan H, Belsher J, Yilmaz M, et al. Fresh-frozen plasma and platelet transfusions are associated with development of acute lung injury in critically ill medical patients. *Chest* 2007; 131:1308–1314.

Levy MM. PEEP in ARDS – how much is enough? *N Engl J Med* 2004; 351:389–391.

Matthay MA, Calfee CS. Therapeutic value of a lung protective ventilation strategy in acute lung injury. *Chest* 2005; 128:3089–3091.

Matthay, MA, Zimmerman GA, Esmon C, et al. Future research directions in acute lung injury: summary of a National Heart, Lung, and Blood Institute working group. *Am J Respir Crit Care Med* 2003; 17:1027–1035.

Meduri GU, Golden E, Freire AX. Methylprednisolone infusion in early severe ARDS: results of a randomized controlled trial. *Chest* 2007; 131:954–963.

Michael JR, Barton RG, Saffle JR, et al. Inhaled nitric oxide versus conventional therapy: effect on oxygenation in ARDS. *Am J Respir Crit Care Med* 1998; 157:1372–1380.

National Heart, Lung and Blood Institute ARDS Clinical Trials Network. Higher versus lower positive end-expiratory pressures in patients with the acute respiratory distress syndrome. *N Engl J Med* 2004; 351:327–336.

Netzer G, Shah CV, Iwashyna TJ, et al. Association of RBC transfusion with mortality in patients with acute lung injury. *Chest* 2007; 132:1116–1123.

Pelosi P, Bottino N, Chiumello D, et al. Sighs in supine and prone position during acute respiratory distress syndrome. *Am J Respir Crit Care Med* 2003; 167:521–527.

Perren A. High versus low PEEP in ARDS. *N Engl J Med* 2004; 351:2128.

Rice TR, Wheeler AP, Bernard GR, et al. Comparison of the SpO$_2$/FiO$_2$ ratio and the PaO$_2$/FiO$_2$ ratio in patients with acute lung injury or ARDS. *Chest* 2007; 132:410–417.

Rouby JJ, Lu Q, Goldstein I. Selecting the right level of positive end-expiratory pressure in patients with acute respiratory distress syndrome. *Am J Respir Crit Care Med* 2002; 165:1182–1186.

Rubenfeld GD, Caldwell E, Peabody E, et al. Incidence and outcomes of acute lung injury. *N Engl J Med* 2005; 353:1685–1693.

Rubenfeld GD, Herridge MS. Epidemiology and outcomes of acute lung injury. *Chest* 2007; 131:554–562.

Spragg RG, Lewis JF, Walmrath HD, et al. Effect of recombinant surfactant protein C-based surfactant on the acute respiratory distress syndrome. *N Engl J Med* 2004; 351:884–892.

Steinberg KP, Hudson LD, Goodman RB, et al. Efficacy and safety of corticosteroids for persistent acute respiratory distress syndrome. *N Engl J Med* 2006; 354:1671–1684.

Stewart TE, Meade MO, Cook DJ, et al. Evaluation of a ventilation strategy to prevent barotrauma in patients at high risk for acute respiratory distress syndrome. *N Engl J Med* 1998; 338:355–361.

Taylor RW, Zimmerman JL, Dellinger RP, et al. Low-dose inhaled nitric oxide in patients with acute lung injury: a randomized controlled trial. *JAMA* 2004; 291:1603–1609.

The acute respiratory distress syndrome network. Ventilation with lower tidal volumes as compared with traditional tidal volumes for acute lung injury and the acute respiratory distress syndrome. *N Engl J Med* 2000; 342:1301–1308.

The National Heart, Lung and Blood Institute ARDS Clinical Trials Network. Higher versus lower positive end-expiratory pressures in patients with the acute respiratory distress syndrome. *N Engl J Med* 2004; 351:327–336.

Ware LB, Matthay MA. The acute respiratory distress syndrome. *N Engl J Med* 2000; 342(18):1334–1349.

Wheeler AP, Bernard GR. Acute lung injury and the acute respiratory distress syndrome: a clinical review. *Lancet* 2007; 369:1553–1565.

Wheeler AP, Bernard GR, Thompson BT, et al. Pulmonary-artery versus central venous catheter to guide treatment of acute lung injury. *N Engl J Med* 2006; 354:2213–2224.

Wiedemann HP, Wheeler AP, Bernard GR, et al. Comparison of two fluid-management strategies in acute lung injury. *N Engl J Med* 2006; 354:2564–2575.

Chapter 160

Nosocomial infections

David Oxman, Shannon S. McKenna, and Gyorgy Frendl

Health care–associated (hereto referred to as *nosocomial*) infections are considered to be infections acquired in acute or chronic health care settings (in hospitals and rehabilitation or chronic care facilities). They are an increasing problem and constitute a major source of morbidity and mortality. In addition, these infections significantly increase the cost and duration of hospital care. Ventilator-associated pneumonia (VAP) and catheter-related bloodstream infections (CRBSI) represent two of the most serious nosocomial infections and will be the focus of this chapter. Both of these infections can easily progress to sepsis and death. Other nosocomial infections, such as urinary tract and wound infections, are typically more easily treatable and less likely to increase patient mortality, and therefore are not discussed here.

A common feature of all these nosocomial infections is that they are preventable, and the most successful strategy for fighting them is prevention. It is essential for the anesthesiologist to be comfortable managing patients who develop these complications and to be aware of proven methods for preventing their occurrence.

Ventilator-associated pneumonia
Incidence, morbidity and, mortality

VAP is one of the most commonly occurring intensive care unit (ICU) infections. Anywhere from 5% to 20% – depending on definitions used – of mechanically ventilated patients develop VAP. Compared to patients with similar initial degrees of illness, patients who acquire VAP stay in the hospital longer, stay on the ventilator more days, and die at a higher rate. Additionally, the costs associated with VAP are significant, with estimated excess hospital costs of at least $40,000 per case.

Pathogenesis

The prolonged presence of an endotracheal tube (greater than 48 hours) is the major contributor to the pathogenesis of VAP. Although other factors contribute to the risk, the endotracheal tube and the alterations in host-defense mechanisms it engenders, as well as the reservoir for pathogenic organisms it creates, are the major causative factors in the development of VAP.

The first protection of the lower respiratory tract against aspiration and microbial colonization are mechanical defenses, including cough reflexes and mucociliary clearance. The presence of an endotracheal tube impairs both of these mechanisms. It also creates a direct conduit by which bacteria from the upper airway and oropharynx can access the lungs. Aspiration of oropharyngeal secretions is the major route by which bacteria gain access to the lower respiratory tract. Although aspiration of gastric contents with bacterial overgrowth plays some role in the acquisition of VAP, it is probably less important. Bacteria can also enter the lungs via other routes: (1) direct extension of a contiguous infection, (2) hematogenous spread from distant sites, and (3) inhalation of contaminated aerosols. The most common route by which organisms enter the lungs is aspiration. The typical organisms causing VAP are listed in Table 160.1.

Clinical manifestations

Signs and symptoms of VAP can be obvious or subtle. Systemic signs such as fever or leukocytosis should, when present in the mechanically ventilated patient, always lead to the consideration of VAP. An increase in the amount of secretions suctioned from the endotracheal tube may also be an early sign of VAP. Changes in a patient's respiratory parameters, such as a decreasing partial pressure of arterial oxygen (PaO_2) as measured by arterial blood gas, or the need to increase the fraction of inspired oxygen content (FiO_2) or positive end-expiratory pressure (PEEP) to maintain normal oxygen saturation, may be the first indication of VAP and should prompt further investigation.

Although chest radiography is often helpful, it is unreliable for ruling in or ruling out the diagnosis of VAP by itself. Other common conditions in mechanically ventilated patients, such as ARDS, atelectasis, or lung contusion, may mimic or obscure VAP (Table 160.2). If the clinical suspicion is high and chest radiograph is inconclusive, CT of the chest may be helpful. A new infiltrate on chest radiograph, however, when

Table 160.1. Typical organisms causing VAP

P. aeruginosa
Klebsiella species
Enterobacter
Acinetobacter species
Burkholderia cepacia
S. aureus (including MRSA)

Table 160.2. Causes other than pneumonia leading to abnormal chest radiograph in mechanically ventilated patients

Pulmonary edema
ARDS
Atelectasis
Pulmonary hemorrhage
Pulmonary contusion
Pulmonary infarct

coupled with other findings (e.g., fever and/or an increase in sputum production or a change in a patient's respiratory status) are together highly suggestive of VAP.

Microbiology of VAP

With critical illness, the microbiologic flora of the oropharynx changes dramatically. In healthy people the oropharynx is overwhelmingly colonized with streptococci and anaerobes. The mouth flora of a critically ill patient becomes colonized with Gram-negative bacteria and *Staphylococcus aureus*. Predictably, Gram-negative organisms and *S. aureus* are the most common pathogens responsible for VAP (Table 160.1). Drug-resistant organisms, such as *Pseudomonas aeruginosa* and methicillin-resistant *S. aureus* (MRSA), pose added danger to critically ill patients. Anaerobic bacteria, *Legionella*, and viruses, such as herpes simplex virus, can cause VAP as well but are much more uncommon.

Diagnosis

Unfortunately, there is no gold standard diagnostic test for VAP, and diagnosis can be challenging. Clinical characteristics, such as fever, sputum production, increased oxygen requirements, and a new infiltrate seen on chest radiograph, are suggestive of VAP, but they are not specific (Table 160.3). Sampling of the lower respiratory tract for pathogenic organisms increases diagnostic accuracy. Several methods exist for obtaining a microbiological specimen – including tracheal aspiration, nonbronchoscopic "min-BALs," and fiber-optic bronchoscopy with bronchoalveolar lavage or a protected brush sampling. Which method is the most accurate and cost-effective is an area of some controversy. Whenever VAP is suspected, however, some type of lower respiratory specimen should be sent for Gram stain and culture.

The Clinical Pulmonary Infection Score (CPIS; Table 160.4) is a prediction tool designed to help make the diagnosis of VAP based on clinical variables. It incorporates variables such as the presence or absence of fever, purulent sputum, or leukocytosis, as well as the degree of hypoxemia, character of radiographic abnormalities, and microbiologic findings. A score of > 6 is typically used to diagnose VAP. Although the CPIS may be helpful in clinical decision making, its positive predictive value is modest – approximately 60% – and should not be overly relied on.

Treatment

Treatment for VAP should begin as soon as VAP is suspected and not be delayed for definitive diagnostic testing, as delays in

Table 160.3. Centers for Disease Control and Prevention surveillance definition for clinical diagnosis of hospital-acquired pneumonia

Radiologic signs
Two or more serial chest radiographs with at least one of the following[a]:
- New or progressive *and* persistent infiltrate
- Consolidation
- Cavitation

Clinical signs
At least one of the following:
- Fever (temperature >38°C) with no other recognized cause
- Leukopenia (leukocyte count <4.0 × 10^9 cells/L) or leukocytosis (leukocyte count >12.0 × 10^9 cells/L)
- For adults ≥70 y, altered mental status with no other recognized cause

And at least two of the following:
- New onset of purulent sputum, change in character of sputum, increased respiratory secretions, or increased suctioning requirements
- New onset or worsening cough, dyspnea, tachypnea
- Rales or bronchial breath sounds
- Worsening gas exchange (e.g., O$_2$ desaturations [e.g., PaO$_2$/FiO$_2$ ≤240], increased oxygen requirements, or increased ventilation demand

[a] In patients without underlying pulmonary or cardiac disease (e.g., respiratory distress syndrome, bronchopulmonary dysplasia, pulmonary edema, or chronic obstructive pulmonary disease), one definitive chest radiograph is acceptable.

Table 160.4. CPIS scoring

Temperature
≥36.5 and ≤38.4 = 0 points
≥38.5 and ≤38.9 = 1 point
≥39 or <36.5 = 2 points

Blood leukocytes, micro/L
≥4000 and ≤11,000 = 0 points
<4000 or >11,000 = 1 point
Band forms ≥50% = add 1 point

Tracheal secretions
Absence of tracheal secretions = 0 point
Presence of nonpurulent tracheal secretions = 1 point
Presence of purulent tracheal secretions = 2 points

Oxygenation
PaO$_2$/FiO$_2$, mm Hg >240 or ARDS (defined as PaO$_2$/FiO$_2$ ≤200, PAWP ≤18 mm Hg and acute bilateral infiltrates) = 0 points
PaO$_2$/FiO$_2$ ≤240 and no ARDS = 2 points

Pulmonary radiography
No infiltrate = 0 points
Diffuse (patchy) infiltrate = 1 point
Localized infiltrate = 2 points

Progression of pulmonary infiltrate
No radiographic progression = 0 points
Radiographic progression (after HF and ARDS excluded) = 2 points

Culture of tracheal aspirate
Pathogenic bacteria cultured in rare or few quantities or no growth = 0 points
Pathogenic bacteria cultured in moderate or heavy quantity = 1 point
Same pathogenic bacteria seen on Gram stain, add 1 point
Total score of >6 suggestive of VAP

PAWP, pulmonary arterial wedge pressure; HF, heart failure. From Pugin J, Auckenthaler R, Mili N, Janssens JP, Lew PD, Suter PM. Diagnosis of ventilator-associated pneumonia by bacteriologic analysis of bronchoscopic and non-bronchoscopic "blind" bronchoalveolar lavage fluid. *Am Rev Respir Dis* 1991;143:1121–112.

Table 160.5. Initial empiric therapy for treatment of VAP

Gram negative coverage			MRSA coverage
Antipseudomonal cephalosporin (cefepime, ceftazidime)	+	Antipseudomonal fluoroquinolone (ciprofloxacin or levofloxacin}	Vancomycin
or Antipseudomonal carbapenem (imipenem or meropenem)	+	**or** Aminoglycoside (amikacin, gentamicin, or tobramycin)	+	**or** Linezolid
or -Lactam/-lactamase inhibitor (piperacillin-tazobactam)			

Adapted from American Thoracic Society/Infectious Diseases Society of America (ATS/IDSA) guidelines, 2005.

Table 160.6. Strategies to prevent VAP

Hand washing before physical examination
Head-of-bed elevation >30°
Limit sedation and perform "daily wake-ups"
Perform daily spontaneous breathing trials
Oropharyngeal decontamination (conflicting evidence)
Continuous subglottic suctioning (some evidence)
Silver-coated endotracheal tubes (some evidence)

treatment lead to poorer outcomes. Initial antibiotic therapy should be broad and directed at the typical nosocomial organisms causing pneumonia in the ICU. VAP is most often caused by Gram-negative bacteria, such as *P. aeruginosa* – but Gram-positive bacteria, particularly *S. aureus*, are increasingly common pathogens. Given the high rates of antibiotic resistance in VAP, combination therapy is almost always indicated initially, and it should include two different classes of antibiotics directed to Gram-negative bacteria and an agent active against MRSA (Table 160.5). After microbiological data become available, antibiotic therapy should be tailored to the specific pathogen and combination therapy can be stopped. Furthermore, in patients who turn out to have an alternative diagnosis and who do not have VAP, antibiotics should be stopped as soon as possible. Exposure to unnecessary antibiotics leads to colonization with drug-resistant organisms in the patient and the entire ICU, and makes future episodes of VAP much more difficult to treat. Adjunctive measures such as lung-protective, low-tidal-volume ventilation strategies may be helpful in patients developing decreased lung compliance from their infection (for details, see Chapter 159).

Prevention

The best way to prevent VAP is to avoid intubation or, if that is not possible, minimize the duration of mechanical ventilation. Therefore, in patients who meet criteria, noninvasive positive pressure ventilation should always be considered. In patients who must be endotracheally intubated, moving toward extubation as soon as the patient is ready prevents many episodes of VAP. Limiting sedation and performing daily spontaneous breathing trials help to identify those patients early who are capable of being liberated from mechanical ventilation.

Several additional simple and inexpensive measures have been proven to reduce rates of VAP. They include maintaining head-of-bed elevation (above 30°) in mechanically ventilated patients, hand washing before physical examination, and limiting respiratory circuit tubing changes. Other measures,

such as continual oral decontamination, continual subglottic suctioning, and the use of silver-coated endotracheal tubes, are promising but not yet definitively proven (Table 160.6).

Catheter-related bloodstream infections
Incidence, morbidity, and mortality

CRBSIs are among the most common hospital-acquired infections. Each year up to 250,000 patients in the United States develop nosocomial bloodstream infections, the majority of which are catheter-related, with an attributable mortality anywhere from 12% to 25%. Understanding the pathogenesis, clinical presentation, and management of CRBSI is vital for the anesthesiologist taking care of patients at risk for CRBSI. Additionally, anesthesiologists should be aware of the state-of-the-art practice for preventing these infections from occurring.

Pathogenesis

Microorganisms causing CRBSI enter the bloodstream via one of four mechanisms. The first is through colonization of the skin at the catheter entry site. Microorganisms can then enter the bloodstream via migration along the catheter itself. The second route of infection is via contamination of the catheter hub or stopcock. These two mechanisms account for the vast majority of all catheter-related bloodstream infections. Seeding of the catheter through the blood from an infection at a distant site, and contamination of intravenous infusates are the two other means by which CRBSI occur, but are much less common. Short-term, noncuffed central venous catheters have the highest rates of infection but arterial catheters and peripherally inserted central venous catheters (PICC lines) can also cause infection at high rates.

Clinical manifestations

The clinical manifestations of CRBSI are generally indistinguishable from bloodstream infections originating from any other source. Fever, rigors, hypotension, or other early signs of sepsis (such as tachycardia or tachypnea) often occur. Catheter entry sites and tunneled catheter tracts should be examined, as infrequently there may be signs such as erythema, local tenderness, or purulent drainage.

Microbiology of CRBSI

S. aureus and coagulase-negative *Staphylococcus* (such as *S. epidermidis*) are the most common organisms responsible for

CRBSI. *Enterococci* and *Candida* species are the next most common with assorted Gram-negative bacteria responsible for most of the remaining infections.

Diagnosis

Blood culture is the definitive diagnostic test for CRBSI. In the patient with an intravascular catheter, if two sets of blood cultures drawn from two separate venopuncture sites are positive, it is highly suggestive of a CRBSI. An additional set drawn from the intravascular catheter may also be helpful in pinpointing the intravascular catheter as the source of the bacteremia. As the lumens of intravascular catheters are frequently colonized with bacteria, sending blood cultures drawn through the catheter alone will lead to a high false-positive rate and the removal of many catheters that are not infected. Differences in the speed at which blood cultures obtained peripherally and those obtained through the intravascular catheter turn positive may help to distinguish between a line-related and a non–line-related bacteremia. Semiquantitative cultures of the tip of the central line, using either the roll plate method or sonication, may help to further define the etiology of a bacteremia. Line tip culture, however, requires removal of the suspected line before a CRBSI is proven. It is important to note that the roll plate method, which is the most commonly used culture technique, examines the outside of the line only and will not identify infections originating from the internal lumen of the line.

Treatment

As CRBSI carries a high rate of morbidity and mortality, treatment should not be delayed until blood cultures become positive. In patients with an intravascular catheter displaying typical signs and symptoms of CRBSI, empiric antibiotics directed at typical pathogens should be started immediately, and, if possible, the catheter should be removed. As Gram-positive organisms, including MRSA, cause the majority of infections, vancomycin is the typical first-line agent. In the immunocompromised or septic patient, empiric treatment should be broadened to cover typical nosocomial Gram-negative organisms. Fungal CRBSI, although increasing in incidence, is still relatively uncommon, and empiric antifungal coverage should be reserved for high-risk patients. After the causative organism is identified, antibiotic therapy should be tailored accordingly and the line should be removed if it has not been already. Exchange of an infected catheter over a guidewire is not effective for managing CRBSI and should be discouraged.

Prevention

Fortunately, CRBSIs are preventable, and recent studies have shown that with careful attention to prevention techniques, rates of CRBSI can be reduced to near zero. When placing intravascular catheters, maximum barrier precautions – including sterile gloves, surgical mask and gown, and a large sterile drape – should be used. Cleansing of the patient's skin with chlorhexidine has been shown to be superior to povidine–iodine. Use of a real-time standardized checklist has been shown to be an effective method of ensuring that appropriate sterile technique is used with each and every line insertion. Standardized sterile technique with maximum barrier precautions should be used for all line insertions, including line insertions in the operating room, emergency department, and ICU. Any central line placed without observance of standard sterile technique should be appropriately identified as such and needs to be removed within 48 hours of placement.

Proper hand hygiene, using either antiseptic soap and water or an alcohol-based hand sanitizer, is essential prior to both line insertion and the handling of catheter hubs and stopcocks and is the backbone of infection prevention. Additionally, access ports must be cleaned with an antiseptic, such as an alcohol swab, immediately prior to use, and only sterile access devices may be used.

Whenever possible, the femoral insertion site should be avoided as this site is associated with higher infection rates. Similarly, several studies have shown that the subclavian approach is associated with a slightly lower risk of infection than is internal jugular catheterization. Although it is true that the longer an intravascular catheter stays in place the higher the risk of bloodstream infection, there is no evidence to support the routine replacement of catheters after an arbitrary duration of time. Any indwelling catheter that is no longer essential for patient care, however, should be removed immediately. When a CRBSI is suspected, or confirmed, the associated line must be removed. If central access is still required, a new line must be inserted at a new site. Ideally, the patient will be given a period of time with antibiotic treatment before the new central venous catheter is inserted to diminish the risk of seeding the new line.

Suggested readings

Barcaulr N, Boulain T. Mortality rate attributable to ventilator-associated nosocomial pneumonia in an adult-intensive care unit: a prospective case-control study. *Crit Care Med* 2001; 29(12):2303–2309.

Chastre J, Fagon J. Ventilator-associated pneumonia. *Am J Respir Crit Care Med* 2002; 165:867–903.

Fartoukh M, Maitre B, Honore S, et al. Diagnosing pneumonia during mechanical ventilation: the clinical pulmonary infection score revisited. *Am J Respir Crit Care Med* 2003; 168(2):173–179.

Guidelines for the management of adults with hospital-acquired, ventilator-associated, and healthcare-associated pneumonia. *Am J Respir Crit Care Med* 2005; 171:388.

Lorente L, Henry C, Martín MM, et al. Central venous catheter-related infection in a prospective and observation study of 2,595 catheters. *Crit Care Med* 2005; 9(6):R631–R635.

Maki DG, Kluger DM, Crnich CJ. The risk of bloodstream infection in adults with different intravascular devices: a systematic review of 200 published prospective studies. *Mayo Clin Proc* 2006; 81(9):1159–1171.

O'Grady NP, Gerberding JL, Weinstein RA, Masur H. Patient safety and the science of prevention: the time for implementing the guidelines for the prevention of intravascular catheter-related infections is now. *Crit Care Med* 2003; 31(1):291–292.

Pittet D, Li N, Woolson RF, Wenzel RP. Microbiological factors influencing the outcome of nosocomial bloodstream infections: a 6-year validated, population-based model. *Clin Infect Dis* 1997; 24(6):1068–1078.

Pronovost P, Needham D, Berenholtz S, et al. An intervention to decrease catheter-related bloodstream infections in the ICU (erratum appears in *N Engl J Med* 2007: 356:2660). *N Engl J Med* 2006; 355:2725–2732.

Safdar N, Dezfulian C, Collard H, Saint S. Clinical and economic consequences of ventilator-associated pneumonia. *Crit Care Med* 2005; 33(10):2184–2193.

Seifert H, Cornely O, Seggewiss K, et al. Bloodstream infection in neutropenic cancer patients related to short-term non-tunneled catheters determined by quantitative blood cultures, differential time to positivity and molecular epidemiological typing with pulsed-gel electrophoresis. *J Clin Microbiol* 2003; 41: 118–123.

Septic shock and sepsis syndromes

Maxwell Weinmann

Introduction

Sepsis and septic shock are causes of substantial morbidity and mortality. Of the 1 million patients diagnosed annually in the United States with septic shock, mortality is approximately 50%, but may increase to as high as 80% in the setting of complicating organ failure. As such, early diagnosis and timely intervention are critical if outcome is to be favorably altered.

Pathogenesis

Pathophysiologically, irrespective of the offending organism, sepsis is a systemic disease with significant involvement of the endothelium. Intravascular recognition of bacterial antigens initiates both inflammatory and procoagulant responses that are intimately associated. Subendothelial injury generates thrombin, which fuels an accelerating and potentially systemic proinflammatory and procoagulant state. Microvascular thrombosis and ischemia ensue with systemic progression of diffuse endovascular inflammation and injury, and, ultimately, vascular autoregulatory collapse. Microvascular thrombosis produces disordered perfusion and oxygen delivery at a time of increased oxygen demand. Unabated, this cycle is self-perpetuating and may culminate in irreversible ischemic organ failure and death. Despite apparent early global stability, the body attempts to shunt blood from nonessential vascular beds to vital organs; a phenomenon known as *compensated shock*. After organ reserve is depleted, systemic failure becomes clinically evident. If therapy is to be successful and either reverse or mitigate the ensuing organ injury and collapse, intervention must be both timely and comprehensive.

Spectrum of disease and definitions

Sepsis presents a spectrum of clinicopathologic phenomena, so a number of clinical definitions have emerged in an attempt to both better understand the phenomena and develop therapeutic strategies. These definitions include the following:

1. Systemic inflammatory response syndrome (SIRS): requires at least two of the following:

    Temperature >38°C or <36°C
    Heart rate >90 bpm
    Respiration >20/min or PCO$_2$ >32 mm Hg

    White cell count >12,000/mm^3
    10% immature neutrophils

2. Sepsis: requires SIRS with a presumed or confirmed septic focus

3. Severe sepsis: requires sepsis with >1 sign of organ dysfunction in the presence of hypotension. Examples include:

Pulmonary	Hypoxia (PaO$_2$/FiO$_2$ <300), tachypnea
Renal	Oliguria (urine output <0.5 ml/kg/h)
	Creatinine increase <0.5 mg/dl
Hematologic	Coagulopathy (international normalized ratio [INR] <1.5, partial thromboplastin time [PTT] >60 s)
	Thrombocytopenia (platelets <100,000/μl)
Hepatic	Elevation in transaminases and bilirubin
Neurologic	Confusion/delirium
Metabolic	Hyperglycemia, lactic acidosis
Cardiac	Tachycardia

As organ systems fail, the potential for reversibility diminishes, and mortality rises. The progressively increasing risk of mortality emphasizes the importance for timely diagnosis and intervention as shown in Fig. 161.1.

4. Septic shock: defined as persistent hypotension, despite adequate fluid resuscitation, which is not explained by other causes. Hypotension is defined as a systolic blood

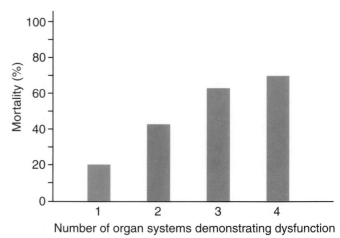

Figure 161.1. Organ system failure and mortality. (*Source:* Angus DC, Linde-Zwirble WT, Lidicker J, et al. Epidemiology of severe sepsis in the United States: analysis of incidence, outcome and associated costs of care. Adapted, with permission, from *Crit Care Med* 2001; 29:1303–1310.)

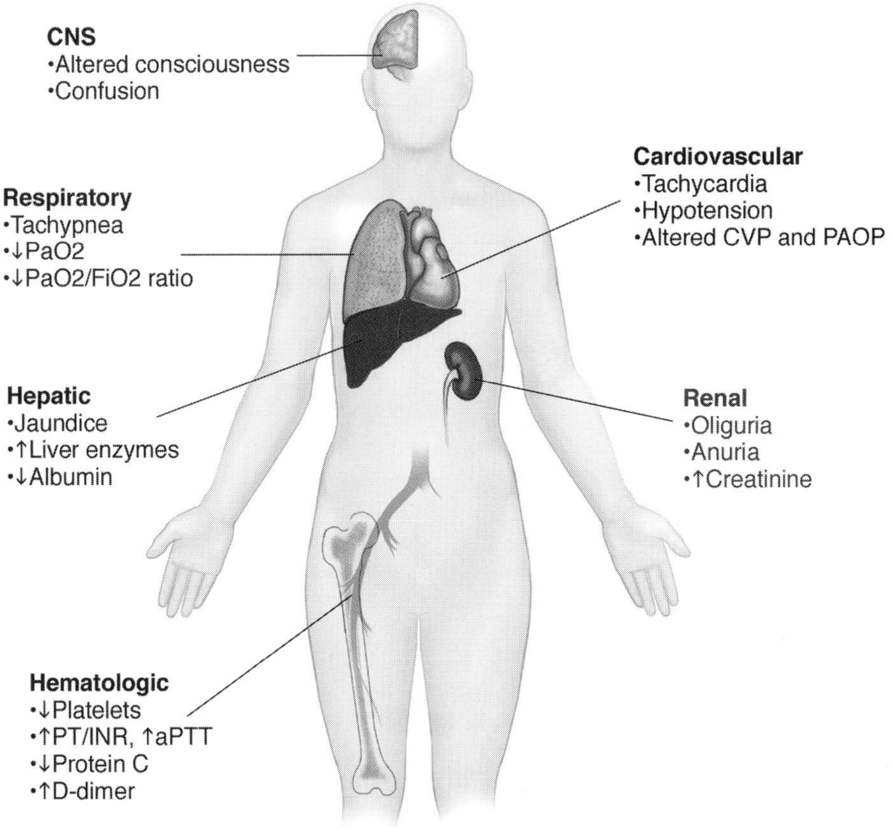

Figure 161.2. Clinical markers of sepsis.

CNS
•Altered consciousness
•Confusion

Respiratory
•Tachypnea
•↓PaO2
•↓PaO2/FiO2 ratio

Hepatic
•Jaundice
•↑Liver enzymes
•↓Albumin

Hematologic
•↓Platelets
•↑PT/INR, ↑aPTT
•↓Protein C
•↑D-dimer

Cardiovascular
•Tachycardia
•Hypotension
•Altered CVP and PAOP

Renal
•Oliguria
•Anuria
•↑Creatinine

pressure (BP) of <90 mm Hg and a mean arterial pressure (MAP) of <60 mm Hg, or a reduction in systolic BP of >40 mm Hg from baseline (Fig. 161.2).

Therapy

The following recommendations emerge largely from the Surviving Sepsis Campaign (SSC), an international effort to decrease the mortality of sepsis consisting of 11 international societies. Recommendations were classified according to literature support or expert opinion.

Fluid resuscitation

The presence of hypotension signals that septic pathophysiology is already well established. If accompanied by systemic lactic acidosis, anaerobic metabolism has commenced (at least in some organ beds) and resuscitation is urgent.

The SSC recommends that resuscitation goals within the first 6 hours include

• Central venous pressure (CVP) 8 to 12 mm Hg,
• MAP >65 mm Hg,
• Urine output >0.5 ml/kg/h,
• Central venous or mixed venous O$_2$ saturation >70%, and
• Consideration of a blood transfusion if venous saturation is unresponsive to fluids alone, despite a CVP of 8 to 12 mm Hg.

However, the clinician must place this information into clinical perspective. Conditions that influence the pressure–volume relationship of the heart will necessitate review of these values. For example, a patient with chronic obstructive pulmonary disease (COPD) and pulmonary hypertension may require a CVP of 14 to 16 mm Hg to achieve the same degree of filling compared to a previously healthy person. Similarly, a venous saturation of >70% may still be a cause of concern in a patient with an increasing lactate, suggesting that shunting or disordered oxygen uptake is persisting despite intervention, requiring a modification of therapeutic strategy.

Additionally, the long-standing controversy over the superiority of either colloid or crystalloid as a resuscitation strategy continues. The Saline versus Albumin Fluid Evaluation Study (SAFE Study) was a prospective analysis of approximately 7000 patients, each patient being randomized to either normal saline or 4% albumin. Results demonstrated that there was no significant difference in mortality, hospital stay, duration of mechanical ventilatory support, incidence of organ failure, or need for continuous renal support between the two therapies. Subgroup analysis suggested a trend toward reduced mortality in patients receiving albumin with severe sepsis but increased mortality when administered with severe head trauma. Whether these effects are through immune modulation, altered microcirculatory performance, and oxygen delivery, both globally and on a microcirculatory level, is yet to be determined (Fig. 161.3).

997

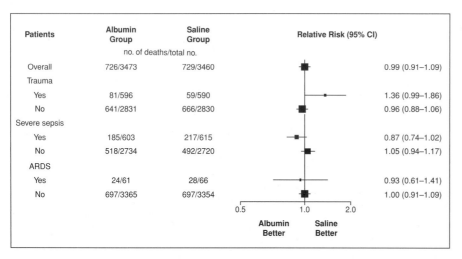

Patients	Albumin Group	Saline Group	Relative Risk (95% CI)	
	no. of deaths/total no.			
Overall	726/3473	729/3460		0.99 (0.91–1.09)
Trauma				
Yes	81/596	59/590		1.36 (0.99–1.86)
No	641/2831	666/2830		0.96 (0.88–1.06)
Severe sepsis				
Yes	185/603	217/615		0.87 (0.74–1.02)
No	518/2734	492/2720		1.05 (0.94–1.17)
ARDS				
Yes	24/61	28/66		0.93 (0.61–1.41)
No	697/3365	697/3354		1.00 (0.91–1.09)

Figure 161.3. Relative mortality risk of administering albumin versus saline during resuscitation. (*Source:* The SAFE Study Investigators. A comparison of albumin and saline for fluid resuscitation in the intensive care unit. *N Engl J Med* 2004; 350(22):2247–2256.)

Diagnosis and source control

Diagnostic procedures should proceed contemporaneously with resuscitation. Two or more blood cultures (preferably drawn from peripheral blood via venipuncture) are advised. Additional blood cultures from the lumen of each intravascular device may be desirable. Other sites should also be cultured, including sputum, urine, and cerebrospinal fluid (CSF), if clinically warranted. Imaging studies should be pursued based on clinical indication, such as recent surgery, premorbid conditions, and preexisting intravascular devices, in order to determine if a distinct focus of infection exists. If so, a determination of the viability of drainage, removal, exploration, and debridement follows. The successful treatment of sepsis hinges on effective source control.

Antibiotic therapy

Antibiotic therapy is considered part of the resuscitative effort and must be instituted as a matter of urgency, ideally within the first hour of arrival. Empiric therapy is therefore often unavoidable. The choice of antibiotics is a function of the clinical scenario encountered: the patient's immunocompetence, clinical history (including recent antibiotic therapy), and susceptibility patterns in the patient's community and hospital of admission.

Typically, broad-spectrum coverage is initiated and tailored to more specific regimens after susceptibilities are determined. This practice helps prevent not only resistance but also superinfection by resistant organisms.

As only 5% of cases of severe sepsis or septic shock have been shown to be due to fungal infection, it is not warranted to commence empiric anti fungal therapy, except when the likelihood of fungal infection is exceedingly high (patient on TPN, immunocompromised patient, and when fungal cultures are positive from multiple sites or fungus is seen on Gram stain of blood).

Vasopressor and inotropic therapy

The mortality of sepsis can be significantly reduced using the early fluid resuscitation strategy (Rivers et al.) combined with the judicious use of inotropic agent (dobutamine) and vasopressors.

If hypotension persists despite fluid resuscitation and adequate circulatory filling as determined by the CVP, vasopressors should be commenced. An ideal vasopressor has yet to emerge, as all have potential side effects, namely exacerbation of ischemia, arrhythmias, etc. Reestablishment of perfusion pressure is vital if organ failure is to be prevented or reversed. The clinician must therefore titrate the dose to effect, while being watchful for any untoward complications. The need to titrate to effect is largely due to the profound alteration of dose–response relationships in severe sepsis.

The drug of first choice is a function of the clinical scenario and the clinician's assessment of the patient's potential to respond (i.e., the patient's clinical reserve). For example, in the setting of associated coronary vascular disease, the physician may be wary of epinephrine's potential for tachycardia and choose phenylephrine. Irrespective of which agent is ultimately selected, restoration of perfusion pressure is the resuscitative goal as long as the intensivist is watchful for the "physiologic cost" of therapy. For example, if the addition of vasopressors produces a decline in venous saturation and raises concerns regarding oxygen dynamics, observation of the lactate response will be a clue to the potential cost of intervention. Elevation of lactate would suggest iatrogenic worsening, requiring a new strategy, whereas a decline in lactate would suggest that the degree of shunting has been reduced. Clinical perspective is the key because, at present, the technology to actually evaluate the microcirculation remains largely in the realm of research.

Vasopressor strategies and ongoing controversies

While no vasopressor agent has been shown to be clearly superior for the management of septic shock, norepinephrine and epinephrine have moderate advantages over the use of dopamine. Phenylephrine appears to have no role (other than a temporizing agent) in the management of septic shock. Studies have shown a moderate benefit of the use of vasopressin (in the 0.04-0.08 U/min range) for the management of early (less severe) septic shock.

Conventional clinical dogma dictates stabilization of systemic BP in resuscitation of the critically ill septic patient. However, despite the efforts to stabilize systolic BP, mortality remains high and prognosis poor. Evaluation of the circulatory response to sepsis has strongly supported that sepsis is primarily a disease of the microcirculation and the endothelium in particular, where endothelial integrity and function are predictive of both organ function and patient survival. Consequently, systemic parameters cannot be considered a reliable reflection of events in key vascular beds.

Traditionally, lactate levels have been the conventional indirect measure of the onset of anaerobic metabolism and organ stress in the intensive care unit (ICU). Sole reliance on lactate, however, is inadequate as a marker of tissue hypoxia, as a critical fraction of tissue must be rendered ischemic before serum lactate levels increase. The absence of lactic acidosis therefore does not exclude the presence of tissue ischemia. Conversely, the presence of lactate does not always confirm ischemia. Lactate elevation is due to biochemical derangements accompanying both sepsis (such as disordered pyruvate dehydrogenase activity) and treatment (such as occurs with the induction of aerobic glycolysis by vasopressor therapy). Thus serum lactate levels may be artificially elevated in the absence of hypoxia. Additionally, lactate levels may continue to increase despite aggressive resuscitation due to a washout effect with the restoration of perfusion. Lactate must therefore be considered a rather late and insensitive marker of ischemia that does not adequately reflect regional or organ-specific events.

Correlation with other markers of oxygen dynamics has included the oximetric pulmonary artery catheter, which has allowed estimation of mixed venous oxygen saturation (SvO_2) in real time. The adequacy of global oxygen use and delivery is determined as outlined by manipulation of the Fick equation:

$$SvO_2 = SaO_2 - VO_2/(CO \times 1.34 \times [Hb])$$

where SaO_2 is arterial oxygen saturation, VO_2 is oxygen consumed per minute, CO is cardiac output, and Hb is hemoglobin concentration.

In the absence of anemia or hypoxia, the measure of SvO_2 will therefore reflect the relationship between VO_2 and CO, or oxygen delivery (DO_2), such that reductions in SvO_2 are presumably due to an imbalance between DO_2 and VO_2:

$$SvO_2 \propto VO_2/CO \text{ or } SvO_2 \propto VO_2/DO_2.$$

Unfortunately, this mathematic expression of a physiologic relationship breaks down in the presence of anemia and hypoxia, which are almost universal in the critically ill. Therefore, regional ischemia and incipient organ failure can occur despite normalization of SvO_2, a *global* measure. Consequently, large studies have not demonstrated a survival advantage to normalization of SvO_2.

By contrast, almost all patients undergoing resuscitation have a central venous catheter placed for fluid management, vasopressor administration, and so forth, as part of the standard of care. As a result, central venous oxygen saturation ($ScvO_2$) has been advocated as a surrogate measure of oxygen dynamics. The validity of the SvO_2–$ScvO_2$ relationship remains in question as the capacity of systemic markers to accurately reflect microcirculatory events is dubious.

Overall, if clinical interventions are to effect morbidity and mortality, they must be initiated prior to irreversibility of organ failure, and titrated according to physiologic reserve to avoid inducing or exacerbating further ischemia and organ injury.

Steroid therapy

The application of steroids in shock has long been debated. Recent studies have demonstrated the secondary adrenal failure of sepsis, where both the synthesis of cortisol is inhibited and its metabolism is enhanced. Evidence of relative adrenal insufficiency is considered present when serum cortisol levels demonstrate a <9 μg/dl increase in response to a 250-μg stimulation of adrenocorticotropic hormone (ACTH) and is also supported by a random basal serum cortisol of <20 μg/dl. Whether or not the decision to commence steroid therapy should be based on this response has been debated, largely because of the variability of the adrenal response in critical illness, the fact that free cortisol (the biologically important hormone) is not measured. Therefore, it is now believed that adrenal testing is unlikely to identify steroid responders and is not warranted.

Where does this leave the clinician in deciding who, if anyone, would benefit from steroids? Review of the latest clinical evidence suggests that, in severe septic shock, where the patient is unresponsive to resuscitation with both fluids and vasopressors, the addition of steroid therapy hastens the reestablishment of hemodynamic stability and reversal of shock. In terms of mortality, however, conflicting results make this an area of ongoing debate.

As for the recommended dose, low dose or physiologic steroid replacement is the current approach (i.e., 200–300 mg of hydrocortisone in three to four divided doses, or by continuous infusion). Higher doses have been associated with worsening mortality and untoward complications including secondary infection, myopathy, and so forth, and are not recommended. The addition of fludrocortisone remains questionable, as hydrocortisone possesses mineralocorticoid activity (20 mg of hydrocortisone is equivalent to 0.05 mg of fludrocortisone), and is currently under investigation.

As to weaning, no clear protocol has emerged due to the phenomenon of *rebound*, where there is a contemporaneous decline in cardiovascular improvements and increased evidence of inflammation with reduction in dose. The clinician must therefore be guided by the clinical picture and consider gradual reduction in dose only after establishment and maintenance of stability.

Recombinant activated protein C

In sepsis, loss of thrombin modulation perpetuates a procoagulant state with systemic progression of diffuse endovascular inflammation and injury, vascular autoregulatory collapse, and organ ischemia. It is therefore apparent that, if outcome is to be effected, one must target the endothelium. The recent therapeutic introduction of exogenous activated protein C in patients with severe sepsis has been associated with a significant reduction in mortality. By restoring levels of protein C, thrombin regulation is reestablished with a subsequent reduction in its systemic inflammatory, procoagulant, and antifibrinolytic activity. As a result, microvascular integrity is restored, attenuating the propagation of inflammatory and ischemic organ injury and culminating in lowered morbidity and enhanced survival in patients with septic shock. It is important to note that activated protein C therapy carries the risk of increased bleeding, and for that reason has not gained wide acceptance in the perioperative setting. Some clinicians have questioned the clinical effectiveness of this intervention, and further large scale clinical trials are under way to confirm the utility of this therapy in sepsis.

Ancillary therapies
Metabolic management

For some time it has been considered intuitive that excellent glycemic control would positively impact morbidity and, possibly, mortality in critically ill patients. However, the relationship between glucose control, the level of hyperglycemia, the amount of administered exogenous insulin, morbidity, and mortality has remained a contentious and hotly debated issue. This debate is emphasized by recent observations of increased mortality despite aggressive insulin regimens in critically ill patients. Additionally, it has been suggested that the role of insulin resistance, the apparent cause of hyperglycemia in critically ill patients, is emerging as a potentially more important predictor and marker of mortality than is glycemic control. This finding has led some researchers to conclude that glucose stability (as opposed to absolute levels) is of greater therapeutic benefit. Indeed, recent meta analyses showed that tight glycemic control did not, in fact, confer any mortality benefit in critically ill patients, in part due to the incidence of hypoglycemic events.

Hypoglycemia may be the physiologic complication of striving for euglycemia, but the clinical cost may often be catastrophic, particularly in those patients with acute neurologic injury. The avoidance of hypoglycemia is therefore critical. The clinician must be aware that many of the clinical signs of hypoglycemia will be masked by intubation, vasoactive agents, sedation, and paralyzing agents, to name a few. Therefore, vigilant biochemical monitoring is often the sole means of avoiding potentially tragic complications.

Ventilator management

Since sepsis is often associated with the injury of multiple organs, it is not uncommon to see acute respiratory distress syndrome or acute lung injury in septic patients. In the absence of any specific pharmacologic intervention in the treatment of acute respiratory distress syndrome and/or acute lung injury (ARDS/ALI), the mainstay of therapy has revolved around mechanical ventilatory strategies. Whereas ARDS/ALI may be diffuse, it is not necessarily uniform. Subsequently, different areas of lung are subjected, and vulnerable to barotrauma and inflammation-mediated alveolar trauma, producing heterogenous injury. Using a lung-protective strategy (i.e., tidal volumes of 6 ml/kg of predicted body weight with a range of 4–8 ml/kg, and plateau pressures of $\leq$30 cm H_2O), mortality has been found to be reduced by 9%. This approach has now become the cornerstone for ventilatory management in these patients. The additional impact of recruitment maneuvers, optimal levels of positive end-expiratory pressure (PEEP), optimal ventilatory mode, and effect of sedation continue to be debated.

Future issues

If sepsis is a disease of the endothelium, then timely intervention will be dependent on moving beyond conventional macrophysiologic monitoring. Real-time assessment of organ-specific microcirculatory events remains largely experimental, but promising. With the evolution of oximetry to near-infrared spectroscopy (NIRS; using near-infrared light of 700–1100 nm wavelength), tissue now becomes virtually translucent. Cytochromes of the respiratory chain now act as chromophores in this spectrum, in relation to their oxidation status allowing real-time assessment of oxygen dynamics at the mitochondrial level.

Similar promise has been demonstrated with reflectance spectrophotometry, optode microsensors, and oxygen electrodes, to name a few.

As such technologies continue to shed light on these clinical syndromes, our understanding of, and the potential for meaningful interventions will continue to evolve.

Summary

1. Sepsis is a significant cause of morbidity and mortality in critically ill patients.
2. Rapid diagnosis and intervention are required if sepsis syndromes are to be successfully treated and organ injury prevented or reversed.
3. It is important to realize that, when clinical evidence of sepsis manifests, the disease process is already well established.
4. The "surviving sepsis guidelines" (see Dillinger 2004) provide the best available evidence for the treatment of sepsis. These guidelines are also evolving as mechanisms of disease and the impact of new therapies are analyzed.
5. Conventional global markers of perfusion are unreliable in evaluating organ injury, since sepsis is a disease of the microcirculation. Therefore, trends of these markers are often more important than their absolute values.

6. There is no clearly superior vasopressor in the treatment of septic shock. The key to the success of resuscitation remains the provision of sufficient perfusion pressure.

7. One must always be aware that dose–response relationships are severely distorted by sepsis. Titrate the dose of the vasoactive agents to effect and be aware of potential side effects.

8. Sepsis is a systemic condition and therefore requires a systemic approach: endocrine, ventilatory, nutritional aspects of care, and so forth should all be carefully monitored and addressed.

Suggested readings

Cohn S, Crookes BA, Proctor KG. Near-infrared spectroscopy in resuscitation. *J Trauma* 2003; 54:S199–S202.

Dillinger RP, Carlet JM, Gerlach H, et al. Surviving Sepsis Campaign guidelines for management of severe sepsis and septic shock. *Int Care Med* 2004; 30:536–555.

Gattinoni L, Pesenti A. The concept of "baby lung." *Intensive Care Med* 2005; 31:776–784.

Griesdale DE, de Souza RJ, van Dam RM, et al. Intensive insulin therapy and mortality among critically ill patients: a meta-analysis including NICE-SUGAR study data. *CMAJ* 2009; 180(8): 821–827.

Hayes M, Timmins AC, Yau E, et al. Elevation of systemic oxygen delivery in the treatment of critically ill patients. *N Engl J Med* 1994; 330:1717–1722.

Ibrahim EH, Sherman G, Ward S, et al. The influence of inadequate antimicrobial treatment in patients with bloodstream infections on patient outcomes in the ICU setting. *Chest* 2000; 118:146–155.

Marik PE, Pastores S, Annane D, et al. Recommendations for the diagnosis and management of corticosteroid insufficiency in critically ill adult patients: consensus statements from an international task force by the American College of Critical Care Medicine. *Crit Care Med* 2008; 36(6):1937–1948.

Park M, Azevedo LC, Maciel AT, et al. Evolutive standard base excess and serum lactate level in severe sepsis and septic shock patients resuscitated with early goal-directed therapy: still outcome markers? *Clinics* 2006; 61(1):47–52.

Rivers E, Nguyen B, Havstad S, et al. Early goal-directed therapy in the treatment of severe sepsis and septic shock. *N Engl J Med* 2001; 345:1368–1377.

The acute respiratory distress syndrome network. Ventilation with lower tidal volumes as compared with traditional tidal volumes for acute lung injury and the acute respiratory distress syndrome. *N Engl J Med* 2000; 342:1301–1308.

The SAFE Study Investigators. A comparison of albumin and saline for fluid resuscitation in the intensive care unit. *N Engl J Med* 2004; 350(22):2247–2256.

Chapter 162

Anesthetic management of the brain-dead organ donor

J. Matthias Walz and Stephen O. Heard

As of August 2010, more than 107,000 individuals were on the waiting list for organ transplantation (Table 162.1). The total number of transplants performed in the Unites States during the preceding year was 28,463, of which 21,854 were from deceased donors, and approximately 6,609 were from living donors. There has been an increasing disparity over the last decade between patients on the waiting list for organ transplantation and available organs, despite governmental, private, and public initiatives to raise awareness about this crisis in health care. One of the most promising strategies to increase the number of available organs for transplantation is to maximize the retrieval of organs from cadaveric donors, which relies on optimal donor management in the preoperative and intraoperative period, because up to 25% of potential organ donors are lost to hemodynamic instability and other complications. Protocol-driven perioperative management has been validated in prospective clinical trials to significantly increase the number of transplantable organs and will be outlined in this chapter.

The legal framework for organ transplantation in the United States is defined in the National Organ Transplant Act (NOTA). Regional agencies under the auspices of the United Network for Organ Sharing (UNOS) are responsible for the allocation of organs and the administration of waiting lists and are called organ procurement organizations (OPOs). For example, the New England Organ Bank (NEOB) is the OPO responsible for the New England region.

The two principal sources of organs for solid organ transplantation are living donors (related or unrelated) and cadavers (cardiac death donors and brain death donors). This chapter will focus on cadaveric transplantation after the brain death of the potential organ donor.

Definition of brain death and management prior to organ donation

The most common cause of brain death in the adult potential organ donor is catastrophic brain injury due to anoxia, trauma, subarachnoid hemorrhage (SAH), or ischemic stroke. In children, the most common causes are abuse, motor vehicle accidents, and asphyxia. The exact definition of brain death may vary from state to state but always requires the absence of brainstem reflexes, motor responses, and respiratory drive in a

comatose patient with irreversible brain injury. Furthermore, the patient has to be normothermic, and metabolic abnormalities and drug intoxication as a cause of coma have to be excluded. In addition to the physical examination, a number of confirmatory tests, including nuclear medicine flow studies and electroencephalogram (EEG), are available to complement the physical examination in the diagnosis. The utility of four-vessel angiography to document lack of blood flow to the brain is limited because of the potential of end organ damage related to the contrast agent (e.g., contrast-induced nephropathy) but may be required for the patient who is in a pentobarbital coma or in situations where the diagnosis of brain death remains in doubt. One example of the key elements of the protocol used for the documentation of brain death shown in Table 162.2 (Source: UMass Memorial Medical Center). The documentation of brain death requires two separate structured examinations documenting the irreversible cessation of all cerebral and brainstem function. The two physical examinations have to be performed at least 6 hours apart, and some centers require that these examinations be performed by two different physicians. In addition to the physical examinations, an apnea test has to be performed to document the absence of any spontaneous breathing activity. For a more detailed discussion of the concept and diagnosis of brain death, see Nathan and Greer. If a patient is declared brain dead according to state and institutional criteria, the focus of critical care therapy shifts from restoring and maintaining brain function (which at this point is irreversibly lost and equates to the death of an individual) to the preservation of end organ function of the potential organ donor. Although patients with overwhelming infection are not

Table 162.1. Patients on transplant waiting lists by organ system

All	107,882
Kidney	85,511
Pancreas	1,434
Kidney/pancreas	2,179
Liver	15,923
Intestine	256
Heart	3,112
Lung	1,772
Heart/lung	75

Source: UNOS, August 10, 2010. http://www.unos.org/data.

Table 162.2. Clinical examination

Motor response	No cerebral motor response to pain in all extremities, sternal rub, supraorbital pressure; no posturing; no grimacing (spinal reflexes do not preclude diagnosis of brain death)
Pupils	No response to bright light; pupils fixed and dilated (rule out preexisting pupillary abnormalities)
Corneal reflex	No response/blink to stimulation of corneas with wisp of cotton
Cough	No cough to deep tracheal/bronchial suctioning
Gag	No gag response to stimulation of posterior pharynx
Oculocephalic	No eye movements to rapid turning of the head (eliminate test if cervical spine injury is suspected)
Oculovestibular	No deviation of eyes to irrigation in each ear with ~30 ml of ice water (allow 1 min after injection and at least 5 min between testing on each side; ensure intact, unobstructed tympanic membrane)
Absence of respiratory drive at a PaCO$_2$ of 60 mm Hg (or 20 mm Hg above patient's baseline values)	Apnea test should be done last, after all other brainstem reflexes are absent, according to institutional guidelines

considered for organ donation, patients with meningitis, bacteremia, or fungemia (as well as hepatitis B or C virus infection) may be eligible. It is important to involve the local OPO early in the process to determine the eligibility of an individual to donate, because eligibility criteria for organ donation are always in flux. Some patients who may not seem to be candidates can go on to successful donation after careful evaluation by a team of experts. For a list of absolute contraindications to organ donation see Table 162.3.

Intraoperative anesthetic management

The progression to brain death will result in a number of pathophysiologic changes that can cause profound hemodynamic instability. Left untreated, this instability would result in multisystem organ failure and cardiovascular collapse in 70% to 80% of brain-dead individuals within 3 to 5 days and include cardiovascular, respiratory, hematologic, and metabolic changes. There is good evidence to support the use of protocol-driven pre- and intraoperative management of the potential organ donor. One of the challenges of providing intraoperative care for the potential organ donor is the competing interests of participating transplant specialties. For example, the team retriev-

Table 162.3. Absolute contraindications to organ donation

HIV infection (donation is possible if recipient is also HIV positive)
Human T-cell leukemia-lymphoma virus infection
Systemic viral infections (e.g., measles, rabies, adenovirus, parvovirus, enterovirus)
Prion-related diseases
Herpetic meningoencephalitis
Advanced malignant disease

ing the kidneys for transplantation will be interested in brisk urine output, whereas the surgeon recovering the lungs may be concerned about volume overload and impaired gas exchange. It is crucially important to maintain excellent communication with the participating providers to prioritize and discuss resuscitation strategies that will result in optimal organ function for the recipients.

Anesthetic management in the operating room is a continuation of therapies started in the intensive care unit with the aim of maintaining end organ perfusion and oxygenation, as well as maintaining optimal electrolyte and acid base status. Monitoring should include American Society of Anesthesiologists (ASA) standard monitors as well as invasive arterial blood pressure management, a central venous catheter, two large-bore peripheral venous catheters, a urinary catheter, blood gas analysis at regular intervals, as well as electrolyte panels as indicated. Because there is no perception of pain in a brain-dead individual (complete loss of cortical function), there is no absolute need for opioids or inhalational anesthetics. Due to the loss of inhibitory signals from the brainstem to the spinal cord, there may be hyperreflexia in response to somatic and visceral stimulation during the surgical procedure. Muscle relaxation should be maintained to optimize surgical conditions, and signs of high sympathetic tone, such as hypertension, tachycardia, and diaphoresis, can be managed with short-acting β-blockers and antihypertensives. After the onset of brain death, the individual is prone to hypothermia due to the loss of hypothalamic thermoregulation. Multimodal warming strategies will help to avoid adverse effects, such as coagulopathy, cardiac dysfunction, arrhythmia, and cold-induced diuresis. Additionally, hypothermia can shift the oxygen–hemoglobin dissociation curve to the left, resulting in impaired oxygen delivery to the tissues. Ideally, core temperature of the potential organ donor should be maintained above 35°C.

Cardiovascular

Ischemia of the brain secondary to irreversible injury results in markedly increased sympathetic tone to maintain cerebral perfusion pressure. This increase in sympathetic outflow can initially lead to hypertension, arrhythmia (bradyarrhythmia), and subendocardial ischemia, predominantly of the left ventricle. After brain herniation is complete, sympathetic outflow will cease, resulting in marked hypotension, often exacerbated by relative hypovolemia as a result of osmotic therapy to lower intracranial pressure. To maintain adequate end organ perfusion prior to organ retrieval, fluid, vasopressor, and inotropic therapy should be titrated to hemodynamic targets as outlined in Table 162.4. Patients eligible for cardiac donation will undergo transthoracic or esophageal echocardiography or cardiac catheterization in the preoperative period to assess cardiac performance or disease. Unstable patients will require advanced hemodynamic monitoring based on thermodilution methods (pulmonary artery catheter), invasive arterial blood pressure monitoring, and/or hemodynamic monitoring based

Table 162.4. Hemodynamic and physiologic endpoints during anesthetic management of the potential organ donor

Systolic/mean arterial blood pressure	≥90 mm Hg / ≥60 mm Hg
Central venous pressure	≤12 mm Hg
Pulmonary capillary wedge pressure	≤12 mm Hg
Cardiac index	>2.5 L/min/M^2
Left ventricular stroke work index	>15 g.m/M^2
Systemic vascular resistance	800–1200 dyn·s·cm^{-5}
Urine output	>1 and <4 ml/kg/h
Core temperature	>35°C
Hematocrit	≥25%
Oxygen saturation	>95%
pH	7.35–7.45

Adapted from Wood KE, et al. Care of the potential organ donor. *N Engl J Med* 2004; 351:2730–2739.

on ultrasound techniques (transesophageal echocardiography, esophageal Doppler ultrasound). For patients who remain hemodynamically unstable despite conventional resuscitative measures as evidenced by poor cardiac output (CO), inadequate end organ perfusion, and increasing lactate levels, three-drug hormonal resuscitation should be initiated. This strategy includes a methylprednisolone bolus and infusion of arginine-vasopressin and thyroid hormone (Table 162.5). Intravenous administration of thyroid hormone appears to improve myocardial contractility, resulting in an increase of mean arterial pressure (MAP) and CO as well as decreased catecholamine requirements and arrhythmias. Although earlier studies have not documented improved cardiac performance with hormone replacement therapy, more recent studies have been encouraging. Rosendale and coworkers were able to show in a group of 701 brain-dead organ donors a 22.5% increase in the number of organs transplanted per donor, and hormonal resuscitation appears to be beneficial for donors both younger and older than 40 years. For a hydraulic model of the circulation in the potential organ donor, see Fig. 162.1.

Fluid management

The principal choice of fluids for intraoperative management of the potential organ donor includes crystalloids, either isotonic or hypotonic, and colloids, including plasma and red cell products. The type of organ(s) scheduled for retrieval will impact the fluid resuscitation strategy. If the lungs are to be procured, a

Table 162.5. Hormone replacement therapy

	Bolus	Infusion
Triiodothyronine	4.0 μg	3.0 μg/h
Alternatively: Thyroxine	20 μg	10 μg/h
In combination with:		
Methylprednisolone	15 mg/kg	Repeat in 24 h
Arginine–vasopressin	1 U	0.5–4.0 U/h

Adapted from Wood KE, et al. Care of the potential organ donor. *N Engl J Med* 2004; 351:2730–2739.

minimally positive fluid balance has been shown to be beneficial for organ function, whereas more aggressive fluid administration results in improved renal function. In cases where both kidneys and lungs are to be procured, targeted hemodynamic management as outlined earlier in the text is advisable. Frequently, patients with devastating head injuries as the cause of brain death will present to the operating room with marked hypernatremia and a free water deficit. These abnormalities should not be corrected with large amounts of dextrose-containing solutions because of resulting hyperglycemia, osmotic diuresis, and other electrolyte abnormalities. Instead, hypotonic solutions should be infused to normalize sodium levels to avoid graft damage (liver) related to high sodium levels. Hyperoncotic colloids containing hydroxyethyl starch have been implicated in renal tubular damage and impaired early graft function and should be avoided. Although there is insufficient evidence to recommend a certain transfusion trigger, it seems reasonable to keep hematocrit levels between 25% and 30% to ensure adequate oxygen delivery and hemodynamic stability. In the case of pronounced metabolic acidosis, sodium bicarbonate may be added to half-normal saline solution (50 mmol/L) to optimize acid–base status. It is important that all fluids be warmed to avoid patient hypothermia.

Respiratory

Respiratory complications are common in the potential organ donor and are related to prolonged mechanical ventilation, neurogenic pulmonary edema secondary to brain death, or aspiration and pulmonary contusion in patients with multiple trauma. In the absence of controlled trials in this patient population, lung-protective ventilation strategies as applied in patients with acute respiratory distress syndrome (ARDS) should be continued through the perioperative period. These strategies include tidal volumes of 6 to 8 ml/kg of ideal body weight and the application of positive end-expiratory pressure to prevent atelectasis and optimize gas exchange. High fractions of inspired oxygen should be avoided, if possible, to prevent oxygen toxicity to the lung. Plateau pressures should not exceed 30 cm H_2O. Bronchoscopy may be necessary to remove airway secretions and evaluate bronchial anatomy prior to transplantation. The use of colloids in patients scheduled for lung retrieval should be considered to avoid a positive fluid balance. Diuresis may be necessary in patients with frank volume overload. Hypocapnia should be avoided after the diagnosis of brain death because it will shift the oxygen–hemoglobin dissociation curve to the left and impair oxygen delivery to the tissues. It is important to remember that a brain-dead individual has a lower metabolic rate, which translates into decreased minute ventilation to maintain normocarbia.

Metabolic

Approximately 80% of patients with brain death will develop diabetes insipidus (DI) due to the destruction of the posterior pituitary gland and the resultant antidiuretic hormone

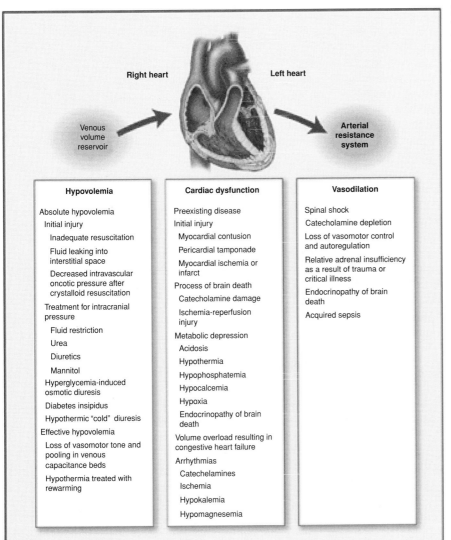

Figure 162.1. Hydraulic model of the circulation in the potential organ donor. Hypotension frequently occurs as a result of many factors and requires a structured approach to the differential diagnosis. Hypovolemia can be either absolute or effective, and an accurate assessment frequently requires the use of invasive monitoring techniques. Cardiac dysfunction and vasodilation commonly occur together, but they can arise from disparate processes that should be sought and corrected. Reprinted with permission from *N Engl J Med* 2004; 351(26):2730–2739.

Hypovolemia

Absolute hypovolemia
  Initial injury
    Inadequate resuscitation
    Fluid leaking into interstitial space
    Decreased intravascular oncotic pressure after crystalloid resuscitation
  Treatment for intracranial pressure
    Fluid restriction
    Urea
    Diuretics
    Mannitol
  Hyperglycemia-induced osmotic diuresis
  Diabetes insipidus
  Hypothermic "cold" diuresis
Effective hypovolemia
  Loss of vasomotor tone and pooling in venous capacitance beds
  Hypothermia treated with rewarming

Cardiac dysfunction

Preexisting disease
Initial injury
  Myocardial contusion
  Pericardial tamponade
  Myocardial ischemia or infarct
Process of brain death
  Catecholamine damage
  Ischemia-reperfusion injury
Metabolic depression
  Acidosis
  Hypothermia
  Hypophosphatemia
  Hypocalcemia
  Hypoxia
  Endocrinopathy of brain death
Volume overload resulting in congestive heart failure
Arrhythmias
  Catechelamines
  Ischemia
  Hypokalemia
  Hypomagnesemia

Vasodilation

Spinal shock
Catecholamine depletion
Loss of vasomotor control and autoregulation
Relative adrenal insufficiency as a result of trauma or critical illness
Endocrinopathy of brain death
Acquired sepsis

(ADH) deficiency. The diagnostic features of DI are outlined in Table 162.6. To avoid hemodynamic instability and marked alterations in electrolyte balance, urine output should be matched with crystalloid infusions while monitoring electrolyte levels. If hourly urine output is greater than 200 ml, pharmacologic treatment with desmopressin acetate (DDAVP), a V_2-receptor agonist causing renal water conservation, is indicated. The drug is available for intravenous (IV), subcutaneous (SC),

Table 162.6. Diagnostic features of DI

Urine output	$\geq$5 ml/kg/h
Urine specific gravity	$\leq$1005
Urine osmolarity	<300 mOsm/L
Serum osmolarity	>310 mOsm/L
Hypernatremia	$\geq$155 mmol/L
Hypovolemia	
Hypokalemia	
Hypomagnesemia	
Hypophosphatemia	
Hypocalcemia	

and intranasal administration. The dose for SC or IV administration is 1 to 2 μg twice daily; the intranasal dose required to maintain normal urine volume is more variable and ranges between 10 and 40 μg daily. A continuous infusion of vasopressin can also be used to treat DI.

Endocrine synthetic function of the pancreas is sufficient after the onset of brain death; however, insulin resistance will result in hyperglycemia in the majority of potential organ donors. Blood glucose levels should be maintained in the range of 80 to 150 mg/dl with a continuous insulin infusion.

Hematologic

Coagulopathy is a common problem in the potential organ donor and can be caused by hypothermia, acidosis, and the release of procoagulant substances from traumatized brain tissue (i.e., thromboplastin and cerebral gangliosides). Disseminated intravascular coagulation (DIC), which can be further exacerbated by dilutional coagulopathy from resuscitation with crystalloid, may ensue. In addition, there is evidence that patients with severe traumatic brain injury (TBI) develop platelet dysfunction, and a bleeding tendency can be present even if circulating platelet counts are normal. The effect of DIC on transplantation appears to be minimal as no significant differences between the number of retrieved organs among donors suffering from severe TBI with or without DIC have been shown. Treatment of clinical coagulopathy should include correction of the international normalized ratio (INR) to < 2.0, maintenance of a platelet count ≥ 80,000 per cubic centimeter, and maintenance of hematocrit levels between 25% and 30%. Thromboelastography may be helpful in addition to routine laboratory testing to guide treatment of coagulopathy in the perioperative period.

In summary, the key elements of anesthetic management for the potential organ donor include maintenance of adequate end organ perfusion by aggressively treating hemodynamic and electrolyte instability. If conventional measures directed at maintaining hemodynamic stability are unsuccessful, the addition of hormonal resuscitation may improve outcomes. The implementation of evidence-based treatment protocols in centers involved in organ donation is recommended to improve function of transplanted organs.

Suggested readings

Goarin JP, Cohen S, Riou B, et al. The effects of triiodothyronine on hemodynamic status and cardiac function in potential heart donors. *Anesth Analg* 1996; 83:41–47.

Mariot J, Sadoune LO, Jacob F, et al. Hormone levels, hemodynamics, and metabolism in brain dead organ donors. *Transplant Proc* 1995; 27:793–794.

Nathan S, Greer DM. Brain death. *Seminars in Anesthesia, Perioperative Medicine and Pain* 2006; 25:225–231.

Nekludov M, Bellander BM, Blomback M, et al. Platelet dysfunction in patients with severe traumatic brain injury. *J Neurotrauma* 2007; 24:1699–1706.

Rosendale JD, Kauffman HM, McBride MA, et al. Aggressive pharmacologic donor management results in more transplanted organs. *Transplantation* 2003; 75:482–487.

Salim A, Martin M, Brown C, et al. Complications of brain death: frequency and impact on organ retrieval. *Am Surg* 2006; 72:377–381.

Salim A, Martin M, Brown C, et al. The effect of a protocol of aggressive donor management: implications for the national organ donor shortage. *J Trauma* 2006; 61:429–433.

Salim A, Martin M, Brown C, et al. Using thyroid hormone in brain-dead donors to maximize the number of organs available for transplantation. *Clin Transplant* 2007; 21:405–409.

Straznicka M, Follette DM, Eisner MD, et al. Aggressive management of lung donors classified as unacceptable: excellent recipient survival one year after transplantation. *J Thorac Cardiovasc Surg* 2002; 124:250–258.

Totsuka E, Fung JJ, Ishii T, et al. Influence of donor condition on postoperative graft survival and function in human liver transplantation. *Transplant Proc* 2000; 32:322–326.

Valdivia M, Chamorro C, Romera MA, et al. Effect of posttraumatic donor's disseminated intravascular coagulation in intrathoracic organ donation and transplantation. *Transplant Proc* 2007; 39:2427–2428.

Chapter 163

Principles of trauma management

Mallory Williams and Selwyn O. Rogers Jr.

Introduction

Trauma is a surgical disease that results in more than 5 million deaths worldwide each year. In the United States, standardized management principles have evolved to address variations in processes of care to improve the outcomes of traumatized patients. The American College of Surgeons developed the Advanced Trauma Life Support (ATLS) and tiered levels of trauma care to improve trauma outcomes across the United States. In many settings, surgeons and emergency medicine physicians participate in the initial workup of trauma patients. The principle of the *golden hour* refers to the limited time available to intervene effectively to salvage life and limb. The golden hour calls for the immediate prioritization and management of the trauma patient according to ATLS principles. The ABCDE mnemonic was developed to enforce prioritization in trauma management in descending order of importance:

Airway and cervical spine protection
Breathing
Circulation and hemorrhage control
Disability and neurologic status
Exposure and environmental aspects

ATLS outlines the fundamental management concepts of the trauma patient:

1. Treat injuries that have the greatest risk to life first.
2. Lack of definitive diagnosis should never impede the application of an indicated treatment.
3. A detailed history is not essential in the evaluation and treatment of the injured patient.

We will review the components of the primary survey in the evaluation of the trauma patient, focusing on what an anesthesiologist should know.

The primary survey

During the primary survey, life-threatening injuries are identified and managed. Careful attention to the ABCDEs provides an opportunity to rapidly evaluate a critically ill trauma patient while stabilizing the patient hemodynamically. This initial assessment must be completed on all trauma patients before moving on to a more detailed history and physical examination, called the secondary survey.

Airway and cervical spine protection

In trauma management, the highest priority is to obtain and maintain a patent airway. Failure to do so leads to increased mortality. The evaluation begins by placing the patient in an appropriately sized cervical spine collar and assessing airway patency. Appropriate voice quality usually indicates a patent airway. A hoarse or breathless response may indicate airway compromise. Disorderly or confused conduct and language may also be indicator of hypoxia, whereas no response may indicate neurologic disturbance. For patients who are unable to protect their own airway, the airway should be inspected for an edematous tongue, foreign body, secretions, and blood. The simple maneuvers of chin lift and jaw thrust can be performed to secure airway patency. For patients with airway compromise or for those in a coma, it is essential to secure a definitive airway. Unless contraindicated, direct laryngoscopy with passage of a cuffed endotracheal tube is the primary approach to securing the airway. Appropriate placement has to be confirmed by both end-tidal carbon dioxide (CO_2) monitor and auscultation of breath sounds. Recent experience indicates that airway patency may be improved by the use of laryngeal mask airways (LMAs); however, these devices should not be considered a secure and definitive airway for the management of trauma patients because of their significant risk of aspiration (due to delayed gastric emptying). In some circumstances, fiberoptic bronchoscopic intubation may be attempted but should not delay the primary survey and the delivery of life-saving interventions. If securing the airway via direct laryngoscopy is unsuccessful in an expeditious manner for patients in need of a definitive airway, surgical airway by cricothyroidotomy has to be performed by an experienced provider. Cricothyroidotomy should be performed at the bedside, preferably by a surgeon. Airway compromise is a threat to life and must be treated emergently. Hypoxia also represents a secondary insult to patients with brain injury and worsens prognosis.

Breathing

The ability to breathe requires a patent airway, functional lung parenchyma, and appropriate chest wall and diaphragm dynamics. Trauma may interfere with all of the above. Pneumothorax or hemothorax both can be life threatening, and should be evacuated with a thoracostomy tube. For patients who present with a deviated trachea, hypotension, distended neck veins, and absent breath sounds, tension pneumothorax should be suspected. Tube thoracotomy should be immediately performed on the side with the absent breath sounds. A tension pneumothorax can be transiently decompressed with the placement of a 14-gauge angiocatheter in the 2nd intercostal space in the midclavicular line. Following this maneuver, a thoracotomy tube has to be placed for continued air evacuation. Occasionally, the chest wall may be violated secondary to penetrating trauma, creating a sucking chest wound. Bandaging this wound with a 4 × 4 gauze taped on three sides will improve chest wall dynamics for breathing.

More commonly, chest wall trauma produces injuries such as pulmonary contusions. A flail chest wall results from multiple contiguous rib fractures along two lines (that are either located bilaterally or in anterior and posterior positions on one side of the chest). Flail chest will lead to poor ventilatory mechanics (due to an unstable chest wall), increased work of breathing, and pain. Although these injuries are not immediately life threatening, they are formidable causes of prolonged intensive care unit (ICU) stay, especially in the elderly population. Pain control is essential. Rib fractures are an important cause of morbidity and mortality, particularly in elderly patients. Elderly patients suffer twice the mortality of younger patients with rib fractures. Rib fractures, due to their accompanying pulmonary compromise, should be identified early as life threatening in the elderly patient. ICU admission for appropriate pain management is recommended, in addition to a thoracic epidural or paravertebral catheter placement, adequate pulmonary toilet, and early mobilization.

Circulation and hemorrhage control

Hypotension is the most ominous sign in the trauma patient. Hypotension is used in the field as a key vital sign to triage patients to Level 1 trauma centers. Prevention and prompt treatment of hypovolemic (hemorrhagic) shock is an essential component of early and successful management of trauma patients. In the hypotensive patient, the primary survey evaluation with ABCDE prioritization is performed with a rapid assessment and correction of life-threatening injuries, such as airway compromise, tension pneumothorax, flail chest, or open exsanguinating wounds. Soft tissue injuries such as scalp lacerations, complex perineal wounds, or vascular bleeding from extremity wounds may all be sources of hypotension. Orthopedic injuries, such as long bone fractures in the lower extremities, can be responsible for two or more units of blood loss per thigh compartment. The primary concern of the trauma surgeon is the rapid identification of the source(s) of hypotension and appropriate therapeutic intervention(s).

The development of trauma systems to rapidly identify and prioritize these patients as critical and rapidly transport them to American College of Surgeons' Committee on Trauma verified trauma centers has been shown to save lives. The hypotensive

trauma patient undergoes a primary survey with ABCDE prioritization. After access has been established, response to bolus crystalloid infusion is evaluated. Appropriate large-bore intravenous access should be established in anticipation of large fluid and blood product requirements. Peripherally placed 14-gauge angiocatheters in bilateral upper extremities should be the minimal standard. Patients may be characterized in the following manner: responders, transient responders, or nonresponders. Patients who are transient or nonresponders and who do not have spinal shock must be assumed to have ongoing hemorrhage. Focused assessment with sonography for trauma (FAST) may be done as an adjunct to the primary survey to rule out intra-abdominal bleeding. Resuscitation should not be delayed due to the lack of crossmatched blood. "Emergency release" O negative blood can be used for blood transfusion of these patients (see more refined details on the rules governing emergency transfusions in Part 12). Early identification of patients who will require large amounts of blood transfusion should prompt activation of a massive transfusion protocol for efficient delivery of blood for transfusion until hemorrhage control has been achieved. Patients with signs and symptoms of intra-abdominal injury, such as a distended and tender abdomen, should undergo emergent celiotomy.

A circumstance needing special discussion is that of the multitrauma patient with pelvic fractures. Pelvic fractures should be appropriately reduced. The patient with a pelvic fracture may have severe hypotension and need angiographic embolization as an initial therapeutic intervention, instead of laparotomy. Patients with pelvic fractures will occasionally require both celiotomy for intra-abdominal injury and embolization for the control of bleeding. Sequencing and timing require surgical judgment as well as timely availability of resources, such as the angiography team.

Compression of actively bleeding open wounds should continue until arrival to the operating room. The radiology suite may not be an appropriate location for unstable patients. Transfusion of red blood cells should prompt an early prioritization of replacing clotting factors with fresh frozen plasma. Massive transfusion can be defined as more than 10 units of packed red blood cells (pRBCs; a patient's total blood volume) over a 24-hour period of time. This definition has been expanded to mean 50 units of pRBCs over 24 to 48 hours. Massive transfusion protocols guide therapy with the aim of rapid restoration of intravascular blood volume with effective oxygen carrying capacity and hemostasis. Dilutional thrombocytopenia becomes a problem after replacement of 1.5 times the blood volume. Thrombocytopenia can occur with smaller transfusion quantities if disseminated intravascular coagulation (DIC) occurs or if there is preexisting thrombocytopenia. Platelets are given when levels fall below 50,000. Fresh frozen plasma is administered concomitantly with the aim of maintaining the prothrombin time (PT) and partial thromboplastin time (PTT) below 1.5 times normal. Cryoprecipitate may be given for fibrinogen levels less than 0.8 g/L. Coagulopathy often results from DIC, metabolic derangements, and hypothermia, which is

Table 163.1. Glasgow Coma Scale

	1	2	3	4	5	6
Eyes	Does not open eyes	Opens eyes in response to painful stimuli	Opens eyes in response to voice	Opens eyes spontaneously	N/A	N/A
Verbal	Makes no sounds	Incomprehensible sounds	Utters inappropriate words	Confused, disoriented	Oriented, converses normally	N/A
Motor	Makes no movements	Extension to painful stimuli	Abnormal flexion to painful stimuli	Flexion/withdrawal to painful stimuli	Localizes painful stimuli	Obeys commands

N/A, not applicable.

further exacerbated by delayed or inadequate resuscitation. New enthusiasm for the use of whole blood has been precipitated by the casualties suffered in the Iraq war. The attractiveness of this approach stems from the fact that whole blood contains all essential clotting factors and maintains oxygen carrying capacity. Retrospective studies suggest the use of fresh frozen plasma and platelets in low ratios with packed red blood cells for resuscitation enhances survival.

Disability and exposure

Assessment of neurologic status is important. Early documentation of neurologic function is valuable, especially for prognostic purposes. The initial neurologic assessment in the trauma bay is often based on the Glasgow Coma Scale (GCS). The GCS is a summation score based on best eye opening, best motor, and best verbal responses (Table 163.1). The GCS can be altered by systematic factors such as drug intoxication, hypoxia, and hypotension.

Trauma patients should be fully exposed to identify all sources of external injury. The exit pathway of projectiles is particularly crucial in establishing whether midline structures have been violated. Ruling out perforation of critical aerodigestive and vascular structures is important, as these missed injuries lead to significant morbidity and delayed mortality. As soon as possible following the secondary survey, the patient's body should be covered. The trauma bay should be maintained at a warm temperature.

Trauma patients are often exposed to the external environment for long periods of time. When the ambient temperature is less than 98.6°F, loss of body heat occurs. Hypothermia by itself increases mortality, contributes to coagulopathy, and must be avoided at all costs. The key factors to consider are body surface area, temperature gradient, and time of exposure.

Conduction, convection, and evaporation are important potential sources of heat loss for trauma patients. Conduction is heat loss through direct contact between objects. Water conducts heat away from the body 25 times faster than air. Wet clothes are an important source of loss of body heat. Convection is a process of conduction during which one of the objects is in motion. Molecules against the surface are heated, move away, and are replaced by new molecules that are also heated. Wind chill is an example of convection heat loss. Finally,

evaporation is heat loss from converting water to a liquid to a gas. Examples of evaporative heat loss are perspiration and respiration.

This chapter has covered the essentials of the initial trauma care in the hospital setting, especially related to the assessment and management of the trauma patient. ATLS addresses the approach to the trauma patient in a structured and systematic manner.

Suggested readings

The American College of Surgeons Committee on Trauma. *Advanced Trauma Life Support for Doctors*. Student Course Manual. 7th ed. Chicago: The American College of Surgeons Committee on Trauma; 2004.

American Society of Anesthesiologists. *Practice Guidelines for Blood Component Therapy*. U.S. Preventive Services Task Force. Baltimore: Williams & Wilkins; 2003.

Bulger EM, Arneson MA, Mock CN, et al. Rib fractures in the elderly. *J Trauma* 2000; 48(6):1040–1046.

Chi JH, Knudson MM, Vasser MJ, et al. Prehospital hypoxia affects outcomes in patients with traumatic brain injury: a prospective multicenter study. *J Trauma* 2006; 61(5):1134–1141.

Codner P, Cinat M. Massive transfusion is appropriate. International Trauma and Critical Care Society. Summer 2005. Available at: www.itaccs.com/traumacare/archive/05_03_Summer_2005/appropriate.pdf.

Hall JR, Reyes HM, Meller JL, et al. The outcome for children with blunt trauma is best at a pediatric trauma center. *J Pediatr Surg* 1996; 31:72.

Holcomb JB, McMullin NR, Kozar RA, et al. Morbidity from rib fractures increases after age 45. *J Am Coll Surg* 2003; 196(4):549–555.

Hunt J, Hill D, Besser M, et al. Outcome of patients with neurotrauma: the effect of a regionalized trauma system. *Aust N Z J Surg* 1995; 65:83.

Kauvar DS, Holcomb JB, Norris GC, Hess JR. Fresh whole blood transfusion: a controversial military practice. *J Trauma* 2006; 61(1):181–184.

Mullins RJ, Mann NC, Hedges JR, et al. Preferential benefit of implementation of a statewide trauma system in one of two adjacent states. *J Trauma* 1998; 44(4):609–616.

Mullins RJ, Veum-Stone J, Hedges JR, et al. Influence of a statewide trauma system on location of hospitalization and outcome of injured patients. *J Trauma* 1996; 40(4):536–545.

Pitts L. Neurotrauma and trauma systems. *New Horiz* 1995; 3:546.

Shreiber M, Tieu B. Hemostasis in Operation Iraqi Freedom. *Surgery* 2007; 142:S61–S66.

Chapter 164

Venous thromboembolic disease in the critically ill patient

Mallory Williams, Naomi Shimizu, and Jonathan D. Gates

Deep venous thrombosis

Rudolf Ludwig Karl Virchow in 1856 described the triad of stasis, injury to the blood vessel (endothelial cell dysfunction), and change in the composition of the blood (hypercoagulability) as factors predisposing patients to pulmonary thromboembolism. He coined the term *embolia* and described the process of emboli breaking off and traveling to the lungs from the deep veins. Virchow understood that the etiology of pulmonary emboli was deep venous thrombosis (DVT). Patients in the intensive care unit (ICU) are at particularly high risk of venous thromboembolic disease. Their overall immobility, high predilection for indwelling venous catheters, and disease processes that induce inflammatory states causing endothelial damage are the basis for a high-risk profile and increased morbidity and mortality from DVT and pulmonary embolism (PE).

Epidemiology

DVT and PE, known collectively as venous thromboembolic events (VTE), are the number one cause of preventable in-hospital mortality. Goldhaber and colleagues reported a 33% incidence of DVT in medical ICU patients despite 61% having prophylaxis. Several studies using Doppler ultrasonography demonstrated that 6.4% of patients had DVT on admission to the ICU. Considering that more than 2 million people are admitted to an ICU each year in the United States, there are possibly 128,000 patients who are admitted to the ICU with DVT. These projections are consistent with the estimated 2 million DVTs per year in the United States. The only study to use contrast venography (the gold standard) to diagnose DVT detected 28% DVT and 8% proximal DVT in the 85 patients with chronic obstructive pulmonary disease (COPD) exacerbations. PE has been reported in 7% to 27% of postmortem examinations of ICU patients.

Pathophysiology

The tendency toward thrombosis occurs when the physiologic balance favors coagulation over anticoagulation. The pathophysiology of venous thrombosis is therefore an accumulation of factors that stimulate coagulation and inhibit anticoagulation and fibrinolysis. Immobility is the principle causative factor

for thrombosis in the ICU. Inactivity inhibits the fibrinolytic system. An overall increase in blood viscosity causes reduced blood flow that facilitates coagulation and venous thrombosis. Tissue damage impairs fibrinolysis through inflammation and cytokine production. Patients who have inherited deficiencies of the circulating anticoagulants, antithrombin and proteins C and S, are more likely to suffer from venous thrombosis. These inherited deficiencies are found in 20% of patients who have a history of venous thrombosis and whose first DVT occurs before age 41. Factor V Leiden deficiency has been established as the most common cause of inherited venous thrombophilia. The second most common cause is a mutation in the prothrombin gene G20210A. Most patients with thromboembolism, however, have no identifiable causes of hypercoagulability.

Venous thrombi are primarily composed of fibrin and red blood cells. Venous thrombus formation principally occurs at sites of vessel damage and at valve cusp pockets in the deep veins of the calves. Veins often do recanalize as the thrombus is resorbed, but they leave behind incompetent venous valves. Destruction of venous valves after venous thrombosis leads to a postphlebitic syndrome that may present as pain, swelling, discoloration, skin pigmentation, and venous ulcers. These veins with damaged valves are susceptible to recurrent thrombosis.

The soleal veins of the lower extremity are the most common sites of thrombosis. Although these thrombi rarely embolize, 15% to 20% do propagate. Venous thrombosis that propagates to the femoral and iliac veins may cause massive swelling, discoloration, and pain. This syndrome is called *phlegmasia cerulean dolans*. If thrombosis is complete in the leg, distal venous pressure will increase to the point at which arterial inflow is reduced and the limb becomes ischemic. This syndrome is called *phlegmasia cerulean albicans* and may be seen with disseminated malignancy and sepsis.

Upper extremity venous thrombosis in the ICU is often related to the presence of indwelling central venous catheters. The expanded use of peripherally inserted central catheters has made secondary thrombosis of the upper extremity more prominent. In a prospective registry of 592 patients, it was found that 324 (or 55%) of patients had central venous catheter–associated DVT, and 268 patients had noncentral venous catheter–associated DVT. PE, however, was as likely in both groups. Upper extremity DVT now accounts for 8% to 10% of all DVTs in the United States. Other causes of upper extremity venous thrombosis are intravenous drug abuse, congenital malformations, neoplasia, or upper extremity trauma.

Diagnosis
Clinical examination

The classic signs of unilateral leg swelling and pain with forced dorsiflexion of the foot (Homan's sign) are only 35% sensitive for DVT. Scoring systems that are often used for outpatients have not been validated in the ICU.

Duplex ultrasonography

The diagnostic test of choice for DVT is duplex ultrasonography. The sensitivity for proximal DVT is 97%, but it decreases to 73% for calf DVT. The specificity for proximal vein DVT is 94% with a negative predictive value of 99%. The overall weakness of this imaging study is in detecting DVT in the calf and DVT proximal to the inguinal ligament. Duplex ultrasonography also cannot detect new clots in patients with known DVT. Ultrasonography has not been found to be cost effective when used as a screening tool for all ICU patients. Only patients with a high degree of clinical suspicion (high pretest probability) should be tested.

The following are the diagnostic criteria of DVT by duplex ultrasonography:

1. Noncompressibility of the vein,
2. Presence of echogenic material in lumen,
3. Loss of phasicity and augmentation of spontaneous flow, and
4. Venous distention.

Contrast venography

Contrast venography is now seldom used in the diagnosis of DVT. The potential for renal toxicity from the contrast dye adds to patient morbidity, which is a concern in the ICU setting. However, it is the accepted gold standard for diagnosis of DVT. Due to its high sensitivity and specificity, only 1.3% of patients with DVT will have negative venography. The morbidity of venography can be reduced by using isotonic radiographic dye.

MRI

Sometimes there are difficulties in obtaining an accurate duplex ultrasound of the extremities for the diagnosis of DVT in ICU patients. Factors such as body habitus, injured extremities, patient hardware, and medical equipment may interfere with the images. While costly and more time consuming, one option is to use MRI, which has a sensitivity of 92% and a specificity of 95% for detecting DVT. Compared to duplex ultrasound, MRI is more sensitive for proximal than distal DVT.

Perioperative management of anticoagulation
Venous thromboembolism

Perioperative management of anticoagulation for venous thromboembolism is determined by the number of months that have passed since the VTE. After an acute episode of venous thromboembolism, the risk of recurrence decreases rapidly over the next 3 months. This risk of recurrent DVT 3 months after a proximal DVT is approximately 50% without anticoagulation therapy. One month of warfarin therapy reduces this risk to 10%, and 3 months of warfarin therapy reduces this risk to 5%. Considering these data, stopping anticoagulants in the first month after an acute DVT is associated with a 40% risk of VTE. Stopping anticoagulants in the second or third month after an acute DVT is associated with a 10% risk of VTE. For patients who are on long-term anticoagulation for multiple episodes of VTE, hypercoagulable state, or cancer, discontinuation of warfarin therapy is associated with a 15% per year risk of thromboembolism.

For patients who present after an acute venous thromboembolism, each day without anticoagulation is associated with a 1% absolute increase in the risk of recurrence. Despite the risk of increasing the rate of bleeding, immediate postoperative intravenous heparin therapy reduces the serious morbidity in these patients because of the extremely high thromboembolic risk. In the second and third months after venous thromboembolism, immediate postoperative intravenous heparin therapy is justified. Three months after a venous thromboembolism, full postoperative anticoagulation measures are no longer required. Only prophylactic measures, such as subcutaneous low-molecular-weight heparin (LMWH) given with or without graduated compression stockings and intermittent pneumatic compression boots, should be used.

Bridge therapy with low-molecular-weight-heparin

Bridge therapy is a therapeutic strategy employed when a patient who is at high risk of VTE needs to have warfarin therapy interrupted for a period of time for surgery. There are no available randomized, prospective trials validating this strategy. Patients would stop taking their warfarin 5 days before their procedure. Full-dose LMWH would be started at this time. On the day of surgery, only a prophylactic LMWH dose would be given. On postoperative day 1, both warfarin and LMWH full-dose therapy would be restarted. Some protocols are more aggressive and start LMWH in the immediate postoperative period.

Prevention and treatment

In the management of patients at high risk for the development of DVT, one should focus on effective prevention. In its 2001 policy statement, the Agency for Healthcare Research and Quality identified DVT prophylaxis as one of the top priorities among 79 patient safety interventions, all based on strong evidence. In 2005, the Institute for Healthcare Improvement developed care bundles, which grouped evidence-based interventions that reduced the morbidity, mortality, and health care costs from a disease process. DVT prophylaxis is now an integral component in the *ventilator bundle* order sets applied to all ventilated ICU patients, unless contraindicated.

Patients at risk for DVT may be identified by surveillance for risk factors and associated comorbidities. One study by Goldhaber and colleagues designed a prospective registry of 5451 patients with ultrasound-confirmed DVT to identify comorbidities. The five most frequent comorbidities were hypertension (50%), surgery within 3 months (38%), immobility within 30 days (34%), cancer (32%), and obesity (27%). Rogers and colleagues used data from the Patient Safety in Surgery Study to develop a predictive model for venous thromboembolism. Fifteen variables were independently associated with increased risk of DVT. These variables included patient gender (female), higher American Society of Anesthesiologists (ASA) class (2–5), ventilator dependence, preoperative dyspnea, wound classification (infected/contaminated), disseminated cancer, chemotherapy within 30 days, transfusion of more than 4 units of packed red blood cells in the 72 hours before operation, preoperative laboratory values (albumin < 3.5 mg/dl, bilirubin > 1.0 mg/dl, sodium > 145 mmol/L, and hematocrit < 38%), and operation characteristics (type of surgical procedure, emergency operation, work relative value units). A multifactorial risk index for DVT may guide our decision on DVT prophylaxis and may improve quality in patient care.

The best method of DVT prevention is early ambulation. Because early ambulation is not an option in the ICU setting, other prophylactic therapy is used.

Compression devices

Compression devices are simple and are without adverse risk. Early studies by Knight and Dawson in 1976 suggested that compression devices work by promoting fibrinolysis. Both pneumatic compression and compression stockings are now used to prevent blood stasis in the deep vein. Although intermittent compression has been thought to work in the prevention of DVT by promoting venous flow, there is no evidence that devices that produce higher velocities are more effective.

Goldhaber and colleagues prospectively studied 330 cardiac surgery patients by using two mechanical regimens of DVT prophylaxis. The primary endpoint in their study was ultrasound assessment of lower extremity DVT on hospital discharge. They found that patients assigned to intermittent pneumatic compression and graduated compression stockings had a DVT rate of 19% versus 22% in patients assigned to graduated compression stockings only.

Chemical prophylaxis

Heparin is the standard of treatment for DVT and for the prevention of DVT and thrombus extension. A more effective chemical prophylaxis for DVT can be accomplished with the use of LMWH, which has been proven to be safe and effective both in prevention and treatment of acute proximal DVT. The advantages of LMWH over unfractionated heparin are better bioavailability, a longer half-life, and more predictable anticoagulant activity. The disadvantages are the higher risk of major bleeding and the inability to monitor and titrate the dosage. Fixed doses of LMWH are used for VTE prophylaxis regardless of body mass index, but weight-based dosing with larger doses for obese patients may be more effective. The even more effective pentasaccharide, fondaparinux, is a synthetic agent introduced for VTE prophylaxis and treatment. Both LMWH and fondaparinux pose an increased risk of bleeding complications with the administration of neuraxial (spinal and epidural) analgesia.

Vena cava filter

There is a subgroup of patients whose risk of thromboembolic complications is high but their treatment with any anticoagulants may increase their risk of bleeding. These patients have either failed previous anticoagulation therapy or have an increased risk of hemorrhage with chemical prophylaxis. One particular subgroup of patients is the trauma population with sustained closed head injury, pelvic fracture, solid organ injury, or spinal cord injury. These patients benefit from a vena cava filter placement early in their hospital course. Other patient subgroups at high risk of VTEs include surgical oncology patients, patients who have a history of hypercoagulable state (Factor V Leiden, lupus anticoagulant, and protein C and S deficiency), and bariatric patients. There is a growing trend in the use of removable preoperative vena cava filters in bariatric patients as a way of reducing morbidity and mortality from PE.

Thrombolytic therapy

Thrombolytic therapy is pursued as a treatment for DVT with the goal of maintaining vein patency and avoiding postthrombotic syndromes. These agents are serine proteases, and they work by converting plasminogen to plasmin, a natural fibrinolytic agent. Plasmin breaks down the fibrinogen and fibrin in the clot. Alteplase, the first recombinant tissue-type plasminogen activator (tPA), is identical to native tPA. Reteplase is a faster-acting second-generation tPA. Because reteplase does not bind fibrin as tightly as native tPA, the drug diffuses more freely through the thrombus. Reteplase also has a faster plasma clearance and shorter half-life (approximately 11–19 min) than does alteplase. Reteplase undergoes renal (and some hepatic) clearance. Both urokinase, a fibrinolytic agent recently reintroduced to the market, and prourokinase, a clot-specific fibrinolytic agent, are also available.

In 2007, the Cochrane Review published results from randomized studies of 668 patients with DVT treated with anticoagulation or thrombolytic therapy. Patients receiving thrombolysis had significantly more bleeding complications

([RR] = 1.73). There was, however, a reduction in postthrombotic syndrome (RR = 0.66) and a complete clot lysis in the thrombolytic group (RR = 0.24). There was no significant effect on mortality.

Long-term treatment

It is important that patients diagnosed with DVT in the ICU have appropriate long-term care. Often the appropriate treatment plans during the hospital course depend on accurate ICU documentation. Guidelines for the treatment of DVT include a short-term course of LMWH or unfractionated heparin therapy plus long-term oral warfarin sodium therapy. LMWH has been shown to be as effective as intravenous unfractionated heparin in the treatment of DVT. The following are recommendations of the American College of Chest Physicians on the treatment of DVT:

1. Patients diagnosed with DVT and who have identifiable risk factors should receive 3 months of anticoagulation therapy.
2. Patients who have an initial episode with an idiopathic cause should receive 6 months of anticoagulation.
3. Patients with symptomatic isolated calf vein thrombosis should receive 6 to 12 weeks of anticoagulation therapy.
4. Patients with recurrent idiopathic venous thromboembolic disease should receive 12 months of anticoagulation therapy.

Accurate documentation of long-term goals and treatment plans before patients leave the ICU setting is a form of quality care.

Pulmonary embolism
Pathophysiology

The circulatory failure secondary to PE is caused by mechanical obstruction of the pulmonary outflow tract. The resulting hypoxemia induces hypoxic vasoconstriction that further reduces the cross-sectional area of the pulmonary vascular bed. This vasoconstriction leads to an increase in both pulmonary artery pressure and right ventricular afterload and, ultimately, to right ventricular strain, increased right ventricular wall tension, and oxygen consumption. Depression of right ventricular function reduces cardiac output and blood pressure despite increased right ventricular end diastolic pressure. Left ventricular filling may also be impeded by an overdistended right ventricle.

Diagnosis

The Prospective Investigation of Pulmonary Embolism Diagnosis II (PIOPED II) showed that the high-resolution multidetector computed tomographic angiography (MDCTA) has sensitivity and specificity comparable to that of contrast pulmonary angiography. The study was performed with a 4-row, 8-row, and

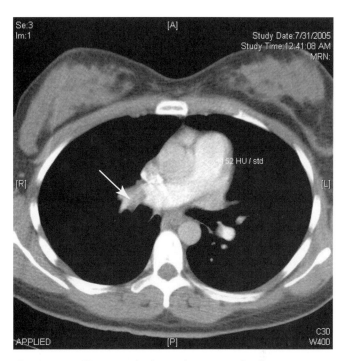

Figure 164.1. CT angiography showing large proximal pulmonary embolism (arrow) in the right pulmonary artery.

16-row multidetector CT. The acquisition time was usually less than 30 seconds. The diagnostic criteria for PE was intraluminal filling defect (Fig. 164.1). The sensitivity of CTA for PE was 83%, and the specificity was 96%. The positive predictive value was 86%, and the negative predictive value was 95%. The positive predictive values for PE were 97% for main or lobar vessel, 68% for segmental vessels, and 25% for subsegmental vessels. The complications from CTA were dye allergy (<1%), urticaria (<1%), and extravasation of contrast material (<1%). Although pulmonary angiography is the gold standard diagnostic modality for PE, it is being replaced by MDCTA, because the latter modality is significantly less invasive, is easier to perform, and offers equal sensitivity and specificity.

Now that CTA has become an accepted diagnostic tool, appropriate hydration and renal protection strategies are important to avoid contrast nephropathy. ICU patients receive large dye loads during diagnostic workup in their first 48 hours in the hospital. They may also be exposed to other pharmacologic agents that are nephrotoxic. The intensivist should be aware of the total contrast load that patients are receiving and provide the maximum intervention for the protection of kidney function for these patients.

D-dimer measures fibrin breakdown products. This laboratory test is highly sensitive (>95%) for the presence of acute venous thrombosis or PE. Because patients in the ICU have many different illnesses, a nonspecific test like D-dimer will often be positive. The utility of this test is in the negative result, which is used to exclude the presence of venous thrombosis or PE.

Prevention and treatment

Vena cava interruption

The idea of placing a barrier in the inferior vena cava (IVC) to prevent PE from a venous thrombus was first introduced by Trousseau in 1868. In 1998, a multicenter group in France conducted the first published, randomized, prospective study of IVC filters in the prevention of PE. They studied 400 patients with known proximal DVT and randomized patients into an IVC filter or no filter group. Additionally, these same patients were randomized to receive LMWH or unfractionated heparin. The primary outcome event was radiographic PE within the first 12 days after randomization and during the 2-year follow-up period. Although they found a statistically significant decrease in the incidence of PE in patients with IVC filter at 12 days, this was not true in the long term. After 2 years, the incidence of symptomatic PE in the filter group was 3.4%. This study suggested that early use of an IVC filter is an effective barrier to PE, yet, over the long term, this protection becomes less effective. After 8 years, although the cumulative incidence of PE was significantly reduced (6% vs. 15%, $P = 0.008$), there was an increased incidence of DVT in the filter group (35% vs. 27%, $P = 0.042$). Studies have also been done to determine whether IVC filters can prevent PE in critically ill trauma patients with known DVTs. In a retrospective review of 200 patients, Carlin and colleagues examined the rate of PE in patients with DVTs, patients with PE, and patients with both DVT and PE. None of the patients with DVT developed a PE. Arguments can be made against the prophylactic use of IVC filters in both trauma and ICU patients. Long-term IVC filters have been associated with risk of thrombosis and postphlebitic venous insufficiency.

Retrievable filters

With the technical advances in the Greenfield IVC filter and percutaneous deployment devices, filters have become easier and safer to place (Fig. 164.2). The newer designs have allowed

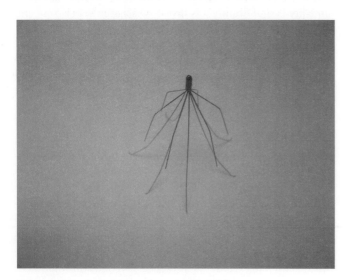

Figure 164.2. Conical shape of a retrievable IVC filter.

retrieval of the filters, which decrease the known complications of caval thrombosis and postphlebitic venous insufficiency. Studies have demonstrated a 51% filter removal rate with no complications. These patients had no proximal thrombus, had a normal venogram prior to filter retrieval, and were anticoagulated with heparin or warfarin. Early retrieval is preferred to decrease the known complications of indwelling filters. These long-term complications include filter migration, occlusion, perforation, IVC thrombosis, and postthrombotic syndrome.

IVC filter placement is now being done in the interventional radiology suite or under ultrasound guidance at the patient's bedside. The safety of IVC filter placement at the bedside using duplex ultrasound in critically ill trauma patients has been proven to be feasible. In one study in 2003, 94 patients with multiple traumas whose injuries precluded them from anticoagulation had temporary IVC filters placed in the ICU. Ninety-six percent had insertions without complications. Complications included hematomas (2%) and filter misplacement (3%). Other reported insertion-related complications include de novo thrombosis (26%) and arteriovenous fistula (<3%). Similar studies in critically ill populations have confirmed the safety of bedside ultrasound-guided insertion of an IVC filter.

Anticoagulation

When a PE is diagnosed, treatment modalities are designed to prevent propagation, worsening obstruction, right ventricular failure, or a second embolism. With PE, the obstruction causes dilation of the right ventricle and displacement of the interventricular septum. As the strain and oxygen demands increase, the ventricle becomes ischemic due to poor oxygen supply. Ischemia eventually leads to cardiac arrest. This fatal progression can be stopped by complete removal of the obstruction to allow normalization of right heart pressures.

Heparin is the first-line of therapy for PE. The effectiveness of heparin is in its prevention of thrombus progression and reduction of embolization. This intervention reduces the mortality rate associated with PE from 30% to 10%. Early anticoagulation is important. Hospital-based heparin protocols were implemented to reduce the number of patients receiving subtherapeutic doses of heparin. In one clinical trial, patients were given either intravenous heparin followed by warfarin or intravenous heparin and simultaneous warfarin. Only 1% to 2% of patients were subtherapeutic for more than 24 hours with respect to the activated partial thromboplastin time (aPTT) level in both groups. When comparing weight-based heparin dosing versus standard-care nomogram, a higher percentage of patients using the weight-based heparin dosing achieved therapeutic range in 24 hours. The weight-based group was dosed with 80 U/kg as a bolus and then 18 U/kg/h infusion. The standard-care nomogram group received a 5000-U bolus followed by 1000 U/h infusion. Eighty-nine percent of weight-based patients achieved the therapeutic range for aPTT (1.5–2.3) versus 75% of standard-care nomogram patients in 24 hours. The risk of recurrent thromboembolism was more frequent in the standard-care group. Subtherapeutic heparin in the initial 24 hours is associated with a higher incidence of recurrences.

In the same study comparing intravenous heparin followed by warfarin versus intravenous heparin and warfarin given concurrently, 69 of 99 (69%) patients had supertherapeutic values (aPTT = 2.5) that persisted for 24 hours. These patients belonged to the group receiving heparin and warfarin together. Despite this more intensive therapy and supertherapeutic values, bleeding complications occurred at similar frequencies in both groups (9.1% combined therapy vs. 12% heparin alone).

Thrombolysis

Thrombolysis is the established treatment for patients with hemodynamic instability following PE because of its ability to lyse the obstructing emboli and improve right ventricular function. There is, however, an ongoing controversy in the use of thrombolytics in patients with hemodynamically stable PE. In 2002, a multicenter, prospective, double-blind, randomized study in Germany studied the effectiveness of heparin and a thrombolytic agent, alteplase, in patients with hemodynamically stable PE. They found that thrombolysis with anticoagulation therapy reduced the need for escalation of therapy (increased heparin dose) and lowered the risk of death threefold.

Embolectomy

Both thrombolytic therapy and catheter-directed fibrinolysis can be used to treat PE. Many critically ill patients are not eligible for thrombolysis, however, because of the risk for bleeding. Suction pulmonary embolectomy is increasingly used to treat PE as it is still less invasive than is an open embolectomy. Although the American College of Chest Physicians recommended against the use of mechanical methods of thrombectomy, many authors agree on the following three criteria for performing catheter thrombectomy in acute PE:

1. Hemodynamic instability, defined as a systolic pressure ≤90 mm Hg, a drop in systolic pressure ≥40 mm Hg for ≥15 minutes, or ongoing administration of vasopressors for the treatment of hypotension;
2. Subtotal or total filling defect in the left and/or right main pulmonary artery; and
3. The presence of one of the following contraindications to thrombolysis: history of intracranial bleeding, head injury, neurosurgery, ischemic stroke, or brain tumor; surgery or organ biopsy; active bleeding, cancer with hemorrhagic risk, gastrointestinal bleeding or major trauma within

15 days; pregnancy or recent delivery; platelet <50,000 cells/μl, international normalized ratio (INR) >2.0.

The goal of embolectomy is to reverse right heart failure. Surgical pulmonary embolectomy is the last resort after less invasive methods have failed or the patient progresses to hemodynamic instability or arrest. The overall survivability and outcomes of embolectomy are better when earlier approaches are chosen. Surgical embolectomy should be considered only when an experienced cardiothoracic team is immediately available.

The overall mortality of pulmonary embolus is between 6% and 8% and increases to as high as 30% when complicated by hypotension. Of those patients with fatal PE, 67% die within 1 hour of onset of symptoms. Early definitive treatment for those patients who are hemodynamically unstable is essential.

Suggested readings

Decousus H, Leizorovicz A, Parent F, et al. A clinical trial of vena caval filters in the prevention of pulmonary embolism in patients with proximal deep-vein thrombosis. *N Engl J Med* 1998; 338:409–415.

Geerts WH, Pineo GF, Heit JA, et al. Prevention of venous thromboembolism: the Seventh ACCP Conference on Antithrombotic and Thrombolytic Therapy. *Chest* 2004; 126(3 Suppl):338S–400S.

Goldhaber SZ, Hirsch DR, MacDougall RC, et al. Prevention of venous thrombosis after coronary artery bypass surgery (a randomized trial comparing two mechanical prophylaxis strategies). *Am J Cardiol* 1995; 76(14):993–996.

Goldhaber SZ, Tapson VF. A prospective registry of 5,451 patients with ultrasound-confirmed deep venous thrombosis. *Am J Cardiol* 2004; 93:259–262.

Hirsch D, Ingenito EP, Goldhaber SZ. Prevalence of deep venous thrombosis among patients in medical intensive care. *JAMA* 1995; 274:335–337.

Joffe HV, Goldhaber SZ. Upper extremity deep vein thrombosis. *Circulation* 2002; 106:1874–1880.

PREPIC Study Group. Eight-year follow-up of patients with permanent vena cava filters in the prevention of pulmonary embolism: the PREPIC (Prevention du Risque d'Embolie Pulmonaire par Interruption Cave) randomized study. *Circulation* 2005; 112(3):416–422.

Rogers SO Jr, Kilaru RK, Hosokawa P, et al. Multivariate predictors of postoperative venous thromboembolic events after general and vascular surgery: results from the Patient Safety in Surgery study. *J Am Coll Surg* 2007; 204(6):1211–1221.

Stein PD, Fowler SE, Goodman LR, et al. Multidetector computed tomography for acute pulmonary embolism. *N Engl J Med* 2006; 354(22):2317–2327.

Watson LI, Armon MP. Thrombolysis for acute deep vein thrombosis. *Cochrane Database Syst Rev* 2007; (4):CD-002783. DOI:10.1002/14651858.CD002783.pub2.

Chapter 165

Traumatic brain injury

Albert H. Kim, Meredith R. Brooks, Ian F. Dunn, Shaheen F. Shaikh, and William B. Gormley

Traumatic brain injury (TBI) remains a significant global health care problem and, in the United States, affects 2% of the population per year. Despite significant advances in our understanding of the pathophysiology of TBI, mortality remains high at 20%, with significant long-term neurologic deficits in 35% of survivors. A joint task force of the Brain Trauma Foundation and the American Association of Neurological Surgeons (AANS) has developed evidence-based guidelines in an attempt to address systematically the care of these patients. The results of such collaborative efforts have focused management on both the primary injury – the initial traumatic insult—and secondary injuries, the pathophysiologic events subsequent to the primary insult.

Our goal is to help practicing anesthesiologists understand the pathophysiology of TBI to allow them to develop perioperative management strategies most consistent with available evidence and current guidelines. TBI is often a key element of multitrauma. Hence, anesthesiologists are often asked to provide care for these patients while surgeons tend to their associated injuries.

In this chapter, we review current concepts in TBI. First, we address the diagnosis and assessment of TBI. Second, we focus on the pathophysiology and management paradigms of both primary and secondary brain injury.

Assessment of traumatic brain injury
Glasgow Coma Score

Developed in 1974 by Jennett and Teasdale, the Glasgow Coma Score (GCS; see Table 163.1) is the most widely used scale for determining the severity of TBI. Included in the scale are the patient's eye opening, verbal response, and motor response. Although the GCS has been widely criticized by many clinicians as being excessively simplistic, it remains the primary assessment tool in this population. In fact, its simplicity allows accurate communication regarding initial impressions of a patient between observers with different levels of expertise.

The GCS helps to classify injuries according to their clinical severity. Two broad categories include minor head injury (GCS 9–15) and severe head injury (GCS 3–8). A simple guide to the management of minor head injuries is highlighted in Fig. 165.1.

Minor head injuries can be further divided into minimal, mild, and moderate head injury. Patients who are neurologically intact, have suffered no amnesia or loss of consciousness, and have a GCS of 15 are categorized as having minimal head injury. These patients generally do not require brain CT scanning except in select cases (Fig. 165.1 for CT indications) and are discharged home with instructions to return should signs or symptoms of brain injury develop. Patients with a GCS of 14 are categorized as having mild brain injury and may experience a brief (<5 minutes) loss of consciousness or memory impairment. Our institution routinely obtains CT scans on these patients. In one of the largest retrospective studies of mild head-injured patients, 16% of patients with a GCS of 14 exhibited abnormal CT scans. A GCS score of 9 to 13 indicates moderate injury. Such patients are able to follow commands at the time of examination but have had longer periods of loss of consciousness (>5 minutes) and have abnormal findings on neurologic examination. This group of patients requires careful monitoring because more than 30% of patients in this subgroup demonstrate abnormal CT scans. Therefore, patients should have emergent CT scans with prompt neurosurgical consultation if findings are abnormal on examination (Fig. 165.1). GCS scores from 3 to 8 indicate severe TBI with worse outcomes. Within this group, nearly 80% of patients with an initial hospital GCS of 3 to 5 eventually die, have severe disability, or are vegetative.

Primary and secondary traumatic brain injury

Significant morbidity and mortality are caused not only by the original insult but also by ensuing pathophysiologic processes evolving over a period of hours to days. This has led to the distinction between primary and secondary brain injury.

Table 165.1. Types of primary brain injury

Focal	Diffuse
Hematoma	Concussion
Epidural	Multifocal contusion
Subdural	DAI
Intraparenchymal	
Contusion	
Concussion	
Lacerations	

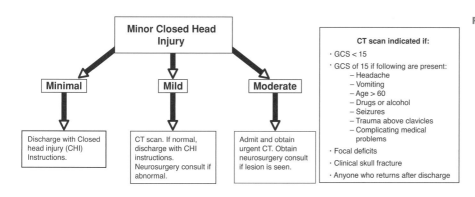

Figure 165.1. Minor head injury management.

Primary brain injury

Primary brain injury can be broadly divided into focal and diffuse injuries (Table 165.1). Focal injuries are related to a narrow force vector delivered to a delimited intracranial region. This type of an injury tends to produce intracranial hemorrhages, including epidural and subdural hematomas, or cerebral contusions and intracerebral hematomas. Diffuse injuries are more often related to wide force vectors and high acceleration or deceleration injuries as seen with motor vehicle accidents. Diffuse injuries range from concussion to diffuse axonal injury (DAI) with widespread long tract signs and posttraumatic coma.

The first critical step in the management of TBI is to determine the nature and severity of the primary injury by using the clinical examination and radiographic evaluation. It is during this assessment of the primary injury that the decision for emergent surgical intervention is made. After the primary injury is considered and addressed, the patient moves into the phase of secondary injury prevention. The general management of TBI can thus be considered in two phases: identification and management of primary brain injury followed by the prevention of secondary brain injury.

Hemorrhages

Acute blood can be readily identified on noncontrast CT of the head, an important component in the initial evaluation of a patient with TBI, as mentioned earlier in the text. The main types of traumatic brain hemorrhage requiring surgery are epidural, subdural, and intracerebral.

Acute epidural hematomas are managed, when surgically appropriate, by craniotomy due to the gelatinous consistency of an acute blood clot, which is difficult to remove without complete bony exposure of the area of bleeding. Expectant management can be an option if mass effect is minimal and the patient's neurologic status is normal, especially in the pediatric population. However, the disadvantage of conservative management is that the patient must be monitored carefully in the intensive care unit (ICU) for several days.

Accumulation of blood in the subdural space can occur in an acute or chronic manner. The acute subdural hematoma can be surgically treated by craniotomy or craniectomy. In a subset of individuals with no neurologic compromise and a stable, limited amount of blood, the subdural collection can be allowed to liquefy over a few weeks and then drained by burr-hole evacuation. In fact, many patients present with a liquefied, subacute or chronic subdural hematoma, often due to (1) persistent oozing or (2) the accumulation of multiple, small subdural bleeds. The advantage of the burr-hole is the low surgical risk, as some cases may even be performed under local anesthesia. The acute-on-chronic subdural hematoma, often the consequence of systemic anticoagulation, can have a significant and sudden acute component on top of an otherwise indolent and inconsequential chronic accumulation. The important first step in the management of these patients is to stop ongoing bleeding by discontinuing anticoagulation and correcting any coagulopathy. Correcting the coagulopathy will become the responsibility of anesthesiologists managing the trauma patient intraoperatively if a decision to perform an emergent operation is made.

Intraparenchymal hemorrhages occur commonly following brain trauma, and most are treated nonoperatively. Often these hemorrhages present as contusions on the surfaces of the inferior frontal lobe and the anterior temporal lobe adjacent to the greater sphenoid wing, sites where the brain strikes bony margins. They may increase dramatically in size over the first few days, creating significant mass lesions where only small lesions were present initially. Therefore, small contusions seen on initial CT scans should be followed closely for the first 3 days. This problem can be much more dramatic in elderly patients on traditional anticoagulation or antiplatelet agents or in patients with a coagulopathy. A recent randomized, controlled trial (Surgical Trial in Intracerebral Haemorrhage [STICH]) suggests that early craniotomy for traumatic intraparenchymal hemorrhages is no better than medical management. Opinion is still divided, however, regarding craniotomy or craniectomy for intraparenchymal hemorrhages associated with refractory, high intracranial pressure (ICP), especially later in the course of the hemorrhage.

Secondary brain injury

Surgery typically is performed in response to the primary brain injury. Secondary brain injury, however, refers to regional cellular processes that take place over hours to days after the initial brain injury. Secondary brain injury results not only from the delayed effects of primary brain injury but also from contributing factors, such as hypotension, hypoxia, intracranial hypertension, and inadequate cerebral perfusion pressure (CPP). Untreated, severe secondary injury ultimately leads to intracranial hypertension and cerebral ischemia, which can significantly compound the effects of the initial injury. Critical care physicians and anesthesiologists play key roles in the prevention of secondary brain injuries as they are most often responsible for managing these patients in this period.

Seizure prophylaxis

TBI clearly increases the risk of seizures, which have been traditionally divided into early (within 1 week) and late posttraumatic seizures. Seizure control is critical in TBI patients, given the effects of epileptiform activity on brain metabolism and the potential systemic complications of seizure, which may exacerbate secondary injury. Temkin and colleagues demonstrated that phenytoin treatment for 7 days in patients with intracranial blood or depressed skull fractures decreased the incidence of early but not late posttraumatic seizures. More recently, levetiracetam, with its favorable side-effect profile, has been employed as prophylaxis against early posttraumatic seizures. Although early seizure control following TBI appears equivalent between phenytoin and levetiracetam, it is important to note that TBI patients on levetiracetam have a higher tendency to exhibit an abnormal electroencephalogram (EEG). Beyond the early posttraumatic period, a TBI patient with seizures is treated as would be any patient with new-onset seizures.

Intracranial hypertension
Pathophysiology

Intracranial hypertension is a common complication of severe head injury, and its management is essential to the control of secondary injury. Nearly half of head-injured patients with intracranial mass lesions have persistently elevated ICP. ICP is determined by the contents of the intracranial vault, the physiology of which was codified by the Monro–Kellie doctrine. An uncompensated increase in one or more compartments in that vault results in ICP above the normal range (5–15 mm Hg). In the absence of a mass, increased ICP in severe TBI can result from aberrations in cerebrospinal fluid (CSF) flow, cerebral blood volume, and the development of vasogenic and cytotoxic edema. When endogenous mechanisms for volume buffering are exhausted, ICP increases in an exponential fashion. The steep nature of the volume–pressure curve complicates ICP management because an increase in ICP signifies a sudden and significant reduction in intracranial compliance (Fig. 165.2). Sustained ICP readings of greater than 20 mm Hg are abnormal. ICP greater than 40 mm Hg represents severe preterminal intracranial hypertension.

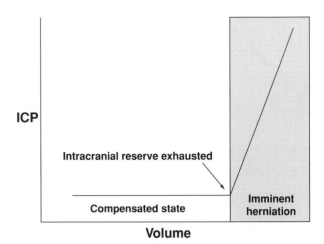

Figure 165.2. ICP–volume relationships.

The two main consequences of elevated ICP are brain herniation and compromised cerebral perfusion (CPP = mean arterial pressure [MAP] – ICP). The three principal forms of herniation are uncal, central diencephalic, and tonsillar herniation. Uncal herniation is produced by medial displacement of the temporal lobe by middle fossa lesions with subsequent midbrain compression, leading to a clinical syndrome involving coma, ipsilateral fixed and dilated pupil, and, commonly, contralateral hemiparesis. Uncal herniation can progress to include brainstem hemorrhages and posterior cerebral artery compression with consequent infarction in this territory. Central diencephalic herniation results from generalized bilateral intracranial hypertension with caudal displacement of the diencephalon through the tentorial incisura, deformation of the brainstem, and progressive decrease in consciousness. In tonsillar herniation, a posterior fossa mass, such as a cerebellar hemorrhage, exerts pressure in the confined space of the posterior fossa, leading to brainstem compression and coma. Cushing's triad of bradycardia, hypertension, and respiratory irregularity may indicate imminent brainstem herniation.

Cerebral perfusion

The management of ischemia focuses on maintaining an adequate CPP and avoiding systemic hypotension, hypoxia, and anemia to ensure adequate cerebral blood flow (CBF). Normally, CBF is relatively constant in a range of CPP between 40 and 160 mm Hg due to autoregulation. At low perfusion pressures within this range, the arteriolar bed dilates to decrease cerebral vascular resistance (CVR) and increase blood flow to normal levels. Below the autoregulatory threshold, arterioles passively collapse and CBF falls. Above the autoregulatory limits, vessels are maximally constricted and CBF increases.

Pressure autoregulation is impaired in many patients following TBI, and even when it is intact, the parameters at which it is operative may be shifted. Most notably, the lower limit of autoregulation may increase from CPPs around 40 to 50 mm

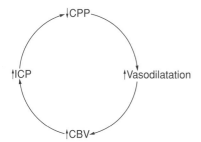

Figure 165.3. CPP–ICP relationship with preserved autoregulation.

Hg, meaning that perfusion pressures that are normally adequate may cause ischemia in these patients. The clinician must assume that, in patients with severe TBI, CBF is directly proportional to CPP, and therefore CPP must be closely monitored and maintained. Prospective studies have demonstrated that mean mortality is reduced by 50% when CPPs are maintained above 70 mm Hg in patients with severe TBI. The Brain Trauma Foundation supports maintaining CPP of 50 mm to 70 mm Hg, whereas other centers, such as ours, advocate a CPP above 70 mm Hg.

Besides the fact that increased ICP can decrease CPP, it is also true that decreases in CPP can increase ICP, leading to a deleterious positive feedback loop. As CPP decreases, pial arterioles dilate to accommodate larger blood volumes (diagrammed in Rosner's vasodilatory cascade; see Fig. 165.3). Increased blood volume can increase ICP. Restoration of CPP can therefore lead to pial arteriolar constriction and decreased ICP.

Systemic hypotension and hypoxia can also contribute to secondary injury by compromising cerebral oxygenation. Miller and others showed a 150% increased risk of mortality in patients with severe TBI who had at least one episode of hypotension as defined by systolic blood pressure < 90 mm Hg when compared with patients without hypotension. Similarly, Stochetti and colleagues showed that severe TBI patients with hypoxic episodes prior to intubation had a 77% mortality rate. Therefore, it is advisable to avoid periods of hypotension and hypoxemia should TBI patients require anesthesia for surgery.

Anemia may also decrease tissue oxygenation, and thus the hematocrit deserves particular attention in the head-injured patient. Kee has suggested that brain tissue oxygen delivery begins to decrease below a hematocrit of 33%, but most centers transfuse packed red blood cells below hematocrits of 30%. These recommendations are similar to those used in acute coronary syndromes and differ with recent reports outside of these two populations where lower hematocrits are felt to be acceptable.

Monitoring

The indications for placing an ICP monitor in patients with TBI are based on the identification of groups at risk for developing intracranial hypertension or for whom a neurologic examination cannot be followed, such as pharmacologically paralyzed patients or patients under general anesthesia. Patients at highest risk are those with GCS ≤ 8 and an abnormal CT scan. All patients with GCS ≤ 8 should have an ICP-monitoring device placed unless there is a coexisting coagulopathy. We also consider ICP monitoring in TBI patients with a GCS > 8 who are undergoing anesthesia for extensive extracranial surgery.

Management of increased intracranial pressure

The goals of intracranial hypertension management are the maintenance of adequate CPP and the avoidance of brain herniation. Elevated ICP is an independent predictor of poor neurologic outcome in patients with severe head injury. The Brain Trauma Foundation supports initiating treatment at ICP readings of 20 to 25 mm Hg with preservation of adequate CBF. A caveat to dogmatic adherence to these values is that herniation may occur at ICP readings below 20 mm Hg, particularly in patients with temporal lesions. Also, a therapeutic CPP target may be reached with ICP readings as high as 25 mm Hg. At our institution, we initiate treatment for ICP readings greater than 25 mm Hg, unless CPP is compromised at lower pressures. We use a stepwise approach, from conservative to more invasive, beginning with head elevation to optimize cerebral venous outflow, followed by pharmacotherapy and CSF drainage (Fig. 165.4).

Specific maneuvers to decrease ICP
Conservative measures: positioning, CO_2, and sedation

We advocate elevating the head of the bed to 30° and maintaining a neutral head position to maximize venous return from the brain and thereby reduce CBV. Additionally, if a cervical collar is present, we confirm that the collar is not so tight as to impede jugular venous flow. This needs to be carefully and repeatedly verified both in the ICU and in the operating room as these

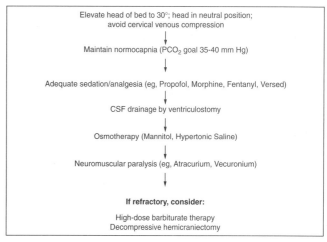

Figure 165.4. Stepwise protocol for ICP management.

patients may require prolonged procedures and passive positioning.

Changes in arterial carbon dioxide (CO_2) are known to affect CBF and vascular caliber. While pressure autoregulation may be dysfunctional in severe TBI, CO_2 reactivity is preserved. Hypoventilation raises $PaCO_2$ and ICP by increasing vascular caliber and CBF, whereas $PaCO_2$ levels below 35 mm Hg may lower ICP but compromise CBF. The ideal $PaCO_2$ level in head-injured patients is thus normocapnia. In emergency situations, such as with acute neurologic deterioration and impending herniation, acute hyperventilation can be considered but should be maintained only until other treatments are expeditiously initiated. The only circumstance in which mild chronic hyperventilation may be considered as a therapy is when cerebral hyperemia (more prevalent in the pediatric population) is shown by either jugular bulb venous saturation ($SjVO_2$) or CBF measurements.

Sedation and analgesia may help to blunt the sympathetic stimulation activated by pain or agitation, endotracheal irritation, or routine nursing care and help to decrease ICP. The short-acting sedative propofol is being used with increasing frequency because its short half-life permits frequent neurologic examinations and because it appears to have superior effects on ICP reduction compared to narcotics. Propofol is a potent vasodilator, however, and careful attention must be paid to MAP and CPP during its administration. Also, propofol is contraindicated in the pediatric population due to the possibility of *propofol syndrome*, characterized by metabolic acidosis, cardiac conduction abnormalities, and rhabdomyolysis. Severe intracranial hypertension may require pharmacologic paralysis by neuromuscular blockade for maximum muscle relaxation.

CSF drainage by ventriculostomy

CSF drainage via an external ventricular drain (EVD) or ventriculostomy is an effective method of ICP reduction in head-injured patients. After placement, the EVD is leveled or "zeroed" to the tragus. With a ventriculostomy in place, we drain CSF to its maximal capacity for increased ICP control prior to starting osmotherapy. We, therefore, recommend the use of a ventricular catheter, whenever possible, prior to the use of osmotherapy and paralysis, and certainly before the initiation of barbiturate coma. When an intraparenchymal monitor without drainage capability is already in place, however, osmotherapy may be instituted before CSF drainage.

Osmotherapy

The osmotic diuretic mannitol is a mainstay in the armamentarium of ICP management. Mannitol was commonly thought to reduce ICP by reducing intracranial water content but is now recognized to also expand plasma volume and decrease viscosity. Experiments have demonstrated that mannitol increases CBF and decreases ICP by autoregulatory vasoconstriction. Furosemide, which can inhibit the production of

CSF, may potentiate the effects of mannitol. When using mannitol, intravascular volume, serum osmolarity, sodium, blood urea nitrogen (BUN), and creatinine must be vigilantly watched for possible adverse effects. When the serum osmolarity is above 320 Osm, mannitol may precipitate acute renal failure, especially in patients with already compromised kidney function. With prolonged use, mannitol can also disrupt the blood–brain barrier and may pass into the brain parenchyma, causing a rebound effect with subsequent increases in ICP.

Hypertonic saline may be used as an adjunct or alternative to mannitol. Hypertonic saline has the advantage of a lower risk of rebound intracranial hypertension and renal failure. At hyperosmolar concentrations, sodium chloride creates a gradient, which drives water from interstitial and intracellular compartments into the intravascular space, reducing brain water and thus ICP. More recent work has suggested that hypertonic saline also exerts anti-inflammatory effects. Qureshi's group has reported that 23.4% saline in doses of 30 to 60 ml over 20 minutes can markedly reduce ICP when standard treatments fail. Hartl and colleagues demonstrated that 7.5% hypertonic saline was particularly effective in ICP reduction and CPP elevation in patients with severe TBI when ICPs were refractory to other measures. Hypernatremia is commonly observed but resolves as renal free water clearance is reduced. Possible adverse consequences include central pontine myelinolysis, seizures, as well as congestive heart failure from fluid shifts and coagulopathy.

Intracranial hypertension refractory to standard treatment

The measures just mentioned are routinely used to manage intracranial hypertension. When ICP begins to increase despite maximal treatment, however, other measures, such as decompressive craniectomy or barbiturate-induced burst suppression, can be considered. We use these measures in select situations only, after careful consideration and discussion with family members regarding the advantages and disadvantages of each.

Barbiturates

Barbiturates potentiate the effects of γ-aminobutyric acid (GABA) at GABA receptors, which inhibit neuronal transmission and thereby reduce the cerebral metabolic rate of oxygen consumption ($CMRO_2$). Barbiturates may also decrease ICP by limiting free radical–mediated lipid peroxidation and resultant cerebral edema. The routine use of barbiturates in the treatment of high ICP is not indicated, especially because outcomes have not been shown to improve with this therapy. Although barbiturates have been shown to decrease ICP, there are important side effects of this therapy. The most clinically significant side effects of barbiturate administration are hypotension and global oligemic hypoxia, followed by hypokalemia, respiratory depression, hepatic dysfunction, and renal dysfunction. For these reasons, this treatment should always be used in conjunction with a

Swan–Ganz catheter. Plasma and CSF pentobarbital levels correlate poorly with physiologic effects; therefore, pentobarbital dosing is best followed by EEG monitoring with titration to achieve burst suppression. Barbiturates, because of their neuroprotective effects, are the first choice for the induction of general anesthesia for TBI patients.

Decompressive hemicraniectomy

In decompressive hemicraniectomy, the bone is removed and the dura is opened to increase the size of the intracranial vault. In a trial consisting of 27 pediatric patients, Taylor and colleagues demonstrated a reduction in risk ratio of 0.54 for death in the acute period as well as for death, vegetative state, and severe disability 6 to 12 months after the event in patients who underwent bitemporal decompressive craniectomy for high ICP. Evidence from the ischemic stroke field also has shown that decompressive craniectomy, especially when performed early, can greatly decrease mortality. Future class I studies in TBI patients are eagerly awaited.

Anesthetic considerations

Analgesia and sedation

Patients with persistent ICP elevation should receive little or no premedication to avoid hypercapnia and hypoxemia. Sedation without control of the airway should be avoided. The agitated patient may require general anesthesia.

Positioning

Please see subsection on conservative measures. In patients who are hypovolemic, elevation of the head may be associated with a decrease in blood pressure; therefore, blood pressure must be maintained so that CPP is not compromised.

Monitoring

Intra-arterial blood pressure monitoring is helpful so that hemodynamic changes may be monitored closely. Central venous pressure or pulmonary artery pressure monitoring may be necessary in patients with significant cardiac or pulmonary comorbidities, but should not delay surgery. The position of the pressure transducers will need to be adjusted to the height of the patient's right atrium to ensure reliable measurements.

Blood pressure management

Hypotension (systolic < 90 mm Hg) at any point during treatment has been identified as one of the primary factors that worsen prognosis. Arterial hypotension attributed to hypovolemia should be rapidly corrected with fluid administration. Placement of two large-bore intravenous (IV) cannulae is necessary. These patients should undergo aggressive fluid resuscitation with isotonic fluids until euvolemia is achieved. Isolated head trauma rarely leads to severe hypotension. Other possible injuries, such as spinal cord trauma and blunt abdominal and/or chest trauma, should be identified and treated. Combined inotropes/vasopressors, such as dopamine or norepinephrine, may be required to sustain arterial pressure in hypotension persisting despite fluid administration, although these agents should be used with caution, as their vasoconstriction effects potentially may impair local CBF despite improving CPP. Norepinephrine may be the vasopressor of choice in these situations.

Induction

All patients with TBI should be regarded as having a full stomach and should have a rapid-sequence induction with cricoid pressure. Intubation without anesthetics may cause coughing and bucking and increase ICP, hence IV anesthetic agents and muscle relaxants must be used to secure the airway. Thiopental at 3 to 5 mg/kg IV or propofol at 1 to 2 mg/kg IV is the drug of choice, along with a short-acting neuromuscular agent. Barbiturates and propofol are effective in lowering ICP by decreasing CBF. Hypotension is a potential side effect of both of these agents and can compromise CPP. The use of succinylcholine in intracranial hypertension is controversial. Animal and human studies have shown an increase in ICP presumably due to fasciculations. This effect can be avoided by using a defasciculating dose of a nondepolarizing drug prior to succinylcholine. Securing the airway promptly with succinylcholine avoids the deleterious effects of hypoxia and hypercarbia and a subsequent increase in ICP. If the airway assessment reveals that intubation may be easy, then rocuronium at 0.6 to 1.2 mg/kg may be used.

Fentanyl, at 3 to 5 μg/kg IV, is administered to blunt the hemodynamic response to laryngoscopy and intubation. Lidocaine, at 1.5 mg/kg IV given 90 seconds before laryngoscopy, can help to prevent the increase in ICP. If a difficult intubation is anticipated, awake fiberoptic intubation, which produces substantial, but transient, increases in ICP, may be necessary, but should be used with caution. Sedation, analgesia, paralysis, and topical tracheal anesthesia do not completely prevent this increase. Blind nasal intubation is contraindicated in patients with a basilar skull fracture, which is suggested in patients with CSF otorrhea, rhinorrhea, hemotympanum, periorbital ecchymosis (raccoon eyes), or ecchymosis behind the ear (Battle's sign).

Sedation, analgesia, and neuromuscular blockade

It is important to maintain neuromuscular blockade during surgery. Care should be taken when suctioning the endotracheal tube because it can increase ICP in the nonrelaxed patient. Coughing and bucking may increase ICP by increasing intrathoracic pressure and obstructing cerebral venous outflow. Agitation and pain may significantly increase blood pressure and ICP. Hence postoperatively adequate sedation and analgesia is an important adjunct treatment. Hypovolemia predisposes to hypotensive side effects and should be treated promptly.

Selection of shorter-acting agents allows for a brief interruption of sedation to examine the neurologic status.

Hyperventilation and PEEP

Hypoxemia is associated with increased morbidity and mortality. Oxygen administration should be generous to maintain an oxygen saturation of hemoglobin (SpO_2) > 90% or PaO_2 > 60 mm Hg. The use of prophylactic hyperventilation therapy ($PaCO_2 \leq 20$–25 mm Hg) during the first 24 hours after severe TBI should be avoided because it can compromise cerebral perfusion during a time when CBF is reduced. High tidal volumes and high respiratory rates are independent predictors of acute lung injury or acute respiratory distress syndrome. Neurogenic pulmonary edema can also contribute to hypoxemia. Alternative ventilator strategies should be considered to protect the lung and maintain tight $PaCO_2$ control. In patients with severe brain injury and acute lung injury, the use of positive end-expiratory pressure (PEEP) is limited by conflicting results on its effect on ICP. With higher levels of PEEP (10–12 cm H_2O), there is a slight increase in ICP in patients with normal ICP. For PEEP to increase cerebral venous pressure to levels that would increase ICP, the cerebral venous pressure must at least equal the ICP. The higher the ICP, the higher the PEEP must be to have such a hydraulic effect on ICP.

Management of brain oxygenation

Therapy following severe TBI is directed toward preventing secondary brain injury. Delivery of oxygen (O_2) to the brain is a function of the oxygen content and CBF. Hypoxemia, usually a PaO_2 below 50 mm Hg or 60 mm Hg, is associated with cerebral vasodilation. The optimal PaO_2 in a brain-injured patient is currently unestablished. Brain tissue monitoring allows one to provide minimal fraction of inspired oxygen (FiO_2) to avoid lung toxicity from hyperoxia that permits the optimal (not too high, not too low) brain tissue oxygen level. Low brain tissue oxygen ($P_{bt}O_2$), less than 15 mm Hg, has been associated with increased mortality.

Glucose management

Glucose is essential to cerebral metabolism, and hypoglycemia should be avoided because, under anaerobic conditions in poorly perfused ischemic areas, lactate levels may increase, contributing to worsening of neuronal damage. Hyperglycemia has been associated with longer length of stay and increased mortality rate. Euglycemia should be maintained.

Temperature management

Hypothermia is associated with better neurologic outcomes. There is evidence of improved neurologic outcome after induced hypothermia to 33°C for 12 to 24 hours in out-of-hospital cardiac arrests. Preliminary studies suggest that decreased mortality may be seen when target temperatures are maintained for more than 48 hours. Clifton and colleagues, however, were unable to show a beneficial effect of induction of hypothermia after TBI.

Fluid management

Please see the earlier sections on hyperosmolar agents and blood pressure management. Hypo-osmolar solutions, such as 5% dextrose in water, reduce serum sodium and increase brain water and ICP. Colloid solutions exert little influence on either variable. Fluid restriction minimally affects cerebral edema and, if pursued to excess, may result in episodes of hypotension, which may increase ICP and worsen neurologic outcome. Although there is no single best fluid for patients with TBI, isotonic crystalloids are widely used.

Systemic sequelae

Fluid therapy used to support CPP may cause visceral edema, increasing intra-abdominal pressure, which increases ICP. Ventilatory maneuvers used to treat respiratory failure may increase intrathoracic pressure, limiting venous return and thereby increasing ICP and decreasing CPP. In severely injured patients with head trauma, treatment decisions may create a cycle that increases pressure in various body compartments.

Antiseizure prophylaxis

Seizures can occur in 15% to 20% of patients after TBI and can increase cerebral metabolic rate and ICP. In patients with severe TBI, 50% of seizures can be subclinical and can be detected only by continuous EEG monitoring. Posttraumatic seizures can occur early (within 7 days) or late (after 7 days) following injury. Anticonvulsants are indicated to decrease the incidence of early seizures. Routine seizure prophylaxis later than 7 days is not recommended.

Postoperative management

If the patient is not responsive to analgesia and sedation alone after surgery, neuromuscular blockade should be considered. The prophylactic use of neuromuscular blockers in patients with intracranial hypertension has not been shown to improve outcome, may be associated with increased risk of pneumonia and sepsis, and may obscure seizure activity.

Conclusion

To conclude, the principal goals of severe TBI management are addressing the primary injury and then limiting secondary brain injury. The avoidance of intracranial hypertension is essential for the latter as it prevents brain herniation and cerebral ischemia. An *ICP-based approach* to patients with severe TBI includes stepwise measures as shown in Fig. 165.4. Just as important is a *CPP-based approach*, in which maintenance of a particular CPP (rather than a particular ICP) guides management.

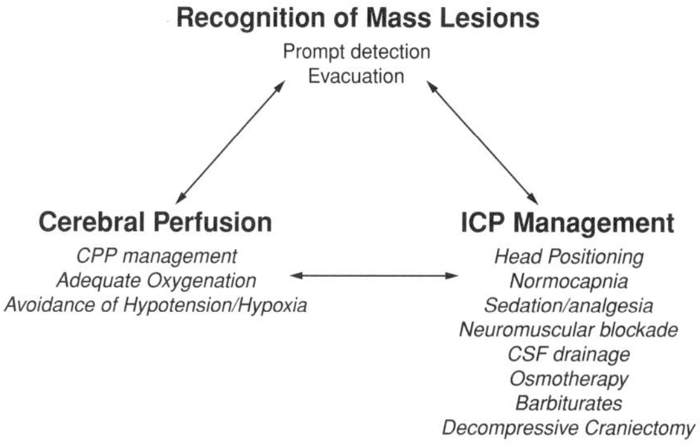

Recognition of Mass Lesions
Prompt detection
Evacuation

Cerebral Perfusion
CPP management
Adequate Oxygenation
Avoidance of Hypotension/Hypoxia

ICP Management
Head Positioning
Normocapnia
Sedation/analgesia
Neuromuscular blockade
CSF drainage
Osmotherapy
Barbiturates
Decompressive Craniectomy

Figure 165.5. Cornerstone of severe TBI management.

An integrated management paradigm that monitors and controls both ICP and CPP is thus strongly recommended. The cornerstones of such a strategy include (1) rapid identification and management of intra- or extradural mass lesions, (2) ICP monitoring and management, and (3) CPP maintenance for avoidance of cerebral ischemia (Fig. 165.5). Finally, meticulous systemic medical management of these patients, including appropriate seizure prophylaxis, is a requirement for successful outcomes.

Suggested readings

Brain Trauma Foundation, American Association of Neurological Surgeons, Joint Section on Neurotrauma and Critical Care. Guidelines for the management of severe head injury. *J Neurotrauma* 2007; 24:S1–S106.

Brain Trauma Foundation, American Association of Neurological Surgeons, Joint Section on Neurotrauma and Critical Care. Trauma systems. *J Neurotrauma* 2000; 17:457–462.

Chesnut RM, Marshall LF, Klauber MR, et al. The role of secondary brain injury in determining outcome from severe head injury. *J Trauma* 1993; 34:216–222.

Ingebrigtsen T, Rise IR, Wester K, et al. [Scandinavian guidelines for management of minimal, mild and moderate head injuries]. *Tidsskr Nor Laegeforen* 2000; 120:1985–1990.

Juul N, Morris GF, Marshall SB, et al. Intracranial hypertension and cerebral perfusion pressure: influence on neurological deterioration and outcome in severe head injury. The Executive Committee of the International Selfotel Trial. *J Neurosurg* 2000; 92:1–6.

Marshall LF, Smith RW, Shapiro HM. The outcome with aggressive treatment in severe head injuries. Part I: the significance of intracranial pressure monitoring. *J Neurosurg* 1979; 50: 20–25.

Mayer SA, Brun NC, Broderick J, et al. Safety and feasibility of recombinant factor VIIa for acute intracerebral hemorrhage. *Stroke* 2005; 36:74–79.

Muizelaar JP, Lutz HA 3rd, Becker DP. Effect of mannitol on ICP and CBF and correlation with pressure autoregulation in severely head-injured patients. *J Neurosurg* 1984; 61:700–706.

Narayan RK, Greenberg RP, Miller JD, et al. Improved confidence of outcome prediction in severe head injury. A comparative analysis of the clinical examination, multimodality evoked potentials, CT scanning, and intracranial pressure. *J Neurosurg* 1981; 54:751–762.

Plum F, Posner J. *Diagnosis of Stupor and Coma*. 3rd ed. New York: Oxford University Press; 1982.

Rosner MJ. Introduction to cerebral perfusion pressure management. *Neurosurg Clin N Am* 1995; 6:761–773.

Servadei F, Ciucci G, Piazza G, et al. A prospective clinical and epidemiological study of head injuries in northern Italy: the commune of Ravenna. *Neurosurg Rev* 1989; 12(Suppl 1): 429–435.

Stein SC, Ross SE. Moderate head injury: a guide to initial management. *J Neurosurg* 1992; 77:562–564.

Suarez JI, Qureshi AI, Bhardwaj A, et al. Treatment of refractory intracranial hypertension with 23.4% saline. *Crit Care Med* 1998; 26:1118–1122.

Teasdale G, Jennett B. Assessment of coma and impaired consciousness. A practical scale. *Lancet* 1974; 2:81–84.

Chapter 166

Burn management

Mark Chrostowski and Edward A. Bittner

Epidemiology

Of the estimated 500,000 patients treated for burns every year in the United States, approximately 40,000 are admitted into the hospital. Of these patients, more than half are sent to specialized regional burn centers. Survival and quality of life for patients with severe thermal injury have significantly improved over the last few decades due to advances in critical care and surgical technique. Today, except for the most severe cases, burn victims are expected to survive their initial injuries. Recent estimates from the American Burn Association show a 94.4% survival rate for all patients admitted to burn centers. As more patients survive, therapy for postburn deformity has increasingly become a major clinical problem. Consequently, more operative cases are now devoted to addressing reconstructive problems. Available data suggest that, by resuscitating patients through postburn shock and managing burn sepsis, patients can survive their burns and maintain a satisfying quality of life.

Pathophysiology

Severe burn injury causes extensive physiologic changes (Table 166.1). Changes begin when significant tissue trauma leads to widespread release of both local and systemic inflammatory mediators. Inflammatory mediators, including histamine, free O_2 radicals, and prostaglandins, cause burn shock through generalized capillary leak, intravascular volume depletion, and myocardial dysfunction. Although evaporative and direct fluid loss from the site of burn injury play a role, it is the extensive systemic capillary leak and protein loss that lead to edema formation and intravascular depletion. This fluid and protein loss occurs both locally at the burn site and at more distant, non-burned tissues. The end result is burn shock that requires large volume resuscitation for stabilization and prevention of tissue ischemia.

To complicate matters further, other mediators, including epinephrine, norepinephrine, vasopressin, angiotensin II, and serotonin, cause an increase in systemic and pulmonary vascular resistance. The vasoconstriction increases afterload and contributes to the decreased cardiac output. This vasoconstriction results in decreased flow to vascular beds that are already underperfused. Tissue ischemia and secondary organ injury can result without early, aggressive fluid resuscitation. After burn shock is successfully treated and capillary integrity is restored, a hypermetabolic response develops with associated fever, tachycardia, and severe fat and muscle wasting. In the hypermetabolic phase of burn injury, resting metabolic rates can double and remain elevated for up to 9 to 12 months post-injury.

Classification of burns

Classification of burns is important because the extent of injury correlates with the severity of pathophysiologic changes and the

Table 166.1. Systemic effects of burn injury

System	Pathophysiologic changes and complications
Respiratory	Airway edema Reduced pulmonary and chest wall compliance Bronchospasm Pneumonia, pulmonary edema, and ARDS
Cardiovascular	Hypovolemia Myocardial dysfunction and decreased cardiac output (early) Increased cardiac output and hypertension (late)
Renal	Decreased renal blood flow (early) Increased renal blood flow (late) Myoglobinemia
Metabolic	Increased metabolic rate Impaired thermoregulation Protein catabolism Electrolyte imbalances (from resuscitation and topical antibiotics)
Gastrointestinal	Curling ulcers Ileus and delayed gastric emptying Impaired intestinal barrier
Hematologic	Hemoconcentration (initially) Chronic anemia (later) Thrombocytopenia (dilutional and consumptive) Coagulopathy and disseminated intravascular coagulopathy (in severe cases)
Infectious	Postburn sepsis
Neurologic	Encephalopathy Acute and chronic pain Cyanide and carbon monoxide poisoning
Skin	Increased fluid and heat loss Need for escharotomy in severe cases Contracture and scar formation
Pharmacologic	Altered pharmacokinetics and pharmacodynamics Increased tolerance to sedatives and opioids Altered response to muscle relaxants

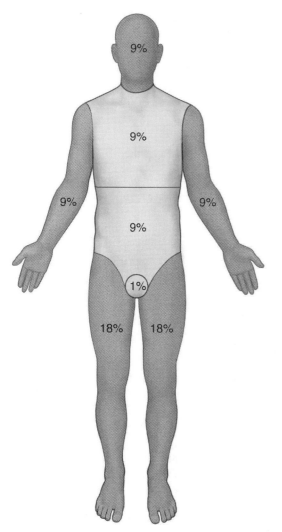

Figure 166.1. The rule of nines for estimating TBSA. *Note:* Not accurate for all age groups.

Table 166.2. Classification of burn depth

Depth	Level of injury	Clinical features
Superficial	Epidermis	Dry, red Blanches Painful
Superficial partial-thickness	Papillary dermis	Blisters Moist, red, weeping Blanches Painful Return to full function
Deep partial-thickness	Reticular dermis	Blisters Wet or waxy dry Does not blanch Absent pain sensation Possible need for surgical excision and grafting
Full thickness	Subcutaneous fat, fascia, muscle, or bone	Waxy white to leathery Dry and inelastic Does not blanch Absent pain sensation Surgical excision and grafting as early as possible

Modified from Bittner EA, Grecu L, Martyn JAJ. Evaluation of the burn patient. In: Longnecker DE, et al., eds. *Anesthesiology.* New York: McGraw-Hill Professional; 2008.

Management

Initial evaluation

Treating patients with burn injuries requires a complex, multidisciplinary approach. As with any other trauma admission, the patient with acute burn injury should be managed to ensure adequate airway, breathing, and circulation. After the airway and hemodynamics are stabilized, a secondary survey is done to look for associated nonthermal injuries, and a comprehensive history and physical examination are performed. The cervical spine should be evaluated for potential injury in the appropriate clinical setting. A Foley catheter, nasogastric tube, and adequate intravenous (IV) access for resuscitation are all needed for major thermal injury.

Patients with electrical injury require immediate hospital admission, often to a specialized burn center. Electrical burns can have massive amounts of tissue destruction that often cannot be predicted by the burn size alone. Although the events that lead to injury can be either obvious or subtle, high-voltage burns cause injury one of three ways: (1) thermal burns to skin, (2) destruction of muscle and nerves, and (3) arrhythmias and cardiac arrest. Extensive deep tissue damage can also cause myoglobinuria and compartment syndromes. Standard resuscitation endpoints must be monitored closely because fluid resuscitation formulae are often inaccurate when hidden, deeper injuries exist.

Airway and respiratory issues

Patients should immediately be assessed for inhalation injury and any evidence of airway compromise. Inhalation injury is a major source of mortality in burn patients. Signs of hoarseness,

need for resuscitation. It also helps to predict how the injury will progress and whether surgical intervention may be needed. The extent of burn injury is assessed in relation to total body surface area (TBSA) involved with either the rule of nines (Fig. 166.1) or Lund and Browder burn diagrams. Although the rule of nines provides useful initial estimates of TBSA in the acute setting for adults, it underestimates the TBSA for children. More accurate characterizations should be obtained through the use of comprehensive and age-specific burn diagrams once the patient is stabilized.

It is also important to assess the depth of burns (Table 166.2). The classical description of burn injury in terms of first, second, and third degree has given way to a new system that is more descriptive of burn depth. The new characterizations (superficial, superficial partial-thickness, deep partial-thickness, and full thickness burns) help to determine the need for inpatient admission and surgical intervention. It often takes 2 to 3 weeks, however, to determine whether the wound will heal primarily or be severe enough to require surgical intervention.

brassy cough, or stridor indicate laryngeal edema and constitute an emergency. Because edema formation occurs in nonburned tissues after major thermal injury, respiratory failure can develop even in the absence of inhalation injury.

The respiratory status often deteriorates in the setting of massive fluid resuscitation. In these cases, it is generally safer to intubate the patient early than risk a difficult intubation later when airway swelling has occurred. With burn injuries of the face or neck, direct laryngoscopy may be difficult or impossible and a surgical airway may be needed. The difficult airway should ideally be managed in the operating room with resources for obtaining a direct surgical airway readily available.

Severe injury complicated by deep, circumferential chest wall wounds can significantly reduce pulmonary and chest wall compliance, causing high airway pressures and significant ventilatory difficulties. Escharotomy should improve ventilation in this situation. Indirect respiratory injury resulting from pulmonary edema, pneumonia, or acute respiratory distress syndrome (ARDS) may develop in the days following the initial burn injury. Many patients are now managed with a low-tidal-volume ventilation of 6 ml/kg. This low-tidal-volume ventilation strategy is thought to help reduce alveolar distention and barotrauma. Permissive hypercapnia is used if not contraindicated by pulmonary hypertension, hemodynamic instability, or intracranial hypertension.

Cardiovascular issues

Hemodynamics in burn injury are initially characterized by a reduction in cardiac output and an increase in systemic and pulmonary vascular resistance. Approximately 3 to 5 days after major burn injury, a hypermetabolic response develops with associated fevers, increased cardiac output, and increased energy expenditure. Severe fat and muscle wasting results.

Although multiple fluid resuscitation formulae exist for estimating fluid needs, no single formula has proved to be superior in improving outcomes. The *Parkland formula* is perhaps the most known and remains a gold standard in guiding fluid resuscitation requirements for burn victims. The formula calls for 4 ml/kg/%TBSA of lactated Ringer's in the first 24 hours, with one half of this amount administered over the first 8 hours. As a general rule, burns of <15% TBSA are not associated with extensive capillary leak and can be managed with fluid of 1.5 times the maintenance rate. Resuscitation formulae should be used only as guidelines. Actual fluid administration should be individualized for each patient and titrated to physiologic endpoints (Table 166.3).

If the total fluid requirement exceeds 6 ml/kg/%TBSA/24 hours, it may be advisable to obtain more information regarding intravascular volume and cardiac function thru measurement of central venous and cardiac filling pressures. After 24 to 48 hours, capillary integrity is restored in nonburned areas and fluid requirements dramatically decrease. It is important to decrease fluid administration at this time because overresuscitation can be associated with substantial morbidity.

Table 166.3. Burn resuscitation endpoints

Arousable and comfortable
Warm extremities
Systolic blood pressure: for infants, 60 mm Hg; for older children, 70–90 + 2 × age (y); for adults, mean arterial pressure > 65 or within 20% of baseline
HR 80–150 bpm (age dependent)
Urine output 0.5 ml/kg/h
Lactate levels < 2 mmol/L

Although the benefits of resuscitation are obvious, the type of fluid used in resuscitation of burn victims has always been controversial. Theoretically, resuscitation with colloid should improve outcomes by preserving plasma oncotic pressure and replacing intravascular volumes with less tissue and pulmonary edema. Clinical studies have not shown improved outcomes, however. Given their significant extra cost but no improvement in survival, many clinicians question the continual use of colloids, especially for burns of < 40% TBSA. If they are used, many advocate waiting until capillary integrity is restored.

Renal issues

Inadequate resuscitation after major thermal injury complicated by hypotension and myoglobinemia contributes to the development of early acute renal failure (ARF). A urine output of at least 0.5 ml/kg/h is one indicator of the adequacy of resuscitation. Late ARF is associated more with multisystem organ failure, sepsis, and the effects of nephrotoxic drugs. The development of ARF is associated with increased mortality in burn patients.

Gastrointestinal and nutritional issues

Patients with severe burns often develop a paralytic ileus and require nasogastric decompression. Gastroduodenal ulceration (Curling ulcers), likely due to reduced splanchnic blood flow, is a risk after severe burn injury. Ulcer prophylaxis with H_2-receptor antagonists or proton pump inhibitors should be initiated early.

The presence of circumferential abdominal burns and accumulation of intraperitoneal fluid and/or bowel edema from large volume resuscitation can lead to abdominal compartment syndrome (ACS). Signs of ACS include diminished urine output, decreased pulmonary compliance, and hemodynamic instability. Bladder pressures can be obtained to make the diagnosis. Surgical decompression may be necessary in some cases.

Severe burn injury results in a hypermetabolic response with profound wasting of lean body mass that can last for more than a year after injury. Strategies used to minimize this catabolic response include early wound excision and grafting, early institution of feeding, prompt treatment of sepsis, and maintenance of high environmental temperature. Nutritional support can partially abate the hypermetabolic response to burns and help maintain muscle mass. Enteral feeding is preferable to parenteral feeding because it maintains gastrointestinal

(GI) motility and reduces bacterial translocation and sepsis. Parenteral nutrition is reserved for patients with intolerance for enteral feeding or prolonged ileus. Some evidence suggests that β-blockade may attenuate this hypermetabolic response and associated muscle wasting. Propranolol has been shown to decrease heart rate (HR) and resting energy expenditures as well as reverse muscle–protein catabolism.

Neurologic and pain issues

Mental status changes can develop in the setting of hypoxia, hypotension, or the inhalation of neurotoxic chemicals. Therapies for anxiety and pain cause sedation and complicate efforts to diagnose the etiology of acute neurologic changes. Signs of central nervous system dysfunction include delirium, hallucinations, personality changes, seizures, and coma. Radiologic imaging should be obtained if intracranial injury is suspected.

Pain management in the burned patient provides many challenges. Nearly every therapy for burn injury is associated with pain. Surgery, dressing changes, physical therapy, and transport exacerbate baseline pain and anxiety levels. Standardized pain and anxiety guidelines are used in many burn centers to provide appropriate and consistent patient comfort. IV morphine and versed are commonly used medications for intubated patients or for those who are NPO. Ketamine has also proved to be a useful adjunct because of its effects as an analgesic acting via the N-methyl-D-aspartate (NMDA) receptor. Transition to oral medications when possible helps to provide more constant therapeutic levels. Burn patients develop tolerance to most opioids and sedatives, so they require higher doses than do patients without thermal injury. Continuous administration of analgesics by themselves can result in opioid-induced hyperalgesia, which will accentuate the need for higher opioid levels.

Infection issues

Infection is a leading cause of morbidity and mortality in burn patients. Sepsis in burn injury can be difficult to diagnose because, even in the absence of sepsis, patients are already hypermetabolic and have hyperdynamic physiology. Prevention, early diagnosis, and treatment of infection is essential. Prophylactic antibiotics have no proven role in burn care and are not routinely given. Topical antimicrobials, however, provide high concentrations of drug at the wound surface, reduce the levels of wound flora, and delay the interval between injury and colonization. Tetanus toxoid should be given to burn patients because all burn injuries have potentially contaminated soft-tissue wounds. Maintaining sterile technique both in the operating room and during transport through the use of a mask and sterile gloves and dressings is essential to preventing infection.

Surgical considerations

Blood loss during burn wound excision can be deceptively large with published estimates ranging from 3.5% to 5% of the blood volume for every 1% TBSA excised. It is not difficult for the surgical team to remove eschar so rapidly that the patient becomes hypovolemic and unstable. Limiting the operative duration and extent of excision can prevent such problems. Techniques to minimize blood loss include intraoperative tourniquets for limb surgery, injection of dilute epinephrine, and brisk operative pace.

Altered pharmacokinetics and pharmacodynamics

The altered physiologic state in burn injury and changes in concentrations of plasma proteins cause changes to the pharmacokinetic and pharmacodynamic response to drugs. Hypotension and low cardiac output decrease hepatic and renal blood flow and function. Standard dosing of drugs should be adjusted accordingly.

Anesthetic considerations
Preoperative evaluation and transport

Given the enormous physiologic changes seen in burn injury, careful planning is essential for safe intraoperative care (Table 166.4). As with any surgical procedure, the preoperative evaluation should consist of gathering information about the patient's history and performing a thorough physical examination. Reviewing details of the patient's burn injury – with special attention to the time since injury, extent of injury, adequacy of resuscitation, and presence of an inhalational component – provides insight into expected physiologic changes and possible anesthetic difficulties. Previous anesthetics, especially those already completed in the postburn period, can provide information on difficulties in airway management, ventilation, hemodynamic stability, or pain control. Coexisting diseases, associated injuries, current medications, and allergies must be reviewed. Standard laboratory tests include electrolytes, blood urea nitrogen (BUN), creatinine, hematocrit, coagulation status, and a blood bank sample. Blood products should be available in the operating room for larger cases where blood loss is expected.

The airway is assessed for the possibility of difficult intubation. Facial wounds often create difficulties for mask ventilation. Likewise, edema formation and scarring can complicate intubating conditions by decreasing neck mobility and mouth opening. There is always a risk for endotracheal tube (ETT) dislodgement during patient transport or intraoperative positioning. Tape alone is usually insufficient to secure the ETT if facial burns are present. Common practices are to either tie the ETT securely around the neck or use wire to secure the tube to a tooth.

The neurologic examination should be focused on baseline mental status and adequacy of anxiety and pain control. The baseline pain and sedation regimen should be known to help guide the need for premedication and intraoperative pain control. Assessment of cardiovascular status should focus on hemodynamic function in response to stage of burn injury (early hypodynamic vs. later hyperdynamic), adequacy of resuscitation, and vasopressor dependence. Given the risk for large

Table 166.4. Perioperative concerns specific to burn patients

Preoperative

Initial evaluation	History and physical examination, including:
	Extent of burn injury (TBSA, depth, and location)
	Mechanism of injury, elapsed time from injury, adequacy of resuscitation
	Associated injuries
	Presence of inhalation injury
	Presence of organ dysfunction
	Presence of infection
	Coexisting diseases
	Surgical plan
Airway	Assess for airway patency and possibility of difficult intubation.
Neurologic	Assess baseline mental status and pain control.
Cardiovascular	Assess adequacy of resuscitation.
	Consider hemodynamic response to injury (hypo- vs. hyperdynamic).
Pulmonary	Assess for evidence of inhalation injury.
	Adequacy of oxygenation and ventilation
	Significant ventilatory support may require ICU ventilator.
Renal	Assess for renal failure and electrolyte imbalances.
Gastrointestinal	Assess NPO status (limit NPO time given increased metabolic requirements).
Laboratory data	CBC, electrolytes, and coagulation studies
	Blood bank sample and availability of blood products
Transport issues	Ensure the ETT is well secured.
	Check all equipment prior to departure.
	Ambu bag, O_2 cylinder, monitors, infusion pumps
	Equipment and medications for reintubation and resuscitation
	Maintain patient comfort and sedation.

Intraoperative

Monitoring	Standard ASA monitors; invasive monitoring as dictated by patient's condition and operative procedure
Airway	Anticipate potential difficulty.
	If injuries do not preclude standard airway management (mask fit, mouth opening, neck extension), direct laryngoscopy and intubation can be performed.
	Gastric emptying may be delayed in burn patients.
IV access	Anticipate difficulty locating vessels; ultrasound guidance can be helpful. Central venous access is usually necessary in patients with large burn injuries.
	Securing adequate vascular access before the surgical procedure begins is necessary because blood loss can be rapid and substantial.
Temperature	Massive heat loss can occur through the open wounds.
	Keep ambient temperature elevated.
	Use warming blankets, radiant warmers, and blood and fluid warmers.
Hemodynamics	Response varies with extent of burn, elapsed time from injury, and adequacy of resuscitation.
	Early (days 1–3): reduction in CO, increased SVR and PVR; later (>3 days): hyperdynamic state with increased CO
Ventilator management	Provide adequate oxygenation and ventilation without inducing further morbidity from oxygen toxicity, hemodynamic compromise, barotrauma, or alveolar overdistension.
Anesthetics	Many anesthetic agents have been used successfully.
	Choice of agent should be based on the patient's hemodynamic and pulmonary status and potential difficulty in securing the patient's airway.
Muscle relaxants	Succinylcholine can result in an exaggerated hyperkalemic response and should be avoided in patients 24 hours after burn injury.
	Dose of nondepolarizing muscle relaxant necessary to achieve paralysis in burn patients can be substantially elevated.
Pain management	Anticipate tolerance to sedatives and opioids.
	Continue baseline pain regimen; multimodal adjuncts (e.g., ketamine) are likely to be useful.

Postoperative

	Assess potential for extubation at end of case.
	Call to the burn unit in adequate time for them to warm the room and obtain necessary supplies and equipment (e.g., infusions, ventilator).
	Ongoing fluid resuscitation and transfusion of blood products is expected after extensive excision and grafting.
	Presence of newly excised tissue and harvested donor sites can be painful and require higher doses of analgesics and sedatives.
	Determine new pain requirements.
	Maintain normothermia.

CBC, complete blood count; PVR, pulmonary vascular resistance; SVR, systemic vascular resistance.

volume blood loss during surgery and significant fluid shifts, in nonurgent cases it is prudent to postpone surgery until hemodynamic stability is achieved. Pulmonary assessment includes evaluation of oxygenation and ventilation, causes of impaired gas exchange, and mechanical ventilatory requirements. Significant pulmonary injury and poor compliance result in auto-PEEP (positive end-expiratory pressure) and breath stacking. Ventilatory requirements may exceed 20 L/min in adults during the hypermetabolic state. The high ventilatory needs combined with high peak inspiratory pressures and PEEP often cannot be sustained on traditional operating room ventilators. An ICU ventilator should be made available in these cases.

The need for aggressive intraoperative resuscitation necessitates adequate IV access. The presence of burn injury, together with tissue edema and hypovolemia, often makes this a challenge. Central lines are not routinely used unless there is a need for administration of vasoactive medications or in severe cases where invasive monitoring is needed. For example, large burns complicated by coexisting heart disease may benefit from the monitoring of central venous pressures, pulmonary artery pressures, or mixed venous oxygen saturation. Because central lines increase the risk for infection and are associated with complications during placement, they should be used only when needed. Most patients with burn injury can safely be managed with only large-bore peripheral IV catheters and invasive arterial pressure monitoring.

Managing the patient during transport is often more complicated. All equipment (including a functioning ambu bag, a full oxygen cylinder, charged batteries for monitors and infusion pumps, and any equipment needed for reintubation) should be checked prior to departure. Fluids and resuscitative medications are also needed. Optimization of the patient's respiratory and hemodynamic status is essential prior to transport. The patient should remain comfortable and sedated to prevent agitation, which can cause ventilator dyssynchrony, hemodynamic changes, and dislodging of lines or tubes. Paralysis during transport is rarely necessary and often undesirable if the patient can breathe spontaneously.

Intraoperative management

Standard American Society of Anesthesiologists (ASA) monitoring including electrocardiogram (ECG), blood pressure, pulse oximetry, capnography, inspired oxygen concentration, and temperature is required. The location of wounds and intraoperative positioning often create difficulties as monitors do not adhere well to injured areas with topical ointments. ECG leads can be secured with staples or placed under dependent portions of the patient's body. A Foley catheter is required to help assess the adequacy of resuscitation.

Given the significant nutritional needs of some patients, careful attention must be paid to scheduling surgeries and limiting NPO status. In patients with suspected ileus and delayed gastric emptying, a rapid-sequence intubation with cricoid pressure is warranted.

It is important to remember that patients have marked changes in their response to muscle relaxants. There is general agreement that succinylcholine administration to patients > 12 hours after injury is unsafe. Significant increases in extrajunctional acetylcholine receptors develop in these cases, placing the patient at risk for severe hyperkalemia and cardiac arrhythmias. This response can exist more than a year after injury. Because burn victims also develop significant resistance to nondepolarizing muscle relaxants, rocuronium may have a delayed onset of action even when dosed at 1.2 mg/kg. Intraoperative monitoring of neuromuscular function must be done frequently.

As stated earlier, tangential excision and grafting of burn wounds leads to significant intraoperative blood loss. The adequacy of resuscitation can usually be monitored by physiologic endpoints (Table 166.3). Blood products should be readily available for transfusion. Fluids should be warmed because burn patients are prone to heat loss. Hypothermia increases the risk for coagulopathies and arrhythmias, and shivering increases metabolic demand and may compromise the viability of newly placed grafts. Other measures to take include increasing ambient temperatures, wrapping the head, and using forced-air warming devices.

Many anesthetic agents have been used successfully in patients with burn injury. Ketamine is frequently used for intraoperative management because of its analgesic properties, relative hemodynamic stability, and tendency to preserve ventilatory efforts. It is a useful adjunct to the patient's baseline pain and sedation regimen, which often consists of morphine and midazolam.

Postoperative care

The potential for extubation is assessed at the end of surgery. Standard extubation criteria are used with significant attention given to the presence of airway edema, hemodynamic stability, need for ongoing resuscitation, and the presence of sepsis. Patients who received significant fluid resuscitation or who were positioned prone for an extended amount of time may benefit from remaining intubated until edema resolves. Chest radiographs may be needed to confirm ETT placement.

As stated earlier, extreme care must be taken during transport. The intensive care unit should have ample time to prepare prior to accepting the patient. Vasoactive medications, blood products, and a ventilator should be available if needed. Both the operating room and the patient's room should be warmed to help maintain normothermia. Finally, changes in the patient's level of pain may develop after extensive excision and grafting. The baseline pain regimen should be adjusted accordingly.

Key points to remember

- Burn injury results in pathophysiologic changes in most organ systems. The perioperative care of burn patients requires knowledge of these pathophysiologic changes from the initial period of injury until wounds have healed.
- The magnitude of burn injury is classified according to the TBSA involved, depth of the burn, and presence of inhalation injury. The rule of nines or age-specific burn diagrams are used to estimate the TBSA burned.
- The Parkland formula is perhaps the most widely used resuscitation formula for burn injury. The formula calls for 4 ml/kg/%TBSA of lactated Ringer's in the first 24 hours, with one half of this amount administered over the first 8 hours. Actual fluid administration should be individualized for each patient and titrated to physiologic endpoints.
- As with any other trauma admission, the patient with acute burn injury should be managed to ensure adequate airway, breathing, and circulation. After the airway and

hemodynamics are stabilized, a secondary survey is done to look for associated nonthermal injuries.

- Severe burn injury results in a hypermetabolic response with profound wasting of lean body mass. Strategies used to minimize this catabolic response include early wound excision and grafting, early aggressive nutritional support, prompt treatment of sepsis, and maintenance of high environmental temperature.

- Pain management in the burned patient provides many challenges. Surgery, dressing changes, physical therapy, and transport exacerbate baseline pain and anxiety levels. Burn patients develop tolerance to most opioids and sedatives, so they require higher doses than do patients without thermal injury.

Suggested readings

Alvarado R, Chung KK, Cancio LC, Wolf SE. Burn resuscitation. *Burns* 2009; 4–14.

American Burn Association. *Burn Incidence and Treatment in the US: 2007 Fact Sheet*. Available at: http://ameriburn.org/resources_factsheet.php.

Bittner EA, Grecu L, Martyn JAJ. Evaluation of the burn patient. In: Longnecker DE, et al., eds. *Anesthesiology*. New York: McGraw-Hill; 2008.

Bittner EA, Grecu L, Martyn JAJ. Management of anesthesia for the burn patient. In: Longnecker DE, et al., eds. *Anesthesiology*. New York: McGraw-Hill; 2008.

Hart DW, Wolf SE, Mlcak RP, et al. Persistence of muscle catabolism after severe burn. *Surgery* 2000; 128:312–319.

Henderson DN, Tompkins RG. Support of the metabolic response in burn injury. *Lancet* 2004; 363:1895–1902.

Herndon DN, Hart DW, Wolf SE, et al. Reversal of catabolism by beta-blockade after severe burns. *N Engl J Med* 2001; 345:1223–1229.

Hobson KG, Young KM, Ciraulo A, et al. Release of abdominal compartment syndrome improves survival in patients with burn injury. *J Trauma* 2002; 53:1129–1134.

Ipaktchi K, Arbabi S. Advances in burn critical care. *Crit Care Med* 2006; 34(Suppl):S239–S244.

Ivy ME, Atweh NA, Palmer J, et al. Intra-abdominal hypertension and abdominal compartment syndrome in burn patients. *J Trauma* 2000; 49:387–391.

Latenser BA. Critical Care of the burn patient: The first 48 hours. *Crit Care Med* 2009; 37:2819–2826.

MacLennan N, Heimbach D, Cullen B. Anesthesia for major thermal injury. *Anesthesiology* 1998; 89(3):749–770.

Monafo W. Initial management of burns. *N Engl J Med* 1996; 335:1581–1586.

Sheridan R. Burns. *Crit Care Med* 2002; 30(Suppl):S500–S514.

Youn Y, LaLonde C, Demling R. The role of mediators in the response to thermal injury. *World J Surg* 1992; 16:30–36.

Chapter 167

Common ethical issues in the intensive care unit

Nicholas Sadovnikoff

Ethical issues, questions, and concerns are common in the intensive care unit (ICU) setting and occur more frequently than in the operative anesthesia setting. The reasons are readily apparent, as patients cared for in the ICU are generally the most ill in the hospital or have undergone the most high-risk surgeries. Mortality in ICU patients varies depending on a hospital's size and the acuity of its population. In major tertiary care teaching hospital settings, ICU mortality may exceed 10%, with a substantial toll in terms of morbidity and loss of function as well. It is no wonder, then, that ethical concerns arise frequently around such issues as decisional capacity, informed consent, surrogate decision making, withdrawing and withholding life-sustaining therapies, and futility. Given the imprecise nature of medical prognostication, decisions must often be made in the context of less than clear-cut parameters and consequences. Compounding the difficulty of such decision making is the profound emotional stress associated with critical illness, on both the caregivers and the decision makers. A rapid decline in a patient's medical condition or a failure to recover well after a surgical intervention can be a sudden event for which little planning or preparation has taken place on the part of the patients or their proxy agents. Fortunately, there has been a recent widespread recognition of the need for guidance and dispassionate appraisal in the context of ethical challenges, and this recognition has resulted in a proliferation of ethics support services. Most hospitals now have an ethics committee, an ethics consultation service, or both; many ethics consultation services are available on a full-time, 24-hour basis. Use of these resources can provide substantial comfort and resolution to caregivers, families, and patients alike.

General principles

Ethics can be distilled in many instances to the body of thought or philosophy that addresses the question "What is the right thing to do?" It is important, however, to recognize that the answer to that question may vary greatly depending on the frame of reference of the questioner or the responder. The pursuit of an absolute set of ethical rules that can be expected to be shared across all cultural and religious contexts has proven challenging, if not an outright failure. It is for this reason that Englehardt is fond of pointing out that the word *ethics* is, in fact, plural. Persons coming from different moral communities

may answer an ethical question differently. The fact of this ethical diversity must be acknowledged a priori when considering ethical questions, and all efforts should be made to understand the ethical context of the individual asking the question without imposing the ethical context of the responder and vice versa.

In the context of moral and ethical diversity, we have, as a society, nevertheless had to achieve enough of a consensus on certain moral questions to write and enforce laws. Legal and ethical questions frequently intersect, but should never be confused for one another. Frequently, an ethics consultation may be accompanied by a consultation with the hospital's legal department, but it is important to clarify the difference between the two. It is important as well to remember that legal statutes in the medical domain often vary substantially from state to state, reflecting the ethical stance of the prevailing communities in the states' legislatures.

In general, the secular ethical community in the United States has embraced a set of four ethical principles popularized by Beauchamp and Childress, often referred to as *the four principles*, which are comprised of autonomy, beneficence, nonmaleficence, and justice.

Autonomy

The right of patients to dictate those medical interventions they will accept and those that they will not is the predominant theme in current ethical practice. This concept is in contradistinction to paternalism, still practiced in many other countries (including some Western societies), wherein physicians may exercise decisions regarding treatments on the basis of the "best interest of the patient." In this line of thinking, physicians' medical knowledge and experience equip them the best to decide on medical interventions.

The argument in favor of autonomy includes the codicil of informed consent, which calls on physicians to use their medical knowledge and experience to fully inform the patient of the potential benefits and risks of an intervention, but then allows patients, in the context of their own predicament, goals, preferences, and culture, to have unimpeded control over what is done to their bodies. As will be explored later in this chapter, patients in the ICU are frequently unable to express their autonomous sentiments. The decision making must then be transferred to a substitute whose duty it is to attempt to advocate for what the patient would want done, given the circumstances, preserving the patient's autonomous wishes.

Beneficence

Beneficence refers to the obligation of physicians to do or promote the most possible good for patients. In instances in which a therapy comports both benefit and harm, the benefit should outweigh the harm. It is thus that it is easy to justify the pain of a surgical incision in order to remove an infected appendix. The concept of beneficence is extended to the obligation to remove harm (e.g., treat pain) as well as to prevent harm (e.g., administer vaccines). Beneficence, which prioritizes the "best interest of the patient," can thus conflict with autonomy. In most cases, the principle of autonomy prevails, as when Jehovah's Witnesses are allowed to refuse blood in situations in which this clearly is not in their best interest. Exceptions occur when there is reason to question the decisional capacity of the patient, such as when suicidal individuals are involuntarily hospitalized for treatment of clinical depression.

Nonmaleficence

Nonmaleficence is the companion concept to beneficence that is summarized by the Latin aphorism *primum non nocere* ("above all, do no harm"). This obligation not to do harm to patients is obviously couched in the same context that the harm cannot exceed the good, and that a certain amount of harm can be acceptable if it is proportionally exceeded by benefit. Unfortunately, quantitating and weighing benefit and harm are at times difficult and sometimes even impossible tasks due to prognostic imprecision. Furthermore, to respect autonomy, patients' preferences must be considered in this calculus. An acceptable harm for one patient may be completely untenable for another (e.g., amputation of a gangrenous leg).

Justice

Justice refers primarily to distributive justice, in which the obligation of the physician, or more widely the health care delivery system, is to ensure that care is delivered fairly, equitably, and appropriately to all individuals. This concept conflicts strongly with the concept of beneficence, which promotes the greatest possible good for the individual patient. This issue is most effectively addressed at the societal and governmental level, rather than through rationing by individual physicians. Unfortunately, despite the fact that health care expenditures constitute an ever-increasing and progressively unaffordable portion of the United States' economic output, there has been, with only a few exceptions, little legislative appetite for limiting health care expenditures. Even the recent legislation passed by the US Congress, mandating certain reforms of the national healthcare delivery system, is characterized by substantial dilution and compromise, such that the net impact on the equitable distribution of health care services is likely to be small. The fact that distributive justice is given so low a national priority is difficult to defend by ethical arguments.

Competence and decisional capacity

The terms *competence* and *decisional capacity* differ in terms of their definition, but for the purpose of this chapter are interchangeable in that neither an incompetent patient nor a patient lacking decisional capacity should dictate his or her own medical decision making. These are conditions in which patients are stripped of their autonomy as a consequence of cognitive impairment that prevents them from fully understanding, considering, and processing information involved in consenting for or refusing medical interventions.

As has previously been noted, a substantial proportion of ICU patients are unable to participate in decision making about their medical treatment. The reasons for this are numerous, but the main issues are now discussed.

Delirium

Delirium is defined as a disturbance of consciousness with inattention accompanied by a change in cognition or perceptual disturbance that develops over a short period of time (hours to days) and fluctuates over time. Depending on how stringently testing is done, delirium is present in as many as 50% to 80% of ICU patients. Risk factors for delirium include advanced age, severity of illness, and medications (in particular, benzodiazepines). Delirium is fairly readily diagnosed by simple testing and, if present, impairs patients from having the capacity to give informed consent or participate in their own health care decisions.

Intubation

Patients who are intubated and receiving mechanical ventilation cannot talk, which substantially impairs discussions regarding medical choices. Although they may be awake and able to write notes, this is a much less rich form of communication as it may not capture emotional content. Furthermore, studies have found that at least 80% of mechanically ventilated patients are delirious, and most are in fact receiving sedative medications. Although there may be exceptions, in general it is prudent to have a proxy decision maker participate in medical decisions for intubated patients.

Dementia

Dementia is defined as the loss (usually progressive) of cognitive and intellectual functions, without impairment of perception or consciousness, caused by a variety of disorders, including severe infections and toxins, but most commonly associated with structural brain disease. It is a diagnosis that needs to have been made before a patient becomes critically ill, as it is a risk factor for, and commonly coexists with, delirium. ICU patients with an established diagnosis of dementia should not be asked to make decisions regarding their medical care.

Depression

Depression frequently coexists with and complicates both chronic and critical illness. It may cause patients to have distorted interpretations of the value of medical therapies and of the value of their own well-being. A formal psychiatric evaluation should be performed if a patient seems to be making decisions that appear not to be made in the best self-interest and are not based on cultural or religious beliefs. A clinical diagnosis of depression may warrant the temporary designation of a proxy decision maker while the depression is treated.

Assessment of competence to consent for treatment can be challenging, and there are no formal guidelines from professional societies regarding this process. There are indeed degrees of impairment that may affect competence, such that it may be reasonable for a moderately impaired patient to give informed consent for procedures where the stakes are low (anesthesia for drainage of a superficial abscess) but not appropriate to give consent for high-risk procedures (organ transplantation). Standardized tools, such as the MacArthur Competence Assessment Tool for Treatment, have been developed that can be administered expeditiously and have shown high inter-rater agreement. Psychiatric evaluation can also be helpful when the question of competency is unclear. Ethics consultations are frequently useful in settings where there is uncertainty, particularly when patients refuse potentially beneficial therapy.

Substituted judgment

When a patient does not possess decisional capacity, the goal is to extend as accurately as possible that person's autonomy through a surrogate decision maker (SDM). The mandate of the SDM is to advocate on behalf of the patient for what the SDM believes that patient wanted when capable of autonomous decision making. SDMs may also have guidance from other documentation, such as living wills and advance directives.

Designated health care proxy agents

Ideally the SDM is someone who was designated by the patient and who has had previous in-depth discussions with the patient regarding wishes and goals for health care. Such a person is called a *designated health care agent*, and there must be a proxy document signed by both parties acknowledging this choice. In the absence of a formal process having taken place to designate a health care agent, there may be a hierarchy of persons to whom that role may fall by default. The exact priority varies from state to state, and some states do not recognize a hierarchy at all. Almost universally, the spouse is the first default, followed by parents, children, siblings, more distant relatives, and close friends. Often the role may be assumed by a less closely related individual (e.g., nephew) who happens to know the patient the best.

Living wills

These documents are generally broad statements completed by patients in anticipation of the possibility of losing decisional capacity. They often contain such conditional language as "if there is no reasonable hope of recovery" or "if I am permanently dependent on machines to stay alive." These phrases are vague and subject to interpretation and the vagaries of prognostication. The instructions often include prohibition of "heroic measures" or other similarly poorly specified interventions. Thus, living wills serve more as indications of the general spirit of the patient's wishes, rather than as detailed instructions for future care.

Advance care directives

Advance care directives are more detailed documents completed by patients in advance of their possibly losing decisional capacity. There is a widespread effort to encourage patients to use advance directives, the purpose of which is to elucidate more clearly than living wills their wishes for their future care. They are useful in that they provide guidance both to physicians and to SDMs. Their strength is that they do not depend on hearsay and are not clouded by the personal bias that an SDM may, whether intentionally or not, impose on the decision-making process. Advance directives are, however, limited by the specifics of their language, which may not apply to the specifics of the predicaments patients ultimately come to face. That is, the more specific are the instructions, the less they are likely to apply to the actual clinical situation that ultimately affects the patient.

The best practical solution is for patients to identify a health care agent who is aware of the spirit (living will) and specifics (advance directive) that characterize that individual's goals for care should decisional capacity be lost. Ideally, decisions are made with advance directive or living will documents and the health care agent present.

Synthetic judgment

There are instances in which critically ill patients have not completed any sort of advance directive or living will and have no known living relatives or close friends who might act as SDM. In these instances, exhaustive efforts should be pursued to learn of the patient's social and medical history, all attempts should be made to identify any previously articulated wishes, the best interests of the patient should be objectively assessed, and all treatment options should be considered. A *synthetic judgment* may then be formulated that takes into account all of the information that has been gathered. In scenarios such as these, consultation of the hospital ethics and legal resources is often of substantial value to help achieve an objective assessment that is free of bias or paternalism and is legally defensible. If consensus as to a reasonable assessment of the patient's wishes cannot be achieved, it may be necessary to engage the legal system to appoint a guardian.

Informed consent

When the issue of who shall consent for treatment decisions is established, it is the ethical duty of a physician to acquaint the patient or proxy with information regarding the risks and benefits of the proposed treatment, so that the autonomy of the patient can be respected in accepting or declining. The exact nature of the information in terms of detail, volume, and exhaustiveness may vary depending on the needs and preferences of the patient or SDM. Clearly, describing every possible outcome of a proposed treatment would be burdensome and potentially frightening to patients, but some important subset of all possible outcomes should be presented to the patient or SDM. Several standards have been proposed to describe this subset.

Reasonable person standard

This standard is used to describe the amount and type of information that a reasonable person would be expected to want to know before deciding on a treatment plan. It assumes that the vast majority of patients would want to hear the same information, and it is somewhat hamstrung as a guide when patients themselves are unreasonable.

Standard of care

This concept, which can also be called the reasonable physician standard, implies that there is a set of information that a prudent, responsible physician in that patient's community should tell a patient or SDM. Although it seems superficially attractive, this concept has been challenged as focusing on the needs of the physician.

Subjective standard

This standard implies a titration of the level and quantity of information given to the patient in proportion to his or her ability to process and use it. The physician decides how much to tell the patient based on the patient's intellectual, emotional, and spiritual characteristics. Some highly intelligent patients may request to be spared a detailed description of potential harm from a treatment; in such cases it is ethical to honor their request, so long as they have a basic understanding of the treatment. Similarly, relatively uneducated patients or SDMs may require risks and benefits described in exquisite detail before they are ready to decide. Here the physician is ethically bound to be thorough but may set limits should the process become overly burdensome.

Waiver of consent

Only under highly stringent conditions is it acceptable to forgo the informed consent process. The most obvious is in the setting of a medical emergency wherein delay in treatment for the purpose of obtaining consent might genuinely risk causing harm to the patient. The more difficult cases occur when the patient has lost decisional capacity and has no health care proxy. Here the terms *presumed consent* and/or *implied consent* have been used. As previously noted in the discussion of competence, these scenarios mandate careful attempts to ascertain the patient's own wishes, and the involvement of hospital ethics resources is often warranted.

End-of-life care

As noted earlier in the text, many patients die in the ICU, often after a long and protracted course during which the clinical picture has changed many times, fostering periods of both optimism and despair. The most common ethical challenges in this setting surround changing the goals of medical care from cure oriented to comfort focused. Several issues frequently arise in this regard.

Withholding life-sustaining therapies

The decision to forgo life-sustaining therapy may be made by a competent patient, in which case the physician is ethically bound to honor this decision. Psychiatric consultation to rule out depression with suicidal ideation may be appropriate in this setting. If a physician feels that he or she cannot ethically continue to care for the patient who refuses a life-sustaining intervention, that physician is ethically obligated to identify and transfer care to a physician who is willing to care for the patient.

The decision to withhold life-sustaining therapy from the incompetent patient is more complicated. Although a SDM may make this decision based on previous discussions with the patient, it is no longer the patient speaking, and a high degree of certainty is warranted given that the consequence of forgoing life-sustaining therapy is usually death. In many states, the power of the SDM is somewhat limited, and decisions to withhold life-sustaining therapy must be supported by "convincing evidence" that this decision accurately reflects the patient's previously stated wishes. On occasion, there may be disagreement between the medical care team and the SDM as to whether life-sustaining therapy should be initiated. The medical care team is not ethically or legally obligated to provide treatment that it does not believe will benefit the patient simply because such treatment is requested; in these instances, ethics consultation is recommended as well as engagement of the hospital legal department to provide an objective assessment of the contradictory opinions. Ethics consultation services are generally not expected to settle decisions, but rather to ensure that all voices have been heard and then to provide non-binding recommendations for ethically defensible courses of action.

Do not resuscitate (DNR) orders constitute a specific proscription of rescue measures taken in a setting of impending or actual cardiac arrest. Cardiopulmonary resuscitation (CPR) and advanced cardiac life support (ACLS) protocols were designed to rescue individuals suffering from reversible medical events such as acute myocardial infarction, yet the concept has been extended to the default assumption that this is desired by all hospitalized patients. That is, unless a patient or SDM requests that resuscitation not be performed, it is assumed that the patient desires or would desire this intervention. The scenario is unusual in that there are few, if any, other interventions that patients are assumed to elect or accept, and yet it is clear that, for a great many critically ill patients, this intervention has no potential for benefit, whether desired or not. Indeed, many patients and SDMs choose to decline CPR and ACLS at the end of life, once they understand the procedures and their potential benefits (or lack thereof). Frank discussions between the care team and the patient or SDM should be held whenever possible to establish the patient's goals and preferences for treatment. Furthermore, it should be clarified that the decision to forego interventions such as CPR and ACLS is not equivalent to declining aggressive care, but rather applies specifically to those particular interventions.

Withdrawing life-sustaining therapies

It is widely accepted both ethically and legally that there is no a priori difference between withholding and withdrawing life-sustaining therapies. That is not to say, however, that there is no difference between the two *processes*. Studies of physician attitudes have shown that physicians have greater misgivings about withdrawing therapies that have already been instituted than about withholding the same therapies to begin with. This distinction naturally extends to family members and SDMs as well. The psychological stigma of taking life-sustaining therapy away – "pulling the plug" – rather than never initiating it in the first place clearly resonates, even if it has no ethical or moral basis. Further complicating the withdrawal of life-sustaining therapies is the fact that this process will often require sedative and/or analgesic medication to ensure the patient's comfort, and the administration of these medications may hasten death.

Providing comfort at the end of life

When the decision is made to seek comfort as a primary goal rather than to pursue a curative therapeutic approach, the objectives become the control of pain and prevention of the discomfort of respiratory distress. Analgesic medications, most commonly opioids, are widely used to achieve these goals, but they comport the additional effect of potentially hastening death through respiratory depression or conceivably hypotension. The tension between the goal of achieving comfort for the patient and the ethical duty not to cause a patient's death is traditionally resolved philosophically by the principle of the *double effect*. First espoused by Roman Catholic theologians in the Middle Ages, this concept permits an otherwise morally unacceptable effect (hastening death) even if it is foreseeable, when the primary intent is inherently good (relief of suffering). The concept of proportionality is important in that the good effect must outweigh the bad, with a net benefit being realized by the patient. This concept is helpful in resolving many ethical dilemmas in end-of-life care, but it must be acknowledged that not all situations lend themselves to being resolved via this line of reasoning. For example, the decision to withdraw mechanical ventilation from a ventilator-dependent patient, an action that would typically be accompanied by heavy sedation to prevent the suffering of respiratory distress (*terminal sedation*), is not permitted under the principle of double effect. The rationale is that the primary act (removal of the ventilator) is not inherently good (results in the death of the patient), hence the use

Table 167.1. The "slippery slope"

Relief of pain and suffering
   Comfort measures only
      Physician-assisted suicide
         Voluntary euthanasia
            Nonvoluntary euthanasia
               Involuntary euthanasia
                  Killing/murder

of sedation to prevent the possibility of suffering is not permissible. Thus the acceptability of a physician potentially hastening a patient's death depends on a number of factors and will vary substantially depending on the moral community within which the physician functions. A gradient of possible behaviors in terms of physicians' hastening of death can be described and is sometimes referred to as a *slippery slope* (see Table 167.1).

Relief of pain and suffering, even while carrying out an aggressive curative treatment approach, is an ethical obligation for the physician to pursue. *Comfort measures only* refers to the abandonment of a curative approach with an emphasis on achieving comfort, though recent data suggest that early palliative care may even prolong life. As mentioned before, such measures may secondarily hasten the death of the patient. Here already, some physicians may feel uncomfortable, believing that every possible effort must be expended to preserve life and that the quest for cure should never be abandoned. *Physician-assisted suicide* refers to a physician aiding a patient who requests assistance in hastening death, usually by providing the patient the means with which to commit suicide. Although this practice is not widely considered ethically acceptable in the United States, it is legal in two states and is known to occur on an undocumented basis with some frequency. *Voluntary euthanasia*, in which a physician commits an act that hastens death at the request of the patient, is illegal and not widely practiced in this country but is permitted in some Western societies, such as the Netherlands. *Nonvoluntary euthanasia* is the hastening of death by a physician of a patient who has not expressed a wish to die, and *involuntary euthanasia* is the hastening of death of a patient who has specifically expressed a wish not to die. Neither of these actions is ethically acceptable in Western societies. Killing and murder are generally morally and ethically forbidden for physicians, but even here societal exceptions may exist in the setting of capital punishment or war.

The concern arises that if hastening death is permissible in the context of providing comfort for terminally ill and suffering patients, then the rather subjective criteria by which such patients are identified (terminal, suffering) might become sufficiently flexible that euthanasia also becomes permissible. Although there is substance to this argument (when taken to the extreme), extending it could prohibit relief of suffering and obstruct the responsibility of the physician to do what is within his or her power to attenuate suffering when cure is not possible. The position taken by most practitioners in this country involves the liberal use of opioids for patients who carry a terminal diagnosis with a life expectancy that is measured in days to weeks, but there is scant legal or professional support for more aggressive measures, such as physician-assisted suicide or euthanasia.

Futility

Much controversy has surrounded the concept of medical futility. Attempts in recent decades to define futility in an objective and non-value-based context have essentially been unsuccessful. The goal of defining futility has at its core the observation that, with advances in life-sustaining therapies, patients could be kept from dying almost indefinitely but could fail as well to make any progress toward recovery. This use of expensive and intensive medical resources tends to have a demoralizing effect on care teams, and efforts to define futile care have been undertaken. A declaration of futility would then justify the withdrawal of aggressive, life-sustaining therapy. The process of defining futility is fraught with problems, however. First, it ignores the generally dominant principle of autonomy. That is, if a patient or SDM desires to continue life-sustaining therapy, the declaration of futility would override this preference; this selective violation of autonomy does not have, in the United States, much traction, although it is accepted and practiced in many other Western countries. Second, a declaration of futility requires some prognostic certainty. It is an uncomfortable truth that physicians' abilities to prognosticate, however refined and aided by advanced technology, are imperfect and subject to error. When the consequences of decisions based on such predictions frequently involve death through withdrawal of life-sustaining therapies, the prognostic certainty must be high indeed. Third, the argument that such use of intensive therapies places a financial burden on the health care system has not been borne out in economic analyses. The number of patients in such predicaments is so small as to have a trivial effect on overall health care expenditures. Finally, inherent in the notion of futility is a predefined assumption of what constitutes a *life worth living*. This is so deeply subjective that it in fact defies definition; existences that many would define as completely intolerable are in fact perfectly acceptable to those inhabiting them.

Keeping all of these issues in mind, there are clear cases of medical futility wherein the likelihood of recovery is so minute as to be dismissed. In these cases, there is often concern on the part of the care team that far more suffering is being inflicted than benefit being obtained by the patient. Typically, these scenarios involve SDMs who insist that the patient would have wanted every attempt made to sustain life. These situations are particularly challenging to care team members, not only because of the sense that they are participating in care that is ultimately more harmful than good, but because, despite their expertise, they are disempowered to change the course of care. Care team members may feel that their integrity is being compromised, leading to resentment and creation of an oppositional relationship with the patient, SDM and/or family members. Given these challenges, most institutions have established futility policies that are to be used when consensus cannot be reached as to the appropriateness of discontinuing life-sustaining therapies. These policies tend, for the reasons just mentioned, to be extremely stringent, requiring objective second medical opinions, extensive involvement of ethics and legal services, and significant mandatory waiting periods. The state of Texas is currently unique in having codified such procedures through legislation; of note is that the law has been called upon only infrequently since its passage, and so far it has not been subjected to judicial challenge.

Truth telling and disclosure

The last decade has seen a sweeping change in attitudes toward disclosure of medical errors, events that occur with higher frequency and with higher stakes in the ICU due to the severity of the patients' conditions. The patient safety movement, spurred by the Institute of Medicine report in 1996 that suggested that between 44,000 and 98,000 patients a year die as a result of medical errors, has revolutionized the approach to medical error. The widespread culture of secrecy and silence in the wake of a medical error was largely fueled by a concern for medicolegal and professional liability. When investigations of errors were performed, the goal was commonly to identify an individual to blame and censure, further reinforcing the desire on the part of physicians for secrecy and evasion. The result of this culture was that the systems of care that were actually to blame were not identified, but rather allowed to persist. Error, rather than being accepted as an inevitable characteristic of human behavior, was reviled and prosecuted. As a more enlightened realm of thought has evolved over the last decade, the attitude toward human error has undergone a complete reversal, and most institutions are now embracing the concept of disclosure of adverse medical events to patients when they occur. Disclosure policies generally consist of three components: a prompt and honest acknowledgment that an error has taken place, an apology or expression of sympathy for its consequences, and a pledge that work is underway to identify the cause of the error and prevent the same event from occurring again. The obvious concern is that this disclosure exposes physicians to the risk of embarrassment, professional censure, and litigation. This risk is felt to be outweighed by the benefits, which begin with the fact that telling patients the truth is the only morally and ethically defensible action. Furthermore, openness and transparency enhance trust on the part of the patient, family, and care team. Reviews of litigation have shown that a majority of patients seek legal redress because of communication failures involving the patient, family, and physician. Ultimately, this act of disclosure begins the process of investigating how the system or process of care can be better designed to prevent similar adverse events from recurring in the future. As this is a relatively new approach within the culture of medicine, it is not yet clear what the overall effect will be on rates of litigation or on overall costs to the health care system.

Middlemen (and women)

No discussion of ethics in the ICU would be complete without acknowledging the position of middlemen. These individuals are members of the health care team, most commonly nurses, fellows, and resident physicians who may be asked to provide patient care that they feel is unethical or causes moral distress, but whose position in the hierarchy does not permit them to express their sentiments or to participate in decisions regarding trajectory of care. This scenario is particularly common in surgical ICUs, where the team in the ICU may have a perspective on a patient's condition that differs from that of the operative surgeon. These conflicts are not easily resolved, for there often is a plethora of ethical viewpoints represented within an ICU care team. Consensus as to what the patient would want, or even what is in the patient's best interest, can be difficult to achieve. In such instances, an institutional mechanism should be available so that individuals who are experiencing moral discomfort or who feel that ethical principles are being violated can express their concerns. In many institutions, use of the ethics consultation service provides such a mechanism; ideally the service can be engaged by anyone, from patient to caregivers to family members to housekeepers, when a question of ethical concern is raised. This resource is extremely important for middlemen, who, due to their intermediary positions in the heirarchy, cannot act as independent agents. Ethics consultation provides a protected and acceptable route for such morally stressed individuals to express their concerns. Again, although ethics consultants do not have the authority to dictate care, they do have the experience and knowledge to consider the concerns of all of the stakeholders and to provide recommendations for ethically defensible plans of care. Even in the absence of a resultant change in the plan for a patient's care, middlemen are often substantially relieved simply to have had their voice heard.

Considerations for the operative anesthesiologist

For the operative anesthesiologist, the ethical issues involving ICU patients come into play most commonly when operative interventions are needed or when assistance with airway management is requested. The circumstances surrounding these events are often characterized by an emergent need for intervention, with little time available for assessment of ethical concerns. In such instances, such as when a patient's wishes regarding endotracheal intubation are unclear, it is ethical for the anesthesiologist to intervene if it appears that the patient is in danger of harm or death in the absence of immediate action. If time permits, however, the anesthesiologist should ascertain that such issues as the goals of therapy and consent for treatment, have been adequately discussed with the patient or SDM. If this is not the case, the process of obtaining informed consent for anesthesia constitutes an opportunity to discuss those issues.

The specific instance of a patient who has asked not to be resuscitated at the end of life (DNR), but who has agreed to a surgical procedure merits specific mention. A clear discussion regarding whether to continue or suspend the DNR status for the time of the procedure and recovery is critical. Patients or surrogates who ask to continue the DNR status while undergoing general anesthesia and surgery present a particular problem for the anesthesiologist. Agreeing to such an arrangement means agreeing to not resuscitating the patient from many potentially reversible complications in the course of surgery and anesthesia. It is ethically defensible for an anesthesiologist to agree to these terms; however, it is also ethically sound for an anesthesiologist to refuse to care for a patient under such circumstances, so long as he or she can identify another anesthesiologist who is willing to assume the care of the patient under those constraints.

Conclusion

This review of common ethical problems in the ICU is meant to be neither exhaustive nor definitive, but rather is meant to highlight the ethical issues commonly faced in this setting. There is a recent overall trend toward identifying and addressing ethical questions head-on within health care institutions, and this has led to the formalization of ethics consultation services and committees in most hospitals. As the volume of this work has increased, so has the skill and experience of its practitioners, and the value of their contributions to the overall medical care environment cannot be overestimated. The fundamental messages of this chapter are simple: the intersection of extreme severity of disease and the diversity of moral communities present in our society will lead to the frequent emergence of complicated ethical questions in the ICU. Although no canonical guidelines for ethical actions can be identified, practical general principles exist, and local expertise in this realm within health care institutions is rapidly burgeoning. Robust use of the guidance provided by ethics services in situations of uncertainty can be of immense value, and their perspective and input should be pursued with impunity.

Suggested readings

Appelbaum PS. Assessment of patients' competence to consent to treatment. *N Engl J Med* 2007; 357:1834–1840.

Attitudes of critical care medicine professionals concerning forgoing life-sustaining treatments. *Crit Care Med* 1992; 20: 320–326.

Beauchamp TL, Childress JF. *Principles of Biomedical Ethics*. 4th ed. New York: Oxford University Press; 1994.

Diagnostic and Statistical Manual of Mental Disorders. 4th ed. text revision (DSM-IV-TR). Arlington, VA: American Psychiatric Association; 2000.

Englehardt HT. *The Foundations of Bioethics*. 2nd ed. New York: Oxford University Press; 1996.

Pandharipande P, Ely EW. Sedative and analgesic medications: risk factors for delirium and sleep disturbances in the critically ill. *Crit Care Clin* 2006; 22(2):313–327, vii.

Index

In this index figures and tables are referred to by f and t, respectively; online content is referred to by w.